	hydrocortisone sodium succinate	insulin (regular)	isoproterenol	lactated Ringer's	lidocaine	methylprednisolone sodium succinate	mezlocillin	multiple vitamin infusion	nafcillin	netilmicin	norepinephrine	normal saline solution	ondansetron	oxacillin	oxytocin	penicillin G potassium	phenytoin	phytonadione	piperacillin	potassium chloride	procainamide	ranitidine	sodium bicarbonate	thiamine	ticarcillin	tobramycin	vancomycin	verapamil	vitamin B complex with C
acyclovir	4			4		4		4	4					4		4			4	4		4	4		4	4	4		
albumin																													
amikacin	24			24							24	24	4	8		8		24		4		24	24				24	24	
amino acid injection	24	24	24		24	24	?	?	24	24	24			24		24		24	?	4		12				24	24		
aminophylline	24			24	24	?			24	2		24								4		24	24						
ampicillin	?	2						24				8						3		4		?	?						4
bretylium		48	3	48	24							48								48	24	24	48					48	
calcium gluconate				24	24					2		24								4						1		48	4
cefamandole												12																24	
cefazolin		2		24				24				24	4									?						24	4
cefoxitin		24		24				24				24	4										24			24		24	24
ceftazidime												24	4									?	6						
cimetidine		24	24		24	24						48	4			24		24		24							24	24	48
ciprofloxacin				48	24														24	24		24				24		24	
clindamycin	24			24		24		24		24		24	4			24			48	24		?	24			48		24	24
corticotropin																													
dexamethasone sodium phosphate	4												4							4		24	4					24	4
dextrose 5% in water (D_5W)	48		24		24	?	24	24	24	24	24		48	6	6	24			24	24	24	48	24	24	24	24	24	24	
D_5W in lactated Ringer's	24		24		24			24						24		24				24				24				24	
D_5W in normal saline solution	48		24		24	?		24	24				48	?		24			24	24			24	24		48		24	
diazepam																						?						24	
diphenhydramine	24									72			4			24				4		1							
dobutamine			24	24	24						24	24								?	24	48						24	
dopamine	18			48	24	18						48		24						24		48						24	4
epinephrine	4			24								24						3		4		24						24	4
erythromycin lactobionate				18				24				22										24	24					24	
esmolol	24			24					24			24				24	24		24	24		24				24	24	24	
gentamicin		2		24				24				24	4									24						24	
heparin sodium	?	2	24		24	?							4	4	4	?		4	6	24	4	24	24		6			24	24
hydrocortisone sodium succinate		4	4	24		?						24	4	4				4	24		4		24					24	
insulin (regular)	4				24										2					4		24	3		2	2	2	48	4
isoproterenol	4			24								24										24						24	
lactated Ringer's	24		24		24	?	72	24	24					24		24			24	24				24	24	24		24	
lidocaine		24		24					48			24									24	24	24					48	
methylprednisolone sodium succinate	?			?								?				24				?		48	2					24	?
mezlocillin				72								48																	
multiple vitamin infusion				24						24		24											24					24	
nafcillin				24	48							24								24			24						?
netilmicin								24				24																	
norepinephrine												24										?						24	
normal saline solution	24		24		24	?	48	24	24	24	24		48	24		24			24	24	24	48	24	24	24	48	24	24	
ondansetron	4											48								4		4			4		4		
oxacillin	4			24								24																	4
oxytocin		2																		4			24					24	4
penicillin G potassium				24		24						24										24						24	
phenytoin																							24					48	
phytonadione	4																			4			24						4
piperacillin	24			24								24								24		4						24	
potassium chloride		4		24		?			24			24	4		4			4	24		4	48	24					24	
procainamide	4				24							24								4		24						48	24
ranitidine		24	24		24	48					?	48	4			24			4	48	24				24	24	24		
sodium bicarbonate	24	3			24	2		24	24			24			24		24	24		24									?
thiamine				24								24																	
ticarcillin		2		24								24	4									24						24	
tobramycin		2		24								48										24						24	
vancomycin		2										24	4									24						24	
verapamil	24	48	24	24	48	24		24			24	24			24	24	48		24	24	48				24	24	24		24
vitamin B complex with C		4				?			?					4	4			4			24		?					24	

SPRINGHOUSE

NURSE'S DRUG GUIDE

FOURTH EDITION

SPRINGHOUSE

NURSE'S DRUG GUIDE

FOURTH EDITION

Springhouse Corporation
Springhouse, Pennsylvania

Staff

Senior Publisher
Donna O. Carpenter

Editorial Director
William J. Kelly

Clinical Director
Marguerite Ambrose, RN, MSN, CS

Design Director
Jake Smith

Art Director
Elaine Kasmer Ezrow

Project Editor
Catherine E. Harold

Clinical Project Editor
Eileen Cassin Gallen, RN, BSN

Associate Editor
Raphe Cheli

Clinical Editors
Joanne M. Bartelmo, RN, MSN; Margaret Friant Creamer, RN, MSN; Christine M. Damico, RN, MSN, CPNP; Lori Musolf Neri, RN, MSN, CRNP; Kimberly A. Zalewski, RN, MSN

Copy Editors
Leslie Dworkin, Elizabeth Hansen, Caryl Knutsen, Dolores Matthews, Beth Pitcher

Designers
Arlene Putterman (associate art director), Joseph John Clark, Donald G. Knauss

Electronic Production Services
Diane Paluba (manager), Joyce Rossi Biletz (technician)

Manufacturing
Patricia K. Dorshaw (manager), Otto Mezei (book production manager)

Editorial Assistants
Carol A. Caputo, Arlene P. Claffee, Beth Janae Orr

Indexer
Deborah Tortulette

Visit our Web site at eDrugInfo.com

SNDG4–D
02 01 10 9 8 7 6 5 4 3 2
ISSN 1088-8063
ISBN 1-58255-124-3

Contents

Consultants and contributors

At the time of publication, the consultants and contributors held the following positions.

Mary E. Bowen, RN, DNS, JD, CNAA
Assistant Professor
Thomas Jefferson University
Philadelphia, Pa.

Alan Caspi, PharmD, MBA, FASHP
Director of Pharmacy
Lenox Hill Hospital
New York, N.Y.

Teresa Dunsworth, PharmD, BCPS
Associate Professor of Clinical Pharmacy
West Virginia University School of Pharmacy
Morgantown, W.Va.

Carmel A. Esposito, RN, MSN, EdD
Coordinator Continuing Education
Nurse Educator
Trinity Health System School of Nursing
Stubenville, Ohio

Nicole T. Galenas, PharmD
Pediatric Clinical Pharmacist
Charleston Area Medical Center
Women & Children's Division
Charleston, W.Va.

Mary Jo Gerlach, RN, MSNEd
Assistant Professor, Adult Nursing (retired)
Medical College of Georgia
School of Nursing, Athens
Athens, Ga.

Edgar Gonzalez, PharmD
Associate Professor
Medical College of Virginia
Richmond, Va.

Tatyana Gurvich, PharmD
Clinical Pharmacologist
Glendale Adventist Family Practice
Residency Program
Glendale, Calif.

Randall A. Lynch, RPh, PharmD
Assistant Director, Pharmacy Services
Presbyterian Medical Center
University of Pennsylvania Health System
Philadelphia, Pa.

Carrie A. McCoy, RN, PhD, MSPH, CEN
Associate Professor of Nursing
Northern Kentucky University
Highland Heights, Ky.

Margaret R. Rateau, RN, MSN
Assistant Professor of Nursing
Kent State University
East Liverpool Regional Campus
East Liverpool, Ohio

Ruthie Robinson, RN, MSN, CEN, CCRN
Instructor of Nursing
Lamar University
Beaumont, Tex.

Linda Roy, RN, MSN, CRNP
Nurse Practitioner
Plumsteadville Family Practice
Plumsteadville, Pa.

Denise A. Vanacore-Netz, RN, MSN CRNP, ANP-CS
Coordinator, Nurse Practitioner Program
Gwynedd Mercy College
Gwynedd Valley, Pa.

Foreword

"Mom, I need a drug book for my clinical courses. What should I get?" asked my daughter, Robin, a nursing student. "Can you recommend a reference that I can *really* use–something that *clearly and directly* provides all the information I'll need to take care of patients? None of us has the time or patience for long, confusing references that we can barely even lift."

"*Springhouse Nurse's Drug Guide*," I replied without hesitation. As a practicing nurse and faculty member for 27 years, I know the importance of understanding medications and being able to quickly find the comprehensive information I need. As the parent of a tuition-paying student, I also know the importance of getting a great value for the price of a book. Since its first edition, the *Springhouse Nurse's Drug Guide* has become a favorite of mine. Current and timely, the *Springhouse Nurse's Drug Guide* provides accurate, essential information in a user-friendly format. It's a respected, easily understood reference written by nurses for nurses and nursing students who care for real patients in all types of settings. The *Springhouse Nurse's Drug Guide*, officially endorsed by the National Student Nurses' Association (NSNA), is a must-have book for everyone who needs drug information, from beginning students like Robin to experienced nurses like me.

The fourth edition of the *Springhouse Nurse's Drug Guide* builds on features that made the first three editions so successful. Developed for use in clinical and study areas, this attractive book has a logical layout, readable print, and a sturdy cover that cleans easily. One of my favorite features continues to be the I.V. drug compatibility chart that is again wisely placed inside the front cover of the book where it can be immediately located—a blessing during stressful times on a clinical unit.

This edition begins with a clear description of how to use the book and a guide to common abbreviations used in the book. Four introductory chapters present crucial drug-related information. Chapter 1, Drug Therapy and the Nursing Process, simply and succinctly explains how the nursing process guides nursing decisions about drug administration to ensure patient safety and medical and legal standards. Chapter 2 presents one of the clearest descriptions of the essentials of adult and pediatric dosage calculations that I have seen in any book. Chapter 3 explains and shows how to administer drugs by various routes. Chapter 4, Avoiding Medication Errors, is an important new feature in this edition. Medication errors can injure or kill patients; this chapter focuses on avoiding common problems related to names of patients and drugs, allergies, orders, routes of administration, staff stress, and medication labels.

Next is an important section that describes need-to-know information about various drug classes. It reviews indications, actions, adverse reactions, contraindications, and nursing considerations (arranged by the nursing process) for each major class of drugs you'll administer. It also shows you which drug is the prototype for each class.

The body of the book presents drugs alphabetically by their generic names, which ensures quick access to information. Each monograph has a consistent, user-friendly format that includes the drug's pronunciation; trade names (including U.S., Canadian, and Australian names); pharmacologic and therapeutic classes; controlled substance schedule, when applicable; pregnancy risk category; indications and dosages; description of how the drug is supplied; pharmacokinetics, including a helpful table showing the route, onset, peak, and duration of action; pharmacodynamics; adverse reactions organized five ways for safety; and contraindications and precautions. This edition of *Springhouse Nurse's Drug Guide* now classifies drug interactions four ways: drug-drug, drug-herb, drug-food, and drug-lifestyle. Also, the popular feature, nursing considerations, now includes new and distinct "alert" logos to draw attention to potential medication errors. As always, the nursing considerations are arranged in keeping with the nursing process.

The increasing use of herbal supplements in the United States makes it crucial for you to understand them; you will undoubtedly care for patients who use herbal remedies alone or in combination with traditional drugs. This book includes a separate section that describes the most commonly used herbal medicines in a consistent format similar to that used for the drug monographs.

An updated, color photoguide helps you identify tablets and capsules in various dosages; this is especially important for situations when patients can't identify their own medications.

The appendices include current information on selected topical, ophthalmic, and otic drugs; a table of equivalents; and a nomogram for estimating body surface area in children. This edition of *Springhouse Nurse's Drug Guide* introduces two new appendices: drugs that shouldn't be crushed and normal laboratory test values. The well-done index is easy to use; it lists the generic and brand drug names, drug classifications, diseases and related drugs, herbal remedies, and drugs pictured in the full color photoguide. The page numbers of the drugs in the photoguide appear in bold type for quick recognition.

The book also includes a free mini-sized CD-ROM, *PharmDisk 4.0*, that works with both Windows and Macintosh operating systems. With an interactive self-test that includes a 200-question bank of pharmacology questions that can be adapted for personal use and a drug-class match game, the mini-CD makes learning important content fun. *Springhouse Nurse's Drug Guide* also provides further support, new developments, and insights available to the book's users through a special Web site: eDrugInfo.com.

Drug administration is a critical aspect of nursing care. When given appropriately, drugs maintain, restore, and promote health. However, no one can recall every essential fact about every common drug. This book offers you quick access to current, accurate information that will help you understand drugs, administer them properly, and teach patients about their proper use.

Springhouse Nurse's Drug Guide is a superb resource to help nursing students, nurses, and other health professionals practice effectively and safely. When a student—such as my daughter—asks for advice in choosing a drug book, I'm confident in recommending a reference I've relied on for my own practice: *Springhouse Nurse's Drug Guide*.

Carol Toussie Weingarten, RN, PhD
Associate Professor, College of Nursing
Villanova University
Villanova, Pennsylvania

How to use *Springhouse Nurse's Drug Guide*

Springhouse Nurse's Drug Guide is the premier drug reference for all nursing students—beginning to advanced. Tightly organized entries offer consistent, practical pharmacologic information about more than 750 common generic drugs, presented in a clear writing style that beginning students can understand. The book is a must-have for advanced students as well; it includes comprehensive pharmacokinetic and pharmacodynamic information and route-onset-peak-duration tables that give readers a clear understanding of drug actions. Because each entry also follows a nursing process organization, the book even helps students formulate accurate care plans. Students of all levels will find that *Springhouse Nurse's Drug Guide* offers a comprehensive, convenient resource for all aspects of drug information.

The book begins with introductory material crucial to safe, accurate drug administration. Chapter 1 discusses drug therapy as it relates to the nursing process. Chapter 2 explains how to calculate dosages and provides examples for each step in the calculations. Chapter 3 discusses how to administer drugs by commonly used routes and includes illustrations to guide students through the steps of each procedure. Chapter 4 focuses on common medication errors and explains how to avoid them.

Drug classifications

Springhouse Nurse's Drug Guide provides complete overviews of 40 pharmacologic and therapeutic drug classifications, from alkylating drugs to xanthine derivatives. Following the class name is an alphabetical list of examples of drugs in that class; the drug highlighted in color represents the prototype drug for the class. The text then provides class-specific information on indications, actions, adverse reactions, contraindications and precautions (including special information for pregnant, breast-feeding, pediatric, and geriatric patients), and nursing considerations.

Alphabetical listing of drugs

Drug entries in this text appear alphabetically by generic name for quick reference. The generic name is followed by a pronunciation guide and an alphabetical list of brand (trade) names. Brands that don't need a prescription are designated with a dagger (†); those available only in Canada with a closed diamond (♦); those available only in Australia with an open diamond (◊); those that contain alcohol with a single asterisk (*); and those that contain tartrazine with a double asterisk (**). The mention of a brand name in no way implies endorsement of that product or guarantees its legality.

Each entry then identifies the drug's pharmacologic and therapeutic classifications; that is, its chemical category and its major clinical use. Listing both classifications helps you grasp the multiple, varying, and sometimes overlapping uses of drugs within a single pharmacologic class and among different classes. Each entry then lists the drug's controlled substance schedule, if applicable, and its pregnancy risk category. (See *Controlled substance schedules* on page xii and *Pregnancy risk categories* on page xiii.)

Indications and dosages

The next section lists the drug's indications and provides dosage information for adults, children, and elderly patients, as applicable. Dosage instructions reflect current clinical trends in therapeutics and can't be considered as absolute or universal recommendations. For individual application, dosage instructions must be considered in light of the patient's clinical condition.

Controlled substance schedules

Drugs regulated under the jurisdiction of the Controlled Substances Act of 1970 are divided into the following groups, or schedules:

- Schedule I (C-I): High abuse potential and no accepted medical use. Examples include heroin, marijuana, and LSD.
- Schedule II (C-II): High abuse potential with severe dependence liability. Examples include narcotics, amphetamines, dronabinol, and some barbiturates.
- Schedule III (C-III): Less abuse potential than schedule II drugs and moderate dependence liability. Examples include nonbarbiturate sedatives, nonamphetamine stimulants, anabolic steroids, and limited amounts of certain narcotics.
- Schedule IV (C-IV): Less abuse potential than schedule III drugs and limited dependence liability. Examples include some sedatives, anxiolytics, and nonnarcotic analgesics.
- Schedule V (C-V): Limited abuse potential. This category includes mainly small amounts of narcotics, such as codeine, used as antitussives or antidiarrheals. Under federal law, limited quantities of certain C-V drugs may be purchased without a prescription directly from a pharmacist if allowed under specific state statutes. The purchaser must be at least age 18 and must furnish suitable identification. All such transactions must be recorded by the dispensing pharmacist.

How supplied

This section lists all available preparations for each drug (for example, tablets, capsules, solutions for injection) and all available dosage forms and strengths. As with the brand names discussed above, over-the-counter dosage forms and strengths are marked with a dagger (†); those available only in Canada with a closed diamond (♦); those available only in Australia with an open diamond (◇); and those that contain alcohol with an asterisk (*).

Pharmacokinetics

This section describes absorption, distribution, metabolism, and excretion, along with the drug's half-life when known. It also provides a quick reference table highlighting onset, peak, and duration for each route of administration. Values for half-life, onset, peak, and duration are for patients with normal renal function, unless specified otherwise.

Pharmacodynamics

This section explains the drug's chemical and therapeutic actions. For example, although all antihypertensives lower blood pressure, they don't all do so by the same pharmacologic process.

Adverse reactions

This section lists adverse reactions to each drug by body system. The most common adverse reactions (those experienced by at least 10% of people taking the drug in clinical trials) are in *italic* type; less common reactions are in roman type; life-threatening reactions are in ***bold italic*** type; and reactions that are common *and* life-threatening are in **BOLD CAPITAL** letters.

Interactions

This section lists each drug's confirmed, clinically significant interactions with other drugs (additive effects, potentiated effects, and antagonistic effects), herbs, foods, and lifestyle (such as alcohol use or smoking).

Drug interactions are listed under the drug that's adversely affected. For example, antacids that contain magnesium may decrease absorption of tetracycline. Therefore, this interaction is listed under tetracycline. To determine the possible effects of using two or more drugs simultaneously, check the interactions section for each of the drugs in question.

Contraindications and precautions

This section specifies conditions in which the drug should not be used and details recommendations for cautious use. For example, a drug that can be given safely to most people may be contraindicated or require cautious use in pregnant or breast-feeding women, in elderly patients or children, in those hypersensitive to the drug, or in those with a disorder that precludes safe administration.

Nursing considerations

This section uses the nursing process as its organizational framework. It also contains an Alert logo to call your attention to vital, need-to-know information or serve as a warning about a common drug error.

- Assessment focuses on observation and monitoring of key patient data, such as vital signs, weight, intake and output, and laboratory values.
- Nursing diagnoses represent those most commonly applied to drug therapy. In actual use, nursing diagnoses must be relevant to an individual patient; therefore, they may not include the listed examples and may include others not listed.
- Planning and implementation offers detailed recommendations for drug administration, including full coverage of P.O., I.V., I.M., S.C., and other routes. Patient teaching focuses on explaining the drug's purpose, promoting compliance, and ensuring proper use and storage of the drug. It also includes instructions for preventing or minimizing adverse reactions.
- Evaluation identifies the expected patient outcomes for the listed nursing diagnoses.

Because nursing considerations in this text emphasize drug-specific recommendations, they don't include standard recommendations that apply to all drugs, such as "assess the five rights of drug therapy before administration" or "teach the patient the name, dose, frequency, route, and strength of the prescribed drug."

Pregnancy risk categories

The Food and Drug Administration has assigned a pregnancy risk category to each systemically absorbed drug based on available clinical and preclinical information. The five categories (A, B, C, D, and X) reflect a drug's potential to cause birth defects. Although drugs are best avoided during pregnancy, this rating system permits rapid assessment of the risk-benefit ratio should drug administration to a pregnant woman become necessary. Drugs in category A are generally considered safe to use in pregnancy; drugs in category X are generally contraindicated.

- A: Adequate studies in pregnant women have failed to show a risk to fetus.
- B: Animal studies haven't shown a risk to fetus, but controlled studies haven't been conducted in pregnant women; or animal studies have shown an adverse effect on fetus, but adequate studies in pregnant women haven't shown a risk to fetus.
- C: Animal studies have shown an adverse effect on fetus, but adequate studies haven't been conducted in humans. The benefits from use in pregnant women may be acceptable despite potential risks.
- D: The drug may cause risk to human fetus, but the potential benefits of use in pregnant women may be acceptable despite the risks (such as in a life-threatening situation or a serious disease for which safer drugs can't be used or are ineffective).
- X: Studies in animals or humans show fetal abnormalities, or adverse reaction reports indicate evidence of fetal risk. The risks involved clearly outweigh potential benefits.
- NR: Not rated.

Photoguide to tablets and capsules

To make drug identification easier and to enhance patient safety, *Springhouse Nurse's Drug Guide* offers a full-color photoguide to the most commonly prescribed tablets and capsules. Shown in their actual sizes, the drugs are arranged alphabetically for quick reference, along with their most common dosage strengths. Page references appear under each drug name so you can turn quickly to information about the drug.

Herbal medicines

Herbal medicine entries appear alphabetically by name, followed by a phonetic spelling and an alphabetical list of common names.

Reported uses

This section lists reported uses of the herbal medicine. Some of these uses are based on anecdotal claims; other uses have been studied. However, a listing in this section should not be considered as a recommendation.

Common forms

This section lists the available preparations for each herbal medicine as well as dosage forms and strengths.

Actions

This section describes the herb's chemical and therapeutic actions.

Dosages

This section lists the routes and general dosage information for each form of the herb and, where available, in accordance with its reported use. This information has been gathered from the herbal literature, anecdotal reports, and available clinical data. However, not all uses have specific dosage information; often, no consensus exists. Dosage notations reflect current clinical trends and should not be considered as recommendations by the publisher.

Adverse reactions

This section lists undesirable effects that may follow use of an herbal supplement. Some of these effects have not been reported but are theoretically possible, given the chemical composition or action of the herb.

Interactions

This section lists each herb's clinically significant interactions, actual or potential, with other herbs, drugs, foods, or lifestyle choices. Each statement describes the effect of the interaction and then offers a specific suggestion for avoiding the interaction. As with adverse reactions, some interactions have not been proven but are theoretically possible.

Cautions

This section lists any condition, especially a disease, in which use of the herbal remedy is undesirable. It also provides recommendations for cautious use, as appropriate.

Nursing considerations

This section offers helpful information, such as monitoring techniques and methods for the prevention and treatment of adverse reactions. Patient teaching tips that focus on educating the patient about the herb's purpose, preparation, administration, and storage are also included, as are suggestions for promoting patient compliance with the therapeutic regimen and steps the patient can take to prevent or minimize the risk or severity of adverse reactions.

Appendices and index

The appendices include five quick-reference charts on topical, ophthalmic, and otic drugs; a table of equivalents; a nomogram for estimating body surface area in children; a list of drugs that shouldn't be crushed; and a list of normal laboratory test values.

The comprehensive index lists drug classifications, all generic drugs, brand names, disorders, and herbal medicines included in this book.

PharmDisk 4.0

The CD-ROM included with this book (inside the back cover) offers two exciting Windows- and Macintosh-based software programs. "Pharmacology Self-test" tests your knowledge with 200 multiple-choice questions. And a challenging interactive game helps you learn drug classifications. *PharmDisk 4.0* also provides a link to eDrugInfo.com.

eDrugInfo.com

This Web site keeps *Springhouse Nurse's Drug Guide* current by providing the following features:

- updates on new drugs, new indications, and new warnings
- patient teaching aids on new drugs
- news summaries of pertinent drug information.

The Web site also gives you:

- clinical pearls of wisdom
- information on herbs
- links to pharmaceutical companies, government agencies, and other drug information sites
- a bookstore full of nursing books, software, and more.

Plus, registering with eDrugInfo.com entitles you to e-mail notifications when new drug updates are posted.

Guide to abbreviations

ACE	angiotensin-converting enzyme
ADH	antidiuretic hormone
AIDS	acquired immunodeficiency syndrome
ALT	alanine transaminase
AST	aspartate transaminase
AV	atrioventricular
b.i.d.	twice daily
BPH	benign prostatic hyperplasia
BUN	blood urea nitrogen
cAMP	cyclic adenosine monophosphate
CBC	complete blood count
CK	creatine kinase
CMV	cytomegalovirus
CNS	central nervous system
COPD	chronic obstructive pulmonary disease
CSF	cerebrospinal fluid
CV	cardiovascular
CVA	cerebrovascular accident
DIC	disseminated intravascular coagulation
D_5W	dextrose 5% in water
DNA	deoxyribonucleic acid
ECG	electrocardiogram
EEG	electroencephalogram
EENT	eyes, ears, nose, throat
FDA	Food and Drug Administration
g	gram
G	gauge
GFR	glomerular filtration rate
GGT	gamma-glutamyltransferase
GI	gastrointestinal
gtt	drops
GU	genitourinary
G6PD	glucose-6-phosphate dehydrogenase
H	histamine
HIV	human immunodeficiency virus
h.s.	at bedtime
ICU	intensive care unit
I.D.	intradermal
I.M.	intramuscular
INR	international normalized ratio
IPPB	intermittent positive-pressure breathing
IU	international unit
I.V.	intravenous
kg	kilogram
L	liter
LD	lactate dehydrogenase
M	molar
m^2	square meter
MAO	monoamine oxidase
mcg	microgram
mEq	milliequivalent
mg	milligram
MI	myocardial infarction
ml	milliliter
mm^3	cubic millimeter
Na	sodium
NG	nasogastric
NSAID	nonsteroidal anti-inflammatory drug

OTC	over-the-counter
PABA	para-aminobenzoic acid
$Paco_2$	carbon dioxide partial pressure
Pao_2	oxygen partial pressure
PCA	patient-controlled analgesia
P.O.	by mouth
P.R.	by rectum
p.r.n.	as needed
PT	prothrombin time
PTT	partial thromboplastin time
PVC	premature ventricular contraction
q	every
q.i.d.	four times daily
RBC	red blood cell
RDA	recommended daily allowance
REM	rapid eye movement
RNA	ribonucleic acid
RSV	respiratory syncytial virus
SA	sinoatrial
S.C.	subcutaneous
SIADH	syndrome of inappropriate antidiuretic hormone
S.L.	sublingual
T_3	triiodothyronine
T_4	thyroxine
t.i.d.	three times daily
USP	United States Pharmacopeia
UTI	urinary tract infection
WBC	white blood cell

1

Drug therapy and the nursing process

Springhouse Nurse's Drug Guide integrates the nursing process into its organizational framework for good reason. The nursing process guides nursing decisions about drug administration to ensure the patient's safety and meet medical and legal standards. This process provides thorough assessment, appropriate nursing diagnoses, effective planning and implementation, and constant evaluation.

Assessment

Data collection begins with a patient history. After taking the patient's history, perform a thorough physical examination. Also, evaluate the patient's knowledge and understanding of the drug therapy he's about to receive.

History

When taking a history, investigate the patient's allergies, use of drugs and herbs, medical history, lifestyle and beliefs, and socioeconomic status.

Allergies

Specify the drug or food to which the patient is allergic. Describe the reaction he has; its situation, time, and setting; and any contributing factors, such as a significant change in eating habits or the concurrent use of stimulants, tobacco, alcohol, or illegal drugs.

Drugs and herbs

Take a complete drug history that includes both prescription and over-the-counter drugs. Also, find out which herbs the patient takes. Investigate the patient's reasons for using a drug or herb and his knowledge of its use. Explore the patient's thoughts and attitudes about drug use to see if he may encounter problems with drug therapy. Note any special procedures he'll need to perform, such as monitoring his blood glucose level or checking his heart rate, and make sure he can perform them correctly.

Discuss the effects of therapy to determine whether new symptoms or adverse drug reactions have developed. Also, talk about measures the patient has taken to recognize, minimize, or avoid adverse drug reactions or accidental overdose. Ask the patient where he stores his medication and what system he uses to help himself remember to take it as prescribed.

Medical history

Note any chronic disorders the patient has, and record the date of diagnosis, the prescribed treatment, and the name of the prescriber. Careful attention during this part of the history can uncover one of the most important problems with drug therapy: conflicting and incompatible drug regimens.

Lifestyle and beliefs

Ask about the patient's support systems, marital status, childbearing status, attitudes toward health and health care, and daily patterns of activity. They all affect patient compliance and, thus, the plan of care.

Also, ask about the patient's diet. Certain foods can influence the efficacy of many drugs. Also, inquire about the patient's use of alcohol, tobacco, caffeine, and such illegal drugs as marijuana, cocaine, and heroin. Note the substance used and the amount and frequency of use.

Socioeconomic status

Note the patient's age, educational level, occupation, and insurance coverage. These characteristics help determine the plan of care, the likelihood of compliance, and the possible need for financial assistance and counseling.

Physical examination

Examine the patient closely for expected drug effects and for adverse reactions. Every drug has a desired effect on one body system, but it may also have one or more undesired effects on that or another body system. For example, chemotherapeutic drugs destroy cancer cells, but they also affect normal cells and typically cause hair loss, diarrhea, or nausea. Besides looking for adverse drug effects, investigate whether the patient has sensory deficits or changes in cognitive status.

Sensory deficits

Assess the patient for sensory deficits that could influence the plan of care. For example, impaired vision or paralysis can hinder the patient's ability to give himself a subcutaneous injection, break a scored tablet, or open a medication container. Hearing impairment can complicate effective patient instruction.

Cognitive status

Note whether the patient is alert, oriented, and able to interact appropriately. Assess whether he can think clearly and converse appropriately. Check his short-term and long-term memory; he needs both to follow a prescribed regimen correctly. Also, determine whether the patient can read and at what level.

Knowledge and understanding of drug therapy

A patient is more likely to comply if he understands the reason for drug therapy. During your assessment, evaluate your patient's understanding of his therapy and the reason for it. Pay particular attention to his emotional acceptance of the need for the drug treatment plan. For instance, a young patient being prescribed an antihypertensive may need more education than an older patient to ensure compliance.

Nursing diagnosis

Using the information you gathered during assessment, define drug-related problems by formulating each problem into a relevant nursing diagnosis. The most common problem statements related to drug therapy are "Deficient knowledge," "Ineffective health maintenance," and "Noncompliance." Nursing diagnoses provide the framework for planning interventions and outcome criteria (patient goals).

Planning and implementation

Make sure that your outcome criteria state the desired patient behaviors or responses that should result from nursing care. Such criteria should have the following characteristics:

- measurable
- objective
- concise
- realistic for the patient
- attainable by nursing management.

Express patient behavior in terms of expectations, and specify a time frame. An example of an acceptable outcome statement is "Before discharge, the patient verbalizes major adverse effects related to his chemotherapy."

After developing outcome criteria, determine the interventions needed to help the patient reach the desired goals. Appropriate interventions may include administration procedures and techniques, legal and ethical concerns, patient teaching, and concerns related to pregnant, breast-feeding, pediatric, or geriatric patients. Interventions may be independent nursing actions, such as turning a bedridden patient every 2 hours, or actions that require a prescriber's order.

Evaluation

The final component of the nursing process is a formal and systematic process for determining the effectiveness of nursing care. This evaluation process lets you determine whether outcome criteria were met, which then helps you make informed decisions about subsequent interventions. If you stated the outcome criteria in measureable terms, then you can easily evaluate the extent to which they were met.

For example, if a patient experiences relief from headache pain within 1 hour after receiving an analgesic, the outcome criterion was met. If the headache was the same or worse, the outcome criterion wasn't met. In that case, you'll need to assess the patient again—a process that may yield a new plan, new data that invalidate the nursing diagnosis, or new nursing interventions that are more specific or more acceptable to the patient. For instance, this reassessment could lead to a higher dosage, a different analgesic, or a reevaluation of the cause of the headache pain.

Evaluation enables you to design and implement a revised plan of care, to continuously reevaluate outcome criteria, and to plan again until each nursing diagnosis is successfully completed.

2

Essentials of dosage calculations

Nurses perform drug and intravenous (I.V.) fluid calculations frequently. That's why you need to know and understand drug weights and measures, how to convert between systems and measures, how to compute drug dosages, and how to make adjustments for pediatric patients.

Systems of drug weights and measures

Prescribers use several systems of measurement when ordering drugs, three in particular: the metric, household, and apothecaries' systems. The metric and household systems are so widely used that most brands of medication cups for liquid measurements are calibrated in both systems. The apothecaries' system isn't widely used but may still be encountered in clinical practice. A fourth system, the avoirdupois system, is rarely used. This system uses solid units of measure, such as the ounce and the pound.

Metric system

The metric system is the international system of measurement, the most widely used system, and the system used by the U.S. Pharmacopoeia. It has units for both liquid and solid measures. Among its many advantages, the metric system enables accuracy in calculating small drug dosages. It uses Arabic numerals, which are commonly used by health care professionals worldwide. And most manufacturers calibrate newly developed drugs in the metric system.

Liquid measures

In the metric system, one liter (L) is about equal to 1 quart in the apothecaries' system. Liters are often used when ordering and administering I.V. solutions. Milliliters are frequently used to administer parenteral and some oral drugs. One milliliter (ml) equals $\frac{1}{1,000}$ of a liter.

Solid measures

The gram (g) is the basis for solid measures or units of weight in the metric system. One milligram (mg) equals $\frac{1}{1,000}$ of a gram. Drugs are frequently ordered in grams, milligrams, or an even smaller unit, the microgram (mcg), depending on the drug. One microgram equals $\frac{1}{1,000}$ of a milligram. Body weight is usually recorded in kilograms (kg). One kilogram equals 1,000 g.

The following are examples of drug orders using the metric system:

- 30 ml milk of magnesia P.O. at bedtime
- Ancef 1 g I.V. every 6 hours
- Lanoxin 0.125 mg P.O. daily.

Household system

Most foods, recipes, over-the-counter drugs, and home remedies use the household system. Health care professionals seldom use this system for drug administration; however, knowledge of household measures may be useful in some clinical situations.

Liquid measures

Liquid measurements in the household system include teaspoons (tsp) and tablespoons (tbs). For clinical purposes, these measurements have been standardized to 5 milliliters and 15 milliliters, respectively. Using these standardized amounts, 3 teaspoons equal 1 tablespoon, 6 teaspoons equal 1 ounce, and so forth. Patients who need to measure doses by teaspoon or tablespoon should do so using calibrated clinical devices to make sure they receive exactly the prescribed amount. Advise against using an ordinary household spoon to measure a teaspoonful of a medication because the amount will most likely be inaccurate. Teaspoon sizes vary from 4 to 6 milliliters or more.

The following are examples of drug orders using the household system:

- 2 tsp Bactrim P.O. twice daily
- Riopan 2 tbs P.O. 1 hour before meals and at bedtime.

Apothecaries' system

Two unique features distinguish the apothecaries' system from other systems: the use of Roman numerals and the placement of the unit of measurement before the Roman numeral. For example, a measurement of 5 grains would be written as *grains v*.

In the apothecaries' system, equivalents among the various units of measure are close approximations of one another. By contrast, equivalents in the metric system are exact. When using apothecaries' equivalents for calculations and conversions, the calculations, although not precise, must fall within acceptable standards.

The apothecaries' system is the only system of measurement that uses both symbols and abbreviations to represent units of measure. Although the use of the apothecaries' system is becoming less common in health care, you must still be able to read dosages that have been written in the apothecaries' system and convert them to the metric system.

Liquid measures

The smallest unit of liquid measurement in the apothecaries' system is the minim (♏), which is about the size of a drop of water. Fifteen to sixteen minims equal about 1 ml.

Solid measures

The grain (gr) is the smallest solid measure or unit of weight in the apothecaries' system. It equals about 60 milligrams. One dram equals about 60 grains.

The following are examples of drug orders using the apothecaries' system:

- Robitussin fʒ (fluidrams) iv P.O. q6h
- Mylanta f℥ (fluidounce) i P.O. 1 hour after meals
- Tylenol gr (grains) X P.O. q4h as needed for headache.

Units, international units, and milliequivalents

For some drugs, you'll need to use a measuring system developed by drug manufacturers. Three of the most common special systems of measurement are units, international units, and milliequivalents.

Units

Insulin is one of several drugs measured in units. Although many types of insulin exist, all are measured in units. The international standard of U-100 insulin means that 1 ml of insulin solution contains 100 units of insulin, regardless of type. Heparin, an anticoagulant, is also measured in units, as are several antibiotics, available in liquid, solid, and powder forms for oral or parenteral use. Each manufacturer of drugs made available in units provides specific information about the measurement of each drug.

The following are examples of drug orders using units:

- Inject 14 units NPH insulin S.C. this a.m.
- Heparin 5,000 units S.C. q12h
- Nystatin 200,000 units P.O. q6h.

The unit is not a standard measure. Thus, different drugs, although each measured in units, may have no relationship to one another in quality or activity.

International units

International units (IU) are used to measure biologicals, such as vitamins, enzymes, and hormones. For instance, the activity of calcitonin, a synthetic hormone used in calcium regulation, is expressed in international units.

The following are examples of drug orders using international units:

- 100 IU calcitonin (salmon) S.C. daily
- 8 IU somatropin S.C. three times a week.

Milliequivalents

Electrolytes may be measured in milliequivalents (mEq). Drug manufacturers provide information about the number of metric units needed to provide a prescribed number of milliequivalents. Potassium chloride (KCl), for example, is usually ordered in milliequivalents.

The following are examples of drug orders using milliequivalents:

- 30 mEq KCl P.O. b.i.d.
- 1 L dextrose 5% in normal saline solution with 40 mEq KCl to be run at 125 ml/hour.

Conversions between measurement systems

Sometimes you may need to convert from one measurement system to another, particularly when a drug is ordered in one system but available only in another system. To perform conversion calculations, you need to know the equivalent measurements for the different systems of measurement. One of the most commonly used methods for converting drug measurements is the fraction method.

Fraction method

The fraction method for converting between measurement systems involves an equation consisting of two fractions. Set up the first fraction by placing the ordered dosage over *x* units of the available dosage.

For example, say a prescriber orders 7.5 ml of acetaminophen elixir to be given by mouth. To find the equivalent in teaspoons, first set up a fraction in which the ml dosage represents the ordered dosage and the teaspoon dosage represents the unknown (*x*) available dosage:

$$\frac{7.5 \text{ ml}}{\text{x tsp}}$$

Then, set up the second fraction, which appears on the right side of the equation. This fraction consists of the standard equivalents between the ordered and the available measures. Because milliliters must be converted to teaspoons, the right side of the equation appears as:

$$\frac{5 \text{ ml}}{1 \text{ tsp}}$$

The same unit of measure should appear in the numerator of both fractions. Likewise, the same unit of measure should appear in both denominators. The entire equation should appear as:

$$\frac{7.5 \text{ ml}}{\text{x tsp}} = \frac{5 \text{ ml}}{1 \text{ tsp}}$$

To solve for *x*, cross multiply.

$$\text{x tsp} \times 5 \text{ ml} = 7.5 \text{ ml} \times 1 \text{ tsp}$$

$$\text{x tsp} = \frac{7.5 \cancel{\text{ml}} \times 1 \text{ tsp}}{5 \cancel{\text{ml}}}$$

$$\text{x tsp} = \frac{7.5 \times 1 \text{ tsp}}{5}$$

$$\text{x tsp} = 1.5 \text{ tsp}$$

The patient should receive 1.5 teaspoons of acetaminophen elixir.

Computing drug dosages

Computing a drug dosage is a two-step process that you complete after verifying the drug order. First, determine whether the ordered drug is available in units in the same system of measurement. If not, then convert the measurement for the ordered drug to the system used for the available drug.

If the ordered units of measurement are available, calculate how much of the available dosage form should be administered. For example, if the prescribed dose is 250 mg, determine the quantity of tablets, powder, or liquid that would equal 250 mg. To determine that quantity, use one of the methods described below.

Fraction method

When using the fraction method to compute a drug dosage, write an equation consisting of two fractions. First, set up a fraction showing the number of units to be given over *x*, which represents the quantity of the dosage form.

On the other side of the equation, set up a fraction showing the number of units of the drug in its dosage form over the quantity of dosage forms that supply that number of units. The number of units and the quantity of dosage forms are specific for each drug. In most cases, the stated quantity equals 1. Information provided on the drug label should supply the details needed to form the second fraction.

For example, if the number of units to be administered equals 250 mg, the first fraction in the equation would appear as:

$$\frac{250\text{ mg}}{\text{x tab}}$$

The drug label states that each tablet contains 125 mg, so the second fraction would appear as:

$$\frac{125\text{ mg}}{1\text{ tab}}$$

Note that the same units of measure appear in the numerators and the same units appear in the denominators. Note also that the units of measure in the denominators differ from the units in the numerators.

The entire equation would appear as:

$$\frac{250\text{ mg}}{\text{x tab}} = \frac{125\text{ mg}}{1\text{ tab}}$$

Solving for *x* determines the quantity of the dosage form—2 tablets, in this example.

Ratio method

To use the ratio method, write the amount of the drug to be given and the quantity of the dose (*x*) as a ratio. Using the example shown above, you'd write:

$$250\text{ mg} : \text{x tab}$$

Next, complete the equation by forming a second ratio from the number of units in each tablet (or whatever form the drug comes in). The manufacturer's label provides this information. Again using the example from above, the entire equation is:

$$250\text{ mg} : \text{x tab} :: 125\text{ mg} : 1\text{ tab}$$

Solve for *x* by multiplying the means (inner portions) and extremes (outer portions) of the equation. The patient should receive 2 tablets.

Desired-available method

You can also use the desired-available method, also known as the dose-over-on hand (D/H) method. This method converts ordered units into available units and computes the drug dosage all in one step. The desired-available equation appears as:

$$\begin{matrix}\text{x}\\\text{quantity}\\\text{to give}\end{matrix} = \frac{\begin{matrix}\text{ordered}\\\text{units}\end{matrix}}{1} \times \begin{matrix}\text{conversion}\\\text{fraction}\end{matrix} \times \frac{\begin{matrix}\text{quantity}\\\text{of dosage}\\\text{form}\end{matrix}}{\begin{matrix}\text{stated}\\\text{quantity of}\\\text{drug within}\\\text{each dosage}\\\text{form}\end{matrix}}$$

For example, say you receive an order for gr x of a drug. The drug is available only in 300-mg tablets. To determine the number of tablets to give the patient, substitute gr x (the ordered number of units) for the first element of the equation. Then use the conversion fraction as the second portion of the formula. The conversion factor is:

$$\frac{60\text{ mg}}{1\text{ gr}}$$

The measure in the denominator must be the same as the measure in the ordered units. In this case, the order specified gr x. As a result, grains appears in the denominator of the conversion fraction.

The third element of the equation shows the dosage form over the stated drug quantity for that dosage form. Because the drug is available in 300-mg tablets, the fraction appears as:

$$\frac{1\text{ tab}}{300\text{ mg}}$$

The dosage form—tablets—should always appear in the numerator, and the quantity of drug in each dosage form should always appear in the denominator. The completed equation is:

$$\text{x tab} = 10\text{ gr} \times \frac{60\text{ mg}}{1\text{ gr}} \times \frac{1\text{ tab}}{300\text{ mg}}$$

Solving for *x* shows that the patient should receive 2 tablets.

The desired-available method has the advantage of using only one equation. However, you need to memorize an equation more elaborate than the one used in the fraction method or the ratio method. Relying on your memorization of a more complicated equation may increase the chance of error.

Dimensional analysis

A variation of the ratio method, dimensional analysis (also known as factor analysis or factor labeling) eliminates the need to memorize formulas and requires only one equation to determine the answer. To compare the two methods at a glance, read the following problem and solutions.

Say a physician prescribes 0.25 g of streptomycin sulfate I.M. The vial reads 2 ml = 1 g. How many milliliters should you give?

Dimensional analysis

$$\frac{0.25 \text{ g}}{1} \times \frac{2 \text{ ml}}{1 \text{ g}} = 0.5 \text{ ml}$$

Ratio method

$$1 \text{ g} : 2 \text{ ml} :: 0.25 \text{ g} : x \text{ ml}$$

$$x = 2 \times 0.25$$

$$x = 0.5 \text{ ml}$$

When using dimensional analysis, you arrange a series of ratios, called factors, in a single (although sometimes lengthy) fractional equation. Each factor, written as a fraction, consists of two quantities and their related units of measurement. For instance, if 1,000 ml of a drug should be given over 8 hours, the relationship between 1,000 and 8 hours is expressed by the fraction

$$\frac{1{,}000 \text{ ml}}{8 \text{ hours}}$$

When a problem includes a quantity and a unit of measurement that are unrelated to any other factor in the problem, they serve as the numerator of the fraction, and 1 (implied) becomes the denominator.

Some mathematical problems contain all of the information needed to identify the factors, set up the equation, and find the solution. Other problems require the use of a conversion factor. Conversion factors are equivalents (for example, 1 g = 1,000 mg) that you can memorize or obtain from a conversion chart. Because the two quantities and units of measurement are equivalent, they can serve as the numerator or the denominator; thus, the conversion factor 1 g = 1,000 mg can be written in fraction form as

$$\frac{1{,}000 \text{ mg}}{1 \text{ g}} \text{ or } \frac{1 \text{ g}}{1{,}000 \text{ mg}}$$

The factors given in the problem plus any conversion factors needed to solve the problem are called *knowns*. The quantity of the answer, of course, is *unknown*. When setting up an equation in dimensional analysis, work backward, beginning with the unit of measurement of the answer. After plotting all the knowns, find the solution by following this sequence:

- Cancel similar quantities and units of measurement.
- Multiply the numerators.
- Multiply the denominators.
- Divide the numerator by the denominator.

Mastering dimensional analysis can take practice, but you may find your efforts well rewarded. To understand more fully how dimensional analysis works, review the following problem and the steps taken to solve it.

A physician prescribes x grains (gr) of a drug. The pharmacy supplies the drug in 300-mg tablets (tab). How many tablets should you administer?

- Write down the unit of measurement of the answer, followed by an "equal to" symbol.

$$\text{tab} =$$

- Search the problem for the quantity with the same unit of measurement (if one doesn't exist, use a conversion factor); place this in the numerator and its related quantity and unit of measurement in the denominator.

$$\text{tab} = \frac{1 \text{ tab}}{300 \text{ mg}}$$

- Separate the first factor from the next with a multiplication symbol.

$$\text{tab} = \frac{1 \text{ tab}}{300 \text{ mg}} \times$$

- Place the unit of measurement of the denominator of the first factor in the numerator of the second factor; search the problem for the quantity with the same unit of measurement (if one doesn't exist, as in this example, use a conversion factor); place this in the numerator and its related quantity and unit of measurement in the denominator, and follow with a multiplication symbol. Repeat this step until all known factors are included in the equation.

$$\text{tab} = \frac{1\text{ tab}}{300\text{ mg}} \times \frac{60\text{ mg}}{1\text{ gr}} \times \frac{10\text{ gr}}{1}$$

• Treat the equation as a large fraction. First, cancel similar units of measurement in the numerator and the denominator (what remains should be what you began with—the unit of measurement of the answer; if not, recheck your equation to find and correct the error). Next, multiply the numerators and then the denominators. Finally, divide the numerator by the denominator.

$$\text{tab} = \frac{1\text{ tab}}{300\text{ }\cancel{\text{mg}}} \times \frac{60\text{ }\cancel{\text{mg}}}{1\text{ }\cancel{\text{gr}}} \times \frac{10\text{ }\cancel{\text{gr}}}{1}$$

$$= \frac{60 \times 10\text{ tab}}{300}$$

$$= \frac{600\text{ tab}}{300}$$

$$= 2\text{ tablets}$$

For more practice, study the following examples, which use dimensional analysis to solve various mathematical problems common to dosage calculations and drug administration.

1. *A patient weighs 140 lb. What is his weight in kilograms (kg)?*
Unit of measurement of the answer: kg

$$\text{1st factor (conversion factor): } \frac{1\text{ kg}}{2.2\text{ lb}}$$

$$\text{2nd factor: } \frac{140\text{ lb}}{1}$$

$$\text{kg} = \frac{1\text{ kg}}{2.2\text{ }\cancel{\text{lb}}} \times 140\text{ }\cancel{\text{lb}}$$

$$= \frac{140\text{ lb}}{2.2\text{ lb}}$$

$$= 63.6\text{ kg}$$

2. *A physician prescribes 75 mg of a drug. The pharmacy stocks a multidose vial containing 100 mg/ml. How many milliliters should you administer?*
Unit of measurement of the answer: ml

$$\text{1st factor: } \frac{1\text{ ml}}{100\text{ mg}}$$

$$\text{2nd factor: } \frac{75\text{ mg}}{1}$$

$$\text{ml} = \frac{1\text{ ml}}{100\text{ }\cancel{\text{mg}}} \times \frac{75\text{ }\cancel{\text{mg}}}{1}$$

$$= \frac{75\text{ ml}}{100}$$

$$= 0.75\text{ ml}$$

3. *A nurse practitioner prescribes 1 teaspoon (tsp) of a cough elixir. The pharmacist sends up a bottle whose label reads 1 ml = 50 mg. How many milligrams should you administer?*
Unit of measurement of the answer: mg

$$\text{1st factor: } \frac{50\text{ mg}}{1\text{ ml}}$$

$$\text{2nd factor (conversion factor): } \frac{50\text{ ml}}{1\text{ tsp}}$$

$$\text{3rd factor: } \frac{1\text{ tsp}}{1}$$

$$\text{mg} = \frac{50\text{ mg}}{1\text{ }\cancel{\text{ml}}} \times \frac{50\text{ }\cancel{\text{ml}}}{1\text{ }\cancel{\text{tsp}}} \times \frac{1\text{ }\cancel{\text{tsp}}}{1}$$

$$= 50\text{ mg} \times \frac{50}{1}$$

$$= 2{,}500\text{ mg}$$

4. *A physician prescribes 1,000 ml of an I.V. solution to be administered over 8 hours. The I.V. tubing delivers 15 gtt/ml/minute. What is the infusion rate in gtt/minute?*
Unit of measurement of the answer: gtt/minute

$$\text{1st factor: } \frac{15\text{ gtt}}{1\text{ ml}}$$

$$\text{2nd factor: } \frac{1{,}000\text{ ml}}{8\text{ hours}}$$

$$\text{3rd factor (conversion factor): } \frac{1\text{ hour}}{60\text{ minutes}}$$

$$\text{gtt/minute} = \frac{15\text{ gtt}}{1\text{ }\cancel{\text{ml}}} \times \frac{1{,}000\text{ }\cancel{\text{ml}}}{8\text{ }\cancel{\text{hours}}} \times \frac{1\text{ }\cancel{\text{hour}}}{60\text{ minutes}}$$

$$= \frac{15\text{ gtt} \times 1{,}000 \times 1}{8 \times 60\text{ minutes}}$$

$$= \frac{15{,}000 \text{ gtt}}{480 \text{ minutes}}$$

$$= 31.3 \text{ or } 31 \text{ gtt/minute}$$

5. *A physician prescribes 10,000 units of heparin added to 500 ml of 5% dextrose and water at 1,200 units/hour. How many drops per minute should you administer if the I.V. tubing delivers 10 gtt/ml?*
Unit of measurement of the answer: gtt/minute

$$\text{1st factor: } \frac{10 \text{ gtt}}{1 \text{ ml}}$$

$$\text{2nd factor: } \frac{500 \text{ ml}}{10{,}000 \text{ units}}$$

$$\text{3rd factor: } \frac{1{,}200 \text{ units}}{1 \text{ hour}}$$

$$\text{4th factor (conversion factor): } \frac{1 \text{ hour}}{60 \text{ minutes}}$$

$$\text{gtt/minute} = \frac{10 \text{ gtt}}{1 \cancel{\text{ml}}} \times \frac{500 \cancel{\text{ml}}}{10{,}000 \cancel{\text{units}}} \times \frac{1{,}200 \cancel{\text{units}}}{1 \cancel{\text{hour}}} \times \frac{1 \cancel{\text{hour}}}{60 \text{ minutes}}$$

$$= \frac{10 \times 500 \times 1{,}200 \text{ gtt}}{10{,}000 \times 60 \text{ minutes}}$$

$$= \frac{6{,}000{,}000 \text{ gtt}}{600{,}000 \text{ minutes}}$$

$$= 10 \text{ gtt/minutes}$$

Special computations

The fraction, ratio, and desired-available methods and dimensional analysis can be used to compute drug dosages when the ordered drug and the available form of the drug occur in the same units of measure. These methods can also be used when the quantity of a particular dosage form differs from the units in which the dosage form is administered.

For example, if a patient is to receive 1,000 mg of a drug available in liquid form and measured in milligrams, with 100 mg contained in 6 ml, how many milliliters should the patient receive? Because the ordered and the available dosages are in milligrams, no initial conversions are needed. The fraction method would be used to determine the number of milliliters the patient should receive, in this case, 60 ml.

Because the drug will be given in ounces, the number of ounces should be determined using a conversion method. For the fraction method of conversion, the equation would appear as:

$$\frac{60 \text{ ml}}{x \text{ oz}} = \frac{30 \text{ ml}}{1 \text{ oz}}$$

Solving for x shows that the patient should receive 2 oz of the drug.

To use the desired-available method, change the order of the elements in the equation to correspond with the situation. The revised equation should appear as:

$$x \text{ quantity to give} = \frac{\text{ordered units}}{1} \times \frac{\text{quantity of dosage form}}{\text{stated quantity of drug within each dosage form}} \times \text{conversion fraction}$$

Placing the given information into the equation results in:

$$x \text{ oz} = \frac{1{,}000 \text{ mg}}{1} \times \frac{6 \text{ ml}}{100 \text{ mg}} \times \frac{1 \text{ oz}}{30 \text{ ml}}$$

Solving for x shows that the patient should receive 2 oz of the drug.

Inexact nature of dosage computations

Converting drug measurements from one system to another and then determining the amount of a dosage form to give can easily produce inexact dosages. A rounding error made during computation or discrepancies in the dosage may occur, depending on the conversion standard used in calculation. Or, you may determine a precise amount to be given, only to find that administering that amount is impossible. For example, precise computations may indicate that a patient should receive 0.97 tablet. Administering such an amount is impossible.

The following general rule helps avoid calculation errors and discrepancies between theoretical and real dosages: *No more than a 10% variation should exist between the dosage ordered and the dosage to be given.* Following this simple rule, if you determine that a patient should receive 0.97 tablet, you can safely give 1 tablet.

Computing parenteral dosages

The methods for computing drug dosages can be used not just for oral but also for parenteral routes. The following example shows how to determine a parenteral drug dosage. Say a prescriber orders 75 mg of Demerol. The package label reads: meperidine (Demerol), 100 mg/ml. Using the fraction method to determine the number of milliliters the patient should receive, the equation should appear as:

$$\frac{75 \text{ mg}}{\text{x ml}} = \frac{100 \text{ mg}}{1 \text{ ml}}$$

To solve for *x*, cross multiply:

$$\text{x ml} \times 100 \text{ mg} = 75 \text{ mg} \times 1 \text{ ml}$$

$$\text{x ml} = \frac{75 \cancel{\text{mg}} \times 1 \text{ ml}}{100 \cancel{\text{mg}}}$$

$$\text{x ml} = \frac{75 \times 1 \text{ ml}}{100}$$

$$\text{x ml} = 0.75 \text{ ml}$$

The patient should receive 0.75 ml.

Reconstituting powders for injection

Although a pharmacist usually reconstitutes powders for parenteral use, nurses sometimes perform this function by following the directions on the drug label. The label gives the total quantity of drug in the vial or ampule, the amount and type of diluent to be added to the powder, and the strength and expiration date of the resulting solution.

When you add diluent to a powder, the powder increases the fluid volume. That's why the label calls for less diluent than the total volume of the prepared solution. For example, a label may tell you to add 1.7 ml of diluent to a vial of powdered drug to obtain a 2-ml total volume of prepared solution.

To determine the amount of solution to administer, use the manufacturer's information about the concentration of the solution. For example, if you want to administer 500 mg of a drug and the concentration of the prepared solution is 1 g (1,000 mg)/10 ml, use the following equation:

$$\frac{500 \text{ mg}}{\text{x ml}} = \frac{1{,}000 \text{ mg}}{10 \text{ ml}}$$

The patient would receive 5 ml of the prepared solution.

Intravenous drip rates and flow rates

Make sure you know the difference between I.V. drip rate and flow rate and also how to calculate each rate. I.V. drip rate refers to the number of drops of solution to be infused per minute. Flow rate refers to the number of milliliters of fluid to be infused over 1 hour.

To calculate an I.V. drip rate, first set up a fraction showing the volume of solution to be delivered over the number of minutes in which that volume should be infused. For example, if a patient should receive 100 ml of solution in 1 hour, the fraction would be written as:

$$\frac{100 \text{ ml}}{60 \text{ min}}$$

Multiply the fraction by the drip factor (the number of drops [gtt] contained in 1 ml) to determine the number of drops per minute to be infused, or the drip rate. The drip factor varies among different I.V. sets and should appear on the package that contains the I.V. tubing administration set.

Following the manufacturer's directions for drip factor is a crucial step. Standard administration sets have drip factors of 10, 15, or 20 gtt/ml. A microdrip, or minidrip, set has a drip factor of 60 gtt/ml.

Use the following equation to determine the drip rate of an I.V. solution:

$$\text{gtt/min} = \frac{\text{total no. of ml}}{\text{total no. of min}} \times \text{drip factor}$$

The equation applies to I.V. solutions that infuse over many hours or to small-volume infusions such as those used for antibiotics, usually administered in less than 1 hour. For example, if an order requires 1,000 ml of 5% dextrose in normal saline solution to infuse over 12 hours and the administration set delivers 15 gtt per ml, what should the drip rate be?

$$x \text{ gtt/min} = \frac{1{,}000 \text{ ml}}{720 \text{ min}} \times 15 \text{ gtt/ml}$$

$$x \text{ gtt/min} = 20.83 \text{ gtt/min}$$

The drip rate would be rounded to 21 gtt per minute.

You'll use flow rate calculations when working with I.V. infusion pumps to set the number of milliliters to be delivered in 1 hour. To perform this calculation, you should know the total volume in milliliters to be infused and the amount of time for the infusion. Use the following equation:

$$\text{flow rate} = \frac{\text{total volume ordered}}{\text{number of hours}}$$

Quick methods for calculating drip rates

Keep in mind that quicker methods exist for computing I.V. solution administration rates. To administer an I.V. solution through a microdrip set, adjust the flow rate (number of milliliters per hour) to equal the drip rate (gtt per minute).

Using this method, the flow rate would be divided by 60 minutes and then multiplied by the drip factor, which also equals 60. Because the flow rate and the drip factor are equal, the two arithmetic operations cancel each other out. For example, if 125 ml/hour represented the ordered flow rate, the equation would be:

$$\text{drip rate (125)} = \frac{125 \text{ ml}}{60 \text{ min}} \times 60$$

Rather than spend time calculating the equation, you can use the number assigned to the flow rate as the drip rate.

For I.V. administration sets that deliver 15 gtt/ml, the flow rate divided by 4 equals the drip rate. For sets with a drip factor of 10, the flow rate divided by 6 equals the drip rate.

Critical care calculations

Many drugs given on the critical care unit are used to treat life-threatening problems; you must be able to perform calculations swiftly and accurately, prepare the drug for infusion, administer it, and then observe the patient closely to evaluate the drug's effectiveness. Three calculations must be performed before administering critical care drugs:

- Calculate the concentration of the drug in the I.V. solution.
- Figure the flow rate needed to deliver the desired dose.
- Determine the needed dosage.

Calculating concentration

To calculate the drug's concentration, use the following formula:

$$\text{concentration in mg/ml} = \text{mg of drug/ml of fluid}$$

To express the concentration in mcg/ml, multiply the answer by 1,000.

Figuring flow rate

To determine the I.V. flow rate per minute, use the following formula:

$$\frac{\text{dose/min}}{x \text{ ml/min}} = \frac{\text{concentration of solution}}{1 \text{ ml of fluid}}$$

To calculate the hourly flow rate, first multiply the ordered dose, given in milligrams or micrograms per minute, by 60 minutes to determine the hourly dose. Then use the following equation to compute the hourly flow rate:

$$\frac{\text{hourly dose}}{x \text{ ml/hr}} = \frac{\text{concentration of solution}}{1 \text{ ml of fluid}}$$

Determining dosage

To determine the dosage in milligrams per kilogram of body weight per minute, first determine the concentration of the solution in milligrams per milliliter. (If a drug is ordered in micrograms, convert milligrams to micrograms by multiplying by 1,000.) To determine the dose in milligrams per hour, multiply the hourly flow rate by the concentration using the formula:

$$\begin{matrix}\text{dose in} \\ \text{mg/hr}\end{matrix} = \begin{matrix}\text{hourly} \\ \text{flow rate}\end{matrix} \times \text{concentration}$$

Then calculate the dose in milligrams per minute. Divide the hourly dose by 60 minutes:

$$\text{dose in mg/min} = \frac{\text{dose in mg/hr}}{60 \text{ min}}$$

Divide the dose per minute by the patient's weight, using the following formula:

$$\text{mg/kg/min} = \frac{\text{mg/min}}{\text{patient's weight in kg}}$$

Finally, make sure that the drug is being given within a safe and therapeutic range. Compare the amount in milligrams per kilogram per minute to the safe range shown in a drug reference book.

The following examples show how to calculate an I.V. flow rate using the different formulas.

Example 1

A patient has frequent runs of ventricular tachycardia that subside after 10 to 12 beats. The prescriber orders 2 g (2,000 mg) of lidocaine in 500 ml of D_5W to infuse at 2 mg/minute. What's the flow rate in milliliters per minute? Milliliters per hour?

First, find the concentration of the solution by setting up a proportion with the unknown concentration in one fraction and the ordered dose in the other fraction:

$$\frac{\text{x mg}}{\text{1 ml}} = \frac{\text{2,000 mg}}{\text{500 ml}}$$

Cross multiply the fractions:

$$\text{x mg} \times \text{500 ml} = \text{2,000 mg} \times \text{1 ml}$$

Solve for *x* by dividing each side of the equation by 500 ml and canceling units that appear in both the numerator and denominator:

$$\frac{\text{x mg} \times \cancel{\text{500 ml}}}{\cancel{\text{500 ml}}} = \frac{\text{2,000 mg} \times 1\ \cancel{\text{ml}}}{500\ \cancel{\text{ml}}}$$

$$\text{x} = \frac{\text{2,000 mg}}{500}$$

$$\text{x} = \text{4 mg}$$

The concentration of the solution is 4 mg/ml. Next, calculate the flow rate per minute needed to deliver the ordered dose of 2 mg/minute. To do this, set up a proportion with the unknown flow rate per minute in one fraction and the concentration of the solution in the other fraction:

$$\frac{\text{2 mg}}{\text{x ml}} = \frac{\text{4 mg}}{\text{1 ml}}$$

Cross multiply the fractions:

$$\text{x ml} \times \text{4 mg} = \text{1 ml} \times \text{2 mg}$$

Solve for *x* by dividing each side of the equation by 4 mg and canceling units that appear in both the numerator and denominator:

$$\frac{\text{x mg} \times \cancel{\text{4 mg}}}{\cancel{\text{4 mg}}} = \frac{\text{2,000 mg} \times 2\ \cancel{\text{mg}}}{4\ \cancel{\text{mg}}}$$

$$\text{x} = \frac{\text{2 ml}}{4}$$

$$\text{x} = \text{0.5 ml}$$

The patient should receive 0.5 ml/minute of lidocaine. Because lidocaine must be given with an infusion pump, compute the hourly flow rate. Set up a proportion with the unknown flow rate per hour in one fraction and the flow rate per minute in the other fraction:

$$\frac{\text{x ml}}{\text{60 min}} = \frac{\text{0.5 ml}}{\text{1 min}}$$

Cross multiply the fractions:

$$\text{x ml} \times \text{1 min} = \text{0.5 ml} \times \text{60 min}$$

Solve for *x* by dividing each side of the equation by 1 minute and canceling units that appear in both the numerator and denominator:

$$\frac{\text{x ml} \times \cancel{\text{1 min}}}{\cancel{\text{1 min}}} = \frac{\text{0.5 ml} \times 60\ \cancel{\text{min}}}{1\ \cancel{\text{min}}}$$

$$\text{x} = \text{30 ml}$$

Set the infusion pump to deliver 30 ml/hour.

Example 2

A 200-lb patient is scheduled to receive an I.V. infusion of dobutamine at 10 mcg/kg/minute. The package insert says to dilute 250 mg of the drug in 50 ml of D_5W. Because the drug vial contains 20 ml of solution, the total to be infused is 70 ml (50 ml of D_5W plus 20 ml of solution). How many micrograms of the drug should the patient receive each minute? Each hour?

First, compute the patient's weight in kilograms. To do this, set up a proportion with the weight in pounds and the unknown weight in kilograms in one fraction and the number of pounds per kilogram in the other fraction:

$$\frac{200\text{ lb}}{x\text{ kg}} = \frac{2.2\text{ lb}}{1\text{ kg}}$$

Cross multiply the fractions:

$$x\text{ kg} \times 2.2\text{ lb} = 1\text{ kg} \times 200\text{ lb}$$

Solve for *x* by dividing each side of the equation by 2.2 lb and canceling units that appear in both the numerator and denominator.

$$\frac{x\text{ kg} \times 2.2\cancel{\text{ lb}}}{2.2\cancel{\text{ lb}}} = \frac{1\text{ kg} \times 200\cancel{\text{ lb}}}{2.2\cancel{\text{ lb}}}$$

$$x = \frac{200\text{ kg}}{2.2}$$

$$x = 90.9\text{ kg}$$

The patient weighs 90.9 kg. Next, determine the dose in micrograms per minute by setting up a proportion with the patient's weight in kilograms and the unknown dose in micrograms per minute in one fraction and the known dose in micrograms per kilogram per minute in the other fraction:

$$\frac{90.9\text{ kg}}{x\text{ mcg/min}} = \frac{1\text{ kg}}{10\text{ mcg/min}}$$

Cross multiply the fractions:

$$x\text{ mcg/min} \times 1\text{ kg} = 10\text{ mcg/min} \times 90.9\text{ kg}$$

Solve for *x* by dividing each side of the equation by 1 kg and canceling units that appear in both the numerator and denominator:

$$\frac{x\text{ mcg/min} \times 1\cancel{\text{kg}}}{1\cancel{\text{kg}}} = \frac{10\text{ mcg/min} \times 90.9\cancel{\text{ kg}}}{1\cancel{\text{ kg}}}$$

$$x = 909\text{ mcg/min}$$

The patient should receive 909 mcg of dobutamine every minute. Finally, determine the hourly dose by multiplying the dose per minute by 60:

$$909\text{ mcg/min} \times 60\text{ min/hr} = 54{,}540\text{ mcg/hr}$$

The patient should receive 54,540 mcg of dobutamine every hour.

Pediatric dosage considerations

To determine the correct pediatric dosage of a drug, prescribers, pharmacists, and nurses usually use two computation methods. One is based on weight in kilograms; the other uses the child's body surface area. Other methods are less accurate and not recommended.

Dosage range per kilogram of body weight

Currently, many pharmaceutical companies provide information on the safe dosage ranges for drugs given to children. The companies usually provide the dosage ranges in milligrams per kilogram of body weight and, in many cases, give similar information for adult dosage ranges. The following example and explanation show how to calculate the safe pediatric dosage range for a drug, using the company's suggested safe dosage range provided in milligrams per kilogram.

For a pediatric patient, a prescriber orders a drug with a suggested dosage range of 10 to 12 mg/kg of body weight/day. The child weighs 12 kg. What is the safe daily dosage range for the child?

You must calculate the lower and upper limits of the dosage range provided by the manufacturer. First, calculate the dosage based on 10 mg/kg of body weight. Then, calculate the dosage based on 12 mg/kg of body weight. The answers represent the lower and upper limits of the daily dosage range, expressed in mg/kg of the child's weight.

Body surface area

A second method for calculating safe pediatric dosages uses the child's body surface area. This method may provide a more accurate calculation because the child's body surface area is thought to parallel the child's organ growth and maturation and metabolic rate.

You can determine the body surface area of a child by using a three-column chart called a nomogram. Mark the child's height in the first column and weight in the third column. Then draw a line between the two marks. The point at which the line intersects the vertical scale in the second column is the child's estimated body surface area in square meters. To calculate the child's approximate dose, use the body surface area measurement in the following equation:

$$\frac{\text{body surface area of child}}{\text{average adult body surface area } (1.73\text{m}^2)} \times \text{average adult dose} = \text{child's dose}$$

The following example illustrates the use of the equation. The nomogram shows that a 25-lb (11.3-kg) child who is 33 inches (84 cm) tall has a body surface area of 0.52 m². To determine the child's dose of a drug with an average adult dose of 100 mg, the equation would appear as:

$$\frac{0.52 \text{ m}^2}{1.73 \text{ m}^2} \times 100 \text{ mg} = \frac{30.06 \text{ mg}}{\text{(child's dose)}}$$

The child should receive 30 mg of the drug. Keep in mind that many facilities have guidelines that determine acceptable calculation methods for pediatric dosages. If you work in a pediatric setting, make sure to familiarize yourself with your facility's policies about pediatric dosages.

3

Drug administration

You may administer drugs by many routes, including topical, oral, buccal, sublingual (S.L.), ophthalmic, otic, respiratory, nasogastric (NG), vaginal, rectal, subcutaneous (S.C.), intramuscular (I.M.), and intravenous (I.V.) routes. No matter which route you use, however, you'll need to follow an established set of precautions to make sure you give the right drug in the right dose to the right patient at the right time and by the right route. These precautions include checking the order and medication record, checking the label, confirming the patient's identity, following standard safety procedures, and addressing any patient questions.

Check the order

Make sure you have a written order for every drug given. Verbal orders should be signed by the prescriber within the time period specified by your facility. If your facility has a computerized order system, it may allow prescribers to order drugs electronically from the pharmacy. The computer may indicate whether the pharmacy has the drug, and it triggers the pharmacy staff to fill the prescription. A computerized order may also generate a patient record on which you can document medication administration. In fact, you may be able to document administration right on the computer.

Computer systems offer several advantages over paper systems. For instance, drugs may arrive on the unit or floor more quickly. Documentation is quicker and easier. Prescribers can see at a glance which drugs have been administered. Errors will no longer result from poor handwriting (although typing mistakes may occur). Finally, computerized records are easier to store than paper records.

Check the medication record

Check the order on the patient's medication record against the prescriber's order.

Check the label

Before administering a drug, check its label three times to make sure you're giving the prescribed drug and the prescribed dose. First, check the label when you take the container from the shelf or drawer. Next, check the label right before pouring the drug into the medication cup or drawing it into the syringe. Finally, check the label again before returning the container to the shelf or drawer. If you're giving a unit-dose drug, you'll be opening the container at the patient's bedside. Check the label for the third time immediately after pouring the drug and again before discarding the wrapper.

Don't administer a drug from a poorly labeled or unlabeled container. Also, don't attempt to label a drug or to reinforce a label; this must be done by a pharmacist.

Confirm the patient's identity

Before giving the drug, ask the patient his full name, and confirm his identity by checking his name and medical record number on his patient identification wristband against the medication administration record. Don't rely on information that can vary during a hospital stay, such as a room or bed number. Check again that you have the correct drug, and make sure the patient has no allergy to it.

If the patient has any drug allergies, check to make sure the chart and medication administration record are labeled accordingly and that the patient is wearing an allergy wristband identifying the allergen.

Follow safety procedures

Whenever you administer a drug, follow these safety procedures:

- Never give a drug poured or prepared by someone else.
- Never allow the medication cart or tray out of your sight once you've prepared a dose.
- Never leave a drug at a patient's bedside.

• Never return unwrapped or prepared drugs to stock containers; instead, dispose of them, and notify the pharmacy.
• Keep the medication cart locked at all times.
• Follow standard precautions, as appropriate.

Respond to questions

If the patient questions you about his drug or dosage, check his medication record again. If the drug you're giving is correct, reassure the patient. Explain any changes in his drug or dosage. Also, instruct him, as appropriate, about possible adverse reactions. And ask him to report anything that he feels may be an adverse reaction.

Topical administration

Topical drugs, such as patches, lotions, and ointments, are applied directly to the skin. They're commonly used for local, rather than systemic, effects. Keep in mind, however, that certain types of topical drugs—known as transdermal drugs—are meant to enter the patient's bloodstream and exert a systemic effect after you apply them.

Equipment

Check the chart and the medication administration record. Gather the prescribed drug, sterile tongue blades, gloves, sterile gloves for open lesions, sterile 4″ × 4″ gauze pads, transparent semipermeable dressing, adhesive tape, normal saline solution, cotton-tipped applicators, cotton gloves, and linen savers, if necessary.

Implementation

• Confirm the patient's identity by asking his full name and checking the name and medical record number on his wristband.
• Explain the procedure to the patient because, after discharge, he may have to apply the drug by himself.
• Premedicate the patient with an analgesic if the procedure is uncomfortable. Give the medication time to take effect.
• Wash your hands to reduce the risk of cross-contamination, and glove your dominant hand.
• Help the patient to a comfortable position, and expose the area to be treated. Make sure the skin or mucous membrane is intact (unless the drug has been ordered to treat a skin lesion). Application of drug to broken or abraded skin may cause unwanted systemic absorption and further irritation.
• If necessary, clean debris from the skin. You may have to change your glove if it becomes soiled.

To apply paste, cream, or ointment

• Open the container. Place the cap upside down to avoid contaminating its inner surface.
• Remove a tongue blade from its sterile wrapper, and cover one end of it with drug from the tube or jar. Then transfer the drug from the tongue blade to your gloved hand.
• Apply the drug to the affected area with long, smooth strokes that follow the direction of hair growth. This technique avoids forcing drug into hair follicles, which can cause irritation and lead to folliculitis. Avoid excessive pressure when applying the drug because it could abrade the skin or cause the patient discomfort.
• When applying drug to the patient's face, use cotton-tipped applicators for small areas, such as under the eyes. For larger areas, use a sterile gauze pad.
• To prevent contamination of the drug, use a new sterile tongue blade each time you remove drug from the container.
• Remove your gloves, and wash your hands.

To apply transdermal ointment

• Choose the application site—usually a dry, hairless spot on the patient's chest or upper arm.
• To promote absorption, wash the site with soap and warm water. Dry it thoroughly.
• Put on gloves.
• If the patient has a previously applied medication strip at another site, remove it and wash this area to clear away any drug residue.

• If the area you choose is hairy, clip excess hair rather than shaving it; shaving causes irritation, which the drug may worsen.
• Squeeze the prescribed amount of ointment onto the application strip or measuring paper. Don't get the ointment on your skin.
• Apply the strip, drug side down, directly to the patient's skin.
• Maneuver the strip slightly to spread a thin layer of the ointment over a 3″ (8-cm) area, but don't rub the ointment into the skin.
• Secure the application strip to the patient's skin by covering it with a semipermeable dressing or plastic wrap.
• Tape the covering securely in place.
• If required by your facility's policy, label the strip with the date, time, and your initials.
• Remove your gloves, and wash your hands.

To apply a transdermal patch

• Remove the old patch.
• Choose a dry, hairless application site.
• As with the transdermal ointment, clip (don't shave) hair from the chosen site. Wash the area with warm water and soap, and dry it thoroughly.
• Open the drug package, and remove the patch.
• Without touching the adhesive surface, remove the clear plastic backing.
• Apply the patch to the site without touching the adhesive.
• If required by your facility's policy, label the patch with the date, time, and your initials.

To remove ointment

• Wash your hands, and put on gloves.
• Gently swab ointment from the patient's skin using a sterile 4″ × 4″ gauze pad saturated with normal saline solution.
• Don't wipe too hard because you could irritate the skin.
• Remove your gloves, and wash your hands.

Nursing considerations

• To prevent skin irritation from drug accumulation, never apply drug without first removing previous applications.
• Always wear gloves to prevent absorption by your skin.
• Never apply ointment to the eyelids or ear canal unless ordered. The ointment may congeal and occlude the tear duct or ear canal.
• Inspect the treated area frequently for allergic or other adverse reactions.
• Don't apply a topical drug to scarred or callused skin because either one may impair absorption.
• Don't place a defibrillator paddle on a transdermal patch. The aluminum on the patch can cause electrical arcing during defibrillation, resulting in smoke and thermal burns. If a patient has a patch on a standard paddle site, remove the patch before applying the paddle.

Oral administration

Because oral drug administration is usually the safest, most convenient, and least expensive, most drugs are administered by this method. Drugs for oral administration are available in many forms: tablets, enteric-coated tablets, capsules, syrups, elixirs, oils, liquids, suspensions, powders, and granules. Some require special preparation before administration, such as mixing with juice to make them more palatable.

Oral drugs are sometimes prescribed in higher dosages than their parenteral equivalents because, after absorption through the gastrointestinal (GI) system, they're broken down by the liver before they reach the systemic circulation.

Equipment

Check the chart and the medication administration record. Gather the prescribed drug and medication cup. If necessary, gather a mortar and pestle for crushing pills and an appropriate vehicle, such as jelly or applesauce for crushed pills or juice, water, or milk for liquid drugs. These variations are commonly used for children or elderly patients.

Implementation

• Wash your hands.
• Confirm the patient's identity by asking his full name and checking the name and medical record number on his wristband.

• Assess the patient's condition, including level of consciousness and vital signs, as needed. Changes in the patient's condition may warrant withholding the drug.
• Give the patient the drug. If appropriate, crush the drug to facilitate swallowing or mix it with an appropriate vehicle or liquid to aid swallowing, minimize adverse effects, or promote absorption.
• Stay with the patient until he has swallowed the drug. If he seems confused or disoriented, check his mouth to make sure he swallowed it. Return and reassess the patient's response within 1 hour after giving the drug.

Nursing considerations

• To avoid damaging or staining the patient's teeth, give acid or iron preparations through a straw. An unpleasant-tasting liquid can usually be made more palatable if taken through a straw because the liquid contacts fewer taste buds.
• If the patient can't swallow a whole tablet or capsule, ask the pharmacist if the drug is available in liquid form or if it can be administered by another route. If not, ask the pharmacist if the tablet can be crushed or if capsules can be opened and mixed with food.
• Don't crush sustained-action drugs, buccal tablets, S.L. tablets, or enteric-coated drugs.

Buccal and sublingual administration

Certain drugs are given buccally (between the cheek and teeth) or S.L. (under the tongue) to bypass the digestive tract and facilitate absorption into the bloodstream. Erythrityl tetranitrate is an example of a drug given buccally. Drugs given S.L. include ergotamine tartrate, erythrityl tetranitrate, isoproterenol hydrochloride, isosorbide dinitrate, and nitroglycerin. When using either administration method, observe the patient carefully to make sure he doesn't swallow the drug or develop mucosal irritation.

Equipment

Check the chart and the medication administration record. Gather the prescribed drug, medication cup, and gloves.

Implementation

• Wash your hands. Put on gloves if you'll be placing the drug into the patient's mouth.
• Confirm the patient's identity by asking his full name and checking the name and medical record number on his wristband.
• For buccal administration, place the tablet in the patient's buccal pouch, between the cheek and teeth, as shown below.

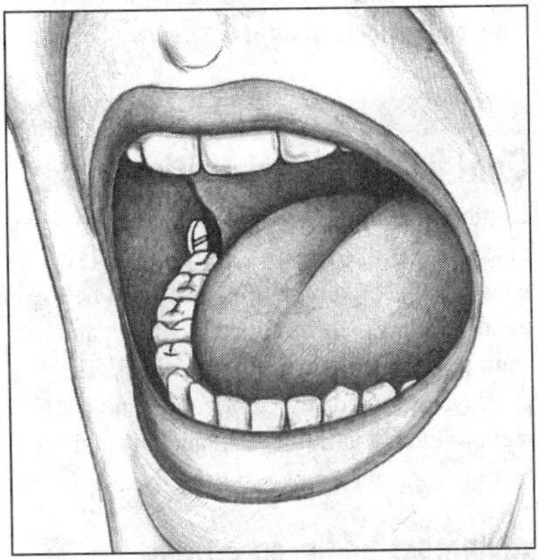

• For S.L. administration, place the tablet under the patient's tongue, as shown below.

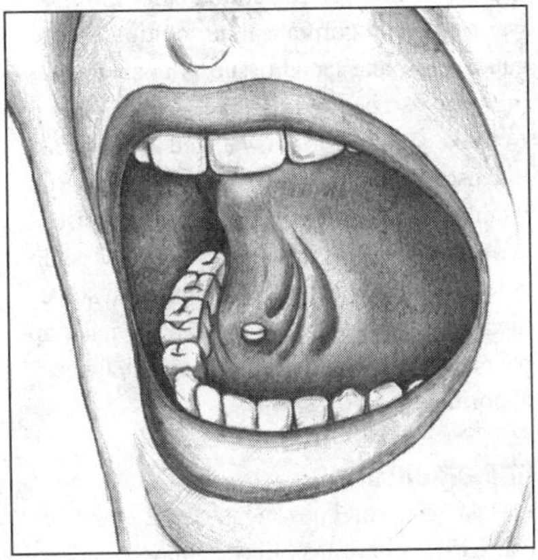

• Remove your gloves, and wash your hands.
• Instruct the patient to keep the drug in place until it dissolves completely to ensure absorp-

tion. Caution the patient against chewing the tablet or touching it with his tongue to prevent accidental swallowing.
• Tell the patient not to smoke before the drug has dissolved because the vasoconstrictive effects of nicotine slow absorption.

Nursing considerations

• Don't give liquids until a buccal tablet is absorbed, in some cases up to 1 hour.
• If the patient has angina, tell him to wet the nitroglycerin tablet with saliva and keep it under his tongue until it's fully absorbed.
• Make sure a patient with angina knows how to take the medication, how many doses to take, and when to call for emergency help.

Ophthalmic administration

Ophthalmic drugs—drops or ointments—serve diagnostic and therapeutic purposes. During an ophthalmic examination, drugs can be used to anesthetize the eye, dilate the pupil, and stain the cornea to identify anomalies. Therapeutic uses include eye lubrication and treatment of such conditions as glaucoma and infections.

Equipment and preparation

Check the chart and the medication administration record. Gather the prescribed ophthalmic medication, sterile cotton balls, gloves, warm water or normal saline solution, sterile gauze pads, and facial tissue. An ocular dressing may also be used.

Make sure the drug is labeled for ophthalmic use. Then check the expiration date. Remember to date the container after first use.

Inspect ocular solutions for cloudiness, discoloration, and precipitation, although some medications are suspensions and normally appear cloudy. Don't use solutions that appear abnormal.

Implementation

• Make sure you know which eye to treat because different drugs or doses may be ordered for each eye.
• Confirm the patient's identity by asking his full name and checking the name and medical record number on his wristband.
• Put on gloves.
• If the patient has an eye dressing, remove it by pulling it down and away from his forehead. Avoid contaminating your hands. Don't apply pressure to the area around the eyes.
• To remove exudates or meibomian gland secretions, clean around the eye with sterile cotton balls or sterile gauze pads moistened with warm water or normal saline solution. Have the patient close his eye; then gently wipe the eyelids from the inner to the outer canthus. Use a fresh cotton ball or gauze pad for each stroke, and use a different cotton ball or pad for each eye.
• Have the patient sit or lie in the supine position. Instruct him to tilt his head back and toward his affected eye so that excess drug can flow away from the tear duct, minimizing systemic absorption through the nasal mucosa.
• Remove the dropper cap from the drug container, and draw the drug into the dropper. Or, if the bottle has a dropper tip, remove the cap and hold or place it upside down to prevent contamination.
• Before instilling eyedrops, instruct the patient to look up and away. This moves the cornea away from the lower lid and minimizes the risk of touching it with the dropper.

To instill eyedrops

• Steady the hand that's holding the dropper by resting it against the patient's forehead. With your other hand, gently pull down the lower lid of the affected eye, and instill the drops in the conjunctival sac. Never instill eyedrops directly onto the eyeball.
• When teaching elderly patients how to instill eyedrops, keep in mind that they may have difficulty sensing drops in the eye. Suggest chilling the drug slightly because the cold drops will be easier to feel when they enter the eye.

To apply eye ointment

• Squeeze a small ribbon of drug on the edge of the conjunctival sac from the inner to the outer canthus. Cut off the ribbon by turning the tube. Don't touch the eye with the tip of the tube.

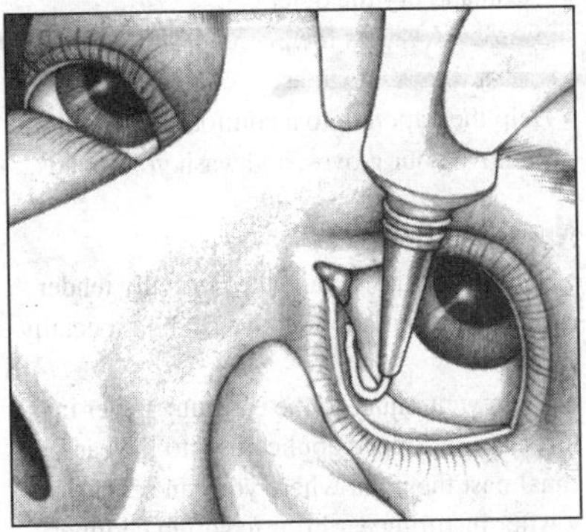

• After instilling eyedrops or applying ointment, instruct the patient to close his eyes gently, without squeezing the lids shut. If you instilled drops, tell the patient to blink. If you applied ointment, tell him to roll his eyes behind closed lids to help distribute the drug over the eyeball.
• Use a clean tissue to remove any excess drug that leaks from the eye. Use a fresh tissue for each eye to prevent cross-contamination.
• Apply a new eye dressing, if necessary.
• Remove and discard your gloves. Wash your hands.

Nursing considerations

• When administering an eye medication that may be absorbed systemically, gently press your thumb on the inner canthus for 1 to 2 minutes after instillation while the patient closes his eyes. Avoid applying pressure around the eye.
• To maintain the drug container's sterility, don't put the cap down after opening the container, and never touch the tip of the dropper or bottle to the eye area. Discard any solution remaining in the dropper before returning it to the bottle. If the dropper or bottle tip has become contaminated, discard it and use another sterile dropper. Never share eye drops from patient to patient.

Otic administration

Eardrops may be instilled to treat infection and inflammation, to soften cerumen for later removal, to produce local anesthesia, or to facilitate removal of an insect trapped in the ear.

Equipment and preparation

Check the chart and the medication administration record. Gather the prescribed eardrops, gloves, a light, and facial tissue or cotton-tipped applicators. Cotton balls and a bowl of warm water may be needed as well.

First, warm the drug to body temperature in the bowl of warm water, or carry the drug in your pocket for 30 minutes before administration. If necessary, test the temperature of the drug by placing a drop on your wrist. (If the drug is too hot, it may burn the patient's eardrum.) To avoid injuring the ear canal, check the dropper before use to make sure it's not chipped or cracked.

Implementation

• Wash your hands, and put on clean gloves.
• Confirm the patient's identity by asking his full name and checking the name and medical record number on his wristband.
• Have the patient lie on the side opposite the affected ear.

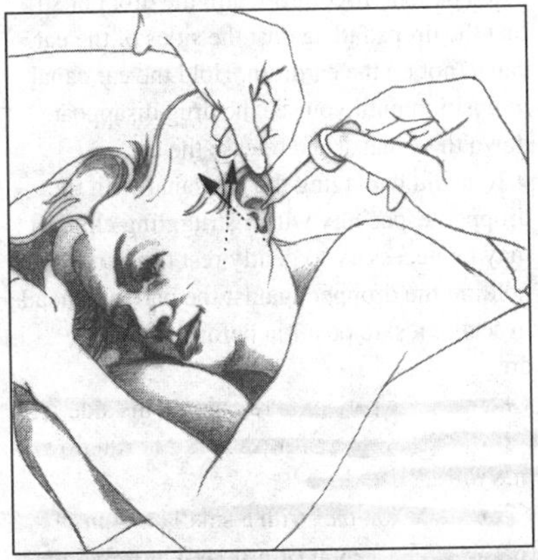

• Straighten the patient's ear canal. For an adult, pull the auricle up and back. For an infant or child under age 3, gently pull the auricle down and back because the ear canal is straighter at this age.

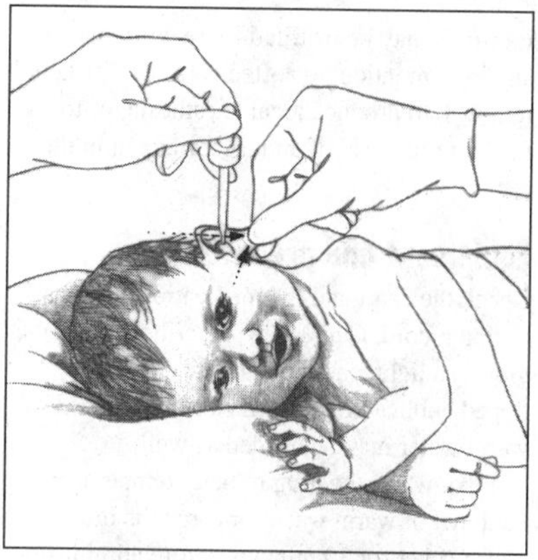

• Using a light, examine the ear canal for drainage. If you see drainage, gently clean the canal with the tissue or cotton-tipped applicators because drainage can reduce the effectiveness of the drug. Never insert an applicator past the point where you can see it.
• Compare the label on the eardrops to the order on the patient's medication record. Check the label again while drawing the drug into the dropper. Check the label for the final time before returning the eardrops to the shelf or drawer.
• Straighten the patient's ear canal once again, and instill the ordered number of drops. To avoid patient discomfort, aim the dropper so that the drops fall against the sides of the ear canal, not on the eardrum. Hold the ear canal in position until you see the drug disappear down the canal. Then release the ear.
• To avoid damaging the ear canal with the dropper, especially with a struggling child, it may be necessary to gently rest the hand holding the dropper against the patient's head to secure a safe position before giving the drug.
• Instruct the patient to remain on his side for 5 to 10 minutes to allow the drug to run down into the ear canal.
• Tuck a cotton ball with a small amount of petroleum jelly on it (if ordered) loosely into the opening of the ear canal to prevent the drug from leaking out. Be careful not to insert it too deeply into the canal because doing so may prevent drainage of secretions and increase pressure on the eardrum.
• Clean and dry the outer ear.
• If ordered, repeat the procedure in the other ear after 5 to 10 minutes.
• Help the patient into a comfortable position.
• Remove your gloves, and wash your hands.

Nursing considerations

• Some conditions make the normally tender ear canal even more sensitive, so be especially gentle.
• To prevent injury to the eardrum, never insert a cotton-tipped applicator into the ear canal past the point where you can see the tip.
• After instilling eardrops to soften cerumen, irrigate the ear as ordered to facilitate its removal. If the patient has vertigo, keep the side rails of his bed up and assist him as necessary during the procedure. Also, move slowly and unhurriedly to avoid worsening his vertigo.
• If necessary, teach the patient to instill the eardrops correctly so that he can continue treatment at home. Review the procedure, and let the patient try it himself while you observe.

Respiratory administration

Hand-held oropharyngeal inhalers include the metered-dose inhaler and the turbo-inhaler. These devices deliver topical drugs to the respiratory tract, producing local and systemic effects. The mucosal lining of the respiratory tract absorbs the inhalant almost immediately. Examples of inhalants are bronchodilators, which improve airway patency and facilitate mucous drainage, and mucolytics, which liquefy tenacious bronchial secretions.

Equipment

Check the chart and the medication administration record. Gather the metered-dose inhaler or turbo-inhaler, prescribed drug, and normal saline solution.

Implementation

• Confirm the patient's identity by asking his full name and checking the name and medical record number on his wristband.

To use a metered-dose inhaler

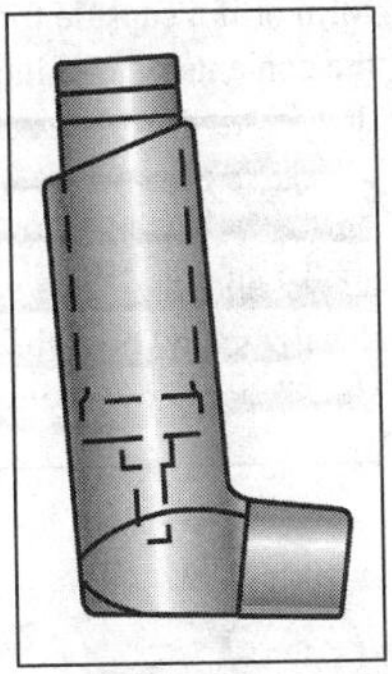

- Shake the inhaler bottle. Remove the cap and insert the stem into the small hole on the flattened portion of the mouthpiece, as shown.
- Place the inhaler about 1″ (2.5 cm) in front of the patient's open mouth.
- Tell the patient to exhale.
- If you're using a spacer, which can make the inhaler more effective, tell the patient to place the mouthpiece of the spacer in his mouth and to press his lips firmly around the mouthpiece.
- As you push the bottle down against the mouthpiece, instruct the patient to inhale slowly through his mouth and to continue inhaling until his lungs feel full. Compress the bottle against the mouthpiece only once.
- Remove the inhaler and tell the patient to hold his breath for several seconds. Then instruct him to exhale slowly through pursed lips to keep distal bronchioles open and allow increased absorption and diffusion of the drug.
- Have the patient gargle with normal saline solution or water to remove the drug from his mouth and the back of his throat. This step helps prevent oral fungal infections. Warn the patient not to swallow after gargling, but rather to spit out the liquid.

To use a turbo-inhaler

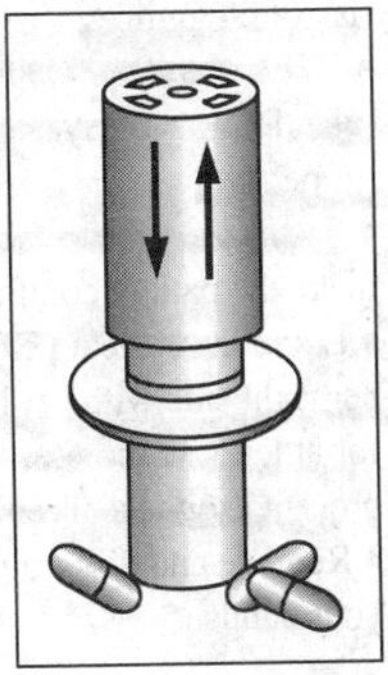

- Hold the mouthpiece in one hand. With the other hand, slide the sleeve away from the mouthpiece as far as possible, as shown.
- Unscrew the tip of the mouthpiece by turning it counterclockwise.
- Press the colored portion of the drug capsule into the propeller stem of the mouthpiece.
- Screw the inhaler together again.
- Holding the inhaler with the mouthpiece at the bottom, slide the sleeve all the way down and then up again to puncture the capsule and release the drug. Do this only once.
- Have the patient exhale completely and tilt his head back. Instruct him to place the mouthpiece in his mouth, close his lips around it, and inhale once. Tell him to hold his breath for several seconds.
- Remove the inhaler from the patient's mouth, and tell him to exhale as much air as possible.
- Repeat the procedure until all the drug in the device is inhaled.
- Have the patient gargle with normal saline solution, if desired.

Nursing considerations

- Teach the patient how to use the inhaler so he can continue treatments after discharge, if necessary. Explain that overdosage can cause the drug to lose its effectiveness. Tell him to record the date and time of each inhalation and his response.
- Be aware that some oral respiratory drugs may cause restlessness, palpitations, nervousness, and other systemic effects. They can also cause hypersensitivity reactions, such as rash, urticaria, or bronchospasm.
- Administer oral respiratory drugs cautiously to patients with heart disease because these drugs may potentiate coronary insufficiency, cardiac arrhythmias, or hypertension. If paradoxical bronchospasm occurs, discontinue the drug and call the prescriber to prescribe another drug.
- If the patient is prescribed a bronchodilator and a corticosteroid, give the bronchodilator first so the air passages can open fully before the patient uses the corticosteroid.
- Instruct the patient to keep an extra inhaler handy.
- Instruct the patiet to discard the inhaler after taking the prescribed number of doses and to then start a new inhaler.

Nasogastric administration

Besides providing an alternate means of nourishment for patients who can't eat normally, a

NG tube allows direct instillation of drugs into the GI system.

Equipment and preparation

Check the chart and the medication administration record. Gather equipment for use at the bedside, including the prescribed drug, a towel or linen-saver pad, 50- or 60-ml piston-type catheter-tip syringe, feeding tubing, two 4″ × 4″ gauze pads, stethoscope, gloves, diluent (juice, water, or a nutritional supplement), cup for mixing drug and fluid, spoon, 50-ml cup of water, and rubber band. Pill-crushing equipment and a clamp (if not already attached to the tube) also may be needed. Make sure that liquids are at room temperature to avoid abdominal cramping and that the cup, syringe, spoon, and gauze are clean.

Implementation

- Wash your hands, and put on gloves.
- Confirm the patient's identity by asking his full name and checking the name and medical record number on his wristband.
- Unpin the tube from the patient's gown. To avoid soiling the sheets during the procedure, fold back the bed linens and drape the patient's chest with a towel or linen-saver pad.
- Help the patient into Fowler's position, if his condition allows.
- After unclamping the tube, auscultate the patient's abdomen about 3″ (8 cm) below the sternum as you gently insert 10 ml of air into the tube with the 50- or 60-ml syringe. You should hear the air bubble entering the stomach. Gently draw back on the piston of the syringe. The appearance of gastric contents implies that the tube is patent and in the stomach.
- If no gastric contents appear or if you meet resistance, the tube may be lying against the gastric mucosa. Withdraw the tube slightly or turn the patient to free it.
- Clamp the tube, detach the syringe, and lay the end of the tube on the 4″ × 4″ gauze pad.
- If the drug is in tablet form, crush it before mixing it with the diluent. Make sure the particles are small enough to pass through the eyes at the distal end of the tube. Keep in mind that some drugs (extended release, enteric-coated, or S.L. medications, for example) shouldn't be crushed. Ask a pharmacist if you aren't sure. Also, check to see if the drug comes in liquid form or if a capsule form may be opened and the contents poured into a diluent. Pour liquid drugs into the diluent and stir well.
- Reattach the syringe, without the piston, to the end of the tube. Holding the tube upright at a level slightly above the patient's nose, open the clamp and pour the drug in slowly and steadily, as shown below.

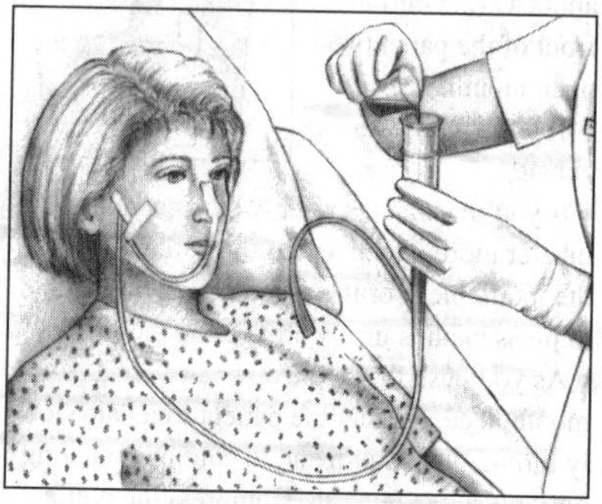

- To keep air from entering the patient's stomach, hold the tube at a slight angle and add more drug before the syringe empties. If the drug flows smoothly, slowly give the entire dose. If it doesn't flow, it may be too thick. If so, dilute it with water. If you suspect that tube placement is inhibiting flow, stop the procedure and reevaluate the placement.
- Watch the patient's reaction. Stop immediately if you see signs of discomfort.
- As the last of the drug flows out of the syringe, start to irrigate the tube by adding 30 to 50 ml of water (15 to 30 ml for a child). Irrigation clears drug from the tube and reduces the risk of clogging.
- When the water stops flowing, clamp the tube. Detach the syringe, and discard it properly.
- Fasten the tube to the patient's gown, and make the patient comfortable.
- Leave the patient in Fowler's position or on her right side with her head partially elevated for at least 30 minutes to facilitate flow and prevent esophageal reflux.
- Remove and discard your gloves, and wash your hands.

Nursing considerations

- If you must give a tube feeding as well as instill a drug, give the drug first to make sure the patient receives it all.
- Certain drugs—such as dilantin—bind with tube feedings, decreasing the availability of the drug. Stop the tube feeding for 2 hours before and after the dose, according to your facility's policy.
- If residual stomach contents exceed 150 ml, withhold the drug and feeding, and notify a prescriber. Excessive stomach contents may indicate intestinal obstruction or paralytic ileus.
- Never crush enteric-coated, buccal, S.L., or sustained-release drugs.
- If the NG tube is on suction, turn it off for 20 to 30 minutes after giving a drug.

Vaginal administration

Vaginal drugs can be inserted as topical treatment for infection, particularly *Trichomonas vaginalis* and vaginal candidiasis or inflammation. Suppositories melt when they contact the vaginal mucosa, and the drug diffuses topically.

Vaginal drugs usually come with a disposable applicator that enables placement of drug in the anterior and posterior fornices. Vaginal administration is most effective when the patient can remain lying down afterward to retain the drug.

Equipment

Check the chart and the medication administration record. Gather the prescribed drug and applicator (if needed), gloves, water-soluble lubricant, and a small sanitary pad.

Implementation

- If possible, plan to give vaginal drugs at bedtime when the patient is recumbent.
- Confirm the patient's identity by asking her full name and checking the name and medical record number on her wristband.
- Wash your hands, explain the procedure to the patient, and provide privacy.
- Ask the patient to void.
- Ask the patient if she would rather insert the drug herself. If so, provide appropriate instructions. If not, proceed with the following steps.
- Help her into the lithotomy position. Drape the patient, exposing only the perineum.
- Remove the suppository from the wrapper and lubricate it with water-soluble lubricant.
- Put on gloves, and expose the vagina by spreading the labia. If you see discharge, wash the area with several cotton balls soaked in warm, soapy water. Clean each side of the perineum and then the center, using a fresh cotton ball for each stroke. While the labia are still separated, insert the suppository or vaginal applicator about 3″ to 4″ (7.6 to 10 cm) into the vagina.

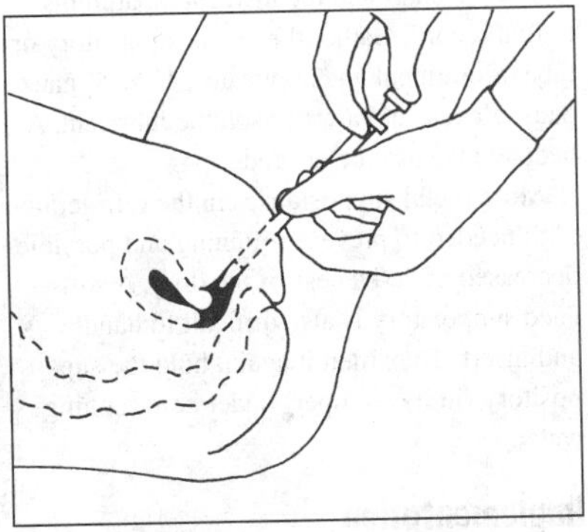

- After insertion, wash the applicator with soap and warm water, and store or discard it, as appropriate. Label it so it will be used only for one patient.
- Remove and discard your gloves.
- To keep the drug from soiling the patient's clothing and bedding, provide a sanitary pad.
- Help the patient return to a comfortable position, and tell her to stay in bed as much as possible for the next several hours.
- Wash your hands thoroughly.

Nursing considerations

- Refrigerate vaginal suppositories that melt at room temperature.
- If possible, teach the patient how to insert the vaginal drug because she may have to administer it herself after discharge. Give her instructions in writing if possible.

• Instruct the patient not to insert a tampon after inserting a vaginal drug because it will absorb the drug and decrease its effectiveness.

Rectal administration

A rectal suppository is a small, solid, medicated mass, usually cone shaped, with a cocoa butter or glycerin base. It may be inserted to stimulate peristalsis and defecation or to relieve pain, vomiting, and local irritation. An ointment is a semisolid drug used to produce local effects. It may be applied externally to the anus or internally to the rectum.

Equipment and preparation

Check the chart and the medication administration record. Gather the rectal suppository or tube of ointment and applicator, 4″ × 4″ gauze pads, gloves, and a water-soluble lubricant. A bedpan may also be needed.

Store rectal suppositories in the refrigerator until needed to prevent softening and possible decreased effectiveness of the drug. A softened suppository is also difficult to handle and insert. To harden it again, hold the suppository (in its wrapper) under cold running water.

Implementation

• Confirm the patient's identity by asking his full name and checking the name and medical record number on his wristband.
• Wash your hands.

To insert a rectal suppository

• Place the patient on his left side in Sims' position. Drape him with the bedcovers, exposing only his buttocks.
• Put on gloves. Unwrap the suppository, and lubricate it with water-soluble lubricant.
• Lift the patient's upper buttock with your nondominant hand to expose the anus.
• Instruct the patient to take several deep breaths through his mouth to relax the anal sphincter and reduce anxiety during drug insertion.
• Using the index finger of your dominant hand, insert the suppository—tapered end first—about 3″ (8 cm) until you feel it pass the internal anal sphincter, as shown.

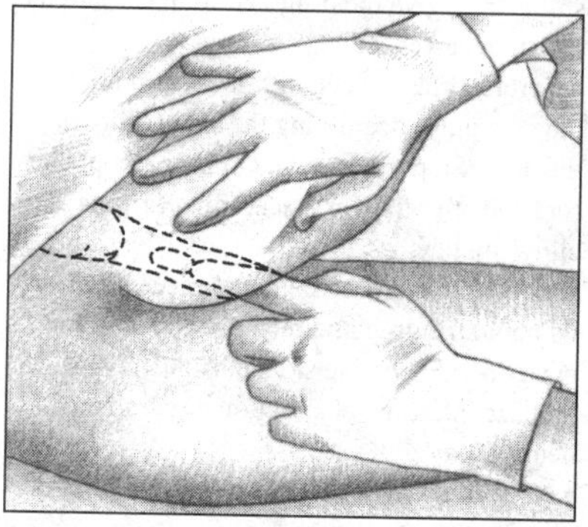

• Direct the tapered end of the suppository toward the side of the rectum so it contacts the membranes.
• Encourage the patient to lie quietly and, if applicable, to retain the suppository for the correct length of time. Press on the patient's anus with a gauze pad, if necessary, until the urge to defecate passes.
• Discard the used equipment and gloves. Wash your hands.

To apply an ointment

• Wash your hands.
• For external application, don gloves and use a gauze pad to spread the drug over the anal area. For internal application, attach the applicator to the tube of ointment, and coat the applicator with water-soluble lubricant.
• Expect to use about 1″ (2.5 cm) of ointment. To gauge how much pressure to use during application, try squeezing a small amount from the tube before you attach the applicator.
• Lift the patient's upper buttock with your nondominant hand to expose the anus.
• Tell the patient to take several deep breaths through his mouth to relax the anal sphincter and reduce discomfort during insertion. Then gently insert the applicator, directing it toward the umbilicus.
• Squeeze the tube to eject drug.
• Remove the applicator, and place a folded 4″ × 4″ gauze pad between the patient's buttocks to absorb excess ointment.
• Disassemble the tube and applicator, and recap the tube. Clean the applicator with soap

and warm water. Remove and discard your gloves. Then wash your hands thoroughly.

Nursing considerations

- Because the intake of food and fluid stimulates peristalsis, a suppository for relieving constipation should be inserted about 30 minutes before mealtime to help soften the stool and facilitate defecation. A medicated retention suppository should be inserted between meals.
- Tell the patient not to expel the suppository. If retaining it is difficult, put the patient on a bedpan.
- Make sure that the patient's call button is handy, and watch for his signal because he may be unable to suppress the urge to defecate.
- Inform the patient that the suppository may discolor his next bowel movement.

Subcutaneous administration

Injection of drug into S.C. tissue allows slower, more sustained administration than I.M. injection. Drugs and solutions delivered by this route are injected through a relatively short needle using meticulous sterile technique.

Equipment and preparation

Check the chart and the medication administration record. Gather gloves, the prescribed drug, a needle of appropriate gauge and length, 1- to 3-ml syringe, and alcohol sponges. Other materials may include an antiseptic cleanser, filter needle, insulin syringe, and insulin pump. Inspect the drug to make sure it's not cloudy and is free of precipitates. Wash your hands.

For single-dose ampules

Wrap the neck of the ampule in an alcohol sponge and snap off the top. If desired, attach a filter needle to the needle and withdraw the drug. Tap the syringe to clear air from it. Cover the needle with the needle sheath by placing the sheath on the counter or medication cart and sliding the needle into the sheath. Before discarding the ampule, check the label against the patient's medication record. Discard the filter needle and the ampule. Attach the appropriate needle to the syringe.

For single-dose or multidose vials

Reconstitute powdered drugs according to the instructions on the label. Clean the rubber stopper on the vial with an alcohol sponge. Pull the syringe plunger back until the volume of air in the syringe equals the volume of drug to be withdrawn from the vial. Insert the needle into the vial. Inject the air, invert the vial, and keep the bevel tip of the needle below the level of the solution as you withdraw the prescribed amount of drug. Tap the syringe to clear air from it. Cover the needle with the needle sheath by placing the sheath on the counter or medication cart and sliding the needle into the sheath. Check the drug label against the patient's medication record before returning the multidose vial to the shelf or drawer or before discarding the single-dose vial.

Implementation

- Confirm the patient's identity by asking her full name and checking the name and medical record number on her wristband.
- Select the injection site from those shown, and tell the patient where you'll be giving the injection.

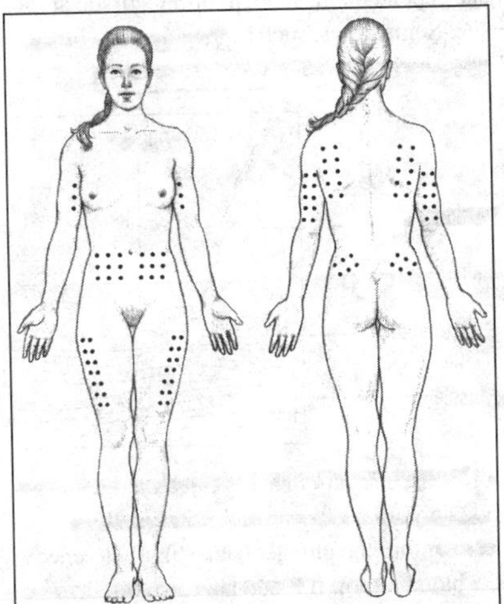

- Put on gloves. Position and drape the patient if necessary.
- Clean the injection site with an alcohol sponge. Loosen the protective needle sheath.
- With your nondominant hand, pinch the skin around the injection site firmly to elevate the

S.C. tissue, forming a 1″ (2.5 cm) fat fold, as shown.

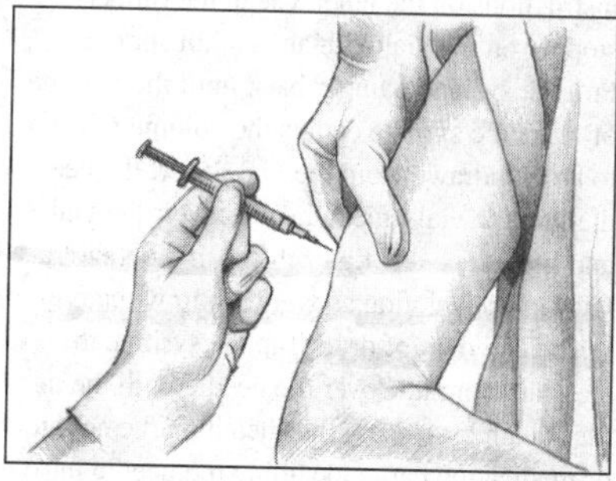

• Holding the syringe in your dominant hand, grip the needle sheath between the fourth and fifth fingers of your nondominant hand (while continuing to pinch the skin around the injection site with the index finger and thumb of your nondominant hand). Pull the sheath back to uncover the needle. Don't touch the needle.
• Position the needle with its bevel up.
• Tell the patient she'll feel a prick as you insert the needle. Do so quickly, in one motion, at a 45-degree or 90-degree angle, as shown below. The needle length and the angle you use depend on the amount of S.C. tissue at the site. Some drugs, such as heparin, should always be injected at a 90-degree angle.

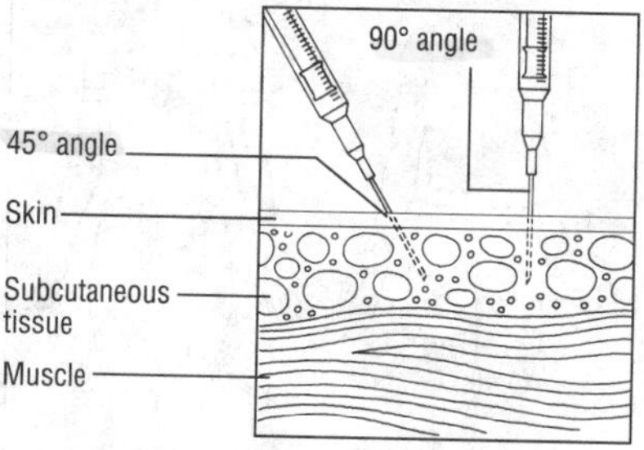

• Release the skin to avoid injecting the drug into compressed tissue and irritating the nerves. Pull the plunger back slightly to check for blood return. If blood appears, withdraw the needle, prepare another syringe, and repeat the procedure. If no blood appears, slowly inject the drug.
• After injection, remove the needle at the same angle you used to insert it. Cover the site with an alcohol sponge, and massage the site gently.
• Remove the alcohol sponge, and check the injection site for bleeding or bruising.
• Don't recap the needle. Follow your facility's policy to dispose of the injection equipment.
• Remove and discard your gloves. Wash your hands.

Nursing considerations

• Don't aspirate for blood return when giving insulin or heparin. It's not necessary with insulin and may cause a hematoma with heparin.
• Don't massage the site after giving heparin.
• Repeated injections in the same site can cause lipodystrophy, a natural immune response. This complication can be minimized by rotating injection sites.

Intramuscular administration

You'll use I.M. injection to deposit up to 5 ml of drug deep into well-vascularized muscle for rapid systemic action and absorption.

Equipment and preparation

Check the chart and the medication administration record. Gather the prescribed drug, diluent or filter needle (if needed), 3- to 5-ml syringe, 20G to 25G 1″ to 3″ needle, gloves, and alcohol sponges.

The prescribed drug must be sterile. The needle may be packaged separately or already attached to the syringe. Needles used for I.M. injections are longer than those used for S.C. injections because they reach deep into the muscle. Needle length also depends on the injection site, the patient's size, and the amount of S.C. fat covering the muscle. A larger needle gauge accommodates viscous solutions and suspensions.

Check the drug for abnormal changes in color and clarity. If in doubt, ask the pharmacist.

Use alcohol to wipe the stopper that tops the drug vial, and draw up the prescribed amount of drug. Provide privacy, and explain the procedure to the patient. Position and drape him appropriately, making sure that the site is well lit and exposed.

Implementation

- Wash your hands.
- Confirm the patient's identity by asking his full name and checking the name and medical record number on his wristband.
- Next, select an appropriate injection site. Avoid any site that looks inflamed, edematous, or irritated. Also, avoid using injection sites that contain moles, birthmarks, scar tissue, or other lesions. The dorsogluteal and ventrogluteal muscles are used most commonly for I.M. injections.

Dorsogluteal muscle

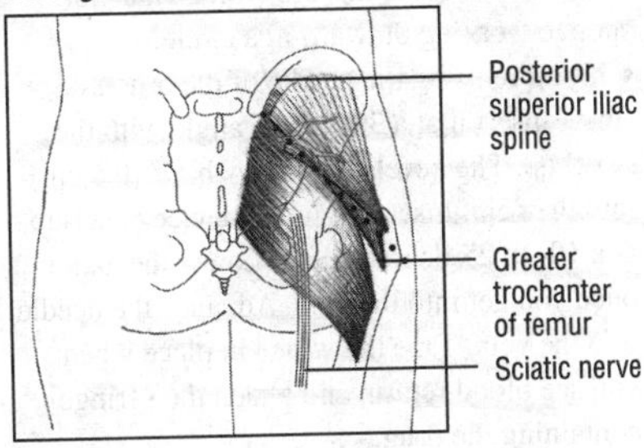

Ventrogluteal muscle

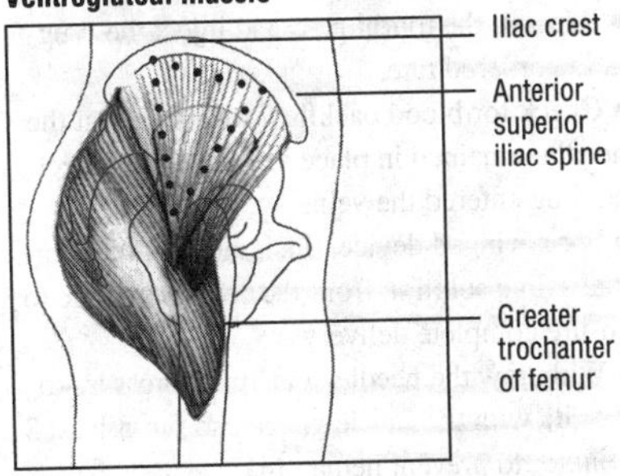

- The deltoid muscle may be used for injections of 2 ml or less.

Deltoid muscle

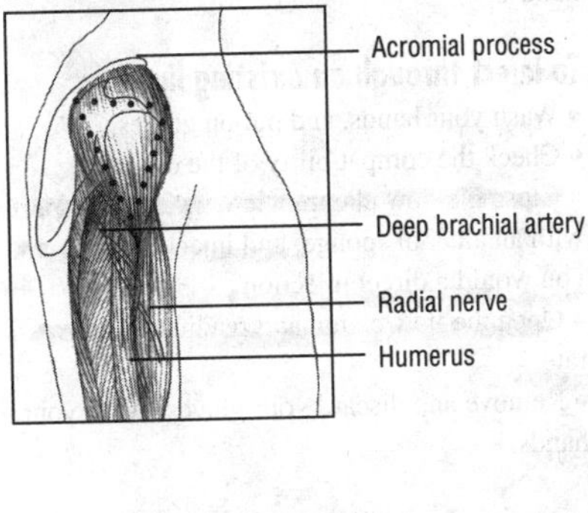

- The vastus lateralis muscle is used most often in children; the rectus femoris may be used in infants.

Vastus lateralis and rectus femoris muscles

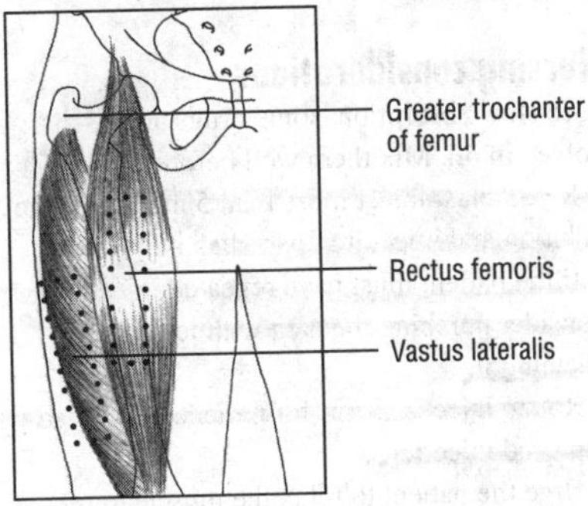

- Loosen, but don't remove, the needle sheath.
- Gently tap the site to stimulate nerve endings and minimize pain.
- Clean the site with an alcohol sponge starting at the site and moving outward in expanding circles to about 2″ (5 cm). Allow the skin to dry because wet alcohol stings in the puncture.
- Put on gloves.
- With the thumb and index finger of your nondominant hand, gently stretch the skin.
- With the syringe in your dominant hand, remove the needle sheath with the free fingers of the other hand.
- Position the syringe perpendicular to the skin surface and a couple of inches from the skin. Tell the patient that he will feel a prick. Then quickly and firmly thrust the needle into the muscle.
- Pull back slightly on the plunger to aspirate for blood. If blood appears, the needle is in a blood vessel. Withdraw it, prepare a fresh syringe, and inject another site. If no blood appears, inject the drug slowly and steadily to let the muscle distend gradually. You should feel little or no resistance. Gently but quickly remove the needle at a 90-degree angle.
- Using a gloved hand, apply gentle pressure to the site with the alcohol sponge. Massage the relaxed muscle, unless contraindicated, to distribute the drug and promote absorption.
- Inspect the site for bleeding or bruising. Apply pressure as necessary.

• Discard all equipment properly. Don't recap needles; put them in an appropriate biohazard container to avoid needle-stick injuries.
• Remove and discard your gloves. Wash your hands.

Nursing considerations

• To slow absorption, some drugs are dissolved in oil. Mix them well before use.
• If you must inject more than 5 ml, divide the solution and inject it at two sites.
• If the patient must have repeated injections, consider numbing the area with ice before cleaning it.
• Rotate injection sites for patients who need repeated injections.
• Urge the patient to relax the muscle to reduce pain and bleeding.
• Never inject into the gluteal muscles of a child who has been walking for less than 1 year.
• Keep in mind that I.M. injections can damage local muscle cells and elevate serum creatine kinase levels, which can be confused with elevated levels caused by myocardial infarction. Diagnostic tests can be used to differentiate between them.

Intravenous bolus administration

In this method, rapid I.V. administration allows drug levels to quickly peak in the bloodstream. This method also may be used for drugs that can't be given I.M. because they're toxic or because the patient has a reduced ability to absorb them. And it may be used to deliver drugs that can't be diluted. Bolus doses may be injected directly into a vein or through an existing I.V. line.

Equipment and preparation

Check the chart and the medication administration record. Gather the prescribed drug, 20G needle and syringe, diluent, if necessary, tourniquet, alcohol sponge, sterile 2″ × 2″ gauze pad, gloves, adhesive bandage, and tape. Other materials may include a winged device primed with normal saline solution and second syringe (and needle) filled with normal saline solution.

Draw the drug into the syringe, and dilute it if necessary.

Implementation

• Confirm the patient's identity by asking his full name and checking the name and medical record number on his wristband.
• Wash your hands, and put on gloves.

To give a direct injection

• Select the largest vein suitable to dilute the drug and minimize irritation.
• Apply a tourniquet above the site to distend the vein, and clean the site with an alcohol sponge working outward in a circle.
• If you're using the needle of the drug syringe, insert it at a 30-degree angle with the bevel up. The bevel should reach ¼″ (0.6 cm) into the vein. Insert a winged device bevel-up at a 10- to 25-degree angle. Lower the angle once you get into the vein. Advance the needle into the vein. Tape the wings in place when you see blood return, and attach the syringe containing the drug.
• Check for blood backflow.
• Remove the tourniquet, and inject the drug at the ordered rate.
• Check for blood backflow to ensure that the needle remained in place and all of the injected drug entered the vein.
• For a winged device, flush the line with normal saline solution from the second syringe to ensure complete delivery.
• Withdraw the needle, and apply pressure to the site with the sterile gauze pad for at least 3 minutes to prevent hematoma.
• Apply an adhesive bandage when the bleeding stops.
• Remove and discard your gloves. Wash your hands.

To inject through an existing line

• Wash your hands, and put on gloves.
• Check the compatibility of the drug.
• Close the flow clamp, wipe the injection port with an alcohol sponge, and inject the drug as you would a direct injection.
• Open the flow clamp and readjust the flow rate.
• Remove and discard your gloves. Wash your hands.

• If the drug isn't compatible with the I.V. solution, flush the line with normal saline solution before and after the injection.

Nursing considerations

• If the existing I.V. line is capped, making it an intermittent infusion device, verify patency and placement of the device before injecting the drug. Then flush the device with normal saline solution, administer the drug, and follow with the appropriate flush.
• Immediately report signs of acute allergic reaction or anaphylaxis. If extravasation occurs, stop the injection, estimate the amount of infiltration, and notify the prescriber.
• When giving diazepam or chlordiazepoxide hydrochloride through a steel needle winged device or an I.V. line, flush with bacteriostatic water to prevent precipitation.

Intravenous administration through a secondary line

A secondary I.V. line is a complete I.V. set connected to the lower Y-port (secondary port) of a primary line instead of to the I.V. catheter or needle. It features an I.V. container, long tubing, and either a microdrip or a macrodrip system, and it can be used for continuous or intermittent drug infusion. When used continuously, it permits drug infusion and titration while the primary line maintains a constant total infusion rate.

A secondary I.V. line used only for intermittent drug administration is called a piggyback set. In this case, the primary line maintains venous access between drug doses. A piggyback set includes a small I.V. container, short tubing, and usually a macrodrip system, and it connects to the primary line's upper Y-port (piggyback port).

Equipment and preparation

Check the chart and the medication administration record. Gather the prescribed I.V. drug, diluent (if necessary), prescribed I.V. solution, administration set with secondary injection port, 22G 1″ needle or a needleless system, alcohol sponges, 1″ (2.5 cm) adhesive tape, time tape, labels, infusion pump, extension hook, and solution for intermittent piggyback infusion.

Wash your hands. Inspect the I.V. container for cracks, leaks, or contamination. Check the expiration date. Check compatibility with the primary solution. Determine whether the primary line has a secondary injection port.

If necessary, add the drug to the secondary I.V. solution (usually 50 to 100 ml "minibags" of normal saline solution or D_5W). To do so, remove any seals from the secondary container and wipe the main port with an alcohol sponge. Inject the prescribed drug and agitate the solution to mix the drug. Label the I.V. mixture. Insert the administration set spike, and attach the needle or needleless system. Open the flow clamp and prime the line. Then close the flow clamp.

Some drugs come in vials for hanging directly on an I.V. pole. In this case, inject diluent directly into the drug vial. Then spike the vial, prime the tubing, and hang the set.

Implementation

• If the drug is incompatible with the primary I.V. solution, replace the primary solution with a fluid that's compatible with both solutions, and flush the line before starting the drug infusion.
• Hang the container of the secondary set and wipe the injection port of the primary line with an alcohol sponge.
• Insert the needle or needleless system from the secondary line into the injection port, and tape it securely to the primary line.
• To run the container of the secondary set by itself, lower the primary set's container with an extension hook. To run both containers simultaneously, place them at the same height.
• Open the clamp, and adjust the drip rate.
• For continuous infusion, set the secondary solution to the desired drip rate; then adjust the primary solution to the desired total infusion rate.
• For intermittent infusion, wait until the secondary solution has completely infused; then adjust the primary drip rate, as required.
• If the secondary solution tubing is being reused, close the clamp on the tubing, and follow your facility's policy: Either remove the needle or needleless system and replace it with

a new one, or leave it taped in the injection port and label it with the time it was first used.

- Leave the empty container in place until you replace it with a new dose of drug at the prescribed time. If the tubing won't be reused, discard it appropriately with the I.V. container.

Nursing considerations

- If institutional policy allows, use a pump for drug infusion. Place a time tape on the secondary container to help prevent an inaccurate administration rate.
- When reusing secondary tubing, change it according to your facility's policy, usually every 48 to 72 hours. Inspect the injection port for leakage with each use; change it more often if needed.
- Except for lipids, don't piggyback a secondary I.V. line to a total parenteral nutrition line because it risks contamination.

4

Avoiding medication errors

In the state where you practice nursing, a number of different health care professionals may be legally permitted to prescribe, dispense, and administer medications—such as doctors, nurse practitioners, dentists, podiatrists, and optometrists. Most often, however, doctors prescribe medications, pharmacists dispense them, and nurses administer them.

That means you're almost always on the front line when it comes to patients and their medications. It also means that you bear a major share of the responsibility for avoiding medication errors. Besides faithfully following your facility's drug administration policies, you can help prevent medication errors by studying common ones and avoiding the slipups that allow them to happen. This chapter outlines some of the more common causes of medication errors.

Name game

Drugs with similar-sounding names can be easy to confuse. What's more, even different-sounding names can look similar when written out rapidly by hand on a medication order: Soriatane and Loxitane, for example, both of which are capsules. Any time a patient's drug order doesn't seem right for his diagnosis, call the prescriber to clarify the order.

ALERT Many nurses have confused an order for morphine with one for hydromorphone (Dilaudid). Both drugs come in 4-mg prefilled syringes. If you give morphine when the prescriber really ordered hydromorphone, the patient could develop respiratory depression or even arrest. Consider posting a prominent notice in your medication room that warns the staff about this common mix-up. Or, try attaching a fluorescent sticker printed with NOT MORPHINE to each hydromorphone syringe.

Drug names aren't the only kinds of words you can confuse. Patient names can cause trouble as well if you fail to verify each person's identity. This problem can be especially troublesome if two patients have the same first name.

Consider this clinical scenario. Robert Brewer, age 5, was hospitalized for measles. Robert Brinson, also age 5, was admitted after a severe asthma attack. The boys were assigned to adjacent rooms on a small pediatric unit. Each had a nonproductive cough. When Robert Brewer's nurse came to give him an expectorant, the child's mother told her that Robert had already inhaled a medication through a mask.

The nurse quickly figured out that another nurse, new to the unit, had given Robert Brinson's medication (acetylcysteine, a mucolytic) to Robert Brewer in error. Fortunately, no harmful adverse effects ensued. Had the nurse checked her patient's identity more carefully, however, no error would have occurred in the first place.

Always check each patient's full name. Also, teach each patient (or parent) to offer an identification bracelet for inspection and to state a full name when anyone enters the room with the intention of giving a medication. (See *Reducing medication errors through patient teaching,* page 34.) Also, urge patients to tell you if an identification bracelet falls off, is removed, or gets lost. Replace it right away.

Allergy alert

Once you've verified your patient's full name, take time to check whether he has any drug allergies—even if he's in distress. Consider this real-life example.

A doctor issued a stat order for chlorpromazine (Thorazine) for a distressed patient. By the time the nurse arrived with it, the patient had grown more distressed and was demanding relief. Unnerved by the patient's demeanor, the nurse gave the drug without checking the patient's medication administration record or documenting the order—and the patient had an allergic reaction to it.

Reducing medication errors through patient teaching

You aren't the only one who's at risk for making medication errors. Patients are at an even higher risk because they know so much less about medications than you do. Indeed, although inpatient deaths from medication errors rose more than twofold from 1983 to 1993, outpatient deaths rose more than eightfold. Clearly, patient teaching is a crucial aspect of your responsibility in minimizing medication errors and their consequences—especially as more patients receive outpatient rather than inpatient care.

To help minimize medication errors, teach your patient about his diagnosis and the purpose of his drug therapy. Make sure he knows the name of each drug in his regimen, how much of each drug he's supposed to take, and when and how he's supposed to take it. Use an interpreter if he doesn't understand English. Ideally, the patient should go home with his drug information in writing.

Remember that some types of drug therapy can be quite confusing for patients. One patient who went home with a warfarin prescription took 2.5 and 5 tablets rather than 2.5 and 5 mg on alternating days. He eventually was hospitalized with gastrointestinal bleeding—a problem that might have been avoided had he better understood his dosage regimen. Likewise, any regimen that requires a patient to take more than one drug greatly increases the complexity of the therapy, along with the chance of confusion and errors. The patient may need special help to establish a practical, workable dosing schedule.

Also, ask if your patient takes over-the-counter medications at home in addition to his prescribed drugs. Make a special point of asking about herbal remedies and other nutritional supplements. Some herbal remedies have druglike effects and could cause or contribute to a drug-related problem. What's more, because these preparations aren't regulated as drugs, government assurance standards don't apply to their labeling or manufacturing, and their ingredients can be misrepresented, substituted, or contaminated.

Finally, tell your patient which kinds of drug-related problems warrant a call to his doctor. And urge him to report anything about his drug therapy that concerns or worries him.

Any time you're in a tense situation with a patient who needs or wants medication fast, resist the temptation to act first and document later. Skipping that crucial assessment step could easily lead to a medication error.

ALERT A patient who is severely allergic to peanuts could have an anaphylactic reaction to ipratropium bromide (Atrovent) aerosol given by metered-dose inhaler. Ask your patient or his parents whether he's allergic to peanuts before you administer this drug. If you find that he has such an allergy, you'll need to use the nasal spray and inhalation solution form of the drug. Because it doesn't contain soy lecithin, it's safe for patients who are allergic to peanuts.

Compound errors

Many medication errors stem from compound problems—a mistake that could have been caught at any of several steps along the way. For a medication to be administered correctly, each member of the health care team must fulfill the appropriate role. The prescriber must write the order correctly and legibly. The pharmacist must evaluate whether the order is appropriate and then fill it correctly. And the nurse must evaluate whether the order is appropriate and then administer it correctly.

A breakdown anywhere along this chain of events can lead to a medication error. That's why it's so important for members of the health care team to act as a real team, checking each other and catching any problems that arise before those problems affect the patient's health. Do your best to foster an environment in which professionals can double-check each other.

For instance, the pharmacist can help clarify the number of times a drug should be given each day. He can help you label drugs in the most appropriate way. He can remind you to always return unused or discontinued medications to the pharmacy.

You can—indeed, you must—clarify any prescriber's order that doesn't seem clear or correct. You also must correctly handle and store any multi-dose vials obtained from the pharmacist. Only administer drugs that you've prepared personally. And never give a drug that has an ambiguous label or no label at all. Here's an actual example of what could happen if you do.

A nurse placed an unlabeled cup of phenol (used in neurolytic procedures) next to a cup of guanethidine (a postganglionic-blocking drug). The doctor accidentally injected the phenol instead of the guanethidine, causing severe tissue damage to a patient's arm. The patient needed emergency surgery and developed neurologic complications.

Obviously, this was a compound problem. The nurse should have labeled each cup clearly, and the doctor shouldn't have given an unlabeled substance to a patient.

Here's another example of a compound problem. In the neonatal intensive care unit, a nurse prepared and administered a dose of aminophylline for an infant. He didn't have anyone else check his work. After receiving the drug, the infant developed tachycardia and other signs of theophylline toxicity. She later died. The nurse thought the order read 7.4 ml of aminophylline; instead, it read 7.4 mg.

This tragedy might have been avoided if the doctor had written a clearer order, if the nurse had clarified the order, if a pharmacist had prepared and dispensed the drug, or if another nurse had checked the dose calculation. To help prevent such problems, many facilities prefer or require that a pharmacist prepare and dispense nonemergency parenteral doses whenever commercial unit doses aren't available.

Here's another example. A container of 5% acetic acid, used to clean tracheostomy tubing, was left near nebulization equipment in the room of a 10-month-old infant. A respiratory therapist mistook the liquid for normal saline solution and used it to dilute albuterol for the child's nebulizer treatment. During treatment, the child experienced bronchospasm, hypercapnic dyspnea, tachypnea, and tachycardia.

Leaving dangerous chemicals near patients is extremely risky, especially when the container labels don't warn of toxicity. To prevent such problems, read the label on every drug you prepare, and never administer anything that isn't labeled or is labeled poorly.

Route trouble

Many medication errors stem at least in part from problems related to the route of administration. The risk of error increases when a patient has several lines running for different purposes. Consider this example.

A nurse prepared a dose of digoxin elixir for a patient who had both a central intravenous (I.V.) line and a jejunostomy tube—and she mistakenly administered the drug into the central I.V. line. Fortunately, the patient had no adverse reaction. To help prevent such mix-ups in route of administration, prepare all oral medications in a syringe that has a tip small enough to fit an abdominal tube but too big to fit a central line.

Here's another error that could have been avoided: To clear air bubbles from a 9-year-old patient's insulin drip, a nurse disconnected the tubing and raised the pump rate to 200 ml/hour to flush the bubbles through quickly. She then reconnected the tubing and restarted the drip, but she forgot to reset the rate back to 2 units/hour. The child received 50 units of insulin before the error was detected. To prevent this kind of error, never increase a drip rate to clear bubbles from a line. Instead, remove the tubing from the pump, disconnect it from the patient, and use the flow-control clamp to establish gravity flow.

Risky abbreviations

Abbreviating drug names is risky, as in this example. Cancer patients with anemia may receive epoetin alfa, commonly abbreviated EPO, to stimulate red blood cell production. In one case, when a cancer patient was admitted to a hospital, the doctor wrote, "May take own supply of EPO." However, the patient wasn't anemic. Sensing that something was wrong, the pharmacist interviewed the patient, who confirmed that he was taking "EPO"—evening primrose oil—to lower his cholesterol level. Ask all prescribers to spell out drug names.

Unclear orders

A patient was supposed to receive one dose of the antineoplastic lomustine to treat brain cancer. (Lomustine is typically given as a single oral dose once every 6 weeks.) The doctor's order read "Administer h.s." Because a nurse misinterpreted the order to mean every night, the patient received nine daily doses, developed severe thrombocytopenia and leukopenia, and died.

If you're unfamiliar with a drug, check a drug book before administering it. If a prescriber uses "h.s." but doesn't specify the frequency of administration, ask him to clarify the order. When documenting orders, note "h.s. nightly" or "h.s. one dose today."

Color changes

In two reports, alert nurses noticed that antineoplastics prepared in the pharmacy didn't look the way they should. The first error involved a 6-year-old child who was to receive 12 mg of methotrexate intrathecally. In the pharmacy, a 1-g vial was mistakenly selected instead of a 20-mg vial, and the drug was reconstituted with 10 ml of normal saline. The vial containing 100 mg/ml was incorrectly labeled as containing 2 mg/ml, and 6 ml of the solution was drawn into a syringe. Although the syringe label indicated 12 mg of drug, the syringe actually contained 600 mg of drug.

When the nurse received the syringe and noted that the drug's color didn't appear right, she returned it to the pharmacy for verification. The pharmacist retrieved the vial used to prepare the dose and drew the remaining solution into another syringe. The solutions in both syringes matched, and no one noticed the vial's 1-g label. The pharmacist concluded that a manufacturing change caused the color difference.

The child received the 600-mg dose and experienced seizures 45 minutes later. A pharmacist responding to the emergency detected the error. The child received an antidote and recovered.

A similar case involved a 20-year-old patient with leukemia who received mitomycin instead of mitoxantrone. The nurse had questioned the drug's unusual bluish tint, but the pharmacist assured her that the color difference was due to a change in manufacturer. Fortunately, the patient didn't suffer any harm.

If a familiar drug seems to have an unfamiliar appearance, investigate the cause. If the pharmacist cites a manufacturing change, ask him to double-check whether he has received verification from the manufacturer. Document the appearance discrepancy, your actions, and the pharmacist's response in the patient record.

Stress levels

A nurse-anesthetist administered the sedative midazolam (Versed) to the wrong patient. When she discovered the error, she reached for what she thought was a vial of the antidote flumazenil (Romazicon), withdrew 2.5 ml of the drug, and administered it. When the patient didn't respond, she realized she'd reached for a vial of ondansetron (Zofran), an antiemetic, instead. Another practitioner assisted with proper I.V. administration of flumazenil, and the patient recovered without harm.

Committing a serious error can cause enormous stress and cloud your judgment. If you're involved in a drug error, ask another professional to administer the antidote.

Clearly, you carry a great deal of responsibility for making sure that the right patient gets the right drug in the right concentration at the right time by the right route. By keeping these common errors in mind, you can minimize your risk of making them and maximize the therapeutic effects of your patients' drug regimens.

Drug Classifications

Alkylating drugs

altretamine
busulfan
carboplatin
carmustine
chlorambucil
cisplatin
cyclophosphamide
dacarbazine
ifosfamide
lomustine
mechlorethamine hydrochloride
melphalan
streptozocin
temozolomide
thiotepa

Indications

▶ Treatment of various tumors, especially those having large volume and slow cell-turnover rate. See individual drugs for specific uses.

Actions

Alkylating drugs appear to act independently of a specific cell-cycle phase. They are polyfunctional compounds that can be divided chemically into five groups: nitrogen mustards, ethylenimines, alkyl sulfonates, triazenes, and nitrosoureas. Highly reactive, they primarily target nucleic acids and form covalent linkages with nucleophilic centers in many different kinds of molecules. Their polyfunctional character allows them to cross-link double-stranded DNA, preventing strands from separating for replication, which appears to contribute more to the cytotoxic effects of these drugs than other results of alkylation.

Adverse reactions

The most common adverse reactions include bone marrow depression, leukopenia, thrombocytopenia, fever, chills, sore throat, nausea, vomiting, diarrhea, flank or joint pain, anxiety, swelling of feet or lower legs, hair loss, and redness or pain at injection site.

Contraindications and precautions

- Contraindicated in patients hypersensitive to drug. See individual drugs for additional contraindications.
- Use cautiously in patients receiving other cytotoxic drugs or radiation therapy. See individual drugs for additional precautions.
- **Breast-feeding patients:** Alkylating drugs appear in breast milk. Breast-feeding should be avoided.
- **Pediatric patients:** Safety and efficacy of many alkylating drugs haven't been established in children. See individual drugs for guidelines.
- **Geriatric patients:** These patients have an increased risk of adverse reactions. Monitor them closely.

NURSING CONSIDERATIONS

Assessment

- Perform a complete assessment before therapy begins.
- Monitor patient for adverse reactions throughout therapy.
- Monitor BUN, hematocrit, platelet count, ALT, AST, LD, serum bilirubin, serum creatinine, uric acid, total and differential leukocyte, and other levels as needed.
- Monitor vital signs and patency of catheter or I.V. line throughout administration.

Key nursing diagnoses

- Ineffective protection related to thrombocytopenia
- Risk for infection related to immunosuppression
- Risk for deficient fluid volume related to adverse GI effects

Planning and implementation

- Follow established procedures for safe and proper handling, administration, and disposal of chemotherapeutic drugs.
- Treat extravasation promptly.
- Keep epinephrine, corticosteroids, and antihistamines available during carboplatin or cisplatin administration. Anaphylactoid reactions may occur.
- Administer ifosfamide with mesna, as prescribed, to prevent hemorrhagic cystitis.

▶ Prototype drug

• Give lomustine 2 to 4 hours after meals. Nausea and vomiting usually last less than 24 hours although loss of appetite may last for several days.
• Administer adequate hydration before and for 24 hours after cisplatin treatment.
• Be aware that allopurinol may be prescribed to prevent drug-induced hyperuricemia.

Patient teaching

• Caution patient to avoid people with bacterial or viral infections because chemotherapy can increase susceptibility. Urge him to report signs of infection promptly.
• Review proper oral hygiene, including cautious use of toothbrush, dental floss, and toothpicks.
• Advise patient to complete dental work before therapy begins or to delay it until blood counts are normal.
• Warn patient that he may bruise easily because of drug's effect on blood count.

☑ Evaluation

• Patient develops no serious bleeding complications.
• Patient remains free from infection.
• Patient maintains adequate hydration.

Alpha-adrenergic blockers

dihydroergotamine mesylate
doxazosin mesylate
ergotamine tartrate
phentolamine mesylate
prazosin hydrochloride
tamsulosin hydrochloride
terazosin hydrochloride

Indications

▶ Peripheral vascular disorders (Raynaud's disease, acrocyanosis, frostbite, acute atrial occlusion, phlebitis, diabetic gangrene), vascular headaches, dermal necrosis, mild to moderate urinary obstruction in men with BPH, hypertension, pheochromocytoma.

Actions

Selective alpha blockers (dihydroergotamine, doxazosin, prazosin, and terazosin) have readily observable effects. They decrease vascular resistance and increase venous capacitance, thereby lowering blood pressure and causing pink warm skin, nasal and scleroconjunctival congestion, ptosis, orthostatic and exercise hypotension, mild to moderate miosis, and interference with ejaculation. They also relax nonvascular smooth muscle, notably in the prostate capsule, thereby reducing urinary symptoms in men with BPH. Because $alpha_1$ blockers don't block $alpha_2$ receptors, they don't cause transmitter overflow.

Nonselective alpha blockers (ergotamine, phentolamine, and tolazoline) antagonize both $alpha_1$ and $alpha_2$ receptors. Generally, alpha blockade results in tachycardia, palpitations, and increased renin secretion because of abnormally large amounts of norepinephrine (transmitter overflow) released from adrenergic nerve endings as a result of the concurrent blockade of $alpha_1$ and $alpha_2$ receptors. Norepinephrine's effects are clinically counterproductive to the major uses of nonselective alpha blockers.

Adverse reactions

Selective alpha blockers may cause severe orthostatic hypotension and syncope, especially with the first dose. The most common adverse effects of $alpha_1$ blockade are dizziness, headache, and malaise.

Nonselective alpha blockers typically cause orthostatic hypotension, tachycardia, palpitations, fluid retention (from excess renin secretion), nasal and ocular congestion, and aggravation of respiratory infection.

Contraindications and precautions

• Contraindicated in patients with MI, coronary insufficiency, or angina.
• **Pregnant patients:** Use cautiously in pregnant women.
• **Breast-feeding patients:** Use cautiously in breast-feeding women.
• **Pediatric patients:** Safety and efficacy of many alpha-adrenergic blockers haven't been established in children. Use caustiously.
• **Geriatric patients:** Hypotensive effects may be more pronounced in elderly patients.

NURSING CONSIDERATIONS

Assessment
- Monitor vital signs, especially blood pressure.
- Monitor patient closely for adverse reactions.

Key nursing diagnoses
- Decreased cardiac output related to hypotension
- Acute pain related to headache
- Excessive fluid volume related to fluid retention

Planning and implementation
- Administer at bedtime to minimize dizziness or light-headedness.
- Begin therapy with small dose, as ordered, to avoid first-dose syncope.

Patient teaching
- Warn patient to avoid rising suddenly from a lying or sitting position.
- Urge patient to avoid hazardous tasks that require mental alertness until the full effects of drug are known.
- Advise patient that alcohol, excessive exercise, prolonged standing, and heat exposure will intensify adverse effects.
- Tell patient to promptly report dizziness or irregular heartbeat.

Evaluation
- Patient maintains adequate cardiac output.
- Patient's headache is relieved.
- Patient has no edema.

Aminoglycosides

amikacin sulfate
gentamicin sulfate
kanamycin sulfate
neomycin sulfate
streptomycin sulfate
tobramycin sulfate

Indications

▶ Septicemia; postoperative, pulmonary, intra-abdominal, and urinary tract infections; infections of skin, soft tissue, bones, and joints; aerobic gram-negative bacillary meningitis (not susceptible to other antibiotics); serious staphylococcal, *Pseudomonas. aeruginosa,* and *Klebsiella* infections; enterococcal infections; nosocomial pneumonia; anaerobic infections involving *Bacteroides fragilis*; tuberculosis; initial empiric therapy in febrile, leukopenic patient.

Actions

Aminoglycosides are bactericidal. They bind directly and irreversibly to 30S ribosomal subunits, inhibiting bacterial protein synthesis. They're active against many aerobic gram-negative and some aerobic gram-positive organisms.

Susceptible gram-negative organisms include *Acinetobacter, Citrobacter, Enterobacter, Escherichia coli, Klebsiella,* indole-positive and indole-negative *Proteus, Providencia, P. aeruginosa, Salmonella, Serratia,* and *Shigella.* Streptomycin is also active against *Brucella, Calymmatobacterium granulomatis, Pasteurella multocida,* and *Yersinia pestis.*

Susceptible gram-positive organisms include *Staphylococcus aureus* and *S. epidermidis.* Streptomycin is also active against *Nocardia, Erysipelothrix,* and some mycobacteria, including *Mycobacterium tuberculosis, M. marinum,* and certain strains of *M. kansasii* and *M. leprae.*

Adverse reactions

Ototoxicity and nephrotoxicity are the most serious complications. Neuromuscular blockade also may occur. Oral forms most commonly cause nausea, vomiting, and diarrhea. Parenteral drugs may cause vein irritation, phlebitis, and sterile abscess.

Contraindications and precautions

- Contraindicated in patients hypersensitive to aminoglycosides.
- Use cautiously in patients with neuromuscular disorder or renal impairment.
- **Pregnant patients:** Use cautiously in pregnant patients.
- **Breast-feeding patients:** Safety hasn't been established in breast-feeding women.
- **Pediatric patients:** The half-life of aminoglycosides is prolonged in neonates and pre-

▶ Prototype drug

mature infants because of their immature renal systems. Dosage adjustment may be needed in infants and children.

• **Geriatric patients:** These patients have an increased risk of nephrotoxicity and commonly need reduced dosages and longer dosing intervals. They're also susceptible to ototoxicity and superinfection.

NURSING CONSIDERATIONS

Assessment

• Obtain patient's history of allergies.
• Monitor patient for adverse reactions.
• Obtain results of culture and sensitivity tests before first dose, and check tests periodically to assess drug efficacy.
• Monitor vital signs, electrolyte levels, hearing ability, and renal function studies before and during therapy.
• Draw blood for peak level 1 hour after I.M. injection (30 minutes to 1 hour after I.V. infusion); for trough level, draw sample just before next dose. Time and date all blood samples. Don't use heparinized tube to collect blood samples because it interferes with results.

Key nursing diagnoses

• Risk for injury related to nephrotoxicity and ototoxicity
• Risk for infection related to drug-induced superinfection
• Risk for deficient fluid volume related to adverse GI reactions

Planning and implementation

• Keep patient well hydrated to minimize chemical irritation of renal tubules.
• Don't add or mix other drugs with I.V. infusions, particularly penicillins, which inactivate aminoglycosides. If other drugs must be given I.V., temporarily stop infusion of primary drug.
• Follow manufacturer's instructions for reconstitution, dilution, and storage of drugs; check expiration dates.
• Shake oral suspensions well before administering.
• Administer I.M. dose deep into large muscle mass (gluteal or midlateral thigh); rotate injection sites to minimize tissue injury. Apply ice to injection site to relieve pain.
• Too rapid I.V. administration may cause neuromuscular blockade. Infuse I.V. drug continuously or intermittently over 30 to 60 minutes for adults, 1 to 2 hours for infants; dilution volume for children is determined individually.

Patient teaching

• Teach signs and symptoms of hypersensitivity and other adverse reactions. Urge patient to report unusual effects promptly.
• Emphasize importance of adequate fluid intake.

Evaluation

• Patient maintains pretreatment renal and hearing functions.
• Patient is free from infection.
• Patient maintains adequate hydration.

Angiotensin-converting enzyme inhibitors

benazepril hydrochloride
captopril
enalapril maleate
fosinopril sodium
lisinopril
moexipril hydrochloride
perindopril erbumine
quinapril hydrochloride
ramipril

Indications

▶ Hypertension, heart failure.

Actions

ACE inhibitors prevent conversion of angiotensin I to angiotensin II, a potent vasoconstrictor. Besides decreasing vasoconstriction and thus reducing peripheral arterial resistance, inhibition of angiotensin II decreases adrenocortical secretion of aldosterone. This reduces sodium and water retention and extracellular fluid volume. ACE inhibition also causes increased levels of bradykinin resulting in vasodilation. This decreases heart rate and systemic vascular resistance.

Adverse reactions

The most common adverse effects of therapeutic doses are headache, fatigue, hypotension, tachycardia, dysgeusia, proteinuria, hyperkalemia, rash, cough, and angioedema of face and limbs. Severe hypotension may occur at toxic drug levels.

Contraindications and precautions

- Contraindicated in patients hypersensitive to ACE inhibitors.
- Use cautiously in patients with impaired renal function or serious autoimmune disease and in those taking other drugs known to depress WBC count or immune response.
- **Pregnant patients:** Women of childbearing age receiving ACE inhibitor therapy should report suspected pregnancy immediately to prescriber. High risks of fetal morbidity and mortality are linked to ACE inhibitor exposure, especially in the second and third trimesters.
- **Breast-feeding patients:** Some ACE inhibitors appear in breast milk. A different feeding method is recommended during therapy.
- **Pediatric patients:** Safety and efficacy in children haven't been established. Give drug only if potential benefit outweighs risk.
- **Geriatric patients:** These patients may need lower doses because of impaired drug clearance.

NURSING CONSIDERATIONS

Assessment

- Observe patient for adverse reactions.
- Monitor vital signs regularly and WBC counts and serum electrolyte levels periodically.

Key nursing diagnoses

- Risk for trauma related to orthostatic hypotension
- Ineffective protection related to hyperkalemia
- Acute pain related to headache

Planning and implementation

- Discontinue diuretic therapy 2 to 3 days before beginning ACE inhibitor therapy, as ordered, to reduce risk of hypotension. If drug doesn't adequately control blood pressure, diuretics may be reinstated.
- Give a reduced dosage, as ordered, if the patient has impaired renal function.
- Give potassium supplements cautiously because ACE inhibitors may cause potassium retention.
- Discontinue ACE inhibitors, as ordered, if patient becomes pregnant. These drugs can cause birth defects or fetal death during second or third trimester.

Patient teaching

- Tell patient that drugs may cause a dry, persistent, tickling cough that stops when therapy stops.
- Urge patient to report light-headedness, especially in the first few days of therapy, so the dosage can be adjusted. Also, tell him to report signs of infection (such as sore throat and fever) because these drugs may decrease WBC count; facial swelling or difficulty breathing because these drugs may cause angioedema; and loss of taste, for which therapy may stop.
- Caution patient to avoid sudden position changes to minimize orthostatic hypotension.
- Warn patient to seek medical approval before taking self-prescribed cold preparations.
- Tell women to report pregnancy at once.

Evaluation

- Patient sustains no injury from orthostatic hypotension.
- Patient's WBC counts remain normal throughout therapy.
- Patient's headache is relieved by mild analgesic.

Antacids

aluminum carbonate
aluminum hydroxide
calcium carbonate
magaldrate
magnesium hydroxide
magnesium oxide
sodium bicarbonate

Indications

▶ Ulcer pain.

Prototype drug

Actions

Antacids reduce the total acid load in the GI tract and elevate gastric pH to reduce pepsin activity. They also strengthen the gastric mucosal barrier and increase esophageal sphincter tone.

Adverse reactions

Aluminum-containing antacids may cause aluminum intoxication, constipation, hypophosphatemia, intestinal obstruction, and osteomalacia. Magnesium-containing antacids may cause diarrhea or hypermagnesemia (in renal failure). Calcium carbonate, magaldrate, magnesium oxide, and sodium bicarbonate may cause milk-alkali syndrome or rebound hyperacidity.

Contraindications and precautions

- Calcium carbonate, magaldrate, and magnesium oxide are contraindicated in severe renal disease. Sodium bicarbonate is contraindicated in patients with hypertension, renal disease, edema, or vomiting; patients receiving diuretics or continuous GI suction; and patients on sodium-restricted diets.
- Give magnesium oxide cautiously in elderly patients and in those with mild renal impairment.
- Give aluminum preparations, calcium carbonate, and magaldrate cautiously in elderly patients; in those receiving antidiarrheals, antispasmodics, or anticholinergics; and in those with dehydration, fluid restriction, chronic renal disease, or suspected intestinal absorption.
- **Breast-feeding patients:** Antacids may be given to breast-feeding women.
- **Pediatric patients:** Serious adverse effects are more likely in infants from changes in fluid and electrolyte balance. Monitor patient closely.
- **Geriatric patients:** These patients have an increased risk of adverse reactions. Monitor them closely.

NURSING CONSIDERATIONS

Assessment

- Assess patient's condition before therapy and regularly thereafter.
- Record number and consistency of stools.
- Observe patient for adverse reactions.
- Monitor patient receiving long-term, high-dose aluminum carbonate and hydroxide for fluid and electrolyte imbalance, especially if patient is on a sodium-restricted diet.
- Monitor serum phosphate levels in a patient receiving aluminum carbonate or hydroxide.
- Watch for signs of hypercalcemia in a patient receiving calcium carbonate.
- Monitor serum magnesium levels in a patient with mild renal impairment who takes magaldrate.

Key nursing diagnoses

- Constipation related to adverse effects of aluminum-containing antacid
- Diarrhea related to adverse effects of magnesium-containing antacid
- Ineffective protection related to drug-induced electrolyte imbalance

Planning and implementation

- Manage constipation with laxatives or stool softeners, or check with prescriber about switching patient to a magnesium preparation.
- Obtain an order for an antidiarrheal, as needed, and check with prescriber about switching patient to aluminum-containing antacid.
- Shake container well, and give with small amount of water or juice to facilitate passage. When administering through a nasogastric tube, make sure the tube is patent and placed correctly. After instilling the drug, flush the tube with water to ensure passage to the stomach and to clear the tube.

Patient teaching

- Warn patient not to take antacids indiscriminately or to switch antacids without prescriber's consent.
- Tell patient not to take calcium carbonate with milk or other foods high in vitamin D.
- Warn patient not to take sodium bicarbonate with milk because doing so could cause hypercalcemia.

Evaluation

- Patient regains normal bowel pattern.
- Patient states that diarrhea is relieved.
- Patient maintains normal electrolyte balance.

Antianginals

Beta blockers
- nadolol
- propranolol hydrochloride

Calcium channel blockers
- amlodipine besylate
- bepridil hydrochloride
- diltiazem hydrochloride
- nicardipine hydrochloride
- nifedipine
- verapamil hydrochloride

Nitrates
- erythrityl tetranitrate
- isosorbide dinitrate
- isosorbide mononitrate
- nitroglycerin

Indications

▶ Moderate to severe angina (beta blockers); classic, effort-induced angina and Prinzmetal's angina (calcium channel blockers); recurrent angina (long-acting nitrates and topical, transdermal, transmucosal, and oral extended-release nitroglycerin); acute angina (S.L. nitroglycerin and S.L. or chewable isosorbide dinitrate); unstable angina (I.V. nitroglycerin).

Actions

Beta blockers block catecholamine-induced increases in heart rate, blood pressure, and myocardial contraction. Calcium channel blockers inhibit influx of calcium through muscle cells, dilating coronary arteries and decreasing afterload. Nitrates decrease left ventricular end-diastolic pressure (preload) and systemic vascular resistance (afterload) and increase blood flow through collateral coronary vessels.

Adverse reactions

Beta blockers may cause bradycardia, heart failure, cough, diarrhea, disturbing dreams, dizziness, dyspnea, fatigue, fever, hypotension, lethargy, nausea, peripheral edema, and wheezing. Calcium channel blockers may cause bradycardia, confusion, constipation, depression, diarrhea, dizziness, edema, elevated liver enzymes (transient), fatigue, flushing, headache, hypotension, insomnia, nervousness, and rash. Nitrates may cause alcohol intoxication (from I.V. preparations containing alcohol), flushing, headache, orthostatic hypotension, reflex tachycardia, rash, syncope, and vomiting.

Contraindications and precautions

- Beta blockers are contraindicated in patients hypersensitive to them and in patients with cardiogenic shock, sinus bradycardia, heart block greater than first degree, bronchial asthma, or heart failure unless failure results from tachyarrhythmia treatable with propranolol. Calcium channel blockers are contraindicated in patients with severe hypotension or heart block greater than first degree (except with functioning pacemaker). Nitrates are contraindicated in patients with severe anemia, cerebral hemorrhage, head trauma, glaucoma, or hyperthyroidism.
- Use beta blockers cautiously in patients with nonallergic bronchospastic disorders, diabetes mellitus, or impaired hepatic or renal function. Use calcium channel blockers cautiously in patients with hepatic or renal impairment, bradycardia, heart failure, or cardiogenic shock. Use nitrates cautiously in patients with hypotension or recent MI.
- **Pregnant patients:** Use beta blockers cautiously in pregnant patients.
- **Breast-feeding patients:** Recommendations for breast-feeding vary by drug. Use beta blockers and calcium channel blockers cautiously.
- **Pediatric patients:** Safety and efficacy haven't been established in children. Check with prescriber before giving these drugs to children.
- **Geriatric patients:** These patients have an increased risk of adverse reactions.

NURSING CONSIDERATIONS

Assessment

- Monitor vital signs. With I.V. nitroglycerin, monitor blood pressure and pulse rate every 5 to 15 minutes while adjusting dosage and every hour thereafter.
- Monitor effectiveness of prescribed drug.
- Observe for adverse reactions.

Prototype drug

Key nursing diagnoses

- Risk for injury related to adverse reactions
- Excessive fluid volume related to adverse CV effects of beta blockers or calcium channel blockers
- Acute pain related to headache

Planning and implementation

- Have patient sit or lie down when receiving the first nitrate dose; take his pulse rate and blood pressure before giving dose and when drug action starts.
- Don't give a beta blocker or calcium channel blocker to relieve acute angina.
- Withhold the dose and notify prescriber if patient's heart rate is below 60 beats/minute or systolic blood pressure is below 90 mm Hg.

Patient teaching

- Warn patient not to discontinue drug abruptly without prescriber's approval.
- Teach patient to take his pulse before taking a beta blocker or calcium channel blocker. Tell him to withhold the dose and alert the prescriber if his pulse rate is below 60 beats/minute.
- Instruct patient taking nitroglycerin S.L. to go to the emergency department if three tablets taken 5 minutes apart don't relieve anginal pain.
- Tell patient to report serious or persistent adverse reactions.

Evaluation

- Patient sustains no injury from adverse reactions.
- Patient maintains normal fluid balance.
- Patient's headache is relieved with mild analgesic.

Antiarrhythmics

Class I
moricizine hydrochloride
Class Ia
disopyramide
procainamide hydrochloride
quinidine bisulfate
quinidine gluconate
quinidine polygalacturonate
quinidine sulfate
Class Ib
lidocaine hydrochloride
mexiletine hydrochloride
phenytoin
phenytoin sodium
tocainide hydrochloride
Class Ic
flecainide acetate
propafenone hydrochloride
Class II (beta blockers)
acebutolol
esmolol hydrochloride
propranolol hydrochloride
sotalol hydrochloride
Class III
amiodarone hydrochloride
bretylium tosylate
dofetilide
ibutilide fumarate
Class IV (calcium channel blocker)
verapamil hydrochloride

Indications

▶ Atrial and ventricular arrhythmias.

Actions

Class I drugs reduce the inward current carried by sodium ions, stabilizing neuronal cardiac membranes. Class Ia drugs depress phase 0, prolong the action potential, and have cardiac membrane–stabilizing effects. Class Ib drugs depress phase 0, shorten the action potential, and have cardiac membrane–stabilizing effects. Class Ic drugs block the transport of sodium ions, decreasing conduction velocity but not repolarization rate. Class II drugs decrease heart rate, myocardial contractility, blood pressure, and AV node conduction. Class III drugs prolong the action potential and refractory period. Class IV drugs decrease myocardial contractility and oxygen demand by inhibiting calcium ion influx; they also dilate coronary arteries and arterioles.

Adverse reactions

Most antiarrhythmics can aggravate existing arrhythmias or cause new ones. They also may produce hypersensitivity reactions; hypotension; GI problems, such as nausea, vomiting, or altered bowel elimination; and CNS disturbances, such as dizziness or fatigue. Some antiarrhythmics may worsen heart failure. Class II drugs may cause bronchoconstriction.

Contraindications and precautions

- Contraindicated in patients hypersensitive to drug.
- Many antiarrhythmics are contraindicated or require cautious use in patients with cardiogenic shock, digitalis toxicity, and second- or third-degree heart block (unless patient has a pacemaker). See individual drugs for specific contraindications and precautions.
- **Breast-feeding patients:** Many antiarrhythmics appear in breast milk. Guidelines for breast-feeding vary with individual drugs.
- **Pediatric patients:** Children have an increased risk of adverse reactions. Monitor them closely.
- **Geriatric patients:** These patients exhibit physiologic alterations in CV system. Use these drugs cautiously.

NURSING CONSIDERATIONS

Assessment
- Monitor ECG continuously when therapy starts and dosage is adjusted.
- Monitor patient's vital signs frequently and assess for signs of toxicity and adverse reactions.
- Measure apical pulse rate before giving drug.
- Monitor serum drug levels as indicated.

Key nursing diagnoses
- Decreased cardiac output related to arrhythmias or myocardial depression
- Ineffective protection related to adverse reactions
- Noncompliance related to long-term therapy

Planning and implementation
- Don't crush sustained-release tablets.
- Take safety precautions if adverse CNS reactions occur.
- Notify prescriber about adverse reactions.

Patient teaching
- Stress the importance of taking drug exactly as prescribed.
- Teach patient to take his pulse before each dose. Tell him to notify prescriber if his pulse is irregular or below 60 beats/minute.
- Instruct patient to avoid hazardous activities that require mental alertness if adverse CNS reactions occur.
- Tell patient to limit fluid and salt intake if his prescribed drug causes fluid retention.

Evaluation
- Patient maintains adequate cardiac output, as evidenced by normal vital signs and adequate tissue perfusion.
- Patient has no serious adverse reactions.
- Patient states importance of compliance with therapy.

Antibiotic antineoplastics

bleomycin sulfate
dactinomycin
daunorubicin hydrochloride
doxorubicin hydrochloride
idarubicin hydrochloride
mitomycin
mitoxantrone hydrochloride
plicamycin
procarbazine hydrochloride
streptozocin

Indications

▶ Treatment of various tumors. See individual drugs for specific uses.

Actions

Although classified as antibiotics, these drugs exert cytotoxic effects, ruling out their use as antimicrobials. They interfere with proliferation of malignant cells through several mechanisms. Their action may be cell-cycle-phase nonspecific, cell-cycle-phase specific, or both. Some exhibit activity resembling alkylating drugs or antimetabolites; for example, streptozocin is considered an alkylating drug because of its therapeutic activity. By binding to or complexing with DNA, antineoplastic antibi-

Prototype drug

otics directly or indirectly inhibit DNA, RNA, and protein synthesis.

Adverse reactions

The most common adverse reactions include nausea, vomiting, diarrhea, fever, chills, sore throat, anxiety, confusion, flank or joint pain, swelling of the feet or lower legs, hair loss, redness or pain at the injection site, bone marrow depression, and leukopenia.

Contraindications and precautions

- Contraindicated in patients hypersensitive to drug.
- See individual drugs for complete listings of contraindications and precautions.
- **Breast-feeding patients:** Breast-feeding is contraindicated in women receiving chemotherapy, including therapy with antibiotic antineoplastic drugs.
- **Pediatric patients:** Safety and efficacy of some drugs haven't been established in children. See individual drugs for specific guidelines.
- **Geriatric patients:** These patients have an increased risk of adverse reactions. Monitor them closely.

NURSING CONSIDERATIONS

Assessment

- Perform a complete assessment before therapy begins.
- Monitor patient for adverse reactions.
- Monitor vital signs and patency of catheter or I.V. line.
- Monitor BUN, hematocrit, platelet count, ALT, AST, LD, serum bilirubin, serum creatinine, uric acid, and total and differential leukocyte counts, as ordered.
- Monitor pulmonary function tests in a patient receiving bleomycin. Assess lung function regularly.
- Monitor ECG before and during treatment with daunorubicin and doxorubicin.

Key nursing diagnoses

- Ineffective protection related to thrombocytopenia
- Risk for infection related to immunosuppression
- Risk for deficient fluid volume related to adverse GI effects

Planning and implementation

- Follow established procedures for safe and proper handling, administration, and disposal of chemotherapeutic drugs.
- Try to ease anxiety in patient and family before treatment.
- Keep epinephrine, corticosteroids, and antihistamines available during bleomycin therapy. Anaphylactoid reactions may occur.
- Treat extravasation promptly.
- Ensure adequate hydration during idarubicin therapy.
- Discontinue procarbazine and notify prescriber if patient becomes confused or neuropathies develop.

Patient teaching

- Warn patient to avoid close contact with persons who have received the oral poliovirus vaccine.
- Caution patient to avoid exposure to persons with bacterial or viral infections because chemotherapy increases susceptibility. Urge him to report signs of infection immediately.
- Review proper oral hygiene, including cautious use of toothbrush, dental floss, and toothpicks. Chemotherapy can increase the risk of microbial infection, delayed healing, and bleeding gums.
- Urge patient to complete dental work before therapy begins or to delay it until blood counts are normal.
- Warn patient that he may bruise easily.
- Tell patient to report redness, pain, or swelling at injection site immediately. Local tissue injury and scarring may result if I.V. infiltration occurs.
- Warn patient taking procarbazine to avoid hazardous activities that require alertness until drug's CNS effects are known. Also advise him to take procarbazine at bedtime and in divided doses to reduce nausea and vomiting.
- Advise patient taking daunorubicin, doxorubicin, or idarubicin that his urine may turn orange or red for 1 to 2 days after therapy begins.

Evaluation
- No serious bleeding complications develop.
- Patient remains free from infection.
- Patient maintains adequate hydration.

Anticholinergics
atropine sulfate
benztropine mesylate
dicyclomine hydrochloride
glycopyrrolate
propantheline bromide
scopolamine
scopolamine butylbromide
scopolamine hydrobromide

Indications
▶ Prevention of motion sickness, preoperative reduction of secretions and blockage of cardiac reflexes, adjunct treatment of peptic ulcers and other GI disorders, blockage of cholinomimetic effects of cholinesterase inhibitors or other drugs, and (for benztropine) various spastic conditions, including acute dystonic reactions, muscle rigidity, parkinsonism, and extrapyramidal disorders.

Actions
Anticholinergics competitively antagonize the actions of acetylcholine and other cholinergic agonists at muscarinic receptors.

Adverse reactions
Therapeutic doses commonly cause dry mouth, decreased sweating or anhidrosis, headache, mydriasis, blurred vision, cycloplegia, urinary hesitancy and retention, constipation, palpitations, and tachycardia.These reactions usually disappear when therapy stops. Toxicity can cause signs and symptoms resembling psychosis (disorientation, confusion, hallucinations, delusions, anxiety, agitation, and restlessness); dilated, nonreactive pupils; blurred vision; hot, dry, flushed skin; dry mucous membranes; dysphagia; decreased or absent bowel sounds; urine retention; hyperthermia; tachycardia; hypertension; and increased respirations.

Contraindications and precautions
- Contraindicated in patients hypersensitive to drug and in those with angle-closure glaucoma, renal or GI obstructive disease, reflux esophagitis, or myasthenia gravis.
- Use cautiously in patients with heart disease, GI infection, open-angle glaucoma, prostatic hypertrophy, hypertension, hyperthyroidism, ulcerative colitis, autonomic neuropathy, or hiatal hernia with reflux esophagitis. Patients over age 40 may be more sensitive to these drugs.
- **Breast-feeding patients:** Anticholinergics may decrease milk production, and some may appear in breast milk, possibly causing infant toxicity. Breast-feeding women should avoid these drugs.
- **Pediatric patients:** Safety and efficacy haven't been established in children.
- **Geriatric patients:** Use cautiously in these patients, and give a reduced dosage as indicated.

NURSING CONSIDERATIONS

Assessment
- Monitor patient regularly for adverse reactions.
- Check vital signs at least every 4 hours.
- Measure urine output; check for urine retention.
- Assess patient for changes in vision and for signs of impending toxicity.

Key nursing diagnoses
- Urinary retention related to adverse effect on bladder
- Constipation related to adverse effect on GI tract
- Acute pain related to headache

Planning and implementation
- Administer drug 30 minutes to 1 hour before meals and at bedtime to maximize therapeutic effects. In some instances, drug should be administered with meals; follow dosage recommendations.
- Provide ice chips, cool drinks, or hard candy to relieve a dry mouth.
- Relieve constipation with stool softeners or bulk laxatives.

• Administer a mild analgesic for headache.
• Notify prescriber of urine retention, and be prepared for catheterization.

Patient teaching
• Teach patient how and when to take the drug; caution him not to take other drugs unless prescribed.
• Warn patient to avoid hazardous tasks if he experiences dizziness, drowsiness, or blurred vision. Inform him that the drug may increase his sensitivity to or intolerance of high temperatures, resulting in dizziness.
• Advise patient to avoid alcohol because it may cause additive CNS effects.
• Urge patient to drink plenty of fluids and to eat a high-fiber diet to prevent constipation.
• Tell patient to notify prescriber promptly if he experiences confusion, rapid or pounding heartbeat, dry mouth, blurred vision, skin rash, eye pain, significant change in urine volume, or pain or difficulty on urination.
• Advise women to report planned or known pregnancy.

Evaluation
• Patient maintains normal voiding pattern.
• Patient regains normal bowel patterns.
• Patient is free from pain.

Anticoagulants

Coumarin derivative
warfarin sodium
Heparin derivatives
dalteparin sodium
danaparoid sodium
enoxaparin sodium
heparin calcium
heparin sodium

Indications

▶ Pulmonary emboli, deep vein thrombosis, thrombus, blood clotting, disseminated intravascular coagulation.

Actions

Heparin derivatives accelerate formation of an antithrombin III-thrombin complex. It inactivates thrombin and prevents conversion of fibrinogen to fibrin. The coumarin derivative, warfarin, inhibits vitamin K–dependent activation of clotting factors II, VII, IX, and X, which are formed in the liver.

Adverse reactions

Anticoagulants commonly cause bleeding and may cause hypersensitivity reactions. Warfarin may cause agranulocytosis, alopecia (long-term use), anorexia, dermatitis, fever, nausea, tissue necrosis or gangrene, urticaria, and vomiting. Heparin derivatives may cause thrombocytopenia and elevated liver enzyme levels.

Contraindications and precautions

• Contraindicated in patients with aneurysm, active bleeding, CV hemorrhage, hemorrhagic blood dyscrasias, hemophilia, severe hypertension, pericardial effusions, or pericarditis; and in patients undergoing neurosurgery, ophthalmic surgery, or major surgery.
• Use cautiously in patients with severe diabetes, renal impairment, severe trauma, ulcerations, or vasculitis.
• **Pregnant patients:** Contraindicated in pregnant women and in women with threatened or complete abortion.
• **Breast-feeding patients:** Women should avoid breast-feeding during therapy, if possible.
• **Pediatric patients:** Infants, especially neonates, may be more susceptible to anticoagulants because of vitamin K deficiency.
• **Geriatric patients:** These patients are more susceptible to anticoagulants and are at greater risk for hemorrhage because of altered hemostatic mechanisms or age-related deterioration of hepatic and renal functions.

NURSING CONSIDERATIONS

Assessment
• Monitor patient closely for bleeding and other adverse reactions.
• Check PT, INR, PTT, or activated PTT, as ordered.
• Monitor vital signs, hemoglobin level, and hematocrit value.

• Assess patient's urine, stools, and emesis for blood.

Key nursing diagnoses

• Ineffective protection related to drug's effects on body's normal clotting and bleeding mechanisms
• Risk for deficient fluid volume related to bleeding
• Noncompliance related to long-term warfarin therapy

Planning and implementation

• Don't administer heparin I.M., and avoid I.M. injections of any anticoagulant, if possible.
• Keep protamine sulfate available to treat severe bleeding caused by heparin. Keep vitamin K available to treat frank bleeding caused by warfarin.
• Notify prescriber about serious or persistent adverse reactions.
• Maintain bleeding precautions throughout therapy.

Patient teaching

• Urge patient to take drug exactly as prescribed. If he's taking warfarin, tell him to take it at night and to have blood drawn for PT or INR in the morning for accurate results.
• Advise patient to consult his prescriber before taking any other drug, including OTC medications or herbal remedies.
• Review bleeding precautions to take in everyday living. Urge patient to make repairs and to remove safety hazards from home to reduce risk of injury.
• Caution patient not to increase his intake of green, leafy vegetables (vitamin K may antagonize anticoagulant effects).
• Instruct patient to report bleeding or other adverse reactions promptly.
• Encourage patient to keep appointments for blood tests and follow-up examinations.
• Advise women to report pregnancy or intent to conceive.

Evaluation

• Patient has no adverse change in health status.
• Patient has no evidence of bleeding.
• Patient demonstrates compliance with therapy, as evidenced by normal bleeding and clotting parameters.

Anticonvulsants

acetazolamide sodium
carbamazepine
clonazepam
clorazepate dipotassium
diazepam
divalproex sodium
ethosuximide
fosphenytoin sodium
gabapentin
lamotrigine
levetiracetam
magnesium sulfate
oxcarbazepine
phenobarbital
phenobarbital sodium
phenytoin
phenytoin sodium
phenytoin sodium (extended)
primidone
tiagabine hydrochloride
topiramate
valproate sodium
valproic acid

Indications

▶ Seizure disorders; acute, isolated seizures not caused by seizure disorders; status epilepticus; prevention of seizures after trauma or craniotomy.

Actions

Anticonvulsants comprise six classes of drugs: selected hydantoin derivatives, barbiturates, benzodiazepines, succinimides, iminostilbene derivatives (carbamazepine), and carboxylic acid derivatives. Two miscellaneous anticonvulsants are acetazolamide and magnesium sulfate. Some hydantoin derivatives and carbamazepine inhibit the spread of seizure activity in the motor cortex. Some barbiturates and succinimides limit seizure activity by increasing the threshold for motor cortex stimuli. Selected benzodiazepines and carboxylic acid derivatives are thought to increase the inhibiting action of gamma-aminobutyric acid in brain neurons. Acetazolamide inhibits carbonic anhydrase. Magnesium sulfate interferes with the release of acetylcholine at the myoneural junction.

Adverse reactions

Anticonvulsants can cause adverse CNS effects, such as confusion, somnolence, tremor, and ataxia. Many anticonvulsants also cause GI effects, such as vomiting; CV disorders, such as arrhythmias and hypotension; and hematologic disorders, such as leukopenia and thrombocytopenia.

Contraindications and precautions

- Contraindicated in patients hypersensitive to anticonvulsants.
- See individual drugs for complete listings of contraindications and precautions.
- **Breast-feeding patients:** The safety of many anticonvulsants hasn't been established in breast-feeding women. See individual drugs for guidelines.
- **Pediatric patients:** Children, especially young ones, are sensitive to CNS depressant effects of some anticonvulsants. Use cautiously.
- **Geriatric patients:** These patients are sensitive to CNS effects and may require lower doses. Also, elimination of some anticonvulsants may be prolonged because of decreased renal function. Parenteral use is more likely to cause apnea, hypotension, bradycardia, and cardiac arrest.

NURSING CONSIDERATIONS

Assessment

- Monitor patient's response to prescribed drug and serum levels as indicated.
- Monitor patient for adverse reactions.
- Assess patient's compliance with therapy at each follow-up visit.

Key nursing diagnoses

- Risk for trauma related to adverse reactions
- Impaired physical mobility related to sedation
- Noncompliance related to long-term therapy

Planning and implementation

- Administer oral forms with food to reduce GI irritation.
- Phenytoin binds with tube feedings, thus decreasing absorption of drug. Turn off tube feedings for 2 hours before and after giving phenytoin, according to your facility's policy.
- Expect to adjust dosage according to patient's response.
- Take safety precautions if patient has adverse CNS reactions.

Patient teaching

- Instruct patient to take drug exactly as prescribed and not to stop drug without medical supervision.
- Urge patient to avoid hazardous activities that require mental alertness if adverse CNS reactions occur.
- Advise patient to wear or carry medical identification at all times.

Evaluation

- Patient sustains no trauma from adverse reactions.
- Patient maintains physical mobility.
- Patient complies with therapy and has no seizures.

Antidepressants, tricyclic

amitriptyline hydrochloride
amitriptyline pamoate
amoxapine
clomipramine hydrochloride
desipramine hydrochloride
doxepin hydrochloride
imipramine hydrochloride
imipramine pamoate
nortriptyline hydrochloride
trimipramine maleate

Indications

▶ Depression, anxiety (doxepin hydrochloride), obsessive-compulsive disorder (clomipramine), enuresis in children over age 6 (imipramine).

Actions

Tricyclic antidepressants (TCAs) may inhibit reuptake of norepinephrine and serotonin in CNS nerve terminals (presynaptic neurons), thus enhancing the concentration and activity of neurotransmitters in the synaptic cleft. TCAs also exert antihistaminic, sedative, anticholinergic, vasodilatory, and quinidine-like effects.

Adverse reactions

Adverse reactions include sedation, anticholinergic effects, and orthostatic hypotension. Tertiary amines (amitriptyline, doxepin, imipramine, and trimipramine) exert the strongest sedative effects; tolerance usually develops in a few weeks. Maprotiline and amoxapine are most likely to cause seizures, especially with overdose.

Contraindications and precautions

- Contraindicated in patients with urine retention, angle-closure glaucoma, or hypersensitivity to TCAs.
- Use cautiously in patients with suicidal tendencies, CV disease, or impaired hepatic function.
- **Breast-feeding patients:** Safety in breast-feeding women hasn't been established. Use cautiously.
- **Pediatric patients:** TCAs aren't recommended for children under age 12.
- **Geriatric patients:** These patients are more sensitive to therapeutic and adverse effects; they need lower dosages.

NURSING CONSIDERATIONS

Assessment

- Observe patient for mood changes to monitor drug effectiveness; benefits may not appear for 3 to 6 weeks.
- Check vital signs regularly for decreased blood pressure or tachycardia; observe patient carefully for other adverse reactions and report changes. Check ECG in patients over age 40 before starting therapy.
- Monitor patient for anticholinergic adverse reactions (urine retention or constipation), which may require dosage reduction.

Key nursing diagnoses

- Disturbed thought processes related to adverse effects
- Risk for injury related to sedation and orthostatic hypotension
- Noncompliance related to long-term therapy

Planning and implementation

- Make sure patient swallows each dose; as depressed patient begins to improve, he may hoard pills for suicide attempt.
- Don't withdraw drug abruptly; gradually reduce dosage over several weeks, as ordered, to avoid rebound effect or other adverse reactions.
- Follow manufacturer's instructions for reconstitution, dilution, and storage of drugs.

Patient teaching

- Explain to patient the rationale for therapy and its anticipated risks and benefits. Inform patient that full therapeutic effect may not occur for several weeks.
- Teach patient how and when to take his drug. Warn him not to increase his dosage, discontinue the drug, or take any other drug (including OTC medicines and herbal remedies) without medical approval.
- Because overdosage with TCAs is commonly fatal, entrust a reliable family member with the medication, and warn him to store drug safely away from children.
- Advise patient not to take drug with milk or food to minimize GI distress. Suggest taking full dose at bedtime if daytime sedation is troublesome.
- Tell patient to avoid beverages and other products containing alcohol.
- Advise patient to avoid hazardous tasks that require mental alertness until full effects of drug are known.
- Warn patient that excessive exposure to sunlight, heat lamps, or tanning beds may cause burns and abnormal hyperpigmentation.
- Urge a diabetic patient to monitor his blood glucose carefully because drug may alter blood glucose levels.
- Recommend sugarless gum or hard candy, artificial saliva, or ice chips to relieve dry mouth.

• Advise patient to report adverse reactions promptly.

Evaluation
• Patient regains normal thought processes.
• Patient sustains no injury from adverse reactions.
• Patient complies with therapy, and his depression is alleviated.

Antidiarrheals

bismuth subgallate
bismuth subsalicylate
calcium polycarbophil
diphenoxylate hydrochloride and atropine sulfate
kaolin and pectin mixtures
loperamide
octreotide acetate
opium tincture
opium tincture, camphorated

Indications

▶ Mild, acute, or chronic diarrhea.

Actions

Bismuth preparations may have a mild water-binding capacity, they may absorb toxins, and they provide a protective coating for the intestinal mucosa. Kaolin and pectin mixtures decrease fluid in the stool by absorbing bacteria and toxins that cause diarrhea. Opium preparations increase smooth muscle tone in the GI tract, inhibit motility and propulsion, and diminish digestive secretions.

Adverse reactions

Bismuth preparations may cause salicylism (with high doses) or temporary darkening of tongue and stools. Kaolin and pectin mixtures may cause constipation and fecal impaction or ulceration. Opium preparations may cause dizziness, light-headedness, nausea, physical dependence (with long-term use), and vomiting.

Contraindications and precautions

• Contraindicated in patients hypersensitive to drug.
• Check individual drug listings for specific recommendations and precautions.
• **Breast-feeding patients:** Some antidiarrheal drugs may appear in breast milk. Check individual drugs for specific recommendations.
• **Pediatric patients:** Consult prescriber before giving bismuth subsalicylate to children or teenagers recovering from flu or chickenpox. Don't give kaolin and pectin mixtures to children under age 2.
• **Geriatric patients:** Use caution when administering antidiarrheal drugs, especially opium preparations.

NURSING CONSIDERATIONS

Assessment
• Assess patient's condition before therapy and regularly thereafter.
• Monitor fluid and electrolyte balance.
• Observe patient for adverse reactions.

Key nursing diagnoses
• Constipation related to adverse effect of bismuth preparations on GI tract
• Risk for injury related to adverse CNS reactions
• Risk for deficient fluid volume related to GI upset

Planning and implementation
• Administer drug exactly as prescribed.
• Take safety precautions if patient experiences adverse CNS reactions.
• Don't substitute opium tincture for paregoric.
• Notify prescriber about serious or persistent adverse reactions.

Patient teaching

• Instruct patient to take drug exactly as prescribed; caution him that excessive use of opium preparations can lead to dependence.
• Instruct patient to notify prescriber if diarrhea lasts for more than 2 days and to report adverse reactions.

• Warn patient to avoid hazardous activities that require alertness if CNS depression occurs.

Evaluation

• Patient doesn't develop constipation.
• Patient remains free from injury.
• Patient maintains adequate hydration.

Antihistamines

azatadine maleate
brompheniramine maleate
chlorpheniramine maleate
clemastine fumarate
cyclizine hydrochloride
cyclizine lactate
cyproheptadine hydrochloride
dimenhydrinate
diphenhydramine hydrochloride
fexofenadine hydrochloride
loratadine
meclizine hydrochloride
promethazine hydrochloride
promethazine theoclate
tripelennamine citrate
tripelennamine hydrochloride
triprolidine hydrochloride

Indications

▶ Rhinitis, urticaria, pruritus, vertigo, nausea and vomiting, sedation, dyskinesia, parkinsonism.

Actions

Antihistamines are structurally related chemicals that compete with histamine for histamine H_1-receptor sites on smooth muscle of bronchi, GI tract, uterus, and large blood vessels, binding to cellular receptors and preventing access to and subsequent activity of histamine. They don't directly alter histamine or prevent its release.

Adverse reactions

Most antihistamines cause drowsiness and impaired motor function early in therapy. They also can cause dry mouth and throat, blurred vision, and constipation. Some antihistamines, such as promethazine, may cause cholestatic jaundice (thought to be a hypersensitivity reaction) and may predispose patients to photosensitivity.

Contraindications and precautions

• Contraindicated in patients hypersensitive to drug and also in breast-feeding women.
• Use cautiously in patients with angle-closure glaucoma, stenosing peptic ulcer, pyloroduodenal obstruction, or bladder neck obstruction.
• **Breast-feeding patients:** Antihistamines should not be used during breast-feeding; many of these drugs appear in breast milk, exposing the infant to unusual excitability. Neonates, especially premature infants, may experience seizures.
• **Pediatric patients:** Children, especially those under age 6, may experience paradoxical hyperexcitability with restlessness, insomnia, nervousness, euphoria, tremors, and seizures. Administer cautiously.
• **Geriatric patients:** These patients usually are more sensitive to the adverse effects of antihistamines, especially dizziness, sedation, hypotension, and urine retention.

NURSING CONSIDERATIONS

Assessment

• Monitor patient for adverse reactions.
• Monitor blood counts during long-term therapy; watch for signs of blood dyscrasia.

Key nursing diagnoses

• Risk for injury related to sedation
• Impaired oral mucous membrane related to dry mouth
• Constipation related to anticholinergic effect of antihistamines

Planning and implementation

• Reduce GI distress by giving antihistamines with food.
• Provide sugarless gum, hard candy, or ice chips to relieve dry mouth.
• Increase fluid intake (if allowed) or humidify air to decrease adverse effect of thickened secretions.

Prototype drug

Patient teaching

- Advise patient to take drug with meals or snacks to prevent gastric upset.
- Suggest that patient use warm water rinses, artificial saliva, ice chips, or sugarless gum or candy to relieve dry mouth. Tell him to avoid overusing mouthwash, which may worsen dryness and destroy normal flora.
- Warn patient to avoid hazardous activities until full CNS effects of drug are known.
- Caution patient to seek medical approval before using alcohol, tranquilizers, sedatives, pain relievers, or sleeping medications.
- Advise patient to stop taking antihistamines 4 days before diagnostic skin tests to preserve accuracy of test results.

☑ Evaluation

- Patient sustains no injury from sedation.
- Patient maintains normal mucous membranes by using preventive measures throughout therapy.
- Patient regains normal bowel function.

Antihypertensives

ACE inhibitors
benazepril hydrochloride
captopril
enalaprilat
enalapril maleate
fosinopril sodium
lisinopril
moexipril hydrochloride
perindopril erbumine
quinapril hydrochloride
ramipril

Alpha-adrenergic blockers
doxazosin mesylate
phentolamine mesylate
prazosin hydrochloride
terazosin hydrochloride

Angiotension II receptor blockers
candesartan cilexetil
eprosartan mesylate
irbesartan
losartan potassium
telmisartan

Beta blockers
acebutolol
atenolol
betaxolol hydrochloride
carteolol hydrochloride
carvedilol
labetalol hydrochloride
metoprolol tartrate
nadolol
penbutolol sulfate
pindolol
propranolol hydrochloride
timolol maleate

Calcium channel blockers
amlodipine besylate
diltiazem hydrochloride
felodipine
isradipine
nicardipine hydrochloride
nifedipine
nisoldipine
verapamil hydrochloride

Centrally acting sympatholytics
clonidine hydrochloride
guanabenz acetate
guanfacine hydrochloride
methyldopa

Rauwolfia alkaloid
reserpine

Vasodilators
diazoxide
hydralazine hydrochloride
minoxidil
nitroprusside sodium

Indications

▶ Essential and secondary hypertension.

Actions

Antihypertensives reduce blood pressure through various mechanisms. For information on the action of ACE inhibitors, alpha blockers, angiotension II receptor blockers, beta blockers, calcium channel blockers, and diuretics, see their drug class entries. Centrally acting sympatholytics stimulate central alpha-adrenergic receptors, reducing cerebral sympathetic outflow, thereby decreasing peripheral vascular resistance and blood pressure. Rauwolfia alkaloids bind to and gradually destroy the norepinephrine-containing storage vesicles in central and peripheral adrenergic neurons. Vasodilators act directly on smooth muscle to reduce blood pressure.

Adverse reactions

Most antihypertensives commonly cause orthostatic hypotension, changes in heart rate, headache, nausea, and vomiting. Other reactions vary greatly among different drug types. Centrally acting sympatholytics may cause constipation, depression, dizziness, drowsiness, dry mouth, headache, palpitations, severe rebound hypertension, and sexual dysfunction; methyldopa may also cause aplastic anemia and thrombocytopenia. Rauwolfia alkaloids may cause anxiety, depression, drowsiness, dry mouth, hyperacidity, impotence, nasal stuffiness, and weight gain. Vasodilators may cause heart failure, ECG changes, diarrhea, dizziness, palpitations, pruritus, and rash.

Contraindications and precautions

- Contraindicated in patients hypersensitive to drug and in those with hypotension.
- Use cautiously in patients with hepatic or renal dysfunction.
- See individual drugs for complete listings of contraindications and precautions.
- **Breast-feeding patients:** Some antihypertensives appear in breast milk. Use cautiously, and see individual drugs for recommendations.
- **Pediatric patients:** Safety and efficacy of many antihypertensives haven't been established in children. Administer these drugs cautiously, and monitor patients closely.
- **Geriatric patients:** These patients are more prone to adverse reactions and may need lower maintenance doses. Monitor them closely.

NURSING CONSIDERATIONS

Assessment

- Obtain baseline blood pressure and pulse rate and rhythm; recheck regularly.
- Monitor patient for adverse reactions.
- Monitor patient's weight and fluid and electrolyte status.
- Monitor patient's compliance with treatment.

Key nursing diagnoses

- Risk for trauma related to orthostatic hypotension
- Risk for deficient fluid volume related to GI upset
- Noncompliance related to long-term therapy or adverse reactions

Planning and implementation

- Administer drug with food or at bedtime, as indicated.
- Follow manufacturer's guidelines when mixing and administering parenteral drugs.
- Take steps to prevent or minimize orthostatic hypotension.
- Maintain patient's nonpharmacologic therapy, such as sodium restriction, calorie reduction, stress management, and exercise program.

Patient teaching

- Instruct patient to take drug exactly as prescribed. Warn him not to stop drug abruptly.
- Review adverse reactions caused by drug, and urge patient to notify prescriber of serious or persistent reactions.
- Advise patient to avoid sudden changes in position to prevent dizziness, light-headedness, or fainting.
- Caution patient to avoid hazardous activities until full effects of drug are known. Also, warn patient to avoid physical exertion, especially in hot weather.
- Advise patient to consult prescriber before taking any OTC medications or herbal remedies; serious drug interactions can occur.
- Encourage patient to comply with therapy.

Evaluation

- Patient sustains no trauma from orthostatic hypotension.
- Patient maintains adequate hydration.
- Patient complies with therapy, as evidenced by normal blood pressure.

Antilipemics

atorvastatin calcium
cerivastatin sodium
cholestyramine
clofibrate
colestipol hydrochloride
fenofibrate
fluvastatin sodium
gemfibrozil
lovastatin
pravastatin sodium
simvastatin

Indications

▶ Hyperlipidemia, hypercholesterolemia.

Actions

Antilipemics lower elevated blood levels of lipids. Bile-sequestering drugs (cholestyramine, colestipol) lower blood levels of low-density lipoproteins by forming insoluble complexes with bile salts, triggering cholesterol to leave the bloodstream and other storage areas to make new bile acids. Fibric acid derivatives (clofibrate, gemfibrozil) reduce cholesterol formation, increase sterol excretion, and decrease lipoprotein and triglyceride synthesis. Cholesterol synthesis inhibitors (fluvastatin, lovastatin, pravastatin, simvastatin) interfere with enzymatic activity that generates cholesterol in the liver.

Adverse reactions

Antilipemics commonly cause GI upset. Bile-sequestering drugs may cause cholelithiasis, constipation, bloating, and steatorrhea. Fibric acid derivatives may cause cholelithiasis and GI or CNS effects. Use of gemfibrozil with lovastatin may cause myopathy. Cholesterol synthesis inhibitors may affect liver function or cause rash, pruritus, increased CK levels, and myopathy.

Contraindications and precautions

• Contraindicated in patients hypersensitive to drug. Also, bile-sequestering drugs are contraindicated in patients with complete biliary obstruction. Fibric acid derivatives are contraindicated in breast-feeding women and in patients with primary biliary cirrhosis or significant hepatic or renal dysfunction. Cholesterol synthesis inhibitors are contraindicated in patients with active liver disease or persistently elevated serum transaminase levels and in pregnant or breast-feeding women.

• Use bile-sequestering drugs cautiously in constipated patients. Use fibric acid derivatives cautiously in patients with peptic ulcer. Use cholesterol synthesis inhibitors cautiously in patients who consume large amounts of alcohol or who have a history of liver disease.

• **Pregnant patients:** Use bile-sequestering drugs and fibric acid derivatives cautiously in pregnant patients.

• **Breast-feeding patients:** Avoid giving fibric acid derivatives and cholesterol synthesis inhibitors to breast-feeding women; give bile-sequestering drugs cautiously.

• **Pediatric patients:** Safety of antilipemic drugs hasn't been established in children.

• **Geriatric patients:** These patients have an increased risk of severe constipation. Use bile-sequestering drugs cautiously, and monitor patients closely.

NURSING CONSIDERATIONS

Assessment

• Monitor blood cholesterol and lipid levels before and periodically during therapy.
• Monitor CK levels when therapy begins and every 6 months thereafter. Also, check CK levels if a paient who takes a cholesterol synthesis inhibitor complains of muscle pain.
• Monitor patient for adverse reactions.

Key nursing diagnoses

• Risk for deficient fluid volume related to adverse GI reactions
• Constipation related to adverse effect on bowel
• Noncompliance related to long-term therapy

Planning and implementation

• Mix powder form of bile-sequestering drugs with 120 to 180 ml of liquid. Never administer dry powder alone because patient may inhale it accidentally.

• Administer daily fibric acid derivative at prescribed times.
• Give lovastatin with evening meal, simvastatin in the evening, and fluvastatin and pravastatin at bedtime.

Patient teaching
• Instruct patient to take his drug exactly as prescribed. If he takes a bile-sequestering drug, warn him never to take the dry form.
• Stress importance of diet in controlling serum lipid levels.
• Advise patient to drink 2 to 3 L of fluid daily and to report persistent or severe constipation.

Evaluation
• Patient maintains adequate fluid volume.
• Patient doesn't experience severe or persistent constipation.
• Patient complies with therapy, as evidenced by normal serum lipid and cholesterol levels.

Antimetabolite antineoplastics

capecitabine
cytarabine
floxuridine
fludarabine phosphate
fluorouracil
hydroxyurea
mercaptopurine
methotrexate
thioguanine

Indications

▶ Treatment of various tumors. See individual drugs for specific uses.

Actions

Antimetabolites are structural analogues of normally occurring metabolites and can be divided into three subcategories: purine analogues, pyrimidine analogues, and folinic acid analogues. Most of these drugs interrupt cell reproduction at a specific phase of the cell cycle. Purine analogues are incorporated into DNA and RNA, interfering with nucleic acid synthesis (via miscoding) and replication. They also may inhibit synthesis of purine bases through pseudo-feedback mechanisms. Pyrimidine analogues inhibit enzymes in metabolic pathways that interfere with biosynthesis of uridine and thymine. Folic acid antagonists prevent conversion of folic acid to tetrahydrofolate by inhibiting the enzyme dihydrofolic acid reductase.

Adverse reactions

The most common adverse effects include nausea, vomiting, diarrhea, fever, chills, hair loss, flank or joint pain, redness or pain at injection site, anxiety, bone marrow depression, leukopenia, and swelling of the feet or lower legs.

Contraindications and precautions

• Contraindicated in patients hypersensitive to drug.
• See individual drugs for complete listings of contraindications and precautions.
• **Pregnant patients:** Pregnant patients should be informed of the risks to the fetus.
• **Breast-feeding patients:** Breast-feeding is contraindicated in women receiving chemotherapy drugs, including antimetabolite antineoplastics.
• **Pediatric patients:** Safety and efficacy of some drugs haven't been established in children. See individual drugs for specific guidelines.
• **Geriatric patients:** These patients have an increased risk of adverse reactions. Monitor them closely.

NURSING CONSIDERATIONS

Assessment
• Perform a complete assessment before therapy begins.
• Monitor patient for adverse reactions.
• Monitor vital signs and patency of catheter or I.V. line throughout administration.
• Monitor BUN, hematocrit, platelet count, ALT, AST, LD, serum bilirubin, serum creatinine, uric acid, total and differential leukocyte, and other values as required.

Key nursing diagnoses
• Ineffective protection related to thrombocytopenia

- Risk for infection related to immunosuppression
- Risk for deficient fluid volume related to adverse GI effects

Planning and implementation
- Follow established procedures for safe and proper handling, administration, and disposal of drugs.
- Try to alleviate or reduce anxiety in the patient and family before treatment.
- Give an antiemetic before administering drug, as ordered, to lessen nausea.
- Administer cytarabine with allopurinol, as ordered, to decrease the risk of hyperuricemia. Promote a high fluid intake.
- Provide diligent mouth care to prevent stomatitis with cytarabine, fluorouracil, or methotrexate therapy.
- Anticipate the need for leucovorin rescue with high-dose methotrexate therapy.
- Treat extravasation promptly.
- Have patient defer immunizations if possible until hematologic stability is confirmed.
- Anticipate diarrhea, possibly severe, with prolonged fluorouracil therapy.

Patient teaching
- Teach patient proper oral hygiene, including cautious use of toothbrush, dental floss, and toothpicks. Chemotherapy can increase the risk of microbial infection, delayed healing, and bleeding gums.
- Advise patient to complete dental work before therapy begins or to delay it until blood counts are normal.
- Warn patient that he may bruise easily because of drug's effect on platelets.
- Advise patient to avoid close contact with persons who have taken oral poliovirus vaccine and to avoid exposure to persons with bacterial or viral infection because chemotherapy may increase susceptibility. Urge patient to notify prescriber promptly if he develops signs or symptoms of infection.
- Instruct patient to report redness, pain, or swelling at injection site. Local tissue injury and scarring may result from tissue infiltration at infusion site.

Evaluation
- Patient develops no serious bleeding complications.
- Patient remains free from infection.
- Patient maintains adequate hydration.

Antiparkinsonians
amantadine hydrochloride
benztropine mesylate
biperiden hydrochloride
biperiden lactate
bromocriptine mesylate
entacapone
levodopa-carbidopa
levodopa
pergolide mesylate
pramipexole dihydrochloride
ropinirole hydrochloride
selegiline hydrochloride
tolcapone
trihexyphenidyl hydrochloride

Indications
▶ Parkinson's disease.

Actions
Antiparkinsonians include synthetic anticholinergic and dopaminergic drugs and the antiviral drug amantadine. Anticholinergics probably prolong the action of dopamine by blocking its reuptake into presynaptic neurons in the CNS and by suppressing central cholinergic activity. Dopaminergic drugs act in the brain by increasing dopamine availability, thus improving motor function. Entacapone is a reversible inhibitor of peripheral catechol-o-methyl-transferase, which is responsible for elimination of various catecholamines, including dopamine. Blocking this pathway when administering levodopa-carbidopa should result in higher serum levels of levodopa, thereby allowing greater dopaminergic stimulation in the CNS and leading to a greater clinical effect in treating parkinsonian symptoms. Amantadine is thought to increase dopamine release in the substantia nigra.

Prototype drug

Adverse reactions

Anticholinergic drugs typically cause decreased sweating or anhidrosis, dry mouth, headache, mydriasis, blurred vision, cycloplegia, urinary hesitancy and urine retention, constipation, palpitations, and tachycardia. Dopaminergic drugs may cause vomiting, orthostatic hypotension, confusion, arrhythmias, and disturbing dreams. Amantadine commonly causes irritability, insomnia, and livedo reticularis (with prolonged use).

Contraindications and precautions

- Contraindicated in patients hypersensitive to drug.
- Use cautiously in patients with prostatic hyperplasia or tardive dyskinesia and in elderly or debilitated patients.
- See individual drugs for complete listings of contraindications and precautions.
- **Breast-feeding patients:** Antiparkinsonians may appear in breast milk; avoid using in breast-feeding women.
- **Pediatric patients:** Safety and efficacy haven't been established in children.
- **Geriatric patients:** These patients have an increased risk for adverse reactions. Monitor them closely.

NURSING CONSIDERATIONS

Assessment

- Obtain baseline assessment of patient's impairment, and reassess regularly to monitor drug effectiveness.
- Monitor patient for adverse reactions.
- Monitor vital signs, especially during dosage adjustments.

Key nursing diagnoses

- Risk for injury related to adverse CNS effects
- Urine retention related to anticholinergic effect on bladder
- Disturbed sleep pattern related to amantadine-induced insomnia

Planning and implementation

- Administer drug with food to prevent GI irritation.
- Adjust dosage, as ordered, according to patient's response and tolerance.
- Never withdraw drug abruptly.
- Institute safety precautions.
- Provide ice chips, drinks, or hard sugarless candy to relieve dry mouth. Increase fluid and fiber intake to prevent constipation, as appropriate.
- Notify prescriber about urine retention, and be prepared to catheterize patient.

Patient teaching

- Instruct patient to take drug exactly as prescribed, and warn him not to stop drug suddenly.
- Advise patient to take drug with food to prevent GI upset.
- Teach patient how to manage anticholinergic effects, if appropriate.
- Caution patient to avoid hazardous tasks if adverse CNS effects occur. Tell him to avoid alcohol during therapy.
- Encourage patient to report severe or persistent adverse reactions.

Evaluation

- Patient remains free from injury.
- Patient has no change in voiding pattern.
- Patient's sleep pattern isn't altered during amantadine therapy.

Antivirals

abacavir sulfate
acyclovir sodium
amantadine hydrochloride
amprenavir
cidofovir
delavirdine mesylate
didanosine
efavirenz
famciclovir
foscarnet sodium
ganciclovir
indinavir sulfate
lamivudine
lamivudine/zidovudine
nelfinavir mesylate

nevirapine
oseltamivir phosphate
ribavirin
rimantadine hydrochloride
ritonavir
saquinavir mesylate
stavudine
valacyclovir hydrochloride
zalcitabine
zanamivir
zidovudine

Indications

▶ Viral infections.

Actions

Acyclovir, cidofovir, didanosine, famciclovir, ganciclovir, valacyclovir, and zalcitabine interfere with DNA synthesis and replication. Amantadine prevents the release of infectious viral nucleic acid into the host cell and possibly interferes with viral penetration into the cells. Foscarnet blocks the pyrophosphate binding site. Ribavirin's mechanism of action is unknown. Rimantadine prevents viral uncoating. Abacavir, amprenavir, indinavir, ritonavir, saquinavir, and stavudine inhibit the activity of HIV protease. Delavirdine, efavirenz, lamivudine, nevirapine, and zidovudine inhibit reverse transcriptase.

Adverse reactions

Antiviral drugs may cause anorexia, chills, confusion, depression, diarrhea, dry mouth, edema, fatigue, hallucinations, headache, nausea, and vomiting. See individual drugs for complete listings of adverse reactions.

Contraindications and precautions

- Contraindicated in patients hypersensitive to drug.
- See individual drugs for complete listings of contraindications and precautions.
- **Breast-feeding patients:** Some antiviral drugs are contraindicated in breast-feeding women; others require cautious use. See individual drugs for specific guidelines.
- **Pediatric patients:** Recommendations vary with the antiviral prescribed. See individual drugs for specific guidelines for use in infants and children.
- **Geriatric patients:** These patients have an increased risk of adverse reactions. Monitor them closely.

NURSING CONSIDERATIONS

Assessment

- Obtain baseline assessment of patient's viral infection, and reassess regularly to monitor drug's effectiveness.
- Monitor renal and hepatic function, CBC, and platelet count regularly. Monitor electrolytes (calcium, phosphate, magnesium, potassium) in patients receiving foscarnet.
- Inspect patient's I.V. site regularly for signs of irritation, phlebitis, inflammation, or extravasation.
- If patient has a history of heart failure, watch closely for exacerbation or recurrence of the condition during amantadine therapy.
- Monitor patient's cardiac status during ribavirin therapy.

Key nursing diagnoses

- Ineffective protection related to adverse hematologic reactions
- Risk for deficient fluid volume related to GI upset
- Noncompliance related to long-term therapy

Planning and implementation

- Adjust dosage of selected antiviral drugs, as ordered, for patient with decreased renal function, especially during parenteral therapy.
- Follow manufacturer's guidelines for reconstituting and administering antiviral drugs.
- Obtain an order for an antiemetic or antidiarrheal drug, if needed.
- Take safety precautions if patient has adverse CNS reactions. For example, place bed in low position, raise bed rails, and supervise ambulation and other activities.
- Notify prescriber about serious or persistent adverse reactions.

Patient teaching

- Instruct patient to take drug exactly as prescribed, even if he feels better.

• Urge patient to notify prescriber promptly about severe or persistent adverse reactions.
• Encourage patient to keep appointments for follow-up care.
• Provide additional teaching as indicated by individual drug.

Evaluation

• Patient has no serious adverse hematologic effects.
• Patient maintains adequate hydration.
• Patient complies with therapy, and viral infection is eradicated.

Barbiturates

amobarbital
amobarbital sodium
pentobarbital sodium
phenobarbital
phenobarbital sodium
primidone
secobarbital sodium

Indications

▶ Insomnia, seizure disorders.

Actions

Barbiturates act throughout the CNS, particularly in the mesencephalic reticular activating system, which controls the CNS arousal mechanism. These drugs decrease presynaptic and postsynaptic membrane excitability, exerting their effects by facilitating the actions of gamma-aminobutyric acid. Barbiturates also exert a central effect, which depresses respiration and GI motility. The main mechanisms of anticonvulsant action are reduction of nerve transmission and decreased excitability of the nerve cell. Barbiturates also raise the seizure threshold.

Adverse reactions

Drowsiness, lethargy, vertigo, headache, and CNS depression are common with barbiturates. After hypnotic doses, a hangover effect, subtle distortion of mood, and impaired judgment and motor skills may continue for many hours. After dosage reduction or discontinuation, rebound insomnia or increased dreaming or nightmares may occur. Barbiturates cause hyperalgesia in subhypnotic doses. They also can cause paradoxical excitement at low doses, confusion in elderly patients, and hyperactivity in children. High fever, severe headache, stomatitis, conjunctivitis, or rhinitis may precede potentially fatal skin eruptions. Withdrawal symptoms may occur after as little as 2 weeks of uninterrupted therapy.

Contraindications and precautions

• Contraindicated in patients hypersensitive to drug and in those with bronchopneumonia or other severe pulmonary insufficiency.
• Use cautiously in patients with blood pressure alterations, pulmonary disease, or CV dysfunction.
• **Pregnant patients:** Use of barbiturates during pregnancy can cause fetal abnormalities. Avoid use.
• **Breast-feeding patients:** Barbiturates appear in breast milk and may result in infant CNS depression. Use cautiously.
• **Pediatric patients:** Premature infants are more susceptible to depressant effects of barbiturates because of their immature hepatic metabolism. Children may experience hyperactivity, excitement, or hyperalgesia.
• **Geriatric patients:** These patients may experience hyperactivity, excitement, or hyperalgesia. Use cautiously.

NURSING CONSIDERATIONS

Assessment

• Assess patient's level of consciousness and sleeping patterns before and during therapy to evaluate drug effectiveness. Monitor neurologic status for alteration or deterioration.
• Assess vital signs frequently, especially during I.V. administration.
• Monitor seizure character, frequency, and duration for changes, as indicated.
• Observe patient to prevent hoarding or self-dosing, especially if patient is depressed, suicidal, or drug dependent.

Key nursing diagnoses
- Risk for injury related to sedation
- Disturbed thought processes related to confusion
- Impaired adjustment related to drug dependence

Planning and implementation
- When administering parenteral drug, avoid extravasation, which may cause local tissue damage and tissue necrosis; inject I.V. or deep I.M. only. Don't exceed 5 ml in any I.M. injection site to avoid tissue damage.
- Keep resuscitative measures available. Too rapid I.V. administration may cause respiratory depression, apnea, laryngospasm, or hypotension.
- Take seizure precautions, as necessary.
- Institute safety measures to prevent falls and injury. Raise side rails, assist patient out of bed, and keep call light within easy reach.
- Stop drug slowly, as ordered. Abrupt discontinuation may cause withdrawal symptoms.

Patient teaching
- Explain that barbiturates can cause physical or psychological dependence.
- Instruct patient to take drug exactly as prescribed. Caution him not to change the dosage or take other drugs, including OTC medications or herbal remedies, without prescriber's approval.
- Reassure patient that a morning hangover is common after therapeutic use of barbiturates.
- Advise patient to avoid hazardous tasks, and review other safety measures to prevent injury.
- Instruct patient to report skin eruption or other significant adverse effects.

Evaluation
- Patient sustains no injury from sedation.
- Patient maintains normal thought processes.
- Patient doesn't develop physical or psychological dependence.

Beta blockers

$Beta_1$ blockers

acebutolol
atenolol
betaxolol hydrochloride
bisoprolol fumarate
esmolol hydrochloride
metoprolol tartrate

$Beta_1$ and $beta_2$ blockers

carteolol hydrochloride
carvedilol
labetalol hydrochloride
nadolol
penbutolol sulfate
pindolol
propranolol hydrochloride
sotalol hydrochloride
timolol maleate

Indications
▶ Hypertension (most drugs), angina pectoris (propranolol, atenolol, nadolol, and metoprolol), arrhythmias (propranolol, acebutolol, sotalol, and esmolol), glaucoma (betaxolol and timolol), prevention of MI (timolol, propranolol, atenolol, and metoprolol), prevention of recurrent migraine and other vascular headaches (propranolol and timolol), pheochromocytomas or essential tremors (selected drugs).

Actions
Beta blockers are chemicals that compete with beta agonists for available beta-receptor sites; individual drugs differ in their ability to affect beta receptors. Some drugs are considered nonselective; that is, they block $beta_1$ receptors in cardiac muscle and $beta_2$ receptors in bronchial and vascular smooth muscle. Several drugs are cardioselective and in lower doses primarily inhibit $beta_1$ receptors. Some beta blockers have intrinsic sympathomimetic activity and stimulate and block beta receptors, decreasing cardiac output; still others also have membrane-stabilizing activity, which affects cardiac action potential.

Adverse reactions

Therapeutic doses may cause bradycardia, fatigue, and dizziness; some may cause other CNS disturbances, such as nightmares, depression, memory loss, and hallucinations. Toxic doses can produce severe hypotension, bradycardia, heart failure, or bronchospasm.

Contraindications and precautions

- Contraindicated in patients hypersensitive to drug and in patients with cardiogenic shock, sinus bradycardia, heart block greater than first degree, bronchial asthma, and heart failure unless failure is caused by tachyarrhythmia treatable with propranolol.
- Use cautiously in patients with nonallergic bronchospastic disorders, diabetes mellitus, or impaired hepatic or renal function.
- **Pregnant patients:** Use cautiously in pregnant patients.
- **Breast-feeding patients:** Beta blockers appear in breast milk. See individual drugs for specific recommendations.
- **Pediatric patients:** Safety and efficacy of beta blockers haven't been established in children; use only if benefit outweighs risk.
- **Geriatric patients:** These patients may need reduced maintenance doses because of increased bioavailability or delayed metabolism; they also may have increased adverse effects.

NURSING CONSIDERATIONS

Assessment

- Check apical pulse rate daily; alert prescriber about extremes (a pulse rate below 60 beats/minute, for example).
- Monitor blood pressure, ECG, and heart rate and rhythm frequently; be alert for progression of AV block or bradycardia.
- If patient has heart failure, weigh him regularly; watch for weight gain of more than 2.25 kg (5 lb) per week.
- Observe diabetic patients for sweating, fatigue, and hunger. Signs of hypoglycemic shock are masked.

Key nursing diagnoses

- Risk for injury related to adverse CNS effects
- Excessive fluid volume related to edema
- Decreased cardiac output related to bradycardia or hypotension

Planning and implementation

- Discontinue a beta blocker, as ordered, before surgery for pheochromocytoma. Before any surgical procedure, notify anesthesiologist that patient is taking a beta blocker.
- Keep glucagon nearby in case prescriber prescribes it to reverse beta blocker overdose.

Patient teaching

- Teach patient to take drug exactly as prescribed, even when he feels better.
- Warn patient not to stop drug suddenly. Abrupt discontinuation can worsen angina or precipitate MI.
- Tell patient not to take OTC cold medications or herbal remedies without medical consent.
- Explain potential adverse reactions, and stress the importance of reporting unusual effects.

Evaluation

- Patient remains free from injury.
- Patient has no signs of edema.
- Patient maintains normal blood pressure and heart rate.

Calcium channel blockers

amlodipine besylate
bepridil hydrochloride
diltiazem hydrochloride
felodipine
isradipine
nicardipine hydrochloride
nifedipine
nimodipine
nisoldipine
verapamil hydrochloride

Indications

▶ Prinzmetal's variant angina, chronic stable angina, unstable angina, mild to moderate hypertension, arrhythmias.

Actions

The main physiologic action of calcium channel blockers is to inhibit calcium influx across the slow channels of myocardial and vascular smooth muscle cells. By inhibiting calcium influx into these cells, calcium channel blockers reduce intracellular calcium concentrations. This, in turn, dilates coronary arteries, peripheral arteries, and arterioles and slows cardiac conduction.

When used to treat Prinzmetal's variant angina, calcium channel blockers inhibit coronary spasm, increasing oxygen delivery to the heart. Peripheral artery dilation decreases total peripheral resistance which reduces afterload, which, in turn, decreases myocardial oxygen consumption. Inhibiting calcium influx into the specialized cardiac conduction cells (specifically, those in the SA and AV nodes) slows conduction through the heart. Of the calcium channel blockers, verapamil and diltiazem have the greatest effect on the AV node, slowing the ventricular rate in atrial fibrillation or flutter and converting supraventricular tachycardia to normal sinus rhythm.

Adverse reactions

Adverse reactions vary with the drug used. Verapamil, for instance, may cause bradycardia, various degrees of heart block, worsening of heart failure, and hypotension after rapid I.V. administration. Prolonged oral verapamil therapy may cause constipation. Nifedipine may cause hypotension, peripheral edema, flushing, light-headedness, and headache. Diltiazem most commonly causes anorexia and nausea and may also induce various degrees of heart block, bradycardia, heart failure, and peripheral edema.

Contraindications and precautions

- Contraindicated in patients hypersensitive to drug.
- **Pregnant patients:** Use cautiously in pregnant women.
- **Breast-feeding patients:** Calcium channel blockers may appear in breast milk. To avoid possible adverse effects in infants, breast-feeding should be discontinued during therapy.
- **Pediatric patients:** Adverse hemodynamic effects of parenteral verapamil have been observed in neonates and infants. Safety and efficacy of other calcium channel blockers haven't been established.
- **Geriatric patients:** The half-life of calcium channel blockers may be increased in elderly patients as a result of decreased clearance. Use cautiously.

NURSING CONSIDERATIONS

Assessment

- Monitor cardiac rate and rhythm and blood pressure carefully when therapy starts or dosage increases.
- Monitor fluid and electrolyte status.
- Monitor patient for adverse reactions.

Key nursing diagnoses

- Decreased cardiac output related to adverse CV reactions
- Constipation related to oral verapamil therapy
- Noncompliance related to long-term therapy

Planning and implementation

- Don't give calcium supplements while patient takes a calcium channel blocker; they may decrease the drug's effectiveness.
- Expect to decrease dosage gradually; don't stop calcium channel blockers abruptly.

Patient teaching

- Teach patient to take drug exactly as prescribed, even if he feels better.
- Instruct patient to take a missed dose as soon as possible, unless it's almost time for his next dose. Warn him never to take a double dose.
- Caution patient not to stop drug suddenly; abrupt discontinuation can produce serious adverse effects.
- Urge patient to report irregular heartbeat, shortness of breath, swelling of hands and feet, pronounced dizziness, constipation, nausea, or hypotension.

Evaluation

- Patient maintains adequate cardiac output throughout therapy, as evidenced by normal blood pressure and pulse rate.
- Patient regains normal bowel pattern.
- Patient complies with therapy, as evidenced by absence of symptoms related to underlying disorder.

Cephalosporins

First generation
cefadroxil monohydrate
cefazolin sodium
cephalexin monohydrate
cephradine
Second generation
cefaclor
cefmetazole sodium
cefonicid sodium
cefotetan disodium
cefoxitin sodium
cefprozil
cefuroxime axetil
cefuroxime sodium
loracarbef
Third generation
cefixime
cefdinir
cefepime hydrochloride
cefoperazone sodium
cefotaxime sodium
cefpodoxime proxetil
ceftazidime
ceftibuten
ceftizoxime sodium
ceftriaxone sodium

Indications

▶ Infections of the lungs, skin, soft tissue, bones, joints, urinary and respiratory tracts, blood, abdomen, and heart; CNS infections caused by susceptible strains of *Neisseria meningitidis, Haemophilus influenzae,* and *Streptococcus pneumoniae;* meningitis caused by *Escherichia coli* or *Klebsiella;* infections that develop after surgical procedures classified as contaminated or potentially contaminated; penicillinase-producing *N. gonorrhoeae;* otitis media and ampicillin-resistant middle ear infection caused by *H. influenzae.*

Actions

Cephalosporins are chemically and pharmacologically similar to penicillin; they act by inhibiting bacterial cell wall synthesis, causing rapid cell lysis. Their sites of action are enzymes known as penicillin-binding proteins. The affinity of certain cephalosporins for these proteins in various microorganisms helps explain the differing spectra of activity in this class of antibiotics. Cephalosporins are bactericidal; they act against many aerobic gram-positive and gram-negative bacteria and some anaerobic bacteria; they don't kill fungi or viruses.

First-generation cephalosporins act against many gram-positive cocci, including penicillinase-producing *Staphylococcus aureus* and *S. epidermidis; S. pneumoniae,* group B streptococci, and group A beta-hemolytic streptococci; susceptible gram-negative organisms include *Klebsiella pneumoniae, E. coli, Proteus mirabilis,* and *Shigella.*

Second-generation cephalosporins are effective against all organisms attacked by first-generation drugs and have additional activity against *Moraxella catarrhalis, H. influenzae, Enterobacter, Citrobacter, Providencia, Acinetobacter, Serratia,* and *Neisseria. Bacteroides fragilis* is susceptible to cefotetan and cefoxitin.

Third-generation cephalosporins are less active than first- and second-generation drugs against gram-positive bacteria, but more active against gram-negative organisms, including those resistant to first- and second-generation drugs; they have the greatest stability against beta-lactamases produced by gram-negative bacteria. Susceptible gram-negative organisms include *E. coli, Klebsiella, Enterobacter, Providencia, Acinetobacter, Serratia, Proteus, Morganella,* and *Neisseria;* some third-generation drugs are active against *B. fragilis* and *Pseudomonas.*

Adverse reactions

Many cephalosporins share a similar profile of adverse effects. Hypersensitivity reactions range from mild rashes, fever, and eosinophilia to fatal anaphylaxis and are more common in patients with penicillin allergy. Hematologic reactions include positive direct and indirect antiglobulin (Coombs' test), thrombocytopenia or thrombocythemia, transient neutropenia, and reversible leukopenia. Adverse renal effects may occur with any cephalosporin; they are most common in older patients, those with decreased renal function, and those taking oth-

Prototype drug

er nephrotoxic drugs. Adverse GI reactions include nausea, vomiting, diarrhea, abdominal pain, glossitis, dyspepsia, and tenesmus; minimal elevation of liver function test results occurs occasionally.

Local venous pain and irritation are common after I.M. injection; such reactions occur more often with higher doses and long-term therapy. Disulfiram-type reactions occur when cefoperazone or cefotetan are administered within 72 hours of alcohol ingestion. Bacterial and fungal superinfections result from suppression of normal flora.

Contraindications and precautions

- Contraindicated in patients hypersensitive to drug.
- Use cautiously in patients with renal or hepatic impairment, history of GI disease, or allergy to penicillins.
- **Breast-feeding patients:** Cephalosporins appear in breast milk; use cautiously in breast-feeding women.
- **Pediatric patients:** Serum half-life is prolonged in neonates and infants.
- **Geriatric patients:** These patients are susceptible to superinfection and coagulopathies. They commonly have renal impairment and may need a lower dosage. Use cautiously.

NURSING CONSIDERATIONS

Assessment

- Review patient's history of allergies. Try to determine whether previous reactions were true hypersensitivity reactions or merely adverse effects (such as GI distress) that patient has interpreted as allergy.
- Monitor patient continuously for possible hypersensitivity reactions or other untoward effects.
- Obtain culture and sensitivity specimen before administering first dose; check test results periodically to assess drug effectiveness.
- Monitor renal function studies; dosages of certain cephalosporins must be lowered in patients with severe renal impairment. In decreased renal function, monitor BUN levels, serum creatinine levels, and urine output for significant changes.
- Monitor PT and platelet counts and assess patient for signs of hypoprothrombinemia, which may occur (with or without bleeding) during therapy with cefoperazone, cefonicid, or cefotetan. It usually occurs in elderly, debilitated, or malnourished patients.
- Monitor patients on long-term therapy for possible bacterial and fungal superinfection, especially elderly and debilitated patients and those receiving immunosuppressants or radiation therapy.
- Monitor susceptible patients receiving sodium salts of cephalosporins for possible fluid retention. (Consult individual drug entry for sodium content.)

Key nursing diagnoses

- Ineffective protection related to hypersensitivity
- Risk for infection related to superinfection
- Risk for deficient fluid volume related to adverse GI reactions

Planning and implementation

- Administer cephalosporins at least 1 hour before bacteriostatic antibiotics (tetracyclines, erythromycins, and chloramphenicol); the latter drugs inhibit bacterial cell growth, decreasing cephalosporin uptake by bacterial cell walls.
- Refrigerate oral suspensions (stable for 14 days); shake well before administering to ensure correct dosage.
- Follow manufacturer's directions for reconstitution, dilution, and storage of drugs; check expiration dates.
- Administer I.M. dose deep into large muscle mass (gluteal or midlateral thigh); rotate injection sites to minimize tissue injury.
- Don't add or mix other drugs with I.V. infusions, particularly aminoglycosides, which will be inactivated if mixed with cephalosporins; if other drugs must be given I.V., temporarily stop infusion of primary drug.
- Ensure adequate dilution of I.V. infusion and rotate site every 48 hours to help minimize local vein irritation; using a small-gauge needle in a larger available vein may be helpful.

Patient teaching

- Make sure patient understands how and when to take drug. Urge him to comply with instructions for around-the-clock dosage and to complete the prescribed regimen.
- Advise patient to take oral drug with food if GI irritation occurs.
- Review proper storage and disposal of drug, and remind him to check drug's expiration date.
- Teach signs and symptoms of hypersensitivity and other adverse reactions, and emphasize importance of reporting unusual effects.
- Teach signs and symptoms of bacterial and fungal superinfection, especially if patient is elderly or debilitated or has low resistance from immunosuppressants or irradiation; emphasize importance of reporting signs and symptoms promptly.
- Warn patient not to ingest alcohol in any form within 72 hours of treatment with cefoperazone or cefotetan.
- Advise patient to add yogurt or buttermilk to diet to prevent intestinal superinfection resulting from suppression of normal intestinal flora.
- Advise diabetic patient to monitor urine glucose level with Diastix and not to use Clinitest.
- Urge patient to keep follow-up appointments.

Evaluation

- Patient has no evidence of hypersensitivity.
- Patient is free from infection.
- Patient maintains adequate hydration.

Corticosteroids

betamethasone
betamethasone sodium phosphate
cortisone acetate
dexamethasone
dexamethasone acetate
dexamethasone sodium phosphate
fludrocortisone acetate
hydrocortisone
hydrocortisone acetate
hydrocortisone cypionate
hydrocortisone sodium phosphate
hydrocortisone sodium succinate
methylprednisolone
methylprednisolone acetate
methylprednisolone sodium succinate
prednisolone
prednisolone acetate
prednisolone sodium phosphate
prednisolone steaglate
prednisolone tebutate
prednisone
triamcinolone
triamcinolone acetonide
triamcinolone diacetate
triamcinolone hexacetonide

Indications

▶ Hypersensitivity; inflammation, particularly of eye, nose, and respiratory tract; induction of immunosuppression; replacement therapy in adrenocortical insufficiency.

Actions

Corticosteroids suppress cell-mediated and humoral immunity by reducing levels of leukocytes, monocytes, and eosinophils; decreasing immunoglobulin binding to cell-surface receptors; and inhibiting interleukin synthesis. They reduce inflammation by preventing hydrolytic enzyme release into the cells, preventing plasma exudation, suppressing polymorphonuclear leukocyte migration, and disrupting other inflammatory processes.

Adverse reactions

Systemic corticosteroid therapy may suppress the hypothalamic-pituitary-adrenal (HPA) axis. Excessive use may cause cushingoid symptoms and various systemic disorders, such as diabetes and osteoporosis. Other effects may include euphoria, insomnia, edema, hypertension, peptic ulcer, increased appetite, fluid and electrolyte imbalances, dermatologic disorders, and immunosuppression.

Contraindications and precautions

- Contraindicated in patients with systemic fungal infection or hypersensitivity to drug or its components.
- Use cautiously in patients with GI ulceration, renal disease, hypertension, osteoporosis, varicella, vaccinia, exanthema, diabetes mellitus, hypothyroidism, thromboembolic disor-

der, seizures, myasthenia gravis, heart failure, tuberculosis, ocular herpes simplex, hypoalbuminemia, emotional instability, or psychosis.

- **Pregnant patients:** Avoid use, if possible, because of risk to fetus.
- **Breast-feeding patients:** Corticosteroids appear in breast milk and could cause serious adverse effects in infants. Women who need corticosteroid therapy should stop breast-feeding.
- **Pediatric patients:** Long-term use should be avoided, if possible, because stunted growth may result.
- **Geriatric patients:** These patients may have an increased risk of adverse reactions. Monitor them closely.

NURSING CONSIDERATIONS

Assessment

- Establish baseline blood pressure, fluid and electrolyte status, and weight; reassess regularly.
- Monitor patient closely for adverse reactions.
- Evaluate drug effectiveness at regular intervals.

Key nursing diagnoses

- Ineffective protection related to suppression of HPA axis with long-term therapy
- Risk for injury related to severe adverse reactions
- Risk for infection related to immunosuppression

Planning and implementation

- Administer drug early in the day to mimic circadian rhythm.
- Give drug with food to prevent GI irritation.
- Take precautions to avoid exposing patient to infection.
- Don't stop drug abruptly.
- Notify prescriber of severe or persistent adverse reactions.

Patient teaching

- Teach patient to take drug exactly as prescribed, and warn him never to stop the drug suddenly.
- Tell patient to notify prescriber if stress level increases; dosage may need to be temporarily increased.
- Instruct patient to take oral drug with food.
- Urge patient to report black tarry stools, bleeding, bruising, blurred vision, emotional changes, or other unusual effects.
- Encourage patient to wear or carry medical identification at all times.

Evaluation

- Patient has no evidence of adrenal insufficiency.
- Patient remains free from injury.
- Patient is free from infection.

Diuretics, loop

bumetanide
ethacrynate sodium
ethacrynic acid
furosemide
torsemide

Indications

▶ Edema from heart failure, hepatic cirrhosis, or nephrotic syndrome; mild to moderate hypertension; adjunct treatment in acute pulmonary edema or hypertensive crisis.

Actions

Loop diuretics inhibit sodium and chloride reabsorption in the ascending loop of Henle, thus increasing renal excretion of sodium, chloride, and water. Like thiazide diuretics, loop diuretics increase excretion of potassium. Loop diuretics produce greater maximum diuresis and electrolyte loss than thiazide diuretics.

Adverse reactions

Therapeutic doses commonly cause metabolic and electrolyte disturbances, particularly potassium depletion. They also may cause hypochloremic alkalosis, hyperglycemia, hyperuricemia, and hypomagnesemia. Rapid parenteral administration may cause hearing loss (including deafness) and tinnitus. High doses can produce profound diuresis, leading to hypovolemia and CV collapse.

Contraindications and precautions

- Contraindicated in patients hypersensitive to drug and in patients with anuria, hepatic coma, or severe electrolyte depletion.
- Use cautiously in patients with severe renal disease.
- **Pregnant patients:** Use cautiously in pregnant women.
- **Breast-feeding patients:** Don't give loop diuretics to breast-feeding women.
- **Pediatric patients:** Use cautiously in neonates. The usual pediatric dose can be used, but dosage intervals should be extended.
- **Geriatric patients:** These patients are more susceptible to drug-induced diuresis. Reduced dosages may be indicated. Monitor patient closely.

NURSING CONSIDERATIONS

Assessment

- Monitor blood pressure and pulse rate (especially during rapid diuresis). Establish baseline values before therapy begins, and watch for significant changes.
- Establish baseline CBC (including WBC count), liver function test results, and levels of serum electrolytes, carbon dioxide, magnesium, BUN, and creatinine. Review periodically.
- Assess patient for evidence of excessive diuresis: hypotension, tachycardia, poor skin turgor, and excessive thirst.
- Monitor patient for edema and ascites. Observe the legs of ambulatory patients and the sacral area of patients on bed rest.
- Weigh patient each morning immediately after voiding and before breakfast, in the same type of clothing and on the same scale. Weight provides a reliable indicator of patient's response to diuretic therapy.

Key nursing diagnoses

- Risk for deficient fluid volume related to excessive diuresis
- Impaired urine elimination related to change in diuresis pattern
- Ineffective protection related to electrolyte imbalance

Planning and implementation

- Give diuretics in morning to make sure that major diuresis occurs before bedtime. To prevent nocturia, don't administer diuretics after 6 p.m.
- If ordered, reduce dosage for patient with hepatic dysfunction, and increase dosage for patient with renal impairment, oliguria, or decreased diuresis. (Inadequate urine output may result in circulatory overload, causing water intoxication, pulmonary edema, and heart failure). If ordered, increase dosage of insulin or oral hypoglycemic in diabetic patient, and reduce dosage of other antihypertensive drugs.
- Take safety measures for all ambulatory patients until response to diuretic is known.
- Consult dietitian about need for potassium supplements.
- Keep urinal or commode readily available to patient.

Patient teaching

- Explain rationale for therapy and importance of following the prescribed regimen.
- Review adverse effects, and urge patient to report symptoms promptly, especially chest, back, or leg pain; shortness of breath; dyspnea; increased edema or weight; or excess diuresis (weight loss of more than 0.9 kg [2 lb] daily).
- Advise patient to eat potassium-rich foods and to avoid high-sodium foods (lunch meat, smoked meats, processed cheeses). Caution him not to add table salt to foods.
- Encourage patient to keep follow-up appointments to monitor effectiveness of therapy.

Evaluation

- Patient maintains adequate hydration.
- Patient states importance of taking diuretic early in the day to prevent nocturia.
- Patient complies with therapy, as evidenced by improvement in underlying condition.

Diuretics, thiazide and thiazide-like

Thiazide
chlorothiazide
hydrochlorothiazide
Thiazide-like
indapamide
metolazone

Indications

▶ Edema from right-sided heart failure, mild to moderate left-sided heart failure, or nephrotic syndrome; edema and ascites caused by hepatic cirrhosis; hypertension; diabetes insipidus, particularly nephrogenic diabetes insipidus.

Actions

Thiazide and thiazide-like diuretics interfere with sodium transport across the tubules of the cortical diluting segment in the nephron, thereby increasing renal excretion of sodium, chloride, water, potassium, and calcium.

Thiazide diuretics also exert an antihypertensive effect. Although the exact mechanism is unknown, direct arteriolar dilation may be partially responsible. In diabetes insipidus, thiazides cause a paradoxical decrease in urine volume and an increase in renal concentration of urine, possibly because of sodium depletion and decreased plasma volume. This increases water and sodium reabsorption in the kidneys.

Adverse reactions

Therapeutic doses cause electrolyte and metabolic disturbances, most commonly potassium depletion. Other abnormalities include hypochloremic alkalosis, hypomagnesemia, hyponatremia, hypercalcemia, hyperuricemia, hyperglycemia, and elevated cholesterol levels.

Contraindications and precautions

- Contraindicated in patients hypersensitive to drug and in those with anuria.
- Use cautiously in patients with severe renal disease, impaired hepatic function, or progressive liver disease.
- **Pregnant patients:** Use cautiously in pregnant patients.
- **Breast-feeding patients:** Thiazides appear in breast milk and are contraindicated in breast-feeding women.
- **Pediatric patients:** Safety and efficacy haven't been established in children.
- **Geriatric patients:** These patients are more susceptible to drug-induced diuresis. Reduced dosages may be needed. Monitor patient closely.

NURSING CONSIDERATIONS

Assessment

- Monitor patient's intake, output, and serum electrolyte levels regularly.
- Weigh patient each morning immediately after voiding and before breakfast, in the same type of clothing and on the same scale. Weight provides a reliable indicator of patient's response to diuretic therapy.
- Monitor blood glucose level in a diabetic patient. Diuretics may cause hyperglycemia.
- Monitor serum creatinine and BUN levels regularly. Drug isn't as effective if these levels are more than twice normal. Also monitor blood uric acid levels.

Key nursing diagnoses

- Risk for deficient fluid volume related to excessive diuresis
- Impaired urine elimination related to change in diuresis pattern
- Ineffective protection related to electrolyte imbalance

Planning and implementation

- Give drug in the morning to prevent nocturia.
- Consult a dietitian to provide a high-potassium diet.
- Administer potassium supplements as prescribed to maintain acceptable serum potassium level.
- Keep urinal or commode readily available to patient.

Patient teaching

- Explain the rationale for therapy and the importance of following the prescribed regimen.
- Tell patient to take drug at same time each day to prevent nocturia. Suggest taking drug with food to minimize gastric irritation.

• Urge patient to seek prescriber's approval before taking any other drug, including OTC medications or herbal remedies.
• Advise patient to record his weight each morning after voiding and before breakfast, in the same type of clothing and on the same scale.
• Review adverse effects, and urge the patient to report symptoms promptly, especially chest, back, or leg pain; shortness of breath; dyspnea; increased edema or weight; or excess diuresis (weight loss of more than 0.9 kg [2 lb] daily). Warn him about photosensitivity reactions (these usually occur 10 to 14 days after initial sun exposure).
• Advise patient to eat potassium-rich foods and to avoid high-sodium foods (lunch meat, smoked meats, processed cheeses). Caution him not to add table salt to foods.
• Encourage patient to keep follow-up appointments to monitor effectiveness of therapy.

☑ Evaluation
• Patient maintains adequate hydration.
• Patient states importance of taking diuretic early in day to prevent nocturia.
• Patient complies with therapy, as evidenced by improvement in underlying condition.

Estrogens
diethylstilbestrol
diethylstilbestrol diphosphate
esterified estrogens
estradiol
estradiol cypionate
estradiol valerate
estrogenic substances, conjugated
estrone
estropipate
ethinyl estradiol

Indications
▶ Prevention of vasomotor symptoms, such as hot flushes and dizziness; stimulation of vaginal tissue development, cornification, and secretory activity; inhibition of hormone-sensitive cancer growth; prevention of bone decalcification; ovulation control; prevention of conception.

Actions
Estrogens promote the development and maintenance of the female reproductive system and secondary sexual characteristics. They inhibit the release of pituitary gonadotropins and have various metabolic effects, including retention of fluid and electrolytes, retention and deposition in bone of calcium and phosphorus, and mild anabolic activity. Of the six naturally occurring estrogens in humans, three (estradiol, estrone, and estriol) are present in significant quantities.

Estrogens and estrogenic substances administered as drugs have effects related to endogenous estrogen's mechanism of action. They can mimic the action of endogenous estrogen when used as replacement therapy and can inhibit ovulation or the growth of certain hormone-sensitive cancers. Conjugated estrogens and estrogenic substances are normally obtained from the urine of pregnant mares. Other estrogens are manufactured synthetically.

Adverse reactions
Acute adverse reactions include changes in menstrual bleeding patterns (spotting, prolongation or absence of bleeding), abdominal cramps, swollen feet or ankles, bloated sensation (fluid and electrolyte retention), breast swelling and tenderness, weight gain, nausea, loss of appetite, headache, photosensitivity, loss of libido.

Chronic effects include elevated blood pressure (sometimes into hypertensive range), cholestatic jaundice, benign hepatomas, endometrial carcinoma (rare), and thromboembolic disease (risk increases markedly with cigarette smoking, especially in women over age 35).

Contraindications and precautions
• Contraindicated in women with thrombophlebitis or thromboembolic disorders, undiagnosed abnormal genital bleeding, or estrogen-dependent neoplasia.
• Use cautiously in patients with hypertension; metabolic bone disease; migraines; seizures; asthma; cardiac, renal, or hepatic impairment;

blood dyscrasia; diabetes; family history of breast cancer; or fibrocystic disease.
• **Pregnant patients:** Contraindicated in pregnant women.
• **Breast-feeding patients:** Estrogens are contraindicated in breast-feeding women.
• **Pediatric patients:** Because of their effects on epiphyseal closure, use estrogens cautiously in adolescents whose bone growth isn't complete.
• **Geriatric patients:** Postmenopausal women with long-term estrogen use have an increased risk of endometrial cancer.

NURSING CONSIDERATIONS

Assessment
• Monitor patient regularly to detect improvement or worsening of symptoms; observe patient for adverse reactions.
• If patient has diabetes mellitus, watch closely for loss of diabetes control.
• Monitor PT of patient receiving warfarin-type anticoagulant. If ordered, adjust anticoagulant dosage.

Key nursing diagnoses
• Excessive fluid volume related to drug-induced fluid retention
• Risk of injury related to adverse effects
• Noncompliance related to long-term therapy

Planning and implementation
• Notify pathologist of patient's estrogen therapy when sending specimens for evaluation.
• Keep in mind that estrogens are usually given cyclically (once daily for 3 weeks, followed by 1 week without drugs; repeated as necessary).

Patient teaching
• Urge patient to read the package insert describing adverse reactions. Follow this with a verbal explanation. Tell patient to keep the package insert for later reference.
• Advise patient to take drug with meals or at bedtime to relieve nausea. Reassure her that nausea usually disappears with continued therapy.
• Teach patient how to apply estrogen ointments or transdermal estrogen. Review symptoms that accompany a systemic reaction to ointments.
• Teach patient how to insert intravaginal estrogen suppository. Advise her to use sanitary pads instead of tampons when using suppository.
• Teach patient how to perform routine breast self-examination.
• Tell patient to stop taking drug immediately if she becomes pregnant because estrogens can harm fetus.
• Remind patient not to breast-feed during estrogen therapy.
• If patient is receiving cyclic therapy for postmenopausal symptoms, explain that withdrawal bleeding may occur during the week off but that fertility hasn't been restored and ovulation doesn't occur.
• Explain that medical supervision is essential during prolonged therapy.
• Tell male patient on long-term therapy about possible gynecomastia and impotence, which will disappear when therapy ends.
• Instruct patient to notify prescriber immediately if she experiences abdominal pain; pain, numbness, or stiffness in legs or buttocks; pressure or pain in chest; shortness of breath; severe headaches; visual disturbances, such as blind spots, flashing lights, or blurriness; vaginal bleeding or discharge; breast lumps; swelling of hands or feet; yellow skin and sclera; dark urine; or light-colored stools.
• Urge diabetic patient to report symptoms of hyperglycemia or glycosuria.

Evaluation
• Patient experiences only minimal fluid retention.
• Serious complications of estrogen therapy don't develop.
• Patient complies with therapy, as evidenced by improvement in underlying condition or absence of pregnancy.

Hematinics, oral

ferrous fumarate
ferrous gluconate
ferrous sulfate

Indications

▶ Prevention and treatment of iron-deficiency anemia.

Actions

Iron is an essential component of hemoglobin. It's needed in adequate amounts for erythropoiesis and for efficient oxygen transport in the blood. After absorption into the blood, iron is immediately bound to transferrin, a plasma protein that transports iron to bone marrow, where it's used during hemoglobin synthesis. Some iron is also used during synthesis of myoglobin and other nonhemoglobin heme units.

Adverse reactions

Because iron is corrosive, GI intolerance is common (5% to 20%); symptoms include nausea, vomiting, anorexia, constipation, and dark stools. Liquid forms may stain teeth.

Contraindications and precautions

- Contraindicated in patients with hemochromatosis, hemolytic anemia, or hemosiderosis.
- Use cautiously in patients with peptic ulcer disease, regional enteritis, ulcerative colitis, or sensitivity to sulfites or tartrazine (some products contain these ingredients).
- **Breast-feeding patients:** Iron supplements are commonly recommended for breast-feeding women; no adverse effects have been documented.
- **Pediatric patients:** Caution parents about possible lethal effects of iron overdose.
- **Geriatric patients:** Iron-induced constipation is common in elderly patients; stress proper diet to minimize this effect. Elderly patients also may need higher doses because reduced gastric secretions and achlorhydria may lower their capacity for iron absorption.

NURSING CONSIDERATIONS

Assessment

- Monitor patient for adverse reactions, especially those related to bowel function.
- Monitor hemoglobin and reticulocyte counts during therapy.

Key nursing diagnoses

- Risk for deficient fluid volume related to GI upset
- Constipation related to adverse effect on bowel
- Noncompliance related to adverse effects or long-term use

Planning and implementation

- Dilute liquid forms in juice (preferably orange juice, which promotes iron absorption) or water, but not in milk or antacids. To avoid staining teeth, give liquid preparations through a straw. Don't give antacids within 1 hour before or 2 hours after an iron product, if possible, to prevent interference with absorption.
- Don't crush tablets or capsules; if patient has trouble swallowing, use a liquid form.

Patient teaching

- Explain rationale for therapy, and urge patient to follow the prescribed regimen.
- Tell patient to continue his regular dosage schedule if he misses a dose, and warn him not to take double doses.
- Advise patient to dilute liquid form in juice (preferably orange juice) or water, not milk or antacids. Suggest that he use a straw to avoid staining his teeth.
- Review possible adverse effects. Tell patient that oral iron may turn stools black, and reassure him that this is harmless. Teach dietary measures to help prevent constipation.
- Explain the toxicity of iron, and emphasize importance of keeping iron away from children to prevent poisoning. As few as three or four tablets can cause serious iron poisoning.
- Urge patient to report diarrhea or constipation because prescriber may want to adjust dosage, modify diet, or order further tests.

• Explain that iron therapy may be required for 4 to 6 months after anemia resolves. Encourage compliance.

Evaluation
• Patient maintains adequate hydration.
• Patient regains normal bowel pattern.
• Patient complies with therapy, as evidenced by return of normal hemoglobin levels and resolution of iron deficiency anemia.

Histamine$_2$-receptor antagonists
cimetidine
famotidine
nizatidine
ranitidine hydrochloride

Indications
▶ Acute duodenal or gastric ulcer, Zollinger-Ellison syndrome, gastroesophageal reflux.

Actions
All H_2-receptor antagonists inhibit the action of H_2 receptors in gastric parietal cells, reducing gastric acid output and concentration, regardless of the stimulatory drug (histamine, food, insulin, caffeine) or basal conditions.

Adverse reactions
H_2-receptor antagonists rarely cause adverse reactions. Mild and transient diarrhea, neutropenia, dizziness, fatigue, cardiac arrhythmias, and gynecomastia have been reported.

Contraindications and precautions
• Contraindicated in patients hypersensitive to drug.
• Use cautiously in patients with impaired renal or hepatic function.
• **Pregnant patients:** Use cautiously in pregnant patients.
• **Breast-feeding patients:** H_2-receptor antagonists may appear in breast milk and are contraindicated in breast-feeding women.
• **Pediatric patients:** Safety and efficacy haven't been established in children.
• **Geriatric patients:** These patients have an increased risk of adverse reactions, particularly those affecting the CNS. Use cautiously.

NURSING CONSIDERATIONS

Assessment
• Monitor patient for adverse reactions, especially hypotension and arrhythmias.
• Periodically monitor laboratory tests, such as CBC and renal and hepatic studies, as ordered.

Key nursing diagnoses
• Risk for infection related to neutropenia
• Decreased cardiac output related to adverse CV effects (cimetidine)
• Fatigue related to drug's CNS effects

Planning and implementation
• Administer once-daily dose at bedtime, twice-daily doses in morning and evening, and multiple doses with meals and at bedtime. Most clinicians prefer once-daily dose at bedtime to promote compliance.
• Don't exceed recommended infusion rates when administering drugs I.V.; doing so increases risk of adverse CV effects. Continuous I.V. infusion may suppress acid secretion more effectively.
• Administer antacids at least 1 hour before or after H_2-receptor antagonists. Antacids can decrease drug absorption.
• Anticipate dosage adjustment for patient with renal disease.
• Avoid discontinuing drug abruptly.

Patient teaching
• Teach patient how and when to take drug, and warn him not to stop drug suddenly.
• Review possible adverse reactions, and urge him to report unusual effects.
• Caution patient to avoid smoking during therapy; smoking stimulates gastric acid secretion and worsens the disease.

Evaluation
• Patient is free from infection.
• Patient maintains a normal heart rhythm.
• Patient states appropriate management plan for combating fatigue.

▶ Prototype drug

Hypoglycemics, oral

acarbose
acetohexamide
chlorpropamide
glimepiride
glipizide
glyburide
metformin hydrochloride
miglitol
pioglitazone hydrochloride
repaglinide
rosiglitazone maleate
tolazamide
tolbutamide

Indications

▶ Mild to moderately severe, stable, nonketotic non-insulin-dependent diabetes mellitus that cannot be controlled by diet alone.

Actions

Oral hypoglycemics come in several types. Sulfonylureas are sulfonamide derivatives that exert no antibacterial activity. They lower blood glucose levels by stimulating insulin release from the pancreas. These drugs work only in the presence of functioning beta cells in the islet tissue of the pancreas. After prolonged administration, they produce hypoglycemia through significant extrapancreatic effects, including reduction of hepatic glucose production and enhanced peripheral sensitivity to insulin. The latter may result from an increased number of insulin receptors or from changes in events after insulin binding. Sulfonylureas are divided into first-generation drugs (acetohexamide, chlorpropamide, tolbutamide, and tolazamide) and second-generation drugs (glyburide, glimepiride, and glipizide). Although their mechanisms of action are similar, the second-generation drugs carry a more lipophilic side chain, are more potent, and cause fewer adverse reactions. Clinically, their most important difference is their duration of action.

Metformin decreases hepatic glucose production, reduces intestinal glucose absorption, and improves insulin sensitivity (increases peripheral glucose uptake and utilization). With metformin therapy, insulin secretion remains unchanged, and fasting insulin levels and day-long plasma insulin response may actually decrease.

Alpha-glucosidase inhibitors such as acarbose and miglitol delay digestion of carbohydrates, resulting in a smaller rise in blood glucose levels.

Rosiglitazone and pioglitazone are thiazolidinediones, which lower blood glucose levels by improving insulin sensitivity. These drugs are potent and highly selective agonists for receptors found in insulin-sensitive tissues, such as adipose tissue, skeletal muscle, and the liver.

Adverse reactions

Sulfonylureas cause dose-related reactions that usually respond to decreased dosage: headache, nausea, vomiting, anorexia, heartburn, weakness, and paresthesia. Hypoglycemia may follow excessive dosage, increased exercise, decreased food intake, or alcohol consumption.

The most serious adverse reaction linked to metformin is lactic acidosis. It's rare and most likely to occur in patients with renal dysfunction. Other reactions to metformin include GI upset, megaloblastic anemia, rash, dermatitis, and unpleasant or metallic taste.

Contraindications and precautions

- Contraindicated in patients hypersensitive to drug and in patients with diabetic ketoacidosis with or without coma. Metformin is also contraindicated in patients with renal disease or metabolic acidosis and generally should be avoided in patients with hepatic disease.
- Use sulfonylureas cautiously in patients with renal or hepatic disease. Use metformin cautiously in patients with adrenal or pituitary insufficiency and in elderly, debilitated, or malnourished patients. Alpha-glucosidase inhibitors should be used cautiously in patients with mild to moderate renal insufficiency. Use thiazolidinediones cautiously in patients with edema or heart failure.
- **Pregnant patients:** Contraindicated in pregnant patients.

• **Breast-feeding patients:** Oral hypoglycemics appear in small amounts in breast milk and may cause hypoglycemia in the breast-feeding infant. They're contraindicated for use in breast-feeding women.
• **Pediatric patients:** Oral hypoglycemics aren't effective in type 1 diabetes mellitus.
• **Geriatric patients:** These patients may be more sensitive to these drugs and usually need lower dosages. What's more, hypoglycemia may be more difficult to recognize, although it usually causes neurologic symptoms in such patients. Monitor these patients closely.

NURSING CONSIDERATIONS

Assessment
• Monitor patient's blood glucose level regularly. Increase monitoring during periods of increased stress (infection, fever, surgery, or trauma).
• Monitor patient for adverse reactions.
• Assess patient's compliance with drug therapy and other aspects of diabetic treatment.

Key nursing diagnoses
• Risk for injury related to hypoglycemia
• Risk for deficient fluid volume related to adverse GI effects
• Noncompliance related to long-term therapy

Planning and implementation
• Give a sulfonylurea 30 minutes before morning meal (once-daily dosing) or 30 minutes before morning and evening meals (twice-daily dosing). Give metformin with morning and evening meals. Alpha-glucosidase inhibitors should be taken with the first bite of each main meal t.i.d.
• Patients who take a thiazolidinedione should have liver enzyme levels measured at the start of therapy, every 2 months for the first year of therapy, and periodically thereafter.
• Keep in mind that patient transferring from one oral hypoglycemic to another (except chlorpropamide) usually needs no transition period.
• Anticipate patient's need for insulin during periods of increased stress.

Patient teaching
• Emphasize the importance of following the prescribed regimen. Urge patient to adhere to diet, weight reduction, exercise, and personal hygiene recommendations.
• Explain that therapy relieves symptoms but doesn't cure the disease.
• Teach patient how to recognize and treat hypoglycemia.

Evaluation
• Patient sustains no injury.
• Patient maintains adequate hydration.
• Patient complies with therapy, as evidenced by normal or near-normal blood glucose levels.

Laxatives

Bulk-forming
calcium polycarbophil
methylcellulose
psyllium
Emollient
docusate calcium
docusate potassium
docusate sodium
Hyperosmolar
glycerin
lactulose
magnesium citrate
magnesium hydroxide
magnesium sulfate
sodium phosphates
Lubricant
mineral oil
Stimulant
bisacodyl
cascara sagrada
castor oil
senna

Indications

▶ Constipation, irritable bowel syndrome, diverticulosis.

Actions

Laxatives promote movement of intestinal contents though the colon and rectum via several modes of action: bulk-forming, emollient, hyperosmolar, lubricant, and stimulant).

Adverse reactions

All laxatives may cause flatulence, diarrhea, abdominal discomfort, weakness, and dependence. Bulk-forming laxatives may cause intestinal obstruction, impaction, or (rarely) esophageal obstruction. Emollient laxatives may cause a bitter taste or throat irritation. Hyperosmolar laxatives may cause fluid and electrolyte imbalances. Lubricant laxatives may cause impaired absorption of fat-soluble vitamins or anal irritation if given rectally. Stimulant laxatives may cause urine discoloration, malabsorption, and weight loss.

Contraindications and precautions

- Contraindicated in patients with GI obstruction or perforation, toxic colitis, megacolon, nausea and vomiting, or acute surgical abdomen.
- Use cautiously in patients with rectal or anal conditions, such as rectal bleeding or large hemorrhoids.
- See individual drugs for complete listings of contraindications and precautions.
- **Breast-feeding patients:** Recommendations vary for use in breast-feeding women. See individual drugs for specific guidelines.
- **Pediatric patients:** Infants and children have an increased risk of fluid and electrolyte disturbances. Use cautiously.
- **Geriatric patients:** Dependence is more likely to develop in elderly patients because of age-related changes in GI function. Monitor these patients closely.

NURSING CONSIDERATIONS

Assessment

- Obtain baseline assessment of patient's bowel patterns and GI history before giving laxative.
- Monitor patient for adverse reactions.
- Monitor bowel pattern throughout therapy. Assess bowel sounds and color and consistency of stools.
- Monitor patient's fluid and electrolyte status during administration.

Key nursing diagnoses

- Diarrhea related to adverse GI effects
- Acute pain related to abdominal discomfort
- Impaired health maintenance related to laxative dependence

Planning and implementation

- Don't crush enteric-coated tablets.
- Time administration so that bowel evacuation doesn't interfere with sleep.
- Make sure patient has easy access to bedpan or bathroom.
- Institute measures to prevent constipation.

Patient teaching

- Advise patient that therapy should be short-term. Point out that abuse or prolonged use can cause nutritional imbalances.
- Tell patient that stool softeners and bulk-forming laxatives may take several days to achieve results.
- Encourage patient to remain active and to drink plenty of fluids if he's taking a bulk-forming laxative.
- Explain that stimulant laxatives may cause harmless urine discoloration.

Evaluation

- Patient regains normal bowel pattern.
- Patient states that pain is relieved with stool evacuation.
- Patient discusses dangers of laxative abuse and importance of limiting laxative use.

Nonsteroidal anti-inflammatory drugs

celecoxib
diflunisal
etodolac
fenoprofen calcium
flurbiprofen
ibuprofen
indomethacin
indomethacin sodium trihydrate
ketoprofen
ketorolac tromethamine
mefenamic acid

meloxicam
nabumetone
naproxen
naproxen sodium
oxaprozin
piroxicam
rofecoxib
sulindac
tolmetin sodium

Indications

▶ Mild to moderate pain, inflammation, stiffness, swelling, or tenderness caused by headache, arthralgia, myalgia, neuralgia, dysmenorrhea, rheumatoid arthritis, juvenile arthritis, osteoarthritis, or dental or surgical procedures.

Actions

The analgesic effect of NSAIDs may result from interference with the prostaglandins involved in pain. Prostaglandins appear to sensitize pain receptors to mechanical stimulation or to other chemical mediators. NSAIDs inhibit synthesis of prostaglandins peripherally and possibly centrally.

Like salicylates, NSAIDs exert an anti-inflammatory effect that may result in part from inhibition of prostaglandin synthesis and release during inflammation. The exact mechanism hasn't been clearly established.

Adverse reactions

Adverse reactions chiefly involve the GI tract, particularly erosion of the gastric mucosa. Most common symptoms are dyspepsia, heartburn, epigastric distress, nausea, and abdominal pain. CNS reactions also may occur. Flank pain with other evidence of nephrotoxicity has occasionally been reported. Fluid retention may aggravate hypertension or heart failure.

Contraindications and precautions

- Contraindicated in patients with GI lesions and in patients hypersensitive to drug.
- Use cautiously in patients with cardiac decompensation, hypertension, fluid retention, or coagulation defects.
- **Breast-feeding patients:** NSAIDs aren't recommended for breast-feeding women.
- **Pediatric patients:** Safety of long-term therapy in children under age 14 hasn't been established.
- **Geriatric patients:** Patients over age 60 may be more susceptible to toxic effects of NSAIDs because of decreased renal function.

NURSING CONSIDERATIONS

Assessment

- Assess patient's level of pain and inflammation before therapy begins, and evaluate drug effectiveness after administration.
- Monitor patient for signs and symptoms of bleeding. Assess bleeding time if patient needs surgery.
- Monitor ophthalmic and auditory function before and periodically during therapy to detect toxicity.
- Monitor CBC, platelets, PT, and hepatic and renal function studies periodically to detect abnormalities.
- Watch for bronchospasm in patients with known "triad" symptoms: aspirin hypersensitivity, rhinitis or nasal polyps, and asthma.

Key nursing diagnoses

- Risk for injury related to adverse reactions
- Excessive fluid volume related to fluid retention
- Disturbed sensory perception (visual and auditory) related to toxicity

Planning and implementation

- Administer oral NSAIDs with 8 oz (240 ml) of water to ensure adequate passage into the stomach. Have patient sit up for 15 to 30 minutes after taking drug to prevent lodging in esophagus.
- As needed, crush tablets or mix with food or fluid to aid swallowing. Administer with antacids to minimize gastric upset.

Patient teaching

- Encourage patient to take drug as directed to achieve desired effect. Explain that he may not notice benefits of drug for 2 to 4 weeks.
- Review methods to prevent or minimize gastric upset.
- Work with patient on long-term therapy to arrange for monitoring of laboratory parame-

ters, especially BUN and serum creatinine levels, liver function tests, and CBC.
• Instruct patient to notify prescriber about severe or persistent adverse reactions.

Evaluation
• Patient remains free from injury.
• Patient shows no signs of edema.
• Patient maintains normal visual and auditory function.

Opioids
alfentanil hydrochloride
codeine phosphate
codeine sulfate
difenoxin
diphenoxylate
fentanyl citrate
hydromorphone hydrochloride
meperidine hydrochloride
methadone hydrochloride
morphine sulfate
oxycodone hydrochloride
oxymorphone hydrochloride
propoxyphene hydrochloride
propoxyphene napsylate
sufentanil citrate

Indications
▶ Moderate to severe pain from acute and some chronic disorders; diarrhea; dry, nonproductive cough.

Actions
Opioids act as agonists at specific opiate-receptor binding sites in the CNS and other tissues, altering the patient's perception of and emotional response to pain.

Adverse reactions
Respiratory depression and circulatory depression (including orthostatic hypotension) are the major hazards of opioids. Other adverse CNS effects include dizziness, visual disturbances, mental clouding or depression, sedation, coma, euphoria, dysphoria, weakness, faintness, agitation, restlessness, nervousness, and seizures. Adverse GI effects include nausea, vomiting, constipation, and biliary colic. Urine retention or hypersensitivity also may occur. Tolerance or psychological or physical dependence may follow prolonged therapy.

Contraindications and precautions
• Contraindicated in patients hypersensitive to drug and in those who have recently taken an MAO inhibitor.
• Use cautiously in patients with head injury, increased intracranial or intraocular pressure, or hepatic or renal dysfunction.
• **Pregnant patients:** Use cautiously in pregnant patients.
• **Breast-feeding patients:** Codeine, meperidine, methadone, morphine, and propoxyphene appear in breast milk and should be used cautiously in breast-feeding women. Methadone causes physical dependence in breast-feeding infants of women maintained on methadone.
• **Pediatric patients:** Safety and efficacy in children haven't been established.
• **Geriatric patients:** These patients may be more sensitive to opioids. Lower doses are usually indicated.

NURSING CONSIDERATIONS

Assessment
• Obtain baseline assessment of patient's pain, and reassess frequently to determine drug effectiveness.
• Evaluate patient's respiratory status before each dose; watch for respiratory rate below patient's baseline level and for restlessness, which may be a compensatory sign of hypoxia. Respiratory depression may last longer than analgesic effect.
• Monitor patient for other adverse reactions.
• Monitor patient for tolerance and dependence. The first sign of tolerance to opioids is usually a shortened duration of effect.

Key nursing diagnoses
• Ineffective breathing pattern related to respiratory depression
• Risk for injury related to orthostatic hypotension
• Ineffective individual coping related to drug dependence

▶ Prototype drug

Planning and implementation

- Keep resuscitative equipment and a narcotic antagonist (naloxone) available.
- Administer I.V. drug by slow injection, preferably in diluted solution. Rapid I.V. injection increases the risk of adverse effects.
- Give I.M. or S.C. injections cautiously to patients with decreased platelet counts and to patients who are chilled, hypovolemic, or in shock; decreased perfusion may lead to drug accumulation and toxicity. Rotate injection sites to avoid induration.
- Carefully note the strength of solution when measuring a dose. Oral solutions of varying concentrations are available.
- For maximum effectiveness, administer on regular dosage schedule rather than p.r.n.
- Institute safety precautions.
- Encourage postoperative patients to turn, cough, and deep-breathe every 2 hours to avoid atelectasis.
- Give oral forms with food if gastric irritation occurs.

Patient teaching

- Teach patient to take drug exactly as prescribed. Urge him to call prescriber if he isn't experiencing desired effect or is experiencing significant adverse reactions.
- Warn patient to avoid hazardous activities until drug's effects are known.
- Advise patient to avoid alcohol while taking opioids; it will cause additive CNS depression.
- Suggest measures to prevent constipation, such as increasing fiber in diet and using a stool softener.
- Instruct patient to breathe deeply, cough, and change position every 2 hours to avoid respiratory complications.

Evaluation

- Patient maintains adequate ventilation, as evidenced by normal respiratory rate and rhythm and pink color.
- Patient remains free from injury.
- Tolerance to therapy doesn't develop.

Penicillins

Natural penicillins
- penicillin G benzathine
- penicillin G potassium
- penicillin G procaine
- penicillin G sodium
- penicillin V potassium

Aminopenicillins
- amoxicillin/clavulanate potassium
- amoxicillin trihydrate
- ampicillin
- ampicillin sodium/sulbactam sodium
- ampicillin trihydrate
- bacampicillin hydrochloride

Penicillinase-resistant penicillins
- cloxacillin sodium
- dicloxacillin sodium
- nafcillin sodium
- oxacillin sodium

Extended-spectrum penicillins
- carbenicillin indanyl sodium
- mezlocillin sodium
- piperacillin sodium
- piperacillin sodium and tazobactam sodium
- ticarcillin disodium
- ticarcillin disodium/clavulanate potassium

Indications

▶ Streptococcal pneumonia; enterococcal and nonenterococcal Group D endocarditis; diphtheria; anthrax; meningitis; tetanus; botulism; actinomycosis; syphilis; relapsing fever; Lyme disease; pneumococcal infections; rheumatic fever; bacterial endocarditis; neonatal Group B streptococcal disease; septicemia; gynecologic infections; infections of urinary, respiratory, and GI tracts; infections of skin, soft tissue, bones, and joints.

Actions

Penicillins are generally bactericidal. They inhibit synthesis of the bacterial cell wall, causing rapid cell lysis. They're most effective against fast-growing susceptible bacteria. Their sites of action are enzymes known as penicillin-binding proteins (PBPs). The affinity of certain penicillins for PBPs in various microorganisms helps explain differing spectra of activity in this class of antibiotics.

Susceptible aerobic gram-positive cocci include *Staphylococcus aureus;* nonenterococcal Group D streptococci; Groups A, B, D, G, H, K, L, and M streptococci; *S. viridans;* and enterococcus (usually in combination with an aminoglycoside). Susceptible aerobic gram-negative cocci include *Neisseria meningitidis* and non-penicillinase-producing *N. gonorrhoeae*.

Susceptible aerobic gram-positive bacilli include *Corynebacterium, Listeria*, and *Bacillus anthracis*. Susceptible anaerobes include *Peptococcus, Peptostreptococcus, Actinomyces, Clostridium, Fusobacterium, Veillonella*, and non-beta-lactamase-producing strains of *S. pneumoniae*. Susceptible spirochetes include *Treponema pallidum, T. pertenue, Leptospira, Borrelia recurrentis*, and, possibly, *Borrelia burgdorferi*.

Aminopenicillins offer a broader spectrum of activity, including many gram-negative organisms. Like natural penicillins, aminopenicillins are vulnerable to inactivation by penicillinase. Their activity spectrum includes *Escherichia coli, Proteus mirabilis, Shigella, Salmonella, S. pneumoniae, N. gonorrhoeae, Haemophilus influenzae, Staphylococcus aureus, Staphylococcus epidermidis* (non-penicillinase-producing *Staphylococcus*), and *Listeria monocytogenes*.

Penicillinase-resistant penicillins are semisynthetic penicillins designed to remain stable against hydrolysis by most staphylococcal penicillinases and thus are the drugs of choice against susceptible penicillinase-producing staphylococci. They also act against most organisms susceptible to natural penicillins.

Extended-spectrum penicillins offer a wider range of bactericidal action than the other three classes and are usually given in combination with aminoglycosides. Susceptible strains include *Enterobacter, Klebsiella, Citrobacter, Serratia, Bacteroides fragilis, Pseudomonas aeruginosa; Proteus vulgaris, Providencia rettgeri*, and *Morganella morganii*. These penicillins are also vulnerable to beta-lactamase and penicillinases.

Adverse reactions

Hypersensitivity reactions occur with all penicillins; they range from mild rash, fever, and eosinophilia to fatal anaphylaxis. Hematologic reactions include hemolytic anemia, transient neutropenia, leukopenia, and thrombocytopenia.

Certain adverse reactions are more common with specific classes: For example, bleeding episodes are usually seen with high doses of extended-spectrum penicillins and GI adverse effects are most common with ampicillin. High doses, especially of penicillin G, irritate the CNS in patients with renal disease, causing confusion, twitching, lethargy, dysphagia, seizures, and coma. Hepatotoxicity is common with penicillinase-resistant penicillins; hyperkalemia and hypernatremia with extended-spectrum penicillins.

Local irritation from parenteral therapy may be severe enough to warrant administration by subclavian or centrally placed catheter or discontinuation of therapy.

Contraindications and precautions

- Contraindicated in patients hypersensitive to drug.
- Use cautiously in pregnant women and in patients with history of asthma or drug allergy, mononucleosis, hemorrhagic condition, or electrolyte imbalance.
- **Breast-feeding patients:** Recommendations vary, depending on drug used. See individual drugs for specific guidelines.
- **Pediatric patients:** Dosage recommendations have been established for most penicillins. See individual drugs for specific guidelines.
- **Geriatric patients:** These patients are susceptible to superinfection and many have renal impairment, which decreases excretion of penicillins. Lower dosage is needed. Use cautiously.

NURSING CONSIDERATIONS

Assessment

- Assess patient's history of allergies. Try to ascertain whether previous reactions were true hypersensitivity reactions or adverse reactions (such as GI distress) that patient has interpreted as allergy.

• Keep in mind that a negative history for penicillin hypersensitivity doesn't preclude future allergic reactions; monitor patient continuously for possible allergic reactions or other untoward effects.
• Obtain culture and sensitivity tests before giving first dose; repeat tests periodically to assess drug's effectiveness.
• Monitor vital signs, electrolytes, and renal function studies.
• Assess level of consciousness and neurologic status when giving high doses; CNS toxicity can occur.
• Coagulation abnormalities, even frank bleeding, can follow high doses, especially of extended-spectrum penicillins. Monitor PT, INR, and platelet counts. Assess patient for signs of occult or frank bleeding.
• Monitor patients receiving long-term therapy for possible superinfection, especially elderly patients, debilitated patients, and patients receiving immunosuppressants or radiation.

Key nursing diagnoses

• Ineffective protection related to hypersensitivity
• Risk for infection related to superinfection
• Risk for deficient fluid volume related to adverse GI reactions

Planning and implementation

• Administer penicillins at least 1 hour before bacteriostatic antibiotics (tetracyclines, erythromycins, and chloramphenicol); these drugs inhibit bacterial cell growth, decreasing rate of penicillin uptake by bacterial cell walls.
• Follow manufacturer's directions for reconstituting, diluting, and storing drugs; check expiration dates.
• Give oral penicillin at least 1 hour before or 2 hours after meals to enhance gastric absorption.
• Refrigerate oral suspensions (stable for 14 days); shake well before administering to ensure correct dosage.
• Administer I.M. dose deep into large muscle mass (gluteal or midlateral thigh); rotate injection sites to minimize tissue injury; don't inject more than 2 g of drug per injection site. Apply ice to injection site to relieve pain.
• Don't add or mix other drugs with I.V. infusions, particularly aminoglycosides, which will be inactivated if mixed with penicillins. If other drugs must be given I.V., temporarily stop infusion of primary drug.
• Infuse I.V. drug continuously or intermittently (over 30 minutes). Rotate infusion site every 48 hours; intermittent I.V. infusion may be diluted in 50 to 100 ml sterile water, normal saline solution, dextrose 5% in water, dextrose 5% in water and half-normal saline, or lactated Ringer's solution.

Patient teaching

• Make sure patient understands how and when to take drug. Urge him to complete the prescribed regimen, comply with instructions for around-the-clock scheduling, and keep follow-up appointments.
• Teach signs and symptoms of hypersensitivity and other adverse reactions. Urge him to report unusual reactions.
• Tell patient to check drug's expiration date and to discard unused drug. Warn him not to share drug with family or friends.

Evaluation

• Patient shows no signs of hypersensitivity.
• Patient is free from infection.
• Patient maintains adequate hydration.

Phenothiazines

chlorpromazine hydrochloride
fluphenazine
mesoridazine besylate
perphenazine
prochlorperazine
promazine hydrochloride
promethazine
thioridazine hydrochloride
thiothixene
trifluoperazine hydrochloride

Indications

▶ Agitated psychotic states, hallucinations, manic-depressive illness, excessive motor and autonomic activity, severe nausea and vomiting induced by CNS disturbances, moderate anxiety, behavioral problems from chronic organic mental syndrome, tetanus, acute intermittent porphyria, intractable hiccups, itching, symptomatic rhinitis.

Actions

Phenothiazines are believed to function as dopamine antagonists, blocking postsynaptic dopamine receptors in various parts of the CNS. Their antiemetic effects result from blockage of the chemoreceptor trigger zone. They also produce varying degrees of anticholinergic and alpha-adrenergic receptor blocking actions.

Adverse reactions

Phenothiazines may produce extrapyramidal symptoms (dystonic movements, torticollis, oculogyric crises, parkinsonian symptoms) ranging from akathisia during early treatment to tardive dyskinesia after long-term use. A neuroleptic malignant syndrome resembling severe parkinsonism may occur (most often in young men taking fluphenazine). Other adverse reactions include orthostatic hypotension with reflex tachycardia, fainting, dizziness, arrhythmias, anorexia, nausea, vomiting, abdominal pain, local gastric irritation, seizures, endocrine effects, hematologic disorders, visual disturbances, skin eruptions, and photosensitivity. Allergic reactions are usually marked by elevated liver enzymes progressing to obstructive jaundice.

Contraindications and precautions

- Contraindicated in patients with CNS depression, bone marrow suppression, heart failure, circulatory collapse, coronary artery or cerebrovascular disorders, subcortical damage, or coma. Contraindicated with use of spinal or epidural anesthetics or adrenergic blockers.
- Use cautiously in debilitated patients and in those with hepatic, renal, or CV disease; respiratory disorders; hypocalcemia; seizure disorders; suspected brain tumor or intestinal obstruction; glaucoma; or prostatic hyperplasia.
- **Breast-feeding patients:** Most phenothiazines appear in breast milk and have a direct effect on prolactin levels. If feasible, patient should not breast-feed during therapy.
- **Pediatric patients:** Unless otherwise specified, phenothiazines aren't recommended for children under age 12. Use cautiously for nausea and vomiting. Acutely ill children (chickenpox, measles, CNS infections, dehydration) have a greatly increased risk of dystonic reactions.
- **Geriatric patients:** These patients are more sensitive to therapeutic and adverse effects, especially cardiac toxicity, tardive dyskinesia, and other extrapyramidal effects. Use cautiously, and give reduced doses as indicated. Adjust dosage to patient response.

NURSING CONSIDERATIONS

Assessment

- Check vital signs regularly for decreased blood pressure (especially before and after parenteral therapy) or tachycardia; observe patient carefully for other adverse reactions.
- Check intake and output for urine retention or constipation, which may require dosage reduction.
- Monitor bilirubin levels weekly for the first 4 weeks. Establish baseline CBC, ECG (for quinidine-like effects), liver and renal function studies, electrolyte levels (especially potassium), and eye examinations. Monitor them periodically thereafter, especially in patients on long-term therapy.
- Observe patient for mood changes to monitor progress.
- Monitor patient for involuntary movements. Check patient receiving prolonged treatment at least once every 6 months.

Key nursing diagnoses

- Risk for injury related to adverse reactions
- Impaired mobility related to extrapyramidal symptoms
- Noncompliance related to long-term therapy

Planning and implementation

- Don't withdraw drug abruptly; although physical dependence doesn't occur with antipsychotic drugs, rebound worsening of psychotic symptoms may occur, and many drug effects persist.
- Follow manufacturer's guidelines for reconstitution, dilution, administration, and storage

of drugs; slightly discolored liquids may or may not be acceptable for use. Check with pharmacist.

Patient teaching

- Teach patient how and when to take drug. Caution him not to increase the dosage or discontinue the drug without prescriber's approval. Suggest taking the full dose at bedtime if daytime sedation is troublesome.
- Explain that full therapeutic effect may not occur for several weeks.
- Teach signs and symptoms of adverse reactions, and urge patient to report unusual effects, especially involuntary movements.
- Instruct patient to avoid beverages and drugs containing alcohol, and warn him not to take other drugs, including OTC or herbal products, without prescriber's approval.
- Advise patient to avoid hazardous tasks until full effects of drug are established. Explain that sedative effects will lessen after several weeks.
- Inform patient that excessive exposure to sunlight, heat lamps, or tanning beds may cause photosensitivity reactions. Advise him to avoid exposure to extreme heat or cold.
- Explain that phenothiazines may cause pink to brown discoloration of urine.

Evaluation

- Patient remains free from injury.
- Extrapyramidal symptoms don't develop.
- Patient complies with therapy, as evidenced by improved thought processes.

Skeletal muscle relaxants

baclofen
carisoprodol
chlorzoxazone
cyclobenzaprine hydrochloride
methocarbamol
orphenadrine citrate

Indications

▶ Painful musculoskeletal disorders, spasticity of multiple sclerosis.

Actions

All skeletal muscle relaxants except baclofen reduce impulse transmission from the spinal cord to skeletal muscle. Baclofen's mechanism of action is unclear.

Adverse reactions

Skeletal muscle relaxants may cause ataxia, confusion, depressed mood, dizziness, drowsiness, dry mouth, hallucinations, headache, hypotension, nervousness, tachycardia, tremor, and vertigo. Baclofen may cause seizures.

Contraindications and precautions

- Contraindicated in patients hypersensitive to drug.
- Use cautiously in patients with impaired renal or hepatic function.
- See individual drugs for complete listings of contraindications and precautions.
- **Breast-feeding patients:** Recommendations vary for use in breast-feeding women. See individual drugs for specific guidelines.
- **Pediatric patients:** Recommendations vary for use in children. See individual drugs for specific guidelines.
- **Geriatric patients:** These patients have an increased risk of adverse reactions. Monitor them carefully.

NURSING CONSIDERATIONS

Assessment

- Monitor patient for hypersensitivity reactions.
- Assess degree of relief obtained to help prescriber determine when dosage can be reduced.
- Watch for increased seizures in epileptic patients receiving baclofen.
- Monitor CBC results closely.
- Monitor platelet counts in patients receiving cyclobenzaprine or orphenadrine.
- Watch for orthostatic hypotension in patient receiving methocarbamol.
- Monitor hepatic function and urinalysis results in patient receiving long-term orphenadrine therapy.

• Assess compliance in patient receiving long-term therapy.

Key nursing diagnoses

• Risk for trauma related to baclofen-induced seizures
• Disturbed thought processes related to confusion
• Noncompliance related to long-term therapy

Planning and implementation

• Don't stop baclofen or carisoprodol abruptly after long-term therapy unless patient has severe adverse reactions.
• Institute safety precautions as needed.
• Give oral forms of drug with meals or milk to prevent GI distress.
• Obtain an order for a mild analgesic to relieve drug-induced headache.

Patient teaching

• Tell patient to take drug exactly as prescribed. Caution him not to stop baclofen or carisoprodol suddenly after long-term therapy.
• Instruct patient to avoid hazardous activities that require mental alertness until CNS effects of drug are known.
• Advise patient to avoid alcohol during therapy.
• Advise patient to follow his prescriber's advice regarding rest and physical therapy.
• Instruct patient receiving cyclobenzaprine or orphenadrine to report urinary hesitancy.
• Inform patient taking methocarbamol or chlorzoxazone that urine may be discolored.

Evaluation

• Patient remains free from seizures.
• Patient exhibits normal thought processes.
• Patient complies with therapy, as evidenced by pain relief or improvement of spasticity.

Sulfonamides

co-trimoxazole (trimethoprim-sulfamethoxazole)
sulfadiazine
sulfamethoxazole
sulfasalazine
sulfisoxazole

Indications

▶ Bacterial infections, nocardiosis, toxoplasmosis, chloroquine-resistant *Plasmodium falciparum* malaria, inflammatory bowel disease.

Actions

Sulfonamides are bacteriostatic. They inhibit biosynthesis of tetrahydrofolic acid, which is needed for bacterial cell growth. They're active against some strains of staphylococci, streptococci, *Nocardia asteroides* and *brasiliensis, Clostridium tetani* and *perfringens, Bacillus anthracis, Escherichia coli,* and *Neisseria gonorrhoeae* and *meningitidis.* They're also active against organisms that cause urinary tract infections, such as *E. coli, Proteus mirabilis* and *vulgaris, Klebsiella, Enterobacter,* and *Staphylococcus aureus,* and genital lesions caused by *Haemophilus ducreyi* (chancroid).

Adverse reactions

Many adverse reactions stem from hypersensitivity, including rash, fever, pruritus, erythema multiforme, erythema nodosum, Stevens-Johnson syndrome, Lyell's syndrome, exfoliative dermatitis, photosensitivity, joint pain, conjunctivitis, leukopenia, and bronchospasm. Hematologic reactions include granulocytopenia, thrombocytopenia, agranulocytosis, hypoprothrombinemia and, in G6PD deficiency, hemolytic anemia. Renal effects usually result from crystalluria (precipitation of sulfonamide in renal system). GI reactions include nausea, vomiting, anorexia, stomatitis, pancreatitis, diarrhea, and folic acid malabsorption.

Contraindications and precautions

• Contraindicated in patients hypersensitive to drug.

• Use cautiously in patients with impaired renal or hepatic function, bronchial asthma, severe allergy, or G6PD deficiency.
• **Pregnant patients:** Contraindicated in pregnant patients at term.
• **Breast-feeding patients:** Sulfonamides appear in breast milk and are contraindicated in breast-feeding women.
• **Pediatric patients:** Sulfonamides are contraindicated in infants under age 2 months unless there is no therapeutic alternative. Use cautiously in children with fragile X chromosome and mental retardation.
• **Geriatric patients:** These patients are susceptible to bacterial and fungal superinfection and have an increased risk of folate deficiency anemia and adverse renal and hematologic effects.

NURSING CONSIDERATIONS

Assessment
• Assess patient's history of allergies, especially to sulfonamides or to any drug containing sulfur (such as thiazides, furosemide, and oral sulfonylureas).
• Monitor patient for adverse reactions; patients with AIDS have a much higher risk of adverse reactions.
• Obtain culture and sensitivity tests before first dose; check test results periodically to assess drug effectiveness.
• Monitor urine cultures, CBC, and urinalysis before and during therapy.
• During long-term therapy, monitor patient for possible superinfection.

Key nursing diagnoses
• Ineffective protection related to hypersensitivity
• Risk for infection related to superinfection
• Risk for deficient fluid volume related to adverse GI reactions

Planning and implementation
• Give oral dose with 8 oz (240 ml) of water. Give 3 to 4 L of fluids daily, depending on drug; patient's urine output should be at least 1,500 ml/day.
• Follow manufacturer's directions for reconstituting, diluting, and storing drugs; check expiration dates.
• Shake oral suspensions well before administering to ensure correct dosage.

Patient teaching
• Urge patient to take drug exactly as prescribed, to complete the prescribed regimen, and to keep follow-up appointments.
• Advise patient to take oral drug with full glass of water and to drink plenty of fluids; explain that tablet may be crushed and swallowed with water to ensure maximal absorption.
• Teach signs and symptoms of hypersensitivity and other adverse reactions. Urge patient to report bloody urine, difficult breathing, rash, fever, chills, or severe fatigue.
• Advise patient to avoid direct sun exposure and to use a sunscreen to help prevent photosensitivity reactions.
• Tell diabetic patient that sulfonamides may increase effects of oral hypoglycemic drugs. Tell him not to use Clinitest to monitor urine glucose levels.
• Inform patient taking sulfasalazine that it may cause an orange-yellow discoloration of urine or skin and may permanently stain soft contact lenses yellow.

Evaluation
• Patient exhibits no signs of hypersensitivity.
• Patient is free from infection.
• Patient maintains adequate hydration.

Tetracyclines

demeclocycline hydrochloride
doxycycline
doxycycline hyclate
doxycycline hydrochloride
minocycline hydrochloride
oxytetracycline hydrochloride
tetracycline hydrochloride

Indications

▶ Bacterial, protozoal, rickettsial, and fungal infections.

Actions

Tetracyclines are bacteriostatic but may be bactericidal against certain organisms. They bind reversibly to 30S and 50S ribosomal subunits, inhibiting bacterial protein synthesis.

Susceptible gram-positive organisms include *Bacillus anthracis, Actinomyces israelii, Clostridium perfringens, C. tetani, Listeria monocytogenes*, and *Nocardia.*

Susceptible gram-negative organisms include *Neisseria meningitidis, Pasteurella multocida, Legionella pneumophila, Brucella, Vibrio cholerae, Yersinia enterocolitica, Y. pestis, Bordetella pertussis, Haemophilus influenzae, H. ducreyi, Campylobacter fetus, Shigella*, and many other common pathogens.

Other susceptible organisms include *Rickettsia akari, R. typhi, R. prowazekii, R. tsutsugamushi, Coxiella burnetii, Chlamydia trachomatis, C. psittaci, Mycoplasma pneumoniae, M. hominis, Leptospira, Treponema pallidum, T. pertenue*, and *Borrelia recurrentis.*

Adverse reactions

The most common adverse effects involve the GI tract and are dose-related; they include anorexia; flatulence; nausea; vomiting; bulky, loose stools; epigastric burning; and abdominal discomfort. Superinfections also commonly occur. Photosensitivity reactions may be severe. Renal failure has been attributed to Fanconi's syndrome after use of outdated tetracycline. Permanent discoloration of teeth occurs if drug is administered during tooth formation (in children younger than age 8).

Contraindications and precautions

- Contraindicated in patients hypersensitive to tetracyclines.
- Use cautiously in patients with impaired renal or hepatic function.
- **Pregnant patients:** Contraindicated in pregnant patients.
- **Breast-feeding patients:** Tetracyclines appear in breast milk and are contraindicated in breast-feeding women.
- **Pediatric patients:** Children under age 8 shouldn't receive tetracyclines. They can cause permanent tooth discoloration, enamel hypoplasia, and a reversible decrease in bone calcification.
- **Geriatric patients:** Some elderly patients have decreased esophageal motility; use these drugs cautiously and monitor patients for local irritation from slow passage of oral forms. Elderly patients are also more susceptible to superinfection.

NURSING CONSIDERATIONS

Assessment

- Assess patient's allergic history.
- Monitor patient for adverse reactions.
- Obtain culture and sensitivity tests before first dose; check cultures periodically to assess drug effectiveness.
- Check expiration dates before administration. Outdated tetracyclines may cause nephrotoxicity.
- Monitor patient for bacterial and fungal superinfection, especially if patient is elderly, debilitated, or receiving immunosuppressants or radiation therapy; watch especially for oral candidiasis.

Key nursing diagnoses

- Ineffective protection related to hypersensitivity
- Risk for infection related to superinfection
- Risk for deficient fluid volume related to adverse GI reactions

Planning and implementation

- Give all oral tetracyclines except doxycycline and minocycline 1 hour before or 2 hours after meals for maximum absorption; don't give drug with food, milk or other dairy products, sodium bicarbonate, iron compounds, or antacids, which may impair absorption.
- Give water with and after oral drug to facilitate passage to stomach because incomplete swallowing can cause severe esophageal irritation. Don't give drug within 1 hour of bedtime to prevent esophageal reflux.
- Follow manufacturer's directions for reconstituting and storing; keep drug refrigerated and away from light.
- Monitor I.V. injection sites and rotate routinely to minimize local irritation. I.V. administration may cause severe phlebitis.

Prototype drug

Patient teaching

- Urge patient to take drug exactly as prescribed, to complete the prescribed regimen, and to keep follow-up appointments.
- Warn patient not to take drug with food, milk or other dairy products, sodium bicarbonate, or iron compounds because they may interfere with absorption. Advise him to wait 3 hours after taking tetracycline before taking an antacid.
- Instruct patient to check expiration dates and to discard any expired drug.
- Teach signs and symptoms of adverse reactions, and urge him to report them promptly.
- Advise patient to avoid direct exposure to sunlight and to use a sunscreen to help prevent photosensitivity reactions.

Evaluation

- Patient shows no signs of hypersensitivity.
- Patient is free from infection.
- Patient maintains adequate hydration.

Thyroid hormones

levothyroxine sodium
liothyronine sodium
thyroid
thyrotropin

Indications

▶ Hypothyroidism, simple goiter, goitrogenesis.

Actions

Thyroid hormones have catabolic and anabolic effects and influence normal metabolism, growth, and development. Affecting every organ system, they are vital to normal CNS function. Thyroid-stimulating hormone increases iodine uptake by the thyroid and increases formation and release of thyroid hormone; it's isolated from bovine anterior pituitary glands.

Adverse reactions

Adverse reactions include nervousness, insomnia, tremor, tachycardia, palpitations, nausea, headache, fever, and sweating.

Contraindications and precautions

- Contraindicated in patients with MI, thyrotoxicosis, or uncorrected adrenal insufficiency.
- Use with extreme caution in patients with angina pectoris, hypertension or other CV disorders, renal insufficiency, or ischemia.
- Use cautiously in patients with myxedema.
- **Breast-feeding patients:** Minimal amounts of exogenous thyroid hormones appear in breast milk. However, problems have not been reported in breast-feeding infants.
- **Pediatric patients:** During first few months of therapy, children may have partial hair loss. Reassure child and parents that this is temporary.
- **Geriatric patients:** In patients over age 60, initial hormone replacement dosage should be 25% less than the usual recommended starting dosage.

NURSING CONSIDERATIONS

Assessment

- Assess patient's thyroid function studies regularly, as ordered.
- Monitor pulse rate and blood pressure.
- Monitor patient for signs of thyrotoxicosis or inadequate dosage, including diarrhea, fever, irritability, listlessness, rapid heartbeat, vomiting, and weakness.
- Monitor PT and INR; patients taking anticoagulants usually need lower doses.

Key nursing diagnoses

- Risk for injury related to adverse CV reactions
- Disturbed sleep pattern related to insomnia
- Noncompliance related to long-term therapy

Planning and implementation

- Thyroid hormone dosage varies widely among patients. As ordered, begin treatment at lowest level, adjusting to higher doses according to patient's symptoms and laboratory data, until euthyroid state is reached.
- Administer thyroid hormones at same time each day. Morning dosage is preferred to prevent insomnia.

Patient teaching

- Instruct patient to take drug exactly as prescribed. Suggest taking dose in morning to prevent insomnia.
- Advise patient to report signs and symptoms of overdose (chest pain, palpitations, sweating, nervousness) or aggravated CV disease (chest pain, dyspnea, tachycardia).
- Tell patient who has achieved a stable response not to change brands.
- Inform parents that child may lose hair during first months of therapy, but reassure them that this is temporary.

Evaluation

- Patient sustains no injury from adverse reactions.
- Patient gets adequate sleep during the night.
- Patient complies with therapy, as evidenced by normal thyroid hormone levels and resolution of underlying disorder.

Xanthine derivatives

aminophylline
caffeine
theophylline

Indications

▶ Asthma and bronchospasm from emphysema and chronic bronchitis.

Actions

Xanthine derivatives are structurally related; they directly relax smooth muscle, stimulate the CNS, induce diuresis, increase gastric acid secretion, inhibit uterine contractions, and exert weak inotropic and chronotropic effects on the heart. Of these drugs, theophylline exerts the greatest effect on smooth muscle.

The action of xanthine derivatives isn't totally mediated by inhibition of phosphodiesterase. Current data suggest that inhibition of adenosine receptors or other as yet unidentified mechanisms may be responsible for therapeutic effects. By relaxing smooth muscle of the respiratory tract, they increase air flow and vital capacity. They also slow onset of diaphragmatic fatigue and stimulate the respiratory center in the CNS.

Adverse reactions

Adverse effects are dose-related, except for hypersensitivity, and can be controlled by dosage adjustment and monitored via serum levels. Common reactions include hypotension, palpitations, arrhythmias, restlessness, irritability, nausea, vomiting, urine retention, and headache.

Contraindications and precautions

- Contraindicated in patients hypersensitive to xanthines.
- Use cautiously in patients with arrhythmias, cardiac or circulatory impairment, cor pulmonale, hepatic or renal disease, active peptic ulcers, hyperthyroidism, and diabetes mellitus.
- **Breast-feeding patients:** Xanthines appear in breast milk and shouldn't be given to breast-feeding women; infants may have serious adverse reactions.
- **Pediatric patients:** Small children may have excessive CNS stimulation. Monitor them closely.
- **Geriatric patients:** Use cautiously in elderly patients.

NURSING CONSIDERATIONS

Assessment

- Monitor theophylline blood levels closely; therapeutic levels range from 10 to 20 mcg/ml.
- Monitor patient closely for adverse reactions, especially toxicity.
- Monitor vital signs.

Key nursing diagnoses

- Disturbed sleep pattern related to CNS effects
- Urine retention related to adverse effects on bladder
- Noncompliance related to long-term therapy

Planning and implementation

- Don't crush or have patient chew timed-release preparations.
- Expect prescriber to calculate dosage from lean body weight because theophylline doesn't distribute into fatty tissue.

Prototype drug

• Anticipate adjustment of daily dosage in elderly patients and in those with heart failure or hepatic disease.
• Provide patient with sleep aids, such as a back rub or milk-based beverage.

Patient teaching

• Tell patient to take drug exactly as prescribed.
• Caution patient to check with prescriber before using any other drug, including OTC or herbal products, or before switching brands.
• If patient smokes, tell him that doing so may decrease theophylline levels. Urge him to notify prescriber if he quits smoking because the dosage will need adjustment to avoid toxicity.

Evaluation

• Patient sleeps usual number of hours without interruption.
• Patient has no change in voiding pattern.
• Patient complies with therapy, as evidenced by maintenance of therapeutic blood levels.

Alphabetical listing of drugs

A

abacavir sulfate

(uh-BACK-ah-veer SUL-fayt)
Ziagen

Pharmacologic class: nucleoside analogue reverse transcriptase inhibitor
Therapeutic class: antiviral
Pregnancy risk category: C

Indications and dosages

▶ **HIV-1 infection.** *Adults:* 300 mg P.O. b.i.d. in combination with other antiretrovirals. *Children ages 3 months to 16 years:* 8 mg/kg P.O. b.i.d. (maximum of 300 mg P.O. b.i.d.) in combination with other antiretrovirals.

How supplied

Tablets: 300 mg
Oral solution: 20 mg/ml

Pharmacokinetics

Absorption: abacavir is rapidly and extensively absorbed after oral administration; the mean absolute bioavailability of the tablet is 83%. Systemic exposure is comparable for oral solution and tablets; they may be used interchangeably.
Distribution: drug is distributed into extravascular space; about 50% binds to plasma proteins.
Metabolism: in the liver, alcohol dehydrogenase and glucuronyl transferase metabolize the drug to form two inactive metabolites. Cytochrome P-450 enzymes don't significantly metabolize the drug.
Excretion: drug is mainly excreted in urine, with 1.2% unchanged. About 16% of a dose is eliminated in feces. *Half-life (elimination):* 1 to 2 hours.

Route	Onset	Peak	Duration
P.O.	Unknown	Unknown	Unknown

Pharmacodynamics

Chemical effect: inhibits the activity of HIV-1 reverse transcriptase after being converted intracellularly to the active metabolite carbovir triphosphate, thereby terminating viral DNA growth.
Therapeutic effect: reduces the symptoms of HIV-1 infection.

Adverse reactions

CNS: insomnia and sleep disorders, headache.
GI: *nausea, vomiting,* diarrhea, loss of appetite, anorexia.
Skin: rash.
Other: ***hypersensitivity reaction,*** fever, *elevated triglyceride levels.*

Interactions

Drug-lifestyle. *Alcohol use:* decreased elimination of abacavir, increasing overall exposure to drug. Monitor alcohol consumption. Discourage concurrent use.

Contraindications and precautions

- Contraindicated in patients hypersensitive to abacavir or its components. Abacavir therapy can cause fatal hypersensitivity reactions. As soon as a patient develops evidence of hypersensitivity—such as fever, rash, fatigue, nausea, vomiting, diarrhea, or abdominal pain—he should stop the drug and seek medical attention immediately.
- Use cautiously when giving drug to patients with risk factors for liver disease. Lactic acidosis and severe hepatomegaly with steatosis, including fatal cases, have been reported with the use of nucleoside analogues alone or in combination, including abacavir and other antiretrovirals. Women are more likely than men to be affected. Obesity and prolonged nucleoside exposure may be risk factors.
- Use cautiously in pregnant women because no adequate studies of drug effect on pregnancy exist. Use during pregnancy only if potential benefits outweigh risk.

NURSING CONSIDERATIONS

Assessment

- Assess patient's condition before therapy and regularly thereafter.

• Watch for hypersensitivity reaction.
• Assess patient for risk factors for liver disease. Lactic acidosis and severe hepatomegaly with steatosis have been reported, especially in women or patients who are obese or have prolonged exposure to nucleosides. Stop treatment, as ordered, if patient develops evidence of lactic acidosis or pronounced hepatotoxicity, which may include hepatomegaly and steatosis even without elevated transaminase levels.
• Evaluate patient's and family's knowledge of drug therapy.

Nursing diagnoses
• Risk for infection secondary to presence of HIV
• Ineffective individual coping related to HIV infection
• Deficient knowledge related to drug therapy

Planning and implementation
• Drug should always be given in combination with other antiretrovirals, never alone.
• Use cautiously in pregnant women and only if potential benefits outweigh risk. Register pregnant women taking abacavir with the Antiretroviral Pregnancy Registry at 1-800-258-4263.
• Don't restart drug after a hypersensitivity reaction because more severe signs and symptoms will recur within hours and may include life-threatening hypotension and death. To facilitate reporting of hypersensitivity reactions, register patients with the Abacavir Hypersensitivity Registry at 1-800-270-0425.
• Drug may cause mildly elevated blood glucose levels. Monitor serum glucose during therapy.

Patient teaching
• Inform patient that abacavir can cause a life-threatening hypersensitivity reaction. Tell patient to stop drug and notify prescriber immediately if evidence of hypersensitivity develops—such as fever, skin rash, severe tiredness, achiness, a generally ill feeling, or GI signs or symptoms such as nausea, vomiting, diarrhea, or stomach pain.
• Give written information about drug with each new prescription and refill. Patient should also receive—and be instructed to carry—a warning card summarizing abacavir hypersensitivity reaction.
• Explain that this drug neither cures HIV infection nor reduces the risk of transmitting HIV to others. Furthermore, its long-term effects are unknown.
• Tell patient to take drug exactly as prescribed.
• Inform patient that drug can be taken with or without food.

Evaluation
• Patient has reduced signs and symptoms of infection.
• Patient demonstrates adequate coping mechanisms.
• Patient and family state understanding of drug therapy.

abciximab
(ab-SIKS-ih-mahb)
ReoPro

Pharmacologic class: fab fragment of chimeric human-murine monoclonal antibody 7E3
Therapeutic class: platelet aggregation inhibitor
Pregnancy risk category: C

Indications and dosages
▶ **Adjunct to percutaneous transluminal coronary angioplasty (PTCA) or atherectomy for prevention of acute cardiac ischemic complications in patients at high risk for abrupt closure of treated coronary vessel.** *Adults:* 0.25 mg/kg as I.V. bolus 10 to 60 minutes before PTCA or atherectomy, followed by continuous I.V. infusion of 10 mcg/minute for 12 hours.

How supplied
Injection: 2 mg/ml

Pharmacokinetics
Absorption: not applicable with I.V. administration.

Distribution: rapidly binds to platelet GPllb/llla receptors.
Metabolism: not reported.
Excretion: not reported. *Half-life:* initially, less than 10 minutes; second phase, about 30 minutes.

Route	Onset	Peak	Duration
I.V.	Almost immediate	Almost immediate	About 24 hr

Pharmacodynamics

Chemical effect: prevents binding of fibrinogen, von Willebrand factor, and other adhesive molecules to GPIIb/IIIa receptor sites on activated platelets.
Therapeutic effect: inhibits platelet aggregation.

Adverse reactions

CNS: hypoesthesia, confusion.
CV: *hypotension, **bradycardia,*** peripheral edema.
EENT: abnormal vision.
GI: *nausea, vomiting.*
Hematologic: bleeding, ***thrombocytopenia,*** anemia, leukocytosis.
Respiratory: pleural effusion, pleurisy, pneumonia.
Other: pain.

Interactions

Drug-drug. *Antiplatelet drugs, heparin, NSAIDs, other anticoagulants, thrombolytics:* increased risk of bleeding. Monitor patient closely.

Contraindications and precautions

- Contraindicated in patients hypersensitive to a drug component or to murine proteins; in those with active internal bleeding, GI or GU bleeding of clinical significance within 6 weeks, history of CVA within 2 years or with significant residual neurologic deficit, bleeding diathesis, thrombocytopenia (less than 100,000/mm^3), major surgery or trauma within 6 weeks, intracranial neoplasm, intracranial arteriovenous malformation, intracranial aneurysm, severe uncontrolled hypertension, or history of vasculitis; when oral anticoagulants have been given within 7 days unless PT is less than or equal to 1.2 times control; or with use of I.V. dextran before PTCA or intent to use it during PTCA.
- Use cautiously in patients at increased risk for bleeding (those who weigh under 75 kg, are over age 65, have history of GI disease, or are receiving thrombolytic drugs). Conditions that also increase risk of bleeding include PTCA within 12 hours of onset of symptoms for acute MI, prolonged PTCA (lasting more than 70 minutes), failed PTCA, and concomitant use of heparin with abciximab.
- Use cautiously in pregnant or breast-feeding women.
- Safety of drug hasn't been established in children.

NURSING CONSIDERATIONS

Assessment

- Note patient's history. Patients at risk for abrupt closure (candidates for abciximab) include those undergoing PTCA with at least one of the following conditions: unstable angina or non-Q wave MI, acute Q wave MI within 12 hours of onset of symptoms, two type B lesions in artery to be dilated, one type B lesion in artery to be dilated in a woman over age 65 or a patient with diabetes, one type C lesion in artery to be dilated, or angioplasty of infarct-related lesion within 7 days of MI.
- Assess vital signs and evaluate bleeding studies before therapy.
- Monitor patient closely for bleeding. Bleeding caused by therapy falls into two broad categories: that observed at arterial access site used for cardiac catheterization and internal bleeding involving GI or GU tract or retroperitoneal sites.
- Be alert for adverse reactions and drug interactions.
- Evaluate patient's and family's knowledge of drug therapy.

Nursing diagnoses

- Ineffective cerebral or cardiopulmonary tissue perfusion related to patient's underlying condition
- Risk for deficient fluid volume related to drug-induced bleeding
- Deficient knowledge related to drug therapy

Planning and implementation
• Inspect solution for particulate matter before administering it. If you see opaque particles, discard solution and obtain new vial. Withdraw necessary amount of abciximab for I.V. bolus injection through sterile, nonpyrogenic, low-protein-binding 0.2- or 0.22-micron filter into syringe. Give I.V. bolus 10 to 60 minutes before procedure.
• Withdraw 4.5 ml of drug for continuous I.V. infusion through sterile, nonpyrogenic, low-protein-binding 0.2- or 0.22-micron filter into syringe. Inject into 250 ml of sterile normal saline solution or D_5W and infuse at 17 ml/hour for 12 hours via continuous infusion pump equipped with in-line filter. Discard unused portion.
• Administer drug in separate I.V. line; don't add other medication to infusion solution.
• Institute bleeding precautions. Keep patient on bed rest for 6 to 8 hours after removing sheath or stopping abciximab infusion, whichever is later.
ALERT Keep epinephrine, dopamine, theophylline, antihistamines, and corticosteroids available in case of anaphylaxis.
• Drug is intended for use with aspirin and heparin.

Patient teaching
• Teach patient about his disease and therapy.
• Stress the importance of reporting signs and symptoms.

Evaluation
• Patient maintains adequate tissue perfusion.
• Patient maintains adequate hydration.
• Patient and family state understanding of drug therapy.

acarbose
(ay-KAR-bohs)
Precose

Pharmacologic class: alpha-glucosidase inhibitor
Therapeutic class: antidiabetic
Pregnancy risk category: B

Indications and dosages
▶ **Adjunct to diet to lower blood glucose in patients with type 2 (non-insulin-dependent) diabetes mellitus whose hyperglycemia can't be managed by diet alone or by diet and a sulfonylurea.** *Adults:* Initially, 25 mg P.O. t.i.d. at start of each main meal. Subsequent dosage adjustment made q 4 to 8 weeks, based on 1-hour postprandial glucose level and tolerance. Maintenance dosage is 50 to 100 mg P.O. t.i.d.
▶ **Adjunct to insulin or metformin therapy in patients with type 2 (non-insulin-dependent) diabetes mellitus whose hyperglycemia can't be managed by diet, exercise, and insulin or metformin alone.** *Adults:* initially, 25 mg P.O. three times daily with first bite of each main meal. Adjust dosage at 4- to 8-week intervals based on 1-hour postprandial glucose levels and tolerance to determine minimum effective dosage of each drug. Maintenance dosage is 50 to 100 mg P.O. three times daily based on patient's weight. Maximum dosage for patients weighing 60 kg (132 lb) or less is 50 mg P.O. three times daily; for patients weighing over 60 kg, maximum dosage is 100 mg P.O. three times daily.

How supplied
Tablets: 25 mg, 50 mg, 100 mg

Pharmacokinetics
Absorption: minimally absorbed.
Distribution: acts locally within GI tract.
Metabolism: metabolized exclusively in the GI tract, primarily by intestinal bacteria and to a lesser extent by digestive enzymes.
Excretion: almost completely excreted by the kidneys. *Half-life:* 2 hours.

Route	Onset	Peak	Duration
P.O.	Unknown	1 hr	2-4 hr

Pharmacodynamics
Chemical effect: an alpha-glucosidase inhibitor that delays digestion of carbohydrates.
Therapeutic effect: delayed glucose absorption and lower postprandial hyperglycemia.

Adverse reactions
GI: *abdominal pain, diarrhea, flatulence.*

Other: elevated serum transaminase levels.

Interactions

Drug-drug. *Calcium channel blockers, corticosteroids, estrogens, isoniazid, nicotinic acid, oral contraceptives, phenothiazines, phenytoin, sympathomimetics, thiazides and other diuretics, thyroid products:* may cause hyperglycemia during concomitant use or hypoglycemia when withdrawn. Monitor blood glucose level.
Digestive enzyme preparations containing carbohydrate-splitting enzymes (such as amylase, pancreatin), intestinal adsorbents (such as activated charcoal): may reduce effect of acarbose. Don't administer concomitantly.
Drug-herb. *Aloe, bitter melon, bilberry leaf, burdock, dandelion, fenugreek, garlic, ginseng:* may improve blood glucose control and allow reduced antidiabetic dosage. Urge patient to discuss herbal products with prescriber before use.

Contraindications and precautions

- Contraindicated in patients hypersensitive to drug and in those with diabetic ketoacidosis, cirrhosis, inflammatory bowel disease, colonic ulceration, partial intestinal obstruction, predisposition to intestinal obstruction, chronic intestinal disease with marked disorder of digestion or absorption, or conditions that may deteriorate because of increased intestinal gas formation.
- Drug isn't recommended in renally impaired patients or pregnant or breast-feeding women.
- Use cautiously in patients receiving a sulfonylurea or insulin. Acarbose may increase the hypoglycemic potential of the sulfonylurea.
- Safety and efficacy of drug haven't been established in children.

NURSING CONSIDERATIONS

Assessment

- Monitor patient's plasma glucose level 1 hour after a meal to determine therapeutic effectiveness of acarbose and to identify appropriate dose. Report hyperglycemia to prescriber.
- Monitor glycosylated hemoglobin every 3 months.
- Monitor serum transaminase level every 3 months in first year of therapy and periodically thereafter in patients receiving doses in excess of 50 mg t.i.d. Report abnormalities.
- Obtain baseline serum creatinine levels; drug isn't recommended in patients with a serum creatinine greater than 2 mg/dl.
- Evaluate patient's and family's knowledge of drug therapy.

Nursing diagnoses

- Risk for imbalanced fluid volume related to adverse GI effect
- Imbalanced nutrition: less than body requirements related to patient's underlying condition
- Deficient knowledge related to drug therapy

Planning and implementation

- In patients weighing less than 60 kg (132 lb), don't exceed 50 mg P.O. t.i.d.
- Watch for elevated serum transaminase and bilirubin levels and low serum calcium and plasma vitamin B_6 levels with doses exceeding 50 mg t.i.d.
- Acarbose may increase hypoglycemic potential of sulfonylureas. Monitor patient receiving both drugs closely. If hypoglycemia occurs, treat with oral glucose (dextrose), I.V. glucose infusion, or glucagon administration. Report hypoglycemia to prescriber.
- Insulin therapy may be needed during increased stress (infection, fever, surgery, or trauma).

Patient teaching

- Tell patient to take drug daily with first bite of each of three main meals.
- Explain that therapy relieves symptoms but doesn't cure the disease.
- Stress importance of adhering to specific diet, weight reduction, exercise, and hygiene programs. Show patient how to monitor blood glucose level and to recognize and treat hyperglycemia.
- Teach patient to recognize hypoglycemia and to treat symptoms with a form of dextrose rather than with a product containing table sugar.
- Urge patient to carry medical identification at all times.

Evaluation
- Patient maintains adequate fluid volume balance.
- Patient doesn't experience hypoglycemic episodes.
- Patient and family state understanding of drug therapy.

acebutolol
(as-ih-BYOO-tuh-lol)
Monitan, Sectral

Pharmacologic class: beta blocker
Therapeutic class: antihypertensive, antiarrhythmic
Pregnancy risk category: B

Indications and dosages
▶ **Hypertension.** *Adults:* 400 mg P.O. as single daily dose or in divided doses b.i.d. Patients may receive as much as 1,200 mg daily.
▶ **Suppression of PVCs.** *Adults:* 400 mg P.O. in divided doses b.i.d. Dosage increased to provide adequate clinical response. Usual dosage is 600 to 1,200 mg daily. In patients with impaired renal function, dosage is reduced. Elderly patients may require lower dosage; dosage shouldn't exceed 800 mg daily.

How supplied
Capsules: 200 mg, 400 mg

Pharmacokinetics
Absorption: well absorbed after oral administration.
Distribution: about 25% protein-bound; minimal quantities detected in CSF.
Metabolism: undergoes extensive first-pass metabolism in liver.
Excretion: from 30% to 40% of dose is excreted in urine; remainder, in feces and bile. *Half-life:* 3 to 4 hours.

Route	Onset	Peak	Duration
P.O.	1-1.5 hr	2.5 hr	Up to 24 hr

Pharmacodynamics
Chemical effect: antihypertensive action unknown. Possible mechanisms include reduced cardiac output, decreased sympathetic outflow to peripheral vasculature, and inhibited renin release. Antiarrhythmic action decreases myocardial contractility and heart rate and has mild intrinsic sympathomimetic activity.
Therapeutic effect: lowers blood pressure and heart rate and restores normal sinus rhythm.

Adverse reactions
CNS: *fatigue,* headache, dizziness, insomnia.
CV: chest pain, edema, ***bradycardia, heart failure, hypotension.***
GI: nausea, constipation, diarrhea, dyspepsia.
Respiratory: dyspnea, ***bronchospasm.***
Skin: rash.
Other: fever, positive antinuclear antibody test.

Interactions
Drug-drug. *Alpha-adrenergic stimulants*: increased hypertensive response. Use together cautiously.
Cardiac glycosides, diltiazem, verapamil: excessive bradycardia and increased depressant effect on myocardium. Use together cautiously.
Insulin, oral antidiabetics: can alter dosage requirements in previously stabilized diabetic patient. Observe patient carefully.
NSAIDs: decreased antihypertensive effect. Monitor blood pressure. Dosage may require adjustment.
Reserpine: additive effect. Monitor patient closely.

Contraindications and precautions
- Contraindicated in breast-feeding women and in patients with persistently severe bradycardia, second- or third-degree heart block, overt heart failure, or cardiogenic shock.
- Use cautiously in pregnant women and in patients with heart failure, peripheral vascular disease, bronchospastic disease, or diabetes.
- Safety of drug hasn't been established in children.

NURSING CONSIDERATIONS

Assessment
- Assess patient's blood pressure and heart rate and rhythm before and during therapy.
- Monitor patient's energy level.

- Be alert for adverse reactions and drug interactions.
- Evaluate patient's and family's knowledge of drug therapy.

Nursing diagnoses

- Risk for injury related to patient's underlying condition
- Fatigue related to drug-induced CNS adverse reactions
- Deficient knowledge related to drug therapy

Planning and implementation

- Dosage should be reduced in elderly patient and patients with decreased renal function.
- Check apical pulse before giving drug; if slower than 60 beats/minute, withhold drug and call prescriber.

ALERT Don't stop drug abruptly; doing so may worsen angina and MI.

- Before surgery, notify anesthesiologist about patient's drug therapy.

Patient teaching

- Teach patient how to take his pulse, and instruct him to withhold dose and notify prescriber if pulse rate is below 60 beats/minute.
- Warn patient that drug may cause dizziness. Instruct him to avoid sudden position changes and to sit down immediately if he feels dizzy.
- Explain the importance of taking drug as prescribed, even when feeling well.

Evaluation

- Patient's blood pressure and heart rate and rhythm are normal.
- Patient effectively combats fatigue.
- Patient and family state understanding of drug therapy.

acetaminophen (APAP, paracetamol)

(as-ee-tuh-MIH-nuh-fin)

Abenol♦ ; Aceta Elixir*†; Acetaminophen Uniserts†; Aceta Tablets†; Actamin†; Actimol♦†; Aminofen†; Anacin-3†; Anacin-3 Children's Elixir*†; Anacin-3 Children's Tablets†; Anacin-3 Extra Strength†; Anacin-3 Infants'†; Apacet Capsules†; Apacet Elixir*†; Apacet Extra Strength Caplets†; Apacet Infants'†; Apo-Acetaminophen♦†; Arthritis Pain Formula Aspirin Free†; Atasol Caplets♦†; Atasol Drops♦†; Atasol Elixir*♦†; Atasol Tablets♦†; Banesin†; Dapa†; Dapa XS†; Datril XS; Dolanex*†; Dorcol Children's Fever and Pain Reducer†; Dymadon◊†; Exdol♦†; Feverall, Children's◊; Feverall Junior Strength◊; Feverall Sprinkle Caps◊; Genapap Children's Elixir†; Genapap Children's Tablets†; Genapap Extra Strength Caplets†; Genapap, Infants'†; Genapap Regular Strength Tablets†; Genebs Extra Strength Caplets†; Genebs Regular Strength Tablets†; Genebs X-Tra†; Halenol Elixir*†; Liquiprin Infants' Drops†; Meda Cap†; Myapap Elixir*†; Myapap, Infants'†; Neopap†; Oraphen-PD†; Panadol†; Panadol, Children's†; Panadol Extra Strength†; Panadol, Infants'†; Panadol Maximum Strength Caplets†; Panamax◊†; Panex†; Panex-500†; Paralgin◊†; Paraspen◊†; Redutemp†; Ridenol Caplets†; Robigesic♦†; Rounox♦†; Setamol-500◊†; Snaplets-FR†; Stanback AF Extra Strength Powder; St. Joseph Aspirin-Free Fever Reducer for Children†; Suppap-120†; Suppap-325†; Suppap-650†; Tapanol Extra Strength Caplets†; Tapanol Extra Strength Tablets†; Tempra†; Tempra D.S.†; Tempra, Infants'†; Tempra Syrup†; Tenol†; Tylenol Children's Elixir†; Tylenol Children's Tablets†; Tylenol Extended Relief†; Tylenol Extra Strength Caplets†; Tylenol Infants'†; Tylenol Junior Strength Caplets†; Ty-Pap†; Ty-Pap, Infants'†; Ty-Pap Syrup†; Ty-Tab Caplets†; Ty-Tab Capsules†; Ty-Tab, Children's†; Ty-Tab Tablets†; Valorin†; Valorin Extra†

Pharmacologic class: para-aminophenol derivative
Therapeutic class: nonnarcotic analgesic, antipyretic
Pregnancy risk category: B

Indications and dosages

▶ **Mild pain or fever.** *Adults and children over age 12:* 325 to 650 mg P.O. or P.R. q 4

hours, p.r.n.; or 1 g P.O. t.i.d. or q.i.d., p.r.n. Alternatively, 2 extended-release caplets P.O. q 8 hours. Maximum, 4 g daily. Dosage for long-term therapy shouldn't exceed 2.6 g daily.
Children ages 11 to 12: 480 mg P.O. or P.R. q 4 to 6 hours.
Children ages 9 to 10: 400 mg P.O. or P.R. q 4 to 6 hours.
Children ages 6 to 8: 320 mg P.O. or P.R. q 4 to 6 hours.
Children ages 4 to 5: 240 mg P.O. or P.R. q 4 to 6 hours.
Children ages 2 to 3: 160 mg P.O. or P.R. q 4 to 6 hours.
Children ages 12 to 23 months: 120 mg P.O. q 4 to 6 hours.
Children ages 4 to 11 months: 80 mg P.O. q 4 to 6 hours.
Children up to age 3 months: 40 mg P.O. q 4 to 6 hours.

How supplied

Tablets: 160 mg†, 325 mg†, 500 mg†, 650 mg†
Tablets (chewable): 80 mg†, 160 mg†
Caplets (extended-release): 650 mg
Capsules: 500 mg†
Oral solution: 48 mg/ml†, 100 mg/ml†
Oral suspension: 120 mg/5 ml ◊, 100 mg/ml†, 160 mg/ml†
Oral liquid: 160 mg/5 ml†, 500 mg/15 ml†
Elixir: 120 mg/5 ml, 130 mg/5 ml*†, 160 mg/5 ml*†, 325 mg/5 ml*†
Granules: 80 mg/packet†, 325 mg/capful†
Powder for solution: 1 g/packet
Sprinkles: 80 mg/capsule, 160 mg/capsule
Tablets for solution: 325 mg
Suppositories: 120 mg†, 125 mg†, 300 mg†, 325 mg†, 650 mg†
Wafers: 120 mg†

Pharmacokinetics

Absorption: absorbed rapidly and completely via GI tract.
Distribution: 25% protein-bound. Plasma levels don't correlate well with analgesic effect but do correlate with toxicity.
Metabolism: from 90% to 95% metabolized in liver.
Excretion: excreted in urine. *Half-life:* 1 to 4 hours.

Route	Onset	Peak	Duration
P.O., P.R.	Unknown	1-3 hr	1-3 hr

Pharmacodynamics

Chemical effect: unknown. May produce analgesia by blocking pain impulses, probably by inhibiting prostaglandin or other substances that sensitize pain receptors. May relieve fever by action in hypothalamic heat-regulating center.
Therapeutic effect: relieves pain and reduces fever.

Adverse reactions

Hematologic: hemolytic anemia, ***neutropenia, leukopenia, pancytopenia, thrombocytopenia.***
Hepatic: ***liver damage*** (with toxic doses), jaundice.
Metabolic: hypoglycemia.
Skin: rash, urticaria.

Interactions

Drug-drug. *Barbiturates, carbamazepine, hydantoins, rifampin, sulfinpyrazone, isoniazid:* high doses or long-term use of these drugs may reduce therapeutic effects and enhance hepatotoxic effects of acetaminophen. Avoid concomitant use.
Warfarin: increased hypoprothrombinemic effects with long-term use with high doses of acetaminophen. Monitor PT and INR closely.
Zidovudine: may increase risk of bone marrow suppression because of impaired zidovudine metabolism. Monitor patient closely.
Drug-food. *Caffeine:* may enhance analgesic effects of acetaminophen. Monitor patient for effect.
Drug-lifestyle. *Alcohol use:* increased risk of hepatic damage. Warn against concomitant use.

Contraindications and precautions

- No known contraindications.
- Use cautiously in patients with history of chronic alcohol abuse; hepatotoxicity has occurred after therapeutic doses.
- Use cautiously in pregnant or breast-feeding women.

NURSING CONSIDERATIONS

Assessment

- Assess patient's pain or temperature before and during therapy.
- Assess patient's medication history. Many OTC products contain acetaminophen; be aware of this when calculating total daily dosage.
- Be alert for adverse reactions and drug interactions.
- Evaluate patient's and family's knowledge of drug therapy.

Nursing diagnoses

- Acute pain related to patient's underlying condition
- Risk for injury related to drug-induced liver damage with toxic doses
- Deficient knowledge related to drug therapy

Planning and implementation

P.O. use: Administer liquid form to children and other patients who have trouble swallowing.

ALERT When giving oral preparations, calculate dosage based on level of drug since drops and elixir have different concentrations.

P.R. use: Use this route in small children and other patients when oral administration isn't feasible.

- Acetaminophen may interfere with laboratory tests for urinary 5-hydroxyindoleacetic acid and may produce false-positive decrease in blood glucose level in home monitoring system.

Patient teaching

- Tell parents to consult prescriber before giving drug to children under age 2.
- Tell patient that drug is for short-term use only. Prescriber should be consulted if administering to children for more than 5 days or to adults for more than 10 days.
- Tell patient not to use drug for marked fever (over 103.1° F [39.5° C]), fever persisting longer than 3 days, or recurrent fever unless directed by prescriber.
- Warn patient that high doses or unsupervised long-term use can cause hepatic damage. Excessive ingestion of alcoholic beverages may increase risk of hepatotoxicity.
- Tell breast-feeding patient that drug is found in breast milk in low levels (less than 1% of dose). Patient may use it safely if therapy is short-term and doesn't exceed recommended doses.

Evaluation

- Patient reports pain relief with drug.
- Patient's liver function studies remain normal.
- Patient and family state understanding of drug therapy.

acetazolamide

(ah-see-tuh-ZOH-luh-mighd)

Acetazolam ♦, Apo-Acetazolamide ♦, Diamox, Diamox Sequels

acetazolamide sodium

Diamox Parenteral, Diamox Sodium

Pharmacologic class: carbonic anhydrase inhibitor

Therapeutic class: adjunct treatment of open-angle glaucoma and perioperative treatment for acute angle-closure glaucoma, anticonvulsant, management of edema, prevention and treatment of acute mountain sickness

Pregnancy risk category: C

Indications and dosages

▶ **Secondary glaucoma and preoperative management of acute angle-closure glaucoma.** *Adults:* 250 mg P.O. q 4 hours, or 250 mg P.O. or I.V. b.i.d. for short-term therapy. I.V. administration (100 to 500 mg/minute) is preferred.

▶ **Edema in heart failure.** *Adults:* 250 to 375 mg (5 mg/kg) P.O. daily in a.m.

▶ **Chronic open-angle glaucoma.** *Adults:* 250 mg to 1 g P.O. daily in divided doses q.i.d., or 500 mg (extended-release) P.O. b.i.d.

▶ **Prevention or amelioration of acute mountain sickness.** *Adults:* 500 mg to 1 g P.O. daily in divided doses q 8 to 12 hours, or 500 mg (extended-release) P.O. b.i.d. Treat-

ment started 24 to 48 hours before ascent and continued for 48 hours while at high altitude.
▶ **Adjunct treatment of myoclonic, refractory generalized tonic-clonic, absence, or mixed seizures.** *Adults and children:* 8 to 30 mg/kg P.O. daily in divided doses. For adults, optimum dosage is 375 mg to 1 g daily. Usually given with other anticonvulsants.

How supplied

Tablets: 125 mg, 250 mg
Capsules (extended-release): 500 mg
Injection: 500 mg/vial

Pharmacokinetics

Absorption: well absorbed from GI tract after oral administration.
Distribution: distributed throughout body tissues.
Metabolism: none.
Excretion: excreted primarily in urine through tubular secretion and passive reabsorption.
Half-life: 10 to 15 hours.

Route	Onset	Peak	Duration
P.O.			
Tablets	1-1.5 hr	2-4 hr	8-12 hr
Capsules	2 hr	8-12 hr	18-24 hr
I.V.	2 min	15 min	4-5 hr

Pharmacodynamics

Chemical effect: blocks action of carbonic anhydrase, promoting renal excretion of sodium, potassium, bicarbonate, and water, and decreases secretion of aqueous humor in eye. As anticonvulsant, may inhibit carbonic anhydrase in CNS and decrease abnormal paroxysmal or excessive neuronal discharge. In acute mountain sickness, carbonic anhydrase inhibitors produce respiratory and metabolic acidosis that may stimulate ventilation, increase cerebral blood flow, and promote release of oxygen from hemoglobin.
Therapeutic effect: lowers intraocular pressure, controls seizure activity, and may improve respiratory function.

Adverse reactions

CNS: drowsiness, paresthesia, confusion.
EENT: transient myopia.
GI: nausea, vomiting, anorexia, altered taste.
GU: crystalluria, renal calculi, hematuria, asymptomatic hyperuricemia
Hematologic: ***aplastic anemia,*** hemolytic anemia, ***leukopenia.***
Metabolic: hyperchloremic acidosis, hypokalemia.
Skin: rash.
Other: *pain at injection site,* sterile abscesses.

Interactions

Drug-drug. *Amphetamines, anticholinergics, mecamylamine, quinidine, tricyclic antidepressants, procainamide:* decreased renal clearance of these drugs, increasing toxicity. Monitor patient closely.
Lithium: increase lithium secretion. Monitor patient.
Methenamine: reduced effectiveness of acetazolamide. Avoid concomitant use.
Salicylates: possible accumulation and toxicity of acetazolamide, including CNS depression and metabolic acidosis. Monitor patient closely.

Contraindications and precautions

• Contraindicated in patients hypersensitive to drug; in those undergoing long-term therapy for chronic noncongestive angle-closure glaucoma; in those with hyponatremia or hypokalemia, renal or hepatic disease or dysfunction, adrenal gland failure, or hyperchloremic acidosis; and in breast-feeding women.
• Use cautiously in patients with respiratory acidosis, emphysema, or chronic pulmonary disease; in patients receiving other diuretics; and in pregnant women.
• Safety of drug hasn't been established in children.

NURSING CONSIDERATIONS

Assessment

• Assess patient's underlying condition before and during therapy, including, as appropriate, eye discomfort and intraocular pressure in those with glaucoma; edema in those with heart failure; and neurologic status in those with seizures. Also monitor intake and output.

• Be alert for adverse reactions and drug interactions.
• Evaluate patient's and family's knowledge of drug therapy.

Nursing diagnoses
• Excessive fluid volume related to patient's underlying condition
• Impaired urine elimination related to diuretic action of drug
• Deficient knowledge related to drug therapy

Planning and implementation
P.O. use: Give oral preparations early in morning to avoid nocturia. Give second doses early in afternoon.
• Check with pharmacist if patient can't swallow oral forms. He may make suspension using crushed tablets in highly flavored syrup, such as cherry, raspberry, or chocolate. Although concentrations up to 500 mg/5 ml are feasible, concentrations of 250 mg/5 ml are more palatable. Refrigeration improves palatability but doesn't improve stability. Suspensions are stable for 1 week.
I.V. use: Reconstitute 500-mg vial with at least 5 ml of sterile water for injection. Use within 24 hours. Inject 100 to 500 mg/minute into large vein, using 21G or 23G needle. Intermittent or continuous infusion isn't recommended.
• Diuretic effect decreases with acidosis but is reestablished by withdrawing drug for several days and then restarting it or by using intermittent administration.
ALERT Don't confuse acetazolamide with acetohexamide.
• Withhold drug and notify prescriber if hypersensitivity or adverse reactions occur.
• Drug may cause false-positive urine protein tests.

Patient teaching
• Advise patient to take drug early in day to avoid interruption of sleep caused by nocturia.
• Teach patient to monitor fluid volume by daily weight and intake and output.
• Encourage patient to avoid high-sodium foods and to choose high-potassium foods.
• Teach patient to recognize and report signs and symptoms of fluid and electrolyte imbalance.

Evaluation
• Patient is free from edema.
• Patient adjusts lifestyle to accommodate altered patterns of urine elimination.
• Patient and family state understanding of drug therapy.

acetohexamide
(ah-see-toh-HEKS-ah-mighd)
Dimelor♦, Dymelor

Pharmacologic class: sulfonylurea
Therapeutic class: antidiabetic
Pregnancy risk category: C

Indications and dosages
▶ **Adjunct to diet to lower blood glucose level in patients with type 2 (non-insulin-dependent) diabetes mellitus.** *Adults:* initially, 250 mg P.O. daily before breakfast; dosage increased q 5 to 7 days (by 250 to 500 mg) as needed to maximum of 1.5 g daily in divided doses b.i.d. or t.i.d. before meals.
▶ **Replacement of insulin therapy in patients with type 2 (non-insulin-dependent) diabetes mellitus.** *Adults:* if insulin dosage is less than 20 units daily, insulin is stopped and oral therapy started with 250 mg P.O. daily, before breakfast, and increased as above if needed. If insulin dosage is 20 to 40 units daily, oral therapy is started with 250 mg P.O. daily, before breakfast, while insulin dosage is reduced 25% to 30% daily or every other day, depending on response to oral therapy.

How supplied
Tablets: 250 mg, 500 mg

Pharmacokinetics
Absorption: absorbed rapidly from GI tract.
Distribution: not fully understood, but probably similar to that of other sulfonylureas; drug is highly protein-bound.
Metabolism: metabolized in liver, primarily to potent active metabolite.

Excretion: about 80% excreted in urine. *Half-life:* about 6 hours.

Route	Onset	Peak	Duration
P.O.	≤ 1 hr	≤ 2 hr	12-24 hr

Pharmacodynamics

Chemical effect: unknown. Probably stimulates insulin release from pancreatic beta cells and reduces glucose output by liver. Increases sensitivity to insulin at cellular level.
Therapeutic effect: lowers blood sugar.

Adverse reactions

GI: nausea, heartburn, vomiting.
Hematologic: ***thrombocytopenia, aplastic anemia, agranulocytosis, leukopenia.***
Metabolic: sodium loss, hypoglycemia.
Skin: rash, pruritus, facial flushing.
Other: hypersensitivity reactions.

Interactions

Drug-drug. *Anabolic steroids, chloramphenicol, clofibrate, guanethidine, ketoconazole, MAO inhibitors, omeprazole, phenylbutazone, probenecid, salicylates, sulfonamides:* increased hypoglycemic activity. Monitor blood glucose level.
Beta blockers, clonidine: prolonged hypoglycemic effect and masked symptoms of hypoglycemia. Use together cautiously.
Corticosteroids, diazoxide, glucagon, hydantoins, rifampin, thiazide diuretics: decreased hypoglycemic response. Monitor blood glucose level.
Oral anticoagulants: increased hypoglycemic activity or enhanced anticoagulant effect. Monitor PT, INR, and blood glucose level.
Drug-herb. *Aloe, bitter melon, bilberry leaf, fenugreek, garlic, ginseng:* May improve blood glucose control and allow a reduced dosage of oral hypoglycemics. Tell patient to consult prescriber before using these herbs.
Drug-lifestyle. *Alcohol use:* possible disulfiram-like reaction. Discourage concomitant use.

Contraindications and precautions

- Contraindicated in patients with type 1 diabetes or diabetes that can be adequately controlled by diet; type 2 diabetes complicated by ketosis, acidosis, or diabetic coma; hyperglycemia with primary renal disease; major surgery; severe infections or trauma; or hypersensitivity to sulfonylureas; and in pregnant or breast-feeding patients.
- Use cautiously in patients with history of porphyria or impaired hepatic or renal function and in debilitated, malnourished, or elderly patients.
- Safety of drug hasn't been established in children.

NURSING CONSIDERATIONS

Assessment
- Assess patient's blood glucose level before and frequently during therapy.
- Monitor patient's glycosylated hemoglobin, as ordered.
- Be alert for adverse reactions and drug interactions.
- Evaluate patient's and family's knowledge of drug therapy.

Nursing diagnoses
- Ineffective health maintenance related to hyperglycemia
- Risk for injury related to drug-induced hypoglycemia
- Deficient knowledge related to drug therapy

Planning and implementation
- Consider that some patients taking drug may be controlled effectively on once-daily regimen, whereas others show better response with divided dosing.
- Administer once-daily doses with breakfast; divided doses, before morning and evening meals.
- Treat hypoglycemic reaction with oral form of rapid-acting glucose if patient is awake or with glucagon or I.V. glucose if patient can't be aroused. Follow treatment with complex carbohydrate snack if mealtime is more than 1 hour away, and determine cause of reaction.
ALERT Don't confuse acetohexamide with acetazolamide.

Patient teaching
- Emphasize importance of following prescribed diet, exercise, and medical regimens.

• Tell patient to take drug at same time each day; to take missed dose immediately, unless it's almost time for next dose; and to refrain from taking double doses.
• Advise patient to avoid alcohol during drug therapy. Remind him that many foods and OTC medications contain alcohol.
• Encourage patient to wear a medical identification bracelet or necklace.
• Tell patient to take drug with food (once-daily dosage with breakfast).
• Teach patient how to monitor blood glucose level.
• Teach patient how to recognize signs and symptoms of hyperglycemia and hypoglycemia and what to do if they occur.
• Stress the importance of compliance with drug therapy.

☑ Evaluation

• Patient's blood glucose level is normal.
• Patient recognizes hypoglycemia early and treats it effectively before injury occurs.
• Patient and family state understanding of drug therapy.

acetylcysteine

(as-ee-til-SIS-teen)

Airbron♦, Mucomyst, Mucomyst 10, Mucosil-10, Mucosil-20, Parvolex♦ ◇

Pharmacologic class: amino acid (l-cysteine) derivative
Therapeutic class: mucolytic, antidote for acetaminophen overdose
Pregnancy risk category: B

Indications and dosages

▶ **Pneumonia, bronchitis, tuberculosis, cystic fibrosis, emphysema, atelectasis (adjunct), complications of thoracic and CV surgery.** *Adults and children:* 1 to 2 ml of 10% or 20% solution by direct instillation into trachea as often as hourly; or 3 to 5 ml of 20% solution or 6 to 10 ml of 10% solution by nebulization q 2 to 3 hours p.r.n. Alternatively, where available, 300 mg/kg by I.V. infusion in divided doses.

▶ **Acetaminophen toxicity.** *Adults and children:* initially, 140 mg/kg P.O., followed by 70 mg/kg P.O. q 4 hours for 17 doses; or, where available, 300 mg/kg by I.V. infusion.

How supplied

Solution: 10%, 20%
Injection: 200 mg/ml♦ ◇

Pharmacokinetics

Absorption: most inhaled acetylcysteine acts directly on mucus in lungs; remainder is absorbed by pulmonary epithelium. After oral administration, drug is absorbed from GI tract.
Distribution: unknown.
Metabolism: metabolized in liver.
Excretion: unknown.

Route	Onset	Peak	Duration
P.O., I.V., inhalation	Unknown	Unknown	Unknown

Pharmacodynamics

Chemical effect: increases production of respiratory tract fluids to help liquefy and reduce viscosity of tenacious secretions. Also restores glutathione in liver to treat acetaminophen toxicity.
Therapeutic effect: thins respiratory secretions and reverses toxic effects of acetaminophen.

Adverse reactions

EENT: *rhinorrhea, hemoptysis.*
GI: *stomatitis, nausea, vomiting.*
Respiratory: ***bronchospasm.***

Interactions

Drug-drug. *Activated charcoal:* limits acetylcysteine's effectiveness. Avoid concomitant use in treating drug toxicity.

Contraindications and precautions

• Contraindicated in patients hypersensitive to drug.
• Use cautiously in elderly or debilitated patients with severe respiratory insufficiency and in pregnant or breast-feeding women.

NURSING CONSIDERATIONS

Assessment
- Assess patient's respiratory secretions before and frequently during therapy.
- Be alert for adverse reactions and drug interactions.
- Evaluate patient's and family's knowledge of drug therapy.

Nursing diagnoses
- Ineffective airway clearance related to patient's underlying condition
- Impaired oral mucous membrane related to drug-induced stomatitis
- Deficient knowledge related to drug therapy

Planning and implementation
P.O. use: Dilute oral doses with cola, fruit juice, or water before administering to treat acetaminophen overdose. Dilute 20% solution to a concentration of 5% (add 3 ml of diluent to each ml of acetylcysteine). If patient vomits within 1 hour of loading or maintenance dose, repeat dose.
I.V. use: To prepare I.V. infusion, dilute calculated dose in D_5W. Dilute initial dose (150 mg/kg) in 200 ml of D_5W and infuse over 15 minutes. Dilute second dose (50 mg/kg) in 500 ml of D_5W and infuse over 4 hours. Dilute final dose (100 mg/kg) in 1,000 ml of D_5W and infuse over 16 hours.
Nebulization use: Use plastic, glass, stainless steel, or another nonreactive metal when administering by nebulization.
– Hand-bulb nebulizers aren't recommended because output is too small and particle size too large.
– Before aerosol administration, have patient clear airway by coughing.
- After opening, store in refrigerator; use within 96 hours.
- Drug is physically or chemically incompatible with tetracyclines, erythromycin lactobionate, amphotericin B, and ampicillin sodium. If administered by aerosol inhalation, these drugs should be nebulized separately. Iodized oil, trypsin, and hydrogen peroxide are physically incompatible with acetylcysteine; don't add to nebulizer.
- Have suction equipment available in case patient can't effectively clear his air passages.

ALERT Acetylcysteine is given to treat acetaminophen overdose within 24 hours after ingestion. Start treatment immediately as ordered; don't wait for results of drug blood levels.
- Alert prescriber if patient's respiratory secretions thicken or become purulent or if bronchospasm occurs.

Patient teaching
- Instruct patient to follow directions on medication label exactly. Explain importance of not using more drug than directed.
- Tell patient to notify prescriber if his condition doesn't improve within 10 days. Drug shouldn't be used for prolonged period without direct medical supervision.
- Teach patient how to use and clean nebulizer.
- Inform patient that drug may have foul taste or smell.
- Instruct patient to clear his airway by coughing before aerosol administration to achieve maximum effect.
- Instruct patient to rinse mouth with water after nebulizer treatment because it may leave sticky coating on oral cavity.

Evaluation
- Patient has clear lung sounds, decreased respiratory secretions, and reduced frequency and severity of cough.
- Patient's oral mucous membranes remain unchanged.
- Patient and family state understanding of drug therapy.

activated charcoal
(AK-tih-vay-ted CHAR-kohl)
Actidose-Aqua†, Charcoaid†, Charcocaps†, Liqui-Char†, Superchar†

Pharmacologic class: adsorbent
Therapeutic class: antidote
Pregnancy risk category: C

Indications and dosages

▶ **Flatulence, dyspepsia.** *Adults:* 600 mg to 5 g P.O. t.i.d. after meals.

▶ **Poisoning.** *Adults:* initially, 1 g/kg (30 to 100 g) P.O. or 5 to 10 times amount of poison ingested as suspension in 180 to 240 ml of water.

Children: 5 to 10 times estimated weight of drug or chemical ingested, with minimum dose being 30 g P.O. in 240 ml of water to make a slurry, preferably within 30 minutes of poisoning. Larger dose is necessary if food is in stomach. Commonly used for treating poisoning or overdose with acetaminophen, aspirin, atropine, barbiturates, cardiac glycosides, poisonous mushrooms, oxalic acid, parathion, phenol, phenylpropanolamine, phenytoin, propantheline, propoxyphene, strychnine, or tricyclic antidepressants. Check with poison control center for use in other types of poisonings or overdoses.

How supplied

Tablets: 200 mg ◊ †, 300 mg ◊ †, 325 mg†, 650 mg†
Capsules: 260 mg†
Powder: 30 g†, 50 g†
Oral suspension: 0.625 g/5 ml†, 0.83 g/5 ml†, 1 g/5 ml†, 1.25 g/5 ml†

Pharmacokinetics

Absorption: none.
Distribution: none.
Metabolism: none.
Excretion: excreted in feces.

Route	Onset	Peak	Duration
P.O.	Immediate	Unknown	Unknown

Pharmacodynamics

Chemical effect: adheres to many drugs and chemicals, inhibiting their absorption from GI tract.
Therapeutic effect: used as antidote for selected poisons and overdoses.

Adverse reactions

GI: black stools, nausea, constipation.

Interactions

Drug-drug. *Acetylcysteine, ipecac:* render charcoal ineffective. Don't administer together, and don't perform gastric lavage until all charcoal is removed.

Contraindications and precautions

- No known contraindications.

NURSING CONSIDERATIONS

Assessment

- Obtain history of substance reportedly ingested, including time of ingestion, if possible. Drug isn't effective for all drugs and toxic substances.
- Be alert for adverse reactions and drug interactions.
- Evaluate patient's and family's knowledge of drug therapy.

Nursing diagnoses

- Risk for injury related to ingestion of toxic substance or overdose
- Risk for deficient fluid volume related to drug-induced vomiting
- Deficient knowledge related to drug therapy

Planning and implementation

- Give after emesis is complete because drug absorbs and inactivates syrup of ipecac.
- Don't give to semiconscious or unconscious persons unless airway is protected and NG tube is in place for instillation.
- Mix powder form (most effective) with tap water to form consistency of thick syrup. Add small amount of fruit juice or flavoring to make mix more palatable.
- Give by NG tube after lavage if necessary.
- Don't give in ice cream, milk, or sherbet, which reduce absorptive capacity.
- Repeat dose if patient vomits shortly after administration.
- Keep airway, oxygen, and suction equipment nearby.
- Follow treatment with stool softener or laxative, as ordered, to prevent constipation.

Patient teaching

- Warn patient that feces will be black.

• Instruct patient to report respiratory difficulty immediately.

Evaluation

• Patient doesn't experience injury because of ingestion of toxic substance or overdose.
• Patient exhibits no signs of deficient fluid volume.
• Patient or family state understanding of drug therapy.

acyclovir sodium

(ay-SIGH-kloh-veer SOH-dee-um)
Zovirax

Pharmacologic class: synthetic purine nucleoside
Therapeutic class: antiviral
Pregnancy risk category: C

Indications and dosages

▶ **Initial and recurrent episodes of mucocutaneous herpes simplex virus (HSV-1 and HSV-2) infections in immunocompromised patients; severe initial episodes of herpes genitalis in nonimmunocompromised patients.** *Adults and children age 12 and over:* 5 mg/kg I.V. at constant rate over 1 hour q 8 hours for 7 days (5 days for herpes genitalis). *Children under age 12:* 250 mg/m² I.V. at constant rate over 1 hour q 8 hours for 7 days (5 days for herpes genitalis).

▶ **Initial genital herpes.** *Adults:* 200 mg P.O. q 4 hours during waking hours (total of 5 capsules daily) for 10 days.

▶ **Intermittent therapy for recurrent genital herpes.** *Adults:* 200 mg P.O. q 4 hours during waking hours (total of 5 capsules daily) for 5 days. Start therapy at first sign of recurrence.

▶ **Chronic suppressive therapy for recurrent genital herpes.** *Adults:* 400 mg P.O. b.i.d. for up to 12 months.

▶ **Chickenpox.** *Adults and children age 2 and over weighing over 40 kg (88 lb):* 800 mg P.O. q.i.d. for 5 days.

▶ **Herpes zoster.** 800 mg P.O. q 4 hours, five times daily for 7 to 10 days.

▶ **Herpes simplex encephalitis.** *Adults:* 10 mg/kg infused at a constant rate over 1 hour, q 8 hours for 10 days. *Children ages 6 months to 12 years:* 500 mg/m² at a constant rate over at least 1 hour, q 8 hours for 10 days.

▶ **Varicella zoster in immunocompromised patients:** *Adults:* 10 mg/kg infused at a constant rate over 1 hour, q 8 hours for 7 days. *Children under age 12:* 500 mg/m² at a constant rate over at least 1 hour, q 8 hours for 7 days. Obese patients should be dosed at 10 mg/kg (ideal body weight). Maximum dose equivalent to 500 mg/m² q 8 hours shouldn't be exceeded.

How supplied

Capsules: 200 mg
Tablets: 400 mg, 800 mg
Suspension: 200 mg/5 ml
Injection: 500 mg/vial, 1 g/vial

Pharmacokinetics

Absorption: with oral administration, drug is absorbed slowly and incompletely (15% to 30%). Absorption isn't affected by food.
Distribution: distributed widely to organ tissues and body fluids. CSF levels equal about 50% of serum levels. From 9% to 33% of dose binds to plasma proteins.
Metabolism: metabolized primarily inside viral cell to its active form. About 10% of dose is metabolized extracellularly.
Excretion: up to 92% of systemically absorbed acyclovir is excreted unchanged by kidneys via glomerular filtration and tubular secretion. *Half-life:* 2 to 3½ hours with normal renal function; up to 19 hours with renal failure.

Route	Onset	Peak	Duration
P.O.	Unknown	Unknown	Unknown
I.V.	Immediate	Immediate	Unknown

Pharmacodynamics

Chemical effect: becomes incorporated into viral DNA and inhibits viral multiplication.
Therapeutic effect: kills susceptible viruses.

Adverse reactions

CNS: *encephalopathic changes including lethargy, obtundation, tremor, confusion, hal-*

lucinations, agitation, ***seizures, coma,*** *headache* (with I.V. dosage).
CV: hypotension.
GI: *nausea, vomiting,* diarrhea.
GU: *transient elevations of serum creatinine level,* hematuria.
Skin: rash, itching, *vesicular eruptions*
Other: *inflammation, phlebitis at injection site.*

Interactions

Drug-drug. *Phenytoin:* possibly decreased phenytoin levels. Monitor patient closely.
Probenecid: increased acyclovir blood level. Monitor patient for possible toxicity.
Valproic acid: decreased valproic acid levels. Monitor patient closely.
Zidovudine: may cause drowsiness or lethargy. Use together cautiously.

Contraindications and precautions

- Contraindicated in patients hypersensitive to drug.
- Use cautiously in patients with underlying neurologic problems, renal disease, or dehydration and in those receiving other nephrotoxic drugs.
- Use cautiously in pregnant or breast-feeding women.
- Safety in children under age 2 hasn't been established.

NURSING CONSIDERATIONS

Assessment

- Assess infection before and regularly during therapy.
- Be alert for adverse reactions and drug interactions.
- Monitor patient for renal toxicity. Bolus injection, dehydration, preexisting renal disease, and concomitant use of other nephrotoxic drugs increase risk.
- Monitor patient's mental status when administering drug I.V. Encephalopathic changes are more likely in patients with neurologic disorders or in those who have had neurologic reactions to cytotoxic drugs.
- Monitor patient's hydration status if adverse GI reactions occur with oral administration.
- Evaluate patient's and family's knowledge of drug therapy.

Nursing diagnoses

- Infection related to presence of virus
- Risk for deficient fluid volume related to adverse GI reactions to oral drug
- Deficient knowledge related to drug therapy

Planning and implementation

P.O. use: Follow normal protocol.
I.V. use: Administer I.V. infusion over at least 1 hour to prevent renal tubular damage.
– Don't give by bolus injection or administer I.M. or S.C.
– Concentrated solutions (10 mg/ml or more) may raise the risk of phlebitis.
- Patients with acute or chronic renal impairment require a dose adjustment.

Patient teaching

- Tell patient that drug effectively manages herpes infection but doesn't eliminate or cure it.
- Warn patient that drug will not prevent spread of infection to others.
- Urge patient to recognize early symptoms of herpes infection (tingling, itching, pain) so he can take acyclovir before infection fully develops.
- Tell patient to alert nurse if pain or discomfort occurs at I.V. injection site.

Evaluation

- Patient's infection is eradicated.
- Patient maintains adequate hydration.
- Patient and family state understanding of drug therapy.

adenosine

(uh-DEN-oh-seen)
Adenocard

Pharmacologic class: nucleoside
Therapeutic class: antiarrhythmic
Pregnancy risk category: C

Indications and dosages

▶ **Conversion of PSVT to sinus rhythm.** *Adults:* 6 mg I.V. by rapid bolus injection over

1 to 2 seconds. If PSVT isn't eliminated in 1 to 2 minutes, 12 mg by rapid I.V. push may be given and repeated (if necessary). Single doses over 12 mg aren't recommended.

How supplied

Injection: 3 mg/ml in 2-ml vials

Pharmacokinetics

Absorption: not applicable with I.V. administration.
Distribution: rapidly taken up by erythrocytes and vascular endothelial cells.
Metabolism: metabolized within tissues to inosine and adenosine monophosphate.
Excretion: unknown. *Half-life:* less than 10 seconds.

Route	Onset	Peak	Duration
I.V.	Immediate	Immediate	Extremely short

Pharmacodynamics

Chemical effect: acts on AV node to slow conduction and inhibit reentry pathways. Adenosine also is useful in treating paroxysmal supraventricular tachycardia (PSVT) with accessory bypass tracts (Wolff-Parkinson-White syndrome).
Therapeutic effect: restores normal sinus rhythm.

Adverse reactions

CNS: apprehension, back pain, blurred vision, burning sensation, dizziness, heaviness in arms, light-headedness, neck pain, numbness, tingling in arms.
CV: chest pain, *facial flushing,* headache, hypotension, palpitations, diaphoresis.
EENT: metallic taste.
GI: nausea.
Respiratory: *chest pressure, dyspnea, shortness of breath,* hyperventilation.
Other: *tightness in throat, groin pressure.*

Interactions

Drug-drug. *Carbamazepine:* higher degrees of heart block may occur. Monitor patient.
Digoxin, verapamil: combined use rarely causes ventricular fibrillation. Use cautiously.
Dipyridamole: may potentiate adenosine's effects. Smaller doses may be necessary.
Methylxanthines: antagonism of adenosine's effects. Patients receiving theophylline or caffeine may require higher doses or may not respond to adenosine therapy.
Drug-herb. *Guarana:* may decrease therapeutic response. Discourage concomitant use.
Drug-food. *Caffeine:* may antagonize adenosine's effects. May require higher doses.

Contraindications and precautions

- Contraindicated in patients hypersensitive to drug and in those with second- or third-degree heart block or sick sinus syndrome unless artificial pacemaker is present. Adenosine decreases conduction through AV node and may produce transient first-, second-, or third-degree heart block. Patients in whom significant heart block develops shouldn't receive additional doses.
- Use cautiously in patients with asthma because bronchoconstriction may occur.
- Safety of drug hasn't been established in pregnant or breast-feeding women or in children.

NURSING CONSIDERATIONS

Assessment

- Monitor patient's heart rate and rhythm before and during therapy.
- Be alert for adverse reactions and drug interactions.
- Evaluate patient's and family's knowledge of drug therapy.

Nursing diagnoses

- Decreased cardiac output related to arrhythmias
- Ineffective protection related to drug-induced proarrhythmias
- Deficient knowledge related to drug therapy

Planning and implementation

- Check solution for crystals, which may form if solution is cold. If crystals are visible, gently warm solution to room temperature. Don't use unclear solutions.
- Administer rapidly for effective drug action. Administer directly into vein if possible; if I.V.

line is used, inject drug into most proximal port and follow with rapid saline flush to ensure that drug reaches systemic circulation quickly.

- Discard unused drug; it contains no preservatives.
- Withhold drug, obtain rhythm strip, and notify prescriber immediately if ECG disturbances occur.

ALERT Have emergency equipment and drugs on hand to treat new arrhythmias.

Patient teaching

- Teach patient about his disease and therapy.
- Stress importance of alerting nurse if chest pain or dyspnea occurs.
- Advise patient to avoid caffeine consumption.

Evaluation

- Patient's arrhythmias are corrected.
- Patient doesn't experience proarrhythmias.
- Patient and family state understanding of drug therapy.

albumin 5%

(al-BYOO-min)

Albuminar 5%, Albutein 5%, Buminate 5%, Plasbumin 5%

albumin 25%

Albuminar 25%, Albumisol 25%, Albutein 25%, Buminate 25%, Plasbumin 25%

Pharmacologic class: blood derivative
Therapeutic class: plasma volume expander
Pregnancy risk category: C

Indications and dosages

▶ **Hypovolemic shock.** *Adults:* initially, 500 ml 5% solution by I.V. infusion, repeated p.r.n. Dosage varies with patient's condition and response. Don't give more than 250 g in 48 hours.
Children: 10 to 20 ml/kg 5% solution by I.V. infusion, repeated in 15 to 30 minutes if response isn't adequate. Alternatively, 2.5 to 5 ml I.V. of 25% solution/kg, repeated after 10 to 30 minutes, if needed.

▶ **Hypoproteinemia.** *Adults:* 1,000 to 1,500 ml 5% solution by I.V. infusion daily, with maximum rate of 5 to 10 ml/minute; or 200 to 300 ml 25% solution by I.V. infusion daily, with maximum rate of 3 ml/minute. Dosage varies with patient's condition and response.

▶ **Hyperbilirubinemia.** *Infants:* 1 g albumin (4 ml 25%)/kg I.V. 1 to 2 hours before transfusion.

How supplied

Injection: 50-ml, 250-ml, 500-ml, 1,000-ml vials (albumin 5%); 10-ml, 20-ml, 50-ml, 100-ml vials (albumin 25%)

Pharmacokinetics

Absorption: not applicable with I.V. administration.
Distribution: albumin accounts for about 50% of plasma proteins; it is distributed into intravascular space and extravascular sites, including skin, muscle, and lungs.
Metabolism: unknown.
Excretion: unknown, although liver, kidneys, or intestines may provide elimination mechanisms for albumin. *Half-life:* 15 to 20 days.

Route	Onset	Peak	Duration
I.V.	≤ 15 min for hydrated patient	≤ 15 min for hydrated patient	Up to several hr with reduced blood volume

Pharmacodynamics

Chemical effect: albumin 5% supplies colloid to blood and expands plasma volume. Albumin 25% provides intravascular oncotic pressure in 5:1 ratio, causing fluid shift from interstitial spaces to circulation and slightly increasing plasma protein level.
Therapeutic effect: relieves shock by increasing plasma volume and corrects plasma protein deficiency.

Adverse reactions

CV: ***vascular overload,*** hypotension, altered pulse rate.
GI: increased salivation, nausea, vomiting.
Respiratory: altered respiration.
Skin: urticaria, rash.
Other: chills, fever.

Interactions

None significant.

Contraindications and precautions

- Contraindicated in patients hypersensitive to drug.
- Use with extreme caution in patients with hypertension, cardiac disease, severe pulmonary infection, severe chronic anemia, or hypoalbuminemia with peripheral edema.
- Use cautiously in pregnant women.

NURSING CONSIDERATIONS

Assessment

- Assess patient's underlying condition.
- Be alert for adverse reactions.
- Monitor fluid intake and output, hemoglobin, hematocrit, and serum protein and electrolytes.
- Evaluate patient's and family's knowledge of drug therapy.

Nursing diagnoses

- Deficient fluid volume related to patient's underlying condition
- Excessive fluid volume related to adverse effects of drug
- Deficient knowledge related to drug therapy

Planning and implementation

- Minimize waste when preparing and administering drug. This product is expensive, and random shortages are common.
- Avoid rapid I.V. infusion. Specific rate is individualized according to patient's age, condition, and diagnosis. Dilute with normal saline solution, or D_5W injection. Use solution promptly; it contains no preservatives. Discard unused solution. Don't use cloudy solutions or those containing sediment. Solution should be clear amber.

ALERT Don't give more than 250 g in 48 hours.

- One volume of 25% albumin is equivalent to five volumes of 5% albumin in producing hemodilution and relative anemia.
- Follow storage instructions on bottle. Freezing may cause bottle to break.
- Withhold fluids in patient with cerebral edema for 8 hours after infusion to avoid fluid overload.

Patient teaching

- Explain how and why albumin is administered.
- Tell patient to report chills, fever, dyspnea, nausea, or rash immediately; normal serum albumin can cause allergic reaction.

Evaluation

- Patient's deficient fluid volume is resolved.
- Patient doesn't experience fluid overload.
- Patient and family state understanding of drug therapy.

albuterol (salbutamol)

(al-BYOO-ter-ohl)

Asmol ◇, Proventil, Respolin ◇, Ventolin

albuterol sulfate (salbutamol sulfate)

Proventil, Proventil Repetabs, Respolin Autohaler Inhalation Device ◇, Respolin Inhaler ◇, Respolin Respirator Solution ◇, Ventolin, Ventolin Obstetric Injection ◇, Ventolin Rotacaps, Volmax

Pharmacologic class: adrenergic
Therapeutic class: bronchodilator
Pregnancy risk category: C

Indications and dosages

▶ **Prevention or treatment of bronchospasm in patients with reversible obstructive airway disease.** *Adults and children ages 12 and over:* dosage and frequency vary with dosage form. *Aerosol inhalation*—1 to 2 inhalations q 4 to 6 hours. More frequent administration or greater number of inhalations isn't recommended. *Solution for inhalation*—2.5 mg t.i.d. or q.i.d. by nebulizer. To prepare solution, use 0.5 ml of 0.5% solution diluted with 2.5 ml of normal saline solution. Alternatively, use 3 ml of 0.083% solution. *Capsules for inhalation*—200 mcg inhaled q 4 to 6 hours using Rotahaler inhalation device. Some

patients may need 400 mcg q 4 to 6 hours.
Oral tablets—2 to 4 mg P.O. t.i.d. or q.i.d. Maximum dosage is 8 mg q.i.d. *Extended-release tablets*—4 to 8 mg P.O. q 12 hours. Maximum dosage is 16 mg b.i.d.
Children ages 6 to 11: 2 mg (1 teaspoonful) P.O. t.i.d. or q.i.d.
Children ages 2 to 5: 0.1 mg/kg P.O. t.i.d., not to exceed 2 mg (1 teaspoonful) t.i.d.
Adults over age 65: 2 mg P.O. t.i.d. or q.i.d.
▶ **Prevention of exercise-induced asthma.** *Adults:* 2 inhalations 15 minutes before exercise.

How supplied

Aerosol inhaler: 90 mcg/metered spray, 100 mcg/metered spray ◇
Capsules for inhalation: 200 mcg
Tablets: 2 mg, 4 mg
Tablets (extended-release): 4 mg, 8 mg
Syrup: 2 mg/5 ml
Solution for inhalation: 0.083%, 0.5%
Injection: 1 mg/ml ◇

Pharmacokinetics

Absorption: after oral inhalation, albuterol appears to be absorbed over several hours from respiratory tract; however, most of dose is swallowed and absorbed through GI tract. After oral administration, drug is well absorbed through GI tract.
Distribution: doesn't cross blood-brain barrier.
Metabolism: extensively metabolized in liver to inactive compounds.
Excretion: rapidly excreted in urine and feces. *Half-life:* about 4 hours.

Route	Onset	Peak	Duration
P.O.	15-30 min	2-3 hr	6-12 hr
I.V.	1-5 min	Unknown	Unknown
Inhalation	5-15 min	1-1.5 hr	3-6 hr

Pharmacodynamics

Chemical effect: relaxes bronchial and uterine smooth muscle by acting on $beta_2$-adrenergic receptors.
Therapeutic effect: improves ventilation.

Adverse reactions

CNS: *tremor, nervousness,* dizziness, insomnia, headache.
CV: tachycardia, palpitations, hypertension.
EENT: drying and irritation of nose and throat.
GI: heartburn, nausea, vomiting.
Metabolic: hypokalemia.
Musculoskeletal: muscle cramps.
Respiratory: ***bronchospasm.***

Interactions

Drug-drug. *CNS stimulants:* increased CNS stimulation. Avoid concomitant use.
Levodopa: risk of arrhythmias. Monitor patient closely.
MAO inhibitors, tricyclic antidepressants: increased adverse CV effects. Monitor patient closely.
Propranolol, other beta blockers: mutual antagonism. Monitor patient carefully.
Drug-food. *Caffeine-containing foods and beverages:* increased CNS stimulation. Avoid concomitant use.

Contraindications and precautions

- Contraindicated in patients hypersensitive to drug or its components and in breast-feeding women.
- Use cautiously in patients with CV disorders (including coronary insufficiency and hypertension), hyperthyroidism, or diabetes mellitus; in those unusually responsive to adrenergics; and during pregnancy.
- Use extended-release tablets cautiously in patients with GI narrowing.
- Safety of drug hasn't been established in children under age 12 for inhalation solution, aerosol, or Repetabs; in those under age 6 for tablets; and in those under age 2 for syrup.

NURSING CONSIDERATIONS

Assessment

- Obtain baseline assessment of patient's respiratory status, and assess frequently throughout therapy.
- Be alert for adverse reactions and drug interactions.

• Evaluate patient's and family's knowledge of drug therapy.

Nursing diagnoses
• Impaired gas exchange related to underlying respiratory condition
• Risk for injury related to drug-induced adverse reactions
• Deficient knowledge related to drug therapy

Planning and implementation
P.O. use: Remember that pleasant-tasting syrup may be taken by children as young as age 2. Syrup contains no alcohol or sugar.
I.V. use: I.V. form may be used, where available, to prepare infusion using saline solution for injection, glucose injection, or saline and glucose injection. Don't administer drug without dilution, and don't mix with other medication. Discard unused diluted solution after 24 hours.
Inhalation use: Wait at least 2 minutes between doses if more than one dose is ordered. If corticosteroid inhaler also is used, first have patient use bronchodilator, wait 5 minutes, and then have patient use corticosteroid inhaler. This permits bronchodilator to open air passages for maximum corticosteroid effectiveness.
– Aerosol form may be prescribed for use 15 minutes before exercise to prevent exercise-induced bronchospasm.
• Patients may use tablets and aerosol concomitantly.

Patient teaching
• Warn patient to stop drug immediately if paradoxical bronchospasm occurs.
• Give patient correct instructions for using metered-dose inhaler: Clear nasal passages and throat. Breathe out, expelling as much air from lungs as possible. Place mouthpiece well into mouth and inhale deeply as dose is released. Hold breath for several seconds, remove mouthpiece, and exhale slowly.
• Advise patient to wait at least 2 minutes before repeating procedure if more than one inhalation is ordered.
• Warn patient to avoid accidentally spraying inhalant form into eyes, which may blur vision temporarily.
• Tell patient to reduce intake of foods containing caffeine, such as coffee, colas, and chocolates, when taking bronchodilator.
• Show patient how to check pulse rate. Instruct him to check pulse before and after using bronchodilator and to call prescriber if pulse rate increases more than 20 to 30 beats/minute.

Evaluation
• Patient's respiratory signs and symptoms improve.
• Patient has no injury from adverse drug reactions.
• Patient and family state understanding of drug therapy.

aldesleukin (interleukin-2, IL-2)
(al-des-LOO-kin)
Proleukin

Pharmacologic class: lymphokine
Therapeutic class: immunoregulatory drug
Pregnancy risk category: C

Indications and dosages
▶ **Metastatic renal cell carcinoma, metastatic melanoma.** *Adults:* 600,000 IU/kg (0.037 mg/kg) I.V. over 15 minutes q 8 hours for 5 days (total of 14 doses). After 9-day rest, sequence is repeated for another 14 doses. After rest period of at least 7 weeks, repeat courses may be administered.

How supplied
Powder for injection: 22 million IU/vial

Pharmacokinetics
Absorption: not applicable with I.V. administration.
Distribution: about 30% of drug is rapidly distributed to plasma; balance is rapidly distributed to liver, kidneys, and lungs. Peak serum levels are proportional to dose.
Metabolism: metabolized by kidneys to amino acids within cells lining proximal convoluted tubules.

Excretion: excreted through kidneys by peritubular extraction and glomerular filtration. *Half-life:* 85 minutes.

Route	Onset	Peak	Duration
I.V.	Unknown	Unknown	Unknown

Pharmacodynamics

Chemical effect: unknown. May stimulate immunologic host reaction to tumor.
Therapeutic effect: eliminates or decreases kidney tumor size.

Adverse reactions

CNS: headache, *mental status changes, dizziness, sensory dysfunction, special senses disorders, syncope, motor dysfunction,* ***coma,*** fatigue, weakness, malaise.
CV: *hypotension, sinus tachycardia, arrhythmias,* ***bradycardia, PVCs,*** *premature atrial contractions, myocardial ischemia,* ***MI, heart failure, cardiac arrest,*** myocarditis, endocarditis, ***CVA,*** pericardial effusion, thrombosis, ***capillary leak syndrome (CLS).***
EENT: conjunctivitis.
GI: *nausea, vomiting, diarrhea, stomatitis, anorexia, bleeding, dyspepsia, constipation.*
GU: *oliguria,* ***anuria,*** *proteinuria, hematuria, dysuria,* urine retention, urinary frequency, UTI, *elevated BUN and serum creatinine levels.*
Hematologic: *anemia,* **THROMBOCYTOPENIA, LEUKOPENIA,** coagulation disorders, leukocytosis, eosinophilia.
Hepatic: *jaundice;* ascites; hepatomegaly; *elevated bilirubin, serum transaminase, alkaline phosphatase levels.*
Metabolic: *hypomagnesemia, acidosis, hypocalcemia, hypophosphatemia, hypokalemia, hyperuricemia, hypoalbuminemia,* hypoproteinemia, hyponatremia, hyperkalemia, weight gain or loss.
Musculoskeletal: abdominal, chest, or back pain; arthralgia; myalgia.
Respiratory: ***pulmonary congestion,*** *dyspnea,* ***pulmonary edema, respiratory failure, pleural effusion, apnea, pneumothorax,*** tachypnea.
Skin: *pruritus, erythema, rash, dryness,* ***exfoliative dermatitis,*** purpura, alopecia, petechiae.
Other: *fever, chills,* edema, infections of catheter tip or injection site, phlebitis, **SEPSIS.**

Interactions

Drug-drug. *Antihypertensives:* increased risk of hypotension. Monitor patient closely.
Cardiotoxic, hepatotoxic, myelotoxic, or nephrotoxic drugs: enhanced toxicity. Avoid concomitant use.
Corticosteroids: decreased antitumor effectiveness of aldesleukin. Avoid concomitant use.
Psychotropic drugs: unpredictable interaction. Use together cautiously.

Contraindications and precautions

- Contraindicated in patients hypersensitive to drug or its components, in those with abnormal cardiac (thallium) stress test or pulmonary function tests or organ allografts, and in breast-feeding women.
- Retreatment is contraindicated in patients who experience the following adverse effects: cardiac tamponade; disturbances in cardiac rhythm that were uncontrolled or unresponsive to intervention; sustained ventricular tachycardia (five beats or more); chest pain accompanied by ECG changes, indicating MI or angina pectoris; renal dysfunction requiring dialysis for 72 hours or more; coma or toxic psychosis lasting 48 hours or more; seizures that were repetitive or difficult to control; ischemia or perforation of bowel; or GI bleeding requiring surgery.
- Don't give drug unless patient has had definitive tests documenting normal cardiac and pulmonary function. Use with extreme caution in patients with normal test results if they have a history of cardiac or pulmonary disease, in patients with a history of seizure disorders because drug may cause seizures, and during pregnancy.
- Use cautiously in patients who require large volumes of fluid (such as patients with hypercalcemia).
- Use cautiously and with close clinical monitoring in all patients because severe adverse effects usually accompany therapy at recommended dosage.
- Safety of drug hasn't been established in children.

NURSING CONSIDERATIONS

Assessment
• Obtain history of patient's renal carcinoma and underlying conditions.
• Assess status of patient's physical condition at onset of aldesleukin therapy and frequently throughout therapy.
• Obtain hematologic tests, serum electrolyte levels, renal and liver function tests, and chest X-ray before therapy and then daily during therapy, as ordered, and monitor results.
• Patient should be neurologically stable with negative computed tomography scan for CNS metastases before therapy is begun. Drug may worsen symptoms in patient with unrecognized or undiagnosed CNS metastases.
• Be alert for adverse reactions and drug interactions.
• Evaluate patient's and family's knowledge of drug therapy.

Nursing diagnoses
• Ineffective health maintenance related to neoplastic disease
• Ineffective protection related to drug-induced adverse reactions
• Deficient knowledge related to drug therapy

Planning and implementation
• Give drug only in a hospital under direction of clinician experienced in use of chemotherapeutic drugs. Intensive care facility and intensive care or cardiopulmonary specialists must be readily available.
• Treat patient with bacterial infections before therapy is begun, as ordered.
• To avoid altering drug's pharmacologic properties, reconstitute and dilute carefully, and follow manufacturer's recommendations. Don't mix with other drugs or albumin.
• Reconstitute vial containing 22 million IU (1.3 mg) with 1.2 ml of sterile water for injection. Don't use bacteriostatic water or normal saline injection; these diluents increase aggregation of drug. Direct stream of sterile water at sides of vial and gently swirl to reconstitute. Don't shake. Reconstituted solution will have concentration of 18 million IU (1.1 mg)/ml. It should be particle-free and colorless to slightly yellow.
• Add ordered dose of reconstituted drug to 50 ml of D_5W and infuse over 15 minutes. Don't use in-line filter. Plastic infusion bags are preferred because they provide consistent drug delivery.
• Discard unused portion. Vials are for single-dose use and contain no preservatives.
• Refrigerate powder for injection. Return drug to room temperature before administering to patient.
ALERT Drug has been linked to CLS, a condition that results from loss of vascular tone, in which plasma proteins and fluids escape into extravascular space. Mean arterial blood pressure begins to drop within 2 to 12 hours of treatment; edema and effusions may be severe, and death can result from hypoperfusion of major organs. Other conditions that accompany CLS include arrhythmias, MI, angina, mental status changes, renal insufficiency, respiratory distress or failure, and GI bleeding or infarction.
• Be prepared to adjust dosage of other drugs, as ordered, to compensate for renal and hepatic impairment occurring during treatment. Modify dosage by withholding dose or interrupting therapy, as ordered, rather than by reducing dose.
• Withhold dose and notify prescriber if moderate to severe lethargy or somnolence develops; continued administration can result in coma.
• Therapy is linked with impaired neutrophil function, which can lead to disseminated infection. Many studies used prophylactic antibiotic therapy with oxacillin, nafcillin, ciprofloxacin, or vancomycin; check protocol and administer antibiotics, as ordered.

Patient teaching
• Make sure patient understands that adverse effects are expected with normal doses and that serious toxicity may occur despite close clinical monitoring.
• Teach patient about specific adverse reactions and how to manage them, including infection and bleeding precautions to take.
• Stress importance of compliance with extensive testing required during aldesleukin therapy.

• Advise patient to alert prescriber when adverse reactions occur.

✓ Evaluation

• Patient's renal studies show positive response to drug.
• Patient exhibits positive response to measures used to limit severity of adverse reactions.
• Patient and family state understanding of drug therapy.

alendronate sodium

(ah-LEN-droh-nayt SOH-dee-um)
Fosamax

Pharmacologic class: inhibitor of osteoclast-mediated bone resorption
Therapeutic class: antiosteoporotic
Pregnancy risk category: C

Indications and dosages

▶ **Treatment of glucocorticoid-induced osteoporosis in men and women who are receiving glucocorticoids equivalent to 7.5 mg or more daily prednisone and who have low bone mineral density.** *Adults:* 5 mg P.O. daily, taken with water only, at least 30 minutes before first food, beverage, or drug of the day. For postmenopausal women not receiving estrogen, the recommended dosage is 10 mg P.O. daily, taken with water only, at least 30 minutes before first food, beverage, or drug of the day.
▶ **Treatment of osteoporosis in postmenopausal women.** *Adults:* 10 mg P.O. daily, at least 30 minutes before first food, beverage, or medication of day, with plain water only.
▶ **Prevention of osteoporosis in postmenopausal women.** *Adults:* 5 mg P.O. daily, at least 30 minutes before first food, beverage, or medication of day, with plain water only.
▶ **Paget's disease of bone.** *Adults:* 40 mg P.O. daily for 6 months, at least 30 minutes before first food, beverage, or medication of day, with plain water only.

How supplied

Tablets: 10 mg, 40 mg

Pharmacokinetics

Absorption: absorbed from GI tract; food or beverages can significantly decrease bioavailability.
Distribution: distributed to soft tissues but is then rapidly redistributed to bone or excreted in urine; about 78% protein–bound.
Metabolism: doesn't appear to be metabolized.
Excretion: excreted in urine.

Route	Onset	Peak	Duration
P.O.	1 mo	3-6 mo	3 wk

Pharmacodynamics

Chemical effect: suppresses osteoclast activity on newly formed resorption surfaces, reducing bone turnover.
Therapeutic effect: increases bone mass.

Adverse reactions

CNS: headache.
GI: abdominal pain, nausea, dyspepsia, constipation, diarrhea, flatulence, acid regurgitation, esophageal ulcer, vomiting, dysphagia, abdominal distention, gastritis, taste perversion.
Musculoskeletal: musculoskeletal pain.

Interactions

Drug-drug. *Antacids, calcium supplements:* interferes with alendronate absorption. Have patient wait 30 minutes after alendronate dose before taking other drugs.
Aspirin, NSAIDs: increased risk of upper GI reactions with alendronate doses over 10 mg/day. Monitor patient closely.
Hormone replacement therapy: not recommended when used with alendronate in treating osteoporosis; evidence of effectiveness is lacking.
Drug-food. *Any food:* decreased absorption of drug. Don't give drug with food.

Contraindications and precautions

• Contraindicated in patients with hypocalcemia, severe renal insufficiency, or hypersensitivity to drug or its component.
• Use cautiously in patients with dysphagia, esophageal diseases, gastritis, duodenitis, ulcers, or mild to moderate renal insufficiency.

• Safety of drug hasn't been established in breast-feeding women and in children.

NURSING CONSIDERATIONS

Assessment

• Obtain history of patient's underlying disorder before therapy.
• Monitor serum calcium and phosphate levels throughout therapy, as ordered.
• Be alert for adverse reactions and drug interactions.
• Evaluate patient's and family's knowledge of drug therapy.

Nursing diagnoses

• Risk for injury related to decreased bone mass
• Risk for deficient fluid volume related to drug-induced GI upset
• Deficient knowledge related to drug therapy

Planning and implementation

• Hypocalcemia and other disturbances of mineral metabolism (such as vitamin D deficiency) should be corrected before therapy begins.
• Administer drug in the morning at least 30 minutes before first meal, fluid, or other oral drug administration.

Patient teaching

ALERT Warn patient not to lie down for at least 30 minutes after taking drug to facilitate delivery to stomach and reduce potential for esophageal irritation.
• Tell patient to take supplemental calcium and vitamin D, if daily dietary intake is inadequate.
• Show patient how to perform weight-bearing exercises, which help increase bone mass.
• Urge patient to limit or restrict smoking and alcohol use, if appropriate.

Evaluation

• Patient remains free from bone fracture.
• Patient maintains adequate hydration.
• Patient and family state understanding of drug therapy.

alfentanil hydrochloride

(al-FEN-tah-nil high-droh-KLOR-ighd)
Alfenta

Pharmacologic class: opioid
Therapeutic class: analgesic, adjunct to anesthesia, anesthetic
Controlled substance schedule: II
Pregnancy risk category: C

Indications and dosages

▶ **Adjunct to general anesthetic.** *Adults:* initially, 8 to 50 mcg/kg I.V.; then increments of 3 to 15 mcg/kg I.V. q 5 to 20 minutes. Reduced dosage needed for elderly and debilitated patients.
▶ **Primary anesthetic.** *Adults:* initially, 130 to 245 mcg/kg I.V.; then 0.5 to 1.5 mcg/kg/minute I.V. Reduced dosage needed for elderly and debilitated patients.

How supplied

Injection: 500 mcg/ml

Pharmacokinetics

Absorption: not applicable with I.V. administration.
Distribution: over 90% is protein-bound.
Metabolism: metabolized in liver.
Excretion: excreted in urine. *Half-life:* about 1½ hours.

Route	Onset	Peak	Duration
I.V.	1 min	1.5-2 min	5-10 min

Pharmacodynamics

Chemical effect: binds with opiate receptors in CNS, altering perception of and emotional response to pain through unknown mechanism.
Therapeutic effect: enhances anesthetic effect and relieves pain.

Adverse reactions

CNS: blurred vision, agitation, anxiety, headache, confusion.
CV: hypotension, hypertension, ***bradycardia***, tachycardia, palpitations, orthostatic hypotension.

GI: nausea, vomiting.
Musculoskeletal: intraoperative muscle movement.
Respiratory: ***chest wall rigidity, bronchospasm, respiratory depression,*** hypercapnia.
Skin: itching.

Interactions

Drug-drug. *Cimetidine:* CNS toxicity. Monitor patient.
CNS depressants: additive effects. Use together cautiously.
Diazepam: CV depression and decreased blood pressure with high doses of alfentanil. Use together cautiously.

Contraindications and precautions

- Contraindicated in patients hypersensitive to drug.
- Use cautiously in patients with head injury, pulmonary disease, decreased respiratory reserve, or hepatic or renal impairment and in pregnant or breast-feeding women.
- Safety of drug hasn't been established in children under age 12.

NURSING CONSIDERATIONS

Assessment
- Assess patient's CV and respiratory status before and during therapy.
- Drug decreases rate and depth of respirations. Monitoring arterial oxygen saturation may aid in assessing effects of respiratory depression.
- Be alert for adverse reactions and drug interactions.
- Evaluate patient's and family's knowledge of drug therapy.

Nursing diagnoses
- Ineffective health maintenance related to need for surgery
- Ineffective breathing pattern related to drug-induced respiratory depression
- Deficient knowledge related to drug therapy

Planning and implementation
- Drug should be administered only by those specifically trained in use of I.V. anesthetics.
- Drug is compatible with D_5W, D_5W in lactated Ringer's solution, and normal saline solution. Most clinicians use infusions containing 25 to 80 mcg/ml.
- Stop infusion 10 to 15 minutes (or more) before surgery ends.
- Use tuberculin syringe to administer small volumes of alfentanil accurately.
- Keep narcotic antagonist (naloxone) and resuscitation equipment available.
- Notify prescriber immediately if assessment findings deviate from expected norm. Patient who has developed tolerance to other opioids may become intolerant to alfentanil as well.

Patient teaching
- Explain anesthetic effect of drug.
- Inform patient that another analgesic will be available after effects of drug have worn off.

Evaluation
- Patient regains health maintenance after alfentanil administration and recovery from surgery.
- Patient's respiratory status returns to normal after effects of drug wear off.
- Patient and family state understanding of drug therapy.

alitretinoin
(a-lih-TREH-tih-noyn)
Panretin

Pharmacologic class: retinoid
Therapeutic class: anti-Kaposi's sarcoma lesions
Pregnancy risk category: D

Indications and dosages

▶ **Topical treatment of cutaneous lesions in patients with Kaposi's sarcoma related to AIDS.** *Adults:* Initially, apply generous coating of gel b.i.d. to lesions only. Frequency may be increased to t.i.d. or q.i.d. based on patient tolerance.

How supplied

Gel: 0.1%

Pharmacokinetics

Absorption: alitretinoin isn't extensively absorbed following topical application.
Distribution: no information available.
Metabolism: although no metabolites are detectable in plasma after topical application, in vitro studies indicate that the drug is metabolized.
Excretion: no information available.

Route	Onset	Peak	Duration
Topical	Unknown	Unknown	Unknown

Pharmacodynamics

Chemical effect: inhibits the growth of Kaposi's sarcoma cells by binding to and activating all known intracellular retinoid receptor subtypes. These activated receptors function as transcription factors that regulate the expression of genes that control cellular differentiation and proliferation in both normal and neoplastic cells.
Therapeutic effect: reduces cutaneous lesions in patients with Kaposi's sarcoma related to AIDS.

Adverse reactions

CNS: paresthesia.
Skin: *rash; burning pain at application site, pruritus;* exfoliative dermatitis, skin disorder, such as excoriation, drainage, fissures, cracking, scabbing, crusting, oozing; edema.

Interactions

Drug-lifestyle. *Exposure to N,N-diethyl-m-toluamide (DEET), a common component of insect repellents:* increased DEET toxicity. Don't use insect repellents containing DEET during alitretinoin treatment.
Sun exposure: possible photosensitizing effect. Minimize exposure of treated areas to sunlight and sunlamps.

Contraindications and precautions

• Contraindicated in pregnant women and in patients hypersensitive to retinoids or to alitretinoin or its components.
• Gel shouldn't be used on patients who need systemic anti-Kaposi's sarcoma therapy, such as those with more than 10 new Kaposi's sarcoma lesions in the previous month, symptomatic lymphedema, symptomatic pulmonary Kaposi's sarcoma, or symptomatic visceral involvement.
• Use cautiously in women of childbearing potential.

NURSING CONSIDERATIONS

Assessment
• Assess patient's skin lesions and surrounding tissue areas before starting treatment.
• Discuss the risk of using this drug in women of childbearing age.
• Be alert for adverse reactions.
• Evaluate patient's and family's knowledge of drug therapy.

Nursing diagnoses
• Risk for infection related to skin lesions
• Impaired skin integrity secondary to adverse reactions of the medication
• Deficient knowledge related to drug therapy

Planning and implementation
• Cover the lesions with a generous coating of gel. Don't apply it to normal skin around the lesions or to (or near) mucosal surfaces because it may cause irritation.
• The gel should be allowed to dry for 3 to 5 minutes before covering with clothing.
• Don't use occlusive dressings with alitretinoin.
• If patient has a toxic reaction at the application site, frequency of application may need to be reduced, as ordered. If severe irritation occurs, notify prescriber; drug may be stopped for a few days until symptoms subside.

Patient teaching
• Tell women of childbearing age that they shouldn't become pregnant while they're taking alitretinoin.
• Inform patient that, although he may respond to drug within 2 weeks of starting treatment, most patients have a longer response time.
• Caution patient to minimize exposure of treated areas to sunlight and sunlamps.
• Tell patient to cover the lesions with a generous coating of gel, but not to apply it to nor-

mal skin around the lesions or to mucosa because it may cause irritation.
- Urge patient to let gel to dry for 3 to 5 minutes before covering with clothing.
- Tell patient that drug has no systemic effect on internal Kaposi's sarcoma and that it doesn't prevent new Kaposi's sarcoma lesions in areas where it hasn't been applied.

Evaluation
- Patient remains free of infection.
- Patient experiences minimal adverse reactions.
- Patient and family state understanding of drug therapy.

allopurinol
(al-oh-PYOOR-ih-nol)
Alloremed ◇, Capurate ◇, Lopurin, Zyloprim

Pharmacologic class: xanthine oxidase inhibitor
Therapeutic class: antigout
Pregnancy risk category: C

Indications and dosages
▶ **Gout, primary or secondary to hyperuricemia; secondary to such diseases as acute or chronic leukemia, polycythemia vera, multiple myeloma, and psoriasis.** Dosage varies with severity of disease; can be given as single dose or in divided doses, but dosages larger than 300 mg should be divided. *Adults:* mild gout, 200 to 300 mg P.O. daily; severe gout with large tophi, 400 to 600 mg P.O. daily. Same dosage for maintenance in gout secondary to hyperuricemia.
▶ **Hyperuricemia secondary to malignancies.** *Children under age 6:* 50 mg P.O. t.i.d. *Children ages 6 to 10:* 300 mg P.O. daily or divided t.i.d.
▶ **Prevention of acute gouty attacks.** *Adults:* 100 mg P.O. daily; increase at weekly intervals by 100 mg without exceeding maximum dose (800 mg), until serum uric acid falls to 6 mg/100 ml or less.
▶ **Prevention of uric acid nephropathy during cancer chemotherapy.** *Adults:* 600 to 800 mg P.O. daily for 2 to 3 days, with high fluid intake.
▶ **Recurrent calcium oxalate calculi.** *Adults:* 200 to 300 mg P.O. daily in single or divided doses.
Adults with impaired renal function: 100 mg q 3 days if creatinine clearance is up to 9 ml/minute; 100 mg q 2 days, 10 to 19 ml/minute; 100 mg daily, 20 to 39 ml/minute; 150 mg daily, 40 to 59 ml/minute; 200 mg daily, 60 to 79 ml/minute; 250 mg daily, 80 ml/minute.

How supplied
Tablets (scored): 100 mg, 300 mg
Capsules: 100 mg ◇, 300 mg ◇

Pharmacokinetics
Absorption: from 80% to 90% of dose is absorbed.
Distribution: distributed widely throughout body except brain, where levels are 50% of those found elsewhere. Allopurinol and oxypurinol aren't bound to plasma proteins.
Metabolism: metabolized to oxypurinol by xanthine oxidase.
Excretion: excreted primarily in urine, with minute amount excreted in feces. *Half-life:* allopurinol, 1 to 2 hours; oxypurinol, about 15 hours.

Route	Onset	Peak	Duration
P.O.	2-3 days (allopurinol) 4.5-5 hr (oxypurinol)	0.5-2 hr	1-2 wk

Pharmacodynamics
Chemical effect: reduces uric acid production by inhibiting biochemical reactions preceding its formation.
Therapeutic effect: alleviates gout symptoms.

Adverse reactions
CNS: drowsiness, headache.
EENT: cataracts, retinopathy.
GI: nausea, vomiting, diarrhea, abdominal pain.
GU: ***renal failure,*** uremia.
Hematologic: ***agranulocytosis,*** anemia, ***aplastic anemia, thrombocytopenia.***
Hepatic: altered liver enzymes, ***hepatitis.***

Skin: *rash, usually maculopapular;* ***exfoliative lesions;*** urticarial and purpuric lesions; ***erythema multiforme;*** severe furunculosis of nose; ichthyosis; ***toxic epidermal necrolysis.***

Interactions

Drug-drug. *ACE inhibitors:* higher risk of hypersensitivity reaction. Monitor patient closely.
Amoxicillin, ampicillin, bacampicillin: increased possibility of skin rash. Avoid concomitant use.
Anticoagulants, dicumarol: potentiation of anticoagulant effect. Dosage adjustments may be necessary.
Antineoplastics: increased potential for bone marrow suppression. Monitor patient carefully.
Azathioprine, mercaptopurine (purinethol): increased serum levels of these drugs. Dosage adjustments may be necessary.
Chlorpropamide: possible increased hypoglycemic effect. Avoid concomitant use.
Diazoxide, diuretics, mecamylamine, pyrazinamide: increased serum acid level. Allopurinol dosage adjustment may be needed.
Ethacrynic acid, thiazide diuretics: increased risk of allopurinol toxicity. Reduce dosage of allopurinol and closely monitor renal function.
Uricosuric drugs: additive effect. May be used to therapeutic advantage.
Urine-acidifying drugs: may increase possibility of kidney stone formation. Monitor patient carefully.
Xanthines: increased serum theophylline level. Adjust dosage of theophylline.
Drug-lifestyle. *Alcohol use:* increased serum uric acid level. Discourage concomitant use.

Contraindications and precautions

- Contraindicated in patients with idiopathic hemochromatosis or hypersensitivity to drug.
- Use cautiously in pregnant and breast-feeding women.

NURSING CONSIDERATIONS

Assessment

- Assess patient's uric acid results, joint stiffness, and pain before and during therapy. Optimal benefits may require 2 to 6 weeks of therapy.
- Monitor fluid intake and output. Daily urine output of at least 2 L and maintenance of neutral or slightly alkaline urine is desirable.
- Monitor CBC and hepatic and renal function at start of therapy and periodically during therapy, as ordered.
- Be alert for adverse reactions and drug interactions.
- Evaluate patient's and family's knowledge of drug therapy.

Nursing diagnoses

- Acute pain (joint) related to patient's underlying condition
- Risk for infection related to drug-induced agranulocytosis
- Deficient knowledge related to drug therapy

Planning and implementation

- Administer drug with or immediately after meals to minimize adverse GI reactions.
- Have patient drink plenty of fluids while taking drug, unless contraindicated.
- Notify prescriber if renal insufficiency occurs during treatment; this usually warrants dosage reduction.

ALERT Don't confuse Zyloprim with ZORprin.

- Administer colchicine with allopurinol, if ordered. This prophylactically treats acute gout attacks that may occur in first 6 weeks of therapy.

Patient teaching

- Advise patient to refrain from driving car or performing hazardous tasks requiring mental alertness until CNS effects of drug are known.
- Advise patient taking allopurinol for treatment of recurrent calcium oxalate stones to reduce intake of animal protein, sodium, refined sugars, oxalate-rich foods, and calcium.
- Tell patient to stop drug at first sign of rash, which may precede severe hypersensitivity or other adverse reaction. Rash is more common in patients taking diuretics and in those with renal disorders. Tell patient to report all adverse reactions immediately.
- Advise patient to avoid alcohol consumption during drug therapy.

☑ Evaluation

- Patient expresses relief of joint pain.
- Patient is free from infection.
- Patient and family state understanding of drug therapy.

alprazolam

(al-PRAH-zoh-lam)

Apo-Alpraz ◆, Novo-Alprazol ◆, Nu-Alpraz ◆, Xanax

Pharmacologic class: benzodiazepine
Therapeutic class: antianxiety
Controlled substance schedule: IV
Pregnancy risk category: D

Indications and dosages

▶ **Anxiety.** *Adults:* usual initial dose, 0.25 to 0.5 mg P.O. t.i.d. Maximum dosage is 4 mg daily in divided doses.
Elderly or debilitated patients or those with advanced liver disease: usual initial dose, 0.25 mg P.O. b.i.d. or t.i.d. Maximum dosage is 4 mg daily in divided doses.
▶ **Panic disorders.** *Adults:* 0.5 mg P.O. t.i.d., increased q 3 to 4 days in increments of no more than 1 mg. Maximum dosage is 10 mg daily in divided doses.

How supplied

Tablets: 0.25 mg, 0.5 mg, 1 mg, 2 mg
Oral solution: 0.5 mg/5 ml, 1 mg/ml (concentrate)

Pharmacokinetics

Absorption: well absorbed.
Distribution: distributed widely throughout body; 80% to 90% of dose is bound to plasma protein.
Metabolism: metabolized in liver equally to alpha-hydroxyalprazolam and inactive metabolites.
Excretion: alpha-hydroxyalprazolam and other metabolites are excreted in urine. *Half-life:* 12 to 15 hours.

Route	Onset	Peak	Duration
P.O.	Unknown	1-2 hr	Unknown

Pharmacodynamics

Chemical effect: unknown. Probably potentiates effects of gamma-aminobutyric acid, an inhibitory neurotransmitter, and depresses CNS at limbic and subcortical levels of brain.
Therapeutic effect: decreases anxiety.

Adverse reactions

CNS: *drowsiness, light-headedness,* headache, confusion, hostility, anterograde amnesia, restlessness, psychosis.
CV: transient hypotension, tachycardia.
EENT: vision disturbances.
GI: dry mouth, nausea, vomiting, constipation, discomfort.
GU: incontinence, urine retention, menstrual irregularities.

Interactions

Drug-drug. *Antihistamines, antipsychotics, CNS depressants:* increased CNS depression. Avoid concomitant use.
Cimetidine: increased sedation. Monitor patient carefully.
Digoxin: may increase serum level of digoxin, increasing toxicity. Monitor patient closely.
Fluoxetine, oral contraceptives: increase serum levels of alprazolam. Watch for toxicity.
Tricyclic antidepressants: increased plasma level of tricyclic antidepressant. Watch for toxicity.
Drug-herb. *Kava*: enhanced CNS sedation. Discourage use together.
Calendula, hops, lemon balm, skullcap, valerian: May enhance sedative effects. Discourage concomitant use.
Drug-lifestyle. *Alcohol use:* increased CNS depression. Discourage concomitant use.
Smoking: decreased effectiveness of benzodiazepine. Advise patient about smoking cessation.

Contraindications and precautions

- Contraindicated in patients with acute angle-closure glaucoma or hypersensitivity to drug or other benzodiazepines and in breast-feeding women.
- Use with extreme caution in pregnant women because infant could be at risk for withdrawal symptoms.

• Use cautiously in patients with hepatic, renal, or pulmonary disease.
• Safety of drug hasn't been established in children.

NURSING CONSIDERATIONS

Assessment
• Assess patient's anxiety before and frequently after therapy.
• Monitor liver, renal, and hematopoietic function studies periodically, as ordered, in patient receiving repeated or prolonged therapy.
• Be alert for adverse reactions and drug interactions.
• Evaluate patient's and family's knowledge of drug therapy.

Nursing diagnoses
• Anxiety related to patient's underlying condition
• Risk for injury related to drug-induced CNS reactions
• Deficient knowledge related to drug therapy

Planning and implementation
• Drug shouldn't be given for everyday stress or for long-term use (more than 4 months).
• When administering drug, make sure patient has swallowed tablets before leaving bedside.
• Expect to administer lower doses at longer intervals in elderly or debilitated patients.
ALERT Don't withdraw drug abruptly after long-term use; withdrawal symptoms may occur. Abuse or addiction is possible.

Patient teaching
• Warn patient to avoid hazardous activities that require alertness and psychomotor coordination until CNS effects of drug are known.
• Tell patient to avoid alcohol consumption and smoking while taking drug.
• Caution patient to take drug as prescribed and not to stop without prescriber's approval. Inform him of potential for dependence if taken longer than directed.
• Teach patient how to manage or avoid troublesome adverse reactions, such as constipation and drowsiness.

Evaluation
• Patient is less anxious.
• Patient doesn't experience injury from adverse CNS reactions.
• Patient and family state understanding of drug therapy.

alprostadil
(al-PROS-tuh-dil)
Prostin VR Pediatric

Pharmacologic class: prostaglandin
Therapeutic class: ductus arteriosus patency adjunct
Pregnancy risk category: NR

Indications and dosages
▶ **Palliative therapy for temporary maintenance of patent ductus arteriosus until surgery can be performed.** *Infants:* 0.05 to 0.1 mcg/kg/minute by I.V. infusion. When therapeutic response is achieved, infusion rate reduced to lowest dosage that will maintain response. Maximum dosage is 0.4 mcg/kg/minute. Alternatively, drug can be administered through umbilical artery catheter placed at ductal opening.

How supplied
Injection: 500 mcg/ml

Pharmacokinetics
Absorption: not applicable with I.V. administration.
Distribution: distributed rapidly throughout body.
Metabolism: about 68% of dose is metabolized in one pass through lung, primarily by oxidation; 100% is metabolized within 24 hours.
Excretion: all metabolites are excreted in urine within 24 hours. *Half-life:* about 5 to 10 minutes.

Route	Onset	Peak	Duration
I.V.	5-10 min	≤ 20 min	1-3 hr

Pharmacodynamics

Chemical effect: relaxes smooth muscle of ductus arteriosus.
Therapeutic effect: improves cardiac circulation.

Adverse reactions

CNS: ***seizures.***
CV: ***bradycardia, cardiac arrest,*** hypotension, tachycardia.
GI: diarrhea.
Hematologic: ***disseminated intravascular coagulation.***
Other: APNEA, *flushing, fever,* ***sepsis.***

Interactions

None significant.

Contraindications and precautions

- Use cautiously in neonates with bleeding tendencies because drug inhibits platelet aggregation.

NURSING CONSIDERATIONS

Assessment

- Obtain baseline assessment of infant's cardiopulmonary status before therapy.
- Measure drug's effectiveness by monitoring blood oxygenation of infants with restricted pulmonary blood flow and by monitoring systemic blood pressure and blood pH of infants with restricted systemic blood flow.
- Be alert for adverse reactions throughout therapy.
- Evaluate parent's knowledge of drug therapy.

Nursing diagnoses

- Ineffective cardiopulmonary tissue perfusion related to underlying condition
- Risk for injury related to drug-induced adverse reactions
- Deficient knowledge related to drug therapy

Planning and implementation

- A differential diagnosis should be made between respiratory distress syndrome and cyanotic heart disease before drug is administered. Don't use drug in neonates with respiratory distress syndrome.
- Dilute drug before administering. Prepare fresh solution daily; discard solution after 24 hours.

ALERT Don't use diluents that contain benzyl alcohol. Fatal toxic syndrome may occur.

- Drug isn't recommended for direct injection or intermittent infusion. Administer by continuous infusion using constant-rate pump. Infuse through large peripheral or central vein or through umbilical artery catheter placed at level of ductus arteriosus. If flushing occurs as a result of peripheral vasodilation, reposition catheter.
- Reduce infusion rate if fever or significant hypotension develops in infant.
- If apnea and bradycardia develop, stop infusion immediately. This may reflect drug overdose.
- Keep respiratory support available.

Patient teaching

- Keep parents informed of infant's status.
- Explain that parents will be allowed as much time and physical contact with infant as feasible.

Evaluation

- Patient demonstrates stable and effective cardiopulmonary status as indicated by adequate cardiac and pulmonary parameters and peripheral systemic perfusion.
- Patient has no injury from adverse drug reactions.
- Parents state understanding of drug therapy.

alteplase (tissue plasminogen activator, recombinant; tPA)

(AL-teh-plays)
Actilyse ◇, Activase

Pharmacologic class: enzyme
Therapeutic class: thrombolytic enzyme
Pregnancy risk category: C

Indications and dosages

▶ **Lysis of thrombi obstructing coronary arteries in acute MI.** *Adults:* 100 mg I.V. infusion over 3 hours as follows: 60 mg in first hour, of which 6 to 10 mg is given as bolus over first 1 to 2 minutes. Then 20 mg/hour infusion for 2 hours. Smaller adults (less than 65 kg) should receive 1.25 mg/kg in similar fashion (60% in first hour with 10% as bolus, then 20% of total dose per hour for 2 hours). Don't exceed 100-mg dose. Higher doses may increase risk of intracranial bleeding.

▶ **Management of acute massive pulmonary embolism.** *Adults:* 100 mg I.V. infusion over 2 hours. Heparin begun at end of infusion when PTT or PT returns to twice normal or less. Don't exceed 100-mg dose. Higher doses may increase risk of intracranial bleeding.

▶ **Management of acute ischemic CVA.** *Adults:* 0.9 mg/kg (maximum 90 mg) I.V. over 60 minutes with 10% of the total dose given as initial bolus over 1 minute.

How supplied

Injection: 20-mg (11.6 million-IU), 50-mg (29 million-IU), 100-mg (58 million-IU) vials

Pharmacokinetics

Absorption: not applicable with I.V. administration.
Distribution: rapidly cleared from plasma by liver (about 80% cleared within 10 minutes after infusion stops).
Metabolism: primarily hepatic.
Excretion: over 85% excreted in urine, 5% in feces. *Half-life:* less than 10 minutes.

Route	Onset	Peak	Duration
I.V.	Immediate	About 45 min	About 4 hr

Pharmacodynamics

Chemical effect: binds to fibrin in thrombus and locally converts plasminogen to plasmin, which initiates local fibrinolysis.
Therapeutic effect: dissolves blood clots in coronary arteries and lungs.

Adverse reactions

CNS: ***cerebral hemorrhage,*** fever.
CV: hypotension, arrhythmias, edema.
GI: nausea, vomiting.
Hematologic: ***severe, spontaneous bleeding.***
Musculoskeletal: arthralgia.
Skin: urticaria.
Other: bleeding at puncture sites, hypersensitivity reactions, ***anaphylaxis.***

Interactions

Drug-drug. *Aspirin, coumarin anticoagulants, dipyridamole, heparin:* increased risk of bleeding. Monitor patient carefully.
Drug-herb. *Dong quai, garlic, ginkgo:* increased risk of bleeding. Discourage concomitant use.

Contraindications and precautions

- Contraindicated in patients with active internal bleeding, intracranial neoplasm, arteriovenous malformation, aneurysm, severe uncontrolled hypertension, history of CVA, intraspinal or intracranial trauma or surgery within past 2 months, or known bleeding diathesis.
- Use cautiously in patients who had major surgery within past 10 days; in pregnancy and first 10 days postpartum; during lactation; in those with organ biopsy; trauma (including cardiopulmonary resuscitation); GI or GU bleeding; cerebrovascular disease; hypertension; mitral stenosis, atrial fibrillation, or other condition that may lead to left-sided heart thrombus; acute pericarditis or subacute bacterial endocarditis; septic thrombophlebitis; or diabetic hemorrhagic retinopathy; in patients receiving anticoagulants; and in patients age 75 and older.
- Safety of drug hasn't been established in children.

NURSING CONSIDERATIONS

Assessment

- Assess patient's cardiopulmonary status (including ECG, vital signs, and coagulation studies) before and during therapy.
- Be alert for adverse reactions and drug interactions.
- Monitor patient for internal bleeding, and frequently check puncture sites.
- Evaluate patient's and family's knowledge of drug therapy.

Nursing diagnoses

- Ineffective cardiopulmonary tissue perfusion related to patient's underlying condition

• Risk for injury related to adverse effects of drug therapy
• Deficient knowledge related to drug therapy

Planning and implementation

• Recanalization of occluded coronary arteries and improvement of heart function require initiation of alteplase as soon as possible after onset of symptoms.
• Reconstitute drug with sterile water for injection (without preservatives) only. Check manufacturer's label for specific information. Don't use vial if vacuum isn't present. Reconstitute with large-bore (18G) needle, directing stream of sterile water at lyophilized cake. Don't shake. Slight foaming is common, and solution should be clear or pale yellow.
• Drug may be administered as reconstituted (1 mg/ml) or diluted with equal volume of normal saline solution or D_5W to make 0.5 mg/ml solution. Adding other drugs to infusion isn't recommended.
• Reconstitute alteplase solution immediately before use and administer within 8 hours because it contains no preservatives. Drug may be temporarily stored at 35° to 86° F (2° to 30° C), but it's only stable for 8 hours at room temperature. Discard unused solution.
• Heparin is frequently initiated after treatment with alteplase to reduce risk of rethrombosis.
• If arterial puncture is necessary, select site on an arm and apply pressure for 30 minutes afterward. Also use pressure dressings, sand bags, or ice packs on recent puncture sites to prevent bleeding.
• Notify prescriber if severe bleeding occurs and doesn't stop with intervention; alteplase and heparin infusions will need to be discontinued.

ALERT Have antiarrhythmic drugs available. Coronary thrombolysis is linked with arrhythmias induced by reperfusion of ischemic myocardium.

• Avoid invasive procedures during thrombolytic therapy.

Patient teaching

• Tell patient to report chest pain, dyspnea, changes in heart rate or rhythm, nausea, or bleeding immediately.

Evaluation

• Patient's cardiopulmonary assessment findings demonstrate improved perfusion.
• Patient has no serious adverse drug reactions.
• Patient and family state understanding of drug therapy.

aluminum carbonate

(uh-LOO-mih-num KAR-buh-nayt)

Basaljel†

Pharmacologic class: inorganic aluminum salt
Therapeutic class: antacid, hypophosphatemic drug
Pregnancy risk category: B

Indications and dosages

▶ **Antacid.** *Adults:* 10 ml of suspension P.O. q 2 hours p.r.n.; or 1 to 2 tablets or capsules P.O. q 2 hours p.r.n. Maximum dosage is 24 capsules, tablets, or teaspoonfuls daily.

▶ **Prevention of urinary phosphate stones (with low-phosphate diet).** *Adults:* 1 g P.O. t.i.d. or q.i.d. Adjust to lowest possible dosage after therapy is initiated, monitoring diet and serum levels.

How supplied

Tablets or capsules: equivalent to aluminum hydroxide 500 mg†
Oral suspension: equivalent to aluminum hydroxide 400 mg/5 ml†

Pharmacokinetics

Absorption: small amounts absorbed systemically.
Distribution: none.
Metabolism: none.
Excretion: excreted in feces.

Route	Onset	Peak	Duration
P.O.	20 min	Unknown if fasting; up to 3 hr if taken 1 hr after meal	20-60 min

Pharmacodynamics

Chemical effect: reduces total acid load in GI tract, elevates gastric pH to reduce pepsin activity, strengthens gastric mucosal barrier, and increases esophageal sphincter tone.
Therapeutic effect: relieves gastric discomfort and prevents phosphate stone formation in urinary tract.

Adverse reactions

GI: anorexia, *constipation,* intestinal obstruction.
Metabolic: hypophosphatemia.

Interactions

Drug-drug. *Allopurinol, antibiotics (including quinolones and tetracyclines), corticosteroids, diflunisal, digoxin, ethambutol, H_2-receptor antagonists, iron, isoniazid, penicillamine, phenothiazines, thyroid hormones:* decreased pharmacologic effect because of possible impaired absorption. Separate administration times.
Enteric-coated drugs: may release prematurely in stomach. Separate doses by at least 1 hour.

Contraindications and precautions

• No known contraindications.
• Use cautiously in patients with chronic renal disease.

NURSING CONSIDERATIONS

Assessment

• Assess patient's discomfort before therapy and regularly thereafter.
• Monitor long-term, high-dose use in patients on restricted sodium intake. Each tablet, capsule, or 5 ml of suspension contains about 3 mg of sodium.
• Be alert for adverse reactions and drug interactions.
• Evaluate patient's and family's knowledge of drug therapy.

Nursing diagnoses

• Acute pain related to gastric hyperacidity
• Constipation related to drug's adverse effects
• Deficient knowledge related to drug therapy

Planning and implementation

• Shake suspension well; give with small amount of water or fruit juice to ease passage.
• When administering through nasogastric tube, make sure tube is patent and placed correctly; after instilling, flush tube with water to ensure passage to stomach and to clear tube.
• Don't give other oral medications within 2 hours of antacid administration. This may cause premature release of enteric-coated drugs in stomach.

Patient teaching

• Caution patient to take aluminum carbonate only as directed, to shake suspension well, and to follow with sips of water or juice.
• Warn patient not to switch antacids without prescriber's advice.
• Warn patient that drug may color stool white or cause white streaks.
• Teach patient how to prevent constipation.

Evaluation

• Patient's pain is relieved.
• Patient maintains normal bowel function.
• Patient and family state understanding of drug therapy.

aluminum hydroxide

(uh-LOO-mih-num high-DROKS-ighd)
AlternaGEL†, Alu-Cap†, Alu-Tab†, Amphojel†, Dialume†, Nephrox†

Pharmacologic class: aluminum salt
Therapeutic class: antacid
Pregnancy risk category: C

Indications and dosages

► **Antacid, hyperphosphatemia.** *Adults:* 500 to 1,500 mg P.O. (tablet or capsule) 1 hour after meals and h.s.; or 5 to 30 ml (suspension) as needed 1 hour after meals and h.s.

How supplied

Tablets: 300 mg†, 500 mg†, 600 mg†
Capsules: 475 mg†, 500 mg†

Oral suspension: 320 mg/5 ml†, 600 mg/5 ml†

Pharmacokinetics

Absorption: small amounts absorbed systemically.
Distribution: none.
Metabolism: none.
Excretion: excreted in feces.

Route	Onset	Peak	Duration
P.O.	Varies: liquids more rapid than tablets or capsules	Unknown	20-60 min if fasting; 3 hr if taken after meal

Pharmacodynamics

Chemical effect: reduces total acid load in GI tract, elevates gastric pH to reduce pepsin activity, strengthens gastric mucosal barrier, and increases esophageal sphincter tone.
Therapeutic effect: relieves gastric discomfort.

Adverse reactions

GI: anorexia, *constipation,* intestinal obstruction.
Other: hypophosphatemia.

Interactions

Drug-drug. *Allopurinol, antibiotics (including quinolones and tetracyclines), corticosteroids, diflunisal, digoxin, ethambutol, H_2-receptor antagonists, iron, isoniazid, penicillamine, phenothiazines, thyroid hormones:* decreased pharmacologic effect because of possible impaired absorption. Separate administration times.
Enteric-coated drugs: may release prematurely in stomach. Separate doses by at least 1 hour.

Contraindications and precautions

- No known contraindications.
- Use cautiously in patients with chronic renal disease.

NURSING CONSIDERATIONS

Assessment

- Assess patient's discomfort before therapy and regularly thereafter.
- Monitor long-term, high-dose use in patient on restricted sodium intake. Each tablet, capsule, or 5 ml of suspension contains 2 to 3 mg of sodium.
- Be alert for adverse reactions and drug interactions.
- Evaluate patient's and family's knowledge of drug therapy.

Nursing diagnoses

- Acute pain related to gastric hyperacidity
- Constipation related to drug's adverse effects
- Deficient knowledge related to drug therapy

Planning and implementation

- Shake suspension well; give with small amount of milk or water to ease passage.
- When administering through nasogastric tube, make sure tube is patent and placed correctly; after instilling, flush tube with water to ensure passage to stomach and to clear tube.
- Don't give other oral medications within 2 hours of antacid administration. This may cause premature release of enteric-coated drugs in stomach.

Patient teaching

- Advise patient not to take aluminum hydroxide indiscriminately or to switch antacids without prescriber's advice.
- Instruct patient to shake suspension well and to follow with sips of water or juice.
- Warn patient that drug may color stool white or cause white streaks.
- Teach patient how to prevent constipation.

Evaluation

- Patient's pain is relieved.
- Patient maintains normal bowel function.
- Patient and family state understanding of drug therapy.

aluminum phosphate

(uh-LOO-mih-num FOS-fayt)
Phosphaljel†

Pharmacologic class: aluminum salt
Therapeutic class: phosphate replacement

Pregnancy risk category: NR

Indications and dosages

▶ **To reduce fecal elimination of phosphate.**
Adults: 15 to 30 ml undiluted P.O. q 2 hours between meals and h.s.

How supplied

Oral suspension: 233 mg/5 ml†

Pharmacokinetics

Absorption: small amounts absorbed systemically.
Distribution: none.
Metabolism: none.
Excretion: excreted in feces.

Route	Onset	Peak	Duration
P.O.	About 20 min	Unknown if fasting; 3 hr if taken with meal	20-60 min

Pharmacodynamics

Chemical effect: reduces fecal excretion of phosphate.
Therapeutic effect: increases phosphate level in body.

Adverse reactions

GI: *constipation,* intestinal obstruction.

Interactions

Drug-drug. *Allopurinol, antibiotics, corticosteroids, diflunisal, digoxin, ethambutol, H_2-receptor antagonists, iron, isoniazid, penicillamine, phenothiazines, thyroid hormones:* decreased pharmacologic effect because of possible impaired absorption. Separate administration times.
Ciprofloxacin, other quinolones, tetracyclines: decreased antibiotic effect. Separate administration times.
Enteric-coated drugs: may release prematurely in stomach. Separate doses by at least 1 hour.

Contraindications and precautions

- No known contraindications.
- Use cautiously in patients with chronic renal disease.

NURSING CONSIDERATIONS

Assessment

- Assess patient's phosphate level before therapy and regularly thereafter.
- Monitor long-term, high-dose use in patient on restricted sodium intake.
- Be alert for adverse reactions and drug interactions.
- Evaluate patient's and family's knowledge of drug therapy.

Nursing diagnoses

- Ineffective protection related to reduced phosphate level
- Constipation related to drug's adverse effects
- Deficient knowledge related to drug therapy

Planning and implementation

- Shake suspension well; give with small amount of milk or water to ease passage.
- When administering through nasogastric tube, make sure tube is patent and placed correctly; after instilling, flush tube with water to ensure passage to stomach and to clear tube.
- Don't give other oral medications within 2 hours of administration.

Patient teaching

- Advise patient not to take drug indiscriminately or to switch antacids without prescriber's advice.
- Instruct patient to shake suspension well and to follow with sips of water or juice.
- Warn patient that drug may color stool white or cause white streaks.
- Teach patient how to prevent constipation.

Evaluation

- Patient's phosphate level is normal.
- Patient maintains normal bowel function.
- Patient and family state understanding of drug therapy.

amantadine hydrochloride

(uh-MAN-tah-deen high-droh-KLOR-ighd)

Antadine ◇, Symadine, Symmetrel

Pharmacologic class: synthetic cyclic primary amine
Therapeutic class: antiviral, antiparkinsonian
Pregnancy risk category: C

Indications and dosages

▶ **Prophylactic or symptomatic treatment of influenza type A virus; respiratory tract illnesses.** *Adults up to age 64 and children ages 10 and over:* 200 mg P.O. daily in single dose or divided b.i.d.
Children ages 1 to 9: 4.4 to 8.8 mg/kg P.O. daily in single dose or divided b.i.d. Maximum dose is 150 mg daily.
Adults over age 64: 100 mg P.O. once daily. Treatment should continue for 24 to 48 hours after symptoms disappear. Prophylaxis should start as soon as possible after initial exposure and continue for at least 10 days. When inactivated influenza A vaccine unavailable, may continue prophylactic treatment for the duration of known influenza A in the community because of repeated or suspected exposures. If used with influenza vaccine, dose is continued for 2 to 4 weeks until protection from vaccine develops.

▶ **Drug-induced extrapyramidal reactions.** *Adults:* 100 mg P.O. b.i.d. Occasionally, patients whose responses aren't optimal may benefit from an increase up to 300 mg P.O. daily in divided doses.

▶ **Idiopathic parkinsonism, parkinsonian syndrome.** *Adults:* 100 mg P.O. b.i.d.; in patients who are seriously ill or receiving other antiparkinsonian drugs, 100 mg daily for at least 1 week, then 100 mg b.i.d., p.r.n.

How supplied

Capsules: 100 mg
Syrup: 50 mg/5 ml

Pharmacokinetics

Absorption: well absorbed from GI tract.
Distribution: distributed widely throughout body; crosses blood-brain barrier.
Metabolism: about 10% of drug is metabolized.
Excretion: about 90% is excreted unchanged in urine, primarily by tubular secretion. Portion of drug may be excreted in breast milk. Excretion rate depends on urine pH. *Half-life:* about 24 hours; with renal dysfunction, may be prolonged to 10 days.

Route	Onset	Peak	Duration
P.O.	48 hr (antidyskinetic)	2-4 hr	Unknown
	Unknown (antiviral)	Unknown	Unknown

Pharmacodynamics

Chemical effect: may interfere with influenza A virus penetration into susceptible cells. In parkinsonism, action unknown.
Therapeutic effect: protects against or reduces symptoms of influenza A viral infection and reduces extrapyramidal symptoms.

Adverse reactions

CNS: depression, fatigue, confusion, dizziness, psychosis, hallucinations, anxiety, *irritability,* ataxia, *insomnia,* weakness, headache, light-headedness, difficulty concentrating.
CV: peripheral edema, orthostatic hypotension, ***heart failure.***
GI: anorexia, nausea, constipation, vomiting, dry mouth.
GU: urine retention.
Skin: *livedo reticularis.*

Interactions

Drug-drug. *Anticholinergics:* increased adverse anticholinergic effects. Use together cautiously.
CNS stimulants: additive CNS stimulation. Use together cautiously.
Hydrochlorothiazide, triamterene: increased levels of amantadine. Use together cautiously.
Quinidine, quinine: reduced renal clearance of amantadine. Use together cautiously.
Sulfamethoxazole, trimethoprim: increased amantadine serum levels. Use together cautiously.
Thioridazine: worsened tremor in elderly patients. Monitor them closely.

Drug-herb. *Jimsonweed:* may adversly affect CV function. Advise against concomitant use.

Contraindications and precautions

- Contraindicated in patients hypersensitive to drug.
- Use cautiously in patients with seizure disorders, heart failure, peripheral edema, hepatic disease, mental illness, eczematoid rash, renal impairment, orthostatic hypotension, or CV disease; in elderly patients; and in pregnant or breast-feeding women. Dosage may need adjustment in patients with renal failure.
- Safety of drug hasn't been established for children under age 1.

NURSING CONSIDERATIONS

Assessment
- Obtain baseline assessment of patient's exposure to influenza A virus or history of Parkinson's disease, as appropriate.
- Be alert for adverse reactions and drug interactions.
- Monitor patient's hydration status if adverse GI reactions occur.
- Evaluate patient's and family's knowledge of drug therapy.

Nursing diagnoses
- Ineffective health maintenance related to patient's underlying condition
- Risk for deficient fluid volume related to adverse GI reactions
- Deficient knowledge related to drug therapy

Planning and implementation
- Elderly patients are more susceptible to neurologic adverse effects. Giving drug in two daily doses rather than as single dose may reduce these effects.
- Administer drug after meals for best absorption.

Patient teaching
- Advise patient to take drug several hours before bedtime to prevent insomnia.
- Advise patient not to stand or change positions too quickly to prevent orthostatic hypotension.
- Instruct patient to report adverse reactions, especially dizziness, depression, anxiety, nausea, and urine retention.
- Warn patient with parkinsonism not to stop drug abruptly; doing so could precipitate a parkinsonian crisis.

Evaluation
- Patient exhibits improved health status.
- Patient maintains adequate hydration.
- Patient and family state understanding of drug therapy.

amifostine
(am-eh-FOS-teen)
Ethyol

Pharmacologic class: organic thiophosphate cytoprotective drug
Therapeutic class: antimetabolite
Pregnancy risk category: C

Indications and dosages

▶ **Reduction of cumulative renal toxicity from repeated administration of cisplatin in patients with advanced ovarian cancer or non-small-cell lung cancer.** *Adults:* 910 mg/m² daily as a 15-minute I.V. infusion, starting 30 minutes before chemotherapy. If hypotension occurs and blood pressure doesn't return to normal within 5 minutes after stopping treatment, subsequent cycles should use 740 mg/m².

▶ **Reduction of moderate to severe xerostomia in patients undergoing postoperative radiation treatment for head or neck cancer.** *Adults:* 200 mg/m² daily as a 3-minute I.V. infusion, starting 15 to 30 minutes before standard fraction radiation therapy. Hydrate patient adequately before infusion. Administer antiemetic before and in conjunction with amifostine infusion. Monitor patient's blood pressure before and immediately after the infusion, and periodically thereafter as indicated.

How supplied

Injection: 500 mg anhydrous base and 500 mg mannitol in 10-ml vial

Pharmacokinetics

Absorption: not applicable.
Distribution: less than 10% remains in plasma 6 minutes after administration.
Metabolism: metabolized to an active free thiol metabolite.
Excretion: renally excreted. *Half-life (elimination):* 8 minutes.

Route	Onset	Peak	Duration
I.V.	5-8 min	Unknown	Unknown

Pharmacodynamics

Chemical effect: dephosphoryated by alkaline phosphatase to pharmacologically active free thiol metabolite. Free thiol in normal tissues is available to bind to and detoxify reactive metabolites of cisplatin.
Therapeutic effect: reduction of toxic effects of cisplatin on renal tissue.

Adverse reactions

CNS: dizziness, somnolence, flushing or feeling of warmth, chills or feeling of coldness.
CV: *hypotension.*
EENT: sneezing.
GI: *nausea, vomiting.*
Metabolic: hypocalcemia.
Respiratory: hiccups.
Other: allergic reactions ranging from rash to rigors.

Interactions

Drug-drug. *Antihypertensive drugs, other drugs that could potentiate hypotension*: may potentiate hypotension. Give special consideration to administration of amifostine in patients receiving these drugs.

Contraindications and precautions

- Contraindicated in patients hypersensitive to aminothiol compounds or mannitol. Don't use drug in patients receiving chemotherapy for potentially curable malignancies (including certain malignancies of germ cell origin), except for patients involved in clinical studies. Also contraindicated in hypotensive or dehydrated patients and in those receiving antihypertensive drugs that can't be stopped during the 24 hours preceding amifostine administration.
- Use cautiously in patients with ischemic heart disease, arrhythmias, heart failure, or history of CVA or transient ischemic attacks.
- Use cautiously in patients for whom common adverse effects (nausea, vomiting, and hypotension) are likely to have serious consequences.
- Use cautiously in elderly patients and in children; safety hasn't been established in these patients.

NURSING CONSIDERATIONS

Assessment

- Patients who receive amifostine should be adequately hydrated before administration. Keep patient supine during infusion.
- Monitor blood pressure every 5 minutes during infusion. If hypotension occurs and requires interrupting therapy, notify prescriber and place patient in Trendelenburg's position. Then give an infusion of normal saline solution, as ordered, using a separate I.V. line. If blood pressure returns to normal within 5 minutes and patient is asymptomatic, restart infusion so full dose of drug can be given. If full dose can't be given, subsequent doses should be limited to 740 mg/m^2.
- Antiemetics, including dexamethasone 20 mg I.V. and a serotonin 5-HT_3 receptor antagonist, should be administered before, and concurrent with, amifostine administration. Additional antiemetics may be needed based on chemotherapeutic drugs administered.
- Monitor patient's fluid balance when drug is given with highly emetogenic chemotherapy.
- Monitor serum calcium level in patients at risk for hypocalcemia, such as those with nephrotic syndrome. If necessary, calcium supplements should be ordered and administered.
- Evaluate patient's and family's knowledge of drug therapy.

Nursing diagnoses

- Ineffective health maintenance related to neoplastic disease
- Deficient knowledge related to drug therapy

Planning and implementation

- Reconstitute each single-dose vial with 9.5 ml of sterile normal saline injection. Don't use other solutions to reconstitute drug. Reconstituted solution (500 mg amifostine/10 ml) is chemically stable for up to 5 hours at room temperature (about 77° F [25° C]) or up to 24 hours under refrigeration (35° to 46° F [2° to 8° C]).

- Drug can be prepared in polyvinyl chloride bags in concentrations of 5 to 40 mg/ml and has the same stability as when it is reconstituted in single-use vial.
- Inspect vial for particulate matter and discoloration before use, if possible. Don't use if cloudiness or precipitate is noted.
- If possible and if ordered, stop antihypertensive therapy 24 hours before drug administration. If antihypertensive therapy can't be stopped, don't use amifostine because severe hypotension may occur.
- Don't infuse for more than 15 minutes; longer infusion raises the risk of adverse reactions.

Patient teaching

- Instruct patient to remain in a supine position throughout infusion.
- Advise patient not to breast-feed; it is unknown whether drug or its metabolites are excreted in breast milk.

Evaluation

- Patient shows positive response to drug.
- Patient and family state understanding of drug therapy.

amikacin sulfate

(am-eh-KAY-sin SUL-fayt)
Amikin

Pharmacologic class: aminoglycoside
Therapeutic class: antibiotic
Pregnancy risk category: D

Indications and dosages

▶ **Serious infections caused by sensitive strains of *Pseudomonas aeruginosa, Escherichia coli, Proteus, Klebsiella, Serratia, Enterobacter, Acinetobacter, Providencia, Citrobacter, Staphylococcus;* meningitis.** *Adults and children:* 15 mg/kg/day divided q 8 to 12 hours I.M. or I.V. infusion.

Neonates: initially, loading dose of 10 mg/kg I.V., followed by 7.5 mg/kg q 12 hours.

▶ **Uncomplicated UTI.** *Adults:* 250 mg I.M. or I.V. b.i.d.

▶ **Adults with impaired renal function.** *Adults:* initially, 7.5 mg/kg I.M. or I.V. Subsequent doses and frequency determined by amikacin blood level and renal function studies.

How supplied

Injection: 50 mg/ml, 250 mg/ml

Pharmacokinetics

Absorption: rapidly absorbed after I.M. administration.

Distribution: distributed widely; protein binding is minimal; drug crosses placenta.

Metabolism: none.

Excretion: excreted primarily in urine by glomerular filtration. *Half-life:* 2 to 3 hours (adults); 30 to 86 hours (patients with severe renal damage).

Route	Onset	Peak	Duration
I.V.	Immediate	Immediate	8-12 hr
I.M.	Unknown	1 hr	8-12 hr

Pharmacodynamics

Chemical effect: inhibits protein synthesis by binding directly to 30S ribosomal subunit. Generally bactericidal.

Therapeutic effect: kills susceptible bacteria. Its spectrum of activity includes many aerobic gram-negative organisms (including most strains of *Pseudomonas aeruginosa*) and some aerobic gram-positive organisms. It is ineffective against anaerobes.

Adverse reactions

CNS: headache, lethargy, ***neuromuscular blockade.***
EENT: *ototoxicity.*
GU: *nephrotoxicity.*
Hepatic: ***hepatic necrosis.***
Other: hypersensitivity reactions, ***anaphylaxis.***

Interactions

Drug-drug. *Acyclovir, amphotericin B, cisplatin, methoxyflurane, other aminoglycosides,*

vancomycin: increased nephrotoxicity. Use together cautiously.
Cephalothin: increased nephrotoxicity. Use together cautiously.
Dimenhydrinate: may mask symptoms of ototoxicity. Use cautiously.
General anesthetics, neuromuscular blocking drugs: may potentiate neuromuscular blockade. Monitor patient.
Indomethacin: may increase serum trough and peak levels of amikacin. Monitor serum amikacin level closely.
I.V. loop diuretics (such as furosemide): increased ototoxicity. Use together cautiously.
Parenteral penicillins (such as ticarcillin): amikacin inactivation in vitro. Don't mix.

Contraindications and precautions

- Contraindicated in breast-feeding women and in patients hypersensitive to drug or other aminoglycosides.
- Use with extreme caution in pregnant women and only if benefit outweighs risk to fetus.
- Use cautiously in patients with impaired renal function or neuromuscular disorders, in neonates and infants, and in elderly patients.

NURSING CONSIDERATIONS

Assessment

- Assess patient's infection, hearing, weight, and renal function studies before therapy and regularly thereafter.
- Watch for signs of ototoxicity, including tinnitus, vertigo, and hearing loss.
- Monitor serum amikacin level. Obtain blood for peak amikacin level 1 hour after I.M. injection and 30 minutes to 1 hour after infusion ends; for trough level, draw blood just before next dose. Don't collect blood in heparinized tube because heparin is incompatible with aminoglycosides. Be aware that peak blood level above 35 mcg/ml and trough level above 10 mcg/ml may raise the risk of toxicity.
- Be alert for signs of nephrotoxicity, including cells or casts in urine, oliguria, proteinuria, decreased creatinine clearance, increased BUN and serum creatinine levels.
- Evaluate patient's and family's knowledge of drug therapy.

Nursing diagnoses

- Risk for infection related to bacteria
- Impaired urine elimination related to amikacin-induced nephrotoxicity
- Deficient knowledge related to drug therapy

Planning and implementation

- Obtain specimen for culture and sensitivity tests before first dose. Therapy may begin pending results.

I.V. use: For adults, dilute in 100 to 200 ml of D_5W or normal saline solution and infuse over 30 to 60 minutes. Volume for pediatric patients depends on dose of drug ordered. Infants should receive a 1- to 2-hour infusion.
– After I.V. infusion, flush line with normal saline solution or D_5W.
I.M. use: Follow normal protocol.

- Therapy usually lasts 7 to 10 days.
- Drug potency isn't affected if solution turns light yellow.
- Encourage adequate fluid intake; patient should be well hydrated while taking drug to minimize chemical irritation of renal tubules.
- If no response occurs after 3 to 5 days, therapy may be stopped and new specimens obtained for culture and sensitivity testing.

Patient teaching

- Tell patient to immediately report changes in hearing or in appearance or elimination pattern of urine. Teach patient how to measure intake and output.
- Emphasize importance of drinking 2 L of fluid daily, if not contraindicated.
- Teach patient to watch for and promptly report signs of superinfection (continued fever and other signs of new infections, especially of upper respiratory tract).

Evaluation

- Patient's infection is eradicated.
- Patient's renal function studies remain unchanged.
- Patient and family state understanding of drug therapy.

amiloride hydrochloride

(uh-MIL-uh-righd high-droh-KLOR-ighd)
Kaluril◇, Midamor

Pharmacologic class: potassium-sparing diuretic
Therapeutic class: diuretic, antihypertensive
Pregnancy risk category: B

Indications and dosages

▶ **Hypertension; edema caused by heart failure, usually in patients also taking thiazide or other potassium-wasting diuretics.** *Adults:* usual dosage is 5 mg P.O. daily. Increased to 10 mg daily, if necessary. Maximum, 20 mg daily.

How supplied

Tablets: 5 mg

Pharmacokinetics

Absorption: about 50% of dose is absorbed from GI tract; food decreases absorption to 30%.
Distribution: has wide extravascular distribution.
Metabolism: insignificant.
Excretion: excreted primarily in urine. *Half-life:* 6 to 9 hours.

Route	Onset	Peak	Duration
P.O.	≤ 2 hr	6-10 hr	24 hr

Pharmacodynamics

Chemical effect: inhibits sodium reabsorption and potassium excretion in distal tubule.
Therapeutic effect: reduces blood pressure; promotes sodium and water excretion while blocking potassium excretion.

Adverse reactions

CNS: *headache,* weakness, dizziness.
CV: orthostatic hypotension.
GI: *nausea, anorexia, diarrhea, vomiting,* abdominal pain, constipation.
GU: impotence.
Hematologic: ***aplastic anemia.***
Metabolic: hyperkalemia.

Interactions

Drug-drug. *ACE inhibitors, potassium-containing salt substitutes, potassium-sparing diuretics, potassium supplements:* possible hyperkalemia. Monitor potassium levels closely.
Lithium: decreased lithium clearance, increasing risk of lithium toxicity. Monitor lithium level.
NSAIDs: decreased diuretic effectiveness. Monitor for lack of therapeutic effect.
Drug-food. *Foods high in potassium, potassium-containing salt substitutes:* possible hyperkalemia. Monitor serum potassium.

Contraindications and precautions

- Contraindicated in patients with elevated serum potassium level (over 5.5 mEq/L); in those receiving other potassium-sparing diuretics, such as spironolactone; in those with anuria, acute or chronic renal insufficiency, diabetic nephropathy, or hypersensitivity to drug; and in breast-feeding women.
- Use with extreme caution, if at all, in patients with diabetes mellitus.
- Use cautiously in patients with severe hepatic insufficiency, in pregnant women, and in elderly or debilitated patients.
- Safety of drug hasn't been established in children.

NURSING CONSIDERATIONS

Assessment

- Assess patient's blood pressure, urine output, weight, serum electrolytes, and degree of edema before therapy and regularly thereafter.
- Be alert for adverse reactions and drug interactions.
- Evaluate patient's and family's knowledge of drug therapy.

Nursing diagnoses

- Excessive fluid volume related to fluid retention
- Risk for injury related to potential for drug-induced hyperkalemia
- Deficient knowledge related to drug therapy

Planning and implementation

- Administer amiloride with meals to prevent nausea.

- Administer early in the day to prevent nocturia.
- Alert prescriber immediately if potassium level exceeds 6.5 mEq/L, and expect drug to be discontinued.
- Choose diet with caution.

Patient teaching
- Advise patient to avoid sudden posture changes and to rise slowly to avoid orthostatic hypotension.
- Warn patient to limit potassium-rich foods (such as oranges and bananas), potassium-containing salt substitutes, and potassium supplements to prevent serious hyperkalemia.
- Teach patient and family to identify and report signs of hyperkalemia.
- Teach patient and family to monitor patient's fluid volume by recording daily weight and intake and output.

Evaluation
- Patient's fluid retention is relieved.
- Patient's serum potassium level remains normal.
- Patient and family state understanding of drug therapy.

amino acid infusions, crystalline
(uh-MEEN-oh AS-id in-FYOO-zhuns)
Aminosyn, Aminosyn II, Aminosyn-PF, FreAmine III, Novamine, Travasol, TrophAmine

amino acid infusions in dextrose
Aminosyn II with Dextrose

amino acid infusions with electrolytes
Aminosyn with Electrolytes, Aminosyn II with Electrolytes, FreAmine III with Electrolytes, ProcalAmine with Electrolytes, Travasol with Electrolytes

amino acid infusions with electrolytes in dextrose
Aminosyn II with Electrolytes in Dextrose

amino acid infusions for hepatic failure
HepatAmine

amino acid infusions for high metabolic stress
Aminosyn-HBC, BranchAmin, FreAmine HBC

amino acid infusions for renal failure
Aminess, Aminosyn-RF, Nephr-Amine, RenAmin

Pharmacologic class: protein substrate
Therapeutic class: parenteral nutritional therapy and caloric
Pregnancy risk category: C

Indications and dosages
▶ **Total parenteral nutrition in patients who can't or won't eat.** *Adults:* 1 to 1.5 g/kg I.V. daily.
Children: 2 to 3 g/kg I.V. daily.
▶ **Nutritional support in patients with cirrhosis, hepatitis, or hepatic encephalopathy.** *Adults:* 80 to 120 g of amino acids (12 to 18 g of nitrogen) I.V. daily using formulation for hepatic failure.
▶ **Nutritional support in patients with high metabolic stress.** *Adults:* 1.5 g/kg I.V. daily using formulation for high metabolic stress.

How supplied
Injection: 250 ml, 500 ml, 1,000 ml, 2,000 ml containing amino acids in varying concentrations. *Crystalline:* Aminosyn, 3.5%, 5%, 7%, 8.5%, 10%. Aminosyn II, 3.5%, 5%, 7%, 8.5%, 10%. Aminosyn-PF, 7%, 10%. FreAmine III, 8.5%, 10%. Novamine, 11.4%, 15%. Travasol, 5.5%, 8.5%, 10%. TrophAmine, 6%, 10%. *In dextrose:* Aminosyn II, 3.5% in 5% dextrose, 3.5% in 25% dextrose, 4.25% in 10% dextrose, 4.25% in 20% dextrose, 4.25% in 25% dextrose, 5% in 25% dextrose. *With electrolytes:* Aminosyn, 3.5%, 7%, 8.5%. Aminosyn II, 3.5%, 7%, 8.5%, 10%. FreAmine III, 3%, 8.5%. ProcalAmine, 3%. Travasol, 3.5%, 5.5%, 8.5%. *With electrolytes in dextrose:* Aminosyn II, 3.5% with electrolytes in 5% dextrose, 4.25%

with electrolytes in 10% dextrose. *For hepatic failure:* HepatAmine, 8%. *For high metabolic stress:* Aminosyn-HBC, 7%. BranchAmin, 4%. FreAmine HBC, 6.9%. *For renal failure:* Aminess, 5.2%. Aminosyn-RF, 5.2%. NephrAmine, 5.4%. RenAmin, 6.5%.

Pharmacokinetics

No information available.

Route	Onset	Peak	Duration
I.V.	Immediate	Immediate	Unknown

Pharmacodynamics

Chemical effect: provides substrate for protein synthesis or enhances conservation of existing body protein. Formulations for hepatic failure and high metabolic stress contain essential and nonessential amino acids, with high levels of branched chain amino acids isoleucine, leucine, and valine. Formulations for renal failure contain histidine and minimal amounts of essential amino acids; nonessential amino acids are synthesized from excess ammonia in blood of uremic patient, thus lowering azotemia.

Therapeutic effect: provides body with needed calories and protein.

Adverse reactions

CNS: mental confusion, unconsciousness, headache, dizziness.

CV: hypervolemia, ***heart failure*** (in susceptible patients), ***pulmonary edema,*** worsening of hypertension (in predisposed patients), thrombophlebitis, thrombosis.

GI: nausea, vomiting.

GU: glycosuria, osmotic diuresis.

Hepatic: fatty liver.

Metabolic: *rebound hypoglycemia,* hyperglycemia, metabolic acidosis, alkalosis, hypophosphatemia, ***hyperosmolar hyperglycemic nonketotic syndrome,*** hyperammonemia, electrolyte imbalances.

Skin: chills, flushing, feeling of warmth.

Other: hypersensitivity reactions, tissue sloughing at infusion site caused by extravasation, *catheter sepsis,* dehydration (if hyperosmolar solutions are used).

Interactions

Drug-drug. *Tetracycline:* may reduce protein-sparing effects of infused amino acids because of its antianabolic activity. Monitor patient.

Contraindications and precautions

- Contraindicated in patients with anuria; inborn errors of amino acid metabolism, such as maple syrup urine disease and isovaleric acidemia; severe uncorrected electrolyte or acid-base imbalances; hyperammonemia; or decreased circulating blood volume.
- Use with extreme caution in pediatric patients and in neonates, especially those of low birth weight.
- Use cautiously in patients with renal insufficiency or failure, cardiac disease, or hepatic impairment.
- Use with caution in diabetic patients; insulin may be required to prevent hyperglycemia. Administer cautiously in cardiac insufficiency; may cause circulatory overload. Patients with fluid restriction may tolerate only 1 to 2 L.

NURSING CONSIDERATIONS

Assessment

- Assess serum electrolyte, glucose, BUN, calcium, and phosphate levels before therapy, as ordered, and regularly thereafter.
- Be alert for adverse reactions and drug interactions.
- Check infusion site frequently for erythema, inflammation, irritation, tissue sloughing, necrosis, and phlebitis.
- Evaluate patient's and family's knowledge of drug therapy.

Nursing diagnoses

- Altered nutrition (less than body requirements) related to patient's underlying condition
- Risk for deficient fluid volume related to adverse drug reactions
- Deficient knowledge related to drug therapy

Planning and implementation

- Control infusion rate carefully with infusion pump. If infusion rate falls behind, notify prescriber; don't increase rate to catch up.

• Peripheral infusions should be limited to 2.5% amino acids and dextrose 10%.
• Prescriber will individualize dosage according to patient's metabolic and clinical response as determined by nitrogen balance and body weight corrected for fluid balance.
• Add vitamins, electrolytes, and trace elements, as ordered.
• If patient has chills, fever, or other signs of sepsis, replace I.V. tubing and bottle and send them to laboratory to be cultured.

Patient teaching
• Tell patient to report discomfort at injection site or unusual symptoms.

Evaluation
• Patient's nutritional status improves.
• Patient maintains adequate hydration.
• Patient and family state understanding of drug therapy.

aminocaproic acid
(uh-mee-noh-kah-PROH-ik AS-id)
Amicar

Pharmacologic class: carboxylic acid derivative
Therapeutic class: fibrinolysis inhibitor
Pregnancy risk category: C

Indications and dosages
▶ **Excessive bleeding from hyperfibrinolysis.** *Adults:* 4 to 5 g I.V. over first hour, followed with constant infusion of 1 g/hour for about 8 hours or until bleeding is controlled. Maximum, 30 g/24 hours.

How supplied
Injection: 5 g/20 ml for dilution, 24 g/96 ml for infusion

Pharmacokinetics
Absorption: rapidly and completely absorbed from GI tract when administered orally.
Distribution: readily permeates human blood cells and other body cells. It isn't protein-bound.
Metabolism: insignificant.
Excretion: from 40% to 60% of single oral dose is excreted unchanged in urine in 12 hours.

Route	Onset	Peak	Duration
I.V.	≤ 1 hr	Unknown	≤ 3 hr

Pharmacodynamics
Chemical effect: inhibits plasminogen activator substances and blocks antiplasmin activity.
Therapeutic effect: promotes blood-clotting activity.

Adverse reactions
CNS: dizziness, headache, delirium, ***seizures,*** weakness, malaise.
CV: hypotension, ***bradycardia, arrhythmias.***
EENT: tinnitus, nasal stuffiness, conjunctival suffusion.
GI: nausea, cramps, diarrhea.
GU: ***acute renal failure.***
Hematologic: generalized thrombosis.
Musculoskeletal: myopathy.
Skin: rash.

Interactions
Drug-drug. *Estrogens, oral contraceptives:* increased probability of hypercoagulability. Use together cautiously.

Contraindications and precautions
• Contraindicated in patients with active intravascular clotting or disseminated intravascular coagulation unless heparin is used concomitantly. Injectable form is contraindicated in newborns.
• Use cautiously in patients with cardiac, hepatic, or renal disease and in pregnant or breast-feeding women.
• Safety of drug hasn't been established in children.

NURSING CONSIDERATIONS

Assessment
• Assess history of blood loss, coagulation studies, blood pressure, and heart rhythm before therapy.
• Monitor coagulation studies throughout therapy, as ordered.

• Observe heart rhythm, especially when giving I.V. dose.
• Be alert for adverse reactions and drug interactions.
• Evaluate patient's and family's knowledge of drug therapy.

Nursing diagnoses
• Deficient fluid volume related to excessive bleeding
• Altered venous tissue perfusion related to drug-induced generalized thrombosis
• Deficient knowledge related to drug therapy

Planning and implementation
• Dilute solution with sterile water for injection, normal saline injection, D_5W, or Ringer's injection. Infuse slowly. Don't give by direct or intermittent injection.
• Keep oxygen and resuscitation equipment nearby.

Patient teaching
• Explain all procedures to patient and family.
• Instruct patient and family to report respiratory difficulty, pain, or changes in mental status immediately.

Evaluation
• Patient regains normal fluid volume status.
• Patient shows no signs of impaired venous tissue perfusion.
• Patient and family state understanding of drug therapy.

aminoglutethimide
(uh-mee-noh-gloo-TETH-ih-mighd)
Cytadren

Pharmacologic class: antiadrenal hormone
Therapeutic class: antineoplastic
Pregnancy risk category: D

Indications and dosages
▶ **Suppression of adrenal function in Cushing's syndrome and adrenal cancer.** *Adults:* 250 mg q.i.d. at 6-hour intervals. Dosage may be increased in increments of 250 mg daily q 1 to 2 weeks to maximum of 2 g daily.

How supplied
Tablets: 250 mg

Pharmacokinetics
Absorption: well absorbed through GI tract.
Distribution: distributed widely into body tissues.
Metabolism: metabolized extensively in liver.
Excretion: excreted primarily through kidneys, mostly as unchanged drug. *Half-life:* 12½ hours (7 hours with prolonged treatment).

Route	Onset	Peak	Duration
P.O.	Unknown	1.5 hr	1.5-3 days

Pharmacodynamics
Chemical effect: blocks conversion of cholesterol to delta-5-pregnenolone in adrenal cortex, inhibiting synthesis of adrenal steroids.
Therapeutic effect: decreases adrenocortical hormone levels.

Adverse reactions
CNS: *drowsiness,* headache, dizziness.
CV: hypotension, tachycardia.
GI: nausea, anorexia.
GU: masculinization.
Hematologic: transient leukopenia, ***agranulocytosis, thrombocytopenia.***
Metabolic: hypothyroidism.
Musculoskeletal: myalgia.
Skin: *morbilliform rash,* pruritus, urticaria, hirsutism.
Other: fever, adrenal insufficiency.

Interactions
Drug-drug. *Dexamethasone, medroxyprogesterone:* increased hepatic metabolism of these drugs. Monitor patient closely.
Digoxin: may increase drug clearance. Monitor patient closely.
Oral anticoagulants: decreased anticoagulant effect. Monitor PT and INR.
Theophylline: reduced action of theophylline. Monitor patient closely.
Drug-lifestyle. *Alcohol use:* may potentiate effects of aminoglutethimide. Discourage concomitant use.

Contraindications and precautions

- Contraindicated in breast-feeding women and in patients hypersensitive to drug or to glutethimide.
- Use with extreme caution in pregnant patients because drug can harm fetus.
- Safety of drug hasn't been established in children.

NURSING CONSIDERATIONS

Assessment

- Assess patient's underlying condition before therapy, and note improvement.
- Watch for adrenal hypofunction, especially under stressful conditions, such as surgery, trauma, or acute illness.
- Be alert for adverse reactions and drug interactions.
- Evaluate patient's and family's knowledge of drug therapy.

Nursing diagnoses

- Ineffective health maintenance related to patient's underlying condition
- Ineffective protection related to drug-induced adrenal suppression
- Deficient knowledge related to drug therapy

Planning and implementation

- Administer on schedule, and alert prescriber if dose is delayed or missed.
- Patient may need more supplements during stress, such as a mineralocorticoid supplement to treat hyponatremia and orthostatic hypotension. Glucocorticoid replacement also may be necessary.

Patient teaching

- Instruct patient to notify prescriber about stress; additional therapy may be needed.
- Caution patient to watch for signs of infection (fever, sore throat, fatigue) and bleeding (easy bruising, nosebleeds, bleeding gums, melena). Tell patient to take temperature daily.
- Warn patient to avoid hazardous activities until full CNS effects of drug are known.
- Advise patient to stand up slowly to minimize orthostatic hypotension.
- Tell patient to report rash that lasts more than 8 days. Reassure patient that drowsiness, nausea, and loss of appetite usually diminish within 2 weeks after start of therapy, but advise him to notify prescriber if symptoms persist.
- Advise patient to avoid alcohol consumption during drug therapy.

Evaluation

- Patient's health is maintained.
- Patient has no hypoadrenalism.
- Patient and family state understanding of drug therapy.

aminophylline (theophylline and ethylenediamine)

(uh-mih-NOF-il-in)

Aminophyllin, Cardophyllin ◇, Corophyllin ♦, Phyllocontin, Phyllocontin-350, Somophyllin, Somophyllin-DF

Pharmacologic class: xanthine derivative
Therapeutic class: bronchodilator
Pregnancy risk category: C

Indications and dosages

▶ **Symptomatic relief of bronchospasm.** *Patients not currently receiving theophylline products who require rapid relief of symptoms:* loading dose is 6 mg/kg (equivalent to 4.7 mg/kg anhydrous theophylline) I.V. (25 mg/minute or less), then maintenance infusion.
Adults (nonsmokers): 0.7 mg/kg/hour I.V. for 12 hours; then 0.5 mg/kg/hour.
Otherwise healthy adult smokers: 1 mg/kg/hour I.V. for 12 hours; then 0.8 mg/kg/hour.
Older patients and adults with cor pulmonale: 0.6 mg/kg/hour I.V. for 12 hours; then 0.3 mg/kg/hour.
Adults with heart failure or liver disease: 0.5 mg/kg/hour I.V. for 12 hours; then 0.1 to 0.2 mg/kg/hour.
Children ages 9 to 16: 1 mg/kg/hour I.V. for 12 hours; then 0.8 mg/kg/hour.
Children ages 6 months to 9 years: 1.2 mg/kg/hour for 12 hours; then 1 mg/kg/hour.

Patients currently receiving theophylline products: aminophylline infusion of 0.63 mg/kg (0.5 mg/kg anhydrous theophylline) increases plasma level of theophylline by 1 mcg/ml. Some clinicians recommend dose of 3.1 mg/kg (2.5 mg/kg anhydrous theophylline) with no obvious signs of theophylline toxicity.

▶ **Chronic bronchial asthma.** Dosage is highly individualized. Rectal dosage is same as that recommended for oral dosage.
Adults: 600 to 1,600 mg P.O. daily in divided doses t.i.d. or q.i.d.
Children: 12 mg/kg P.O. daily in divided doses t.i.d. or q.i.d.

How supplied

Tablets: 100 mg, 200 mg
Tablets (extended-release): 225 mg, 350 mg ♦
Oral liquid: 105 mg/5 ml
Injection: 250 mg/10 ml, 500 mg/20 ml, 500 mg/2 ml, 100 mg/100 ml in half-normal saline solution, 200 mg/100 ml in half-normal saline solution
Rectal suppositories: 250 mg, 500 mg

Pharmacokinetics

Absorption: well absorbed except for suppository form, which is unreliable and slow. Food may alter rate but not extent of absorption of oral doses.
Distribution: distributed in all tissues and extracellular fluids except fatty tissue.
Metabolism: converted to theophylline, then metabolized to inactive compounds.
Excretion: excreted in urine as theophylline (10%). *Half-life:* depends on many variables, including smoking status, concurrent illness, age, and formulation used.

Route	Onset	Peak	Duration
P.O.			
Tablets	15-60 min	2 hr	Varies
Extended-release	Unknown	4-7 hr	Varies
Solution	15-60 min	≤ 1 hr	Varies
I.V.	15 min	Immediate	Varies
P.R.	Varies	Varies	Varies

Pharmacodynamics

Chemical effect: inhibits phosphodiesterase, the enzyme that degrades cAMP, thereby relaxing smooth muscle of bronchial airways and pulmonary blood vessels.
Therapeutic effect: eases breathing.

Adverse reactions

CNS: *nervousness, restlessness, dizziness,* headache, *insomnia,* light-headedness, ***seizures,*** muscle twitching.
CV: *palpitations, tachycardia,* extrasystole, flushing, marked hypotension, increased respiratory rate, ***arrhythmias.***
GI: *nausea, vomiting, anorexia,* dyspepsia, heavy feeling in stomach, diarrhea, bitter aftertaste.
Respiratory: ***respiratory arrest.***
Skin: urticaria, local irritation with rectal suppositories.

Interactions

Drug-drug. *Adenosine:* decreased antiarrhythmic effectiveness. Higher doses of adenosine may be necessary.
Alkali-sensitive drugs: reduced activity. Don't add to I.V. fluids containing aminophylline.
Allopurinol (high doses), cimetidine, influenza virus vaccine, macrolide antibiotics (such as erythromycin), oral contraceptives, quinolone antibiotics (such as ciprofloxacin): decreased hepatic clearance of theophylline; elevated theophylline blood level. Monitor patient for toxicity.
Amiodarone, ticlopidine, verapamil: increase theophylline levels. Use together cautiously.
Barbiturates, carbamazepine, nicotine, phenytoin, rifampin: enhanced metabolism and decreased theophylline blood level. Monitor patient for decreased aminophylline effect.
Beta blockers: antagonism. Propranolol and nadolol, especially, may cause bronchospasm in sensitive patients. Use together cautiously.
Ephedrine, other sympathomimetics: theophylline may exhibit synergistic toxicity with these drugs, predisposing patient to arrhythmias. Monitor patient closely.
Isoniazid, ketoconazole: decrease theophylline absorption.
Lithium: theophylline may increase lithium level. Monitor patient closely.
Drug-herb. *St. John's wort:* may lower blood levels of drug making it less effective. Monitor

patient for lack of therapeutic effect. Discourage concomitant use.

Drug-lifestyle. *Smoking:* may increase clearance and decrease half-life of theophylline. Higher doses may be needed to achieve desired effect.

Contraindications and precautions

- Contraindicated in patients with active peptic ulcer disease, seizure disorders (unless anticonvulsant therapy is given), and hypersensitivity to xanthine compounds (caffeine, theobromine) or ethylenediamine.
- Use cautiously in neonates, infants, young children, elderly patients, pregnant or breast-feeding women, and patients with heart failure or other cardiac or circulatory impairment, COPD, cor pulmonale, renal or hepatic disease, hyperthyroidism, diabetes mellitus, peptic ulcer, severe hypoxemia, or hypertension.

NURSING CONSIDERATIONS

Assessment

- Assess patient's underlying respiratory condition.
- Monitor drug effectiveness by regularly auscultating lungs and noting respiratory rate and results of laboratory studies, such as arterial blood gas analysis.
- Monitor patient's hydration status if adverse GI reactions occur.
- Be alert for adverse reactions and drug interactions.
- Evaluate patient's and family's knowledge of drug therapy.

Nursing diagnoses

- Impaired gas exchange related to bronchospasm
- Risk for deficient fluid volume related to drug-induced adverse GI reactions
- Deficient knowledge related to drug therapy

Planning and implementation

- Make sure that patient hasn't had recent theophylline therapy before giving loading dose.

P.O. use: Give oral drug with full glass of water at meals. Food in stomach delays absorption. Enteric-coated tablets may delay and impair absorption.

I.V. use: Because I.V. drug can burn, dilute with compatible I.V. solution and inject at no more than 25 mg/minute. Exceeding recommended I.V. infusion rates increases the risk of adverse reactions. Drug is compatible with most I.V. solutions except invert sugar, fructose, and fat emulsions.

P.R. use: Suppositories are slowly and erratically absorbed. Administer suppository if patient can't take drug orally, as ordered. Schedule after evacuation, if possible; may be retained better if given before meal. Have patient remain recumbent 15 to 20 minutes after insertion.

- Aminophylline is a soluble salt of theophylline. Dosage is adjusted by monitoring response, tolerance, pulmonary function, and serum theophylline level. Theophylline concentration should range from 10 to 20 mcg/ml; toxicity has been reported with level above 20 mcg/ml.

Patient teaching

- Supply instructions for home care and dosage schedule. Some patients may need an around-the-clock schedule.
- Warn elderly patients that dizziness is common at start of therapy.
- Warn patient to check with prescriber or pharmacist before combining aminophylline with other drugs; OTC products and herbal remedies may contain ephedrine. Excessive CNS stimulation may result.
- Advise patient to avoid switching brands without consulting prescriber.
- Tell patient to notify prescriber if he quits smoking. Dosage may need to be reduced.

Evaluation

- Patient's appearance, vital signs, and laboratory test results demonstrate improved gas exchange.
- Patient remains hydrated throughout therapy.
- Patient and family state understanding of drug therapy.

amiodarone hydrochloride

(am-ee-OH-dah-rohn high-droh-KLOR-ighd)

Aratac ◇, Cordarone, Cordarone X ◇

Pharmacologic class: benzofuran derivative
Therapeutic class: ventricular antiarrhythmic
Pregnancy risk category: D

Indications and dosages

▶ **Recurrent ventricular fibrillation and unstable ventricular tachycardia.** *Adults:* loading dose of 800 to 1,600 mg P.O. daily for 1 to 3 weeks until initial therapeutic response occurs, then 650 to 800 mg P.O. daily for 1 month, then 200 to 600 mg P.O. daily as maintenance dosage. Or, for first 24 hours, 150 mg I.V. over 10 minutes (mixed in 100 ml D_5W); then 360 mg I.V. over 6 hours (mix 900 mg in 500 ml D_5W); then maintenance of 540 mg I.V. over 18 hours at a rate of 0.5 mg/minute. After first 24 hours, continue a maintenance infusion of 0.5 mg/minute in a 1 to 6 mg/ml concentration. For infusions longer than 1 hour, concentrations shouldn't exceed 2 mg/ml unless you use a central venous catheter. Don't use for more than 3 weeks.

How supplied

Tablets: 100 mg ♦ ◇, 200 mg
Injection: 50 mg/ml ◇

Pharmacokinetics

Absorption: slow, variable absorption with oral administration.
Distribution: distributed widely, accumulating in adipose tissue and in organs with marked perfusion, such as lungs, liver, and spleen. It is highly protein-bound (96%).
Metabolism: metabolized extensively in liver to active metabolite, desethyl amiodarone.
Excretion: main excretory route is hepatic through biliary tree. *Half-life:* 25 to 110 days (usually, 40 to 50 days).

Route	Onset	Peak	Duration
P.O.	2-21 days	3-7 hr	Varies
I.V.	Unknown	Unknown	Unknown

Pharmacodynamics

Chemical effect: unknown; thought to prolong refractory period and action potential duration and decrease repolarization.
Therapeutic effect: abolishes ventricular arrhythmia.

Adverse reactions

CNS: peripheral neuropathy, extrapyramidal symptoms, headache, *malaise, fatigue.*
CV: ***bradycardia,*** hypotension, ***arrhythmias, heart failure, heart block, sinus arrest.***
EENT: *corneal microdeposits,* vision disturbances.
GI: *nausea, vomiting,* constipation.
Hepatic: *altered liver enzymes,* hepatic dysfunction.
Metabolic: hypothyroidism, hyperthyroidism.
Musculoskeletal: muscle weakness.
Respiratory: **SEVERE PULMONARY TOXICITY (PNEUMONITIS, ALVEOLITIS).**
Skin: *photosensitivity,* blue-gray skin.
Other: gynecomastia.

Interactions

Drug-drug. *Antiarrhythmics:* amiodarone may reduce hepatic or renal clearance of certain antiarrhythmics (especially flecainide, procainamide, or quinidine); concomitant use of amiodarone with other antiarrhythmics (especially mexiletine, propafenone, quinidine, disopyramide, or procainamide) may induce torsades de pointes. Monitor ECG closely.
Antihypertensives: increased hypotensive effect. Use together cautiously.
Beta blockers, calcium channel blockers: increased cardiac depressant effects; may potentiate slowing of sinus node and AV conduction. Use together cautiously.
Cardiac glycosides: increased serum digoxin level (average of 70% to 100%). Monitor digoxin level closely.
Cimetidine: interferes with action of amiodarone causing increased amiodarone levels. Avoid concomitant use.
Cholestyramine: decreased serum levels and half-life of amiodarone. Avoid concomitant use.
Cyclosporine: increased levels of cyclosporine. Monitor serum creatinine.

Phenytoin: may decrease phenytoin metabolism. Monitor serum phenytoin level.
Theophylline: increased theophylline level with toxicity may occur. Monitor serum theophylline level.
Warfarin: increased INR (average of 100% within 1 to 4 weeks of therapy). Warfarin dosage should be decreased 33% to 50% when amiodarone is initiated. Monitor patient closely.
Drug-herb. *Pennyroyal:* may change the rate at which toxic metabolites of pennyroyal form. Discourage concomitant use.
Drug-lifestyle. *Sun exposure:* photosensitivity reaction may occur. Advise against prolonged or unprotected sun exposure.

Contraindications and precautions

- Contraindicated in patients hypersensitive to drug, in those with severe sinus node disease and bradycardia, in those with second- or third-degree AV block (unless artificial pacemaker is present), in those in whom bradycardia has caused syncope, and in breast-feeding women.
- Use with extreme caution in patients receiving other antiarrhythmics and in pregnant women.
- Use cautiously in patients with pulmonary or thyroid disease.
- Safety of drug hasn't been established in children.

NURSING CONSIDERATIONS

Assessment

- Assess CV status before therapy.
- Review pulmonary, liver, and thyroid function test results before and regularly during therapy.
- Continuously monitor cardiac status of patient receiving I.V. amiodarone to evaluate its effectiveness.
- Be alert for adverse reactions and drug interactions.
- Monitor patient carefully for pulmonary toxicity, which can be fatal. Risk increases in patients receiving more than 400 mg/day.
- Monitor serum electrolytes, particularly potassium and magnesium levels.
- Evaluate patient's and family's knowledge of drug therapy.

Nursing diagnoses

- Decreased cardiac output related to ventricular arrhythmia
- Risk for injury related to drug-induced adverse reactions
- Deficient knowledge related to drug therapy

Planning and implementation

- Adverse reactions commonly limit drug's use.

ALERT Drug poses major and potentially life-threatening management problems in patients at risk for sudden death and should be used only in patients with documented, life-threatening, recurrent ventricular arrhythmias nonresponsive to documented adequate doses of other antiarrhythmics or when alternative drugs can't be tolerated. Amiodarone can cause fatal toxicities, including hepatic and pulmonary toxicity.
P.O. use: Divide oral loading dose into three equal doses and give with meals to decrease GI intolerance. Maintenance dosage may be given once daily or divided into two doses taken with meals if GI intolerance occurs.
I.V. use: Amiodarone may be given I.V. where facilities for close monitoring of cardiac function and resuscitation are available. Initial dosage of 5 mg/kg should be mixed in 250 ml of D_5W. Repeat doses preferably should be administered through central venous catheter. Patient should receive maximum of 1.2 g in up to 500 ml of D_5W daily.

- Maintain ECG monitoring during initiation and alteration of dosage. Notify prescriber of any significant change.
- Recommend instillation of methylcellulose ophthalmic solution during amiodarone therapy to minimize corneal microdeposits.

Patient teaching

- Stress importance of taking medication exactly as prescribed.
- Emphasize importance of close follow-up and regular diagnostic studies to monitor drug action and assess for adverse reactions.

• Warn patient that drug may cause blue-gray skin pigmentation.
• Advise patient to use sunscreen to prevent photosensitivity reaction (burning or tingling skin followed by erythema and possible skin blistering).
• Inform patient that adverse effects are more prevalent at high doses but are generally reversible when therapy stops. Resolution of adverse reactions may take up to 4 months.

☑ Evaluation

• Patient's arrhythmia is corrected.
• Patient has no injury from adverse reactions.
• Patient and family state understanding of drug therapy.

amitriptyline hydrochloride

(am-ih-TRIP-tuh-leen high-droh-KLOR-ighd)
Apo-Amitriptyline♦, Elavil, Emitrip, Endep, Enovil, Levate♦, Novotriptyn♦, PMS-Amitriptyline, Tryptanol◇

amitriptyline pamoate

Elavil♦

Pharmacologic class: tricyclic antidepressant
Therapeutic class: antidepressant
Pregnancy risk category: C

Indications and dosages

▶ **Depression.** *Adults:* 50 to 100 mg P.O. h.s., increasing to 150 mg daily; maximum dosage is 300 mg daily, if needed. Or 20 to 30 mg I.M. q.i.d.
Elderly patients and adolescents: 10 mg P.O. t.i.d. and 20 mg h.s. daily.

How supplied

Tablets: 10 mg, 25 mg, 50 mg, 75 mg, 100 mg, 150 mg
Injection: 10 mg/ml
Syrup: 10 mg/5 ml

Pharmacokinetics

Absorption: absorbed rapidly from GI tract after oral administration and from muscle tissue after I.M. administration.
Distribution: distributed widely into body, including CNS and breast milk. Drug is 96% protein-bound.
Metabolism: metabolized by liver to active metabolite nortriptyline; significant first-pass effect may account for variable serum concentrations in different patients taking same dosage.
Excretion: most of drug is excreted in urine.

Route	Onset	Peak	Duration
P.O., I.M.	Unknown	2-12 hr	Unknown

Pharmacodynamics

Chemical effect: unknown, but tricyclic antidepressant (TCA) increases norepinephrine, serotonin, or both in CNS by blocking their reuptake by presynaptic neurons.
Therapeutic effect: relieves depression.

Adverse reactions

CNS: *drowsiness, dizziness,* excitation, tremors, weakness, confusion, headache, nervousness, EEG alterations, ***seizures,*** extrapyramidal reactions.
CV: *orthostatic hypotension, tachycardia, ECG changes,* hypertension, ***MI, CVA, arrhythmias.***
EENT: *blurred vision,* tinnitus, mydriasis.
GI: *dry mouth, constipation,* nausea, vomiting, anorexia, paralytic ileus.
GU: *urine retention.*
Hematologic: ***agranulocytosis, thrombocytopenia.***
Skin: diaphoresis, rash, urticaria, photosensitivity.
Other: hypersensitivity reactions.

Interactions

Drug-drug. *Barbiturates, CNS depressants:* enhanced CNS depression. Avoid concomitant use.
Cimetidine, methylphenidate: increased TCA blood levels. Watch for enhanced antidepressant effect.
Clonidine: hypertensive crises have occurred. Avoid concomitant use.
Epinephrine, norepinephrine: increased hypertensive effect. Use cautiously.
Guanethidine: antagonize the antihypertensive action of guanethidine. Monitor patient.

MAO inhibitors: may cause severe excitation, hyperpyrexia, or seizures, usually with high dosage. Use cautiously.
Drug-herb. *St. John's wort, SAMe, yohimbe:* may elevate serotonin levels too high. Discourage concomitant use.
Drug-lifestyle. *Alcohol use:* enhanced CNS depression. Avoid concomitant use.
Smoking: may lower plasma levels of drug. Monitor patient for lack of effect.
Sun exposure: increased risk of photosensitivity reactions. Advise against prolonged or unprotected sun exposure.

Contraindications and precautions

- Contraindicated during acute recovery phase of MI, in patients hypersensitive to drug, in patients who have received an MAO inhibitor within past 14 days, and in breast-feeding women.
- Use cautiously in patients with history of seizures, urine retention, angle-closure glaucoma, or increased intraocular pressure; in those with hyperthyroidism, CV disease, diabetes, or impaired liver function; in those receiving thyroid medications; and during pregnancy.
- Don't use drug in children under age 12.

NURSING CONSIDERATIONS

Assessment
- Assess patient's depression before therapy.
- Be alert for adverse reactions and drug interactions.
- Evaluate patient's and family's knowledge of drug therapy.

Nursing diagnoses
- Ineffective individual coping related to depression
- Risk for injury related to adverse CNS reactions
- Deficient knowledge related to drug therapy

Planning and implementation
P.O. use: Oral therapy should replace injection as soon as possible.
I.M. use: Follow normal protocol. Effects may appear more rapidly than with oral administration.
- Administer full dose at bedtime when possible.
- Expect reduced dosage in elderly or debilitated patients and adolescents.
- Don't withdraw drug abruptly.
- Expect prescriber to reduce dosage if signs of psychosis occur or increase. Allow patient only minimum supply of drug.
- Because hypertensive episodes have occurred during surgery in patients receiving TCAs, be aware that drug should be gradually stopped several days before surgery.

Patient teaching
- Advise patient to take full dose at bedtime, but warn him of possible morning orthostatic hypotension.
- Tell patient to avoid alcohol and smoking while taking drug.
- Warn patient to avoid hazardous activities until full CNS effects of drug are known. Drowsiness and dizziness usually subside after a few weeks.
- Advise patient to consult prescriber before taking other prescription drugs, OTC medications, or herbal remedies.
- Teach patient to relieve dry mouth with sugarless hard candy or gum. Saliva substitutes may be necessary.
- Advise patient to use sunblock, wear protective clothing, and avoid prolonged exposure to strong sunlight.
- Warn patient not to stop drug therapy abruptly. After abrupt withdrawal of long-term therapy patient may experience nausea, headache, and malaise. These symptoms don't indicate addiction.
- Tell patient to watch for urine retention and constipation. Instruct him to increase fluids and suggest stool softener or high-fiber diet as needed.
- Advise patient that effects of the drug may not be apparent for 2 to 3 weeks.

Evaluation
- Patient behavior and communication indicate improvement of depression.
- Patient doesn't experience injury from CNS adverse reactions.
- Patient and family state understanding of drug therapy.

amlodipine besylate
(am-LOH-dih-peen BES-eh-layt)
Norvasc

Pharmacologic class: dihydropyridine calcium channel blocker
Therapeutic class: antianginal, antihypertensive
Pregnancy risk category: C

Indications and dosages

▶ **Chronic stable angina; vasospastic angina (Prinzmetal's [variant] angina).** *Adults:* initially, 10 mg P.O. daily.
Small, frail, or elderly patients or patients with hepatic insufficiency: should begin therapy at 5 mg daily. Most patients need 10 mg daily for adequate results.
▶ **Hypertension.** *Adults:* initially, 5 mg P.O. daily. Small, frail, or elderly patients; patients currently receiving other antihypertensives, and patients with hepatic insufficiency, should begin therapy at 2.5 mg daily. Dosage adjusted based on patient response and tolerance. Maximum, 10 mg daily.

How supplied

Tablets: 2.5 mg, 5 mg, 10 mg

Pharmacokinetics

Absorption: absolute bioavailability from 64% to 90%.
Distribution: about 93% of circulating drug is bound to plasma proteins.
Metabolism: extensively metabolized in liver; about 90% of drug converted to inactive metabolites.
Excretion: excreted primarily in urine. *Half-life:* 30 to 50 hours.

Route	Onset	Peak	Duration
P.O.	Unknown	6-9 hr	24 hr

Pharmacodynamics

Chemical effect: inhibits calcium ion influx across cardiac and smooth-muscle cells, thus decreasing myocardial contractility and oxygen demand. Also dilates coronary arteries and arterioles.
Therapeutic effect: reduces blood pressure and prevents anginal pain.

Adverse reactions

CNS: *headache,* fatigue, somnolence.
CV: *edema,* dizziness, flushing, palpitations.
GI: nausea, abdominal pain.

Interactions

None reported.

Contraindications and precautions

- Contraindicated in patients hypersensitive to drug and in breast-feeding women.
- Use cautiously in patients receiving other peripheral vasodilators (especially those with severe aortic stenosis), in those with heart failure, and in pregnant women. Because drug is metabolized by liver, also use cautiously and in reduced dosage in patients with severe hepatic disease.
- Safety of drug hasn't been established in children.

NURSING CONSIDERATIONS

Assessment

- Assess patient's blood pressure or anginal condition before therapy and regularly thereafter.
- Monitor patient carefully for pain. In some patients, especially those with severe obstructive coronary artery disease, increased frequency, duration, or severity of angina or even acute MI has developed after initiation of calcium channel blocker therapy or at time of dosage increase.
- Be alert for adverse reactions.
- Evaluate patient's and family's knowledge of drug therapy.

Nursing diagnoses

- Acute pain related to increased oxygen demand in cardiac tissue
- Risk for injury related to hypertension
- Deficient knowledge related to drug therapy

Planning and implementation

- Dosage should be adjusted by prescriber based on patient response and tolerance.

• Administer S.L. nitroglycerin as needed for acute anginal symptoms.

Patient teaching
• Tell patient that S.L. nitroglycerin may be taken as needed for acute angina. If patient continues nitrate therapy during titration of amlodipine dosage, urge continued compliance.
• Caution patient to continue taking drug even when feeling better.

Evaluation
• Patient's blood pressure is normal.
• Patient states anginal pain occurs with less frequency and severity.
• Patient and family state understanding of drug therapy.

ammonia, aromatic spirits†
(uh-MOH-nee-uh, ar-oh-MAT-ik SPIR-its)

Pharmacologic class: miscellaneous antagonist
Therapeutic class: antifainting drug
Pregnancy risk category: NR

Indications and dosages

▶ **Treatment or prevention of fainting.** *Adults and children:* 1 broken capsule inhaled until awake or no longer faint; or 2 to 4 ml P.O. diluted in at least 30 ml of water.

How supplied

Solution: 30 ml†, 60 ml†, 120 ml†; pints†; gallons†
Inhalant: 0.33 ml†, 0.4 ml†

Pharmacokinetics

No information available.

Route	Onset	Peak	Duration
Inhalation	Immediate	Unknown	Unknown

Pharmacodynamics

Chemical effect: irritates sensory receptors in nasal membranes, producing reflex stimulation of respiratory centers.
Therapeutic effect: prevents fainting or awakens person from fainting.

Adverse reactions

EENT: irritation.

Interactions

None significant.

Contraindications and precautions

• No known contraindications or precautions.

NURSING CONSIDERATIONS

Assessment
• Determine that patient has palpable pulse and visible respirations.
• Evaluate patient's and family's knowledge of drug therapy.

Nursing diagnoses
• Deficient knowledge related to drug therapy

Planning and implementation
• Avoid inhaling vapors when administering drug.
• Keep bottle tightly capped when not in use.
• Notify prescriber if patient doesn't respond to drug.

Patient teaching
• Teach family when and how to administer drug.
• Instruct patient to notify prescriber if drug is required so he can determine cause of fainting.

Evaluation
• Patient and family state understanding of drug therapy.

amoxapine
(uh-MOKS-uh-peen)
Asendin

Pharmacologic class: dibenzoxazepine, tricyclic antidepressant
Therapeutic class: antidepressant
Pregnancy risk category: C

Indications and dosages

▶ **Depression.** *Adults:* initially, 50 mg P.O. b.i.d. or t.i.d. Increased to 100 mg b.i.d. or t.i.d. by the end of the first week. Increases above 300 mg daily are made only if 300 mg daily has been ineffective during trial period of at least 2 weeks. When effective dosage is established, entire dosage (not to exceed 300 mg) may be given h.s.

How supplied

Tablets: 25 mg, 50 mg, 100 mg, 150 mg

Pharmacokinetics

Absorption: absorbed rapidly and completely from GI tract.
Distribution: distributed widely. Drug is 92% protein-bound.
Metabolism: metabolized by liver to active metabolite; significant first-pass effect may explain variable serum levels in different patients taking same dosage.
Excretion: excreted in urine and feces (7% to 18%); about 60% of dose is excreted as conjugated form within 6 days. *Half-life:* 8 hours for amoxapine, 30 hours for its metabolite.

Route	Onset	Peak	Duration
P.O.	2-4 wk	About 90 min	Unknown

Pharmacodynamics

Chemical effect: increases amount of norepinephrine, serotonin, or both in CNS by blocking their reuptake by presynaptic neurons.
Therapeutic effect: relieves depression.

Adverse reactions

CNS: *drowsiness, dizziness,* excitation, tremors, weakness, confusion, headache, nervousness, *tardive dyskinesia*; EEG changes, ***seizures, neuroleptic malignant syndrome.***
CV: *orthostatic hypotension, tachycardia, ECG changes,* hypertension.
EENT: *blurred vision,* tinnitus, mydriasis.
GI: *dry mouth, constipation,* nausea, vomiting, anorexia, paralytic ileus.
GU: *urine retention,* ***acute renal failure.***
Metabolic: weight gain and craving for sweets.
Skin: *diaphoresis,* photosensitivity, rash, urticaria.
Other: hypersensitivity reaction.

Interactions

Drug-drug. *Barbiturates:* decreased tricyclic antidepressant blood level. Monitor patient for decreased antidepressant effect.
Cimetidine, methylphenidate, oral contraceptives: may increase amoxapine serum level. Monitor patient for increased adverse effects.
Clonidine, epinephrine, norepinephrine: increased hypertensive effect. Use cautiously.
CNS depressants: enhanced CNS depression. Avoid concomitant use.
MAO inhibitors: may cause severe excitation, hyperpyrexia, or seizures, usually with high dosage. Use cautiously.
Drug-herb. *St. John's wort, SAMe, yohimbe:* may increase serotonin levels. Discourage concomitant use.
Drug-lifestyle. *Alcohol use:* enhanced CNS depression. Avoid concomitant use.
Sun exposure: increased risk of photosensitivity. Avoid prolonged or unprotected sun exposure.

Contraindications and precautions

- Contraindicated in patients hypersensitive to drug, patients in acute recovery phase of MI, patients who have received an MAO inhibitor within past 14 days, and breast-feeding women.
- Use with extreme caution in patients with history of seizure disorder or those with overt or latent seizure disorders.
- Use cautiously in patients with history of urine retention, angle-closure glaucoma, or increased intraocular pressure, as well as patients with CV disease or during pregnancy.
- Don't use drug in children under age 12.

NURSING CONSIDERATIONS

Assessment

- Assess patient's depression before therapy and regularly thereafter.
- Be alert for adverse reactions and drug interactions.
- Watch for evidence of tardive dyskinesia, especially in elderly women.
- Evaluate patient's and family's knowledge of drug therapy.

Nursing diagnoses

- Ineffective individual coping related to patient's underlying condition
- Risk for injury related to drug-induced adverse reactions
- Deficient knowledge related to drug therapy

Planning and implementation

- Administer full dose at bedtime when possible. Expect delay of 2 weeks or more before noticeable effect. Full effect may take 4 weeks or more.
- Dosage should be reduced in elderly or debilitated persons and adolescents.
- Don't withdraw drug abruptly. After abrupt withdrawal of long-term therapy patient may experience nausea, headache, and malaise, though this doesn't indicate addiction.
- Because hypertensive episodes have occurred during surgery in patients receiving tricyclic antidepressants, be aware that drug should be gradually stopped several days before surgery.
- If signs of psychosis occur or increase, expect prescriber to reduce dosage. Allow patient only minimum supply of drug.

Patient teaching

- Warn patient not to stop therapy abruptly.
- Advise patient that effects of drug may not be apparent for 2 to 4 weeks.
- Teach patient signs and symptoms of neuroleptic malignant syndrome including high fever, tachycardia, tachypnea, and profuse diaphoresis.
- Caution patient to avoid hazardous activities until full CNS effects of drug are known. Drowsiness and dizziness usually subside after a few weeks.
- Tell patient to avoid alcohol consumption while on drug therapy.
- Advise patient to use sunblock, wear protective clothing, and avoid prolonged exposure to strong sunlight.

Evaluation

- Patient behavior and communication indicate improvement of depression.
- Patient doesn't experience injury from adverse CNS reactions.
- Patient and family state understanding of drug therapy.

amoxicillin/clavulanate potassium

(uh-moks-uh-SIL-in/KLAV-yoo-lan-ayt poh-TAH-see-um)

Augmentin, Clavulin♦

Pharmacologic class: aminopenicillin, beta-lactamase inhibitor
Therapeutic class: antibiotic
Pregnancy risk category: B

Indications and dosages

▶ **Lower respiratory tract infections, otitis media, sinusitis, skin and skin structure infections, and UTI caused by susceptible strains of gram-positive and gram-negative organisms.** *Adults:* 250 mg (based on amoxicillin component) P.O. q 8 hours. For more severe infections, 500 mg q 8 hours, or 875 mg P.O. q 12 hours.
Children: 20 to 40 mg/kg (based on amoxicillin component) P.O. daily in divided doses q 8 hours.

How supplied

Tablets (chewable): 125 mg amoxicillin trihydrate, 31.25 mg clavulanic acid; 250 mg amoxicillin trihydrate, 62.5 mg clavulanic acid
Tablets (film-coated): 250 mg amoxicillin trihydrate, 125 mg clavulanic acid; 500 mg amoxicillin trihydrate, 125 mg clavulanic acid; 875 mg amoxicillin trihydrate, 125 mg clavulanic acid
Oral suspension: 125 mg amoxicillin trihydrate and 31.25 mg clavulanic acid/5 ml (after reconstitution); 250 mg amoxicillin trihydrate and 62.5 mg clavulanic acid/5 ml (after reconstitution)

Pharmacokinetics

Absorption: well absorbed.
Distribution: both drugs distribute into pleural fluid, lungs, and peritoneal fluid; high urine levels are attained. Amoxicillin also distributes into synovial fluid, liver, prostate, muscle, and

gallbladder and penetrates into middle ear effusions, maxillary sinus secretions, tonsils, sputum, and bronchial secretions. Both drugs have minimal protein binding.
Metabolism: amoxicillin is metabolized only partially; clavulanate potassium appears to undergo extensive metabolism.
Excretion: amoxicillin is excreted principally in urine by renal tubular secretion and glomerular filtration; clavulanate potassium is excreted by glomerular filtration. *Half-life:* amoxicillin, 1 to 1½ hours (7½ hours in severe renal impairment); clavulanate, about 1 to 1½ hours (4½ hours in severe renal impairment).

Route	Onset	Peak	Duration
P.O.	Unknown	1-2.5 hr	6-8 hr

Pharmacodynamics

Chemical effect: prevents bacterial cell-wall synthesis during replication. Clavulanic acid increases amoxicillin's effectiveness by inactivating beta lactamases, which destroy amoxicillin.
Therapeutic effect: kills susceptible bacteria. Active against penicillinase-producing gram-positive bacteria, *Neisseria gonorrhoeae, N. meningitidis, Haemophilus influenzae, Escherichia coli, Proteus mirabilis, Citrobacter diversus, Klebsiella pneumoniae, P. vulgaris, Salmonella,* and *Shigella.*

Adverse reactions

GI: *nausea,* vomiting, *diarrhea.*
Hematologic: anemia, ***thrombocytopenia,*** thrombocytopenic purpura, eosinophilia, ***leukopenia, agranulocytopenia.***
Other: hypersensitivity reactions (erythematous maculopapular rash, urticaria, ***anaphylaxis),*** overgrowth of nonsusceptible organisms.

Interactions

Drug-drug. *Allopurinol:* increased risk of skin rash. Monitor patient.
Probenecid: increased blood level of amoxicillin and other penicillins. Probenecid may be used for this purpose.

Contraindications and precautions

- Contraindicated in patients hypersensitive to drug or other penicillins and in those with a history of amoxicillin-related cholestatic jaundice or hepatic dysfunction.
- Use cautiously in patients with other drug allergies, especially to cephalosporins (possible cross-sensitivity); in those with mononucleosis (high risk of maculopapular rash); and in pregnant or breast-feeding women.

NURSING CONSIDERATIONS

Assessment

- Before therapy begins, assess patient's infection, ask him about allergic reactions to penicillin (negative history is no guarantee against allergic reaction), and obtain specimen for culture and sensitivity tests. Therapy may begin pending results.
- Be alert for adverse reactions and drug interactions.
- Monitor hydration status if adverse GI reactions occur.
- Evaluate patient's and family's knowledge of drug therapy.

Nursing diagnoses

- Infection related to susceptible bacteria
- Risk for deficient fluid volume related to drug-induced adverse GI reactions
- Deficient knowledge related to drug therapy

Planning and implementation

- Give drug with food to prevent GI distress. Adverse effects, especially diarrhea, are more common than with amoxicillin alone.
- Give drug at least 1 hour before bacteriostatic antibiotics.
- Both 250-mg and 500-mg tablets contain same amount of clavulanic acid (125 mg). Therefore, two 250-mg tablets don't equal one 500-mg tablet.
- This drug combination is particularly useful with amoxicillin-resistant organisms.
- After reconstitution, refrigerate oral suspension and discard after 10 days.
- Urine glucose determinations may be false-positive with copper sulfate tests (Benedict's solution, Clinitest); glucose enzymatic tests (Diastix) aren't affected.

Patient teaching

- Tell patient to take entire quantity of drug exactly as prescribed, even after he feels better.
- Tell patient to call prescriber if rash develops (sign of allergic reaction).
- Instruct patient to take drug with food to prevent GI distress.

Evaluation

- Patient is free from infection.
- Patient maintains adequate hydration.
- Patient and family state understanding of drug therapy.

amoxicillin trihydrate (amoxycillin trihydrate)

(uh-moks-uh-SIL-in trigh-HIGH-drayt)

Alphamox, Amoxil, Apo-Amoxi, Cilamox, Ibiamox, Larotid, Moxacin, Novamoxin, Nu-Amoxi, Polymox, Trimox, Wymox

Pharmacologic class: aminopenicillin
Therapeutic class: antibiotic
Pregnancy risk category: B

Indications and dosages

▶ **Systemic infections, acute and chronic UTI caused by susceptible strains of gram-positive and gram-negative organisms.** *Adults:* 250 mg P.O. q 8 hours. In adults and children over 20 kg who have severe infections or those caused by susceptible organisms, 500 mg P.O. q 8 hours or 875 mg P.O. q 12 hours may be needed.
Children: 20 to 40 mg/kg P.O. daily, divided into doses given q 8 hours.

▶ **Uncomplicated gonorrhea.** *Adults:* 3 g P.O. as a single dose.
Children over age 2: 50 mg/kg given with 25 mg/kg probenecid as a single dose.

▶ **Endocarditis prophylaxis for dental procedures.** *Adults:* initially, 3 g P.O. 1 hour before procedure; then 1.5 g 6 hours later.
Children: initially, 50 mg/kg P.O. 1 hour before procedure; then half initial dose 6 hours later.

▶ ***H. pylori*** **eradication to reduce the risk of duodenal ulcer in combination with clarithromycin or lansoprazole. Triple therapy.** *Adults:* amoxicillin 1 g P.O., clarithromycin 500 mg P.O., lansoprazole 30 mg P.O.; each q 12 hours for 14 days.
Dual therapy. *Adults:* amoxicillin 1 g P.O. and lansoprazole 30 mg P.O., each q 8 hours for 14 days.

How supplied

Tablets: 500 mg, 875 mg
Tablets (chewable): 125 mg, 250 mg
Capsules: 250 mg, 500 mg
Oral suspension: 50 mg/ml (pediatric drops), 125 mg/5 ml, 250 mg/5 ml (after reconstitution)

Pharmacokinetics

Absorption: about 80% absorbed after oral administration.
Distribution: distributed into pleural, peritoneal, and synovial fluids; lungs; prostate; muscle; liver; and gallbladder. Also penetrates middle ear, maxillary sinus and bronchial secretions, tonsils, and sputum. Amoxicillin readily crosses placenta and is 17% to 20% protein-bound.
Metabolism: only partially metabolized.
Excretion: excreted principally in urine by renal tubular secretion and glomerular filtration; also excreted in breast milk. *Half-life:* 1 to 1½ hours (7½ hours in severe renal impairment).

Route	Onset	Peak	Duration
P.O.	Unknown	1-2 hr	6-8 hr

Pharmacodynamics

Chemical effect: inhibits cell-wall synthesis during bacterial multiplication.
Therapeutic effect: kills susceptible bacteria (*Streptococcus, Pneumococcus, Enterococcus, Haemophilus influenzae, Escherichia coli, Proteus mirabilis, Neisseria meningitidis, N. gonorrhoeae, Shigella, Salmonella, Borrelia burgdorferi*).

Adverse reactions

CNS: ***seizures.***
GI: *nausea,* vomiting, *diarrhea.*
Hematologic: anemia, ***thrombocytopenia,*** thrombocytopenic purpura, eosinophilia, ***leukopenia, agranulocytosis.***

*Liquid form contains alcohol. **May contain tartrazine. ♦Canada ◇Australia †OTC

Other: hypersensitivity reactions (erythematous maculopapular rash, urticaria, ***anaphylaxis***), overgrowth of nonsusceptible organisms.

Interactions

Drug-drug. *Allopurinol:* increased risk of rash. Monitor patient.
Probenecid: increased blood level of amoxicillin and other penicillins. Probenecid may be used for this purpose.

Contraindications and precautions

- Contraindicated in patients hypersensitive to drug or other penicillins.
- Use cautiously in patients with other drug allergies, especially to cephalosporins (possible cross-sensitivity); in those with mononucleosis (high risk of maculopapular rash); and in pregnant or breast-feeding women.

NURSING CONSIDERATIONS

Assessment

- Before therapy, assess patient's infection, ask him about allergic reactions to drug or other forms of penicillin (negative history doesn't guarantee future safety), and obtain specimen for culture and sensitivity tests. Therapy may begin pending test results.
- Be alert for adverse reactions and drug interactions.
- Monitor patient's hydration status if adverse GI reactions occur.
- Evaluate patient's and family's knowledge of drug therapy.

Nursing diagnoses

- Infection related to susceptible bacteria
- Risk for deficient fluid volume related to drug-induced adverse GI reactions
- Deficient knowledge related to drug therapy

Planning and implementation

- Give amoxicillin at least 1 hour before bacteriostatic antibiotics.
- Administer with food to prevent GI distress.
- Trimox oral suspension may be stored at room temperature for up to 2 weeks. Check individual product labels for storage information.
- Drug may cause false-positive urine glucose determinations with copper sulfate tests (Clinitest); drug doesn't affect glucose enzymatic tests (Diastix).

Patient teaching

- If drug allergy develops, advise patient to wear or carry medical identification stating penicillin allergy.
- Tell patient to take entire quantity of drug exactly as ordered, even after he feels better.
- Tell patient to call prescriber if rash (most common), fever, or chills develop.
- Instruct patient to take drug with food to prevent GI distress.
- Warn patient never to use leftover amoxicillin for a new illness or to share it with others.

Evaluation

- Patient is free from infection.
- Patient maintains adequate hydration.
- Patient and family state understanding of drug therapy.

amphetamine sulfate

(am-FET-ah-meen SUL-fayt)

Pharmacologic class: amphetamine
Therapeutic class: CNS stimulant, short-term adjunct anorexigenic drug, sympathomimetic amine
Controlled substance schedule: II
Pregnancy risk category: C

Indications and dosages

▶ **Attention deficit hyperactivity disorder (ADHD).** *Children ages 3 to 5:* 2.5 mg P.O. daily, with 2.5-mg increments weekly, p.r.n. *Children age 6 and older:* 5 mg P.O. daily, with 5-mg increments weekly, p.r.n. Give first dose on awakening; additional doses (one or two) at 4- to 6-hour intervals.
▶ **Narcolepsy.** *Adults:* 5 to 60 mg P.O. daily in divided doses.
▶ **Short-term adjunct in exogenous obesity.** *Adults:* 5 to 30 mg P.O. daily in divided doses 30 to 60 minutes before meals.

How supplied

Tablets: 5 mg, 10 mg

Pharmacokinetics

Absorption: absorbed completely within 3 hours.
Distribution: distributed widely throughout body, with high levels in brain.
Metabolism: metabolized in liver.
Excretion: excreted in urine. *Half-life:* 10 to 30 hours.

Route	Onset	Peak	Duration
P.O.	Unknown	Unknown	Unknown

Pharmacodynamics

Chemical effect: unknown; probably promotes nerve impulse transmission by releasing stored norepinephrine from nerve terminals in brain. Main sites of activity appear to be cerebral cortex and reticular activating system.
Therapeutic effect: improves behavior in ADHD, helps prevent falling asleep, and aids in weight loss.

Adverse reactions

CNS: *restlessness,* tremors, *hyperactivity, talkativeness, insomnia,* irritability, dizziness, headache, chills, dysphoria.
CV: *tachycardia, palpitations,* hypertension, hypotension, ***arrhythmias.***
GI: dry mouth, nausea, vomiting, cramps, diarrhea, constipation, anorexia, weight loss, metallic taste.
GU: impotence.
Skin: urticaria.
Other: altered libido.

Interactions

Drug-drug. *Acetazolamide, antacids, sodium bicarbonate:* increased renal reabsorption. Monitor patient for enhanced effect.
Ammonium chloride, ascorbic acid: decreased serum levels and increased renal excretion of amphetamine. Monitor patient for decreased amphetamine effect.
Antihypertensives: reversal of antihypertensive action. Monitor blood pressure.
Haloperidol, phenothiazines, tricyclic antidepressants: increased CNS effect. Avoid concomitant use.
Insulin, oral antidiabetics: may decrease antidiabetic drug requirements. Monitor blood glucose level.
MAO inhibitors: severe hypertension; possibly hypertensive crisis. Don't use together or within 14 days after an MAO inhibitor has been discontinued.
Drug-food. *Caffeine:* may increase amphetamine and relate amine effects. Avoid concomitant use.

Contraindications and precautions

- Contraindicated in patients hypersensitive or idiosyncrasy to sympathomimetic amines, symptomatic CV disease, hyperthyroidism, moderate to severe hypertension, glaucoma, advanced arteriosclerosis, or history of drug abuse; within 14 days of MAO inhibitor therapy; and in agitated patients.
- Use cautiously in elderly, debilitated, or hyperexcitable patients and in those with psychopathic personalities or history of suicidal or homicidal tendencies; and in pregnant or breast-feeding women.
- Drug isn't recommended for treating obesity in children under age 12 or for treating ADHD in children under age 3.

NURSING CONSIDERATIONS

Assessment

- Obtain history of patient's underlying condition.
- Be alert for adverse reactions and drug interactions.
- Monitor dietary intake when drug is used to treat obesity.
- Evaluate patient's and family's knowledge of drug therapy.

Nursing diagnoses

- Ineffective health maintenance related to underlying disorder
- Disturbed sleep pattern related to drug-induced insomnia
- Deficient knowledge related to drug therapy

Planning and implementation

- Drug isn't recommended for first-line treatment of obesity or for treatment of obesity in

children under age 12. Use as an anorexigenic drug is prohibited in some states.
- Drug shouldn't be used to combat fatigue.
- Give drug at least 6 hours before bedtime to avoid interference with sleep.
- When used for obesity, administer drug 30 to 60 minutes before meals.
- Don't give drug for a prolonged period because psychological dependence may occur. When used long term, reduce dosage gradually, as ordered, to prevent acute rebound depression.
- If tolerance to anorexigenic effect develops, therapy should be stopped. Notify prescriber.
- Make sure obese patient is on a weight-reduction program.

Patient teaching
- Tell patient to take drug at least 6 hours before bedtime to avoid sleep pattern disturbance. If used to treat obesity, tell patient to take drug 30 to 60 minutes before meals.
- Warn patient to avoid hazardous activities until full CNS effects of drug are known.
- Tell patient to avoid drinks or foods containing caffeine, which increase effects of amphetamines and related amines.
- Tell patient to report signs of excess stimulation.
- Inform patient that fatigue may result as drug effects wear off. He'll need more rest.
- Tell patient that when tolerance to anorexigenic effect develops, dosage shouldn't be increased, but drug discontinued. He should report decreased effectiveness of drug. Warn patient against stopping drug abruptly.

☑ Evaluation
- Patient's health is maintained during amphetamine sulfate therapy.
- Patient can sleep without difficulty.
- Patient and family state an understanding of drug therapy.

amphotericin B
(am-foh-TER-ah-sin bee)
Fungilin Oral ◇, Fungizone Intravenous

Pharmacologic class: polyene macrolide
Therapeutic class: antifungal
Pregnancy risk category: B

Indications and dosages
▶ **Systemic fungal infections (histoplasmosis, coccidioidomycosis, blastomycosis, cryptococcosis, disseminated candidiasis, aspergillosis, mucormycosis); meningitis.** *Adults:* test dose of 1 mg I.V. in 20 ml of D_5W infused over 20 to 30 minutes may be recommended. If tolerated, daily dosage is then started as 0.25 to 0.3 mg/kg by slow I.V. infusion (0.1 mg/ml) over 2 to 6 hours. Dose is gradually increased, as patient tolerance develops, to maximum of 1 mg/kg daily. Therapy must not exceed 1.5 mg/kg daily. If drug is discontinued for 1 week or more, drug is resumed with initial dose and increased gradually.
▶ **Infections of GI tract caused by *Candida albicans*.** *Adults:* 100 mg P.O. q.i.d. for 2 weeks.
▶ **Oral and perioral candidal infections.** *Adults:* 1 lozenge q.i.d. for 7 to 14 days. Lozenge should be allowed to dissolve slowly.

How supplied
Tablets: 100 mg ◇
Oral suspension: 100 mg/ml ◇
Lozenges: 10 mg ◇
Injection: 50-mg lyophilized cake

Pharmacokinetics
Absorption: absorbed poorly from GI tract.
Distribution: distributed well into pleural cavities and joints; less so into aqueous humor, bronchial secretions, pancreas, bone, muscle, and parotid gland. Drug is 90% to 95% bound to plasma proteins.
Metabolism: not well defined.
Excretion: up to 5% excreted unchanged in urine. *Half-life:* initially, 24 hours; second phase, about 15 days.

Route	Onset	Peak	Duration
P.O.	Unknown	Unknown	Unknown
I.V.	Immediate	Immediate	Unknown

Pharmacodynamics
Chemical effect: may bind to sterol in fungal cell membrane and alter cell permeability, allowing leakage of intracellular components.

Therapeutic effect: decreases activity of or kills susceptible fungi, such as *Histoplasma capsulatum, Coccidioides immitis, Blastomyces dermatitidis, Cryptococcus neoformans, Candida, Aspergillus fumigatus, Mucor, Rhizopus, Absidia, Entomophthora, Basidiobolus, Paracoccidioides brasiliensis, Sporothrix schenckii,* and *Rhodotorula.*

Adverse reactions

CNS: malaise, headache, peripheral neuropathy, ***seizures;*** peripheral nerve pain, paresthesia (with I.V. use).
CV: hypotension, ***arrhythmias, asystole,*** phlebitis, thrombophlebitis.
GI: *anorexia, weight loss, nausea,* vomiting, dyspepsia, diarrhea, epigastric cramps, ***hemorrhagic gastroenteritis.***
GU: abnormal renal function with hypokalemia, azotemia, hyposthenuria, hypomagnesemia, renal tubular acidosis, nephrocalcinosis; ***permanent renal impairment***, anuria, oliguria.
Hematologic: normochromic normocytic anemia, ***thrombocytopenia, agranulocytosis.***
Hepatic: ***acute liver failure.***
Metabolic: hypokalemia.
Musculoskeletal: arthralgia, myalgia.
Skin: burning, stinging, irritation, tissue damage with extravasation, pain at injection site.
Other: *fever, chills,* generalized pain; ***anaphylactoid reactions.***

Interactions

Drug-drug. *Cardiac glycosides:* increased risk of digitalis toxicity in potassium-depleted patients. Monitor patient closely.
Corticosteroids: potassium depletion. Monitor potassium level.
Flucytosine: may increase flucytosine toxicity. Monitor patient closely.
Other nephrotoxic drugs (such as antibiotics, antineoplastic drugs): increased risk of nephrotoxicity. Administer cautiously.

Contraindications and precautions

- Contraindicated in patients hypersensitive to drug and in breast-feeding women.
- Use cautiously in patients with impaired renal function and in pregnant women.
- Safety of drug hasn't been established in children.

NURSING CONSIDERATIONS

Assessment

- Obtain history of fungal infection and samples for culture and sensitivity tests before first dose. Reevaluate condition during therapy.
- Be alert for adverse reactions and drug interactions.
- Monitor patient's pulse, respiratory rate, temperature, and blood pressure every 30 minutes for at least 4 hours after administering drug I.V.; fever, shaking chills, and hypotension may appear 1 to 2 hours after start of I.V. infusion and should subside within 4 hours of discontinuation.
- Monitor BUN, serum creatinine (or creatinine clearance), and serum electrolyte levels; CBC; and liver function studies at least weekly, as ordered.
- Evaluate patient's and family's knowledge of drug therapy.

Nursing diagnoses

- Infection related to presence of susceptible fungal infection
- Risk for injury related to drug-induced adverse reactions
- Deficient knowledge related to drug therapy

Planning and implementation

P.O. use: Lozenge form of drug should be dissolved slowly.
I.V. use: Give drug parenterally only in hospitalized patients, under close supervision, when diagnosis of potentially fatal fungal infection has been confirmed. Be prepared to administer an initial test dose, as ordered; 1 mg is added to 20 ml of D_5W and infused over 20 to 30 minutes.
– Use an infusion pump and in-line filter with a mean pore diameter larger than 1 micron. Infuse over 2 to 6 hours; rapid infusion may cause CV collapse.
– Use I.V. sites in distal veins. If thrombosis occurs, alternate sites.
– Reconstituted solution is stable for 1 week in refrigerator or 24 hours at room temperature. It has 8-hour stability in room light.

– Give antibiotics separately; don't mix or piggyback with amphotericin B.
– Amphotericin B appears to be compatible with limited amounts of heparin sodium, hydrocortisone sodium succinate, and methylprednisolone sodium succinate.
– Store dry form at 36° to 46° F (2° to 8° C). Protect from light. Reconstitute with 10 ml of sterile water only. To avoid precipitation, don't mix with solutions containing sodium chloride, other electrolytes, or bacteriostatic drugs (such as benzyl alcohol). Don't use if solution contains precipitate or foreign matter.
– If BUN level exceeds 40 mg/dl, or if serum creatinine level exceeds 3 mg/dl, prescriber may reduce or stop drug until renal function improves. Drug may be stopped if alkaline phosphatase or bilirubin level increases.
– To reduce severe adverse reactions, patient may receive premedication with antipyretics, antihistamines, antiemetics, or small doses of corticosteroids; addition of phosphate buffer and heparin to solution; or an alternate-day schedule. For severe reactions, discontinue drug and notify prescriber.

Patient teaching

- Teach patient signs and symptoms of hypersensitivity, and stress importance of reporting them immediately.
- Warn patient that therapy may take several months; teach personal hygiene and other measures to prevent spread and recurrence of lesions.
- Urge patient to comply with prescribed regimen and recommended follow-up.
- With oral form, instruct patient to let lozenges dissolve slowly.
- With I.V. therapy, warn patient that discomfort at injection site and adverse reactions may occur during therapy, which may last several months.

☑ Evaluation

- Patient is free from fungal infection.
- Patient doesn't experience injury as a result of drug-induced adverse reactions.
- Patient and family state understanding of drug therapy.

amphotericin B lipid complex

(am-foe-TER-ah-sin bee LIP-id KOM-pleks)
Abelcet

Pharmacologic class: polyene antibiotic
Therapeutic class: antifungal
Pregnancy risk category: B

Indications and dosages

▶ **Treatment of invasive fungal infections including *Aspergillus fumigatus, Candida albicans, C. guillermondii, C. stellatoideae, and C. tropicalis, Coccidioidomyces* sp., *Cryptococcus* sp., *Histoplasma* sp., and *Blastomyces* sp. in patients refractory to or intolerant of conventional amphotericin B therapy.** *Adults and children:* 5 mg/kg daily as a single I.V. infusion. Administer by continuous I.V. infusion at 2.5 mg/kg/hr.

How supplied

Suspension for injection: 100 mg/20 ml vial

Pharmacokinetics

Absorption: unknown.
Distribution: well distributed. The distribution volume increases with increasing dose. Abelcet yields measurable amphotericin B levels in spleen, lung, liver, lymph nodes, kidney, heart, and brain.
Metabolism: unknown.
Excretion: although rapidly cleared from blood, Abelcet has a long terminal half-life (173½ hr), probably because of slow elimination from tissues.

Route	Onset	Peak	Duration
I.V.	Unknown	Unknown	Unknown

Pharmacodynamics

Chemical effect: the active component of Abelcet, amphotericin B, binds to sterols in fungal cell membranes, resulting in enhanced cellular permeability and cell damage. Amphotericin B has fungistatic or fungicidal effects depending on fungal susceptibility.
Therapeutic effect: decreases activity of or kills susceptible fungi including *Aspergillus fumigatus, Candida albicans, C. guiller-*

mondii, C. stellatoideae, and C.tropicalis, Cryptococcus sp., *Coccidioidomyces* sp., *Histoplasma* sp., and *Blastomyces* sp.

Adverse reactions

CNS: headache, pain.
CV: chest pain, ***cardiac arrest,*** hypertension, hypotension.
GI: abdominal pain, diarrhea, ***hemorrhage,*** nausea, vomiting.
GU: *increased serum creatinine,* ***kidney failure.***
Hematologic: anemia, ***leukopenia, thrombocytopenia.***
Hepatic: bilirubinemia.
Metabolic: hypokalemia.
Respiratory: dyspnea, respiratory disorder, ***respiratory failure.***
Skin: rash.
Other: *chills, fever,* infection, **MULTIPLE ORGAN FAILURE,** ***sepsis.***

Interactions

Drug-drug: *Antineoplastics:* increased risk of renal toxicity, bronchospasm, and hypotension. Use cautiously.
Corticosteroids, corticotropin: enhanced hypokalemia, which may lead to cardiac dysfunction. Monitor serum electrolytes and cardiac function.
Cyclosporin A: increased renal toxicity. Monitor patient closely.
Cardiac glycosides: increased risk of digitalis toxicity and induced hypokalemia. Monitor serum potassium levels closely.
Flucytosine: increased risk of flucytosine toxicity due to increased cellular uptake or impaired renal excretion. Use cautiously.
Imidazoles (clotrimazole, fluconazole, itraconazole, ketoconazole, miconazole): decreased efficacy of amphotericin B due to inhibition of ergosterol synthesis. Clinical significance is unknown.
Leukocyte transfusions: acute pulmonary toxicity. Avoid concurrent use.
Nephrotoxic drugs (aminoglycosides, pentamidine): increased risk of renal toxicity. Use cautiously. Monitor renal function closely.
Skeletal muscle relaxants: enhanced effects of skeletal muscle relaxants, due to amphotericin B induced hypokalemia. Monitor serum potassium levels closely.
Zidovudine: increased myelotoxicity and nephrotoxicity. Monitor renal and hematologic function.

Contraindications and precautions

- Contraindicated in patients hypersensitive to amphotericin B or any of its components.
- Use cautiously in patients with renal impairment.

NURSING CONSIDERATIONS

Assessment

- Obtain history of fungal infection and samples for culture and sensitivity tests before therapy. Reevaluate condition during therapy.
- Be alert for adverse reactions and drug interactions.
- Assess renal function before therapy starts.
- Monitor serum creatinine, liver function, electrolytes (especially magnesium and potassium), and CBC during therapy, as ordered.
- Evaluate patient's and family's knowledge of drug therapy.

Nursing diagnoses

- Risk for infection related to presence of susceptible fungal infection
- Risk for injury related to drug-induced adverse reactions
- Deficient knowledge related to drug therapy

Planning and implementation

- To prepare, shake the vial gently until you see no yellow sediment. Using aseptic technique, draw the calculated dose into one or more 20 ml syringes, using an 18-gauge needle. You'll need more than one vial. Attach a 5-micron filter needle to the syringe and inject the dose into an I.V. bag of D_5W. One filter needle can be used for up to four vials of drug. The volume of D_5W should be sufficient to yield a final concentration of 1 mg/ml.
- For pediatric patients and patients with CV disease, the recommended final concentration is 2 mg/ml.
- Shake the bag and check the contents for any foreign matter. Discard any unused drug; it doesn't contain a preservative.

• Don't mix with saline solution or infuse in the same I.V. line as other drugs. Don't use an in-line filter.
• If infusing through an existing I.V. line, flush first with D_5W.
• Infusions are stable for up to 48 hours when refrigerated (2° to 8° C) and up to 6 hours at room temperature.
• Refrigerate (2° to 8° C) and protect from light. Don't freeze.
ALERT Note that different amphotericin B preparations aren't interchangable and that dosages vary.
• Premedicate with acetaminophen, antihistamines, and corticosteroids as ordered, to prevent or lessen the severity of infusion-related reactions, such as fever, chills, nausea, and vomiting, which occur 1 to 2 hours after the start of the infusion.
• Slowing the infusion rate may also decrease the risk of infusion-related reactions.
• For infusions lasting more than 2 hours, shake the I.V. bag every 2 hours to ensure an even suspension.
• If severe respiratory distress develops, stop the infusion, provide supportive therapy for anaphylaxis, and notify the prescriber. Don't resume the infusion.

Patient teaching

• Inform patient that fever, chills, nausea, and vomiting may occur during the infusion and that these reactions usually subside with subsequent doses.
• Instruct patient to report any redness or pain at the infusion site.
• Teach patient to recognize and report any symptoms of acute hypersensitivity, such as respiratory distress.
• Tell patient to expect frequent laboratory testing to monitor kidney and liver function.

Evaluation

• Patient is free from fungal infection.
• Patient has no injury from adverse drug reactions.
• Patient and family state understanding of drug therapy.

amphotericin B liposomal

(am-foh-TER-ah-sin bee lye po SO mal)
AmBisome

Pharmacologic class: polyene antibiotic
Therapeutic class: antifungal
Pregnancy risk category: B

Indications and dosages

▶ **Empirical therapy for presumed fungal infection in febrile, neutropenic patients.** *Adults and children:* 3 mg/kg IV infusion daily.
▶ **Treatment of systemic fungal infections caused by *Aspergillus* sp., *Candida* sp., or *Cryptococcus* sp. refractory to amphotericin B deoxycholate or in patients where renal impairment or unacceptable toxicity precludes the use of amphotericin B deoxycholate.** *Adults and children:* 3 to 5 mg/kg IV infusion daily.
▶ **Treatment of visceral leishmaniasis in immunocompetent patients.** *Adults and children:* 3 mg/kg IV infusion daily on days 1 to 5, 14 and 21. A repeat course of therapy may be beneficial if initial treatment fails to achieve parasitic clearance.
▶ **Treatment of visceral leishmaniasis in immunocompromised patients.** *Adults and children:* 4 mg/kg IV infusion daily on days 1 to 5, 10, 17, 24, 31 and 38. Expert advice regarding further treatment is recommended if initial therapy fails or patient experiences a relapse.

How supplied

Injection: 50 mg vial

Pharmacokinetics

Absorption: drug is given I.V.
Distribution: unknown.
Metabolism: unknown.
Excretion: initial half-life is 7 to10 hours with 24 hour dosing; terminal elimination half-life is 100 to 153 hours.

Route	Onset	Peak	Duration
I.V.	Unknown	Unknown	Unknown

Pharmacodynamics

Chemical effect: amphotericin B, the active component of Ambisome, binds to the sterol component of a fungal cell membrane leading to alterations in cell permeability and cell death.

Therapeutic effect: decreases activity of or kills susceptible fungi including *Aspergillus* species, *Candida* species, or *Cryptococcus* species refractory to amphotericin B deoxycholate or in patients where renal impairment or unacceptable toxicity precludes the use of amphotericin B deoxycholate; treatment of visceral protozoal infections caused by the leishmania species.

Adverse reactions

CNS: *anxiety, confusion, headache, insomnia, asthenia.*

CV: *chest pain, hypotension, tachycardia,* hypertension, *edema,* vasodilitation.

EENT: *epistaxis, rhinitis.*

GI: *nausea, vomiting, abdominal pain, diarrhea,* ***hemorrhage.***

GU: *hematuria, elevated creatinine and BUN.*

Hepatic: *hepatomegaly, elevated ALT and AST levels, increased alkaline phosphatase, bilirubinemia.*

Metabolic: *hyperglycemia,* hypernatremia, *hypocalcemia, hypokalemia, hypomagnesemia.*

Musculoskeletal: *back pain.*

Respiratory: *cough increased, dyspnea,* hypoxia, *pleural effusion, lung disorder,* hyperventilation.

Skin: *pruritus, rash,* sweating.

Other: *chills, infection,* ***anaphylaxis,*** *pain,* ***sepsis,*** *fever, blood product infusion reaction.*

Interactions

Drug-drug. *Antineoplastics:* may enhance potential for renal toxicity, bronchospasm, and hypotension. Use cautiously.

Cardiac glycosides: Increased risk of digitalis toxicity in potassium-depleted patients. Monitor serum potassium closely.

Corticosteroids, corticotropin: may potentiate hypokalemia, which could result in cardiac dysfunction. Monitor serum potassium level and cardiac function.

Flucytosine: may increase flucytosine toxicity by increasing cellular uptake or impairing renal excretion of flucytosine. Monitor renal function closely.

Imidazole antifungals (ketoconazole, miconazole, clotrimazole): imidazoles may induce fungal resistance to amphotericin B. Use combination therapy with caution.

Leukocyte transfusions: Risk of acute pulmonary toxicity. Avoid concomitant use.

Other nephrotoxic drugs (antibiotics, antineoplastics): increased risk of nephrotoxicity. Administer cautiously. Monitor renal function closely.

Skeletal muscle relaxants: enhanced effects of skeletal muscle relaxants, due to amphotericin induced hypokalemia. Monitor serum potassium levels.

Contraindications and precautions

- Contraindicated in patients hypersensitive to drug or any of its components. Use cautiously in patients with impaired renal function, in elderly patients, and in pregnant women.

NURSING CONSIDERATIONS

Assessment

- Obtain history of fungal infection and samples for culture and sensitivity tests before therapy. Reevaluate condition during therapy.
- Assess patients concomitantly receiving chemotherapy or bone marrow transplantation carefully as they are at greater risk for additional adverse reactions including seizures, arrhythmias, thrombocytopenia and respiratory failure.
- Monitor serum creatinine and BUN, liver function studies and CBC and serum electrolytes (particularly magnesium and potassium).
- Monitor patient for signs of hypokalemia (ECG changes, muscle weakness, cramping, drowsiness).
- Watch for adverse reactions. Patients who receive drug may have fewer chills, lower blood urea nitrogen, a lower risk of hypokalemia, and less vomiting than patients who receive regular amphotericin B.
- Evaluate patient's and family's knowledge of drug therapy.

Nursing diagnoses

- Risk for infection related to presence of susceptible fungal or parasite infections
- Risk for injury related to drug-induced adverse reactions
- Deficient knowledge related to drug therapy

Planning and implementation

ALERT Different amphotericin B preparations aren't interchangeable and dosages will vary.

- Reconstitute each 50-mg vial of amphotericin B liposomal with 12 ml of sterile water for injection to yield 4 mg amphotericin B/ml. Don't reconstitute with bacteriostatic water for injection, and don't allow bacteriostatic drug into the solution. Don't reconstitute with saline solution, add saline solution to the reconstituted concentration, or mix with other drugs. After reconstitution, shake vial vigorously for 30 seconds or until particulate matter is dispersed. Withdraw calculated amount of reconstituted solution into a sterile syringe and inject through a 5-micron filter into the appropriate amount of D_5W to a final concentration of 1 to 2 mg/mL. Lower concentrations (0.2 to 0.5 mg/ml) may be appropriate for children to provide sufficient volume for infusion.
- Flush existing I.V. line with D_5W before infusing drug. If this isn't feasible, give drug through a separate line.
- Use a controlled infusion device and an in-line filter with a mean pore diameter larger than 1 micron. Initially, infuse drug over at least 2 hours. Infusion time may be reduced to 1 hour if the treatment is well-tolerated. If the patient has discomfort during infusion, the duration of infusion may be increased.
- Observe patient closely for adverse reactions during infusion. If anaphylaxis occurs, stop the infusion immediately, provide supportive therapy, and notify the prescriber.
- Refrigerate unopened drug at 2° to 8° C (36°to 46° F). Once reconstituted, the vial of the reconstituted product concentrate may be stored for up to 24 hours at 2° to 8° C (36°to 46° F). Don't freeze.
- To lessen the risk or severity of adverse reactions, premedicate patient with antipyretics, antihistamines, antiemetics or corticosteroids, as ordered.
- Therapy may take several weeks to months.

Patient teaching

- Teach patient signs and symptoms of hypersensitivity, and stress importance of reporting them immediately.
- Warn patient that therapy may take several months; teach personal hygiene and other measures to prevent spread and recurrence of lesions.
- Instruct the patient to report any adverse reactions that occur while receiving the medication.
- Instruct patient to watch for and report any signs of hypokalemia (muscle weakness, cramping, drowsiness).
- Advise patient that frequent laboratory testing will be performed.

Evaluation

- Patient is free from fungal or parasite infection.
- Patient doesn't experience injury as a result of drug-induced adverse reactions.
- Patient and family state understanding of drug therapy.

ampicillin

(am-pih-SIL-in)

Apo-Ampi ♦, Novo-Ampicillin ♦, Nu-Ampi ♦, Omnipen, Principen

ampicillin sodium

Ampicin ♦, Ampicyn Injection ◇, Omnipen-N, Penbritin ♦, Polycillin-N, Totacillin-N

ampicillin trihydrate

Ampicyn Oral ◇, D-Amp, Omnipen, Penbritin ◇, Polycillin, Principen-250, Principen-500, Totacillin

Pharmacologic class: aminopenicillin
Therapeutic class: antibiotic
Pregnancy risk category: B

Indications and dosages

▶ **Systemic infections and acute and chronic UTI caused by susceptible gram-positive and gram-negative organisms.** *Adults and*

children weighing 20 kg (44 lb) and over: 250 to 500 mg P.O. q 6 hours; or 2 to 12 g I.M. or I.V. daily in divided doses q 4 to 6 hours.
Children weighing under 20 kg: 50 to 100 mg/kg P.O. daily in divided doses q 6 hours; or 100 to 200 mg/kg I.M. or I.V. daily in divided doses q 6 hours.
▶ **Meningitis.** *Adults:* 8 to 14 g I.V. daily in divided doses q 3 to 4 hours.
Children ages 2 months to 12 years: up to 400 mg/kg I.V. daily for 3 days; then up to 300 mg/kg I.M. divided q 4 hours.
▶ **Uncomplicated gonorrhea.** *Adults and children weighing over 45 kg (99 lb):* 3.5 g P.O. with 1 g probenecid in a single dose.
▶ **Endocarditis prophylaxis for dental procedures.** *Adults:* 2 g I.V. or I.M. 30 minutes before procedure.
Children: 50 mg/kg I.V. or I.M. 30 minutes before procedure.

How supplied

Capsules: 250 mg, 500 mg
Oral suspension: 100 mg/ml (pediatric drops), 125 mg/5 ml, 250 mg/5 ml, 500 mg/5 ml (after reconstitution)
Injection: 125 mg, 250 mg, 500 mg, 1 g, 2 g
Infusion: 500 mg, 1 g, 2 g

Pharmacokinetics

Absorption: about 42% is absorbed after an oral dose; unknown after I.M. administration.
Distribution: distributes into pleural, peritoneal and synovial fluids; lungs; prostate; liver; and gallbladder. Also penetrates middle ear effusions, maxillary sinus and bronchial secretions, tonsils, and sputum. Ampicillin is minimally protein-bound at 15% to 25%.
Metabolism: metabolized only partially.
Excretion: excreted in urine by renal tubular secretion and glomerular filtration. *Half-life:* about 1 to 1½ hours (10 to 24 hours in severe renal impairment).

Route	Onset	Peak	Duration
P.O.	Unknown	≤ 2 hr	6-8 hr
I.V.	Immediate	Immediate	Unknown
I.M.	Unknown	≤ 1 hr	Unknown

Pharmacodynamics

Chemical effect: inhibits cell-wall synthesis during microorganism multiplication.
Therapeutic effect: kills susceptible bacteria. Its spectrum of action includes non-penicillinase-producing gram-positive bacteria. It is also effective against many gram-negative organisms, including *Neisseria gonorrhoeae, N. meningitidis, Haemophilus influenzae, Escherichia coli, Proteus mirabilis, Salmonella,* and *Shigella.*

Adverse reactions

CNS: *seizures.*
CV: vein irritation, thrombophlebitis.
GI: *nausea,* vomiting, *diarrhea,* glossitis, stomatitis.
Hematologic: anemia, ***thrombocytopenia,*** thrombocytopenic purpura, eosinophilia, ***leukopenia, agranulocytosis.***
Other: hypersensitivity reactions (maculopapular rash, urticaria, ***anaphylaxis***), overgrowth of nonsusceptible organisms, pain at injection site.

Interactions

Drug-drug. *Allopurinol:* increased risk of rash.
Probenecid: increased blood level of ampicillin and other penicillins. Probenecid may be used for this purpose.

Contraindications and precautions

- Contraindicated in patients hypersensitive to drug or other penicillins.
- Use cautiously in patients with other drug allergies, especially to cephalosporins (possible cross-sensitivity); in those with mononucleosis (high risk of maculopapular rash); and in pregnant or breast-feeding women.

NURSING CONSIDERATIONS

Assessment

- Obtain history of patient's infection before therapy, and reassess for improvement regularly thereafter.
- Before giving drug, ask patient about previous allergic reaction to penicillin. Keep in mind that a negative history of penicillin aller-

gy doesn't guarantee freedom from future reaction.
• Obtain specimen for culture and sensitivity tests before administering first dose.
• Be alert for adverse reactions and drug interactions.
• Monitor patient's hydration status if adverse GI reactions occur.
• Evaluate patient's and family's knowledge of drug therapy.

Nursing diagnoses

• Risk for infection related to presence of susceptible bacterial infection
• Risk for deficient fluid volume related to drug-induced adverse GI reactions
• Deficient knowledge related to drug therapy

Planning and implementation

P.O. use: Give 1 hour before or 2 hours after meals. When given orally, drug may cause adverse GI reactions. Food may interfere with absorption.
I.V. use: Reconstitute with bacteriostatic water for injection. Use 5 ml for 125-mg, 250-mg, or 500-mg vials; 7.4 ml for 1-g vials; and 14.8 ml for 2-g vials. Give direct I.V. injections over 3 to 5 minutes for doses of 500 mg or less; over 10 to 15 minutes for larger doses. Don't exceed a rate of 100 mg/minute. Alternatively, dilute in 50 to 100 ml of normal saline injection and give by intermittent infusion over 15 to 30 minutes. Don't mix with solutions containing dextrose or fructose because these solutions promote rapid breakdown of ampicillin.
– Use initial dilution within 1 hour. Follow manufacturer's directions for stability data when ampicillin is further diluted for I.V. infusion.
– Give intermittently to prevent vein irritation. Change site every 48 hours.
– Don't give I.V. unless prescribed and infection is severe or patient can't take oral dose.
I.M. use: Don't give I.M. unless prescribed and infection is severe or patient can't take oral dose.
• Dosage should be altered in patients with impaired renal function.
• Give ampicillin at least 1 hour before bacteriostatic antibiotics.
• In pediatric meningitis, ampicillin may be given concurrently with parenteral chloramphenicol for 24 hours pending culture results.
• Drug may cause false-positive urine glucose determinations with copper sulfate tests (Clinitest); drug doesn't affect glucose enzymatic tests (Diastix).
• Stop drug immediately if anaphylactic shock occurs. Notify prescriber and prepare to administer immediate treatment (such as epinephrine, corticosteroids, antihistamines, and other resuscitative measures), as indicated.

Patient teaching

• Tell patient to take entire quantity of drug exactly as ordered, even after he feels better.
• Tell patient to call prescriber if a rash (most common), fever, or chills develop.
• Warn patient never to use leftover ampicillin for a new illness or to share it with others.
• Tell patient to take oral ampicillin 1 hour before or 2 hours after meals for best absorption.

Evaluation

• Patient is free from infection.
• Patient maintains adequate hydration.
• Patient and family state understanding of drug therapy.

ampicillin sodium/sulbactam sodium

(am-pih-SIL-in SOH-dee-um/sul-BAC-tam SOH-dee-um)
Unasyn

Pharmacologic class: aminopenicillin/beta-lactamase inhibitor combination
Therapeutic class: antibiotic
Pregnancy risk category: B

Indications and dosages

▶ **Intra-abdominal, gynecologic, and skin structure infections caused by susceptible strains.** *Adults:* dosage expressed as total drug (each 1.5-g vial contains 1 g ampicillin sodium and 0.5 g sulbactam sodium)—1.5 to 3 g I.M. or I.V. q 6 hours. Maximum daily dosage is 4 g sulbactam (12 g of combined drugs).

How supplied

Injection: vials and piggyback vials containing 1.5 g (1 g ampicillin sodium with 0.5 g sulbactam sodium) and 3 g (2 g ampicillin sodium with 1 g sulbactam sodium)

Pharmacokinetics

Absorption: unknown.
Distribution: both drugs distribute into pleural, peritoneal, and synovial fluids; lungs; prostate; liver; and gallbladder. They also penetrate middle ear effusions, maxillary sinus and bronchial secretions, tonsils, and sputum. Ampicillin is minimally protein-bound at 15% to 25%; sulbactam is about 38% bound.
Metabolism: both drugs are metabolized only partially.
Excretion: both drugs excreted in urine by renal tubular secretion and glomerular filtration. *Half-life:* 1 to 1½ hours (10 to 24 hours in severe renal impairment).

Route	Onset	Peak	Duration
I.V.	Immediate	Immediate	Unknown
I.M.	Unknown	Unknown	Unknown

Pharmacodynamics

Chemical effect: ampicillin inhibits cell-wall synthesis during microorganism multiplication; sulbactam inactivates bacterial beta-lactamase, the enzyme that inactivates ampicillin and provides bacterial resistance to it.
Therapeutic effect: kills susceptible bacteria. Spectrum of activity includes beta-lactamase-producing strains of *Staphylococcus aureus, Escherichia coli, Klebsiella, Proteus mirabilis, Bacteroides, Enterobacter,* and *Acinetobacter calcoaceticus.*

Adverse reactions

CV: vein irritation, thrombophlebitis.
GI: *nausea,* vomiting, *diarrhea,* glossitis, stomatitis.
Hematologic: anemia, ***thrombocytopenia,*** thrombocytopenic purpura, eosinophilia, ***leukopenia, agranulocytosis.***
Other: hypersensitivity reactions (erythematous maculopapular rash, urticaria, ***anaphylaxis), overgrowth of nonsusceptible organisms,*** pain at injection site.

Interactions

Drug-drug. *Allopurinol:* increased risk of rash. Monitor patient.
Probenecid: increased blood level of ampicillin. Probenecid may be used for this purpose.
Oral contraceptives: efficacy of oral contraceptives may be decreased. Advise patient to use barrier contraception until course of therapy is complete.

Contraindications and precautions

- Contraindicated in patients hypersensitive to drug or other penicillins.
- Use cautiously in patients with other drug allergies, especially to cephalosporins (possible cross-sensitivity); in those with mononucleosis (high risk of maculopapular rash); and in pregnant or breast-feeding women.
- Safety of drug hasn't been established in children under age 12.

NURSING CONSIDERATIONS

Assessment

- Obtain history of patient's infection before therapy, and observe for improvement in condition throughout therapy.
- Before giving drug, ask patient about previous allergic reaction to penicillin. Be aware that a negative history of penicillin allergy is no guarantee against a future reaction.
- Obtain specimen for culture and sensitivity tests before administering first dose.
- Be alert for adverse reactions and drug interactions.
- Monitor patient's hydration status if adverse GI reactions occur.
- Evaluate patient's and family's knowledge of drug therapy.

Nursing diagnoses

- Risk for infection related to presence of susceptible bacterial infection
- Risk for deficient fluid volume related to drug-induced adverse GI reactions
- Deficient knowledge related to drug therapy

Planning and implementation

I.V. use: When preparing injection, reconstitute powder with any of the following diluents: normal saline solution, D_5W, lactated Ringer's

injection, 1/6 M sodium lactate, dextrose 5% in half-normal saline solution for injection, and 10% invert sugar. Stability varies with diluent, temperature, and concentration of solution.
– After reconstitution, allow vials to stand for a few minutes for foam to dissipate to permit visual inspection of contents for particles.
– Give dose by slow injection (over 10 to 15 minutes), or dilute in 50 to 100 ml of a compatible diluent and infuse over 15 to 30 minutes. If permitted, give intermittently to prevent vein irritation. Change site every 48 hours.
– Don't add or mix with other drugs because they might prove physically or chemically incompatible.
I.M. use: Reconstitute with sterile water for injection or 0.5% or 2% lidocaine hydrochloride injection. Add 3.2 ml to a 1.5-g vial (or 6.4 ml to a 3-g vial) to yield a concentration of 375 mg/ml. Administer deeply.
• Dosage should be altered in patients with impaired renal function.
• Give drug at least 1 hour before bacteriostatic antibiotics.
• Drug may cause false-positive urine glucose determinations with copper sulfate tests (Clinitest); drug doesn't affect glucose enzymatic tests (Diastix).
• Stop drug immediately if anaphylactic shock occurs. Notify prescriber, and prepare to administer immediate treatment (such as epinephrine, corticosteroids, antihistamines, and other resuscitative measures), as indicated.

Patient teaching
• Tell patient to call prescriber if rash (most common), fever, or chills develop.
• Advise women to use an additional form of contraception with oral contraceptives during drug therapy.

☑ Evaluation
• Patient is free from infection.
• Patient maintains adequate hydration.
• Patient and family state understanding of drug therapy.

amprenavir
(am-PREH-nah-veer)
Agenerase

Pharmacologic class: HIV protease inhibitor
Therapeutic class: antiviral
Pregnancy risk category: C

Indications and dosages
▶ **Treatment of HIV-1 infection in combination with other antiretrovirals.** *Adults and adolescents ages 13 to 16 weighing more than 50 kg (110 lb):* 1,200 mg (eight 150-mg capsules) P.O. b.i.d. in combination with other antiretrovirals.
Children ages 4 to 12 and adolescents ages 13 to 16 weighing less than 50 kg: For capsules, give 20 mg/kg P.O. b.i.d. or 15 mg/kg P.O. t.i.d. (maximum, 2,400 mg daily) in combination with other antiretrovirals. For oral solution, give 22.5 mg/kg (1.5 ml/kg) P.O. b.i.d. or 17 mg/kg (1.1ml/kg) P.O. t.i.d. (maximum, 2,800 mg daily) in combination with other antiretrovirals.
▶ **For patients with hepatic impairment.** *Patients with a Child-Pugh score of 5 to 8:* For capsule, reduce dosage to 450 mg P.O. b.i.d. *Patients with a Child-Pugh score of 9 to 12:* For capsules, reduce dosage to 300 mg P.O. b.i.d.

How supplied
Capsules: 50 mg, 150 mg
Oral solution: 15 mg/ml

Pharmacokinetics
Absorption: rapidly absorbed. Level peaks in 1 to 2 hours.
Distribution: apparent volume of distribution is about 430 L. In vitro, about 90% of drug binds to plasma proteins.
Metabolism: cytochrome P-450 CYP3A4 enzyme system metabolizes the drug in the liver.
Excretion: minimal excretion of unchanged drug in urine and feces. *Half-life (plasma elimination):* 7 to 10½ hours.

Route	Onset	Peak	Duration
P.O.	Unknown	1-2 hr	Unknown

Pharmacodynamics

Chemical effect: amprenavir inhibits HIV-1 protease by binding to the active site of HIV-1 protease, which causes immature noninfectious viral particles to form.
Therapeutic effect: reduces the symptoms of HIV-1 infection.

Adverse reactions

CNS: *paresthesia,* depressive or mood disorders.
GI: *nausea, vomiting, diarrhea or loose stools,* taste disorders.
Hepatic: *hypertriglyceridemia,* hypercholesterolemia.
Metabolic: *hyperglycemia.*
Skin: *rash,* ***Stevens-Johnson syndrome.***

Interactions

Drug-drug. *Amiodarone, lidocaine, quinidine, tricyclic antidepressants:* inhibited metabolism of these drugs. Monitor drug levels closely.
Antacids, didanosine: decreased absorption. Separate administration by at least 1 hour.
Anticonvulsants, such as carbamazepine, phenobarbital, and phenytoin: potentially decreased amprenavir levels. Monitor patient closely and adjust dosage as needed.
Bepridil, dihydroergotamine, ergotamine, midazolam, triazolam: inhibited metabolism of these drugs, which may cause serious or life-threatening adverse reactions. Don't use together.
Rifabutin: decreased amprenavir levels and increased rifabutin levels. Reduce rifabutin dosage to at least half the recommended dosage. Monitor CBC weekly for neutropenia.
Rifampin: 90% reduced plasma amprenavir levels. Don't use together.
Sildenafil: increased sildenafil levels, which may increase the frequency of sildenafil-related adverse reactions, such as hypotension, visual changes, and priapism. Use together cautiously.
Warfarin: inhibited metabolism of warfarin, which may cause serious or life-threatening adverse reactions. Monitor INR closely.
Drug-herb. *St. John's wort:* may cause substantial reduction of serum blood levels of protease inhibitors. Discourage concomitant use.
Drug-food. *High-fat foods:* decreased absorption of the drug. Discourage taking the drug with high-fat foods.

Contraindications and precautions

- Contraindicated in patients hypersensitive to amprenavir or its components.
- Use cautiously in patients with moderate or severe hepatic impairment, diabetes mellitus, sulfonamide allergy, or hemophilia A or B; also, use cautiously in pregnant patients.
- Drug can cause severe or life-threatening rash, including Stevens-Johnson syndrome. Therapy should be stopped if patient develops a severe or life-threatening rash or a moderate rash with systemic signs and symptoms.

NURSING CONSIDERATIONS

Assessment

- Assess patient for appropriateness of drug therapy.
- Because drug may interact with many drugs, obtain patient's complete drug history. Ask patient to show you the drugs he takes.
- Patients with moderate or severe hepatic impairment, diabetes mellitus, a known sulfonamide allergy, or hemophilia A or B must be monitored very closely while taking this drug.
- Determine if patient is pregnant or plans to become pregnant. No adequate studies exist regarding effects of amprenavir given during pregnancy. Use during pregnancy only if potential benefits outweigh the risks.
- Monitor patient for adverse reactions. A patient taking a protease inhibitor may experience a redistribution of body fat, including central obesity, dorsocervical fat enlargement (buffalo hump), peripheral wasting, breast enlargement, and cushingoid appearance.
- Evaluate patient's and family's knowledge about drug therapy.

Nursing diagnoses

- Risk for infection secondary to presence of HIV
- Ineffective individual coping related to HIV infection
- Deficient knowledge related to drug therapy

Planning and implementation

- Don't give patient high-fat foods because they may decrease absorption of oral drug.

ALERT Amprenavir capsules aren't interchangeable with amprenavir oral solution on a milligram-per-milligram basis.

- Monitor coagulation studies. Drug provides high daily doses of vitamin E.
- Protease inhibitors have caused spontaneous bleeding in some patients with hemophilia A or B. In some patients, additional factor VIII was required. In many of the reported cases, treatment with protease inhibitors was continued or restarted.

Patient teaching

- Inform patient that drug doesn't cure HIV infection and that opportunistic infections and other complications may continue to develop. Also, explain that drug doesn't reduce the risk of transmitting HIV to others.
- Tell patient that drug can be taken with or without food, but that he shouldn't take it with a high-fat meal because doing so may decrease drug absorption.
- Urge patient to report adverse reactions, especially rash.
- Advise patient to take drug every day as prescribed, always in combination with other antiretrovirals. Warn against changing the dosage or stoping the drug without prescriber's approval.
- If patient takes an antacid or didanosine, tell him to do so 1 hour before or after amprenavir to avoid interfering with amprenavir absorption.
- If patient misses a dose by more than 4 hours, tell him to wait and take the next dose at the regularly scheduled time. If he misses a dose by less than 4 hours, tell him to take the dose as soon as possible and then take the next dose at the regularly scheduled time. Caution against doubling the dose.
- Caution patient not to take supplemental vitamin E because high levels of this vitamin may worsen the blood coagulation defect of vitamin K deficiency that anticoagulant therapy or malabsorption causes.
- If patient uses a hormonal contraceptive, warn her to use another contraceptive during therapy with amprenavir.
- Urge patient to notify prescriber about planned, suspected, or known pregnancy during therapy.

Evaluation

- Patient exhibits reduced signs and symptoms of infection.
- Patient demonstrates adequate coping mechanisms.
- Patient and family state understanding of drug therapy.

anastrozole

(uh-NAS-truh-zohl)
Arimidex

Pharmacologic class: nonsteroidal aromatase inhibitor
Therapeutic class: antineoplastic
Pregnancy risk category: D

Indications and dosages

▶ **Treatment of advanced breast cancer in postmenopausal women with disease progression after tamoxifen therapy.** *Adults:* 1 mg P.O. daily.

How supplied

Tablets: 1 mg

Pharmacokinetics

Absorption: absorbed from GI tract. Food affects extent of absorption.
Distribution: 40% bound to plasma proteins in therapeutic range.
Metabolism: metabolized in liver.
Excretion: about 11% excreted in urine as parent drug; about 60% excreted in urine as metabolites. *Half-life:* about 50 hours.

Route	Onset	Peak	Duration
P.O.	Unknown	Unknown	Unknown

Pharmacodynamics

Chemical effect: significantly lowers serum estradiol levels.
Therapeutic effect: hinders breast cancer cell growth.

Adverse reactions

CNS: *asthenia, headache,* dizziness, depression, paresthesia.
CV: chest pain, edema, thromboembolic disease, peripheral edema.
EENT: pharyngitis.
GI: *nausea,* vomiting, diarrhea, constipation, dry mouth, abdominal pain, anorexia.
GU: pelvic pain, vaginal hemorrhage, vaginal dryness.
Metabolic: weight gain, increased appetite.
Musculoskeletal: *back pain,* bone pain.
Respiratory: dyspnea, increased cough.
Skin: *hot flushes,* rash, sweating.
Other: *pain.*

Interactions

None reported.

Contraindications and precautions

- Drug isn't recommended for use in pregnant women.
- Use cautiously in breast-feeding women.
- Safety of drug hasn't been established in children.

NURSING CONSIDERATIONS

Assessment
- Obtain history of patient's neoplastic disease before therapy.
- Be alert for adverse reactions.
- Evaluate patient's and family's knowledge of drug therapy.

Nursing diagnoses
- Ineffective health maintenance related to neoplastic disease
- Risk for deficient fluid volume related to drug-induced adverse GI reactions
- Deficient knowledge related to drug therapy

Planning and implementation
- Pregnancy must be ruled out before treatment can begin.
- Give drug under supervision of a qualified clinician experienced in using anticancer drugs.

Patient teaching
- Instruct patient to report adverse reactions.
- Stress importance of follow-up care.

Evaluation
- Patient has positive response to therapy.
- Patient maintains adequate hydration.
- Patient and family state understanding of drug therapy.

anistreplase (anisoylated plasminogen-streptokinase activator complex; APSAC)

(an-ih-STREP-layz)
Eminase

Pharmacologic class: thrombolytic enzyme
Therapeutic class: thrombolytic enzyme
Pregnancy risk category: C

Indications and dosages

▶ **Lysis of coronary artery thrombi after acute MI.** *Adults:* 30 units I.V. over 2 to 5 minutes by direct injection.

How supplied

Injection: 30 units/vial

Pharmacokinetics

Absorption: not applicable with I.V. administration.
Distribution: information not available.
Metabolism: immediately after injection, drug is deacylated by a nonenzymatic process to form active streptokinase-plasminogen complex.
Excretion: unknown. *Half-life:* 88 to 112 minutes.

Route	Onset	Peak	Duration
I.V.	Immediate	About 45 min	6 hr-2 days

Pharmacodynamics

Chemical effect: anistreplase, derived from Lys-plasminogen and streptokinase, is formulated into a fibrinolytic enzyme plus activator complex with activator temporarily blocked by an anisoyl group. Drug is activated in vivo by a nonenzymatic process that removes the anisoyl group. The active Lys-plasminogen—

streptokinase activator complex is progressively formed in bloodstream or within thrombus.
Therapeutic effect: dissolves blood clots in coronary arteries.

Adverse reactions

CNS: ***intracranial hemorrhage.***
CV: ARRHYTHMIAS, conduction disorders, hypotension, edema.
GI: ***bleeding,*** gum or mouth hemorrhage.
GU: hematuria.
Hematologic: ***bleeding tendency,*** eosinophilia.
Musculoskeletal: arthralgia.
Respiratory: hemoptysis.
Skin: hematomas, urticaria, itching, flushing.
Other: bleeding at puncture sites, ***anaphylaxis or anaphylactoid reactions***

Interactions

Drug-drug. *Heparin, oral anticoagulants, drugs that alter platelet function (including aspirin, dipyridamole):* may increase risk of bleeding. Use together cautiously.
Drug-herb. *St. John's wort, ginger, ginkgo:* may increase the risk of bleeding. Discourage concomitant use.

Contraindications and precautions

- Contraindicated in patients with history of severe allergic reaction to anistreplase or streptokinase and in those with active internal bleeding, CVA, recent (within past 2 months) intraspinal or intracranial surgery or trauma, aneurysm, arteriovenous malformation, intracranial neoplasm, uncontrolled hypertension, or known bleeding diathesis.
- Use cautiously in patients with recent (within 10 days) major surgery; trauma (including CPR); GI or GU bleeding; cerebrovascular disease; hypertension; mitral stenosis, atrial fibrillation, or other conditions that may lead to left-sided heart thrombus; acute pericarditis or subacute bacterial endocarditis; septic thrombophlebitis; diabetic hemorrhagic retinopathy; in pregnant women and during first 10 days postpartum; in breast-feeding women; in patients receiving anticoagulants; and in patients age 75 or older.
- Safety of drug hasn't been established in children.

NURSING CONSIDERATIONS

Assessment

- Obtain history of patient's underlying cardiac condition before therapy.
- Monitor drug's effectiveness by carefully checking ECG and vital signs.
- Drug's efficacy may be limited if antistreptokinase antibodies are present. Antibody levels may be elevated if more than 5 days have elapsed since treatment with anistreplase or streptokinase or if patient has recently had a streptococcal infection.
- Be alert for adverse reactions and drug interactions.
- Evaluate patient's and family's knowledge about drug therapy.

Nursing diagnoses

- Ineffective tissue perfusion related to presence of coronary thrombosis
- Risk for injury related to drug-induced adverse reactions
- Deficient knowledge related to drug therapy

Planning and implementation

- Reconstitute drug by slowly adding 5 ml of sterile water for injection. Direct stream against side of vial, not at drug itself. Gently roll vial to mix dry powder and water. To avoid excessive foaming, don't shake vial. Reconstituted solution should be colorless to pale yellow. Inspect for precipitate. If drug isn't administered within 30 minutes of reconstituting, discard vial.

ALERT Unlike other thrombolytics that must be infused, anistreplase should be given by direct injection over 2 to 5 minutes.

- Don't mix anistreplase with other drugs; don't dilute solution after reconstitution.
- Be prepared to treat bradycardia or ventricular irritability. Thrombolytic therapy is linked with reperfusion arrhythmias that may signify successful thrombolysis.
- Avoid I.M. injections and nonessential handling or moving of patient.
- If arterial puncture is necessary, select a compressible site (such as an arm), and apply pressure for 30 minutes afterward. Also, use pressure dressings, sandbags, or ice packs on recent puncture sites to prevent bleeding.

• Heparin therapy is frequently initiated after treatment with anistreplase to decrease risk of rethrombosis.
• In vitro coagulation tests are affected by presence of anistreplase. This can be attenuated if blood samples are collected in presence of aprotinin (150 to 200 units/ml).

Patient teaching
• Teach patient to recognize signs of internal bleeding, and tell him to report them immediately. Advise patient about proper dental care to avoid excessive gum trauma.
• Advise patient to report shortness of breath or palpitations.

Evaluation
• Patient's ECG and vital signs reflect improvement in cardiopulmonary perfusion.
• Patient has no injury from anistreplase therapy.
• Patient and family state understanding of drug therapy.

antihemophilic factor (AHF)
(an-tigh-hee-moh-FIL-ik FAK-tor)
Bioclate, Hemofil M, Helixate, Humate-P, Hyate:C, Koate-HP, Koate-HS, Kogenate, Monoclate, Monoclate-P, Profilate OSD, Recombinate

Pharmacologic class: blood derivative
Therapeutic class: antihemophilic
Pregnancy risk category: C

Indications and dosages
▶ **Hemophilia A (factor VIII deficiency).**
Adults and children: dosage is highly individualized and depends on patient weight, severity of the deficiency, severity of the hemorrhage, presence of inhibitors, and level of factor VIII desired.

How supplied
Injection: vials, with diluent. Units specified on label.

Pharmacokinetics
Absorption: not applicable with I.V. administration.
Distribution: equilibrates intravascular and extravascular compartments.
Metabolism: cleared rapidly from plasma.
Excretion: consumed during blood clotting.
Half-life: 4 to 24 hours (averages 12 hours).

Route	Onset	Peak	Duration
I.V.	Immediate	1-2 hr	Unknown

Pharmacodynamics
Chemical effect: directly replaces deficient clotting factor that converts prothrombin to thrombin.
Therapeutic effect: causes blood clotting.

Adverse reactions
CNS: headache, paresthesia, clouding or loss of consciousness, somnolence, lethargy.
CV: tachycardia, hypotension, tightness in chest.
EENT: visual disturbances.
GI: nausea, vomiting.
Hematologic: ***hemolysis*** (in patients with blood type A, B, or AB).
Respiratory: wheezing.
Skin: *erythema,* urticaria.
Other: *chills, fever, backache, flushing,* ***hypersensitivity reactions,*** rigor, stinging at injection site, risk of hepatitis B and HIV.

Interactions
None significant.

Contraindications and precautions
• Contraindicated in patients hypersensitive to murine (mouse) protein or to drug.
• Use cautiously in neonates, infants, pregnant women, and patients with hepatic disease because of susceptibility to hepatitis, which may be transmitted in AHF.
• Safety of drug hasn't been established in breast-feeding women.

NURSING CONSIDERATIONS

Assessment
• Obtain thorough history of patient's underlying condition (including hematocrit, results

of coagulation studies, and vital signs) before therapy begins and regularly throughout therapy.
- Inhibitors to factor VIII develop in some patients. This can eventually result in decreased response to drug.
- Assess patient for adverse reactions to drug.
- Evaluate patient's and family's knowledge of drug therapy.

Nursing diagnoses
- Ineffective health maintenance related to bleeding caused by underlying condition
- Risk for injury related to drug-induced adverse reactions
- Deficient knowledge related to drug therapy

Planning and implementation
- As ordered, give hepatitis B vaccine before giving drug.

ALERT One AHF unit equals the activity present in 1 ml normal pooled human plasma less than 1 hour old. Don't confuse commercial product with blood bank-produced cryoprecipitated factor VIII from individual human donors. Drug is designed for I.V. use only; use plastic syringe, because solution adheres to glass surfaces.
- Take baseline pulse rate before giving drug. If pulse rate increases significantly, flow rate should be reduced or administration stopped.
- Refrigerate concentrate until ready to use. Warm concentrate and diluent bottles to room temperature before reconstituting. To mix drug, gently roll vial between your hands.
- Use reconstituted solution within 3 hours. Store away from heat, and don't refrigerate. Refrigeration after reconstitution may cause active ingredient to precipitate. Don't shake or mix with other I.V. solutions.
- Don't give by S.C. or I.M. routes.
- A porcine product is available for patients with congenital hemophilia A who have antibodies to human factor VIII:C.

Patient teaching
- Educate patient about drug therapy.
- Inform patient about risks of drug therapy, such as contracting hepatitis or HIV.
- Instruct patient to call prescriber if adverse reactions develop.

Evaluation
- Patient's vital signs and blood studies are within normal parameters with cessation of bleeding.
- Patient doesn't experience injury as a result of drug therapy.
- Patient and family state understanding of drug therapy.

anti-inhibitor coagulant complex
(an-tigh-in-HIB-eh-tor koh-AG-yoo-lant KOM-pleks)
Autoplex T, Feiba VH Immuno

Pharmacologic class: blood derivative
Therapeutic class: antihemophilic
Pregnancy risk category: C

Indications and dosages
▶ **Prevention and control of hemorrhagic episodes in certain patients with hemophilia A in whom inhibitor antibodies to antihemophilic factor have developed; management of bleeding in patients with acquired hemophilia who have spontaneously acquired inhibitors to factor VIII.** *Adults and children:* highly individualized and varies among manufacturers. For Autoplex T, 25 to 100 units/kg I.V., depending on severity of hemorrhage. If no hemostatic improvement occurs within 6 hours after administration, dosage repeated. For Feiba VH Immuno, 50 to 100 units/kg I.V. q 6 or 12 hours until clear signs of improvement.

How supplied
Injection: number of units of factor VIII correctional activity indicated on label of vial

Pharmacokinetics

Route	Onset	Peak	Duration
I.V.	10-30 min	Unknown	Unknown

Pharmacodynamics
Chemical effect: unknown. Efficacy may be related in part to presence of activated factors, which leads to more complete factor X activation in conjunction with tissue factor, phos-

pholipid, and ionic calcium and allows coagulation process to proceed beyond those stages where factor VIII is needed.
Therapeutic effect: causes blood clotting.

Adverse reactions

CNS: dizziness, headache, lethargy, drowsiness.
CV: hypotension, transient chest discomfort, changes in pulse rate, ***acute MI, thromboembolic events.***
GI: nausea.
Hematologic: ***DIC.***
Respiratory: dyspnea.
Skin: flushing, rash, urticaria.
Other: fever, chills, hypersensitivity reactions, ***risk of hepatitis B and HIV.***

Interactions

Drug-drug. *Antifibrinolytic drugs:* may alter effects of anti-inhibitor coagulant complex. Don't use together.

Contraindications and precautions

- Contraindicated in patients with signs of fibrinolysis, in those with disseminated intravascular coagulation and in those with a normal coagulation mechanism.
- Use cautiously in pregnant women and patients with liver disease.
- Safety of drug hasn't been established in breast-feeding women.

NURSING CONSIDERATIONS

Assessment

- Obtain history of patient's underlying condition (including hematocrit, coagulation studies, and vital signs) before therapy and regularly throughout therapy.
- Be alert for adverse reactions and drug interactions.
- Evaluate patient's and family's knowledge of drug therapy.

Nursing diagnoses

- Ineffective health maintenance related to bleeding caused by underlying condition
- Risk for injury related to drug-induced adverse reactions
- Deficient knowledge related to drug therapy

Planning and implementation

- As ordered, give hepatitis B vaccine before giving drug.
- Warm drug and diluent to room temperature before reconstitution. Reconstitute according to manufacturer's directions. Use filter needle provided by manufacturer to withdraw reconstituted solution from vial into syringe; filter needle should then be replaced with a sterile injection needle for administration. Administer as soon as possible. Autoplex T infusions should be completed within 1 hour after reconstitution; Feiba VH Immuno infusions, within 3 hours.
- The rate of administration should be individualized according to patient's response. Autoplex T infusions may begin at a rate of 1 ml/minute; if well tolerated, infusion rate may be increased gradually to 10 ml/minute. Feiba VH Immuno infusion rate shouldn't exceed 2 units/kg.
- Keep epinephrine readily available to treat anaphylaxis.
- If flushing, lethargy, headache, transient chest discomfort, or changes in blood pressure or pulse rate develop because of a rapid rate of infusion, stop drug and notify prescriber. These symptoms usually disappear when infusion stops. The infusion may then be resumed at a slower rate, as ordered.

Patient teaching

- Educate patient about anti-inhibitor coagulant complex therapy.
- Reassure patient that because of manufacturing process, risk of HIV transmission is extremely low.

Evaluation

- Patient's vital signs and blood studies are within normal parameters with cessation of bleeding.
- Patient doesn't experience injury as a result of anti-inhibitor coagulant complex therapy.
- Patient and family state understanding of drug therapy.

antithrombin III, human (ATIII, heparin cofactor I)

(an-tigh-THROM-bin three, HYOO-mun)
ATnativ, Thrombate III

Pharmacologic class: glycoprotein
Therapeutic class: anticoagulant, antithrombotic
Pregnancy risk category: C

Indications and dosages

▶ **Thromboembolism from hereditary ATIII deficiency.** *Adults and children:* initial dose individualized to quantity needed to increase ATIII activity to 120% of normal activity as determined 30 minutes after administration. Usual dose is 50 to 100 IU/minute I.V., not to exceed 100 IU/minute. Dose calculated based on anticipated 1% increase in plasma ATIII activity produced by 1 IU/kg of body weight using the formula: Dose (Units) is equal to desired activity (%) minus baseline activity (%) times weight (kg) divided by 1.4 (IU/kg). Maintenance dosage individualized to quantity required to increase ATIII activity to 80% of normal activity and is administered at 24-hour intervals. To calculate dosage, multiply desired ATIII activity (as % of normal) minus baseline ATIII activity (as % of normal) by body weight (in kg). Divide by actual increase in ATIII activity (in %) produced by 1 IU/kg as determined 30 minutes after administration of initial dose. Treatment usually continues for 2 to 8 days but may be prolonged in pregnancy or when used with surgery or immobilization.

How supplied

Injection: 500 IU

Pharmacokinetics

Absorption: not applicable with I.V. administration.
Distribution: binding to epithelium and redistribution into extravascular compartment removes ATIII from blood. Special receptors on hepatocytes bind ATIII clotting factor complexes, rapidly removing them from circulation.
Metabolism: unknown.
Excretion: unknown. *Half-life:* 2 to 3 days.

Route	Onset	Peak	Duration
I.V.	Immediate	Unknown	About 4 days

Pharmacodynamics

Chemical effect: replaces deficient ATIII in patients with hereditary ATIII deficiency, normalizing coagulation inhibition and inhibiting thromboembolism. Also deactivates plasmin (to lesser extent than clotting factor).
Therapeutic effect: prevents or decreases blood clotting.

Adverse reactions

CV: vasodilation, lowered blood pressure.
GU: diuresis.

Interactions

Drug-drug. *Heparin:* increased anticoagulant effect of both drugs. Heparin dose reduction may be necessary.

Contraindications and precautions

• No known contraindications.
• Use with extreme caution in children and neonates because safety and efficacy haven't been established.

NURSING CONSIDERATIONS

Assessment

• Obtain history of patient's underlying condition before therapy, and reassess regularly throughout therapy.
• Because of risk of neonatal thromboembolism (sometimes fatal) in children of parents with hereditary ATIII deficiency, anticipate determining ATIII levels immediately after birth.
• Obtain ATIII activity levels twice daily until dosage requirement has stabilized, then daily immediately before dose. Functional assays are preferred because quantitative immunologic test results may be normal despite decreased ATIII activity.
• Be alert for adverse reactions and drug interactions.
• Watch for dyspnea and increased blood pressure, which may occur if administration rate is too rapid (1,500 IU in 5 minutes).

• Evaluate patient's and family's understanding of drug therapy.

Nursing diagnoses

• Ineffective tissue perfusion related to underlying condition
• Deficient knowledge related to drug therapy

Planning and implementation

• Reconstitute drug using 10 ml of sterile water (provided), normal saline solution, or D_5W. Don't shake vial. Dilute further in same diluent solution, if desired.
• Keep in mind that 1 IU is equivalent to quantity of endogenous ATIII present in 1 ml of normal human plasma.
• Drug isn't recommended for long-term prophylaxis of thrombotic episodes.
• Store drug at 36° to 46° F (2° to 8° C).

Patient teaching

• Tell patient to report difficulty breathing and any other sudden symptoms immediately while drug is being administered because a rate adjustment may be necessary.
• Inform patient that risk of hepatitis or HIV contraction is minimal.

Evaluation

• Patient has adequate tissue perfusion.
• Patient and family state understanding of drug therapy.

aprotinin

(uh-proh-TIN-in)
Trasylol

Pharmacologic class: naturally occurring protease inhibitor
Therapeutic class: systemic hemostatic drug
Pregnancy risk category: B

Indications and dosages

▶ **To reduce blood loss or need for transfusion in patients undergoing coronary artery bypass grafts.** *Adults:* start with 10,000 KIU test dose at least 10 minutes before loading dose. If no allergic reaction is evident, anesthesia may be induced while loading dose of 2 million KIU is given slowly over 20 to 30 minutes. When loading dose is complete, sternotomy may be performed. Before bypass is initiated, cardiopulmonary bypass circuit is primed with 2 million KIU of drug by replacing an aliquot of priming fluid with drug. A continuous infusion at a rate of 500,000 KIU/hour is then given until patient leaves operating room. This is known as regimen A. A second regimen called regimen B may be given, which is half the dosage of regimen A (except for test dose).

How supplied

Injection: 10,000 KIU (kallikrein inactivator units)/ml (1.4 mg/ml) in 100-ml and 200-ml vials

Pharmacokinetics

Absorption: not applicable with I.V. administration.
Distribution: rapidly distributed into total extracellular space, leading to a rapid initial decrease in plasma levels.
Metabolism: unknown.
Excretion: 25% to 40% excreted in urine over 48 hours. *Half-life:* about 10 hours.

Route	Onset	Peak	Duration
I.V.	Unknown	Unknown	Unknown

Pharmacodynamics

Chemical effect: acts as systemic hemostatic drug, decreasing bleeding and turnover of coagulation factors. Aprotinin inhibits fibrinolysis by affecting kallikrein and plasmin, prevents triggering of contact phase of coagulation pathway, and increases resistance of platelets to damage from mechanical injury and high plasmin levels that occur during cardiopulmonary bypass.
Therapeutic effect: decreases bleeding.

Adverse reactions

CNS: ***cerebral embolism, CVA.***
CV: ***cardiac arrest, heart failure, MI, heart failure, ventricular tachycardia,*** atrial fibrillation, atrial flutter, hypotension, supraventricular tachycardia.
GU: ***nephrotoxicity, renal failure.***

Respiratory: pneumonia, respiratory disorder, ***bronchospasm, pulmonary edema.***
Other: hypersensitivity reactions, ***anaphylaxis,*** fever.

Interactions

None significant.

Contraindications and precautions

- Contraindicated in patients hypersensitive to beef because drug is prepared from bovine lung.
- Use cautiously in pregnant women.
- Safety of drug hasn't been established in breast-feeding women and in children.

NURSING CONSIDERATIONS

Assessment

- Obtain history of allergies. Patients with a history of allergic reactions to drugs or other substances may be at higher risk of development of an allergic reaction to aprotinin.
- Obtain history of patient's bleeding status before therapy and reassess regularly thereafter.
- Be alert for adverse reactions.
- Monitor laboratory studies, as ordered. Aprotinin prolongs activated clotting time and PTT. It may increase CK and transaminase levels and may falsely prolong whole blood clotting times when determined by surface activation methods.
- Evaluate patient's and family's understanding of drug therapy.

Nursing diagnoses

- Risk for deficient fluid volume related to potential bleeding during surgery
- Risk for injury related to drug-induced adverse reactions
- Deficient knowledge related to drug therapy

Planning and implementation

- Be prepared to give a test dose, particularly to patients who have previously received drug. They have a higher risk of anaphylaxis. In such patients, pretreat with an antihistamine, as ordered.
- Aprotinin is incompatible with amino acids, corticosteroids, fat emulsions, heparin, and tetracyclines. Don't add any drugs to I.V. container, and use a separate I.V. line.
- Administer all doses through a central line.
- To avoid hypotension, make sure patient is supine during loading dose.
- Store drug between 36° and 77° F (2° and 25° C). Protect from freezing.
- If symptoms of hypersensitivity occur (skin eruptions, itching, dyspnea, nausea, tachycardia), stop infusion immediately, call prescriber, and provide supportive treatment.

Patient teaching

- Inform patient and family about aprotinin's use with cardiopulmonary bypass surgery and its potential adverse reactions.

Evaluation

- Patient's bleeding during surgery is kept to a minimum as a result of aprotinin therapy.
- Patient doesn't experience injury as a result of aprotinin therapy.
- Patient and family state understanding of drug therapy.

asparaginase (L-asparaginase)

(as-PAR-ah-jin-ays)
Elspar, Kidrolase♦

Pharmacologic class: enzyme (L-asparagine amidohydrolase), cell cycle-phase specific, G1 phase
Therapeutic class: antineoplastic
Pregnancy risk category: C

Indications and dosages

▶ **Acute lymphocytic leukemia (in combination with other drugs).** *Adults and children:* 1,000 IU/kg I.V. daily for 10 days, injected over 30 minutes or by slow I.V. push; or 6,000 IU/m^2 I.M. at intervals specified in protocol.

▶ **Sole induction drug for acute lymphocytic leukemia.** *Adults:* 200 IU/kg I.V. daily for 28 days.

How supplied

Injection: 10,000-unit vial

Pharmacokinetics

Absorption: unknown for I.M. administration.
Distribution: distributes primarily within intravascular space, with detectable levels in thoracic and cervical lymph. Minimal drug crosses blood-brain barrier.
Metabolism: hepatic sequestration by reticuloendothelial system may occur.
Excretion: unknown. *Half-life:* 8 to 30 hours.

Route	Onset	Peak	Duration
I.V.	Almost immediate	Almost immediate	23-33 days after stopping drug
I.M.	Almost immediate	4-24 hr after stopping drug	23-33 days

Pharmacodynamics

Chemical effect: destroys amino acid asparagine, which is needed for protein synthesis in acute lymphocytic leukemia. This leads to death of leukemic cell.
Therapeutic effect: kills leukemic cells.

Adverse reactions

CNS: confusion, drowsiness, depression, hallucinations, nervousness, lethargy, somnolence.
GI: *vomiting* , *anorexia, nausea,* cramps, weight loss, **HEMMORHAGIC PANCREATITIS.**
GU: azotemia, ***renal failure,*** uric acid nephropathy, glycosuria, polyuria, *increased blood ammonia level.*
Hematologic: *anemia,* ***hypofibrinogenemia,*** depression of other clotting factors, ***thrombocytopenia, leukopenia,*** depressed serum albumin level.
Hepatic: elevated AST and ALT levels, ***hepatotoxicity,*** elevated bilirubin levels.
Metabolic: increase or decrease in total lipid level, *hyperuricemia, hyperglycemia.*
Skin: rash, urticaria.
Other: **ANAPHYLAXIS,** chills, fever, ***fatal hyperthermia.***

Interactions

Drug-drug. *Methotrexate:* decreased methotrexate effectiveness when administered immediately prior to or with the methotrexate dose. Monitor serum levels and for loss of therapeutic effect.
Prednisone, vincristine: increased toxicity. Monitor patient closely.

Contraindications and precautions

- Contraindicated in patients with pancreatitis or history of pancreatitis and previous hypersensitivity unless desensitized. Drug should also not be used in breast-feeding women.
- Use cautiously in patients with preexisting hepatic dysfunction and in pregnant women.

NURSING CONSIDERATIONS

Assessment

- Obtain history of patient's leukemic condition.
- Monitor effectiveness by evaluating CBC and bone marrow function tests, as ordered. Bone marrow regeneration may take 5 to 6 weeks.
- Be alert for adverse reactions and drug interactions.
- Evaluate patient's and family's knowledge of drug therapy.

Nursing diagnoses

- Ineffective health maintenance related to leukemic condition
- Ineffective protection related to drug-induced adverse reactions
- Deficient knowledge related to drug therapy

Planning and implementation

- Give drug in a hospital under close supervision.
- Follow facility policy to reduce risks. Preparation and administration of parenteral form is linked with carcinogenic, mutagenic, and teratogenic risks for personnel.
- Prevent occurrence of tumor lysis, which can result in uric acid nephropathy, by increasing fluid intake. Allopurinol should be started before therapy begins.

ALERT The risk of hypersensitivity reaction increases with repeated doses. An intradermal skin test should be performed before initial dose and when drug is given after an interval of a week or more between doses. To perform skin test, give 2 IU of drug intradermally, as

ordered. Observe site for at least 1 hour for erythema or a wheal, which indicates a positive response. An allergic reaction to the drug may still develop in a patient with a negative skin test.
• A desensitization dose of 1 IU I.V. may be ordered. Dose is doubled q 10 minutes if no reaction occurs until total amount given equals patient's total dose for that day.
I.V. use: Give injection over 30 minutes through a running infusion of normal saline solution for injection or D_5W dextrose injection.
I.M. use: Limit dose at single injection site to 2 ml.
• Reconstitute with 2 to 5 ml of either sterile water for injection or normal saline solution for injection. Don't shake vial. Don't use cloudy solutions.
• Drug shouldn't be used as sole drug to induce remission unless combination therapy is inappropriate. Not recommended for maintenance therapy.
• Refrigerate unopened dry powder. Reconstituted solution is stable for 8 hours if refrigerated.
• If drug contacts skin or mucous membranes, wash with copious amounts of water for at least 15 minutes.
• Keep epinephrine, diphenhydramine, and I.V. corticosteroids available for treating anaphylaxis.
• Because of vomiting, administer parenteral fluids, as ordered, for 24 hours or until oral fluids are tolerated.

Patient teaching
• Tell patient to watch for signs of infection (fever, sore throat, fatigue) and bleeding (easy bruising, nosebleeds, bleeding gums, melena). Instruct patient to take temperature daily.
• Encourage patient to maintain an adequate fluid intake to increase urine output and facilitate excretion of uric acid.
• Tell patient that drowsiness may occur during therapy or for several weeks after treatment has ended. Warn patient to avoid hazardous activities requiring mental alertness.

☑ Evaluation
• Patient is free of leukemic cells after asparaginase therapy.
• Patient doesn't experience injury as a result of drug-induced adverse reactions.
• Patient and family state understanding of drug therapy.

aspirin (acetylsalicylic acid)
(AS-prin)

Ancasal♦†, Arthrinol♦†, Artria S.R.†, ASA†, ASA Enseals†, Aspergum†, Aspro◊, Astrin♦†, Bayer Aspirin†, Bex◊, Coryphen♦†, Easprin†, Ecotrin†, Empirin†, Entrophen♦†, Halfprin, Measurin†, Norwich Aspirin Extra Strength†, Novasen♦†, Riphen-10♦†, Sal-Adult♦†, Sal-Infant♦†, Sloprin◊, Supasa♦†, Triaphen-10♦†, Vincent's Powders◊, Winsprin Capsules◊, ZORprin†

Pharmacologic class: salicylate
Therapeutic class: nonnarcotic analgesic, antipyretic, anti-inflammatory, antiplatelet
Pregnancy risk category: C (D in third trimester)

Indications and dosages
▶ **Arthritis.** *Adults:* initially, 2.4 to 3.6 g P.O. daily in divided doses. Maintenance dosage is 3.6 to 5.4 g P.O. daily in divided doses.
Children: 80 to 130 mg/kg P.O. daily in divided doses.
▶ **Mild pain or fever.** *Adults:* 325 to 650 mg P.O. or P.R. q 4 hours, p.r.n.
Children: (for mild pain only) 65 mg/kg P.O. or P.R. daily in four to six divided doses.
▶ **Prevention of thrombosis.** *Adults:* 1.3 g P.O. daily in two to four divided doses.
▶ **Reduction of risk of heart attack in patients with previous MI or unstable angina.** *Adults:* 160 to 325 mg P.O. daily.
▶ **Kawasaki syndrome (mucocutaneous lymph node syndrome).** *Adults:* 80 to 100 mg/kg P.O. daily in four divided doses during febrile phase. Some patients may need up to 120 mg/kg. When fever subsides, decrease dosage to 3 to 8 mg/kg once daily, adjusted according to serum salicylate level.

How supplied
Tablets†: 325 mg, 500 mg, 600 mg, 650 mg

Tablets (chewable): 81 mg†
Tablets (enteric-coated): 165 mg, 325 mg†, 500 mg†, 650 mg†, 975 mg
Tablets (extended-release): 800 mg
Tablets (timed-release): 650 mg†
Capsules: 325 mg†, 500 mg†
Chewing gum: 227.5 mg†
Suppositories: 60 mg†, 65 mg†, 120 mg†, 125 mg†, 130 mg†, 195 mg†, 200 mg†, 300 mg†, 325 mg†, 600 mg†, 650 mg†

Pharmacokinetics

Absorption: absorbed rapidly and completely from GI tract.
Distribution: distributed widely into most body tissues and fluids. Protein-binding to albumin is concentration-dependent; ranges from 75% to 90%, and decreases as serum level increases.
Metabolism: hydrolyzed partially in GI tract to salicylic acid with almost complete metabolism in liver.
Excretion: excreted in urine as salicylate and its metabolites. *Half-life:* 15 to 20 minutes.

Route	Onset	Peak	Duration
P.O.			
Solution	5-30 min	15-60 min	1-4 hr
Regular	5-30 min	25-40 min	1-4 hr
Buffered	5-30 min	1-2 hr	1-4 hr
Extended-release	5-30 min	1-2 hr	1-4 hr
Enteric-coated	5-30 min	4-8 hr	1-4 hr
P.R.	5-30 min	3-4 hr	1-4 hr

Pharmacodynamics

Chemical effect: produces analgesia by blocking prostaglandin synthesis (peripheral action). Aspirin and other salicylates may prevent lowering of pain threshold that occurs when prostaglandins sensitize pain receptors to mechanical and chemical stimulation. Exerts its anti-inflammatory effect by inhibiting prostaglandin synthesis; also may inhibit synthesis or action of other mediators of inflammatory response. Relieves fever by acting on hypothalamic heat-regulating center to cause peripheral vasodilation. This increases peripheral blood supply and promotes sweating, which leads to heat loss and to cooling by evaporation. In low doses, aspirin also appears to impede clotting by blocking prostaglandin synthesis, which prevents formation of platelet-aggregating substance thromboxane A_2.
Therapeutic effect: relieves pain, reduces fever and inflammation, and decreases risk of transient ischemic attacks and MI.

Adverse reactions

EENT: *tinnitus, hearing loss.*
GI: *nausea, vomiting, GI distress, occult bleeding,* dyspepsia, ***GI bleeding.***
Hematologic: *prolonged bleeding time,* ***thrombocytopenia.***
Hepatic: altered liver function enzyme levels, ***hepatitis.***
Skin: *rash,* bruising, urticaria.
Other: ***angioedema,*** hypersensitivity reactions, (***anaphylaxis,*** asthma), ***Reye's syndrome.***

Interactions

Drug-drug. *Ammonium chloride, other urine acidifiers:* increased blood levels of aspirin products. Watch for aspirin toxicity.
Antacids in high doses (and other urine alkalinizers): decreased blood levels of aspirin products. Watch for decreased aspirin effect.
Beta blockers: decreased antihypertensive effect. Avoid long-term aspirin use if patient is taking antihypertensives.
Corticosteroids: enhanced salicylate elimination. Watch for decreased salicylate effect.
Heparin, oral anticoagulants: increased risk of bleeding. Monitor for signs of bleeding.
Methotrexate: increased risk of methotrexate toxicity. Monitor patient closely.
NSAIDs, steroids: increased risk of GI bleeding. Monitor patient closely.
NSAIDs, including diflunisal, fenoprofen, ibuprofen, indomethacin, piroxicam, meclofenamate, naproxen: altered pharmacokinetics of these drugs, leading to lowered serum levels and decreased effectiveness. Avoid concomitant use.
Oral antidiabetics: increased hypoglycemic effect. Monitor patient closely.
Probenecid, sulfinpyrazone: decreased uricosuric effect. Avoid aspirin during therapy with these drugs.

Drug-herb. *Dong quai, feverfew, garlic, ginger, horse chestnut, red clover:* possible increased risk of bleeding. Monitor patient for increased effects, and discourage concomitant use.

Drug-food. *Caffeine:* may increase the absorption of aspirin. Monitor patient for increased effects.

Drug-lifestyle. *Alcohol use:* increased risk of GI bleeding. Discourage concomitant use.

Contraindications and precautions

- Contraindicated in patients with G6PD deficiency; bleeding disorders such as hemophilia, von Willebrand's disease, or telangiectasia; NSAID-induced sensitivity reactions; or hypersensitivity to drug.
- Use cautiously in patients with GI lesions, impaired renal function, hypoprothrombinemia, vitamin K deficiency, thrombocytopenia, thrombotic thrombocytopenic purpura, or severe hepatic impairment.
- Use cautiously in pregnant women. Safety hasn't been established in breast-feeding women.

ALERT Because of the link with Reye's syndrome, the Centers for Disease Control and Prevention recommends not giving salicylates to children or teenagers with chickenpox or flulike illness.

NURSING CONSIDERATIONS

Assessment

- Obtain history of patient's pain or fever before therapy, and monitor patient throughout therapy.
- Be alert for adverse reactions and drug interactions.
- During chronic therapy, monitor serum salicylate level. Therapeutic level in arthritis is 10 to 30 mg/dl. With long-term therapy, mild toxicity may occur at plasma levels of 20 mg/dl. Tinnitus may occur at plasma levels of 30 mg/dl and above but doesn't reliably indicate toxicity, especially in very young patients and those over age 60.
- Evaluate patient's and family's knowledge of drug therapy.

Nursing diagnoses

- Acute pain related to underlying condition.
- Risk for injury related to drug-induced adverse GI reactions
- Deficient knowledge related to drug therapy

Planning and implementation

P.O. use: Give aspirin with food, milk, antacid, or large glass of water to reduce adverse GI reactions.

- If patient has trouble swallowing, crush aspirin, combine it with soft food, or dissolve it in liquid. Administer aspirin immediately after mixing it with liquid because drug doesn't stay in solution. Don't crush enteric-coated aspirin.
- Remember that enteric-coated products are slowly absorbed and not suitable for acute effects. They cause less GI bleeding and may be more suited for long-term therapy, such as arthritis.

P.R. use: Absorption following P.R. administration is slow and variable depending on how long suppository is retained. If retained for 2 to 4 hours, absorption of dose is 20% to 60%; if retained for at least 10 hours, absorption is 70% to 100%.

- Hold dose and notify prescriber if bleeding, salicylism (tinnitus, hearing loss), or adverse GI reactions develop.
- Stop aspirin 5 to 7 days before elective surgery, as ordered.

Patient teaching

- Advise patient receiving high-dose prolonged treatment to watch for petechiae, bleeding gums, and signs of GI bleeding and to maintain adequate fluid intake. Encourage use of a soft toothbrush.
- Because of many possible drug interactions involving aspirin, warn patient who takes prescription form to check with prescriber or pharmacist before taking OTC combinations containing aspirin or herbal preparations.
- Explain that various OTC preparations contain aspirin. Warn patient to read labels carefully to avoid overdose.
- Advise patient to avoid alcohol consumption during drug therapy.
- Advise patient to restrict intake of caffeine during drug therapy.

• Instruct patient to take aspirin with food or milk.
• Instruct patient not to chew enteric-coated products.
• Emphasize safe storage of medications in the home. Teach patient to keep aspirin and other drugs out of children's reach. Aspirin is a leading cause of poisoning in children. Encourage use of child-resistant containers in households that include children, even if only as occasional visitors.

Evaluation
• Patient states that aspirin has relieved pain.
• Patient remains free of adverse GI effects throughout drug therapy.
• Patient and family state understanding of drug therapy.

atenolol
(uh-TEN-uh-lol)
Apo-Atenolol ♦, Noten ◇, Nu-Atenol ♦, Tenormin

Pharmacologic class: beta blocker
Therapeutic class: antihypertensive, antianginal
Pregnancy risk category: D

Indications and dosages
▶ **Hypertension.** *Adults:* initially, 50 mg P.O. daily as a single dose. Dosage increased to 100 mg once daily after 7 to 14 days. Doses over 100 mg are unlikely to produce further benefit. Dosage adjustment required in patients with creatinine clearance below 35 ml/minute.
▶ **Angina pectoris.** *Adults:* 50 mg P.O. once daily. Increased as needed to 100 mg daily after 7 days for optimal effect. Maximum dosage is 200 mg daily.
▶ **Reduction of CV mortality rate and risk of reinfarction in patients with acute MI.** *Adults:* 5 mg I.V. over 5 minutes, followed by another 5 mg 10 minutes later. After another 10 minutes, 50 mg P.O., followed by 50 mg P.O. in 12 hours. Thereafter, 100 mg P.O. daily (as a single dose or 50 mg b.i.d.) for at least 7 days.

How supplied
Tablets: 25 mg, 50 mg, 100 mg
Injection: 5 mg/10 ml

Pharmacokinetics
Absorption: about 50% to 60% of oral dose is absorbed.
Distribution: distributes into most tissues and fluids except brain and CSF. About 5% to 15% protein-bound.
Metabolism: minimal.
Excretion: from 40% to 50% of dose is excreted unchanged in urine; remainder is excreted as unchanged drug and metabolites in feces. *Half-life:* 6 to 7 hours (increases as renal function decreases).

Route	Onset	Peak	Duration
P.O.	1 hr	2-4 hr	24 hr
I.V.	5 min	5 min	12 hr

Pharmacodynamics
Chemical effect: selectively blocks $beta_1$-adrenergic receptors; decreases cardiac output, peripheral resistance, and cardiac oxygen consumption; and depresses renin secretion.
Therapeutic effect: decreases blood pressure, relieves anginal symptoms, and reduces CV mortality rate and risk of reinfarction after acute MI.

Adverse reactions
CNS: fatigue, lethargy.
CV: ***bradycardia***, *hypotension*, ***heart failure***, intermittent claudication.
GI: nausea, vomiting, diarrhea.
Respiratory: dyspnea, ***bronchospasm.***
Skin: rash.
Other: fever.

Interactions
Drug-drug. *Antihypertensives:* enhanced hypotensive effect. Use together cautiously.
Cardiac glycosides, diltiazem, verapamil: excessive bradycardia and increased depressant effect on myocardium. Use together cautiously.
Insulin, oral antidiabetics: can alter dosage requirements in previously stabilized diabetic patients. Observe patient carefully.

Reserpine: may cause hypotension. Use with caution.

Contraindications and precautions

- Contraindicated in patients with sinus bradycardia, greater than first-degree heart block, overt cardiac failure, or cardiogenic shock.
- Don't use in pregnant women unless absolutely necessary because fetal harm can occur.
- Use cautiously in patients at risk for heart failure and in patients with bronchospastic disease, diabetes, and hyperthyroidism. Also use cautiously in breast-feeding women.
- Safety of drug hasn't been established in children.

NURSING CONSIDERATIONS

Assessment

- Obtain history of patient's underlying condition.
- Monitor effectiveness by frequently checking blood pressure if prescribed for hypertension, frequency and severity of anginal pain if prescribed for angina pectoris, and signs of reinfarction if prescribed to reduce CV mortality rate and risk of reinfarction after acute MI. Be aware that full antihypertensive effect may not appear for 1 to 2 weeks after therapy starts.
- Be alert for adverse reactions and drug interactions.
- Evaluate patient's and family's understanding of drug therapy.

Nursing diagnoses

- Risk for injury related to underlying condition
- Decreased cardiac output related to drug-induced adverse CV reactions
- Deficient knowledge related to drug therapy

Planning and implementation

- Patients with renal insufficiency and those on hemodialysis require a dosage adjustment.
- Check patient's apical pulse before giving drug; if slower than 60 beats/minute, withhold drug and call prescriber.

P.O. use: Administer as a single daily dose.
I.V. use: Give by slow injection, not to exceed 1 mg/minute. Doses may be mixed with D_5W, normal saline solution, or dextrose and sodium chloride solutions. Solution is stable for 48 hours after mixing.

- Be prepared to treat shock or hypoglycemia because this drug masks common signs of these conditions.
- Notify prescriber immediately if patient shows signs of decreased cardiac output.

Patient teaching

- Caution patient that stopping drug abruptly can worsen angina and MI. Drug should be withdrawn gradually over a 2-week period.
- Counsel patient to take drug at same time every day.
- Tell woman to notify prescriber if pregnancy occurs. Drug will need to be discontinued.
- Teach patient how to take his pulse. Tell patient to withhold drug and call prescriber if pulse rate is below 60 beats/minute.

Evaluation

- Patient's underlying condition improves with drug therapy.
- Patient's cardiac output remains unchanged throughout drug therapy.
- Patient and family state understanding of drug therapy.

atorvastatin calcium

(uh-TOR-vah-stah-tin KAL-see-um)
Lipitor

Pharmacologic class: 3-hydroxy-3-methylglutaryl-coenzyme A (HMG-CoA) reductase inhibitor
Therapeutic class: antilipemic
Pregnancy risk category: X

Indications and dosages

▶ **Adjunct to diet to reduce low-density lipoprotein (LDL), total cholesterol, apo B, and triglyceride levels in patients with primary hypercholesterolemia and mixed dyslipidemia (Fredrickson types Iia and Iib); primary dysbetalipoproteinemia (Fredrickson type III) that doesn't respond adequately to diet; adjunctive therapy to diet for elevated serum triglyceride levels**

(Fredrickson type IV). Adjunct to diet to increase high-density lipoprotein cholesterol in patients with primary hypercholesterolemia (heterozygous familial and nonfamilial) and mixed dyslipidemia (Fredrickson types IIa and IIb). *Adults:* initially, 10 mg P.O. once daily. Increased p.r.n. to maximum of 80 mg daily as single dose. Dosage based on blood lipid levels drawn within 2 to 4 weeks after starting therapy.

▶ **Alone or as an adjunct to lipid-lowering treatments, such as LDL apheresis, in patients with homozygous familial hypercholesterolemia.** *Adults and children age 9 and older:* 10 to 80 mg P.O. once daily.

How supplied

Tablets: 10 mg, 20 mg, 40 mg

Pharmacokinetics

Absorption: rapidly absorbed.
Distribution: 98% is bound to plasma proteins.
Metabolism: metabolized by liver.
Excretion: eliminated in bile.

Route	Onset	Peak	Duration
P.O.	Unknown	1-2 hr	Unknown

Pharmacodynamics

Chemical effect: selective inhibitor of HMG-CoA reductase, which converts HMG-CoA to mevalonate, a precursor of sterols.
Therapeutic effect: lowers plasma cholesterol and lipoprotein levels.

Adverse reactions

CNS: *headache,* asthenia.
EENT: sinusitis, pharyngitis.
GI: abdominal pain, constipation, diarrhea, dyspepsia, flatulence.
Musculoskeletal: back pain, arthralgia, myalgia.
Skin: rash.
Other: *infection,* accidental injury, flulike syndrome, hypersensitivity reaction.

Interactions

Drug-drug. *Antacids:* decrease bioavailability. Administer separately.
Azole antifungals, cyclosporine, erythromycin, fibric acid derivatives, niacin: may cause rhabdomyolysis. Avoid use together.
Digoxin: may increase digoxin levels. Monitor serum digoxin levels.
Erythromycin: increases plasma drug levels. Monitor patient.
Oral contraceptives: increases hormone levels. Consider when selecting an oral contraceptive.
Drug-herb. *Red yeast:* herb contains similar components to statin drugs, which increases the risk of adverse reactions or toxicity. Discourage concomitant use.

Contraindications and precautions

- Contraindicated in patients with active liver disease, conditions linked with unexplained persistent increases in serum transaminases, or hypersensitivity to drug; in pregnant or breast-feeding women; and in women of childbearing potential.

NURSING CONSIDERATIONS

Assessment

- Withhold or stop drug in patients with serious, acute conditions that suggest myopathy or in those at risk for renal failure caused by rhabdomyolysis from trauma; major surgery; severe metabolic, endocrine, and electrolyte disorders; severe acute infection; hypotension; or uncontrolled seizures.
- Evaluate patient's and family's understanding of drug therapy.

Nursing diagnoses

- Risk for injury related to elevated cholesterol levels
- Deficient knowledge related to drug therapy

Planning and implementation

- Use drug only after diet and other nonpharmacologic treatments prove ineffective. Patient should follow a standard low-cholesterol diet before and during therapy.
- Before starting treatment, perform a baseline lipid profile to exclude secondary causes of hypercholesterolemia. Liver function tests and lipid levels should be done before therapy, after 6 and 12 weeks, or following an increase

in dosage and periodically thereafter, as ordered.

Patient teaching

- Teach patient about proper dietary management, weight control, and exercise and explain their role in controlling elevated serum lipid levels.
- Warn patient to avoid alcohol.
- Tell patient to inform prescriber of adverse reactions.
- Urge woman to notify prescriber immediately if pregnancy is suspected.

Evaluation

- Patient's blood cholesterol level is within normal limits.
- Patient and family state understanding of drug therapy.

atovaquone
(uh-TOH-vuh-kwohn)
Mepron

Pharmacologic class: ubiquinone analogue
Therapeutic class: antiprotozoal
Pregnancy risk category: C

Indications and dosages

▶ **Prevention of *Pneumocystis carinii* pneumonia in patients who are intolerant to co-trimoxazole.** *Adults and adolescents ages 13 and older:* 1,500 mg (10 ml) P.O. daily with a meal.

▶ **Treatment of mild to moderate *P. carinii* in patients who can't tolerate co-trimoxazole.** *Adults:* 750 mg P.O. t.i.d. for 21 days.

How supplied

Tablets: 250 mg

Pharmacokinetics

Absorption: limited. Bioavailability is increased threefold when administered with meals. Fat enhances absorption significantly.
Distribution: extensively bound (99.9%) to plasma proteins.
Metabolism: not metabolized.
Excretion: undergoes enterohepatic cycling and is primarily excreted in feces. Less than 0.6% is excreted in urine. *Half-life:* 2 to 3 days.

Route	Onset	Peak	Duration
P.O.	Unknown	1-8 hr (1st peak) 1-4 days (2nd peak)	Unknown

Pharmacodynamics

Chemical effect: unknown; appears to interfere with electron transport in protozoal mitochondria, inhibiting enzymes needed for synthesis of nucleic acids and adenosine triphosphate.
Therapeutic effect: kills *Pneumocystis carinii* protozoa.

Adverse reactions

CNS: *headache, insomnia,* asthenia, dizziness.
GI: *nausea, diarrhea, vomiting,* oral candidiasis, constipation, abdominal pain.
Respiratory: cough.
Skin: *rash,* pruritus.
Other: *fever.*

Interactions

Drug-drug. *Highly protein-bound drugs (phenytoin, coumadin):* may compete for receptor sites affecting drug levels. Use cautiously.
Rifampin, rifabutin: decreased atovaquone's steady-state levels. Avoid concurrent use.

Contraindications and precautions

- Contraindicated in patients hypersensitive to drug.
- Use cautiously in pregnant or breast-feeding women. Because drug is highly bound to plasma protein (greater than 99.9%), also use cautiously with other highly protein-bound drugs.
- Safety of drug hasn't been established in children.

NURSING CONSIDERATIONS

Assessment

- Obtain history of patient's protozoal respiratory infection and reassess regularly.
- Be alert for adverse reactions.

• Monitor patient's hydration status if adverse GI reactions occur.
• Evaluate patient's and family's knowledge of drug therapy.

Nursing diagnoses

• Infection related to presence of susceptible protozoal organisms
• Risk for deficient fluid volume related to drug-induced adverse GI reactions
• Deficient knowledge related to drug therapy

Planning and implementation

• Administer drug with food to improve bioavailability.

Patient teaching

• Instruct patient to take drug with meals because food enhances absorption significantly.
• Warn patient not to perform hazardous activities if dizziness occurs.
• Emphasize importance of taking drug as prescribed, even if patient is feeling better.
• Tell patient to notify prescriber if serious adverse reactions occur.

Evaluation

• Patient's infection is eradicated.
• Patient remains adequately hydrated throughout therapy.
• Patient and family state understanding of drug therapy.

atracurium besylate

(uh-trah-KYOO-ree-um BES-eh-layt)
Tracrium

Pharmacologic class: nondepolarizing neuromuscular blocker
Therapeutic class: skeletal muscle relaxant
Pregnancy risk category: C

Indications and dosages

▶ **Adjunct to general anesthesia, to facilitate endotracheal intubation and cause skeletal muscle relaxation during surgery or mechanical ventilation.** Dosage depends on anesthetic used, individual needs, and response. Dosages given here are representative and must be adjusted.
Adults and children over age 2: 0.4 to 0.5 mg/kg by I.V. bolus. Maintenance dosage of 0.08 to 0.10 mg/kg within 20 to 45 minutes of initial dose should be administered during prolonged surgical procedures. Maintenance dosages may be administered q 15 to 25 minutes in patients receiving balanced anesthesia. For prolonged surgical procedures, a constant infusion of 5 to 9 mcg/kg/minute may be used after initial bolus.
Children ages 1 month to 2 years: initial dose, 0.3 to 0.4 mg/kg. Frequent maintenance doses may be needed.

How supplied

Injection: 10 mg/ml

Pharmacokinetics

Absorption: not applicable with I.V. administration.
Distribution: distributed into extracellular space. About 82% protein-bound.
Metabolism: rapidly metabolized by Hofmann elimination and by nonspecific enzymatic ester hydrolysis. The liver doesn't appear to play a major role.
Excretion: atracurium and its metabolites are excreted in urine and feces. *Half-life:* 20 minutes.

Route	Onset	Peak	Duration
I.V.	≤ 2 min	3-5 min	35-70 min

Pharmacodynamics

Chemical effect: prevents acetylcholine from binding to receptors on muscle end plate, thus blocking depolarization and resulting in skeletal muscle paralysis.
Therapeutic effect: relaxes skeletal muscles.

Adverse reactions

CV: increased heart rate, ***bradycardia,*** hypotension.
Respiratory: ***prolonged dose-related apnea,*** wheezing, increased bronchial secretions.
Skin: *flushing,* erythema, pruritus, urticaria.
Other: ***anaphylaxis.***

Interactions

Drug-drug. *Aminoglycoside antibiotics (including amikacin, gentamicin, kanamycin, neomycin, streptomycin); polymyxin antibiotics (polymyxin B sulfate, colistin); clindamycin; quinidine; general anesthetics (such as enflurane, halothane, isoflurane):* potentiated neuromuscular blockade, leading to increased skeletal muscle relaxation and prolongation of effect. Use cautiously during surgical and postoperative periods.
Lithium, magnesium salts, opioid analgesics: potentiated neuromuscular blockade, leading to increased skeletal muscle relaxation and, possibly, respiratory paralysis. Reduce dose of atracurium.

Contraindications and precautions

- Contraindicated in patients hypersensitive to drug.
- Use cautiously in patients with CV disease; severe electrolyte disorders; bronchogenic carcinoma; hepatic, renal, or pulmonary impairment; neuromuscular diseases; or myasthenia gravis.
- Also use cautiously in pregnant women, breast-feeding women, and elderly or debilitated patients.

NURSING CONSIDERATIONS

Assessment
- Obtain history of patient's neuromuscular status before therapy and reassess regularly.
- Be alert for adverse reactions and interactions.
- Monitor respirations closely until patient is fully recovered from neuromuscular blockade, as evidenced by tests of muscle strength (hand grip, head lift, and ability to cough).
- A nerve stimulator and train-of-four monitoring are recommended to confirm antagonism of neuromuscular blockade and recovery of muscle strength. Before attempting pharmacologic reversal with neostigmine, some evidence of spontaneous recovery should be seen.
- Evaluate patient's and family's understanding of drug therapy.

Nursing diagnoses
- Risk for injury related to underlying condition
- Impaired spontaneous ventilation related to drug-induced respiratory paralysis
- Deficient knowledge related to drug therapy

Planning and implementation
- Administer sedatives or general anesthetics before neuromuscular blockers, as ordered. Neuromuscular blockers don't obtund consciousness or alter pain threshold.

ALERT Use this drug only under direct medical supervision by personnel skilled in use of neuromuscular blockers and techniques for maintaining a patent airway. Don't use unless facilities and equipment for mechanical ventilation, oxygen therapy, and intubation as well as an antagonist are immediately available.

- Drug usually is given by rapid I.V. bolus injection but may be given by intermittent infusion or continuous infusion. At 0.2 mg/ml to 0.5 mg/ml, atracurium is compatible for 24 hours in D_5W, normal saline injection, or dextrose 5% in normal saline injection.
- Don't use lactated Ringer's solution. In lactated Ringer's injection, atracurium is stable for 8 hours at a concentration of 0.5 mg/ml. Because of an increased rate of drug degradation in this solution, it isn't recommended.
- Don't administer by I.M. injection.
- Don't mix with acidic or alkaline solutions (precipitate may form).
- Prior administration of succinylcholine doesn't prolong duration of action but quickens onset and may deepen neuromuscular blockade.
- Explain all events and happenings to patient because he can still hear.
- Administer analgesics, as ordered, for pain. Remember that patient can have pain but not be able to express it.
- Keep airway clear. Have emergency equipment and drugs immediately available.
- Once spontaneous recovery starts, be prepared to reverse atracurium-induced neuromuscular blockade with an anticholinesterase drug (such as neostigmine or edrophonium), as ordered. Such a drug usually is administered together with an anticholinergic (such as atropine).

Patient teaching

- Instruct patient and family about drug therapy.
- Reassure both patient and family that patient will be monitored at all times and that respiratory life-support will be used during paralysis.
- Reassure patient that pain medication will be given as needed.

☑ Evaluation

- Patient's underlying condition is resolved without causing injury.
- Patient is able to sustain spontaneous ventilation after effects of atracurium besylate wear off.
- Patient and family state understanding of drug therapy.

atropine sulfate

(AH-troh-peen SUL-fayt)

Pharmacologic class: anticholinergic, belladonna alkaloid
Therapeutic class: antiarrhythmic, vagolytic
Pregnancy risk category: C

Indications and dosages

▶ **Symptomatic bradycardia, bradyarrhythmia (junctional or escape rhythm).** *Adults:* usually 0.5 to 1 mg I.V. push; repeated q 3 to 5 minutes to maximum of 2 mg, p.r.n. Lower doses (less than 0.5 mg) can cause bradycardia.
Children: 0.02 mg/kg I.V. up to maximum of 1 mg; or 0.3 mg/m^2; may repeat q 5 minutes.

▶ **Antidote for anticholinesterase insecticide poisoning.** *Adults and children:* 1 to 2 mg I.M. or I.V. repeated q 20 to 30 minutes until muscarinic symptoms disappear or signs of atropine toxicity appear. Severe poisoning may require up to 6 mg q hour.

▶ **Preoperatively for decreasing secretions and blocking cardiac vagal reflexes.** *Adults and children weighing 20 kg or more:* 0.4 mg I.M. or S.C. 30 to 60 minutes before anesthesia.
Children weighing less than 20 kg: 0.1 mg I.M. for 3 kg, 0.2 mg I.M. for 4 to 9 kg, 0.3 mg I.M. for 10 to 20 kg 30 to 60 minutes before anesthesia.

▶ **Adjunct treatment of peptic ulcer disease; treatment of functional GI disorders such as irritable bowel syndrome.** *Adults:* 0.4 to 0.6 mg P.O. q 4 to 6 hours.
Children: 0.01 mg/kg or 0.3 mg/m^2 (not to exceed 0.4 mg) q 4 to 6 hours.

How supplied

Tablets: 0.4 mg, 0.6 mg
Injection: 0.05 mg/ml, 0.1 mg/ml, 0.3 mg/ml, 0.4 mg/ml, 0.5 mg/ml, 0.6 mg/ml, 0.8 mg/ml, 1 mg/ml, 1.2 mg/ml

Pharmacokinetics

Absorption: well absorbed after P.O. and I.M. administration; unknown for S.C. administration.
Distribution: distributed throughout body, including CNS. Only 18% binds with plasma protein.
Metabolism: metabolized in liver to several metabolites.
Excretion: excreted primarily through kidneys; small amount may be excreted in feces and expired air. *Half-life:* initial, 2 hours; second phase, 12½ hours.

Route	Onset	Peak	Duration
P.O.	0.5-1 hr	2 hr	4 hr
I.V.	Immediate	2-4 min	4 hr
I.M.	30 min	1-1.6 hr	4 hr
S.C.	Unknown	Unknown	4 hr

Pharmacodynamics

Chemical effect: inhibits acetylcholine at parasympathetic neuroeffector junction, blocking vagal effects on SA node; this enhances conduction through AV node and speeds heart rate.
Therapeutic effect: increases heart rate; antidote for anticholinesterase insecticide poisoning; decreases secretions preoperatively; and slows GI motility.

Adverse reactions

CNS: *headache, restlessness,* ataxia, disorientation, hallucinations, delirium, ***coma,*** *insomnia, dizziness;* excitement, agitation, and confusion.
CV: *tachycardia, palpitations, angina.*

EENT: *slight mydriasis,* photophobia, *blurred vision, mydriasis.*
GI: *dry mouth,* thirst, *constipation,* nausea, vomiting.
GU: urine retention.
Hematologic: leukocytosis.
Skin: flushing.
Other: ***anaphylaxis.***

Interactions

Drug-drug. *Antacids:* decreased absorption of anticholinergics. Separate administration times by at least 1 hour.
Anticholinergics, drugs with anticholinergic effects (such as amantadine, glutethimide, meperidine, antiarrhythmics, antiparkinsonians, phenothiazines, tricyclic antidepressants): additive anticholinergic effects. Use together cautiously.
Ketoconazole, levodopa: decreased absorption. Avoid concomitant use.
Methotrimeprazine: may produce extrapyramidal symptoms. Monitor patient carefully.
Potassium chloride wax matrix tablets: increased risk of mucosal lesions. Use cautiously.

Contraindications and precautions

- Contraindicated in patients with acute angle-closure glaucoma, obstructive uropathy, obstructive disease of GI tract, paralytic ileus, toxic megacolon, intestinal atony, unstable CV status in acute hemorrhage, asthma, myasthenia gravis, or hypersensitivity to drug. Also not recommended for use in breast-feeding women.
- Use cautiously in patients with Down syndrome and in pregnant women.

NURSING CONSIDERATIONS

Assessment

- Obtain history of patient's underlying condition and reassess regularly.
- Be alert for adverse reactions and drug interactions.
- Monitor patients for paradoxical initial bradycardia, especially those receiving small doses (0.4 to 0.6 mg) caused by a drug effect in CNS and usually disappears within 2 minutes.

ALERT Watch for tachycardia in cardiac patients because it may precipitate ventricular fibrillation.
- Evaluate patient's and family's knowledge of drug therapy.

Nursing diagnoses

- Ineffective health maintenance related to underlying condition
- Risk for injury related to drug-induced adverse reactions
- Deficient knowledge related to drug therapy

Planning and implementation

P.O. use: Drug may be taken with or without food.
I.V. use: Administer by direct I.V. into a large vein or I.V. tubing over 1 to 2 minutes.
I.M. and S.C. use: Follow normal protocol.
- If ECG disturbances occur, withhold drug, obtain a rhythm strip, and notify prescriber immediately.
- Have emergency equipment and drugs on hand to treat new arrhythmias. Be aware that other anticholinergic drugs may increase vagal blockage.
- Use physostigmine salicylate as antidote for atropine overdose.

Patient teaching
- Teach patient about atropine sulfate therapy.
- Instruct patient to ask for assistance with activities if adverse CNS reactions occur.
- Teach patient how to handle distressing anticholinergic effects.

Evaluation

- Patient's underlying condition improves.
- Patient has no injury as a result of therapy.
- Patient and family state understanding of drug therapy.

auranofin
(or-AN-uh-fin)
Ridaura

Pharmacologic class: gold salt
Therapeutic class: antiarthritic
Pregnancy risk category: C

Indications and dosages

▶ **Rheumatoid arthritis.** *Adults:* 6 mg P.O. daily, either as 3 mg b.i.d. or 6 mg once daily. After 4 to 6 months, dosage may be increased to 9 mg daily.

How supplied

Capsules: 3 mg

Pharmacokinetics

Absorption: 25% absorbed through GI tract.
Distribution: distributed widely in body tissues. Synovial fluid levels are about 50% of blood levels. Drug is 60% protein-bound.
Metabolism: unknown.
Excretion: 60% of absorbed drug excreted in urine and remainder in feces. *Half-life:* 26 days.

Route	Onset	Peak	Duration
P.O.	1-3 mo	≤ 2 hr	Unknown

Pharmacodynamics

Chemical effect: unknown. Anti-inflammatory effects in rheumatoid arthritis are probably caused by inhibition of sulfhydryl systems, which alters cellular metabolism. Auranofin may also alter enzyme function and immune response and suppress phagocytic activity.
Therapeutic effect: relieves symptoms of rheumatoid arthritis.

Adverse reactions

CNS: confusion, ***seizures.***
EENT: metallic taste.
GI: *diarrhea, abdominal pain, nausea, vomiting,* stomatitis, enterocolitis, anorexia, dyspepsia, flatulence.
GU: proteinuria, hematuria, glomerulonephritis, ***acute renal failure,*** nephrotic syndrome.
Hematologic: ***thrombocytopenia, aplastic anemia, agranulocytosis, leukopenia,*** eosinophilia.
Hepatic: jaundice, elevated liver enzymes.
Respiratory: interstitial pneumonitis.
Skin: *rash, pruritus, dermatitis,* ***exfoliative dermatitis.***

Interactions

Drug-drug. *Phenytoin:* may raise phenytoin blood levels. Watch for toxicity.

Contraindications and precautions

- Contraindicated in patients with history of severe gold toxicity, necrotizing enterocolitis, pulmonary fibrosis, exfoliative dermatitis, bone marrow aplasia, severe hematologic disorders, or history of severe toxicity resulting from previous exposure to other heavy metals. Also contraindicated in patients with urticaria, eczema, colitis, severe debilitation, hemorrhagic conditions, or systemic lupus erythematosus and in patients who have recently received radiation therapy.
- Use in breast-feeding women isn't recommended.
- Use cautiously with other drugs that cause blood dyscrasia. Also use cautiously in patients who have renal, hepatic, or inflammatory bowel disease; rash; or a history of bone marrow depression.
- Safety of drug hasn't been established in children.

NURSING CONSIDERATIONS

Assessment

- Obtain history of patient's joint pain and stiffness before therapy and reassess regularly thereafter.
- Be alert for adverse reactions and drug interactions.
- Monitor patient's hydration status if adverse GI reactions occur.
- Monitor patient's platelet count and CBC regularly, as ordered.
- Evaluate patient's and family's knowledge of drug therapy.

Nursing diagnoses

- Acute pain related to presence of rheumatoid arthritis
- Risk for deficient fluid volume related to drug-induced adverse GI reactions
- Deficient knowledge related to drug therapy

Planning and implementation

- Store at controlled room temperature and in a light-resistant container.
- Administer concomitant drug therapy, such as NSAIDs, as ordered.
- Notify prescriber and expect to stop drug if patient's platelet count falls below 100,000/mm^3,

if hemoglobin drops suddenly, if granulocytes are below 1,500/mm³, and if leukopenia (WBC count below 4,000/mm³) or eosinophilia (eosinophils greater than 75%) occurs.

Patient teaching

- Encourage patient to take drug as prescribed and not to alter dosage schedule.
- Tell patient to continue taking concomitant drug therapy, such as NSAIDs, if prescribed.
- Remind patient to see prescriber monthly to monitor platelet counts. Auranofin should be stopped if platelet count falls below 100,000/mm³, if hemoglobin drops suddenly, if granulocytes are below 1,500/mm³, or if leukopenia (WBC count below 4,000/mm³) or eosinophilia (eosinophils more than 75%) is present.
- Advise patient to have regular urinalysis. If proteinuria or hematuria is detected, stop drug because it can produce a nephrotic syndrome or glomerulonephritis, and notify prescriber.
- Tell patient to continue taking drug if he experiences mild diarrhea and to contact prescriber immediately if blood isn't in stool. Diarrhea is the most common adverse reaction.
- Advise patient to report any rashes or other skin problems immediately. Pruritus often precedes dermatitis; any pruritic skin eruption while patients are receiving auranofin should be considered a reaction to this drug until proven otherwise. Advise patient to stop therapy until reaction subsides and notify prescriber.
- Advise patient that stomatitis is often preceded by a metallic taste, which should be reported to prescriber immediately. Promote careful oral hygiene during therapy.
- Reassure patient that beneficial drug effect may be delayed as long as 3 months. If response is inadequate and maximum dosage has been reached, expect prescriber to stop drug.
- Warn patient not to give drug to others. Auranofin, like injectable gold preparations, should be prescribed only for selected rheumatoid arthritis patients.

✔ Evaluation

- Patient expresses that his arthritic pain is relieved.
- Patient maintains fluid volume balance throughout therapy.
- Patient and family state understanding of drug therapy.

aurothioglucose

(or-oh-thigh-oh-GLOO-kohs)
Gold-50 ◊, Solganal

gold sodium thiomalate

(gohld SOH-dee-um thee-oh-MAH-layt)
Myochrysine

Pharmacologic class: gold salt
Therapeutic class: antiarthritic
Pregnancy risk category: C

Indications and dosages

▶ **Rheumatoid arthritis. Aurothioglucose.** *Adults:* initially, 10 mg I.M., followed by 25 mg for second and third doses at weekly intervals. Then, 50 mg weekly until 0.8 to 1 g has been given. If improvement occurs without toxicity, 50 mg is continued at 3- to 4-week intervals indefinitely as maintenance therapy.
Children ages 6 to 12: one-fourth usual adult dosage, not to exceed 25 mg per dose.
Gold sodium thiomalate. *Adults:* initially, 10 mg I.M., followed by 25 mg in 1 week. Then, 25 to 50 mg weekly until 14 to 20 doses have been given. If improvement occurs without toxicity, 25 to 50 mg is continued q 2 weeks for four doses; then, 25 to 50 mg q 3 weeks for four doses; then, 25 to 50 mg every month indefinitely as maintenance therapy. If relapse occurs during maintenance therapy, injections are resumed at weekly intervals.
Children: 1 mg/kg I.M. weekly for 20 weeks. If response is good, may be given q 3 to 4 weeks indefinitely.

How supplied

Injection (suspension): 50 mg/ml in sesame oil with aluminum monostearate 2% and propylparaben 0.1% in 10-ml container (aurothioglucose)
Injection: 25 mg/ml, 50 mg/ml with benzyl alcohol (gold sodium thiomalate)

Pharmacokinetics

Absorption: slow and erratic because drug is in oil suspension.
Distribution: distributed widely throughout body in lymph nodes, bone marrow, kidneys, liver, spleen, and tissues. About 85% to 90% is protein-bound.
Metabolism: not broken down into elemental form.
Excretion: about 70% excreted in urine; 30% in feces. *Half-life:* 14 to 40 days.

Route	Onset	Peak	Duration
I.M.	Unknown	3-6 hr	Unknown

Pharmacodynamics

Chemical effect: unknown. Anti-inflammatory effects in rheumatoid arthritis are probably caused by inhibition of sulfhydryl systems, which alters cellular metabolism. Gold salts may also alter enzyme function and immune response and suppress phagocytic activity.
Therapeutic effect: relieves signs and symptoms of rheumatoid arthritis.

Adverse reactions

CNS: *dizziness,* syncope, ***seizures.***
CV: ***bradycardia***, hypotension.
EENT: corneal gold deposition, corneal ulcers.
GI: *stomatitis,* difficulty swallowing, nausea, vomiting, metallic taste.
GU: albuminuria, proteinuria, nephrotic syndrome, nephritis, ***acute tubular necrosis, acute renal failure.***
Hematologic: ***thrombocytopenia, aplastic anemia, agranulocytosis, leukopenia,*** eosinophilia.
Hepatic: hepatitis, jaundice.
Skin: diaphoresis, photosensitivity, *rash and dermatitis.*
Other: ***anaphylaxis, angioedema.***

Interactions

None significant.

Contraindications and precautions

- Contraindicated in patients hypersensitive to drug or with a history of severe toxicity from exposure to gold or other heavy metals, hepatitis, or exfoliative dermatitis; severe, uncontrollable diabetes; renal disease; hepatic dysfunction; uncontrolled heart failure; systemic lupus erythematosus; colitis; Sjögren's syndrome; urticaria; eczema; hemorrhagic conditions; severe hematologic disorders; or recent radiation therapy.
- Drug isn't recommended for breast-feeding women.
- Use with extreme caution, if at all, in patients with rash, marked hypertension, compromised cerebral or CV circulation, or history of renal or hepatic disease, drug allergies, or blood dyscrasia.
- Use cautiously in pregnant women.
- Safety of drug hasn't been established in children under age 6.

NURSING CONSIDERATIONS

Assessment

- Obtain history of patient's rheumatoid arthritis before therapy and reassess regularly thereafter.
- Be alert for adverse reactions.
- Analyze urine for protein and sediment changes before each injection.
- Monitor CBC, including platelet count, before every second injection, as ordered.
- Evaluate patient's and family's knowledge of drug therapy.

Nursing diagnoses

- Acute pain (joint) related to presence of rheumatoid arthritis
- Risk for injury related to drug-induced adverse reactions
- Deficient knowledge related to drug therapy

Planning and implementation

- Administer only under constant supervision of prescriber who is thoroughly familiar with drug's toxicities and benefits.

ALERT Rash and dermititis occur in 20% of patients and may lead to fatal exfoliative dermatitis if drug not stopped.

- Gold compounds are typically used only in active rheumatoid arthritis that hasn't responded adequately to salicylates, rest, and physical therapy. Some clinicians advocate earlier use before disease progresses.

• Administer all gold salts I.M., as ordered, preferably intragluteally. Drug is pale yellow; don't use if it darkens.
• Immerse aurothioglucose (a suspension) vial in warm water, and shake vigorously before injecting.
• When giving gold sodium thiomalate, have patient lie down and remain recumbent for 10 to 20 minutes after injection to minimize hypotension.
• Observe patient for 30 minutes after administration because of possible anaphylactoid reaction.
• If adverse reactions develop and are mild, some rheumatologists resume gold therapy after 2 to 3 weeks' rest.
• Monitor platelet count if patient develops purpura or ecchymoses, as ordered.
• Keep dimercaprol on hand to treat acute toxicity.

Patient teaching
• Inform patient that benefits of therapy may not appear for 3 to 4 months or longer.
• Advise patient that increased joint pain may occur for 1 to 2 days after injection but usually subsides after a few injections.
• Advise patient to report any rashes or skin problems immediately. Pruritus often precedes dermatitis; pruritic skin eruptions that develop while patient is receiving gold salt therapy should be considered a reaction to therapy until proven otherwise. Advise patient to stop therapy until reaction subsides and to notify prescriber.
• Advise patient that stomatitis is often preceded by metallic taste, which should be reported to prescriber immediately. Promote careful oral hygiene during therapy.
• Tell patients to avoid sunlight and artificial ultraviolet light to minimize risk of photosensitivity.
• Stress need for close medical follow-ups and frequent blood and urine tests during therapy.

☑ Evaluation
• Patient expresses relief of joint stiffness and pain.
• Patient doesn't experience injury as result of drug-induced adverse reactions.
• Patient and family state understanding of drug therapy.

azathioprine
(ay-zuh-THIGH-oh-preen)
Imuran, Thioprine ◇

Pharmacologic class: purine antagonist
Therapeutic class: immunosuppressive
Pregnancy risk category: D

Indications and dosages
▶ **Immunosuppression in kidney transplantation.** *Adults and children:* initially, 3 to 5 mg/kg P.O. or I.V. daily, usually beginning on day of transplantation. Maintained at 1 to 3 mg/kg daily (dosage varies considerably according to patient response).
▶ **Severe, refractory rheumatoid arthritis.** *Adults:* initially, 1 mg/kg P.O. as single dose or as two doses. If patient response isn't satisfactory after 6 to 8 weeks, dosage may be increased by 0.5 mg/kg daily (up to maximum of 2.5 mg/kg daily) at 4-week intervals.

How supplied
Tablets: 50 mg
Injection: 100 mg

Pharmacokinetics
Absorption: oral dose absorbed well from GI tract.
Distribution: azathioprine and its major metabolite, mercaptopurine, are distributed throughout body; both are 30% protein-bound.
Metabolism: metabolized primarily to mercaptopurine.
Excretion: small amounts of azathioprine and mercaptopurine are excreted in urine intact; most of given dose is excreted in urine as secondary metabolites. *Half-life:* about 5 hours.

Route	Onset	Peak	Duration
P.O., I.V.	4-8 wk	1-2 hr	Unknown

Pharmacodynamics
Chemical effect: unknown.

Therapeutic effect: suppresses immune system activity.

Adverse reactions

EENT: esophagitis.
GI: nausea, vomiting, anorexia, ***pancreatitis,*** steatorrhea, mouth ulceration.
Hematologic: **LEUKOPENIA,** ***bone marrow suppression,*** anemia, ***pancytopenia,*** **THROMBOCYTOPENIA.**
Hepatic: ***hepatotoxicity,*** jaundice.
Musculoskeletal: arthralgia, muscle wasting.
Skin: rash, alopecia, pruritus.
Other: ***immunosuppression, infections, neoplasia.***

Interactions

Drug-drug. *ACE inhibitors:* combination may cause severe leukopenia. Monitor patient closely.
Allopurinol: impaired inactivation of azathioprine. Decrease azathioprine dose to one-fourth or one-third normal dose.
Vaccines: decreased immune response. Postpone routine immunization.
Warfarin: may inhibit the anticoagulant effect of warfarin. Monitor PT and INR.

Contraindications and precautions

- Contraindicated in patients hypersensitive to drug.
- Drug isn't recommended for breast-feeding women.
- Use cautiously in patients with hepatic or renal dysfunction.
- Don't use drug for treating rheumatoid arthritis in pregnant women.

NURSING CONSIDERATIONS

Assessment

- Obtain history of patient's immune status before therapy.
- Monitor effectiveness by observing for signs of organ rejection. Be aware that therapeutic response usually occurs within 8 weeks.
- Be alert for adverse reactions and drug interactions.
- Monitor hemoglobin, WBC, and platelet counts at least once monthly, as ordered—more often at beginning of treatment.
- Evaluate patient's and family's knowledge of drug therapy.

Nursing diagnoses

- Ineffective protection related to threat of organ rejection
- Risk for infection related to drug-induced immunosuppression
- Deficient knowledge related to drug therapy

Planning and implementation

P.O. use: Administer drug in divided doses or after meals to minimize adverse GI effects.
I.V. use: Reconstitute 100-mg vial with 10 ml of sterile water for injection. Visually inspect for particles before giving. Drug may be administered by direct I.V. injection or further diluted in normal saline injection or D_5W and infused over 30 to 60 minutes. Use only for patients unable to tolerate P.O. medications.

- Benefits must be weighed against risks with systemic viral infections, such as chickenpox and herpes zoster.
- Patients with rheumatoid arthritis previously treated with alkylating drugs, such as cyclophosphamide, chlorambucil, and melphalan, may have prohibitive risk of neoplasia if treated with azathioprine.
- Drug should be stopped immediately when WBC count is less than 3,000/mm^3 to prevent irreversible bone marrow suppression. Notify prescriber.
- To prevent bleeding, avoid I.M. injections when platelet count is below 100,000/mm^3.

Patient teaching

- Warn patient to report even mild infections (colds, fever, sore throat, and malaise) because drug is potent immunosuppressant.
- Instruct woman to avoid conception during therapy and for 4 months after stopping therapy.
- Warn patient that some thinning of hair is possible.
- Tell patient taking this drug for refractory rheumatoid arthritis that it may take up to 12 weeks to be effective.

Evaluation

- Patient exhibits no signs of organ rejection.

• Patient demonstrates no signs and symptoms of infection.
• Patient and family state understanding of drug therapy.

azelastine hydrochloride
(ah-zuh-LAST-een high-droh-KLOR-ighd)
Astelin

Pharmacologic class: H_1-receptor agonist
Therapeutic class: antihistamine
Pregnancy risk category: C

Indications and dosages

▶ **Seasonal allergic rhinitis.** *Adults and children age 12 and older:* two sprays per nostril b.i.d.

How supplied

Aerosol inhaler: 137 mcg/metered spray

Pharmacokinetics

Absorption: undefined.
Distribution: systemic bioavailability is 40%.
Metabolism: after dosing to a steady-state, plasma level ranges from 20% to 50%.
Excretion: oral dosage excreted in feces. *Half-life:* 22 hours.

Route	Onset	Peak	Duration
Inhalation	1-3 hr	2-3 hr	12 hr

Pharmacodynamics

Chemical effect: exhibited histamine H_1-receptor agonist activity.
Therapeutic effect: relief of seasonal allergic rhinitis.

Adverse reactions

CNS: *headache, somnolence,* fatigue, dizziness.
EENT: epistaxis, nasal burning, pharyngitis, rhinitis.
GI: *bitter taste,* dry mouth, nausea.
Musculoskeletal: myalgia.
Respiratory: paroxysmal sneezing.
Other: weight increase.

Interactions

Drug-drug. *Cimetidine:* increased plasma levels of azelastine. Avoid concomitant use.
CNS depressants: increased sedation. Avoid concomitant use.
Drug-lifestyle. *Alcohol use*: increased sedation. Discourage concomitant use.

Contraindications and precautions

• Contraindicated in patients hypersensitive to drug.

NURSING CONSIDERATIONS

Assessment

• Obtain history of patient's allergy condition before therapy begins and reassess regularly thereafter.
• Be alert for adverse reactions and drug interactions.
• Evaluate patient's and family's knowledge of drug therapy.

Nursing diagnoses

• Ineffective health maintenance related to underlying allergic condition
• Deficient knowledge related to drug therapy

Planning and implementation

• Drug should be used in pregnancy only if benefit justifies potential risk to fetus. Breast-feeding women shouldn't take drug.
• Safety and effectiveness in patients under age 12 haven't been established.

Patient teaching

• Warn patient not to drive or perform hazardous activities if somnolence occurs.
• Advise patient not to use alcohol, CNS depressants, or other antihistamines while taking drug.
• Teach patient proper usage of nasal spray. Instruct patient to replace child-resistant screw top on bottle with pump unit. Prime delivery system with four sprays or until a fine mist appears. Reprime system with two sprays or until a fine mist appears if 3 or more days have elapsed since last use. Store bottle upright at room temperature with pump closed tightly. Keep unit away from children.
• Tell patient to avoid getting spray in eyes.

☑ **Evaluation**

- Patient's allergic symptoms are relieved with drug therapy.
- Patient and family state understanding of drug therapy.

azithromycin

(uh-zith-roh-MIGH-sin)

Zithromax

Pharmacologic class: azalide macrolide
Therapeutic class: antibiotic
Pregnancy risk category: B

Indications and dosages

▶ **Acute bacterial exacerbations of COPD caused by *Haemophilus influenzae, Moraxella catarrhalis,* or *Streptococcus pneumoniae*; uncomplicated skin and skin-structure infections caused by *Staphylococcus aureus, Streptococcus pyogenes,* or *Streptococcus agalactiae*; second-line therapy of pharyngitis or tonsillitis caused by *S. pyogenes.*** *Adults and adolescents age 16 and older:* 500 mg P.O. as a single dose on day 1, followed by 250 mg P.O. daily on days 2 through 5. Total dose is 1.5 g.

▶ **Community-acquired pneumonia caused by *Chlamydia pneumoniae, H. influenzae, Mycoplasma pneumoniae, S. pneumoniae*; I.V. form can also be used for *Legionella pneumophila, M. catarrhalis, and S. aureus.*** *Adults and adolescents age 16 or older:* 500 mg P.O. as a single dose on day 1, followed by 250 mg P.O. daily on days 2 through 5. Total dose is 1.5 g. For patients requiring initial I.V. therapy, 500 mg I.V. as a single daily dose for 2 days, followed by 500 mg P.O. as a single daily dose to complete a 7-to 10-day course of therapy. Switch from I.V. to P.O. therapy should be done at prescriber's discretion and based on patient's clinical response.

▶ **Nongonococcal urethritis or cervicitis caused by *Chlamydia trachomatis.*** *Adults and adolescents age 16 and older:* 1 g P.O. as a single dose.

▶ **Prevention of disseminated *Mycobacterium avium* complex disease in patients with advanced HIV infection.** *Adults:* 1,200 mg P.O. once weekly, as indicated.

▶ **Urethritis and cervicitis due to *Neisseria gonorrhoeae.*** *Adults:* 2 g P.O. as a single dose.

▶ **Pelvic inflammatory disease caused by *C. trachomatis, N. gonorrhoeae, or Mycoplasma hominis* in patients who require initial I.V. therapy.** *Adults:* 500 mg I.V. as a single daily dose for 1 to 2 days, followed by 250 mg P.O. daily to complete a 7-day course of therapy. Switch from I.V. to P.O. therapy should be done at prescriber's discretion and based on patient's clinical response.

▶ **Genital ulcer disease in men due to *Haemophilus ducreyi (chancroid).*** *Adults:* 1 g P.O. as a single dose.

▶ **Acute otitis media.** *Children over age 6 months:* 10 mg/kg (maximum 500 mg) P.O. on day 1, followed by 5 mg/kg (maximum 250 mg) on days 2 to 5.

▶ **Pharyngitis, tonsillitis.** *Children over age 2:* 12 mg/kg (maximum 500 mg) P.O. daily for 5 days.

How supplied

Tablets: 250 mg
Capsules: 250 mg
Injection: 500mg
Oral suspension: 100 mg/5 ml, 200 mg/5 ml
Single dose powder for oral suspension: 1 g

Pharmacokinetics

Absorption: rapidly absorbed from GI tract; food decreases both maximum plasma levels and amount of drug absorbed.
Distribution: rapidly distributed throughout body and readily penetrates cells; it doesn't readily enter CNS. Drug concentrates in fibroblasts and phagocytes. Significantly higher levels are reached in tissues compared with plasma.
Metabolism: not metabolized.
Excretion: excreted mostly in feces after excretion into bile. Less than 10% is excreted in urine. Terminal elimination *half-life:* 68 hours.

Route	Onset	Peak	Duration
P.O.	Unknown	2.5-4.4 hr	Unknown
I.V.	Unknown	Unknown	Unknown

Pharmacodynamics

Chemical effect: binds to 50S subunit of bacterial ribosomes, blocking protein synthesis; bacteriostatic or bactericidal, depending on concentration.
Therapeutic effect: hinders or kills susceptible bacteria. Spectrum of activity includes many gram-positive and gram-negative aerobic and anaerobic bacteria, such as *Haemophilus influenzae, Moraxella catarrhalis, Staphylococcus aureus, Streptococcus agalactiae, Streptococcus pneumoniae, Streptococcus pyogenes,* and *Chlamydia trachomatis.*

Adverse reactions

CNS: dizziness, vertigo, headache, fatigue, somnolence.
CV: palpitations, chest pain.
GI: *nausea, vomiting, diarrhea, abdominal pain,* dyspepsia, flatulence, melena, cholestatic jaundice, ***pseudomembranous colitis.***
GU: candidiasis, vaginitis, nephritis.
Skin: rash, photosensitivity.
Other: ***angioedema.***

Interactions

Drug-drug. *Aluminum- and magnesium-containing antacids:* lowered peak plasma levels of azithromycin. Separate administration times by at least 2 hours.
Digoxin: elevated digoxin levels. Monitor patient closely.
Dihydroergotamine, ergotamine: acute ergot toxicity. Avoid concomitant use.
Drugs metabolized by cytochrome P-450 system: elevations of serum carbamazepine, cyclosporine, hexobarbital, and phenytoin levels. Monitor patient closely.
Theophylline: possibly increased plasma theophylline levels with other macrolides; effect of azithromycin is unknown. Monitor theophylline levels carefully.
Triazolam: increased pharmacologic effect of triazolam. Use cautiously.
Warfarin: possibly increased PT with other macrolides; effect of azithromycin is unknown. Monitor PT and INR carefully.
Drug-food. *Any food:* decreased absorption. Give at least 1 hour before or 2 hours after a meal.
Drug-lifestyle. *Sun exposure:* photosensitivity reactions may occur. Advise against prolonged or unprotected sun exposure.

Contraindications and precautions

• Contraindicated in patients hypersensitive to erythromycin or other macrolides.
• Use cautiously in patients with impaired hepatic function and in pregnant or breast-feeding women.

NURSING CONSIDERATIONS

Assessment
• Obtain history of patient's infection before therapy and reassess regularly thereafter.
• Obtain specimen for culture and sensitivity tests before first dose. Therapy may begin pending test results.
• Be alert for adverse reactions and drug interactions.
• Evaluate patient's and family's knowledge of drug therapy.

Nursing diagnoses
• Infection related to presence of susceptible bacteria
• Ineffective protection related to drug-induced superinfection
• Deficient knowledge related to drug therapy

Planning and implementation
P.O. use: Administer 1 hour before or 2 hours after meals; don't administer with antacids.
I.V. use: Reconstitute drug by adding 4.8 ml sterile water for injection to 500-mg vial and shake until all the drug is dissolved. Further dilute in 250 to 500 ml D_5W, normal saline solution, or other compatible solution. Infuse over 1 to 3 hours. Reconstituted solution is stable for 7 days if stored in refrigerator (41°F [5° C]).

Patient teaching
• Tell patient that drug should always be taken on an empty stomach because food or antacids decrease absorption.

• Tell patient to take all medication as prescribed, even after he feels better.
• Instruct patient to use sunblock and avoid prolonged exposure to the sun, to decrease risk of photosensitivity reactions.

☑ Evaluation

• Patient's infection is eradicated.
• Patient doesn't experience superinfection during therapy.
• Patient and family state understanding of drug therapy.

aztreonam

(az-TREE-oh-nam)
Azactam

Pharmacologic class: monobactam
Therapeutic class: antibiotic
Pregnancy risk category: B

Indications and dosages

▶ **UTI, lower respiratory tract infections, septicemia, skin and skin-structure infections, intra-abdominal infections, surgical infections, and gynecologic infections caused by various aerobic organisms.**
Adults: 500 mg to 2 g I.V. or I.M. q 8 to 12 hours. For severe systemic or life-threatening infections, 2 g q 6 to 8 hours may be given. Maximum dosage is 8 g daily.

How supplied

Injection: 500-mg, 1-g, 2-g vials

Pharmacokinetics

Absorption: absorbed rapidly and completely after I.M. administration.
Distribution: distributed rapidly and widely to all body fluids and tissues, including bile, breast milk, and CSF.
Metabolism: from 6% to 16% metabolized to inactive metabolites by nonspecific hydrolysis of beta-lactam ring; 56% to 60% protein-bound, less if renal impairment is present.
Excretion: excreted primarily unchanged in urine by glomerular filtration and tubular secretion; 1.5% to 3.5% excreted unchanged in feces. *Half-life:* averages 1.7 hours.

Route	Onset	Peak	Duration
I.V.	Immediate	Immediate	Unknown
I.M.	Unknown	0.6-1.3 hr	Unknown

Pharmacodynamics

Chemical effect: inhibits bacterial cell-wall synthesis, ultimately causing cell wall destruction; bactericidal.
Therapeutic effect: kills susceptible bacteria. Spectrum of activity is narrow and includes *Enterobacter, Escherichia coli, Klebsiella pneumoniae, Proteus mirabilis,* and *Pseudomonas aeruginosa.* It has limited activity against *Citrobacter, Haemophilus influenzae, Hafnia, Klebsiella oxytoca, Moraxella catarrhalis, Neisseria gonorrhoeae, Providencia,* and *Serratia margaris.*

Adverse reactions

CNS: ***seizures,*** headache, insomnia, confusion.
CV: hypotension.
EENT: halitosis, altered taste.
GI: diarrhea, nausea, vomiting.
Hematologic: ***neutropenia,*** anemia, ***thrombocytopenia, pancytopenia.***
Hepatic: transient elevation of ALT and AST levels.
Other: hypersensitivity reactions (rash, ***anaphylaxis***); rash, thrombophlebitis at I.V. site; discomfort, swelling at I.M. injection site.

Interactions

Drug-drug. *Aminoglycosides, beta-lactam antibiotics, other anti-infectives:* synergistic effect. Monitor patient closely.
Cefoxitin, imipenem: possible antagonistic effect. Don't use together.
Furosemide, probenecid: increased serum aztreonam levels. Avoid concomitant use.

Contraindications and precautions

• Contraindicated in patients hypersensitive to drug.
• Drug isn't recommended for breast-feeding women.

• Use cautiously in elderly patients and in those with impaired renal function. Dosage adjustment may be necessary.
• Safety of drug hasn't been established in children.

NURSING CONSIDERATIONS

Assessment
• Obtain history of patient's infection before therapy, and reassess regularly thereafter.
• Obtain urine specimen for culture and sensitivity tests before giving first dose. Therapy may begin pending test results.
• Be aware of adverse reactions and drug interactions.
• Be aware that patients allergic to penicillins or cephalosporins may not be allergic to aztreonam. However, closely monitor patients who have had an immediate hypersensitivity reaction to these antibiotics.
• Evaluate patient's and family's understanding of drug therapy.

Nursing diagnoses
• Infection related to presence of susceptible bacteria
• Ineffective protection related to drug-induced superinfection
• Deficient knowledge related to drug therapy

Planning and implementation
I.V. use: To administer bolus of aztreonam, inject drug slowly (over 3 to 5 minutes), directly into vein or I.V. tubing. Give infusion over 20 minutes to 1 hour.
I.M. use: Administer I.M. injection deep into large muscle mass, such as upper outer quadrant of gluteus maximus or lateral aspect of thigh. Give doses large than 1 g by I.V. route.

Patient teaching
• Tell patient to report pain or discomfort at I.V. site.
• Warn patient receiving drug I.M. that pain and swelling may develop at injection site.
• Instruct patient to report signs or symptoms that suggest superinfection.

Evaluation
• Patient is free of infection.
• Patient doesn't develop superinfection as a result of therapy.
• Patient and family state understanding of drug therapy.

B

bacillus Calmette-Guérin (BCG), live intravesical
(bah-SIL-us kal-MET geh-RAN, in-trah-VES-ih-kal)
ImmuCyst♦, TheraCys, TICE BCG

Pharmacologic class: bacterial agent
Therapeutic class: antineoplastic
Pregnancy risk category: C

Indications and dosages
▶ **In situ carcinoma of urinary bladder (primary and relapsed).** *Adults:* consult published protocols, specialized references, and manufacturer's recommendations.

How supplied
Suspension (freeze-dried) for bladder instillation: 2-ml vial containing 1 to 8 × 10^8 colony-forming units, equivalent to about 50 mg

Pharmacokinetics
No information available.

Route	Onset	Peak	Duration
Intravesical	Unknown	Unknown	Unknown

Pharmacodynamics
Chemical effect: unknown. Instillation of live bacterial suspension causes local inflammatory response. Local infiltration of histiocytes and leukocytes is followed by decrease in superficial tumors in bladder.
Therapeutic effect: decreases risk of superficial bladder tumors.

Adverse reactions
CNS: malaise.

GI: nausea, vomiting, anorexia, diarrhea, mild abdominal pain.
GU: *dysuria, urinary frequency, hematuria,* cystitis, urinary urgency, urinary incontinence, urinary tract infection, cramps, pain, decreased bladder capacity, tissue in urine, local infection, nephrotoxicity, genital pain.
Hematologic: anemia, ***leukopenia, thrombocytopenia, disseminated intravascular coagulapathy (DIC).***
Hepatic: elevated liver enzyme levels.
Musculoskeletal: myalgia, arthralgia.
Other: ***hypersensitivity reaction,*** *fever above 101°F (38.3°C),* chills.

Interactions

Drug-drug. *Antibiotics:* may attenuate response to BCG intravesical. Avoid concomitant use.
Bone marrow suppressants, immunosuppressants, radiation therapy: may impair response to BCG intravesical by decreasing immune response; also may increase risk of osteomyelitis or disseminated BCG infection. Avoid concomitant use.

Contraindications and precautions

- Contraindicated in immunocompromised patients, in those receiving immunosuppressive therapy (because of risk of bacterial infection), and in those with urinary tract infection (because of risk of increased bladder irritation or disseminated BCG infection).
- Also contraindicated in patients with fever of unknown origin. If fever is caused by an infection, withhold drug until patient has recovered.
- Pregnant or breast-feeding women should use with caution.
- Safety of drug hasn't been established in children.

NURSING CONSIDERATIONS

Assessment

- Obtain history of patient's bladder cancer.
- Monitor drug's effectiveness by regularly checking tumor size and rate of growth through appropriate studies, as ordered, and by noting results of follow-up diagnostic tests and overall physical status.
- Be alert for adverse reactions and drug interactions.
- Closely monitor patient for evidence of systemic BCG infection. Such infections are seldom detected by positive cultures.
- Evaluate patient's and family's understanding of drug therapy.

Nursing diagnoses

- Risk for injury related to underlying condition
- Risk for trauma related to instillation procedure for drug therapy
- Deficient knowledge related to drug therapy

Planning and implementation

- Drug isn't used as an immunizing agent to prevent cancer or tuberculosis; drug shouldn't be confused with BCG vaccine.
- Drug shouldn't be handled or administered by caregiver with known immunologic deficiency.

ALERT Don't administer BCG intravesical within 7 to 14 days of transurethral resection or biopsy. Fatal disseminated BCG infection has occurred after traumatic catheterization.

- To administer TheraCys or ImmuCyst, reconstitute with 1 ml of provided diluent per vial, just before use. Don't remove rubber stopper to prepare solution. Use immediately. Add contents of three reconstituted vials to 50 ml of sterile, preservative-free saline solution (final volume, 53 ml). Instill urethral catheter into bladder under aseptic conditions, drain bladder, and infuse 53 ml of prepared solution by gravity feed. Remove catheter and properly dispose of unused drug.
- To administer TICE BCG, use thermosetting plastic or sterile glass containers and syringes. Draw 1 ml of sterile, preservative-free saline solution into 3-ml syringe. Add to 1 ampule of drug; gently expel back into ampule three times to mix thoroughly. Use immediately. Dispense cloudy suspension into top end of catheter-tipped syringe that contains 49 ml of saline solution. Gently rotate syringe. Properly dispose of unused drug.
- Handle drug and all material used for instillation of drug as infectious material because they contain live attenuated mycobacteria.

Dispose of all materials (syringes, catheters, and containers) as biohazardous waste.

- Use strict aseptic technique to administer drug to minimize trauma to GU tract and to prevent introduction of other contaminants.
- If patient has evidence of traumatic catheterization, don't administer drug, and alert prescriber. Treatment may resume after 1 week.
- Therapy should be withheld if systemic infection is suspected (short-term fever above 103° F [39.4° C], persistent fever above 101° F [38.3° C] over 2 days, or severe malaise). Prescriber may contact an infectious disease specialist for initiation of fast-acting antituberculosis therapy.
- Be prepared to treat symptoms of bladder irritation with phenazopyridine, acetaminophen, and propantheline, as ordered. Systemic hypersensitivity can be treated with diphenhydramine. To minimize risk of systemic infection, some clinicians give isoniazid for 3 days starting on first day of treatment.

Patient teaching

- Tell patient to retain drug in bladder for 2 hours after instillation (if possible). For the first hour, have patient lie prone for 15 minutes, supine for 15 minutes, and on each side for 15 minutes; the second hour may be spent in sitting position.
- Instruct patient to sit when voiding to avoid splashing of urine.
- Instruct patient to disinfect urine for 6 hours after instillation of drug. Tell him to add undiluted household bleach (5% sodium hypochlorite solution) in equal volume to voided urine in toilet and let stand for 15 minutes before flushing.
- Tell patient to call prescriber if symptoms worsen or if the following symptoms develop: blood in urine, frequent urge to urinate, painful urination, fever and chills, nausea, vomiting, joint pain, or rash.
- Tell patient to notify prescriber immediately if cough develops after therapy because it may indicate life-threatening BCG infection.

☑ Evaluation

- Patient exhibits no further evidence of superficial bladder tumors.
- Patient doesn't experience trauma as result of drug use.
- Patient and family state understanding of drug therapy.

bacitracin

(bas-uh-TRAY-sin)
Baci-IM

Pharmacologic class: polypeptide antibiotic
Therapeutic class: antibiotic
Pregnancy risk category: NR

Indications and dosages

▶ **Treatment of infants with pneumonia or empyema caused by susceptible staphylococci.** *Infants weighing over 2.5 kg (5.5 lb):* 500 units/kg I.M. b.i.d. q 8 to 12 hours. *Infants weighing under 2.5 kg:* 450 units/kg I.M. b.i.d. q 8 to 12 hours.

How supplied

Injection: 10,000-unit, 50,000-unit vials

Pharmacokinetics

Absorption: absorbed rapidly and completely after I.M. injection.
Distribution: distributed widely throughout all body organs and fluids except CSF (unless meninges are inflamed). Drug binds to plasma proteins only minimally.
Metabolism: not significantly metabolized.
Excretion: 10% to 40% of dose excreted by kidneys.

Route	Onset	Peak	Duration
I.M.	Unknown	≤ 1 hr	Unknown

Pharmacodynamics

Chemical effect: hinders bacterial cell wall synthesis, damaging bacterial plasma membrane and making cell more vulnerable to osmotic pressure.
Therapeutic effect: hinders bacterial activity. Drug is effective against many gram-positive organisms, including *Clostridium difficile.* Drug is minimally effective against gram-negative organisms.

Adverse reactions

EENT: ototoxicity.
GI: nausea, vomiting, anorexia, diarrhea, rectal itching or burning.
GU: ***nephrotoxicity*** (*albuminuria,* cylindruria, oliguria, anuria, increased BUN, ***tubular and glomerular necrosis***).
Hematologic: blood dyscrasia, eosinophilia.
Musculoskeletal: ***neuromuscular blockade.***
Skin: urticaria, rash.
Other: superinfection, fever, ***anaphylaxis,*** pain at injection site.

Interactions

Drug-drug. *Inhaled anesthetics, neuromuscular blockers:* prolonged muscle weakness. Monitor patient for excessive muscle weakness or respiratory distress.
Nephrotoxic drugs (such as aminoglycosides): increased nephrotoxicity. Use together cautiously.

Contraindications and precautions

- Contraindicated in pregnant women, in patients hypersensitive to drug, and in patients with impaired renal function.
- Use cautiously in patients with myasthenia gravis or neuromuscular disease.

NURSING CONSIDERATIONS

Assessment

- Obtain history of patient's infection before therapy, and reassess regularly thereafter.
- Assess baseline renal function studies before starting therapy.
- Obtain urine specimen for culture and sensitivity tests before first dose. Therapy may begin pending test results.
- Be alert for adverse reactions and drug interactions.
- Evaluate family's understanding of drug therapy.

Nursing diagnoses

- Infection related to presence of susceptible bacteria
- Impaired urinary elimination related to drug-induced nephrotoxicity
- Deficient knowledge related to drug therapy

Planning and implementation

- Dissolve in saline solution for injection containing 2% procaine to a bacitracin concentration between 5,000 and 10,000 units/ml. Don't dilute with solutions containing parabens.
- Administer by deep I.M. injection only.
- Store in refrigerator. Drug is inactivated if stored at room temperature.
- Provide measures to keep urine pH above 6 and reduce the risk of nephrotoxicity, such as alkalinizing agents, as ordered, and adequate fluid intake.

Patient teaching

- Warn parent that injection may be painful.
- Instruct parents to report unusual signs or symptoms because drug causes many adverse reactions.
- Advise parent that child should maintain adequate fluid intake.

Evaluation

- Patient is free of infection.
- Patient's kidney function remains normal throughout therapy.
- Caregivers state understanding of drug therapy.

baclofen

(BAH-kloh-fen)
Clofen ◇, Lioresal, Lioresal Intrathecal

Pharmacologic class: chlorophenyl derivative
Therapeutic class: skeletal muscle relaxant
Pregnancy risk category: C

Indications and dosages

▶ **Spasticity in multiple sclerosis, spinal cord injury.** *Adults:* initially, 5 mg P.O. t.i.d. for 3 days. Dosage may be increased based on response at 3-day intervals by 15 mg (5 mg/dose) daily up to maximum of 80 mg daily (20 mg q.i.d.).
▶ **Management of severe spasticity in patients who don't respond to or cannot tolerate oral baclofen therapy.** *Adults (screening phase):* after test dose to check responsiveness, administer drug by an implantable infusion pump. The test dose is 1 ml of 50-mcg/ml

dilution administered into intrathecal space by barbotage over 1 minute or more. Significantly decreased severity or frequency of muscle spasm or reduced muscle tone should be evident in 4 to 8 hours. If response is inadequate, give second test dose of 75 mcg/1.5 ml 24 hours after the first. If response is still inadequate, give final test dose of 100 mcg/2 ml 24 hours later. Patients unresponsive to 100-mcg dose shouldn't be considered candidates for implantable pump.
Adults (maintenance therapy): initial dose titrated based on screening dose that elicited an adequate response. This effective dose is doubled and administered over 24 hours. If screening dose efficacy is maintained for 8 hours or more, dosage isn't doubled. After first 24 hours, increase dose slowly, as needed and tolerated, by 10% to 30% daily until desired clinical effects are obtained.

How supplied

Tablets: 10 mg, 20 mg, 25 mg◆
Intrathecal injection: 500 mcg/ml, 2,000 mcg/ml

Pharmacokinetics

Absorption: rapidly and extensively absorbed from GI tract with P.O. administration; may vary.
Distribution: widely distributed throughout body, with small amounts crossing blood-brain barrier. It's about 30% plasma protein–bound.
Metabolism: about 15% metabolized in liver via deamination.
Excretion: 70% to 80% excreted in urine unchanged or as metabolites; remainder excreted in feces. *Half-life:* 2½ to 4 hours.

Route	Onset	Peak	Duration
P.O.	Hrs-wk	2-3 hr	Unknown
Intrathecal	0.5-1 hr	About 4 hr	4-8 hr

Pharmacodynamics

Chemical effect: unknown; appears to reduce transmission of impulses from spinal cord to skeletal muscle.
Therapeutic effect: relieves muscle spasms.

Adverse reactions

CNS: *drowsiness, dizziness,* headache, *weakness, fatigue,* hypotonia, confusion, insomnia, dysarthria, SEIZURES.
CV: hypotension.
EENT: nasal congestion, blurred vision.
GI: *nausea,* constipation, vomiting.
GU: urinary frequency.
Metabolic: hyperglycemia, weight gain.
Hepatic: increased AST and alkaline phosphatase levels.
Respiratory: dyspnea.
Skin: rash, pruritus, excessive perspiration.
Other: ankle edema.

Interactions

Drug-drug. *CNS depressants:* increased CNS depression. Avoid concomitant use.
MAO inhibitors, tricyclic antidepressants: CNS and respiratory depression, hypotension. Avoid concomitant use.
Drug-lifestyle. *Alcohol use:* increased CNS depression. Discourage concomitant use.

Contraindications and precautions

- Contraindicated in patients hypersensitive to drug.
- Use cautiously in patients with impaired renal function or seizure disorder or when spasticity is used to maintain motor function. Also use cautiously in pregnant or breast-feeding women.
- Safety of oral or intrathecal use of drug hasn't been established in children under age 12 or 4, respectively.

NURSING CONSIDERATIONS

Assessment

- Obtain history of patient's pain and muscle spasms from underlying condition before therapy, and reassess regularly thereafter.
- Be alert for adverse reactions and drug interactions.
- Watch for increased risk of seizures in patient with seizure disorder.
- Evaluate patient's and family's understanding of drug therapy.

Nursing diagnoses

- Acute pain related to spasticity

• Risk for injury related to drug-induced adverse CNS reactions
• Deficient knowledge related to drug therapy

Planning and implementation

P.O. use: Give with meals or milk to prevent GI distress.
– Drug shouldn't be given orally to treat muscle spasm caused by rheumatic disorders, cerebral palsy, Parkinson's disease, or CVA because efficacy hasn't been established.
– Treatment for oral overdose is supportive; emesis shouldn't be induced and respiratory stimulant shouldn't be used in obtunded patient.
Intrathecal use: Implantable pump or catheter failure can result in sudden loss of effectiveness of intrathecal baclofen.
– Don't administer intrathecal injection by I.V., I.M., S.C., or epidural route.
• The amount of relief determines if dose (and drowsiness) can be reduced.
• Don't withdraw drug abruptly after long-term use unless required by severe adverse reactions; abrupt withdrawal may precipitate hallucinations or rebound spasticity.
• About 10% of patients may develop tolerance to drug. In some cases, this may be treated by hospitalizing patient and slowly withdrawing drug over 2-week period.
• Institute safety precautions if patient develops adverse CNS reactions.

Patient teaching
• Tell patient to avoid activities that require alertness until drug's CNS effects are known. Drowsiness usually is transient.
• Tell patient to avoid alcohol while taking drug.
• Advise patient to follow prescriber's orders about rest and physical therapy.
• Advise patient to take drug with food or milk to prevent GI distress.

Evaluation

• Patient reports that pain and muscle spasms have ceased with drug therapy.
• Patient doesn't experience injury as a result of drug-induced drowsiness.
• Patient and family state understanding of drug therapy.

basiliximab

(ba-sil-IK-si-mab)
Simulect

Pharmacologic class: recombinant chimeric human monoclonal antibody IgG_{1k}
Therapeutic class: immunosuppressant
Pregnancy risk category: B

Indications and dosages

▶ **Prevention of acute organ rejection in patients receiving renal transplantation when used as part of an immunosuppressive regimen that includes cyclosporine and corticosteroids.** *Adults and children over age 15:* 20 mg I.V. given within 2 hours before transplant surgery and 20 mg I.V. given 4 days after transplantation.
Children ages 2 to 15: 12 mg/m² (to maximum of 20 mg) I.V. given within 2 hours before transplant surgery and 12 mg/m² (to maximum of 20 mg) I.V. given 4 days after transplantation.

How supplied

Injection: 20-mg vials

Pharmacokinetics

Absorption: drug is administered I.V.
Distribution: unknown.
Metabolism: unknown.
Excretion: *half-life:* about 7.2 days in adults, 11.5 days in children.

Route	Onset	Peak	Duration
I.V.	Unknown	Immediate	Unknown

Pharmacodynamics

Chemical effect: binds specifically to and blocks the interleukin (IL)-2 receptor alpha chain on the surface of activated T lymphocytes, inhibiting IL-2–mediated activation of lymphocytes, a critical pathway in the cellular immune response involved in allograft rejection.

Therapeutic effect: prevents organ rejection.

Adverse reactions

CNS: agitation, anxiety, *asthenia,* depression, *dizziness, headache,* hypoesthesia, *insomnia,* neuropathy, paresthesia, *tremor,* fatigue.
CV: angina pectoris, ***arrhythmias,*** atrial fibrillation, ***heart failure,*** chest pain, abnormal heart sounds, aggravated hypertension, *hypertension,* hypotension, tachycardia.
EENT: abnormal vision, cataract, conjunctivitis, *rhinitis,* sinusitis, *pharyngitis.*
GI: *abdominal pain, candidiasis, constipation, diarrhea, dyspepsia,* esophagitis, enlarged abdomen, flatulence, gastroenteritis, GI disorder, ***GI hemorrhage,*** gum hyperplasia, melena, *nausea,* ulcerative stomatitis, *vomiting.*
GU: abnormal renal function, albuminuria, bladder disorder, *dysuria,* frequent micturition, genital edema, hematuria, *increased nonprotein nitrogen,* oliguria, renal tubular necrosis, surgery, ureteral disorder, *urinary tract infection,* urine retention, impotence.
Hematologic: *anemia*, hematoma, ***hemorrhage,*** polycythemia, purpura, ***thrombocytopenia,*** thrombosis.
Metabolic: *acidosis,* dehydration, diabetes mellitus, fluid overload, hypercalcemia, *hypercholesterolemia, hyperglycemia, hyperkalemia,* hyperlipemia, *hyperuricemia, hypocalcemia, hypokalemia,* hypomagnesemia, *hypophosphatemia,* hypoproteinemia, *weight gain.*
Musculoskeletal: arthralgia, arthropathy, *back pain,* bone fracture, cramps, hernia, *leg pain,* myalgia.
Respiratory: abnormal chest sounds, bronchitis, ***bronchospasm,*** *cough, dyspnea,* pneumonia, pulmonary disorder, ***pulmonary edema,*** *upper respiratory tract infection.*
Skin: *acne,* cyst, herpes simplex, herpes zoster, hypertrichosis, pruritus, rash, skin disorder or ulceration.
Other: accidental trauma, *viral infection, leg or peripheral edema,* general edema, infection, ***sepsis,*** *fever, surgical wound complications.*

Interactions

None significant.

Contraindications

- Contraindicated in patients hypersensitive to drug or its components.

NURSING CONSIDERATIONS

Assessment

- Monitor patient for anaphylactoid reactions. Be sure that drugs for treating severe hypersensitivity reactions are available for immediate use.
- Check for electrolyte imbalances and acidosis during drug therapy.
- Monitor patient's intake and output, vital signs, hemoglobin level, and hematocrit during therapy.
- Be alert for signs and symptoms of opportunistic infections during drug therapy.
- Evaluate patient's and family's knowledge of drug therapy.

Nursing diagnoses

- Risk for injury related to potential for organ rejection
- Ineffective protection related to drug-induced immunosuppression
- Deficient knowledge related to drug therapy

Planning and implementation

- Reconstitute with 5 ml sterile water for injection. Shake vial gently to dissolve powder. Dilute reconstituted solution to volume of 50 ml with normal saline solution or D_5W for infusion. When mixing solution, gently invert bag to avoid foaming. Don't shake.
- Infuse over 20 to 30 minutes via a central or peripheral vein. Don't add or infuse other drugs simultaneously through same I.V. line.
- Use reconstituted solution immediately; may be refrigerated between 36° to 46° F (2° to 8° C) for up to 24 hours or kept at room temperature for 4 hours.
- Drug must be used only under supervision of prescriber qualified and experienced in immunosuppressive therapy and management of organ transplantation.
- Drug must be used cautiously in elderly patients.

Patient teaching

- Inform patient of potential benefits and risks of immunosuppressive therapy, including decreased risk of graft loss or acute rejection. Advise patient that immunosuppressive therapy increases risks of developing lymphoproliferative disorders and opportunistic infections. Tell him to report signs and symptoms of infection promptly.
- Tell women of childbearing age to use effective contraception before therapy starts and for 2 months after therapy ends.
- Instruct patient to report adverse effects to prescriber immediately.
- Explain that drug is used with cyclosporine and corticosteroids.

Evaluation

- Patient doesn't experience organ rejection while taking this drug.
- Patient is free from infection and serious bleeding episodes throughout drug therapy.
- Patient and family state understanding of drug therapy.

becaplermin

(be-KAP-ler-min)

Regranex Gel

Pharmacologic class: recombinant human platelet-derived growth factor (rh-PDGF-BB)
Therapeutic class: wound repair agent
Pregnancy risk category: C

Indications and dosages

▶ **Diabetic neuropathic leg ulcers that extend into the subcutaneous tissue or beyond and have adequate blood supply.** *Adults:* apply daily in 1⁄16-inch even thickness to entire surface of wound. Use following table to calculate the length of gel to apply in inches or centimeters, which is dependent on wound size and tube size.

Tube size	Inches	Centimeters
2 g	Ulcer length × ulcer width × 1.3	(Ulcer length × ulcer width) ÷ 2
7.5 g, 15 g	Ulcer length × ulcer width × 0.6	(Ulcer length × ulcer width) ÷ 4

How supplied

Gel: 100 mcg/g in tubes of 2 g, 7.5 g, 15 g

Pharmacokinetics

Absorption: minimal systemic absorption.
Distribution: unknown.
Metabolism: unknown.
Excretion: unknown.

Route	Onset	Peak	Duration
Topical	Unknown	Unknown	Unknown

Pharmacodynamics

Chemical effect: thought to promote chemotactic recruitment and proliferation of cells involved in wound repair and formation of new granulation tissue.
Therapeutic effect: wound repair.

Adverse reactions

Musculoskeletal: osteomyelitis.
Skin: erythematous rash.
Other: cellulitis, infection.

Interactions

None significant.

Contraindications

- Contraindicated in patients hypersensitive to drug or its components (such as parabens or m-cresol) and in those with neoplasms at application site.

NURSING CONSIDERATIONS

Assessment

- Obtain history of patient's underlying condition before therapy, and reassess regularly thereafter.
- Ask woman if she's breast-feeding; use cautiously in breast-feeding women.
- Monitor wound size and healing; recalculate amount of drug to be applied at least once weekly. If ulcer doesn't decrease in size by about one-third after 10 weeks, or if complete healing hasn't occurred within 20 weeks, reassess treatment.
- Watch for application site reactions. Sensitization or irritation caused by parabens or m-cresol should be considered.

• Evaluate patient's and family's knowledge of drug therapy.

Nursing diagnoses

• Impaired skin integrity related to leg ulcer
• Acute pain related to presence of skin wound
• Deficient knowledge related to drug therapy

Planning and implementation

• When using the dosage formula, measure ulcer at its greatest length and width. Squeeze the gel onto clean measuring surface such as waxed paper. Use cotton swab or other application aid to transfer and spread drug over entire ulcer area in a 1/16-inch continuous layer. Place a saline-moistened dressing over site and leave in place for about 12 hours. After 12 hours, remove dressing and rinse away residual gel with normal saline solution or water, and apply a fresh moist dressing, without becaplermin, for rest of day.
• Drug is for external use only.
ALERT Don't use drug in wounds that close by primary intention.
• Treatment efficacy hasn't been evaluated for diabetic neuropathic ulcers that don't extend through the dermis into subcutaneous tissue or for ischemic diabetic ulcers.
• Drug facilitates complete healing of diabetic ulcers when used as an adjunct to good ulcer care practices, which include initial sharp debridement, infection control, and pressure relief.

Patient teaching

• Instruct patient to wash hands thoroughly before applying gel.
• Advise patient not to touch tip of tube against ulcer or any other surfaces.
• Instruct patient on proper procedure for wound care, including applying gel and changing dressings.
• Stress need to keep area covered with a wet dressing at all times.
• Tell patient to store drug in refrigerator (36° to 46° F [2° to 8° C]).
• Instruct patient not to use drug after expiration date.

Evaluation

• Patient experiences healing of ulcer.
• Patient doesn't experience pain.
• Patient and family state understanding of drug therapy.

beclomethasone dipropionate

(bek-loh-METH-eh-sohn digh-proh-PIGH-uh-nayt)

Aldecin Inhaler ◊, Beclodisk ♦, Becloforte Inhaler ◊, Beclovent, Beclovent Rotacaps ♦, Vanceril, Vanceril Double Strength Inhalation

Pharmacologic class: glucocorticoid
Therapeutic class: anti-inflammatory, antiasthmatic
Pregnancy risk category: C

Indications and dosages

▶ **Steroid-dependent asthma.** *Adults and children age 12 and over:* for regular strength, 2 inhalations t.i.d. or q.i.d or 4 inhalations b.i.d.; for double strength, 2 inhalations b.i.d. Maximum dosage is 840 mcg daily.
Children ages 6 to 12: for regular strength, 1 to 2 inhalations t.i.d. or q.i.d; for double strength, 2 inhalations b.i.d. Maximum dosage is 420 mcg daily.

How supplied

Oral inhalation aerosol: 42 mcg/metered spray, 50 mcg /metered spray ◊, 84 mcg/metered spray

Pharmacokinetics

Absorption: after oral inhalation, absorbed rapidly from lungs and GI tract.
Distribution: no evidence of tissue storage of beclomethasone or its metabolites. About 10% to 25% of an orally inhaled dose is deposited in respiratory tract. The remainder, deposited in mouth and oropharynx, is swallowed. When absorbed, it's 87% bound to plasma proteins.
Metabolism: most of drug is metabolized in liver.
Excretion: unknown, although when drug is administered systemically, its metabolites are

excreted mainly in feces and, to a lesser extent, in urine. *Half-life:* average 15 hours.

Route	Onset	Peak	Duration
Inhalation	1-4 wk	Unknown	Unknown

Pharmacodynamics

Chemical effect: decreases inflammation, mainly by stabilizing leukocyte lysosomal membranes.
Therapeutic effect: helps alleviate asthma symptoms.

Adverse reactions

EENT: hoarseness, fungal infections of throat, throat irritation, irritation of nasal mucosa.
GI: dry mouth, fungal infections of mouth.
Respiratory: ***bronchospasm.***
Other: ***angioedema, adrenal insufficiency.***

Interactions

None significant.

Contraindications and precautions

- Contraindicated in patients hypersensitive to drug or its components (fluorocarbons, oleic acid) and in those with status asthmaticus.
- Don't use in patients with asthma controlled by bronchodilators or other noncorticosteroids alone or in those with nonasthmatic bronchial diseases.
- Use with extreme caution, if at all, in patients with tuberculosis, fungal or bacterial infections, ocular herpes simplex, or systemic viral infections.
- Use with caution in patients receiving systemic corticosteroid therapy and in pregnant or breast-feeding women.
- Safety of drug hasn't been established in children under age 6.

NURSING CONSIDERATIONS

Assessment

- Obtain history of patient's asthma before therapy, and reassess regularly thereafter.
- Be alert for adverse reactions.
- Monitor patient closely during times of stress (trauma, surgery, or infection) because systemic corticosteroids may be needed to prevent adrenal insufficiency in previously steroid-dependent patients.
- Periodic measurement of growth and development may be necessary during high-dose or prolonged therapy in children.
- Evaluate patient's and family's understanding of drug therapy.
- Check for irritation of nasal mucosa.

Nursing diagnoses

- Impaired gas exchange related to asthma
- Impaired oral mucous membranes related to drug-induced fungal infections
- Deficient knowledge related to drug therapy

Planning and implementation

ALERT Never administer drug to relieve an emergency asthma attack because onset of action is too slow.

- Administer prescribed bronchodilators several minutes before beclomethasone.
- Have patient hold breath for a few seconds after each puff and rest 1 minute between puffs to enhance drug action.
- Spacer device may help ensure delivery of proper dose, although use of such a device with Becloforte Inhaler isn't recommended.
- Taper oral glucocorticoid therapy slowly, as ordered. Acute adrenal insufficiency and death have occurred in asthmatics who changed abruptly from oral corticosteroids to beclomethasone.
- Notify prescriber if decreased response is noted after administration of drug.
- Have patient gargle and rinse mouth with water after inhalations to help prevent oral fungal infections.
- Keep inhaler clean and unobstructed by washing it with warm water and drying it thoroughly after each use.

Patient teaching

- Inform patient that drug doesn't relieve acute asthma attacks.
- Tell patient who needs a bronchodilator to use it several minutes before drug.
- Instruct patient to wear or carry medical identification indicating need for supplemental systemic glucocorticoid during stress.
- Instruct patient to contact prescriber if response to therapy decreases or if symptoms

don't improve within 3 weeks; dosage may need to be adjusted. Tell patient not to exceed recommended dose on his own.
- Tell patient to keep inhaler clean and unobstructed by washing it with warm water and drying it thoroughly.
- Tell patient to prevent oral fungal infections by gargling or rinsing mouth with water after each use but not to swallow water.
- Tell patient to report symptoms of corticosteroid withdrawal, including fatigue, weakness, arthralgia, orthostatic hypotension, and dyspnea.
- Instruct patient to store drug between 36° and 86° F (2° and 30° C). Advise him to ensure delivery of proper dose by gently warming canister to room temperature before using. He may carry canister in pocket to keep it warm.

☑ Evaluation
- Patient's lungs are clear, and breathing and skin color are normal.
- Patient doesn't exhibit an oral fungal infection during therapy.
- Patient and family state understanding of drug therapy.

beclomethasone dipropionate monohydrate
(bek-loh-METH-eh-sohn digh-proh-PIGH-uh-nayt mon-oh-HIGH-drayt)

Beconase AQ Nasal Spray, Beconase Nasal Inhaler, Vancenase AQ Nasal Spray, Vancenase AQ 84 mcg, Vancenase Nasal Inhaler

Pharmacologic class: glucocorticoid
Therapeutic class: anti-inflammatory
Pregnancy risk category: C

Indications and dosages
▶ **Relief of symptoms of seasonal or perennial rhinitis; prevention of recurrence of nasal polyps after surgical removal.** *Adults and children over age 6:* for 42 mcg/metered spray, usual dosage is 1 or 2 sprays in each nostril, b.i.d. Maximum dosage is 336 mcg daily. For 84 mcg/metered spray, usual dosage is 1 to 2 inhalations daily. Maximum dosage is 336 mcg daily.

How supplied
Nasal aerosol: 42 mcg/metered spray
Nasal spray: 42 mcg/metered spray, 84 mcg/metered spray

Pharmacokinetics
Absorption: after nasal inhalation, drug is absorbed primarily through nasal mucosa with minimal systemic absorption.
Distribution: unknown.
Metabolism: most of drug is metabolized in liver.
Excretion: unknown, although when drug is administered systemically, its metabolites are excreted mainly in feces and, to a lesser extent, in urine. *Biological half-life:* average 15 hours.

Route	Onset	Peak	Duration
Inhalation	5-7 days	≤ 3 wk	Unknown

Pharmacodynamics
Chemical effect: decreases nasal inflammation, mainly by stabilizing leukocyte lysosomal membranes.
Therapeutic effect: helps relieve nasal allergy symptoms.

Adverse reactions
CNS: headache.
EENT: *mild, transient nasal burning and stinging;* nasal congestion; sneezing; epistaxis; watery eyes; nasopharyngeal fungal infections; irritation of nasal mucosa.
GI: nausea, vomiting.

Interactions
None significant.

Contraindications and precautions
- Contraindicated in patients hypersensitive to drug and in those experiencing status asthmaticus or other acute episodes of asthma.
- Use cautiously, if at all, in patients with active or quiescent respiratory tract tubercular infections or untreated fungal, bacterial, systemic viral, or ocular herpes simplex infec-

tions. Also use cautiously in patients who've recently had nasal septal ulcers, nasal surgery, or trauma.

- Use cautiously in pregnant or breast-feeding women.
- Safety of drug hasn't been established in children under age 6.

NURSING CONSIDERATIONS

Assessment

- Obtain history of patient's allergy symptoms and nasal congestion before therapy, and reassess regularly thereafter.
- Be alert for adverse reactions.
- Monitor patient's hydration status if adverse GI reactions occur.
- Evaluate patient's and family's understanding of drug therapy.
- Check for irritation of nasal mucosa.

Nursing diagnoses

- Ineffective health maintenance related to allergy-induced nasal congestion
- Risk for deficient fluid volume related to drug-induced adverse GI reactions
- Deficient knowledge related to drug therapy

Planning and implementation

- Drug isn't effective for acute exacerbations of rhinitis. Decongestants or antihistamines may be needed.
- Shake container and invert. Have patient clear his nasal passages and then tilt his head back. Insert nozzle into nostril (pointed away from septum), holding other nostril closed. Deliver spray while patient inhales. Shake container, and repeat in other nostril.
- Notify prescriber if relief isn't obtained or signs of infection appear.

Patient teaching

- Instruct patient to shake container before using, to blow nose to clear nasal passages, and to tilt head slightly forward and insert nozzle into nostril, pointing away from septum. Tell him to hold other nostril closed and then to inhale gently and spray. Next, have him shake container again and repeat in other nostril.
- Advise patient to pump new nasal spray three or four times before first use and then once or twice before first use each day thereafter. Also tell patient to clean cap and nosepiece of activator in warm water every day and then air-dry them.
- Advise patient to use drug regularly, as prescribed, because its effectiveness depends on regular use.
- Explain that drug's therapeutic effects, unlike those of decongestants, aren't immediate. Most patients achieve benefit within a few days, but some may require 2 to 3 weeks.
- Warn patient not to exceed recommended doses because of risk of hypothalamic-pituitary-adrenal function suppression.
- Tell patient to notify prescriber if symptoms don't improve within 3 weeks or if nasal irritation persists.
- Teach patient good nasal and oral hygiene.

Evaluation

- Patient's nasal congestion subsides with therapy.
- Patient maintains adequate hydration throughout therapy.
- Patient and family state understanding of drug therapy.

benazepril hydrochloride

(ben-AY-zuh-pril high-droh-KLOR-ighd)
Lotensin

Pharmacologic class: ACE inhibitor
Therapeutic class: antihypertensive
Pregnancy risk category: C (D in second and third trimesters)

Indications and dosages

▶ **Hypertension.** *Adults not taking diuretics:* initially, 10 mg P.O. daily. Dose adjusted, as needed and tolerated; most patients take 20 to 40 mg daily, divided into one or two doses.
Adults taking diuretics: discontinue diuretic 2 to 3 days before starting benazepril hydrochloride to minimize hypotension. If unable to discontinue diuretic, starting dose should be 5 mg daily.
In patients with renal insufficiency: starting dose is 5 mg daily.

How supplied

Tablets: 5 mg, 10 mg, 20 mg, 40 mg

Pharmacokinetics

Absorption: at least 37% is absorbed.
Distribution: serum protein binding of benazepril is about 96.7%; that of benazeprilat, 95.3%.
Metabolism: almost completely metabolized in liver to benazeprilat, which has much greater ACE inhibitory activity than benazepril, and to glucuronide conjugates of benazepril and benazeprilat.
Excretion: primarily in urine. *Half-life:* benazepril, 0.6 hours; benazeprilat, 10 to 12 hours.

Route	Onset	Peak	Duration
P.O.	≤ 1 hr	2-4 hr	24 hr

Pharmacodynamics

Chemical effect: inhibits ACE, preventing conversion of angiotensin I to angiotensin II, a potent vasoconstrictor. Reduced formation of angiotensin II decreases peripheral arterial resistance, thus decreasing aldosterone secretion. This reduces sodium and water retention and lowers blood pressure. Benazepril also has antihypertensive activity in patients with low-renin hypertension.
Therapeutic effect: lowers blood pressure.

Adverse reactions

CNS: asthenia, headache, dizziness, lightheadedness, anxiety, amnesia, depression, insomnia, nervousness, neuralgia, neuropathy, paresthesia, somnolence.
CV: symptomatic hypotension, syncope, angina, ***arrhythmias,*** palpitations, edema.
GI: nausea, vomiting, abdominal pain, constipation, dyspepsia, gastritis, dysphagia, increased salivation.
GU: impotence.
Metabolic: hyperkalemia, weight gain.
Musculoskeletal: arthralgia, arthritis, myalgia.
Respiratory: dry, persistent, tickling, nonproductive cough; dyspnea.
Skin: hypersensitivity reactions, rash, dermatitis, increased diaphoresis, pruritus, photosensitivity, purpura.
Other: ***angioedema.***

Interactions

Drug-drug. *ACE inhibitors, diuretics, other antihypertensives:* risk of excessive hypotension. Discontinue diuretic or lower dose of benazepril, as directed.
Digoxin: may increase plasma digoxin levels. Monitor patient for toxicity.
Indomethacin: may reduce hypotensive effects. Monitor blood pressure.
Lithium: increased serum lithium levels and lithium toxicity. Avoid concomitant use.
Potassium-sparing diuretics, potassium supplements: risk of hyperkalemia. Monitor patient closely.
Drug-herb. *Capsaicin*: may aggravate or cause ACE-induced cough. Discourage concomitant use.
Licorice: may cause sodium retention thus decreasing ACE effects. Discourage concomitant use.
Drug-food. *Foods, especially those high in fat:* can impair drug absorption. Instruct patient to take drug on an empty stomach.
Sodium substitutes containing potassium: risk of hyperkalemia. Monitor patient closely.

Contraindications and precautions

- Contraindicated in patients hypersensitive to ACE inhibitors.
- Use in pregnant women only if absolutely necessary and then with extreme caution. Drug is usually discontinued during pregnancy.
- Use cautiously in patients with impaired hepatic or renal function and in breast-feeding women.
- Safety of drug hasn't been established in children.

NURSING CONSIDERATIONS

Assessment

- Obtain history of patient's blood pressure before therapy, and reassess regularly thereafter. Measure blood pressure when drug levels are at peak (2 to 6 hours after dose) and at trough (just before dose) to verify adequate blood pressure control.
- Be alert for adverse reactions and drug interactions.
- Monitor patient's ECG.

• Monitor renal and hepatic function periodically, as ordered. Also monitor serum potassium levels.
• Monitor patient's CBC with differential every 2 weeks for first 3 months of therapy and periodically thereafter, as ordered. Other ACE inhibitors have been linked to agranulocytosis and neutropenia.
• Evaluate patient's and family's understanding of drug therapy.

Nursing diagnoses
• Risk for injury related to hypertension
• Decreased cardiac output related to drug-induced arrhythmias
• Deficient knowledge related to drug therapy

Planning and implementation
• If patient is taking a diuretic, dose should be lower than if patient isn't taking a diuretic; excessive hypotension can occur when drug is given with diuretics.
• Dosage adjustment may be necessary in patients with renal impairment.
• Administer at about same time every day to maintain consistent effect on blood pressure.
• Administer drug when patient's stomach is empty.

Patient teaching
• Instruct patient to take drug on an empty stomach; meals, particularly those high in fat, can impair absorption.
• Tell patient to avoid sodium substitutes; such products may contain potassium, which can cause hyperkalemia in patients taking drug.
• Tell patient to rise slowly to minimize risk of dizziness, which may occur during first few weeks of therapy. If dizziness does occur, he should stop taking drug and call prescriber immediately.
• Tell patient to use caution in hot weather and during exercise. Inadequate fluid intake, vomiting, diarrhea, and excessive perspiration can lead to light-headedness and syncope.
• Urge patient to report signs of infection, such as fever and sore throat. Also tell him to call prescriber if the following signs or symptoms occur: easy bruising or bleeding; swelling of tongue, lips, face, eyes, mucous membranes, or limbs; difficulty swallowing or breathing; and hoarseness.
• Tell women to notify prescriber if pregnancy occurs. Drug will need to be discontinued.

Evaluation
• Patient's blood pressure is normal.
• Patient maintains adequate cardiac output during drug therapy.
• Patient and family state understanding of drug therapy.

benzonatate
(ben-ZOH-nuh-tayt)
Tessalon

Pharmacologic class: local anesthetic (ester)
Therapeutic class: nonnarcotic antitussive
Pregnancy risk category: C

Indications and dosages
▶ **Symptomatic relief of cough.** *Adults and children over age 10:* 100 mg P.O. t.i.d., increased as needed to maximum of 600 mg daily.

How supplied
Capsules: 100 mg

Pharmacokinetics
Unknown.

Route	Onset	Peak	Duration
P.O.	15-20 min	Unknown	≤ 8 hr

Pharmacodynamics
Chemical effect: suppresses cough reflex by direct action on cough center in medulla. Also has local anesthetic action.
Therapeutic effect: relieves cough.

Adverse reactions
CNS: dizziness, drowsiness, headache, restlessness.
EENT: nasal congestion, burning sensation in eyes.
GI: nausea, constipation.
Skin: rash.
Other: chills.

Interactions

None significant.

Contraindications and precautions

- Contraindicated in patients hypersensitive to drug.
- Use cautiously in pregnant women and in patients hypersensitive to para-aminobenzoic acid anesthetics (procaine, tetracaine) because cross-sensitivity reactions may occur.
- Safety of drug hasn't been established in breast-feeding women and in children under age 10.

NURSING CONSIDERATIONS

Assessment

- Obtain history of patient's cough before therapy, and reassess regularly thereafter.
- Be alert for adverse reactions.
- Evaluate patient's and family's understanding of drug therapy.

Nursing diagnoses

- Ineffective airway clearance related to underlying condition producing nonproductive cough
- Risk for injury related to drug-induced adverse CNS reactions
- Deficient knowledge related to drug therapy

Planning and implementation

- Don't use benzonatate when cough is a valuable diagnostic sign or is beneficial (such as after thoracic surgery).
- Use with percussion and chest vibration.
- Maintain fluid intake to help liquefy sputum.

Patient teaching

ALERT Warn patient not to chew capsules or let them dissolve in his mouth because resulting local anesthesia may cause aspiration.
- Warn patient about increased risk of choking.
- Instruct patient not to take more of drug than directed.
- Tell patient to call prescriber if cough persists more than 7 days.
- Caution patient against performing hazardous activities that require alertness until CNS effects of drug are known.
- Explain importance of consuming 2,000 to 3,000 ml of fluid daily to liquefy sputum.

Evaluation

- Patient's cough is resolved.
- Patient doesn't experience injury as result of drug-induced adverse CNS reactions.
- Patient and family state understanding of drug therapy.

benztropine mesylate

(BENZ-troh-peen MES-ih-layt)

Apo-Benztropine♦, Cogentin

Pharmacologic class: anticholinergic
Therapeutic class: antiparkinsonian
Pregnancy risk category: NR

Indications and dosages

▶ **Drug-induced extrapyramidal disorders (except tardive dyskinesia).** *Adults:* 1 to 4 mg P.O. or I.V. once or twice daily.

▶ **Acute dystonic reaction.** *Adults:* 1 to 2 mg I.V. or I.M., followed by 1 to 2 mg P.O. b.i.d. to prevent recurrence.

▶ **Parkinsonism.** *Adults:* 0.5 to 6 mg P.O. daily. Initial dose is 0.5 to 1 mg. Increased by 0.5 mg q 5 to 6 days. Adjust dosage to meet individual requirements.

How supplied

Tablets: 0.5 mg, 1 mg, 2 mg
Injection: 1 mg/ml in 2-ml ampules

Pharmacokinetics

Absorption: absorbed from GI tract when administered P.O.
Distribution: largely unknown; however, drug crosses blood-brain barrier.
Metabolism: unknown.
Excretion: excreted in urine as unchanged drug and metabolites. After P.O. therapy, small amounts may be excreted in feces as unabsorbed drug.

Route	Onset	Peak	Duration
P.O.	1-2 hr	Unknown	24 hr
I.V., I.M.	≤ 15 min	Unknown	24 hr

Pharmacodynamics

Chemical effect: unknown; thought to block central cholinergic receptors, helping to balance cholinergic activity in basal ganglia.
Therapeutic effect: improves capability for voluntary movement.

Adverse reactions

CNS: disorientation, restlessness, irritability, incoherence, hallucinations, headache, sedation, depression.
CV: palpitations, tachycardia, ***paradoxical bradycardia.***
EENT: dilated pupils, blurred vision, photophobia, difficulty swallowing.
GI: dry mouth, *constipation,* nausea, vomiting, epigastric distress.
GU: urinary hesitancy, urine retention.
Musculoskeletal: muscle weakness.
Skin: flushing.

Interactions

Drug-drug. *Amantadine, phenothiazines, tricyclic antidepressants:* additive anticholinergic adverse reactions, such as confusion and hallucinations. Reduce dose before administering.

Contraindications and precautions

- Contraindicated in patients with acute angle-closure glaucoma, in patients hypersensitive to drug or its components, in children under age 3, and in breast-feeding women.
- Use cautiously in patients exposed to hot weather, in those with mental disorders, in pregnant women, and in children age 3 and older.

NURSING CONSIDERATIONS

Assessment

- Obtain history of patient's dyskinetic movements and underlying condition before therapy.
- Monitor effectiveness by regularly checking body movements for signs of improvement; full effect of drug may take 2 to 3 days.
- Be alert for adverse reactions and drug interactions. Some adverse reactions may result from atropine-like toxicity and are dose-related.
- Evaluate patient's and family's understanding of drug therapy.

Nursing diagnoses

- Impaired physical mobility related to dyskinetic movements
- Risk for injury related to drug-induced adverse CNS reactions
- Deficient knowledge related to drug therapy

Planning and implementation

P.O. use: Administer drug after meals to help prevent GI distress.
I.V. use: Drug is seldom used I.V. because of small difference in onset compared with I.M. route.
I.M. use: The I.M. route is preferred for parenteral administration.
- Give drug at bedtime if patient is to receive single daily dose.

ALERT Never discontinue drug abruptly; reduce dose gradually.

Patient teaching

- Warn patient to avoid activities requiring alertness until CNS effects of drug are known.
- If patient is to receive single daily dose, tell him to take it at bedtime.
- If patient is to receive drug orally, tell him to take it after meals.
- Advise patient to report signs of urinary hesitancy or urine retention.
- Tell patient to relieve dry mouth with cool drinks, ice chips, sugarless gum, or hard candy.
- Advise patient to limit activities during hot weather because drug-induced anhidrosis may result in hyperthermia.
- In general, elderly and thin patients can't tolerate larger dosages of this medication.

Evaluation

- Patient exhibits improved mobility with reduction in muscle rigidity, akinesia, and tremors.
- Patient doesn't experience injury as result of drug-induced adverse CNS reactions.
- Patient and family state understanding of drug therapy.

bepridil hydrochloride

(BEH-prih-dil high-droh-KLOR-ighd)
Vascor

Pharmacologic class: calcium channel blocker
Therapeutic class: antianginal
Pregnancy risk category: C

Indications and dosages

▶ **Chronic stable angina in patients who can't tolerate or who fail to respond to other drugs.** *Adults:* initially, 200 mg P.O. daily. After 10 days, increase dosage based on response. Maintenance dosage in most patients is 300 mg/day. Maximum daily dosage is 400 mg.

How supplied

Tablets: 200 mg, 300 mg, 400 mg

Pharmacokinetics

Absorption: rapidly and completely absorbed.
Distribution: more than 99% is plasma protein–bound.
Metabolism: metabolized in liver.
Excretion: over 10 days, 70% is excreted in urine, 22% in feces as metabolites. *Half-life:* after multiple doses, averages 42 hours.

Route	Onset	Peak	Duration
P.O.	Unknown	2-3 hr	24 hr

Pharmacodynamics

Chemical effect: inhibits calcium ion influx across cardiac and smooth muscle cells. This action dilates coronary arteries, peripheral arteries, and arterioles; it may reduce heart rate, decrease myocardial contractility, and slow AV node conduction.
Therapeutic effect: prevents anginal pain.

Adverse reactions

CNS: dizziness.
CV: edema; flushing; palpitations; tachycardia; ***ventricular arrhythmias, including torsades de pointes, ventricular tachycardia, and ventricular fibrillation.***
GI: nausea, diarrhea.
Hematology: ***agranulocytosis.***
Respiratory: dyspnea.
Skin: rash.

Interactions

Drug-drug. *Antiarrhythmics, tricyclic antidepressants:* could prolong QT interval. Use together cautiously.
Cardiac glycosides: could exaggerate AV nodal conduction. Use together cautiously.

Contraindications and precautions

- Contraindicated in patients hypersensitive to drug and in those with uncompensated cardiac insufficiency, sick sinus syndrome, or second- or third-degree AV block unless pacemaker is present; hypotension; congenital QT interval prolongation; or history of serious ventricular arrhythmias. Also contraindicated in those receiving other drugs that prolong QT interval.
- Use cautiously in pregnant women and in patients with left bundle branch block, sinus bradycardia (less than 50 beats/minute), impaired renal or hepatic function, or heart failure.
- Risk-benefit ratio must be assessed for use in breast-feeding women because of risk of serious adverse reactions in infants.
- Safe use of drug hasn't been established in children.

NURSING CONSIDERATIONS

Assessment

- Obtain history of patient's angina before therapy; reassess regularly thereafter.
- Be alert for adverse reactions and drug interactions.
- Monitor patient's ECG, heart rate, and rhythm regularly; use of bepridil may cause severe ventricular arrhythmias, including torsades de pointes.
- Monitor patient's CBC and differential; use of drug is linked to agranulocytosis.
- Evaluate patient's and family's understanding of drug therapy.
- Elderly patients don't need a reduced dosage but do need frequent monitoring for hepatic impairment.

Nursing diagnoses
• Acute pain related to presence of angina
• Ineffective protection related to drug-induced ventricular arrhythmias
• Deficient knowledge related to drug therapy

Planning and implementation
• Give drug following usual protocol for P.O. administration.
• Consult prescriber if patient doesn't experience pain relief.

Patient teaching
• Tell patient to report unusual bruising, bleeding, or signs of persistent infection promptly.
• Stress the importance of taking drug exactly as prescribed, even when feeling well.
• Tell patient to schedule activities to allow adequate rest.
• Encourage patient to restrict fluid and sodium intake to minimize edema.

Evaluation
• Patient states that angina is relieved.
• Patient's ECG, heart rate, and rhythm are unchanged with therapy.
• Patient and family state understanding of drug therapy.

beractant (natural lung surfactant)
(beh-RAK-tant)
Survanta

Pharmacologic class: bovine lung extract
Therapeutic class: lung surfactant
Pregnancy risk category: NR

Indications and dosages
▶ **Prevention and rescue treatment of respiratory distress syndrome (RDS, or hyaline membrane disease), in premature infants weighing 1,250 g (2.75 lb) or less at birth or having symptoms of surfactant deficiency.** *Infants:* 4 ml/kg administered by intratracheal instillation through a #5 French end-hole catheter inserted into the neonate's endotracheal tube with the tip of the catheter protruding just beyond the end of the tube above the carina. Length of catheter should be shortened before inserting it through the tube. Drug shouldn't be instilled into a mainstem bronchus. Use the following dosing table:

BERACTANT DOSING CHART

Weight (g)	Total dose (ml)
600 to 650	2.6
651 to 700	2.8
701 to 750	3
751 to 800	3.2
801 to 850	3.4
851 to 900	3.6
901 to 950	3.8
951 to 1,000	4
1,001 to 1,050	4.2
1,051 to 1,100	4.4
1,101 to 1,150	4.6
1,151 to 1,200	4.8
1,201 to 1,250	5
1,251 to 1,300	5.2
1,301 to 1,350	5.4
1,351 to 1,400	5.6
1,401 to 1,450	5.8
1,451 to 1,500	6
1,501 to 1,550	6.2
1,551 to 1,600	6.4
1,601 to 1,650	6.6
1,651 to 1,700	6.8
1,701 to 1,750	7
1,751 to 1,800	7.2
1,801 to 1,850	7.4
1,851 to 1,900	7.6
1,901 to 1,950	7.8
1,951 to 2,000	8

How supplied
Suspension for intratracheal instillation: 25 mg/ml

Pharmacokinetics
Absorption: most of dose becomes lung-associated within hours.
Distribution: distributed across alveolar surface.

Metabolism: lipids enter endogenous surfactant pathway of recycling and reutilization.
Excretion: alveolar clearance of lipid components is rapid.

Route	Onset	Peak	Duration
Intratracheal	0.5-2 hr	Unknown	2-3 days

Pharmacodynamics

Chemical effect: lowers surface tension of alveoli during respiration and stabilizes alveoli against collapse. An extract of bovine lung containing neutral lipids, fatty acids, surfactant-associated proteins, and phospholipids that mimics naturally occurring surfactant; palmitic acid, tripalmitin, and colfosceril palmitate are added to standardize solution's composition.
Therapeutic effect: prevents RDS in premature neonates with specific characteristics.

Adverse reactions

CV: ***bradycardia,*** vasoconstriction, hypotension.
Respiratory: endotracheal tube reflux or blockage, ***apnea,*** decreased oxygen saturation, hypocapnia, hypercapnia.
Other: pallor.

Interactions

None significant.

Contraindications and precautions

No known contraindications.

NURSING CONSIDERATIONS

Assessment

- Obtain history of neonate's respiratory status before therapy.
- Continuously monitor neonate before, during, and after beractant administration for effectiveness.
- Continuously monitor ECG and transcutaneous oxygen saturation; also, frequently monitor arterial blood pressure and sample arterial blood gas. Transient bradycardia and oxygen desaturation are common after dosing.
- Evaluate parent's understanding of drug therapy.

Nursing diagnoses

- Risk for injury related to potential for RDS
- Deficient knowledge related to drug therapy

Planning and implementation

ALERT Beractant should be administered only by personnel experienced in care of clinically unstable premature neonates. Such personnel should have knowledge of neonatal intubation and airway management.
- Accurate determination of weight is essential to ensure proper measurement of dose.
- Endotracheal tube may be suctioned before giving drug; allow neonate to stabilize before proceeding with administration.
- Refrigerate drug at 36° to 46° F (2° to 8° C). Warm before administration by allowing drug to stand at room temperature for at least 20 minutes or by holding in hand for at least 8 minutes. Don't use artificial warming methods. Unopened vials that have been warmed to room temperature may be returned to refrigerator within 8 hours; warm and return drug to refrigerator only once. Vials are for single use only; discard unused drug.
- Beractant doesn't need sonication or reconstitution before use. Inspect contents before giving; ensure that color is off-white to light brown and that contents are uniform. If settling occurs, swirl vial gently; don't shake. Some foaming is normal.
- Homogeneous distribution of drug is important. In clinical trials, each dose of drug was given in four quarter-doses, with patient positioned differently after each administration. Each quarter-dose was given over 2 to 3 seconds; the catheter was removed and patient ventilated between quarter-doses. With head and body inclined slightly downward, first quarter-dose was given with head turned to right; second quarter-dose, with head turned to left. Then head and body were inclined slightly upward; third quarter-dose was given with head turned to right; fourth quarter-dose, with head turned to left.
- Moist breath sounds and crackles can occur immediately after administration. Don't suction neonate for 1 hour unless other signs of airway obstruction are evident.

• Audiovisual materials that describe dose and administration procedures are available from manufacturer.
• Beractant can rapidly affect oxygenation and lung compliance. Peak ventilator inspiratory pressures may need to be adjusted if chest expansion improves substantially after drug administration. Notify prescriber and adjust immediately, as directed, because lung overdistention and fatal pulmonary air leakage may result.
• For prevention, beractant should be administered within 15 minutes of birth.
• For active rescue treatment, administer first dose within 8 hours of birth.

Patient teaching
• Teach parents about beractant therapy.
• Reassure parents that neonate will be monitored at all times.

☑ Evaluation
• Patient doesn't develop RDS.
• Parents state understanding of drug therapy.

17 beta-estradiol/norgestimate
(SEV-en-tene bay-ta-s-tra-dye-ol nor-JES-ti-mate)
Ortho-Prefest

Pharmacologic class: combined synthetic estrogen and progestin
Therapeutic class: hormone replacement
Pregnancy risk category: X

Indications and dosages
▶ **Treatment of moderate to severe vasomotor symptoms and vulvar and vaginal atrophy caused by menopause; prevention of osteoporosis in women with an intact uterus.** *Adults:* 1 mg estradiol (pink tablet) P.O. daily for 3 days; then 1 mg estradiol/0.09 mg norgestimate (white tablet) P.O. daily for 3 days. Repeat cycle until blister card is empty.

How supplied
Tablets: blister card of 15 pink and 15 white tablets, for a total of 30 tablets
Pink tablets: 1 mg estradiol
White tablets: 1 mg estradiol and 0.09 mg norgestimate

Pharmacokinetics
Absorption: estradiol reaches peak serum levels about 7 hours after a dose. The metabolite of norgestimate, 17-deacetylnorgestimate, reaches peak serum levels about 2 hours after a dose. When given with a high-fat meal, peak serum levels of estrone and estrone sulfate were increased by 14% and 24% respectively; peak serum level of 17-deacetylnorgestimate was decreased by 16%.
Distribution: estrogens are widely distributed throughout the body. Estradiol is bound mainly to sex hormone–binding globulin, and to albumin. The primary active metabolite of norgestimate, 17-deacetylnorgestimate, is about 99% protein-bound.
Metabolism: estrogens are mainly metabolized in the liver. Estradiol is converted reversibly to estrone, and both can be converted to estriol, which is the major urinary metabolite. Estrogens also undergo enterohepatic recirculation via sulfate and glucuronide conjugation in the liver, biliary secretion of conjugates in the intestine, and hydrolysis in the gut followed by reabsorption. Norgestimate is extensively metabolized by first-pass metabolism to 17-deacetylnorgestimate in the GI tract or liver.
Excretion: estradiol, estrone, and estriol are excreted in the urine. Norgestimate metabolites are eliminated in the urine or feces. *Half-life:* about 16 hours for estradiol and 37 hours for 17-deacetylnorgestimate in postmenopausal women.

Route	Onset	Peak	Duration
P.O.	Unknown	7 hr (estradiol) 2 hr (norgestimate)	Unknown

Pharmacodynamics
Chemical effect: mimics the action of endogenous estrogen and natural progesterone. Circulating estrogens modulate pituitary secretion of gonadotropins, luteinizing hormone, and follicle-stimulating hormone through a negative feedback mechanism. They also contribute to the shaping of the skeleton. Estrogen replacement therapy reduces elevated levels of

these hormones in postmenopausal women. Estradiol is more potent than its metabolites estrone and estriol.

Norgestimate mimics the natural hormone progesterone. Progestins counter estrogenic effects by decreasing the number of nuclear estradiol receptors and suppressing epithelial DNA synthesis in endometrial tissue.
Therapeutic effect: relieves menopausal vasomotor symptoms and vaginal dryness; reduces the severity of osteoporosis.

Adverse reactions

CNS: depression, dizziness, fatigue, pain, *headache.*
EENT: pharyngitis, sinusitis.
GI: flatulence, nausea, *abdominal pain.*
GU: dysmenorrhea, vaginal bleeding, vaginitis.
Musculoskeletal: arthralgia, myalgia, *back pain.*
Respiratory: cough, *upper respiratory tract infection.*
Other: *flulike symptoms,* viral infection, *breast pain,* tooth disorder.

Interactions

None reported.

Contraindications and precautions

- Contraindicated in patients hypersensitive to any component of Ortho-Prefest and in patients with known or suspected pregnancy, cancer of the breast, estrogen-dependent neoplasia, undiagnosed abnormal vaginal bleeding, or active or previous thrombophlebitis or thromboembolic disorders.
- Use cautiously in women who have have had a hysterectomy, who are overweight, who have abnormal lipid profiles, or who have impaired liver function.

NURSING CONSIDERATIONS

Assessment

- Obtain history of patient's underlying condition before therapy, and reassess regularly thereafter.
- Make sure patient has a thorough physical examination before starting drug therapy.
- Assess patient's risks for venous thromboembolism.
- Assess patient's risk for cancer; hormone replacement therapy may increase the risk of breast cancer in postmenopausal women.
- Stay alert for adverse reactions.
- Evaluate patient's and family's knowledge of drug therapy.

Nursing diagnoses

- Ineffective peripheral tissue perfusion related to drug-induced thromboembolism
- Ineffective health maintenance related to underlying condition
- Deficient knowledge related to drug therapy

Planning and implementation

- Reassess patient at 6-month intervals to make sure treatment is still needed.
- Estrogens may induce malignant neoplasms. Combining progestin therapy with estrogen therapy significantly reduces this risk.
- Monitor patient for hypercalcemia if she has breast cancer and bone metastases. If severe hypercalcemia occurs, notify the prescriber and stop the drug; take the appropriate measures to reduce serum calcium level, as ordered.
- These test results may be elevated: thyroid-binding globulin; platelet count; factors II, VII antigen, VIII antigen, VIII coagulant activity, IX, X, XII, VII-X complex, and II-VII-X complex; beta-thromboglobulin; high-density lipoproteins; triglycerides; corticosteroids; sex steroids; angiotensinogen/renin substrate; alpha$_1$-antitrypsin; ceruloplasmin; fibrinogen; and plasminogen antigen. Also, PT, PTT, and platelet aggregation time may be accelerated.
- The following test results may be decreased: T_3 resin uptake, serum folate, metyrapone, glucose tolerance, low-density lipoproteins, anti-factor Xa, and antithrombin III.

Patient teaching

- Explain the risk of taking estrogen therapy, such as breast cancer, cancer of the uterus, abnormal blood clotting and gallbladder disease.
- Tell patient to immediately report any undiagnosed, persistent, or recurring abnormal vaginal bleeding.

• Instruct women taking this drug to perform monthly breast examinations. Also, recommend a mammogram if patient is over age 50.
• Tell patient to immediately report pain in the calves or chest, sudden shortness of breath, coughing blood, severe headache, vomiting, dizziness, faintness, changes in vision or speech, and weakness or numbness in arms or legs. These are warning signals of blood clots.
• Urge patient to report evidence of liver problems, such as yellowing of skin or eyes and upper right quadrant pain.
• Instruct patient to report pain, swelling, or tenderness in abdomen, which may indicate gallbladder problems.
• Tell patient to store drug at room temperature away from excessive heat and moisture. It remains stable for 18 months.

Evaluation
• Patient has no thromboembolic event during therapy.
• Patient's underlying condition improves.
• Patient and family state understanding of drug therapy.

betamethasone
(bay-tuh-METH-uh-sohn)
Betnesol♦, Celestone*

betamethasone acetate and betamethasone sodium phosphate
Celestone Chronodose◇, Celestone Soluspan

betamethasone sodium phosphate
Celestone Phosphate, Selestoject

Pharmacologic class: glucocorticoid
Therapeutic class: anti-inflammatory
Pregnancy risk category: NR

Indications and dosages
▶ **Conditions of severe inflammation or that need immunosuppression.** *Adults:* 0.6 to 7.2 mg P.O. daily. Or, 0.5 to 9 mg I.V., I.M., or injected into joint or soft tissue daily. Or, 0.5 to 2 ml of sodium phosphate-acetate suspension injected into joint or soft tissue q 1 to 2 weeks, p.r.n.

How supplied
betamethasone
Tablets: 600 mcg
Tablets (extended-release): 1 mg
Tablets (effervescent): 500 mcg♦
Syrup: 600 mcg/5 ml
betamethasone acetate and betamethasone sodium phosphate
Injection (suspension): betamethasone acetate 3 mg and betamethasone sodium phosphate (equivalent to 3-mg base) per ml
betamethasone sodium phosphate
Tablets (effervescent): 500 mcg
Injection: 4 mg (equivalent to 3-mg base)/ml in 5-ml vials

Pharmacokinetics
Absorption: absorbed readily after P.O. administration. Systemic absorption occurs slowly after intra-articular injections.
Distribution: removed rapidly from blood and distributed to muscle, liver, skin, intestines, and kidneys. Bound weakly to plasma proteins. Only unbound portion is active.
Metabolism: metabolized in liver to inactive glucuronide and sulfate metabolites.
Excretion: inactive metabolites and small amounts of unmetabolized drug are excreted in urine. Insignificant quantities of drug are also excreted in feces. *Half-life:* 36 to 54 hours.

Route	Onset	Peak	Duration
P.O.	Unknown	1-2 hr	3.25 days
I.V., I.M., intra-articular	Rapid	Unknown	7-14 days

Pharmacodynamics
Chemical effect: not completely defined. Decreases inflammation, mainly by stabilizing leukocyte lysosomal membranes; suppresses immune response; stimulates bone marrow; and influences protein, fat, and carbohydrate metabolism.
Therapeutic effect: causes immunosuppression.

Adverse reactions

CNS: *euphoria, insomnia,* psychotic behavior, pseudotumor cerebri, ***seizures.***
CV: ***heart failure,*** hypertension, edema, ***thromboembolism.***
EENT: cataracts, glaucoma.
GI: *peptic ulceration,* GI irritation, increased appetite, pancreatitis.
Metabolic: hypokalemia, hyperglycemia, carbohydrate intolerance.
Musculoskeletal: muscle weakness, osteoporosis, growth suppression in children.
Skin: hirsutism, delayed wound healing, acne, various skin eruptions.
Other: susceptibility to infections, ***acute adrenal insufficiency*** after stress (infection, surgery, or trauma) or abrupt withdrawal after long-term therapy.

Interactions

Drug-drug. *Aspirin, indomethacin, other NSAIDs:* increased risk of GI distress and bleeding. Give together cautiously.
Barbiturates, phenytoin, rifampin: decreased corticosteroid effect. Corticosteroid dosage may need to be increased.
Oral anticoagulants: altered dosage requirements. Monitor PT and INR closely.
Potassium-depleting drugs (such as thiazide diuretics): enhanced potassium-depleting effects of betamethasone. Monitor serum potassium levels.
Skin test antigens: decreased response. Defer skin testing until therapy is completed.
Toxoids, vaccines: decreased antibody response and increased risk of neurologic complications. Avoid concomitant use. Delay vaccines if possible.

Contraindications and precautions

- Contraindicated in patients hypersensitive to drug and in those with viral or bacterial infections (except in life-threatening situations) or systemic fungal infections.
- Use with extreme caution, and only in life-threatening situations, in patients with recent MI or peptic ulcer.
- Use cautiously in patients with renal disease, hypertension, osteoporosis, diabetes mellitus, hypothyroidism, cirrhosis, diverticulitis, nonspecific ulcerative colitis, recent intestinal anastomoses, thromboembolic disorders, seizures, myasthenia gravis, heart failure, tuberculosis, ocular herpes simplex, emotional instability, or psychotic tendencies. Because some formulations contain sulfite preservatives, use cautiously in patients sensitive to sulfites. Also use cautiously in pregnant women.
- Breast-feeding women should discontinue breast-feeding if drug is given.
- Safety of drug hasn't been established in children under age 12.

NURSING CONSIDERATIONS

Assessment

- Obtain history of patient's underlying condition and current health status, including vital signs and weight.
- Be alert for adverse reactions and drug interactions. Most adverse reactions are dose- or duration-dependent.
- Monitor patient's weight, blood pressure, and blood glucose and serum potassium levels regularly, as ordered.
- Monitor patient for early signs of adrenal insufficiency or cushingoid symptoms. Adrenal suppression may last up to 1 year after drug is stopped.
- Monitor patient's stress level. Stress (fever, trauma, surgery, or emotional problems) may increase adrenal insufficiency.
- Evaluate patient's and family's understanding of drug therapy.

Nursing diagnoses

- Ineffective health maintenance related to underlying condition
- Risk for injury related to drug-induced adverse reactions
- Deficient knowledge related to drug therapy

Planning and implementation

P.O. use: Give drug with milk or food to reduce GI irritation.
I.V. use: Drug is compatible with normal saline solution, D_5W, lactated Ringer's injection, dextrose 5% in lactated Ringer's injection, and dextrose 5% in Ringer's injection. Suspension for injection isn't for I.V. use.

I.M. use: Give I.M. injection deeply to prevent muscle atrophy. Rotate injection sites.
Intra-articular use: Prepare drug for prescriber to administer, as directed.
- Drug shouldn't be used for alternate-day therapy.
- Give once-daily dose in the morning for best results and least toxicity.
- Drug should always be adjusted to lowest effective dose.

ALERT Gradually reduce drug dosage after long-term therapy, as ordered. After abrupt withdrawal patient may experience rebound inflammation, fatigue, weakness, arthralgia, fever, dizziness, lethargy, depression, fainting, orthostatic hypotension, dyspnea, anorexia, and hypoglycemia. After prolonged use, sudden withdrawal may be fatal.
- Expect to increase dose, as ordered, during times of physiologic stress (surgery, trauma, or infection).
- Potassium supplements may be necessary for patients receiving long-term therapy.

Patient teaching
- Tell patient not to stop drug abruptly or without prescriber's consent.
- Tell patient using effervescent tablets to dissolve them in water immediately before ingestion.
- Teach patient about drug's effects. Warn patient receiving long-term therapy about cushingoid symptoms; instruct him to report sudden weight gain or swelling to prescriber.
- Instruct patient to report symptoms of corticosteroid withdrawal, including fatigue, weakness, arthralgia, orthostatic hypotension, and dyspnea.
- Tell patient to contact prescriber if symptoms worsen or drug is no longer effective. Also tell him not to increase dose without prescriber's consent.
- Advise elderly patient receiving long-term therapy to consider exercise or physical therapy. Tell him to ask prescriber about vitamin D or calcium supplements.
- Advise patient receiving prolonged therapy to have periodic ophthalmic examinations.
- Tell patient to report slow healing.
- Instruct patient to wear or carry medical identification indicating his need for supplemental corticosteroids during stress.

☑ Evaluation
- Patient's underlying condition improves.
- Patient doesn't experience injury as a result of drug-induced adverse reactions.
- Patient and family state understanding of drug therapy.

betaxolol hydrochloride
(beh-TAKS-oh-lol high-droh-KLOR-ighd)
Betoptic, Betoptic S, Kerlone

Pharmacologic class: beta blocker
Therapeutic class: antihypertensive
Pregnancy risk category: C

Indications and dosages
▶ **Hypertension**. *Adults:* initially, 10 mg P.O. once daily. 20 mg P.O. once daily if desired response not achieved in 7 to 14 days.
▶ **Elevated intraocular pressure, occular hypertension, chronid open-angle glaucoma.** *Adults:* 1 to 2 drops in affected eye(s) b.i.d.

How supplied
Tablets: 10 mg, 20 mg

Pharmacokinetics
Absorption: absorbed completely. Small first-pass effect reduces bioavailability by about 10%.
Distribution: about 50% bound to plasma proteins.
Metabolism: metabolized in liver.
Excretion: excreted primarily in urine (about 80%) as metabolites. *Half-life:* 14 to 22 hours.

Route	Onset	Peak	Duration
P.O.	≤ 3 hr	2-4 hr (antihypertensive effects peak in 7-14 days)	24-48 hr

Pharmacodynamics
Chemical effect: unknown.

Therapeutic effect: reduces blood pressure.

Adverse reactions

CNS: dizziness, fatigue, headache, lethargy, anxiety.
CV: ***bradycardia,*** chest pain, hypotension, worsening of angina, peripheral vascular insufficiency, ***heart failure,*** edema, syncope, orthostatic hypotension, conduction disturbances.
GI: flatulence, constipation, nausea, diarrhea, vomiting, anorexia, dry mouth.
Respiratory: ***bronchospasm,*** dyspnea, wheezing.
Skin: rash.

Interactions

Drug-drug. *Calcium channel blockers:* increased risk of hypotension, left ventricular failure, and AV conduction disturbances. Use I.V. calcium channel blockers with caution.
Catecholamine-depleting drugs, reserpine: may have an additive effect. Monitor patient closely.
General anesthetics: increased hypotensive effects. Watch carefully for excessive hypotension, bradycardia, and orthostatic hypotension.
Lidocaine: may increase the effects of lidocaine. Monitor patient closely.

Contraindications and precautions

- Contraindicated in patients hypersensitive to drug and in those with severe bradycardia, greater than first-degree heart block, cardiogenic shock, or uncontrolled heart failure.
- Use cautiously in patient with heart failure controlled by cardiac glycosides and diuretics because he may show signs of cardiac decompensation with beta blocker therapy.
- Use with caution in pregnant or breast-feeding women.
- Safety of drug hasn't been established in children.

NURSING CONSIDERATIONS

Assessment

- Obtain history of patient's blood pressure before therapy, and reassess regularly thereafter.
- Be alert for adverse reactions and drug interactions.
- Monitor blood glucose levels regularly in diabetic patients. Beta blockade may inhibit glycogenolysis and signs and symptoms of hypoglycemia (such as tachycardia and blood pressure changes).
- Evaluate patient's and family's understanding of drug therapy.

Nursing diagnoses

- Risk for injury related to presence of hypertension
- Decreased cardiac output related to drug-induced adverse CV reactions
- Deficient knowledge related to drug therapy

Planning and implementation

ALERT Never discontinue drug abruptly; angina pectoris may occur in patients with unrecognized coronary artery disease. Obtain guidelines from prescriber for how dose should be tapered before discontinuing drug.

- Advise anesthesiologist when surgical patient is receiving a beta blocker so that isoproterenol or dobutamine can be made readily available for reversal of drug's cardiac effects.
- Beta blockers may mask tachycardia caused by hyperthyroidism. In patients with suspected thyrotoxicosis, withdraw beta blocker gradually, as ordered, to avoid thyroid storm.

Patient teaching

- Explain importance of taking drug as prescribed, even when feeling well. Tell patient not to discontinue drug suddenly but to call prescriber if unpleasant adverse reactions occur.
- Teach patient signs and symptoms of heart failure, including shortness of breath or difficulty breathing, unusually fast heartbeat, cough, or fatigue with exertion, and tell patient to report them immediately.
- If patient uses ophthalmic drops, tell him to shake well before administration and to store at room temperature.

Evaluation

- Patient's blood pressure is within normal limits.
- Patient's cardiac output remains unchanged throughout therapy.

• Patient and family state understanding of drug therapy.

bethanechol chloride

(beh-THAN-eh-kol KLOR-ighd)
Duvoid, Urecholine, Urocarb Liquid ◇, Urocarb Tablets ◇

Pharmacologic class: cholinergic agonist
Therapeutic class: urinary tract stimulant
Pregnancy risk category: C

Indications and dosages

▶ **Acute postoperative and postpartum nonobstructive (functional) urine retention, neurogenic atony of urinary bladder with urine retention.** *Adults:* 10 to 50 mg P.O. b.i.d. to q.i.d. Or, 2.5 to 5 mg S.C. Never give I.V. or I.M. When used for urine retention, some patients may need 50 to 100 mg P.O. per dose. Use such doses with extreme caution.

Test dose is 2.5 mg S.C. repeated at 15- to 30-minute intervals to total of four doses to determine minimal effective dose; then use minimal effective dose q 6 to 8 hours. All doses must be adjusted individually.

How supplied

Tablets: 5 mg, 10 mg, 25 mg, 50 mg
Injection: 5.15 mg/ml

Pharmacokinetics

Absorption: poorly absorbed from GI tract after P.O. administration; unknown after S.C. administration.
Distribution: unknown.
Metabolism: unknown.
Excretion: unknown.

Route	Onset	Peak	Duration
P.O.	30-90 min	About 1 hr	≤ 6 hr
S.C.	5-15 min	5-30 min	About 2 hr

Pharmacodynamics

Chemical effect: directly stimulates cholinergic receptors, mimicking action of acetylcholine.
Therapeutic effect: relieves urine retention.

Adverse reactions

CNS: headache, malaise.
CV: ***bradycardia,*** hypotension, reflex tachycardia.
EENT: lacrimation, miosis.
GI: *abdominal cramps, diarrhea,* excessive salivation, nausea, vomiting, belching, borborygmi, esophageal spasms.
GU: urinary urgency.
Respiratory: ***bronchoconstriction,*** increased bronchial secretions.
Skin: flushing, sweating.

Interactions

Drug-drug. *Anticholinergics, atropine, procainamide, quinidine:* may reverse cholinergic effects. Watch for lack of drug effect.
Anticholinesterases, cholinergic agonists: may cause additive effects or increase toxicity. Avoid concomitant use.
Ganglionic blockers: may cause severe abdominal pain followed by a critical drop in blood pressure. Avoid concomitant use.

Contraindications and precautions

• Contraindicated for I.V. or I.M. use and when increased muscle activity of GI or urinary tract is harmful. Also contraindicated in patients hypersensitive to drug or its components and in those with hyperthyroidism, peptic ulceration, latent or active bronchial asthma, pronounced bradycardia or hypotension, vasomotor instability, cardiac or coronary artery disease, seizure disorder, Parkinson's disease, spastic GI disturbances, acute inflammatory lesions of GI tract, peritonitis, mechanical obstruction of GI or urinary tract, marked vagotonia, or uncertain strength or integrity of bladder wall.
• Use cautiously in pregnant women.
• Breast-feeding should be discontinued if drug must be administered to breast-feeding women.
• Safety of drug hasn't been established in children or pregnant or breast-feeding women.

NURSING CONSIDERATIONS

Assessment
- Obtain history of patient's bladder condition before therapy, and reassess regularly throughout therapy.
- Be alert for adverse reactions and drug interactions.
- Evaluate patient's and family's understanding of drug therapy.

Nursing diagnoses
- Impaired urinary elimination related to underlying bladder condition
- Ineffective breathing pattern related to drug-induced bronchoconstriction
- Deficient knowledge related to drug therapy

Planning and implementation
P.O. use: Give drug on empty stomach to prevent nausea and vomiting.
S.C. use: Onset of action is more rapid and duration is shorter than with P.O. use. P.O. and S.C. doses aren't interchangeable.
ALERT Never give I.V. or I.M.; doing so could cause circulatory collapse, hypotension, severe abdominal cramping, bloody diarrhea, shock, or cardiac arrest.
- Always have atropine injection readily available, and be prepared to give 0.5 mg S.C. or slow I.V. push, as ordered. Provide respiratory support, as necessary.

Patient teaching
- Advise patient to take oral dose on an empty stomach.
- Tell patient to report breathing difficulty immediately.

Evaluation
- Patient is able to void without urine retention.
- Patient's respiratory function remains normal during therapy.
- Patient and family state understanding of drug therapy.

bexarotene
(bex-AHR-oh-teen)
Targretin

Pharmacologic class: retinoid (selective retinoid X receptor activator)
Therapeutic class: tumor cell growth inhibitor
Pregnancy risk category: X

Indications and dosages
▶ **Cutaneous effects of cutaneous T-cell lymphoma in patients refractory to at least one previous systemic therapy.** *Adults:* 300 mg/m²/day P.O. as a single dose with a meal. If no response after 8 weeks, increase to 400 mg/m²/day. Adjust dose to 200 mg/m²/day, and then to 100 mg/m²/day if toxicity occurs, or drug may be temporarily suspended. When toxicity is controlled, dosage may be carefully readjusted upward.

How supplied
Capsules: 75 mg

Pharmacokinetics
Absorption: absorbed from the GI tract. Absorption is increased if given with a meal that contains fat.
Distribution: drug is more than 99% bound to plasma proteins.
Metabolism: metabolized through oxidative pathways, primarily by the cytochrome P-450 3A4 system, to four metabolites. These may maintain retinoid receptor activity.
Excretion: thought to be eliminated primarily through the hepatobiliary system. *Terminal half-life:* 7 hours.

Route	Onset	Peak	Duration
P.O.	Unknown	Unknown	Unknown

Pharmacodynamics
Chemical effect: selectively binds and activates retinoid X receptor subtypes. Once activated, these receptors function as transcription factors that regulate the expression of genes that control cellular differentiation and proliferation. In vitro, bexarotene inhibits the

growth of some tumor cell lines of hematopoietic and squamous cell origin; in vivo, it induces tumor cell regression in some animal models. The exact mechanism of action in the treatment of cutaneous T-cell lymphoma is unknown.
Therapeutic effect: inhibits tumor growth in cutaneous T-cell lymphoma.

Adverse reactions

CNS: *headache,* insomnia, *asthenia,* fatigue, syncope, depression, agitation, ataxia, ***CVA,*** confusion, dizziness, hyperesthesia, hypoesthesia, neuropathy.
CV: *peripheral edema*, chest pain, ***hemorrhage,*** hypertension, angina, ***heart failure,*** tachycardia.
EENT: cataracts, pharyngitis, rhinitis, dry eyes, conjunctivitis, ear pain, blepharitis, corneal lesion, keratitis, otitis externa, visual field defect.
GI: *nausea,* diarrhea, vomiting, anorexia, ***pancreatitis,*** *abdominal pain,* elevated amylase level, constipation, dry mouth, flatulence, colitis, dyspepsia, cheilitis, gastroenteritis, gingivitis, melena.
GU: elevated creatinine level, albuminuria, hematuria, incontinence, urinary tract infection, urinary urgency, dysuria, abnormal kidney function.
Hematologic: ***leukopenia,*** anemia, eosinophilia, thrombocythemia, lymphocytosis, ***thrombocytopenia.***
Hepatic: increased LD, aspartate transaminase, and alanine transaminase levels; bilirubinemia, ***liver failure.***
Metabolic: *hyperlipemia, hypercholesteremia, hypothyroidism,* hyperglycemia, hypoproteinemia, hypocalcemia, hyponatremia, weight change.
Musculoskeletal: arthralgia, myalgia, back pain, bone pain, myasthenia, arthrosis.
Respiratory: pneumonia, dyspnea, hemoptysis, pleural effusion, bronchitis, cough, lung edema, hypoxia.
Skin: *rash, dry skin,* ***exfoliative dermatitis,*** *alopecia, photosensitivity,* pruritus, cellulitis, acne, skin ulcer, skin nodule.
Other: breast pain, *infection,* chills, fever, flu syndrome, ***sepsis.***

Interactions

Drug-drug. *Erythromycin, gemfibrozil, itraconazole, ketoconazole, other inhibitors of cytochrome P-450 3A4:* increased plasma levels of bexarotene. Avoid concomitant use.
Insulin, sulfonylureas: enhanced hypoglycemic action of these drugs, resulting in hypoglycemia in patients with diabetes mellitus. Use together cautiously.
Phenobarbital, phenytoin, rifampin, other inducers of cytochrome P-450 3A4: decreased plasma levels of bexarotene. Avoid concomitant use.
Vitamin A preparations: increased potential for vitamin A toxicity. Avoid vitamin A supplements.
Drug-food. *Any food:* enhances drug absorption. Administer with food.
Grapefruit juice: may inhibit cytochrome P-450 3A4. Don't give concomitantly.
Drug-lifestyle. *Sun exposure:* retinoids may cause photosensitivity. Minimize exposure to sunlight and artificial ultraviolet light.

Contraindications and precautions

- Contraindicated in patients hypersensitive to drug or its components and in pregnant women.
- Drug isn't recommended for patients taking drugs that increase triglyceride levels or cause pancreatic toxicity. Also not recommended for patients who have risk factors for pancreatitis, such as prior pancreatitis, uncontrolled hyperlipidemia, excessive alcohol consumption, uncontrolled diabetes mellitus, or biliary tract disease.
- Use cautiously in women of childbearing potential, in patients with hepatic insufficiency, and in patients hypersensitive to retinoids.

NURSING CONSIDERATIONS

Assessment

- Assess women of childbearing potential carefully; they should use effective contraception at least one month before therapy starts, during therapy, and for at least one month after therapy stops. During therapy, patient should use two reliable forms of contraception simultaneously unless abstinence is the chosen method. A negative pregnancy test should be

obtained within one week before therapy starts and monthly during therapy.
• Men with sexual partners who are pregnant, who could be pregnant, or who could become pregnant must use condoms during sexual intercourse during therapy and for at least one month after therapy ends.
• Obtain total cholesterol, high-density lipoprotein, and triglyceride levels when therapy starts, weekly until the lipid response is established (2 to 4 weeks) and at 8-week intervals thereafter. Elevated triglycerides during treatment should be treated with antilipemic therapy, as ordered, and the dose of bexarotene reduced or suspended as needed.
• Obtain baseline thyroid function tests, and monitor results during treatment.
• Monitor WBC with differential at baseline and periodically during treatment.
• Monitor liver function test results at baseline and after 1, 2, and 4 weeks of treatment. If patient is stable, monitor test results every 8 weeks during treatment. The prescriber may consider suspending treatment if results are three times the upper limit of normal.
• Obtain ophthalmologic evaluation for cataracts in patients who experience visual difficulties.
• Evaluate patient's and family's knowledge of drug therapy.

Nursing diagnoses

• Ineffective health maintenance related to underlying condition
• Risk for injury related to drug-induced adverse reactions
• Deficient knowledge related to drug therapy

Planning and implementation

• Lower doses may be needed for patients with hepatic insufficiency.
• Administer drug with food for better absorption, although not with grapefruit or grapefruit juice.
• Start therapy on the second or third day of a normal menstrual period.
• No more than a one-month supply of bexarotene should be given to a patient of childbearing potential so the results of pregnancy testing can be assessed regularly and the patient can be reminded to avoid pregnancy.
• Bexarotene therapy may increase CA 125 assay values in patients with ovarian cancer.

Patient teaching

• Advise patient to minimize exposure to sunlight and artificial ultraviolet light and to take appropriate precautions.
• Teach patient that it may take several capsules to make the necessary dose and that these capsules should all be taken at the same time and with a meal.
• Teach women of childbearing potential the dangers of becoming pregnant while taking bexarotene and the need for monthly pregnancy tests.
• Explain the need for obtaining baseline laboratory tests and for periodic monitoring of these tests.
• Tell patient to report any visual changes.

Evaluation

• Patient exhibits positive response to therapy.
• Patient has no injury as a result of drug-induced adverse reactions.
• Patient and family state understanding of drug therapy.

bicalutamide

(bigh-kah-LOO-tuh-mighd)
Casodex

Pharmacologic class: nonsteroidal antiandrogen
Therapeutic class: antineoplastic
Pregnancy risk category: X

Indications and dosages

▶ **Adjunct therapy for treatment of advanced prostate cancer.** *Adults:* 50 mg P.O. once daily in morning or evening.

How supplied

Tablets: 50 mg

Pharmacokinetics

Absorption: well absorbed from GI tract.
Distribution: 96% protein-bound.
Metabolism: undergoes stereo-specific metabolism. The S (inactive) isomer is metabolized

primarily by glucuronidation. The R (active) isomer also undergoes glucuronidation but is mainly oxidized to an inactive metabolite.
Excretion: excreted in urine and feces.

Route	Onset	Peak	Duration
P.O.	Unknown	Unknown	Unknown

Pharmacodynamics

Chemical effect: competitively inhibits action of androgens by binding to cytosol androgen receptors in target tissue.
Therapeutic effect: counteracts the effect of androgen or removes its source.

Adverse reactions

CNS: *asthenia,* headache, dizziness, paresthesia, insomnia.
CV: *hot flushes,* hypertension, chest pain, peripheral edema.
GI: *constipation, nausea, diarrhea,* abdominal pain, flatulence, increased liver enzyme levels, vomiting, weight loss.
GU: nocturia, hematuria, urinary tract infection, impotence, urinary incontinence.
Hematologic: hypochromic anemia, iron deficiency anemia.
Metabolic: hyperglycemia.
Musculoskeletal: *back, pelvic,* and bone pain.
Respiratory: dyspnea.
Skin: rash, diaphoresis.
Other: *general pain, infection,* flu syndrome, gynecomastia.

Interactions

Drug-drug. *Coumarin anticoagulants:* displacement of these drugs from protein-binding sites. Monitor PT and INR closely; adjust anticoagulant dosage, as necessary.

Contraindications and precautions

- Contraindicated in patients hypersensitive to drug or its components.
- Use cautiously in patients with moderate to severe hepatic impairment; drug is extensively metabolized by liver.
- Safety of drug hasn't been established in children.

NURSING CONSIDERATIONS

Assessment

- Obtain history of patient's cancer before therapy.
- Regularly monitor serum prostate specific antigen (PSA) levels, as ordered.
- Monitor liver function studies, as ordered.
- Be alert for adverse reactions and drug interactions.
- Evaluate patient's and family's understanding of drug therapy.

Nursing diagnoses

- Ineffective health maintenance related to neoplastic disease
- Acute pain related to drug-induced adverse reactions
- Deficient knowledge related to drug therapy

Planning and implementation

ALERT Bicalutamide is used with a luteinizing hormone-releasing hormone analogue. Treatment should be started at the same time for both.

- Administer drug at the same time each day.
- Report elevated PSA levels to prescriber, who should evaluate patient to determine disease progression.
- Bicalutamide should be discontinued if patient develops jaundice or exhibits laboratory evidence of liver injury in absence of liver metastases. Abnormalities are usually reversible by discontinuing drug.

Patient teaching

- Inform patient that drug may be taken without regard to meals.
- Advise patient to take drug at same time each day.
- Tell patient not to interrupt or stop drug without consulting prescriber.

Evaluation

- Patient shows positive response to drug.
- Patient states that he is pain free.
- Patient and family state understanding of drug therapy.

biperiden hydrochloride

(bih-PEH-rih-den high-droh-KLOR-ighd)
Akineton

biperiden lactate

Akineton

Pharmacologic class: anticholinergic
Therapeutic class: antiparkinsonian
Pregnancy risk category: C

Indications and dosages

▶ **Drug-induced extrapyramidal disorders.** *Adults:* 2 mg P.O. once daily, b.i.d., or t.i.d., depending on severity. Or, 2 mg I.M. or I.V. q 30 minutes until symptoms resolve. Don't exceed four consecutive doses in a 24-hour period.

▶ **Parkinsonism.** *Adults:* 2 mg P.O. t.i.d. or q.i.d., not to exceed 16 mg/day.

How supplied

biperiden hydrochloride
Tablets: 2 mg
biperiden lactate
Injection: 5 mg/ml in 1-ml ampules

Pharmacokinetics

Absorption: well absorbed from GI tract.
Distribution: well distributed throughout body.
Metabolism: unknown.
Excretion: excreted in urine as unchanged drug and metabolites.

Route	Onset	Peak	Duration
P.O.	≤ 1 hr	Unknown	6-12 hr
I.V.	≤ 30 min	Unknown	1–8 hr
I.M.	Unknown	Unknown	Unknown

Pharmacodynamics

Chemical effect: blocks central cholinergic receptors, helping to balance cholinergic activity in basal ganglia.
Therapeutic effect: improves voluntary movement.

Adverse reactions

CNS: disorientation, euphoria, restlessness, irritability, incoherence, dizziness, increased tremors.
CV: transient orthostatic hypotension.
EENT: blurred vision.
GI: dry mouth, *constipation,* nausea, vomiting, epigastric distress.
GU: urinary hesitancy, urine retention.
Skin: rash, urticaria.

Interactions

Drug-drug. *Amantadine, phenothiazines, tricyclic antidepressants:* excessive CNS anticholinergic effects. Avoid concomitant use.
Drug-lifestyle. *Alcohol use:* increased sedative affect. Discourage concomitant use.

Contraindications and precautions

- Contraindicated in patients hypersensitive to drug and in those with angle-closure glaucoma, bowel obstruction, or megacolon.
- Use cautiously in patients with prostatic hyperplasia, arrhythmias, open-angle glaucoma, and seizure disorder.
- Use cautiously in pregnant or breast-feeding women.
- Safety of drug hasn't been established in children.

NURSING CONSIDERATIONS

Assessment

- Obtain history of patient's underlying condition.
- Monitor effectiveness by regularly checking body movements for signs of improvement. However, in severe parkinsonism, tremors may increase as spasticity is relieved.
- Be alert for adverse reactions and drug interactions. Adverse reactions are dose-related and may resemble those of atropine toxicity.
- Evaluate patient's and family's understanding of drug therapy.

Nursing diagnoses

- Impaired physical mobility related to underlying parkinsonism or other extrapyramidal disorders

• Risk for injury related to drug-induced adverse CNS reactions
• Deficient knowledge related to drug therapy

Planning and implementation

P.O. use: Give oral doses with or after meals to decrease adverse GI effects.
I.V. use: Administer drug very slowly.
I.M. use: Follow normal protocol. No local tissue reactions have been reported with I.M. use.
• When giving parenterally, keep patient in supine position. Parenteral administration may cause transient orthostatic hypotension and coordination disturbances.
• Notify prescriber if tolerance to drug develops; dose will need to be increased.
• Notify prescriber if patient develops serious adverse reactions that may require dosage reduction.

Patient teaching
• Warn patient to avoid activities that require alertness until CNS effects of drug are known.
• Tell patient to report urinary hesitancy or urine retention.
• Advise patient to relieve dry mouth with cool drinks, ice chips, or sugarless gum or hard candy.

Evaluation

• Patient exhibits improved mobility with reduced muscle rigidity and tremors.
• Patient doesn't experience injury as result of drug-induced adverse CNS reactions.
• Patient and family state understanding of drug therapy.

bisacodyl

(bigh-suh-KOH-dil)

Bisac-Evac†, Bisacolax◆†, Bisalax◇, Bisco-Lax**†, Biscodyl Uniserts†, Carter's Little Pills†, Correctal†, Dacodyl†, Deficol†, Dulcolax†, Durolax◇, Feen-A-Mint†, Fleet Bisacodyl†, Fleet Bisacodyl Prep†, Fleet Laxative†, Laxit◆†, Modane†, Theralax†

Pharmacologic class: diphenylmethane derivative
Therapeutic class: stimulant laxative
Pregnancy risk category: B

Indications and dosages

▶ **Chronic constipation; preparation for childbirth, surgery, or rectal or bowel examination.** *Adults and children age 12 and over:* 10 to 15 mg P.O. in evening or before breakfast; maximum 30 mg P.O. For evacuation before examination or surgery, 10 mg P.R.
Children ages 6 to 12: 5 mg P.O. or P.R. h.s. or before breakfast.

How supplied

Tablets (enteric-coated): 5 mg†
Enema: 0.33 mg/dl†, 10 mg/5 ml (microenema)◇, 10 mg/30 ml
Powder for rectal solution (bisacodyl tannex): 1.5 mg bisacodyl and 2.5 g tannic acid
Suppositories: 10 mg†

Pharmacokinetics

Absorption: minimal.
Distribution: distributed locally.
Metabolism: up to 15% of P.O. dose may enter enterohepatic circulation.
Excretion: excreted primarily in feces; some excreted in urine.

Route	Onset	Peak	Duration
P.O.	6-12 hr	Variable	Variable
P.R.	15-60 min	Variable	Variable

Pharmacodynamics

Chemical effect: increases peristalsis, probably by acting directly on smooth muscle of intestine. Thought to irritate musculature or stimulate colonic intramural plexus. Also promotes fluid accumulation in colon and small intestine.
Therapeutic effect: relieves constipation.

Adverse reactions

GI: *nausea, vomiting, abdominal cramps,* diarrhea (with high doses), *burning sensation in rectum* (with suppositories), protein-losing enteropathy (with excessive use), laxative dependence (with long-term or excessive use).
Metabolic: alkalosis, hypokalemia, fluid and electrolyte imbalance.

Musculoskeletal: tetany, muscle weakness (with excessive use).

Interactions

Drug-drug. *Antacids:* gastric irritation or dyspepsia from premature dissolution of enteric coating. Avoid concurrent use.
Drug-food. *Milk:* gastric irritation or dyspepsia from premature dissolution of enteric coating. Avoid concurrent use.

Contraindications and precautions

- Contraindicated in patients hypersensitive to drug and in those with rectal bleeding, gastroenteritis, intestinal obstruction, or symptoms of appendicitis or acute surgical abdomen, such as abdominal pain, nausea, or vomiting.
- Use cautiously in pregnant women.

NURSING CONSIDERATIONS

Assessment

- Obtain history of bowel disorder, GI status, fluid intake, nutritional status, exercise habits, and normal patterns of elimination.
- Monitor effectiveness by checking frequency and characteristics of stools.
- Be alert for adverse reactions and drug interactions.
- Auscultate bowel sounds at least once a shift. Check for pain and cramping.
- Evaluate patient's and family's understanding of drug therapy.

Nursing diagnoses

- Constipation related to interruption of normal pattern of elimination
- Acute pain related to drug-induced abdominal cramps
- Deficient knowledge related to drug therapy

Planning and implementation

P.O. use: Don't give tablets within 60 minutes of milk or antacid.
P.R. use: Insert suppository as high as possible into rectum and try to position suppository against rectal wall. Avoid embedding within fecal material because this may delay onset of action.
- Time administration of drug so as not to interfere with scheduled activities or sleep. Soft, formed stool usually produced 15 to 60 minutes after P.R. administration.
- Tablets and suppositories are used together to clean colon before and after surgery and before barium enema.
- Store tablets and suppositories below 86° F (30° C).

Patient teaching

- Advise patient to swallow enteric-coated tablet whole to avoid GI irritation. Tell him not to take tablet within 1 hour of milk or antacid.
- Advise patient to report adverse effects to prescriber.
- Teach patient about dietary sources of bulk, including bran and other cereals, fresh fruit, and vegetables.
- Caution patient against excessive use of drug.

Evaluation

- Patient reports return of normal bowel pattern of elimination.
- Patient is free from abdominal pain and cramping.
- Patient and family state understanding of drug therapy.

bismuth subgallate

(BIS-muth sub-GAL-ayt)
Devrom

bismuth subsalicylate

Maximum Strength Pepto-Bismol Liquid†, Pepto-Bismol†

Pharmacologic class: adsorbent
Therapeutic class: antidiarrheal
Pregnancy risk category: NR

Indications and dosages

▶ **Mild, nonspecific diarrhea.** *Adults and children over age 12:* 1 to 2 tablets (subgallate) P.O. t.i.d. with meals. Or, 30 ml or 2 tablets (subsalicylate) P.O. q 30 to 60 minutes up to maximum of eight doses and for no longer than 2 days.
Children ages 3 to 6: 5 ml or ⅓ tablet P.O.

Children ages 6 to 9: 10 ml or ⅔ tablet P.O.
Children ages 9 to 12: 15 ml or 1 tablet P.O.

How supplied

bismuth subgallate
Tablets (chewable): 200 mg†
bismuth subsalicylate
Tablets (chewable): 262.5 mg†
Oral suspension: 262.5 mg/15 ml†, 525 mg/15 ml†

Pharmacokinetics

Absorption: absorbed poorly; significant salicylate absorption may occur after using bismuth subsalicylate.
Distribution: distributed locally in gut.
Metabolism: metabolized minimally.
Excretion: bismuth subsalicylate is excreted in urine.

Route	Onset	Peak	Duration
P.O.	≤ 1 hr	Unknown	Unknown

Pharmacodynamics

Chemical effect: unknown; has mild water-binding capacity. Also may adsorb toxins and provide protective coating for mucosa.
Therapeutic effect: relieves diarrhea.

Adverse reactions

GI: temporary darkening of tongue and stools.
Other: salicylism (with high doses).

Interactions

Drug-drug. *Aspirin, other salicylates:* risk of salicylate toxicity. Monitor patient closely.
Oral anticoagulants, oral antidiabetics: theoretical risk of increased effects of these drugs after high doses of bismuth subsalicylate. Monitor patient closely.
Probenecid: theoretical risk of decreased uricosuric effects after high doses of bismuth subsalicylate. Monitor patient closely.
Tetracycline: decreased tetracycline absorption. Separate administration times by at least 2 hours.

Contraindications and precautions

- Contraindicated in patients hypersensitive to salicylates.
- Use cautiously in patients already taking aspirin and in pregnant or breast-feeding women.

NURSING CONSIDERATIONS

Assessment

- Obtain history of patient's bowel disorder, GI status, and frequency of loose stools before therapy.
- Monitor effectiveness by checking frequency and characteristics of stools.
- Be alert for adverse reactions and drug interactions.
- Check patient's hearing if he takes drug in large doses.
- Evaluate patient's and family's understanding of drug therapy.

Nursing diagnoses

- Diarrhea related to underlying GI condition
- Disturbed sensory perception (auditory) related to drug-induced salicylism
- Deficient knowledge related to drug therapy

Planning and implementation

- Avoid use before GI radiologic procedures because bismuth is radiopaque and may interfere with X-rays.
- Read label carefully because dosage varies with form of drug.
- Discontinue therapy and notify prescriber if tinnitus occurs.

Patient teaching

- Advise patient that drug contains large amount of salicylate. (Each tablet contains 102 mg; regular-strength liquid contains 130 mg/15 ml, and extra-strength liquid contains 230 mg/15 ml.)
- Instruct patient to chew tablets well or to shake liquid before measuring dose.
- Tell patient to report diarrhea that persists for more than 2 days or is accompanied by high fever.
- Tell patient to consult with prescriber before giving bismuth subsalicylate to children or teenagers who have or are recovering from flu or chickenpox.
- Inform patient that both liquid and tablet forms of Pepto-Bismol are effective against

traveler's diarrhea. Tablets may be more convenient to carry.

Evaluation
• Patient reports decrease or absence of loose stools.
• Patient remains free from signs and symptoms of salicylism.
• Patient and family state understanding of drug therapy.
• Patient reports being free from heartburn and indigestion.

bisoprolol fumarate
(bis-OP-roh-lol FYOO-muh-rayt)
Zebeta

Pharmacologic class: beta blocker
Therapeutic class: antihypertensive
Pregnancy risk category: C

Indications and dosages
▶ **Hypertension.** *Adults:* initially, 5 mg P.O. once daily. If response is inadequate, increase to 10 mg once daily or to 20 mg P.O. daily; 20 mg is maximum recommended dosage. *Patients with renal or hepatic impairment:* 2.5 mg P.O. daily. Subsequent dosage adjustment is done cautiously.

How supplied
Tablets: 5 mg, 10 mg

Pharmacokinetics
Absorption: bioavailability after 10-mg dose is about 80%.
Distribution: about 30% of drug binds to serum proteins.
Metabolism: first-pass metabolism of drug is about 20%.
Excretion: excreted equally by renal and nonrenal pathways, with about 50% of dose appearing unchanged in urine and remainder appearing as inactive metabolites. Less than 2% of dose is excreted in feces. *Half-life:* 9 to 12 hours.

Route	Onset	Peak	Duration
P.O.	Unknown	2-4 hr	About 24 hr

Pharmacodynamics
Chemical effect: not completely defined. Bisoprolol is a $beta_1$-selective blocker that decreases myocardial contractility, heart rate, and cardiac output; lowers blood pressure; and reduces myocardial oxygen consumption.
Therapeutic effect: decreases blood pressure.

Adverse reactions
CNS: asthenia, fatigue, dizziness, headache, hypoesthesia, vivid dreams, depression, insomnia.
CV: ***bradycardia,*** peripheral edema, chest pain, ***heart failure.***
EENT: pharyngitis, rhinitis, sinusitis.
GI: nausea, vomiting, diarrhea, dry mouth.
Musculoskeletal: arthralgia.
Respiratory: cough, dyspnea.
Skin: sweating.

Interactions
Drug-drug. *Beta blockers:* can cause extreme hypotension. Don't use together.
Calcium channel blockers: can cause myocardial depression and AV conductive inhibition. Monitor ECG closely.
Guanethidine, reserpine: can cause hypotension. Monitor patient closely.
NSAIDs: decreased antihypertensive effect. Monitor blood pressure and adjust dosage.
Rifampin: increased metabolic clearance of bisoprolol. Monitor patient.

Contraindications and precautions
• Contraindicated in patients hypersensitive to drug and in those with cardiogenic shock, overt cardiac failure, marked sinus bradycardia, or second- or third-degree AV block.
• Use cautiously in patients with bronchospastic disease. These patients should avoid beta blockers because blockade of $beta_1$-receptors isn't absolute and blockage of pulmonary $beta_2$-receptors may result in worsening of symptoms. A bronchodilator should be made available.
• Also use cautiously in patients with diabetes, peripheral vascular disease, or thyroid disease; in those with history of heart failure; and in pregnant or breast-feeding women.
• Safety of drug has not been established in children.

NURSING CONSIDERATIONS

Assessment
- Obtain history of patient's hypertensive status before therapy, and check blood pressure regularly throughout therapy.
- Be alert for adverse reactions and drug interactions.
- Monitor patient's hydration status if adverse GI reactions occur.
- Closely monitor blood glucose levels in diabetic patients. Beta blockers may mask some evidence of hypoglycemia, such as tachycardia.
- Evaluate patient's and family's understanding of drug therapy.

Nursing diagnoses
- Risk for injury related to presence of hypertension
- Risk for deficient fluid volume related to drug-induced adverse GI reactions
- Deficient knowledge related to drug therapy

Planning and implementation
- A $beta_2$-agonist (bronchodilator) should be available for patients with bronchospastic disease.

ALERT Don't discontinue drug abruptly because angina may occur in patients with unrecognized coronary artery disease.

Patient teaching
- Tell patient to take drug as prescribed, even when he's feeling well. Warn him that abruptly discontinuing drug can worsen angina and precipitate MI. Explain that drug must be withdrawn gradually over 1 to 2 weeks.
- Instruct patient to call prescriber if adverse reactions occur.
- Tell diabetic patient to closely monitor blood glucose levels.
- Tell patient to check with prescriber or pharmacist before taking OTC medications or herbal remedies.

Evaluation
- Patient's blood pressure is normal.
- Patient maintains adequate fluid balance throughout therapy.
- Patient and family state understanding of drug therapy.

bleomycin sulfate
(blee-oh-MIGH-sin SUL-fayt)
Blenoxane

Pharmacologic class: antibiotic, antineoplastic (specific to G_2 and M phases of cell cycle)
Therapeutic class: antineoplastic
Pregnancy risk category: D

Indications and dosages

Indications and dosage may vary. Check treatment protocol with prescriber.

▶ **Hodgkin's lymphoma, squamous cell carcinoma, non-Hodgkin's lymphoma, testicular cancer.** *Adults:* 10 to 20 units/m^2 (0.25 to 0.5 units/kg) I.V., I.M., or S.C. once or twice weekly. After 50% response in patients with Hodgkin's disease, maintenance dosage is 1 unit I.V. or I.M. daily or 5 units I.V. or I.M. weekly.

▶ **Malignant pleural effusion.** *Adults:* 60 units administered as a single-dose bolus by intrapleural injection through a thoracostomy tube. Leave in for 4 hours then drain and resume suction.

How supplied

Injection: 15- and 30-unit vials (1 unit=1 mg)

Pharmacokinetics

Absorption: I.M. administration results in lower serum levels than those produced by equivalent I.V. doses.
Distribution: distributed widely into total body water, mainly in skin, lungs, kidneys, peritoneum, and lymphatic tissue.
Metabolism: unknown; however, extensive tissue inactivation occurs in liver and kidneys, with much less in skin and lungs.
Excretion: drug and its metabolites excreted primarily in urine. *Half-life:* 2 hours.

Route	Onset	Peak	Duration
I.V., I.M., S.C.	Unknown	Unknown	Unknown
Intrapleural	Unknown	Unknown	Unknown

Pharmacodynamics

Chemical effect: unknown; thought to inhibit DNA synthesis and cause scission of single- and double-stranded DNA.
Therapeutic effect: kills selected types of cancer cells.

Adverse reactions

CNS: hyperesthesia of scalp and fingers, headache.
GI: *stomatitis, prolonged anorexia, nausea, vomiting,* diarrhea.
Hematologic: leukocytosis.
Musculoskeletal: swelling of interphalangeal joints.
Respiratory: **PNEUMONITIS,** ***pulmonary fibrosis,*** *fine crackles, dyspnea, nonproductive cough.*
Skin: *reversible alopecia; erythema; vesiculation; hardening and discoloration of palmar and plantar skin;* desquamation of hands, feet, and pressure areas; *hyperpigmentation; acne.*
Other: ***hypersensitivity reaction*** *(fever up to 106° F [41.1° C] with chills up to 5 hours after injection,* ***anaphylaxis****)*, fever.

Interactions

Drug-drug. *Cardiac glycosides:* decreased serum digoxin levels. Monitor patient closely for loss of therapeutic effect.
Phenytoin: decreased serum phenytoin levels. Monitor patient closely.

Contraindications and precautions

- Contraindicated in patients hypersensitive to drug.
- Use cautiously in patients with renal or pulmonary impairment.
- Safety of drug hasn't been established in children or in pregnant or breast-feeding women.

NURSING CONSIDERATIONS

Assessment

- Obtain history of patient's overall physical status (especially respiratory status, CBC, and pulmonary and renal function tests) before therapy and reassess regularly thereafter.
- Be alert for adverse reactions and drug interactions.
- Adverse pulmonary reactions are common in patients over age 70. Fatal pulmonary fibrosis occurs in 1% of patients, especially when cumulative dose exceeds 400 units.
- Monitor for bleomycin-induced fever, which is common and usually occurs within 3 to 6 hours after administering drug.
- Watch for hypersensitivity reactions, which may be delayed for several hours, especially in patients with lymphoma.
- Evaluate patient's and family's understanding of drug therapy.
- Watch for development of fine crackles and dyspnea.

Nursing diagnoses

- Risk for injury related to underlying neoplastic condition
- Impaired gas exchange related to drug-induced adverse pulmonary reactions
- Deficient knowledge related to drug therapy

Planning and implementation

- Follow institutional policy for administration of drug to reduce risks. Preparation and administration of parenteral form of this drug cause carcinogenic, mutagenic, and teratogenic risks for personnel.

I.V. use: Reconstitute drug with 5 ml or more of normal saline solution for injection. For I.V. infusion, dilute with 50 to 100 ml of normal saline solution for injection. Administer slowly over 10 minutes. Bleomycin may adsorb to plastic I.V. bags. For prolonged stability, use glass containers.
I.M. use: Dilute drug in 1 to 5 ml of sterile water for injection, bacteriostatic water for injection, or normal saline solution for injection.
Intrapleural use: Dissolve drug in 50 to 100 ml normal saline solution injection. Administer through a thoracotomy tube after excess intrapleural fluid has been drained and complete lung expansion has been confirmed.
S.C. use: Follow manufacturer's guidelines for administering bleomycin S.C.

- Refrigerate unopened vials containing dry powder.
- Refrigerated, reconstituted solution is stable for 4 weeks; at room temperature, it's stable for 2 weeks.

• Drug should be stopped if pulmonary function test shows a marked decline.
• To prevent linear streaking from drug concentrating in keratin of squamous epithelium, don't use adhesive dressings on skin.
• In patients prone to post-treatment fever, give acetaminophen, as ordered, before treatment and for 24 hours after treatment.
• If ordered after treatment, give supplemental oxygen at an FIO_2 no higher than 25% to avoid potential lung damage.

Patient teaching
• Explain the risks of drug therapy, especially the danger of serious pulmonary reactions in high-risk patients.
• Explain the need for monitoring and the type of monitoring to be done.
• Tell patient that alopecia may occur, but that it's usually reversible.

☑ Evaluation
• Patient exhibits positive response to therapy, as evidenced by follow-up diagnostic test results.
• Patient's gas exchange remains normal throughout therapy.
• Patient and family state understanding of drug therapy.

bretylium tosylate
(breh-TIL-ee-um TOH-si-layt)
Bretylate ◇

Pharmacologic class: adrenergic blocker
Therapeutic class: ventricular antiarrhythmic
Pregnancy risk category: C

Indications and dosages
▶ **Ventricular fibrillation or hemodynamically unstable ventricular tachycardia unresponsive to other antiarrhythmics.** *Adults:* 5 mg/kg by I.V. push over 1 minute. If necessary, increase dose to 10 mg/kg and repeat q 15 to 30 minutes until 35 to 40 mg/kg have been given. For continuous suppression, administer diluted solution at 1 to 2 mg/minute continuously, or give 5 to 10 mg/kg diluted solution over more than 8 minutes q 6 hours. If unable to obtain I.V. access, may administer 5 to 10 mg/kg undiluted I.M. q 1 to 2 hours if the arrhythmia persists or q 6 to 8 hours for maintenance therapy.

How supplied
Injection: 50 mg/ml

Pharmacokinetics
Absorption: not applicable with I.V. administration.
Distribution: distributed widely throughout body. Only about 1% to 10% is bound to plasma.
Metabolism: no metabolites have been identified.
Excretion: excreted in urine. *Half-life:* 5 to 10 hours (longer in patients with renal impairment).

Route	Onset	Peak	Duration
I.V.	3 min-2 hr	6-9 hr	6-24 hr

Pharmacodynamics
Chemical effect: unknown; considered a class III antiarrhythmic that initially exerts transient adrenergic stimulation through release of norepinephrine. Subsequent depletion of norepinephrine causes adrenergic blocking actions to predominate, prolonging repolarization and increasing duration of action potential and effective refractory period.
Therapeutic effect: abolishes ventricular arrhythmias.

Adverse reactions
CNS: *vertigo, dizziness, light-headedness, syncope.*
CV: **SEVERE HYPOTENSION** (especially orthostatic), ***bradycardia,*** angina, ***transient arrhythmias,*** transient hypertension.
GI: severe nausea, vomiting (with rapid infusion).
Musculoskeletal: muscle atrophy, tissue necrosis (with repeated injections).

Interactions
Drug-drug. *Antihypertensives:* may potentiate hypotension. Monitor blood pressure.

Other antiarrhythmics: additive or antagonistic antiarrhythmic effects. Monitor patient for additive toxicity.
Sympathomimetics: bretylium may potentiate effects of drugs given to correct hypotension. Monitor blood pressure.

Contraindications and precautions

- Safety and efficacy of drug haven't been established in children.
- Contraindicated in patients taking a cardiac glycoside unless arrhythmia is life-threatening, not caused by digitalis, and unresponsive to other antiarrhythmics.
- Use with extreme caution in patients with fixed cardiac output (aortic stenosis and pulmonary hypertension). Drug may cause severe and sudden drop in blood pressure.
- Use with caution in pregnant or breast-feeding women.

NURSING CONSIDERATIONS

Assessment

- Obtain history of patient's heart rate and rhythm before therapy.
- Monitor effectiveness by evaluating continuous ECG recordings, blood pressure, and heart rate. Initial drug-induced release of norepinephrine may cause transient hypertension and arrhythmias.
- Be alert for adverse reactions and drug interactions.
- Evaluate patient's and family's understanding of drug therapy.

Nursing diagnoses

- Decreased cardiac output related to presence of ventricular arrhythmia
- Ineffective cerebral tissue perfusion related to drug-induced severe hypotension
- Deficient knowledge related to drug therapy

Planning and implementation

- When used in maintenance therapy, dilute with dextrose or saline solution for injection before administering. Follow manufacturer's guidelines for specific dilution (varies according to dosage). When administering as direct I.V. injection, use 20G to 22G needle and inject over 1 minute into vein or I.V. line containing free-flowing compatible solution.
- Drug is used with other cardiac life-support measures, such as cardiopulmonary resuscitation, defibrillation, epinephrine, sodium bicarbonate, and lidocaine.
- To prevent nausea and vomiting, follow dosage directions carefully.
- Keep patient in supine position until tolerance to hypotension develops. Have patient avoid sudden position changes.
- If supine systolic blood pressure falls below 75 mm Hg, prescriber may order norepinephrine, dopamine, or volume expanders to raise blood pressure.

Patient teaching

- Tell patient to report chest pain or dyspnea immediately.
- Tell patient to avoid sudden position changes.

Evaluation

- Patient's ECG reveals that arrhythmia has been corrected.
- Patient's blood pressure remains normal throughout therapy.
- Patient and family state understanding of drug therapy.

bromocriptine mesylate

(broh-moh-KRIP-teen MES-ih-layt)
Parlodel, Parlodel Snap Tabs

Pharmacologic class: dopamine receptor agonist
Therapeutic class: semisynthetic ergot alkaloid, dopaminergic agonist, antiparkinsonian, inhibitor of prolactin and growth hormone release
Pregnancy risk category: NR

Indications and dosages

▶ **Parkinson's disease.** *Adults:* 1.25 to 2.5 mg P.O. b.i.d. with meals. Increase dosage q 14 to 28 days, up to 100 mg daily, as needed.
▶ **Acromegaly.** *Adults:* 1.25 to 2.5 mg P.O. with h.s. snack for 3 days. An additional 1.25 to 2.5 mg may be added q 3 to 7 days until

patient receives therapeutic benefit. Maximum dosage is 100 mg/day.

▶ **Amenorrhea and galactorrhea related to hyperprolactinemia; infertility or hypogonadism in women.** *Adults:* 1.25 to 2.5 mg P.O. daily. Increase by 2.5 mg daily at 3- to 7-day intervals until desired effect is achieved. Maintenance dosage is usually 5 to7.5 mg/day, but may be 2.5 to 15 mg/day.

How supplied

Tablets: 2.5 mg
Capsules: 5 mg

Pharmacokinetics

Absorption: 28% absorbed.
Distribution: 90% to 96% bound to serum albumin.
Metabolism: first-pass metabolism occurs with more than 90% of absorbed dose. Drug is metabolized completely in liver.
Excretion: major route of excretion is through bile. Only 2.5% to 5.5% of dose excreted in urine. *Half-life:* 15 hours.

Route	Onset	Peak	Duration
P.O.	0.5-2 hr	1-3 hr	12-24 hr

Pharmacodynamics

Chemical effect: inhibits secretion of prolactin and acts as dopamine-receptor agonist by activating postsynaptic dopamine receptors.
Therapeutic effect: reverses amenorrhea and galactorrhea caused by hyperprolactinemia, increases fertility in women, improves voluntary movement, and inhibits prolactin and growth hormone release.

Adverse reactions

CNS: confusion, hallucinations, uncontrolled body movements, *dizziness, headache,* fatigue, mania, delusions, nervousness, insomnia, depression, ***seizures.***
CV: *hypotension,* orthostatic hypotension, hypertension, ***CVA,*** syncope, ***acute MI.***
EENT: nasal congestion, tinnitus, blurred vision.
GI: *nausea,* vomiting, *abdominal cramps,* constipation, diarrhea.
GU: urine retention, urinary frequency.
Skin: coolness and pallor of fingers and toes.

Interactions

Drug-drug. *Antihypertensives:* increased hypotensive effects. Adjust dosage of antihypertensive, as directed.
Ergot alkaloids, estrogens, oral contraceptives, progestins: interfere with effects of bromocriptine. Don't use concomitantly.
Erythromycin: increased serum bromocriptine levels. Adjust bromocriptine, as directed.
Haloperidol, loxapine, MAO inhibitors, methyldopa, metoclopramide, phenothiazines, reserpine: interfere with effects of bromocriptine. Increase bromocriptine dosage, as directed.
Levodopa: additive effects. Adjust levodopa dosage, as directed.
Drug-lifestyle. *Alcohol use:* disulfiram-like reaction. Discourage concurrent use.

Contraindications and precautions

- Contraindicated in patients hypersensitive to ergot derivatives and in those with uncontrolled hypertension and toxemia of pregnancy.
- Use cautiously in patients with impaired renal or hepatic function or history of MI with residual arrhythmias.
- Because drug inhibits lactation, it shouldn't be used in women who intend to breast-feed.
- Safety of drug hasn't been established in children under age 15.

NURSING CONSIDERATIONS

Assessment

- Obtain history of patient's underlying condition before therapy, and reassess regularly thereafter.
- Perform baseline and periodic evaluations of cardiac, hepatic, renal, and hematopoietic function during prolonged therapy.
- Be alert for adverse reactions and drug interactions. Risk of adverse reactions is high (about 68%), particularly at beginning of therapy; most are mild to moderate, with nausea being most common. Adverse reactions are more frequent when drug is used for Parkinson's disease.
- Evaluate patient's and family's understanding of drug therapy.

Nursing diagnoses
- Ineffective health maintenance related to underlying condition
- Risk for injury related to drug-induced adverse CNS or CV reactions
- Deficient knowledge related to drug therapy

Planning and implementation
- Patients with impaired renal function may require dosage adjustments.
- Give drug with meals.
- Gradually adjust doses to effective levels, as ordered, to minimize adverse reactions.
- For Parkinson's disease, bromocriptine usually is given with either levodopa or carbidopa-levodopa.

Patient teaching
- Advise patient to use contraceptive methods other than oral contraceptives or subdermal implants during treatment.
- Advise patient to rise slowly to an upright position and avoid sudden position changes to avoid dizziness and fainting.
- Advise patient that resumption of menses and suppression of galactorrhea may take 6 weeks or longer.
- Warn patient to avoid hazardous activities that require alertness until CNS and CV effects of drug are known.
- Tell patient to take drug with meals to minimize GI distress.

Evaluation
- Patient exhibits improvement in underlying condition.
- Patient doesn't experience injury as a result of drug-induced adverse reactions.
- Patient and family state understanding of drug therapy.

brompheniramine maleate
(brom-fen-IR-ah-meen MAL-ee-ayt)
Bromphen*†, Dimetane*†, Dimetane Extentabs†, Dimetapp Allergy†, Nasahist B, ND-Stat

Pharmacologic class: alkylamine antihistamine
Therapeutic class: antihistamine (H_1-receptor antagonist)
Pregnancy risk category: C

Indications and dosages
▶ **Rhinitis, allergy symptoms.** *Adults:* 4 to 8 mg P.O. t.i.d. or q.i.d. Or, 8 to 12 mg extended-release P.O. b.i.d. or t.i.d. Or, 5 to 20 mg q 6 to 12 hours I.V., I.M., or S.C. Maximum dosage is 40 mg daily.
Children age 6 and over: 2 to 4 mg P.O. t.i.d. or q.i.d. Or, 8 to 12 mg extended-release P.O. q 12 hours. Or, 0.5 mg/kg I.V., I.M., or S.C. daily in divided doses t.i.d. or q.i.d.
Children under age 6: 0.5 mg/kg P.O., I.V., I.M., or S.C. daily in divided doses t.i.d. or q.i.d.

How supplied
Tablets: 4 mg†
Tablets (extended-release): 12 mg†
Elixir: 2 mg/5 ml*†
Injection: 10 mg/ml

Pharmacokinetics
Absorption: absorbed readily from GI tract; unknown for parenteral administration.
Distribution: distributed widely throughout body.
Metabolism: about 90% to 95% metabolized by liver.
Excretion: drug and its metabolites excreted primarily in urine; small amount excreted in feces. *Half-life:* 12 to 34½ hours.

Route	Onset	Peak	Duration
P.O., I.V. I.M., S.C.	15-60 min	2-5 hr	4-8 hr (longer for P.O. extended-release)

Pharmacodynamics
Chemical effect: competes with histamine for H_1-receptor sites on effector cells. Prevents but doesn't reverse histamine-mediated responses.
Therapeutic effect: relieves allergy symptoms.

Adverse reactions

CNS: dizziness, tremors, irritability, insomnia, syncope, *drowsiness, stimulation* (especially in elderly patients).
CV: hypotension, palpitations.
GI: anorexia, nausea, vomiting, *dry mouth and throat.*
GU: urine retention.
Hematologic: ***thrombocytopenia, agranulocytosis.***
Skin: urticaria, rash.
Other: local stinging, diaphoresis.

Interactions

Drug-drug. *CNS depressants:* increased sedation. Use together cautiously.
MAO inhibitors: increased anticholinergic effects. Don't use together.

Contraindications and precautions

- Contraindicated in patients hypersensitive to drug's ingredients and in those with acute asthmatic attacks, severe hypertension, coronary artery disease, angle-closure glaucoma, urine retention, or peptic ulcer. Also contraindicated in breast-feeding women and within 14 days of MAO inhibitor therapy.
- Use cautiously in pregnant women, elderly patients, and those with increased intraocular pressure, diabetes, ischemic heart disease, hyperthyroidism, hypertension, bronchial asthma, or prostatic hyperplasia.
- Drug isn't recommended for neonates. Children, especially those under age 6, may experience paradoxical hyperexcitability. Extended-release tablets aren't recommended for children age 11 and under.

NURSING CONSIDERATIONS

Assessment
- Assess patient's allergy symptoms before therapy and regularly thereafter.
- Be alert for adverse reactions and drug interactions.
- Monitor CBC during long-term therapy, as ordered; watch for signs of blood dyscrasias.
- Monitor patient's hydration status if adverse GI reactions occur.
- Evaluate patient's and family's understanding of drug therapy.

Nursing diagnoses
- Ineffective health maintenance related to allergy symptoms
- Risk for deficient fluid volume related to drug-induced adverse GI reactions
- Deficient knowledge related to drug therapy

Planning and implementation
P.O. use: Give drug with food or milk to reduce GI distress.
I.V. use: Injectable form containing 10 mg/ml can be given diluted or undiluted very slowly I.V. Don't give 100 mg/ml injection I.V.
I.M. and S.C. use: Follow normal protocol.
- Alert prescriber if patient appears to be developing tolerance to drug. A different antihistamine may need to be substituted.

Patient teaching
- Tell patient to reduce GI distress by taking drug with food or milk.
- Warn patient to avoid alcohol and activities that require alertness until CNS effects of drug are known.
- Tell patient that coffee or tea may reduce drug-induced drowsiness, although drug causes less drowsiness than some other antihistamines.
- Tell patient to relieve dry mouth with ice chips, sugarless gum, or hard candy.
- Instruct patient to notify prescriber if tolerance develops because different antihistamine may need to be ordered.
- Instruct patient to stop drug 4 days before skin tests to preserve accuracy of tests.
- If patient operates machinery or motor vehicles, explain that drug has sedative effects.

Evaluation
- Patient's allergy symptoms are relieved.
- Patient maintains adequate hydration throughout therapy.
- Patient and family state understanding of drug therapy.

budesonide

(byoo-DES-oh-nighd)
Rhinocort

Pharmacologic class: glucocorticoid
Therapeutic class: anti-inflammatory
Pregnancy risk category: C

Indications and dosages

▶ **Symptoms of seasonal or perennial allergic rhinitis and non-allergic perennial rhinitis.** *Adults:* two sprays (64 mcg) in each nostril in morning and evening or four sprays (128 mcg) in each nostril in morning. Maintenance dosage should be fewest number of sprays needed to control symptoms.

▶ **Symptoms of seasonal or perennial allergic rhinitis.** *Children age 6 and older:* two sprays (64 mcg) in each nostril in morning and evening or four sprays (128 mcg) in each nostril in morning. Maintenance dosage should be fewest number of sprays needed to control symptoms.

How supplied

Nasal spray: 32 mcg/metered spray (7-g canister)

Pharmacokinetics

Absorption: amount of intranasal dose that reaches systemic circulation is typically low (approximately 20%).
Distribution: 88% protein-bound in plasma.
Metabolism: rapidly and extensively metabolized in liver.
Excretion: excreted in urine (about 67%) and feces (about 33%). *Half-life:* about 2 hours.

Route	Onset	Peak	Duration
Inhalation	Unknown	Unknown	Unknown

Pharmacodynamics

Chemical effect: unknown; probably decreases nasal inflammation, mainly by inhibiting activities of specific cells and mediators involved in allergic response.
Therapeutic effect: decreases nasal congestion.

Adverse reactions

CNS: nervousness.
EENT: *nasal irritation, epistaxis, pharyngitis,* reduced sense of smell, nasal pain, hoarseness.
GI: bad taste, dry mouth, dyspepsia, nausea.
Musculoskeletal: myalgia.
Respiratory: *cough,* candidiasis, wheezing, dyspnea.
Skin: facial edema, rash, pruritus, contact dermatitis.
Other: ***hypersensitivity reactions.***

Interactions

None significant.

Contraindications and precautions

- Contraindicated in patients hypersensitive to drug or its components and in those who have had recent septal ulcers, nasal surgery, or nasal trauma, until total healing has occurred.
- Use cautiously in pregnant or breast-feeding women and in patients with tuberculous infections, ocular herpes simplex, or untreated fungal, bacterial, or systemic viral infections.
- Safety of drug hasn't been established in children under age 6.

NURSING CONSIDERATIONS

Assessment

- Obtain history of patient's allergy symptoms and nasal congestion before therapy, and reassess regularly thereafter.
- Be alert for adverse reactions.
- Evaluate patient's and family's understanding of drug therapy.

Nursing diagnoses

- Ineffective health maintenance related to allergy-induced nasal congestion
- Impaired gas exchange related to drug-induced wheezing
- Deficient knowledge related to drug therapy

Planning and implementation

- Before giving drug, shake container and invert. Have patient clear his nasal passages and then tilt his head back. Insert nozzle into nostril (pointed away from septum), holding other nostril closed. Deliver spray while patient inhales. Repeat in other nostril.

• Notify prescriber if relief isn't obtained or signs of infection appear.
• Obtain specimen for culture, as ordered, if signs of nasal infection occur.

Patient teaching
• Instruct patient to shake container before using, blow nose to clear nasal passages, and insert nozzle into nostril, pointing away from septum. Tell him to hold other nostril closed and inhale gently while spraying; then shake container again and repeat in other nostril.
• Tell patient that product should be used by only one person to prevent spread of infection.
• Advise patient not to break, incinerate, or store canister in extreme heat; contents are under pressure.
• Warn patient not to exceed prescribed dose or use for long periods because of risk of hypothalamic-pituitary-adrenal axis suppression.
• Tell patient to report worsened condition or symptoms that don't improve in 3 weeks.
• Teach patient good nasal and oral hygiene.

☑ Evaluation
• Patient's nasal congestion subsides.
• Patient has adequate gas exchange.
• Patient and family state understanding of drug therapy.

bumetanide
(byoo-MEH-tuh-nighd)
Bumex, Burinex ◇

Pharmacologic class: loop diuretic
Therapeutic class: diuretic
Pregnancy risk category: C

Indications and dosages

▶ **Edema in heart failure or hepatic or renal disease.** *Adults:* 0.5 to 2 mg P.O. once daily. If diuretic response isn't adequate, second or third dose may be given at 4- to 5-hour intervals. Maximum dosage is 10 mg/day. May be administered parenterally if P.O. not feasible. Usual initial dose is 0.5 to 1 mg given I.V. over 1 to 2 minutes or I.M. If response isn't adequate, second or third dose may be given at 2- to 3-hour intervals. Maximum dosage is 10 mg/day.

How supplied

Tablets: 0.5 mg, 1 mg, 2 mg
Injection: 0.25 mg/ml

Pharmacokinetics

Absorption: after P.O. administration, 85% to 95% absorbed; food delays absorption of P.O. dose. I.M. bumetanide is completely absorbed.
Distribution: about 92% to 96% protein-bound; unknown if drug enters CSF.
Metabolism: metabolized by liver to at least five metabolites.
Excretion: excreted in urine (80%) and feces (10% to 20%). *Half-life:* 1 to 1½ hours.

Route	Onset	Peak	Duration
P.O.	30-60 min	1-2 hr	4-6 hr
I.V.	3 min	15-30 min	3.5-4 hr
I.M.	40 min	Unknown	Unknown

Pharmacodynamics

Chemical effect: inhibits sodium and chloride reabsorption at ascending portion of loop of Henle.
Therapeutic effect: promotes sodium and water excretion.

Adverse reactions

CNS: dizziness, headache.
CV: volume depletion and dehydration, orthostatic hypotension, ECG changes.
EENT: transient deafness.
GI: nausea.
GU: ***renal failure,*** nocturia, polyuria, frequent urination, oliguria.
Hematologic: azotemia, ***thrombocytopenia.***
Metabolic: hypokalemia; hypochloremic alkalosis; asymptomatic hyperuricemia; fluid and electrolyte imbalances, including dilutional hyponatremia, hypocalcemia, and hypomagnesemia; hyperglycemia; impaired glucose tolerance.
Musculoskeletal: muscle pain and tenderness.
Skin: rash.

Interactions

Drug-drug. *Aminoglycoside antibiotics:* potentiated ototoxicity. Use together cautiously.
Antihypertensives: increased risk of hypotension. Use together cautiously.
Cardiac glycosides: increased risk of digitalis toxicity from bumetanide-induced hypokalemia. Monitor potassium and digoxin levels.
Indomethacin, NSAIDs, probenecid: inhibited diuretic response. Use together cautiously.
Lithium: decreased lithium clearance, increasing risk of lithium toxicity. Monitor lithium level.
Metolazone: profound diuresis and potential electrolyte loss. Monitor patient for fluid and electrolyte imbalances.
Other potassium-wasting drugs: increased risk of hypokalemia. Use together cautiously.
Drug-herb. *Licorice:* may contribute to excessive potassium loss. Discourage concomitant use.

Contraindications and precautions

- Contraindicated in patients hypersensitive to drug or sulfonamides (possible cross-sensitivity), in those with anuria or hepatic coma, in those with severe electrolyte depletion, and in breast-feeding women.
- Use cautiously in pregnant women and in patients with depressed renal function or hepatic cirrhosis or ascites.
- Safety of drug hasn't been established in children.

NURSING CONSIDERATIONS

Assessment

- Obtain history of patient's urine output, vital signs, serum electrolyte levels, breath sounds, peripheral edema, and weight before therapy, and reassess regularly thereafter.
- Be alert for adverse reactions and drug interactions.
- Evaluate patient's and family's understanding of drug therapy.

Nursing diagnoses

- Excessive fluid volume related to underlying condition
- Impaired urinary elimination related to therapeutic effect of drug therapy
- Deficient knowledge related to drug therapy

Planning and implementation

P.O. and I.M. use: Follow normal protocol.
I.V. use: Give I.V. doses directly using 21G or 23G needle over 1 to 2 minutes. For intermittent infusion, give diluted drug through an intermittent infusion device or piggyback into an I.V. line containing free-flowing compatible solution. Infuse at ordered rate. Continuous infusion not recommended.

- To prevent nocturia, give in morning. If second dose is necessary, give in early afternoon.
- The safest and most effective dosage schedule for control of edema is intermittent dosage either given on alternate days or given for 3 to 4 days with 1- or 2-day rest periods.
- Drug can be used safely in patients allergic to furosemide; 1 mg of bumetanide equals 40 mg of furosemide. Bumetanide may be less ototoxic than furosemide, but clinical relevance hasn't been determined.
- If oliguria or azotemia develops or increases, anticipate that prescriber may stop drug.
- Notify prescriber if drug-related hearing changes occur.

Patient teaching

- Advise patient to stand up slowly to prevent dizziness; also, tell him to limit alcohol intake and strenuous exercise in hot weather to avoid exacerbating orthostatic hypotension.
- Teach patient to monitor fluid volume by measuring weight and fluid intake and output daily.
- Advise patient to take drug early in day to avoid sleep interruption caused by nocturia.
- Tell diabetic patient receiving bumetanide to monitor blood glucose levels closely.

Evaluation

- Patient is free from edema.
- Patient demonstrates adjustment of lifestyle to deal with altered patterns of urinary elimination.
- Patient and family state understanding of drug therapy.

buprenorphine hydrochloride

(byoo-preh-NOR-feen high-droh-KLOR-ighd)
Buprenex

Pharmacologic class: narcotic agonist-antagonist, opioid partial agonist
Therapeutic class: analgesic
Controlled substance schedule: V
Pregnancy risk category: C

Indications and dosages

▶ **Moderate to severe pain.** *Adults and children age 13 and over:* 0.3 mg I.M. or slow I.V. q 6 hours, p.r.n., or around clock; may repeat 0.3 mg or increase to 0.6 mg, if needed, 30 to 60 minutes after initial dose.
Children ages 2 to 12: 2 to 6 mcg/kg I.V. or I.M. q 4 to 6 hours.

How supplied

Injection: 0.324 mg (equivalent to 0.3 mg base/ml).

Pharmacokinetics

Absorption: absorbed rapidly after I.M. administration.
Distribution: about 96% protein-bound.
Metabolism: metabolized in liver.
Excretion: excreted primarily in feces as unchanged drug; about 30% excreted in urine.
Half-life: 1.2 to 7.2 hours.

Route	Onset	Peak	Duration
I.V., I.M.	≤ 15 min	≤ 1 hr	About 6 hr

Pharmacodynamics

Chemical effect: binds with opiate receptors in CNS, altering both perception of and emotional response to pain through an unknown mechanism.
Therapeutic effect: relieves pain.

Adverse reactions

CNS: dizziness, sedation, headache, confusion, nervousness, euphoria, ***increased intracranial pressure.***
CV: *hypotension,* ***bradycardia,*** tachycardia, hypertension.
EENT: *miosis,* blurred vision.
GI: *nausea,* vomiting, constipation.
GU: urine retention.
Respiratory: ***respiratory depression,*** hypoventilation.
Skin: pruritus, *sweating.*

Interactions

Drug-drug. *CNS depressants, MAO inhibitors:* additive effects. Use together cautiously.
Narcotic analgesics: possible decreased analgesic effect. Avoid concomitant use.
Drug-lifestyle. *Alcohol use:* additive effects. Discourage concurrent use.

Contraindications and precautions

- Contraindicated in patients hypersensitive to drug.
- Use cautiously in elderly or debilitated patients and in pregnant or breast-feeding women. Also use cautiously in patients with head injury; intracranial lesions; increased intracranial pressure; severe respiratory, liver, or kidney impairment; CNS depression or coma; thyroid irregularities; adrenal insufficiency; prostatic hyperplasia; urethral stricture; acute alcoholism; alcohol withdrawal syndrome; or kyphoscoliosis.

NURSING CONSIDERATIONS

Assessment

- Obtain history of patient's pain before and after drug use.
- Be alert for adverse reactions and drug interactions.
- Monitor respiratory status frequently for at least 1 hour after administration, and notify prescriber about evidence of respiratory depression.
- Evaluate patient's and family's understanding of drug therapy.

Nursing diagnoses

- Acute pain related to underlying condition
- Ineffective breathing pattern related to drug-induced respiratory depression
- Deficient knowledge related to drug therapy

Planning and implementation

I.V. use: Give by direct I.V. injection slowly into vein or through tubing of free-flowing compatible I.V. solution over not less than 2 minutes.

I.M. use: Follow normal protocol.

- S.C. administration isn't recommended.
- Analgesic potency of 0.3 mg of buprenorphine is equal to that of 10 mg of morphine and 75 mg of meperidine; buprenorphine has longer duration of action than morphine or meperidine.
- Notify prescriber, and anticipate increasing dose or frequency of drug if pain isn't relieved.
- If patient's respiratory rate falls below 8 breaths/minute, withhold dose, arouse patient to stimulate breathing, and notify prescriber.
- Naloxone won't completely reverse respiratory depression caused by buprenorphine overdose; mechanical ventilation may be necessary. Larger-than-usual doses of naloxone (more than 0.4 mg) and doxapram also may be ordered.
- Drug's narcotic antagonist properties may precipitate withdrawal syndrome in narcotic-dependent patients.
- If dependence occurs, withdrawal symptoms may appear up to 14 days after drug is stopped.

Patient teaching

- Caution ambulatory patient about getting out of bed or walking because of dizziness or hypotension.
- When drug is used postoperatively, encourage patient to turn, cough, and deep-breathe to prevent atelectasis.

☑ Evaluation

- Patient reports pain relief.
- Patient's respiratory status is within normal limits.
- Patient and family state understanding of drug therapy.

bupropion hydrochloride

(byoo-PROH-pee-on high-droh-KLOR-ighd)

Wellbutrin, Wellbutrin SR

Pharmacologic class: aminoketone
Therapeutic class: antidepressant
Pregnancy risk category: B

Indications and dosages

▶ **Depression.** *Adults:* initially, 100 mg P.O. b.i.d. Increase dosage after 3 days to 100 mg P.O. t.i.d., if needed. If no response occurs after several weeks of therapy, increase dosage to 150 mg t.i.d. For sustained-release tablets, 150 mg P.O. q morning; increased to target dose of 150 mg P.O. b.i.d., as tolerated, as early as day 4 of dosing. Usual adult dose is 300 mg/day; maximum dose is 450 mg daily.

How supplied

Tablets: 75 mg, 100 mg
Tablets (sustained-release): 100 mg, 150 mg

Pharmacokinetics

Absorption: unknown.
Distribution: at plasma levels up to 200 mcg/ml, drug appears to be about 80% bound to plasma proteins.
Metabolism: probably metabolized in liver; several active metabolites have been identified.
Excretion: primarily excreted in urine. *Half-life:* 8 to 24 hours.

Route	Onset	Peak	Duration
P.O.	1-3 wk	$\leq$ 2 hr	Unknown

Pharmacodynamics

Chemical effect: unknown. Drug isn't a tricyclic antidepressant, doesn't inhibit MAO, and is a weak inhibitor of norepinephrine, dopamine, and serotonin reuptake.
Therapeutic effect: relieves depression.

Adverse reactions

CNS: *headache,* akathisia, ***seizures, agitation,*** anxiety, *confusion,* delusions, euphoria, hostility, impaired sleep quality, insomnia, sedation, sensory disturbance, tremors.
CV: ***arrhythmias,*** hypertension, hypotension, palpitations, syncope, tachycardia.
EENT: auditory disturbance, blurred vision.
GI: dry mouth, taste disturbance, increased appetite, constipation, dyspepsia, nausea, vomiting.
GU: impotence, menstrual complaints, urinary frequency.
Musculoskeletal: arthritis.
Skin: pruritus, rash, cutaneous temperature disturbance, diaphoresis.

Other: fever, chills, decreased libido.

Interactions

Drug-drug. *Carbamazepine:* May decrease bupropion levels. Monitor patient for loss of therapeutic effect.
Levodopa, MAO inhibitors, phenothiazines, tricyclic antidepressants; recent and rapid withdrawal of benzodiazepines: increased risk of adverse reactions, including seizures. Monitor patient closely.
Ritonavir: increased serum bupropion levels, increasing toxicity risk. Monitor patient closely.
Drug-lifestyle. *Alcohol use:* increased risk of adverse reactions, including seizures. Monitor patient closely.

Contraindications and precautions

- Contraindicated in patients hypersensitive to drug, in those with seizure disorders or a history of bulimia or anorexia nervosa, and in those who have taken MAO inhibitors during previous 14 days.
- Use cautiously in pregnant women, patients with renal or hepatic impairment, and patients with recent MI or unstable heart disease.
- Breast-feeding should be discontinued if drug must be administered to breast-feeding woman.
- Safety of drug hasn't been established in children.

NURSING CONSIDERATIONS

Assessment

- Obtain history of patient's depression before therapy, and reassess regularly thereafter.
- Be alert for adverse reactions and drug interactions.
- Monitor patient with history of bipolar disorder closely. Antidepressants can cause manic episodes during depressed phase of bipolar disorder.
- Evaluate patient's and family's understanding of drug therapy.

Nursing diagnoses

- Ineffective individual coping related to underlying condition
- Risk for injury related to drug-induced adverse CNS reactions
- Deficient knowledge related to drug therapy

Planning and implementation

ALERT Risk of seizures may be minimized by not exceeding 450 mg/day and by administering daily amount in three to four equally divided doses. Many patients who experience seizures have predisposing factors, including history of head trauma, seizures, or CNS tumors, or they may be taking a drug that lowers seizure threshold.

- Make sure patient has swallowed dose before leaving bedside.
- Patient may experience period of increased restlessness, agitation, insomnia, and anxiety, especially at beginning of therapy.

Patient teaching

- Advise patient to take drug as scheduled and to take each day's amount in three divided doses to minimize risk of seizures.
- Tell patient to avoid alcohol while taking drug because alcohol may contribute to development of seizures.
- Advise patient to avoid hazardous activities that require alertness and good psychomotor coordination until CNS effects of drug are known.

ALERT Advise patient not to take Wellbutrin in combination with Zyban and to seek medical advice before taking other prescription drugs, OTC medications, or herbal remedies.

- Tell patient not to crush, chew, or divide sustained-release tablets.

Evaluation

- Patient's behavior and communication indicate improvement of depression.
- Patient doesn't experience injury from drug-induced adverse CNS reactions.
- Patient and family state understanding of drug therapy.

buspirone hydrochloride

(byoo-SPEER-ohn high-droh-KLOR-ighd)
BuSpar

Pharmacologic class: azaspirodecanedione derivative

Therapeutic class: antianxiety agent
Pregnancy risk category: B

Indications and dosages

▶ **Anxiety disorders, short-term relief of anxiety.** *Adults:* initially, 5 mg P.O. t.i.d. Increase dosage at 2- to 4-day intervals in 5-mg/day increments. Usual maintenance dosage is 15 to 30 mg daily in 2 or 3 divided doses. Don't exceed 60 mg daily.

How supplied

Tablets: 5 mg, 10 mg, 15 mg

Pharmacokinetics

Absorption: absorbed rapidly and completely, but extensive first-pass metabolism limits absolute bioavailability to between 1% and 13% of P.O. dose. Food slows absorption but increases amount of unchanged drug in systemic circulation.
Distribution: 95% protein-bound; doesn't displace other highly protein-bound medications.
Metabolism: metabolized in liver, resulting in at least one active metabolite.
Excretion: 29% to 63% excreted in urine in 24 hours, primarily as metabolites; 18% to 38% excreted in feces. *Half-life:* 2 to 3 hours.

Route	Onset	Peak	Duration
P.O.	Unknown	40-90 min	Unknown

Pharmacodynamics

Chemical effect: unknown; may inhibit neuronal firing and reduce serotonin turnover in cortical, amygdaloid, and septohippocampal tissue.
Therapeutic effect: relieves anxiety.

Adverse reactions

CNS: *dizziness, drowsiness,* nervousness, excitement, insomnia, headache.
GI: dry mouth, nausea, diarrhea.
Other: fatigue.

Interactions

Drug-drug. *CNS depressants:* increased CNS depression. Avoid concomitant use.
MAO inhibitors: may elevate blood pressure. Avoid concomitant use.
Drug-lifestyle. *Alcohol use:* may increase CNS depression. Discourage concurrent use.

Contraindications and precautions

- Contraindicated in patients hypersensitive to drug and in those who have taken an MAO inhibitor within 14 days.
- Avoid use in breast-feeding women, if possible.
- Use cautiously in patients with hepatic or renal failure and in pregnant women.
- Safety of drug hasn't been established in children.

NURSING CONSIDERATIONS

Assessment

- Obtain history of patient's anxiety before therapy, and reassess regularly thereafter.
- Signs of improvement usually appear within 7 to 10 days; optimal results occur after 3 to 4 weeks of therapy.
- Be alert for adverse reactions and drug interactions.
- Evaluate patient's and family's understanding of drug therapy.

Nursing diagnoses

- Anxiety related to underlying condition
- Fatigue related to drug-induced adverse reactions
- Deficient knowledge related to drug therapy

Planning and implementation

- Although drug has shown no potential for abuse and hasn't been classified as a controlled substance, it isn't recommended for relief of everyday stress.
- Before starting therapy in patient already being treated with a benzodiazepine, make sure he doesn't stop benzodiazepine abruptly; withdrawal reaction may occur.
- Administer drug with food or milk.
- Dosage may be increased, as ordered, in 2- to 4-day intervals.

Patient teaching

- Tell patient to take drug with food.
- Warn patient to avoid hazardous activities that require alertness and psychomotor coordination until CNS effects of drug are known.

• Review energy-saving measures with patient and family.
• If patient is already being treated with a benzodiazepine, warn him not to abruptly discontinue it because withdrawal reaction can occur. Teach him how and when benzodiazepine can be withdrawn safely.

Evaluation

• Patient's anxiety is reduced.
• Patient states that energy-saving measures help combat fatigue caused by therapy.
• Patient and family state understanding of drug therapy.

busulfan

(byoo-SUL-fan)
Myleran

Pharmacologic class: alkylating agent (not specific to cell cycle phase)
Therapeutic class: antineoplastic
Pregnancy risk category: D

Indications and dosages

Dosage and indications may vary. Check current literature for recommended protocol.

▶ **Chronic myelocytic (granulocytic) leukemia.** *Adults:* for remission induction, 4 to 8 mg P.O. daily (0.06 mg/kg or 1.8 mg/m^2). For maintenance therapy, 1 to 3 mg P.O. daily. *Children:* 0.06 mg/kg or 1.8 mg/m^2 P.O. daily.

How supplied

Tablets: 2 mg

Pharmacokinetics

Absorption: well absorbed from GI tract.
Distribution: unknown.
Metabolism: metabolized in liver.
Excretion: cleared rapidly from plasma and excreted in urine. *Half-life:* about 2½ hours.

Route	Onset	Peak	Duration
P.O.	1-2 wk	Unknown	Unknown

Pharmacodynamics

Chemical effect: unknown; thought to cross-link strands of cellular DNA and interfere with RNA transcription, causing an imbalance of growth that leads to cell death.
Therapeutic effect: kills selected type of cancer cell.

Adverse reactions

CNS: ***seizures,*** unusual tiredness or weakness.
GI: nausea, vomiting, diarrhea, cheilosis, glossitis.
GU: amenorrhea, testicular atrophy, impotence.
Hematologic: ***leukocytopenia, thrombocytopenia, anemia, severe pancytopenia.***
Respiratory: persistent cough; dyspnea; ***irreversible pulmonary fibrosis,*** commonly termed "busulfan lung."
Skin: transient hyperpigmentation, rash, urticaria, anhidrosis, alopecia.
Other: gynecomastia, Addison-like wasting syndrome, profound hyperuricemia caused by increased cell lysis.

Interactions

Drug-drug. *Acetaminophen:* busulfan levels increase with concurrent administration or if given within 72 hours. Avoid concurrent use.
Anticoagulants, aspirin: increased risk of bleeding. Avoid concomitant use.
Itraconazole: decreases busulfan clearance by 25%. Avoid concomitant use.
Phenytoin: increases busulfan clearance by 18%. Monitor patient for reduced effectiveness.
Thioguanine: may cause hepatotoxicity, esophageal varices, or portal hypertension. Use together cautiously.

Contraindications and precautions

• Contraindicated in patients with chronic myelogenous leukemia, which is known to be resistant to drug, and in breast-feeding women.
• Use with extreme caution, if at all, in pregnant women.
• Use cautiously in patients recently given other myelosuppressive drugs or radiation therapy and in those with depressed neutrophil or platelet count. Because high-dose therapy has been linked to seizures, use such therapy cautiously in patients with history of head trauma or seizures and in patients receiving other drugs that lower seizure threshold.

NURSING CONSIDERATIONS

Assessment

- Obtain history of patient's underlying neoplastic disease.
- Monitor effectiveness by noting results of follow-up diagnostic tests and overall physical status. Note patient response (increased appetite and sense of well-being, decreased total WBC count, reduced size of spleen), which usually begins within 1 to 2 weeks.
- Monitor WBC and platelet counts weekly while patient is receiving drug. WBC count falls about 10 days after the start of therapy and continues to fall for 2 weeks after stopping drug.
- Monitor serum uric acid level.

ALERT Be alert for adverse reactions and drug interactions. Pulmonary fibrosis may occur as late as 4 to 6 months after treatment.

- Evaluate patient's and family's understanding of drug therapy.

Nursing diagnoses

- Ineffective health maintenance related to presence of neoplastic disease
- Risk for infection related to drug-induced immunosuppression
- Deficient knowledge related to drug therapy

Planning and implementation

- Follow facility policy regarding preparation and handling of drug. Label as hazardous drug.
- Administer drug at same time each day.
- Make sure patient is adequately hydrated.
- Dosage is adjusted based on patient's weekly WBC counts, and the prescriber may temporarily stop drug therapy if severe leukocytopenia develops. Therapeutic effects are often accompanied by toxicity.
- Drug is usually administered with allopurinol in addition to adequate hydration to prevent hyperuricemia with resulting uric acid nephropathy.

Patient teaching

- Warn patient to watch for signs of infection (fever, sore throat, fatigue) and bleeding (easy bruising, nosebleeds, bleeding gums, melena) and to take temperature daily.

ALERT Instruct patient to report symptoms of toxicity so that dosage adjustments can be made. Symptoms include persistent cough and progressive dyspnea with alveolar exudate, suggestive of pneumonia.

- Instruct patient to avoid OTC products that contain aspirin.
- Advise woman of childbearing age to avoid becoming pregnant during therapy. Recommend that patient consult with prescriber before becoming pregnant.
- Advise breast-feeding woman to discontinue breast-feeding because of possible risk of toxicity in infant.

Evaluation

- Patient exhibits positive response to drug therapy.
- Patient remains free from infection.
- Patient and family state understanding of drug therapy.

butorphanol tartrate

(byoo-TOR-fah-nohl TAR-trayt)

Stadol, Stadol NS

Pharmacologic class: narcotic agonist-antagonist; opioid partial agonist

Therapeutic class: analgesic, adjunct to anesthesia

Pregnancy risk category: C

Indications and dosages

▶ **Moderate to severe pain.** *Adults:* 0.5 to 2 mg I.V. q 3 to 4 hours, p.r.n. or around the clock. Or, 1 to 4 mg I.M. q 3 to 4 hours, p.r.n. or around the clock. Maximum 4 mg per dose. Alternatively, 1 mg by nasal spray q 3 to 4 hours (1 spray in one nostril); repeated in 60 to 90 minutes if pain relief is inadequate.

▶ **Labor for pregnant women at full term and in early labor.** *Adults:* 1 to 2 mg I.V. or I.M., repeated after 4 hours, p.r.n.

▶ **Preoperative anesthesia or preanesthesia.** *Adults:* 2 mg I.M. 60 to 90 minutes before surgery.

▶ **Adjunct to balanced anesthesia**. *Adults:* 2 mg I.V. shortly before induction or 0.5 to 1 mg I.V. in increments during anesthesia.

How supplied

Injection: 1 mg/ml, 2 mg/ml
Nasal spray: 10 mg/ml

Pharmacokinetics

Absorption: well absorbed after I.M. administration; unknown after nasal administration.
Distribution: about 80% bound to plasma proteins. After I.V. administation, mean volume of distribution is about 500 L. Drug rapidly crosses placenta, and neonatal serum levels are 0.4 to 1.4 times maternal levels.
Metabolism: extensively metabolized in liver to inactive metabolites.
Excretion: excreted in inactive form, mainly by kidneys. About 11% to 14% of parenteral dose excreted in feces.

Route	Onset	Peak	Duration
I.V.	2-3 min	0.5-1 hr	2-4 hr
I.M.	10-30 min	0.5-1 hr	3-4 hr
Intranasal	≤ 15 min	1-2 hr	4-5 hr

Pharmacodynamics

Chemical effect: binds with opiate receptors in CNS, altering both perception of and emotional response to pain through unknown mechanism.
Therapeutic effect: relieves pain and enhances anesthesia.

Adverse reactions

CNS: *sedation, headache, vertigo, floating sensation,* lethargy, *confusion,* nervousness, unusual dreams, agitation, euphoria, hallucinations, flushing, increased intracranial pressure.
CV: palpitations, fluctuation in blood pressure.
EENT: diplopia, blurred vision, *nasal congestion* (with nasal spray).
GI: nausea, vomiting, constipation, *dry mouth.*
Respiratory: ***respiratory depression.***
Skin: rash, urticaria, *clamminess, excessive sweating.*

Interactions

Drug-drug. *CNS depressants:* additive effects. Use together cautiously.
Narcotic analgesics: possible decreased analgesic effect. Avoid concomitant use.
Drug-lifestyle. *Alcohol use:* additive depressant effects. Discourage concomitant use.

Contraindications and precautions

- Contraindicated in patients with narcotic addiction; may precipitate withdrawal syndrome. Also contraindicated in breast-feeding women and in patients hypersensitive to drug or to preservative (benzethonium chloride).
- Use with extreme caution, if at all, in pregnant women.
- Use cautiously in patients with head injury, increased intracranial pressure, acute MI, ventricular dysfunction, coronary insufficiency, respiratory disease or depression, or renal or hepatic dysfunction. Also use cautiously in patients who have recently received repeated doses of narcotic analgesic.
- Use cautiously in children; drug may cause paradoxical excitement.

NURSING CONSIDERATIONS

Assessment

- Obtain history of patient's pain before and after drug administration.
- Be alert for adverse reactions and drug interactions.
- Periodically monitor postoperative vital signs and bladder function. Because drug decreases both rate and depth of respirations, monitoring arterial oxygen saturation may aid in assessing respiratory depression.
- Evaluate patient's and family's understanding of drug therapy.

Nursing diagnoses

- Acute pain related to underlying condition
- Risk for injury related to drug-induced adverse CNS reactions
- Deficient knowledge related to drug therapy

Planning and implementation

I.V. use: Give drug by direct I.V. injection into vein or into I.V. line containing free-flowing compatible solution.
I.M. use: Follow normal protocol.
Intranasal use: Have patient clear nasal passages before administering drug. Shake container. Tilt patient's head slightly backward; insert nozzle into nostril, pointing away from

septum. Have patient hold other nostril closed, and then spray while patient inhales gently.
- S.C. route isn't recommended.
- Psychological and physical addiction may occur.
- Notify prescriber and discuss increasing dose or frequency if pain persists.
- Keep narcotic antagonist (naloxone) and resuscitative equipment readily available.

Patient teaching
- Caution ambulatory patient about getting out of bed or walking. Warn outpatient to refrain from driving and performing other activities that require mental alertness until drug's CNS effects are known.
- Warn patient that drug can cause physical and psychological dependence. Tell him that he should use drug only as directed and that abrupt withdrawal after prolonged use produces intense withdrawal symptoms.

Evaluation
- Patient reports relief of pain.
- Patient doesn't experience injury as a result of therapy.
- Patient and family state understanding of drug therapy.

C

caffeine
(ka-FEEN)
Caffedrine Caplets†, NoDoz†, Quick Pep†, Vivarin†

Pharmacologic class: methylxanthine
Therapeutic class: CNS stimulant
Pregnancy risk category: B

Indications and dosages
▶ **CNS stimulant.** *Adults:* 100 to 200 mg P.O. q 4 hours, p.r.n.

How supplied
Tablets: 100 mg†, 150 mg†, 200 mg†
Capsules (timed-release): 200 mg†

Pharmacokinetics
Absorption: well absorbed from GI tract.
Distribution: distributed rapidly throughout body; crosses blood-brain barrier; about 17% protein-bound.
Metabolism: metabolized by liver.
Excretion: excreted in urine. *Half-life:* 3 to 7 hours.

Route	Onset	Peak	Duration
P.O.	Unknown	50-75 min	Unknown

Pharmacodynamics
Chemical effect: inhibits phosphodiesterase, the enzyme that degrades cAMP.
Therapeutic effect: stimulates CNS.

Adverse reactions
CNS: *stimulation, insomnia,* restlessness, nervousness, mild delirium, headache, excitement, agitation, twitches.
CV: *tachycardia, palpitations.*
GI: nausea, vomiting.
GU: *diuresis.*
Metabolic: hyperglycemia.
Musculoskeletal: muscle tremors.
Skin: hyperesthesia.
Other: dehydration, fever, abrupt withdrawal symptoms (headache, irritability).

Interactions
Drug-drug. *Beta-adrenergic agonists, cimetidine, fluoroquinolones, oral contraceptives, theophylline:* excessive CNS stimulation. Avoid concomitant use.
Drug-food. *Caffeine-containing foods and beverages:* excessive CNS stimulation. Discourage concomitant use.

Contraindications and precautions
- Contraindicated in patients hypersensitive to drug.
- Use cautiously in pregnant women, patients in the first several days to weeks after an acute MI, and patients with a history of peptic ulcer, symptomatic arrhythmias, or palpitations.
- Avoid use of caffeine tablets or capsules in breast-feeding women.

• Safety of drug hasn't been established in children.

NURSING CONSIDERATIONS

Assessment
• Assess patient's CNS depression before therapy and regularly thereafter.
• Be alert for adverse reactions and drug interactions.
• Monitor patient for tolerance or psychological dependence.
• Evaluate patient's and family's knowledge of drug therapy.

Nursing diagnoses
• Ineffective health maintenance related to patient's underlying condition
• Fatigue related to caffeine-induced CNS stimulation
• Deficient knowledge related to drug therapy

Planning and implementation
• Single dose shouldn't exceed 1 g.
• Sudden discontinuation may cause headache and irritability.
• Caffeine doesn't reverse alcohol intoxication or CNS-depressant effects of alcohol.
• Restrict caffeine-containing beverages in patients who experience palpitations. Caffeine content per 180 ml: cola, 17 to 55 mg; tea, 40 to 100 mg; instant coffee, 60 to 180 mg; brewed coffee, 100 to 150 mg; decaffeinated coffee, 1 to 6 mg.

Patient teaching
• Caution patient not to use drug excessively; tolerance or psychological dependence may occur.
• Tell patient to restrict caffeine-containing beverages.
• Instruct patient to stop using drug and notify prescriber if palpitations occur.

Evaluation
• Patient exhibits CNS stimulation.
• Patient doesn't develop fatigue.
• Patient and family state understanding of drug therapy.

calcifediol
(kal-sih-fih-DIGH-al)
Calderol

Pharmacologic class: vitamin D analogue
Therapeutic class: antihypocalcemic
Pregnancy risk category: C

Indications and dosages

▶ **Metabolic bone disease related to chronic renal failure.** *Adults:* initially, 300 to 350 mcg/week P.O. daily or every other day. Dosage increased at 4-week intervals if necessary.

How supplied

Capsules: 20 mcg, 50 mcg

Pharmacokinetics

Absorption: absorbed readily from small intestine.
Distribution: distributed widely; highly protein-bound.
Metabolism: metabolized in liver and kidney.
Excretion: excreted in urine and bile. *Half-life:* 16 days.

Route	Onset	Peak	Duration
P.O.	Unknown	4 hr	15-20 days

Pharmacodynamics

Chemical effect: stimulates calcium absorption from GI tract; promotes calcium secretion from bone to blood.
Therapeutic effect: raises blood calcium level.

Adverse reactions

Vitamin D intoxication caused by hypercalcemia:
CNS: headache, somnolence.
EENT: conjunctivitis, rhinorrhea.
GI: nausea, vomiting, constipation, metallic taste, dry mouth, anorexia, diarrhea.
GU: polyuria.
Musculoskeletal: weakness, bone and muscle pain.
Skin: photosensitivity reactions.

Interactions

Drug-drug. *Cholestyramine, colestipol:* decreased absorption of orally administered vitamin D analogues. Avoid concomitant use.
Cardiac glycosides: increased risk of arrhythmias. Avoid concomitant use.
Magnesium-containing antacids: possible hypermagnesemia, especially in patients with chronic renal failure. Avoid concomitant use.
Other vitamin D analogues: increased toxicity. Avoid concomitant use.

Contraindications and precautions

- Contraindicated in patients with hypercalcemia or vitamin D toxicity.
- Use cautiously in pregnant or breast-feeding women.
- Safety of drug hasn't been established in children.

NURSING CONSIDERATIONS

Assessment

- Assess patient's metabolic bone disease before therapy and regularly thereafter.
- Monitor drug effectiveness by regularly checking serum calcium level, as ordered: serum calcium times serum phosphate shouldn't exceed 70. During dosage adjustment, determine serum calcium level at least weekly.
- Be alert for adverse reactions and drug interactions.
- Evaluate patient's and family's knowledge of drug therapy.

Nursing diagnoses

- Risk for injury related to patient's underlying bone condition
- Ineffective protection related to potential for drug-induced vitamin D intoxication
- Deficicent knowledge related to drug therapy

Planning and implementation

- Optimal dosage is highly individualized.
- Notify prescriber if hypercalcemia occurs; drug should be discontinued until serum calcium level returns to normal.
- Ensure that patient's daily calcium intake is adequate.

Patient teaching

- Advise patient to adhere to diet and calcium supplementation and to avoid OTC drugs.
- Teach patient to report signs and symptoms of hypercalcemia.

Evaluation

- Patient's underlying condition improves and serum calcium level rises.
- Patient doesn't experience drug-induced vitamin D intoxication.
- Patient and family state understanding of drug therapy.

calcitonin (human)

(kal-sih-TOH-nin)
Cibacalcin

calcitonin (salmon)

Calcimar, Miacalcin, Osteocalcin, Salmonine

Pharmacologic class: thyroid hormone
Therapeutic class: hypocalcemic
Pregnancy risk category: C

Indications and dosages

▶ **Paget's disease of bone (osteitis deformans).** *Adults:* initially, 100 IU of calcitonin (salmon) daily I.M. or S.C.; maintenance dosage is 50 to 100 IU daily or every other day. Calcitonin (human) 0.5 mg S.C. daily, maximum 1 mg daily. If patient improves sufficiently, dosage reduced to 0.25 mg daily two or three times weekly.

▶ **Hypercalcemia.** *Adults:* 4 IU/kg of calcitonin (salmon) q 12 hours I.M. or S.C. If response is inadequate after 1 or 2 days, dosage increased to 8 IU/kg I.M. q 12 hours. If response remains unsatisfactory after 2 more days, dosage increased to maximum of 8 IU/kg q 6 hours.

▶ **Postmenopausal osteoporosis.** *Adults:* 100 IU of calcitonin (salmon) daily I.M. or S.C. 200 IU (one activation) of calcitonin (salmon) daily intranasally, alternating nostrils daily. Patients should receive adequate vitamin D and calcium supplements.

How supplied

calcitonin (human)
Injection: 0.5 mg/vial
calcitonin (salmon)
Injection: 100 IU/ml, 1-ml ampules; 200 IU/ml, 2-ml ampules
Nasal spray: 200 IU/activation in 2-ml bottle

Pharmacokinetics

Absorption: unknown.
Distribution: unknown.
Metabolism: rapidly metabolized in kidneys; additional activity in blood and peripheral tissues.
Excretion: excreted in urine as inactive metabolites. *Half-life:* calcitonin human, 60 minutes; calcitonin salmon, 70 to 90 minutes.

Route	Onset	Peak	Duration
I.M., S.C.	≤ 15 min	≤ 4 hr	8-24 hr
Intranasal	Rapid	30 min	1 hr

Pharmacodynamics

Chemical effect: decreases osteoclastic activity by inhibiting osteocytic osteolysis; decreases mineral release and matrix or collagen breakdown in bone.
Therapeutic effect: prohibits bone and kidney (tubular) resorption of calcium.

Adverse reactions

CNS: headache.
GI: transient nausea, unusual taste, diarrhea, anorexia.
GU: transient diuresis.
Metabolic: hypocalcemia, hyperglycemia.
Other: inflammation at injection site; rash; *facial flushing;* hand swelling, tingling, and tenderness; hypersensitivity reactions, ***anaphylaxis.***

Interactions

None significant.

Contraindications and precautions

- Calcitonin may inhibit lactation and shouldn't be used in breast-feeding women.
- Calcitonin salmon is contraindicated in patients hypersensitive to drug.
- Use cautiously in pregnant women.
- Safety of drug hasn't been established in children.

NURSING CONSIDERATIONS

Assessment

- Assess patient's serum calcium level before therapy and regularly thereafter.
- Monitor serum alkaline phosphatase and 24-hour urine hydroxyproline levels to evaluate drug effectiveness, as ordered.
- Periodic examinations of urine sediment are advisable.
- Be alert for adverse reactions.
- Evaluate patient's and family's knowledge of drug therapy.

Nursing diagnoses

- Risk for trauma related to patient's underlying bone condition
- Ineffective protection related to potential for drug-induced anaphylaxis
- Deficient knowledge related to drug therapy

Planning and implementation

- Skin test is usually performed before therapy.
- Calcitonin (human) is especially indicated in patients who have developed resistance to calcitonin (salmon). Calcitonin (human) is linked to risk of diminishing efficacy caused by antibody formation or hypersensitivity reactions.
- Administer drug at bedtime when possible to minimize nausea and vomiting.

I.M. use: I.M. route is preferred if volume of dose to be administered exceeds 2 ml. Follow normal protocol.
S.C. use: S.C. route is the preferred route for outpatient self-administration. Follow normal protocol.
Intranasal use: Alternate nostrils daily.

- Use freshly reconstituted solution within 2 hours.
- Keep parenteral calcium available during first doses in case hypocalcemic tetany occurs.
- Store calcitonin human at room temperature (77° F [25° C]); refrigerate calcitonin salmon at 36° to 46° F (2° to 8° C). Store open nasal spray at room temperature.

• In patients who relapse after a positive initial response, expect to evaluate for antibody response to hormone protein.
• Keep epinephrine handy; systemic allergic reactions are possible because hormone is protein.
• If symptoms have been relieved after 6 months, treatment may be discontinued until symptoms or radiologic signs recur.

Patient teaching
• Teach patient how to take drug.
• Teach patient to activate nasal spray before first use. He should hold bottle upright and depress side arms six times until a faint mist occurs. This signifies that pump is ready for use.
• Instruct patient to report signs of nasal irritation with nasal spray.
• Tell patient to handle missed doses as follows: With daily dosing, take as soon as possible, but don't double the dose. With alternate-day dosing, take missed dose as soon as possible, and then restart alternate days from this dose.
• Reassure patient that facial flushing and warmth (which occur in 20% to 30% of patients within minutes of injection) usually subside in about 1 hour.
• Remind patient with postmenopausal osteoporosis to take adequate calcium and vitamin D supplements.
• Inform patient that further drug treatment or increased dosages will be of no value in those where the drug loses its hypocalcemic activity.

Evaluation
• Patient's serum calcium levels are normal.
• Patient doesn't experience anaphylaxis.
• Patient and family state understanding of drug therapy.

calcitriol (1,25-dihydroxycholecalciferol)
(kal-SIH-tree-ohl)
Rocaltrol, Calcijex

Pharmacologic class: vitamin D analogue
Therapeutic class: antihypocalcemic
Pregnancy risk category: C

Indications and dosages
▶ **Hypocalcemia in patients undergoing long-term dialysis.** *Adults:* initially, 0.25 mcg P.O. daily, increased by 0.25 mcg daily at 4- to 8-week intervals. Maintenance dosage is 0.25 mcg every other day up to 1.25 mcg daily, or 1 to 2 mcg I.V. three times weekly approximately every other day. Dosages from 0.5 to 4 mcg three times weekly have been used initially. If response to initial dose is inadequate, may increase by 0.5 to 1 mcg at 2- to 4-week intervals. Maintenance dosage is 0.5 to 3 mcg I.V. three times weekly.
▶ **Hypoparathyroidism and pseudohypoparathyroidism.** *Adults and children age 6 and older:* initially, 0.25 mcg P.O. daily. Dosage may be increased at 2- to 4-week intervals. Maintenance dosage is 0.25 to 2 mcg daily.
▶ **Hypoparathyroidism**. *Children ages 1 to 5 years:* 0.25 to 0.75 mcg P.O. daily.
▶ **Management of secondary hyperparathyroidism and resulting metabolic bone disease in predialysis patients (moderate to severe chronic renal failure with creatinine clearance of 15 to 55 ml/minute).** *Adults and children age 3 and older:* initially, 0.25 mcg P.O. daily. Dosage may be increased to 0.5 mcg/day if necessary.
Children younger than age 3: initially, 10 to 15 ng/kg P.O. daily.

How supplied
Capsules: 0.25 mcg, 0.5 mcg
Injection: 1 mcg/ml, 2 mcg/ml
Oral solution: 1 mcg/ml

Pharmacokinetics
Absorption: absorbed readily.
Distributed: distributed widely; protein-bound.
Metabolism: metabolized in liver and kidney.
Excretion: excreted primarily in feces. *Half-life:* 3 to 6 hours.

Route	Onset	Peak	Duration
P.O.	2-6 hr	3-6 hr	3-5 days
I.V.	Immediate	Unknown	3-5 days

Pharmacodynamics

Chemical effect: stimulates calcium absorption from GI tract; promotes calcium secretion from bone to blood.
Therapeutic effect: raises blood calcium levels.

Adverse reactions

Vitamin D intoxication related to hypercalcemia:
CNS: headache, somnolence.
EENT: conjunctivitis, photophobia, rhinorrhea.
GI: nausea, vomiting, constipation, metallic taste, dry mouth, anorexia.
GU: polyuria.
Musculoskeletal: weakness, bone and muscle pain.

Interactions

Drug-drug. *Cardiac glycosides:* increased risk of arrhythmias. Avoid concomitant use.
Cholestyramine, colestipol, excessive use of mineral oil: decreased absorption of orally administered vitamin D analogues. Avoid concomitant use.
Corticosteroids: counteracts vitamin D analogue effects. Don't use together.
Magnesium-containing antacids: may induce hypermagnesemia, especially in patients with chronic renal failure. Avoid concomitant use.
Phenytoin, phenobarbital: may reduce plasma calcitriol levels. Higher doses may be needed.
Thiazides: may induce hypercalcemia. Monitor serum calcium levels and patient closely.

Contraindications and precautions

- Contraindicated in patients with hypercalcemia or vitamin D toxicity.
- Use cautiously in pregnant or breast-feeding women.

NURSING CONSIDERATIONS

Assessment

- Assess patient's serum calcium level before therapy, and reassess regularly thereafter to monitor drug effectiveness; serum calcium level times serum phosphate level shouldn't exceed 70. During dosage adjustment, determine serum calcium level twice weekly.
- Be alert for adverse reactions and drug interactions.
- Evaluate patient's and family's knowledge of drug therapy.

Nursing diagnoses

- Risk for injury related to patient's underlying condition
- Ineffective protection related to potential for drug-induced vitamin D intoxication
- Deficient knowledge related to drug therapy

Planning and implementation

P.O. use: Follow normal protocol.
I.V. use: Administer I.V. dose by rapid injection via dialysis catheter at end of hemodialysis treatment.

- Keep drug away from heat and light.
- Administer drug at same time daily.
- Discontinue drug and notify prescriber if hypercalcemia occurs; resume drug after serum calcium level returns to normal. Patient should receive 1,000 mg of calcium daily.

Patient teaching

- Tell patient to immediately report early symptoms of vitamin D intoxication: weakness, nausea, vomiting, dry mouth, constipation, muscle or bone pain, or metallic taste.
- Instruct patient to adhere to diet and calcium supplements and to avoid unapproved OTC drugs and magnesium-containing antacids.
- Warn patient that calcitriol is most potent form of vitamin D available; severe toxicity can occur if ingested by anyone for whom it wasn't prescribed.
- Teach patient to protect medication from light.

Evaluation

- Patient's serum calcium level is normal.
- Patient doesn't experience injury from drug-induced vitamin D toxicity.
- Patient and family state understanding of drug therapy.

calcium acetate
(KAL-see-um AS-ih-tayt)
Calphron, Phos-Ex , Phos-Lo

calcium carbonate
Apo-Cal ♦ †, Cal-Carb-HD†, Calci-Chew†, Calciday 667†, Calci-Mix†, Calcite 500 ♦ †, Calcium 500 ♦ †, Calcium 600†, Cal-Plus†, Calsan ♦ †, Caltrate†, Caltrate 600 ♦ †, Chooz†, Fem Cal†, Florical†, Gencalc 600†, Mallamint†, Nephro-Calci†, Nu-Cal ♦ †, Os-Cal ♦ †, Os-Cal 500†, Os-Cal Chewable ♦ †, Oysco†, Oysco 500 Chewable†, Oyst-Cal 500†, Oystercal 500†, Oyster Shell Calcium-500†, Rolaids Calcium Rich†, Super Calcium 1200†, Titralac†, Tums†, Tums 500†, Tums E-X†

calcium chloride†
Calciject ♦

calcium citrate†
Citrical†, Citrical Liquitabs ♦ †

calcium glubionate†
Calcium-Sandoz ♦, Neo-Calglucon

calcium gluceptate†

calcium gluconate

calcium lactate†

calcium phosphate, dibasic†

calcium phosphate, tribasic
Posture†

Pharmacologic class: calcium supplement
Therapeutic class: therapeutic agent for electrolyte balance, cardiotonic
Pregnancy risk category: C

Indications and dosages

▶ **Hypocalcemic emergency.** *Adults:* 7 to 14 mEq calcium I.V. May be given as 10% calcium gluconate solution, 2% to 10% calcium chloride solution, or 22% calcium gluceptate solution. (Calcium gluceptate sodium may be given I.M. only in emergencies.)
Children: 1 to 7 mEq calcium I.V. *Infants:* up to 1 mEq calcium I.V.

▶ **Hypocalcemic tetany.** *Adults:* 4.5 to 16 mEq calcium I.V. Repeated until tetany is controlled.
Children: 0.5 to 0.7 mEq calcium I.V. t.i.d. or q.i.d. until tetany is controlled.
Neonates: 2.4 mEq I.V. daily in divided doses.

▶ **Adjunct treatment of cardiac arrest.** *Adults:* 0.027 to 0.054 mEq calcium chloride I.V., 4.5 to 6.3 mEq calcium gluceptate I.V., or 2.3 to 3.7 mEq calcium gluconate I.V.
Children: 0.27 mEq/kg calcium chloride I.V. Repeated in 10 minutes if necessary; determine serum calcium levels before administering further doses.

▶ **Adjunct treatment of magnesium intoxication.** *Adults:* initially, 7 mEq I.V. Subsequent doses based on patient's response.

▶ **During exchange transfusions.** *Adults:* 1.35 mEq concurrently with each 100 ml citrated blood.
Neonates: 0.45 mEq after each 100 ml citrated blood.

▶ **Hyperphosphatemia in end-stage renal failure.** *Adults:* 2 to 4 tablets calcium acetate P.O. with each meal.

▶ **Dietary supplement.** *Adults:* 800 mg to 1.2 g P.O. daily.

How supplied

calcium acetate
Contains 253 mg or 12.7 mEq of elemental calcium/g
Tablets: 250 mg†, 500 mg†, 667 mg, 668 mg†, 1,000 mg†
Injection: 0.5 mEq Ca^{++} per ml

calcium carbonate
Contains 400 mg or 20 mEq of elemental calcium/g
Tablets: 650 mg†, 667 mg†, 750 mg†, 1.25 g†, 1.5 g†
Tablets (chewable): 350 mg†, 420 mg†, 500 mg†, 625 mg†, 750 mg†, 850 mg†, 1.25 g†
Capsules: 364 mg†, 1.25 g†
Oral suspension: 1.25 g/5 ml†
Powder packets: 6.5 g (2,400 mg calcium) per packet†

calcium chloride
Contains 270 mg or 13.5 mEq of elemental calcium/g
Injection: 10% solution in 10-ml ampules, vials, and syringes
calcium citrate
Contains 211 mg or 10.6 mEq of elemental calcium/g
Tablets: 950 mg†
Effervescent tablets: 2,376 mg†
calcium glubionate
Contains 64 mg or 3.2 mEq of elemental calcium/g
Syrup: 1.8 g/5 ml
calcium gluceptate
Contains 82 mg or 4.1 mEq of elemental calcium/g
Injection: 1.1 g/5 ml in 5-ml ampules or 10-ml vials
calcium gluconate
Contains 90 mg or 4.5 mEq of elemental calcium/g
Tablets: 500 mg†, 650 mg†, 975 mg†, 1 g†
Injection: 10% solution in 10-ml ampules and vials, 10-ml or 50-ml vials
calcium lactate
Contains 130 mg or 6.5 mEq of elemental calcium/g
Tablets: 325 mg, 650 mg
calcium phosphate, dibasic
Contains 230 mg or 11.5 mEq of elemental calcium/g
Tablets: 468 mg†
calcium phosphate, tribasic
Contains 400 mg or 20 mEq of elemental calcium/g
Tablets: 600 mg†

Pharmacokinetics

Absorption: absorbed actively in duodenum and proximal jejunum and, to lesser extent, in distal part of small intestine after oral administration. Pregnancy and reduced calcium intake may enhance absorption. Vitamin D in active form is required for absorption.
Distribution: enters extracellular fluid and is incorporated rapidly into skeletal tissue. Bone contains 99% of total calcium; 1% is distributed equally between intracellular and extracellular fluids. Levels in CSF are about half those in serum.
Metabolism: insignificant.
Excretion: excreted mainly in feces, minimally in urine.

Route	Onset	Peak	Duration
P.O., I.M.	Unknown	Unknown	Unknown
I.V.	Immediate	Immediate	0.5-2 hr

Pharmacodynamics

Chemical effect: replaces and maintains calcium.
Therapeutic effect: raises blood calcium level.

Adverse reactions

CNS: tingling sensations, sense of oppression or heat waves with I.V. use; syncope with rapid I.V. injection.
CV: mild decrease in blood pressure; vasodilation, ***bradycardia, arrhythmias, and cardiac arrest*** with rapid I.V. injection.
GI: irritation, hemorrhage, *constipation* with oral use; chalky taste with I.V. use; hemorrhage, nausea, vomiting, thirst, abdominal pain with oral calcium chloride.
GU: hypercalcemia, polyuria, renal calculi.
Skin: local reactions including burning, necrosis, tissue sloughing, cellulitis, soft-tissue calcification with I.M. use.
Other: pain, irritation (with S.C. injection); *vein irritation* with I.V. use.

Interactions

Drug-drug. *Atenolol, fluoroquinolones, tetracyclines:* decreased bioavailability of these drugs and calcium when oral forms are taken together. Separate administration times.
Calcium channel blockers: decreased calcium effectiveness. Avoid concomitant use.
Cardiac glycosides: increased digitalis toxicity. Administer calcium cautiously (if at all) to digitalized patients.
Sodium polystyrene sulfonate: risk of metabolic acidosis in patients with renal disease. Avoid concomitant use.
Thiazide diuretics: risk of hypercalcemia. Avoid concomitant use.
Drug-food. *Foods containing oxalic acid (rhubarb, spinach), phytic acid (bran, whole cereals), or phosphorus (milk, dairy products):* may interfere with calcium absorption. Tell patient to avoid these foods.

Contraindications and precautions

• Contraindicated in patients with ventricular fibrillation, hypercalcemia, hypophosphatemia, or renal calculi.
• Use all calcium products with extreme caution in digitalized patients and in patients with sarcoidosis and renal or cardiac disease. Use calcium chloride cautiously in patients with cor pulmonale, respiratory acidosis, and respiratory failure.
• Use I.V. route cautiously in children.

NURSING CONSIDERATIONS

Assessment

• Assess patient's serum calcium level before therapy, and reassess frequently thereafter to monitor drug effectiveness. Hypercalcemia may result after large doses in chronic renal failure.
• Be alert for adverse reactions and drug interactions.
• Evaluate patient's and family's knowledge of drug therapy.

Nursing diagnoses

• Ineffective protection related to calcium deficiency
• Risk for injury related to drug-induced adverse reactions
• Deficient knowledge related to drug therapy

Planning and implementation

P.O. use: If GI upset occurs, give oral calcium products 1 to 1½ hours after meals.
I.V. use: Administer direct injection slowly through small needle into large vein or through I.V. line containing free-flowing, compatible solution at no more than 1 ml/minute (1.5 mEq/minute) for calcium chloride, 1.5 to 5 ml/minute for calcium gluconate, and 2 ml/minute for calcium gluceptate. Don't use scalp veins in children.
– When giving intermittent infusion, infuse diluted solution through I.V. line containing compatible solution. Maximum rate of 200 mg/minute suggested for calcium gluceptate and calcium gluconate.
ALERT Make sure prescriber specifies calcium form to administer because code carts usually contain both calcium gluconate and calcium chloride.
– Give calcium chloride only by I.V. route. When adding to parenteral solutions that contain other additives (especially phosphorus or phosphate), observe solution closely for precipitate. Use in-line filter.
– Warm solutions to body temperature before administration.
– After injection, make sure patient remains recumbent for 15 minutes.
– Monitor ECG when giving calcium I.V. Stop if patient complains of discomfort, and notify prescriber.
– Stop drug immediately if extravasation occurs (severe necrosis and tissue sloughing), and change I.V. site before continuing drug.
I.M. use: Give injection in gluteal region in adults; lateral thigh in infants. Only calcium gluceptate can be given via the I.M. route in emergencies when no I.V. route available.
• Withhold drug and notify prescriber if hypercalcemia occurs. Be prepared to provide emergency supportive care as needed until calcium level returns to normal.

Patient teaching

• Tell patient to take oral calcium 1 to 1½ hours after meals if GI upset occurs.
• Warn patient to avoid oxalic acid (found in rhubarb and spinach), phytic acid (in bran and whole cereals), and phosphorus (in milk and dairy products) because these substances may interfere with calcium absorption.
• Teach patient to recognize and report signs and symptoms of hypercalcemia.
• Stress importance of follow-up care and regular blood samples to monitor calcium level.

Evaluation

• Patient's calcium level is normal.
• Patient doesn't experience injury from calcium-induced adverse reactions.
• Patient and family state understanding of drug therapy.

calcium carbonate

(KAL-see-um KAR-buh-nayt)

Alka-Mints†, Amitone†, Calcimax◇, Cal-Sup◇, Chooz†, Effercal-600◇, Equilet†, Mallamint†, Rolaids Calcium Rich†, Titralac†, Titralac Extra Strength†, Titralac Plus†, Tums†, Tums E-X†, Tums Liquid Extra Strength†

Pharmacologic class: calcium supplement
Therapeutic class: therapeutic agent for electrolyte balance, antacid
Pregnancy risk category: NR

Indications and dosages

▶ **Antacid, calcium supplement.** *Adults:* 350 mg to 1.5 g P.O. or two pieces of chewing gum 1 hour after meals and h.s. p.r.n.

How supplied

Calcium carbonate contains 40% calcium; 20 mEq calcium/g.
Tablets (chewable): 350 mg†, 420 mg†, 500 mg†, 750 mg, 850 mg, 1,000 mg, 1,250 mg◇
Tablets: 500 mg†, 600 mg†, 650 mg†, 1,000 mg†, 1,250 mg†
Chewing gum: 500 mg/piece
Oral suspension: 1 g/5 ml†, 250 mg/5 ml
Lozenges: 600 mg†

Pharmacokinetics

Absorption: absorbed actively in small intestine. Pregnancy and reduced calcium intake may enhance absorption. Vitamin D in its active form is required for absorption.
Distribution: enters extracellular fluid and is incorporated rapidly into skeletal tissue. Bone contains 99% of total calcium; 1% is distributed equally between intracellular and extracellular fluids. Levels in CSF are about half those of serum.
Metabolism: insignificant.
Excretion: excreted mainly in feces, minimally in urine.

Route	Onset	Peak	Duration
P.O.	≤ 20 min	Unknown	20-60 min (fasting) 3 hr (nonfasting)

Pharmacodynamics

Chemical effect: reduces total acid load in GI tract, elevates gastric pH to reduce pepsin activity, strengthens gastric mucosal barrier, and increases esophageal sphincter tone.
Therapeutic effect: raises blood calcium level and relieves mild gastric discomfort.

Adverse reactions

GI: *constipation,* gastric distention, flatulence, rebound hyperacidity, *nausea.*

Interactions

Drug-drug. *Antibiotics (including quinolones and tetracyclines), hydantoins, iron, isoniazid, salicylates:* decreased effects of these drugs because of possible impaired absorption. Separate administration times.
Enteric-coated drugs: may release prematurely in stomach. Separate doses by at least 1 hour.
Drug-food. *Milk, other foods high in vitamin D:* possible milk-alkali syndrome (headache, confusion, distaste for food, nausea, vomiting, hypercalcemia, hypercalciuria, calcinosis, and hypophosphatemia). Discourage concomitant use.

Contraindications and precautions

- Contraindicated in patients with ventricular fibrillation or hypercalcemia.
- Use cautiously, if at all, in patients receiving cardiac glycosides and in patients with sarcoidosis or renal or cardiac disease.

NURSING CONSIDERATIONS

Assessment

- Assess patient's underlying condition before therapy and regularly thereafter.
- Monitor serum calcium level, especially in patient with mild renal impairment.
- Be alert for adverse reactions and drug interactions.

• Evaluate patient's and family's knowledge of drug therapy.

Nursing diagnoses
• Imbalanced nutrition: less than body requirements related to insufficient calcium intake
• Risk for injury related to calcium-induced hypercalcemia
• Deficient knowledge related to drug therapy

Planning and implementation
• Administer 1 hour after meals as needed.
• Make sure patient with calcium deficiency is receiving adequate calcium in diet.

Patient teaching
• Advise patient not to take calcium carbonate indiscriminately or to switch antacids without consulting prescriber.
• Tell patient to take drug 1 hour after meals and at bedtime, as needed.

Evaluation
• Patient's symptoms are alleviated.
• Patient's blood calcium level is normal.
• Patient and family state understanding of drug therapy.

calcium polycarbophil
(KAL-see-um pah-lee-KAR-boh-fil)
Equalactin†, Fiberall†, FiberCon†, Fiber-Lax†, FiberNorm†, Mitrolan†

Pharmacologic class: hydrophilic agent
Therapeutic class: bulk laxative, antidiarrheal
Pregnancy risk category: NR

Indications and dosages
▶ **Constipation.** *Adults and children age 12 and over:* 1 g P.O. q.i.d. as required. Maximum dosage is 6 g daily.
Children ages 6 to 12: 500 mg P.O. one to three times daily as required. Maximum dosage is 3 g daily.
Children ages 3 to 6: 500 mg P.O. b.i.d. as required. Maximum dosage is 1.5 g daily. Use must be directed by prescriber.

▶ **Diarrhea related to irritable bowel syndrome; acute nonspecific diarrhea.** *Adults and children age 12 and over:* 1 g P.O. q.i.d. as required. Maximum dosage is 6 g daily.
Children ages 6 to 12: 500 mg P.O. t.i.d. as required. Maximum dosage is 3 g daily.
Children ages 2 to 6: 500 mg P.O. b.i.d. as required. Maximum dosage is 1.5 g daily. Use must be directed by prescriber.

How supplied
Tablets: 500 mg†, 625 mg†, 1,250 mg†
Tablets (chewable): 500 mg†

Pharmacokinetics
Absorption: none.
Distribution: none.
Metabolism: none.
Excretion: excreted in feces.

Route	Onset	Peak	Duration
P.O.	12-24 hr	≤ 3 days	Varies

Pharmacodynamics
Chemical effect: as laxative, absorbs water and expands to increase bulk and moisture content of stool, which encourages peristalsis and bowel movement. As antidiarrheal, absorbs free fecal water, thereby producing formed stools.
Therapeutic effect: relieves constipation; relieves diarrhea caused by irritable bowel syndrome.

Adverse reactions
GI: abdominal fullness, increased flatus, intestinal obstruction.
Other: laxative dependence with long-term or excessive use.

Interactions
Drug-drug. *Tetracyclines:* impaired tetracycline absorption. Avoid use together.

Contraindications and precautions
• Contraindicated in patients with signs of GI obstruction.

NURSING CONSIDERATIONS

Assessment
- Assess patient's bowel condition.
- Before giving drug for constipation, determine if patient has adequate fluid intake, exercise, and diet.
- Monitor drug effectiveness by evaluating frequency and characteristics of patient's stools.
- Be alert for adverse reactions and drug interactions.
- Evaluate patient's and family's knowledge of drug therapy.

Nursing diagnoses
- Constipation related to underlying condition
- Diarrhea related to irritable bowel syndrome
- Deficient knowledge related to drug therapy

Planning and implementation
- Give drug with full glass of water when used to treat constipation. Don't give drug with water when used for diarrhea.
- Dose may be repeated every 30 minutes, if ordered, for severe diarrhea, but maximum daily dosage shouldn't be exceeded.
- Don't give to patient who has signs of GI obstruction.

Patient teaching
- Advise patient to chew Equalactin or Mitrolan tablets thoroughly before swallowing and to drink a full glass of water with each dose. If drug is used as an antidiarrheal, tell patient not to drink water with dose.
- Teach patient about dietary sources of bulk, including bran and other cereals, fresh fruit, and vegetables.
- For severe diarrhea, advise patient to repeat dose every 30 minutes, but tell him not to exceed maximum daily dosage.

Evaluation
- Patient's elimination pattern returns to normal.
- Patient and family state understanding of drug therapy.

calfactant
(kal-FAK-tant)
Infasurf

Pharmacologic class: surfactant
Therapeutic class: respiratory distress syndrome (RDS) agent
Pregnancy risk category: NR

Indications and dosages
▶ **Prevention of RDS in premature infants under 29 weeks' gestational age at high risk for RDS; treatment of infants under 72 hours of age in whom RDS develops (confirmed by clinical and radiologic findings) and who need endotracheal intubation.** *Newborns:* 3 ml/kg body weight at birth intratracheally, administered in two aliquots of 1.5 ml/kg each, q 12 hours for total of three doses.

How supplied
Intratracheal suspension: 35 mg phospholipids and 0.65 mg proteins/ml; 6-ml vial

Pharmacokinetics
No information available.

Route	Onset	Peak	Duration
Intratracheal	24-48 hr	Unknown	Unknown

Pharmacodynamics
Chemical effect: nonpyrogenic lung surfactant that modifies alveolar surface tension, thereby stabilizing the alveoli.
Therapeutic effect: prevention of RDS in premature infants or infants with specific characteristics.

Adverse reactions
CV: BRADYCARDIA.
Respiratory: AIRWAY OBSTRUCTION, APNEA, ***reflux of drug into endotracheal tube,*** dislodgment of endotracheal tube, *hypoventilation, cyanosis.*

Interactions
None significant.

Contraindications

None reported.

NURSING CONSIDERATIONS

Assessment

- Obtain history of patient's underlying condition before therapy, and reassess regularly thereafter.
- Monitor patient for reflux of drug into endotracheal tube, cyanosis, bradycardia, or airway obstruction during the dosing procedure. If these occur, stop drug and take appropriate measures to stabilize infant. After infant is stable, resume dosing with appropriate monitoring.
- After giving drug, carefully monitor infant so that oxygen therapy and ventilatory support can be modified in response to improvements in oxygenation and lung compliance.
- Evaluate patient's and family's knowledge of drug therapy.

Nursing diagnoses

- Risk for injury related to potential for RDS
- Impaired gas exchange related to presence of RDS
- Deficient knowledge related to drug therapy

Planning and implementation

- Drug should be given under supervision of a prescriber experienced in the acute care of newborn infants with respiratory failure who need intubation.
- Drug is intended only for intratracheal use; administer for prophylaxis of RDS as soon as possible after birth, preferably within 30 minutes.
- Suspension settles during storage. Gentle swirling or agitation of the vial is often needed for redispersion, but don't shake. Visible flecks in the suspension and foaming at the surface are normal.
- Withdraw dose into a syringe from single-use vial using a 20G or larger needle; avoid excessive foaming.
- Each single-use vial should be entered only once; discard unused material after use.
- Administer through a side-port adapter into the endotracheal tube. Two medical personnel should be present during dosing. Administer dose in two aliquots of 1.5 ml/kg each. Administer while ventilation continues over 20 to 30 breaths for each aliquot, with small bursts timed only during the inspiratory cycles. Evaluate respiratory status and reposition infant between each aliquot.
- Store drug at 36° to 46° F (2° to 8° C). It isn't necessary to warm drug before use. Unopened, unused vials that have warmed to room temperature can be returned to refrigerated storage within 24 hours for future use. Avoid repeated warming to room temperature.

Patient teaching

- Explain to parents the reason for using drug to prevent or treat RDS.
- Notify parents that although infant may improve rapidly after treatment, he may continue to need intubation and mechanical ventilation.
- Notify parents of the potential adverse effects of drug, including bradycardia, reflux into endotracheal tube, airway obstruction, cyanosis, dislodgment of endotracheal tube, and hypoventilation.
- Reassure parents that infant will be carefully monitored.

Evaluation

- Premature infant doesn't develop RDS.
- Patient's gas exchange improves because of oxygenation and increased lung compliance.
- Family states understanding of drug therapy.

candesartan cilexetil

(kan-dih-SAR-ten se-LEKS-ih-til)
Atacand

Pharmacologic class: angiotensin II receptor antagonist
Therapeutic class: antihypertensive
Pregnancy risk category: C (D in second and third trimesters)

Indications and dosages

▶ **Treatment of hypertension (alone or with other antihypertensives).** *Adults:* initially, 16 mg P.O. once daily when used as monotherapy; usual dosage is 8 to 32 mg P.O. daily as single dose or divided b.i.d.

How supplied

Tablets: 4 mg, 8 mg, 16 mg, 32 mg

Pharmacokinetics

Absorption: absolute bioavailability is about 15%.
Distribution: more than 99% binds to plasma protein and doesn't penetrate RBCs.
Metabolism: rapidly and completely bioactivated by ester hydrolysis to candesartan.
Excretion: about 33% is recovered in urine (26% unchanged) and 67% in feces. *Half-life:* 9 hours.

Route	Onset	Peak	Duration
P.O.	Unknown	3-4 hr	24 hr

Pharmacodynamics

Chemical effect: inhibits the vasoconstrictive action of angiotensin II by blocking the angiotensin II receptor on the surface of vascular smooth muscle and other tissue cells.
Therapeutic effect: dilates blood vessels and decreases blood pressure.

Adverse reactions

CNS: dizziness, fatigue, headache.
CV: chest pain, peripheral edema.
EENT: pharyngitis, rhinitis, sinusitis.
GI: abdominal pain, diarrhea, nausea, vomiting.
GU: albuminuria.
Musculoskeletal: arthralgia, back pain.
Respiratory: coughing, bronchitis, upper respiratory tract infection.

Interactions

None reported.

Contraindications and precautions

- Contraindicated in patients hypersensitive to drug or its components.
- Use cautiously in patients whose renal function depends on the renin-angiotensin-aldosterone system (such as patients with heart failure) because of risk of oliguria and progressive azotemia with acute renal failure or death.
- Use cautiously in patients who are volume- or salt-depleted because of risk of symptomatic hypotension.
- Drugs that act directly on the renin-angiotension system (such as candesartan) can cause fetal and neonatal harm and death when given to pregnant women. These problems haven't been detected when exposure has been limited to first trimester. If pregnancy is suspected, notify prescriber because drug should be discontinued.

NURSING CONSIDERATIONS

Assessment

- Monitor patient's electrolytes, and assess patient for volume or salt depletion (as from vigorous diuretic use) before starting drug.
- Carefully monitor therapeutic response and adverse reactions, especially in elderly patients and patients with renal impairment.
- Evaluate patient's and family's knowledge of drug therapy.

Nursing diagnoses

- Decreased cardiac output related to risk for symptomatic hypotension in volume- or salt-depleted patients
- Risk for imbalanced fluid volume in patients with impaired renal function related to drug-induced oliguria
- Deficient knowledge related to drug therapy

Planning and implementation

- Make sure patient is adequately hydrated before starting therapy.
- Observe patient for hypotension. If it occurs after a dose of candesartan, place patient in supine position and, if necessary, give an I.V. infusion of normal saline, as ordered.
- Most of antihypertensive effect is present within 2 weeks. Maximal antihypertensive effect is obtained within 4 to 6 weeks. Diuretic may be added if blood pressure isn't controlled by drug alone.
- Drug can't be removed by hemodialysis.

Patient teaching

- Advise woman of childbearing age about risk of second and third trimester exposure to drug. If pregnancy is suspected, tell her to notify prescriber immediately.

• Advise breast-feeding patient about risk for adverse drug effects on infant and need to stop either breast-feeding or drug.
• Tell patient to store drug at room temperature and to keep container tightly sealed.
• Inform patient to report adverse reactions promptly.
• Instruct patient to take drug exactly as directed.
• Tell patient that drug may be taken without regard to meals.

Evaluation

• Patient's volume or salt depletion is corrected so that symptomatic hypotension doesn't occur.
• Patient maintains fluid balance.
• Patient and family state understanding of drug therapy.

capecitabine

(ka-pe-SITE-a-been)
Xeloda

Pharmacologic class: fluoropyrimidine carbamate
Therapeutic class: antineoplastic
Pregnancy risk category: D

Indications and dosages

▶**Patients with metastatic breast cancer who are resistant to both paclitaxel and an anthracycline-containing chemotherapy regimen or resistant to paclitaxel and for whom further anthracycline therapy isn't indicated.** *Adults:* 1,250 mg/m^2 P.O. b.i.d. (about 12 hours apart) with food for 2 weeks, followed by a 1-week rest period. Adjust dosage as directed according to the National Cancer Institute of Canada (NCIC) Common Toxicity Criteria:

NCIC grade 2: First appearance, interrupt treatment until resolved to grade 0 to 1; then restart at 100% of starting dose for next cycle. Second appearance, interrupt treatment until resolved to grade 0 to 1 and use 75% of starting dose for next cycle. Third appearance, interrupt treatment until resolved to grade 0 to 1 and use 50% of starting dose for next cycle. Fourth appearance, discontinue treatment permanently.

NCIC grade 3: First appearance, interrupt treatment until resolved to grade 0 to 1 and use 75% of starting dose for next cycle. Second appearance, interrupt treatment until resolved to grade 0 to 1 and use 50% of starting dose for next cycle. Third appearance, discontinue treatment permanently.

NCIC grade 4: First appearance, discontinue treatment permanently or interrupt treatment until resolved to grade 0 to 1 and use 50% of starting dose for next cycle.

Toxicity criteria relate to degrees of severity of diarrhea, nausea, vomiting, stomatitis, and hand-and-foot syndrome. Refer to drug package insert for specific toxicity definitions.

How supplied

Tablets: 150 mg, 500 mg

Pharmacokinetics

Absorption: drug is readily absorbed from the GI tract. Levels of parent drug peak in 1½ hours; levels of active metabolite peak in 2 hours. Rate and extent of absorption is decreased by food.
Distribution: about 60% is bound to plasma proteins.
Metabolism: drug is extensively metabolized to 5-fluorouracil (5-FU), an active metabolite.
Excretion: 70% excreted in urine. *Half-life:* about 45 minutes.

Route	Onset	Peak	Duration
P.O.	Unknown	1.5-2 hr	Unknown

Pharmacodynamics

Chemical effect: drug is converted to active drug 5-FU, which is metabolized by both normal and tumor cells to metabolites that cause cellular injury via two different mechanisms: interference with DNA synthesis to inhibit cell division and interference with RNA processing and protein synthesis.
Therapeutic effect: inhibits cell growth of selected cancer.

Adverse reactions

CNS: dizziness, *fatigue,* headache, insomnia, *paresthesia.*

CV: edema.
EENT: eye irritation.
GI: *diarrhea, nausea, vomiting, stomatitis, abdominal pain, constipation, anorexia,* intestinal obstruction, *dyspepsia.*
Hematologic: NEUTROPENIA, THROMBOCYTOPENIA, *anemia, lymphopenia.*
Hepatic: *hyperbilirubinemia.*
Musculoskeletal: myalgia, limb pain.
Skin: *hand-and-foot syndrome, dermatitis,* nail disorder.
Other: *pyrexia,* dehydration.

Interactions

Drug-drug. *Leucovorin:* increased levels of 5-FU with enhanced toxicity. Monitor patient carefully.

Contraindications and precautions

Contraindicated in patients hypersensitive to 5-FU.

NURSING CONSIDERATIONS

Assessment

- Obtain history of patient's underlying condition before therapy, and reassess regularly thereafter.
- Assess patient for coronary artery disease, mild to moderate hepatic dysfunction caused by liver metastases, hyperbilirubinemia, renal insufficiency.
- Monitor patient for severe diarrhea, and notify prescriber if it occurs.
- Monitor patient for hand-and-foot syndrome (numbness, paresthesia, tingling, painless or painful swelling, erythema, desquamation, blistering, and severe pain of hands or feet), hyperbilirubinemia, and severe nausea. Drug therapy will need to be immediately adjusted.
- Evaluate patient's and family's knowledge of drug therapy.

Nursing diagnoses

- Risk for infection related to adverse effects of drug
- Risk for impaired skin integrity related to potential for hand-and-foot syndrome
- Deficient knowledge related to drug therapy

Planning and implementation

- If diarrhea occurs and patient becomes dehydrated, give fluid and electrolyte replacement, as ordered. Drug may need to be immediately interrupted until diarrhea resolves or decreases in intensity.
- Patients over age 80 may have a greater risk of GI adverse effects.
- Hyperbilirubinemia may require stopping drug.
- Monitor patient carefully for toxicity. Toxicity may be managed by symptomatic treatment, dose interruptions, and dosage adjustments, as ordered.

Patient teaching

- Inform patient and caregiver of expected adverse effects of drug, especially nausea, vomiting, diarrhea, and hand-and-foot syndrome (pain, swelling or redness of hands or feet). Explain that patient-specific dose adaptations during therapy are expected and needed.

ALERT Instruct patient to stop taking drug and to contact prescriber immediately if the following occur: diarrhea (more than four bowel movements daily or diarrhea at night), vomiting (two to five episodes in 24 hours), nausea, appetite loss or decrease in amount of food taken each day, stomatitis (pain, redness, swelling or sores in mouth), hand-and-foot syndrome, fever of 100.5° F (38° C) or more, or other evidence of infection.

- Tell patient that most adverse effects improve within 2 or 3 days after stopping drug. If improvement doesn't occur, tell him to contact prescriber.
- Tell patient how to take drug. Dosage cycle is usually to take drug for 14 days followed by 7-day rest period. Prescriber determines number of treatment cycles.
- Instruct patient to take drug with water within 30 minutes after breakfast and dinner end.
- If a combination of tablets is prescribed, teach patient importance of correctly identifying the tablets to avoid possible misdosing.
- For missed doses, instruct patient not to take the missed dose and not to double the next one. Instead, he should continue with regular dosing schedule and check with prescriber.
- Instruct patient to inform prescriber if he's taking folic acid.

• Advise woman of childbearing age to avoid becoming pregnant during therapy.
• Advise breast-feeding woman to discontinue breast-feeding during therapy.

☑ Evaluation
• Patient doesn't develop infection.
• Patient doesn't develop hand-and-foot syndrome.
• Patient and family state understanding of drug therapy.

captopril
(KAP-toh-pril)
Apo-Capto ♦, Capoten, Novo-Captopril ♦

Pharmacologic class: ACE inhibitor
Therapeutic class: antihypertensive, adjunct treatment of heart failure and diabetic nephropathy
Pregnancy risk category: C (D in second and third trimesters)

Indications and dosages
▶ **Hypertension.** *Adults:* initially, 25 mg P.O. b.i.d. or t.i.d. If blood pressure isn't controlled in 1 to 2 weeks, dosage increased to 50 mg b.i.d. or t.i.d. If not controlled after another 1 to 2 weeks, expect a thiazide diuretic to be added to regimen. If further blood pressure reduction is necessary, dosage may be raised to as high as 150 mg t.i.d. while continuing diuretic. Maximum daily dose is 450 mg.
▶ **Heart failure; to reduce risk of death and to slow development of heart failure after MI.** *Adults:* 6.25 to 12.5 mg P.O. t.i.d. initially. Gradually increased to 50 to 100 mg t.i.d. as needed. Maximum daily dosage is 450 mg.
▶ **Diabetic nephropathy.** *Adults:* 25 mg P.O. t.i.d.

How supplied
Tablets: 12.5 mg, 25 mg, 50 mg, 100 mg

Pharmacokinetics
Absorption: absorbed through GI tract; food may reduce absorption by up to 40%.
Distribution: distributed into most body tissues except CNS; 25% to 30% protein-bound.
Metabolism: about 50% metabolized in liver.
Excretion: excreted primarily in urine, minimally in feces. *Half-life:* less than 2 hours.

Route	Onset	Peak	Duration
P.O.	15-60 min	30-90 min	6-12 hr

Pharmacodynamics
Chemical effect: thought to inhibit ACE, preventing conversion of angiotensin I to angiotensin II. Reduced formation of angiotensin II decreases peripheral arterial resistance, thus decreasing aldosterone secretion.
Therapeutic effect: reduces sodium and water retention, lowers blood pressure, and helps improve renal function adversely affected by diabetes.

Adverse reactions
CNS: dizziness, fainting.
CV: *tachycardia, hypotension,* angina pectoris, ***heart failure,*** pericarditis.
GI: anorexia, *dysgeusia.*
GU: *proteinuria, nephrotic syndrome, membranous glomerulopathy,* ***renal failure*** (in patients with renal disease or those receiving high dosages), urinary frequency.
Hematologic: ***leukopenia, agranulocytosis, pancytopenia, thrombocytopenia.***
Hepatic: transient increase in hepatic enzymes.
Metabolic: hyperkalemia.
Respiratory: dry, persistent, tickling, nonproductive cough.
Skin: urticarial rash, maculopapular rash, pruritus.
Other: fever, ***angioedema of face and limbs.***

Interactions
Drug-drug. *Antacids:* decreased captopril effect. Separate administration times.
Cardiac glycosides: may increase serum digoxin levels by 15% to 30%. Monitor patient for toxicity.
Diuretics, other antihypertensives: risk of excessive hypotension. Diuretic may need to be discontinued or captopril dosage lowered.
Insulin, oral antidiabetics: risk of hypoglycemia when captopril therapy starts. Monitor patient closely.

Lithium: increased lithium levels and symptoms of toxicity may occur. Monitor patient closely.
NSAIDs: may reduce antihypertensive effect. Monitor blood pressure.
Potassium supplements, potassium-sparing diuretics: increased risk of hyperkalemia. Avoid these drugs unless hypokalemic blood levels are confirmed.
Probencid: Increased blood capotopril level. Avoid concomitant use.
Drug-herb. *Black catechu:* additional hypotensive effect of catechu. Discourage concomitant use.
Capsaicin: may cause or worsen coughing linked to ACE inhibitors. Discourage concomitant use.
Licorice: may cause sodium retention, which counteracts ACE effects. Monitor blood pressure.
Drug-food. *Any food:* may reduce absorption. Administer drug 1 hour before meals.

Contraindications and precautions

- Contraindicated in patients hypersensitive to drug or other ACE inhibitors.
- Use with extreme caution, if at all, in pregnant women. Drug usually is discontinued if patient becomes pregnant.
- Use cautiously in patients with impaired renal function or serious autoimmune disease (particularly systemic lupus erythematosus), in patients exposed to other drugs known to affect WBC counts or immune response, and in breast-feeding women.
- Safety of drug hasn't been established in children.

NURSING CONSIDERATIONS

Assessment

- Assess patient's underlying condition before therapy and regularly thereafter.
- Monitor blood pressure and pulse rate frequently.
- Monitor WBC and differential counts before therapy, every 2 weeks for first 3 months of therapy, and periodically thereafter, as ordered.
- Monitor serum potassium level and renal function (BUN and creatinine clearance levels, urinalysis), as ordered.
- Be alert for adverse reactions and drug interactions.
- Evaluate patient's and family's knowledge of drug therapy.

Nursing diagnoses

- Risk for injury related to patient's underlying condition
- Ineffective protection related to drug-induced blood disorder
- Deficient knowledge related to drug therapy

Planning and implementation

- Administer 1 hour before meals because food may reduce absorption.
- Because antacids decrease drug's effect, separate administration times.
- Withhold dose and notify prescriber if patient develops fever, sore throat, leukopenia, hypotension, or tachycardia.
- Notify prescriber of abnormal laboratory studies.

Patient teaching

- Instruct patient to take drug 1 hour before meals.
- Inform patient that light-headedness can occur, especially during first few days of therapy. Tell patient to rise slowly to minimize this effect and to report symptoms to prescriber. Tell patient who experiences syncope to stop taking drug and call prescriber immediately.
- Tell patient to use caution in hot weather and during exercise. Inadequate fluid intake, vomiting, diarrhea, and excessive perspiration can lead to light-headedness and syncope.
- Advise patient to report signs of infection, such as fever and sore throat.
- Tell woman to notify prescriber if pregnancy occurs. Drug should be discontinued.

Evaluation

- Patient's underlying condition improves.
- Patient's WBC and differential counts are normal.
- Patient and family state understanding of drug therapy.

carbamazepine

(kar-buh-MEH-zuh-peen)

Apo-Carbamazepine ♦, Atretol, Carbamazepine Chewable Tablets, Carbatrol, Epitol, Novocarbamaz ♦, Tegretol, Tegretol CR ♦, Tegretol-XR

Pharmacologic class: iminostilbene derivative
Therapeutic class: anticonvulsant, analgesic
Pregnancy risk category: D

Indications and dosages

▶ **Generalized tonic-clonic and complex partial seizures, mixed seizure patterns.** *Adults and children over age 12:* initially, 200 mg P.O. b.i.d. for tablets or 100 mg of suspension P.O. q.i.d. May be increased at weekly intervals by 200 mg P.O. daily, in divided doses at 6- to 8-hour intervals. Adjusted to minimum effective level when control is achieved. Maximum daily dosage is 1 g in children ages 12 to 15, or 1.2 g in patients over age 15.
Children ages 6 to 12: initially, 100 mg P.O. b.i.d. or 50 mg of suspension P.O. q.i.d. Increased at weekly intervals by 100 mg P.O. daily. Maximum daily dosage is 1 g.

▶ **Trigeminal neuralgia.** *Adults:* initially, 100 mg P.O. b.i.d. or 50 mg of suspension P.O. q.i.d. with meals. Increased by 100 mg q 12 hours for tablets or 50 mg of suspension q.i.d. until pain is relieved. Maximum daily dosage is 1,200 mg. Maintenance dosage is 200 to 1,200 mg P.O. daily. Decrease dose to minimum effective level or discontinue drug at least once q 3 months.

How supplied

Tablets: 200 mg
Tablets (chewable): 100 mg
Tablets (extended-release): 100 mg, 200 mg, 400 mg
Capsules (extended-release): 200 mg, 300 mg
Oral suspension: 100 mg/5 ml

Pharmacokinetics

Absorption: absorbed slowly from GI tract.
Distribution: distributed widely throughout body; about 75% protein-bound.
Metabolism: metabolized by liver to active metabolite; may also induce its own metabolism.
Excretion: excreted in urine (70%) and feces (30%). *Half-life:* 25 to 65 hours with single dosing; 8 to 29 hours with chronic dosing.

Route	Onset	Peak	Duration
P.O.	Hrs-days	1.5 hr (suspension) 4-12 hr (tablets)	Unknown

Pharmacodynamics

Chemical effect: may stabilize neuronal membranes and limit seizure activity by increasing efflux or decreasing influx of sodium ions across cell membranes in motor cortex during generation of nerve impulses.
Therapeutic effect: prevents seizure activity; eliminates pain caused by trigeminal neuralgia.

Adverse reactions

CNS: *dizziness, vertigo, drowsiness,* fatigue, *ataxia,* ***worsening of seizures*** (usually in patients with mixed seizure disorders, including atypical absence seizures).
CV: ***heart failure,*** hypertension, hypotension, aggravation of coronary artery disease.
EENT: conjunctivitis, dry mouth and pharynx, blurred vision, diplopia, nystagmus.
GI: *nausea, vomiting,* abdominal pain, diarrhea, anorexia, stomatitis, glossitis.
GU: urinary frequency, urine retention, impotence, albuminuria, glycosuria, elevated BUN.
Hematologic: ***aplastic anemia, agranulocytosis,*** eosinophilia, leukocytosis, ***thrombocytopenia.***
Hepatic: abnormal liver function test results, ***hepatitis.***
Respiratory: pulmonary hypersensitivity.
Skin: excessive sweating, rash, urticaria, erythema multiforme, ***Stevens-Johnson syndrome.***
Other: fever, chills, water intoxication.

Interactions

Drug-drug. *Cimetidine, danazol, diltiazem, macrolides (such as erythromycin), isoniazid, propoxyphene, valproic acid, verapamil:* may

increase carbamazepine blood levels. Use cautiously.
Doxycycline, haloperidol, oral contraceptives, phenytoin, theophylline, warfarin: carbamazepine may decrease blood levels of these drugs. Monitor patient for decreased effect.
Lithium: increased CNS toxicity of lithium. Avoid concomitant use.
MAO inhibitors: increased depressant and anticholinergic effects. Don't use together.
Phenobarbital, phenytoin, primidone: may decrease carbamazepine levels. Monitor patient for decreased effect.
Drug-herb. *Plantains:* psyllium seed has been reported to inhibit GI absorption. Discourage concomitant use.

Contraindications and precautions

- Contraindicated in patients hypersensitive to drug or tricyclic antidepressants, in patients with previous bone marrow suppression, and in patients who have taken an MAO inhibitor within 14 days of therapy.
- Breast-feeding should be discontinued if drug must be used in breast-feeding women.
- Use cautiously in patients with mixed seizure disorders (they may have increased risk of seizures, usually atypical absence or generalized) and in pregnant women.

NURSING CONSIDERATIONS

Assessment

- Assess patient's seizure disorder or trigeminal neuralgia before therapy and regularly thereafter.
- Obtain baseline determinations of urinalysis, BUN level, liver function, CBC, platelet and reticulocyte counts, and serum iron level. Reassess regularly, as ordered.
- Monitor blood levels and effects closely (therapeutic carbamazepine blood level is 4 to 12 mcg/ml).
- Be alert for adverse reactions and drug interactions.
- Evaluate patient's and family's knowledge of drug therapy.

Nursing diagnoses

- Risk for injury related to seizure disorder
- Acute pain related to trigeminal neuralgia
- Deficient knowledge related to drug therapy

Planning and implementation

- Administer drug in divided doses, when possible, to maintain consistent blood levels.
- Administer drug with food to minimize GI distress.
- Shake oral suspension well before measuring dose.
- When administering by nasogastric tube, mix dose with equal volume of water, normal saline solution, or D_5W. Flush tube with 100 ml of diluent after administering dose.
- Never discontinue suddenly when treating seizures or status epilepticus. Notify prescriber immediately if adverse reactions occur. Expect prescriber to increase dosage gradually to minimize adverse reactions.

Patient teaching

- Tell patient to take drug with food to minimize GI distress.
- Tell patient to keep tablets in original container, tightly closed, and away from moisture. Some formulations may harden when exposed to excess moisture, resulting in decreased bioavailability and loss of seizure control.
- Inform patient with trigeminal neuralgia that prescriber may attempt to decrease dosage or withdraw drug every 3 months.

ALERT Tell patient to notify prescriber immediately about fever, sore throat, mouth ulcers, or easy bruising or bleeding.

- Warn patient that drug may cause mild to moderate dizziness and drowsiness when first taken. Advise patient to avoid hazardous activities until effects disappear (usually within 3 to 4 days).
- Advise patient to have periodic ophthalmic examinations.

Evaluation

- Patient remains free from seizures.
- Patient reports pain relief.
- Patient and family state understanding of drug therapy.

carbidopa-levodopa
(kar-bih-DOH-puh LEE-vuh-doh-puh)
Sinemet, Sinemet CR

Pharmacologic class: decarboxylase inhibitor-dopamine precursor combination
Therapeutic class: antiparkinsonian
Pregnancy risk category: C

Indications and dosages

▶ **Idiopathic Parkinson's disease, postencephalitic parkinsonism, and symptomatic parkinsonism resulting from carbon monoxide or manganese intoxication.** *Adults:* 1 tablet of 25 mg carbidopa/100 mg levodopa or carbidopa 10 mg/levodopa 100 mg P.O. daily t.i.d. followed by increase of 1 tablet daily or every other day as necessary; maximum daily dosage 8 tablets. 25 mg carbidopa/250 mg levodopa or 10 mg carbidopa/100 mg levodopa tablets are substituted as required to obtain maximum response. Optimum daily dosage must be determined by careful titration for each patient. Patients treated with conventional tablets may receive extended-release tablets; dosage is calculated on current levodopa intake. Initially, extended-release tablets given equal to 10% more levodopa per day; increased as needed and tolerated to 30% more levodopa per day. Administered in divided doses at intervals of 4 to 8 hours.

How supplied

Tablets: carbidopa 10 mg with levodopa 100 mg (Sinemet 10-100), carbidopa 25 mg with levodopa 100 mg (Sinemet 25-100), carbidopa 25 mg with levodopa 250 mg (Sinemet 25-250)
Tablets (extended-release): carbidopa 25 mg with levodopa 100 mg, carbidopa 50 mg with levodopa 200 mg, (Sinemet CR)

Pharmacokinetics

Absorption: 40% to 70% of dose absorbed.
Distribution: distributed widely in body tissues except CNS.
Metabolism: carbidopa isn't metabolized extensively. It inhibits metabolism of levodopa in GI tract, thus increasing its absorption from GI tract and its concentration in plasma.
Excretion: 30% of dose excreted unchanged in urine within 24 hours. When given with carbidopa, amount of levodopa excreted unchanged in urine is increased by about 6%.
Half-life: 1 to 2 hours.

Route	Onset	Peak	Duration
P.O.	Unknown	40 min (regular-release) 2.5 hr (extended-release)	Unknown

Pharmacodynamics

Chemical effect: unknown for levodopa. Thought to be decarboxylated to dopamine, countering depletion of striatal dopamine in extrapyramidal centers. Carbidopa inhibits peripheral decarboxylation of levodopa without affecting levodopa's metabolism within CNS. Therefore, more levodopa is available to be decarboxylated to dopamine in brain.
Therapeutic effect: improves voluntary movement.

Adverse reactions

CNS: *choreiform, dystonic, dyskinetic movements; involuntary grimacing, head movements, myoclonic body jerks, ataxia,* tremors, muscle twitching; bradykinetic episodes; psychiatric disturbances, memory loss, nervousness, anxiety, disturbing dreams, euphoria, malaise, fatigue; severe depression, suicidal tendencies, dementia, delirium, hallucinations.
CV: *orthostatic hypotension, **cardiac irregularities,*** flushing, hypertension, phlebitis.
EENT: blepharospasm, blurred vision, diplopia, mydriasis or miosis, widening of palpebral fissures, activation of latent Horner's syndrome, oculogyric crises, nasal discharge, excessive salivation.
GI: dry mouth, bitter taste, nausea, vomiting, anorexia, and weight loss at start of therapy; constipation; flatulence; diarrhea; epigastric pain.
GU: urinary frequency, urine retention, urinary incontinence, darkened urine, excessive and inappropriate sexual behavior, priapism.

Hematologic: ***hemolytic anemia.***
Hepatic: ***hepatotoxicity.***
Respiratory: hyperventilation, hiccups.
Skin: dark perspiration.

Interactions

Drug-drug. *Antihypertensives:* additive hypotensive effects. Use together cautiously.
Antacids: may increase absorption of levodopa components. Monitor patient closely.
MAO inhibitors: risk of severe hypertension. Avoid concomitant use.
Papaverine, phenytoin: antagonism of antiparkinsonian actions. Don't use together.
Phenothiazines, other antipsychotics: may antagonize antiparkinsonian actions. Use together cautiously.
Drug-herb. *Octacosanol:* may worsen dyskinesia. Discourage concomitant use.
Kava: could interfere with action of levodopa and natural dopamine, worsening Parkinson's symptoms. Discourage concomitant use.
Drug-food. *Foods high in protein:* decreased absorption of levodopa. Don't give levodopa with high-protein foods.

Contraindications and precautions

- Contraindicated in patients hypersensitive to drug; in patients with acute angle-closure glaucoma, melanoma, or undiagnosed skin lesions; in patients who have taken an MAO inhibitor within 14 days; and in breast-feeding women.
- Use with extreme caution, if at all, in pregnant women.
- Use cautiously in patients with severe CV, renal, hepatic, endocrine, or pulmonary disorders; history of peptic ulcer; psychiatric illness; MI with residual arrhythmias; bronchial asthma; emphysema; or well-controlled, chronic, open-angle glaucoma.
- Safety of drug hasn't been established in children.

NURSING CONSIDERATIONS

Assessment

- Assess patient's underlying condition before therapy and regularly thereafter; therapeutic response usually follows each dose and disappears within 5 hours; may vary considerably.
- Be alert for adverse reactions and drug interactions.

ALERT Immediately report muscle twitching and blepharospasm (twitching of eyelids), which may be early signs of drug overdose.

- Patients receiving long-term therapy should be tested regularly for diabetes and acromegaly and should have periodic tests of liver, renal, and hematopoietic function, as ordered.
- Evaluate patient's and family's knowledge of drug therapy.

Nursing diagnoses

- Impaired physical mobility related to underlying parkinsonian syndrome
- Disturbed thought processes related to drug-induced CNS adverse reactions
- Deficient knowledge related to drug therapy

Planning and implementation

- If patient is being treated with levodopa, drug should be discontinued at least 8 hours before starting carbidopa-levodopa.
- Administer drug with food to minimize adverse GI reactions.
- Be aware that dosage will be adjusted according to patient's response and tolerance.
- Withhold dose and notify prescriber if vital signs or mental status change significantly. Reduced dosage or discontinuation may be necessary.
- Depending on reagent and test method used, expect possible false-positive increases in levels of uric acid, urine ketones, urine catecholamines, and urine vanillylmandelic acid.
- False-positive tests for urine glucose can occur with reagents using copper sulfate; false-negative results can occur with tests that use glucose enzymatic methods. An accurate measure can be obtained if paper strip is only partially immersed in urine sample. Urine will migrate up strip, as with an ascending chromatographic system. Read only top of strip.
- Be aware of patients with open-angle glaucoma and treat with caution. Monitor patient closely. Watch for change in intraocular pressure and arrange for periodic eye exams.

Patient teaching

- Tell patient to take drug with food to minimize GI upset.

• Caution patient and family not to increase dosage without prescriber's orders.
• Warn patient of possible dizziness and orthostatic hypotension, especially at start of therapy. Tell patient to change positions slowly and to dangle legs before getting out of bed. Elastic stockings may control this adverse reaction in some patients.
• Instruct patient to report adverse reactions and therapeutic effects.
• Inform patient that pyridoxine (vitamin B_6) doesn't reverse beneficial effects of carbidopa-levodopa. Multivitamins can be taken without losing control of symptoms.

Evaluation

• Patient exhibits improved mobility with reduction of muscular rigidity and tremor.
• Patient remains mentally alert.
• Patient and family state understanding of drug therapy.

carboplatin

(KAR-boh-plat-in)

Paraplatin, Paraplatin-AQ ♦

Pharmacologic class: alkylating agent (not specific to cell cycle phase)
Therapeutic class: antineoplastic
Pregnancy risk category: D

Indications and dosages

▶ **Palliative treatment of ovarian cancer.**
Adults: 360 mg/m² I.V. on day 1 q 4 weeks; doses shouldn't be repeated until platelet count exceeds 100,000/mm³ and neutrophil count exceeds 2,000/mm³. Subsequent doses are based on blood counts.
Patients with renal dysfunction: starting dose is 250 mg/m² in patients with creatinine clearance of 41 to 59 ml/minute or 200 mg/m² in those with creatinine clearance of 16 to 40 ml/minute. Recommended dosage adjustments aren't available for patients with creatinine clearance of 15 ml/minute or less.
▶ **Concomitant use with cyclosporine.**
Adults: the initial dose is 300 mg/m².

How supplied

Injection: 50-mg, 150-mg, 450-mg vials

Pharmacokinetics

Absorption: not applicable with I.V. administration.
Distribution: volume distributed is about equal to that of total body water; no significant protein binding occurs.
Metabolism: hydrolyzed to form hydroxylated and aquated species.
Excretion: 65% excreted by kidneys within 12 hours, 71% within 24 hours. *Half-life:* 5 hours.

Route	Onset	Peak	Duration
I.V.	Unknown	Unknown	Unknown

Pharmacodynamics

Chemical effect: probably produces cross-linking of DNA strands.
Therapeutic effect: impairs ovarian cancer cells.

Adverse reactions

CNS: dizziness, confusion, peripheral neuropathy, ototoxicity, central neurotoxicity, ***CVA.***
CV: ***cardiac failure, embolism.***
GI: constipation, diarrhea, *nausea, vomiting.*
GU: increased BUN and creatinine levels.
Hematologic: **THROMBOCYTOPENIA,** *leukopenia,* **NEUTROPENIA,** *anemia,* **BONE MARROW SUPPRESSION.**
Hepatic: ***hepatotoxicity***, increased AST or alkaline phosphatase levels.
Skin: alopecia.
Other: ***hypersensitivity reactions.***

Interactions

Drug-drug. *Bone marrow depressants, including radiation therapy:* increased hematologic toxicity. Monitor patient closely.
Nephrotoxic agents: enhanced nephrotoxicity of carboplatin. Monitor patient closely.

Contraindications and precautions

• Contraindicated in patients hypersensitive to cisplatin, platinum-containing compounds, or mannitol. Also contraindicated in patients with severe bone marrow suppression or bleeding.

• Drug shouldn't be used during pregnancy if at all possible because fetal harm may occur.
• Safety of drug hasn't been established in breast-feeding women and children.

NURSING CONSIDERATIONS

Assessment

• Assess patient's condition before therapy and regularly thereafter.
• Determine serum electrolyte, creatinine, and BUN levels; creatinine clearance; CBC; and platelet count before first infusion and before each course of treatment. WBC and platelet count nadirs usually occur by day 21. Levels usually return to baseline by day 28.
• Be alert for adverse reactions and drug interactions.
• Patients over age 65 are at greater risk for neurotoxicity.
• Evaluate patient's and family's knowledge of drug therapy.

Nursing diagnoses

• Ineffective health maintenance related to ovarian cancer
• Ineffective protection related to drug-induced adverse reactions
• Deficient knowledge related to drug therapy

Planning and implementation

• Follow facility policy to reduce risks because preparation and administration of parenteral form is linked to mutagenic, teratogenic, and carcinogenic risks for personnel.
• Check ordered dose against laboratory test results carefully. Only one increase in dosage is recommended. Subsequent doses shouldn't exceed 125% of starting dose.
• Reconstitute with D_5W, normal saline solution, or sterile water for injection to make 10 mg/ml. Add 5 ml of diluent to 50-mg vial, 15 ml of diluent to 150-mg vial, or 45 ml of diluent to 450-mg vial. It can then be further diluted for infusion with normal saline solution or D_5W. Concentration as low as 0.5 mg/ml can be prepared. Give drug by continuous or intermittent infusion over at least 15 minutes.
• Don't use needles or I.V. administration sets that contain aluminum to administer carboplatin; precipitation and loss of drug's potency may occur.
• Bone marrow suppression may be more severe in patients with creatinine clearance below 60 ml/minute; dosage adjustments are recommended for such patients.
• Dose shouldn't be repeated unless platelet count exceeds 100,000/mm^3.
• Store unopened vials at room temperature. Once reconstituted and diluted as directed, drug is stable at room temperature for 8 hours. Discard unused drug after 8 hours.
ALERT Have epinephrine, corticosteroids, and antihistamines available when administering carboplatin because anaphylactoid reactions may occur within minutes of administration.
• Administer antiemetic therapy as ordered. Carboplatin can produce severe vomiting.

Patient teaching

• Warn patient to watch for signs of infection (fever, sore throat, fatigue) and bleeding (easy bruising, nosebleeds, bleeding gums, melena). Take temperature daily.
• Instruct patient to avoid OTC products that contain aspirin.
• Advise woman of childbearing age to avoid pregnancy during therapy and to consult prescriber before becoming pregnant.
• Advise breast-feeding patient to discontinue breast-feeding because of risk of toxicity in infant.

Evaluation

• Patient has positive response to carboplatin as evidenced by follow-up diagnostic tests.
• Patient doesn't experience injury from drug therapy.
• Patient and family state understanding of drug therapy.

carboprost tromethamine

(KAR-boh-prost troh-METH-ah-meen)
Hemabate

Pharmacologic class: prostaglandin
Therapeutic class: oxytocic
Pregnancy risk category: C

Indications and dosages

▶ **Abortion between 13th and 20th weeks of gestation.** *Adults:* initially, 250 mcg deep I.M. Subsequent doses of 250 mcg administered at intervals of 1½ to 3½ hours, depending on uterine response. Dosage may be increased in increments to 500 mcg if contractility is inadequate after several 250-mcg doses. Total dosage shouldn't exceed 12 mg.

▶ **Postpartum hemorrhage caused by uterine atony not managed by conventional methods.** *Adults:* 250 mcg by deep I.M. injection. Repeat doses administered at 15- to 90-minute intervals, p.r.n. Maximum total dosage is 2 mg.

How supplied

Injection: 250 mcg/ml

Pharmacokinetics

Absorption: unknown.
Distribution: unknown.
Metabolism: enzymatic deactivation occurs in maternal tissues.
Excretion: excreted primarily in urine.

Route	Onset	Peak	Duration
I.M.	Unknown	15-60 min	16-24 hr

Pharmacodynamics

Chemical effect: produces strong, prompt contractions of uterine smooth muscle, possibly mediated by calcium and cAMP.
Therapeutic effect: aborts fetus and stops postpartum hemorrhage.

Adverse reactions

CV: ***arrhythmias.***
GI: *vomiting, diarrhea,* nausea.
GU: uterine rupture.
Other: *fever,* chills, flushing.

Interactions

Drug-drug. *Other oxytocics:* may potentiate action. Avoid concomitant use.

Contraindications and precautions

- Contraindicated in patients hypersensitive to drug and in those with acute pelvic inflammatory disease or active cardiac, pulmonary, renal, or hepatic disease.
- Use cautiously in patients with history of asthma; hypotension; hypertension; CV, adrenal, renal, or hepatic disease; anemia; jaundice; diabetes; seizure disorders; or previous uterine surgery.

NURSING CONSIDERATIONS

Assessment

- Assess patient's pregnancy status before therapy.
- Monitor drug effectiveness by evaluating uterine contractions, expulsion of products of conception, or cessation of postpartum hemorrhage.
- Be alert for adverse reactions.
- Evaluate patient's and family's knowledge of drug therapy.

Nursing diagnoses

- Impaired adjustment related to pregnancy
- Risk for altered body temperature related to drug-induced fever
- Deficient knowledge related to drug therapy

Planning and implementation

- Unlike other prostaglandin abortifacients, carboprost is administered by I.M. injection. Injectable form avoids risk of expelling vaginal suppositories, which may occur with profuse vaginal bleeding.
- Drug should be used only by trained personnel in hospital setting.
- Consult prescriber if uterine contractions are ineffective or postpartum bleeding persists.

Patient teaching

- Explain importance of follow-up care.
- Tell patient to report adverse reactions immediately.

Evaluation

- Patient aborts successfully.
- Patient's temperature remains normal.
- Patient and family state understanding of drug therapy.

carisoprodol

(kar-ih-soh-PROH-dol)

Soma

Pharmacologic class: caramate derivative
Therapeutic class: skeletal muscle relaxant
Pregnancy risk category: NR

Indications and dosages

▶ **Adjunct in acute, painful musculoskeletal conditions.** *Adults:* 350 mg P.O. t.i.d. and h.s.

How supplied

Tablets: 350 mg

Pharmacokinetics

Absorption: unknown.
Distribution: widely distributed throughout body.
Metabolism: metabolized in liver.
Excretion: excreted in urine mainly as metabolites; less than 1% of dose excreted unchanged. *Half-life:* 8 hours.

Route	Onset	Peak	Duration
P.O.	≤ 30 min	≤ 4 hr	4-6 hr

Pharmacodynamics

Chemical effect: appears to modify central perception of pain without modifying pain reflexes. Blocks interneuronal activity in descending reticular activating system and in spinal cord.
Therapeutic effect: relieves musculoskeletal pain.

Adverse reactions

CNS: *drowsiness, dizziness,* vertigo, ataxia, tremor, agitation, irritability, headache, depressive reactions, insomnia.
CV: orthostatic hypotension, tachycardia, facial flushing.
GI: nausea, vomiting, increased bowel activity, epigastric distress.
Hematologic: eosinophilia.
Respiratory: asthmatic episodes, hiccups.
Skin: rash, erythema multiforme, pruritus.
Other: fever, ***angioedema, anaphylaxis.***

Interactions

Drug-drug. *CNS depressants:* increased CNS depression. Avoid concomitant use.
Drug-lifestyle. *Alcohol use:* increased CNS depression. Discourage concurrent use.

Contraindications and precautions

- Contraindicated in patients hypersensitive to related compounds (such as meprobamate, tybamate) and in patients with intermittent porphyria.
- Use cautiously in patients with impaired hepatic or renal function.

NURSING CONSIDERATIONS

Assessment

- Assess patient's pain before and after drug administration.
- Monitor drug effectiveness by regularly assessing severity and frequency of muscle spasms.
- Be alert for adverse reactions and drug interactions.

ALERT Watch for idiosyncratic reactions after first to fourth doses (weakness, ataxia, visual and speech difficulties, fever, skin eruptions, and mental changes) and for severe reactions (bronchospasm, hypotension, and anaphylactic shock).

- Evaluate patient's and family's knowledge of drug therapy.

Nursing diagnoses

- Acute pain related to patient's underlying condition
- Risk for injury related to drug-induced drowsiness
- Deficient knowledge related to drug therapy

Planning and implementation

- Give drug with meals or milk to prevent GI distress.
- Amount of pain relief obtained determines if dosage can be reduced.
- Withhold dose and notify prescriber immediately if unusual reactions occur.
- Don't stop drug abruptly; mild withdrawal effects (such as insomnia, headache, nausea, and abdominal cramps) may result.

Patient teaching

- Warn patient to avoid activities that require alertness until drug's CNS effects are known. Drowsiness is transient.
- Advise patient to avoid combining drug with alcohol or other CNS depressants.
- Advise patient to follow prescriber's orders about rest and physical therapy.
- Tell patient to take drug with meals or milk to prevent GI distress.
- Warn patient that carisoprodol may impair ability to preform hazardous activities requiring mental alertness or physical dexterity, such as operating machinery or a motor vehicle.

Evaluation

- Patient reports pain has ceased.
- Patient doesn't experience injury from drug-induced CNS adverse reactions.
- Patient and family state understanding of drug.

carmustine (BCNU)

(kar-MUHS-teen)

BiCNU, Gliadel

Pharmacologic class: alkylating agent; nitrosourea (not specific to cell cycle phase)
Therapeutic class: antineoplastic
Pregnancy risk category: D

Indications and dosages

▶ **Brain tumors, Hodgkin's disease, non-Hodgkin's lymphoma, and multiple myeloma.** *Adults:* 150 to 200 mg/m^2 I.V. by slow infusion as single dose, repeated q 6 weeks or 75 to 100 mg/m^2 I.V. by slow infusion daily for 2 days; repeated q 6 weeks if platelet count is above 100,000/mm^3 and WBC count is above 4,000/mm^3. Dosage is reduced by 30% when WBC count is 2,000 to 3,000/mm^3 and platelet count is 25,000 to 75,000/mm^3. Dosage is reduced by 50% when WBC count is below 2,000/mm^3 and platelet count is below 25,000/mm^3.

▶ **Recurrent glioblastoma and metastatic brain tumors (adjunct to surgery to prolong survival):** *Adults:* implant 8 wafers into resection cavity as size of cavity allows.

How supplied

Injection: 100-mg vial (lyophilized), with 3-ml vial of absolute alcohol supplied as diluent
Wafer: 7.7 mg

Pharmacokinetics

Absorption: not applicable with I.V. administration.
Distribution: distributed rapidly into CSF.
Metabolism: metabolized extensively in liver.
Excretion: from 60% to 70% excreted in urine within 96 hours, 6% to 10% excreted as carbon dioxide by lungs, and 1% excreted in feces. *Half-life:* 15 to 30 minutes.

Route	Onset	Peak	Duration
I.V., wafer	Unknown	Unknown	Unknown

Pharmacodynamics

Chemical effect: inhibits enzymatic reactions involved with DNA synthesis, cross-links strands of cellular DNA, and interferes with RNA transcription, causing growth imbalance that leads to cell death.
Therapeutic effect: kills selected cancer cells.

Adverse reactions

CNS: ataxia, drowsiness.
GI: *nausea beginning in 2 to 6 hours (can be severe), vomiting, anorexia, dysphagia, esophagitis, diarrhea.*
GU: ***nephrotoxicity, renal failure.***
Hematologic: ***cumulative bone marrow suppression*** (delayed 4 to 6 weeks, lasting 1 to 2 weeks), ***leukopenia, thrombocytopenia, acute leukemia or bone marrow dysplasia*** (may occur after long-term use).
Hepatic: ***hepatotoxicity.***
Respiratory: ***pulmonary fibrosis.***
Skin: facial flushing, hyperpigmentation (if drug contacts skin).
Other: *intense pain* (at infusion site from venous spasm), possible hyperuricemia (in lymphoma patients when rapid cell lysis occurs).

Interactions

Drug-drug. *Anticoagulants, aspirin:* increased risk of bleeding. Avoid concomitant use.

Cimetidine: may increase carmustine's bone marrow toxicity. Avoid concomitant use if possible.
Digoxin, phenytoin: serum levels of these drugs may be reduced. Use together cautiously.

Contraindications and precautions

- Contraindicated in patients hypersensitive to drug and in pregnant or breast-feeding women.
- Safety of drug hasn't been established in children.

NURSING CONSIDERATIONS

Assessment

- Assess patient's neoplastic disorder before therapy and regularly thereafter.
- Obtain baseline pulmonary function tests as ordered before therapy because pulmonary toxicity appears to be dose-related. Be sure to evaluate results of liver, renal, and pulmonary function tests periodically thereafter.
- Monitor CBC and serum uric acid level, as ordered.
- Be alert for adverse reactions and drug interactions.
- Evaluate patient's and family's knowledge of drug therapy.

Nursing diagnoses

- Ineffective health maintenance related to neoplastic disease
- Risk for injury related to drug-induced adverse reactions
- Deficient knowledge related to drug therapy

Planning and implementation

- Follow facility policy to reduce risks because preparation and administration of parenteral form is linked to carcinogenic, mutagenic, and teratogenic risks for personnel.
- To reduce nausea, give antiemetic before administering drug, as ordered.

I.V. use: To reconstitute, dissolve 100 mg of carmustine in 3 ml of absolute alcohol provided by manufacturer. Dilute solution with 27 ml of sterile water for injection. Resulting solution contains 3.3 mg of carmustine/ml in 10% alcohol. Dilute in normal saline solution or D_5W for I.V. infusion. Give at least 250 ml over 1 to 2 hours. To reduce pain on infusion, dilute further or slow infusion rate.
– Discard drug if powder liquefies or appears oily (decomposition has occurred).
– Administer only in glass containers. Solution is unstable in plastic I.V. bags.
– Don't mix with other drugs during administration.
– Store reconstituted solution in refrigerator for 48 hours. May decompose at temperatures above 80° F (27° C).
– Avoid contact with skin because carmustine will cause brown stain. If drug contacts skin, wash off thoroughly.

Wafer use: Unopened foil packs are stable at room temperature for 6 hours. Store below -4° F.
– Use double gloves if handling wafer in operating room.

- Allopurinol may be used with adequate hydration to prevent hyperuricemia and uric acid nephropathy.

Patient teaching

- Warn patient to watch for signs of infection (fever, sore throat, fatigue) and bleeding (easy bruising, nosebleeds, bleeding gums, melena). Take temperature daily.
- Instruct patient to avoid OTC products containing aspirin.
- Advise breast-feeding women to discontinue breast-feeding during therapy because of possible infant toxicity.
- Advise women of childbearing age to avoid pregnancy during therapy and to consult prescriber before becoming pregnant.

Evaluation

- Patient shows positive response to drug therapy as evidenced by follow-up diagnostic studies.
- Patient doesn't experience injury from drug-induced adverse reactions.
- Patient and family state understanding of drug therapy.

carteolol hydrochloride
(KAR-tee-oh-lol high-dro-KLOR-ide)
Cartrol

Pharmacologic class: beta blocker
Therapeutic class: antihypertensive
Pregnancy risk category: C

Indications and dosages

▶ **Hypertension.** *Adults:* initially, 2.5 mg P.O. daily. Gradually increased to 5 or 10 mg daily, as needed. Dosages exceeding 10 mg daily don't produce greater response and may decrease response.
Patients with substantial renal failure: if creatinine clearance is over 60 ml/minute, administer drug at 24-hour intervals; 20 to 60 ml/minute, at 48-hour intervals; below 20 ml/minute, at 72-hour intervals.

How supplied

Tablets: 2.5 mg, 5 mg

Pharmacokinetics

Absorption: bioavailability is about 85%.
Distribution: 20% to 30% bound to plasma proteins.
Metabolism: 30% to 50% metabolized in liver to active and inactive metabolites.
Excretion: excreted primarily by kidneys.
Half-life: about 6 hours.

Route	Onset	Peak	Duration
P.O.	Unknown	1-3 hr	Unknown

Pharmacodynamics

Chemical effect: unknown. Nonselective beta blocker with intrinsic sympathomimetic activity. Antihypertensive effects probably caused by decreased sympathetic outflow from brain and decreased cardiac output. Carteolol doesn't have consistent effect on renin output.
Therapeutic effect: lowers blood pressure.

Adverse reactions

CNS: lassitude, tiredness, fatigue, somnolence, *asthenia.*
CV: conduction disturbances.
Musculoskeletal: *muscle cramps.*

Interactions

Drug-drug. *Calcium channel blockers:* increased risk of hypotension, left ventricular failure, and AV conduction disturbances. Use I.V. calcium antagonists with caution.
Cardiac glycosides: may produce additive effects on slowing AV node conduction. Avoid concomitant use.
Catecholamine-depleting drugs, reserpine: may have additive effect. Monitor patient.
General anesthetics: increased hypotensive effects. Observe patient carefully for excessive hypotension, bradycardia, or orthostatic hypotension.
Insulin, oral antidiabetics: may alter hypoglycemic response. Adjust dosage as necessary.

Contraindications and precautions

- Contraindicated in patients with bronchial asthma, severe bradycardia, greater than first-degree heart block, cardiogenic shock, or uncontrolled heart failure.
- Use cautiously in patients with heart failure controlled by cardiac glycosides and diuretics (patient may exhibit signs of cardiac decompensation with beta-blocker therapy) and in pregnant or breast-feeding women.
- Safety of drug hasn't been established in children.

NURSING CONSIDERATIONS

Assessment

- Assess patient's blood pressure before therapy and regularly thereafter.
- Be alert for adverse reactions and drug interactions.
- Patients with unrecognized coronary artery disease may exhibit signs of angina pectoris on withdrawal of drug. Monitor patient closely.
- Evaluate patient's and family's knowledge of drug therapy.

Nursing diagnoses

- Risk for injury related to hypertension
- Acute pain related to drug-induced muscle cramps
- Deficient knowledge related to drug therapy

Planning and implementation

- Patients with significant renal failure should receive usual dose of carteolol at longer intervals.
- Withdrawal of beta-blocker therapy before surgery is controversial. Advise anesthesiologist that isoproterenol or dobutamine is readily available for reversal of drug's cardiac effects.
- Gradually withdraw beta-blocker therapy, as ordered, to avoid thyroid storm in patients with suspected thyrotoxicosis.

Patient teaching

- Explain importance of taking drug as prescribed, even when feeling well. Tell patient not to discontinue drug suddenly, but to notify prescriber of distressing reactions, such as muscle cramps.
- Emphasize importance of reporting signs of heart failure, including shortness of breath, difficulty breathing, unusually fast heartbeat, cough, and fatigue with exertion.

Evaluation

- Patient's blood pressure is normal.
- Patient doesn't experience muscle cramps.
- Patient and family state understanding of drug therapy.

carvedilol

(kar-VAY-deh-lol)
Coreg

Pharmacologic class: $alpha_1$-adrenergic and beta blocker
Therapeutic class: antihypertensive, adjunct treatment for heart failure
Pregnancy risk category: C

Indications and dosages

▶ **Hypertension.** *Adults:* dosage highly individualized. Initially, 6.25 mg P.O. b.i.d. with food. Obtain a standing blood pressure 1 hour after initial dose. If tolerated, continue dosage for 7 to 14 days. May increase to 12.5 mg P.O. b.i.d. for 7 to 14 days, following blood pressure monitoring protocol noted above. Maximum dosage is 25 mg P.O. b.i.d. as tolerated.

▶ **Heart failure.** *Adults:* dosage highly individualized and adjusted carefully. Initially, 3.125 mg P.O. b.i.d. with food for 2 weeks; if tolerated, can increase to 6.25 mg P.O. b.i.d. Dosage may be doubled q 2 weeks as tolerated. At start of new dosage, observe patient for dizziness or light-headedness for 1 hour. Maximum dosage for patients weighing less than 85 kg (187 lb) is 25 mg P.O. b.i.d.; for those weighing over 85 kg, dosage is 50 mg P.O. b.i.d.

How supplied

Tablets: 3.125 mg, 6.25 mg, 12.5 mg, 25 mg

Pharmacokinetics

Absorption: rapidly and extensively absorbed with absolute bioavailability of 25% to 35% because of significant first-pass metabolism.
Distribution: extensively distributed into extravascular tissues; about 98% bound to plasma proteins.
Metabolism: primarily metabolized by aromatic ring oxidation and glucuronidation.
Excretion: metabolites are primarily excreted via bile in the feces. Less than 2% is excreted unchanged in urine. *Half-life:* 7 to 10 hours.

Route	Onset	Peak	Duration
P.O.	Unknown	1-2 hr	7-10 hr

Pharmacodynamics

Chemical effect: nonselective beta-adrenergic blocker with $alpha_1$-blocking activity causes significant reductions in systemic blood pressure, pulmonary arterial pressure, pulmonary capillary wedge pressure, and heart rate.
Therapeutic effect: lowers blood pressure and heart rate.

Adverse reactions

CNS: *dizziness, fatigue,* headache, hypesthesia, insomnia, pain, paresthesia, somnolence, vertigo, malaise.
CV: aggravated angina pectoris, edema, ***AV block, bradycardia,*** *chest pain,* fluid overload, hypertension, hypotension, orthostatic hypotension, syncope.
EENT: abnormal vision, rhinitis, pharyngitis, sinusitis.

GI: abdominal pain, *diarrhea,* melena, nausea, periodontitis, vomiting.
GU: abnormal renal function, albuminuria, hematuria, impotence, urinary tract infection.
Hematologic: decreased PT, purpura, ***thrombocytopenia.***
Hepatic: increased ALT and AST levels.
Metabolic: dehydration, glycosuria, gout, hypercholesterolemia, *hyperglycemia,* hypertriglyceridemia, hypervolemia, hypovolemia, hyperuricemia, hypoglycemia, hyponatremia, weight gain.
Musculoskeletal: arthralgia, myalgia, back pain.
Respiratory: bronchitis, dyspnea, *upper respiratory tract infection.*
Skin: increased sweating.
Other: allergy, fever, peripheral edema, viral infection.

Interactions

Drug-drug. *Calcium channel blockers:* can cause isolated conduction disturbances. Monitor patient's heart rhythm and blood pressure.
Catecholamine-depleting drugs (such as reserpine, MAO inhibitors): may cause bradycardia or severe hypotension. Monitor patient closely.
Cimetidine: increased bioavailability of carvedilol. Monitor vital signs carefully.
Clonidine: may potentiate blood pressure and heart rate–lowering effects. Monitor vital signs closely.
Digoxin: increased of digoxin level by about 15% during concurrent therapy. Monitor digoxin levels and vital signs carefully.
Insulin, oral antidiabetics: concomitant use may enhance hypoglycemic properties. Monitor blood glucose levels.
Rifampin: reduced plasma levels of carvedilol by 70%. Monitor vital signs closely.
Drug-food. *Any food:* delays rate of carvedilol absorption but doesn't alter extent of bioavailability. Advise patient to take drug with food to minimize orthostatic effects.

Contraindications and precautions

- Contraindicated in patients hypersensitive to drug and in those with New York Heart Association class IV decompensated cardiac failure requiring I.V. inotropic therapy, bronchial asthma or related bronchospastic conditions, second- or third- degree AV block, sick sinus syndrome (unless a permanent pacemaker is in place), cardiogenic shock, or severe bradycardia. Drug isn't recommended for patients with symptomatic hepatic impairment.
- Use cautiously in hypertensive patients with left ventricular failure, perioperative patients who receive anesthetics that depress myocardial function, diabetic patients who receive insulin or oral antidiabetics, and patients subject to spontaneous hypoglycemia. Also use cautiously in patients with thyroid disease, pheochromocytoma, Prinzmetal's variant angina, bronchospastic disease, or peripheral vascular disease.
- Safety and efficacy in patients under age 18 haven't been established.

NURSING CONSIDERATIONS

Assessment

- Monitor patient for decreased PT and increased serum alkaline phosphatase, BUN, ALT, and AST levels.
- Assess patient with heart failure for worsened condition, renal dysfunction, or fluid retention; diuretics may need to be increased, as ordered.
- Monitor diabetic patient closely; drug may mask signs of hypoglycemia, or hyperglycemia may be worsened.
- Observe patient for dizziness or lightheadedness for 1 hour after giving each dose.
- Evaluate patient's and family's knowledge of drug therapy.

Nursing diagnoses

- Ineffective health maintenance related to underlying disorder
- Ineffective cerebral tissue perfusion secondary to therapeutic action of drug
- Deficient knowledge related to drug therapy

Planning and implementation

- Before starting drug, dosages of digoxin, diuretics, or ACE inhibitors should be stabilized.
- Plasma levels are about 50% higher in elderly patients; monitor these patients closely.
- Give drug with food to reduce risk of orthostatic hypotension.

• Notify prescriber if pulse drops below 55 beats/minute; dosage may need to be reduced.

Patient teaching

• Tell patient not to interrupt or discontinue drug without medical approval. Drug should be withdrawn gradually over 1 to 2 weeks.
• Advise heart failure patient to call prescriber if weight gain or shortness of breath occurs.
• Inform patient that he may experience low blood pressure when standing. If he's dizzy or faints, advise him to sit or lie down.
• Caution patient against driving or performing hazardous tasks until CNS effects of drug are known.
• Tell patient to notify prescriber if dizziness or faintness occurs; dosage may need to be adjusted.
• Inform breast-feeding patient that effects on the infant are unknown. Breast-feeding should be discontinued during drug therapy.
• Advise diabetic patient to report changes in blood glucose promptly.
• Inform patient who wears contact lenses that decreased lacrimation may occur.

☑ Evaluation

• Patient responds well to therapy.
• Patient doesn't experience dizziness or lightheadedness.
• Patient and family state understanding of drug therapy.

cascara sagrada†

(kas-KAR-uh suh-GRAH-duh)

cascara sagrada aromatic fluidextract†*

cascara sagrada fluidextract†*

Pharmacologic class: anthraquinone glycoside mixture
Therapeutic class: laxative
Pregnancy risk category: C

Indications and dosages

▶ **Acute constipation; preparation for bowel or rectal examination.** *Adults and children over age 12:* 1 tablet P.O. h.s.; 0.5 to 1 ml fluidextract P.O. daily; or 5 ml aromatic fluidextract P.O. daily. *Children ages 2 to 12:* half of adult dosage. *Children under age 2:* one-quarter adult dosage.

How supplied

Tablets: 325 mg†
Aromatic fluidextract: 1 g/ml†*
Fluidextract: 1 g/ml†*

Pharmacokinetics

Absorption: minimally absorbed in small intestine.
Distribution: distributed in bile, saliva, colonic mucosa, and breast milk.
Metabolism: hydrolyzed by colonic flora enzymes to active free anthraquinones, which are metabolized in liver.
Excretion: excreted in feces via biliary elimination, in urine, or both.

Route	Onset	Peak	Duration
P.O.	6-10 hr	Varies	Varies

Pharmacodynamics

Chemical effect: increases peristalsis, probably by direct effect on smooth muscle of intestine. Thought to irritate musculature or stimulate colonic intramural plexus. Also promotes fluid accumulation in colon and small intestine.
Therapeutic effect: relieves constipation.

Adverse reactions

GI: *nausea,* vomiting, diarrhea, and loss of normal bowel function with excessive use; *abdominal cramps,* especially in severe constipation; malabsorption of nutrients; "cathartic colon" (syndrome resembling ulcerative colitis radiologically and pathologically) in chronic misuse; discoloration of rectal mucosa after long-term use; protein enteropathy; laxative dependence with long-term or excessive use.
Metabolic: hypokalemia, electrolyte imbalance with excessive use.

Interactions

None significant.

Contraindications and precautions

• Contraindicated in patients with evidence of appendicitis or acute surgical abdomen (such as abdominal pain, nausea, and vomiting), acute surgical delirium, fecal impaction, or intestinal obstruction or perforation.
• Use cautiously in patients with rectal bleeding, in pregnant or breast-feeding women, and in children.

NURSING CONSIDERATIONS

Assessment

• Assess patient's constipation before therapy, and evaluate drug effectiveness after administration.
• Determine if patient has adequate fluid intake, exercise, and diet before giving for constipation.
• Monitor patient for adverse reactions.
• Monitor serum electrolytes during prolonged use.
• Evaluate patient's and family's knowledge of drug therapy.

Nursing diagnoses

• Constipation related to patient's underlying condition
• Acute pain related to drug-induced abdominal cramps
• Deficient knowledge related to drug therapy

Planning and implementation

• Check prescriber's orders and read drug label carefully to ensure administration of correct drug form.
• Cascara sagrada aromatic fluidextract is less active and less bitter than nonaromatic fluidextract.
• Liquid preparations are more reliable than solid dosage forms.

Patient teaching

• Discourage excessive use of laxatives.
• Warn patient that drug may turn alkaline urine red-pink and acidic urine yellow-brown.
• Teach patient about dietary sources of bulk, including bran and other cereals, fresh fruit, and vegetables.
• Warn patient that abdominal cramping may occur because cascara works by increasing intestinal peristalsis.

Evaluation

• Patient's elimination pattern returns to normal.
• Patient remains free from pain.
• Patient and family state understanding of drug therapy.

castor oil

(KAS-tir oyl)
Emulsoil†, Purge†

Pharmacologic class: glyceride, *Ricinus communis* derivative
Therapeutic class: stimulant laxative
Pregnancy risk category: NR

Indications and dosages

▶ **Preparation for rectal or bowel examination or for surgery.** For all patients, administered as single dose about 16 hours before surgery or procedure.
Adults and children age 12 and older: 15 to 60 ml P.O.
Children ages 2 to 12: 5 to 15 ml P.O.
Children under age 2: 2.5 to 7.5 ml P.O. Increased dose produces no greater effect.

How supplied

Oral liquid: 95% (Emulsoil†, Purge†)

Pharmacokinetics

Absorption: unknown.
Distribution: distributed locally, primarily in small intestine.
Metabolism: metabolized by intestinal enzymes into its active form, ricinoleic acid.
Excretion: excreted in feces.

Route	Onset	Peak	Duration
P.O.	2-6 hr	Varies	Varies

Pharmacodynamics

Chemical effect: increases peristalsis, probably by direct effect on smooth muscle of intestine. Thought to irritate musculature or stimulate colonic intramural plexus. Also promotes fluid accumulation in colon and small intestine.
Therapeutic effect: cleans bowel.

Adverse reactions

GI: *nausea,* vomiting, diarrhea, and loss of normal bowel function with excessive use; *abdominal cramps,* especially in severe constipation; malabsorption of nutrients; "cathartic colon" (syndrome resembling ulcerative colitis radiologically and pathologically) with chronic misuse; laxative dependence with long-term or excessive use; protein-losing enteropathy. May cause constipation after catharsis.
GU: pelvic congestion (in menstruating women).
Metabolic: hypokalemia, other electrolyte imbalances (with excessive use).

Interactions

Drug-herb. *Male fern:* may increase absorption and increase risk of toxicity. Discourage concomitant use.

Contraindications and precautions

- Contraindicated in menstruating or pregnant patients and in patients with evidence of appendicitis or acute surgical abdomen (such as abdominal pain, nausea, vomiting), ulcerative bowel lesions, anal or rectal fissures, fecal impaction, or intestinal obstruction or perforation.
- Use cautiously in patients with rectal bleeding.
- Breast-feeding women should seek medical approval before using castor oil.

NURSING CONSIDERATIONS

Assessment

- Assess patient's underlying condition.
- Monitor drug effectiveness by noting if diagnostic testing provides accurate results.
- Failure to respond to drug may indicate acute condition requiring surgery.
- Be alert for adverse reactions and drug interactions.
- Evaluate patient's and family's knowledge of drug therapy.

Nursing diagnoses

- Health-seeking behavior (seeking diagnostic testing) related to underlying condition
- Acute pain related to drug-induced abdominal cramps
- Deficient knowledge related to drug therapy

Planning and implementation

- Have patient suck on ice before drug administration and give drug with juice or carbonated beverage to mask oily taste. Stir mixture and have patient drink it promptly.
- Shake emulsion well before measuring dose. Emulsion is better tolerated but more expensive. Store below 40° F (4.4° C). Don't freeze.
- Time drug administration so it doesn't interfere with scheduled activities or sleep.
- Give drug on empty stomach for best results.
- Increased intestinal motility lessens absorption of concomitantly administered oral drugs. Separate administration times.

Patient teaching

- Tell patient not to expect another bowel movement for 1 to 2 days after castor oil has emptied bowel.

Evaluation

- Patient obtains accurate results of diagnostic testing.
- Patient doesn't experience pain from therapy.
- Patient and family state understanding of drug therapy.

cefaclor

(SEH-fuh-klor)
Ceclor, Ceclor CD

Pharmacologic class: second-generation cephalosporin
Therapeutic class: antibiotic
Pregnancy risk category: B

Indications and dosages

▶ **Respiratory, urinary tract, skin, and soft-tissue infections and otitis media caused by *Haemophilus influenzae, Streptococcus pneumoniae, S. pyogenes, Escherichia coli, Proteus mirabilis, Klebsiella* species, and staphylococci.** *Adults:* 250 to 500 mg P.O. q 8 hours. Total daily dosage shouldn't exceed 4 g. For extended-release forms, 500 mg P.O. q 12 hours for 7 days for bronchitis. For pharyngitis or skin and skin-structure infections, 375 mg P.O. q 12 hours for 10 days and 7 to 10 days respectively.
Children: 10 mg/kg P.O. b.i.d. q 8 hours. For pharyngitis or otitis media, b.i.d. q 12 hours. For more serious infections, 40 mg/kg daily are recommended, not to exceed 1 g daily. If given for otitis media, dose can be divided equally and given every 12 hours.

How supplied

Tablets: (extended-release): 375 mg, 500 mg
Capsules: 250 mg, 500 mg
Oral suspension: 125 mg/5 ml, 250 mg/5 ml, 187 mg/5 ml, 375 mg/5 ml

Pharmacokinetics

Absorption: well absorbed from GI tract. Food will delay but not prevent complete GI tract absorption.
Distribution: distributed widely into most body tissues and fluids; CSF penetration is poor. Drug is 25% protein-bound.
Metabolism: none.
Excretion: excreted primarily in urine by renal tubular secretion and glomerular filtration. *Half-life:* 0.5 to 1 hour.

Route	Onset	Peak	Duration
P.O.	Unknown	30-60 min	Unknown

Pharmacodynamics

Chemical effect: inhibits cell-wall synthesis, promoting osmotic instability; usually bactericidal.
Therapeutic effect: hinders or kills susceptible bacteria: many gram-positive cocci, including penicillinase-producing *Staphylococcus aureus, S. epidermidis, S. pneumoniae,* group B streptococci, and group A beta-hemolytic streptococci; gram-negative organisms, including *K. pneumoniae, E. coli, P. mirabilis,* and *Shigella;* and other organisms, such as *Moraxella catarrhalis, H. influenzae, Enterobacter, Citrobacter, Providencia, Acinetobacter, Serratia,* and *Neisseria.*

Adverse reactions

CNS: dizziness, headache, somnolence, malaise.
GI: *nausea,* vomiting, *diarrhea,* anorexia, dyspepsia, abdominal cramps, pseudomembranous colitis, oral candidiasis.
GU: red and white cells in urine, vaginal candidiasis, vaginitis.
Hematologic: ***transient leukopenia,*** lymphocytosis, anemia, eosinophilia, ***thrombocytopenia.***
Hepatic: transient increases in liver enzyme levels.
Skin: *maculopapular rash,* dermatitis.
Other: hypersensitivity reactions (serum sickness, ***anaphylaxis***), fever.

Interactions

Drug-drug. *Chloramphenicol:* antagonistic effect. Don't use together.
Probenecid: may inhibit excretion and increase blood levels of cefaclor. Monitor patient.

Contraindications and precautions

- Contraindicated in patients hypersensitive to other cephalosporins.
- Use cautiously in pregnant patients, breast-feeding patients, and patients with impaired renal function or history of sensitivity to penicillin.
- Watch renal function; administer cautiously to patients with renal impairment.

NURSING CONSIDERATIONS

Assessment

- Assess patient's infection before therapy and regularly thereafter.
- Obtain specimen for culture and sensitivity tests before first dose. Therapy may begin pending test results.
- Ask patient about previous reactions to cephalosporins or penicillin before administering first dose.

• Be alert for adverse reactions and drug interactions.
• Monitor patient's hydration status if adverse GI reactions occur.
• Evaluate patient's and family's knowledge of drug therapy.

Nursing diagnoses
• Infection related to bacteria susceptible to drug
• Risk for deficient fluid volume related to drug-induced adverse GI reactions
• Deficient knowledge related to drug therapy

Planning and implementation
• Administer drug with food to prevent or minimize GI upset.
• Store reconstituted suspension in refrigerator (stable for 14 days). Keep tightly closed and shake well before using.
• Urine glucose determinations may be false-positive with copper sulfate tests (Clinitest); glucose enzymatic tests (Diastix or Chemstrip uG) aren't affected.
ALERT Don't confuse with other cephalosporins with similar sounding names.

Patient teaching
• Tell patient that drug may be taken with meals.
• Advise patient to take drug exactly as prescribed, even after he feels better.
• Instruct patient to call prescriber if rash develops.
• Teach patient how to store drug.

Evaluation
• Patient is free from infection.
• Patient maintains adequate hydration.
• Patient and family state understanding of drug therapy.

cefadroxil monohydrate
(seh-fuh-DROKS-il MON-oh-HIGH-drayt)
Duricef, Cefadroxil

Pharmacologic class: first-generation cephalosporin
Therapeutic class: antibiotic
Pregnancy risk category: B

Indications and dosages
▶ **Urinary tract infections caused by *Escherichia coli, Proteus mirabilis,* and *Klebsiella* species; skin and soft-tissue infections; and streptococcal pharyngitis.** *Adults:* 1 to 2 g P.O. daily, depending on infection treated, usually once or twice daily.
Children: 30 mg/kg P.O. daily in two divided doses. Course of treatment is usually at least 10 days.

How supplied
Tablets: 1 g
Capsules: 500 mg
Oral suspension: 125 mg/5 ml, 250 mg/5 ml, 500 mg/5 ml

Pharmacokinetics
Absorption: absorbed rapidly and completely from GI tract.
Distribution: distributed widely into most body tissues and fluids; CSF penetration is poor. Drug is 20% protein-bound.
Metabolism: none.
Excretion: excreted primarily unchanged in urine. *Half-life:* about 1 to 2 hours.

Route	Onset	Peak	Duration
P.O.	Unknown	1-2 hr	Unknown

Pharmacodynamics
Chemical effect: inhibits cell-wall synthesis, promoting osmotic instability; usually bactericidal.
Therapeutic effect: hinders or kills susceptible bacteria: many gram-positive cocci, including penicillinase-producing *Staphylococcus aureus, S. epidermidis, Streptococcus pneumoniae,* group B streptococci, and group A beta-hemolytic streptococci; and gram-negative organisms, including *K. pneumoniae, E. coli, P. mirabilis,* and *Shigella.*

Adverse reactions
CNS: dizziness, headache, malaise, paresthesia.
GI: pseudomembranous colitis, *nausea,* anorexia, vomiting, *diarrhea,* glossitis, *dyspep-*

sia, abdominal cramps, anal pruritus, tenesmus, oral candidiasis.
GU: genital pruritus, candidiasis.
Hematologic: ***transient neutropenia,*** eosinophilia, ***leukopenia,*** anemia, ***agranulocytosis, thrombocytopenia.***
Hepatic: transient increases in liver enzyme levels.
Respiratory: dyspnea.
Skin: *maculopapular and erythematous rashes.*
Other: hypersensitivity reactions (serum sickness, ***anaphylaxis***).

Interactions

Drug-drug. *Probenecid:* may inhibit excretion and increase blood levels of cefadroxil. Monitor patient.

Contraindications and precautions

- Contraindicated in patients hypersensitive to drug or other cephalosporins.
- Use cautiously in pregnant patients, breast-feeding patients, and patients with impaired renal function (dosage adjustments may be necessary) or a history of sensitivity to penicillin.

NURSING CONSIDERATIONS

Assessment

- Assess patient's infection before therapy and regularly thereafter.
- Obtain specimen for culture and sensitivity tests before first dose. Therapy may begin pending test results.
- Be alert for adverse reactions and drug interactions.
- Monitor patient's hydration status if adverse GI reactions occur.
- Evaluate patient's and family's knowledge of drug therapy.

Nursing diagnoses

- Infection related to bacteria susceptible to drug
- Risk for deficient fluid volume related to drug-induced adverse GI reactions
- Deficient knowledge related to drug therapy

Planning and implementation

- Drug's half-life permits once- or twice-daily dosing.
- Expect prescriber to lengthen dosage interval to prevent drug accumulation if creatinine clearance is below 50 ml/minute.
- Store reconstituted suspension in refrigerator. Keep container tightly closed and shake well before using.
- About 40% to 75% of patients receiving cephalosporins show false-positive direct Coombs' test.
- Urine glucose determinations may be false-positive with copper sulfate tests (Clinitest); glucose enzymatic tests (Diastix or Chemstrip uG) aren't affected.

ALERT Don't confuse with other cephalosporins with similar sounding names.

Patient teaching

- Tell patient to take drug exactly as prescribed, even after he feels better.
- Advise patient to take drug with food or milk to lessen GI discomfort.
- Tell patient to call prescriber if rash develops.
- Inform patient using oral suspension to shake it well before using and to refrigerate mixture in tightly closed container.

Evaluation

- Patient is free from infection.
- Patient maintains adequate hydration.
- Patient and family state understanding of drug therapy.

cefazolin sodium

(sef-EH-zoh-lin SOH-dee-um)
Ancef, Kefzol, Zolicef

Pharmacologic class: first-generation cephalosporin
Therapeutic class: antibiotic
Pregnancy risk category: B

Indications and dosages

▶ **Serious infections of respiratory, biliary, and GU tracts; skin, soft-tissue, bone, and joint infections; septicemia; and endocarditis caused by *Escherichia coli,* Entero-**

bacteriaceae, gonococci, *Haemophilus influenzae, Klebsiella, Proteus mirabilis, Staphylococcus aureus, Streptococcus pneumoniae,* and group A beta-hemolytic streptococci. *Adults:* 250 mg I.V. or I.M. q 8 hours to 1 g q 6 hours. Maximum 12 g/day in life-threatening situations.
Children over age 1 month: 50 to 100 mg/kg or 1.25 g/m^2 daily I.V. or I.M. in three or four divided doses.
▶ **Perioperative prophylaxis in contaminated surgery.** *Adults:* 1 g I.V. or I.M. 30 to 60 minutes before surgery; then 0.5 to 1 g I.V. or I.M. q 6 to 8 hours for 24 hours. In operations lasting over 2 hours, another 0.5- to 1-g dose may be administered intraoperatively. In cases where infection would be devastating, prophylaxis may be continued for 3 to 5 days. After initial dose, dosage should be adjusted in patients with renal failure.

How supplied

Injection (parenteral): 250 mg, 500 mg, 1 g
Infusion: 500 mg/50 ml or 100 ml vial, 1 g/50 ml or 100 ml vial, 500 mg or 1 g RediVials, Faspaks, or ADD-Vantage vials

Pharmacokinetics

Absorption: unknown after I.M. administration.
Distribution: distributed widely into most body tissues and fluids; CSF penetration is poor; 74% to 86% protein-bound.
Metabolism: none.
Excretion: excreted primarily in urine. *Half-life:* about 1 to 2 hours.

Route	Onset	Peak	Duration
I.V.	Immediate	Immediate	Unknown
I.M.	Unknown	1-2 hr	Unknown

Pharmacodynamics

Chemical effect: inhibits cell-wall synthesis, promoting osmotic instability; usually bactericidal.
Therapeutic effect: hinders or kills susceptible bacteria: many gram-positive cocci, including penicillinase-producing *Staphylococcus aureus, S. pneumoniae,* group A beta-hemolytic streptococci, *Klebsiella, E. coli, Enterobacteriaceae,* gonococci, *P. mirabilis,* and *H. influenzae.*

Adverse reactions

CNS: dizziness, headache, malaise, paresthesia.
GI: pseudomembranous colitis, nausea, anorexia, vomiting, *diarrhea,* glossitis, dyspepsia, abdominal cramps, anal pruritus, tenesmus, oral candidiasis.
GU: genital pruritus and candidiasis, vaginitis.
Hematologic: ***transient neutropenia, leukopenia,*** eosinophilia, anemia, ***thrombocytopenia.***
Hepatic: transient increases in liver enzyme levels.
Respiratory: dyspnea.
Skin: *maculopapular and erythematous rashes, urticaria,* ***Stevens-Johnson syndrome.***
Other: hypersensitivity reactions (serum sickness, ***anaphylaxis***).

Interactions

Drug-drug. *Probenecid:* may inhibit excretion and increase blood levels of cefazolin. Monitor patient.

Contraindications and precautions

- Contraindicated in patients hypersensitive to other cephalosporins.
- Use cautiously in pregnant patients, breast-feeding patients, patients with a history of sensitivity to penicillin, and patients with renal failure (dosage adjustments may be needed).

NURSING CONSIDERATIONS

Assessment

- Assess patient's infection before therapy and regularly thereafter.
- Obtain specimen for culture and sensitivity tests. Therapy may begin pending test results.
- Ask patient about previous reactions to cephalosporins or penicillin before administering first dose.
- Be alert for adverse reactions and drug interactions.
- Monitor patient's hydration status if adverse GI reactions occur.
- Evaluate patient's and family's knowledge of drug therapy.

Nursing diagnoses

- Infection related to bacteria susceptible to drug
- Risk for deficient fluid volume related to drug-induced adverse GI reactions
- Deficient knowledge related to drug therapy

Planning and implementation

I.V. use: Reconstitute with sterile water, bacteriostatic water, or normal saline solution as follows: 2 ml to 500-mg vial to yield 225 mg/ml or 2.5 ml to 1-g vial to yield 330 mg/ml. Shake well until dissolved.

– For direct injection, further dilute Ancef with 5 ml of sterile water (Kefzol with 10 ml). Inject into large vein or into tubing of free-flowing I.V. solution over 3 to 5 minutes. For intermittent infusion, add reconstituted drug to 50 to 100 ml of compatible solution or use premixed solution. Commercially available frozen solutions of cefazolin in D_5W should be given only by intermittent or continuous I.V. infusion.

– Alternate injection sites if I.V. therapy lasts longer than 3 days. Use of small I.V. needles in larger available veins may be preferable.

I.M. use: After reconstitution, inject I.M. drug without further dilution (not as painful as other cephalosporins). Inject deep into large muscle mass, such as gluteus maximus or lateral aspect of thigh.

- Reconstituted drug is stable for 24 hours at room temperature and 96 hours if refrigerated.
- Dose and dosing interval will be adjusted if creatinine clearance is below 55 ml/minute.
- Because of long duration of effect, most infections can be treated with dose every 8 hours.
- Urine glucose determinations may be false-positive with copper sulfate tests (Clinitest); glucose enzymatic tests (Diastix or Chemstrip uG) aren't affected.

ALERT Don't confuse with other cephalosporins with similar sounding names.

Patient teaching

- Tell patient to report adverse reactions.

Evaluation

- Patient is free from infection.
- Patient maintains adequate hydration.
- Patient and family state understanding of drug therapy.

cefdinir

(SEF-dih-neer)
Omnicef

Pharmacologic class: third-generation cephalosporin
Therapeutic class: antibiotic
Pregnancy risk category: B

Indications and dosages

▶ **Treatment of mild to moderate infections caused by susceptible strains of microorganisms for conditions of community-acquired pneumonia, acute exacerbations of chronic bronchitis, acute maxillary sinusitis, acute bacterial otitis media, and uncomplicated skin and skin-structure infection.** *Adults and children age 13 and older:* 300 mg P.O. q 12 hours or 600 mg P.O. q 24 hours for 10 days. (Use q-12-hour dosages for pneumonia and skin infections.)

Children ages 6 months to 12 years: 7 mg/kg P.O. q 12 hours or 14 mg/kg P.O. q 24 hours for 10 days; maximum daily dose 600 mg. (Use q-12-hour dosages for skin infections.) Dosage is adjusted for patients with impaired renal function and is based on creatinine clearance.

▶ **Treatment of pharyngitis and tonsillitis.** *Adults and children age 13 and older:* 300 mg P.O. q 12 hours for 5 to 10 days or 600 mg P.O. q 24 hours for 10 days.

Children ages 6 months to 12 years: 7 mg/kg P.O. q 12 hours for 5 to 10 days or 14 mg/kg P.O. q 24 hours for 10 days, up to a maximum dose of 600 mg daily.

How supplied

Capsules: 300 mg
Suspension: 125 mg/5 ml

Pharmacokinetics

Absorption: bioavailability of drug is about 21% after 300-mg capsule dose, 16% after 600-mg capsule dose, and 25% for suspension.

Distribution: 60% to 70% bound to plasma proteins.
Metabolism: not appreciably metabolized; activity results mainly from parent drug.
Excretion: eliminated primarily by renal excretion. *Half-life:* 1.7 hours.

Route	Onset	Peak	Duration
P.O.	Unknown	2-4 hr	Unknown

Pharmacodynamics

Chemical effect: bactericidal activity results from inhibition of cell-wall synthesis.
Therapeutic effect: is stable in the presence of some beta-lactamase enzymes, causing some microorganisms resistant to penicillins and cephalosporins to be susceptible to cefdinir. Excluding *Pseudomonas, Enterobacter, Enterococcus,* and methicillin-resistant *Staphylococcus* species, cefdinir's spectrum of activity includes a broad range of gram-positive and gram-negative aerobic microorganisms.

Adverse reactions

CNS: headache.
GI: abdominal pain, *diarrhea*, nausea, vomiting.
GU: vaginal candidiasis, vaginitis, increased urine proteins and RBCs.
Skin: rash.

Interactions

Drug-drug. *Antacids (magnesium- and aluminum-containing), iron supplements, multivitamins containing iron:* decrease cefdinir's rate of absorption and bioavailability. Administer such preparations 2 hours before or after cefdinir dose.
Probenecid: inhibits the renal excretion of cefdinir. Monitor patient.

Contraindications and precautions

- Contraindicated in patients hypersensitive to cephalosporins.
- Use cautiously in patients hypersensitive to penicillin because of risk of cross-sensitivity with other beta-lactam antibiotics.
- Use cautiously in patients with history of colitis or renal insufficiency.

NURSING CONSIDERATIONS

Assessment

- Ask patient about previous reactions to cephalosporins or penicillin before administering first dose.
- Obtain specimen for culture and sensitivity tests as ordered before giving first dose.
- Monitor patient for symptoms of superinfection.
- Assess patient with diarrhea carefully; pseudomembranous colitis has been reported with drug.
- Evaluate patient's and family's knowledge of drug therapy.

Nursing diagnoses

- Infection related to susceptible bacteria
- Risk for deficient fluid volume related to drug-induced adverse GI reactions
- Deficient knowledge related to drug therapy

Planning and implementation

- Begin therapy pending culture and sensitivity test results.
- Patients with renal insufficiency require reduced dosage.
- Notify prescriber if allergic reaction is suspected; drug should be discontinued and emergency treatment given as needed.

ALERT Don't confuse with other cephalosporins with similar sounding names.

Patient teaching

- Instruct patient to take antacids and iron supplements 2 hours before or after dose of cefdinir.
- Inform diabetic patient that each teaspoon of suspension contains 2.86 g of sucrose.
- Tell patient that drug may be taken without regard to meals.
- Advise patient to report severe diarrhea or diarrhea accompanied by abdominal pain.
- Tell patient to report adverse reactions or symptoms of superinfection promptly.

Evaluation

- Patient is free from infection.
- Patient maintains adequate hydration.
- Patient and family state understanding of drug therapy.

cefixime
(sef-IKS-eem)
Suprax

Pharmacologic class: third-generation cephalosporin
Therapeutic class: antibiotic
Pregnancy risk category: B

Indications and dosages

▶ **Uncomplicated urinary tract infections caused by *Escherichia coli* and *Proteus mirabilis;* otitis media caused by *Haemophilus influenzae* (beta-lactamase positive and negative strains), *Moraxella catarrhalis,* and *Streptococcus pyogenes*; pharyngitis and tonsillitis caused by *S. pyogenes;* acute bronchitis and acute exacerbations of chronic bronchitis caused by *S. pneumoniae* and *H. influenzae* (beta-lactamase positive and negative strains).** *Adults and children over age 12 or weighing over 50 kg (110 lb):* 400 mg/day P.O. as single 400-mg tablet or 200 mg q 12 hours.
Children age 12 and younger or weighing 50 kg or less: 8 mg/kg P.O. daily dose in one or two divided doses. For otitis media, use suspension only.

▶ **Uncomplicated gonorrhea caused by *Neisseria gonorrhoeae*.** *Adults:* 400 mg P.O. as single dose.

How supplied

Tablets: 200 mg, 400 mg
Oral suspension: 100 mg/5 ml (after reconstitution)

Pharmacokinetics

Absorption: well absorbed from GI tract.
Distribution: widely distributed; enters CSF in patients with inflamed meninges; about 65% bound to plasma proteins.
Metabolism: about 50% of drug is metabolized.
Excretion: excreted primarily in urine. *Half-life:* 3 to 4 hours.

Route	Onset	Peak	Duration
P.O.	Unknown	3.1-4.4 hr	Unknown

Pharmacodynamics

Chemical effect: inhibits cell-wall synthesis, promoting osmotic instability; usually bactericidal.
Therapeutic effect: hinders or kills bacteria, including *H. influenzae, M. catarrhalis, S. pyogenes, S. pneumoniae, E. coli,* and *P. mirabilis.*

Adverse reactions

CNS: headaches, dizziness, nervousness, malaise, fatigue, somnolence, insomnia.
GI: *diarrhea,* loose stools, abdominal pain, nausea, vomiting, dyspepsia, flatulence, pseudomembranous colitis.
GU: genital pruritus, vaginitis, genital candidiasis, transient increases in BUN and serum creatinine levels.
Hematologic: ***thrombocytopenia, leukopenia,*** eosinophilia.
Hepatic: transient increases in liver enzyme levels.
Skin: pruritus, rash, urticaria, ***Stevens-Johnson syndrome.***
Other: drug fever, hypersensitivity reactions (serum sickness, ***anaphylaxis***).

Interactions

Drug-drug. *Probenecid:* may inhibit excretion and increase blood levels of cefixime. Monitor patient.
Salicylates: may displace cefixime from plasma protein–binding sites. Clinical significance is unknown.
Nifedepine: Concommitant use increases cefixime levels. Avoid concomitant use.

Contraindications and precautions

- Contraindicated in patients hypersensitive to drug or other cephalosporins.
- Use cautiously in pregnant or breast-feeding women and in patients with renal dysfunction (reduced dosage necessary with creatinine clearance below 60 ml/minute) or history of sensitivity to penicillin.

NURSING CONSIDERATIONS

Assessment

- Assess patient's infection before therapy and regularly thereafter.

• Obtain specimen for culture and sensitivity tests before first dose. Therapy may begin pending test results.
• Ask patient about previous reactions to cephalosporins or penicillin before administering first dose.
• Be alert for adverse reactions and drug interactions.
• Monitor patient's hydration status if adverse GI reactions occur.
• Evaluate patient's and family's knowledge of drug therapy.

Nursing diagnoses
• Infection related to bacteria susceptible to drug
• Risk for deficient fluid volume related to drug-induced adverse GI reactions
• Deficient knowledge related to drug therapy

Planning and implementation
• To prepare oral suspension, add required amount of water to powder in two portions. Shake well after each addition. After mixing, suspension is stable for 14 days (no need to refrigerate). Keep tightly closed. Shake well before using.
• Urine glucose determinations may be false-positive with copper sulfate tests (Clinitest); glucose enzymatic tests (Diastix or Chemstrip uG) aren't affected.
ALERT Don't confuse with other cephalosporins with similar sounding names.

Patient teaching
• Tell patient to take drug exactly as prescribed, even after he feels better.
• Tell patient to call prescriber if rash develops.
• Teach patient how to store drug.

Evaluation
• Patient is free from infection.
• Patient maintains adequate hydration.
• Patient and family state understanding of drug therapy.

cefmetazole sodium (cefmetazone)
(sef-MET-ah-zohl SOH-dee-um)
Zefazone

Pharmacologic class: second-generation cephalosporin
Therapeutic class: antibiotic
Pregnancy risk category: B

Indications and dosages
▶ **Lower respiratory tract infections caused by *Streptococcus pneumoniae, Staphylococcus aureus* (penicillinase- and non-penicillinase–producing strains), *Escherichia coli,* and *Haemophilus influenzae* (non-penicillinase–producing strains); intra-abdominal infections caused by *E. coli* or *Bacteroides fragilis;* skin and skin-structure infections caused by *S. aureus* (penicillinase- and non-penicillinase–producing strains), *S. epidermidis, S. pyogenes, S. agalactiae, E. coli, Proteus mirabilis, Klebsiella pneumoniae,* and *B. fragilis.*** *Adults:* 2 g I.V. q 6 to 12 hours for 5 to 14 days.
▶ **Urinary tract infections caused by *E. coli.*** *Adults:* 2 g I.V. q 12 hours.
▶ **Prophylaxis in patients undergoing vaginal hysterectomy.** *Adults:* 2 g I.V. 30 to 90 minutes before surgery as single dose; or 1 g I.V. 30 to 90 minutes before surgery, repeated after 8 and 16 hours.
▶ **Prophylaxis in patients undergoing abdominal hysterectomy.** *Adults:* 1 g I.V. 30 to 90 minutes before surgery, repeated after 8 and 16 hours.
▶ **Prophylaxis in patients undergoing cesarean section.** *Adults:* 2 g I.V. as single dose after clamping cord; or 1 g I.V. after clamping cord, repeated after 8 and 16 hours.
▶ **Prophylaxis in patients undergoing colorectal surgery.** *Adults:* 2 g I.V. as single dose 30 to 90 minutes before surgery. Some clinicians follow with additional 2-g doses after 8 and 16 hours.
▶ **Prophylaxis in patients undergoing cholecystectomy (high risk).** *Adults:* 1 g I.V.

30 to 90 minutes before surgery, repeated after 8 and 16 hours.

How supplied

Injection: 1 g, 2 g

Pharmacokinetics

Absorption: not applicable with I.V. administration.
Distribution: distributed widely into most body tissues and fluids; CSF penetration is P.O.; 65% protein-bound.
Metabolism: about 15% of dose is metabolized, probably in liver.
Excretion: excreted primarily in urine. *Half-life:* about 1.5 hours.

Route	Onset	Peak	Duration
I.V.	Unknown	Immediate	Unknown

Pharmacodynamics

Chemical effect: inhibits cell-wall synthesis, promoting osmotic instability; usually bactericidal.
Therapeutic effect: hinders or kills susceptible bacteria: many gram-positive organisms and enteric gram-negative bacilli, including *S. aureus, S. epidermidis,* streptococci, *Klebsiella, E. coli* and other coliform bacteria, *H. influenzae,* and *Bacteroides* species.

Adverse reactions

CNS: headache.
CV: *shock,* hypotension, phlebitis.
EENT: altered color perception, epistaxis.
GI: nausea, vomiting, *diarrhea,* epigastric pain, pseudomembranous colitis.
GU: vaginitis.
Respiratory: pleural effusion, dyspnea, respiratory distress.
Skin: rash, pruritus, generalized erythema.
Other: fever, bacterial or fungal superinfection, hypersensitivity reactions (serum sickness, ***anaphylaxis***), pain at injection site.

Interactions

Drug-drug. *Aminoglycosides:* possible increased risk of nephrotoxicity. Monitor patient closely.
Probenecid: may inhibit excretion and increase blood levels of cefmetazole. Sometimes used for this effect.
Drug-lifestyle. *Alcohol use:* possible disulfiram-like reaction. Discourage alcohol consumption for 24 hours before and after cefmetazole.

Contraindications and precautions

- Contraindicated in patients hypersensitive to drug or other cephalosporins.
- Use cautiously in pregnant women and in patients with history of sensitivity to penicillin.
- Traces of drug have been detected in breast milk. Breast-feeding should be discontinued temporarily during therapy.
- Safety of drug hasn't been established in children.

NURSING CONSIDERATIONS

Assessment

- Assess patient's infection before therapy and regularly thereafter.
- Obtain specimen for culture and sensitivity tests before first dose. Therapy may begin pending test results.
- Ask patient about previous reactions to cephalosporins or penicillin before administering first dose.
- Be alert for adverse reactions and drug interactions. Watch for superinfection, especially in elderly patients or those with chronic conditions.
- Monitor patient's hydration status for adverse GI reactions.
- Evaluate patient's and family's knowledge of drug therapy.

Nursing diagnoses

- Infection related to bacteria susceptible to drug
- Risk for deficient fluid volume related to drug-induced adverse GI reactions
- Deficient knowledge related to drug therapy.

Planning and implementation

- Reconstitute with bacteriostatic water for injection, sterile water for injection, or normal saline solution for injection. After reconstitution, drug may be further diluted to concentrations ranging from 1 to 20 mg/ml by adding it to normal saline solution for injection, D_5W, or lactated Ringer's injection. Reconstituted or dilute solutions are stable for 24 hours at room temperature (77° F [25° C]) or 1 week if refrigerated at 46° F (8° C).

• Urine glucose determinations may be false-positive with copper sulfate tests (Clinitest); glucose enzymatic tests (Diastix or Chemstrip uG) aren't affected.

ALERT Don't confuse with other cephalosporins with similar sounding names.

Patient teaching

• Instruct patient to report adverse reactions.

Evaluation

• Patient is free from infection.
• Patient maintains adequate hydration.
• Patient and family state understanding of drug therapy.

cefonicid sodium

(sef-ON-eh-sid SOH-dee-um)
Monocid

Pharmacologic class: second-generation cephalosporin
Therapeutic class: antibiotic
Pregnancy risk category: B

Indications and dosages

▶ **Perioperative prophylaxis in contaminated surgery.** *Adults:* 1 g I.M. or I.V. 60 minutes before surgery.

▶ **Serious infections of lower respiratory and urinary tracts, skin and skin-structure infections, septicemia, bone and joint infections, and perioperative prophylaxis. Susceptible microorganisms include *Streptococcus pneumoniae, S. pyogenes, Klebsiella pneumoniae, Escherichia coli, Haemophilus influenzae, Proteus mirabilis, Staphylococcus aureus, and S. epidermidis.*** *Adults:* usual dosage is 1 g I.V. or I.M. q 24 hours. In life-threatening infections, 2 g q 24 hours.

How supplied

Injection: 1 g
Infusion: 1 g/100 ml

Pharmacokinetics

Absorption: unknown after I.M. administration.
Distribution: distributed widely into most body tissues and fluids; CSF penetration is poor; 90% to 98% protein-bound.
Metabolism: none.
Excretion: excreted primarily in urine. *Half-life:* about 3½ to 6 hours.

Route	Onset	Peak	Duration
I.V.	Immediate	Immediate	Unknown
I.M.	Unknown	1-2 hr	Unknown

Pharmacodynamics

Chemical effect: inhibits cell-wall synthesis, promoting osmotic instability; usually bactericidal.
Therapeutic effect: hinders or kills susceptible bacteria: many gram-positive organisms and enteric gram-negative bacilli, such as *S. aureus, S. epidermidis, S. pyogenes, S. pneumoniae, K. pneumoniae, E. coli, P. mirabilis,* and *H. influenzae.*

Adverse reactions

CNS: dizziness, headache, malaise, paresthesia.
GI: pseudomembranous colitis, nausea, anorexia, vomiting, diarrhea, glossitis, dyspepsia, abdominal cramps, anal pruritus, tenesmus, oral candidiasis.
GU: genital pruritus and candidiasis, vaginitis, ***acute renal failure.***
Hematologic: ***transient neutropenia, leukopenia***, eosinophilia, anemia, ***thrombocytopenia.***
Respiratory: dyspnea.
Skin: *maculopapular and erythematous rashes, urticaria.*
Other: hypersensitivity reactions (serum sickness, ***anaphylaxis***); *pain, induration, sterile abscesses, tissue sloughing* (at injection site); *phlebitis, thrombophlebitis* (with I.V. injection).

Interactions

Drug-drug. *Aminoglycosides:* potential increased risk of nephrotoxicity. Monitor patient's renal function closely.
Probenecid: may inhibit excretion and increase blood levels of cefonicid. Monitor patient.

Contraindications and precautions

- Contraindicated in patients hypersensitive to drug or other cephalosporins.
- Use cautiously in patients with history of sensitivity to penicillin, in pregnant or breast-feeding women, and in patients with renal failure (may need dosage adjustment).
- Safety of drug hasn't been established in children.

NURSING CONSIDERATIONS

Assessment

- Assess patient's infection before therapy and regularly thereafter.
- Obtain specimen for culture and sensitivity tests before first dose. Therapy may begin pending test results.
- Ask patient about previous reactions to cephalosporins or penicillin before administering first dose.
- Be alert for adverse reactions and drug interactions. Monitor patient for superinfection.
- Monitor patient's hydration status if adverse GI reactions occur.
- Evaluate patient's and family's knowledge of drug therapy.

Nursing diagnoses

- Infection related to bacteria susceptible to drug
- Risk for deficient fluid volume related to drug-induced adverse GI reactions
- Deficient knowledge deficit related to drug therapy

Planning and implementation

I.V. use: Reconstitute 500-mg vial with 2 ml of sterile water for injection (yields 225 mg/ml) and 1-g vial with 2.5 ml of sterile water for injection (yields 325 mg/ml). Shake well. Reconstitute piggyback vials with 50 to 100 ml of D_5W or normal saline solution.

I.M. use: When administering 2-g I.M. doses once daily, divide dose equally and inject deeply into large muscle mass, such as gluteus maximus or lateral aspect of thigh.

- Dosing interval will be adjusted for patients with renal impairment.
- Urine glucose determinations may be false-positive with copper sulfate tests (Clinitest); glucose enzymatic tests (Diastix or Chemstrip uG) aren't affected.

ALERT Don't confuse with other cephalosporins with similar sounding names.

Patient teaching

- Tell patient to report adverse reactions.

Evaluation

- Patient is free from infection.
- Patient maintains adequate hydration.
- Patient and family state understanding of drug therapy.

cefoperazone sodium

(sef-oh-PER-ah-zohn SOH-dee-um)
Cefobid

Pharmacologic class: third-generation cephalosporin
Therapeutic class: antibiotic
Pregnancy risk category: B

Indications and dosages

▶ **Serious infections of respiratory tract; intra-abdominal, gynecologic, and skin infections; bacteremia; and septicemia. Susceptible microorganisms include *Streptococcus pneumoniae* and *S. pyogenes; Staphylococcus aureus* (penicillinase- and non-penicillinase–producing) and *S. epidermidis;* enterococci; *Escherichia coli; Klebsiella; Haemophilus influenzae; Enterobacter; Citrobacter; Proteus;* some *Pseudomonas,* including *P. aeruginosa;* and *Bacteroides fragilis.*** *Adults:* usual dosage is 1 to 2 g q 12 hours I.V. or I.M. In severe infections or those caused by less sensitive organisms, total daily dosage may be increased to 16 g/day.

How supplied

Infusion: 1 g, 2 g piggyback
Parenteral: 1 g, 2 g

Pharmacokinetics

Absorption: unknown after I.M. administration.
Distribution: distributed widely into most body tissues and fluids; CSF penetration in patients with inflamed meninges; 82% to 93% protein-bound.
Metabolism: insubstantial.
Excretion: excreted primarily in urine. *Half-life:* about 1.5 to 2.5 hours.

Route	Onset	Peak	Duration
I.V.	Immediate	Immediate	Unknown
I.M.	Unknown	1-2 hr	Unknown

Pharmacodynamics

Chemical effect: inhibits cell-wall synthesis, promoting osmotic instability; usually bactericidal.
Therapeutic effect: hinders or kills susceptible bacteria: some gram-positive organisms and many enteric gram-negative bacilli, including *S. pneumoniae* and *S. pyogenes, S. aureus, S. epidermidis,* enterococcus, *E. coli, Klebsiella, H. influenzae, Enterobacter, Citrobacter, Proteus,* some *Pseudomonas* species (including *P. aeruginosa*), and *B. fragilis.*

Adverse reactions

CNS: headache, malaise, paresthesia, dizziness.
GI: pseudomembranous colitis, nausea, anorexia, vomiting, *diarrhea,* glossitis, dyspepsia, abdominal cramps, tenesmus, anal pruritus, oral candidiasis.
GU: genital pruritus and candidiasis.
Hematologic: ***transient neutropenia,*** eosinophilia, hemolytic anemia, hypoprothrombinemia, bleeding.
Hepatic: mildly elevated liver enzyme levels.
Respiratory: dyspnea.
Skin: *maculopapular and erythematous rashes, urticaria.*
Other: hypersensitivity reactions (serum sickness, ***anaphylaxis***); *pain, induration, sterile abscesses, warmth, tissue sloughing* at injection site; *phlebitis, thrombophlebitis* with I.V. injection.

Interactions

Drug-drug. *Anticoagulants:* effects of anticoagulant may be increased. Use with caution.
Probenecid: may inhibit excretion and increase blood levels of cefoperazone. Monitor patient.
Drug-lifestyle. *Alcohol use:* possible disulfiram-like reaction. Caution patient to avoid alcohol consumption for several days after discontinuing cefoperazone.

Contraindications and precautions

- Contraindicated in patients hypersensitive to drug or other cephalosporins.
- Use cautiously in pregnant patients, breast-feeding patients, patients with impaired renal function, and patients with a history of sensitivity to penicillin.
- Safety of drug hasn't been established in children under age 12.

NURSING CONSIDERATIONS

Assessment

- Assess patient's infection before therapy and regularly thereafter.
- Obtain specimen for culture and sensitivity tests before first dose. Therapy may begin pending test results.
- Ask patient about previous reactions to cephalosporins or penicillin before administering first dose.
- Be alert for adverse reactions and drug interactions.
- Monitor hydration status if patient develops adverse GI reactions. Cefoperazone may increase risk of diarrhea over other cephalosporins.
- Evaluate patient's and family's knowledge of drug therapy.

Nursing diagnoses

- Infection related to bacteria susceptible to drug
- Risk for deficient fluid volume related to drug-induced adverse GI reactions
- Deficient knowledge related to drug therapy

Planning and implementation

• Administer doses of 4 g/day cautiously to patients with hepatic disease or biliary obstruction. Higher dosages require monitoring of serum levels.

I.V. use: Reconstitute 1- or 2-g vial with minimum of 2.8 ml of compatible I.V. solution; manufacturer recommends using 5 ml/g.

– Give by direct injection into large vein or into tubing of free-flowing I.V. solution over 3 to 5 minutes.

– When giving by intermittent infusion, add reconstituted drug to 20 to 40 ml of compatible I.V. solution and infuse over 15 to 30 minutes.

I.M. use: To prepare drug for I.M. injection, using 1-g vial, dissolve drug with 2 ml of sterile water for injection; add 0.6 ml of 2% lidocaine hydrochloride for final concentration of 333 mg/ml. Alternatively, dissolve drug with 2.8 ml of sterile water for injection; then add 1 ml of 2% lidocaine hydrochloride for final concentration of 250 mg/ml. When using 2-g vial, dissolve drug with 3.8 ml of sterile water for injection; then add 1.2 ml of 2% lidocaine hydrochloride for final concentration of 333 mg/ml. Alternatively, dissolve drug with 5.4 ml of sterile water for injection; then add 1.8 ml of 2% lidocaine hydrochloride for final concentration of 250 mg/ml.

– Inject deeply into large muscle mass, such as gluteus maximus or lateral aspect of thigh.

• Urine glucose determinations may be false-positive with copper sulfate tests (Clinitest); glucose enzymatic tests (Diastix or Chemstrip uG) aren't affected.

ALERT Don't confuse with other cephalosporins with similar sounding names.

Patient teaching

• Tell patient to report adverse reactions.

Evaluation

• Patient is free from infection.
• Patient maintains adequate hydration.
• Patient and family state understanding of drug therapy.

cefotaxime sodium
(sef-oh-TAKS-eem SOH-dee-um)
Claforan

Pharmacologic class: third-generation cephalosporin
Therapeutic class: antibiotic
Pregnancy risk category: B

Indications and dosages

▶ **Perioperative prophylaxis in contaminated surgery.** *Adults:* 1 g I.V. or I.M. 30 to 60 minutes before surgery. Patients undergoing cesarean section should receive 1 g I.V. or I.M. as soon as umbilical cord is clamped, followed by 1 g I.V. or I.M. 6 and 12 hours later.

▶ **Serious infections of lower respiratory and urinary tracts, CNS, skin, bone, and joints; gynecologic and intra-abdominal infections; bacteremia; and septicemia. Susceptible microorganisms include streptococci, including *Streptococcus pneumoniae* and *S. pyogenes; Staphylococcus aureus* (penicillinase- and non-penicillinase–producing) and *S. epidermidis; Escherichia coli; Klebsiella; Haemophilus influenzae; Enterobacter; Proteus*; and *Peptostreptococcus*.** *Adults:* usual dosage is 1 g I.V. or I.M. q 6 to 12 hours. Up to 12 g daily can be administered in life-threatening infections.
Children weighing at least 50 kg (110 lb): usual adult dose but dosage shouldn't exceed 12 g daily.
Children ages 1 month to 12 years weighing under 50 kg: 50 to 180 mg/kg/day I.V. or I.M. in four to six divided doses.
Neonates ages 1 to 4 weeks: 50 mg/kg I.V. q 8 hours. *Neonates up to age 1 week:* 50 mg/kg I.V. q 12 hours.

How supplied

Injection: 500 mg, 1 g, 2 g
Infusion: 1 g, 2 g

Pharmacokinetics

Absorption: unknown after I.M. administration.
Distribution: distributed widely into most body tissues and fluids; adequate CSF penetra-

tion when meninges are inflamed; 13% to 38% protein-bound.
Metabolism: partially metabolized to active metabolite, desacetylcefotaxime.
Excretion: excreted primarily in urine. *Half-life:* 1 to 2 hours.

Route	Onset	Peak	Duration
I.V.	Immediate	Immediate	Unknown
I.M.	Unknown	30 min	Unknown

Pharmacodynamics

Chemical effect: inhibits cell-wall synthesis, promoting osmotic instability; usually bactericidal.
Therapeutic effect: hinders or kills susceptible bacteria: some gram-positive organisms and many enteric gram-negative bacilli, including streptococci (*S. pneumoniae* and *pyogenes*), *S. aureus, S. epidermidis, E. coli, Klebsiella* species, *H. influenzae, Enterobacter* species, *Proteus* species, *Peptostreptococcus* species, and some strains of *Pseudomonas aeruginosa.*

Adverse reactions

CNS: headache, malaise, paresthesia, dizziness.
GI: pseudomembranous colitis, nausea, anorexia, vomiting, *diarrhea,* glossitis, dyspepsia, abdominal cramps, tenesmus, anal pruritus, oral candidiasis.
GU: genital pruritus and candidiasis.
Hematologic: ***transient neutropenia,*** eosinophilia, hemolytic anemia, ***thrombocytopenia, agranulocytosis.***
Hepatic: transient increases in liver enzyme levels.
Respiratory: dyspnea.
Skin: *maculopapular and erythematous rashes, urticaria.*
Other: hypersensitivity reactions (serum sickness, ***anaphylaxis***); elevated temperature; *pain, induration, sterile abscesses, warmth, tissue sloughing* at injection site; *phlebitis, thrombophlebitis* with I.V. injection.

Interactions

Drug-drug. *Aminoglycosides:* may increase risk of nephrotoxicity. Monitor renal function closely.
Probenecid: may inhibit excretion and increase blood levels of cefotaxime. Use together cautiously.

Contraindications and precautions

- Contraindicated in patients hypersensitive to drug or other cephalosporins.
- Use cautiously in pregnant patients, breast-feeding patients, patients with history of sensitivity to penicillin, and patients with renal failure (may need dosage adjustment).

NURSING CONSIDERATIONS

Assessment

- Assess patient's infection before therapy and regularly thereafter.
- Obtain specimen for culture and sensitivity tests. Therapy may begin before test results are known.
- Ask patient about previous reactions to cephalosporins or penicillin before administering first dose.
- Be alert for adverse reactions and drug interactions.
- Monitor patient's hydration status if adverse GI reactions occur.
- Evaluate patient's and family's knowledge of drug therapy.

Nursing diagnoses

- Infection related to bacteria susceptible to drug
- Risk for deficient fluid volume related to drug-induced adverse GI reactions
- Deficient knowledge related to drug therapy

Planning and implementation

I.V. use: For direct injection, reconstitute 500-mg, 1-g, or 2-g vials with 10 ml of sterile water for injection. Solutions containing 1 g/ 14 ml are isotonic.
– Inject drug into large vein or into tubing of free-flowing I.V. solution over 3 to 5 minutes.
– For I.V. infusion, reconstitute infusion vials with 50 to 100 ml of D_5W or normal saline solution. Infuse drug over 20 to 30 minutes. Interrupt flow of primary I.V. solution during infusion.

I.M. use: Inject deeply into large muscle mass, such as gluteus maximus or lateral aspect of thigh.

- Urine glucose determinations may be false-positive with copper sulfate tests (Clinitest); glucose enzymatic tests (Diastix or Chemstrip uG) aren't affected.

ALERT Don't confuse with other cephalosporins with similar sounding names.

Patient teaching

- Tell patient to report adverse reactions.
- Teach patient to report decrease in urinary output. May have to decrease total daily dosage.

Evaluation

- Patient is free from infection.
- Patient maintains adequate hydration.
- Patient and family state understanding of drug therapy.

cefotetan disodium

(SEF-oh-teh-tan die-SOH-dee-um)

Cefotan

Pharmacologic class: second-generation cephalosporin

Therapeutic class: antibiotic

Pregnancy risk category: B

Indications and dosages

▶ **Serious urinary tract infections, lower respiratory tract infections, and gynecologic, skin and skin-structure, intra-abdominal, and bone and joint infections caused by susceptible streptococci, *Staphylococcus aureus* and *S. epidermidis, Escherichia coli, Klebsiella, Enterobacter, Proteus, Haemophilus influenzae, Neisseria gonorrhoeae,* and *Bacteroides,* including *B. fragilis.*** *Adults:* 1 mg to 2 g I.V. or I.M. q 12 hours for 5 to 10 days. In life-threatening infections, up to 6 g daily.

▶ **Perioperative prophylaxis.** *Adults:* 1 to 2 g I.V. given once 30 to 60 minutes before surgery. In cesarean section, dose should be administered as soon as umbilical cord is clamped.

How supplied

Injection: 1 g, 2 g

Infusion: 1 g, 2 g piggyback

Pharmacokinetics

Absorption: unknown after I.M. administration.

Distribution: distributed widely into most body tissues and fluids; CSF penetration is poor; 75% to 90% protein-bound.

Metabolism: none.

Excretion: excreted primarily in urine. *Half-life:* about 3 to 4.5 hours.

Route	Onset	Peak	Duration
I.V.	Immediate	Immediate	Unknown
I.M.	Unknown	1.5-2 hr	Unknown

Pharmacodynamics

Chemical effect: inhibits cell-wall synthesis, promoting osmotic instability; usually bactericidal.

Therapeutic effect: hinders or kills susceptible bacteria: many gram-positive organisms and enteric gram-negative bacilli, such as streptococci, *S. aureus* and *S. epidermidis, E. coli, Klebsiella* species, *Enterobacter* species, *Proteus* species, *H. influenzae, N. gonorrhoeae,* and *Bacteroides* species.

Adverse reactions

CNS: headache, malaise, paresthesia, dizziness.

GI: pseudomembranous colitis, nausea, anorexia, vomiting, *diarrhea,* glossitis, dyspepsia, abdominal cramps, tenesmus, anal pruritus.

GU: genital pruritus and candidiasis, ***nephrotoxicity.***

Hematologic: ***transient neutropenia,*** eosinophilia, hemolytic anemia, hypoprothrombinemia, bleeding, ***agranulocytosis, thrombocytopenia.***

Hepatic: transient increases in liver enzyme levels.

Respiratory: dyspnea.

Skin: *maculopapular and erythematous rashes, urticaria.*

Other: hypersensitivity reactions (serum sickness, ***anaphylaxis***); elevated temperature; *pain, induration, sterile abscesses, tissue* *sloughing* at injection site; *phlebitis, thrombophlebitis* with I.V. injection.

Interactions

Drug-drug. *Aminoglycosides:* possible synergistic effect and possible increased risk of nephrotoxicity. Use with caution.
Anticoagulants: effects of anticoagulants may be increased. Use with caution.
Probenecid: may inhibit excretion and increase blood levels of cefotetan. Sometimes used for this effect.
Drug-lifestyle. *Alcohol use:* possible disulfiram-like reaction. Tell patient to avoid alcohol for several days after stopping cefotetan.

Contraindications and precautions

- Contraindicated in patients hypersensitive to drug or other cephalosporins.
- Use cautiously in pregnant patients, breast-feeding patients, patients with history of sensitivity to penicillin, and patients with renal failure (may need dosage adjustment).
- Safety of drug hasn't been established in children.

NURSING CONSIDERATIONS

Assessment

- Assess patient's infection before therapy and regularly thereafter.
- Obtain specimen for culture and sensitivity tests before first dose. Therapy may begin pending test results.
- Ask patient about previous reactions to cephalosporins or penicillin before administering first dose.
- Be alert for adverse reactions and drug interactions.
- Monitor patient's hydration status if adverse GI reactions occur.
- Evaluate patient's and family's knowledge of drug therapy.

Nursing diagnoses

- Infection related to bacteria susceptible to drug
- Risk for deficient fluid volume related to drug-induced adverse GI reactions
- Deficient knowledge related to drug therapy

Planning and implementation

I.V. use: Reconstitute drug with sterile water for injection. Then may be mixed with 50 to 100 ml of D_5W or normal saline solution.
– Interrupt flow of primary I.V. solution during drug infusion.
– For direct injection, give solutions containing 1 or 2 g of solution over 3 to 5 minutes.
I.M. use: Reconstitute I.M. injection with sterile water or bacteriostatic water for injection, normal saline solution for injection, or 0.5% or 1% lidocaine hydrochloride.
– Shake to dissolve and let stand until clear.

- Reconstituted solution remains stable for 24 hours at room temperature or 96 hours if refrigerated.
- Urine glucose determinations may be false-positive with copper sulfate tests (Clinitest); glucose enzymatic tests (Diastix or Chemstrip uG) aren't affected.

ALERT Don't confuse with other cephalosporins with similar sounding names.

Patient teaching

- Tell patient to report adverse reactions.
- Alert patient to signs of superinfection. Careful observation by patient is essential.

Evaluation

- Patient is free from infection.
- Patient maintains adequate hydration.
- Patient and family state understanding of drug therapy.

cefoxitin sodium

(sef-OKS-ih-tin SOH-dee-um)
Mefoxin

Pharmacologic class: second-generation cephalosporin
Therapeutic class: antibiotic
Pregnancy risk category: B

Indications and dosages

▶ **Serious infections of respiratory and GU tracts; skin, soft-tissue, bone, and joint infections; bloodstream and intra-abdominal infections caused by susceptible *Escherichia coli* and other coliform bacte-**

ria, *Staphylococcus aureus* (penicillinase- and non-penicillinase–producing), *S. epidermidis*, streptococci, *Klebsiella, Haemophilus influenzae*, and *Bacteroides*, including *B. fragilis;* and perioperative prophylaxis.
Adults: 1 to 2 g I.V. q 6 to 8 hours for uncomplicated forms of infection. In life-threatening infections, up to 12 g daily.
Children over age 3 months: 80 to 160 mg/kg I.V. or I.M. daily given in four to six equally divided doses. Maximum daily dose is 12 g.
▶ **Prophylactic use in surgery.** *Adults:* 2 g I.V. 30 to 60 minutes before surgery; then 2 g I.M. or I.V. q 6 hours for 24 hours.
Children age 3 months and older: 30 to 40 mg/kg I.M. or I.V. 30 to 60 minutes before surgery; then 30 mg/kg q 6 hours for 24 hours.

How supplied

Injection: 1 g, 2 g
Infusion: 1 g, 2 g in 50-ml or 100-ml container

Pharmacokinetics

Absorption: unknown after I.M. administration.
Distribution: distributed widely into most body tissues and fluids; CSF penetration is poor; 50% to 80% protein-bound.
Metabolism: insignificant (about 2%).
Excretion: excreted primarily in urine. *Half-life:* about 0.5 to 1 hours.

Route	Onset	Peak	Duration
I.V.	Immediate	Immediate	Unknown

Pharmacodynamics

Chemical effect: inhibits cell-wall synthesis, promoting osmotic instability; usually bactericidal.
Therapeutic effect: hinders or kills susceptible bacteria: many gram-positive organisms and enteric gram-negative bacilli, such as *E. coli* and other coliform bacteria, streptococci, *S. aureus, S. epidermidis, Klebsiella, H. influenzae,* and *Bacteroides* species.

Adverse reactions

CNS: headache, malaise, paresthesia, dizziness.
GI: pseudomembranous colitis, nausea, anorexia, vomiting, *diarrhea,* glossitis, dyspepsia, abdominal cramps, tenesmus, anal pruritus, oral candidiasis.
GU: genital pruritus and candidiasis, ***acute renal failure.***
Hematologic: transient neutropenia, eosinophilia, ***hemolytic anemia, thrombocytopenia.***
Hepatic: transient increases in liver enzyme levels.
Respiratory: dyspnea.
Skin: *maculopapular and erythematous rashes, urticaria.*
Other: hypersensitivity reactions (serum sickness, ***anaphylaxis***), elevated temperature, *phlebitis, thrombophlebitis* (with I.V. injection).

Interactions

Drug-drug. *Nephrotoxic drugs:* possible increased risk of nephrotoxicity. Monitor renal function closely.
Probenecid: may inhibit excretion and increase blood levels of cefoxitin. Sometimes used for this effect.

Contraindications and precautions

- Contraindicated in patients hypersensitive to drug or other cephalosporins.
- Use cautiously in pregnant patients, breast-feeding patients, patients with history of sensitivity to penicillin, and patients with renal failure (may need dosage adjustment).

NURSING CONSIDERATIONS

Assessment

- Assess patient's infection before therapy and regularly thereafter.
- Obtain specimen for culture and sensitivity tests before first dose. Therapy may begin pending test results.
- Ask patient about previous reactions to cephalosporins or penicillin before administering first dose.
- Be alert for adverse reactions and drug interactions.
- Assess I.V. site frequently for thrombophlebitis.
- Monitor patient's hydration status if adverse GI reactions occur.
- Evaluate patient's and family's knowledge of drug therapy.

Nursing diagnoses
- Infection related to bacteria susceptible to drug
- Risk for deficient fluid volume related to drug-induced adverse GI reactions
- Deficient knowledge related to drug therapy

Planning and implementation
- Reconstitute 1 g with at least 10 ml of sterile water for injection and 2 g with 10 to 20 ml of sterile water for injection. Solutions of D_5W and normal saline solution for injection can also be used.
- For direct injection, inject drug into large vein or into tubing of free-flowing I.V. solution over 3 to 5 minutes.
- For intermittent infusion, add reconstituted drug to 50 or 100 ml of dextrose 5% or 10% in water or normal saline solution for injection. Interrupt flow of primary I.V. solution during infusion.
- After reconstitution, drug may be stored for 24 hours at room temperature or refrigerated for 1 week.
- Urine glucose determinations may be false-positive with copper sulfate tests (Clinitest); glucose enzymatic tests (Diastix or Chemstrip uG) aren't affected.
- Patients with renal dysfunction require dosage adjustment.

ALERT Don't confuse with other cephalosporins with similar sounding names.

Patient teaching
- Tell patient to report adverse reactions and signs and symptoms of superinfection promptly.
- Instruct patient to notify prescriber if he experiences loose stools or diarrhea.

Evaluation
- Patient is free from infection.
- Patient maintains adequate hydration.
- Patient and family state understanding of drug therapy.

cefpodoxime proxetil
(sef-poh-DOKS-eem PROKS-eh-til)
Vantin

Pharmacologic class: third-generation cephalosporin
Therapeutic class: antibiotic
Pregnancy risk category: B

Indications and dosages
▶ **Acute, community-acquired pneumonia caused by non-beta-lactamase–producing strains of *Haemophilus influenzae* or *Streptococcus pneumoniae*.** *Adults and children age 12 and older:* 200 mg P.O. q 12 hours for 14 days.

▶ **Acute bacterial exacerbation of chronic bronchitis caused by *S. pneumoniae, H. influenzae* (non-beta-lactamase–producing strains), or *Moraxella catarrhalis*.** *Adults and children age 12 and older:* 200 mg P.O. q 12 hours for 10 days.

▶ **Uncomplicated gonorrhea in men and women; rectal gonococcal infections in women.** *Adults and children age 12 and older:* 200 mg P.O. as single dose. Follow with doxycycline 100 mg P.O. b.i.d. for 7 days.

▶ **Uncomplicated skin and skin-structure infections caused by *S. aureus or S. pyogenes*.** *Adults and children age 12 and older:* 400 mg P.O. q 12 hours for 7 to 14 days.

▶ **Acute otitis media caused by *S. pneumoniae, H. influenzae,* or *M. catarrhalis*.** *Children age 6 months and over:* 5 mg/kg (not to exceed 200 mg) P.O. q 12 hours or 10 mg/kg (not to exceed 400 mg) P.O. daily for 10 days.

▶ **Pharyngitis or tonsillitis caused by *S. pyogenes*.** *Adults and children age 12 and older:* 100 mg P.O. q 12 hours for 5 to 10 days. *Children ages 2 months to 12 years:* 5 mg/kg (not to exceed 100 mg) P.O. q 12 hours for 10 days.

▶ **Uncomplicated urinary tract infections caused by *E. coli, Klebsiella pneumoniae, Proteus mirabilis,* or *S. saprophyticus*.** *Adults:* 100 mg P.O. q 12 hours for 7 days.

▶ **Mild to moderate acute maxillary sinusitis caused by *H. influenzae, S. pneumoniae,* or *M. catarrhalis*.** *Adults and children age 12*

and older: 200 mg P.O. every 12 hours for 10 days.
Children ages 2 months to 11 years: 5 mg/kg P.O. every 12 hours for 10 days; maximum dosage is 200 mg/dose.
Patients with renal failure: if creatinine clearance is below 30 ml/minute, dosage interval should be increased to q 24 hours. Patients receiving dialysis should get drug three times weekly, after dialysis.

How supplied

Tablets (film-coated): 100 mg, 200 mg
Oral suspension: 50 mg/5 ml, 100 mg/5 ml in 100-ml bottles

Pharmacokinetics

Absorption: absorbed from GI tract.
Distribution: distributed widely into most body tissues and fluids except CSF; 22% to 33% protein-bound in serum and 21% to 29% protein-bound in plasma.
Metabolism: drug is de-esterified to its active metabolite, cefpodoxime.
Excretion: excreted primarily in urine. *Half-life:* 2.1 to 2.8 hours.

Route	Onset	Peak	Duration
P.O.	Unknown	2-3 hr	Unknown

Pharmacodynamics

Chemical effect: inhibits cell-wall synthesis, promoting osmotic instability; usually bactericidal.
Therapeutic effect: hinders or kills susceptible bacteria: many gram-positive aerobes, such as *S. aureus, S. saprophyticus, S. pneumoniae,* and *S. pyogenes;* and gram-negative aerobes, including *K. pneumoniae, E. coli, P. mirabilis, M. catarrhalis, H. influenzae,* and *N. gonorrhoeae.*

Adverse reactions

CNS: headache.
GI: *diarrhea,* nausea, vomiting, abdominal pain.
GU: vaginal fungal infections.
Skin: rash.
Other: hypersensitivity reactions (***anaphylaxis***).

Interactions

Drug-drug. *Antacids, H_2-receptor antagonists:* decreased absorption of cefpodoxime. Avoid concomitant use.
Probenecid: decreased excretion of cefpodoxime. Monitor patient for toxicity.
Drug-food. *Any food:* increases drug absorption. Give drug with food.

Contraindications and precautions

- Contraindicated in patients hypersensitive to drug or other cephalosporins.
- Use cautiously in pregnant patients, breast-feeding patients, patients with history of hypersensitivity to penicillin (risk of cross-sensitivity), and patients receiving nephrotoxic drugs (other cephalosporins have had nephrotoxic potential).

NURSING CONSIDERATIONS

Assessment

- Assess patient's infection before therapy and regularly thereafter.
- Obtain specimen for culture and sensitivity tests before first dose. Therapy may begin pending test results.
- Ask patient about previous reactions to cephalosporins or penicillin before administering first dose.
- Be alert for adverse reactions and drug interactions.
- Monitor patient's hydration status if adverse GI reactions occur.
- Evaluate patient's and family's knowledge of drug therapy.

Nursing diagnoses

- Infection related to bacteria susceptible to drug
- Risk for deficient fluid volume related to drug-induced adverse GI reactions
- Deficient knowledge related to drug therapy

Planning and implementation

- Administer drug with food to minimize adverse GI reactions. Shake well before using.
- Store suspension in refrigerator (36° to 46° F [2° to 8° C]). Discard unused portion after 14 days.

• Urine glucose determinations may be false-positive with copper sulfate tests (Clinitest); glucose enzymatic tests (Diastix or Chemstrip uG) aren't affected.
ALERT Don't confuse with other cephalosporins with similar sounding names.

Patient teaching
• Advise patient to take drug with meals to minimize adverse GI reactions.
• Tell patient to take drug exactly as prescribed, even after he feels better.
• Instruct patient to notify prescriber if rash develops.
• Teach patient how to store drug.
• Instruct patient to notify prescriber about a reduction in urinary output, especially if patient takes a diuretic.

Evaluation
• Patient is free from infection.
• Patient maintains adequate hydration.
• Patient and family state understanding of drug therapy.

cefprozil
(SEF-pruh-zil)
Cefzil

Pharmacologic class: second-generation cephalosporin
Therapeutic class: antibiotic
Pregnancy risk category: B

Indications and dosages
▶ **Pharyngitis or tonsillitis caused by *Streptococcus pyogenes*.** *Adults and children age 13 and older:* 500 mg P.O. daily for 10 days.
▶ **Otitis media caused by *Streptococcus pneumoniae, Haemophilus influenzae,* or *Moraxella catarrhalis*.** *Infants and children age 6 months to 12 years:* 15 mg/kg P.O. q 12 hours for 10 days.
▶ **Secondary bacterial infections of acute bronchitis and acute bacterial exacerbation of chronic bronchitis caused by *S. pneumoniae, H. influenzae,* and *M. catarrhalis*.** *Adults and children age 13 and older:* 500 mg P.O. q 12 hours for 10 days.
▶ **Uncomplicated skin and skin-structure infections caused by *Staphylococcus aureus* or *S. pyogenes*.** *Adults and children age 13 and older:* 250 mg P.O. b.i.d., or 500 mg daily to b.i.d. for 10 days.

How supplied
Tablets: 250 mg, 500 mg
Oral suspension: 125 mg/5 ml, 250 mg/5 ml

Pharmacokinetics
Absorption: about 95% absorbed from GI tract.
Distribution: about 35% protein-bound; distributed into various body tissues and fluids.
Metabolism: probably metabolized by the liver.
Excretion: excreted primarily in urine. *Half-life:* 1.3 hours in patients with normal renal function; 2 hours in patients with impaired hepatic function; and 5.2 to 5.9 hours in patients with end-stage renal disease.

Route	Onset	Peak	Duration
P.O.	Unknown	Unknown	Unknown

Pharmacodynamics
Chemical effect: inhibits cell-wall synthesis, promoting osmotic instability; usually bactericidal.
Therapeutic effect: hinders or kills susceptible bacteria: *S. aureus, S. pyogenes, S. pneumoniae, M. catarrhalis,* and *H. influenzae.*

Adverse reactions
CNS: dizziness, hyperactivity, headache, nervousness, insomnia.
GI: *diarrhea, nausea,* vomiting, abdominal pain.
GU: elevated BUN level, elevated serum creatinine level, genital pruritus, vaginitis.
Hematologic: decreased leukocyte count, eosinophilia.
Hepatic: elevated liver enzyme levels.
Skin: rash, urticaria.
Other: superinfection, hypersensitivity reactions (serum sickness, ***anaphylaxis***).

Interactions
Drug-drug. *Aminoglycosides:* increased risk of nephrotoxicity. Monitor patient closely.

Probenecid: may inhibit excretion and increase blood levels of cefprozil. Monitor patient.

Contraindications and precautions

- Contraindicated in patients hypersensitive to drug or other cephalosporins.
- Use cautiously in pregnant patients, breast-feeding patients, patients with history of sensitivity to penicillin, and patients with impaired hepatic or renal function.

NURSING CONSIDERATIONS

Assessment

- Assess patient's infection before therapy and regularly thereafter.
- Obtain specimen for culture and sensitivity tests before first dose. Therapy may begin pending test results.
- Ask patient about previous reactions to cephalosporins or penicillin before giving first dose.
- Be alert for adverse reactions and drug interactions.
- Monitor patient's hydration status if adverse GI reactions occur.
- Evaluate patient's and family's knowledge of drug therapy.
- Monitor patient's renal function.

Nursing diagnoses

- Infection related to bacteria susceptible to drug
- Risk for deficient fluid volume related to drug-induced adverse GI reactions
- Deficient knowledge related to drug therapy

Planning and implementation

- Patients with creatinine clearance less than 30 ml/minute should receive 50% of usual dose.
- Administer drug after hemodialysis treatment is completed; drug is removed by hemodialysis.
- Refrigerate reconstituted suspension (stable for 14 days). Keep tightly closed and shake well before using.
- Urine glucose determinations may be false-positive with copper sulfate tests (Clinitest); glucose enzymatic tests (Diastix or Chemstrip uG) aren't affected.

ALERT Don't confuse with other cephalosporins with similar sounding names.

Patient teaching

- Tell patient to shake suspension well before measuring dose.
- Advise patient to take drug as prescribed, even after he feels better.
- Inform patient that oral suspensions contain drug in bubble-gum flavor to improve palatability and promote compliance in children. Tell him to refrigerate reconstituted suspension and to discard unused portion after 14 days.
- Advise elderly patients receiving concurrent diuretic therapy to notify prescriber of decreased urine output.

Evaluation

- Patient is free from infection.
- Patient maintains adequate hydration.
- Patient and family state understanding of drug therapy.

ceftazidime

(sef-TAZ-ih-deem)

Ceptaz, Fortaz, Tazicef, Tazidime

Pharmacologic class: third-generation cephalosporin
Therapeutic class: antibiotic
Pregnancy risk category: B

Indications and dosages

▶ **Serious infections of lower respiratory and urinary tracts; gynecologic, intra-abdominal, CNS, and skin infections; bacteremia; and septicemia. Among susceptible microorganisms are streptococci, including *Streptococcus pneumoniae* and *S. pyogenes, Staphylococcus aureus, Escherichia coli, Klebsiella, Proteus, Enterobacter, Haemophilus influenzae, Pseudomonas,* and some strains of *Bacteroides*.** *Adults and children age 12 and older:* 1 g I.V. or I.M. q 8 to 12 hours; maximum 6 g daily for life-threatening infections.

Children age 1 month to 12 years: 30 to 50 mg/kg I.V. q 8 hours. Maximum 6 g daily.
Neonates up to 4 weeks: 30 mg/kg I.V. q 12 hours.
▶ **Uncomplicated urinary tract infections.**
Adults: 250 mg I.V. or I.M. q 12 hours.
▶ **Complicated urinary tract infections.**
Adults: 500 mg I.V. or I.M. q 8 to 12 hours.

How supplied

Injection (with sodium carbonate): 500 mg, 1 g, 2 g
Injection (with arginine): 1 g, 2 g, 6 g
Infusion: 1 g, 2 g in 50-ml and 100-ml vials (premixed)

Pharmacokinetics

Absorption: unknown after I.M. administration.
Distribution: distributed widely into most body tissues and fluids, including CSF (unlike most other cephalosporins); 5% to 24% protein-bound.
Metabolism: none.
Excretion: excreted primarily in urine. *Half-life:* about 1.5 to 2 hours.

Route	Onset	Peak	Duration
I.V.	Immediate	Immediate	Unknown
I.M.	Unknown	≤ 1 hr	Unknown

Pharmacodynamics

Chemical effect: inhibits cell-wall synthesis, promoting osmotic instability; usually bactericidal.
Therapeutic effect: hinders or kills susceptible bacteria: some gram-positive organisms and many enteric gram-negative bacilli, as well as streptococci *(S. pneumoniae* and *S. pyogenes); S. aureus; E. coli; Klebsiella* species; *Proteus* species; *Enterobacter* species; *H. influenzae; Pseudomonas* species; and some strains of *Bacteroides.*

Adverse reactions

CNS: headache, dizziness, ***seizures.***
GI: pseudomembranous colitis, nausea, vomiting, diarrhea, dysgeusia, abdominal cramps.
GU: genital pruritus, candidiasis.
Hematologic: eosinophilia, thrombocytosis, leukopenia, ***agranulocytosis.***
Hepatic: transient elevation in liver enzyme levels.
Respiratory: dyspnea.
Skin: *maculopapular and erythematous rashes, urticaria.*
Other: hypersensitivity reactions (serum sickness, ***anaphylaxis***); elevated temperature; *pain, induration, sterile abscesses, tissue sloughing* at injection site; *phlebitis, thrombophlebitis* with I.V. injection.

Interactions

Drug-drug. *Chloramphenicol:* antagonistic effect. Avoid concomitant use.

Contraindications and precautions

- Contraindicated in patients hypersensitive to drug or other cephalosporins.
- Use cautiously in pregnant patients, breast-feeding patients, patients with history of sensitivity to penicillin, and patients with renal failure (dosage adjustment may be needed).

ALERT Commercially available preparations contain either sodium carbonate (Fortaz, Tazicef, Tazidime) or arginine (Ceptaz) to facilitate dissolution of drug. Safety and efficacy of arginine-containing solutions in children age 12 and younger haven't been established.

NURSING CONSIDERATIONS

Assessment

- Assess patient's infection before therapy and regularly thereafter.
- Obtain specimen for culture and sensitivity tests before first dose. Therapy may begin pending test results.
- Ask patient about previous reactions to cephalosporins or penicillin before administering first dose.
- Be alert for adverse reactions and drug interactions.
- Monitor patient's hydration status if adverse GI reactions occur.
- Evaluate patient's and family's knowledge of drug therapy.

Nursing diagnoses

- Infection related to bacteria susceptible to drug

• Risk for deficient fluid volume related to drug-induced adverse GI reactions
• Deficient knowledge related to drug therapy

Planning and implementation

I.V. use: Reconstitute sodium carbonate-containing solutions with sterile water for injection. Add 5 ml to 500-mg vial; 10 ml to 1-g or 2-g vial. Shake well to dissolve drug. Carbon dioxide is released during dissolution, and positive pressure will develop in vial. Reconstitute arginine-containing solutions with 10 ml of sterile water for injection; this formulation won't release gas bubbles. Each brand of ceftazidime includes specific instructions for reconstitution. Read and follow these instructions carefully.
I.M. use: Inject deeply into large muscle mass, such as gluteus maximus or lateral aspect of thigh.
• Ceftazidime is removed by hemodialysis; supplemental dose of drug is indicated after each dialysis period, as directed.
• Urine glucose determinations may be false-positive with copper sulfate tests (Clinitest); glucose enzymatic tests (Diastix or Chemstrip uG) aren't affected.
ALERT Don't confuse with other cephalosporins with similar sounding names.

Patient teaching

• Tell patient to report adverse reactions.
• Instruct patient to report any change in urinary output to prescriber immediately. Dosage may need to be decreased to compensate for decreased excretion.

Evaluation

• Patient is free from infection.
• Patient maintains adequate hydration.
• Patient and family state understanding of drug therapy.

ceftibuten

(sef-tih-BYOO-tin)
Cedax

Pharmacologic class: third-generation cephalosporin
Therapeutic class: antibiotic
Pregnancy risk category: B

Indications and dosages

▶ **Acute bacterial exacerbation of chronic bronchitis caused by *Haemophilus influenzae, Moraxella catarrhalis,* or penicillin-susceptible strains of *Streptococcus pneumoniae*.** *Adults and children age 12 and over:* 400 mg P.O. daily for 10 days.
▶ **Pharyngitis and tonsillitis caused by *Streptococcus pyogenes,* acute bacterial otitis media caused by *H. influenzae, M. catarrhalis*, or *S. pyogenes*.** *Adults and children age 12 and over:* 400 mg P.O. daily for 10 days.
Children under age 12: 9 mg/kg P.O. daily for 10 days.
Children weighing over 45 kg (99 lb): 400 mg P.O. daily for 10 days.
Patients with renal impairment: if creatinine clearance is 30 to 49 ml/minute, 4.5 mg/kg or 200 mg P.O. q 24 hours; if it's 5 to 29 ml/minute, 2.25 mg/kg or 100 mg P.O. q 24 hours.

How supplied

Capsules: 400 mg
Oral suspension: 90 mg/5 ml, 180 mg/5 ml

Pharmacokinetics

Absorption: rapidly absorbed.
Distribution: 65% bound to plasma proteins.
Metabolism: by kidneys.
Excretion: mainly in urine.

Route	Onset	Peak	Duration
P.O.	Unknown	2-4 hr	Unknown

Pharmacodynamics

Chemical effect: exerts its bacterial action by binding to essential target proteins of the bacterial cell wall, thus inhibiting cell-wall synthesis.
Therapeutic effect: hinders or kills susceptible bacteria.

Adverse reactions

CNS: headache, dizziness, aphasia, psychosis.

GI: nausea, vomiting, diarrhea, dyspepsia, abdominal pain, loose stools, pseudomembranous colitis.
GU: elevated BUN levels, toxic nephropathy, renal dysfunction.
Hematologic: elevated eosinophil levels, decreased hemoglobin levels, altered platelet count, aplastic anemia, hemolytic anemia, ***hemorrhage, neutropenia, agranulocytosis, pancytopenia.***
Hepatic: hepatic cholestasis, elevated liver enzyme and bilirubin levels.
Skin: ***Stevens-Johnson syndrome.***
Other: allergic reaction, ***anaphylaxis,*** drug fever.

Interactions

Drug-food. *Any food:* decreases bioavailability of drug. Administer drug 2 hours before or 1 hour after a meal.

Contraindications and precautions

- Contraindicated in patients hypersensitive to cephalosporins.
- Use cautiously in elderly patients, patients with history of hypersensitivity to penicillin, and patients with GI disease or impaired renal function.

NURSING CONSIDERATIONS

Assessment

- Obtain specimen for culture and sensitivity tests before starting drug.
- Evaluate patient's and family's knowledge of drug therapy.
- Monitor patient for superinfection.
- Monitor elderly patient's renal function. Dosage may need to be adjusted.
- Obtain specimen for *Clostridium difficile,* as ordered, in patient who develops diarrhea after therapy.

Nursing diagnoses

- Infection related to bacteria susceptible to drug
- Deficient knowledge related to drug therapy

Planning and implementation

- To prepare oral suspension, tap bottle to loosen powder. Follow chart supplied by manufacturer for mixing instructions. Suspension is stable for 14 days if refrigerated.
- Shake suspension well before use.
- Stop drug and notify prescriber if allergic reaction occurs.

ALERT Don't confuse with other cephalosporins with similar sounding names.

Patient teaching

- Instruct patient to take drug as prescribed, even if he feels better.
- Instruct patient using oral suspension to shake bottle before use and to take it at least 2 hours before or 1 hour after a meal.
- Instruct patient to store oral suspension in the refrigerator, with lid tightly closed, and to discard unused drug after 14 days.
- Warn breast-feeding patient that it's unclear if drug appears in breast milk.
- Tell diabetic patient that suspension has 1 g sucrose per teaspoon.

Evaluation

- Patient is free from infection.
- Patient and family state understanding of drug therapy.

ceftizoxime sodium

(sef-tih-ZOKS-eem SOH-dee-um)
Cefizox

Pharmacologic class: third-generation cephalosporin
Therapeutic class: antibiotic
Pregnancy risk category: B

Indications and dosages

▶ **Serious infections of lower respiratory and urinary tracts, gynecologic infections, bacteremia, septicemia, meningitis, intra-abdominal infections, bone and joint infections, and skin infections. Among susceptible microorganisms are streptococci, including *Streptococcus pneumoniae* and *S. pyogenes, Staphylococcus aureus* (penicillinase- and non-penicillinase–producing), and *S. epidermidis, Escherichia coli, Klebsiella, Haemophilus influenzae, Enterobacter, Proteus,* some *Pseudomonas,* and *Peptostrepto-***

coccus. Adults: 1 g to 2 g I.V. or I.M. q 8 to 12 hours. In life-threatening infections, 3 to 4 g I.V. q 8 hours.
Children over age 6 months: 50 mg/kg I.V. q 6 to 8 hours. For serious infections, up to 200 mg/kg/day in divided doses may be used, maximum 12 g/day.
▶ **Acute bacterial otitis media.** *Children:* 50 mg/kg (not to exceed 1 gram) I.M. as a single dose.

How supplied

Injection: 500 mg, 1 g, 2 g
Infusion: 1 g, 2 g in 100-mg vials or in 50 ml of D_5W

Pharmacokinetics

Absorption: unknown after I.M. administration.
Distribution: distributed widely into most body tissues and fluids; unlike many other cephalosporins, ceftizoxime has good CSF penetration and achieves adequate concentration in inflamed meninges. Drug is 28% to 31% protein-bound.
Metabolism: none.
Excretion: excreted primarily in urine. *Half-life:* about 1.5 to 2 hours.

Route	Onset	Peak	Duration
I.V.	Immediate	Immediate	Unknown
I.M.	Unknown	0.5-1.5 hr	Unknown

Pharmacodynamics

Chemical effect: inhibits cell-wall synthesis, promoting osmotic instability; usually bactericidal.
Therapeutic effect: hinders or kills susceptible bacteria: some gram-positive organisms and many enteric gram-negative bacilli, as well as streptococci (*S. pneumoniae* and *S. pyogenes*); *S. aureus; E. coli; Klebsiella* species; *Proteus* species; *Enterobacter* species; *H. influenzae; Pseudomonas* species; and some strains of *Bacteroides*.

Adverse reactions

CNS: headache, malaise, paresthesia, dizziness.
GI: pseudomembranous colitis, nausea, anorexia, vomiting, *diarrhea,* glossitis, dyspepsia, abdominal cramps, tenesmus, anal pruritus.
GU: genital pruritus and candidiasis.
Hematologic: ***transient neutropenia,*** eosinophilia, hemolytic anemia, ***thrombocytopenia.***
Respiratory: dyspnea.
Skin: *maculopapular and erythematous rashes, urticaria.*
Other: hypersensitivity reactions (serum sickness, ***anaphylaxis***); fever; *pain, induration, sterile abscesses, tissue sloughing* at injection site; *phlebitis, thrombophlebitis* with I.V. injection.

Interactions

Drug-drug. *Probenecid:* may inhibit excretion and increase blood levels of ceftizoxime. Sometimes used for this effect.

Contraindications and precautions

- Contraindicated in patients hypersensitive to drug or other cephalosporins.
- Use cautiously in pregnant patients, breast-feeding patients, patients with history of sensitivity to penicillin, and patients with renal failure (may need dosage adjustment).
- Safety of drug hasn't been established in infants under age 6 months.

NURSING CONSIDERATIONS

Assessment

- Assess patient's infection before therapy and regularly thereafter.
- Obtain specimen for culture and sensitivity tests before giving first dose. Therapy may begin pending test results.
- Ask patient about previous reactions to cephalosporins or penicillin before giving first dose.
- Be alert for adverse reactions and drug interactions.
- Monitor patient's hydration status if adverse GI reactions occur.
- Evaluate patient's and family's knowledge of drug therapy.

Nursing diagnoses

- Infection related to bacteria susceptible to drug

- Risk for deficient fluid volume related to drug-induced adverse GI reactions
- Deficient knowledge related to drug therapy

Planning and implementation

I.V. use: To reconstitute powder, add 5 ml of sterile water to 500-mg vial, 10 ml to 1-g vial, or 20 ml to 2-g vial. Reconstitute piggyback vials with 50 to 100 ml of normal saline solution or D_5W. Shake vial well.
I.M. use: Inject deeply into large muscle mass, such as gluteus maximus or lateral aspect of thigh. Larger doses (2 g) should be divided and administered at two separate sites.
- Urine glucose determinations may be false-positive with copper sulfate tests (Clinitest); glucose enzymatic tests (Diastix or Chemstrip uG) aren't affected.

ALERT Don't confuse with other cephalosporins with similar sounding names.

Patient teaching

- Tell patient to report adverse reactions and signs and symptoms of superinfection promptly.
- Instruct patient to report discomfort at the I.V. site.
- Tell patient to notify prescriber if loose stools or diarrhea occur.

Evaluation

- Patient is free from infection.
- Patient maintains adequate hydration.
- Patient and family state understanding of drug therapy.

ceftriaxone sodium
(sef-trigh-AKS-ohn SOH-dee-um)
Rocephin

Pharmacologic class: third-generation cephalosporin
Therapeutic class: antibiotic
Pregnancy risk category: B

Indications and dosages

▶ **Uncomplicated gonococcal vulvovaginitis.** *Adults:* 125 to 250 mg I.M. as single dose, followed by 100 mg of doxycycline P.O. q 12 hours for 7 days.

▶ **Serious infections of lower respiratory and urinary tracts; gynecologic, bone, joint, intra-abdominal, and skin infections; Lyme disease; bacteremia; and septicemia caused by such susceptible microorganisms as streptococci (including *Streptococcus pneumoniae* and *S. pyogenes*), *Staphylococcus aureus*, *S. epidermidis*, *Escherichia coli*, *Klebsiella*, *Haemophilus influenzae*, *Neisseria meningitides*, *N. gonorrhoeae*, *Enterobacter*, *Proteus*, *Pseudomonas*, *Peptostreptococcus*, and *Serratia marcescens*.** *Adults and children over age 12:* 1 to 2 g I.V. or I.M. daily or in equally divided doses, maximum 4 g. *Children age 12 and under:* 50 to 75 mg/kg, maximum 2 g/day, given in divided doses q 12 hours.

▶ **Meningitis**. *Adults and children:* initially, 100 mg/kg I.M. or I.V. (maximum 4 g); thereafter, 100 mg/kg I.M. or I.V. given once daily or in divided doses q 12 hours. Maximum 4 g , for 7 to 14 days.

▶ **Preoperative prophylaxis.** *Adults:* 1 g I.V. as single dose 30 minutes to 2 hours before surgery.

▶ **Acute bacterial otitis media**. *Children:* 50 mg/kg I.M. as a single dose, maximum 1 g I.M./dose.

How supplied

Injection: 250 mg, 500 mg, 1 g, 2 g
Infusion: 1 g, 2 g

Pharmacokinetics

Absorption: unknown after I.M. administration.
Distribution: distributed widely into most body tissues and fluids; unlike many other cephalosporins, ceftriaxone has good CSF penetration. Drug is 58% to 96% protein-bound.
Metabolism: partially metabolized.
Excretion: excreted primarily in urine, minimally in bile. *Half-life:* about 5.5 to 11 hours.

Route	Onset	Peak	Duration
I.V.	Immediate	Immediate	Unknown
I.M.	Unknown	1.5-4 hr	Unknown

Pharmacodynamics

Chemical effect: inhibits cell-wall synthesis, promoting osmotic instability; usually bactericidal.

Therapeutic effect: hinders or kills susceptible bacteria: some gram-positive organisms and many enteric gram-negative bacilli, as well as streptococci, *S. epidermidis, E. coli, Klebsiella* species, *Proteus* species, *Enterobacter* species, *H. influenzae,* some strains of *Pseudomonas* species, *Peptostreptococcus* species, and spirochetes such as *Borrelia burgdorferi*.

Adverse reactions

CNS: headache, dizziness.
GI: pseudomembranous colitis, nausea, vomiting, diarrhea, dysgeusia.
GU: genital pruritus and candidiasis.
Hematologic: eosinophilia, thrombocytosis, leukopenia.
Skin: pain, induration, and tenderness at injection site; phlebitis; *rash.*
Other: hypersensitivity reactions (serum sickness, ***anaphylaxis***), fever.

Interactions

Drug-drug. *Probenecid:* high doses may shorten half-life of ceftriaxone. Avoid concomitant use.
Aminoglycosides: concurrent use has additive effect. Monitor drug levels and adjust dosage as required.
Quinolones: synergistic effect against *S. pneumoniae.* Concurrent use recommended against this organism.
Drug-lifestyle. *Alcohol use:* a disulfiram-like reaction can occur. Discourage concomitant use.

Contraindications and precautions

- Contraindicated in patients hypersensitive to drug or other cephalosporins.
- Use cautiously in pregnant patients, breast-feeding patients, and patients with history of sensitivity to penicillin.

NURSING CONSIDERATIONS

Assessment

- Assess patient's infection before therapy and regularly thereafter.
- Obtain specimen for culture and sensitivity tests. Therapy may begin before test results are known.
- Ask patient about previous reactions to cephalosporins or penicillin before giving first dose.
- Be alert for adverse reactions and drug interactions.
- Monitor patient's hydration status if adverse GI reactions occur.
- Evaluate patient's and family's knowledge of drug therapy.

Nursing diagnoses

- Infection related to bacteria susceptible to drug
- Risk for deficient fluid volume related to drug-induced adverse GI reactions
- Deficient knowledge related to drug therapy

Planning and implementation

I.V. use: Reconstitute with sterile water for injection, normal saline solution for injection, D_5W or $D_{10}W$ injection, or combination of saline and dextrose injection and other compatible solutions. Reconstitute by adding 2.4 ml of diluent to 250-mg vial, 4.8 ml to 500-mg vial, 9.6 ml to 1-g vial, and 19.2 ml to 2-g vial. All reconstituted solutions yield concentration that averages 100 mg/ml. After reconstitution, dilute further for intermittent infusion to desired concentration. I.V. dilutions are stable for 24 hours at room temperature.
I.M. use: Inject deeply into large muscle mass, such as gluteus maximus or lateral aspect of thigh. May use lidocaine 1% without epinephrine to dilute for I.M. use if ordered by the prescriber.

- Urine glucose determinations may be false-positive with copper sulfate tests (Clinitest); glucose enzymatic tests (Diastix or Chemstrip uG) aren't affected.

ALERT Don't confuse with other cephalosporins with similar sounding names.

Patient teaching

- Tell patient to report adverse reactions and signs and symptoms of superinfection promptly.
- Instruct patient to report pain at the I.V. site.

• Tell patient to notify prescriber if loose stools or diarrhea occur.

Evaluation

• Patient is free from infection.
• Patient maintains adequate hydration.
• Patient and family state understanding of drug therapy.

cefuroxime axetil

(sef-yoor-OKS-eem AKS-eh-til)
Ceftin

cefuroxime sodium

Kefurox, Zinacef

Pharmacologic class: second-generation cephalosporin
Therapeutic class: antibiotic
Pregnancy risk category: B

Indications and dosages

▶ **Injectable form: Serious infections of lower respiratory and urinary tracts, skin and skin-structure infections, bone and joint infections, septicemia, meningitis, gonorrhea, and perioperative prophylaxis.**
Oral form: Otitis media, pharyngitis, tonsillitis, infections of urinary and lower respiratory tracts, and skin and skin-structure infections. Among susceptible organisms are *Streptococcus pneumoniae* and *S. pyogenes, Haemophilus influenzae, Klebsiella, Staphylococcus aureus, Escherichia coli, Enterobacter,* and *Neisseria gonorrhoeae*. *Adults and children age 12 and older:* 750 mg to 1.5 g I.V. or I.M. q 8 hours for 5 to 10 days. For life-threatening infections and infections caused by less susceptible organisms, 1.5 g I.V. or I.M. q 6 hours; for bacterial meningitis, up to 3 g I.V. q 8 hours. Alternatively, 250 mg cefuroxime axetil P.O. q 12 hours for 10 days. For severe infections, dosage may be increased to 500 mg q 12 hours.
Children and infants over age 3 months: 50 to 100 mg/kg/day cefuroxime sodium I.V. or I.M. in equally divided doses q 6 to 8 hours. Higher doses of 100 mg/kg/day (not to exceed adult maximum dosage) should be used for more severe or serious infections. For bacterial meningitis, 200 to 240 mg/kg I.V. in divided doses q 6 to 8 hours. For other infections, 125 to 250 mg or cefuroxime axetil P.O. q 12 hours for a child who can swallow pills.
▶ **Uncomplicated urinary tract infections.** *Adults:* 125 to 250 mg P.O. q 12 hours for 10 days.
▶ **Otitis media.** *Children age 3 months to 12 years:* 30 mg/kg/day oral suspension P.O. divided in two doses (maximum dose, 1 g), or 250-mg tablet P.O. b.i.d. for 10 days.
▶ **Perioperative prophylaxis.** *Adults:* 1.5 g I.V. 30 to 60 minutes before surgery; in lengthy operations, 750 mg I.V. or I.M. q 8 hours. For open-heart surgery, 1.5 g I.V. at induction of anesthesia and q 12 hours; total dosage 6 g.
▶ **Acute bacterial maxillary sinusitis caused by *S. pneumoniae* or *H. influenzae* in pediatric patients.** *Adults and children age 13 and older:* 250 mg (tablet) P.O. twice daily for 10 days.
Infants and children 3 months to 12 years: 30 mg/kg (suspension) by mouth daily in two divided doses for 10 days. Maximum daily suspension dose is 1,000 mg. For children who can swallow tablets whole, give 250 mg (tablet) by mouth twice daily for 10 days.

How supplied

cefuroxime axetil
Tablets: 125 mg, 250 mg, 500 mg
Suspension: 125 mg/5 ml, 250 mg/5 ml
cefuroxime sodium
Injection: 750 mg, 1.5 g
Infusion: 750 mg, 1.5 g premixed, frozen solution

Pharmacokinetics

Absorption: cefuroxime axetil is absorbed from GI tract with 37% to 52% of oral dose reaching systemic circulation. Food appears to enhance absorption. Cefuroxime sodium isn't well absorbed from GI tract; absorption from I.M. administration is unknown.
Distribution: distributed widely into most body tissues and fluids; CSF penetration is greater than that of most first- and second-generation cephalosporins and achieves ade-

quate therapeutic levels in inflamed meninges. It's 33% to 50% protein-bound.
Metabolism: none.
Excretion: excreted primarily in urine. *Half-life:* 1 to 2 hours.

Route	Onset	Peak	Duration
P.O.	Unknown	2 hr	Unknown
I.V.	Unknown	Immediate	Unknown
I.M.	Unknown	15-60 min	Unknown

Pharmacodynamics

Chemical effect: inhibits cell-wall synthesis, promoting osmotic instability; usually bactericidal.
Therapeutic effect: hinders or kills susceptible bacteria, including many gram-positive organisms and enteric gram-negative bacilli.

Adverse reactions

CNS: headache, malaise, paresthesia, dizziness.
GI: pseudomembranous colitis, nausea, anorexia, vomiting, *diarrhea,* glossitis, dyspepsia, abdominal cramps, tenesmus, anal pruritus.
GU: genital pruritus and candidiasis.
Hematologic: ***transient neutropenia,*** eosinophilia, ***hemolytic anemia***, decrease in hemoglobin level and hematocrit, ***thrombocytopenia.***
Hepatic: transient increases in liver enzyme levels.
Respiratory: dyspnea.
Skin: *maculopapular and erythematous rashes, urticaria.*
Other: hypersensitivity reactions (serum sickness, ***anaphylaxis***); *pain, induration, sterile abscesses, warmth, tissue sloughing* at injection site; *phlebitis, thrombophlebitis* with I.V. injection.

Interactions

Drug-drug. *Diuretics:* increased risk of adverse renal reactions. Monitor renal function closely.
Probenecid: may inhibit excretion and increase blood levels of cefuroxime. Sometimes used for this effect.
Drug-food. *Any food:* increased absorption. Give drug with food.

Contraindications and precautions

- Contraindicated in patients hypersensitive to drug or other cephalosporins.
- Use cautiously in pregnant patients, breast-feeding patients, patients with history of sensitivity to penicillin, and patients with impaired renal function (may need reduced dosage).
- Safety of drug hasn't been established in infants under age 3 months.

NURSING CONSIDERATIONS

Assessment

- Assess patient's infection before therapy and regularly thereafter.
- Obtain specimen for culture and sensitivity tests before first dose. Therapy may begin pending test results.
- Ask patient about previous reactions to cephalosporins or penicillin before giving first dose.
- Be alert for adverse reactions and drug interactions.
- Monitor patient's hydration status if adverse GI reactions occur.
- Evaluate patient's and family's knowledge of drug therapy.

Nursing diagnoses

- Infection related to bacteria susceptible to drug
- Risk for deficient fluid volume related to drug-induced adverse GI reactions
- Deficient knowledge related to drug therapy

Planning and implementation

P.O. use: Food enhances absorption of cefuroxime axetil.
- Cefuroxime axetil is available only in tablet form, which may be crushed for patients who can't swallow tablets. Tablets may be allowed to dissolve in small amounts of apple, orange, or grape juice or chocolate milk. However, drug has bitter taste that is difficult to mask, even with food.

ALERT Cefuroxime tablets and oral suspensions aren't bioequivalent and can't be substituted on a mg/mg basis.
I.V. use: For each 750-mg vial of Kefurox, reconstitute with 9 ml of sterile water for injection. Withdraw 8 ml from vial for proper dose. For each 1.5-g vial of Kefurox, reconstitute with 14 ml of sterile water for injection; withdraw entire contents of vial for dose. For each 750-mg vial of Zinacef, reconstitute with 8 ml of sterile water for injection; for each 1.5-g vial, reconstitute with 16 ml. In each case, withdraw entire contents of vial for dose.
- To give by direct injection, inject into large vein or into tubing of free-flowing I.V. solution over 3 to 5 minutes.
- For intermittent infusion, add reconstituted drug to 100 ml D_5W, normal saline solution for injection, or other compatible I.V. solution. Infuse over 15 to 60 minutes.

I.M. use: Inject deeply into large muscle mass, such as gluteus maximus or lateral aspect of thigh.
- Urine glucose determinations may be false-positive with copper sulfate tests (Clinitest); glucose enzymatic tests (Diastix or Chemstrip uG) aren't affected.

ALERT Don't confuse with other cephalosporins with similar sounding names.

Patient teaching
- Instruct patient to take drug exactly as prescribed, even after he feels better.
- Advise patient to take oral drug with food to enhance absorption. Explain that tablets may be crushed, but drug has bitter taste that is difficult to mask, even with food.
- Tell patient to report adverse reactions.

Evaluation
- Patient is free from infection.
- Patient maintains adequate hydration.
- Patient and family state understanding of drug therapy.

celecoxib
(sel-eh-COKS-ib)
Celebrex

Pharmacologic classification: cyclooxygenase-2 inhibitor
Therapeutic classification: anti-inflammatory
Pregnancy risk category: C

Indications, route, and dosages
▶ **Relief of signs and symptoms of osteoarthritis.** *Adults:* 200 mg P.O. daily as a single dose or divided equally b.i.d.
▶ **Relief of signs and symptoms of rheumatoid arthritis.** *Adults:* 100 to 200 mg P.O. b.i.d.
▶ **Adjunct to treatment for familial adenomatous polyposis to reduce the number of adenomatous colorectal polyps.** *Adults:* 400 mg P.O. b.i.d. with food for up to 6 months.

How supplied
Capsules: 100 mg, 200 mg

Pharmacokinetics
Absorption: following oral administration, plasma levels peak in about 3 hours. Steady-state plasma levels can be expected within 5 days if celecoxib is given in multiple dosages. Elderly patients have higher serum levels than younger adult patients.
Distribution: drug is highly protein-bound, primarily to albumin. It also has extensive distribution into the tissues.
Metabolism: in the liver, cytochrome P-450 2C9 metabolizes the drug. No active metabolites of celecoxib have been identified.
Excretion: drug is eliminated primarily through hepatic metabolism, with less than 3% as unchanged drug excreted in urine and feces. Elimination half-life is about 11 hours.

Route	Onset	Peak	Duration
P.O.	Unknown	3 hr	Unknown

Pharmacodynamics
Chemical use: Celecoxib is thought to selectively inhibit cyclooxygenase-2, resulting in decreased prostaglandin synthesis. Its anti-

inflammatory effects along with its analgesic and antipyretic properties are thought to be related to a decrease in prostaglandin synthesis.
Therapeutic use: relief of osteoarthritis and rheumatoid arthritis symptoms.

Adverse reactions

CNS: dizziness, *headache*, insomnia.
CV: peripheral edema.
EENT: pharyngitis, rhinitis, sinusitis.
GI: abdominal pain, diarrhea, dyspepsia, flatulence, nausea.
GU: elevated BUN level.
Hepatic: elevated liver enzyme levels.
Metabolic: hyperchloremia, hypophosphatemia.
Musculoskeletal: back pain.
Respiratory: upper respiratory tract infection.
Skin: rash.
Other: accidental injury.

Interactions

Drug-drug. *ACE inhibitors:* diminished antihypertensive effects. Monitor patient's blood pressure.
Aluminum- and magnesium-containing antacids: reduced celecoxib levels. Separate administration times.
Aspirin: increased risk of ulcers; low aspirin dosages can be used safely to prevent CV events. Monitor patient for signs and symptoms of GI bleeding.
Fluconazole: increased celecoxib levels. Reduce dosage of celecoxib to minimal effective level.
Furosemide: NSAIDs can reduce sodium excretion caused by diuretics, leading to sodium retention. Monitor patient for swelling and increased blood pressure.
Lithium: increased lithium level. Monitor plasma lithium levels closely during treatment.
Warfarin: increased PT and bleeding complications. Monitor PT and INR, and check for signs and symptoms of bleeding.
Drug-herb. *Dong quai, ginkgo, feverfew, garlic, ginger, horse chestnut, red clover*: may increase the risk of bleeding. Discourage concomitant use.
Drug-lifestyle. *Chronic alcohol use, smoking:* increased risk of GI irritation or bleeding. Check for signs and symptoms of bleeding, and discourage concurrent use.

Contraindications and precautions

- Contraindicated in patients hypersensitive to celecoxib, sulfonamides, aspirin, or other NSAIDs; patients with severe hepatic impairment; and patients in the third trimester of pregnancy.
- Use cautiously in patients with known or suspected history of poor P-450 2C9 metabolization and in patients with history of ulcers, GI bleeding, advanced renal disease, dehydration, anemia, symptomatic liver disease, hypertension, edema, heart failure, or asthma.
- Use cautiously in patients who smoke or drink alcohol frequently, in those who take oral corticosteroids or anticoagulants, and in elderly or debilitated patients because of the increased risk of GI bleeding.

NURSING CONSIDERATIONS

Assessment

- Assess patient for appropriateness of therapy. Drug must be used cautiously in patients with history of ulcers or GI bleeding, advanced renal disease, dehydration, anemia, symptomatic liver disease, hypertension, edema, heart failure, or asthma.
- Obtain accurate list of patient's allergies. Patients may be allergic to celecoxib if they're allergic and have had anaphylactic reactions to sulfonamides, aspirin, or other NSAIDs.
- Assess patients for risk factors for GI bleeding including treatment with corticosteroids or anticoagulants, longer duration of NSAID treatment, smoking, alcoholism, older age, and poor overall health. Patients with a history of ulcers or GI bleeding are at higher risk for GI bleeding while taking NSAIDs such as celecoxib.
- Monitor patient for signs and symptoms of overt and occult bleeding.
- Celecoxib may be hepatotoxic; monitor patient for signs and symptoms of liver toxicity.
- Evaluate patient's and family's knowledge of drug therapy.

Nursing diagnoses
- Acute pain related to underlying condition
- Risk for injury related to drug-induced adverse reactions
- Deficient knowledge related to drug therapy

Planning and implementation
- In patients weighing below 50 kg (110 lb), therapy should start at lowest recommended dosage. In patients with moderate hepatic impairment (Child-Pugh Class II), start therapy with reduced dosage.
- Although drug can be given without regard to meals, food may decrease GI upset.
- Before starting treatment with celecoxib, be sure to rehydrate patient.
- Although celecoxib may be used with low aspirin dosages, the combination may increase the risk of GI bleeding.
- NSAIDs such as celecoxib can cause fluid retention; closely monitor patient who has hypertension, edema, or heart failure while taking this drug.

Patient teaching
- Tell patient to report history of allergic reactions to sulfonamides, aspirin, or other NSAIDs before starting therapy.
- Instruct patient to report signs of GI bleeding—such as bloody vomitus, blood in urine or stool, and black, tarry stools—to prescriber immediately.

ALERT Advise patient to report skin rash, unexplained weight gain, or edema to prescriber immediately.
- Tell woman to notify prescriber if she becomes pregnant or is planning to become pregnant while taking this drug.
- Instruct patient to take drug with food if stomach upset occurs.
- Teach patient that all NSAIDs including celecoxib may adversely affect the liver. Signs and symptoms of liver toxicity include nausea, fatigue, lethargy, itching, jaundice, right upper quadrant tenderness, and flulike syndrome. Advise patient to stop therapy and seek immediate medical advice if he experiences any of these signs or symptoms.
- Inform patient that it may take several days before he feels consistent pain relief.

Evaluation
- Patient is free from pain.
- Patient doesn't experience injury as a result of drug-induced adverse reactions.
- Patient and family state understanding of drug therapy.

cephalexin hydrochloride
(sef-uh-LEK-sin high-droh-KLOR-ighd)

Keftab

cephalexin monohydrate
Apo-Cephalex♦, Cefanex, Keflex, Novo-Lexin♦, Nu-Cephalex◇

Pharmacologic class: first-generation cephalosporin
Therapeutic class: antibiotic
Pregnancy risk category: B

Indications and dosages
▶ **Respiratory tract, GI tract, skin, soft-tissue, bone, and joint infections and otitis media caused by *Escherichia coli* and other coliform bacteria, group A beta-hemolytic streptococci, *Haemophilus influenzae, Klebsiella, Moraxella catarrhalis, Proteus mirabilis, Streptococcus pneumoniae,* and staphylococci.** *Adults:* 250 mg to 1 g P.O. q 6 hours or 500 mg q 12 hours; maximum 4 g/day. *Children:* 6 to 12 mg/kg P.O. q 6 hours (monohydrate only); maximum 25 mg/kg q 6 hours.

How supplied
cephalexin hydrochloride
Tablets: 500 mg
cephalexin monohydrate
Tablets: 250 mg, 500 mg, 1 g
Capsules: 250 mg, 500 mg
Oral suspension: 125 mg/5 ml, 250 mg/5 ml

Pharmacokinetics
Absorption: absorbed rapidly and completely from GI tract. Food delays but doesn't prevent complete absorption.
Distribution: distributed widely into most body tissues and fluids; CSF penetration is poor. Drug is 6% to 15% protein-bound.

Metabolism: none.
Excretion: excreted primarily unchanged in urine. *Half-life:* about 30 minutes to 1 hour.

Route	Onset	Peak	Duration
P.O.	Unknown	≤ 1 hr	Unknown

Pharmacodynamics

Chemical effect: inhibits cell-wall synthesis, promoting osmotic instability; usually bactericidal.
Therapeutic effect: hinders or kills susceptible bacteria: many gram-positive cocci, including penicillinase-producing *S. aureus* and *S. epidermidis, S. pneumoniae,* group B streptococci, and group A beta-hemolytic streptococci; and gram-negative organisms, including *Klebsiella pneumoniae, E. coli, P. mirabilis,* and *Shigella.*

Adverse reactions

CNS: dizziness, headache, malaise, paresthesia.
GI: pseudomembranous colitis, *nausea, anorexia,* vomiting, *diarrhea,* glossitis, dyspepsia, abdominal cramps, anal pruritus, tenesmus, oral candidiasis.
GU: genital pruritus, candidiasis, vaginitis.
Hematologic: transient neutropenia, eosinophilia, anemia, ***thrombocytopenia.***
Hepatic: transient increases in liver enzyme levels.
Respiratory: dyspnea.
Skin: *maculopapular and erythematous rashes, urticaria.*
Other: hypersensitivity reactions (serum sickness, ***anaphylaxis***).

Interactions

Drug-drug. *Probenecid:* may increase blood levels of cephalosporins. Sometimes used for this effect.

Contraindications and precautions

- Contraindicated in patients hypersensitive to cephalosporins.
- Use cautiously in pregnant patients, breast-feeding patients, patients hypersensitive to penicillin, and patients with impaired renal function.

NURSING CONSIDERATIONS

Assessment

- Assess patient's infection before therapy and regularly thereafter.
- Obtain specimen for culture and sensitivity tests before giving first dose. Therapy may begin pending test results.
- Ask patient about previous reactions to cephalosporins or penicillin before administering first dose.
- Be alert for adverse reactions and drug interactions.
- Monitor patient's hydration status if adverse GI reactions occur.
- Evaluate patient's and family's knowledge of drug therapy.

Nursing diagnoses

- Infection related to bacteria susceptible to drug
- Risk for deficient fluid volume related to drug-induced adverse GI reactions
- Deficient knowledge related to drug therapy

Planning and implementation

- To prepare oral suspension, first add required amount of water to powder in two portions. Shake well after each addition. After mixing, store in refrigerator (stable for 14 days without significant loss of potency). Keep tightly closed and shake well before using.
- Administer drug with food or milk to minimize adverse GI reactions.
- Group A beta-hemolytic streptococcal infections should be treated for minimum of 10 days.
- Urine glucose determinations may be false-positive with copper sulfate tests (Clinitest); glucose enzymatic tests (Diastix or Chemstrip uG) aren't affected.

ALERT Don't confuse with other cephalosporins with similar sounding names.

Patient teaching

- Inform patient that drug may be taken with meals.
- Instruct patient to take drug exactly as prescribed, even after he feels better.
- Tell patient to call prescriber if rash develops.
- Teach patient how to store drug.

Evaluation

- Patient is free from infection.
- Patient maintains adequate hydration.
- Patient and family state understanding of drug therapy.

cephradine

(SEF-ruh-deen)
Velosef**

Pharmacologic class: first-generation cephalosporin
Therapeutic class: antibiotic
Pregnancy risk category: B

Indications and dosages

▶ **Serious infections of respiratory, GU, or GI tract; skin and soft-tissue infections; bone and joint infections; septicemia; endocarditis; and otitis media caused by such susceptible organisms as *Escherichia coli* and other coliform bacteria, group A beta-hemolytic streptococci, *Haemophilus influenzae, Klebsiella, Proteus mirabilis, Staphylococcus aureus, Streptococcus pneumoniae, S. viridans*, and staphylococci; and perioperative prophylaxis.** *Adults:* 250 to 500 mg P.O. q 6 hours or 500 mg to 1 g q 12 hours. For severe or chronic infections, larger doses may be needed, maximum dose 4 g/day.
Children over age 9 months: 25 to 50 mg/kg/day P.O. given in equally divided doses q 6 to 12 hours. For otitis media, usual dosage is 75 to 100 mg/kg/day P.O. in equally divided doses q 6 to 12 hours, maximum dose 4g/day.
Otitis media. *Children:* 75 to 100 mg/kg P.O. daily in equally divided doses q 6 to 12 hours; maximum dose 4 g daily.

How supplied

Capsules: 250 mg, 500 mg
Oral suspension: 125 mg/5 ml, 250 mg/5 ml

Pharmacokinetics

Absorption: absorbed rapidly and completely from GI tract.
Distribution: distributed widely into most body tissues and fluids; CSF penetration is poor. Drug is 6% to 20% protein-bound.
Metabolism: none.
Excretion: excreted primarily in urine. *Half-life:* about 0.5 to 2 hours.

Route	Onset	Peak	Duration
P.O.	Unknown	≤ 1 hr	Unknown

Pharmacodynamics

Chemical effect: inhibits cell-wall synthesis, promoting osmotic instability; usually bactericidal.
Therapeutic effect: hinders or kills susceptible bacteria: many gram-positive organisms and some gram-negative organisms, such as *E. coli* and other coliform bacteria, group A beta-hemolytic streptococci, *H. influenzae, Klebsiella, P. mirabilis, S. aureus,* staphylococci, *S. pneumoniae*, and *S. viridans*.

Adverse reactions

CNS: dizziness, headache, malaise, paresthesia.
GI: pseudomembranous colitis, *nausea, anorexia,* vomiting, heartburn, glossitis, dyspepsia, abdominal cramping, *diarrhea,* tenesmus, anal pruritus, oral candidiasis.
GU: genital pruritus and candidiasis, vaginitis.
Hematologic: ***transient neutropenia,*** eosinophilia, ***thrombocytopenia.***
Hepatic: transient increases in liver enzyme levels.
Respiratory: dyspnea.
Skin: *maculopapular and erythematous rashes, urticaria.*
Other: hypersensitivity reactions (serum sickness, ***anaphylaxis***).

Interactions

Drug-drug. *Probenecid:* may increase blood levels of cephalosporins. Sometimes used for this effect.

Contraindications and precautions

- Contraindicated in patients hypersensitive to drug and other cephalosporins.
- Use cautiously in pregnant patients, breast-feeding patients, patients with impaired renal

function, and patients with history of sensitivity to penicillin.

NURSING CONSIDERATIONS

Assessment
- Assess patient's infection before therapy and regularly thereafter.
- Obtain specimen for culture and sensitivity tests before first dose. Therapy may begin pending test results.
- Ask patient about previous reactions to cephalosporins or penicillin before giving first dose.
- Be alert for adverse reactions and drug interactions.
- Monitor patient's hydration status if adverse GI reactions occur.
- Evaluate patient's and family's knowledge of drug therapy.

Nursing diagnoses
- Infection related to bacteria susceptible to drug
- Risk for deficient fluid volume related to drug-induced adverse GI reactions
- Deficient knowledge related to drug therapy

Planning and implementation
- Administer drug with food to prevent or minimize GI upset.
- Group A beta-hemolytic streptococcal infections should be treated for minimum of 10 days.
- Store reconstituted suspension for 7 days at room temperature or 14 days if refrigerated. Keep tightly closed, and shake well before using.
- Urine glucose determinations may be false-positive with copper sulfate tests (Clinitest); glucose enzymatic tests (Diastix or Chemstrip uG) aren't affected.

ALERT Don't confuse with other cephalosporins with similar sounding names.

Patient teaching
- Inform patient that drug may be taken with meals.
- Instruct patient to take drug exactly as prescribed, even after he feels better.
- Tell patient to call prescriber if rash develops.
- Teach patient how to store drug.

Evaluation
- Patient is free from infection.
- Patient maintains adequate hydration.
- Patient and family state understanding of drug therapy.

cerivastatin sodium
(seh-rih-vah-STAH-tin SOH-dee-um)
Baycol

Pharmacologic class: 3-hydroxy-3-methylglutaryl-coenzyme A (HMG-CoA) reductase inhibitor
Therapeutic class: antilipemic
Pregnancy risk category: X

Indications and dosages
▶ **Adjunct to diet to reduce total and low-density cholesterol levels in patients with primary hypercholesterolemia or mixed dyslipidemia (Fredrickson types IIa and IIb) when diet and other nonpharmacologic measures have been inadequate. Adjunct to diet for treatment of elevated triglycerides and apolipoprotein B levels in patients with primary hypercholesterolemia and mixed dyslipidemia (Fredrickson types IIa and IIb) when diet and other nonpharmacologic measures have been inadequate.** *Adults:* 0.4 mg P.O. daily in the evening.

How supplied
Tablets: 0.2 mg, 0.3 mg

Pharmacokinetics
Absorption: mean absolute bioavailability is 60% following administration of 0.2-mg dose.
Distribution: more than 99% is bound to plasma protein, primarily albumin.
Metabolism: converted to two active metabolites, M1 and M23, with relative potencies of 50% and 80% of parent compound, respectively. Cholesterol-lowering effect is primarily caused by parent drug.
Excretion: M1 and M23 metabolites are excreted about 24% in urine and 70% in feces;

none of parent compound is excreted in urine or feces. *Half-life:* 2 to 3 hours.

Route	Onset	Peak	Duration
P.O.	Unknown	2.5 hr	Unknown

Pharmacodynamics

Chemical effect: competitive inhibitor of HMG-CoA reductase that is responsible for converting HMG-CoA to mevalonate, a precursor of sterols including cholesterol.
Therapeutic effect: reduction in plasma cholesterol level.

Adverse reactions

CNS: asthenia, dizziness, *headache*.
CV: chest pain, peripheral edema.
EENT: *pharyngitis, rhinitis,* sinusitis.
GI: abdominal pain, constipation, diarrhea, dyspepsia, flatulence, nausea.
GU: urinary tract infection.
Musculoskeletal: arthralgia, back or leg pain, myalgia.
Respiratory: increased cough.
Skin: rash.
Other: flu syndrome.

Interactions

Drug-drug. *Azole antifungals, cyclosporine, erythromycin, fibric acid derivatives, niacin:* may increase the risk of myopathy. Use cautiously together.
Cholestyramine: when given within 4 hours of drug, results in decreased absorption and decreased peak plasma levels of cerivastatin. Use cautiously together.
Erythromycin: may decrease hepatic metabolism of drug; has resulted in increases of cerivastatin of up to 50%. Monitor liver function closely.
Drug-herb. *Red yeast rice:* contains ingredients similar to those of statin drugs, possibly increasing the risk of adverse reactions or toxicity. Discourage concomitant use.

Contraindications and precautions

- Contraindicated in pregnant patients, breast-feeding patients, patients hypersensitive to drug, and patients with active liver disease or unexplained persistent elevations of serum transaminases.
- Use cautiously in patients with history of liver disease or chronic alcohol use.
- Safety and efficacy in children haven't been established.
- Drug should be given to women of child-bearing age only if conception is highly unlikely and they have been warned of risks to fetus.

NURSING CONSIDERATIONS

Assessment

- Monitor lipid levels and liver function test results before starting treatment and at no less than 4-week intervals thereafter as ordered.
- Make sure woman of childbearing age is using effective birth control methods. Drug is contraindicated in pregnancy because of risk of fetal harm.
- Evaluate patient's and family's knowledge of drug therapy.

Nursing diagnoses

- Imbalanced nutrition: less than body requirements related to drug-induced adverse GI reactions
- Risk for injury related to underlying condition
- Deficient knowledge related to drug therapy

Planning and implementation

- Counsel patient regarding appropriate diet, exercise, and weight reduction before starting therapy.
- Patients with moderate or severe renal dysfunction need a reduced dosage.
- Withhold drug temporarily in patients experiencing an acute or serious condition predisposing them to renal failure secondary to rhabdomyolysis.

Patient teaching

- Tell patient to take drug in the evening with or without food.
- Inform patient that it may take up to 4 weeks for full therapeutic effect to occur.
- Caution women to stop drug and notify prescriber if pregnancy occurs or is suspected.
- Advise breast-feeding patient to discontinue breast feeding during drug therapy.

• Tell patient to notify prescriber about unexplained muscle pain, tenderness, or weakness (particularly if accompanied by fever or malaise).

☑ Evaluation

• Patient maintains adequate nutritional intake.
• Patient remains free from injury and shows improvement of underlying condition.
• Patient and family state understanding of drug therapy.

cevimeline hydrochloride

(seh-vih-MEH-leen high-dro-KLOR-ide)
Evoxac

Pharmacologic class: Cholinergic agonist
Therapeutic class: Pro-secretory
Pregnancy risk category: C

Indications and dosages

▶ **Dry mouth in patients with Sjögren's syndrome.** Adults: 30 mg P.O. t.i.d.

How supplied

Tablets: 30 mg

Pharmacokinetics

Absorption: rapidly absorbed, reaching peak plasma levels at 1.5 to 2 hours. Food decreases the rate of absorption, and peak level is reduced by 17.3%.
Distribution: less than 20% protein-bound.
Metabolism: liver enzymes CYP2D6, CYP3A3, and CYP3A4 are involved in the metabolism of cevimeline. The drug is metabolized to a number of metabolites.
Excretion: mostly excreted in urine. *Half-life:* about 5 hours.

Route	Onset	Peak	Duration
P.O.	Unknown	1.5 to 2 hours	Unknown

Pharmacodynamics

Chemical effect: as a cholinergic agonist, cevimeline binds to and stimulates muscarinic receptors. This results in increased secretion of exocrine glands that cause salivation, sweating, and increased tone of smooth muscles in the GI and GU tracts.
Therapeutic effect: helps counteract the dry mouth linked to Sjögren's syndrome.

Adverse reactions

CNS: anxiety, depression, dizziness, fatigue, *headache,* hypoesthesia, insomnia, migraine, pain, tremor, vertigo.
CV: chest pain, palpitations, peripheral edema, edema.
EENT: abnormal vision, conjunctivitis, earache, epistaxis, eye infection, eye pain, otitis media, pharyngitis, *rhinitis, sinusitis,* xeropthalmia, eye abnormality.
GI: abdominal pain, anorexia, constipation, *diarrhea,* dry mouth, eructation, excessive salivation, flatulence, gastroesophageal reflux, *nausea,* salivary gland enlargement and pain, sialoadenitis, ulcerative stomatitis, vomiting, dyspepsia.
GU: cystitis, candidiasis, urinary tract infection, vaginitis.
Hematologic: anemia.
Hepatic: increased amylase.
Musculoskeletal: arthralgia, back pain, hypertonia, hyporeflexia, leg cramps, myalgia, rigors, skeletal pain.
Respiratory: *upper respiratory infection,* bronchitis, pneumonia, coughing, hiccups.
Skin: rash, pruritus, skin disorder, erythematous rash, *excessive sweating.*
Other: fever, fungal infections, flulike symptoms, injury, surgical intervention, hot flushes, postoperative pain, ***allergic reaction***, infection, abscess, tooth disorder, toothache.

Interactions

Drug-drug. *Beta blockers:* possible conduction disturbances. Use cautiously.
Drugs with parasympathomimetic effects: additive effects. Use cautiously.
Drugs that inhibit CYP2D6, CYP3A4, CYP3A3: inhibited metabolism of cevimeline. Monitor patient closely.

Contraindications and precautions

• Contraindicated in patients hypersensitive to drug. Also contraindicated in patients with uncontrolled asthma and when miosis is un-

desirable, as in acute iritis or angle-closure glaucoma.
- Use cautiously in patients with significant CV disease, evidenced by angina pectoris or MI, because it can alter cardiac conduction and heart rate. Use cautiously in patients with controlled asthma, chronic bronchitis, or COPD, because it can cause bronchial constriction and increase bronchial secretions.
- Use cautiously in patients with a history of nephrolithiasis because an increase in ureteral smooth muscle tone could cause renal colic or ureteral reflux.
- Use cautiously in patients with cholelithiasis because contractions of the gallbladder or biliary smooth muscle could cause cholecystitis, cholangitis, and biliary obstruction.

NURSING CONSIDERATIONS

Assessment
- Make sure patient has a thorough physical examination before starting drug therapy.
- Assess patient's fluid balance before therapy.
- Be alert for adverse reactions and drug interactions.
- Monitor liver function test results during therapy if patient has risk of liver dysfunction.
- Evaluate patient's and family's knowledge of drug therapy.

Nursing diagnoses
- Impaired oral mucus membrane related to Sjögren's syndrome
- Risk for injury related to drug-induced adverse reactions
- Deficient knowledge related to drug therapy

Planning and implementation
- Rehydrate patient who is dehydrated, as needed and directed.
- Monitor patient with a history of asthma, COPD, or chronic bronchitis for an increase in symptoms (such as wheezing, sputum production, or cough) during therapy.
- Monitor patient with a history of cardiac disease for increased frequency, severity, or duration of angina or changes in heart rate during therapy.

Patient teaching
- Tell patient not to interrupt or stop treatment without medical approval.
- Tell patient that sweating is a common effect of the drug. Fluid intake is important to prevent dehydration.
- Inform patient that cevimeline may cause visual disturbances, especially at night, that can impair driving ability.

Evaluation
- Increased salivation as a result of drug therapy.
- Patient doesn't experience injury as a result of drug-induced adverse reactions.
- Patient and family state understanding of drug therapy.

chloral hydrate
(KLOR-ul HIGH-drayt)
Aquachloral Supprettes, Noctec
Novo-Chlorhydrate ♦

Pharmacologic class: general CNS depressant
Therapeutic class: sedative-hypnotic
Controlled substance schedule: IV
Pregnancy risk category: C

Indications and dosages
▶ **Sedation.** *Adults:* 250 mg P.O. or P.R. t.i.d. after meals.
Children: 25 mg/kg P.O. or P.R. t.i.d.; maximum 500 mg per single dose per day; doses may be divided.
▶ **Insomnia.** *Adults:* 500 mg to 1 g P.O. or P.R. 15 to 30 minutes before bedtime.
Children: 50 mg/kg P.O. or P.R. 15 to 30 minutes before bedtime; maximum single dose 1 g.
▶ **Preoperatively.** *Adults:* 500 mg to 1 g P.O. or P.R. 30 minutes before surgery.
▶ **Premedication for EEG.** *Children:* 20 to 25 mg/kg P.O. or P.R.

How supplied
Capsules: 250 mg, 500 mg
Syrup: 250 mg/5 ml, 500 mg/5 ml
Suppositories: 324 mg, 500 mg, 648 mg

Pharmacokinetics

Absorption: absorbed well after oral and rectal administration.
Distribution: distributed throughout body tissue and fluids; trichloroethanol (the active metabolite) is 35% to 41% protein-bound.
Metabolism: metabolized rapidly and nearly completely in liver and erythrocytes to trichloroethanol; further metabolized in liver and kidneys to trichloroacetic acid and other inactive metabolites.
Excretion: inactive metabolites are excreted primarily in urine, minimally in bile. *Half-life:* 8 to 10 hours for trichloroethanol.

Route	Onset	Peak	Duration
P.O.	≤ 30 min	Unknown	4-8 hr
P.R.	Unknown	Unknown	4-8 hr

Pharmacodynamics

Chemical effect: unknown; sedative effects may be caused by trichloroethanol.
Therapeutic effect: promotes sleep and calmness.

Adverse reactions

CNS: hangover, drowsiness, nightmares, dizziness, ataxia, paradoxical excitement.
GI: *nausea, vomiting, diarrhea,* flatulence.
Hematologic: eosinophilia, leukopenia.
Skin: hypersensitivity reactions.

Interactions

Drug-drug. *Alkaline solutions:* incompatible with aqueous solutions of chloral hydrate. Don't mix.
CNS depressants, including narcotic analgesics: excessive CNS depression or vasodilation reaction. Use together cautiously.
Furosemide I.V.: sweating, flushes, variable blood pressure, and uneasiness. Use together cautiously or use different hypnotic drug.
Oral anticoagulants: increased risk of bleeding. Monitor patient closely.
Phenytoin: decreased phenytoin levels. Monitor serum levels closely.
Drug-lifestyle. *Alcohol use:* excessive CNS depression or vasodilation reaction. Discourage concomitant use.

Contraindications and precautions

- Contraindicated in patients hypersensitive to chloral hydrate and in those with hepatic or renal impairment. Oral administration contraindicated in patients with gastric disorders.
- Avoid use in breast-feeding women because small amounts of drug pass into breast milk and may cause drowsiness in infants.
- Use with extreme caution in patients with severe cardiac disease.
- Use cautiously in patients with mental depression, suicidal tendencies, or history of drug abuse.

NURSING CONSIDERATIONS

Assessment

- Assess patient's underlying condition.
- Evaluate drug effectiveness after administration.
- Monitor BUN levels as ordered. Large dosage may raise BUN levels.
- Be alert for adverse reactions and drug interactions.
- Evaluate patient's and family's knowledge of drug therapy.

Nursing diagnoses

- Disturbed sleep pattern related to patient's underlying condition
- Risk for trauma related to adverse CNS reactions
- Deficient knowledge related to drug therapy

Planning and implementation

ALERT There are two strengths of oral liquid form; double-check dose, especially when administering to children. Fatal overdoses have occurred.
- To minimize unpleasant taste and stomach irritation, dilute or administer drug with liquid. Drug should be taken after meals.

P.R. use: Store rectal suppositories in refrigerator.
- Long-term use isn't recommended; drug loses its efficacy in promoting sleep after 14 days of continued use. Long-term use may cause drug dependence, and patient may experience withdrawal symptoms if drug is suddenly stopped.

• Drug may interfere with fluorometric tests for urine catecholamines and Reddy-Jenkins-Thorn test for urine 17-hydroxycorticosteroids. Don't administer drug for 48 hours before fluorometric test as ordered. May also cause false-positive tests for urine glucose when using copper sulfate tests (Clinitest). Use glucose enzymatic tests (Diastix or Chemstrip uG) instead.

Patient teaching
• Caution patient about performing activities that require mental alertness or physical coordination. For inpatients, supervise walking and raise bed rails, particularly for elderly patients.
• Tell patient to store capsules or syrup in dark container; store suppositories in refrigerator.
• Explain that drug may cause morning hangover. Encourage patient to report severe hangover or feelings of oversedation so prescriber can be consulted to adjust dosage or change drug.

☑ Evaluation
• Patient states drug effectively induced sleep.
• Patient's safety is maintained.
• Patient and family state understanding of drug therapy.

chlorambucil
(klor-AM-byoo-sil)
Leukeran

Pharmacologic class: alkylating agent (not specific to cell cycle phase)
Therapeutic class: antineoplastic
Pregnancy risk category: D

Indications and dosages

▶ **Chronic lymphocytic leukemia; malignant lymphomas, including lymphosarcoma, giant follicular lymphoma, and Hodgkin's disease.** *Adults:* 0.1 to 0.2 mg/kg P.O. daily for 3 to 6 weeks; then adjusted for maintenance (usually 4 to 10 mg daily).

How supplied

Tablets: 2 mg

Pharmacokinetics

Absorption: well absorbed from GI tract.
Distribution: not well understood; drug and its metabolites are highly bound to plasma and tissue proteins.
Metabolism: metabolized in liver; primary metabolite, phenylacetic acid mustard, also possesses cytotoxic activity.
Excretion: metabolites are excreted in urine.
Half-life: 2 hours for parent compound; 2.5 hours for phenylacetic acid metabolite.

Route	Onset	Peak	Duration
P.O.	3-4 wk	1 hr	Unknown

Pharmacodynamics

Chemical effect: cross-links strands of cellular DNA and interferes with RNA transcription, causing growth imbalance that leads to cell death.
Therapeutic effect: kills selected cancer cells.

Adverse reactions

CNS: ***seizures***.
GI: *nausea, vomiting, stomatitis.*
GU: *azoospermia, infertility.*
Hematologic: ***neutropenia*** (delayed up to 3 weeks, lasting up to 10 days after last dose), ***thrombocytopenia, anemia, myelosuppression*** (usually moderate, gradual, and rapidly reversible).
Hepatic: ***hepatotoxicity***.
Metabolic: hyperuricemia.
Respiratory: interstitial pneumonitis, ***pulmonary fibrosis***.
Skin: exfoliative dermatitis, rash, ***Stevens-Johnson syndrome.***
Other: allergic febrile reaction.

Interactions

Drug-drug. *Anticoagulants, aspirin:* increased risk of bleeding. Avoid concomitant use.

Contraindications and precautions

• Contraindicated in breast-feeding patients and patients hypersensitive or resistant to previous therapy (those hypersensitive to other alkylating agents also may be hypersensitive to chlorambucil).
• Use with extreme caution, if at all, in pregnant women because fetal harm may occur.

• Use cautiously in patients with history of head trauma or seizures and in patients receiving other drugs that lower seizure threshold.
• Safety of drug hasn't been established in children.

NURSING CONSIDERATIONS

Assessment
• Assess patient's underlying neoplastic disorder before therapy and reassess regularly throughout therapy.
• Monitor CBC and serum uric acid level, as ordered.
• Be alert for adverse reactions and drug interactions.
• Evaluate patient's and family's knowledge of drug therapy.

Nursing diagnoses
• Ineffective health maintenance related to presence of neoplastic disease
• Ineffective protection related to drug-induced hematologic adverse reactions
• Deficient knowledge related to drug therapy

Planning and implementation
• Dose is individualized according to patient's response.
• Give drug 1 hour before breakfast and at least 2 hours after evening meal.
• Nausea and vomiting caused by drug use can usually be controlled with antiemetics.
• Allopurinol may be used with adequate hydration to prevent hyperuricemia with resulting uric acid nephropathy,
• Follow institutional policy for infection control in immunocompromised patients if WBC count falls below 2,000/mm^3 or granulocyte count falls below 1,000/mm^3. Severe neutropenia is reversible up to cumulative dosage of 6.5 mg/kg in single course.

Patient teaching
• Warn patient to watch for signs of infection (fever, sore throat, fatigue) and bleeding (easy bruising, nosebleeds, bleeding gums, melena). Tell him to take temperature daily.
• Instruct patient to avoid OTC products that contain aspirin.
• Tell patient to take drug 1 hour before breakfast and 2 hours after evening meal if bothered by nausea and vomiting.
• Instruct patient to maintain fluid intake of 2,400 to 3,000 ml/day, if not contraindicated.

Evaluation
• Patient shows improvement in underlying neoplastic condition on follow-up diagnostic tests.
• Patient remains infection free and doesn't bleed abnormally.
• Patient and family state understanding of drug therapy.

chloramphenicol sodium succinate
(klor-am-FEN-eh-kol SOH-dee-um SUK-seh-nayt)
Chloromycetin, Chloromycetin Sodium Succinate, Pentamycetin ♦

Pharmacologic class: dichloroacetic acid derivative
Therapeutic class: antibiotic
Pregnancy risk category: NR

Indications and dosages

▶ ***Haemophilus influenzae*** **meningitis; acute** ***Salmonella typhi*** **infection; meningitis, bacteremia, or other severe infection caused by sensitive** ***Salmonella*** **species,** ***Rickettsia,*** **or various sensitive gram-negative organisms; lymphogranuloma; or psittacosis.** *Adults and children:* 50 to 100 mg/kg P.O. or I.V. daily (depending on the severity of infection), divided q 6 hours. Maximum dosage is 100 mg/kg daily.
Full-term infants over age 2 weeks with normal metabolic processes: up to 50 mg/kg I.V. daily, divided q 6 hours.
Premature infants, neonates age 2 weeks or younger, and children and infants with immature metabolic processes: 25 mg/kg I.V. once daily. I.V. route must be used to treat meningitis.

How supplied

Capsules: 250 mg
Oral suspension: 150 mg/5ml (as palmitate)

Injection: 100 mg/ml (as sodium succinate)

Pharmacokinetics

Absorption: well absorbed from GI tract after oral administration.
Distribution: distributed widely to most body tissues and fluids. About 50% to 60% bound to plasma protein.
Metabolism: parent drug is metabolized primarily by hepatic glucuronyl transferase to inactive metabolites.
Excretion: 8% to 12% of dose is excreted by kidneys as unchanged drug; remainder is excreted as inactive metabolites. *Half-life:* about 1.5 to 4.5 hours.

Route	Onset	Peak	Duration
P.O.	Unknown	1-3 hr	Unknown
I.V.	Immediate	Immediate	Unknown

Pharmacodynamics

Chemical effect: inhibits bacterial protein synthesis by binding to 50S subunit of ribosome; bacteriostatic.
Therapeutic effect: inhibits growth of susceptible bacteria. Spectrum of activity includes *Rickettsia, Chlamydia, Mycoplasma,* and certain *Salmonella* strains, as well as most gram-positive and gram-negative organisms.

Adverse reactions

CNS: headache, mild depression, confusion, delirium; peripheral neuropathy (with prolonged therapy).
EENT: optic neuritis (in patients with cystic fibrosis), glossitis, decreased visual acuity.
GI: nausea, vomiting, stomatitis, diarrhea, enterocolitis.
Hematologic: ***aplastic anemia, hypoplastic anemia, thrombocytopenia, agranulocytosis.***
Other: infection with nonsusceptible organisms, hypersensitivity reactions (fever, rash, urticaria, ***anaphylaxis***), jaundice, ***gray syndrome in neonates.***

Interactions

Drug-drug. *Chlorpropamide, dicumarol, phenobarbital, phenytoin, tolbutamide:* increased blood levels possible. Monitor patient for toxicity.
Folic acid, iron supplements, vitamin B_{12}: possible delayed response in patients with anemia. Monitor patient closely.

Contraindications and precautions

- Contraindicated in patients hypersensitive to drug.
- Breast-feeding women should temporarily stop breast-feeding during therapy because drug appears in breast milk, posing risk of bone marrow depression and slight risk of gray syndrome.
- Use cautiously in patients with impaired hepatic or renal function, acute intermittent porphyria, or G6PD deficiency; in those taking other drugs that cause bone marrow suppression or blood disorders; and in pregnant women.

NURSING CONSIDERATIONS

Assessment

- Assess patient's infection before therapy and reassess regularly throughout therapy.
- Obtain specimen for culture and sensitivity tests before first dose. Therapy may begin pending results.
- Monitor plasma drug levels. Therapeutic plasma levels are 5 to 25 mcg/ml.
- Monitor CBC, platelets, serum iron, and reticulocytes before and every 2 days during therapy, as ordered.
- Be alert for adverse reactions and drug interactions.

ALERT Signs and symptoms of gray syndrome in neonates include abdominal distention, gray cyanosis, vasomotor collapse, respiratory distress, and death within few hours after onset of symptoms.

- Evaluate patient's and family's knowledge about drug therapy.

Nursing diagnoses

- Infection related to presence of bacteria susceptible to drug
- Impaired protection related to drug-induced aplastic anemia
- Deficient knowledge related to drug therapy

Planning and implementation

P.O. use: Administer oral drug forms on empty stomach 1 hour before or 2 hours after

meals. (If patient develops adverse GI effects, administer with food.)
I.V. use: Give I.V. slowly over at least 1 minute. Check injection site daily for phlebitis and irritation.
– Reconstitute 1-g vial of powder for injection with 10 ml of sterile water for injection. Concentration will be 100 mg/ml. Stable for 30 days at room temperature, but refrigeration recommended. Don't use cloudy solutions.
- Stop drug immediately and notify prescriber if anemia, reticulocytopenia, leukopenia, or thrombocytopenia develops.
- If patient's serum drug level exceeds 25 mcg/ml, take bleeding precautions and infection-control measures because bone marrow suppression can occur.

Patient teaching
- Instruct patient to report adverse reactions to prescriber, especially nausea, vomiting, diarrhea, fever, confusion, sore throat, or mouth sores.
- Stress importance of having frequent blood tests to monitor therapeutic effectiveness and adverse reactions.

☑ Evaluation
- Patient is free from infection after drug therapy.
- Patient's hematologic status remains unchanged with drug therapy.
- Patient and family state understanding of drug therapy.

chlordiazepoxide
(klor-digh-eh-zuh-POKS-ighd)
Libritabs

chlordiazepoxide hydrochloride
Apo-Chlordiazepoxide ♦, Librium, Novopoxide ♦

Pharmacologic class: benzodiazepine
Therapeutic class: antianxiety agent, sedative-hypnotic
Controlled substance schedule: IV
Pregnancy risk category: NR

Indications and dosages
▶ **Mild to moderate anxiety.** *Adults:* 5 to 10 mg P.O. t.i.d. or q.i.d.
Children over age 6: 5 mg P.O. b.i.d. to q.i.d. Maximum dosage 10 mg P.O. b.i.d. or t.i.d.
▶ **Severe anxiety**. *Adults:* 20 to 25 mg P.O. t.i.d. or q.i.d.
Elderly patients: 5 mg P.O. b.i.d. to q.i.d.
▶ **Withdrawal symptoms of acute alcoholism.** *Adults:* 50 to 100 mg P.O., I.V., or I.M. Repeated in 2 to 4 hours, p.r.n. Maximum dosage is 300 mg daily.
▶ **Preoperative apprehension and anxiety.** *Adults:* 5 to 10 mg P.O. t.i.d. or q.i.d. on day preceding surgery. Or, 50 to 100 mg I.M. 1 hour before surgery.

How supplied
chlordiazepoxide
Tablets: 10 mg, 25 mg
chlordiazepoxide hydrochloride
Capsules: 5 mg, 10 mg, 25 mg
Powder for injection: 100 mg/ampule

Pharmacokinetics
Absorption: when given orally, drug is absorbed well through GI tract; unknown after I.M. administration.
Distribution: distributed widely throughout body. Drug is 80% to 90% protein-bound.
Metabolism: metabolized in liver to several active metabolites.
Excretion: most metabolites of drug are excreted in urine. *Half-life:* 5 to 30 hours.

Route	Onset	Peak	Duration
P.O., I.V., I.M.	Unknown	0.5-4 hr	Unknown

Pharmacodynamics
Chemical effect: unknown. Thought to depress CNS at limbic and subcortical levels of brain.
Therapeutic effect: relieves anxiety and promotes sleep and calmness.

Adverse reactions
CNS: *drowsiness, lethargy, hangover,* fainting, restlessness, psychosis, ***suicidal tendencies.***
CV: *thrombophlebitis,* transient hypotension.

EENT: visual disturbances.
GI: nausea, vomiting, abdominal discomfort.
GU: incontinence, urine retention, menstrual irregularities.
Hematologic: ***agranulocytosis.***
Skin: *swelling, pain at injection site.*

Interactions

Drug-drug. *Cimetidine:* increased sedation. Monitor patient carefully.
CNS depressants: increased CNS depression. Avoid concomitant use.
Digoxin: increased serum digoxin levels and risk of toxicity. Monitor patient closely.
Drug-herb. *Kava*: can lead to excessive sedation. Discourage concurrent use.
Drug-lifestyle. *Alcohol use:* increased CNS depression. Discourage concurrent use.
Smoking: increased clearance of benzodiazepines. Monitor patient for lack of effect.

Contraindications and precautions

- Contraindicated in pregnant patients and patients hypersensitive to drug.
- Drug shouldn't be given to breast-feeding women because of risk of adverse effects in infant.
- Use cautiously in patients with mental depression, porphyria, or hepatic or renal disease.
- Safety of drug hasn't been established in children under age 6; parenteral use in children under age 12 isn't recommended.

NURSING CONSIDERATIONS

Assessment

- Assess patient's underlying condition before therapy, and reassess regularly thereafter.
- Monitor respirations every 5 to 15 minutes after I.V. administration and before each repeated I.V. dose.
- Monitor liver, renal, and hematopoietic function studies periodically in patients receiving repeated or prolonged therapy as ordered.
- Monitor patient for abuse and addiction.
- Be alert for adverse reactions and drug interactions.
- Evaluate patient's and family's knowledge of drug therapy.
- In elderly patient, use smallest effective dose to avoid ataxia and oversedation.

Nursing diagnoses

- Anxiety related to patient's underlying condition
- Risk for injury related to drug-induced CNS reactions
- Deficient knowledge related to drug therapy

Planning and implementation

- Dosage should be reduced in elderly or debilitated patients.
- Drug shouldn't be prescribed regularly for everyday stress.

P.O. use: Make sure patient has swallowed tablets before you leave the bedside.
ALERT Chlordiazepoxide 5 mg and 25 mg unit-dose capsules may appear similar in color when viewed through the package. Verify contents and read label carefully.
I.V. use: Use 5 ml of normal saline solution or sterile water for injection as diluent. Administer over 1 minute.
ALERT Don't give packaged diluent I.V. because air bubbles may form when using prepackaged diluent.
– Be sure equipment and personnel needed for emergency airway management are available.
I.M. use: Add 2 ml of diluent to powder and agitate gently until clear. Use immediately. I.M. form may be erratically absorbed.
– Recommended for I.M. use only, but may be given I.V.
– Injectable form (as hydrochloride) comes in two types of ampules—as diluent and as powdered drug. Read directions carefully.
– Don't mix injectable form with any other parenteral drug.

- Refrigerate powder and keep away from light; mix just before use and discard remainder.
- Drug shouldn't be withdrawn abruptly after long-term administration; withdrawal symptoms may occur.
- May cause false-positive reaction in Gravindex pregnancy test. Drug may also interfere with certain tests for urine 17-ketosteroids.

Patient teaching
- Warn patient to avoid hazardous activities that require alertness and good psychomotor coordination until CNS effects of drug are known.
- Tell patient to avoid alcohol while taking drug.
- Warn patient to take this drug only as directed and not to discontinue it without prescriber's approval. Inform patient of drug's potential for dependence if taken longer than directed.

Evaluation
- Patient says he is less anxious.
- Patient's safety is maintained.
- Patient and family state understanding of drug therapy.

chloroquine hydrochloride
(KLOR-uh-qwin high-droh-KLOR-ighd)
Aralen HCl

chloroquine phosphate
Aralen Phosphate, Chlorquin ◇

Pharmacologic class: 4-amino-quinoline
Therapeutic class: antimalarial, amebicide
Pregnancy risk category: C

Indications and dosages
▶ **Acute malarial attacks caused by *Plasmodium vivax, P. malariae, P. ovale,* and susceptible strains of *P. falciparum.*** *Adults:* 1 g (600-mg base) P.O. followed by 500 mg (300-mg base) P.O. after 6 to 8 hours; for next 2 days a single dose of 500 (300-mg base) P.O. or 4 to 5 ml (160- to 200-mg base) I.M., repeated in 6 hours, if needed, changing to P.O. as soon as possible.
Children: initially, 10 mg (base)/kg P.O.; then 5 mg (base)/kg at 6, 24, and 48 hours (don't exceed adult dose). Or, 5 mg (base)/kg I.M. initially; repeated in 6 hours p.r.n. Don't exceed 10 mg (base)/kg/24 hours. Patient should be switched to oral therapy as soon as possible.
▶ **Malaria prophylaxis.** *Adults:* 500 mg (300-mg base) P.O. on same day once weekly, beginning 2 weeks before exposure. Continue for 4 weeks after leaving endemic area.
Children: 5 mg (base)/kg P.O. on the same day once weekly (not to exceed adult dosage), beginning 2 weeks before exposure.
▶ **Extraintestinal amebiasis.** *Adults:* 1 g (600-mg base) chloroquine phosphate P.O. daily for 2 days; then 500 mg (300-mg base) daily for at least 2 to 3 weeks. Treatment is usually combined with intestinal amebicide.

How supplied
chloroquine hydrochloride
Injection: 50 mg/ml (40-mg/ml base)
chloroquine phosphate
Tablets: 250 mg (150-mg base), 500 mg (300-mg base)

Pharmacokinetics
Absorption: absorbed readily and almost completely.
Distribution: concentrates in liver, spleen, kidneys, heart, and brain and is strongly bound in melanin-containing cells.
Metabolism: about 30% of dose is metabolized by liver to monodesethylchloroquine and bidesethylchloroquine.
Excretion: about 70% of administered dose is excreted unchanged in urine; unabsorbed drug is excreted in feces. Small amounts of drug may be present in urine for months after drug is discontinued. Renal excretion is enhanced by urine acidification. *Half-life:* 1 to 2 months.

Route	Onset	Peak	Duration
P.O.	Unknown	1-3 hr	Unknown
I.M.	Unknown	30 min	Unknown

Pharmacodynamics
Chemical effect: unknown. As antimalarial, chloroquine may bind to and alter properties of DNA in susceptible parasites.
Therapeutic effect: prevents or eradicates malarial infections; eradicates amebiasis.

Adverse reactions
CNS: mild and transient headache, neuromyopathy, psychic stimulation, fatigue, irritability, nightmares, ***seizures,*** dizziness.
CV: hypotension, ECG changes.

EENT: *visual disturbances* (blurred vision; difficulty in focusing; reversible corneal changes; typically irreversible, sometimes progressive or delayed retinal changes, such as narrowing of arterioles; macular lesions; pallor of optic disk; optic atrophy; patchy retinal pigmentation, typically leading to blindness), ototoxicity (nerve deafness, vertigo, tinnitus).
GI: anorexia, abdominal cramps, diarrhea, nausea, vomiting, stomatitis.
Hematologic: ***agranulocytosis, aplastic anemia,*** hemolytic anemia, ***thrombocytopenia.***
Skin: pruritus, lichen planus eruptions, skin and mucosal pigmentary changes, pleomorphic skin eruptions.

Interactions

Drug-drug. *Cimetidine:* decreased hepatic metabolism of chloroquine. Monitor patient for toxicity.
Kaolin, magnesium and aluminum salts: decreased GI absorption. Separate administration times.
Drug-lifestyle. *Sun exposure:* may worsen drug-induced dermatomes. Tell patient to avoid excessive sun exposure.

Contraindications and precautions

- Contraindicated in patients hypersensitive to drug and in patients with retinal changes, visual field changes, or porphyria. Use during pregnancy isn't recommended except for suppression or treatment of malaria (since malaria poses greater danger to mother and fetus than prophylactic administration) or hepatic amebiasis.
- Use with extreme caution in patients with severe GI, neurologic, or blood disorders.
- Use cautiously in patients with hepatic disease or alcoholism (drug concentrates in liver), in those with G6PD deficiency or psoriasis (drug may exacerbate these conditions), and in breast-feeding women.

NURSING CONSIDERATIONS

Assessment

- Assess patient's infection before therapy, and reassess regularly throughout therapy.
- Ensure that baseline and periodic ophthalmic examinations are performed. Check periodically for ocular muscle weakness after long-term use.
- Assist patient with obtaining audiometric examinations before, during, and after therapy, especially if long-term.
- Monitor CBC and liver function studies periodically during long-term therapy, as ordered.
- Be alert for adverse reactions and drug interactions.
- Assess patient for possible overdose, which can quickly lead to toxic symptoms: headache, drowsiness, visual disturbances, CV collapse, and seizures, followed by cardiopulmonary arrest. Children are extremely susceptible to toxicity.
- Evaluate patient's and family's knowledge of drug therapy.

Nursing diagnoses

- Infection related to presence of organisms susceptible to drug
- Disturbed sensory perception (visual or auditory) related to adverse reactions to drug
- Deficient knowledge related to drug therapy

Planning and implementation

- Administer drug at same time of same day each week.
- Missed doses should be given as soon as possible. To avoid doubling doses in regimens requiring more than one dose per day, administer missed dose within 1 hour of scheduled time or omit dose.

P.O. use: Administer drug with milk or meals to minimize GI distress. Tablets may be crushed and mixed with food or chocolate syrup for patients who have trouble swallowing; however drug has bitter taste and patients may find mixture unpleasant. Crushed tablets may be placed inside empty gelatin capsules, which are easier to swallow.
I.M. use: Replace with oral administration as soon as possible.

- Store drug in amber-colored containers to protect from light.
- Prophylactic antimalarial therapy should begin 2 weeks before exposure and should continue for 4 weeks after patient leaves endemic area.

• Monitor patient's weight for significant changes because dosage is calculated by patient's weight.
• Notify prescriber if patient develops severe blood disorder not attributable to disease; drug may need to be discontinued.

Patient teaching
• Tell patient to take drug with food at same time on same day each week.
• Instruct patient to avoid excessive sun exposure to prevent exacerbation of drug-induced dermatoses.
• Tell patient to report blurred vision, increased sensitivity to light, and muscle weakness.
• Warn patient to avoid alcohol while taking drug.
• Teach patient how to take missed doses.

Evaluation
• Patient is free from infection.
• Patient maintains normal visual and auditory function.
• Patient and family state understanding of drug therapy.

chlorothiazide
(klor-oh-THIGH-uh-zighd)
Chlotride ◇, Diurigen, Diuril

chlorothiazide sodium
Sodium Diuril

Pharmacologic class: thiazide diuretic
Therapeutic class: diuretic, antihypertensive
Pregnancy risk category: D

Indications and dosages
▶ **Edema, hypertension.** *Adults:* 500 mg to 2 g P.O. or I.V. daily or in divided doses.
▶ **Diuresis, hypertension.** *Children age 6 months and over:* 20 mg/kg P.O. or I.V. daily in divided doses.
Children under age 6 months: May require 30 mg/kg P.O. or I.V. daily in two divided doses.

How supplied
Tablets: 250 mg, 500 mg
Oral suspension: 250 mg/5 ml
Injection: 500-mg vial

Pharmacokinetics
Absorption: absorbed incompletely and variably from GI tract.
Distribution: unknown.
Metabolism: none.
Excretion: excreted unchanged in urine. *Half-life:* 1 to 2 hours.

Route	Onset	Peak	Duration
P.O.	≤ 2 hr	About 4 hr	6-12 hr
I.V.	≤ 15 min	30 min	6-12 hr

Pharmacodynamics
Chemical effect: increases sodium and water excretion by inhibiting sodium reabsorption in nephron's cortical diluting site.
Therapeutic effect: promotes sodium and water excretion.

Adverse reactions
CV: orthostatic hypotension.
GI: anorexia, nausea, ***pancreatitis.***
GU: impotence, nocturia, polyuria, frequent urination, ***renal failure.***
Hematologic: ***aplastic anemia, agranulocytosis,*** leukopenia, thrombocytopenia.
Hepatic: hepatic encephalopathy.
Metabolic: asymptomatic hyperuricemia; hypokalemia; hyperglycemia and impaired glucose tolerance; fluid and electrolyte imbalances, including dilutional hyponatremia and hypochloremia, metabolic alkalosis, and hypercalcemia; gout.
Skin: dermatitis, photosensitivity, rash.
Other: hypersensitivity reactions.

Interactions
Drug-drug. *Barbiturates, opiates:* increased orthostatic hypotensive effect. Monitor patient closely.
Cardiac glycosides: increased risk of digitalis toxicity from chlorothiazide-induced hypokalemia. Monitor potassium and digitalis levels.
Cholestyramine, colestipol: decreased intestinal absorption of thiazides. Separate doses.
Diazoxide: increased antihypertensive, hyperglycemic, and hyperuricemic effects. Use together cautiously.

Lithium: decreased lithium clearance, increasing risk of lithium toxicity. Monitor lithium level.
NSAIDs: increased risk of NSAID-induced renal failure. Monitor patient for renal failure.
Drug-herb. *Licorice root:* could worsen the potassium depletion caused by thiazides. Discourage concomitant use.
Drug-lifestyle. *Alcohol use:* increased orthostatic hypotensive effect. Monitor patient closely.

Contraindications and precautions

- Contraindicated in patients hypersensitive to other thiazides or other sulfonamide-derived drugs and in patients with anuria.
- Use cautiously in patients with severe renal disease and impaired hepatic function.
- Safety of drug hasn't been established in pregnant or breast-feeding women.

NURSING CONSIDERATIONS

Assessment

- Assess patient's underlying condition.
- Monitor effectiveness by regularly checking blood pressure, fluid intake and urine output, blood pressure, and weight.
- Expect that therapeutic response may be delayed several days in patients with hypertension
- Monitor serum electrolyte and blood glucose levels.
- Monitor serum creatinine and BUN levels regularly. Drug not as effective if these levels are more than twice normal.
- Monitor blood uric acid level, especially in patients with history of gout.
- Be alert for adverse reactions and drug interactions.
- Evaluate patient's and family's knowledge about drug therapy.

Nursing diagnoses

- Excessive fluid volume related to patient's underlying condition
- Impaired urinary elimination related to drug therapy
- Deficient knowledge related to drug therapy

Planning and implementation

- To prevent nocturia, give drug in the morning.

P.O. use: Don't give more than 250 mg P.O. per dose. Bioavailability studies show that 250 mg P.O. every 6 hours is absorbed better than single dose of 1 g.
I.V. use: Reconstitute 500 mg with 18 ml of sterile water for injection. Inject reconstituted drug directly into vein, through I.V. line containing free-flowing, compatible solution, or through intermittent infusion device. Compatible with I.V. dextrose or saline solutions.
– Store reconstituted solutions at room temperature up to 24 hours.
– Avoid I.V. infiltration, as it can be very painful.
– Avoid simultaneous administration with whole blood and its derivatives.
– Stop administering drug and notify prescriber if hypersensitivity reactions occur.

- Never inject I.M. or S.C.
- Drug may be used with potassium-sparing diuretic to prevent potassium loss.
- As ordered, discontinue thiazides and thiazide-like diuretics before parathyroid function tests are performed.

Patient teaching

- Teach patient and family to identify and report signs of hypersensitivity and hypokalemia.
- Teach patient to monitor fluid intake and output and daily weight.
- Instruct patient to avoid high-sodium foods and to choose high-potassium foods.
- Tell patient to take drug early in day to avoid nocturia.
- Advise patient to avoid sudden posture changes and to rise slowly to avoid orthostatic hypotension.
- Advise patient to use sunblock to prevent photosensitivity reactions.
- Teach patient the importance of periodic laboratory tests to detect possible electrolyte imbalances.

Evaluation

- Patient is free from edema.
- Patient adjusts lifestyle to cope with altered patterns of urine elimination.

• Patient and family state understanding of drug therapy.

chlorpheniramine maleate

(klor-fen-EER-uh-meen MAL-ee-ayt)

Aller-Chlor*†, Chlo-Amine†, Chlor-100†, Chlorate†, Chlor-Niramine†, Chlor-Pro, Chlor-Pro 10, Chlor-Trimeton*†, Chlor-Trimeton Allergy 12 Hour†, Chlor-Tripolon ♦†, Gen-Allerate†, Novopheniram ◇†, Pfeiffer's Allergy†, Phenetron*, Teldrin†

Pharmacologic class: propylamine-derivative antihistamine

Therapeutic class: antihistamine (H_1-receptor antagonist)

Pregnancy risk category: B

Indications and dosages

▶ **Rhinitis, allergy symptoms.** *Adults and children age 12 and older:* 4 mg P.O. q 4 to 6 hours or 8 to 12 mg timed-release P.O. q 8 to 12 hours; maximum 24 mg/day. Or, 10 to 20 mg I.M. or S.C. as single dose.

Children ages 6 to 11: 2 mg P.O. q 4 to 6 hours; maximum 12 mg/day. Or, may give 8 mg timed-release P.O. h.s.

Children ages 2 to 6: 1 mg P.O. q 4 to 6 hours; maximum 4 mg daily.

How supplied

Tablets: 4 mg†

Tablets (chewable): 2 mg†

Tablets (timed-release): 8 mg†, 12 mg†

Capsules (timed-release): 8 mg†, 12 mg†

Syrup: 2 mg/5 ml*†

Injection: 10 mg/ml, 100 mg/ml

Pharmacokinetics

Absorption: well absorbed from GI tract after oral administration. Food delays absorption but doesn't affect bioavailability. Unknown for I.M. or S.C. administration.

Distribution: distributed extensively into body; drug is about 72% protein-bound.

Metabolism: metabolized largely in GI mucosal cells and liver (first-pass effect).

Excretion: drug and metabolites are excreted in urine. *Half-life:* 12 to 43 hours in adults; 10 to 13 hours in children.

Route	Onset	Peak	Duration
P.O.	15-60 min	2-6 hr	< 24 hr
I.V.	15-60 min	Immediate	24 hr
I.M., S.C.	15-60 min	Unknown	< 24 hr

Pharmacodynamics

Chemical effect: competes with histamine for H_1-receptor sites on effector cells. Prevents, but doesn't reverse, histamine-mediated responses.

Therapeutic effect: relieves allergy symptoms.

Adverse reactions

CNS: *stimulation,* sedation, *drowsiness* (especially in elderly patients), excitability in children.

CV: hypotension, palpitations.

GI: epigastric distress, *dry mouth.*

GU: urine retention.

Respiratory: thick bronchial secretions.

Skin: rash, urticaria.

Other: local stinging, burning sensation, pallor, weak pulse, transient hypotension after parenteral administration.

Interactions

Drug-drug. *CNS depressants:* increased sedation. Use together cautiously.

MAO inhibitors: increased anticholinergic effects. Don't use together.

Drug-lifestyle. *Alcohol use:* increased sedation. Tell patient to use together cautiously.

Contraindications and precautions

• Contraindicated in patients with acute asthmatic attacks.

• Antihistamines aren't recommended for breast-feeding patients because small amounts of drug appear in breast milk. Also not recommended for premature or newborn infants.

• Use cautiously in elderly patients and in those with increased intraocular pressure, hyperthyroidism, CV or renal disease, hypertension, bronchial asthma, urine retention, prostatic hyperplasia, bladder-neck obstruction, and stenosing peptic ulcerations.

• Safety of drug hasn't been established for use in pregnant women.

NURSING CONSIDERATIONS

Assessment

• Assess patient's underlying allergy condition, and reassess regularly thereafter.
• Be alert for adverse reactions and drug interactions.
• Evaluate patient's and family's knowledge about drug therapy.

Nursing diagnoses

• Ineffective health maintenance related to underlying allergy condition
• Risk for injury related to drug-induced CNS adverse reactions
• Deficient knowledge related to drug therapy

Planning and implementation

P.O. use: Give drug with food or milk to reduce GI distress.
I.V. use: Drug is available in 10 mg/ml ampules for I.V., I.M., or S.C. administration; drug is compatible with most I.V. solutions. Check with pharmacist before mixing with other I.V. solutions to verify specific compatibilities. Give injection over 1 minute.
ALERT Don't give the 100 mg/ml strength I.V.
I.M. and S.C. use: Follow normal protocol.
• Notify prescriber if patient develops tolerance. Prescriber may substitute another antihistamine.
• If symptoms occur during or after parenteral dose, discontinue drug. Notify prescriber.

Patient teaching

• Instruct patient to take oral drug with food or milk.
• Warn patient to avoid alcohol and other CNS depressants and driving or other activities that require alertness until drug's CNS effects are known.
• Tell patient that coffee or tea may reduce drowsiness. Also, recommend sugarless gum, sugarless sour hard candy, or ice chips to relieve dry mouth.
• Advise patient to stop drug 4 days before allergy skin tests to preserve accuracy of tests.
• Tell patient to notify prescriber if tolerance develops because different antihistamine may need to be prescribed.
• Tell parents that drug, including extended-release product, shouldn't be used in children under age 12 unless directed by prescriber.

Evaluation

• Patient's allergic symptoms are relieved with drug therapy.
• Patient doesn't experience injury as a result of drug-induced adverse reactions.
• Patient and family state understanding of drug therapy.

chlorpromazine hydrochloride

(klor-PROH-meh-zeen high-droh-KLOR-ighd)
Chlorpromanyl-5 ♦, Chlorpromanyl-20 ♦, Chlorpromanyl-40 ♦, Largactil ♦ ◇, Novo-Chlorpromazine ♦, Thorazine

Pharmacologic class: aliphatic phenothiazine
Therapeutic class: antipsychotic, antiemetic
Pregnancy risk category: C

Indications and dosages

▶ **Psychosis.** *Adults:* initially, 30 to 75 mg P.O. daily in two to four divided doses. Increase dosage by 20 to 50 mg twice weekly until symptoms are controlled. Some patients may need up to 800 mg daily. Switch to oral therapy as soon as possible.
Children age 6 months and older: 0.55 mg/kg P.O. q 4 to 6 hours or I.M. q 6 to 8 hours. Or, 1.1 mg/kg P.R. q 6 to 8 hours. Maximum I.M. dose in children under age 5 or weighing less than 22.7 kg (50 lb) is 40 mg. Maximum I.M. dose in children ages 5 to 12 or weighing 22.7 to 45.5 kg (100 lb) is 75 mg.
▶ **Nausea and vomiting.** *Adults:* 10 to 25 mg P.O. q 4 to 6 hours, p.r.n. Or, 50 to 100 mg P.R. q 6 to 8 hours, p.r.n. Or, 25 mg I.M. If no hypotension occurs, give 25 to 50 mg I.M. q 3 to 4 hours p.r.n. until vomiting stops.
Children age 6 months and older: 0.55 mg/kg P.O. q 4 to 6 hours or I.M. q 6 to 8 hours. Or, 1.1 mg/kg P.R. q 6 to 8 hours. Maximum I.M. dose in children under age 5 or weighing less than 22.7 kg is 40 mg. Maximum I.M. dose in

children ages 5 to 12 or weighing 22.7 to 45.5 kg is 75 mg.

▶ **Intractable hiccups, acute intermittent porphyria.** *Adults:* 25 to 50 mg P.O. t.i.d. or q.i.d. If symptoms persist for 2 to 3 days, 25 to 50 mg I.M. If symptoms still persist, 25 to 50 mg diluted in 500 to 1,000 ml of normal saline solution and infused slowly.

▶ **Tetanus.** *Adults:* 25 to 50 mg I.V. or I.M. t.i.d. or q.i.d.

Children age 6 months or older: 0.55 mg/kg I.M. or I.V. q 6 to 8 hours. Maximum parenteral dosage in children weighing less than 22.7 kg is 40 mg daily; in children weighing 22.7 to 45.5 kg, 75 mg daily, except in severe cases.

▶ **Relief of apprehension and nervousness before surgery.** *Adults:* preoperatively, 25 to 50 mg P.O. 2 to 3 hours before surgery or 12.5 to 25 mg I.M. 1 to 2 hours before surgery. During surgery, 12.5 mg I.M. repeated after 30 minutes if needed or fractional 2-mg doses I.V. at 2-minute intervals; maximum dose 25 mg. Postoperatively, 10 to 25 mg P.O. q 4 to 6 hours or 12.5 mg to 25 mg I .M. repeated in 1 hour if needed.

Children age 6 months and older: preoperatively, 0.55 mg/kg P.O. 2 to 3 hours before surgery or I.M. 1 to 2 hours before surgery. During surgery, 0.275 mg/kg I.M. repeated after 30 minutes if needed or fractional 1-mg doses I.V. at 2-minute intervals, maximum dose 0.275 mg/kg. May repeat fractional I.V. regimen in 30 minutes if needed; postoperatively, 0.55 mg/kg P.O. q 4 to 6 hours or 0.55 mg/kg I.M. repeated in 1 hour if needed and hypotension doesn't occur.

How supplied

Tablets: 10 mg, 25 mg, 50 mg, 100 mg, 200 mg
Capsules (controlled-release): 30 mg, 75 mg, 150 mg, 200 mg, 300 mg
Oral concentrate: 30 mg/ml, 100 mg/ml
Syrup: 10 mg/5 ml
Injection: 25 mg/ml
Suppositories: 25 mg, 100 mg

Pharmacokinetics

Absorption: absorption of oral administration is erratic and variable. Absorption of I.M. administration is rapid.
Distribution: distributed widely into body; concentration is usually higher in CNS than plasma. Drug is 91% to 99% protein-bound.
Metabolism: metabolized extensively by liver and forms 10 to 12 metabolites; some are pharmacologically active.
Excretion: most of drug is excreted as metabolites in urine; some is excreted in feces. Chlorpromazine may undergo enterohepatic circulation.

Route	Onset	Peak	Duration
All	Varies	Varies	Varies

Pharmacodynamics

Chemical effect: unknown. Probably blocks postsynaptic dopamine receptors in brain and inhibits medullary chemoreceptor trigger zone.
Therapeutic effect: relieves nausea and vomiting; hiccups; and signs and symptoms of psychosis, acute intermittent porphyria, and tetanus. Produces calmness and sleep preoperatively.

Adverse reactions

CNS: *extrapyramidal reactions, sedation,* ***seizures,*** *tardive dyskinesia,* pseudoparkinsonism, dizziness, ***neuroleptic malignant syndrome.***
CV: *orthostatic hypotension,* tachycardia, ECG changes.
EENT: ocular changes, blurred vision.
GI: *dry mouth, constipation.*
GU: *urine retention,* menstrual irregularities, inhibited ejaculation.
Hematologic: transient leukopenia, *agranulocytosis,* hyperprolactinemia, *aplastic anemia,* ***thrombocytopenia.***
Hepatic: cholestatic jaundice, abnormal liver function test results.
Skin: *mild photosensitivity.*
Other: gynecomastia, allergic reactions, *I.M. injection site pain,* sterile abscess.

Interactions

Drug-drug. *Antacids:* inhibited absorption of oral phenothiazines. Separate antacid and phenothiazine doses by at least 2 hours.
Anticholinergics, including antidepressants and antiparkinsonians: increased anticholinergic activity, aggravated parkinsonian symptoms. Use with caution.

Barbiturates, lithium: may decrease phenothiazine effect. Observe patient.
Centrally acting antihypertensives: decreased antihypertensive effect. Monitor patient.
CNS depressants: increased CNS depression. Avoid concomitant use.
Propranolol: increased levels of both propranolol and chlorpromazine. Monitor patient.
Warfarin: decreased effect of oral anticoagulants. Monitor PT and INR.
Drug-herb. *Kava:* can increase the risk or severity of dystonic reactions. Discourage concomitant use.
Dong quai, St. John's wort: increased risk of photosensitivity. Advise patient to avoid prolonged or unprotected exposure to sunlight.
Yohimbe: increased risk of toxicity. Discourage concomitant use.
Drug-lifestyle. *Alcohol use:* increased CNS depression. Discourage concomitant use.
Sun exposure: increased risk of photosensitivity. Discourage prolonged or unprotected exposure to sun. Encourage protective sunglasses.

Contraindications and precautions

- Contraindicated in patients hypersensitive to drug and in patients with CNS depression, bone marrow suppression, subcortical damage, and coma. Also not recommended for pregnant or breast-feeding women.
- Use cautiously in elderly or debilitated patients and in those with hepatic or renal disease, severe CV disease (may cause sudden drop in blood pressure), exposure to extreme heat or cold (including antipyretic therapy), exposure to organophosphate insecticides, respiratory disorders, hypocalcemia, seizure disorders (may lower seizure threshold), severe reactions to insulin or electroconvulsive therapy, glaucoma, or prostatic hyperplasia.
- Use cautiously in acutely ill or dehydrated children.

NURSING CONSIDERATIONS

Assessment

- Assess patient's underlying condition and reassess regularly thereafter.
- Be alert for adverse reactions and drug interactions.
- Monitor blood pressure regularly. Watch for orthostatic hypotension, especially with parenteral administration. Monitor blood pressure before and after I.M. administration.
- Monitor patient for tardive dyskinesia, which may occur after prolonged use. It may not appear until months or years later and may disappear spontaneously or persist for life despite discontinuation of drug.
- Watch for symptoms of neuroleptic malignant syndrome. It's rare, but commonly fatal. It isn't necessarily related to length of drug use or type of neuroleptic, but over 60% of affected patients are men.
- Monitor therapy with weekly bilirubin tests during first month, periodic blood tests (CBC and liver function), and ophthalmic tests (long-term use), as ordered.
- Evaluate patient's and family's knowledge about drug therapy.

Nursing diagnoses

- Ineffective health maintenance related to patient's underlying condition
- Impaired physical mobility related to drug-induced extrapyramidal reactions
- Deficient knowledge related to drug therapy

Planning and implementation

- Wear gloves when preparing solutions, and prevent any contact with skin and clothing. Oral liquid and parenteral forms can cause contact dermatitis.
- Slight yellowing of injection or concentrate is common; potency isn't affected. Discard markedly discolored solutions.

P.O. use: Protect liquid concentrate from light.
– Dilute with fruit juice, milk, or semisolid food just before administration.
– Sustained-release preparations shouldn't be crushed but administered whole.
– Shake syrup before administration.
I.V. use: For direct injection, drug may be diluted with normal saline solution for injection and administered into large vein or through tubing of free-flowing I.V. solution. Don't exceed 1 mg/minute for adults or 0.5 mg/minute for children.
– Drug also may be given as I.V. infusion; dilute with 500 or 1,000 ml of normal saline solution and administer slowly.

– Chlorpromazine is compatible with most common I.V. solutions, including D_5W, Ringer's injection, lactated Ringer's injection, and normal saline solution for injection.
I.M. use: Give deep I.M. only in upper outer quadrant of buttocks. Massage slowly afterward to prevent sterile abscess. Injection stings.
P.R. use: Follow normal protocol for administering suppository.
– Store suppositories in cool place.
• Keep patient supine for 1 hour after parenteral administration and advise him to get up slowly.
• Don't withdraw drug abruptly unless required by severe adverse reactions. After abrupt withdrawal from long-term therapy patient may experience gastritis, nausea, vomiting, dizziness, and tremors.
• Withhold dose and notify prescriber if patient develops jaundice, symptoms of blood dyscrasia (fever, sore throat, infection, cellulitis, weakness), persistent extrapyramidal reactions (longer than a few hours), or any such reaction in pregnancy or in children.
• Dystonic reactions may be treated with diphenhydramine.

Patient teaching
• Warn patient to avoid activities that require alertness or good psychomotor coordination until CNS effects of drug are known. Drowsiness and dizziness usually subside after first few weeks.
• Instruct patient to avoid alcohol while taking drug.
• Tell patient to notify prescriber if urine retention or constipation occurs.
• Tell patient to use sunblock and wear protective clothing to avoid photosensitivity reactions. Chlorpromazine causes higher risk of photosensitivity than other drugs in its class.
• Tell patient to use sugarless gum or hard candy to relieve dry mouth.
• Tell patient not to stop taking drug suddenly but to take it exactly as prescribed and not to double doses to compensate for missed ones.
• Instruct patient about which fluids are appropriate for diluting concentrate, and show dropper technique for measuring dose. Warn patient to avoid spilling liquid on skin because it may cause rash and irritation.
• Advise patient that injection stings.

☑ Evaluation
• Patient's has reduced signs and symptoms.
• Patient maintains physical mobility throughout drug therapy.
• Patient and family state understanding of drug therapy.

chlorpropamide
(klor-PROH-puh-mighd)
Apo-Chlorpropamide ♦, Diabinese, Novo-Propamide ♦

Pharmacologic class: sulfonylurea
Therapeutic class: antidiabetic
Pregnancy risk category: C

Indications and dosages
▶ **Adjunct to diet to lower blood glucose level in patients with type 2 non-insulin-dependent diabetes mellitus.** *Adults:* 250 mg P.O. daily with breakfast or in divided doses if GI disturbances occur. First dosage increased after 5 to 7 days because of extended duration of action; then increased q 3 to 5 days by 50 to 125 mg, if needed, to maximum of 750 mg daily. Some patients with mild diabetes respond well to dosages of 100 mg or less daily. *Adults over age 65:* initially, 100 to 125 mg P.O. daily.
▶ **To change from insulin to oral therapy.** *Adults:* if insulin dosage is less than 40 units daily, insulin stopped and oral therapy started as above. If insulin dosage is 40 units or more daily, oral therapy started as above with insulin reduced 50%. Insulin dosage reduced further based on patient response.

How supplied
Tablets: 100 mg, 250 mg

Pharmacokinetics
Absorption: absorbed readily from GI tract.
Distribution: unknown, although it's highly protein-bound.

Metabolism: about 80% of drug is metabolized by liver.
Excretion: excreted in urine. Rate of excretion depends on urinary pH; it increases in alkaline urine and decreases in acidic urine. *Half-life:* 36 hours.

Route	Onset	Peak	Duration
P.O.	1 hr	3-6 hr	< 60 hr

Pharmacodynamics

Chemical effect: unknown. A sulfonylurea that may stimulate insulin release from pancreatic beta cells, reduce glucose output by liver, and increase peripheral sensitivity to insulin. Also exerts antidiuretic effect in patients with diabetes insipidus.
Therapeutic effect: lowers blood glucose level; also promotes water excretion in patients with diabetes insipidus.

Adverse reactions

GI: nausea, heartburn, vomiting.
GU: tea-colored urine.
Hematologic: ***thrombocytopenia, aplastic anemia, agranulocytosis.***
Metabolic: ***prolonged hypoglycemia, dilutional hyponatremia.***
Skin: rash, pruritus, facial flushing.
Other: ***hypersensitivity reactions.***

Interactions

Drug-drug. *Anabolic steroids, chloramphenicol, clofibrate, guanethidine, MAO inhibitors, phenylbutazone, salicylates, sulfonamides:* increased hypoglycemic activity. Monitor blood glucose level.
Beta blockers, clonidine: prolonged hypoglycemic effect and masked symptoms of hypoglycemia. Use together cautiously.
Corticosteroids, glucagon, rifampin, thiazide diuretics: decreased hypoglycemic response. Monitor blood glucose level.
Hydantoins: increased blood levels of hydantoins. Monitor patient closely.
Oral anticoagulants: increased hypoglycemic activity or enhanced anticoagulant effect. Monitor blood glucose level and PT and INR.
Drug-herb. *Aloe, bitter melon, bilberry leaf, burdock, dandelion, fenugreek, garlic, ginseng:* may improve blood glucose control and allow reduced dosage of oral antidiabetic. Tell patient to discuss use of herbal remedies with prescriber before using them.
Drug-lifestyle. *Alcohol use:* possible disulfiram-like reaction. Discourage concurrent use.

Contraindications and precautions

- Contraindicated in patients with type 1 (insulin-dependent) diabetes mellitus or diabetes that can be adequately controlled by diet. Also contraindicated in patients with type 2 diabetes complicated by ketosis, acidosis, diabetic coma, major surgery, severe infections, or severe trauma.
- Contraindicated in pregnant patients, breast-feeding patients, and patients hypersensitive to drug.
- Use cautiously in debilitated patients, malnourished patients, elderly patients, and patients with porphyria or impaired hepatic or renal function.
- Safety of drug hasn't been established in children.

NURSING CONSIDERATIONS

Assessment

- Assess patient's diabetes mellitus before therapy.
- Monitor effectiveness by checking patient's blood glucose level regularly and monitoring patient for signs and symptoms of hyperglycemia which may indicate drug is ineffective.
- Monitor patient's hemoglobin A_{1C} regularly as ordered.
- Monitor serum alkaline phosphatase levels routinely, as ordered. Progressive increases may indicate need to discontinue drug.
- Be alert for adverse reactions and drug interactions. Be aware adverse effects of chlorpropamide, especially hypoglycemia, may be more frequent or severe than with some other sulfonylureas because of its long duration of action.
- If hypoglycemia occurs, monitor patient closely for at least 3 to 5 days.
- Evaluate patient's and family's knowledge of drug therapy.

Nursing diagnoses
- Ineffective health maintenance related to hyperglycemia
- Risk for injury related to drug-induced hypoglycemia
- Deficient knowledge related to drug therapy

Planning and implementation
- Administer once-daily doses with breakfast; divided doses are usually given before morning and evening meals.
- Notify prescriber if blood glucose levels remain elevated or frequent episodes of hypoglycemia occur.
- Treat hypoglycemic reaction with oral form of rapid-acting glucose if patient can swallow or with glucagon or I.V. glucose if patient can't swallow. Give complex carbohydrate snack when patient is awake and determine cause of reaction.

ALERT Don't confuse chlorpropamide with chlorpromazine.

Patient teaching
- Instruct patient about nature of disease, importance of following therapeutic regimen, adhering to specific diet, losing weight, getting exercise, following personal hygiene programs, and avoiding infection. Explain how and when to monitor blood glucose level, and teach recognition of and intervention for hypoglycemia and hyperglycemia.
- Make sure patient understands that therapy relieves symptoms but doesn't cure disease.
- Tell patient not to change dosage without prescriber's consent, and to report abnormal blood or urine glucose test results.
- Instruct patient to carry candy or other simple sugars to treat mild hypoglycemic episodes. Severe episodes may need hospital treatment.
- Advise patient not to take other medications, including OTC drugs, without first checking with prescriber.
- Advise patient to avoid alcohol. Chlorpropamide-alcohol flush is characterized by facial flushing, light-headedness, headache, and occasional breathlessness. Even very small amounts of alcohol can produce this reaction.
- Advise patient to wear or carry medical identification indicating that he has diabetes.
- Teach patient about hypoglycemia; symptoms may be especially difficult to recognize in elderly patients and in patients taking beta blockers.

Evaluation
- Patient's blood glucose level is normal with drug therapy.
- Patient doesn't experience injury as a result of drug-induced hypoglycemia.
- Patient and family state understanding of drug therapy.

chlorzoxazone
(klor-ZOKS-uh-zohn)
Paraflex, Parafon Forte DSC, Remular-S

Pharmacologic class: benzoxazole derivative
Therapeutic class: skeletal muscle relaxant
Pregnancy risk category: C

Indications and dosages
▶ **As adjunct in acute, painful musculoskeletal conditions.** *Adults:* 250 to 750 mg P.O. t.i.d. or q.i.d.

How supplied
Tablets: 250 mg, 500 mg
Caplets: 500 mg

Pharmacokinetics
Absorption: rapidly and completely absorbed from GI tract.
Distribution: widely distributed in body.
Metabolism: metabolized in liver to inactive metabolites.
Excretion: excreted in urine as glucuronide metabolite. *Half-life:* 1 to 2 hours.

Route	Onset	Peak	Duration
P.O.	1 hr	1-2 hr	3-4 hr

Pharmacodynamics
Chemical effect: unknown. Appears to modify central perception of pain without modifying pain reflexes. Blocks interneuronal activity in

descending reticular activating system and in spinal cord.
Therapeutic effect: relaxes skeletal muscles.

Adverse reactions

CNS: *drowsiness, dizziness, light-headedness,* malaise, headache, overstimulation, tremor.
GI: anorexia, nausea, vomiting, heartburn, abdominal distress, constipation, diarrhea.
GU: urine discoloration (orange or purple-red).
Hematologic: anemia, ***agranulocytosis.***
Hepatic: hepatic dysfunction.
Skin: urticaria, redness, itching, petechiae, bruising.
Other: ***anaphylaxis.***

Interactions

Drug-drug. *CNS depressants:* increased CNS depression. Avoid concomitant use.
Drug-lifestyle. *Alcohol use:* increased CNS depression. Discourage use together.

Contraindications and precautions

- Contraindicated in patients hypersensitive to drug and in those with impaired hepatic function.
- Use cautiously in patients with history of drug allergies and in pregnant or breast-feeding women.

NURSING CONSIDERATIONS

Assessment

- Assess patient's underlying condition before therapy.
- Monitor effectiveness by regularly assessing severity and frequency of muscle spasms.
- Amount of relief determines if dosage (and drowsiness) can be reduced.
- Be alert for adverse reactions and drug interactions.
- Evaluate patient's and family's knowledge of drug therapy.

Nursing diagnoses

- Acute pain related to patient's underlying condition
- Risk for injury related to drug-induced adverse CNS reactions
- Deficient knowledge related to drug therapy

Planning and implementation

- Administer drug with meals or milk to prevent GI distress.
- Withhold dose and notify prescriber of unusual reactions.

Patient teaching

- Tell patient to avoid activities that require mental alertness, such as driving, until full CNS effects of drug are known.
- Advise patient to avoid combining drug with alcohol or other CNS depressants.
- Instruct patient to take drug with food or milk to prevent GI distress.
- Tell patient that drug may discolor urine orange or purple-red.
- Advise patient to follow prescriber's orders regarding physical activity.

Evaluation

- Patient reports that pain has decreased or ceased as result of chlorzoxazone therapy.
- Patient doesn't experience injury as result of drug-induced adverse CNS reactions.
- Patient and family state understanding of drug therapy.

cholestyramine

(koh-leh-STIGH-ruh-meen)
LoCHOLEST, Prevalite, Questran**, Questran Light, Questran Lite ◇

Pharmacologic class: anion exchange resin
Therapeutic class: antilipemic, bile acid sequestrant
Pregnancy risk category: C

Indications and dosages

▶ **Primary hyperlipidemia or pruritus caused by partial bile obstruction; adjunct for reduction of elevated serum cholesterol level in patients with primary hypercholesterolemia.** *Adults:* 4 g P.O. once or twice daily. Maintenance dosage is 8 to 16 g P.O. daily. Maximum daily dosage is 24 g P.O.

How supplied

Powder: 78-g cans, 9-g single-dose packets. Each scoop of powder or single-dose packet contains 4 g of cholestyramine resin.

Pharmacokinetics

Absorption: drug isn't absorbed.
Distribution: none.
Metabolism: none.
Excretion: insoluble cholestyramine with bile acid complex is excreted in feces.

Route	Onset	Peak	Duration
P.O.	1-2 wk	Unknown	2-4 wk

Pharmacodynamics

Chemical effect: a bile-acid sequestrant that combines with bile acid to form insoluble compound that is excreted. The liver must synthesize new bile acid from cholesterol, which reduces low-density-lipoprotein cholesterol levels.
Therapeutic effect: lowers blood cholesterol levels and relieves itching caused by partial bile obstruction.

Adverse reactions

GI: *constipation,* fecal impaction, hemorrhoids, *abdominal discomfort,* flatulence, *nausea,* vomiting, steatorrhea.
Metabolic: *vitamin A, D, E, and K deficiency;* hyperchloremic acidosis (with long-term use or very high dosage).
Skin: *rash;* irritation of skin, tongue, and perianal area.

Interactions

Drug-drug. *Acetaminophen, beta blockers, cardiac glycosides, corticosteroids, fat-soluble vitamins (A, D, E, and K), iron preparations, thiazide diuretics, thyroid hormones, warfarin and other coumarin derivatives:* absorption may be substantially decreased by cholestyramine. Administer at least 2 hours apart.

Contraindications and precautions

- Contraindicated in patients hypersensitive to bile-acid sequestering resins and in patients with complete biliary obstruction.
- Use cautiously in patients at risk for constipation and those with conditions aggravated by constipation, such as severe, symptomatic coronary artery disease.
- Use cautiously in pregnant or breast-feeding women because of possible interference with fat-soluble vitamin absorption.
- Safety of drug hasn't been established for children.

NURSING CONSIDERATIONS

Assessment

- Assess patient's blood cholesterol level and pruritus before therapy.
- Monitor effectiveness by checking serum cholesterol and triglyceride levels every 4 weeks, as ordered, or asking patient if pruritus has diminished or abated.
- Be alert for adverse reactions and drug interactions.
- Monitor patient for fat-soluble vitamin deficiency because long-term use may be linked to deficiency of vitamins A, D, E, and K and folic acid.
- Evaluate patient's and family's knowledge of drug therapy.

Nursing diagnoses

- Risk for injury related to elevated cholesterol levels
- Constipation related to drug-induced adverse GI reactions
- Deficient knowledge related to drug therapy

Planning and implementation

- To mix powder, sprinkle on surface of preferred beverage or wet food (soup, applesauce, crushed pineapple). Let stand a few minutes, then stir to obtain uniform suspension. Mixing with carbonated beverages may result in excess foaming. Use large glass and mix slowly.
- Administer drug before meals and at bedtime.
- If drug therapy is discontinued, adjust dosage of cardiac glycosides, as ordered and applicable, to avoid toxicity.
- If severe constipation develops, decrease dosage, add stool softener, or discontinue drug, as ordered.
- Administer all other drugs at least 1 hour before or 4 to 6 hours after cholestyramine to avoid blocking their absorption.

Patient teaching

- Instruct patient never to take drug in its dry form; esophageal irritation or severe constipation may result. Using large glass, patient should sprinkle powder on surface of preferred beverage; let mixture stand a few minutes; then stir thoroughly. The best diluents are water, milk, and juice (especially pulpy fruit juice). Mixing with carbonated beverages may result in excess foaming. After drinking this preparation, patient should swirl small additional amount of liquid in same glass and then drink it to ensure ingestion of entire dose.
- Advise patient to take all other drugs at least 1 hour before or 4 to 6 hours after cholestyramine to avoid blocking their absorption.
- Teach patient about proper dietary management of serum lipids (restricting total fat and cholesterol intake), as well as measures to control other cardiac disease risk factors.
- When appropriate, recommend weight control, exercise, and smoking cessation programs.

☑ Evaluation

- Patient's blood cholesterol level is normal with drug therapy.
- Patient maintains normal bowel patterns throughout drug therapy.
- Patient and family state understanding of drug therapy.

cidofovir

(sigh-doh-FOH-veer)

Vistide

Pharmacologic class: inhibitor of viral DNA synthesis
Therapeutic class: antiviral
Pregnancy risk category: C

Indications and dosages

▶ **CMV retinitis in patients with AIDS.** *Adults:* 5 mg/kg I.V. infused over 1 hour once weekly for 2 consecutive weeks, followed by a maintenance dose of 5 mg/kg I.V. infused over 1 hour once q 2 weeks. Probenecid and prehydration with normal saline solution I.V. must be given concomitantly and may reduce risk of nephrotoxicity. Dosage may need adjustment in patients with renal impairment.

How supplied

Injection: 75 mg/ml in 5-ml ampule

Pharmacokinetics

Absorption: not applicable with I.V. administration.
Distribution: less than 6% plasma protein–bound.
Metabolism: mainly by kidneys.
Excretion: by renal tubular secretion.

Route	Onset	Peak	Duration
I.V.	Unknown	Unknown	Unknown

Pharmacodynamics

Chemical effect: selective inhibition of CMV DNA polymerase; inhibits DNA viral synthesis.
Therapeutic effect: reduces rate of CMV replication.

Adverse reactions

CNS: *asthenia, headache*, amnesia, anxiety, confusion, ***seizures,*** depression, dizziness, malaise, abnormal gait, hallucinations, insomnia, neuropathy, paresthesia, somnolence.
CV: hypotension, orthostatic hypotension, pallor, syncope, tachycardia, vasodilation.
EENT: amblyopia, conjunctivitis, eye disorders, *ocular hypotony*, iritis, pharyngitis, retinal detachment, rhinitis, sinusitis, uveitis, abnormal vision.
GI: *nausea, vomiting, diarrhea, anorexia, abdominal pain,* dry mouth, taste perversion, colitis, constipation, tongue discoloration, dyspepsia, dysphagia, flatulence, gastritis, melena, oral candidiasis, rectal disorders, stomatitis, aphthous stomatitis, mouth ulcerations.
GU: *elevated creatinine levels, nephrotoxicity, proteinuria,* decreased creatinine clearance levels, glycosuria, hematuria, urinary incontinence, urinary tract infection.
Hematologic: ***neutropenia, thrombocytopenia,*** *anemia.*
Hepatic: hepatomegaly, abnormal liver function test results, increased alkaline phosphatase levels.

Respiratory: asthma, bronchitis, coughing, *dyspnea*, hiccups, increased sputum, lung disorders, pneumonia.
Metabolic: fluid imbalance, hyperglycemia, hyperlipemia, hypocalcemia, hypokalemia, weight loss, decreased serum bicarbonate level.
Musculoskeletal: arthralgia, myasthenia, myalgia, pain in back, chest, or neck.
Skin: *rash, alopecia*, acne, skin discoloration, dry skin, herpes simplex, pruritus, sweating, urticaria.
Other: *fever, infections, chills,* allergic reactions, facial edema, ***sarcoma, sepsis***.

Interactions

Drug-drug. *Nephrotoxic drugs (such as aminoglycosides, amphotericin B, foscarnet, I.V. pentamidine):* may increase nephrotoxicity. Avoid concomitant use.
Probenecid: interacts with metabolism or renal tubular excretion of many drugs. Monitor patient closely.

Contraindications and precautions

- Contraindicated in patients hypersensitive to drug and in those with history of clinically severe hypersensitivity to probenecid or other sulfa-containing drug. Don't give drug to breast-feeding women or as intraocular injection.
- Use cautiously in patients with impaired renal function.

NURSING CONSIDERATIONS

Assessment

- Monitor WBC counts with differential and renal function before each dose.
- Monitor intraocular pressure, visual acuity, and ocular symptoms periodically.
- Don't use drug in patients with baseline serum creatinine above 1.5 mg/dl or calculated creatinine clearance of 55 ml/minute or below unless potential benefits outweigh risks.
- Evaluate patient's and family's knowledge of drug therapy.

Nursing diagnoses

- Infection related to presence of virus
- Ineffective protection related to adverse renal reactions
- Deficient knowledge related to drug therapy

Planning and implementation

- Use I.V. prehydration with normal saline solution, and give probenecid with each cidofovir infusion, as ordered.
- Administer 1 L of normal saline solution, as ordered, usually over 1- to 2-hour period immediately before each cidofovir infusion.
- To prepare drug for infusion, remove appropriate amount of drug from vial using syringe, and transfer dose to an infusion bag containing 100 ml of normal saline solution. Infuse entire volume I.V. at constant rate over 1 hour. Use a standard infusion pump.
- Prepare drug in a class II laminar flow biological safety cabinet.
- Cidofovir infusion admixtures should be given within 24 hours of preparation. Let drug reach room temperature before use.

Patient teaching

- Inform patient that drug doesn't cure CMV retinitis and that regular ophthalmologic follow-up examinations are needed.
- Explain that close monitoring of renal function is critical.
- Tell patient to take probenecid with food to reduce drug-related nausea and vomiting.
- Advise men to practice barrier contraception during and for 3 months after drug treatment.

Evaluation

- Patient's infection is eradicated.
- Patient doesn't experience serious renal reactions.
- Patient and family state understanding of drug therapy.

cilostazol

(sil-OS-tah-zol)
Pletal

Pharmacologic class: quinolinone phosphodiesterase inhibitor
Therapeutic class: antiplatelet drug
Pregnancy risk category: C

Indications and dosages

▶ **Reduction of symptoms of intermittent claudication.** *Adults:* 100 mg P.O. b.i.d. taken at least 30 minutes before or 2 hours after breakfast and dinner. Decrease dosage to 50 mg P.O. b.i.d during coadministration with drugs that may interact to increase serum cilostazol levels.

How supplied

Tablets: 50 mg, 100 mg

Pharmacokinetics

Absorption: cilostazol is absorbed following oral administration. Absolute bioavailability is unknown.
Distribution: drug is highly protein-bound, primarily to albumin.
Metabolism: in the liver, cytochrome P-450 enzyme system (primarily CYP3A4) extensively metabolizes the drug. There are two active metabolites, one of which accounts for at least 50% of pharmacologic activity.
Excretion: drug is eliminated primarily through urine excretion of metabolites (74%). The remainder of the drug is eliminated in feces (20%). The half-life of cilostazol and its active metabolites is 11 to 13 hours.

Route	Onset	Peak	Duration
P.O.	Unknown	2-4 hr	Unknown

Pharmacodynamics

Chemical effect: not fully understood. Drug is thought to inhibit the enzyme phosphodiesterase III, causing an increase of cAMP in platelets and blood vessels, thus inhibiting platelet aggregation. Cilostazol reversibly inhibits the aggregation of platelets induced by various stimuli. Drug also has a vasodilating effect that's greatest in the femoral vascular beds.
Therapeutic effect: reduction of symptoms of intermittent claudication.

Adverse reactions

CNS: *headache, dizziness,* vertigo.
CV: *palpitations,* tachycardia, peripheral edema.
EENT: *pharyngitis, rhinitis.*
GI: *abnormal stools, diarrhea,* dyspepsia, abdominal pain, flatulence, nausea.
Musculoskeletal: back pain, myalgia.
Respiratory: increased cough.
Other: *infection.*

Interactions

Drug-drug. *Diltiazem:* increased plasma cilostazol levels. Reduce cilostazol dosage to 50 mg b.i.d. as directed.
Erythromycin, other macrolides: increased levels of serum cilostazol and one of the metabolites. Reduce cilostazol dosage to 50 mg b.i.d. as directed.
Omeprazole: increased serum levels of active cilostazol metabolite. Reduce cilostazol dosage to 50 mg b.i.d. as directed.
Strong inhibitors of CYP3A4, such as fluconazole, fluoxetine, fluvoxamine, itraconazole, ketoconazole, miconazole, nefazodone, sertraline: possible increased levels of cilostazol and its metabolites. Reduce cilostazol dosage to 50 mg b.i.d. as directed.
Drug-food. *Grapefruit juice:* increased cilostazol levels. Tell patient to avoid grapefruit juice during therapy.
Drug-lifestyle. *Smoking:* may decrease cilostazol exposure by about 20%. Monitor patient closely.

Contraindications and precautions

- Contraindicated in patients with heart failure and in those hypersensitive to cilostazol or its components.
- Use cautiously in patients with severe underlying heart disease and in combination with other drugs that have antiplatelet activity.

NURSING CONSIDERATIONS

Assessment

- Obtain history of patient's underlying condition before therapy, and reassess regularly thereafter.
- Cilostazol and similar drugs that inhibit the enzyme phosphodiesterase decrease the likelihood of survival in patients with class III and IV heart failure. Cilostazol is contraindicated in patients with heart failure of any severity.
- Make sure patient has a thorough physical examination before therapy starts.
- Be alert for adverse reactions and drug interactions.
- Evaluate patient's and family's knowledge of drug therapy.

Nursing diagnoses
- Acute pain related to underlying disease
- Ineffective peripheral tissue perfusion secondary to underlying disease
- Deficient knowledge related to drug therapy

Planning and implementation
- Give drug at least 30 minutes before or 2 hours after breakfast and dinner.
- Use cautiously in patients with severe underlying heart disease and in combination with other drugs having antiplatelet activity.
- Beneficial effects may not be apparent for up to 12 weeks following start of therapy.
- Dosage of cilostazol can be reduced or discontinued without such rebound effects as platelet hyperaggregability. Notify prescriber of coagulation studies.
- Drug may cause reduced triglyceride levels and increased high-density lipoprotein levels.

Patient teaching
- Instruct patient to take cilostazol on an empty stomach, at least 30 minutes before or 2 hours after breakfast and dinner.
- Tell patient that the beneficial effect of cilostazol on intermittent claudication isn't likely to be noticed for 2 to 4 weeks and that it may take as long as 12 weeks.
- Instruct patient to avoid consuming grapefruit juice while taking this drug.
- Inform patient that CV risk is unknown in patients who use the drug on a long-term basis and in patients who have severe underlying heart disease.
- Tell patient that drug may cause dizziness. Caution patient not to drive or perform other activities that require alertness until response to drug is known.

Evaluation
- Patient experiences a decrease in pain.
- Patient has adequate tissue perfusion.
- Patient and family state understanding of drug therapy.

cimetidine
(sih-MEH-tih-deen)
Tagamet, Cimetatidine, Tagamet HB†

Pharmacologic class: H_2-receptor antagonist
Therapeutic class: antiulcer agent
Pregnancy risk category: B

Indications and dosages
▶ **Duodenal ulcer (short-term treatment).** *Adults and children age 16 and over:* 800 mg P.O. h.s. Or, 400 mg P.O. b.i.d. or 300 mg q.i.d. (with meals and h.s.). Treatment continued for 4 to 6 weeks unless endoscopy shows healing. For maintenance therapy, 400 mg h.s. For parenteral therapy, 300 mg diluted to 20 ml with normal saline solution or other compatible I.V. solution by I.V. push over at least 5 minutes q 6 hours. Or, 300 mg diluted in 100 ml D_5W or other compatible I.V. solution by I.V. infusion over 15 to 20 minutes q 6 hours. Or, 300 mg I.M. q 6 hours (no dilution necessary). Parenteral dosage increased by giving 300-mg doses more frequently to maximum daily dosage of 2,400 mg as needed. Or, 900 mg/day (37.5 mg/hour) I.V. diluted in 100 to 1,000 ml of compatible solution by continuous I.V. infusion.

▶ **Active benign gastric ulceration.** *Adults:* 800 mg P.O. h.s., or 300 mg P.O. q.i.d., with meals and h.s., for up to 8 weeks.

▶ **Pathologic hypersecretory conditions (such as Zollinger-Ellison syndrome, systemic mastocytosis, and multiple endocrine adenomas).** *Adults and children age 16 and over:* 300 mg P.O. q.i.d. with meals and h.s.; adjusted to patient needs. Maximum oral daily dosage is 2,400 mg. For parenteral therapy, 300 mg diluted to 20 ml with normal saline solution or other compatible I.V. solution by I.V. push over at least 5 minutes q 6 hours. Or, 300 mg diluted in 100 ml D_5W or other compatible I.V. solution by I.V. infusion over 15 to 20 minutes q 6 hours. Parenteral dosage increased by giving 300-mg doses more frequently to maximum daily dosage of 2,400 mg as needed.

▶ **Gastroesophageal reflux disease.** *Adults:* 800 mg P.O. b.i.d. or 400 mg q.i.d. before meals and h.s. for up to 12 weeks.

▶ **Prevention of upper GI bleeding in critically ill patients.** *Adults:* 50 mg/hour by continuous I.V. infusion for up to 7 days; 25 mg/hour to patients with creatinine clearance below 30 ml/minute.

▶ **Heartburn.** Adults: 200 mg (Tagamet HB only) P.O. with water as symptoms occur, or as directed, up to b.i.d. Maximum 400 mg/day. Drug shouldn't be taken daily for more than 2 weeks.

How supplied

Tablets: 200 mg ◇, 300 mg, 400 mg, 800 mg
Oral liquid: 300 mg/5 ml
Injection: 150 mg/ml; 300 mg in 50 ml normal saline solution for injection

Pharmacokinetics

Absorption: 60% to 75% of oral dose is absorbed. Absorption rate but not extent may be affected by food. Degree of absorption unknown after I.M. administration.
Distribution: distributed to many body tissues. About 15% to 20% of drug is protein-bound.
Metabolism: 30% to 40% of dose is metabolized in liver.
Excretion: excreted primarily in urine (48% of oral dose, 75% of parenteral dose); 10% of oral dose excreted in feces. Half-life: 2 hours.

Route	Onset	Peak	Duration
P.O.	Unknown	45-90 min	4-5 hr
I.V.	Unknown	Immediate	Unknown
I.M.	Unknown	Unknown	Unknown

Pharmacodynamics

Chemical effect: competitively inhibits action of H_2 at receptor sites of parietal cells, decreasing gastric acid secretion.
Therapeutic effect: lessens upper GI irritation caused by increased gastric acid secretion.

Adverse reactions

CNS: confusion, dizziness, headaches, peripheral neuropathy.
CV: ***bradycardia.***
GI: *mild and transient diarrhea.*
GU: transient elevations in serum creatinine levels.
Hematologic: ***agranulocytosis, neutropenia, thrombocytopenia, aplastic anemia.***
Hepatic: jaundice.
Musculoskeletal: muscle pain.
Skin: acnelike rash, urticaria.
Other: hypersensitivity reactions, mild gynecomastia (if used longer than 1 month).

Interactions

Drug-drug. *Antacids:* interference with cimetidine absorption. Separate administration by at least 1 hour if possible.
Lidocaine, phenytoin, propranolol, some benzodiazepines, warfarin: inhibited hepatic microsomal enzyme metabolism of these drugs. Monitor serum levels of these drugs.
Drug-herb. *Pennyroyal:* may change the rate at which toxic metabolites of pennyroyal form.
Yerba maté: may decrease clearance of yerba maté methylxanthines and cause toxicity. Tell patient to use together cautiously.

Contraindications and precautions

- Contraindicated in patients hypersensitive to drug and in breast-feeding women.
- Use cautiously in pregnant women and in elderly or debilitated patients because they may be more susceptible to drug-induced confusion.
- Safety of drug hasn't been established in children under age 16.

NURSING CONSIDERATIONS

Assessment

- Assess patient's underlying upper GI condition before therapy, and reassess regularly throughout therapy.
- Be alert for adverse reactions and drug interactions.
- Identify tablet strength when obtaining drug history.
- Monitor patient's CV status during I.V. administration; drug can cause profound bradycardia and other cardiotoxic effects when given too rapidly I.V.
- Evaluate patient's and family's knowledge of drug therapy.

Nursing diagnoses

- Impaired tissue integrity related to patient's underlying condition
- Diarrhea related to drug-induced adverse reaction
- Deficient knowledge related to drug therapy

Planning and implementation

P.O. use: Give tablets with meals to ensure more consistent therapeutic effect.
I.V. use: Dilute drug before direct injection and give over 5 minutes.
ALERT Rapid I.V. injection may result in arrhythmias and hypotension. Infuse drug over at least 30 minutes to minimize risk of adverse cardiac effects.
– If cimetidine is given as continuous I.V. infusion, use infusion pump if giving in a total volume of 250 ml over 24 hours or less.
– Don't dilute with sterile water for injection.
I.M. use: I.M. administration may be painful.
- Schedule cimetidine dose at end of hemodialysis treatment. Hemodialysis reduces blood levels of cimetidine. Adjust dosage as ordered in patients with renal failure.

ALERT Don't confuse cimetidine with simethicone.

Patient teaching

- Remind patient taking drug once daily to take it at bedtime for best results.
- Warn patient to take drug as directed and to continue taking it even after pain subsides, to allow for adequate healing.
- Remind patient not to take antacid within 1 hour of taking drug.
- Urge patient to avoid cigarette smoking because it may increase gastric acid secretion and worsen disease.
- Instruct patient to immediately report black tarry stools, diarrhea, confusion, or rash.

Evaluation

- Patient experiences decrease in or relief of upper GI symptoms with drug therapy.
- Patient maintains normal bowel habits throughout drug therapy.
- Patient and family state understanding of drug therapy.

cinoxacin

(sin-OKS-uh-sin)
Cinobac

Pharmacologic class: fluoroquinolone antibiotic
Therapeutic class: urinary tract antiseptic
Pregnancy risk category: B

Indications and dosages

▶ **Initial and recurrent urinary tract infections caused by susceptible strains of *Escherichia coli, Klebsiella, Enterobacter, Proteus mirabilis, P. vulgaris,* and *Citrobacter.*** *Adults and children over age 12:* 1 g P.O. daily, in two to four divided doses for 7 to 14 days.

How supplied

Capsules: 250 mg, 500 mg

Pharmacokinetics

Absorption: well absorbed from GI tract. Food decreases peak levels but not total absorption.
Distribution: drug concentrates in renal tissue; it's 60% to 80% protein-bound and has only fair prostatic penetration (30% to 60% of plasma levels).
Metabolism: 30% to 40% of drug is metabolized in liver to inactive compounds.
Excretion: inactive metabolites and unchanged drug are excreted in urine. *Half-life:* 1 to 1.5 hours.

Route	Onset	Peak	Duration
P.O.	Unknown	≤ 2 hr	≤ 12 hr (plasma) 2-4 hr (urine)

Pharmacodynamics

Chemical effect: inhibits microbial DNA synthesis.
Therapeutic effect: hinders or kills susceptible bacteria in urine. Spectrum of activity includes most strains of *E. coli, Klebsiella, Enterobacter, P. mirabilis,* and *P. vulgaris.*

Adverse reactions

CNS: *dizziness, headache,* drowsiness, insomnia, ***seizures.***
EENT: tinnitus.
GI: nausea, vomiting, abdominal pain, *diarrhea, distorted taste.*
Hematologic: ***thrombocytopenia.***
Hepatic: elevated liver enzyme levels.
Skin: rash, urticaria, pruritus, photosensitivity, ***Stevens-Johnson syndrome.***
Other: ***anaphylaxis.***

Interactions

Drug-drug. *Oral anticoagulants:* increased anticoagulant effect. Monitor patient for bleeding.
Probenecid: may decrease urine levels of cinoxacin by inhibiting renal tubular secretion. Monitor patient for increased toxicity and reduced antibacterial effectiveness.
Theophylline: increased effects of these drugs. Monitor theophylline levels.
Drug-lifestyle. *Caffeine:* increased effects of these drugs. Monitor patient for toxicity.

Contraindications and precautions

- Contraindicated in patients hypersensitive to drug or other fluoroquinolones; also contraindicated in breast-feeding women.
- Use cautiously in pregnant women and in patients with impaired renal and hepatic function.
- Safety of drug hasn't been established and isn't recommended for children under age 12.

NURSING CONSIDERATIONS

Assessment

- Assess patient's urinary tract infection before therapy, and reassess regularly throughout therapy.
- Obtain clean-catch urine specimen for culture and sensitivity tests before starting therapy, and repeat as needed. Therapy may begin pending results.
- Be alert for adverse reactions and drug interactions.
- Monitor patient's hydration status if adverse GI reactions occur.
- Evaluate patient's and family's knowledge of drug therapy.

Nursing diagnoses

- Infection related to presence of bacteria susceptible to drug therapy
- Risk for deficient fluid volume related to drug-induced adverse GI reactions
- Deficient knowledge related to drug therapy

Planning and implementation

- Give cinoxacin with meals to help decrease adverse GI reactions.
- High urine levels permit twice-daily dosing.
- Report adverse CNS reactions immediately, which indicate toxicity and usually mean that patient should stop taking drug.

Patient teaching

- Remind patient to take entire amount of this drug as prescribed, even when he feels better.
- Warn patient about photosensitizing effects of drug, and advise him to avoid bright sunlight and to wear sunblock.
- Warn patient to avoid driving and other hazardous tasks that require alertness until CNS effects of drug are known or until effects abate. Tell patient to notify prescriber if CNS reactions occur because drug may need to be discontinued.

Evaluation

- Patient is free from infection after drug therapy.
- Patient maintains adequate hydration throughout drug therapy.
- Patient and family state understanding of drug therapy.

ciprofloxacin

(sih-proh-FLOKS-uh-sin)
Cipro, Cipro I.V., Ciproxin ◇

Pharmacologic class: fluoroquinolone antibiotic
Therapeutic class: antibiotic
Pregnancy risk category: C

Indications and dosages

▶ **Mild to moderate urinary tract infections.** *Adults:* 250 mg P.O. or 200 mg I.V. q 12 hours.

▶ **Severe or complicated urinary tract infections; mild to moderate bone and joint infections; mild to moderate respiratory tract infections; mild to moderate skin and skin-structure infections; infectious diarrhea.** *Adults:* 500 mg P.O. or 400 mg I.V. q 12 hours.

▶ **Severe or complicated bone or joint infections; severe respiratory tract infections; severe skin and skin-structure infections.** *Adults:* 750 mg P.O. q 12 hours.

▶ **Treatment of mild to moderate acute sinusitis caused by *Haemophilus influenzae, Streptococcus pneumoniae,* or *Moraxella catarrhalis*; mild to moderate chronic bacterial prostatitis caused by *Escherichia coli* or *Proteus mirabilis*.** *Adults:* 400 mg I.V. infusion given over 60 minutes every 12 hours.

How supplied

Tablets: 250 mg, 500 mg, 750 mg
Infusion (premixed): 200 mg in 100 ml D_5W, 400 mg in 200 ml D_5W
Injection: 200 mg, 400 mg

Pharmacokinetics

Absorption: about 70% of drug absorbed after oral administration. Food delays rate of absorption but not extent.
Distribution: drug is 20% to 40% protein-bound. CSF levels are only about 10% of plasma levels.
Metabolism: unknown but probably hepatic. Four metabolites have been identified; each has less antimicrobial activity than parent compound.
Excretion: primarily renal. *Half-life:* about 4 hours.

Route	Onset	Peak	Duration
P.O.	Unknown	0.5-2.3 hr	Unknown
I.V.	Immediate	Immediate	Unknown

Pharmacodynamics

Chemical effect: unknown. Bactericidal effects may result from inhibition of bacterial DNA gyrase and prevention of replication in susceptible bacteria.
Therapeutic effect: kills susceptible bacteria. Spectrum of activity includes *Campylobacter jejuni, Citrobacter diversus, Citrobacter freundii, Enterobacter cloacae, E.coli, H. influenzae, Klebsiella pneumoniae, Morganella organii, P. mirabilis, P. vulgaris, Providencia stuartii, P. rettgeri, Pseudomonas aeruginosa, Serratia marcescens, Shigella flexneri, S. sonnei, Staphylococcus aureus, S. epidermidis, Streptococcus faecalis,* and *S. pyogenes.*

Adverse reactions

CNS: headache, restlessness, tremor, lightheadedness, confusion, hallucinations, ***seizures,*** paresthesia.
GI: *nausea, diarrhea,* vomiting, abdominal pain or discomfort, oral candidiasis.
GU: crystalluria, increased serum creatinine and BUN levels, interstitial nephritis.
Hematologic: eosinophilia, ***leukopenia, neutropenia, thrombocytopenia.***
Hepatic: elevated liver enzymes.
Musculoskeletal: arthralgia, joint or back pain, joint inflammation, joint stiffness, achiness, neck or chest pain.
Skin: *rash,* photosensitivity, ***Stevens-Johnson syndrome.***
Other: thrombophlebitis, burning, pruritus, erythema, swelling with I.V. administration.

Interactions

Drug-drug. *Antacids containing magnesium hydroxide or aluminum hydroxide, sucralfate, iron supplements:* decreased ciprofloxacin absorption. Separate administration by at least 2 hours.
Probenecid: may elevate serum level of ciprofloxacin. Monitor patient for toxicity.
Theophylline: increased plasma theophylline levels and prolonged theophylline half-life. Monitor blood levels of theophylline, and observe patient for adverse effects.
Drug-herb. *Yerba maté:* may decrease clearance of yerba maté methylxanthines and cause toxicity. Discourage concomitant use.
Drug-lifestyle. *Caffeine:* increased effect of caffeine. Monitor patient for toxicity.

Contraindications and precautions

- Contraindicated in breast-feeding women and in patients hypersensitive to fluoroquinolones.
- Use cautiously in patients with CNS disorders, such as severe cerebral arteriosclerosis or seizure disorders, and in those at increased risk for seizures. May cause CNS stimulation. Also, use cautiously in pregnant women.
- Safety of drug hasn't been established in children under age 18.

NURSING CONSIDERATIONS

Assessment

- Assess patient's infection before therapy, and reassess regularly throughout therapy.
- Obtain specimen for culture and sensitivity tests before first dose. Therapy may begin pending results.
- Be alert for adverse reactions and drug interactions.
- Monitor patient's hydration status if adverse GI reactions occur.
- Evaluate patient's and family's knowledge of drug therapy.

Nursing diagnoses

- Infection related to presence of bacteria susceptible to drug
- Risk for deficient fluid volume related to drug-induced adverse GI reactions
- Deficient knowledge related to drug therapy

Planning and implementation

P.O. use: Administer oral form 2 hours after meal or 2 hours before or after taking antacids, sucralfate, or products that contain iron (such as vitamins with mineral supplements). Food doesn't affect absorption but may delay peak serum levels.

I.V. use: Dilute drug using D_5W or normal saline solution for injection to final concentration of 1 to 2 mg/ml before use. Infuse slowly (over 1 hour) into large vein.

- Dosage adjustments are necessary in patients with renal dysfunction.
- Have patient drink plenty of fluids to reduce risk of crystalluria.

Patient teaching

- Tell patient to take drug 2 hours after meal and to take prescribed antacids at least 2 hours after taking drug.
- Advise patient to drink plenty of fluids to reduce risk of crystalluria.
- Warn patient to avoid hazardous tasks that require alertness, such as driving, until CNS effects of drug are known.
- Advise patient to avoid caffeine while taking drug because of potential for cumulative caffeine effects.
- Advise patient that hypersensitivity reactions may occur even after first dose. If he notices rash or other allergic reactions, tell him to stop drug immediately and notify prescriber.
- Instruct patient to either discontinue breast-feeding during treatment or take a different drug. Drug appears in breast milk.

Evaluation

- Patient is free from infection after drug therapy.
- Patient maintains adequate hydration throughout drug therapy.
- Patient and family state understanding of drug therapy.

cisplatin (cis-platinum)

(sis-PLAH-tin)

Platinol AQ

Pharmacologic class: alkylating agent (not specific to cell cycle phase)
Therapeutic class: antineoplastic
Pregnancy risk category: D

Indications and dosages

▶ **Adjunct therapy in metastatic testicular cancer.** *Adults:* 20 mg/m² I.V. daily for 5 days. Repeated q 3 weeks for three cycles or longer.
▶ **Adjunct therapy in metastatic ovarian cancer.** *Adults:* 100 mg/m² I.V.; repeated q 4 weeks. Or, 50 to 100 mg/m² I.V. once q 4 weeks in combination with cyclophosphamide.
▶ **Advanced bladder cancer.** *Adults:* 50 to 70 mg/m² I.V. q 3 to 4 weeks. Patients who have received other antineoplastic drugs or

radiation therapy should receive 50 mg/m^2 q 4 weeks.

How supplied

Injection: 0.5 mg/ml, 1 mg/ml

Pharmacokinetics

Absorption: not applicable.
Distribution: distributes widely into tissues, with highest levels in kidneys, liver, and prostate. Drug doesn't readily cross blood-brain barrier. Drug is extensively and irreversibly bound to plasma and tissue proteins.
Metabolism: unknown.
Excretion: excreted primarily unchanged in urine. *Half-life:* initial phase, 25 to 79 minutes; terminal phase, 58 to 78 hours.

Route	Onset	Peak	Duration
I.V.	Unknown	Unknown	Several days

Pharmacodynamics

Chemical effect: unknown. Probably cross-links strands of cellular DNA and interferes with RNA transcription, causing imbalance of growth that leads to cell death.
Therapeutic effect: kills selected cancer cells.

Adverse reactions

CNS: *peripheral neuritis,* ***seizures.***
EENT: *tinnitus, hearing loss.*
GI: *nausea and vomiting beginning 1 to 4 hours after dose and lasting 24 hours,* diarrhea, loss of taste, metallic taste.
GU: *more prolonged and* **SEVERE RENAL TOXICITY** *with repeated courses of therapy.*
Hematologic: **MILD MYELOSUPPRESSION,** ***leukopenia, thrombocytopenia, anemia,*** nadirs in circulating platelet and WBC counts on days 18 to 23 with recovery by day 39.
Metabolic: *hypomagnesemia,* hypokalemia, hypocalcemia.
Other: ***anaphylactoid reaction.***

Interactions

Drug-drug. *Aminoglycoside antibiotics:* additive nephrotoxicity. Monitor renal function studies carefully.
Bumetanide, ethacrynic acid, furosemide: additive ototoxicity. Avoid concomitant use.
Phenytoin: decreased serum phenytoin levels. Monitor serum levels.

Contraindications and precautions

- Contraindicated in patients hypersensitive to drug or other platinum-containing compounds. Also contraindicated in patients with severe renal disease, hearing impairment, or myelosuppression. Also not recommended for use in breast-feeding patients.
- Use with extreme caution and only when absolutely necessary in pregnant women because fetal harm may occur.
- Safety of drug hasn't been established in children.

NURSING CONSIDERATIONS

Assessment

- Assess patient's underlying neoplastic disease before therapy, and reassess regularly throughout therapy.
- Monitor CBC, electrolyte levels (especially potassium and magnesium), platelet count, and renal function studies before initial and subsequent dosages, as ordered.
- To detect permanent hearing loss, obtain audiometry test results before initial dose and subsequent courses, as ordered.
- Be alert for adverse reactions and drug interactions.
- Evaluate patient's and family's knowledge of drug therapy.

Nursing diagnoses

- Ineffective health maintenance related to presence of neoplastic disease
- Ineffective protection related to drug-induced adverse reactions
- Deficient knowledge related to drug therapy

Planning and implementation

- Follow facility policy to reduce risks because preparation and administration of parenteral form of drug is linked to carcinogenic, mutagenic, and teratogenic risks for personnel.
- As ordered, administer mannitol or furosemide boluses or infusions before and with cisplatin infusion to maintain diureses of 100 to

400 ml/hour during and for 24 hours after therapy. Prehydration and diuresis may reduce renal toxicity and ototoxicity significantly.
- Manufacturer recommends administering drug as I.V. infusion in 2 L of normal saline solution with 37.5 g of mannitol over 6 to 8 hours.
- Dilute with D_5W in one-third normal saline solution for injection or dextrose 5% in half-normal saline solution for injection. Solutions are stable for 20 hours at room temperature. Don't refrigerate.
- Infusions are most stable in chloride-containing solutions (such as normal, half-normal, and one-quarter saline solution).
- Don't use needles or I.V. administration sets that contain aluminum because it will displace platinum, causing loss of potency and formation of black precipitate.
- Renal toxicity is cumulative. Renal function must return to normal before next dose can be given.
- Dosage shouldn't be repeated unless platelet count is over 100,000/mm^3, WBC count is over 4,000/mm^3, creatinine level is under 1.5 mg/dl, or BUN level is under 25 mg/dl.
- Check current protocol. Some clinicians use I.V. sodium thiosulfate to minimize toxicity.
- Administer antiemetics as ordered. Nausea and vomiting may be severe and protracted (up to 24 hours). Provide I.V. hydration as ordered until patient can tolerate adequate oral intake.
- Ondansetron, granisetron, and high-dose metoclopramide have been used effectively to prevent and treat nausea and vomiting. Some clinicians combine metoclopramide with dexamethasone and antihistamines, or ondansetron or granisetron with dexamethasone.
- Delayed-onset vomiting (3 to 5 days after treatment) has been reported. Patients may need prolonged antiemetic treatment.
- To prevent hypokalemia, potassium chloride (10 to 20 mEq/L) is commonly added to I.V. fluids before and after cisplatin therapy.
- Immediately administer epinephrine, corticosteroids, or antihistamines for anaphylactoid reactions, as ordered.

ALERT Don't confuse cisplatin with carboplatin.

Patient teaching
- Warn patient to watch for signs of infection (fever, sore throat, fatigue) and bleeding (easy bruising, nosebleeds, bleeding gums, melena). Tell him to take his temperature daily.
- Tell patient to report tinnitus immediately.
- Instruct patient to avoid OTC products that contain aspirin.
- Teach patient to record intake and output on daily basis and to report edema or decrease in urine output.
- Encourage patient to notify prescriber if any concerns arise during drug therapy.

✓ Evaluation
- Patient exhibits positive response to cisplatin therapy according to follow-up diagnostic studies.
- Patient doesn't experience permanent injury as a result of drug-induced adverse reactions.
- Patient and family state understanding of drug therapy.

citalopram hydrobromide
(sih-TAL-oh-pram high-droh-BROH-mighd)
Celexa

Pharmacologic class: selective serotonin reuptake inhibitor (SSRI)
Therapeutic class: antidepressant
Pregnancy risk category: C

Indications and dosages
▶ **Depression.** *Adults:* initially, 20 mg P.O. once daily, increasing to maximum dose of 40 mg daily after no less than 1 week. *Elderly patients:* 20 mg P.O. daily with adjustment to 40 mg daily only for nonresponding patients.

How supplied
Tablets: 20 mg, 40 mg

Pharmacokinetics
Absorption: absolute bioavailability is 80%.
Distribution: about 80% bound to plasma proteins.
Metabolism: metabolized primarily by the liver.

Excretion: about 10% of drug is recovered in urine. *Half-life:* 35 hours.

Route	Onset	Peak	Duration
P.O.	Unknown	4 hr	Unknown

Pharmacodynamics

Chemical effect: probably enhances serotonergic activity in CNS resulting from its inhibition of CNS neuronal reuptake of serotonin.
Therapeutic effect: relieves depression.

Adverse reactions

CNS: tremor, *somnolence, insomnia*, anxiety, agitation, dizziness, paresthesia, migraine, impaired concentration, amnesia, depression, apathy, ***suicide attempt,*** confusion, fatigue.
CV: tachycardia, orthostatic hypotension, hypotension.
EENT: rhinitis, sinusitis, abnormal accommodation.
GI: *nausea, dry mouth,* diarrhea, anorexia, dyspepsia, vomiting, abdominal pain, increased saliva, taste perversion, flatulence, decreased and increased weight, increased appetite.
GU: dysmenorrhea, amenorrhea, ejaculation disorder, impotence, polyuria.
Musculoskeletal: arthralgia, myalgia.
Respiratory: upper respiratory tract infection, coughing.
Skin: rash, pruritus, *increased sweating*.
Other: fever, yawning, decreased libido.

Interactions

Drug-drug. *Carbamazepine:* may increase citalopram clearance. Monitor patient for toxicity.
CNS drugs: Increased CNS effects. Use together cautiously.
Drugs that inhibit cytochrome P-450 isoenzymes 3A4 (such as ketoconazole, erythromycin, fluconazole, itraconazole) and 2C19 (such as omeprazole): decreased citalopram clearance.
Imipramine, other tricyclic antidepressants: concentration of imipramine metabolite desipramine increased by about 50%. Use together cautiously.
Lithium: may enhance serotonergic effect of citalopram. Use with caution, and monitor lithium levels.
MAO inhibitors: serious, sometimes fatal, reactions may occur. Don't use drug with MAO inhibitors or within 14 days of stopping MAO inhibitor use.
Warfarin: PT increased by 5%. Monitor patient carefully.
Drug-herb. *St. John's wort:* serotonin levels may rise too high, causing serotonin syndrome. Discourage concomitant use.
Drug-lifestyle. *Alcohol use:* increased CNS effects. Discourage concomitant use.

Contraindications and precautions

- Contraindicated in patients taking MAO inhibitors or within 14 days of stopping MAO inhibitor therapy. Also contraindicated in patients hypersensitive to drug or its inactive ingredients.
- Use cautiously in patients with history of mania, seizures, suicidal ideation, hepatic impairment, or renal impairment.
- Safety and effectiveness haven't been established in children.

NURSING CONSIDERATIONS

Assessment

- Assess patient's underlying condition before therapy, and reassess regularly thereafter.
- Check vital signs regularly for decreased blood pressure or tachycardia.
- Closely supervise high-risk patients at start of drug therapy.
- Evaluate patient's and family's knowledge of drug therapy.

Nursing diagnoses

- Risk for injury related to patient's underlying condition
- Ineffective individual coping related to patient's underlying condition
- Deficient knowledge related to drug therapy

Planning and implementation

- A reduced dosage is indicated for elderly patients and in those with hepatic impairment.
- Don't give until at least 14 days have elapsed between stopping MAO inhibitor therapy and starting citalopram therapy.

ALERT Don't confuse Celexa with Celebrex or Cerebyx.

Patient teaching

- Inform patient that although improvement may occur within 1 to 4 weeks, he should continue therapy as prescribed.
- Instruct patient to exercise caution when operating hazardous machinery, including automobiles, because psychoactive drugs can impair judgment, thinking, and motor skills.
- Advise patient to consult prescriber before breast-feeding an infant or taking other prescription drugs, OTC medicines, or herbal remedies.

ALERT If the patient wishes to switch from an SSRI to St. John's wort, tell him to wait a few weeks for the SSRI to wash out of his system before he starts the herb. Urge him to ask his prescriber for advice.

- Warn patient not to consume alcohol during therapy.
- Instruct woman of childbearing age to use birth control during drug therapy and to notify prescriber immediately if she suspects pregnancy.

Evaluation

- Patient's safety is maintained.
- Patient's condition is improved with drug.
- Patient and family state understanding of drug therapy.

cladribine (2-chlorodeoxyadenosine)

(klah-DRIGH-been)

Leustatin

Pharmacologic class: purine nucleoside analogue
Therapeutic class: antineoplastic
Pregnancy risk category: D

Indications and dosages

▶ **Active hairy cell leukemia.** *Adults:* 0.09 mg/kg daily by continuous I.V. infusion for 7 days.

How supplied

Injection: 1 mg/ml

Pharmacokinetics

Absorption: not applicable .
Distribution: about 20% of drug is bound to plasma proteins.
Metabolism: unknown.
Excretion: unknown. *Half-life:* 5.4 hours.

Route	Onset	Peak	Duration
I.V.	4 mo	Unknown	> 8 mo

Pharmacodynamics

Chemical effect: unknown. A purine nucleoside analogue that enters tumor cells, is phosphorylated by deoxycytidine kinase, and is subsequently converted into active triphosphate deoxynucleotide. This metabolite probably impairs synthesis of new DNA, inhibits repair of existing DNA, and disrupts cellular metabolism.
Therapeutic effect: kills selected cancer cells.

Adverse reactions

CNS: headache, fatigue, dizziness, insomnia, asthenia, malaise.
CV: tachycardia, edema.
EENT: epistaxis.
GI: nausea, decreased appetite, vomiting, diarrhea, constipation, abdominal pain.
GU: acute renal insufficiency.
Hematologic: NEUTROPENIA, ***anemia, thrombocytopenia.***
Metabolic: hyperuricemia.
Musculoskeletal: trunk pain, myalgia, arthralgia.
Respiratory: abnormal breath or chest sounds, cough, shortness of breath.
Skin: *rash, pruritus, erythema,* purpura, petechiae, diaphoresis.
Other: fever, **INFECTION,** local reactions at the injection site, chills.

Interactions

None significant.

Contraindications and precautions

- Contraindicated in patients hypersensitive to drug and in breast-feeding women.
- Use with extreme caution and only if absolutely necessary in pregnant women because fetal harm may occur.

• Use cautiously in patients with renal or hepatic impairment.
• Safety of drug hasn't been established in children.

NURSING CONSIDERATIONS

Assessment

• Assess patient's underlying neoplastic disease before therapy and reassess regularly throughout therapy.
• Monitor hematologic function closely as ordered, especially during first 4 to 8 weeks of therapy.
• Be alert for adverse reactions and drug interactions.
• Evaluate patient's and family's knowledge of drug therapy.

Nursing diagnoses

• Ineffective health maintenance related to presence of neoplastic disease
• Ineffective protection related to drug-induced hematologic adverse reactions
• Deficient knowledge related to drug therapy

Planning and implementation

• For 24-hour infusion, add calculated dose to 500-ml infusion bag of normal saline solution for injection. Once diluted, administer promptly or begin administration within 8 hours. Don't use solution that contains dextrose because it may increase degradation of drug. Because drug doesn't contain bacteriostatic agents, use strict aseptic technique to prepare admixture. Repeat daily for 7 consecutive days.
• Alternatively, prepare 7-day infusion solution using bacteriostatic saline injection, which contains 0.9% benzyl alcohol. Studies have shown acceptable physical and chemical stability using Pharmacia Deltec medication cassettes. First, pass calculated amount of drug through disposable 0.22-micron hydrophilic syringe filter into sterile infusion reservoir. Next, add sufficient bacteriostatic saline injection to bring total volume to 100 ml. Clamp line; then disconnect and discard filter. If necessary, aseptically aspirate air bubbles from reservoir using new filter or sterile vent filter assembly.
• Because calculated dose dilutes benzyl alcohol preservative, 7-day infusion solutions prepared for patients weighing more than 85 kg (187 lb) may have reduced preservative effectiveness.
• Refrigerate unopened vials at 36° to 46° F (2° to 8° C) and protect from light. Although freezing doesn't adversely affect drug, precipitate may form; it will disappear if drug is allowed to warm to room temperature gradually and vial is vigorously shaken. Don't heat or microwave; don't refreeze.
• Because of risk of hyperuricemia from tumor lysis, administer allopurinol as ordered during therapy.
• Fever is commonly observed during first month of therapy. In clinical trials, virtually all patients received parenteral antibiotics.

Patient teaching

• Warn patient to watch for signs of infection (fever, sore throat, fatigue) and bleeding (easy bruising, nosebleeds, bleeding gums, melena). Tell patient to take his temperature daily.
• Teach patient about infection control and bleeding precautions.
• Instruct patient to notify prescriber if other adverse reactions occur.

Evaluation

• Patient shows positive response to drug therapy on follow-up diagnostic studies.
• Patient doesn't experience injury as a result of drug-induced hematologic adverse reactions.
• Patient and family state understanding of drug therapy.

clarithromycin

(klah-rith-roh-MIGH-sin)
Biaxin

Pharmacologic class: macrolide
Therapeutic class: antibiotic
Pregnancy risk category: C

Indications and dosages

▶ **Pharyngitis or tonsillitis caused by *Streptococcus pyogenes*.** *Adults:* 250 mg P.O. q 12 hours for 10 days.
Children: 7.5 mg/kg/day P.O. b.i.d. q 12 hours for 10 days.
▶ **Acute maxillary sinusitis caused by *S. pneumoniae*.** *Adults:* 500 mg P.O. q 12 hours for 14 days.
Children: 7.5 mg/kg/day P.O. b.i.d. q 12 hours for 10 days.
▶ **Acute exacerbations of chronic bronchitis caused by *Moraxella catarrhalis* or *S. pneumoniae*; pneumonia caused by *S. pneumoniae* or *Mycoplasma pneumoniae*.** *Adults:* 250 mg P.O. q 12 hours for 7 to 14 days.
▶ **Acute exacerbations of chronic bronchitis caused by *Haemophilus influenzae*.** *Adults:* 500 mg P.O. q 12 hours for 7 to 14 days.
▶ **Uncomplicated skin and skin-structure infections caused by *Staphylococcus aureus* or *S. pyogenes*.** *Adults:* 250 mg P.O. q 12 hours for 7 to 14 days.
Children: 7.5 mg/kg P.O. q 12 hours for 10 days.
▶ **Acute otitis media.** *Children:* 7.5 mg/kg P.O. q 12 hours for 10 days.
▶ **Active duodenal ulcer linked to *Helicobacter pylori* infection.** *Adults:* 500 mg P.O. t.i.d. for 14 days with omeprazole 40 mg P.O. each morning. Omeprazole should continue at 20 mg P.O. each morning for days 15-28. Or, 500 mg P.O. t.i.d. for 14 days with ranitidine bismuth citrate 400 mg P.O. b.i.d. Ranitidine bismuth citrate therapy continues for days 15-28.
▶ **Eradication of *H. pylori* infection in patients with duodenal ulcer disease** *Adults:* 500 mg P.O. plus lansoprazole 30 mg P.O. and amoxicillin 1 g P.O. each q 12 hours for 14 days.

How supplied

Tablets: 250 mg, 500 mg
Suspension: 125 mg/5 ml, 250 mg/5 ml

Pharmacokinetics

Absorption: rapidly absorbed from GI tract.
Distribution: widely distributed. Because it readily penetrates cells, tissue levels are higher than plasma levels.
Metabolism: drug's major metabolite, 14-hydroxy clarithromycin, has significant antimicrobial activity; it's about twice as active against *H. influenzae* as parent drug.
Excretion: 20% to 30% excreted in urine unchanged. The major metabolite accounts for about 15% of drug in urine. *Half-life:* 5 to 6 hours with 250 mg q 12 hours; 7 hours with 500 mg q 12 hours.

Route	Onset	Peak	Duration
P.O.	Unknown	2-3 hr	Unknown

Pharmacodynamics

Chemical effect: binds to 50S subunit of bacterial ribosomes, blocking protein synthesis; bacteriostatic or bactericidal, depending on concentration.
Therapeutic effect: hinders or kills susceptible bacteria. Spectrum of activity includes *S. pyogenes, S. pneumoniae, M. catarrhalis, M. pneumoniae, H. influenzae,* and *S. aureus.*

Adverse reactions

CNS: headache.
CV: ***ventricular arrhythmias.***
GI: *diarrhea, nausea, abnormal taste,* dyspepsia, abdominal pain or discomfort.
Hematologic: ***leukopenia, thrombocytopenia.***
Skin: ***Stevens-Johnson syndrome.***

Interactions

Drug-drug. *Carbamazepine:* may increase serum levels of carbamazepine. Monitor blood levels.
Theophylline: increased plasma theophylline levels possible with other macrolides; effect of clarithromycin is unknown. Monitor theophylline levels carefully.
Warfarin: increased PT and INR possible with other macrolides; effect of clarithromycin is unknown. Monitor PT and INR carefully.

Contraindications and precautions

- Contraindicated in patients hypersensitive to erythromycin or other macrolides.
- Use cautiously in patients with hepatic or renal impairment and in pregnant or breast-feeding women.

• Safety of drug hasn't been established in children under age 6 months.

NURSING CONSIDERATIONS

Assessment

• Assess patient's infection before therapy, and reassess regularly throughout therapy.
• Obtain urine specimen for culture and sensitivity tests before first dose. Therapy may begin pending results.
• Be alert for adverse reactions and drug interactions.
• Monitor patient's hydration status if adverse GI reactions occur.
• Evaluate patient's and family's knowledge of drug therapy.

Nursing diagnoses

• Infection related to presence of bacteria susceptible to drug
• Risk for deficient fluid volume related to drug-induced adverse GI reactions
• Deficient knowledge related to drug therapy

Planning and implementation

• Administer drug with or without food.

Patient teaching

• Tell patient to take all of drug, as prescribed, even after he feels better.
• Tell patient to notify prescriber if adverse reactions occur.

Evaluation

• Patient is free from infection after drug therapy.
• Patient maintains adequate hydration throughout drug therapy.
• Patient and family state understanding of drug therapy.

clemastine fumarate

(KLEM-eh-steen FOO-muh-rayt)
Tavist, Tavist Allergy†, Dayhist-1

Pharmacologic class: ethanolamine-derivative antihistamine
Therapeutic class: antihistamine (H_1-receptor antagonist)
Pregnancy risk category: B

Indications and dosages

▶ **Rhinitis, allergy symptoms.** *Adults and children age 12 and over:* 1.34 mg P.O. q 12 hours, or 2.68 mg P.O. once daily to t.i.d. as needed.
Children ages 6 to 12: 0.67 to 1.34 mg P.O. b.i.d.

How supplied

Tablets: 1.34 mg†, 2.68 mg
Syrup: 0.67 mg per 5 ml

Pharmacokinetics

Absorption: absorbed readily from GI tract.
Distribution: unknown.
Metabolism: drug is extensively metabolized, probably in liver.
Excretion: excreted in urine.

Route	Onset	Peak	Duration
P.O.	15-60 min	2-4 hr	12 hr

Pharmacodynamics

Chemical effect: competes with histamine for H-receptor sites on effector cells. Prevents, but doesn't reverse, histamine-mediated responses.
Therapeutic effect: relieves allergy symptoms.

Adverse reactions

CNS: *sedation, drowsiness,* ***seizures.***
CV: hypotension, palpitations, tachycardia.
GI: epigastric distress, anorexia, nausea, vomiting, constipation, *dry mouth.*
GU: urine retention.
Hematologic: hemolytic anemia, ***thrombocytopenia, agranulocytosis.***
Respiratory: thick bronchial secretions.
Skin: rash, urticaria.
Other: ***anaphylactic shock.***

Interactions

Drug-drug. *CNS depressants:* increased sedation. Use together cautiously.
MAO inhibitors: increased anticholinergic effects. Don't use together.
Drug-lifestyle. *Sun exposure:* photosensitivity may occur. Urge patient to take precautions.

Contraindications and precautions

- Contraindicated in patients hypersensitive to drug or other antihistamines of similar chemical structure, in patients with acute asthma attacks, in breast-feeding patients, and in neonates and premature infants.
- Use cautiously in elderly patients and in those with angle-closure glaucoma, increased intraocular pressure, hyperthyroidism, CV disease, hypertension, bronchial asthma, prostatic hyperplasia, bladder-neck obstruction, pyloroduodenal obstruction, and stenosing peptic ulcerations. Also use cautiously in pregnant women.

NURSING CONSIDERATIONS

Assessment
- Assess patient's allergy condition before therapy, and reassess regularly thereafter.
- Monitor blood counts during long-term therapy, as ordered; watch for signs of blood dyscrasias.
- Be alert for adverse reactions and drug interactions.
- Evaluate patient's and family's knowledge of drug therapy.

Nursing diagnoses
- Ineffective health maintenance related to patient's underlying allergy condition
- Ineffective airway clearance related to drug-induced thickening of bronchial secretions
- Deficient knowledge related to drug therapy

Planning and implementation
- Children under age 12 should use only as directed by prescriber.
- Administer drug with food or milk to minimize GI distress.
- Notify prescriber if tolerance occurs because another antihistamine may need to be substituted for clemastine.

Patient teaching
- Warn patient to avoid driving or other activities that require alertness until drug's CNS effects are known.
- Warn patient to avoid alcohol while taking drug; it will increase drowsiness.
- Tell patient that coffee or tea may reduce drowsiness and that sugarless gum, sugarless sour hard candy, or ice chips may relieve dry mouth.
- Advise patient to stop drug 4 days before allergy skin tests to preserve accuracy of tests.
- Tell patient to notify prescriber if tolerance develops because different antihistamine may need to be prescribed.
- Advise patient to increase fluid intake, if not contraindicated, to help keep bronchial secretions thin.

Evaluation
- Patient's allergy symptoms are relieved with drug therapy.
- Patient maintains adequate air exchange throughout drug therapy.
- Patient and family state understanding of drug therapy.

clindamycin hydrochloride
(klin-duh-MIGH-sin high-droh-KLOR-ighd)
Cleocin HCl, Dalacin C♦ ◇

clindamycin palmitate hydrochloride
Cleocin Pediatric

clindamycin phosphate
Cleocin Phosphate

Pharmacologic class: lincomycin derivative
Therapeutic class: antibiotic
Pregnancy risk category: B

Indications and dosages

▶ **Infections caused by sensitive staphylococci, streptococci, pneumococci, *Bacteroides, Fusobacterium, Clostridium perfringens*, and other sensitive aerobic and anaerobic organisms.** *Adults:* 150 to 450 mg P.O. q 6 hours. Or, 300 to 600 mg I.M. or I.V. q 6, 8, or 12 hours.
Children over age 1 month: 4 to 10 mg/kg P.O. daily b.i.d. q 6 to 8 hours. Or, 15 to 40 mg/kg I.M. or I.V. daily, in divided doses q 6 hours.

▶ **Endocarditis prophylaxis for dental procedures in patients allergic to penicillin.** *Adults:* initially, 300 mg P.O. 1 hour before procedure; then 150 mg 6 hours later.
Children: initially, 10 mg/kg P.O. 1 hour before procedure; then 5 mg/kg 6 hours later.

How supplied

clindamycin hydrochloride
Capsules: 75 mg, 150 mg, 300 mg
clindamycin palmitate hydrochloride
Oral solution: 75 mg/5 ml
clindamycin phosphate
Injection: 150 mg/ml

Pharmacokinetics

Absorption: when administered orally, drug is absorbed rapidly and almost completely from GI tract. Drug is absorbed well after I.M. administration.
Distribution: distributed widely to most body tissues and fluids (except CSF). Drug is about 93% bound to plasma proteins.
Metabolism: metabolized partially to inactive metabolites.
Excretion: about 10% of clindamycin dose is excreted unchanged in urine; rest is excreted as inactive metabolites. *Half-life:* 2.5 to 3 hours.

Route	Onset	Peak	Duration
P.O.	Unknown	0.75-1 hr	Unknown
I.V.	Immediate	Immediate	Unknown
I.M.	Unknown	3 hr	Unknown

Pharmacodynamics

Chemical effect: inhibits bacterial protein synthesis by binding to 50S subunit of ribosome.
Therapeutic effect: hinders or kills susceptible bacteria. Spectrum of activity includes most aerobic gram-positive cocci and anaerobic gram-negative and gram-positive organisms. It's considered first-line drug in treating *Bacteroides fragilis* and most other gram-positive and gram-negative anaerobes. It's also effective against *Mycoplasma pneumoniae, Leptotrichia buccalis,* and some gram-positive cocci and bacilli.

Adverse reactions

CV: thrombophlebitis.
GI: unpleasant or bitter taste, *nausea,* vomiting, abdominal pain, ***diarrhea, pseudomembranous colitis,*** esophagitis, flatulence, anorexia, *bloody or tarry stools, dysphagia.*
Hematologic: ***transient leukopenia,*** eosinophilia, ***thrombocytopenia.***
Hepatic: elevated alkaline phosphatase, AST, bilirubin.
Skin: maculopapular rash, urticaria.
Other: ***anaphylaxis;*** *pain,* induration, *sterile abscess* (with I.M. injection); erythema, pain (after I.V. administration).

Interactions

Drug-drug. *Erythromycin:* may block clindamycin site of action. Don't use together.
Kaolin: decreased absorption of oral clindamycin. Separate administration times.
Neuromuscular blockers: potentiated neuromuscular blockade possible. Monitor patient closely.
Drug-food. *Diet foods with sodium cyclamate:* decreased serum drug level. Discourage use together.

Contraindications and precautions

- Contraindicated in patients hypersensitive to antibiotic congener lincomycin.
- Breast-feeding women should use a different feeding method during drug therapy.
- Use cautiously in neonates and patients with renal or hepatic disease, asthma, history of GI disease, or significant allergies.

NURSING CONSIDERATIONS

Assessment

- Assess patient's infection before therapy, and reassess regularly throughout therapy.
- Obtain urine specimen for culture and sensitivity tests before first dose. Therapy may begin pending results.
- Monitor renal, hepatic, and hematopoietic functions during prolonged therapy, as ordered.
- Be alert for adverse reactions and drug interactions.
- Monitor patient's hydration status if adverse GI reactions occur.

• Evaluate patient's and family's knowledge about drug therapy.

Nursing diagnoses
• Infection related to presence of bacteria susceptible to drug
• Risk for deficient fluid volume related to drug-induced adverse GI reactions
• Deficient knowledge related to drug therapy

Planning and implementation
P.O. use: Don't refrigerate reconstituted oral solution because it will thicken. Drug is stable for 2 weeks at room temperature.
– Administer capsule form with full glass of water to prevent dysphagia.
I.V. use: When giving I.V., check site daily for phlebitis and irritation. For I.V. infusion, dilute each 300 mg in 50 ml solution, and give no faster than 30 mg/minute (over 10 to 60 minutes). Never give undiluted as bolus.
I.M. use: Inject drug deeply. Rotate sites. Warn patient that I.M. injection may be painful. Doses over 600 mg per injection are not recommended.
– I.M. injection may raise CK in response to muscle irritation.
ALERT Don't give opioid antidiarrheals to treat drug-induced diarrhea; they may prolong and worsen diarrhea.

Patient teaching
• Advise patient taking capsule form to take with full glass of water to prevent dysphagia.
• Teach patient how to store oral solution.
• Instruct patient to take drug for as long as prescribed, exactly as directed.
• Tell patient to take entire amount prescribed even after he feels better.
• Warn patient that I.M. injection may be painful.
• Instruct patient to report diarrhea and to avoid self-treatment.
• Tell patient receiving drug I.V. to report discomfort at infusion site.

Evaluation
• Patient is free from infection after drug therapy.
• Patient maintains adequate hydration during drug therapy.
• Patient and family state understanding of drug therapy.

clofazimine
(kloh-FAH-zih-meen)
Lamprene

Pharmacologic class: substituted iminophenazine dye
Therapeutic class: leprostatic
Pregnancy risk category: C

Indications and dosages
▶ **Dapsone-resistant leprosy (Hansen's disease).** *Adults:* 100 mg P.O. daily with other antileprotics for 3 years. Then, clofazimine alone, 100 mg daily.
▶ **Erythema nodosum leprosum.** *Adults:* 100 to 200 mg P.O. daily for up to 3 months. Dosage is tapered to 100 mg daily as soon as possible. Dosages above 200 mg daily aren't recommended.

How supplied
Capsules: 50 mg

Pharmacokinetics
Absorption: absorption is variable (45% to 62%) after oral administration.
Distribution: highly lipophilic, drug is distributed widely into fatty tissues and is taken up by macrophages into reticuloendothelial system. Little, if any, crosses blood-brain barrier or enters CNS.
Metabolism: not totally known; some evidence exists of enterohepatic cycling.
Excretion: most is excreted in feces; some in sputum, sebum, and sweat; very little in urine.
Half-life: up to 70 days.

Route	Onset	Peak	Duration
P.O.	Unknown	1-6 hr	Unknown

Pharmacodynamics
Chemical effect: unknown. Thought to inhibit mycobacterial growth by binding preferentially to mycobacterial DNA. Also has anti-inflammatory effects that suppress skin reactions of erythema nodosum leprosum.

Therapeutic effect: adjunct leprosy therapy. Relieves inflammation of erythema nodosum leprosum.

Adverse reactions

EENT: conjunctival and corneal pigmentation.
GI: *epigastric pain, diarrhea, nausea, vomiting, GI intolerance,* ***bowel obstruction, GI bleeding,*** discolored feces.
Skin: *pink to brownish black pigmentation, ichthyosis and dryness,* rash, itching.
Other: ***splenic infarction,*** discolored body fluids.

Interactions

Drug-drug. *Dapsone:* impaired anti-inflammatory effects of clofazimine. No intervention appears necessary.
Isoniazid: may decrease skin levels and increase serum and urine levels of clofazimine. Monitor patient for decreased effectiveness.
Rifampin: decreased rifampin bioavailability. Monitor patient for decreased effectiveness.

Contraindications and precautions

- No known contraindications, although drug shouldn't be administered to breast-feeding women unless potential benefit to mother outweighs risk to infant.
- Use cautiously in pregnant women and in patients with GI dysfunction, such as abdominal pain and diarrhea.
- Safety of drug hasn't been established in children.

NURSING CONSIDERATIONS

Assessment

- Assess patient's leprosy or erythema nodosum leprosum before therapy, and reassess regularly thereafter.
- Be alert for adverse reactions and drug interactions.
- Monitor patient's hydration status if adverse GI reactions occur.
- Evaluate patient's and family's knowledge of drug therapy.

Nursing diagnoses

- Ineffective health maintenance related to patient's underlying condition
- Risk for deficient fluid volume related to drug-induced adverse GI reactions
- Deficient knowledge related to drug therapy

Planning and implementation

- Administer drug with food or milk.

ALERT Doses that exceed 100 mg daily should be given for as short a period as possible and only under close medical supervision.

- If patient complains of colic, burning abdominal pain, or other GI symptoms, notify prescriber, who may reduce dose or increase interval between doses.

Patient teaching

- Advise patient to take drug with meals or milk.
- Warn patient that drug may discolor skin, body fluids, and stool. The color ranges from red to brownish black. Reassure patient that skin discoloration is reversible but may not disappear until several months or years after drug treatment ends.
- Recommend application of skin oil or cream to help reverse skin dryness or ichthyosis.

Evaluation

- Patient exhibits improvement of underlying condition with drug therapy.
- Patient maintains adequate hydration throughout drug therapy.
- Patient and family state understanding of drug therapy.

clofibrate

(kloh-FIGH-brayt)
Atromid-S

Pharmacologic class: fibric acid derivative
Therapeutic class: antilipemic
Pregnancy risk category: C

Indications and dosages

▶ **Hyperlipidemia.** *Adults:* 1 g P.O. b.i.d. Some patients may respond to lower doses as assessed by serum lipid monitoring.

How supplied

Capsules: 500 mg

Pharmacokinetics

Absorption: absorbed slowly but completely from GI tract.
Distribution: distributed into extracellular space as its active form, clofibric acid, which is up to 98% protein-bound.
Metabolism: drug is hydrolyzed by serum enzymes to clofibric acid, which is metabolized by liver.
Excretion: 20% of clofibric acid is excreted unchanged in urine; 70% is eliminated in urine as conjugated metabolite. *Half-life:* 6 to 25 hours.

Route	Onset	Peak	Duration
P.O.	2-5 days	3 wk	≤ 3 wk

Pharmacodynamics

Chemical effect: unknown. Seems to inhibit biosynthesis of cholesterol at early stage.
Therapeutic effect: lowers blood cholesterol levels.

Adverse reactions

CNS: fatigue, weakness.
CV: ***arrhythmias.***
GI: *nausea, diarrhea, vomiting,* stomatitis, *dyspepsia,* flatulence.
GU: impotence, ***acute renal failure.***
Hematologic: leukopenia, anemia.
Hepatic: gallstones, ***transient and reversible elevations of liver function test results.***
Metabolic: *weight gain, polyphagia.*
Musculoskeletal: myalgia and arthralgia resembling flulike syndrome.
Skin: rash, urticaria, pruritus, dry skin and hair.
Other: decreased libido, fever.

Interactions

Drug-drug. *Furosemide, sulfonylureas:* clofibrate may potentiate clinical effects of these drugs. Monitor patient closely.
Lovastatin, pravastatin, simvastatin: risk of myositis, rhabdomyolysis, and renal failure. Avoid concomitant use.
Oral anticoagulants: clofibrate may potentiate anticoagulant effects of warfarin or dicumarol. Decrease anticoagulant dosage.
Oral contraceptives, rifampin: may antagonize clofibrate's lipid-lowering effect. Monitor serum lipids.
Probenecid: increased clofibrate effect. Monitor patient for toxicity.

Contraindications and precautions

- Contraindicated in pregnant patients, breast-feeding patients, patients hypersensitive to drug, and patients with significant hepatic or renal dysfunction or primary biliary cirrhosis.
- Use cautiously in patients with peptic ulcer.
- Safety of drug hasn't been established in children.

NURSING CONSIDERATIONS

Assessment

- Assess patient's blood cholesterol level before therapy.
- Monitor effectiveness by evaluating serum cholesterol and triglyceride levels regularly during therapy.
- Monitor renal and hepatic function, blood counts, and serum electrolyte and blood glucose levels.
- Be alert for adverse reactions and drug interactions.
- Evaluate patient's and family's knowledge of drug therapy.

Nursing diagnoses

- Risk for injury related to elevated blood cholesterol
- Impaired urine elimination related to drug-induced acute renal failure
- Deficient knowledge related to drug therapy

Planning and implementation

- Drug may be discontinued if liver function tests show steady rise.
- Drug typically is discontinued if lipids aren't lowered significantly within 3 months.

Patient teaching

- Teach patient about proper dietary management of serum lipids (restricting total fat and cholesterol intake) as well as measures to control other cardiac disease risk factors. When appropriate, recommend weight control, exercise, and smoking cessation programs.

• Advise patient to report flulike symptoms immediately because they may indicate rhabdomyolysis-induced renal failure.

Evaluation

• Patient's blood cholesterol level is normal with drug therapy.
• Patient maintains normal urine elimination pattern throughout drug therapy.
• Patient and family state understanding of drug therapy.

clomiphene citrate

(KLOH-meh-feen SIGH-trayt)
Clomid, Serophene

Pharmacologic class: chlorotrianisene derivative
Therapeutic class: ovulation stimulant
Pregnancy risk category: X

Indications and dosages

▶ **Induction of ovulation.** *Adults:* 50 mg P.O. daily for 5 days starting on day 5 of menstrual cycle if bleeding occurs (first day of menstrual flow is day 1), or at any time if patient hasn't had recent uterine bleeding. If ovulation doesn't occur, may increase dose to 100 mg P.O. daily for 5 days as soon as 30 days after previous course. Repeated until conception occurs or until three courses of therapy are completed.

How supplied

Tablets: 50 mg

Pharmacokinetics

Absorption: absorbed readily from GI tract.
Distribution: may undergo enterohepatic recirculation or may be stored in body fat.
Metabolism: metabolized by liver.
Excretion: excreted principally in feces via biliary elimination. *Half-life:* about 5 days.

Route	Onset	Peak	Duration
P.O.	Unknown	Unknown	Unknown

Pharmacodynamics

Chemical effect: unknown. Appears to stimulate release of pituitary gonadotropins, follicle-stimulating hormone, and luteinizing hormone. This results in maturation of ovarian follicle, ovulation, and development of corpus luteum.
Therapeutic effect: causes women to ovulate.

Adverse reactions

CNS: headache, restlessness, insomnia, dizziness, light-headedness, depression, fatigue, tension.
CV: hypertension.
EENT: blurred vision, diplopia, scotoma, photophobia.
GI: nausea, vomiting, bloating, distention.
GU: urinary frequency and polyuria; ovarian enlargement and cyst formation, which regress spontaneously when drug is stopped.
Metabolic: *hyperglycemia,* increased appetite, weight gain.
Skin: reversible alopecia, urticaria, rash, dermatitis.
Other: *hot flushes, breast discomfort.*

Interactions

None significant.

Contraindications and precautions

• Contraindicated in pregnant patients and in patients with undiagnosed abnormal genital bleeding, ovarian cyst not caused by polycystic ovarian syndrome, hepatic disease or dysfunction, uncontrolled thyroid or adrenal dysfunction, or organic intracranial lesion (such as pituitary tumor).

NURSING CONSIDERATIONS

Assessment

• Assess patient's underlying condition before therapy.
• Monitor effectiveness by assessing ovulation through biphasic body temperature measurement, postovulatory urinary levels of pregnanediol, estrogen excretion, and changes in endometrial tissues.
• Be alert for adverse reactions. The most common is nausea.

• Evaluate patient's and family's knowledge of drug therapy.

Nursing diagnoses

• Excessive fluid volume related to drug-induced fluid retention
• Sexual dysfunction related to underlying condition
• Deficient knowledge related to drug therapy

Planning and implementation

• Prepare administration instructions for patient: Begin daily dosage on fifth day of menstrual flow for 5 consecutive days.
• No more than three courses of therapy should be given to attempt conception.

Patient teaching

• Tell patient about risk of multiple births with drug use; risk increases with higher doses.
• Teach patient how to take and chart basal body temperature and to ascertain whether ovulation has occurred.
• Reassure patient that ovulation typically occurs after first course of therapy. If pregnancy doesn't occur, course of therapy may be repeated twice.

ALERT Advise patient to stop drug and contact prescriber immediately if pregnancy is suspected because drug may have teratogenic effect.

• Advise patient to stop drug and contact prescriber immediately if abdominal symptoms or pain occurs because these may indicate ovarian enlargement or ovarian cyst.
• Tell patient to immediately report signs of impending visual toxicity, such as blurred vision, diplopia, scotoma, or photophobia.
• Warn patient to avoid hazardous activities until CNS effects of drug are known. Drug may cause dizziness or visual disturbances.

Evaluation

• Patient is free from fluid retention at end of drug therapy.
• Patient ovulates with drug therapy.
• Patient and family state understanding of drug therapy.

clomipramine hydrochloride

(kloh-MIH-pruh-meen high-droh-KLOR-ighd)
Anafranil

Pharmacologic class: tricyclic antidepressant (TCA)
Therapeutic class: antiobsessional agent
Pregnancy risk category: C

Indications and dosages

▶ **Obsessive-compulsive disorder.** *Adults:* initially, 25 mg P.O. daily in divided doses with meals, gradually increased to 100 mg daily during first 2 weeks. Thereafter, increased to maximum dosage of 250 mg daily in divided doses with meals as needed. After dosage adjustment, total daily dosage may be given h.s.
Children and adolescents: initially, 12.5 mg P.O. b.i.d. with meals, gradually increased to daily maximum of 3 mg/kg or 100 mg P.O., whichever is smaller. Maximum daily dosage is 3 mg/kg or 200 mg, whichever is smaller; may be given h.s. after adjustment. Periodic reassessment and adjustment necessary.

How supplied

Capsules: 25 mg, 50 mg, 75 mg

Pharmacokinetics

Absorption: well absorbed from the GI tract, but extensive first-pass metabolism limits bioavailability to about 50%.
Distribution: distributes well into lipophilic tissues; about 98% bound to plasma proteins.
Metabolism: primarily hepatic. Several metabolites have been identified; desmethylclomipramine is primary active metabolite.
Excretion: about 66% is excreted in urine; remainder in feces. *Half-life:* parent compound, about 36 hours; desmethylclomipramine, 4 to 233 days.

Route	Onset	Peak	Duration
P.O.	≥ 2 wk	Unknown	Unknown

Pharmacodynamics

Chemical effect: unknown but a TCA that selectively inhibits reuptake of serotonin.

Therapeutic effect: relieves obsessive-compulsive behaviors.

Adverse reactions

CNS: *somnolence, tremors, dizziness,* headache, insomnia, *nervousness, myoclonus, fatigue, EEG changes,* ***seizures,*** extrapyramidal reactions, asthenia, aggressiveness.
CV: orthostatic hypotension, palpitations, tachycardia.
EENT: otitis media in children, abnormal vision, laryngitis, pharyngitis, rhinitis.
GI: dry mouth, constipation, nausea, dyspepsia, diarrhea, anorexia, abdominal pain, eructation, *nausea.*
GU: *urinary hesitancy,* urinary tract infection, dysmenorrhea, *ejaculation failure,* impotence.
Hematologic: anemia, bone marrow suppression.
Metabolic: increased appetite, weight gain.
Musculoskeletal: myalgia.
Skin: *diaphoresis,* rash, pruritus, photosensitivity, dry skin.
Other: *altered libido.*

Interactions

Drug-drug. *Barbiturates:* decreased TCA blood levels. Monitor patient for decreased antidepressant effect.
Cimetidine, methylphenidate: increased TCA blood levels. Monitor patient for enhanced antidepressant effect.
Clonidine, epinephrine, norepinephrine: increased hypertensive effect. Use with caution.
CNS depressants: enhanced CNS depression. Avoid concomitant use.
MAO inhibitors: may cause hyperpyretic crisis, seizures, coma, or death. Don't use together.
Drug-herb. *St. John's wort:* serotonin levels may rise too high, causing serotonin syndrome. Discourage concomitant use.
Drug-lifestyle. *Alcohol use:* enhanced CNS depression. Discourage use together.
Sun exposure: photosensitivity may occur. Urge patient to take precautions.

Contraindications and precautions

- Contraindicated in patients hypersensitive to drug or other TCAs, in those who have taken MAO inhibitors within the previous 14 days, and in patients in acute recovery period after MI.
- Use cautiously in patients with history of seizure disorders or with brain damage of varying etiology; in those receiving other seizure threshold–lowering drugs; in patients at risk for suicide; in patients with history of urine retention or angle-closure glaucoma, increased intraocular pressure, CV disease, impaired hepatic or renal function, or hyperthyroidism; in patients with tumors of the adrenal medulla; in patients receiving thyroid drug or electroconvulsive therapy; and in those undergoing elective surgery.
- Also use cautiously in pregnant or breast-feeding women.

NURSING CONSIDERATIONS

Assessment

- Assess patient's underlying condition before therapy, and reassess regularly throughout therapy.
- Evaluate patient's and family's knowledge of drug therapy.

Nursing diagnoses

- Ineffective individual coping related to patient's underlying condition
- Risk for injury related to drug-induced adverse reactions
- Deficient knowledge related to drug therapy

Planning and implementation

- Total daily dose may be taken at bedtime after dosage adjustment. During dosage adjustment, dosage may be divided and given with meals to minimize GI effects.
- Don't withdraw drug abruptly.
- Because hypertensive episodes have occurred during surgery in patients receiving TCAs, drug should be gradually discontinued several days before surgery.

ALERT Don't confuse clomipramine with chlorpromazine or clomiphene; don't confuse Anafranil with enalapril, nafarelin, or alfentanil.

Patient teaching

- Warn patient to avoid hazardous activities requiring alertness and good psychomotor

coordination, especially during dosage adjustment. Daytime sedation and dizziness may occur.
• Tell patient to avoid alcohol while taking drug.
• Warn patient not to withdraw drug suddenly.
• Advise patient to use sunblock, wear protective clothing, and avoid prolonged exposure to strong sunlight to prevent photosensitivity reactions.

☑ Evaluation

• Patient's behavior and communication indicate improvement of obsessive-compulsive pattern.
• Patient doesn't experience injury from drug-induced adverse CNS reactions.
• Patient and family state understanding of drug therapy.

clonazepam

(kloh-NEH-zuh-pam)
Klonopin, Rivotril ◇ ♦

Pharmacologic class: benzodiazepine
Therapeutic class: anticonvulsant
Controlled substance schedule: IV
Pregnancy risk category: C

Indications and dosages

▶ **Lennox-Gastaut syndrome; atypical absence seizures; akinetic and myoclonic seizures.** *Adults:* initially, not to exceed 1.5 mg P.O. t.i.d. May be increased by 0.5 to 1 mg q 3 days until seizures are controlled. If given in unequal doses, largest dose given h.s. Maximum daily dosage is 20 mg.
Children up to age 10 or 30 kg (66 lb): initially, 0.01 to 0.03 mg/kg P.O. daily (maximum 0.05 mg/kg daily), in two or three divided doses. Increased by 0.25 to 0.5 mg q third day to maximum maintenance dosage of 0.1 to 0.2 mg/kg daily as needed.
▶ **Status epilepticus (where parenteral form is available).** *Adults:* 1 mg by slow I.V. infusion.
Children: 0.5 mg by slow I.V. infusion.
▶ **Panic disorder**. *Adults*: initially, 0.25 mg P.O. b.i.d.; increase to target dose of 1 mg/day after 3 days. Some patients may benefit from doses up to maximum of 4 mg/day. To achieve 4 mg/day, increase dosage in increments of 0.125 to 0.25 mg b.i.d. q 3 days as tolerated until panic disorder is controlled. Discontinue drug gradually with decrease of 0.125 mg b.i.d. q 3 days until drug is stopped.

How supplied

Tablets: 0.5 mg, 1 mg, 2 mg
Injection: 1mg/ml ◇

Pharmacokinetics

Absorption: well absorbed from GI tract.
Distribution: distributed widely throughout body; about 47% protein-bound.
Metabolism: metabolized by liver to several metabolites.
Excretion: excreted in urine. *Half-life:* 18 to 50 hours.

Route	Onset	Peak	Duration
P.O.	Unknown	1-2 hr	Unknown
I.V.	Unknown	Unknown	Unknown

Pharmacodynamics

Chemical effect: unknown. A benzodiazepine that probably acts by facilitating effects of inhibitory neurotransmitter gamma-aminobutyric acid.
Therapeutic effect: prevents or stops seizure activity.

Adverse reactions

CNS: *drowsiness, ataxia, behavioral disturbances* (especially in children), slurred speech, tremor, confusion, psychosis, agitation.
EENT: *increased salivation,* diplopia, nystagmus, abnormal eye movements, sore gums.
GI: constipation, gastritis, nausea, abnormal thirst.
GU: dysuria, enuresis, nocturia, urine retention.
Hematologic: ***leukopenia, thrombocytopenia,*** eosinophilia.
Metabolic: change in appetite.
Musculoskeletal: muscle weakness or pain.
Respiratory: ***respiratory depression.***
Skin: rash.

Interactions

Drug-drug. *CNS depressants:* increased CNS depression. Monitor patient closely.
Drug-herb. *Catnip, kava, lady's slipper, lemon balm, passion flower, sassafras, skullcap, valerian:* sedative effects of clonazepam may be enhanced. Discourage use together.
Drug-lifestyle. *Alcohol use:* increased CNS depression. Discourage use together.

Contraindications and precautions

- Contraindicated in patients hypersensitive to benzodiazepines and in those with acute angle-closure glaucoma or significant hepatic disease.
- Use cautiously in patients with mixed type of seizure because drug may precipitate generalized tonic-clonic seizures. Also, use cautiously in children and in patients with chronic respiratory disease or open-angle glaucoma.
- Safety of drug hasn't been established in breast-feeding women.

NURSING CONSIDERATIONS

Assessment

- Assess patient's seizure condition before therapy, and reassess regularly thereafter.
- Monitor blood levels. Therapeutic blood level is 20 to 80 ng/ml.
- Monitor CBC and liver function tests, as ordered.
- Be alert for adverse reactions and drug interactions.
- Evaluate patient's and family's knowledge of drug therapy.

Nursing diagnoses

- Risk for injury related to potential for seizure activity
- Activity intolerance related to drug-induced sedation
- Deficient knowledge related to drug therapy

Planning and implementation

P.O. use: Dosage should be increased gradually, as ordered.
I.V. use: Give slowly by direct injection or by slow I.V. infusion. Drug may be diluted with D_5W, dextrose 2.5% in water, normal saline solution, or half-normal saline solution.

- Mix solutions in glass bottles because drug binds to polyvinyl chloride plastics. If polyvinyl chloride infusion bags are used, administer immediately and infuse at rate of 60 ml/hour or greater.

ALERT Never withdraw therapy suddenly because seizures may worsen. Call prescriber at once if adverse reactions develop.

- Withdrawal symptoms are similar to those of barbiturates.
- Maintain seizure precautions.

Patient teaching

- Advise patient to avoid driving or other potentially hazardous activities until CNS effects of drug are known.
- Instruct parents to monitor child's school performance because drug may interfere with attentiveness in school.
- Instruct patient and family never to stop drug abruptly because seizures may occur.
- Instruct patient or family to notify prescriber if oversedation or other adverse reactions develop or questions arise about drug therapy.

Evaluation

- Patient is free from seizure activity during drug therapy.
- Patient is able to meet daily activity needs.
- Patient and family state understanding of drug therapy.

clonidine hydrochloride

(KLON-uh-deen high-droh-KLOR-ighd)
Catapres, Catapres-TTS, Dixarit◆ ◇, Duraclon

Pharmacologic class: centrally acting antiadrenergic
Therapeutic class: antihypertensive
Pregnancy risk category: C

Indications and dosages

▶ **Essential, renal, and malignant hypertension.** *Adults:* initially, 0.1 mg P.O. b.i.d. Then increased by 0.1 to 0.2 mg/day q week. Usual dosage range is 0.1 to 0.3 mg b.i.d.; infrequently, dosages as high as 2.4 mg daily are used. Or, transdermal patch applied to nonhairy area of intact skin on upper arm or torso q 7 days. Start with 0.1-mg system and adjust after 1 to 2 weeks with another 0.1-mg system or larger system if increases are needed to maintain normal pressure.

How supplied

Tablets: 0.025 mg ♦ ◇, 0.1 mg, 0.2 mg, 0.3 mg
Transdermal: TTS-1 (releases 0.1 mg/24 hours), TTS-2 (releases 0.2 mg/24 hours), TTS-3 (releases 0.3 mg/24 hours)
Injectable: 100 mg/ml

Pharmacokinetics

Absorption: absorbed well from GI tract when administered orally. Also absorbed well percutaneously after transdermal topical administration.
Distribution: distributed widely into body.
Metabolism: metabolized in liver, where nearly 50% is transformed to inactive metabolites.
Excretion: about 65% of drug is excreted in urine; 20% in feces. *Half-life:* 6 to 20 hours.

Route	Onset	Peak	Duration
P.O.	15-30 min	1.5-2.5 hr	6-8 hr
Trans-dermal	2-3 days	2-3 days	Several days

Pharmacodynamics

Chemical effect: unknown. Thought to inhibit central vasomotor centers, thereby decreasing sympathetic outflow to heart, kidneys, and peripheral vasculature; this results in decreased peripheral vascular resistance, decreased systolic and diastolic blood pressure, and decreased heart rate.
Therapeutic effect: lowers blood pressure.

Adverse reactions

CNS: *drowsiness, dizziness,* fatigue, sedation, nervousness, headache, vivid dreams.
CV: orthostatic hypotension, ***bradycardia, severe rebound hypertension.***
GI: *constipation, dry mouth,* nausea, vomiting.
GU: urine retention, impotence.
Metabolic: transient glucose intolerance.
Skin: *pruritus and dermatitis* with transdermal patch.

Interactions

Drug-drug. *CNS depressants:* enhanced CNS depression. Use together cautiously.
MAO inhibitors, tricyclic antidepressants: may decrease antihypertensive effect. Use together cautiously.
Propranolol, other beta blockers: severe rebound hypertension. Monitor patient carefully.
Drug-herb. *Capsicum, yohimbe:* May reduce antihypertensive effectiveness. Discourage concomitant use.

Contraindications and precautions

- Contraindicated in patients hypersensitive to drug. Transdermal form is contraindicated in patients hypersensitive to any component of adhesive layer.
- Use cautiously in patients with severe coronary insufficiency, recent MI, cerebrovascular disease, chronic renal failure, or impaired liver function. Also, use cautiously in breast-feeding women.
- Safety of drug hasn't been established in children or pregnant women.

NURSING CONSIDERATIONS

Assessment

- Assess patient's blood pressure before therapy, and reassess regularly thereafter.
- Antihypertensive effects of transdermal clonidine may take 2 to 3 days to become apparent. Oral antihypertensive therapy may have to be continued in interim.
- Be alert for adverse reactions and drug interactions.
- Observe for patient tolerance to drug's therapeutic effects, which may require increased dosage.
- Periodic eye examinations are recommended.
- Monitor site of transdermal patch for dermatitis. Ask patient about pruritus.
- Evaluate patient's and family's knowledge about drug therapy.

Nursing diagnoses

- Risk for injury related to presence of hypertension

• Ineffective protection related to severe rebound hypertension caused by abrupt cessation of drug
• Deficient knowledge related to drug therapy

Planning and implementation
• Drug may be given to lower blood pressure rapidly in some hypertensive emergency situations.
• Dosage is usually adjusted to patient's blood pressure and tolerance.
• Administer last dose of day at bedtime.
P.O. use: Follow normal protocol.
Transdermal use: To improve adherence of patch, apply adhesive overlay. Place patch at different site each week.
– Remove transdermal patch before defibrillation to prevent arcing.
• When stopping therapy in patients receiving both clonidine and beta blocker, gradually withdraw beta blocker first to minimize adverse reactions, as ordered.
• Discontinuation of clonidine for surgery isn't recommended.

Patient teaching
• Advise patient that abrupt discontinuation of drug may cause severe rebound hypertension. Reduce dosage gradually over 2 to 4 days, as ordered.
• Tell patient to take last dose of day immediately before bedtime.
• Reassure patient that transdermal patch usually adheres despite showering and other routine daily activities. Instruct him on use of adhesive overlay to improve skin adherence if necessary. Also tell patient to place patch at different site each week.
• Caution patient that drug can cause drowsiness, but that tolerance to this adverse effect will develop.
• Inform patient that orthostatic hypotension can be minimized by rising slowly and avoiding sudden position changes.

Evaluation
• Patient's blood pressure is normal with drug therapy.
• Patient states understanding of need to not stop drug abruptly.
• Patient and family state understanding of drug therapy.

clopidogrel bisulfate
(kloh-PIH-doh-grel bigh-SUL-fayt)
Plavix

Pharmacologic class: inhibitor of adenosine diphosphate (ADP) induced platelet aggregation
Therapeutic class: antiplatelet
Pregnancy risk category: B

Indications and dosages
▶ To reduce atherosclerotic events in patients with atherosclerosis documented by recent CVA, MI, or peripheral arterial disease. *Adults:* 75 mg P.O. daily.

How supplied
Tablets: 75 mg

Pharmacokinetics
Absorption: rapidly absorbed following oral administration.
Distribution: highly bound to plasma protein.
Metabolism: extensively metabolized by the liver.
Excretion: about 50% is excreted in urine and 46% in feces. *Half-life:* 8 hours

Route	Onset	Peak	Duration
P.O.	2 hr	Unknown	5 days

Pharmacodynamics
Chemical effect: inhibits binding of ADP to its platelet receptor, which inhibits ADP-mediated activation and subsequent platelet aggregation. Because clopidogrel acts by irreversibly modifying the platelet ADP receptor, platelets exposed to drug are affected for their lifespan.
Therapeutic effect: prevent clot formation.

Adverse reactions
CNS: headache, dizziness, fatigue, depression.
CV: chest pain, edema, hypertension.
EENT: epistaxis, rhinitis.

GI: ***hemorrhage,*** abdominal pain, dyspepsia, gastritis, constipation, diarrhea, ulcers.
GU: urinary tract infection.
Hematologic: purpura.
Musculoskeletal: arthralgia, back pain.
Respiratory: bronchitis, coughing, dyspnea, upper respiratory infection.
Skin: *rash,* pruritus.
Other: flulike symptoms, pain.

Interactions

Drug-drug. *Aspirin, NSAIDs:* may increase risk for GI bleeding. Use together cautiously. *Heparin, warfarin:* safety hasn't been established. Use together cautiously.
Drug-herb. *Dong quai, feverfew, garlic, ginger, horse chestnut, red clover:* possible increased risk of bleeding. Monitor patient closely.

Contraindications and precautions

- Contraindicated in patients hypersensitive to drug or its components and in those with pathologic bleeding, such as peptic ulcer or intracranial hemorrhage.
- Use cautiously in patients with hepatic impairment and in those at risk for increased bleeding from trauma, surgery, or other pathologic conditions.

NURSING CONSIDERATIONS

Assessment

- Assess concurrent use of OTC drugs, such as aspirin or NSAIDs, and herbal remedies.
- Assess patient for increased bleeding or bruising tendencies before and during drug therapy.
- Evaluate patient's and family's knowledge of drug therapy.

Nursing diagnoses

- Risk for injury related to potential for atherosclerotic events from underlying condition
- Ineffective protection related to increased risk of bleeding
- Deficient knowledge related to drug therapy

Planning and implementation

- Platelet aggregation will return to normal 5 days after drug has been discontinued.
- Withhold drug from patients with hepatic impairment and those at increased risk for bleeding from trauma, surgery, or other pathologic conditions.

Patient teaching

- Inform patient it may take longer than usual to stop bleeding. Tell him to refrain from activities in which trauma and bleeding may occur; encourage use of seat belt when in a car.
- Instruct patient to notify prescriber if unusual bleeding or bruising occurs.
- Tell patient to inform prescriber or dentist that he is taking drug before having surgery or starting new drug therapy.
- Inform patient that drug may be taken without regard to meals.

Evaluation

- Patient has reduced risk of CVA, MI, and vascular death.
- Patient states appropriate bleeding precautions to take.
- Patient and family state understanding of drug therapy.

clorazepate dipotassium

(klor-AYZ-eh-payt digh-po-TAH-see-um)
Apo-Clorazepate ♦, Gen-XENE, Novoclopate ♦, Tranxene, Tranxene-SD, Tranxene-T-Tab, Clorazecaps

Pharmacologic class: benzodiazepine
Therapeutic class: antianxiety, anticonvulsant, sedative-hypnotic agent
Controlled substance schedule: IV
Pregnancy risk category: D

Indications and dosages

▶ **Acute alcohol withdrawal.** *Adults:* day 1—30 mg P.O. initially, followed by 30 to 60 mg P.O. in divided doses; day 2—45 to 90 mg P.O. in divided doses; day 3—22.5 to 45 mg P.O. in divided doses; day 4—15 to 30 mg P.O. in divided doses; then gradually reduce dosage to 7.5 to 15 mg daily. Maximum daily dose is 90 mg.

▶ **Anxiety.** *Adults:* 15 to 60 mg P.O. daily. *Elderly patients:* initially, 7.5 to 15 mg daily in divided doses or as a single dose.

▶ **Adjunct in partial seizure disorder.** *Adults and children over age 12:* maximum recommended initial dosage is 7.5 mg P.O. t.i.d. Maximum dosage increase 7.5 mg/week; maximum dosage 90 mg daily.
Children ages 9 to 12: maximum recommended initial dosage is 7.5 mg P.O. b.i.d. Maximum dosage increase 7.5 mg/week; maximum dosage 60 mg daily.

How supplied

Tablets: 3.75 mg, 7.5 mg, 11.25 mg, 15 mg, 22.5 mg
Capsules: 3.75 mg, 7.5 mg, 15 mg

Pharmacokinetics

Absorption: absorbed completely and rapidly after being hydrolyzed in stomach to desmethyldiazepam.
Distribution: distributed widely throughout body. About 80% to 95% of drug is bound to plasma protein.
Metabolism: metabolized in liver to oxazepam.
Excretion: inactive glucuronide metabolites are excreted in urine. *Half-life:* 30 to 200 hours.

Route	Onset	Peak	Duration
P.O.	Unknown	0.5-2 hr	Unknown

Pharmacodynamics

Chemical effect: unknown. A benzodiazepine that probably facilitates action of inhibitory neurotransmitter gamma-aminobutyric acid. Depresses CNS at limbic and subcortical levels of brain and suppresses spread of seizure activity produced by epileptogenic foci in cortex, thalamus, and limbic structures.
Therapeutic effect: relieves anxiety, prevents seizure activity, and promotes sleep and calmness.

Adverse reactions

CNS: *drowsiness, lethargy, hangover,* fainting, restlessness, psychosis.
CV: transient hypotension.
EENT: visual disturbances.
GI: nausea, vomiting, abdominal discomfort, dry mouth.
GU: urine retention, incontinence.

Interactions

Drug-drug. *Cimetidine:* increased sedation. Monitor patient carefully.
CNS depressants: increased CNS depression. Avoid concomitant use.
Digoxin: may increase serum levels of digoxin, increasing toxicity. Monitor patient closely.
Drug-herb. *Catnip, kava, lady's slipper, lemon balm, passion flower, sassafras, skullcap, valerian:* sedative effects may be enhanced. Discourage using together.
Drug-lifestyle. *Alcohol use:* increased CNS depression. Don't use together.
Smoking: increased clearance of benzodiazepines. Monitor patient for lack of effect.

Contraindications and precautions

- Contraindicated in patients hypersensitive to drug and in those with acute angle-closure glaucoma.
- Avoid drug during pregnancy, especially first trimester.
- Use cautiously in patients with suicidal tendencies, renal or hepatic impairment, or history of drug abuse.
- Safety of drug hasn't been established for children under age 9.

NURSING CONSIDERATIONS

Assessment

- Assess patient's underlying condition before therapy, and reassess regularly thereafter.
- Monitor liver, renal, and hematopoietic function studies periodically in patients receiving repeated or prolonged therapy as ordered.
- Be alert for adverse reactions and drug interactions.
- Evaluate patient's and family's knowledge of drug therapy.

Nursing diagnoses

- Anxiety related to patient's underlying condition
- Risk of injury related to drug-induced adverse CNS reactions

• Deficient knowledge related to drug therapy

Planning and implementation

• Dosage should be reduced in elderly or debilitated patients.
• Possibility of abuse and addiction exists. Don't withdraw drug abruptly after prolonged use; withdrawal symptoms may occur.
ALERT Don't confuse clorazepate with clofibrate.

Patient teaching

• Warn patient to avoid activities that require alertness and good psychomotor coordination until CNS effects of drug are known.
• Tell patient to avoid alcohol while taking drug.
• Suggest sugarless chewing gum or hard candy to relieve dry mouth.
• Warn patient to take drug only as directed and not to stop without prescriber's approval. Inform patient of drug's potential for dependence if taken longer than directed.

Evaluation

• Patient says he is less anxious after taking drug therapy.
• Patient doesn't experience injury as a result of drug-induced adverse CNS reactions.
• Patient and family state understanding of drug therapy.

cloxacillin sodium

(kloks-uh-SIL-in SOH-dee-um)

Alclox◇, Apo-Cloxi◆, Cloxapen, Novocloxin◆, Nu-Cloxi◆, Orbenin◆

Pharmacologic class: penicillinase-resistant penicillin
Therapeutic class: antibiotic
Pregnancy risk category: B

Indications and dosages

▶ **Systemic infections caused by penicillinase-producing staphylococci.** *Adults and children weighing over 20 kg (44 lb):* 250 to 500 mg P.O. q 6 hours.
Children weighing 20 kg or less: 50 to 100 mg/kg P.O. daily, in divided doses q 6 hours.

How supplied

Capsules: 250 mg, 500 mg
Oral solution: 125 mg/5 ml (after reconstitution)

Pharmacokinetics

Absorption: absorbed rapidly but incompletely (37% to 60%) from GI tract. Food may decrease both rate and extent of absorption.
Distribution: distributed widely. CSF penetration is poor but enhanced in meningeal inflammation. Drug is 90% to 96% protein-bound.
Metabolism: only partially metabolized.
Excretion: drug and metabolites are excreted in urine. *Half-life:* 0.5 to 1 hour.

Route	Onset	Peak	Duration
P.O.	Unknown	0.5-2 hr	About 6 hr

Pharmacodynamics

Chemical effect: a penicillinase-resistant penicillin that inhibits cell-wall synthesis during microorganism multiplication; bacteria resist penicillins by producing penicillinases—enzymes that convert penicillins to inactive penicilloic acid. Cloxacillin resists these enzymes.
Therapeutic effect: hinders bacterial activity. Spectrum of activity includes many strains of penicillinase-producing bacteria of which most pronounced activity occurs against penicillinase-producing staphylococci. Also active against gram-positive aerobic and anaerobic bacilli.

Adverse reactions

CNS: ***seizures.***
GI: *nausea,* vomiting, *epigastric distress, diarrhea.*
Hematologic: eosinophilia, ***thrombocytopenia, agranulocytosis, leukopenia.***
Hepatic: intrahepatic cholestasis.
Other: hypersensitivity reactions (rash, urticaria, chills, fever, sneezing, wheezing, ***anaphylaxis***, overgrowth of nonsusceptible organisms).

Interactions

Drug-drug. *Probenecid:* increased blood levels of cloxacillin. Probenecid may be used for this purpose.
Drug-food. *Any food:* may interfere with absorption. Give 1 to 2 hours before or 2 to 3 hours after meals.
Carbonated beverages, fruit juice: will inactivate drug. Don't give together.

Contraindications and precautions

- Contraindicated in patients hypersensitive to drug or other penicillins.
- Use cautiously in patients with mononucleosis (high risk of maculopapular rash) or other drug allergies, especially to cephalosporins (possible cross-sensitivity).
- Also use cautiously in pregnant or breast-feeding women.

NURSING CONSIDERATIONS

Assessment

- Assess patient's infection before therapy, and reassess regularly throughout therapy.
- Before giving, ask patient about any allergic reactions to penicillin. However, negative history of penicillin allergy is no guarantee against future allergic reaction.
- Obtain specimen for culture and sensitivity tests before first dose. Therapy may begin pending results.
- Periodically assess renal, hepatic, and hematopoietic function in patients receiving long-term therapy, as ordered.
- Be alert for adverse reactions and drug interactions.
- Monitor patient's hydration status if adverse GI reactions occur.
- Evaluate patient's and family's knowledge of drug therapy.

Nursing diagnoses

- Infection related to presence of bacteria susceptible to drug
- Risk for deficient fluid volume related to drug-induced adverse GI reactions
- Deficient knowledge related to drug therapy

Planning and implementation

- Give drug 1 to 2 hours before or 2 to 3 hours after meals to avoid GI disturbances. Food may interfere with absorption. Give each dose with full glass of water, not fruit juice or carbonated beverage because acid will inactivate drug.
- Give drug at least 1 hour before bacteriostatic antibiotics.
- Drug may falsely elevate or cause false-positive results with certain tests for urine or serum proteins.

Patient teaching

- Tell patient to take entire quantity of drug exactly as prescribed, even after he feels better. Also tell him to take drug on empty stomach.
- Tell patient to call prescriber if rash, fever, or chills develop. A rash is most common allergic reaction.

ALERT Instruct patient to take each dose with full glass of water, not with fruit juice or carbonated beverage, because acid inactivates drug.

- Warn patient never to use leftover drug for new illness or to share it with anyone.

Evaluation

- Patient is free from infection after therapy.
- Patient maintains adequate hydration throughout drug therapy.
- Patient and family state understanding of drug therapy.

clozapine

(KLOH-zuh-peen)
Clozaril

Pharmacologic class: tricyclic dibenzodiazepine derivative
Therapeutic class: antipsychotic
Pregnancy risk category: B

Indications and dosages

▶ **Schizophrenia in severely ill patients unresponsive to other therapies.** *Adults:* initially, 12.5 mg P.O. once daily or b.i.d., adjusted upward at 25 to 50 mg daily (if tolerated) to 300 to 450 mg daily by end of 2 weeks. Individual dosage based on clinical response, patient tolerance, and adverse reactions. Dosage shouldn't be increased more than once or twice weekly and shouldn't exceed 100 mg. Many patients respond to 300 to 600 mg daily, but some may need as much as 900 mg daily. Don't exceed 900 mg daily.

How supplied

Tablets: 25 mg, 100 mg

Pharmacokinetics

Absorption: thought to be absorbed from GI tract.
Distribution: about 95% bound to serum proteins.
Metabolism: metabolism is nearly complete.
Excretion: about 50% of drug appears in urine and 30% in feces, mostly as metabolites. *Half-life:* appears proportional to dose and may range from 8 to 12 hours.

Route	Onset	Peak	Duration
P.O.	Unknown	2.5 hr	4-12 hr

Pharmacodynamics

Chemical effect: unknown. Binds to dopaminergic receptors (both D_1 and D_2) within limbic system of CNS and may interfere with adrenergic, cholinergic, histaminergic, and serotoninergic receptors.
Therapeutic effect: relieves psychotic signs and symptoms.

Adverse reactions

CNS: *drowsiness, sedation,* ***seizures,*** dizziness, syncope, vertigo, headache, tremor, disturbed sleep or nightmares, restlessness, hypokinesia or akinesia, agitation, rigidity, akathisia, confusion, fatigue, insomnia, hyperkinesia, weakness, lethargy, ataxia, slurred speech, depression, myoclonus, anxiety.
CV: tachycardia, hypotension, hypertension, chest pain, ECG changes, orthostatic hypotension.
GI: dry mouth, constipation, nausea, vomiting, *excessive salivation*, heartburn, constipation.
GU: urinary frequency, urinary urgency, urine retention, incontinence, abnormal ejaculation.
Hematologic: ***leukopenia, agranulocytosis.***
Metabolic: weight gain.
Musculoskeletal: muscle pain or spasm, muscle weakness.
Skin: rash.
Other: fever.

Interactions

Drug-drug. *Anticholinergics:* may potentiate anticholinergic effects of clozapine. Avoid concomitant use.
Antihypertensives: may potentiate hypotensive effects. Monitor blood pressure.
Bone marrow suppressants: may increase bone marrow toxicity. Don't use together.
Digoxin, warfarin, other highly protein-bound drugs: may increase serum levels of these drugs. Monitor patient closely for adverse reactions.
Psychoactive drugs: may produce additive effects. Use together cautiously.
Drug-herb. *St. John's wort:* may reduce blood levels causing a loss of symptom control in patients taking an antipsychotic. Discourage concomitant use.
Drug-food. *Caffeine-containing beverages:* may inhibit antipsychotic effects of clozapine. Monitor patient closely.
Drug-lifestyle. *Alcohol use:* increased CNS depression. Discourage use together.

Contraindications and precautions

- Contraindicated in patients with uncontrolled epilepsy, history of drug-induced agranulocytosis, myelosuppressive disorders, severe CNS depression or coma, or WBC count below 3,500/mm^3; in those taking other drugs that suppress bone marrow function; and in breast-feeding women.
- Use cautiously in patients with prostatic hyperplasia or angle-closure glaucoma because clozapine has potent anticholinergic effects. Also use cautiously in pregnant women, patients receiving general anesthesia, and patients with hepatic, renal, or cardiac disease.
- Safety of drug hasn't been established in children.

NURSING CONSIDERATIONS

Assessment

- Assess patient's psychotic condition before therapy, and reassess regularly thereafter.
- Baseline WBC and differential counts are required before therapy and weekly thereafter.
- Be alert for adverse reactions and drug interactions.
- Monitor WBC counts weekly for at least 4 weeks after drug therapy is discontinued, as ordered, and monitor patient closely for recurrence of psychotic symptoms.
- Evaluate patient's and family's knowledge about drug therapy.

Nursing diagnoses

- Disturbed thought processes related to patient's underlying condition
- Risk of infection related to potential for drug-induced agranulocytosis
- Deficient knowledge related to drug therapy

Planning and implementation

- Drug carries significant risk of agranulocytosis. If possible, patients should receive at least two trials of standard antipsychotic drug therapy before clozapine therapy begins.
- Give drug with meals if patient develops GI distress.
- Give no more than a 1-week supply of drug.
- WBC count is used to help determine safety of therapy. If WBC count drops below 3,500/mm^3 after therapy starts or it drops substantially from baseline, monitor patient closely for signs of infection. If WBC count is 3,000 to 3,500/mm^3 and granulocyte count is above 1,500/mm^3, obtain WBC and differential count twice weekly as directed. If WBC count drops below 3,000/mm^3 and granulocyte count drops below 1,500/mm^3, interrupt therapy, notify prescriber, and monitor patient for signs of infection. Therapy may be restarted cautiously if WBC count returns to above 3,000/mm^3 and granulocyte count returns above 1,500/mm^3. Continue monitoring of WBC and differential counts twice weekly until WBC count exceeds 3,500/mm^3, as ordered.
- Follow usual guidelines for dosage increase if therapy is reinstated in patients withdrawn from drug. However, reexposure of patient to drug may increase severity and risk of adverse reactions. If therapy was withdrawn for WBC counts below 2,000/mm^3 or granulocyte counts below 1,000/mm^3, don't expect drug to be continued.
- Monitor patient for seizures, especially if he receives high doses.
- Some patients experience transient fevers (temperature over 100.4° F [38° C]), especially in first 3 weeks of therapy. Monitor patient closely.
- If WBC count drops below 2,000/mm^3 and granulocyte count drops below 1,000/mm^3, patient may require protective isolation. If patient develops infection, prepare cultures according to institutional policy and administer antibiotics as ordered. Some clinicians may perform bone marrow aspiration to assess bone marrow function. Future clozapine therapy is contraindicated in such patients.

ALERT Drug usually is withdrawn gradually (over 1- to 2-week period) if it must be discontinued. However, changes in patient's medical condition (including development of leukopenia) may require abrupt discontinuation of drug. Abrupt withdrawal of long-term therapy may cause an abrupt recurrence of psychotic symptoms.

- Severe hypoglycemia has been reported in patients without a history of hypoglycemia while receiving this therapy.

ALERT If medication levels were adjusted for a patient already taking St. John's wort, stopping the herb could cause these levels to rise, potentially causing dangerous toxic symptoms.

Patient teaching

- Warn patient about risk of agranulocytosis. Tell him drug is available only through special monitoring program that requires weekly blood tests to monitor for agranulocytosis. Advise patient to report flulike symptoms, fever, sore throat, lethargy, malaise, or other signs of infection.
- Warn patient to avoid hazardous activities that require alertness and good psychomotor coordination while taking drug.
- Tell patient to rise slowly to avoid orthostatic hypotension.

• Advise patient to check with prescriber before taking OTC medicines, herbal remedies, or alcohol.
• Recommend ice chips or sugarless candy or gum to help relieve dry mouth.

☑ Evaluation

• Patient demonstrates reduction in psychotic symptoms with drug therapy.
• Patient doesn't develop infection throughout drug therapy.
• Patient and family state understanding of drug therapy.

codeine phosphate
(KOH-deen FOS-fayt)
Paveral ♦

codeine sulfate

Pharmacologic class: opioid
Therapeutic class: analgesic, antitussive
Controlled substance schedule: II
Pregnancy risk category: C

Indications and dosages

▶ **Mild to moderate pain.** *Adults:* 15 to 60 mg P.O. or 15 to 60 mg (phosphate) S.C., I.M., or I.V. q 4 to 6 hours, p.r.n.
Children over age 1: 0.5 mg/kg P.O., I.M., or S.C. q 4 hours, p.r.n.
▶ **Nonproductive cough.** *Adults:* 10 to 20 mg P.O. q 4 to 6 hours. Maximum dosage is 120 mg/24 hours.
Children ages 6 to 12: 5 to 10 mg P.O. q 4 to 6 hours. Maximum dosage is 60 mg/24 hours.
Children ages 2 to 6: 2.5 to 5 mg P.O. q 6 hours. Maximum dosage is 30 mg/24 hours.

How supplied

codeine phosphate
Oral solution: 15 mg/5 ml, 10 mg/ml ♦
Injection: 15 mg/ml, 30 mg/ml, 60 mg/ml
Soluble tablets: 30 mg, 60 mg
codeine sulfate
Tablets: 15 mg, 30 mg, 60 mg

Pharmacokinetics

Absorption: well absorbed after oral or parenteral administration. About two-thirds as potent orally as parenterally.
Distribution: distributed widely throughout body.
Metabolism: metabolized mainly in liver.
Excretion: excreted mainly in urine. *Half-life:* 2.5 to 4 hours.

Route	Onset	Peak	Duration
P.O.	30-45 min	1-2 hr	4-6 hr
I.V.	Immediate	Immediate	4-6 hr
I.M.	10-30 min	0.5-1 hr	4-6 hr
S.C.	10-30 min	Unknown	4-6 hr

Pharmacodynamics

Chemical effect: binds with opiate receptors in CNS, altering both perception of and emotional response to pain through unknown mechanism. Also suppresses cough reflex by direct action on cough center in medulla.
Therapeutic effect: relieves pain and cough.

Adverse reactions

CNS: *sedation, clouded sensorium, euphoria,* dizziness, ***seizures***.
CV: *hypotension,* ***bradycardia***.
GI: *nausea, vomiting, constipation, dry mouth,* ileus.
GU: *urine retention.*
Respiratory: ***respiratory depression.***
Skin: pruritus, flushing.
Other: physical dependence.

Interactions

Drug-drug. *CNS depressants, general anesthetics, hypnotics, MAO inhibitors, other narcotic analgesics, sedatives, tranquilizers, tricyclic antidepressants:* additive effects. Use together with extreme caution. Monitor patient response.
Drug-lifestyle. *Alcohol use:* additive effects. Use together with extreme caution. Monitor patient response.

Contraindications and precautions

• Contraindicated in patients hypersensitive to drug.

• Use with extreme caution in patients with head injury, increased intracranial pressure, increased CSF pressure, hepatic or renal disease, hypothyroidism, Addison's disease, acute alcoholism, seizures, severe CNS depression, bronchial asthma, COPD, respiratory depression, and shock. Also use with extreme caution in elderly or debilitated patients.
• Use cautiously in pregnant or breast-feeding women and in children.

NURSING CONSIDERATIONS

Assessment
• Assess patient's pain or cough before and after drug administration.
• Be alert for adverse reactions and drug interactions.
• Evaluate patient's and family's knowledge of drug therapy.

Nursing diagnoses
• Acute pain related to patient's underlying condition
• Fatigue related to presence of cough
• Deficient knowledge related to drug therapy

Planning and implementation
• For full analgesic effect, administer drug before patient has intense pain.
• Drug is an antitussive and shouldn't be used when cough is valuable diagnostic sign or is beneficial (as after thoracic surgery).
P.O. use: Administer drug with food or milk to minimize adverse GI reactions.
I.V. use: Give drug by direct injection into large vein. Administer very slowly. Don't mix with other solutions because codeine phosphate is incompatible with many drugs.
ALERT Don't give drug to children by I.V. route.
I.M. and S.C. use: Follow normal protocol.
– Don't administer discolored injection solution.
• Codeine and aspirin or acetaminophen are often prescribed together to provide enhanced pain relief.
• Codeine's abuse potential is much lower than that of morphine.
• Notify prescriber if patient doesn't experience pain or cough relief after codeine administration.
• Keep narcotic antagonist (naloxone) and resuscitative equipment available if administering drug intravenously.

Patient teaching
• Advise patient to take drug with milk or meals to minimize GI distress caused by oral administration.
• Advise patient to ask for or take drug (if at home) before pain becomes severe.
• Caution ambulatory patient about getting out of bed or walking. Warn outpatient to avoid driving and other hazardous activities until CNS effects of drug are known.
• Tell patient to report adverse drug reactions.

Evaluation
• Patient is free of pain after drug administration.
• Patient's cough is suppressed after drug administration.
• Patient and family state understanding of drug therapy.

colchicine
(KOHL-chih-seen)
Colchicine MR ◇, Colgout ◇

Pharmacologic class: *Colchicum autumnate* alkaloid
Therapeutic class: antigout agent
Pregnancy risk category: C (P.O.), D (I.V.)

Indications and dosages

▶ **Prevention of acute gout attacks as prophylactic or maintenance therapy.** *Adults:* 0.5 or 0.6 mg P.O. daily. Patients who normally have one attack per year or fewer should receive drug only 1 to 4 days per week; patients who have more than one attack per year should receive drug daily. In severe cases, 1 to 1.8 mg daily.
▶ **Prevention of gout attacks in patients undergoing surgery.** *Adults:* 0.5 to 0.6 mg P.O. t.i.d. 3 days before and 3 days after surgery.

▶ **Acute gout, acute gouty arthritis.** *Adults:* initially, 0.5 to 1.2 mg P.O.; then 0.5 or 0.6 mg q 1 to 2 hours until pain is relieved, nausea, vomiting, or diarrhea ensues, or a maximum dose of 8 mg is reached. Or, 2 mg I.V. followed by 0.5 mg I.V. q 6 hours if necessary. (Some clinicians prefer to give a single injection of 3 mg I.V.) Total I.V. dosage over 24 hours (one course of treatment) shouldn't exceed 4 mg.

How supplied

Tablets: 0.5 mg (1/120 grain), 0.6 mg (1/100 grain) as sugar-coated granules
Injection: 0.5 mg/ml

Pharmacokinetics

Absorption: rapidly absorbed from GI tract when orally administered. Unchanged drug may be reabsorbed from intestine by biliary processes.
Distribution: distributed rapidly into various tissues. Concentrated in leukocytes and distributed into kidneys, liver, spleen, and intestinal tract, but absent in heart, skeletal muscle, and brain.
Metabolism: metabolized partially in liver and also slowly metabolized in other tissues.
Excretion: drug and its metabolites are excreted primarily in feces, with lesser amounts excreted in urine. *Half-life:* 1 to 10.5 hours.

Route	Onset	Peak	Duration
P.O.	≤ 12 hr	0.5-2 hr	Unknown
I.V.	6-12 hr	0.5-2 hr	Unknown

Pharmacodynamics

Chemical effect: unknown. As antigout agent, apparently decreases WBC motility, phagocytosis, and lactic acid production, decreasing urate crystal deposits and reducing inflammation. As antiosteolytic agent, apparently inhibits mitosis of osteoprogenitor cells and decreases osteoclast activity.
Therapeutic effect: relieves gout signs and symptoms.

Adverse reactions

CNS: peripheral neuritis.
GI: *nausea, vomiting, abdominal pain, diarrhea.*
Hematologic: ***aplastic anemia, thrombocytopenia, agranulocytosis*** (with prolonged use); nonthrombocytopenic purpura.
Hepatic: ***hepatic necrosis.***
Skin: alopecia, urticaria, dermatitis.
Other: severe local irritation (if extravasation occurs), ***hypersensitivity, anaphylaxis.***

Interactions

Drug-drug. *Loop diuretics:* may decrease efficacy of colchicine prophylaxis. Avoid concomitant use.
Phenylbutazone: may increase risk of leukopenia or thrombocytopenia. Avoid concomitant use.
Vitamin B_{12}: impaired absorption of vitamin B_{12}. Avoid concomitant use.
Drug-lifestyle. *Alcohol use:* may impair efficacy of colchicine prophylaxis. Don't use together.

Contraindications and precautions

- Contraindicated in elderly patients, debilitated patients, and patients with serious cardiac disease, renal disease, or GI disorders.
- Use with extreme caution, if at all, in pregnant women because fetal harm may occur.
- Use cautiously in elderly or debilitated patients or in patients with early evidence of cardiac, renal, or GI disease.
- Safety of drug hasn't been established in children or breast-feeding women.

NURSING CONSIDERATIONS

Assessment

- Assess patient's underlying condition before therapy, and reassess regularly thereafter.
- Obtain baseline laboratory studies, including CBC and uric acid levels, before therapy and repeat regularly, as ordered.
- Be alert for adverse reactions and drug interactions.
- Evaluate patient's and family's knowledge of drug therapy.

Nursing diagnoses

- Acute pain related to presence of gout
- Ineffective protection related to drug-induced hematologic adverse reactions
- Deficient knowledge related to drug therapy

Planning and implementation

P.O. use: Give drug with meals to reduce GI effects as maintenance therapy. May be used with uricosuric agents.
I.V. use: Give drug by slow I.V. push over 2 to 5 minutes. Avoid extravasation because colchicine is very irritating to tissues.
– Don't dilute colchicine injection with D_5W injection or other fluids that might change pH of colchicine solution. If lower concentration of colchicine injection is needed, dilute with normal saline solution or sterile water for injection and administer over 2 to 5 minutes by direct injection. Preferably, inject into tubing of free-flowing I.V. solution. However, don't inject if diluted solution becomes turbid.
ALERT After full course of I.V. colchicine (4 mg), no more colchicine should be given by any other route for at least 7 days. Colchicine is toxic and death can result from overdose.
- Don't administer I.M. or S.C.; severe local irritation occurs.
- Store drug in tightly closed, light-resistant container.
- Discontinue drug as soon as gout pain is relieved or at first sign of GI symptoms, as ordered.
- Force fluids to maintain output at 2,000 ml daily.

Patient teaching
- Teach patient how to take drug.
- Advise patient to report rash, sore throat, fever, unusual bleeding, bruising, fatigue, weakness, numbness, or tingling.
- Instruct patient on when drug should be discontinued.
- Tell patient to avoid alcohol during drug therapy because it may inhibit drug action.
- Advise patient to avoid all drugs containing aspirin because they may precipitate gout.

Evaluation
- Patient becomes pain free after drug therapy.
- Patient's CBC and platelet counts remain normal throughout drug therapy.
- Patient and family state understanding of drug therapy.

colestipol hydrochloride
(koh-LEH-stih-pohl high-droh-KLOR-ighd)
Colestid

Pharmacologic class: anion exchange resin
Therapeutic class: antilipemic
Pregnancy risk category: B

Indications and dosages
▶ **Primary hypercholesterolemia.** *Adults:* initially, 5 g P.O. daily or b.i.d.; increased in 5-mg increments q 1 to 2 months, p.r.n. Usual dose is 5 to 30 g (granules) P.O. once daily or in divided doses. Or, 2 to 16 g (tablets) P.O. daily given once or in divided doses.

How supplied
Granules: 300-g and 500-g bottles, 5-g packets
Tablets: 1 g

Pharmacokinetics
Absorption: not absorbed.
Distribution: distributed locally in intestines.
Metabolism: none.
Excretion: excreted in feces.

Route	Onset	Peak	Duration
P.O.	1-2 days	1 mo	≤ 1 mo

Pharmacodynamics
Chemical effect: combines with bile acid to form insoluble compound that is excreted. The liver must synthesize new bile acid from cholesterol; this leads to reduced low-density lipoprotein levels.
Therapeutic effect: lowers low-density lipoprotein levels.

Adverse reactions
CNS: headache, dizziness.
GI: constipation, fecal impaction, hemorrhoids, abdominal discomfort, flatulence, nausea, vomiting, steatorrhea.
Skin: rash; irritation of tongue and perianal area.
Other: vitamin A, D, E, and K deficiency (from decreased absorption); hyperchloremic acidosis (with long-term use or high dosage).

Interactions

Drug-drug. *Orally administered drugs:* colestipol may decrease absorption. Separate administration times; give other drugs at least 1 hour before or 4 hours after colestipol.
Oral antidiabetics: may antagonize response to colestipol. Monitor serum lipids.

Contraindications and precautions

- Contraindicated in patients hypersensitive to bile-acid sequestering resins.
- Use cautiously in patients predisposed to constipation and in those with conditions aggravated by constipation, such as severe, symptomatic coronary artery disease. Also use cautiously in pregnant women.
- Safety of drug hasn't been established in children or breast-feeding women.

NURSING CONSIDERATIONS

Assessment
- Assess patient's blood cholesterol level before therapy.
- Monitor effectiveness by evaluating serum cholesterol and triglyceride levels regularly during therapy.
- Be alert for adverse reactions and drug interactions.
- Monitor patient for signs of fat-soluble vitamin deficiencies.
- Evaluate patient's and family's knowledge of drug therapy.

Nursing diagnoses
- Risk for injury related to elevated blood cholesterol
- Constipation related to drug-induced adverse GI reactions
- Deficient knowledge related to drug therapy

Planning and implementation
- To prepare granules, use large glass containing water, milk, or juice (preferably pulpy fruit juice). Sprinkle powder on surface of beverage; let mixture stand few minutes; then stir thoroughly to obtain uniform suspension. After patient drinks this preparation, swirl small additional amount of liquid in same glass and then have him drink it to ensure ingestion of entire dose.
- If severe constipation develops, decrease dosage or add stool softener as ordered. Encourage diet high in fiber and fluids.
- Administer all other drugs at least 1 hour before or 4 to 6 hours after colestipol to avoid blocking their absorption.

Patient teaching
- Instruct patient never to take drug in its dry form; esophageal irritation or severe constipation may result.
- Teach patient how to mix and take drug. To enhance palatability, tell him to mix and refrigerate the next daily dose the previous evening.
- Advise patient to take all other drugs at least 1 hour before or 4 to 6 hours after colestipol to avoid blocking their absorption.
- Teach patient about proper dietary management of serum lipids (restricting total fat and cholesterol intake) as well as measures to control other cardiac disease risk factors. When appropriate, recommend weight control, exercise, and smoking cessation programs.
- Inform patient that long-term use may be linked to deficiency of vitamins A, D, E, and K and folic acid. Instruct patient to report unusual signs and symptoms and to ask prescriber about taking multivitamins.

Evaluation
- Patient's blood cholesterol level is normal.
- Patient's constipation is relieved.
- Patient and family state understanding of drug therapy.

corticotropin (adrenocorticotropic hormone, ACTH)
(kor-teh-koh-TROH-pin)
ACTH, Acthar

repository corticotropin
Acthar Gel (H.P.)♦, ACTH Gel, Acthar Gel

Pharmacologic class: anterior pituitary hormone

Therapeutic class: diagnostic aid, replacement hormone
Pregnancy risk category: C

Indications and dosages

▶ **Diagnostic test of adrenocortical function.** *Adults:* 40 units repository form I.M. or S.C. q 12 hours for 1 to 2 days. Or, 10 to 25 units aqueous form in 500 ml of D_5W I.V. over 8 hours, between blood samplings. Individual dosages generally vary with adrenal glands' sensitivity to stimulation as well as with specific disease. Infants and younger children require larger doses per kilogram than older children and adults.

▶ **For therapeutic use.** *Adults:* 20 units aqueous form S.C. or I.M. in four divided doses. Or, 40 to 80 units q 24 to 72 hours (repository form).

How supplied

Aqueous injection: 25 units/vial, 40 units/vial
Repository injection: 40 units/ml, 80 units/ml

Pharmacokinetics

Absorption: absorbed rapidly after I.M. administration; unknown for S.C. administration.
Distribution: unknown.
Metabolism: unknown.
Excretion: excreted by kidneys. *Half-life:* about 15 minutes.

Route	Onset	Peak	Duration
I.V, I.M., S.C.	Rapid	Varies	2 hr (zinc form) ≤ 3 days (repository)

Pharmacodynamics

Chemical effect: by replacing body's own tropic hormone, stimulates secretion of adrenal cortex hormones.
Therapeutic effect: diagnosis or treatment of adrenocortical hormonal deficiency.

Adverse reactions

CNS: ***seizures,*** *dizziness,* ***papilledema,*** headache, *euphoria, insomnia,* mood swings, personality changes, depression, psychosis, ***increased intracranial pressure.***
CV: ***shock.***
EENT: cataracts, glaucoma.
GI: peptic ulceration (with perforation and hemorrhage), ***pancreatitis,*** abdominal distention, ulcerative esophagitis, nausea, vomiting.
GU: menstrual irregularities.
Metabolic: activation of latent diabetes mellitus, *sodium and fluid retention,* calcium and potassium loss, hypokalemic alkalosis, negative nitrogen balance.
Musculoskeletal: muscle weakness, steroid myopathy, loss of muscle mass, osteoporosis, vertebral compression fractures, suppression of growth in children.
Skin: impaired wound healing, thin and fragile skin, petechiae, ecchymoses, facial erythema, diaphoresis, acne, hyperpigmentation, allergic skin reactions, hirsutism.
Other cushingoid symptoms, progressive increase in antibodies, loss of corticotropin stimulatory effect, hypersensitivity reactions (rash, ***bronchospasm***).

Interactions

Drug-drug. *Anticonvulsants, barbiturates, rifampin:* increased metabolism of corticotropin and decreased effectiveness. Monitor patient for lack of effect.
Estrogens: may potentiate effects of cortisol. Dosage adjustments may be necessary.
NSAIDs, salicylates: increased risk of GI bleeding. Avoid concomitant use.
Oral anticoagulants: altered PT. Monitor PT and INR. Dosage adjustments may be necessary.
Potassium-wasting diuretics: increased risk of hypokalemia. Monitor serum potassium levels.

Contraindications and precautions

- Contraindicated in patients hypersensitive to pork and pork products and in patients with peptic ulcer, scleroderma, osteoporosis, systemic fungal infections, ocular herpes simplex, peptic ulceration, heart failure, hypertension, adrenocortical hyperfunction or primary insufficiency, or Cushing's syndrome. Also contraindicated in those who have had recent surgery.
- Use cautiously in pregnant women and in women of childbearing age. Also use cautiously in patients being immunized and in those with latent tuberculosis or tuberculin reactivi-

ty, hypothyroidism, cirrhosis, acute gouty arthritis, psychotic tendencies, renal insufficiency, diverticulitis, nonspecific ulcerative colitis, thromboembolic disorders, seizures, uncontrolled hypertension, or myasthenia gravis.
• Also use cautiously in children because prolonged use of drug will inhibit skeletal growth. Intermittent administration is recommended.
• Safety of drug hasn't been established in breast-feeding women.

NURSING CONSIDERATIONS

Assessment
• Assess patient's underlying condition before therapy, and reassess regularly during therapy.
• Corticotropin treatment should be preceded by verification of adrenal responsiveness and test for hypersensitivity and allergic reactions.
• Be alert for adverse reactions and drug interactions.
• Note and record weight changes, fluid exchange, and resting blood pressures until minimal effective dosage is achieved.
• Watch neonates of corticotropin-treated mothers for signs of hypoadrenalism.
• Monitor patient for stress.
• Evaluate patient's and family's knowledge about drug test or therapy.

Nursing diagnoses
• Ineffective protection related to underlying condition
• Risk for injury related to drug-induced adverse reactions
• Deficient knowledge related to drug test or therapy

Planning and implementation
• Corticotropin should be adjunct, not sole, therapy. Oral form is preferred for long-term therapy.
I.V. use: Use only aqueous form for I.V. administration. Dilute in 500 ml of D_5W and infuse over 8 hours.
I.M. use: If administering gel, warm it to room temperature, draw into large needle, and give slowly as deep I.M. injection with 21G or 22G needle. Warn patient that injection is painful.
• Refrigerate reconstituted solution and use within 24 hours.
• Counteract edema with low-sodium, high-potassium intake; nitrogen loss with a high-protein diet; and psychotic changes with a reduction in corticotropin dosage or use of sedatives as ordered.
• Unusual stress may require additional use of rapidly acting corticosteroids. When possible, gradually reduce corticotropin dosage to smallest effective dose as ordered to minimize induced adrenocortical insufficiency. Therapy can be reinstituted if stressful situation (trauma, surgery, severe illness) occurs shortly after stopping drug.

Patient teaching
• Stress importance of informing health care team members about corticotropin use because unusual stress may need additional use of rapidly acting corticosteroids. If corticotropin was recently stopped, therapy may have to be reinstituted.
• Tell patient to restrict sodium intake and consume high-protein, high-potassium diet.
• Advise patient to have close follow-up care.
• Warn patient that injections, especially I.M. injections, are painful.

Evaluation
• Patient's underlying condition improves with drug therapy.
• Patient doesn't experience injury as result of drug-induced adverse reactions.
• Patient and family state understanding of drug test or therapy.

cortisone acetate
(KOR-tih-sohn AS-ih-tayt)
Cortone Acetate, Cortisone Acetate

Pharmacologic class: glucocorticoid, mineralocorticoid
Therapeutic class: anti-inflammatory, replacement therapy
Pregnancy risk category: C

Indications and dosages

▶ **Adrenal insufficiency, allergy, inflammation.** *Adults:* 25 to 300 mg P.O. or 20 to 300 mg I.M. daily or on alternate days. Dosages are highly individualized, depending on severity of disease.

How supplied

Tablets: 5 mg, 10 mg, 25 mg
Injection (suspension): 50 mg/ml

Pharmacokinetics

Absorption: absorbed readily after oral administration; unknown for I.M. administration.
Distribution: distributed rapidly to muscle. liver, skin, intestines, and kidneys. Cortisone is extensively bound to plasma proteins. Only unbound portion is active.
Metabolism: metabolized in liver to active metabolite hydrocortisone, which is metabolized to inactive glucuronide and sulfate metabolites.
Excretion: inactive metabolites and small amounts of unmetabolized drug are excreted by kidneys. Insignificant quantities of drug also excreted in feces. *Half-life:* 8 to 12 hours.

Route	Onset	Peak	Duration
P.O.	Rapid	2 hr	1.25-1.5 days
I.M.	Slow	20-48 hr	Varies

Pharmacodynamics

Chemical effect: not completely defined. Decreases inflammation, mainly by stabilizing leukocyte lysosomal membranes; suppresses immune response; stimulates bone marrow; and influences protein, fat, and carbohydrate metabolism.
Therapeutic effect: reduces inflammation; raises corticosteroid therapy.

Adverse reactions

Most adverse reactions are dose- or duration-dependent.
CNS: *euphoria, insomnia,* psychotic behavior, pseudotumor cerebri, ***seizures.***
CV: ***arrhythmias, heart failure, thromboembolism,*** hypertension, edema.
EENT: cataracts, glaucoma.
GI: *peptic ulceration,* GI irritation, increased appetite, pancreatitis.
Metabolic: possible hypokalemia, hyperglycemia, and carbohydrate intolerance.
Musculoskeletal: muscle weakness, osteoporosis, growth suppression in children.
Skin: hirsutism, delayed wound healing, acne, various skin eruptions, atrophy at I.M. injection site.
Other: susceptibility to infections, ***acute adrenal insufficiency following increased stress (infection, surgery, or trauma) or abrupt withdrawal after long-term therapy.***

Interactions

Drug-drug. *Aspirin, indomethacin, other NSAIDs:* increased risk of GI distress and bleeding. Give together cautiously.
Barbiturates, phenytoin, rifampin: decreased corticosteroid effect. Increase corticosteroid dosage, as ordered.
Live-attenuated virus vaccines, other toxoids and vaccines: decreased antibody response and increased risk of neurologic complications. Avoid concomitant use.
Oral anticoagulants: altered dosage requirements. Monitor PT closely.
Potassium-depleting drugs (such as thiazide diuretics): enhanced potassium-wasting effects of cortisone. Monitor serum potassium levels.
Skin-test antigens: decreased response. Defer skin testing until therapy is completed.
Drug-lifestyle. *Alcohol use:* increased risk of gastric irritation. Discourage concomitant use.

Contraindications and precautions

- Contraindicated in patients hypersensitive to drug or its ingredients and in those with systemic fungal infections.
- Use with extreme caution in patient with recent MI.
- Use cautiously in patients with GI ulcer, renal disease, hypertension, osteoporosis, diabetes mellitus, hypothyroidism, cirrhosis, diverticulitis, nonspecific ulcerative colitis, recent intestinal anastomoses, thromboembolic disorders, seizures, myasthenia gravis, heart failure, tuberculosis, ocular herpes simplex, emotional instability, and psychotic tendencies.
- Use cautiously in pregnant or breast-feeding women.

• Long-term use of drug in children isn't recommended because growth and maturation may be delayed.

NURSING CONSIDERATIONS

Assessment

• Assess patient's underlying condition before therapy, and reassess regularly thereafter.
• Monitor serum electrolyte and blood glucose levels as ordered. Check patient's weight and vital signs regularly.
• Monitor patient's stress level.
• Be alert for adverse reactions and drug interactions.
• Evaluate patient's and family's knowledge of drug therapy.

Nursing diagnoses

• Ineffective protection related to underlying condition
• Risk for injury related to drug-induced adverse reactions
• Deficient knowledge related to drug therapy

Planning and implementation

P.O. use: Give drug with milk or food to reduce GI irritation.
– Give once-daily dose in morning for best results and least toxicity.
I.M. use: I.M. route causes slow onset of action. Shouldn't be used in acute conditions where rapid effect is required. May be used on twice-daily schedule matching diurnal variation. Rotate injection sites to prevent muscle atrophy.
– Mixing or diluting parenteral suspension may alter absorption rate and decrease drug's effectiveness.
• Drug isn't for I.V. use.
• Drug should always be adjusted to lowest effective dose.
• Gradually reduce drug dosage after long-term therapy, as ordered.
• Notify prescriber if signs of adrenal insufficiency increase. Unusual stress may require additional use of rapidly acting corticosteroids.

Patient teaching

ALERT Tell patient not to discontinue drug abruptly or without prescriber's consent. Abrupt withdrawal may cause rebound inflammation, fatigue, weakness, arthralgia, fever, dizziness, lethargy, depression, fainting, orthostatic hypotension, dyspnea, anorexia, and hypoglycemia. After prolonged use, sudden withdrawal may be fatal.
• Advise patient receiving long-term therapy to consider exercise or physical therapy. Also tell him to ask prescriber about vitamin D or calcium supplements.
• Tell patient to restrict sodium intake and consume high-protein, high-potassium diet.
• Tell patient to report slow healing.
• Warn patient receiving long-term therapy about cushingoid symptoms and the need to report sudden weight gain or swelling to prescriber.
• Instruct patient to wear or carry medical identification indicating his need for supplemental glucocorticoids during stress.

Evaluation

• Patient shows improvement in underlying condition with drug therapy.
• Patient doesn't experience injury as result of drug-induced adverse reactions.
• Patient and family state understanding of drug therapy.

cosyntropin

(koh-sin-TROH-pin)
Cortrosyn

Pharmacologic class: anterior pituitary hormone
Therapeutic class: diagnostic agent
Pregnancy risk category: C

Indications and dosages

▶ **Diagnostic test of adrenocortical function.** *Adults and children age 2 and older:* 0.25 to 1 mg I.M. or I.V. over 2 minutes (unless label prohibits I.V. administration) between blood samplings.
Children under age 2: 0.125 mg I.V. or I.M.

How supplied

Injection: 0.25 mg/vial

Pharmacokinetics

Absorption: absorbed rapidly after I.M. administration.
Distribution: unknown.
Metabolism: unknown.
Excretion: thought to be excreted by kidneys.

Route	Onset	Peak	Duration
I.V.	≤ 5 min	1 hr	Unknown
I.M.	Unknown	1 hr	Unknown

Pharmacodynamics

Chemical effect: by replacing body's own tropic hormone, stimulates secretion of adrenal cortex hormones.
Therapeutic effect: aid in diagnosing adrenocortical dysfunction.

Adverse reactions

CNS: ***seizures, increased intracranial pressure with papilledema.***
Skin: pruritus.
Other: flushing, hypersensitivity reactions.

Interactions

Drug-drug. *Blood and plasma products:* inactivate cosyntropin. Avoid concomitant administration.
Cortisone, hydrocortisone: may interfere with test results of cortisol levels if administered on test day.
Spironolactone: may interfere with fluorometric analysis of cortisol levels. Avoid concomitant use.

Contraindications and precautions

- Contraindicated in patients hypersensitive to drug.
- Use cautiously in patients hypersensitive to natural corticotropin.
- Safety of drug hasn't been established in pregnant or breast-feeding women and children under age 2.

NURSING CONSIDERATIONS

Assessment

- Assess patient's reason for test before administration. Evaluate test results.
- Be alert for adverse reactions and drug interactions.
- Monitor patients for allergic reactions, rashes, dyspnea, wheezing, or evidence of anaphylaxis.
- Evaluate patient's and family's knowledge about drug test.

Nursing diagnoses

- Risk for injury related to potential for cosyntropin to cause hypersensitivity reactions
- Deficient knowledge related to drug test

Planning and implementation

I.V. use: Reconstitute drug with 1 ml of supplied diluent. For direct injection, administer over at least 2 minutes. May be further diluted with D_5W or normal saline solution and infused at 0.04 mg/hr over 6 hours. Solution is stable for 12 hours at room temperature.
I.M. use: Follow normal protocol.
- Notify prescriber if hypersensitivity occurs, and be prepared to administer emergency care.

Patient teaching

- Instruct patient to notify prescriber immediately if pruritus or other signs of hypersensitivity occur.
- Explain how drug test is performed.

Evaluation

- Patient doesn't have hypersensitivity reaction to drug.
- Patient and family state understanding of drug test.

co-trimoxazole (sulfamethoxazole-trimethoprim)

(koh-trigh-MOX-uh-zohl)

Apo-Sulfatrim ♦, Apo-Sulfatrim DS ♦, Bactrim*, Bactrim DS, Bactrim I.V. Infusion, Cotrim, Cotrim D.S., Novotrimel ♦, Novotrimel DS ♦, Resprim ◊, Roubac ♦, Septra*, Septra DS, Septra I.V. Infusion, Septrin ◊, SMZ-TMP

Pharmacologic class: sulfonamide and folate antagonist
Therapeutic class: antibiotic

Pregnancy risk category: C (contraindicated at term)

Indications and dosages

▶ **Urinary tract infections and shigellosis.** *Adults:* 160 mg trimethoprim/800 mg sulfamethoxazole (double-strength tablet) P.O. q 12 hours for 10 to 14 days in urinary tract infections and for 5 days in shigellosis. If indicated, I.V. infusion is given at 8 to 10 mg/kg/day (based on trimethoprim component) in two to four divided doses q 6, 8, or 12 hours for up to 14 days. Maximum dose is 960 mg/day trimethoprim.
Children age 2 months and over: 8 mg/kg trimethoprim/40 mg/kg sulfamethoxazole P.O. per 24 hours, in two divided doses q 12 hours (10 days for urinary tract infections; 5 days for shigellosis). If indicated, I.V. infusion is given at 8 to 10 mg/kg/day (based on trimethoprim component) in two to four divided doses q 6, 8, or 12 hours. Don't exceed adult dose.

▶ **Otitis media in patients with penicillin allergy or penicillin-resistant infections.** *Children age 2 months and over:* 8 mg/kg/day (based on trimethoprim component) P.O., in two divided doses q 12 hours for 10 days.

▶ ***Pneumocystis carinii* pneumonia.** *Adults and children age 2 months and over:* 20 mg/kg trimethoprim/100 mg/kg sulfamethoxazole P.O. per 24 hours, in equally divided doses q 6 hours for 14 days. If indicated, I.V. infusion may be given 15 to 20 mg/kg/day (based on trimethoprim component) in three or four divided doses q 6 to 8 hours for up to 14 days.

▶ **Chronic bronchitis.** *Adults:* 160 mg trimethoprim/800 mg sulfamethoxazole P.O. q 12 hours for 10 to 14 days.

▶ **Traveler's diarrhea.** *Adults:* 160 mg trimethoprim/800 mg sulfamethoxazole P.O. b.i.d. for 3 to 5 days. Some patients may require 2 days of therapy or less.

▶ **Urinary tract infections in men with prostatitis.** *Adults:* 160 mg trimethoprim/800 mg sulfamethoxazole P.O. b.i.d. for 3 to 6 months.

▶ **Chronic urinary tract infections.** *Adults:* 40 mg trimethoprim/200 mg sulfamethoxazole (½ tablet) or 80 mg trimetoprim/400 mg sulfamethoxazole P.O. daily or three times week for 3 to 6 months.

How supplied

Tablets: trimethoprim 80 mg and sulfamethoxazole 400 mg; trimethoprim 160 mg and sulfamethoxazole 800 mg
Oral suspension: trimethoprim 40 mg and sulfamethoxazole 200 mg/5 ml
Injection: trimethoprim 16 mg and sulfamethoxazole 80 mg/ml (5 ml/ampule)

Pharmacokinetics

Absorption: well absorbed from GI tract after oral administration.
Distribution: distributed widely into body tissues and fluids, including middle ear fluid, prostatic fluid, bile, aqueous humor, and CSF. Protein binding is 44% for trimethoprim, 70% for sulfamethoxazole.
Metabolism: both components of drug are metabolized by liver.
Excretion: both components of drug are excreted primarily in urine. *Half-life:* trimethoprim, 8 to 11 hours; sulfamethoxazole, 10 to 13 hours.

Route	Onset	Peak	Duration
P.O.	Unknown	1-4 hr	Unknown
I.V.	Immediate	Immediate	Unknown

Pharmacodynamics

Chemical effect: sulfamethoxazole component inhibits formation of dihydrofolic acid from PABA; trimethoprim component inhibits dihydrofolate reductase. Both decrease bacterial folic acid synthesis.
Therapeutic effect: inhibits susceptible bacterial activity. Spectrum of activity include *Escherichia coli, Klebsiella, Enterobacter, Proteus mirabilis, Haemophilus influenzae, Streptococcus pneumoniae, Staphylococcus aureus, Acinetobacter, Salmonella, Shigella,* and *P.carinii.*

Adverse reactions

CNS: headache, mental depression, ***seizures,*** hallucinations, ataxia, nervousness, fatigue, vertigo, insomnia.
CV: thrombophlebitis.
GI: *nausea, vomiting, diarrhea,* abdominal pain, anorexia, stomatitis.
GU: ***toxic nephrosis with oliguria and anuria,*** crystalluria, hematuria.

Hematologic: ***agranulocytosis, aplastic anemia,*** megaloblastic anemia, ***thrombocytopenia, leukopenia, hemolytic anemia.***
Hepatic: jaundice, ***hepatic necrosis.***
Musculoskeletal: muscle weakness.
Skin: ***erythema multiforme, Stevens-Johnson syndrome,*** *generalized skin eruption,* ***epidermal necrolysis, exfoliative dermatitis,*** photosensitivity, urticaria, pruritus.
Other: hypersensitivity reactions (serum sickness, drug fever, ***anaphylaxis***).

Interactions

Drug-drug. *Oral anticoagulants:* increased anticoagulant effect. Monitor patient for bleeding.
Oral antidiabetics: increased hypoglycemic effect. Monitor blood glucose levels.
Oral contraceptives: decreased contraceptive effectiveness and increased risk of breakthrough bleeding. Suggest nonhormonal form of contraception.
Phenytoin: may inhibit hepatic metabolism of phenytoin. Monitor phenytoin levels.
Drug-herb. *Dong quai, St. John's wort:* increased risk of photosensitivity. Advise patient to avoid unprotected exposure to sunlight.
Drug-lifestyle. *Sun exposure:* Photosensitivity reactions may occur. Urge patient to take precautions.

Contraindications and precautions

- Contraindicated in patients with megaloblastic anemia caused by folate deficiency, porphyria, severe renal impairment (creatinine clearance less than 15 ml/minute), or hypersensitivity to trimethoprim or sulfonamides; in pregnant women at term; and in breast-feeding women.
- Use cautiously and in reduced dosages in patients with impaired hepatic or renal function (creatinine clearance of 15 to 30 ml/minute), severe allergy or bronchial asthma, G6PD deficiency, and blood dyscrasia.
- Safety of drug hasn't been established in infants under age 2 months.

NURSING CONSIDERATIONS

Assessment

- Assess patient's infection before therapy, and reassess regularly thereafter.
- Obtain specimen for culture and sensitivity tests before first dose. Therapy may begin pending results.
- Be alert for adverse reactions and drug interactions.
- Monitor patient's hydration status if adverse GI reactions occur.
- Monitor intake and output. Urine output should be at least 1,500 ml/day to ensure proper hydration. Inadequate urine output can lead to crystalluria or tubular deposits of drug.
- Evaluate patient's and family's knowledge of drug therapy.

Nursing diagnoses

- Infection related to presence of bacteria susceptible to drug
- Risk for deficient fluid volume related to drug induced adverse GI reactions
- Deficient knowledge related to drug therapy

Planning and implementation

P.O. use: Administer drug with full glass of water at least 1 hour before or 2 hours after meals for maximum absorption. Shake oral suspension thoroughly before administering.
I.V. use: Dilute contents of 5-ml ampule of drug in 125 ml of D_5W before administration. If patient is on a fluid restriction, dilute 5 ml of drug in 75 ml D_5W. Don't mix with other drugs or solutions. Infuse slowly over 60 to 90 minutes. Don't give by rapid infusion or bolus injection. Don't refrigerate.
- Never administer I.M.
- Note that DS in product name means double strength.

Patient teaching

- Tell patient to take entire amount of medication exactly as prescribed, even if he feels better.
- Tell patient to take drug with full glass of water and to drink at least 3 to 4 L/day of water.

• Advise patient to avoid exposure to direct sunlight because of risk of photosensitivity reaction.
• Tell patient to report signs of rash, sore throat, fever, or mouth sores because drug may need to be discontinued.

Evaluation
• Patient is free from infection after drug therapy.
• Patient maintains adequate hydration after drug therapy.
• Patient and family state understanding of drug therapy.

cromolyn sodium (sodium cromoglycate)

(KROH-moh-lin SOH-dee-um)
Crolom, Gastrocrom, Intal, Intal Aerosol Spray, Intal Nebulizer Solution, Nasalcrom, Rynacrom ♦

Pharmacologic class: chromone derivative
Therapeutic class: mast cell stabilizer, antiasthmatic
Pregnancy risk category: B

Indications and dosages

▶ **Mild to moderate persistent asthma.** *Adults and children age 5 and over:* 2 metered sprays using inhaler q.i.d. at regular intervals. Or, 20 mg via nebulization q.i.d. at regular intervals.

▶ **Prevention and treatment of allergic rhinitis.** *Adults and children over age 6:* 1 spray in each nostril t.i.d or q.i.d. Maximal administration is six times daily.

▶ **Prevention of exercise-induced bronchospasm.** *Adults and children age 5 and over:* 2 metered sprays inhaled no more than 1 hour before anticipated exercise.

▶ **Conjunctivitis.** *Adults and children age 4 and older:* 1 to 2 drops in each eye four to six times daily at regular intervals.

▶ **Systemic mastocytosis.** *Adults and children over age 12:* 200 mg P.O. q.i.d. before meals and h.s.
Children ages 2 to 12: 100 mg P.O. q.i.d. 30 minutes before meals or h.s.

How supplied

Capsules (for oral solution): 100 mg
Aerosol: 800 mcg/metered spray
Nasal solution: 5.2 mg/metered spray (40 mg/ml)
Solution (for nebulization): 20 mg/2 ml
Ophthalmic solution: 4% (with benzalkonium chloride 0.01%, EDTA 0.01%, and phenylethyl ethanol 0.4%)

Pharmacokinetics

Absorption: only 0.5% to 2% of oral dose, 7% of intranasal dose, and 0.03% of ophthalmic dose is absorbed.
Distribution: drug doesn't cross most biological membranes.
Metabolism: none significant.
Excretion: excreted unchanged in urine (50%) and bile (about 50%). Small amounts may be excreted in feces or exhaled. *Half-life:* 81 minutes.

Route	Onset	Peak	Duration
All routes	Unknown	Unknown	Unknown

Pharmacodynamics

Chemical effect: inhibits degranulation of sensitized mast cells that occurs after patient's exposure to specific antigens. Also inhibits release of histamine and slow-reacting substance of anaphylaxis.
Therapeutic effect: adjunct to preventing bronchospasms and allergy symptoms.

Adverse reactions

CNS: dizziness, headache.
EENT: *irritation of throat and trachea,* nasal congestion, pharyngeal irritation, lacrimation.
GI: nausea, esophagitis.
GU: dysuria, urinary frequency.
Respiratory: ***bronchospasm*** (after inhalation of dry powder), *cough,* wheezing, *eosinophilic pneumonia.*
Skin: rash, urticaria.
Other: joint swelling and pain, swollen parotid gland, ***angioedema.***

Interactions

None significant.

Contraindications and precautions

• Contraindicated in patients hypersensitive to drug and in those experiencing acute asthma attacks and status asthmaticus.
• Use with caution in pregnant or breast-feeding women.
• Administer drug with caution in children. Use of cromolyn oral inhalation solution isn't recommended in children under age 2; cromolyn powder or aerosol for oral inhalation not recommended in children under age 5; and cromolyn nasal solution not recommended in children under age 6.
• Use inhalation form cautiously in patients with coronary artery disease or history of arrhythmias.

NURSING CONSIDERATIONS

Assessment

• Assess patient's underlying condition before therapy, and reassess regularly thereafter.
• Monitor pulmonary function tests to demonstrate bronchodilator-reversible component of airway obstruction.
• Monitor patient for eosinophilic pneumonia.
• Watch for recurrence of asthma symptoms when dosage is decreased, especially when corticosteroids are also used.
• Be alert for adverse reactions.
• Evaluate patient's and family's knowledge of drug therapy.

Nursing diagnoses

• Impaired gas exchange related to patient's underlying condition
• Impaired tissue integrity related to drug-induced adverse EENT reactions
• Deficient knowledge related to drug therapy

Planning and implementation

• Drug should be used only when acute episode of asthma has been controlled, airway is cleared, and patient can inhale independently.
P.O. use: Dissolve powder in capsules for oral dose in hot water and further dilute with cold water before ingestion. Don't mix with fruit juice, milk, or food.
– Oral cromolyn sodium should be used in full-term neonates and infants only for severe, incapacitating disease when benefits clearly outweigh risks.
Inhalation use: Insert inhalation capsule into inhalation device as described in manufacturer's directions. Have patient exhale completely. Then place mouthpiece between patient's lips; have him inhale deeply and rapidly with a steady, even breath; remove inhaler from mouth, have patient hold his breath for few seconds, and then exhale. Repeat until all powder has been inhaled.
Intranasal and ophthalmic use: Follow normal protocol.
• Discontinue drug if patient develops eosinophilic pneumonia, indicated by eosinophilia and infiltrates on chest X-ray.
• Aid in relief of esophagitis by use of antacids, as ordered, or milk.

Patient teaching

• Instruct patient on how to administer form of drug prescribed. Warn him to avoid excessive handling of capsules for inhalation.
• Tell patient that esophagitis may be relieved by antacids or milk.
• Instruct patient to notify prescriber if adverse reactions occur frequently or become troublesome or severe.

Evaluation

• Patient exhibits adequate air exchange with drug therapy.
• Patient demonstrates appropriate management of adverse EENT reactions.
• Patient and family state understanding of drug therapy.

cyanocobalamin (vitamin B_{12})

(sigh-an-oh-koh-BAH-luh-meen)

Anacobin♦, Bedoz♦, Crystamine, Crysti 1000, Cyanocobalamin, Cyanoject, Cyomin

hydroxocobalamin (vitamin B_{12})

Hydro-Cobex, LA-12

Pharmacologic class: water-soluble vitamin

Therapeutic class: vitamin, nutrition supplement
Pregnancy risk category: A (C if used in doses above RDA)

Indications and dosages

▶ **RDA for cyanocobalamin.** *Adults and children age 11 and over:* 2 mcg.
Pregnant women: 2.2 mcg.
Breast-feeding women: 2.6 mcg.
Children ages 7 to 10: 1.4 mcg.
Children ages 4 to 6: 1 mcg.
Children over age 1 to age 3: 0.7 mcg.
Infants ages 6 months to 1 year: 0.5 mcg.
Neonates and infants to age 6 months: 0.3 mcg.
▶ **Vitamin B_{12} deficiency caused by inadequate diet, subtotal gastrectomy, or any other condition, disorder, or disease except malabsorption related to pernicious anemia or other GI disease.** *Adults:* 30 mcg hydroxocobalamin I.M. daily for 5 to 10 days, depending on severity of deficiency. Maintenance dosage is 100 to 200 mcg I.M. once monthly. For subsequent prophylaxis, advise adequate nutrition and daily RDA vitamin B_{12} supplements.
Children: 1 to 5 mg hydroxocobalamin spread over 2 or more weeks in doses of 100 mcg I.M., depending on severity of deficiency. Maintenance dosage is 30 to 50 mcg/month I.M. For subsequent prophylaxis, advise adequate nutrition and daily RDA vitamin B_{12} supplements.
▶ **Pernicious anemia or vitamin B_{12} malabsorption.** *Adults:* initially, 100 mcg cyanocobalamin I.M. or S.C. daily for 6 to 7 days; then 100 mcg I.M. or S.C. once monthly.
Children: 30 to 50 mcg I.M. or S.C. daily over 2 or more weeks; then 100 mcg I.M. or S.C. monthly for life.
▶ **Methylmalonic aciduria.** *Neonates:* 1,000 mcg cyanocobalamin I.M. daily.
▶ **Schilling test flushing dose.** *Adults and children:* 1,000 mcg hydroxocobalamin I.M. in single dose.

How supplied

cyanocobalamin
Tablets: 25 mcg†, 50 mcg†, 100 mcg†, 250 mcg†, 500 mcg†, 1,000 mcg†
Injection: 1,000 mcg/ml
hydroxocobalamin
Injection: 1,000 mcg/ml

Pharmacokinetics

Absorption: after oral administration, vitamin B_{12} is absorbed irregularly from distal small intestine. Vitamin B_{12} is protein-bound. Absorption depends on sufficient intrinsic factor and calcium. Vitamin B_{12} is absorbed rapidly from I.M. and S.C. administration sites.
Distribution: distributed into liver, bone marrow, and other tissues.
Metabolism: metabolized in liver.
Excretion: amount of vitamin B_{12} needed by body is reabsorbed; excess is excreted in urine. *Half-life:* about 6 days.

Route	Onset	Peak	Duration
P.O.	Unknown	8-12 hr	Unknown
I.M.	Unknown	60 min	Unknown
S.C.	Unknown	Unknown	Unknown

Pharmacodynamics

Chemical effect: coenzyme that stimulates metabolic functions. Necessary for cell replication, hematopoiesis, and nucleoprotein and myelin synthesis.
Therapeutic effect: increases vitamin B_{12} level.

Adverse reactions

CV: peripheral vascular thrombosis, pulmonary edema, heart failure.
GI: transient diarrhea.
Skin: itching, transitory exanthema, urticaria.
Other: ***anaphylaxis, anaphylactoid reactions*** (with parenteral administration); pain, burning (at S.C. or I.M. injection sites).

Interactions

Drug-drug. *Aminoglycosides, chloramphenicol, colchicine, para-aminosalicylic acid and salts:* malabsorption of vitamin B_{12}. Don't use concomitantly.
Drug-lifestyle. *Alcohol use:* malabsorption of vitamin B_{12}. Don't use together.

Contraindications and precautions

- Contraindicated in patients with early Leber's disease or hypersensitivity to vitamin B_{12} or cobalt.
- Use cautiously in anemic patients with coexisting cardiac, pulmonary, or hypertensive disease and in those with severe vitamin B_{12}-dependent deficiencies.
- Use cautiously in premature infants. Some products contain benzyl alcohol which may cause gasping syndrome.

NURSING CONSIDERATIONS

Assessment

- Assess patient's vitamin B_{12} deficiency before therapy.
- Determine reticulocyte count, hematocrit, and B_{12}, iron, and folate levels before beginning therapy, as ordered.
- Monitor effectiveness by assessing patient for improvement in signs and symptoms of vitamin B_{12} deficiency. Also monitor reticulocyte count, hematocrit, and B_{12}, iron, and folate levels between fifth and seventh day of therapy and periodically thereafter, as ordered.
- Infection, tumors, and renal, hepatic, and other debilitating diseases may reduce therapeutic response.
- Closely monitor serum potassium levels for first 48 hours. Be alert for adverse reactions and drug interactions.
- Evaluate patient's and family's knowledge of drug therapy.

Nursing diagnoses

- Ineffective health maintenance related to underlying vitamin B_{12} deficiency
- Risk for injury related to parenteral administration of drug-induced hypersensitivity reactions
- Deficient knowledge related to drug therapy

Planning and implementation

- Don't mix parenteral liquids in same syringe with other medications.
- Drug is physically incompatible with dextrose solutions, alkaline or strongly acidic solutions, oxidizing or reducing agents, heavy metals, chlorpromazine, phytonadione, prochlorperazine, and many other drugs.

P.O. use: Don't administer large oral doses of vitamin B_{12} routinely because drug is lost through excretion.
I.M. use: Follow normal protocol. Hydroxocobalamin is approved only for I.M. use.
S.C. use: Follow normal protocol.

- Protect vitamin from light. Don't refrigerate or freeze.
- Give potassium supplement if necessary, as ordered.
- Drug may cause false-positive intrinsic factor antibody test.

Patient teaching

- Stress need for patient with pernicious anemia to return for monthly injections. Although total body stores may last 3 to 6 years, anemia will recur without monthly treatment.
- Emphasize importance of well-balanced diet.
- Tell patient to store oral tablets in tightly closed container at room temperature.

Evaluation

- Patient's vitamin B_{12} deficiency is resolved with drug therapy.
- Patient doesn't experience hypersensitivity reactions following parenteral administration of drug.
- Patient and family state understanding of drug therapy.

cyclizine hydrochloride

(SIGH-klih-zeen high-droh-KLOR-ighd)
Marezine†

cyclizine lactate

Pharmacologic class: piperazine-derivative antihistamine
Therapeutic class: antiemetic, antivertigo agent
Pregnancy risk category: B

Indications and dosages

▶ **Prevention or treatment of motion sickness.** *Adults and children age 12 and older:* 50 mg P.O. (hydrochloride) 30 minutes before travel, then q 4 to 6 hours, p.r.n., maximum 200 mg/day. Or, 50 mg I.M. (lactate) q 4 to 6 hours, p.r.n.
Children ages 6 to 12: 25 mg (hydrochloride) P.O. q 4 to 6 hours, p.r.n., maximum 75 mg/day.

How supplied

cyclizine hydrochloride
Tablets: 50 mg†
cyclizine lactate
Injection: 50 mg/ml

Pharmacokinetics

Absorption: unknown after oral administration.
Distribution: well distributed throughout body.
Metabolism: metabolized in liver.
Excretion: unknown.

Route	Onset	Peak	Duration
P.O., I.M.	0.5-1 hr	Unknown	4-6 hr

Pharmacodynamics

Chemical effect: unknown. An antihistamine that may affect neural pathways originating in labyrinth to inhibit nausea and vomiting.
Therapeutic effect: prevents or relieves motion sickness.

Adverse reactions

CNS: *drowsiness,* dizziness, auditory and visual hallucinations.
CV: hypotension.
EENT: blurred vision.
GI: constipation, dry mouth.
GU: urine retention.

Interactions

Drug-drug. *CNS depressants:* additive CNS depression. Avoid concomitant use.
Drug-lifestyle. *Alcohol use:* additive CNS depression. Don't use together.

Contraindications and precautions

- Contraindicated in patients hypersensitive to drug and in breast-feeding women.
- Use cautiously in patients with severe heart failure, patients with recent surgery, and pregnant women.
- Safety of drug hasn't been established in children under age 6.

NURSING CONSIDERATIONS

Assessment

- Assess patient's motion sickness before and after drug administration.
- Be alert for adverse reactions and drug interactions.
- Evaluate patient's and family's knowledge of drug therapy.

Nursing diagnoses

- Ineffective health maintenance related to motion sickness
- Risk for injury related to drug-induced adverse CNS reactions
- Deficient knowledge related to drug therapy

Planning and implementation

P.O. and I.M. use: Follow normal protocol.
- Drug should be administered 30 minutes before anticipated motion sickness.
- Store drug in cool place. When stored at room temperature, injection may turn slightly yellow; this change doesn't indicate loss of potency.

Patient teaching
- Advise patient to avoid driving and other activities that require alertness until CNS effects of drug are known.
- Advise patient that repeat doses may be necessary in 4 to 6 hours.
- Tell patient to store drug in a cool place; drug may turn slightly yellow at room temperature, but this doesn't indicate loss of potency.

Evaluation

- Patient's motion sickness is relieved or prevented with drug therapy.
- Patient doesn't experience injury as result of drug-induced adverse CNS reactions.
- Patient and family state understanding of drug therapy.

cyclobenzaprine hydrochloride

(sigh-kloh-BEN-zah-preen high-droh-KLOR-ighd)
Flexeril

Pharmacologic class: tricyclic antidepressant derivative
Therapeutic class: skeletal muscle relaxant
Pregnancy risk category: B

Indications and dosages

▶ **Short-term treatment of muscle spasm.** *Adults:* 10 mg P.O. t.i.d. for 7 days. Maximum dosage 60 mg/day; maximum duration 2 to 3 weeks.

How supplied

Tablets: 10 mg

Pharmacokinetics

Absorption: almost completely absorbed during first pass through GI tract.
Distribution: 93% plasma protein–bound.
Metabolism: during first pass through GI tract and liver, drug and metabolites undergo enterohepatic recycling.
Excretion: excreted primarily in urine as conjugated metabolites; also in feces via bile as unchanged drug. *Half-life:* 1 to 3 days.

Route	Onset	Peak	Duration
P.O.	≤ 1 hr	3-8 hr	12-24 hr

Pharmacodynamics

Chemical effect: unknown.
Therapeutic effect: relieves muscle spasms.

Adverse reactions

CNS: *drowsiness,* euphoria, weakness, headache, insomnia, nightmares, paresthesia, dizziness, depression, visual disturbances, ***seizures.***
CV: tachycardia, ***arrhythmias.***
EENT: blurred vision.
GI: dry mouth, abdominal pain, dyspepsia, abnormal taste, constipation.
GU: urine retention.
Skin: rash, urticaria, pruritus.

Interactions

Drug-drug. *Anticholinergics:* additive anticholinergic effects. Avoid concomitant use.
CNS depressants: may cause additive CNS depression. Avoid concomitant use.
MAO inhibitors: may exacerbate CNS depression or anticholinergic effects. Don't give within 14 days after discontinuing MAO inhibitors.
Drug-lifestyle. *Alcohol use:* may cause additive CNS depression. Discourage concurrent use.

Contraindications and precautions

- Contraindicated in patients hypersensitive to drug, patients who have received MAO inhibitors within 14 days, patients in the acute recovery phase of MI, and patients with hyperthyroidism, heart block, arrhythmias, conduction disturbances, or heart failure.
- Use cautiously in elderly patients, debilitated patients, and patients with history of urine retention, acute angle-closure glaucoma, or increased intraocular pressure.
- Safety of drug hasn't been established in pregnant or breast-feeding women or children.
- Caution use in patients taking anticholinergics.

NURSING CONSIDERATIONS

Assessment

- Assess patient's underlying condition before therapy.
- Monitor effectiveness by assessing severity and frequency of patient's muscle spasms.
- Be alert for nausea, headache, and malaise, which may occur if drug is stopped abruptly after long-term use.
- Evaluate patient's and family's knowledge about drug therapy.

Nursing diagnoses

- Acute pain related to presence of muscle spasms
- Risk for injury related to potential for drug-induced CNS adverse reactions
- Deficient knowledge related to drug therapy

Planning and implementation

ALERT Watch for symptoms of overdose, including cardiac toxicity. Keep physostigmine available, and notify prescriber immediately if you suspect toxicity.
- Don't administer drug with other CNS depressants.
- With high doses, watch for adverse reactions similar to those of other TCAs.

ALERT Don't confuse Flexeril with Flaxedil.

Patient teaching
- Advise patient to report urinary hesitancy or urine retention. If constipation occurs, tell him to increase fluid intake and suggest use of a stool softener.
- Warn patient to avoid activities that require alertness until drug's CNS effects are known.
- Warn patient to avoid combining drug with alcohol or other CNS depressants.
- Tell patient that dry mouth may be relieved with sugarless candy or gum.

Evaluation
- Patient is free from pain with drug therapy.
- Patient doesn't experience injury as a result of drug-induced adverse CNS reactions.
- Patient and family state understanding of drug therapy.

cyclophosphamide
(sigh-kloh-FOS-fuh-mighd)
Cycloblastin ◊, Cytoxan**, Cytoxan Lyophilized, Endoxan-Asta ◊, Neosar, Procytox ♦

Pharmacologic class: alkylating agent (not specific to cell cycle phase)
Therapeutic class: antineoplastic
Pregnancy risk category: D

Indications and dosages

▶ **Breast, head, neck, prostate, lung, and ovarian cancers; Hodgkin's disease; chronic lymphocytic leukemia; chronic myelocytic leukemia; acute lymphoblastic leukemia; acute myelocytic leukemia; neuroblastoma; retinoblastoma; non-Hodgkin's lymphoma; multiple myeloma; mycosis fungoides; sarcoma.** *Adults and children:* initially, 40 to 50 mg/kg I.V. in divided doses over 2 to 5 days. Or, 10 to 15 mg/kg I.V. q 7 to 10 days, 3 to 5 mg/kg I.V. twice weekly, or 1 to 5 mg/kg P.O. daily, based on patient tolerance. Subsequent dosage adjusted according to evidence of antitumor activity or leukopenia.

▶ **"Minimal change" nephrotic syndrome in children.** *Children:* 2.5 to 3 mg/kg P.O. daily for 60 to 90 days.

How supplied

Tablets: 25 mg, 50 mg
Injection: 100-mg, 200-mg, 500-mg, 1-g, 2-g vials

Pharmacokinetics

Absorption: almost completely absorbed from GI tract at oral doses of 100 mg or less. Higher doses (300 mg) are about 75% absorbed.
Distribution: distributed throughout body, although only minimal amounts have been found in saliva, sweat, and synovial fluid. Active metabolites are about 50% bound to plasma proteins.
Metabolism: metabolized to its active form by hepatic microsomal enzymes. Activity of these metabolites is terminated by metabolism to inactive forms.
Excretion: drug and its metabolites are eliminated primarily in urine, with 15% to 30% excreted as unchanged drug. *Half-life:* 4 to 6.5 hours.

Route	Onset	Peak	Duration
P.O., I.V.	Unknown	Unknown	Unknown

Pharmacodynamics

Chemical effect: cross-links strands of cellular DNA and interferes with RNA transcription, causing imbalance of growth that leads to cell death.
Therapeutic effect: kills specific types of cancer cells; improves renal function in mild nephrotic syndrome in children.

Adverse reactions

CV: *cardiotoxicity* (with very high doses and in combination with doxorubicin).
GI: anorexia, *nausea and vomiting beginning within 6 hours,* stomatitis, mucositis.

GU: gonadal suppression (may be irreversible), **HEMORRHAGIC CYSTITIS,** bladder fibrosis.
Hematologic: ***leukopenia,*** nadir between days 8 and 15, recovery in 17 to 28 days; ***thrombocytopenia; anemia.***
Respiratory: ***pulmonary fibrosis*** (with high doses).
Skin: *reversible alopecia in 50% of patients, especially with high doses.*
Other: ***secondary malignancies; anaphylaxis;*** hyperuricemia; SIADH (with high doses).

Interactions

Drug-drug. *Barbiturates:* increased pharmacologic effect and enhanced cyclophosphamide toxicity caused by induction of hepatic enzymes. Monitor patient closely.
Cardiotoxic drugs: additive adverse cardiac effects. Monitor patient closely.
Chloramphenicol, corticosteroids: reduced activity of cyclophosphamide. Use cautiously.
Digoxin: may decrease serum digoxin levels. Monitor levels closely.
Succinylcholine: prolonged neuromuscular blockade. Don't use together.

Contraindications and precautions

- Contraindicated in patients hypersensitive to drug, in breast-feeding women, and in patients with severe bone marrow depression.
- Use with extreme caution, if at all, in pregnant women because fetal harm may occur.
- Use cautiously in patients who have recently undergone radiation therapy or chemotherapy and in patients with leukopenia, thrombocytopenia, malignant cell infiltration of bone marrow, or hepatic or renal disease.

NURSING CONSIDERATIONS

Assessment

- Assess patient's underlying condition before therapy, and reassess regularly during therapy.
- Monitor CBC, serum uric acid levels, and renal and liver function tests, as ordered.
- Monitor patient for cyclophosphamide toxicity if corticosteroid therapy is discontinued.
- Be alert for adverse reactions and drug interactions.
- Evaluate patient's and family's knowledge of drug therapy.

Nursing diagnoses

- Ineffective health maintenance related to underlying condition
- Risk for injury related to drug-induced adverse reactions
- Deficient knowledge related to drug therapy

Planning and implementation

- Follow facility policy to reduce risks. Preparation and administration of parenteral form of this drug is linked to carcinogenic, mutagenic, and teratogenic risks for personnel.

P.O. use: Tablets are used for children with "minimal change" nephrotic syndrome and not to treat neoplastic disease.
I.V. use: Reconstitute powder using sterile water for injection or bacteriostatic water for injection that contains only parabens. For nonlyophilized product, add 5 ml to 100-mg vial, 10 ml to 200-mg vial, 25 ml to 500-mg vial, 50 ml to 1-g vial, or 100 ml to 2-g vial to produce solution containing 20 mg/ml. Shake to dissolve; this may take up to 6 minutes and it may be difficult to completely dissolve drug. Lyophilized preparation is much easier to reconstitute; check package insert for quantity of diluent needed to reconstitute drug.
– After reconstitution, administer as ordered by direct I.V. injection or infusion. For I.V. infusion, further dilute with D_5W, dextrose 5% in normal saline injection, dextrose 5% in Ringer's injection, lactated Ringer's injection, sodium lactate injection, or half-normal saline injection.
– Check reconstituted solution for small particles. Filter solution if necessary.
– Reconstituted solution is stable for 6 days refrigerated or 24 hours at room temperature. However, use stored solutions cautiously because drug contains no preservatives.

- To prevent hyperuricemia with resulting uric acid nephropathy, allopurinol may be used with adequate hydration.

Patient teaching

- Warn patient that alopecia is likely to occur but that it's reversible.
- Warn patient to watch for signs of infection (fever, sore throat, fatigue) and bleeding (easy bruising, nosebleeds, bleeding gums, melena), and to take temperature daily.

• Instruct patient to avoid OTC products that contain aspirin.
• Encourage patient to void every 1 to 2 hours while awake and to drink at least 3 L of fluid daily to minimize risk of hemorrhagic cystitis. Tell patient not to take drug at bedtime; infrequent urination during night may increase possibility of cystitis. If cystitis occurs, tell him to discontinue drug and notify prescriber. Cystitis can occur months after therapy ceases. Mesna may be given to lower risk and severity of bladder toxicity.
• Advise both men and women to practice contraception while taking drug and for 4 months after; drug is potentially teratogenic.
• Advise women of childbearing age to avoid becoming pregnant during therapy. Also recommend consulting with prescriber before becoming pregnant.

☑ Evaluation

• Patient shows positive response to drug therapy.
• Patient doesn't experience injury as a result of drug-induced adverse reactions.
• Patient and family state understanding of drug therapy.

cycloserine
(sigh-kloh-SER-een)
Seromycin

Pharmacologic class: isoxizolidone, d-alanine analogue
Therapeutic class: antituberculotic
Pregnancy risk category: C

Indications and dosages

▶ **Adjunct treatment in pulmonary or extrapulmonary tuberculosis.** *Adults:* initially, 250 mg P.O. q 12 hours for 2 weeks; then, if blood levels are below 25 to 30 mcg/ml and no toxicity has developed, 250 mg q 8 hours for 2 weeks. If optimum blood levels aren't achieved and no toxicity has developed, dose is increased to 250 mg q 6 hours. Maximum dosage is 1 g/day. If CNS toxicity occurs, drug is discontinued for 1 week, and then resumed at 250 mg daily for 2 weeks. If no serious toxic effects occur, dosage is increased by 250-mg increments q 10 days until blood level is 25 to 30 mcg/ml.

How supplied

Capsules: 250 mg

Pharmacokinetics

Absorption: about 80% is absorbed from GI tract.
Distribution: distributed widely into body tissues and fluids, including CSF. It doesn't bind to plasma proteins.
Metabolism: may be metabolized partially.
Excretion: excreted primarily in urine. *Half-life:* 10 hours.

Route	Onset	Peak	Duration
P.O.	Unknown	3-4 hr	Unknown

Pharmacodynamics

Chemical effect: inhibits cell-wall biosynthesis by interfering with bacterial use of amino acids (bacteriostatic).
Therapeutic effect: aids in eradicating tuberculosis.

Adverse reactions

CNS: ***seizures,*** drowsiness, headache, tremor, dysarthria, vertigo, confusion, loss of memory, ***possible suicidal tendencies*** and other psychotic symptoms, *nervousness, hallucinations, depression,* hyperirritability, paresthesia, paresis, hyperreflexia, ***coma.***
Other: hypersensitivity reactions (allergic dermatitis).

Interactions

Drug-drug. *Ethionamide, isoniazid:* increased risk of CNS toxicity (seizures, dizziness, or drowsiness). Monitor patient closely.
Drug-lifestyle. *Alcohol use:* increased risk of CNS toxicity. Advise patient to refrain from alcohol consumption during therapy.

Contraindications and precautions

• Contraindicated in patients hypersensitive to drug, patients who concurrently consume excessive amounts of alcohol, and patients with seizure disorders, depression, severe anxiety, psychosis, or severe renal insufficiency.

• Use cautiously in patients with impaired renal function; reduced dosage is required. Also use cautiously in pregnant or breast-feeding women.
• Safety of drug hasn't been established in children.

NURSING CONSIDERATIONS

Assessment
• Assess patient's underlying condition before therapy.
• Obtain specimen for culture and sensitivity tests before therapy begins and periodically thereafter to detect possible resistance.
• Monitor effectiveness by evaluating culture and sensitivity results; watch for improvement in patient's underlying condition.
• Monitor serum cycloserine levels periodically as ordered, especially in patients receiving high doses (more than 500 mg daily) because toxic reactions may occur with blood levels above 30 mcg/ml.
• Monitor results of hematologic tests and renal and liver function studies.
• Be alert for adverse reactions and drug interactions.
• Evaluate patient's and family's knowledge of drug therapy.

Nursing diagnoses
• Ineffective health maintenance related to presence of tuberculosis
• Risk for injury related to drug-induced CNS adverse reactions
• Deficient knowledge related to drug therapy

Planning and implementation
• Cycloserine is considered second-line drug in treatment of tuberculosis and should always be administered with other antituberculotics to prevent development of resistant organisms.
• Expect to adjust dosage according to blood levels, clinical toxicity, or ineffectiveness, as ordered.
• Administer pyridoxine, anticonvulsants, tranquilizers, or sedatives, as ordered, to relieve adverse reactions.

Patient teaching
• Warn patient to avoid alcohol, which may cause serious neurologic reactions.
• Instruct patient to take drug exactly as prescribed; warn against discontinuing drug without prescriber's approval.
• Stress importance of having laboratory studies done as ordered to monitor drug effectiveness and toxicity.

Evaluation
• Patient maintains health after drug therapy.
• Patient has no injury as a result of drug-induced adverse reactions.
• Patient and family state understanding of drug therapy.

cyclosporine (cyclosporin)
(sigh-kloh-SPOOR-een)
Neoral, Sandimmun ◇, Sandimmune

Pharmacologic class: polypeptide antibiotic
Therapeutic class: immunosuppressant
Pregnancy risk category: C

Indications and dosages

▶ **Prophylaxis of organ rejection in kidney, liver, or heart transplantation.** *Adults and children:* 15 mg/kg P.O. 4 to 12 hours before transplantation and continued daily postoperatively for 1 to 2 weeks. Dosage is reduced by 5% each week to maintenance level of 5 to 10 mg/kg/day. Or, 5 to 6 mg/kg I.V. concentrate 4 to 12 hours before transplantation. Postoperatively, dosage repeated daily until patient can tolerate P.O. forms. For microemulsion, oral doses are the same and dosage adjustments are made according to a predefined cyclosporine blood level.
▶ **Severe, active rheumatoid arthritis that hasn't adequately responded to methotrexate (Neoral only).** *Adults:* 1.25 mg/kg/day P.O. b.i.d.
▶ **Recalcitrant, plaque psoriasis that isn't adequately responsive to at least one systemic therapy or in patients for whom other systemic therapy is contraindicated or isn't tolerated (Neoral only).** *Adults*: initially 2.5 mg/kg/day P.O. divided b.i.d. Initially dose

should be maintained for 4 weeks. If dosage increase is necessary, increase at 2-week intervals, 0.5 mg/kg/day to a maximum of 4 mg/kg/day.

How supplied

Oral solution: 100 mg/ml
Injection: 50 mg/ml
Capsules: 25 mg, 50 mg, 100 mg
Capsules for microemulsion: 25 mg, 100 mg

Pharmacokinetics

Absorption: absorption varies widely after oral administration between patients and in same patients. Only 30% of Sandimmune oral dose reaches systemic circulation, while 60% of Neoral reaches systemic circulation.
Distribution: distributed widely outside blood volume. In plasma, about 90% is bound to proteins.
Metabolism: metabolized extensively in liver.
Excretion: excreted primarily in feces with only 6% of drug found in urine. *Half-life:* 10 to 27 hours.

Route	Onset	Peak	Duration
P.O.			
Sandimmune	Unknown	3.5 hr	Unknown
Neoral	Unknown	1.5-2 hr	Unknown
I.V.	Unknown	Unknown	Unknown

Pharmacodynamics

Chemical effect: inhibits proliferation of T lymphocytes.
Therapeutic effect: prevents organ rejection.

Adverse reactions

CNS: *tremor,* headache, ***seizures.***
CV: hypertension.
EENT: sinusitis.
GI: *gum hyperplasia,* oral thrush, nausea, vomiting, diarrhea.
GU: **NEPHROTOXICITY.**
Hematologic: anemia, *leukopenia, thrombocytopenia.*
Hepatic: ***hepatotoxicity.***
Metabolic: increased low-density lipoprotein levels.
Skin: *hirsutism,* acne.
Other: flushing, ***infections, anaphylaxis.***

Interactions

Drug-drug. *Aminoglycosides, amphotericin B, co-trimoxazole, NSAIDs:* increased risk of nephrotoxicity. Monitor patient for toxicity.
Amphotericin B, cimetidine, diltiazem, erythromycin, imipenem, cilastatin, ketoconazole, metoclopramide, prednisolone: may increase blood levels of cyclosporine. Monitor patient for increased toxicity.
Azathioprine, corticosteroids, cyclophosphamide, verapamil: increased immunosuppression. Monitor patient closely.
Carbamazepine, isoniazid, phenobarbital, phenytoin, rifampin: possible decreased immunosuppressant effect. May need to increase cyclosporine dosage.
Vaccines: decreased immune response; postpone routine immunization.
Drug-herb. *St. John's wort*: may significantly lower cyclosporine levels in the blood, contributing to organ rejection. Strongly advise against concomitant use.
Pill-bearing spurge: may inhibit CYP3A enzymes affecting drug metabolism. Discourage concurrent use.
Drug-food. *Grapefruit juice:* slows metabolism of drug. Avoid concomitant use.

Contraindications and precautions

- Contraindicated in patients hypersensitive to drug or to polyoxyethylated castor oil (found in injectable form). Neoral contraindicated in patients with psoriasis or rheumatoid arthritis who also have abnormal renal function, uncontrolled hypertension, or malignancies.
- Use cautiously in pregnant women.
- Safety of drug hasn't been established in breast-feeding women.

NURSING CONSIDERATIONS

Assessment

- Assess patient's organ transplant before therapy.
- Monitor effectiveness by evaluating patient for signs and symptoms of organ rejection.
- Monitor cyclosporine blood levels at regular intervals.
- Monitor BUN and serum creatinine levels because nephrotoxicity may develop 2 to 3

months after transplant surgery, possibly requiring dosage reduction.
- Monitor liver function tests, as ordered, for hepatotoxicity, which usually occurs during first month after transplant.
- Monitor CBC and platelet counts regularly.
- Be alert for adverse reactions and drug interactions.
- Evaluate patient's and family's knowledge of drug therapy.

Nursing diagnoses
- Risk for injury related to potential for organ rejection
- Ineffective protection related to drug-induced immunosuppression
- Deficient knowledge related to drug therapy

Planning and implementation
P.O. use: Measure oral doses carefully in oral syringe. To increase palatability, mix with whole milk, chocolate milk, or fruit juice (except grapefruit juice). Oral cyclosporine solution for emulsion is less palatable when mixed with milk. Use glass container to minimize adherence to container walls.
– Administer drug with meals to minimize GI distress.
I.V. use: Administer cyclosporine I.V. concentrate at one-third oral dose and dilute before use. Dilute each milliliter of concentrate in 20 to 100 ml of D_5W or normal saline for injection. Dilute immediately before administration; infuse over 2 to 6 hours. Usually reserved for patients who cannot tolerate oral drugs.
- Sandimmune and Neoral aren't bioequivalent and cannot be used interchangeably without prescriber supervision. Conversion from Neoral to Sandimmune should be made with increased monitoring as ordered to avoid underdosing.
- Psoriasis patients who are treated with Neoral shouldn't receive concomitant PUVA or UVB therapy, methotrexate or other immunosuppressive agents, coal tar, or radiation therapy.
- Always give drug with adrenal corticosteroids, as ordered.
- Drug is used for rheumatoid arthritis but not in patients with abnormal renal function or uncontrolled hypertension.

Patient teaching
- Encourage patient to take drug at same times each day.
- Advise patient to take Neoral on an empty stomach and not to mix with grapefruit juice.
- Advise patient to take with meals if drug causes nausea. Anorexia, nausea, and vomiting are usually transient and most frequently occur at start of therapy.
- Stress that therapy shouldn't be stopped without prescriber's approval.
- Instruct patient to swish and swallow nystatin four times daily to prevent oral thrush.
- Instruct patient on infection control and bleeding precautions, as indicated by CBC and platelet count results.

Evaluation
- Patient doesn't experience organ rejection while taking drug.
- Patient is free from infection and serious bleeding episodes throughout drug therapy.
- Patient and family state understanding of drug therapy.

cyproheptadine hydrochloride
(sigh-proh-HEP-tah-deen high-droh-KLOR-ighd)
Periactin

Pharmacologic class: piperidine-derivative antihistamine
Therapeutic class: antihistamine (H_1-receptor antagonist), antipruritic
Pregnancy risk category: B

Indications and dosages
▶ **Allergy symptoms, pruritus.** *Adults:* 4 to 20 mg P.O. daily in divided doses. Maximum dosage is 0.5 mg/kg daily.
Children ages 7 to 14: 4 mg P.O. b.i.d. or t.i.d. Maximum dosage is 16 mg daily.
Children ages 2 to 6: 2 mg P.O. b.i.d. or t.i.d. Maximum dosage is 12 mg daily.

How supplied
Tablets: 4 mg
Syrup: 2 mg/5 ml

Pharmacokinetics

Absorption: well absorbed from GI tract.
Distribution: unknown.
Metabolism: appears to be almost completely metabolized in liver.
Excretion: metabolites are excreted primarily in urine; unchanged drug isn't excreted in urine but small amounts of unchanged cyproheptadine and metabolites are excreted in feces.

Route	Onset	Peak	Duration
P.O.	15-60 min	6-9 hr	8 hr

Pharmacodynamics

Chemical effect: competes with histamine for H_1-receptor sites on effector cells. Prevents, but doesn't reverse, histamine-mediated responses.
Therapeutic effect: relieves allergy symptoms and itching.

Adverse reactions

CNS: *drowsiness,* dizziness, headache, fatigue, ***seizures*** (especially in elderly patients).
GI: nausea, vomiting, epigastric distress, *dry mouth.*
GU: urine retention.
Hematologic: ***agranulocytosis, thrombocytopenia.***
Metabolic: weight gain.
Skin: rash.
Other: ***anaphylactic shock.***

Interactions

Drug-drug. *CNS depressants:* increased sedation. Use together cautiously.
MAO inhibitors: increased anticholinergic effects. Don't use together.
Drug-lifestyle. *Sun exposure:* photosensitivity reactions may occur. Urge patient to take precautions.

Contraindications and precautions

- Contraindicated in patients hypersensitive to drug or other drugs of similar chemical structure; in those with acute asthmatic attacks, angle-closure glaucoma, stenosing peptic ulcer, symptomatic prostatic hypertrophy, bladder-neck obstruction, and pyloroduodenal obstruction; in patients taking MAO inhibitors; in neonates or premature infants; in elderly or debilitated patients; and in breast-feeding patients.
- Use cautiously in pregnant women and in patients with increased intraocular pressure, hyperthyroidism, CV disease, hypertension, or bronchial asthma.

NURSING CONSIDERATIONS

Assessment

- Assess patient's underlying condition before therapy and reassess regularly during therapy.
- Be alert for adverse reactions and drug interactions.
- Evaluate patient's and family's knowledge of drug therapy.

Nursing diagnoses

- Ineffective health maintenance related to underlying condition
- Risk for injury related to potential for drug-induced adverse CNS reactions
- Deficient knowledge related to drug therapy

Planning and implementation

- Reduce GI distress by giving drug with food or milk.
- Notify prescriber if tolerance is suspected; another antihistamine may need to be used.

Patient teaching

- Instruct patient to take drug with food or milk to reduce GI distress.
- Warn patient to avoid alcohol and hazardous activities until CNS effects of drug are known.
- Tell patient that coffee or tea may reduce drowsiness. Sugarless gum, sugarless sour hard candy, or ice chips may relieve dry mouth.
- Advise patient to stop drug 4 days before allergy skin tests to preserve accuracy of tests.
- Instruct patient to notify prescriber if tolerance develops; different antihistamine may be needed.

Evaluation

- Patient is free from allergy symptoms or pruritus with drug therapy.

• Patient has no injury as result of drug-induced CNS adverse reactions.
• Patient and family state understanding of drug therapy.

cytarabine (ara-C, cytosine arabinoside)

(sigh-TAR-uh-been)

Cytosar♦, Cytosar-U, Cytarbine injection

Pharmacologic class: antimetabolite (specific to S phase of cell cycle)
Therapeutic class: antineoplastic
Pregnancy risk category: D

Indications and dosages

▶ **Acute nonlymphocytic leukemia, acute lymphocytic leukemia, blast phase of chronic myelocytic leukemia.** *Adults and children:* 100 mg/m² daily by continuous I.V. infusion or 100 mg/m² I.V. q 12 hours, given for 5 days and repeated q 2 weeks. For maintenance, 1 mg/kg S.C. once or twice weekly.

▶ **Meningeal leukemia.** *Adults and children:* highly variable from 5 to 75 mg/m² intrathecally. Frequency also varies from once a day for 4 days to once q 4 days. Most common dosage is 30 mg/m², q 4 days until CSF is normal, followed by one more dose.

How supplied

Injection: 100-mg, 500-mg, 1-g, 2-g vials

Pharmacokinetics

Absorption: unknown after S.C. administration.
Distribution: rapidly distributes widely throughout body. About 13% of drug is bound to plasma proteins. Drug penetrates the blood-brain barrier only slightly after rapid I.V. dose; however, when drug is administered by continuous I.V. infusion, CSF levels achieve 40% to 60% of that of plasma levels.
Metabolism: metabolized primarily in liver but also in kidneys, GI mucosa, and granulocytes.
Excretion: drug and its metabolites are excreted in urine. Less than 10% of dose is excreted as unchanged drug in urine. *Half-life:* elimination of cytarabine is biphasic, with initial half-life of 8 minutes and terminal phase half-life of 1 to 3 hours.

Route	Onset	Peak	Duration
I.V.	Unknown	Unknown	Unknown
S.C.	Unknown	20-60 min	Unknown
Intrathecal	Unknown	Unknown	Unknown

Pharmacodynamics

Chemical effect: inhibits DNA synthesis.
Therapeutic effect: kills selected cancer cells.

Adverse reactions

CNS: neurotoxicity, including ataxia and cerebellar dysfunction (with high doses).
EENT: keratitis, nystagmus.
GI: nausea, vomiting, diarrhea, dysphagia; reddened area at juncture of lips, followed by sore mouth and oral ulcers in 5 to 10 days; high dose given by rapid I.V. may cause projectile vomiting.
GU: urate nephropathy.
Hematologic: ***leukopenia,*** with initial WBC count nadir 7 to 9 days after drug is stopped and second (more severe) nadir 15 to 24 days after drug is stopped; anemia; reticulocytopenia; ***thrombocytopenia,*** with platelet count nadir occurring on day 10; *megaloblastosis.*
Hepatic: hepatotoxicity (usually mild and reversible).
Metabolic: hyperuricemia.
Skin: rash.
Other: flu syndrome, ***anaphylaxis.***

Interactions

Drug-drug. *Digoxin:* may decrease serum digoxin levels. Monitor digoxin levels.
Flucytosine: decreased flucytosine activity. Monitor closely.
Gentamicin: decreased activity against *Klebsiella pneumoniae.* Don't use concomitantly.

Contraindications and precautions

• Contraindicated in patients hypersensitive to drug and in breast-feeding women.
• Drug isn't recommended for use in pregnant women because fetal harm may occur.

• Use cautiously in patients with hepatic disease.

NURSING CONSIDERATIONS

Assessment

• Assess patient's underlying condition before therapy, and reassess regularly throughout therapy.
• Monitor serum uric acid level, hepatic and renal function studies, and CBC, as ordered.
• Be alert for adverse reactions and drug interactions.
• If patient receives high doses, watch for neurotoxicity, which may first appear as nystagmus but can progress to ataxia and cerebellar dysfunction.
• Evaluate patient's and family's knowledge of drug therapy.

Nursing diagnoses

• Ineffective health maintenance related to underlying condition
• Risk for injury related to drug-induced adverse hematologic reactions
• Deficient knowledge related to drug therapy

Planning and implementation

• Follow facility policy to reduce risks. Preparation and administration of parenteral form of this drug are linked to carcinogenic, mutagenic, and teratogenic risks for personnel.
I.V. use: To reduce nausea, give antiemetic before drug, as ordered. Nausea and vomiting are more frequent when large doses are administered rapidly by I.V. push. These reactions are less frequent when given by infusion.
– Reconstitute drug using provided diluent, which is bacteriostatic water for injection containing benzyl alcohol. Avoid this diluent when preparing drug for neonates or for intrathecal use. Reconstitute 100-mg vial with 5 ml of diluent or 500-mg vial with 10 ml of diluent. Reconstituted solution is stable for 48 hours. Discard cloudy reconstituted solution.
– For I.V. infusion, further dilute using normal saline solution for injection, D_5W, or sterile water for injection.
S.C. use: Follow manufacturer guidelines.
Intrathecal use: Use preservative-free normal saline solution. Add 5 ml to 100-mg vial or 10 ml to 500-mg vial. Use immediately after reconstitution. Discard unused drug.
• Maintain high fluid intake and give allopurinol, if ordered, to avoid urate nephropathy in leukemia induction therapy.
• Therapy may be modified or stopped if granulocyte count is below 1,000/mm^3 or if platelet count is below 50,000/mm^3.
• Corticosteroid eye drops are prescribed to prevent drug-induced keratitis.
• Prescriber must judge possible benefit against known adverse effects.

Patient teaching

• Warn patient to watch for signs of infection (fever, sore throat, fatigue) and bleeding (easy bruising, nosebleeds, bleeding gums, melena). Tell patient to take temperature daily.
• Instruct patient on infection control and bleeding precautions.
• Advise woman of childbearing age to avoid becoming pregnant during therapy. Also recommend consulting with prescriber before becoming pregnant.
• Encourage patient to drink at least 3 L of fluids daily.
• Instruct patient about need for frequent oral hygiene.

Evaluation

• Patient demonstrates positive response to drug therapy.
• Patient doesn't experience injury as result of drug therapy.
• Patient and family state understanding of drug therapy.

cytomegalovirus immune globulin, intravenous (CMV-IGIV)

(sigh-toh-meh-GEH-loh VIGH-rus ih MYOON GLOH-byoo-lin)
CytoGam

Pharmacologic class: immune globulin
Therapeutic class: immune serum
Pregnancy risk category: C

Indications and dosages

▶ **To attenuate primary CMV disease in seronegative kidney transplant recipients who receive kidney from a CMV seropositive donor.** *Adults:* administered I.V. according to following schedule based on time after transplantation:

within 72 hours: 150 mg/kg
2 weeks after: 100 mg/kg
4 weeks after: 100 mg/kg
6 weeks after: 100 mg/kg
8 weeks after: 100 mg/kg
12 weeks after: 50 mg/kg
16 weeks after: 50 mg/kg.

Initial dose administered at 15 mg/kg/hour. Increased to 30 mg/kg/hour, after 30 minutes if no untoward reactions occur, then increased to 60 mg/kg/hour after another 30 minutes if no untoward reactions occur. Volume shouldn't exceed 75 ml/hour. Subsequent doses may be administered at 15 mg/kg/hour for 15 minutes, increasing at 15-minute intervals in stepwise fashion to 60 mg/kg/hour.

▶ **Prophylaxis of CMV disease related to lung, liver, pancreas, and heart transplants.** *Adults:* used with ganciclovir in organ transplants from CMV seropositive donors into seronegative recipients. Maximum total dosage per infusion is 150 mg/kg I.V. administered as follows based on time after transplantation:

within 72 hours: 150 mg/kg
2 weeks after: 150 mg/kg
4 weeks after: 150 mg/kg
6 weeks after: 150 mg/kg
8 weeks after: 150 mg/kg
12 weeks after: 100 mg/kg
16 weeks after: 100 mg/kg.

Administer initial dose at 15 mg/kg/hour. If no adverse reactions occur after 30 minutes, increase rate to 30 mg/kg/hour. If no adverse reactions occur after another 30 minutes, infusion may be increased to 60 mg/kg/hour (volume shouldn't exceed 75 ml/hour). Subsequent doses may be given at 15 mg/kg/hour for 15 minutes, increasing every 15 minutes in a stepwise fashion to a maximum of 60 mg/kg/hour (volume shouldn't exceed 75 ml/hour). Monitor patient closely during and after each rate change.

How supplied

Solution for injection: 50 ± 10 mg/ml.

Pharmacokinetics

Unknown.

Route	Onset	Peak	Duration
I.V.	Unknown	Unknown	Unknown

Pharmacodynamics

Chemical effect: supplies relatively high concentration of immunoglobulin G (IgG) antibodies against CMV. Increasing these antibody levels in CMV-exposed patients may attenuate or reduce risk of serious CMV disease.

Therapeutic effect: provides passive immunity to CMV.

Adverse reactions

CVS: hypotension.
GI: nausea, vomiting.
Musculoskeletal: muscle cramps, back pain.
Respiratory: wheezing
Other: ***anaphylaxis,*** flushing, chills, fever.

Interactions

Drug-drug. *Live-virus vaccines:* may interfere with immune response to live-virus vaccines. Defer vaccination for at least 3 months.

Contraindications and precautions

• Contraindicated in patients with selective IgA deficiency or history of sensitivity to other human immunoglobulin preparations.
• Use with caution in pregnant women.
• Safety of drug hasn't been established for breast-feeding women or children.

NURSING CONSIDERATIONS

Assessment

• Assess patient's kidney transplant before therapy.
• Take vital signs before starting therapy and then midinfusion, postinfusion, and before any increase in infusion rate.
• Monitor effectiveness by evaluating kidney function.
• Be alert for adverse reactions and drug interactions.

• Evaluate patient's and family's knowledge of drug therapy.

Nursing diagnoses

• Risk for injury related to potential for organ rejection
• Decreased cardiac output related to drug-induced hypotension
• Deficient knowledge related to drug therapy

Planning and implementation

• Remove tab portion of vial cap and clean rubber stopper with 70% alcohol or equivalent. Don't shake vial; avoid foaming. Infuse solution only if it is colorless, free of particulate matter, and not turbid. Pre-dilution before infusion isn't recommended.
• If possible, administer through separate I.V. line using constant infusion pump. Filters are unnecessary. If unable to administer through separate line, piggyback into existing line of saline solution injection or one of following dextrose solutions with or without saline: dextrose 2.5% in water, D_5W, dextrose 10% in water, or dextrose 20% in water. Don't dilute more than 1:2 with any of these solutions.
• Refrigerate drug at 36° to 46° F (2° to 8° C).
• If patient develops anaphylaxis or if blood pressure drops, discontinue infusion, notify prescriber, and be prepared to administer CPR and such drugs as diphenhydramine and epinephrine.

Patient teaching

• Teach patient about drug therapy.
• Instruct patient to notify prescriber immediately if adverse reactions develop.

Evaluation

• Patient doesn't reject transplanted kidney during drug therapy.
• Patient maintains normal cardiac output throughout drug therapy.
• Patient and family state understanding of drug therapy.

D

dacarbazine (DTIC)

(deh-KAR-buh-zeen)
DTIC♦, DTIC-Dome

Pharmacologic class: alkylating agent (cell cycle–phase nonspecific)
Therapeutic class: antineoplastic
Pregnancy risk category: C

Indications and dosages

▶ **Metastatic malignant melanoma.** *Adults:* 2 to 4.5 mg/kg I.V. daily for 10 days; then repeated q 4 weeks as tolerated. Or 250 mg/m^2 I.V. daily for 5 days, repeated at 3-week intervals.
▶ **Hodgkin's disease.** *Adults:* 150 mg/m^2 I.V. daily (combined with other drugs) for 5 days, repeated q 4 weeks. Or, 375 mg/m^2 on first day of combination regimen, repeated q 15 days.

How supplied

Injection: 100-mg, 200-mg vials

Pharmacokinetics

Absorption: not applicable with I.V. administration.
Distribution: thought to localize in body tissues, especially the liver; minimally bound to plasma proteins.
Metabolism: rapidly metabolized in liver to several compounds, some of which may be active.
Excretion: about 30% to 45% of dose excreted in urine. *Half-life:* initial, 19 minutes; terminal, 5 hours.

Route	Onset	Peak	Duration
I.V.	Unknown	Unknown	Unknown

Pharmacodynamics

Chemical effect: unknown; probably cross-links strands of cellular DNA and interferes

with RNA transcription, causing imbalance of growth that leads to cell death.
Therapeutic effect: kills selected cancer cells.

Adverse reactions

GI: *severe nausea and vomiting, anorexia.*
Hematologic: ***leukopenia, thrombocytopenia*** (nadir at 3 to 4 weeks).
Hepatic: transient increase in liver enzyme levels.
Metabolic: hyperuricemia.
Skin: alopecia, phototoxicity.
Other: *flulike syndrome* (fever, malaise, myalgia beginning 7 days after treatment and possibly lasting 7 to 21 days), ***anaphylaxis,*** severe pain with concentrated solution or extravasation, tissue damage.

Interactions

Drug-drug. *Allopurinol:* additive hypouricemic effects. Monitor patient closely.
Anticoagulants, aspirin: increased risk of bleeding. Avoid concomitant use.
Bone marrow suppressants: additive toxicity. Monitor patient closely.
Phenobarbital, phenytoin, other drugs that induce hepatic metabolism: enhanced dacarbazine metabolism. Dosage adjustment may be needed.
Drug-lifestyle. *Sun exposure:* photosensitivity reactions may occur, especially during the first 2 days of therapy. Advise precautions.

Contraindications and precautions

- Contraindicated in patients hypersensitive to drug and in breast-feeding women.
- Use with extreme caution and only when absolutely necessary in pregnant women because fetus may be harmed.
- Use cautiously if patient has impaired bone marrow function.
- Safety of drug hasn't been established in children.

NURSING CONSIDERATIONS

Assessment

- Obtain history of patient's underlying neoplastic disease before therapy, and reassess regularly throughout therapy.
- Monitor CBC, platelet count, and liver enzyme levels, as ordered.
- Be alert for adverse reactions and drug interactions.
- Evaluate patient's and family's knowledge of drug therapy.

Nursing diagnoses

- Ineffective health maintenance related to presence of neoplastic disease
- Risk for injury related to risk of drug-induced adverse reactions
- Deficient knowledge related to drug therapy

Planning and implementation

- Follow facility policy to reduce risks. Preparation and administration of parenteral form raises risk of carcinogenic, mutagenic, and teratogenic effects for personnel.
- Administer antiemetics, as ordered, before giving dacarbazine to help decrease nausea. Nausea and vomiting may subside after several doses.
- Reconstitute drug with sterile water for injection. Add 9.9 ml to 100-mg vial or 19.7 ml to 200-mg vial. The resulting solution is colorless to clear yellow. For infusion, further dilute, using up to 250 ml of normal saline injection or D_5W. Infuse over 30 minutes.
- During infusion, protect bag from direct sunlight to avoid drug breakdown. Solution may be diluted further or infusion slowed to decrease pain at infusion site.
- Reconstituted solutions are stable for 8 hours at room temperature and under normal lighting conditions, up to 3 days if refrigerated. Diluted solutions are stable for 8 hours at room temperature and normal light, up to 24 hours if refrigerated. If solutions turn pink, decomposition has occurred; discard drug.
- Take care to avoid extravasation during infusion. If I.V. solution infiltrates, discontinue immediately, apply ice to area for 24 to 48 hours, and notify prescriber.
- For Hodgkin's disease, drug is usually given with bleomycin, vinblastine, and doxorubicin.

Patient teaching

- Warn patient to watch for signs of infection (fever, sore throat, fatigue) and bleeding (easy

bruising, nosebleeds, bleeding gums, melena). Tell patient to take temperature daily.
- Instruct patient to avoid OTC products containing aspirin.
- Advise patient to avoid sunlight and sunlamps for first 2 days after treatment.
- Reassure patient that flulike syndrome may be treated with mild antipyretics, such as acetaminophen.

☑ Evaluation

- Patient exhibits positive response to therapy, as evidenced on follow-up diagnostic studies and overall physical status.
- Patient has no injury from drug-induced adverse reactions.
- Patient and family state understanding of drug therapy.

daclizumab

(da-KLIZ-yoo-mab)
Zenapax

Pharmacologic class: humanized immunoglobulin G_1 monoclonal antibody
Therapeutic class: immunosuppressant
Pregnancy risk category: C

Indications and dosages

▶ **Prevention of acute organ rejection in patients receiving renal transplants with an immunosuppressive regimen that includes cyclosporine and corticosteroids.** *Adults:* 1 mg/kg I.V. Standard course of therapy is five doses. Give first dose no more than 24 hours before transplantation; give remaining four doses at 14-day intervals.

How supplied

Injection: 25 mg/5 ml

Pharmacokinetics

Absorption: serum levels increase between first and fifth doses.
Distribution: unknown.
Metabolism: unknown.
Excretion: estimated terminal elimination half-life is 20 days (480 hours).

Route	Onset	Peak	Duration
I.V.	Unknown	Unknown	Unknown

Pharmacodynamics

Chemical effect: an interleukin (IL)-2 receptor antagonist that inhibits IL-2 binding to prevent IL-2–mediated activation of lymphocytes, a critical pathway in the cellular immune response against allografts. Once in circulation, drug impairs response of immune system to antigenic challenges.
Therapeutic effect: prevents organ rejection.

Adverse reactions

CNS: tremor, headache, dizziness, insomnia, generalized weakness, prickly sensation, fever, pain, fatigue, depression, anxiety.
CV: tachycardia, hypertension, hypotension, aggravated hypertension, edema, fluid overload, chest pain.
EENT: blurred vision, pharyngitis, rhinitis.
GI: constipation, nausea, diarrhea, vomiting, abdominal pain, dyspepsia, pyrosis, abdominal distention, epigastric pain, flatulence, gastritis, hemorrhoids.
GU: ***oliguria,*** dysuria, ***renal tubular necrosis,*** renal damage, urine retention, hydronephrosis, urinary tract bleeding, urinary tract disorder, renal insufficiency.
Hematologic: lymphocele, bleeding.
Metabolic: diabetes mellitus, dehydration.
Musculoskeletal: musculoskeletal or back pain, arthralgia, myalgia, leg cramps.
Respiratory: dyspnea, coughing, atelectasis, congestion, ***hypoxia,*** rales, abnormal breath sounds, pleural effusion, pulmonary edema.
Skin: acne, impaired wound healing without infection, pruritus, hirsutism, rash, night sweats, increased sweating.
Other: shivering, limb edema.

Interactions

None significant.

Contraindications and precautions

- Contraindicated in patients hypersensitive to daclizumab and its components.

NURSING CONSIDERATIONS

Assessment
- Obtain history of patient's underlying condition before therapy, and reassess regularly thereafter.
- Check for lipoproliferative disorders and opportunistic infections.
- Monitor patient for anaphylactoid reactions.
- Evaluate patient's and family's knowledge of drug therapy.

Nursing diagnoses
- Risk for injury related to potential for organ rejection
- Ineffective protection related to drug-induced immunosuppression
- Deficient knowledge related to drug therapy

Planning and implementation
- Drug should be used only under supervision of a prescriber experienced in immunosuppressant therapy and management of organ transplantation.
- Drug is used as part of an immunosuppressant regimen that includes corticosteroids and cyclosporine.
- Keep drugs used to treat anaphylactic reactions immediately available.
- Don't use drug as a direct I.V. injection. Dilute in 50 ml of sterile normal saline solution before administration. To avoid foaming, don't shake. Inspect for particulates or discoloration before use; don't use if either occurs.
- Administer over 15 minutes via a central or peripheral line. Don't add or infuse other drugs simultaneously through the same line.
- Drug may be refrigerated at 36° to 46° F (2° to 8° C) for 24 hours and is stable at room temperature for 4 hours. Discard solution if not used within 24 hours.
- Protect undiluted solution from direct light.

Patient teaching
- Tell patient to consult prescriber before taking other drugs during therapy.
- Advise patient to take precautions against infection.
- Inform patient that neither he nor any household member should receive vaccinations unless medically approved.
- Tell patient to report immediately wounds that fail to heal, unusual bruising or bleeding, or fever.
- Advise patient to drink plenty of fluids during therapy and to report painful urination, blood in the urine, or a decrease in urine amount.
- Instruct woman of childbearing age to use effective contraception before starting therapy and to continue until 4 months after completing therapy.

Evaluation
- Patient doesn't experience organ rejection while taking drug.
- Patient is free from infection and serious bleeding episodes throughout drug therapy.
- Patient and family state understanding of drug therapy

dactinomycin (actinomycin-D)
(dak-tih-noh-MIGH-sin)
Cosmegen

Pharmacologic class: antibiotic antineoplastic (cell cycle–phase nonspecific)
Therapeutic class: antineoplastic
Pregnancy risk category: C

Indications and dosages
Indications and dosages may vary. Check treatment protocol with prescriber.

▶ **Sarcoma, trophoblastic tumors in women, testicular cancer.** *Adults:* 500 mcg (0.5 mg) I.V. daily for 5 days. Maximum, 15 mcg/kg/day or 400 to 600 mcg/m^2/day for 5 days. Course may be repeated after 3 weeks if all signs of toxicity have disappeared.

▶ **Wilms' tumor, rhabdomyosarcoma, Ewing's sarcoma.** *Children:* 10 to 15 mcg/kg or 450 mcg/m^2/day I.V. for 5 days. Maximum, 500 mcg/day or 2.5 mg/m^2 I.V. in equally divided daily doses over 7-day period. Course may be repeated after 3 weeks if all signs of toxicity have disappeared.

How supplied
Injection: 500 mcg/vial

Pharmacokinetics

Absorption: not applicable with I.V. administration.
Distribution: widely distributed in body tissues, with highest levels found in bone marrow and nucleated cells.
Metabolism: minimally metabolized in liver.
Excretion: drug and its metabolites excreted in urine and bile. *Half-life:* 36 hours.

Route	Onset	Peak	Duration
I.V.	Unknown	Unknown	Unknown

Pharmacodynamics

Chemical effect: unknown; thought to interfere with DNA-dependent RNA synthesis by intercalation.
Therapeutic effect: kills selected cancer cells.

Adverse reactions

CNS: malaise, fatigue, lethargy.
GI: *anorexia, nausea, vomiting,* abdominal pain, diarrhea, *stomatitis,* ulceration, proctitis.
Hematologic: *anemia, **leukopenia, thrombocytopenia, pancytopenia, aplastic anemia, agranulocytosis.***
Hepatic: ***hepatotoxicity.***
Metabolic: hypocalcemia.
Musculoskeletal: myalgia.
Skin: reversible alopecia, *erythema,* desquamation, *hyperpigmentation of skin (especially in previously irradiated areas), acnelike eruptions (reversible).*
Other: phlebitis and severe damage to soft tissue at injection site, fever, ***anaphylaxis.***

Interactions

Drug-drug. *Bone marrow suppressants:* additive toxicity. Monitor patient closely.
Vitamin K derivatives: decreased effectiveness. Monitor patient closely.

Contraindications and precautions

- Contraindicated in breast-feeding women and in patients with chickenpox or herpes zoster.
- Use in pregnant women with extreme caution and only when absolutely necessary because fetal harm may occur.

NURSING CONSIDERATIONS

Assessment

- Obtain history of patient's underlying cancer before therapy, and reassess regularly throughout therapy.
- Monitor CBC, platelet count, and kidney and liver function tests, as ordered.
- Be alert for adverse reactions and drug interactions.
- Evaluate patient's and family's knowledge of drug therapy.

Nursing diagnoses

- Ineffective health maintenance related to presence of cancer
- Risk for injury related to risk of drug-induced adverse reactions
- Deficient knowledge related to drug therapy

Planning and implementation

- Follow facility policy to reduce risks. Preparation and administration of parenteral form carry risk of carcinogenic, mutagenic, and teratogenic effects for staff.
- If accidental skin contact occurs, irrigate area with copious amounts of water for at least 15 minutes.
- Give antiemetics, as ordered, before giving drug to help decrease nausea.
- Use only sterile water (without preservatives) as diluent for reconstitution. Add 1.1 ml to vial to yield gold-colored solution containing 0.5 mg/ml. Give by direct injection into vein or through I.V. line of free-flowing compatible I.V. solution of normal saline injection or D_5W.
- For I.V. infusion, dilute with up to 50 ml of D_5W or normal saline solution for injection, and infuse over 15 minutes.
- Administer drug through running I.V. line with good blood return.
- Dosage must be reduced if patient has recently been treated with or will receive concomitant treatment with radiation therapy or other chemotherapy drugs.
- If drug spills, manufacturer recommends using a solution of trisodium phosphate 5% to inactivate it.
- Discard unused portions of solutions because they contain no preservative.

• Stomatitis, diarrhea, leukopenia, and thrombocytopenia may indicate that dosage and schedule should be modified.
• Dactinomycin is a vesicant. If infiltration occurs, apply cold compresses to area and notify prescriber.

Patient teaching
• Warn patient to watch for signs of infection (fever, sore throat, fatigue) and bleeding (easy bruising, nosebleeds, bleeding gums, melena). Tell patient to take temperature daily.
• Instruct patient to avoid OTC products containing aspirin.
• Tell patient that alopecia may occur but that it's usually reversible.

Evaluation
• Patient has positive response to therapy, as evidenced by follow-up diagnostic studies and overall physical status.
• Patient has no injury from drug-induced adverse reactions.
• Patient and family state understanding of drug therapy.

dalteparin sodium
(dal-TEH-peh-rin SOH-dee-um)
Fragmin

Pharmacologic class: low-molecular-weight heparin
Therapeutic class: anticoagulant
Pregnancy risk category: B

Indications and dosages
▶ **Prevention of deep vein thrombosis (DVT) in patients undergoing abdominal surgery or hip replacement surgery who are at risk for thromboembolic complications.** *Adults:* 2,500 IU S.C. daily, starting 1 to 2 hours before surgery and repeated once daily for 5 to 10 days postoperatively until patient is mobile Or, 5,000 IU S.C. the evening before surgery, repeated once daily every evening for 5-10 days until patient is mobile
▶ **Treatment of unstable angina/non-Q wave MI.** *Adults:* 120 IU/kg up to 10,000 IU S.C. every 12 hours with concurrent oral aspirin (75-165 mg/day) therapy. Continue until patient is stable.

How supplied
Syringe: 2,500 anti-factor Xa IU/0.2 ml; 5,000 anti-factor Xa IU/0.2 ml
Multidose vial: 10,000 anti-factor Xa IU/ml

Pharmacokinetics
Absorption: unknown.
Distribution: unknown.
Metabolism: unknown.
Excretion: excreted in urine. *Half-life:* 3 to 5 hours after S.C. administration.

Route	Onset	Peak	Duration
S.C.	Unknown	About 4 hr	Unknown

Pharmacodynamics
Chemical effect: enhances inhibition of factor Xa and thrombin by antithrombin.
Therapeutic effect: prevents DVT in selected patients.

Adverse reactions
Hematologic: ***hemorrhage,*** ecchymosis, bleeding complications, ***thrombocytopenia.***
Skin: pruritus, rash.
Local: *hematoma at injection site,* pain at injection site.
Other: fever, ***anaphylaxis.***

Interactions
Drug-drug. *Antiplatelet drugs, oral anticoagulants:* may increase risk of bleeding. Use together cautiously.

Contraindications and precautions
• Contraindicated in patients hypersensitive to drug, heparin, or pork products and in patients with active major bleeding or thrombocytopenia with positive in vitro tests for antiplatelet antibody in presence of drug.
• Use with extreme caution in patients with a history of heparin-induced thrombocytopenia; in patients with an increased risk of hemorrhage, such as those with severe uncontrolled hypertension, bacterial endocarditis, congenital or acquired bleeding disorders, active ulceration, angiodysplastic GI disease, or hemor-

rhagic CVA; and in those who recently underwent brain, spinal, or ophthalmologic surgery.
• Use cautiously in patients with bleeding diathesis, thrombocytopenia, platelet defects, severe liver or kidney insufficiency, hypertensive or diabetic retinopathy, or recent GI bleeding. Also use cautiously in pregnant or breast-feeding women.
• Safety of drug hasn't been established in children.

NURSING CONSIDERATIONS

Assessment
• Obtain history of patient's underlying condition before starting therapy.
• Monitor effectiveness by assessing patient for evidence of DVT.
• Routine CBCs (including platelet count) and fecal occult blood tests are recommended during treatment. Patient doesn't need regular monitoring of PT, INR, or PTT.
• Watch for adverse reactions and drug interactions.
• Evaluate patient's and family's knowledge of drug therapy.

Nursing diagnoses
• Risk for injury related to risk of DVT as result of underlying condition
• Ineffective protection related to drug-induced adverse hematologic reactions
• Deficient knowledge related to drug therapy

Planning and implementation
• Candidates for dalteparin therapy are at risk for DVT. Patients at risk include those who are over age 40 or obese and those having surgery lasting longer than 30 minutes under general anesthesia or having additional risk factors (such as cancer or a history of DVT or pulmonary embolism).
• Place patient in sitting or supine position when giving drug. Administer S.C. injection deeply. Injection sites include U-shaped area below navel, upper outer side of thigh, and upper outer quadrangle of buttock. Rotate sites daily. When area around navel or thigh is used, use thumb and forefinger to lift up fold of skin while giving injection. The entire length of needle should be inserted at a 45- to 90-degree angle.
• Never administer drug I.M.
• Don't mix with other injections or infusions unless specific compatibility data are available that support such mixing.
ALERT Drug isn't interchangeable (unit for unit) with unfractionated heparin or other low-molecular-weight heparin derivatives.
• Stop drug and notify prescriber if a thromboembolic event occurs despite dalteparin therapy.

Patient teaching
• Instruct patient and family to watch for signs of bleeding and notify prescriber immediately.
• Tell patient to avoid OTC medications containing aspirin or other salicylates.

Evaluation
• Patient doesn't develop DVT.
• Patient maintains hematologic function.
• Patient and family state understanding of drug therapy.

danaparoid sodium
(dan-eh-PEH-royd SOH-dee-um)
Organan

Pharmacologic class: heparinoid derivative
Therapeutic class: antithrombotic
Pregnancy risk category: B

Indications and dosages
▶ **Prevention of postoperative deep vein thrombosis (DVT) in patients undergoing elective hip replacement surgery.** *Adults:* 750 units S.C. b.i.d. starting 1 to 4 hours preoperatively; then no sooner than 2 hours after surgery. Continue treatment for 7 to 14 days postoperatively or until risk of DVT has diminished.

How supplied
Ampule: 750 anti-Xa units/0.6 ml
Syringe: 750 anti-Xa units/0.6 ml

Pharmacokinetics
Absorption: 100% bioavailability.

Distribution: nonspecific.
Metabolism: unknown.
Excretion: excreted in urine.

Route	Onset	Peak	Duration
S.C.	Unknown	2-5 hr	Unknown

Pharmacodynamics

Chemical effect: prevents fibrin formation in the coagulation pathway via thrombin generation inhibition by anti-Xa and anti-IIa effects.
Therapeutic effect: prevents DVT.

Adverse reactions

CNS: insomnia, headache, asthenia, dizziness.
CV: peripheral edema, ***hemorrhage.***
GI: *nausea, constipation,* vomiting.
GU: urinary tract infection, urine retention.
Hematologic: anemia.
Musculoskeletal: joint disorder.
Skin: rash, pruritus.
Other: fever, injection site pain, infection.

Interactions

Drug-drug. *Oral anticoagulants, platelet inhibitors:* may increase risk of bleeding. Use together cautiously.

Contraindications and precautions

- Contraindicated in patients hypersensitive to drug or to pork products and in patients with severe hemorrhagic diathesis, active major bleeding, or thrombocytopenia with a positive in vitro test for antiplatelet antibody in the presence of drug.
- Use cautiously in breast-feeding patients and patients with impaired renal function or an increased risk of bleeding.

NURSING CONSIDERATIONS

Assessment

- Drug contains sodium sulfite, which can cause allergic reactions in some patients.
- Periodically monitor CBCs (including platelet count) and fecal occult blood tests during therapy; PT and PTT aren't needed.
- Monitor patient's hematocrit and blood pressure closely.
- Evaluate patient's and family's knowledge of drug therapy.

Nursing diagnoses

- Risk for injury related to risk of blood clot formation
- Ineffective protection related to increased risk of bleeding
- Deficient knowledge related to drug therapy

Planning and implementation

- Alternate abdominal wall injection sites; don't rub the site.

ALERT Drug isn't interchangeable (unit for unit) with heparin or low-molecular-weight heparin.

- Store ampules at room temperature, away from light. Refrigerate syringes at 36° to 46° F (2° to 8° C).

Patient teaching

- Instruct patient and family to watch for and report signs of bleeding.
- Tell patient to avoid OTC drugs or herbal remedies containing aspirin or other salicylates.

Evaluation

- Patient develops no blood clots.
- Patient explains appropriate bleeding precautions.
- Patient and family state understanding of drug therapy.

danazol

(DAN-ah-zol)
Cyclomen◆, Danocrine

Pharmacologic class: androgen
Therapeutic class: antiestrogen, androgen
Pregnancy risk category: X

Indications and dosages

▶ **Mild endometriosis.** *Women:* initially, 100 to 200 mg P.O. b.i.d. Subsequent dosage based on patient response.

▶ **Moderate to severe endometriosis.** *Women:* 400 mg P.O. b.i.d. uninterrupted for 3 to 6 months; may be continued for 9 months.

▶ **Fibrocystic breast disease.** *Women:* 100 to 400 mg P.O. daily in two divided doses uninterrupted for 6 months or until symptoms disappear, whichever comes first. If symptoms recur within 1 year of discontinuing therapy, therapy may be restarted. Begin on day 1 of menstruation, if possible.

▶ **Prevention of hereditary angioedema.**
Adults: 200 mg P.O. b.i.d to t.i.d., continued until favorable response occurs. Then dosage decreased 50% at 1- to 3-month intervals.

How supplied

Capsules: 50 mg, 100 mg, 200 mg

Pharmacokinetics

Absorption: amount absorbed by body isn't proportional to administered dose.
Distribution: unknown.
Metabolism: metabolized to 2-hydroxymethylethisterone.
Excretion: unknown. *Half-life:* about 4½ hours.

Route	Onset	Peak	Duration
P.O.	≤ 1 mo	1.5-3 mo	Unknown

Pharmacodynamics

Chemical effect: not clearly defined; inhibits gonadotropins, suppresses pituitary-ovarian axis, and inhibits estrogenic effects.
Therapeutic effect: relieves symptoms of endometriosis and fibrocystic breast disease; prevents hereditary angioedema.

Adverse reactions

CNS: dizziness, headache, sleep disorders, fatigue, tremors, irritability, excitation, lethargy, depression, paresthesia.
CV: elevated blood pressure.
EENT: visual disturbances.
GI: gastric irritation, nausea, vomiting, diarrhea, constipation, change in appetite.
GU: hematuria.
Hematologic: ***thrombocytopenia,*** elevated serum lipid levels.
Hepatic: reversible jaundice, peliosis hepatis, elevated liver enzyme levels, ***liver cell tumors.***
Musculoskeletal: muscle cramps or spasms.
Other: androgenic effects in women, such as *weight gain, hirsutism,* hoarseness, clitoral enlargement, *decreased breast size,* changes in libido, *oily skin or hair,* voice deepening; *hypoestrogenic effects, such as flushing, diaphoresis, vaginitis (including itching, dryness, and burning); vaginal bleeding; nervousness; emotional lability; menstrual irregularities;* chills; *allergic reactions.*

Interactions

Drug-drug. *Carbamazepine:* may increase carbamazepine levels. Monitor patient closely.
Cyclosporine: can increase cyclosporine levels and increase chance of nephrotoxicity. Monitor patient closely.
Insulin, oral hypoglycemics: increased blood glucose level and insulin resistance. Dosage adjustment may be needed. Monitor blood glucose level.
Tacrolimus: may increase tacrolimus levels and risk of nephrotoxicity. Monitor patient closely.
Warfarin: may prolong PT in patients stabilized on warfarin. Monitor PT and INR.

Contraindications and precautions

- Contraindicated in pregnant women, breastfeeding women, and patients with undiagnosed abnormal genital bleeding, porphyria, or impaired renal, cardiac, or hepatic function. Avoid use in women of childbearing age until pregnancy is ruled out.
- Use cautiously in patients with seizure disorder or migraine headache.
- Safety of drug hasn't been established in children.

NURSING CONSIDERATIONS

Assessment

- Obtain history of patient's underlying condition before therapy.
- Monitor effectiveness by assessing severity of pain and other evidence of underlying condition.
- Periodically evaluate liver function, as ordered. Semen evaluation is performed every 3 to 4 months, especially in adolescent boys.
- Be alert for adverse reactions.
- Monitor patient closely for signs of virilization. Some androgenic effects, such as deepening of voice, may not be reversible when therapy stops.
- Evaluate patient's and family's knowledge of drug therapy.

- Monitor INR in patients who take Coumadin.
- Monitor blood glucose levels carefully in diabetic patients.

Nursing diagnoses
- Acute pain related to underlying condition
- Disturbed body image related to drug-induced adverse androgenic reactions
- Deficient knowledge related to drug therapy

Planning and implementation
- For treatment of endometriosis, therapy should start on day 1 of menstruation and typically lasts for at least 3 months and up to 9 months. Therapy may be restarted if symptoms reappear.
- Periodic dosage decreases or gradual drug withdrawal is best.
- Notify prescriber about signs of virilization in women.
- Have patient seek counseling if body image disturbance is serious.

Patient teaching
- Make sure patient understands the importance of using effective nonhormonal contraceptive during therapy.
- Tell patient that ovulation and cyclic menstrual bleeding usually return 2 to 3 months after treatment stops; fibrocystic disease symptoms return within 1 year in 50% of patients.
- If patient takes danazol for fibrocystic breast disease, urge her to examine her breasts regularly and to call prescriber immediately if a breast nodule enlarges during treatment.
- Instruct patient to wash after intercourse to decrease the risk of vaginitis. Tell patient to wear only cotton underwear.
- Prepare woman for possible changes in appearance as a result of virilization, and instruct her to report any changes immediately to prescriber.

Evaluation
- Patient is free from pain.
- Patient states acceptance of body image throughout therapy.
- Patient and family state understanding of drug therapy.

dantrolene sodium
(DAN-troh-leen SOH-dee-um)
Dantrium, Dantrium Intravenous

Pharmacologic class: hydantoin derivative
Therapeutic class: skeletal muscle relaxant
Pregnancy risk category: C

Indications and dosages

▶ **Spasticity and sequelae from severe chronic disorders (such as multiple sclerosis, cerebral palsy, spinal cord injury, CVA).** *Adults:* 25 mg P.O. daily. Increased in 25-mg increments up to 100 mg b.i.d. to q.i.d. Maximum, 400 mg daily. Maintain each dosage level for 4-7 days to determine response. *Children:* initially, 0.5 mg/kg P.O. b.i.d., increased to t.i.d. and then to q.i.d. Dosage increased as needed by 0.5 mg/kg daily to 3 mg/kg b.i.d. to q.i.d. Maximum, 100 mg q.i.d.

▶ **Management of malignant hyperthermic crisis.** *Adults and children:* 1 mg/kg I.V. initially, repeated as needed up to a cumulative dose of 10 mg/kg.

▶ **Prevention or attenuation of malignant hyperthermia in susceptible patients who need surgery.** *Adults:* 4 to 8 mg/kg P.O. daily in three or four divided doses for 1 or 2 days before procedure. Final dose administered 3 to 4 hours before procedure. Or, 2.5 mg/kg I.V. infused over 1 hour about 1 hour before anesthesia. Additional doses, which must be individualized, may be given intraoperatively if necessary.

▶ **Prevention of recurrence of malignant hyperthermia.** *Adults:* 4 to 8 mg/kg/day P.O. in four divided doses for up to 3 days after hyperthermic crisis.

How supplied

Capsules: 25 mg, 50 mg, 100 mg
Injection: 20 mg/vial

Pharmacokinetics

Absorption: 35% of P.O. dose absorbed through GI tract.
Distribution: substantially bound to plasma protein, mainly albumin.

Metabolism: metabolized in liver to its less active 5-hydroxy derivatives and to its amino derivative by reductive pathways.
Excretion: excreted in urine as metabolites.
Half-life: P.O., 9 hours; I.V., 4 to 8 hours.

Route	Onset	Peak	Duration
P.O.	≤ 1 wk	5 hr	Unknown
I.V.	Unknown	Unknown	Unknown

Pharmacodynamics

Chemical effect: acts directly on skeletal muscle to interfere with intracellular calcium movement.
Therapeutic effect: relieves muscle spasms.

Adverse reactions

CNS: *muscle weakness, drowsiness, dizziness,* light-headedness, *malaise,* headache, confusion, nervousness, insomnia, hallucinations, ***seizures.***
CV: tachycardia, blood pressure changes.
EENT: excessive tearing, auditory or visual disturbances.
GI: anorexia, constipation, cramping, dysphagia, metallic taste, severe diarrhea, drooling, bleeding.
GU: urinary frequency, hematuria, incontinence, nocturia, dysuria, crystalluria, difficulty achieving erection.
Hepatic: ***hepatitis.***
Musculoskeletal: myalgia.
Respiratory: pleural effusion.
Skin: diaphoresis, abnormal hair growth, eczematous eruption, pruritus, urticaria, photosensitivity.
Other: chills, fever.

Interactions

Drug-drug. *CNS depressants:* increased CNS depression. Avoid concomitant use.
Estrogens: may increase risk of hepatotoxicity. Use together cautiously.
I.V. verapamil: may result in CV collapse. Stop verapamil before administering I.V. dantrolene.
Drug-lifestyle. *Alcohol use:* increased CNS depression. Discourage concomitant use.
Sunlight: Photosensitivity may occur. Urge precautions.

Contraindications and precautions

- Contraindicated in breast-feeding women, in patients whose spasticity is used to maintain motor function, and in patients with upper motor neuron disorders, spasms from rheumatic disorders, or active hepatic disease.
- Use cautiously in women (including pregnant women), in patients over age 35, and in patients with hepatic disease or severely impaired cardiac or pulmonary function.

NURSING CONSIDERATIONS

Assessment

- Obtain history of patient's spasticity disorder before therapy.
- Obtain liver function tests at start of therapy.
- Monitor effectiveness by evaluating severity of spasticity.
- Be alert for adverse reactions and drug interactions.
- Evaluate patient's and family's knowledge of drug therapy.

Nursing diagnoses

- Acute pain related to presence of spasticity disorder
- Risk for injury related to drug-induced adverse reactions
- Deficient knowledge related to drug therapy

Planning and implementation

- For optimum drug effect, give daily amount in four divided doses.

P.O. use: Give drug with meals or milk to prevent GI distress.
– Prepare oral suspension for single dose by dissolving capsule contents in juice or other suitable liquid. For multiple doses, use acid vehicle, such as citric acid in USP syrup. Refrigerate, and use within several days.
I.V. use: Administer as soon as malignant hyperthermia reaction is recognized, as ordered. Reconstitute each vial with 60 ml of sterile water for injection and shake vial until clear. Don't use diluent that contains bacteriostatic agent. Protect contents from light, and use within 6 hours. Be careful to avoid extravasation.

- Amount of relief determines whether dosage (and drowsiness) can be reduced.

• If hepatitis, severe diarrhea, severe weakness, or sensitivity reactions occur, withhold dose and notify prescriber.

Patient teaching
• Tell patient to use caution when eating to avoid choking. Some patients may have trouble swallowing during therapy.
• Warn patient to avoid hazardous activities until full CNS effects of drug are known.
• Advise patient to avoid combining dantrolene with alcohol or other CNS depressants.
• Tell patient to use sunblock and wear protective clothing, to report GI problems immediately, and to follow prescriber's orders regarding rest and physical therapy.

Evaluation
• Patient states that pain from muscle spasticity has lessened.
• Patient has no injury from drug-induced adverse reactions.
• Patient and family state understanding of drug therapy.

dapsone (DDS)
(DAP-sohn)
Avlosulfon ♦, Dapsone 100 ◇

Pharmacologic class: synthetic sulfone
Therapeutic class: antileprotic, antimalarial
Pregnancy risk category: C

Indications and dosages
▶ **Treatment of multibacillary leprosy.** *Adults:* 100 mg P.O. daily plus rifampin and clofazimine given for 12 months.
Children ages 10 to 14: 50 mg P.O. daily plus rifampin and clofazimine given for 12 months.
▶ **Treatment of paucibacillary leprosy.** *Adults:* 100 mg P.O. daily plus rifampin for 6 months.
Children ages 10 to 14: 50 mg P.O. daily plus rifampin given for 6 months.
▶ **Dermatitis herpetiformis.** *Adults:* Initially, 50 mg P.O. daily, increased to 300 mg daily if symptoms aren't completely controlled. Dose should be reduced to lowest effective level as soon as possible.

How supplied
Tablets: 25 mg, 100 mg

Pharmacokinetics
Absorption: absorbed completely but rather slowly from GI tract.
Distribution: distributed widely in most body tissues and fluids; 50% to 80% protein-bound.
Metabolism: undergoes acetylation by liver enzymes; rate varies and is genetically determined. Almost 50% of blacks and whites are slow acetylators, whereas more than 80% of Chinese, Japanese, and Eskimos are fast acetylators. Dosage adjustment may be needed.
Excretion: dapsone and metabolites excreted primarily in urine; small amounts excreted in feces. *Half-life:* 10 to 50 hours.

Route	Onset	Peak	Duration
P.O.	Unknown	4-8 hr	Unknown

Pharmacodynamics
Chemical effect: unknown; may inhibit folic acid biosynthesis in susceptible organisms (bacteriostatic).
Therapeutic effect: hinders or kills selected bacteria. Spectrum of activity includes *Mycobacterium leprae* and *Mycobacterium tuberculosis*. Drug has some activity against *Pneumocystis carinii* and *Plasmodium*.

Adverse reactions
CNS: insomnia, psychosis, headache, dizziness, lethargy, severe malaise, paresthesia, peripheral neuropathy, vertigo.
CV: tachycardia.
EENT: tinnitus, blurred vision, allergic rhinitis.
GI: anorexia, abdominal pain, ***pancreatitis,*** nausea, vomiting.
GU: albuminuria, nephrotic syndrome, renal papillary necrosis, male infertility.
Hematologic: ***aplastic anemia, agranulocytosis, hemolytic anemia, methemoglobinemia, leukopenia.***
Hepatic: ***hepatitis,*** cholestatic jaundice.
Respiratory: pulmonary eosinophilia.
Skin: allergic dermatitis, lupus erythematosus, phototoxicity, ***exfoliative dermatitis, toxic erythema, erythema multiforme, toxic epidermal***

necrolysis, morbilliform and scarlatiniform reactions, urticaria, ***erythema nodosum.***

Other: fever, infectious mononucleosis–like syndrome, ***sulfone syndrome***, lymphadenopathy.

Interactions

Drug-drug. *Folic acid antagonists (such as methotrexate):* increased risk of adverse hematologic reactions. Avoid concomitant use.

Didanosine: may increase dapsone absorption, leading to therapeutic failure and an increase in infection. Administer at least 2 hours before or after didanosine.

Rifampin: increased hepatic metabolism and renal excretion of dapsone. Monitor patient closely. Clinical significance hasn't been determined.

Drug-lifestyle: *Sunlight:* Photosensitivity may occur. Advise precautions.

Contraindications and precautions

- Contraindicated in breast-feeding women and patients hypersensitive to drug.
- Use cautiously in patients with chronic renal, hepatic, or CV disease; refractory types of anemia; or G6PD deficiency.
- Also use cautiously in pregnant women.

NURSING CONSIDERATIONS

Assessment

- Obtain history of patient's underlying infection and CBC before therapy.
- Monitor effectiveness by assessing for improvement of infection and evaluating culture and sensitivity test results, as ordered.
- Monitor CBC weekly for first month, monthly for 6 months, and semiannually thereafter.
- Be alert for adverse reactions and drug interactions.
- Evaluate patient's and family's knowledge of drug therapy.

Nursing diagnoses

- Infection related to presence of susceptible bacteria
- Risk of impaired skin integrity related to drug-induced adverse dermatologic reactions
- Deficient knowledge related to drug therapy

Planning and implementation

- Be prepared to reduce dosage or temporarily discontinue drug if hemoglobin falls below 9 g/dl, if WBC count falls below 5,000/mm³, or if RBC count falls below 2.5 million/mm³ or remains low.
- If generalized diffuse dermatitis occurs, notify prescriber and prepare to interrupt therapy regimen.
- Administer antihistamines, as ordered, to combat drug-induced allergic dermatitis.
- In severe erythema nodosum, therapy should be stopped and glucocorticoids given cautiously.
- Evidence of sulfone syndrome includes fever, malaise, and jaundice with hepatic necrosis.

Patient teaching

- Inform patient of need for periodic laboratory studies.
- Teach patient to watch for and promptly report adverse dermatologic changes because such reactions may necessitate stopping drug.
- Warn patient to avoid hazardous activities that require alertness if adverse CNS reactions occur.

Evaluation

- Patient is free from infection.
- Patient maintains normal skin integrity throughout therapy.
- Patient and family state understanding of drug therapy.

daunorubicin citrate liposomal

(daw-noh-roo-BYE-sin SIH-trayt li-po-SOE-mul)

DaunoXome

Pharmacologic class: anthracycline
Therapeutic class: antineoplastic
Pregnancy risk category: D

Indications and dosages

▶ **First-line cytotoxic therapy for advanced HIV-related Kaposi's sarcoma.** *Adults:* 40 mg/m² I.V. over 60 minutes once every 2 weeks. Treatment should continue until patient has evidence of progressive disease or until other complications of HIV preclude continuation of therapy.

How supplied

Injection: 2 mg/ml (equivalent to 50 mg daunorubicin base)

Pharmacokinetics

Absorption: must be given I.V. because it's a vesicant.
Distribution: thought to distribute primarily in the vascular fluid volume.
Metabolism: metabolized by the liver into active metabolites.
Excretion: apparent elimination half-life is 4.4 hours.

Route	Onset	Peak	Duration
I.V.	Unknown	Unknown	Unknown

Pharmacodynamics

Chemical effect: Daunorubicin exerts cytotoxic effects by intercalating between DNA base pairs and uncoiling the DNA helix. This inhibits DNA synthesis and DNA-dependent RNA synthesis. Drug may also inhibit polymerase activity. The liposomal preparation maximizes the selectivity of daunorubicin for solid tumors in situ. After penetrating the tumor, daunorubicin is released over time to exert antineoplastic effects.
Therapeutic effect: decreased tumor growth for advanced HIV-related Kaposi's sarcoma.

Adverse reactions

CNS: *headache, neuropathy,* depression, dizziness, insomnia, amnesia, anxiety, ataxia, confusion, ***seizures,*** hallucinations, tremor, hypertonia, meningitis, *fatigue,* malaise, emotional lability, abnormal gait, hyperkinesia, somnolence, abnormal thinking.
CV: ***cardiomyopathy,*** chest pain, hypertension, palpitations, syncope, ***arrhythmias, pericardial effusion, cardiac tamponade, cardiac arrest,*** angina pectoris, ***pulmonary hypertension,*** flushing, edema, tachycardia, ***MI.***
EENT: *rhinitis,* sinusitis, abnormal vision, conjunctivitis, tinnitus, eye pain, deafness, taste disturbances, earache, gingival bleeding, tooth caries, dry mouth.
GI: *nausea, diarrhea, abdominal pain, vomiting, anorexia,* constipation, ***GI hemorrhage,*** gastritis, dysphagia, stomatitis, increased appetite, melena, hemorrhoids, tenesmus.
GU: dysuria, nocturia, polyuria.
Hematologic: NEUTROPENIA.
Hepatic: hepatomegaly.
Musculoskeletal: *rigors, back pain,* arthralgia, myalgia.
Respiratory: *cough, dyspnea,* hemoptysis, hiccups, pulmonary infiltration, increased sputum.
Skin: alopecia, pruritus, *increased sweating,* dry skin, seborrhea, folliculitis.
Other: *fever,* splenomegaly, lymphadenopathy, *opportunistic infections, allergic reactions,* flulike symptoms, dehydration, thirst, injection site inflammation.

Interactions

None reported.

Contraindications and precautions

- Contraindicated in patients who have had a severe hypersensitivity reaction to daunorubicin citrate liposomal or its constituents.
- Use cautiously in patients with myelosuppression, cardiac disease, previous radiotherapy involving the heart, pevious anthracycline use (doxorubicin > 300 mg/m^2 or equivalent), or hepatic or renal dysfunction.

NURSING CONSIDERATIONS

Assessment

- Obtain history of patient's underlying condition before therapy, and reassess regularly thereafter.
- Obtain hepatic and renal studies before therapy.
- Monitor cardiac function regularly and before giving each dose because of the risk of cardiac toxicity and heart failure. Left ventricular ejection fraction should be determined at a total cumulative dose of 320 mg/m^2 and every 160 mg/m^2 thereafter.
- Monitor patient closely for signs of opportunistic infections, especially since patients with HIV infection are immunocompromised.
- Be alert for adverse reactions and drug interactions.

• Evaluate patient's and family's knowledge of drug therapy.

Nursing diagnoses

• Risk for injury related to drug-induced adverse reactions
• Risk for infection related to myelosupression
• Deficient knowledge related to drug therapy

Planning and implementation

• Patients with hepatic or renal insufficiency may need a reduced dosage.
• Drug should be diluted with D_5W—and only D_5W—before administration.
• Withdraw the calculated volume of drug from the vial and transfer it into an equivalent amount of D_5W. The recommended concentration after dilution is 1 mg/ml.
• Don't mix daunorubicin citrate liposomal with other drugs, saline solution, bacteriostatic agents, or any other solution.
• After dilution, immediately administer I.V. over 60 minutes. If unable to use drug immediately, refrigerate at 2° to 8°C (36° to 46°F) for a maximum of 6 hours.
• Because local tissue necrosis is possible, monitor I.V. site closely to avoid extravasation.
• Don't use in-line filters for I.V. infusion.
• Follow proper procedures for handling and disposing of antineoplastics.
• Administer only under the supervision of a prescriber specializing in cancer chemotherapy.
• Monitor patient for adverse reactions. A triad of back pain, flushing, and chest tightness may occur within the first 5 minutes of the infusion. This triad subsides after stopping the infusion and typically doesn't recur when the infusion resumes at a slower rate.
• Monitor hematologic status closely because severe myelosuppression may occur. Blood counts should be repeated and checked before each dose. Withhold treatment if absolute granulocyte count is below 750 cells/mm^3.

Patient teaching

• Inform patient that alopecia may occur but usually is reversible.
• Tell patient to notify prescriber about sore throat, fever, or other signs of infection. Tell patient to avoid exposure to people with infections.
• Advise patient to report suspected or known pregnancy during therapy.
• Tell patient to report back pain, flushing, and chest tightness during the infusion.

Evaluation

• Patient has no injury as a result of drug-induced adverse reactions.
• Patient remains free of infection.
• Patient and family state understanding of drug therapy.

daunorubicin hydrochloride

(daw-noh-ROO-buh-sin high-droh-KLOR-ighd)
Cerubidine

Pharmacologic class: antibiotic antineoplastic (cell cycle–phase nonspecific)
Therapeutic class: antineoplastic
Pregnancy risk category: D

Indications and dosages

Indications and dosages may vary. Check treatment protocol with prescriber.
▶ **Remission induction in acute nonlymphocytic (myelogenous, monocytic, erythroid) leukemia.** *Adults:* in combination, 30 to 45 mg/m^2/day I.V. on days 1, 2, and 3 of first course and on days 1 and 2 of subsequent courses with cytarabine infusions.
▶ **Remission induction in acute lymphocytic leukemia.** *Adults:* 45 mg/m^2/day I.V. on days 1, 2, and 3.
Children age 2 and older: 25 mg/m^2 I.V. on day 1 every week for up to 6 weeks, if needed.
Children under age 2 or with body surface area of less than 0.5 mg/m^2: dose should be calculated based on body weight (1 mg/kg) rather than body surface area.

How supplied

Injection: 20 mg/vial

Pharmacokinetics

Absorption: not applicable with I.V. administration.
Distribution: widely distributed in body tissues; drug doesn't cross blood-brain barrier.

Metabolism: extensively metabolized in liver. One of metabolites has cytotoxic activity.
Excretion: daunorubicin and its metabolites primarily excreted in bile, with small portion excreted in urine. *Half-life:* initial, 45 minutes; terminal, 18½ hours.

Route	Onset	Peak	Duration
I.V.	Unknown	Unknown	Unknown

Pharmacodynamics

Chemical effect: unknown; thought to interfere with DNA-dependent RNA synthesis by intercalation.
Therapeutic effect: kills selected cancer cells.

Adverse reactions

CV: ***irreversible cardiomyopathy,*** ECG changes, ***arrhythmias,*** pericarditis, myocarditis.
GI: *nausea, vomiting, stomatitis, esophagitis,* anorexia, diarrhea.
GU: red urine.
Hematologic: ***bone marrow suppression.***
Hepatic: ***hepatotoxicity.***
Metabolic: hyperuricemia.
Skin: rash, pigmentation of fingernails and toenails, *generalized alopecia, tissue sloughing* with extravasation.
Other: *severe cellulitis,* fever, chills, ***anaphylaxis.***

Interactions

Drug-drug. *Doxorubicin:* additive cardiotoxicity. Monitor patient closely.
Bone marrow suppressants: additive toxicity. Monitor patient closely.
Hepatotoxic drugs: increased risk of additive hepatotoxicity. Monitor patient closely.

Contraindications and precautions

- No known contraindications. However, breast-feeding isn't recommended during therapy.
- Use with extreme caution, if at all, in pregnant women.
- Use cautiously in patients with myelosuppression and in those with impaired cardiac, renal, or hepatic function.

NURSING CONSIDERATIONS

Assessment

- Obtain history of patient's underlying neoplastic disease before therapy, and reassess regularly throughout therapy.
- Check ECG before treatment.
- Monitor CBC and liver function tests, as ordered; monitor ECG every month during therapy.
- Monitor pulse rate closely.
- Be alert for adverse reactions and drug interactions.
- Monitor patient for nausea and vomiting, which may be severe and may last 24 to 48 hours. Monitor patient's hydration status during episodes of nausea and vomiting.
- Evaluate patient's and family's knowledge of drug therapy.

Nursing diagnoses

- Risk for injury related to presence of neoplastic disease
- Risk for deficient fluid volume related to drug-induced nausea and vomiting
- Deficient knowledge related to drug therapy

Planning and implementation

- Follow institutional policy to reduce risks. Preparation and administration of parenteral form have carcinogenic, mutagenic, and teratogenic risks for staff.
- Reconstitute drug using 4 ml of sterile water for injection to produce a 5-mg/ml solution.
- Withdraw desired dose into syringe containing 10 to 15 ml of normal saline solution for injection. Inject into I.V. line containing free-flowing compatible solution of D_5W or normal saline solution for injection over 2 to 3 minutes. Or, dilute in 50 ml of normal saline solution and infuse over 10 to 15 minutes. Or, dilute in 100 ml and infuse over 30 to 45 minutes.
- Avoid extravasation. If it occurs, discontinue I.V. infusion immediately, notify prescriber, and apply ice to area for 24 to 48 hours.
- Don't infuse with dexamethasone or heparin; a precipitate may form.
- Never give drug I.M. or S.C.

• Cumulative dosage is limited to 500 to 600 mg/m² (450 mg/m² if patient also receives or has received cyclophosphamide or radiation therapy to cardiac area).

ALERT Color is similar to that of doxorubicin. Don't confuse these two drugs.

• Optimally, use within 8 hours of preparation. Reconstituted solution is stable 24 hours at room temperature, 48 hours if refrigerated.

• Notify prescriber if adverse cardiac reactions occur. Stop drug immediately and notify prescriber if signs of heart failure or cardiomyopathy develop.

• Give antiemetics to help control nausea and vomiting.

Patient teaching

• Warn patient to watch for signs of infection and bleeding.

• Advise patient that red urine for 1 to 2 days is normal and doesn't indicate blood in urine.

• Inform patient that alopecia may occur but that it's usually reversible.

• Advise woman of childbearing age to avoid becoming pregnant during therapy. Recommend that she consult with prescriber before becoming pregnant.

• Instruct patient about need for protective measures, including conservation of energy, balanced diet, adequate rest, personal cleanliness, clean environment, and avoidance of people with infections.

Evaluation

• Patient shows positive response to therapy as evidenced by reports of follow-up diagnostic tests and improved physical status.

• Patient maintains adequate hydration throughout therapy.

• Patient and family state understanding of drug therapy.

deferoxamine mesylate

(deh-fer-OKS-uh-meen MES-ih-layt)

Desferal

Pharmacologic class: chelating agent

Therapeutic class: heavy metal antagonist

Pregnancy risk category: C

Indications and dosages

▶ **Adjunct treatment of acute iron intoxication.** *Adults and children:* 1 g I.M. or I.V. followed by 500 mg I.M. or I.V. for two doses q 4 hours; then 500 mg I.M. or I.V. q 4 to 12 hours based on response. Maximum, 6 g in 24 hours.

▶ **Chronic iron overload from multiple transfusions.** *Adults and children:* 500 mg to 1 g I.M. daily, and 2 g by slow I.V. infusion in separate solution along with each unit of blood transfused. Maximum, 6 g daily with transfusion, 1 g without transfusion. Or, 20 to 40 mg/kg by S.C. infusion pump daily.

How supplied

Powder for injection: 500 mg

Pharmacokinetics

Absorption: unknown after S.C. or I.M. administration.

Distribution: distributed widely in body after parenteral administration.

Metabolism: small amounts of drug metabolized by plasma enzymes.

Excretion: excreted in urine as unchanged drug or as ferrioxamine, deferoxamine-iron complex. *Half-life:* about 6 hours.

Route	Onset	Peak	Duration
All routes	Unknown	Unknown	Unknown

Pharmacodynamics

Chemical effect: chelates iron by binding ferric ions.

Therapeutic effect: abolishes acute iron intoxication.

Adverse reactions

CV: tachycardia, *hypotension.*

EENT: blurred vision, cataracts, hearing loss.

GI: diarrhea, abdominal discomfort.

GU: dysuria.

Musculoskeletal: leg cramps.

Skin: pain and induration at injection site, *erythema, urticaria.*

Other: ***hypersensitivity reaction,*** fever, ***shock*** (after rapid I.V. administration).

Interactions

Drug-drug. *Ascorbic acid:* may enhance effects of deferoxamine and increase tissue toxicity of iron. Use together with extreme caution and close monitoring.

Contraindications and precautions

- Contraindicated in patients with severe renal disease, heart failure, or anuria.
- Use cautiously in patients with impaired kidney function and in pregnant women.
- Safety of drug hasn't been established in breast-feeding women.

NURSING CONSIDERATIONS

Assessment

- Obtain history of patient's iron intoxication before therapy.
- Monitor effectiveness by monitoring serum iron levels and assessing patient for decreased signs of iron intoxication.
- Observe for signs of anaphylactic reaction immediately after injection.
- Check respiratory status and vital signs frequently until stable.
- Be alert for adverse reactions and drug interactions.
- Evaluate patient's and family's knowledge of drug therapy.

Nursing diagnoses

- Risk for poisoning related to iron intoxication
- Risk for injury related to drug-induced hypersensitivity reactions
- Deficient knowledge related to drug therapy

Planning and implementation

I.V. use: To reconstitute, add 2 ml of sterile water for injection to each ampule. Make sure drug is dissolved completely. After reconstitution, add to normal saline solution, D_5W, or lactated Ringer's solution, and infuse at rate not exceeding 15 mg/kg hourly. Reconstituted solution is good for 1 week at room temperature. Protect from light. Change to I.M. route as soon as possible, as ordered.

I.M. use: Preferred method of administration is I.M. injection. Follow normal protocol.

S.C. use: Follow normal protocol.

- Have epinephrine 1:1,000 readily available to treat hypersensitivity reaction.
- Apply ice or cold compresses to injection site to alleviate local discomfort.
- Long-term use can lead to tachycardia, diarrhea, abdominal discomfort, and dysuria.

Patient teaching

- Instruct patient to report respiratory difficulty or decreased urine output immediately.
- Warn patient that urine may turn red.
- Advise patient to have eye examinations regularly during long-term therapy.
- Warn patient that pain and induration may occur at injection site.

Evaluation

- Patient's iron intoxication is resolved.
- Patient shows no hypersensitivity to therapy.
- Patient and family state understanding of drug therapy.

delavirdine mesylate

(deh-luh-VEER-deen MES-ih-layt)

Rescriptor

Pharmacologic class: nonnucleoside reverse transcriptase inhibitor

Therapeutic class: antiviral

Pregnancy risk category: C

Indications and dosages

▶ **Treatment of HIV-1 infection.** *Adults:* 400 mg P.O. t.i.d. in combination with other appropriate antiretroviral agents.

How supplied

Tablets: 100 mg

Pharmacokinetics

Absorption: rapidly absorbed after oral administration.

Distribution: 98% bound to plasma protein.

Metabolism: extensively converted to inactive metabolites. Primarily metabolized in liver by cytochrome enzyme systems.

Excretion: 51% excreted in the urine (less than 5% unchanged), 44% excreted in the feces. *Half-life:* 5.8 hours.

Route	Onset	Peak	Duration
P.O.	Unknown	1 hr	Unknown

Pharmacodynamics

Chemical effect: drug binds directly to reverse transcriptase and blocks RNA- and DNA-dependent DNA polymerase activities.
Therapeutic effect: inhibits HIV replication.

Adverse reactions

CNS: headache, fatigue.
GI: *nausea,* vomiting, diarrhea.
Hepatic: increased ALT and AST levels.
Skin: *rash,* maculopapular rash, pruritus.

Interactions

Drug-drug. *Amphetamines, benzodiazepines, calcium channel blockers, ergot alkaloid preparations, quinidine:* may result in serious or life-threatening adverse events. Avoid concomitant use.
Antacids: reduced delavirdine absorption. Separate doses by at least 1 hour.
Carbamazepine, phenobarbital, phenytoin, rifampin: substantially decreased plasma delavirdine levels. Avoid coadministration.
Clarithromycin: increased levels of both drugs. Monitor patient carefully.
Dapsone, warfarin: delavirdine increases plasma concentrations of these drugs. Monitor patient carefully.
Didanosine: coadministration with delavirdine results in a 20% decrease in absorption of both drugs. Separate administration by at least 1 hour.
Fluoxetine, ketoconazole: increased delavirdine trough levels. Monitor patient.
H_2-receptor antagonists: may reduce absorption of delavirdine. Long-term use of these drugs with delavirdine isn't recommended.
Indinavir: increased plasma levels of indinavir. May require lower dose of indinavir.
Rifabutin: decreased delavirdine levels and increased rifabutin levels. Monitor patient closely.
Saquinavir: fivefold increase in systemic levels of saquinavir. Monitor AST and ALT levels frequently when used together.

Contraindications and precautions

• Contraindicated in patients hypersensitive to drug's formulation.
• Use cautiously in patients with impaired hepatic function.

NURSING CONSIDERATIONS

Assessment
• Assess patient's underlying condition before therapy and regularly thereafter.
• Be alert for adverse reactions and drug interactions.
• Monitor patient for drug-induced rash.
• Evaluate patient's and family's knowledge of drug therapy.

Nursing diagnoses
• Risk for impaired skin integrity related to potential adverse effects of medication
• Risk for infection related to patient's underlying condition
• Deficient knowledge related to drug therapy

Planning and implementation
• If rash develops, give diphenhydramine, hydroxyzine, or topical corticosteroids as ordered to relieve symptoms.
• Resistance develops rapidly when drug is used as monotherapy. Always give in combination with appropriate antiretroviral therapy.
• Drug may be dispersed in water before ingestion. Add tablets to at least 3 oz (90 ml) of water, let stand for a few minutes; then stir well. Have patient drink promptly, rinse glass, and swallow the rinse to make sure entire dose is consumed.

Patient teaching
• Tell patient to stop drug and call prescriber if he develops severe rash or rash accompanied by such symptoms as fever, blistering, oral lesions, conjunctivitis, swelling, or muscle or joint aches.
• Tell patient that drug doesn't cure HIV-1 infection and that he may continue to acquire illnesses related to HIV-1 infection.

• Urge patient to remain under medical supervision when taking drug because long-term effects aren't known.
• Tell patient to take drug as prescribed and not to alter doses without prescriber's approval. If a dose is missed, tell him to take the next dose as soon as possible but not to double the next dose.
• Inform patient that drug may be taken without regard to food.
• Tell patient with achlorhydria to take drug with an acidic beverage, such as orange or cranberry juice.
• Advise patient to report use of other prescription drugs, OTC medicines, or herbal remedies.

Evaluation
• Patient's skin integrity is maintained.
• Patient is free from opportunistic infections.
• Patient and family state understanding of drug therapy.

demeclocycline hydrochloride
(dee-meh-kloh-SIGH-kleen high-droh-KLOR-ighd)
Declomycin

Pharmacologic class: tetracycline antibiotic
Therapeutic class: antibiotic
Pregnancy risk category: D

Indications and dosages
▶ **Infections caused by susceptible gram-negative and gram-positive organisms, including *Campylobacter fetus, Haemophilus ducreyi*, rickettsiae, *Mycoplasma pneumoniae, Yersinia pestis.* Also indicated for organisms causing psittacosis, lymphogranuloma venereum, granuloma inguinale, relapsing fever, and trachoma.** *Adults:* 150 mg P.O. q 6 hours or 300 mg P.O. q 12 hours.
Children over age 8: 6 to 12 mg/kg P.O. daily in divided doses q 6 to 12 hours.
▶ **Gonorrhea.** *Adults:* initially, 600 mg P.O.; then 300 mg P.O. q 12 hours for 4 days (total 3 g).

How supplied
Tablets: 150 mg, 300 mg
Capsules: 150 mg

Pharmacokinetics
Absorption: 60% to 80% absorbed from GI tract. Food or milk reduces absorption by 50%.
Distribution: distributed widely in body tissues and fluids; however, CSF penetration is poor. Drug is 36% to 91% protein-bound.
Metabolism: not metabolized.
Excretion: excreted primarily unchanged in urine. *Half-life:* 10 to 17 hours.

Route	Onset	Peak	Duration
P.O.	Unknown	3-4 hr	Unknown

Pharmacodynamics
Chemical effect: unknown; thought to exert bacteriostatic effect by binding to 30S ribosomal subunit of microorganisms, thus inhibiting protein synthesis.
Therapeutic effect: inhibits bacterial activity. Spectrum of activity includes many gram-negative and gram-positive organisms, *Mycoplasma, Rickettsia, Chlamydia*, and spirochetes.

Adverse reactions
CNS: ***intracranial hypertension*** (***pseudotumor cerebri***), dizziness.
CV: pericarditis.
EENT: dysphagia, glossitis, tinnitus, visual disturbances.
GI: anorexia, *nausea, vomiting, diarrhea,* enterocolitis, anogenital inflammation, dysphagia, glossitis, ***pancreatitis.***
GU: *increased BUN level.*
Hematologic: ***neutropenia,*** eosinophilia, ***thrombocytopenia, hemolytic anemia.***
Hepatic: elevated liver enzyme levels.
Musculoskeletal: permanent tooth discoloration or bone growth retardation if used in children under age 8.
Skin: *maculopapular and erythematous rashes, photosensitivity, increased pigmentation, urticaria.*
Other: hypersensitivity reactions, ***anaphylaxis,*** diabetes insipidus syndrome (polyuria, polydipsia, weakness).

Interactions

Drug-drug. *Antacids (including sodium bicarbonate) and laxatives containing aluminum, magnesium, or calcium; antidiarrheals:* decreased antibiotic absorption. Give antibiotic 1 hour before or 2 hours after any of above.
Digoxin: may increase serum digoxin levels in a small portion of patients. Monitor patient for signs of toxicity.
Ferrous sulfate and other iron products, zinc: decreased antibiotic absorption. Give antibiotic 3 hours after or 2 hours before iron.
Methoxyflurane: may cause nephrotoxicity with tetracyclines. Monitor patient carefully.
Oral anticoagulants: increased anticoagulant effect. Monitor PT and INR and adjust dosage, as ordered.
Oral contraceptives: decreased contraceptive effectiveness and increased risk of breakthrough bleeding. Recommend nonhormonal birth control.
Penicillins: may interfere with bactericidal action of penicillins. Avoid using together.
Drug-food. *Food, dairy products:* decreased antibiotic absorption. Give antibiotic 1 hour before or 2 hours after any of above.
Drug-lifestyle. *Sun exposure:* photosensitivity reactions may occur. Advise precautions.

Contraindications and precautions

- Contraindicated in patients hypersensitive to drug or other tetracyclines and in breast-feeding women.
- Use cautiously in patients with impaired kidney or liver function.
- Use of these drugs during last half of pregnancy and in children under age 8 may cause permanent discoloration of teeth, enamel defects, and bone growth retardation.

NURSING CONSIDERATIONS

Assessment

- Obtain history of patient's infection before therapy, and reassess regularly throughout therapy.
- Obtain specimen for culture and sensitivity tests before giving first dose. Therapy may begin pending test results.
- Be alert for adverse reactions and drug interactions.
- Monitor patient's hydration status if adverse GI reactions occur.
- Evaluate patient's and family's knowledge of drug therapy.

Nursing diagnoses

- Infection related to presence of susceptible organism
- Risk for deficient fluid volume related to drug-induced adverse GI reactions
- Deficient knowledge related to drug therapy

Planning and implementation

- Check expiration date. Outdated or deteriorated tetracyclines have been linked to reversible nephrotoxicity (Fanconi's syndrome).
- Don't expose these drugs to light or heat; store in tight container.
- Don't give drug with milk or other dairy products, food, antacids, or iron products because they reduce effectiveness.
- Give drug with full glass of water at least 1 hour before meals or 2 hours afterward. Give at least 1 hour before bedtime to prevent esophagitis.
- Demeclocycline may cause a false-negative reading in urine tests that use glucose oxidase reagent (Diastix, Chemstrip uG).
- Notify prescriber if patient develops superinfection. Drug may need to be discontinued and another antibiotic substituted.

Patient teaching

- Tell patient to take each dose with full glass of water at least 1 hour before or 2 hours after meals and to remain standing for 90 seconds after ingestion. Tell patient to take drug at least 1 hour before bedtime to prevent esophagitis.
- Explain that drug effectiveness is reduced when taken with milk or other dairy products, food, antacids, or iron products.
- Instruct patient to take entire amount of medication, exactly as prescribed, even after he feels better.
- Stress good oral hygiene.
- Warn patient to avoid direct sunlight and ultraviolet light. A sunscreen may help prevent photosensitivity reactions. Photosensitivity persists for some time after therapy ends.

• Tell patient to check expiration date and discard outdated demeclocycline because it may become toxic.
• Advise woman taking oral contraceptive to use alternative means of contraception during drug therapy and for 1 week afterward.

Evaluation
• Patient is free from infection.
• Patient maintains adequate hydration throughout therapy.
• Patient and family state understanding of drug therapy.

desipramine hydrochloride
(deh-SIP-rah-meen high-droh-KLOR-ighd)
Norpramin**

Pharmacologic class: dibenzazepine tricyclic antidepressant (TCA)
Therapeutic class: antidepressant
Pregnancy risk category: C

Indications and dosages
▶ **Depression.** *Adults:* initially, 100 to 200 mg P.O. daily in divided doses; increased to maximum of 300 mg daily. Or entire dosage can be given h.s.
Elderly patients and adolescents: 25 to 100 mg P.O. daily in divided doses; increased gradually to maximum of 150 mg daily, if needed.

How supplied
Tablets: 10 mg, 25 mg, 50 mg, 75 mg, 100 mg, 150 mg

Pharmacokinetics
Absorption: absorbed rapidly from GI tract.
Distribution: distributed widely throughout body, including CNS; 90% protein-bound.
Metabolism: metabolized by liver; significant first-pass effect may explain variability of serum levels in different patients taking same dosage.
Excretion: excreted primarily in urine.

Route	Onset	Peak	Duration
P.O.	2-4 wk	4-6 hr	Unknown

Pharmacodynamics
Chemical effect: unknown; increases amount of norepinephrine, serotonin, or both in CNS by blocking their reuptake by neurons.
Therapeutic effect: relieves depression.

Adverse reactions
CNS: *drowsiness, dizziness,* excitation, tremors, weakness, confusion, headache, nervousness, EEG changes, ***seizures,*** extrapyramidal reactions.
CV: orthostatic hypotension, *tachycardia, ECG changes,* hypertension.
EENT: *blurred vision,* tinnitus, mydriasis.
GI: *dry mouth, constipation,* nausea, vomiting, anorexia, paralytic ileus.
GU: *urine retention.*
Skin: rash, urticaria, *diaphoresis,* photosensitivity.
Other: ***hypersensitivity reaction.***

Interactions
Drug-drug. *Anticholinergics:* Enhanced anticholinergic effects. Monitor patient closely.
Barbiturates, CNS depressants: enhanced CNS depression. Avoid concomitant use.
Cimetidine, methylphenidate: may increase desipramine serum levels. Monitor patient for adverse reactions.
Clonidine, epinephrine, norepinephrine: increased hypertensive effect. Use cautiously.
MAO inhibitors: may cause severe excitation, hyperpyrexia, or seizures, usually with high dosage. Use cautiously.
Selective serotonin reuptake inhibitors (SSRIs): may inhibit the metabolism of TCAs, causing toxicity. Symptoms of TCA toxicity may persist for several weeks after stopping SSRI. At least 5 weeks may be necessary when switching from fluoxetine to a TCA because of the long half-life of the active and parent metabolite.
Drug-lifestyle. *Alcohol use:* enhanced CNS depression. Discourage concomitant use.
Smoking: may lower plasma desipramine levels. Monitor patient for lack of effect, and encourage smoking cessation.
Sun exposure: increased risk of photosensitivity. Advise against unprotected or prolonged sun exposure.

Contraindications and precautions

• Contraindicated in patients hypersensitive to drug, in those who have taken an MAO inhibitor within previous 14 days, and in patients in acute recovery phase of MI.
• Use with extreme caution in patients taking thyroid medication and in those with CV disease, seizure disorder, glaucoma, thyroid disorder, or history of urine retention.
• Use cautiously in pregnant or breast-feeding women.
• Safety of drug hasn't been established in children under age 12.

NURSING CONSIDERATIONS

Assessment

• Obtain history of patient's depression before therapy, and reassess regularly thereafter.
• Be alert for adverse reactions and drug interactions.
• Evaluate patient's and family's knowledge of drug therapy.

Nursing diagnoses

• Ineffective individual coping related to depression
• Risk for injury related to drug-induced adverse reactions
• Deficient knowledge related to drug therapy

Planning and implementation

• Don't withdraw drug abruptly. After abrupt withdrawal of long-term therapy, patient may experience nausea, headache, and malaise. This doesn't indicate addiction.
• Because desipramine produces fewer anticholinergic effects than other TCAs, it's prescribed often for patients with cardiac problems.
• Because hypertensive episodes have occurred during surgery in patients receiving TCAs, this drug should be discontinued gradually several days before surgery.
ALERT Although the cause isn't clearly defined, this drug may cause sudden death in children.
• If signs of psychosis occur or increase, expect prescriber to reduce dosage.

Patient teaching

• Warn patient to avoid hazardous activities until CNS effects of drug are known. Drowsiness and dizziness usually subside after a few weeks.
• Tell patient to avoid alcohol during therapy because it may antagonize effects of desipramine.
• Warn patient not to stop drug suddenly.
• Advise patient to consult prescriber before taking other prescription drugs, OTC medications, or herbal remedies.
• Instruct patient to use sunblock, wear protective clothing, and avoid prolonged exposure to strong sunlight.

Evaluation

• Patient behavior and communication indicate improvement of depression.
• Patient has no injury as a result of drug-induced adverse reactions.
• Patient and family state understanding of drug therapy.

desmopressin acetate

(dez-moh-PREH-sin AS-ih-tayt)
DDAVP, Stimate

Pharmacologic class: posterior pituitary hormone
Therapeutic class: antidiuretic, hemostatic agent
Pregnancy risk category: B

Indications and dosages

▶ **Nonnephrogenic diabetes insipidus, temporary polyuria and polydipsia from pituitary trauma.** *Adults:* 10 to 40 mcg/day intranasally in one to three divided doses daily. Morning and evening doses adjusted separately for adequate diurnal rhythm of water turnover. Or, 0.05 mg P.O. b.i.d. Each dose should be adjusted separately for an adequate diurnal rhythm of water turnover. Total oral daily dosage should be increased or decreased as needed to achieve desired response. Doses may range from 0.1 to 1.2 mg divided into two or three daily doses. Oral therapy should start

12 hours after last intranasal dose. Or, injectable form at 2 to 4 mcg/day I.V. or S.C. daily, usually in two equally divided doses.
Children ages 3 months to 12 years (nasal spray): 0.05 to 0.3 ml intranasally daily in one or two doses.
Children age 4 and older (oral form): begin with 0.05 mg P.O. b.i.d. Each dose should be adjusted separately for an adequate diurnal rhythm of water turnover. Total oral daily dosage should be increased or decreased as necessary to achieve desired response. Doses may range from 0.1 to 1.2 mg divided into two or three daily doses. Oral therapy should start 12 hours after the last intranasal dose.
Children under age 4 (oral form): dosage must be individually adjusted to prevent an excessive decrease in plasma osmolality.

▶ **Hemophilia A and von Willebrand's disease.** *Adults and children:* 0.3 mcg/kg diluted in normal saline solution and infused I.V. over 15 to 30 minutes. Dose repeated if necessary based on laboratory response and patient's condition. Intranasal dose is 1 spray (of solution containing 1.5 mg/ml) into each nostril to provide total of 300 mcg. In patients weighing less than 50 kg (110 lb), use 1 spray into a single nostril (150 mcg).

▶ **Primary nocturnal enuresis.** *Children age 6 and over:* initially, 20 mcg intranasally h.s. Dosage adjusted according to response. Maximum recommended dosage is 40 mcg daily. Or, 0.2 mg P.O. h.s. Dose may be adjusted up to 0.6 mg P.O. to achieve desired response. Oral therapy may start 24 hours after last intranasal dose.

How supplied

Nasal solution: 0.1 mg/ml, 1.5 mg/ml
Injection: 4 mcg/ml, 15 mcg/ml
Tablets: 0.1 mg, 0.2 mg

Pharmacokinetics

Absorption: after intranasal administration, 10% to 20% of dose absorbed through nasal mucosa. Absorption after S.C. administration is unknown. Following P.O. administration, drug is minimally absorbed from the GI tract.
Distribution: unknown.
Metabolism: unknown.
Excretion: unknown. *Half-life:* fast phase, about 8 minutes; slow phase, 75½ minutes.

Route	Onset	Peak	Duration
P.O.	1 hr	4-7 hr	Unknown
I.V.	15-30 min	1.5-2 hr	4-12 hr
S.C.	Unknown	Unknown	Unknown
Intranasal	≤ 1 hr	1-5 hr	8-12 hr

Pharmacodynamics

Chemical effect: increases permeability of renal tubular epithelium to adenosine monophosphate and water; epithelium promotes reabsorption of water and produces concentrated urine (ADH effect). Desmopressin also increases factor VIII activity by releasing endogenous factor VIII from plasma storage sites.
Therapeutic effect: decreases diuresis and promotes clotting.

Adverse reactions

CNS: headache.
CV: slight rise in blood pressure.
EENT: nasal congestion, rhinitis, epistaxis, sore throat.
GI: nausea, abdominal cramps.
GU: vulvar pain.
Respiratory: cough.
Other: flushing, local erythema, swelling or burning after injection.

Interactions

Drug-drug. *Clofibrate:* enhanced and prolonged effects of desmopressin. Monitor patient carefully.
Demeclocycline, epinephrine, heparin, lithium: Decreased response to desmopression. Monitor patient closely.
Drug-lifestyle. *Alcohol use:* increased risk of adverse effects. Discourage concomitant use.

Contraindications and precautions

• Contraindicated in patients hypersensitive to drug and in those with type IIB von Willebrand's disease.

• Use cautiously in patients with coronary artery insufficiency or hypertensive CV disease and in those with conditions linked to fluid and electrolyte imbalance, such as cystic fibrosis, because these patients are prone to hyponatremia. Also use cautiously in pregnant or breast-feeding women.
• Use of drug in infants under age 3 months isn't recommended because of their increased tendency to develop fluid imbalance.
• Safety of parenteral form of drug hasn't been established for management of diabetes insipidus in children under age 12.

NURSING CONSIDERATIONS

Assessment
• Obtain history of patient's underlying condition before therapy.
• Monitor effectiveness by checking patient's fluid intake and output, serum and urine osmolality, and urine specific gravity for treatment of diabetes insipidus or relief of symptoms of other disorders.
• Be alert for adverse reactions and drug interactions.
• Monitor patient carefully for hypertension during high-dose treatment.
• Evaluate patient's and family's knowledge of drug therapy.

Nursing diagnoses
• Deficient fluid volume related to underlying condition
• Acute pain related to drug-induced headache
• Deficient knowledge related to drug therapy

Planning and implementation
P.O. use: Follow normal protocol.
I.V. use: Dilute drug with normal saline solution according to prescriber's instructions when administering I.V. for treatment of hemophilia A and von Willebrand's disease.
S.C. use: Follow normal protocol. Rotate injection sites.
Intranasal use: Follow manufacturer's instructions exactly for administration.
• Desmopressin injection shouldn't be used to treat hemophilia A with factor VIII levels of 0% to 5%, or severe cases of von Willebrand's disease.
• When drug is used to treat diabetes insipidus, dosage or frequency of administration may be adjusted according to patient's fluid output. Morning and evening doses are adjusted separately for adequate diurnal rhythm of water turnover.
• Intranasal use can cause changes in nasal mucosa, resulting in erratic, unreliable absorption. Report worsening condition to prescriber, who may prescribe injectable DDAVP.

Patient teaching
• Instruct patient to clear nasal passages before using drug intranasally.
• Patient may have trouble measuring and inhaling drug into nostrils. Teach patient and caregiver correct method of administration.
• Advise patient to report conditions such as nasal congestion, allergic rhinitis, or upper respiratory tract infection; dosage adjustment may be required.
• Teach patient using S.C. desmopressin to rotate injection sites to avoid tissue damage.
• Warn patient to drink only enough water to satisfy thirst.
• Inform patient that when treating hemophilia A and von Willebrand's disease, giving desmopressin may avoid hazards of using blood products.
• Advise patient to wear or carry medical identification indicating use of drug.

Evaluation
• Patient achieves normal fluid and electrolyte balance.
• Patient states that headache is relieved with mild analgesic.
• Patient and family state understanding of drug therapy.

dexamethasone
(deks-ah-METH-uh-sohn)
Decadron*, Dronil♦, DexaMeth, Dexamethasone Intensol*, Dexasone♦, Dexone 0.5, Dexone 0.75, Dexone 1.5, Dexone 4, Hexadrol*, Mymethasone*, Oradexon♦

dexamethasone acetate
Cortostat LA, Dalalone D.P., Dalalone L.A., Decadron-LA, Decaject-L.A., Dexacen LA-8, Dexasone-L.A., Dexone L.A., Solurex-LA

dexamethasone sodium phosphate
Ak-Dex, Cortastat, Cortastat 10, Dalalone, Decadrol, Decadron Phosphate, Decaject, Dexacen-4, Dexacorten, Dexone, Hexadrol Phosphate, Primethasone, Solurex

Pharmacologic class: glucocorticoid
Therapeutic class: anti-inflammatory, immunosuppressant
Pregnancy risk category: NR

Indications and dosages

▶ **Cerebral edema (Phosphate).** *Adults:* initially, 10 mg I.V. Then 4 mg I.M. q 6 hours until symptoms subside (usually 2 to 4 days). Then tapered over 5 to 7 days.

▶ **Inflammatory conditions, allergic reactions, neoplasias (Phosphate).** *Adults:* 4 mg I.M. as a single dose. Continue maintenance therapy with dexamethasone tablets, 1.5 mg P.O. b.i.d. for 2 days, and then 0.75 mg P.O. b.i.d. for 1 day, and then 0.75 mg P.O. once daily for 2 days, and then discontinue drug. (**Acetate.**) *Adults:* 4 to 16 mg I.M. into joint or soft tissue q 1 to 3 weeks. Or, 0.8 to 1.6 mg into lesions q 1 to 3 weeks.

▶ **Shock (Phosphate).** *Adults:* 1 to 6 mg/kg I.V. as single dose or 40 mg I.V. q 2 to 6 hours, p.r.n. Or, 20 mg I.V. as a single dose followed by continuous infusion of 3 mg/kg per 24 hours.

▶ **Dexamethasone suppression test for Cushing's syndrome.** *Adults:* after determining baseline 24-hour urine levels of 17-hydroxycorticosteroids, 0.5 mg P.O. q 6 hours for 48 hours; 24-hour urine collection made for determination of 17-hydroxycorticosteroid excretion again during second 24 hours of dexamethasone administration. Or, 1 mg P.O. as a single dose at 11 p.m. Draw plasma cortisol level at 8 a.m. the following day.

How supplied

dexamethasone
Tablets: 0.25 mg, 0.5 mg, 0.75 mg, 1 mg, 1.5 mg, 2 mg, 4 mg, 6 mg
Oral solution: 0.5 mg/5 ml, 1 mg/ml*
Elixir: 0.5 mg/5 ml*
dexamethasone acetate
Injection: 8 mg/ml, 16 mg/ml suspension
dexamethasone sodium phosphate
Injection: 4 mg/ml, 10 mg/ml, 20 mg/ml, 24 mg/ml

Pharmacokinetics

Absorption: absorbed readily after P.O. administration. Absorption of suspension for injection depends on whether it is injected into an intra-articular space, a muscle, or blood supply to a muscle.
Distribution: distributed to muscle, liver, skin, intestines, and kidneys. Drug is bound weakly to plasma proteins (transcortin and albumin). Only unbound portion is active.
Metabolism: metabolized in liver to inactive glucuronide and sulfate metabolites.
Excretion: inactive metabolites and small amounts of unmetabolized drug excreted by kidneys. Insignificant quantities of drug also are excreted in feces. *Half-life:* 36 to 54 hours.

Route	Onset	Peak	Duration
P.O.	1-2 hr	1-2 hr	2.5 days
I.V., I.M.	≤ 1 hr	1 hr	2 days-3 wk

Pharmacodynamics

Chemical effect: not clearly defined; decreases inflammation, mainly by stabilizing leukocyte lysosomal membranes; suppresses immune response; stimulates bone marrow; and influences protein, fat, and carbohydrate metabolism.
Therapeutic effect: relieves cerebral edema, reduces inflammation and immune response, and reverses shock.

Adverse reactions

CNS: *euphoria, insomnia,* psychotic behavior, pseudotumor cerebri, ***seizures.***
CV: ***heart failure,*** hypertension, edema, ***arrhythmias, thromboembolism.***
EENT: cataracts, glaucoma.
GI: *peptic ulceration,* GI irritation, increased appetite, ***pancreatitis.***
GU: menstrual irregularities.
Metabolic: hypokalemia, hyperglycemia, carbohydrate intolerance.
Musculoskeletal: muscle weakness, osteoporosis, growth suppression in children.
Skin: hirsutism, delayed wound healing, acne, skin eruptions, atrophy at I.M. injection sites.
Other: cushingoid state (moonface, buffalo hump, central obesity), susceptibility to infections, ***acute adrenal insufficiency may follow increased stress (infection, surgery, or trauma) or abrupt withdrawal after long-term therapy.***

Interactions

Drug-drug. *Antidiabetics, including insulin:* decreased response. May need dosage adjustment.
Aspirin, indomethacin, other NSAIDs: increased risk of GI distress and bleeding. Give together cautiously.
Barbiturates, phenytoin, rifampin: decreased corticosteroid effect. Increase corticosteroid dosage, as ordered.
Cardiac glycosides: increased possibility of arrhythmia from hypokalemia. May warrant dosage adjustment.
Oral anticoagulants: altered dosage requirements. Monitor PT and INR closely.
Potassium-depleting drugs: enhanced potassium-wasting effects of dexamethasone. Monitor serum potassium levels.
Salicylates: decreased serum salicylate levels. Monitor patient for lack of therapeutic effects.
Skin-test antigens: decreased response. Defer skin testing until therapy is completed.
Toxoids, vaccines: decreased antibody response and increased risk of neurologic complications. Avoid concomitant use.
Drug-lifestyle. *Alcohol use:* increased risk of gastric irritation and GI ulceration. Discourage concomitant use.

Contraindications and precautions

- Contraindicated in patients hypersensitive to drug or its components and in those with systemic fungal infections.
- Drug isn't recommended for use in breast-feeding women.
- Use with extreme caution in patient with recent MI.
- Use cautiously in pregnant women and in patients with GI ulcer, renal disease, hypertension, osteoporosis, diabetes mellitus, hypothyroidism, cirrhosis, diverticulitis, nonspecific ulcerative colitis, recent intestinal anastomoses, thromboembolic disorders, seizures, myasthenia gravis, heart failure, tuberculosis, ocular herpes simplex, emotional instability, or psychotic tendencies. Because some forms contain sulfite preservatives, also use cautiously in patients sensitive to sulfites.
- Long-term use of drug in children and adolescents may delay growth and maturation.

NURSING CONSIDERATIONS

Assessment

- Obtain history of patient's underlying condition before therapy.
- Monitor patient's weight, blood pressure, blood glucose level, and serum electrolyte levels.
- Be alert for adverse reactions and drug interactions. Most adverse reactions to corticosteroids are dose- or duration-dependent.
- Watch for depression or psychotic episodes, especially in high-dose therapy.
- Evaluate patient's and family's knowledge of drug therapy.

Nursing diagnoses

- Ineffective health maintenance related to underlying condition
- Risk for injury related to drug-induced adverse reactions
- Deficient knowledge related to drug therapy

Planning and implementation

- For better results and less toxicity, give once-daily dose in morning.

P.O. use: Give with food when possible.
I.V. use: When giving as direct injection, inject undiluted over at least 1 minute. When

giving as intermittent or continuous infusion, dilute solution according to manufacturer's instructions and give over prescribed duration. If given by continuous infusion, change solution every 24 hours.
I.M. use: Give I.M. injection deeply into gluteal muscle. Rotate injection sites to prevent muscle atrophy.
• Avoid S.C. injection because atrophy and sterile abscesses may occur.
• Always adjust to lowest effective dose, as ordered.
ALERT Gradually reduce dosage after long-term therapy, as ordered. Abrupt withdrawal may cause rebound inflammation, fatigue, weakness, arthralgia, fever, dizziness, lethargy, depression, fainting, orthostatic hypotension, dyspnea, anorexia, and hypoglycemia. After prolonged use, abrupt withdrawal may be fatal.
• Unless contraindicated, give patient low-sodium diet high in potassium and protein. Also, give potassium supplements as directed.
• Notify prescriber if patient has increased stress (physical or psychological) because dosage may need to be increased.
• Notify prescriber if patient develops adverse reactions, and be prepared to provide supportive and symptomatic treatment, as prescribed.

Patient teaching
• Tell patient not to stop drug abruptly or without prescriber's consent because abrupt withdrawal may be fatal.
• Teach patient signs of early adrenal insufficiency: fatigue, muscle weakness, joint pain, fever, anorexia, nausea, dyspnea, dizziness, and fainting.
• Instruct patient to wear or carry medical identification that indicates need for supplemental systemic glucocorticoids during stress, especially as dosage is decreased.
• Warn patient receiving long-term therapy about cushingoid symptoms and the need to notify prescriber about sudden weight gain or swelling.
• Warn patient about easy bruising.
• Advise patient receiving long-term therapy to consider exercise or physical therapy. Give vitamin D or calcium supplements, as ordered.
• Advise patient receiving long-term therapy to have periodic ophthalmologic examinations.

Evaluation
• Patient's condition being treated with drug therapy shows improvement.
• Patient has no injury as a result of drug therapy.
• Patient and family state understanding of drug therapy.

dexmedetomidine hydrochloride
(DEX-meh-dih-TOE-mih-deen high-droh-KLOR-ighd)
Precedex

Pharmacologic class: selective alpha$_2$-adenoreceptor agonist with sedative properties
Therapeutic class: sedative
Pregnancy risk category: C

Indications and dosages
▶ **Sedation of initially intubated and mechanically ventilated patients in ICU setting.** *Adults:* loading infusion of 1 mcg/kg I.V. over 10 minutes; then a maintenance infusion of 0.2 to 0.7 mcg/kg/hr for up to 24 hours, adjusted to achieve the desired level of sedation.

How supplied
Injection: 100 mcg/ml in 2-ml vials and 2-ml ampules

Pharmacokinetics
Absorption: given parenterally.
Distribution: after I.V. administration, drug is rapidly and widely distributed. Drug is 94% protein bound.
Metabolism: almost completely hepatically metabolized to inactive metabolites.
Excretion: inactive metabolites are 95% renally eliminated and 4% fecally eliminated. *Elimination half-life:* about 2 hours.

Route	Onset	Peak	Duration
I.V.	Unknown	Unknown	Unknown

Pharmacodynamics

Chemical effect: selectively stimulates $alpha_2$-adenoceptor in the CNS.
Therapeutic effect: produces sedation of initially intubated and mechanically ventilated patients in ICU setting.

Adverse reactions

CV: *hypotension, **bradycardia**, **arrhythmias**.*
GI: *nausea,* thirst.
GU: oliguria.
Hematologic: anemia, leukocytosis.
Respiratory: ***hypoxia,*** pleural effusion, pulmonary edema.
Other: pain, infection.

Interactions

Drug-drug. *Anesthetics, hypnotics, opioids, sedatives:* possible enhancement of effects. A reduction of dexmedetomidine dose may be needed.

Contraindications and precautions

- Use cautiously in elderly patients and those with advanced heart block or renal or hepatic impairment.

NURSING CONSIDERATIONS

Assessment

- Assess renal and hepatic function before administration, particularly in elderly patients.
- Assess patient's response to drug. Some patients receiving dexmedetomidine have been observed to be arousable and alert when stimulated. This alone shouldn't be considered evidence of lack of efficacy in the absence of other clinical signs and symptoms.
- Be alert for adverse reactions and drug interactions.
- Evaluate patient's and family's knowledge about drug therapy.

Nursing diagnoses

- Risk for injury related to drug-induced adverse reactions
- Impaired spontaneous ventilation related to underlying disease process
- Deficient knowledge related to drug therapy

Planning and implementation

- Elderly patients and those with renal or hepatic failure may need a reduced dosage.
- Dexmedetomidine must be diluted in normal saline solution before administration. To prepare the infusion, withdraw 2 ml of dexmedetomidine and add to 48 ml of normal saline injection to a total of 50 ml. Shake gently to mix well.
- Don't coadminister through the same I.V. catheter with blood or plasma because physical compatibility hasn't been established. Dexmedetomidine infusion is compatible with lactated Ringer's solution, D_5W, normal saline solution, and 20% mannitol. It's also compatible with thiopental sodium, etomidate, vecuronium bromide, pancuronium bromide, succinylcholine, atracurium besylate, mivacurium chloride, glycopyrrolate bromide, phenylephrine hydrochloride, atropine sulfate, midazolam, morphine sulfate, fentanyl citrate, and plasma substitute. Administer using a controlled infusion device at the rate calculated for body weight.
- Don't administer infusion for longer than 24 hours.
- Continuously monitor cardiac status.
- Dexmedetomidine has been continuously infused in mechanically ventilated patients before, during, and after extubation. It isn't necessary to stop dexmedetomidine before extubation.

Patient teaching

- Tell patient that he'll be sedated while the drug is administered, but that he may arouse when stimulated.
- Tell patient that he'll be closely monitored and attended while sedated.

Evaluation

- Patient has no injury as a result of drug-induced adverse reactions.
- Patient regains spontaneous ventilation.
- Patient and family state understanding of drug therapy.

dexrazoxane

(deks-rah-ZOKS-ayn)
Zinecard

Pharmacologic class: intracellular chelating agent
Therapeutic class: cardioprotective agent
Pregnancy risk category: C

Indications and dosages

▶ **Reduction of occurrence and severity of doxorubicin-induced cardiomyopathy in women with metastatic breast cancer who have received a cumulative doxorubicin dose of 300 mg/m² but would benefit from continued therapy with doxorubicin.** *Adults:* dosage ratio of dexrazoxane to doxorubicin must be 10:1, such as 500 mg/m² of dexrazoxane to 50 mg/m² of doxorubicin. After reconstitution, dexrazoxane should be given by slow I.V. push or rapid drip I.V. infusion. After completion of dexrazoxane administration (and less than 30 minutes from the beginning of this administration), I.V. injection of doxorubicin should be given.

How supplied

Injection: 250 mg, 500 mg

Pharmacokinetics

Absorption: not applicable with I.V. administration.
Distribution: not bound to plasma proteins.
Metabolism: not thought to be metabolized.
Excretion: excreted primarily in urine.

Route	Onset	Peak	Duration
I.V.	Unknown	15 min	Unknown

Pharmacodynamics

Chemical effect: unknown; cyclic derivative of ethylenediamine tetra-acetic acid that readily penetrates cell membranes and may be converted to ring-opened chelating agent that interferes with iron-mediated free radical generation.
Therapeutic effect: prevents doxorubicin-induced cardiomyopathy or reduces its severity.

Adverse reactions

CNS: *fatigue, malaise,* ***neurotoxicity.***
GI: *nausea, vomiting, anorexia, stomatitis, diarrhea,* esophagitis, dysphagia.
Hematologic: ***immunosuppression, hemorrhage.***
Skin: *alopecia,* erythema, urticaria, skin reaction.
Other: *fever, infection, pain on injection,* ***sepsis,*** streaking at I.V. insertion site, phlebitis, extravasation.

Interactions

None reported.

Contraindications and precautions

- Contraindicated in patients not receiving chemotherapy regimens that contain an anthracycline.
- Drug isn't recommended for use in pregnant or breast-feeding women.
- Use cautiously in all patients. Additive effects of immunosuppression may result from required concomitant administration of cytotoxic drugs.
- Safety of drug hasn't been established in children.

NURSING CONSIDERATIONS

Assessment

- Obtain history of patient's underlying condition before drug administration.
- Monitor CBC closely, as ordered. Dexrazoxane is always used with other cytotoxic drugs, and it may add to their myelosuppressive effects.
- Be alert for adverse reactions.
- The adverse reactions listed, with the exception of pain on injection, may be attributed to the regimen given shortly after dexrazoxane, which includes fluorouracil, doxorubicin, and cyclophosphamide.
- Evaluate patient's and family's knowledge of drug therapy.

Nursing diagnoses

- Risk for injury related to doxorubicin-induced cardiomyopathy

• Ineffective protection related to immunosuppression induced by dexrazoxane and concomitant cardiotoxic drug therapy
• Deficient knowledge related to drug therapy

Planning and implementation

• Dexrazoxane is recommended only when patient has already received an accumulated doxorubicin dose of 300 mg/m^2 and continuation of doxorubicin is desired.
• Drug must be diluted with the diluent supplied with drug (0.167 molar sodium lactate injection) to yield 10 mg dexrazoxane for each milliliter of sodium lactate. Reconstituted solution should be given by slow I.V. push or rapid drip I.V. infusion from a bag.
• Reconstituted solution, when transferred to an empty infusion bag, is stable for 6 hours from the time of reconstitution when stored at controlled room temperature (59° to 86° F [15° to 30° C]) or refrigerated (36° to 46° F [2° to 8°C]). Discard unused solution.
• Reconstituted drug may be diluted with either normal saline solution or D_5W to a range of 1.3 to 5 mg/ml in I.V. infusion bags. Resulting solution is stable for 6 hours under the same storage conditions as the diluted drug.
• Dexrazoxane shouldn't be mixed with other drugs because of possible incompatibility.
• When handling and preparing reconstituted solution, use the same precautions as those for handling antineoplastic drugs. Use of gloves is recommended.
• If drug powder or solution contacts skin or mucosa, immediately wash thoroughly with soap and water.
• Institute infection-control and bleeding precautions, as indicated by CBC results.

Patient teaching

• Inform patient of the need for drug during continued doxorubicin therapy.
• Warn patient to watch for signs of infection (fever, sore throat, fatigue) and bleeding (easy bruising, nosebleeds, bleeding gums, melena). Emphasize importance of infection-control and bleeding precautions. Tell patient to take temperature daily.
• Warn patient that alopecia may occur but that it's usually reversible.

Evaluation

• Patient has no evidence of cardiomyopathy (or, if present before dexrazoxane therapy, it doesn't worsen).
• Patient develops no serious complications from drug-induced immunosuppression.
• Patient and family state understanding of drug therapy.

dextran, high-molecular-weight (dextran 70, dextran 75)

(DEKS-tran, high moh-LEH-kyoo-ler wayt)
Dextran 70, Dextran 75, Gentran 70, Gendex 75, Macrodex

Pharmacologic class: glucose polymer
Therapeutic class: plasma volume expander
Pregnancy risk category: C

Indications and dosages

▶ **Plasma expander.** *Adults:* 30 g (500 ml of 6% solution) I.V. In emergencies, may be given at 1.2 to 2.4 g (20 to 40 ml)/minute. In normovolemic or nearly normovolemic patients, rate of infusion shouldn't exceed 240 mg (4 ml)/minute. Total dosage during first 24 hours shouldn't exceed 1.2 g/kg. Actual dosage depends on amount of fluid loss and resulting hemoconcentration and must be determined for each patient.

How supplied

Injection: dextran 70 in normal saline solution or D_5W; 6% dextran 75 in normal saline solution or D_5W

Pharmacokinetics

Absorption: not applicable with I.V. administration.
Distribution: distributed throughout vascular system.
Metabolism: dextran molecules with molecular weights above 50,000 are enzymatically degraded by dextranase to glucose at rate of about 70 to 90 mg/kg/day. This process is variable.

Excretion: dextran molecules with molecular weights below 50,000 are eliminated by renal excretion.

Route	Onset	Peak	Duration
I.V.	Immediate	Immediate	Unknown

Pharmacodynamics

Chemical effect: expands plasma volume by way of colloidal osmotic effect, drawing fluid from interstitial to intravascular space, providing fluid replacement.
Therapeutic effect: expands plasma volume.

Adverse reactions

CV: fluid overload, thrombophlebitis.
EENT: nasal congestion.
GI: nausea, vomiting.
GU: increased specific gravity and viscosity of urine, tubular stasis and blocking, oliguria, anuria.
Hematologic: decreased hemoglobin level and hematocrit; prolonged bleeding time and significant suppression of platelet function with doses of 15 ml/kg.
Hepatic: increased AST and ALT levels.
Musculoskeletal: arthralgia.
Skin: hypersensitivity reactions, urticaria.
Other: fever, ***anaphylaxis.***

Interactions

Drug-drug. *Abciximab, aspirin, heparin, thrombolytics, warfarin:* increased bleeding if given in combination. Use together with extreme caution.

Contraindications and precautions

- Contraindicated in patients hypersensitive to dextran and in those with marked hemostatic defects, marked cardiac decompensation, renal disease with severe oliguria or anuria, hypervolemic conditions, or severe bleeding disorders.
- Breast-feeding women should stop breast-feeding or shouldn't use drug.
- Use cautiously in patients with active hemorrhage, thrombocytopenia, impaired renal clearance, chronic liver disease, or abdominal conditions and in patients undergoing bowel surgery. Also use cautiously in pregnant women.
- Safety of drug hasn't been established in children.

NURSING CONSIDERATIONS

Assessment

- Obtain history of patient's underlying condition and hydration status before therapy, and reassess regularly throughout therapy. Frequently assess vital signs, fluid intake and output, and urine or serum osmolarity levels, as ordered.
- Be alert for adverse reactions.
- Observe patient closely during early phase of infusion, when most anaphylactic reactions occur.
- Watch for circulatory overload and rise in central venous pressure. Plasma expansion is slightly greater than volume infused.
- Check hemoglobin and hematocrit levels, as ordered.
- Evaluate patient's and family's knowledge of drug therapy.

Nursing diagnoses

- Decreased cardiac output related to underlying condition
- Risk for injury related to potential for drug-induced hypersensitivity reaction
- Deficient knowledge related to drug therapy

Planning and implementation

ALERT As ordered, use D_5W instead of normal saline solution because drug is hazardous for patients with heart failure, especially when given in normal saline solution.

- Prescriber may order dextran 1, a dextran adjunct, to protect against drug-induced anaphylaxis. Administer 20 ml of dextran 1 (containing 150 mg/ml) I.V. over 60 seconds 1 to 2 minutes before I.V. infusion of dextran.
- Store drug at constant 77° F (25° C). Dextran may precipitate in storage, but it can be heated to dissolve, if necessary.
- If oliguria or anuria occurs or isn't relieved by infusion, stop dextran and give loop diuretic, as ordered.
- If hematocrit values fall below 30% by volume, notify prescriber.

• Drug may interfere with analyses of blood grouping, crossmatching, and bilirubin, blood glucose, and protein levels.

Patient teaching
• Inform patient, if alert, and family about dextran therapy.
• Instruct patient to notify prescriber if adverse reactions occur, such as itching.

Evaluation
• Patient's vital signs and urine output return to normal.
• Patient doesn't develop hypersensitivity reaction to drug.
• Patient and family state understanding of drug therapy.

dextran, low-molecular-weight (dextran 40)

(DEKS-tran, loh moh-LEH-kyoo-ler wayt)
Dextran 40, Gentran 40, 10% LMD, Rheomacrodex

Pharmacologic class: glucose polymer
Therapeutic class: plasma volume expander
Pregnancy risk category: C

Indications and dosages

▶ **Plasma volume expansion.** *Adults:* dosage by I.V. infusion depends on amount of fluid loss. Initially, 10 ml/kg of dextran infused rapidly with central venous pressure monitoring; remainder of dose administered slowly. Total dosage not to exceed 20 ml/kg in the first 24 hours. If therapy is continued longer than 24 hours, don't exceed 10 ml/kg daily. Continued for no longer than 5 days.
▶ **Prevention of venous thrombosis.** *Adults:* 10 ml/kg (500 to 1,000 ml) I.V. on day of procedure; 500 ml on days 2 and 3.
▶ **Hemodiluent in extracorporeal circulation.** *Adults:* 10 to 20 ml/kg added to perfusion circuit. Total dosage not to exceed 20 ml/kg.

How supplied

Injection: 10% dextran 40 in D_5W or normal saline solution

Pharmacokinetics

Absorption: not applicable with I.V. administration.
Distribution: distributed throughout vascular system.
Metabolism: dextran molecules with molecular weights above 50,000 are enzymatically degraded by dextranase to glucose at a rate of about 70 to 90 mg/kg/day. This is a variable process.
Excretion: drug molecules with molecular weights below 50,000 are excreted by kidneys.

Route	Onset	Peak	Duration
I.V.	Immediate	Immediate	≤ 3 hr

Pharmacodynamics

Chemical effect: expands plasma volume by way of colloidal osmotic effect, drawing fluid from interstitial to intravascular space, providing fluid replacement.
Therapeutic effect: expands plasma volume.

Adverse reactions

CV: thrombophlebitis.
GI: nausea, vomiting.
GU: tubular stasis and blocking, increased urine viscosity.
Hematologic: *decreased hemoglobin and hematocrit levels,* increased bleeding time.
Hepatic: increased AST and ALT levels.
Skin: ***hypersensitivity reactions,*** urticaria.
Other: ***anaphylaxis***.

Interactions

None significant.

Contraindications and precautions

• Contraindicated in patients hypersensitive to drug and in those with marked hemostatic defects, marked cardiac decompensation, and renal disease with severe oliguria or anuria.
• Breast-feeding women should stop breast-feeding or shouldn't use drug.
• Use cautiously in patients with active hemorrhage, thrombocytopenia, or diabetes mellitus. Also use cautiously in pregnant women.

• Safety of drug hasn't been established in children.

NURSING CONSIDERATIONS

Assessment
• Obtain history of patient's underlying condition and hydration status before therapy, and reassess regularly throughout therapy. Frequently assess vital signs, fluid intake and output, and urine or serum osmolarity levels, as ordered.
• Be alert for adverse reactions.
• Observe patient closely during early phase of infusion, when most anaphylactic reactions occur.
• Watch for circulatory overload and rise in central venous pressure. Plasma expansion is slightly greater than volume infused.
• Check hemoglobin and hematocrit levels, as ordered.
• Evaluate patient's and family's knowledge of drug therapy.

Nursing diagnoses
• Decreased cardiac output related to underlying condition
• Risk for injury related to potential for drug-induced hypersensitivity reaction
• Deficient knowledge related to drug therapy

Planning and implementation
ALERT As ordered, use D_5W solution instead of normal saline solution because drug is hazardous for patients with heart failure, especially when given in normal saline solution.
• Prescriber may order dextran 1, a dextran adjunct, to protect against drug-induced anaphylaxis. Administer 20 ml of dextran 1 (containing 150 mg/ml) I.V. over 60 seconds 1 to 2 minutes before I.V. infusion of dextran.
• Store at constant 77° F (25° C). Dextran may precipitate in storage, but it can be heated to dissolve, if necessary.
• If oliguria or anuria occurs or isn't relieved by infusion, stop dextran and give loop diuretic, as ordered.
• If hematocrit values fall below 30% by volume, notify prescriber.
• Drug may interfere with analyses of blood grouping, crossmatching, and bilirubin, blood glucose, and protein levels.

Patient teaching
• Inform patient, if alert, and family about dextran therapy.
• Instruct patient to notify prescriber if adverse reactions, such as itching, occur.

Evaluation
• Patient's vital signs and urine output return to normal.
• Patient has no hypersensitivity reaction to drug.
• Patient and family state understanding of drug therapy.

dextroamphetamine sulfate
(deks-troh-am-FET-uh-meen SUL-fayt)
Dexedrine* **, Dexedrine Spansule, Dextrosts**, Ferndex, Oxydess II, Spancap #1

Pharmacologic class: amphetamine
Therapeutic class: CNS stimulant, sympathomimetic amine
Controlled substance schedule: II
Pregnancy risk category: C

Indications and dosages

▶ **Narcolepsy.** *Adults:* 5 to 60 mg P.O. daily in divided doses.
Children age 12 and older: 10 mg P.O. daily, increased by 10-mg increments weekly until desired response occurs or adult dose is reached.
Children ages 6 to 12: 5 mg P.O. daily, increased by 5-mg increments weekly until desired response occurs. Give first dose on awakening, additional doses (one or two) at intervals of 4 to 6 hours.
▶ **Attention deficit hyperactivity disorder.** *Children age 6 and older:* 5 mg P.O. once daily or b.i.d., increased by 5-mg increments weekly, p.r.n.
Children ages 3 to 5: 2.5 mg P.O. daily, increased by 2.5-mg increments weekly, p.r.n.

Only in rare cases is it necessary to exceed 40 mg/day.

How supplied

Tablets: 5 mg, 10 mg
Capsules (sustained-release): 5 mg, 10 mg, 15 mg
Elixir: 5 mg/5 ml

Pharmacokinetics

Absorption: rapidly absorbed from GI tract; longer-acting capsules are absorbed more slowly.
Distribution: distributed widely throughout body.
Metabolism: unknown.
Excretion: excreted in urine. *Half-life:* 10 to 12 hours.

Route	Onset	Peak	Duration
P.O.	Unknown	Unknown	Unknown

Pharmacodynamics

Chemical effect: unknown; probably promotes nerve impulse transmission by releasing stored norepinephrine from nerve terminals in brain. Main sites of activity appear to be the cerebral cortex and reticular activating system. In children with hyperkinesis, amphetamines have paradoxical calming effect.
Therapeutic effect: helps prevent sleep and calms hyperactive children.

Adverse reactions

CNS: *restlessness,* tremors, *insomnia,* dizziness, headache, overstimulation, dysphoria.
CV: *tachycardia, palpitations,* hypertension, ***arrhythmias.***
GI: dry mouth, unpleasant taste, diarrhea, constipation, anorexia, weight loss, and other GI disturbances.
GU: impotence.
Skin: urticaria.
Other: altered libido, chills.

Interactions

Drug-drug. *Acetazolamide, alkalizing agents, antacids, sodium bicarbonate:* increased renal reabsorption. Monitor patient for enhanced amphetamine effects.
Acidifying agents, ammonium chloride, ascorbic acid: decreased blood levels and increased renal clearance of dextroamphetamine. Monitor patient for decreased amphetamine effects.
Adrenergic blockers: adrenergic blockers inhibited by amphetamines. Avoid concomitant use.
Antihistamines: amphetamines may counteract sedative effects of antihistamines. Monitor patient for loss of therapeutic effects.
Chlorpromazine: inhibits central stimulant effects of amphetamines; may be used to treat amphetamine poisoning. Monitor patient closely.
Haloperidol, phenothiazines, tricyclic antidepressants: decreased amphetamine effect. Increased dose may be needed.
Insulin, oral antidiabetics: may decrease antidiabetic requirement. Monitor blood glucose levels.
Lithium carbonate: may inhibit antiobesity and stimulating effects of amphetamines. Monitor patient closely.
MAO inhibitors: severe hypertension; possibly hypertensive crisis. Don't use together or within 14 days after MAO inhibitor.
Meperidine: amphetamines potentiate analgesic effect. Use together cautiously.
Methenamine: increased urinary excretion and reduced efficacy of amphetamines. Monitor effects.
Norepinephrine: amphetamines enhance adrenergic effect of norepinephrine. Monitor patient closely.
Phenobarbital, phenytoin: amphetamines may delay absorption. Monitor patient closely.
Propoxyphene: in cases of propoxyphene overdose, amphetamine CNS stimulation is potentiated and fatal seizures can occur. Avoid concominant use.
Drug-food. *Caffeine:* may increase amphetamine and related amine effects. Monitor patient closely.

Contraindications and precautions

- Contraindicated in patients hypersensitive to sympathomimetic amines, patients with idiosyncratic reactions to them, patients who took an MAO inhibitor within 14 days, and patients with hyperthyroidism, moderate to severe hypertension, symptomatic CV disease, glauco-

ma, advanced arteriosclerosis, or a history of drug abuse.
- Use cautiously in patients with motor and phonic tics, Tourette syndrome, and agitated states. Also use cautiously in pregnant women.
- Safety of drug hasn't been established in breast-feeding women.

NURSING CONSIDERATIONS

Assessment
- Obtain history of patient's underlying condition before therapy, and reassess regularly throughout therapy.
- Be alert for adverse reactions and drug interactions.
- Monitor sleeping pattern, and observe patient for signs of excessive stimulation.
- Evaluate patient's and family's knowledge of drug therapy.

Nursing diagnoses
- Ineffective health maintenance related to underlying condition
- Disturbed sleep pattern related to drug-induced insomnia
- Deficient knowledge related to drug therapy

Planning and implementation
- Give at least 6 hours before bedtime to avoid sleep interference.
- Prolonged administration may cause psychological dependence or habituation, especially in patients with history of drug addiction. After prolonged use, reduce dosage gradually to prevent acute rebound depression, as ordered.

Patient teaching
- Warn patient to avoid hazardous activities until CNS effects of drug are known.
- Tell patient to avoid drinks containing caffeine, which increases effects of amphetamines and related amines.
- Inform patient that fatigue may result as drug effects wear off. He'll need more rest.
- Instruct patient to report signs of excessive stimulation.
- Inform patient that when tolerance to anorexigenic effect develops, dosage shouldn't be increased, but drug discontinued. Tell him to report decreased effectiveness of drug. Warn patient against stopping drug abruptly.

Evaluation
- Patient shows improvement in underlying condition.
- Patient can sleep without difficulty.
- Patient and family state understanding of drug therapy.

dextromethorphan hydrobromide
(deks-troh-meth-OR-fan high-droh-BROH-mighd)

Balminil D.M.†♦, Benylin DM†, Broncho-Grippol-DM♦, Children's Hold†, Hold†, Koffex♦, Pertussin Cough Suppressant†, Pertussin CS†, Pertussin ES*†, Robitussin Pediatric†, St. Joseph Cough Suppressant for Children†, Sucrets Cough Control Formula†, Trocal†, Vicks Formula 44 Pediatric Formula†

More commonly available in combination products such as: Anti-Tuss DM Expectorant†, Cheracol D Cough†, Extra Action Cough†, Glycotuss dm†, Guiamid D.M. Liquid†, Guiatuss-DM†, Halotussin-DM Expectorant†, Kolephrin GG/DM†, Mytussin DM†, Naldecon Senior DX†, Pertussin All-Night CS†, Rhinosyn-DMX Expectorant†, Robitussin-DM†, Silexin Cough†, Tolu-Sed DM†, Tuss-DM†, Unproco†, Vicks Children's Cough Syrup†, Vicks DayQuil Liqicaps†

Pharmacologic class: levorphanol derivative (dextrorotatory methyl ether)
Therapeutic class: antitussive (nonnarcotic)
Pregnancy risk category: C

Indications and dosages

▶ **Nonproductive cough.** *Adults and children age 12 and over:* 10 to 20 mg P.O. q 4 hours, or 30 mg q 6 to 8 hours. Or, 60 mg extended-release liquid b.i.d. Maximum, 120 mg daily. *Children ages 6 to 12:* 5 to 10 mg P.O. q 4 hours, or 15 mg q 6 to 8 hours. Or, 30 mg extended-release liquid b.i.d. Maximum, 60 mg daily.

Children ages 2 to 6: 2.5 to 5 mg P.O. q 4 hours, or 7.5 mg q 6 to 8 hours. Or, 15 mg extended-release liquid b.i.d. Maximum, 30 mg daily. Dosages for children under age 2 must be individualized.

How supplied

Liquid (extended-release): 30 mg/5 ml†
Lozenges: 2.5 mg, 5 mg†, 7.5 mg†, 15 mg†
Solution: 3.5 mg/5 ml, 5 mg/5 ml*†, 7.5 mg/5 ml*†, 10 mg/5 ml*†, 15 mg/5 ml*†, 10 mg/15 ml* **

Pharmacokinetics

Absorption: absorbed readily from GI tract.
Distribution: unknown.
Metabolism: metabolized extensively by liver.
Excretion: small amount excreted unchanged. Metabolites excreted primarily in urine; about 7% to 10% excreted in feces. *Half-life:* about 11 hours.

Route	Onset	Peak	Duration
P.O.	≤ 30 min	Unknown	3-12 hr

Pharmacodynamics

Chemical effect: suppresses cough reflex by direct action on cough center in medulla.
Therapeutic effect: prevents cough.

Adverse reactions

CNS: drowsiness, dizziness.
GI: nausea, vomiting, stomach pain.

Interactions

Drug-drug. *MAO inhibitors:* risk of hypotension, coma, hyperpyrexia, and death. Avoid concomitant use; don't use within 2 weeks of dextromethorphan hydrobromide.
Selegiline: risk of confusion, coma, hyperpyrexia. Avoid concurrent use.
Drug-herb. *Parsley:* May promote or produce serotonin syndrome. Discourage concomittant use.

Contraindications and precautions

- Contraindicated in patients taking MAO inhibitors or within 2 weeks of stopping an MAO inhibitor.
- Use cautiously in atopic children, sedated or debilitated patients, and patients confined to supine position. Also, use cautiously in patients with aspirin sensitivity and in pregnant women.
- Safety of drug hasn't been established in breast-feeding women.

NURSING CONSIDERATIONS

Assessment

- Obtain history of patient's cough before and after drug administration.
- Be alert for adverse reactions and drug interactions.
- Evaluate patient's and family's knowledge of drug therapy.

Nursing diagnoses

- Fatigue related to presence of nonproductive cough
- Risk for injury related to drug-induced adverse CNS reactions
- Deficient knowledge related to drug therapy

Planning and implementation

- Don't use drug when cough is valuable diagnostic sign or is beneficial (as after thoracic surgery).
- As an antitussive, 15 to 30 mg of dextromethorphan is equivalent to 8 to 15 mg of codeine.
- Use drug with chest percussion and vibration.
- Notify prescriber if cough isn't relieved by drug.

Patient teaching

- Instruct patient to follow directions on medication bottle exactly; stress importance of not taking more drug than directed.
- Tell patient to call prescriber if cough persists more than 7 days.
- Suggest sugarless throat lozenges to decrease throat irritation and resulting cough.
- Advise patient to use humidifier to moisten air and ionizer or air filter to filter dust, smoke, and air pollutants.

Evaluation

- Patient's cough is relieved.
- Patient has no injury as a result of therapy.
- Patient and family state understanding of drug therapy.

dextrose (d-glucose)
(DEKS-trohs)

Pharmacologic class: carbohydrate
Therapeutic class: total parenteral nutrition (TPN) component, caloric agent, fluid volume replacement
Pregnancy risk category: C

Indications and dosages

▶ **Fluid replacement and calorie supplement in patients who can't maintain adequate oral intake or who are restricted from doing so.** *Adults and children:* dosage depends on fluid and calorie requirements. Peripheral I.V. infusion of 2.5%, 5%, or 10% solution or central I.V. infusion of 20% solution is used for minimal fluid needs; 25% solution is used to treat acute hypoglycemia in neonate or older infant; 50% solution is used to treat insulin-induced hypoglycemia; 10%, 20%, 30%, 40%, 50%, 60%, and 70% solutions diluted in admixtures, normally amino acid solutions, for TPN are given through the central vein.

How supplied

Injection: 3-ml ampule (10%); 5-ml ampule (10%); 10 ml (25%); 50 ml (5% and 50% available in vial, ampule, and Bristoject); 70-ml pin-top vial (70% for additive use only); 100 ml (5%); 250 ml (5%, 10%); 500 ml (5%, 10%, 20%, 30%, 40%, 50%, 60%, 70%); 1,000 ml (2.5%, 5%, 10%, 20%, 30%, 40%, 50%, 60%, 70%)

Pharmacokinetics

Absorption: not applicable with I.V. administration.
Distribution: distributed throughout plasma volume.
Metabolism: metabolized to carbon dioxide and water.
Excretion: excess excreted in urine.

Route	Onset	Peak	Duration
I.V.	Immediate	Immediate	Unknown

Pharmacodynamics

Chemical effect: simple water-soluble sugar that minimizes glyconeogenesis and promotes anabolism in patient who can't receive sufficient oral caloric intake.
Therapeutic effect: provides supplemental calories and fluid.

Adverse reactions

CNS: confusion, ***unconsciousness in hyperosmolar hyperglycemic nonketotic syndrome.***
CV: ***pulmonary edema, worsened hypertension, heart failure*** (with fluid overload in susceptible patients), *phlebitis, venous sclerosis.*
GU: glycosuria, osmotic diuresis.
Metabolic: hyperglycemia, hypervolemia, hyperosmolarity (with rapid infusion of concentrated solution or prolonged infusion), hypoglycemia from rebound hyperinsulinemia (rapid termination of long-term infusions).
Skin: sloughing, tissue necrosis with prolonged or concentrated infusions or extravasation, especially with peripheral administration.

Interactions

None significant.

Contraindications and precautions

- Contraindicated in patients in diabetic coma while blood glucose level remains excessively high. Use of concentrated solutions is contraindicated in patients with intracranial or intraspinal hemorrhage, in dehydrated patients with delirium tremens, and in patients with severe dehydration, anuria, hepatic coma, or glucose-galactose malabsorption syndrome.
- Use cautiously in patients with cardiac or pulmonary disease, hypertension, renal insufficiency, urinary obstruction, or hypovolemia.

NURSING CONSIDERATIONS

Assessment

- Obtain history of patient's underlying condition before therapy, and reassess regularly throughout therapy.
- Be alert for adverse reactions.
- Evaluate patient's and family's knowledge of drug therapy.

Nursing diagnoses

- Imbalanced nutrition: less than body requirements related to underlying condition
- Ineffective health maintenance related to drug-induced hyperglycemia
- Deficient knowledge related to drug therapy

Planning and implementation

- Control infusion rate carefully; maximal rate is 0.5 g/kg/hour. Use infusion pump when infusing with amino acids for TPN. Never infuse concentrated solutions rapidly; this may cause hyperglycemia and fluid shift.
- Don't give dextrose solutions without saline solution in blood transfusions; this may cause clumping of RBCs. Use central veins to infuse dextrose solutions with concentrations greater than 10%.

ALERT Verify percentage before administering. Concentrations aren't interchangeable.

- Take care to prevent extravasation.
- Never stop hypertonic solutions abruptly. If necessary, have $D_{10}W$ available to treat hypoglycemia if rebound hyperinsulinemia occurs.

Patient teaching

- Inform patient of need for dextrose therapy, method by which it will be administered, and adverse reactions that should be reported.

Evaluation

- Patient shows improvement of underlying condition.
- Patient maintains normal blood glucose level throughout therapy.
- Patient and family state understanding of drug therapy.

diazepam

(digh-AZ-uh-pam)

Diastat, Apo-Diazepam♦, Diazemuls♦ ◇, Diazepam Intensol, Novo-Dipam♦, PMS-Diazepam♦, Valium, Vivol♦

Pharmacologic class: benzodiazepine
Therapeutic class: antianxiety, skeletal muscle relaxant, anticonvulsant, sedative-hypnotic agent
Controlled substance schedule: IV
Pregnancy risk category: D

Indications and dosages

▶ **Anxiety.** *Adults:* depending on severity, 2 to 10 mg P.O. b.i.d. to q.i.d. Or, 2 to 10 mg I.M. or I.V. q 3 to 4 hours, if needed.
Elderly patients: 2 to 2.5 mg P.O. once or twice daily, increased gradually as needed.
Children age 6 months and older: 1 to 2.5 mg P.O. t.i.d or q.i.d., increased gradually as needed and tolerated.

▶ **Acute alcohol withdrawal.** *Adults:* 10 mg P.O. t.i.d. or q.i.d. for the first 24 hours, reduced to 5 mg P.O. t.i.d. or q.i.d., p.r.n. Or, initially, 10 mg I.M. or I.V.; then 5 to 10 mg I.M. or I.V. in 3 to 4 hours, if necessary.

▶ **Before endoscopic procedures.** *Adults:* I.V. dose titrated to desired sedative response (up to 20 mg). Or, 5 to 10 mg I.M. 30 minutes before procedure.

▶ **Muscle spasm.** *Adults:* 2 to 10 mg P.O. b.i.d. to q.i.d. daily. Or, 5 to 10 mg I.M. or I.V. initially; then 5 to 10 mg I.M. or I.V. in 3 to 4 hours, p.r.n. For tetanus, larger doses may be required.
Elderly patients: 2 to 2.5 mg I.M. or I.V. once or twice daily, increased as needed.
Children age 5 and older: 5 to 10 mg I.M. or I.V. q 3 to 4 hours, p.r.n.
Infants over age 30 days to children age 5 years: 1 to 2 mg I.M. or I.V. slowly repeated q 3 to 4 hours, p.r.n.

▶ **Preoperative sedation.** *Adults:* 10 mg I.M. (preferred) or I.V. before surgery.

▶ **Cardioversion.** *Adults:* 5 to 15 mg I.V. 5 to 10 minutes before procedure.

▶ **Adjunct in seizure disorders.** *Adults:* 2 to 10 mg P.O. b.i.d. to q.i.d.
Elderly patients: 2 to 2.5 mg P.O. once or twice daily, increased as needed.
Children age 6 months and older: 1 to 2.5 mg P.O. t.i.d. or q.i.d initially; increased as tolerated and needed.

▶ **Status epilepticus.** *Adults:* 5 to 10 mg I.V. (preferred) or I.M. initially. Repeated q 10 to 15 minutes, p.r.n., up to maximum dose of 30 mg. Repeated in 2 to 4 hours, p.r.n.

Children age 5 and older: 1 mg I.V. q 2 to 5 minutes up to maximum of 10 mg. Repeated in 2 to 4 hours, p.r.n.
Children over age 30 days to 5 years: 0.2 to 0.5 mg I.V. slowly q 2 to 5 minutes up to maximum of 5 mg. Repeated in 2 to 4 hours, p.r.n.
▶ **Control of acute repetitive seizure activity in patients already taking anticonvulsants.** *Adults and children age 12 and older:* 0.2 mg/kg P.R. using applicator. A second dose may be given 4 to 12 hours after the first dose, if needed.
Children ages 6 to 11: 0.3 mg/kg P.R. using applicator. A second dose may be given 4 to 12 hours after the first dose, if needed.
Children ages 2 to 5: 0.5 mg/kg P.R. using applicator. A second dose may be given 4 to 12 hours after the first dose, if needed.

How supplied

Tablets: 2 mg, 5 mg, 10 mg
Oral solution: 5 mg/ml, 5 mg/5 ml
Injection: 5 mg/ml
Rectal gel: 2.5 mg*, 5 mg*, 10 mg*, 15 mg*, 20 mg*
Sterile emulsion for injection: 5 mg/ml ♦

Pharmacokinetics

Absorption: when administered P.O., absorbed through GI tract. Administration by I.M. route results in erratic absorption.
Distribution: distributed widely throughout body; about 85% to 95% bound to plasma protein.
Metabolism: metabolized in liver to active metabolite, desmethyldiazepam.
Excretion: most metabolites of diazepam excreted in urine, with only small amount excreted in feces. *Half-life:* 30 to 200 hours.

Route	Onset	Peak	Duration
P.O.	30 min	0.5-2 hr	3-8 hr
I.V.	1-5 min	≤ 15 min	15-60 min
I.M.	Unknown	2 hr	Unknown
P.R.	Unknown	1-5 hr	Unknown

Pharmacodynamics

Chemical effect: unknown; probably depresses CNS at limbic and subcortical levels of brain; suppresses spread of seizure activity produced by epileptogenic foci in cortex, thalamus, and limbic structures.
Therapeutic effect: relieves anxiety, muscle spasms, and seizures (parenteral form); promotes calmness and sleep.

Adverse reactions

CNS: *drowsiness, lethargy, hangover, ataxia,* fainting, depression, restlessness, anterograde amnesia, psychosis, slurred speech, tremors, headache, insomnia.
CV: transient hypotension, ***bradycardia, CV collapse.***
EENT: diplopia, blurred vision, nystagmus.
GI: nausea, vomiting, abdominal discomfort, constipation.
GU: incontinence, urine retention.
Respiratory: ***respiratory depression.***
Skin: rash, urticaria, desquamation.
Other: physical or psychological dependence, ***acute withdrawal syndrome*** after sudden discontinuation in physically dependent people, *pain, phlebitis at injection site.*

Interactions

Drug-drug. *Cimetidine:* increased sedation. Monitor patient carefully.
CNS depressants: increased CNS depression. Avoid concomitant use.
Digoxin: may increase serum levels of digoxin, increasing toxicity. Monitor patient closely.
Phenobarbital: increased effects of both drugs. Use together cautiously.
Phenytoin: may increase serum levels of phenytoin. Monitor patient for toxicity.
Rantidine: may decrease absorption. Monitor patient for decreased effect.
Drug-herb. *Kava, sassafras, valerian:* sedative effects may be enhanced. Discourage concomitant use.
Drug-lifestyle. *Alcohol use:* increased CNS depression. Discourage concomitant use.
Smoking: increased benzodiazepine clearance. Monitor patient for lack of drug effect.

Contraindications and precautions

- Contraindicated in children under age 6 months (oral form), in patients hypersensitive to drug, and in those with angle-closure glaucoma, shock, coma, or acute alcohol intoxication (parenteral form).

• Avoid use of drug in pregnant women, especially during the first trimester, and in breast-feeding women.
• Use cautiously in patients with hepatic or renal impairment, depression, or chronic open-angle glaucoma.
• Also use cautiously in elderly and debilitated patients. Dosage should be reduced because these patients may be more susceptible to adverse CNS effects of drug.

NURSING CONSIDERATIONS

Assessment
• Obtain history of patient's underlying condition before therapy, and reassess regularly thereafter.
• Monitor respirations every 5 to 15 minutes and before each repeated I.V. dose.
• Periodically monitor liver, kidney, and hematopoietic function studies in patient receiving repeated or prolonged therapy, as ordered.
• Be alert for adverse reactions and drug interactions.
• Evaluate patient's and family's knowledge of drug therapy.

Nursing diagnoses
• Ineffective health maintenance related to underlying condition
• Risk for injury related to drug-induced adverse CNS reactions
• Deficient knowledge related to drug therapy

Planning and implementation
P.O. use: When oral concentrate solution is used, dilute dose just before administering. Use water, juice, or carbonated beverages, or mix with semisolid food such as applesauce or pudding.
P.R. use: Avoid P.R. use of Diastat for more than 5 episodes per month or one episode every 5 days.
ALERT Diastat rectal gel should be given only by caregivers who can distinguish the distinct cluster of seizures or events from the patient's ordinary seizure activity, who have been instructed and can administer the treatment competently, who understand which seizure characteristics may or may not be treated with Diastat, and who can monitor the clinical response and recognize when immediate professional medical evaluation is needed.
I.V. use: Give drug at no more than 5 mg/minute. When injecting, administer directly into vein. If this is impossible, inject slowly through infusion tubing as near to venous insertion site as possible. Watch daily for phlebitis at injection site.
– Avoid extravasation. Don't inject into small veins.
– Have emergency resuscitation equipment and oxygen at bedside when administering drug I.V.
I.M. use: I.M. administration isn't recommended because absorption is variable and injection is painful. Used only when I.V. route and P.O. route are not applicable.
• Don't mix injectable form with other drugs because diazepam is incompatible with most drugs.
• Don't store parenteral solution in plastic syringes.
• Parenteral emulsion—a stabilized oil-in-water emulsion—should appear milky white and uniform. Avoid mixing with any other drugs or solutions, and avoid infusion sets or containers made from polyvinyl chloride. If dilution is necessary, drug may be mixed with I.V. fat emulsion. Use admixture within 6 hours.
• Possibility of abuse and addiction exists. Don't withdraw drug abruptly after long-term use; withdrawal symptoms may occur.
• Institute safety measures.

Patient teaching
• Warn patient to avoid hazardous activities until CNS effects of drug are known.
• Tell patient to avoid alcohol during drug therapy.
• Warn patient to take drug only as directed and not to discontinue it without prescriber's approval.
• Warn patient about risk of physical and psychological dependence.

Evaluation
• Patient shows improvement in underlying condition.

• Patient has no injury as result of drug-induced adverse CNS reactions.
• Patient and family state understanding of drug therapy.

diazoxide
(digh-uz-OKS-ighd)
Hyperstat IV

Pharmacologic class: peripheral vasodilator
Therapeutic class: antihypertensive
Pregnancy risk category: C

Indications and dosages

▶ **Hypertensive crisis.** *Adults and children:* 1 to 3 mg/kg by I.V. bolus (maximum, 150 mg) q 5 to 15 minutes until adequate response occurs. Repeat at 4- to 24-hour intervals, p.r.n.

How supplied

Injection: 15 mg/ml, 300 mg/20 ml

Pharmacokinetics

Absorption: not applicable with I.V. administration.
Distribution: distributed throughout body; about 90% protein-bound.
Metabolism: metabolized partially in liver.
Excretion: diazoxide and its metabolites excreted slowly by kidneys. *Half-life:* 21 to 36 hours.

Route	Onset	Peak	Duration
I.V.	≤ 1 min	2-5 min	2-12 hr

Pharmacodynamics

Chemical effect: unknown; directly relaxes arteriolar smooth muscle and decreases peripheral vascular resistance.
Therapeutic effect: lowers blood pressure.

Adverse reactions

CNS: *headache,* dizziness, light-headedness, euphoria, ***cerebral ischemia, seizures, paralysis.***
CV: *orthostatic hypotension,* diaphoresis, flushing, warmth, angina, myocardial ischemia, ***arrhythmias,*** ECG changes, ***shock, MI.***
GI: *nausea, vomiting,* abdominal discomfort, dry mouth, constipation, diarrhea.
Hematologic: ***thrombocytopenia.***
Metabolic: *sodium and water retention, hyperglycemia,* hyperuricemia.
Other: inflammation, pain (with extravasation).

Interactions

Drug-drug. *Antihypertensives:* may cause severe hypotension. Use together cautiously.
Hydantoins: may decrease levels of hydantoins, resulting in decreased anticonvulsant action. Monitor patient closely.
Sulfonylureas: may cause hyperglycemia. Monitor serum glucose levels.
Thiazide diuretics: may increase diazoxide effects. Use together cautiously.

Contraindications and precautions

• Contraindicated in patients hypersensitive to drug, other thiazides, or other sulfonamide-derived drugs. Also contraindicated in treatment of compensatory hypertension (as in coarctation of the aorta or arteriovenous shunt).
• Use of drug not recommended in breast-feeding women.
• Use cautiously in pregnant women and patients with impaired cerebral or cardiac function or uremia.

NURSING CONSIDERATIONS

Assessment

• Obtain history of patient's blood pressure before therapy.
• Monitor effectiveness by monitoring blood pressure and ECG continuously during drug administration.
• Weigh patient daily.
• Monitor blood glucose level daily; watch closely for signs of severe hyperglycemia or hyperosmolar nonketotic syndrome.
• Check patient's uric acid levels frequently, as ordered.
• Be alert for adverse reactions and drug interactions.
• Evaluate patient's and family's knowledge of drug therapy.

Nursing diagnoses
- Risk for injury related to presence of hypertension
- Excessive fluid volume related to drug-induced fluid retention
- Deficient knowledge related to drug therapy

Planning and implementation
- Place patient in supine or Trendelenburg position during and for 1 hour after infusion.
- Protect I.V. solutions from light. Darkened I.V. solutions of diazoxide are subpotent and shouldn't be used.
- Take care to avoid extravasation.
- Check patient's standing blood pressure before stopping drug.
- Notify prescriber immediately if severe hypotension develops, and keep norepinephrine available.
- If fluid or sodium retention develops, prescriber may order diuretics.

ALERT Don't confuse diazoxide with diamox.

Patient teaching
- Inform patient that orthostatic hypotension can be minimized by rising slowly and avoiding sudden position changes.
- Instruct patient to remain in supine position for 30 minutes after injection.

Evaluation
- Patient's blood pressure returns to normal.
- Patient maintains normal fluid and electrolyte balance during therapy.
- Patient and family state understanding of drug therapy.

diclofenac potassium
(digh-KLOH-fen-ek poh-TAH-see-um)
Cataflam

diclofenac sodium
Voltaren, Voltaren SR♦, Voltaren-XR

Pharmacologic class: NSAID
Therapeutic class: antiarthritic, anti-inflammatory
Pregnancy risk category: B

Indications and dosages
▶ **Ankylosing spondylitis.** *Adults:* 25 mg P.O. q.i.d. (and h.s., p.r.n.).
▶ **Osteoarthritis (diclofenac sodium).** *Adults:* 50 mg P.O. b.i.d. or t.i.d. Or, 75 mg P.O. b.i.d. Or, 100 mg P.O. a day of extended release.
▶ **Rheumatoid arthritis.** *Adults:* 50 mg P.O. t.i.d. or q.i.d. Or, 75 mg P.O. b.i.d. (diclofenac sodium). Or, 50 to 100 mg P.R. (where available) h.s. as substitute for last P.O. dose of day. Not to exceed 225 mg daily.
▶ **Analgesia and primary dysmenorrhea (diclofenac potassium).** *Adults:* 50 mg P.O. t.i.d. If necessary, 100 mg may be administered for first dose only.

How supplied
diclofenac potassium
Tablets: 50 mg
diclofenac sodium
Tablets (delayed-release/enteric-coated): 25 mg, 50 mg, 75 mg
Tablets (extended-release): 100 mg♦
Suppositories: 50 mg♦, 100 mg♦

Pharmacokinetics
Absorption: after P.O. or P.R. administration, rapidly and almost completely absorbed. Absorption is delayed by food.
Distribution: highly (nearly 100%) protein-bound.
Metabolism: undergoes first-pass metabolism, with 60% of unchanged drug reaching systemic circulation.
Excretion: about 40% to 60% excreted in urine; balance is excreted in bile. *Half-life:* 1.2 to 1.8 hours after P.O. dose.

Route	Onset	Peak	Duration
P.O., P.R.	30 min	Unknown	8 hr
P.O. (enteric-coated)	30 min	2-3 hr	8 hr

Pharmacodynamics
Chemical effect: unknown; produces anti-inflammatory, analgesic, and antipyretic effects, possibly by inhibiting prostaglandin synthesis.

Therapeutic effect: relieves inflammation, pain, and fever.

Adverse reactions

CNS: anxiety, depression, dizziness, drowsiness, insomnia, irritability, myoclonus, migraine, *headache.*
CV: ***heart failure,*** hypertension, edema, fluid retention.
EENT: *tinnitus,* ***laryngeal edema***, swelling of lips and tongue, blurred vision, eye pain, night blindness, epistaxis, reversible hearing loss.
GI: taste disorder, *abdominal pain or cramps, constipation, diarrhea, indigestion, nausea,* abdominal distention, flatulence, peptic ulceration, ***bleeding,*** melena, bloody diarrhea, appetite change, colitis.
GU: azotemia, proteinuria, ***acute renal failure,*** oliguria, interstitial nephritis, papillary necrosis, ***nephrotic syndrome,*** *fluid retention.*
Hepatic: elevated liver enzyme levels, jaundice, ***hepatitis, hepatotoxicity.***
Metabolic: hypoglycemia, hyperglycemia.
Musculoskeletal: back, leg, or joint pain.
Respiratory: asthma.
Skin: rash, pruritus, urticaria, eczema, dermatitis, alopecia, photosensitivity, bullous eruption, ***Stevens-Johnson syndrome***, allergic purpura.
Other: ***anaphylaxis, angioedema.***

Interactions

Drug-drug. *Anticoagulants, including warfarin:* possible increased risk of bleeding. Monitor patient closely.
Aspirin: may increase risk of bleeding. Concomitant use not recommended by manufacturer.
Beta blockers: antihypertensive effect may be blunted. Monitor blood pressure closely.
Cyclosporine, digoxin, lithium, methotrexate: diclofenac may reduce renal clearance of these drugs and increase risk of toxicity. Monitor patient closely.
Diuretics: decreased effectiveness of diuretics. Monitor patient closely.
Insulin, oral antidiabetics: diclofenac may alter antidiabetic requirement. Monitor patient closely.
Potassium-sparing diuretics: enhanced potassium retention and increased serum potassium levels. Monitor patient for hyperkalemia.
Drug-herb. *Dong quai, feverfew, garlic, ginger, horse chestnut, red clover:* possible increased risk of bleeding. Discourage concomitant use.
St. John's wort: increased risk of photosensitivity. Advise patient to avoid unprotected exposure to sunlight.
Drug-lifestyle. *Sun exposure:* may cause photosensitivity reactions. Urge precautions.

Contraindications and precautions

- Contraindicated in patients hypersensitive to drug and in those with hepatic porphyria or a history of asthma, urticaria, or other allergic reactions after taking aspirin or other NSAIDs. Drug isn't recommended for use during late pregnancy or while breast-feeding.
- Use cautiously in patients with history of peptic ulcer disease, hepatic dysfunction, cardiac disease, hypertension, conditions that cause fluid retention, or impaired kidney function.
- Safety of drug hasn't been established in children.

NURSING CONSIDERATIONS

Assessment

- Obtain history of patient's underlying condition before therapy.
- Monitor effectiveness by assessing patient for pain relief.
- Liver function test results may become elevated during therapy. Monitor serum transaminase levels, especially ALT levels, periodically in patients undergoing long-term therapy, as ordered. First serum transaminase measurement should be no later than 8 weeks after therapy starts.
- Be alert for adverse reactions and drug interactions.
- Evaluate patient's and family's knowledge of drug therapy.

Nursing diagnoses

- Acute pain related to underlying condition
- Risk for injury related to drug-induced adverse reactions

• Deficient knowledge related to drug therapy

Planning and implementation

P.O. use: Administer drug with milk or food if GI distress occurs.

– Notify prescriber immediately if patient develops signs of GI bleeding, hepatotoxicity, or other adverse reactions.

P.R. use: Not commercially available in the United States. May be substituted for the last oral dose of the day.

Patient teaching

• Tell patient to take drug with milk or food to minimize GI distress.

• Instruct patient not to crush, break, or chew enteric-coated tablets.

• Teach patient signs and symptoms of GI bleeding, and tell him to contact prescriber immediately if they occur.

• Teach patient signs and symptoms of hepatotoxicity, including nausea, fatigue, lethargy, pruritus, jaundice, right upper quadrant tenderness, and flulike symptoms. Tell him to contact prescriber immediately if these symptoms appear.

• Tell pregnant patient not to take drug during last trimester or while breast-feeding.

Evaluation

• Patient is free from pain.

• Patient has no injury as result of drug-induced adverse reactions.

• Patient and family state understanding of drug therapy.

dicloxacillin sodium

(digh-kloks-uh-SIL-in SOH-dee-um)

Dycill, Dynapen, Pathocil

Pharmacologic class: penicillinase-resistant penicillin

Therapeutic class: antibiotic

Pregnancy risk category: B

Indications and dosages

▶ **Systemic infection with penicillinase-producing staphylococci.** *Adults and children weighing more than 40 kg (88 lb):* 125 to 250 mg P.O. q 6 hours.

Children weighing 40 kg or less: 25 to 50 mg/kg P.O. daily in divided doses q 6 hours.

How supplied

Capsules: 125 mg, 250 mg, 500 mg

Oral suspension: 62.5 mg/5 ml (after reconstitution)

Pharmacokinetics

Absorption: absorbed rapidly but incompletely (35% to 76%) from GI tract; food may decrease rate and extent of absorption.

Distribution: distributed widely in bone, bile, and pleural and synovial fluids. CSF penetration is poor but is enhanced by meningeal inflammation. Drug is 95% to 99% protein-bound.

Metabolism: metabolized only partially.

Excretion: dicloxacillin and metabolites excreted in urine. *Half-life:* 30 to 60 minutes.

Route	Onset	Peak	Duration
P.O.	Unknown	0.5-2 hr	About 6 hr

Pharmacodynamics

Chemical effect: inhibits cell wall synthesis during microorganism multiplication. Bacteria resist penicillins by producing penicillinases—enzymes that convert penicillins to inactive penicilloic acid. Dicloxacillin resists these enzymes.

Therapeutic effect: kills susceptible bacteria. Spectrum of activity includes many strains of penicillinase-producing bacteria. This activity is most important against penicillinase-producing staphylococci; some strains may remain resistant. Dicloxacillin is also active against a few gram-positive aerobic and anaerobic bacilli but has no significant effect on gram-negative bacilli.

Adverse reactions

CNS: neuromuscular irritability, ***seizures,*** lethargy, hallucinations, anxiety, confusion, agitation, depression, dizziness, fatigue.

GI: *nausea,* vomiting, *epigastric distress,* flatulence, *diarrhea,* enterocolitis, ***pseudomem-***

branous colitis, black "hairy" tongue, abdominal pain.
Hematologic: eosinophilia, anemia, ***thrombocytopenia, agranulocytosis, leukopenia,*** hemolytic anemia.
Other: ***hypersensitivity reactions*** (pruritus, urticaria, rash, ***anaphylaxis***), overgrowth of nonsusceptible organisms.

Interactions

Drug-drug. *Oral contraceptives:* contraceptive efficacy may be decreased. Additional form of contraception recommended during penicillin therapy.
Probenecid: increased blood levels of dicloxacillin and other penicillins. Probenecid may be used for this purpose.

Contraindications and precautions

- Contraindicated in patients hypersensitive to drug or other penicillins.
- Use cautiously in patients with other drug allergies, especially to cephalosporins (possible cross-sensitivity), and in those with mononucleosis (high risk of maculopapular rash).
- Also use cautiously in pregnant or breast-feeding women.

NURSING CONSIDERATIONS

Assessment

- Obtain history of patient's infection before therapy, and reassess regularly thereafter.
- Before giving drug, ask patient about any allergic reactions to penicillin. Negative history of penicillin allergy is no guarantee against future allergic reactions.
- Obtain specimen for culture and sensitivity tests before first dose. Therapy may begin pending test results.
- As ordered, periodically assess renal, hepatic, and hematopoietic function in patients receiving long-term therapy.
- Be alert for adverse reactions and drug interactions.
- Monitor patient's hydration status if adverse GI reactions occur.
- Evaluate patient's and family's knowledge of drug therapy.

Nursing diagnoses

- Infection related to presence of susceptible bacteria
- Risk for deficient fluid volume related to drug-induced adverse GI reactions
- Deficient knowledge related to drug therapy

Planning and implementation

- Give drug 1 to 2 hours before or 2 to 3 hours after meals. It may cause GI disturbances. Food may interfere with absorption.
- Give drug at least 1 hour before bacteriostatic antibiotics.
- Notify prescriber if adverse reactions occur, especially rash, because dicloxacillin may need to be discontinued and another antibiotic substituted.

ALERT Don't confuse dicloxacillin with cloxacillin.

Patient teaching

- Tell patient to take entire quantity of medication exactly as prescribed, even after he feels better.
- Tell patient to call prescriber if rash develops.
- Warn patient not to use leftover drug for new illness or share it with others.
- Teach patient that oral contraceptive may be ineffective.

Evaluation

- Patient is free from infection.
- Patient maintains adequate hydration throughout therapy.
- Patient and family state understanding of drug therapy.

dicyclomine hydrochloride

(digh-SIGH-kloh-meen high-droh-KLOR-ighd)
Antispas, Bemote, Bentyl, Bentylol ♦, Byclomine, Dibent, Dilomine, Di-Spaz, Formulex ♦, Lomine ♦, Merbentyl ◇, Or-Tyl, Spasmoban ♦

Pharmacologic class: anticholinergic
Therapeutic class: antimuscarinic, GI antispasmodic
Pregnancy risk category: B

Indications and dosages

▶ **Irritable bowel syndrome and other functional GI disorders.** *Adults:* initially, 20 mg P.O. q.i.d., increased to 40 mg q.i.d. Or, 20 mg I.M. q 4 to 6 hours.
Children age 2 and older: 10 mg P.O. t.i.d. or q.i.d.
Children ages 6 months to 2 years: 5 to 10 mg P.O. t.i.d. or q.i.d.

How supplied

Tablets: 10 mg ◇, 20 mg
Capsules: 10 mg, 20 mg
Syrup: 5 mg/5 ml ◇, 10 mg/5 ml
Injection: 10 mg/ml

Pharmacokinetics

Absorption: about 67% of P.O. dose absorbed from GI tract; unknown after I.M. administration.
Distribution: unknown.
Metabolism: unknown.
Excretion: after P.O. administration, 80% excreted in urine and 10% in feces; unknown after I.M. administration. *Half-life:* initial, 1.8 hours; secondary, 9 to 10 hours.

Route	Onset	Peak	Duration
P.O.	Unknown	1-1.5 hr	Unknown
I.M.	Unknown	Unknown	Unknown

Pharmacodynamics

Chemical effect: unknown; appears to exert nonspecific, nondirect spasmolytic action on smooth muscle. Dicyclomine also possesses local anesthetic properties that may be partly responsible for spasmolysis.
Therapeutic effect: relieves GI spasms.

Adverse reactions

CNS: *headache, dizziness,* insomnia, drowsiness; nervousness, confusion, excitement (in elderly patients).
CV: *palpitations,* tachycardia.
EENT: blurred vision, increased intraocular pressure, mydriasis.
GI: nausea, vomiting, *constipation, dry mouth,* abdominal distention, heartburn, paralytic ileus.
GU: *urinary hesitancy, urine retention,* impotence.
Skin: urticaria, decreased sweating or possibly anhidrosis, other dermal changes.
Other: fever, allergic reactions.

Interactions

Drug-drug. *Amantadine, antihistamines, antiparkinsonians, disopyramide, glutethimide, meperidine, phenothiazines, procainamide, quinidine, tricyclic antidepressants:* additive adverse effects. Avoid concomitant use.
Antacids: decreased absorption of oral anticholinergics. Separate administration times by 2 to 3 hours.
Ketoconazole: anticholinergics may interfere with ketoconazole absorption. Administer at least 2 hours after ketoconazole.

Contraindications and precautions

- Contraindicated in patients hypersensitive to anticholinergices and in those with obstructive uropathy, obstructive disease of GI tract, reflux esophagitis, severe ulcerative colitis, myasthenia gravis, unstable CV status in acute hemorrhage, or glaucoma. Also contraindicated in breast-feeding women and in children under age 6 months.
- Use cautiously in pregnant patients and those with autonomic neuropathy, hyperthyroidism, coronary artery disease, arrhythmias, heart failure, hypertension, hiatal hernia, hepatic or renal disease, prostatic hypertrophy, or ulcerative colitis.

NURSING CONSIDERATIONS

Assessment

- Obtain history of patient's underlying condition before therapy.
- Monitor effectiveness by regularly assessing patient for pain relief and improvement of underlying condition.
- Be alert for adverse reactions and drug interactions.
- Evaluate patient's and family's knowledge of drug therapy.

Nursing diagnoses

- Acute pain related to underlying condition
- Risk for injury related to drug-induced adverse CNS reactions
- Deficient knowledge related to drug therapy

Planning and implementation

ALERT Drug is synthetic tertiary derivative that may have atropine-like adverse reactions. Overdose may cause curare-like effects, such as respiratory paralysis.

P.O. use: Give 30 to 60 minutes before meals and at bedtime. Bedtime dose can be larger; give at least 2 hours after last meal of day.

I.M. use: Follow normal protocol.

- Don't give by S.C. or I.V. route.
- Be prepared to adjust dosage according to patient's needs and response, as ordered. Doses up to 40 mg P.O. q.i.d. have been used in adults, but safety and efficacy for more than 2 weeks haven't been established.

Patient teaching

- Instruct patient to refrain from driving and performing other hazardous activities if he is drowsy or dizzy or has blurred vision.
- Tell him to drink plenty of fluids to help prevent constipation.
- Urge patient to report rash or skin eruption.
- Tell patient to use sugarless gum or hard candy to relieve dry mouth.

Evaluation

- Patient is free from pain.
- Patient doesn't experience injury as a result of drug-induced adverse CNS reactions.
- Patient and family state understanding of drug therapy.

didanosine (ddI)

(digh-DAN-uh-zeen)
Videx

Pharmacologic class: purine analogue
Therapeutic class: antiviral
Pregnancy risk category: B

Indications and dosages

▶ **Treatment of HIV infection when antiretroviral therapy is warranted.** *Adults weighing 60 kg (132 lb) and over:* 200 mg (tablets) P.O. q 12 hours or 400 mg (tablets) P.O. once daily. Or, 250 mg buffered powder q 12 hours.

Adults weighing below 60 kg: 125 mg (one 100-mg tablet and one 25-mg tablet) P.O. q 12 hours or 250 mg P.O. once daily. Or, 167 mg buffered powder q 12 hours.

Children: 120 mg/m^2 P.O. q 12 hours.

How supplied

Tablets (chewable): 25 mg, 50 mg, 100 mg, 150 mg, 200 mg

Powder for oral solution (buffered): 100 mg/packet, 167 mg/packet, 250 mg/packet, 375 mg/packet

Powder for oral solution (pediatric): 10 mg/ml in 2- and 4-g bottles

Pharmacokinetics

Absorption: degrades rapidly in gastric acid. Commercially available preparations contain buffers to raise stomach pH. Bioavailability averages about 33%; tablets may exhibit better bioavailability than buffered powder for oral solution. Food can decrease absorption by 50%.

Distribution: widely distributed; drug penetration into CNS varies, but CSF levels average 46% of concurrent plasma levels.

Metabolism: not fully understood; probably similar to that of endogenous purines.

Excretion: excreted in urine. *Half-life:* 0.8 hours.

Route	Onset	Peak	Duration
P.O.	Unknown	0.5-1 hr	Unknown

Pharmacodynamics

Chemical effect: unknown; appears to inhibit replication of HIV by preventing DNA replication.

Therapeutic effect: inhibits replication of HIV.

Adverse reactions

CNS: *headache,* insomnia, *dizziness,* ***seizures,*** confusion, anxiety, nervousness, hypertonia, abnormal thinking, twitching, depression, asthenia, pain, *peripheral neuropathy.*

CV: hypertension, edema, hyperlipemia, ***heart failure.***

GI: *diarrhea, nausea, vomiting, abdominal pain,* ***pancreatitis,*** dry mouth, dyspepsia, flatulence.

Hematologic: ***thrombocytopenia, leukopenia,*** granulocytosis, anemia.
Hepatic: liver abnormalities, ***hepatic failure.***
Metabolic: increased serum uric acid levels.
Musculoskeletal: myalgia, arthritis, myopathy.
Respiratory: cough, dyspnea, pneumonia.
Skin: rash, pruritus, alopecia.
Other: infection, sarcoma, ***allergic reaction,*** *chills, fever.*

Interactions

Drug-drug. *Antacids containing magnesium or aluminum hydroxides:* enhanced adverse effects of antacid component (including diarrhea or constipation) when administered with didanosine tablets or pediatric suspension. Avoid concomitant use.
Dapsone, ketoconazole, drugs that require gastric acid for adequate absorption: decreased absorption from buffering action. Administer these drugs 2 hours before didanosine.
Fluoroquinolones, tetracyclines: decreased absorption from buffering agents in didanosine tablets or antacids in pediatric suspension. Monitor patient for decreased effectiveness.
Itraconazole: decreased serum levels of itraconazole. Avoid concomitant use.
Drug-food. *Any food:* increased rate of absorption. Give drug on an empty stomach.

Contraindications and precautions

- Contraindicated in patients hypersensitive to drug or its components.
- Use of drug isn't recommended in breast-feeding women.
- Use cautiously in pregnant women, patients with a history of pancreatitis, and patients with peripheral neuropathy, renal or hepatic impairment, or hyperuricemia.

NURSING CONSIDERATIONS

Assessment

- Obtain history of patient's underlying condition before therapy, and reassess regularly thereafter.
- Be alert for adverse reactions and drug interactions.
- Evaluate patient's and family's knowledge of drug therapy.

Nursing diagnoses

- Infection related to presence of HIV infection
- Diarrhea related to drug-induced adverse effect on bowel
- Deficient knowledge related to drug therapy

Planning and implementation

- Administer drug on empty stomach, regardless of dosage form used; administering drug with meals can decrease absorption by 50%.
- Most patients should receive two tablets per dose.
- To administer single-dose packets containing buffered powder for oral solution, pour contents into 4 oz of water. Don't use fruit juice or other beverages that may be acidic. Stir for 2 to 3 minutes until powder dissolves completely. Administer immediately.
- Use care when preparing powder or crushing tablets to avoid excessive dispersal of powder into air.
- Pediatric powder for oral solution must be prepared by pharmacist before dispensing. It must be constituted with Purified Water, USP, and then diluted with antacid (either Mylanta Double Strength Liquid or Maalox TC Suspension) to final concentration of 10 mg/ml. The admixture is stable for 30 days if refrigerated (at 36° to 46° F [2° to 8° C]). Shake solution well before measuring dose.
- Notify prescriber if patient taking powder form develops diarrhea; in early clinical trials, powder for oral solution raised the risk of diarrhea. The manufacturer suggests switching to tablet form if diarrhea is a problem, although no evidence suggests that other forms have a lower risk of diarrhea.

Patient teaching

- Instruct patient to chew tablets thoroughly before swallowing and to drink at least 1 oz of water with each dose because tablets contain buffers that raise stomach pH to levels that prevent degradation of active drug. If tablets are manually crushed, stir them thoroughly in 1 oz of water to disperse particles uniformly; then have patient drink mixture immediately.

• Inform patient on sodium-restricted diet that each two-tablet dose of didanosine contains 529 mg of sodium; each single packet of buffered powder for oral solution contains 1.38 g of sodium.

• Warn patient about adverse CNS reactions and tell patient to take safety precautions.

• Tell patient to notify prescriber if adverse GI reactions occur.

☑ Evaluation

• Patient improves with therapy.

• Patient regains normal bowel pattern.

• Patient and family state understanding of drug therapy.

diflunisal

(digh-FLOO-neh-sol)
Dolobid

Pharmacologic class: NSAID, salicylic acid derivative
Therapeutic class: nonnarcotic analgesic, antipyretic, anti-inflammatory
Pregnancy risk category: C

Indications and dosages

▶ **Mild to moderate pain, osteoarthritis, rheumatoid arthritis.** *Adults:* 500 to 1,000 mg P.O. daily in two divided doses, usually q 12 hours. Maximum, 1,500 mg daily.
Adults over age 65: half the usual adult dose.

How supplied

Tablets: 250 mg, 500 mg

Pharmacokinetics

Absorption: absorbed rapidly and completely by way of GI tract.
Distribution: highly protein-bound.
Metabolism: metabolized in liver.
Excretion: excreted in urine. *Half-life:* 8 to 12 hours.

Route	Onset	Peak	Duration
P.O.	1 hr	2-3 hr	8-12 hr

Pharmacodynamics

Chemical effect: unknown; probably related to inhibition of prostaglandin synthesis.
Therapeutic effect: relieves inflammation and pain; reduces body temperature.

Adverse reactions

CNS: *dizziness,* somnolence, insomnia, *headache,* fatigue.
EENT: *tinnitus,* visual disturbances.
GI: *nausea, dyspepsia, GI pain, diarrhea,* vomiting, constipation, flatulence.
GU: renal impairment, hematuria, ***interstitial nephritis.***
Skin: rash, pruritus, sweating, stomatitis, ***erythema multiforme, Stevens-Johnson syndrome.***
Other: dry mucous membranes.

Interactions

Drug-drug. *Acetaminophen, hydrochlorothiazide, indomethacin:* diflunisal may substantially increase blood levels of these drugs, increasing risk of toxicity. Avoid concomitant use.
Antacids: decreased diflunisal blood levels. Monitor patient for possible decreased therapeutic effect.
Aspirin: increased adverse effects. Monitor patient closely.
Cyclosporine: diflunisal may increase nephrotoxicity of cyclosporine. Avoid concomitant use.
Methotrexate: diflunisal may increase toxicity of methotrexate. Avoid concomitant use.
Oral anticoagulants, thrombolytics: diflunisal may enhance effects of these drugs. Use together cautiously.
Sulindac: diflunisal decreases blood levels of sulindac's active metabolite. Monitor patient for decreased effect.
Drug-herb. *Dong quai, feverfew, garlic, ginger, horse chestnut, red clover:* possible increased risk of bleeding. Discourage concomitant use.

Contraindications and precautions

• Contraindicated in patients hypersensitive to drug and in those who develop acute asthmatic attacks, urticaria, or rhinitis after taking aspirin or other NSAIDs.

• Drug isn't recommended for breast-feeding women.
• Because of epidemiologic connection to Reye's syndrome, Centers for Disease Control and Prevention recommends not giving salicylates to children and teenagers with chickenpox or flulike illness.
• Use cautiously in patients with GI bleeding, history of peptic ulcer disease, renal impairment, compromised cardiac function, hypertension, or other conditions predisposing patient to fluid retention.

NURSING CONSIDERATIONS

Assessment
• Obtain history of patient's underlying condition before therapy, and reassess regularly thereafter.
• Be alert for adverse reactions and drug interactions.
• Evaluate patient's and family's knowledge of drug therapy.

Nursing diagnoses
• Acute pain related to underlying condition
• Risk for deficient fluid volume related to drug-induced adverse reactions
• Deficient knowledge related to drug therapy

Planning and implementation
• Administer drug with milk or food to minimize adverse GI reactions.

Patient teaching
• Advise patient to take with water, milk, or meals.
• Warn patient to check with prescriber or pharmacist before taking OTC medications or herbal remedies to avoid possible interactions with drugs, such as those containing aspirin or salicylates.

Evaluation
• Patient is free from pain.
• Patient maintains adequate hydration throughout therapy.
• Patient and family state understanding of drug therapy.

digoxin
(dih-JOKS-in)
Digoxin, Lanoxicaps, Lanoxin*

Pharmacologic class: cardiac glycoside
Therapeutic class: antiarrhythmic, inotropic
Pregnancy risk category: C

Indications and dosages

▶ Heart failure, atrial fibrillation and flutter, paroxysmal atrial tachycardia
Tablets, elixir
Adults: For rapid digitalization, give 0.75 to 1.25 mg P.O. over 24 hours in two or more divided doses q 6 to 8 hours. For slow digitalization, give 0.125 to 0.5 mg daily for 5 to 7 days. Maintenance dosage is 0.125 to 0.5 mg daily.
Children age 10 and older: 10 to 15 mcg/kg P.O. over 24 hours in two or more divided doses q 6 to 8 hours. Maintenance dosage is 25% to 35% of total digitalizing dose.
Children ages 5 to 10: 20 to 35 mcg/kg P.O. over 24 hours in two or more divided doses q 6 to 8 hours. Maintenance dosage is 25% to 35% of total digitalizing dose.
Children ages 2 to 5: 30 to 40 mcg/kg P.O. over 24 hours in two or more divided doses q 6 to 8 hours. Maintenance dosage is 25% to 35% of total digitalizing dose.
Infants ages 1 month to 2 years: 35 to 60 mcg/kg P.O. over 24 hours in two or more divided doses q 6 to 8 hours. Maintenance dosage is 25% to 35% of total digitalizing dose.
Neonates: 25 to 35 mcg/kg P.O. over 24 hours in two or more divided doses q 6 to 8 hours. Maintenance dosage is 25% to 35% of total digitalizing dose.
Premature infants: 20 to 30 mcg/kg P.O. over 24 hours in two or more divided doses q 6 to 8 hours. Maintenance dosage is 20% to 30% of total digitalizing dose.
Capsules
Adults: For rapid digitalization, give 0.4 to 0.6 mg P.O. initially, followed by 0.1 to 0.3 mg q 6 to 8 hours, as needed and tolerated, for 24 hours. For slow digitalization, give 0.05 to 0.35 mg daily in two divided doses for 7 to 22 days, as needed, until therapeutic serum

levels are reached. Maintenance dosage is 0.05 to 0.35 mg daily in one or two divided doses.

Children: Digitalizing dose is based on child's age and is administered in three or more divided doses over the first 24 hours. Initial dose should be 50% of the total dose; subsequent doses are given q 4 to 8 hours as needed and tolerated.

Children age 10 and older: For rapid digitalization, give 8 to 12 mcg/kg P.O. over 24 hours, divided as above. Maintenance dosage is 25% to 35% of total digitalizing dose, given daily as a single dose.

Children ages 5 to 10: For rapid digitalization, give 15 to 30 mcg/kg P.O. over 24 hours, divided as above. Maintenance dosage is 25% to 35% of total digitalizing dose, divided and given in two or three equal portions daily.

Children ages 2 to 5: For rapid digitalization, give 25 to 35 mcg/kg P.O. over 24 hours, divided as above. Maintenance dosage is 25% to 35% of total digitalizing dose, divided and given in two or three equal portions daily.

Injection

Adults: For rapid digitalization, give 0.4 to 0.6 mg I.V. initially, followed by 0.1 to 0.3 mg I.V. q 4 to 8 hours, as needed and tolerated, for 24 hours. For slow digitalization, give appropriate daily maintenance dosage for 7 to 22 days as needed until therapeutic serum levels are reached. Maintenance dosage is 0.125 to 0.5 mg I.V. daily in one or two divided doses.

Children: Digitalizing dose is based on child's age and is administered in three or more divided doses over the first 24 hours. Initial dose should be 50% of total dose; subsequent doses are given q 4 to 8 hours as needed and tolerated.

Children age 10 and older: For rapid digitalization, give 8 to 12 mcg/kg I.V. over 24 hours, divided as above. Maintenance dosage is 25% to 35% of total digitalizing dose, given daily as a single dose.

Children ages 5 to 10: For rapid digitalization, give 15 to 30 mcg/kg I.V. over 24 hours, divided as above. Maintenance dosage is 25% to 35% of total digitalizing dose, divided and given in two or three equal portions daily.

Children ages 2 to 5: For rapid digitalization, give 25 to 35 mcg/kg I.V. over 24 hours, divided as above. Maintenance dosage is 25% to 35% of total digitalizing dose, divided and given in two or three equal portions daily.

Infants ages 1 month to 2 years: For rapid digitalization, give 30 to 50 mcg/kg I.V. over 24 hours, divided as above. Maintenance dosage is 25% to 35% of total digitalizing dose, divided and given in two or three equal portions daily.

Neonates: For rapid digitalization, give 20 to 30 mcg/kg I.V. over 24 hours, divided as above. Maintenance dosage is 25% to 35% of the total digitalizing dose, divided and given in two or three equal portions daily.

Premature infants: For rapid digitalization, give 15 to 25 mcg/kg I.V. over 24 hours, divided as above. Maintenance dosage is 20% to 30% of the total digitalizing dose, divided and given in two or three equal portions daily.

How supplied

Tablets: 0.125 mg, 0.25 mg, 0.5 mg
Capsules: 0.05 mg, 0.1 mg, 0.2 mg
Elixir: 0.05 mg/ml
Injection: 0.05 mg/ml ♦, 0.1 mg/ml (pediatric), 0.25 mg/ml

Pharmacokinetics

Absorption: with tablet or elixir form, 60% to 85% of dose is absorbed. With capsule form, bioavailability increases, with about 90% to 100% of dose absorbed.

Distribution: distributed widely in body tissues; about 20% to 30% bound to plasma proteins.

Metabolism: small amount of digoxin is thought to be metabolized in liver and gut by bacteria. This metabolism varies and may be substantial in some patients. Drug undergoes some enterohepatic recirculation (also variable). Metabolites have minimal cardiac activity.

Excretion: most of dose excreted by kidneys as unchanged drug, although some patients excrete a substantial amount of metabolized or reduced drug. In patients with renal failure, biliary excretion is more important excretion route. *Half-life:* 30 to 40 hours.

Route	Onset	Peak	Duration
P.O.	0.5-2 hr	2-6 hr	3-4 days
I.V.	5-30 min	1-4 hr	3-4 days

Pharmacodynamics

Chemical effect: inhibits sodium-potassium-activated adenosine triphosphatase, thereby promoting movement of calcium from extracellular to intracellular cytoplasm and strengthening myocardial contraction. Digoxin also acts on CNS to enhance vagal tone, slowing conduction through SA and AV nodes and providing antiarrhythmic effect.
Therapeutic effect: strengthens myocardial contractions and slows conduction through SA and AV nodes.

Adverse reactions

CNS: *fatigue, generalized muscle weakness, agitation, hallucinations,* headache, malaise, dizziness, vertigo, stupor, paresthesia.
CV: ***arrhythmias, heart failure,*** hypotension.
EENT: yellow-green halos around visual images, blurred vision, light flashes, photophobia, diplopia.
GI: *anorexia, nausea,* vomiting, diarrhea.

Interactions

Drug-drug. *Amiloride:* inhibited digoxin effect and increased digoxin excretion. Monitor patient for altered digoxin effect.
Amiodarone, diltiazem, nifedipine, quinidine, verapamil: increased digoxin levels. Monitor patient for toxicity.
Amphotericin B, carbenicillin, corticosteroids, diuretics (including loop diuretics, chlorthalidone, metolazone, and thiazides), ticarcillin: hypokalemia, predisposing patient to digitalis toxicity. Monitor serum potassium levels.
Antacids, kaolin-pectin: decreased digoxin absorption. Schedule doses as far as possible from P.O. digoxin administration.
Cholestyramine, colestipol, metoclopramide: decreased absorption of P.O. digoxin. Monitor patient for decreased effect and low blood levels. Increase dosage, if necessary, as directed.
Parenteral calcium, thiazides: hypercalcemia and hypomagnesemia, predisposing patient to digitalis toxicity. Monitor serum calcium and magnesium levels.
Drug-herb. *Betel palm, fumitory, goldenseal, lily-of-the-valley, motherwort, rue, shepherd's purse:* Possible increased cardiac effect. Discourage concurrent use.
Horse tail, licorice: may deplete potassium stores, leading to digitalis toxicity. Monitor serum potassium level closely.
Oleander, siberian ginseng, squill: Possible enhanced toxicity. Discourage concurrent use.
St. John's wort: may reduce therapeutic effect of digoxin, requiring an increased dosage. Monitor patient for loss of therapeutic effect, and advise patient to avoid this herb.
Drug-lifestyle. *Alcohol use*: increased CNS effects. Discourage concurrent use.

Contraindications and precautions

- Contraindicated in patients hypersensitive to drug and in those with digitalis-induced toxicity, ventricular fibrillation, or ventricular tachycardia unless caused by heart failure.
- Use with extreme caution in elderly patients and in those with acute MI, incomplete AV block, sinus bradycardia, PVCs, chronic constrictive pericarditis, hypertrophic cardiomyopathy, renal insufficiency, severe pulmonary disease, or hypothyroidism. Reduce dosage in patients with renal impairment.
- Use cautiously in pregnant or breast-feeding women.

NURSING CONSIDERATIONS

Assessment

- Obtain history of patient's underlying condition before therapy.
- Monitor effectiveness by taking apical pulse for 1 full minute before each dose. Evaluate ECG when ordered, and regularly assess patient's cardiopulmonary status for signs of improvement.
- Monitor serum digoxin levels. Therapeutic blood levels of digoxin range from 0.5 to 2 ng/ml. Obtain blood for digoxin levels 8 hours after last P.O. dose.
- Monitor serum potassium level carefully.

• Be alert for adverse reactions and drug interactions.
• Evaluate patient's and family's knowledge of drug therapy.

Nursing diagnoses
• Decreased cardiac output related to underlying condition
• Ineffective protection related to digitalis toxicity caused by drug
• Deficient knowledge related to drug therapy

Planning and implementation
• Hypothyroid patients are extremely sensitive to glycosides; hyperthyroid patients may need larger doses. Reduce dosage in patients with impaired renal function.
• Before administering loading dose, obtain baseline data (heart rate and rhythm, blood pressure, and electrolyte levels), and question patient about recent use of cardiac glycosides (within previous 2 to 3 weeks).
• Loading dose is always divided over first 24 hours unless clinical situation indicates otherwise.
• Before giving drug, take apical pulse for 1 full minute. Record and report to prescriber significant changes (sudden increase or decrease in pulse rate, pulse deficit, irregular beats, and regularization of previously irregular rhythm). If these changes occur, check blood pressure and obtain 12-lead ECG.
• Withhold drug and notify prescriber if pulse rate slows to 60 beats/minute or less.
P.O. use: Because absorption of digoxin from parenteral route and from liquid-filled capsules is superior to absorption from tablets or elixir, expect dosage reduction of 20% to 25% when changing from tablets or elixir to liquid-filled capsules or parenteral therapy.
I.V. use: Infuse drug slowly over at least 5 minutes.
• For digitalis toxicity, administer agents that bind drug in intestine (for example, colestipol or cholestyramine). Treat arrhythmias with phenytoin I.V. or lidocaine I.V. and potentially life-threatening toxicity with specific antigen-binding fragments (such as digoxin immune Fab), as ordered.
• Withhold drug for 1 to 2 days before elective cardioversion, as ordered. Adjust dose after cardioversion, as ordered.
ALERT Be careful when calculating doses. Ten-fold errors have been reported in children.

Patient teaching
• Instruct patient and responsible family member about drug action, dosage regimen, pulse taking, reportable signs, and follow-up plans.
• Instruct patient not to substitute one brand of digoxin for another.
• Tell patient to eat potassium-rich foods.

Evaluation
• Patient has adequate cardiac output.
• Patient has no digitalis toxicity.
• Patient and family state understanding of drug therapy.

digoxin immune Fab (ovine)
(dih-JOKS-in ih-MYOON Fab)
Digibind

Pharmacologic class: antibody fragment
Therapeutic class: cardiac glycoside antidote
Pregnancy risk category: C

Indications and dosages
▶ **Potentially life-threatening digoxin or digitoxin intoxication.** *Adults and children:* I.V. dosage varies according to amount of digoxin or digitoxin to be neutralized. Each vial binds about 0.5 mg of digoxin or digitoxin. Average dosage is 6 vials (228 mg). If toxicity resulted from acute digoxin ingestion and neither serum digoxin level nor estimated ingestion amount is known, 20 vials (760 mg) may be required. See package insert for complete, specific dosage instructions.

How supplied
Injection: 38-mg vial

Pharmacokinetics
Absorption: not applicable with I.V. administration.
Distribution: unknown.

Metabolism: unknown.
Excretion: excreted in urine. *Half-life:* 15 to 20 hours.

Route	Onset	Peak	Duration
I.V.	Varies	On completion of I.V. dose	2-6 hr

Pharmacodynamics

Chemical effect: binds molecules of digoxin and digitoxin, making them unavailable for binding at site of action on cells.
Therapeutic effect: reverses digitalis intoxication.

Adverse reactions

CV: ***heart failure,*** rapid ventricular rate.
Metabolic: hypokalemia.
Other: ***hypersensitivity reactions, anaphylaxis.***

Interactions

None reported.

Contraindications and precautions

- No known contraindications.
- Use cautiously in patients allergic to ovine proteins. In these high-risk patients, skin testing is recommended because drug is derived from digoxin-specific antibody fragments obtained from immunized sheep. Also use cautiously in pregnant or breast-feeding women.

NURSING CONSIDERATIONS

Assessment

- Obtain history of patient's digitalis intoxication before therapy.
- Monitor effectiveness by watching for decreased signs and symptoms of digitalis toxicity; in most patients, signs of digitalis toxicity disappear within a few hours.
- Because drug interferes with digitalis immunoassay measurements, standard serum digoxin levels are misleading until drug is cleared from body (about 2 days).
- Be alert for adverse reactions.
- Evaluate patient's and family's knowledge of drug therapy.

Nursing diagnoses

- Ineffective health maintenance related to digitalis intoxication
- Decreased cardiac output related to drug-induced heart failure
- Deficient knowledge related to drug therapy

Planning and implementation

- Refrigerate powder for injection. Reconstitute drug immediately before use. Reconstituted solutions may be refrigerated for 4 hours.
- Reconstitute 38-mg vial with 4 ml of sterile water for injection. Gently roll vial to dissolve powder. Reconstituted solution contains 9.5 mg/ml. Drug may be given by direct injection if cardiac arrest seems imminent. Or, dilute with normal saline solution injection to appropriate volume and give by intermittent infusion.
- Infuse drug through 0.22-micron membrane filter.
- Drug is used only for life-threatening overdose in patients with shock or cardiac arrest; ventricular arrhythmias, such as ventricular tachycardia or fibrillation; progressive bradycardia, such as severe sinus bradycardia; or second- or third-degree AV block not responsive to atropine.
- Administer oxygen, as ordered. Keep resuscitation equipment nearby.

Patient teaching

- Instruct patient to report respiratory difficulty, chest pain, or dizziness immediately.

Evaluation

- Patient exhibits improved health with alleviation of digitalis toxicity.
- Patient demonstrates adequate cardiac output through normal vital signs and urine output and clear mental status.
- Patient and family state understanding of drug therapy.

dihydroergotamine mesylate

(digh-high-droh-er-GAH-tuh-meen MES-ih-layt)

D.H.E. 45, Dihydroergotamine-Sandoz♦, Migranal

Pharmacologic class: ergot alkaloid
Therapeutic class: vasoconstrictor
Pregnancy risk category: X

Indications and dosages

▶ **To prevent or abort vascular or migraine headache.** *Adults:* 1 mg I.M. or I.V. Repeated q 1 to 2 hours, p.r.n., up to total of 2 mg I.V. or 3 mg I.M. per attack. Maximum, 6 mg weekly. For nasal spray, 1 spray into each nostril; repeated in 15 minutes for total of 4 sprays (2 mg). Maximum, 8 sprays (4 mg) weekly.

How supplied

Injection: 1 mg/ml
Intranasal solution: 0.5 mg/metered spray (4 mg/ml)

Pharmacokinetics

Absorption: unknown for S.C. and I.M. administration.
Distribution: 90% plasma protein–bound.
Metabolism: extensively metabolized, probably in liver (extensive first-pass metabolism).
Excretion: 10% excreted in urine as metabolites; rest in feces by biliary elimination.

Route	Onset	Peak	Duration
I.V.	≤ 5 min	≤ 15 min	8 hr
I.M.	15-30 min	≤ 30 min	8 hr
S.C.	Unknown	15-45 min	8 hr
Intranasal	Rapid	0.5-1 hr	Unknown

Pharmacodynamics

Chemical effect: causes peripheral vasoconstriction primarily by stimulating alpha-adrenergic receptors; may abort vascular headaches by direct vasoconstriction of dilated carotid artery bed with decline in amplitude of pulsations.
Therapeutic effect: prevents or relieves vascular or migraine headache.

Adverse reactions

CNS: dizziness.
CV: numbness and tingling in fingers and toes, transient tachycardia or ***bradycardia,*** precordial distress and pain, increased arterial pressure.
EENT: rhinitis, application site reaction, pharyngitis, sinusitis.
GI: taste perversion, dry mouth, *nausea, vomiting.*
GU: uterine contractions.
Musculoskeletal: weakness in legs, muscle pain in limbs, localized edema.
Skin: itching.

Interactions

Drug-drug. *Erythromycin, other macrolides:* may cause symptoms of ergot toxicity. Vasodilators (nitroprusside, nifedipine, or prazosin) may be ordered to treat such an attack. Monitor patient closely.
Nitrates: decreased antianginal effects may occur. Monitor patient.
Propranolol, other beta blockers: blocked natural pathway for vasodilation in patients receiving ergot alkaloids; may result in excessive vasoconstriction and cold limbs. Watch closely if drugs are used together.
Drug-lifestyle. *Smoking:* nicotine may promote vasoconstriction, predisposing patient to a greater ischemic response. Discourage concomitant use.

Contraindications and precautions

- Contraindicated in pregnant or breast-feeding patients, patients hypersensitive to drug, and patients with peripheral and occlusive vascular disease, coronary artery disease, uncontrolled hypertension, severe hepatic or renal dysfunction, or sepsis.
- Don't use drug in patients with hemiplegic or basilar migraines.
- Safety of drug hasn't been established in children.

NURSING CONSIDERATIONS

Assessment

- Obtain history of patient's vascular or migraine headache before therapy, and reassess regularly thereafter.

• Be alert for adverse reactions and drug interactions.
• Be alert for ergotamine rebound or increase in frequency and duration of headache, which may occur when drug is stopped.
• Evaluate patient's and family's knowledge of drug therapy.

Nursing diagnoses

• Acute pain related to vascular or migraine headache
• Disturbed sensory perception (tactile) related to drug-induced adverse reactions
• Deficient knowledge related to drug therapy

Planning and implementation

• Drug is most effective when used at first sign of migraine or soon after onset.
I.V. use: Directly inject solution into vein over 3 minutes. Continuous or intermittent infusion isn't recommended.
I.M. and S.C. use: Follow normal protocol.
Intranasal use: Pump spray four times before using to prepare unit for administration. Discard spray ampule 8 hours after opening.
• Don't give drug within 24 hours of a 5-HT agonist (sumatriptan), ergotamine-containing or ergot-type medication, or methysergide.
• Avoid prolonged administration; don't exceed recommended dosage, as ordered. Adjust to minimum effective dosage, as ordered, for best results.
• Protect ampules from heat and light. Discard if solution is discolored.
• Protect limbs, fingers, and toes from injury if tactile adverse reactions occur.

Patient teaching

• Tell patient not to tilt head back when using intranasal spray and not to sniff while spraying drug.
• Instruct patient to lie down and relax in quiet, low-light environment after taking drug.
• Tell patient to report coldness in limbs or tingling in fingers and toes. Severe vasoconstriction may result in tissue damage. Keep limbs warm and administer vasodilators, as ordered.
• Help patient to evaluate underlying causes of stress, which may precipitate attacks.

Evaluation

• Patient's pain is relieved.
• Patient has no injury as result of drug-induced adverse tactile reactions.
• Patient and family state understanding of drug therapy.

dihydrotachysterol

(digh-high-droh-tak-ES-ster-ol)
DHT, DHT Intensol*, Hytakerol

Pharmacologic class: vitamin D analogue
Therapeutic class: antihypocalcemic
Pregnancy risk category: C

Indications and dosages

▶ **Hypocalcemia related to hypoparathyroidism and pseudohypoparathyroidism.** *Adults:* initially, 0.75 to 2.5 mg P.O. daily for several days. Maintenance, 0.2 to 1 mg daily. *Children:* initially, 1 to 5 mg P.O. for 4 days. Dosage is then continued or reduced to one-fourth the initial amount. Maintenance, 0.5 to 1.5 mg daily.
▶ **Prevention of hypocalcemic tetany after thyroid surgery.** *Adults:* 0.25 mg P.O. daily (with calcium supplements).

How supplied

Tablets: 0.125 mg, 0.2 mg, 0.4 mg
Capsules: 0.125 mg
Oral solution: 0.2 mg/5 ml, 0.2 mg/ml* (DHT Intensol*), 0.25 mg/ml (in sesame oil)
Note: 1 mg of dihydrotachysterol is equal to 120,000 units of ergocalciferol (vitamin D_2).

Pharmacokinetics

Absorption: absorbed readily from small intestine.
Distribution: distributed widely; largely protein-bound.
Metabolism: metabolized in liver.
Excretion: excreted in urine and bile.

Route	Onset	Peak	Duration
P.O.	Several hr	1-2 wk	< 9 wk

Pharmacodynamics

Chemical effect: stimulates calcium absorption from GI tract and promotes secretion of calcium from bone to blood.
Therapeutic effect: raises blood calcium level.

Adverse reactions

CNS: headache, somnolence, vertigo, irritability.
CV: hypertension, ***arrhythmias.***
EENT: conjunctivitis, photophobia, rhinorrhea, tinnitus.
GI: nausea, vomiting, constipation, metallic taste, dry mouth, thirst, anorexia, diarrhea, ***pancreatitis.***
GU: nephrocalcinosis, polyuria, nocturia.
Metabolic: weight loss.
Musculoskeletal: weakness, bone and muscle pain.
Other: decreased libido, hyperthermia.

Interactions

Drug-drug. *Cholestyramine, colestipol, excessive use of mineral oil:* decreased absorption of orally administered vitamin D analogues. Avoid concomitant use.
Corticosteroids: counteract vitamin D analogue effects. Don't use together.
Cardiac glycosides: increased risk of arrhythmias. Avoid concomitant use.
Magnesium-containing antacids: possibly hypermagnesemia, especially in patients with chronic renal failure. Monitor patient.
Other vitamin D analogues: increased toxicity. Avoid concomitant use.
Thiazide diuretics: may cause hypercalcemia. Monitor patient for muscle twitching and weakness.

Contraindications and precautions

- Contraindicated in patients with hypercalcemia or vitamin D toxicity.
- Drug isn't recommended for breast-feeding women.
- Use cautiously in pregnant women.

NURSING CONSIDERATIONS

Assessment

- Obtain history of patient's blood calcium level before therapy.
- Monitor effectiveness by checking serum and urine calcium levels, as ordered; serum calcium level multiplied by serum phosphate level shouldn't exceed 70. During dosage adjustment, determine serum calcium level twice weekly.
- Be alert for adverse reactions and drug interactions.
- Evaluate patient's and family's knowledge of drug therapy.

Nursing diagnoses

- Ineffective health maintenance related to hypocalcemia
- Ineffective protection related to potential for vitamin D intoxication caused by drug therapy
- Deficient knowledge related to drug therapy

Planning and implementation

- Optimal dosage is highly individualized.
- Store in tightly closed, light-resistant container. Don't refrigerate.
- Discontinue if hypercalcemia occurs, and notify prescriber. Drug can be resumed after serum calcium level returns to normal.
- Make sure patient is consuming adequate daily calcium (1,000 mg).

Patient teaching

- Advise patient to adhere to diet and calcium supplementation and to avoid OTC drugs (especially those containing magnesium).
- Teach patient the signs and symptoms of hypercalcemia, and instruct him to report them if they occur.
- Tell patient how to store drug properly.

Evaluation

- Patient's serum and urine calcium levels are within normal range.
- Patient has no drug-induced adverse reactions.
- Patient and family state understanding of drug therapy.

diltiazem hydrochloride

(dil-TIGH-uh-zem high-droh-KLOR-ighd)

Cardizem, Cardizem CD, Cardizem SR, Dilacor XR, Tiamate, Tiazac

Pharmacologic class: calcium channel blocker
Therapeutic class: antianginal
Pregnancy risk category: C

Indications and dosages

▶ **Vasospastic angina (Prinzmetal's [variant] angina), classic chronic stable angina pectoris.** *Adults:* 30 mg P.O. t.i.d. or q.i.d. before meals and h.s. Dosage increased gradually to maximum of 360 mg/day in divided doses.Or, 120 to 180 mg (extended-release) P.O. once daily. Dosage may be adjusted up to 480 mg once daily, if necessary.

▶ **Hypertension.** *Adults:* 60 to 120 mg P.O. b.i.d. (sustained-release capsule). Adjusted to effect. Maximum recommended dosage is 360 mg/day. Or, 180 to 240 mg/day (extended-release capsule) initially. Dosage adjusted as necessary.

▶ **Atrial fibrillation or flutter; paroxysmal supraventricular tachycardia.** *Adults:* 0.25 mg/kg as I.V. bolus injection over 2 minutes. If response is inadequate, 0.35 mg/kg I.V. after 15 minutes, followed with continuous infusion of 10 mg/hour. May be increased in increments of 5 mg/hour. Maximum, 15 mg/hour.

How supplied

Tablets: 30 mg, 60 mg, 90 mg, 120 mg
Capsules (extended-release [Cardizem CD, Dilacor XR, Tiazac]): 120 mg, 180 mg, 240 mg, 300 mg (Cardizem CD only), 360 mg (Tiazac only)
Capsules (sustained-release [Cardizem SR]): 60 mg, 90 mg, 120 mg
Injection: 5 mg/ml

Pharmacokinetics

Absorption: about 80% of dose is absorbed rapidly from GI tract. Only about 40% of drug enters systemic circulation because of significant first-pass effect in liver.
Distribution: about 70% to 85% of circulating diltiazem is bound to plasma proteins.
Metabolism: metabolized in liver.
Excretion: about 35% excreted in urine and about 65% in bile as unchanged drug and inactive and active metabolites. *Half-life:* 3 to 9 hours.

Route	Onset	Peak	Duration
P.O.	0.5-3 hr	2-14 hr	6-24 hr
I.V.	3 min	Immediate	1-3 hr (bolus); < 10 hr (infusion)

Pharmacodynamics

Chemical effect: inhibits calcium ion influx across cardiac and smooth-muscle cells, decreasing myocardial contractility and oxygen demand; also dilates coronary arteries and arterioles.
Therapeutic effect: relieves anginal pain, lowers blood pressure, and restores normal sinus rhythm.

Adverse reactions

CNS: *headache,* somnolence, dizziness, insomnia, asthenia.
CV: *edema, **arrhythmias,*** flushing, ***bradycardia,*** hypotension, conduction abnormalities, ***heart failure, AV block,*** abnormal ECG.
GI: *nausea, constipation,* vomiting, diarrhea, abdominal discomfort.
GU: nocturia, polyuria.
Hepatic: transient elevation of liver enzyme levels.
Skin: rash, pruritus, photosensitivity.

Interactions

Drug-drug. *Anesthetics:* effects may be potentiated. Monitor patient.
Cimetidine: may inhibit diltiazem metabolism. Monitor patient for toxicity.
Cyclosporine: diltiazem may increase serum cyclosporine levels, possibly by decreasing its metabolism, leading to increased risk of cyclosporine toxicity. Avoid concomitant use.

Digoxin: diltiazem may increase serum levels of digoxin. Monitor patient and serum digoxin levels.
Propranolol, other beta blockers: may precipitate heart failure or prolong cardiac conduction time. Use together cautiously.
Drug-lifestyle. *Sunlight:* photosensitivity may occur. Advise precautions.

Contraindications and precautions

- Contraindicated in patients hypersensitive to drug and in those with sick sinus syndrome, second- or third-degree AV block in absence of artificial pacemaker, hypotension (systolic blood pressure below 90 mm Hg), acute MI, or pulmonary congestion (documented by X-ray).
- Breast-feeding should be discontinued during drug use.
- Use cautiously in elderly patients, patients with heart failure, and those with impaired liver or kidney function. Also use cautiously in pregnant women.
- Safety of drug hasn't been established in children.

NURSING CONSIDERATIONS

Assessment

- Obtain history of patient's underlying condition before therapy, and reassess regularly thereafter.
- Monitor blood pressure when therapy starts and when dosage changes.
- Monitor patient's ECG and heart rate and rhythm regularly.
- Be alert for adverse reactions and drug interactions.
- Evaluate patient's and family's knowledge of drug therapy.

Nursing diagnoses

- Ineffective health maintenance related to underlying condition
- Decreased cardiac output related to drug-induced adverse reactions
- Deficient knowledge related to drug therapy

Planning and implementation

P.O. use: Administer tablets before meals and at bedtime.
I.V. use: Infusions lasting longer than 24 hours aren't recommended.
- Furosemide forms a precipitate when mixed with diltiazem injection. Administer through separate I.V. lines.
- If systolic blood pressure is below 90 mm Hg or heart rate is below 60 beats/minute, withhold dose and notify prescriber.
- Assist patient with ambulation during start of therapy because dizziness may occur.
- Restrict patient's fluid and sodium intake to minimize edema.

Patient teaching

- If nitrate therapy is prescribed during adjustment of diltiazem dosage, urge patient compliance. Tell patient that S.L. nitroglycerin, especially, may be taken concomitantly as needed and ordered when angina is acute.
- Instruct patient to call prescriber with chest pain, shortness of breath, dizziness, palpitations, or swelling of the limbs.
- Tell patient to swallow extended- and sustained-release capsules whole and not to open, crush, or chew them.
- Instruct patient to take drug exactly as prescribed, even when feeling well.
- Advise patient to minimize exposure to direct sunlight and to take precautions when in sun because of drug-induced photosensitivity.
- Instruct patient to limit fluid and sodium intake to minimize edema.

Evaluation

- Patient exhibits improvement in underlying condition.
- Patient maintains adequate cardiac output throughout therapy.
- Patient and family state understanding of drug therapy.

dimenhydrinate

(digh-men-HIGH-drih-nayt)

Apo-Dimenhydrinate ♦, Calm X†, Children's Dramamine†, Dimetabs, Dinate, Dramamine†*, Dramamine Chewable†**, Dramamine Liquid†*, Dymenate, Gravol ♦, Gravol L/A ♦, Hydrate, PMS-Dimenhydrinate ♦, Triptone Caplets†

Pharmacologic class: ethanolamine derivative antihistamine
Therapeutic class: antihistamine (H_1-receptor antagonist), antiemetic, antivertigo agent
Pregnancy risk category: B

Indications and dosages

▶ **Prevention and treatment of motion sickness.** *Adults and children age 12 and over:* 50 to 100 mg P.O. q 4 to 6 hours. Or, 50 mg I.M., p.r.n. Or, 50 mg I.V. diluted in 10 ml sodium chloride injection, injected over 2 minutes. Maximum, 400 mg daily.
Children ages 6 to 12: 25 to 50 mg P.O. q 6 to 8 hours, not to exceed 150 mg in 24 hours.
Children ages 2 to 6: 12.5 to 25 mg P.O. q 6 to 8 hours, not to exceed 75 mg in 24 hours.

How supplied

Tablets: 50 mg†
Tablets (chewable): 50 mg†
Capsules: 75 mg†
Elixir: 15 mg/5 ml ♦
Syrup: 12.5 mg/4 ml*†, 15.62 mg/5 ml
Injection: 50 mg/ml

Pharmacokinetics

Absorption: well absorbed after P.O. and I.M. administration.
Distribution: well distributed throughout body.
Metabolism: metabolized in liver.
Excretion: excreted in urine. *Half-life:* 1 to 4 hours.

Route	Onset	Peak	Duration
P.O.	20-30 min	Unknown	3-6 hr
I.V.	Immediate	Unknown	3-6 hr
I.M.	15-20 min	Unknown	3-6 hr

Pharmacodynamics

Chemical effect: unknown; may affect neural pathways originating in labyrinth.
Therapeutic effect: prevents and relieves motion sickness.

Adverse reactions

CNS: *drowsiness,* headache, confusion, nervousness, insomnia, vertigo, tingling and weakness of hands, lassitude, excitation, incoordination, dizziness.
CV: palpitations, hypotension, tachycardia.
EENT: blurred vision, diplopia, nasal congestion, tinnitus, dry respiratory passages.
GI: dry mouth, nausea, vomiting, diarrhea, epigastric distress, constipation, anorexia.
Respiratory: wheezing, thickened bronchial secretions.
Skin: photosensitivity, urticaria, rash.
Other: ***anaphylaxis,*** tightness of chest.

Interactions

Drug-drug. *CNS depressants:* additive CNS depression. Avoid concomitant use.
Drug-lifestyle. *Alcohol use:* additive CNS depression. Discourage concomitant use.

Contraindications and precautions

- No known contraindications, although drug isn't recommended for use in breast-feeding women.
- Use cautiously in patients with seizures, acute angle-closure glaucoma, enlarged prostate gland, or in patients receiving ototoxic drugs. Also use cautiously in pregnant women.

NURSING CONSIDERATIONS

Assessment

- Obtain history of patient's underlying condition before therapy.
- Monitor effectiveness by evaluating patient for nausea and vomiting.
- Be alert for adverse reactions and drug interactions.
- Evaluate patient's and family's knowledge of drug therapy.

Nursing diagnoses
- Risk for deficient fluid volume related to nausea and vomiting induced by motion sickness
- Risk for injury related to drug-induced adverse CNS reactions
- Deficient knowledge related to drug therapy

Planning and implementation
P.O. use: To prevent motion sickness, give drug at least 30 minutes before patient travels.
I.V. use: Before administration, dilute each milliliter of drug with 10 ml of sterile water for injection, D_5W, or normal saline solution injection. Give by direct injection over not less than 2 minutes.
– Undiluted solution is irritating to veins and may cause sclerosis.
I.M. use: Follow normal protocol.
- Because incompatibilities are common, avoid mixing parenteral form with other drugs.

Patient teaching
- Advise patient to avoid hazardous activities until CNS effects of drug are known.
- Tell patient to take drug at least 30 minutes before beginning travel.

Evaluation
- Patient maintains adequate hydration.
- Patient has no injury as result of drug-induced adverse CNS reactions.
- Patient and family state understanding of drug therapy.

dimercaprol
(digh-mer-KAP-rohl)
BAL in Oil

Pharmacologic class: chelating agent
Therapeutic class: heavy metal antagonist
Pregnancy risk category: C

Indications and dosages
▶ **Severe arsenic or gold poisoning.** *Adults and children:* 3 mg/kg deep I.M. q 4 hours for 2 days; then q.i.d. on third day; then b.i.d. for 10 days.
▶ **Mild arsenic or gold poisoning.** *Adults and children:* 2.5 mg/kg deep I.M. q.i.d. for 2 days; then b.i.d. on third day; then once daily for 10 days.
▶ **Mercury poisoning.** *Adults and children:* initially, 5 mg/kg deep I.M.; then 2.5 mg/kg daily or b.i.d. for 10 days.
▶ **Acute lead encephalopathy or lead level exceeding 100 mcg/dl.** *Adults and children:* 4 mg/kg deep I.M.; then q 4 hours with edetate calcium disodium (250 mg/m2 I.M.). Use separate sites. Maximum, 5 mg/kg per dose.

How supplied
Injection: 100 mg/ml

Pharmacokinetics
Absorption: unknown.
Distribution: distributed to all tissues, mainly intracellular space.
Metabolism: uncomplexed dimercaprol is metabolized rapidly to inactive products.
Excretion: most dimercaprol metal complexes and inactive metabolites are excreted in urine and feces.

Route	Onset	Peak	Duration
I.M.	Unknown	30-60 min	4 hr

Pharmacodynamics
Chemical effect: forms complexes with heavy metals.
Therapeutic effect: treats heavy metal intoxication.

Adverse reactions
CNS: headache, paresthesia.
CV: *transient increase in blood pressure, tachycardia.*
EENT: blepharospasm, conjunctivitis, lacrimation, rhinorrhea, excessive salivation.
GI: *halitosis; nausea; vomiting; burning sensation in lips, mouth, and throat; abdominal pain.*
GU: *dysuria,* renal damage.
Musculoskeletal: muscle pain or weakness.
Skin: diaphoresis, sterile abscess, pain at injection site.
Other: *fever;* pain or tightness in throat, chest, or hands; decreased iodine uptake; pain in teeth.

Interactions

Drug-drug. *Iron:* toxic metal complex formed; concurrent therapy contraindicated. Wait 24 hours after last dimercaprol dose.

Contraindications and precautions

- Contraindicated in patients with hepatic dysfunction (except postarsenical jaundice).
- Use cautiously in patients with hypertension or oliguria.
- Safety of drug hasn't been established in pregnant or breast-feeding women.

NURSING CONSIDERATIONS

Assessment

- Obtain history of patient's toxicity before therapy.
- Assess effectiveness by monitoring serum level of substance ingested and for improvement in patient's condition.
- Be alert for adverse reactions and drug interactions.
- Monitor patient's hydration status if adverse GI reactions occur.
- Observe injection site for local reaction.
- Evaluate patient's and family's knowledge of drug therapy.

Nursing diagnoses

- Risk for poisoning related to exposure to toxic substance
- Risk for deficient fluid volume related to drug-induced nausea and vomiting
- Deficient knowledge related to drug therapy

Planning and implementation

- Don't give I.V.; give by deep I.M. route only. Massage injection site after administration.
- Be careful not to let drug come in contact with skin because it may cause skin reaction.
- Don't schedule patient for ^{131}I uptake thyroid tests during therapy because dimercaprol decreases results.
- Solution with slight sediment is usable.
- Drug is ineffective in arsine gas poisoning.

ALERT Don't use for iron, cadmium, or selenium toxicity. Complex formed is highly toxic, even fatal.

- Use ephedrine or antihistamine, as ordered, to prevent or relieve mild adverse reactions.
- Keep urine alkaline to prevent renal damage. Oral sodium bicarbonate may be ordered.
- Apply ice or cold compresses to injection site to alleviate local discomfort.

Patient teaching

- Warn patient that drug has unpleasant garlic-like odor.
- Advise patient that drug may cause pain at injection site.
- Instruct patient to report changes in urine output, fever, pain, nausea, or vomiting immediately.

Evaluation

- Patient's toxicity is eliminated.
- Patient maintains adequate hydration throughout therapy.
- Patient and family state understanding of drug therapy.

dinoprostone

(digh-noh-PROS-tohn)

Cervidil, Prepidil, Prostin E2

Pharmacologic class: prostaglandin
Therapeutic class: oxytocic
Pregnancy risk category: C

Indications and dosages

▶ **To abort second-trimester pregnancy; to evacuate uterus in missed abortion, intrauterine fetal deaths up to 28 weeks of gestation, or benign hydatidiform mole (Suppository).** *Adults:* 20-mg suppository inserted high into posterior vaginal fornix. Repeated q 3 to 5 hours until abortion is complete.

▶ **Ripening of unfavorable cervix in pregnant patients at or near term (Gel).** *Adults:* contents of one syringe administered intravaginally; if cervix remains unfavorable after 6 hours, dosage repeated. No more than 1.5 mg (three applications) should be given per 24 hours. **(Vaginal insert).** *Adults:* one insert with retrieval system placed intravaginally. Remove the insert upon onset of active labor or 12 hours after insertion.

How supplied

Vaginal suppositories: 20 mg
Vaginal insert: 10 mg
Endocervical gel: 0.5 mg/application (2.5-ml syringe)

Pharmacokinetics

Absorption: after vaginal insertion, drug diffuses slowly into maternal blood. There's also some local absorption into uterus through cervix or local vascular and lymphatic channels, but this accounts for only small portion of dose.
Distribution: distributed widely in mother.
Metabolism: metabolized in lungs, liver, kidneys, spleen, and other maternal tissues.
Excretion: drug and metabolites are excreted primarily in urine, with small amounts in feces. *Half-life:* less than 1 minute.

Route	Onset	Peak	Duration
Intra-vaginal	10-60 min	Unknown	About 17 hr (suppositories); unknown (gel); 12 hr (insert)

Pharmacodynamics

Chemical effect: produces strong, prompt contractions of uterine smooth muscle, possibly mediated by calcium and cAMP.
Therapeutic effect: causes abortion.

Adverse reactions

CNS: *headache, dizziness,* anxiety, hot flushes, paresthesia, weakness, syncope.
CV: chest pain, ***arrhythmias,*** hypotension.
EENT: blurred vision, eye pain.
GI: *nausea, vomiting, diarrhea.*
GU: vaginal pain, vaginitis, endometritis.
Musculoskeletal: *nocturnal leg cramps,* backache, muscle cramps.
Respiratory: coughing, dyspnea, ***bronchospasm.***
Skin: rash, diaphoresis.
Other: *fever, shivering, chills,* breast tenderness.

Interactions

Drug-drug. *Other oxytocics:* may potentiate action. Avoid concomitant use.

Contraindications and precautions

- Gel form contraindicated when prolonged contractions of uterus are considered inappropriate. Also contraindicated in patients hypersensitive to prostaglandins or constituents of gel and in patients with placenta previa or unexplained vaginal bleeding during this pregnancy and in whom vaginal delivery isn't indicated (that is, because of vasa previa or active herpes genitalia).
- Suppository form contraindicated in patients hypersensitive to drug and in those with acute pelvic inflammatory disease or active cardiac, pulmonary, renal, or hepatic disease.
- Use suppository form cautiously in patients with asthma; seizure disorders; anemia; diabetes; hypertension or hypotension; jaundice; CV, renal, or hepatic disease; scarred uterus; cervicitis; or acute vaginitis.
- Use gel form cautiously in patients with ruptured membranes and in those with asthma or history of asthma, glaucoma or raised intraocular pressure, or renal or hepatic dysfunction.

NURSING CONSIDERATIONS

Assessment

- Obtain history of patient's pregnancy status before therapy.
- Monitor effectiveness by observing patient for desired response to drug. Keep in mind that abortion should be complete within 30 hours when suppository form is used.
- Be alert for adverse reactions and drug interactions.
- Monitor patient's hydration status if adverse GI reactions occur.
- Evaluate patient's and family's knowledge of drug therapy.

Nursing diagnoses

- Risk for deficient fluid volume related to potential drug-induced adverse GI reactions
- Risk for altered body temperature related to possible drug-induced fever
- Deficient knowledge related to drug therapy

Planning and implementation

- Administer only when critical care facilities are readily available.

• Just before use, warm dinoprostone suppositories in their wrappers to room temperature. After administration, patient should remain supine for 10 minutes.
• When used for cervical ripening, make sure patient is lying on her back, with cervix visualized using speculum. Assist with insertion. Using aseptic technique, catheter provided with drug is used to administer gel into cervical canal just below level of internal os.
• When gel form is used, contents of syringe are used for one patient only. Discard syringe, catheter, and unused drug after administration; don't attempt to administer small amount of drug remaining in catheter.
• Freeze suppositories at –4° F (–20° C).
• When using drug as abortifacient, be prepared to pretreat patient with antiemetic and antidiarrheal.
• Treat dinoprostone-induced fever (self-limiting and transient and occurs in about 50% of patients) with water or alcohol sponging and increased fluid intake, not with aspirin.
• A dosing interval of at least 30 minutes is recommended for sequential use of oxytocin following the removal of a vaginal insert.
ALERT Don't confuse Prostin E2 with Prostin VR (alprastadil), which is used to maintain patency of ductus arteriosus in neonates with congenital heart defects.

Patient teaching

• Instruct patient to remain supine for 10 minutes after administration.

Evaluation

• Patient maintains adequate hydration throughout therapy.
• Patient's body temperature returns to normal.
• Patient and family state understanding of drug therapy.

diphenhydramine hydrochloride

(digh-fen-HIGH-drah-meen high-droh-KLOR-ighd)

Allerdryl ♦ †, AllerMax Caplets†, Allermed†, Banophen†, Banophen Caplets†, Beldin†, Belix†, Benadryl†, Benadryl 25†, Benadryl Kapseals†, Benylin Cough†, Bydramine Cough†, Compoz†, Diphenadryl†, Diphen Cough†, Diphenhist†, Diphenhist Captabs†, Genahist†, Hyrexin-50, Nytol Maximum Strength†, Nytol with DPH†, Sleep-Eze 3†, Sominex Formula 2†, Tusstat†, Twilite Caplets†, Uni-Bent Cough†

Pharmacologic class: ethanolamine derivative antihistamine
Therapeutic class: antihistamine (H_1-receptor antagonist), antiemetic, antivertigo, antitussive, sedative-hypnotic, antidyskinetic (anticholinergic)
Pregnancy risk category: B

Indications and dosages

▶ **Rhinitis, allergy symptoms, motion sickness, Parkinson's disease.** *Adults and children age 12 and over:* 25 to 50 mg P.O. t.i.d. or q.i.d. Or, 10 to 50 mg deep I.M. or I.V. Maximum I.M. or I.V. dosage is 400 mg daily.
Children under age 12: 5 mg/kg daily P.O., deep I.M., or I.V. in divided doses q.i.d. Maximum, 300 mg daily.
▶ **Sedation.** *Adults:* 25 to 50 mg P.O. or deep I.M., p.r.n.
▶ **Nighttime sleep aid.** *Adults:* 50 mg P.O. h.s.
▶ **Nonproductive cough.** *Adults:* 25 mg P.O. q 4 to 6 hours (up to 150 mg daily).
Children ages 6 to 12: 12.5 mg P.O. q 4 to 6 hours (up to 75 mg daily).
Children ages 2 to 6: 6.25 mg P.O. q 4 to 6 hours (up to 25 mg daily).

How supplied

Tablets: 25 mg†, 50 mg†
Chewable tablets: 12.5 mg†
Capsules: 25 mg†, 50 mg†
Elixir: 12.5 mg/5 ml*†
Syrup: 12.5 mg/5 ml†, 6.25 mg/5 ml†
Injection: 10 mg/ml, 50 mg/ml

Pharmacokinetics

Absorption: well absorbed from GI tract after P.O. administration; unknown after I.M. administration.
Distribution: distributed widely throughout body, including CNS; about 82% protein-bound.
Metabolism: metabolized in liver.
Excretion: drug and metabolites excreted primarily in urine. *Half-life:* about 3½ hours.

Route	Onset	Peak	Duration
P.O.	≤ 15 min	1-4 hr	6-8 hr
I.V.	Immediate	1-4 hr	6-8 hr
I.M.	Unknown	1-4 hr	6-8 hr

Pharmacodynamics

Chemical effect: competes with histamine for H_1-receptor sites on effector cells. Diphenhydramine prevents but doesn't reverse histamine-mediated responses, particularly histamine's effects on smooth muscle of bronchial tubes, GI tract, uterus, and blood vessels. Structurally related to local anesthetics, diphenhydramine provides local anesthesia by preventing initiation and transmission of nerve impulses. It also suppresses cough reflex by direct effect in medulla of brain.
Therapeutic effect: relieves allergy symptoms, motion sickness, and cough; improves voluntary movement; and promotes sleep and calmness.

Adverse reactions

CNS: *drowsiness,* confusion, insomnia, headache, vertigo, *sedation, sleepiness, dizziness,* incoordination, fatigue, restlessness, tremor, nervousness, ***seizures.***
CV: palpitations, hypotension, tachycardia.
EENT: diplopia, blurred vision, nasal congestion, tinnitus.
GI: *nausea,* vomiting, diarrhea, *dry mouth,* constipation, *epigastric distress,* anorexia.
GU: dysuria, urine retention, urinary frequency.
Hematologic: *hemolytic anemia,* ***thrombocytopenia, agranulocytosis.***
Respiratory: thickening of bronchial secretions.
Skin: urticaria, photosensitivity, rash.
Other: ***anaphylactic shock.***

Interactions

Drug-drug. *CNS depressants:* increased sedation. Use together cautiously.
MAO inhibitors: increased anticholinergic effects. Don't use together.
Drug-lifestyle. *Alcohol use:* may increase adverse CNS effects. Discourage concomitant use.
Sun exposure: photosensitivity reactions may occur. Urge precautions.

Contraindications and precautions

- Contraindicated in patients hypersensitive to drug, patients having acute asthmatic attacks, newborns, premature neonates, and breast-feeding women.
- Use with extreme caution in patients with angle-closure glaucoma, prostatic hyperplasia, pyloroduodenal and bladder-neck obstruction, asthma or COPD, increased intraocular pressure, hyperthyroidism, CV disease, hypertension, or stenosing peptic ulcer.
- Use cautiously in pregnant women.
- Children under age 12 should use only as directed by prescriber.

NURSING CONSIDERATIONS

Assessment
- Obtain history of patient's underlying condition before therapy, and reassess regularly thereafter.
- Be alert for adverse reactions and drug interactions.
- Evaluate patient's and family's knowledge of drug therapy.

Nursing diagnoses
- Ineffective health maintenance related to underlying condition
- Risk for injury related to drug-induced adverse CNS reactions
- Deficient knowledge related to drug therapy

Planning and implementation
P.O. use: Reduce GI distress by giving drug with food or milk.

I.V. use: Follow manufacturer's guidelines.
I.M. use: Alternate injection sites to prevent irritation. Administer I.M. injection deep into large muscle.
• Notify prescriber if tolerance is observed because another antihistamine may need to be substituted.

Patient teaching
• Instruct patient to take drug 30 minutes before travel to prevent motion sickness.
• Warn patient to avoid alcohol and to refrain from driving or performing other hazardous activities that require alertness until drug's CNS effects are known.
• Tell patient that coffee or tea may reduce drowsiness.
• Inform patient that ice chips or sugarless gum or sour hard candy may relieve dry mouth.
• Advise patient to stop drug 4 days before allergy skin tests to preserve accuracy of tests.
• Tell patient to notify prescriber if tolerance develops because different antihistamine may need to be prescribed.
• Warn patient of possible photosensitivity. Advise use of sunblock.

☑ Evaluation
• Patient shows improvement in underlying condition.
• Patient has no injury as result of therapy.
• Patient and family state understanding of drug therapy.

diphenoxylate hydrochloride and atropine sulfate
(digh-fen-OKS-ul-ayt high-droh-KLOR-ighd and AH-troh-peen SUL-fayt)
Logen, Lomanate, Lomotil*, Lonox

Pharmacologic class: opioid
Therapeutic class: antidiarrheal
Controlled substance schedule: V
Pregnancy risk category: C

Indications and dosages
▶ **Acute, nonspecific diarrhea.** *Adults:* initially, 5 mg P.O. q.i.d.; then dosage adjusted as needed.
Children ages 2 to 12: 0.3 to 0.4 mg/kg liquid form P.O. daily in four divided doses. Maintenance dosage may be one-fourth of original dose.

How supplied
Tablets: 2.5 mg (with atropine sulfate 0.025 mg)
Liquid: 2.5 mg/5 ml (with atropine sulfate 0.025 mg/5 ml)*

Pharmacokinetics
Absorption: about 90% absorbed.
Distribution: unknown.
Metabolism: metabolized extensively by liver.
Excretion: metabolites excreted mainly in feces with lesser amounts excreted in urine. *Half-life:* diphenoxylate, 2½ hours; its major metabolite, diphenoxylic acid, 4½ hours; atropine, 2½ hours.

Route	Onset	Peak	Duration
P.O.	45-60 min	About 3 hr	3-4 hr

Pharmacodynamics
Chemical effect: unknown; probably increases smooth-muscle tone in GI tract, inhibits motility and propulsion, and diminishes secretions.
Therapeutic effect: relieves diarrhea.

Adverse reactions
CNS: *sedation, dizziness,* headache, drowsiness, lethargy, restlessness, depression, euphoria, malaise, confusion, numbness in limbs.
CV: tachycardia.
EENT: mydriasis.
GI: *dry mouth,* nausea, vomiting, abdominal discomfort or distention, ***paralytic ileus,*** anorexia, fluid retention in bowel, possible physical dependence with long-term use, ***pancreatitis.***
GU: urine retention.
Respiratory: ***respiratory depression.***
Skin: pruritus, rash.
Other: ***angioedema, anaphylaxis.***

Interactions

Drug-drug. *Barbiturates, CNS depressants, narcotics, tranquilizers:* enhanced CNS depression. Monitor patient closely.
MAO inhibitors: possibly hypertensive crisis. Avoid concomitant use.
Drug-lifestyle. *Alcohol use:* enhanced CNS depression. Discourage concomitant use.

Contraindications and precautions

- Contraindicated in patients hypersensitive to diphenoxylate or atropine and in those with acute diarrhea from poison (until toxic material is eliminated from GI tract), acute diarrhea caused by organisms that penetrate the intestinal mucosa, or diarrhea from antibiotic-induced pseudomembranous enterocolitis. Also contraindicated in jaundiced patients and in children under age 2.
- Drug isn't recommended for use in breast-feeding women.
- Use cautiously in children age 2 and over; in patients with hepatic disease, narcotic dependence, or acute ulcerative colitis; and in pregnant women. Stop therapy immediately if abdominal distention or other signs of toxic megacolon develop, and notify prescriber.

NURSING CONSIDERATIONS

Assessment

- Assess patient's diarrhea before and regularly during therapy.
- Be alert for adverse reactions and drug interactions.
- Evaluate patient's and family's knowledge of drug therapy.

Nursing diagnoses

- Diarrhea related to underlying condition
- Ineffective breathing pattern related to drug-induced respiratory depression
- Deficient knowledge related to drug therapy

Planning and implementation

- Fluid retention in the bowel may mask depletion of extracellular fluid and electrolytes, especially in young children treated for acute gastroenteritis. Correct fluid and electrolyte disturbances before starting drug. Dehydration may increase risk of delayed toxicity.
- Keep in mind that 2.5-mg dose is as effective as 5 ml of camphorated opium tincture.
- Drug isn't indicated for treating antibiotic-induced diarrhea.
- Drug is unlikely to be effective if no response occurs within 48 hours.
- Risk of physical dependence increases with high dosage and long-term use. Atropine sulfate helps discourage abuse.
- Use naloxone, as ordered, to treat respiratory depression caused by overdose.

Patient teaching

- Tell patient not to exceed recommended dosage.
- Warn patient not to use drug to treat acute diarrhea for longer than 2 days. Encourage him to seek medical attention if diarrhea continues.
- Advise patient to avoid hazardous activities, such as driving, until CNS effects of drug are known.

Evaluation

- Patient regains normal bowel pattern.
- Patient maintains normal breathing pattern throughout therapy.
- Patient and family state understanding of drug therapy.

dipyridamole

(digh-peer-IH-duh-mohl)

Apo-Dipyridamole ♦, Novo-Dipiradol ♦, Persantin ◇, Persantin 100 ◇, Persantine**

Pharmacologic class: pyrimidine analogue
Therapeutic class: coronary vasodilator, platelet aggregation inhibitor
Pregnancy risk category: B

Indications and dosages

▶ **Inhibition of platelet adhesion in prosthetic heart valves (in combination with warfarin or aspirin).** *Adults:* 75 to 100 mg P.O. q.i.d.

▶ **Alternative to exercise in evaluation of coronary artery disease during thallium-201 myocardial perfusion scintigraphy.**

Adults: 0.57 mg/kg as I.V. infusion at constant rate over 4 minutes (0.142 mg/kg/minute).

How supplied

Tablets: 25 mg, 50 mg, 75 mg
Injection: 10 mg/2 ml

Pharmacokinetics

Absorption: variable and slow; bioavailability ranges from 27% to 59%.
Distribution: wide distribution in body tissues. Protein binding ranges from 91% to 97%.
Metabolism: metabolized by liver.
Excretion: elimination occurs by way of biliary excretion of glucuronide conjugates. Some dipyridamole and conjugates may undergo enterohepatic circulation and fecal excretion; small amount is excreted in urine.
Half-life: 1 to 12 hours.

Route	Onset	Peak	Duration
P.O.	Unknown	45-150 min	Unknown
I.V.	Unknown	2 min after infusion completed	Unknown
I.M.	Unknown	Unknown	Unknown

Pharmacodynamics

Chemical effect: unknown; may involve its ability to increase adenosine, which is a coronary vasodilator and platelet aggregation inhibitor.
Therapeutic effect: dilates coronary arteries and helps prevent clotting.

Adverse reactions

CNS: *headache, dizziness,* weakness.
CV: flushing, fainting, hypotension, chest pain, ECG abnormalities, blood pressure lability, hypertension (with I.V. infusion).
GI: *nausea,* vomiting, diarrhea, abdominal distress.
Skin: rash, irritation (with undiluted injection), pruritus.

Interactions

Drug-drug. *Heparin:* may cause increased bleeding. Monitor patient closely.
Theophylline: may prevent coronary vasodilation by I.V. dipyridamole. Avoid concomitant use.
Drug-herb. *Dong quai, feverfew, garlic, ginger, horse chestnut, red clover:* possible increased risk of bleeding. Discourage concomitant use.

Contraindications and precautions

- No known contraindications.
- Use cautiously in patients with hypotension and in pregnant women.
- Safety of drug hasn't been established in breast-feeding women or in children.

NURSING CONSIDERATIONS

Assessment

- Obtain history of patient's underlying condition before therapy, and reassess regularly thereafter.
- Be alert for adverse reactions and drug interactions.
- Evaluate patient's and family's knowledge of drug therapy.

Nursing diagnoses

- Ineffective cardiopulmonary tissue perfusion related to underlying condition
- Acute pain related to drug-induced headache
- Deficient knowledge related to drug therapy

Planning and implementation

P.O. use: Administer drug 1 hour before meals. If patient develops adverse GI reactions, administer drug with meals.
I.V. use: If administering drug as diagnostic agent, dilute in half-normal or normal saline solution or D_5W in at least a 1:2 ratio for total volume of 20 to 50 ml. Inject thallium-201 within 5 minutes after completing 4-minute dipyridamole infusion.
I.M. use: Follow normal protocol.

Patient teaching

- Instruct patient when to take drug.
- Tell patient to have his blood pressure checked frequently.
- Advise patient to take mild analgesic if headache occurs.
- Instruct patient to notify prescriber if chest pain occurs.

Evaluation

- Patient maintains adequate tissue perfusion and cellular oxygenation.
- Patient obtains relief from drug-induced headache with use of mild analgesic.
- Patient and family state understanding of drug therapy.

dirithromycin

(digh-rith-roh-MIGH-sin)
Dynabac

Pharmacologic class: macrolide
Therapeutic class: antibiotic
Pregnancy risk category: C

Indications and dosages

▶ **Acute bacterial exacerbations of chronic bronchitis caused by *Moraxella catarrhalis* or *Streptococcus pneumoniae;* secondary bacterial infection of acute bronchitis caused by *M. catarrhalis* or *S. pneumoniae;* uncomplicated skin and skin-structure infections caused by *Staphylococcus aureus* (methicillin-susceptible strains only).** *Adults and children age 12 and older:* 500 mg P.O. daily with food for 7 days.

▶ **Acute bacterial exacerbations of chronic bronchitis caused by *Haemophilus influenzae* and uncomplicated skin and skin-structure infections caused by *Streptococcus pyogenes.*** *Adults and children age 12 and older:* 500 mg P.O. daily with food (or within 1 hour of a meal) for 5 to 7 days.

▶ **Community-acquired pneumonia caused by *Legionella pneumophila, Mycoplasma pneumoniae,* or *S. pneumoniae.*** *Adults and children age 12 and older:* 500 mg P.O. daily with food for 14 days.

▶ **Pharyngitis or tonsillitis caused by *S. pyogenes.*** *Adults and children age 12 and older:* 500 mg P.O. daily with food for 10 days.

How supplied

Tablets (enteric-coated): 250 mg

Pharmacokinetics

Absorption: rapidly absorbed from GI tract and converted by nonenzymatic hydrolysis to the microbiologically active compound erythromycyclamine. Food slightly increases bioavailability.
Distribution: widely distributed throughout body; protein binding ranges from 15% to 30%.
Metabolism: undergoes little to no hepatic metabolism.
Excretion: eliminated primarily in bile; small amount excreted in urine. *Half-life:* about 8 hours.

Route	Onset	Peak	Duration
P.O.	Unknown	About 4 hr	Unknown

Pharmacodynamics

Chemical effect: inhibits bacterial RNA-dependent protein synthesis by binding to 50S subunit of ribosome.
Therapeutic effect: hinders susceptible bacteria. Spectrum of activity includes gram-positive aerobes, such as *S. aureus* (methicillin-susceptible strains only), *S. pneumoniae,* and *S. pyogenes;* gram-negative aerobes, such as *L. pneumophila* and *M. catarrhalis;* and other bacteria, such as *M. pneumoniae.*

Adverse reactions

CNS: asthenia, headache, dizziness, vertigo, insomnia.
GI: abdominal pain, nausea, diarrhea, vomiting, dyspepsia, GI disorder, flatulence.
Hematologic: increased platelet, eosinophil, and neutrophil counts.
Hepatic: increased CK and liver enzyme levels.
Metabolic: hyperkalemia, decreased bicarbonate levels.
Respiratory: increased cough, dyspnea.
Skin: rash, pruritus, urticaria.
Other: pain.

Interactions

Drug-drug. *Alfentanil, bromocriptine, carbamazepine, cyclosporine, digoxin, disopyramide, ergotamine, hexobarbital, lovastatin, oral anticoagulants, phenytoin, triazolam, and valproate:* have been reported to interact with

erythromycin products. It isn't known whether these same drug interactions occur with dirithromycin. Until further data are available, caution should be used during coadministration.
Antacids, H_2-receptor antagonists: absorption slightly enhanced when dirithromycin is administered immediately after these drugs. May give concomitantly.
Theophylline: may alter steady-state plasma level of theophylline. Monitor theophylline plasma levels. Dosage adjustments may be needed.
Drug-food. *Any food:* increased absorption. Administer drug with food.

Contraindications and precautions

- Contraindicated in patients hypersensitive to drug, erythromycin, or other macrolide antibiotics.
- Use cautiously in patients with hepatic insufficiency and in pregnant or breast-feeding women.
- Safety of drug hasn't been established in children under age 12.

NURSING CONSIDERATIONS

Assessment

- Obtain history of patient's infection before therapy.
- Obtain culture and sensitivity tests before first dose. Therapy may begin pending test results.
- Be alert for adverse reactions and drug interactions.
- Evaluate patient's and family's knowledge of drug therapy.

Nursing diagnoses

- Infection related to susceptible bacteria
- Risk for deficient fluid volume related to adverse GI reactions
- Deficient knowledge related to drug therapy

Planning and implementation

- Drug shouldn't be used in patient with known, suspected, or potential bacteremia; serum levels are inadequate to provide antibacterial coverage of the bloodstream.
- Administer drug with food or within 1 hour of food intake.

Patient teaching

- Tell patient to take all of drug, as ordered, even if he feels better.
- Advise him to take drug with food or within 1 hour of having eaten. Tell him not to cut, chew, or crush the tablet.

Evaluation

- Patient is free from infection.
- Patient maintains adequate hydration.
- Patient and family state understanding of drug therapy.

disopyramide

(digh-so-PEER-uh-mighd)
Rythmodan ♦ ◇

disopyramide phosphate

Norpace, Norpace CR, Rythmodan LA ♦

Pharmacologic class: pyridine derivative
Therapeutic class: antiarrhythmic
Pregnancy risk category: C

Indications and dosages

▶ **Symptomatic PVCs (unifocal, multifocal, or coupled); ventricular tachycardia not severe enough to require cardioversion.**
Adults weighing over 50 kg (110 lb): 150 mg q 6 hours with conventional capsules or 300 mg q 12 hours with controlled-release forms.
Adults weighing 50 kg or less: 100 mg P.O. every 6 hours as conventional capsules or 200 mg P.O. q 12 hours with controlled-release capsules.
Children ages 12 to 18: 6 to 15 mg/kg P.O. daily.
Children ages 4 to 12: 10 to 15 mg/kg P.O. daily.
Children ages 1 to 4: 10 to 20 mg/kg P.O. daily.
Children under age 1: 10 to 30 mg/kg P.O. daily.
For pediatric dosages, divide into equal amounts and give q 6 hours.

Administer until arrhythmia is eliminated or patient has received 150 mg. Repeat dosage if conversion is successful but arrhythmia returns. Total I.V. dosage shouldn't exceed 300 mg in first hour. Follow with I.V. infusion of 0.4 mg/kg/hour (usually 20 to 30 mg/hour) to maximum of 800 mg/day.
Recommended dosages in advanced renal insufficiency: if creatinine clearance is 30 to 40 ml/minute, 100 mg q 8 hours; if creatinine clearance is 15 to 30 ml/minute, 100 mg q 12 hours; if creatinine clearance is less than 15 ml/minute, 100 mg q 24 hours.

How supplied

disopyramide
Capsules: 100 mg ♦, 150 mg ♦
disopyramide phosphate
Tablets (sustained-release): 150 mg ♦
Capsules: 100 mg, 150 mg
Capsules (controlled-release): 100 mg, 150 mg
Injection: 10 mg/ml ♦ ◇

Pharmacokinetics

Absorption: rapidly and well absorbed from GI tract with P.O. administration.
Distribution: well distributed throughout extracellular fluid but not extensively bound to tissues. Plasma protein–binding varies but generally ranges from about 50% to 65%.
Metabolism: metabolized in liver.
Excretion: excreted in urine. *Half-life:* about 7 hours.

Route	Onset	Peak	Duration
P.O.	0.5-3.5 hr	2-2.5 hr	1.5-8.5 hr
I.V.	Unknown	Unknown	Unknown

Pharmacodynamics

Chemical effect: unknown; considered class Ia antiarrhythmic that depresses phase 0 and prolongs action potential. All class I drugs have membrane-stabilizing effects.
Therapeutic effect: restores normal sinus rhythm.

Adverse reactions

CNS: dizziness, agitation, depression, fatigue, headache, acute psychosis.
CV: ***hypotension,*** syncope, ***heart failure, heart block,*** edema, ***arrhythmias,*** chest pain.
EENT: blurred vision, dry eyes, dry nose.
GI: nausea, vomiting, anorexia, bloating, abdominal pain, constipation, dry mouth, diarrhea.
GU: urine retention, urinary hesitancy.
Hepatic: cholestatic jaundice.
Metabolic: weight gain.
Musculoskeletal: aches, pain, muscle weakness.
Respiratory: shortness of breath.
Skin: rash, pruritus, dermatosis.

Interactions

Drug-drug. *Antiarrhythmics:* possibly additive or antagonized antiarrhythmic effects. Monitor patient closely.
Erythromycin: increased disopyramide levels may occur, causing arrhythmias and prolonged QTc interval. Monitor ECG closely.
Phenytoin: increased metabolism of disopyramide. Monitor patient for decreased antiarrhythmic effect.
Rifampin: disopyramide levels may be decreased. Monitor patient for decreased effectiveness.
Drug-herb. *Jimson weed:* May adversely affect CV function. Discourage concomitant use.

Contraindications and precautions

- Contraindicated in patients hypersensitive to drug and in those with cardiogenic shock or second- or third-degree heart block without an artificial pacemaker.
- Drug isn't recommended for use in breast-feeding women.
- Use with extreme caution and avoid, if possible, in patients with heart failure. Use cautiously in patients with underlying conduction abnormalities, urinary tract diseases (especially prostatic hypertrophy), hepatic or renal impairment, myasthenia gravis, or acute angle-closure glaucoma.
- Also use cautiously in pregnant women.

NURSING CONSIDERATIONS

Assessment

- Obtain history of patient's arrhythmia before therapy.

• Monitor effectiveness by assessing patient's ECG pattern and apical pulse rate.
• Be alert for adverse reactions and drug interactions.
• Evaluate patient's and family's knowledge of drug therapy.

Nursing diagnoses
• Decreased cardiac output related to underlying arrhythmia
• Ineffective protection related to drug-induced proarrhythmias
• Deficient knowledge related to drug therapy

Planning and implementation
• Correct any underlying electrolyte abnormalities before therapy begins, as ordered.
• Check apical pulse before giving drug. Notify prescriber if pulse rate is slower than 60 beats/minute or faster than 120 beats/minute.
P.O. use: Sustained-release and controlled-release preparations shouldn't be used for rapid control of ventricular arrhythmias, when therapeutic blood levels must be rapidly attained; in patients with cardiomyopathy or possible cardiac decompensation; or in those with severe renal impairment.
– For administration to young children, pharmacist may prepare disopyramide suspension from 100-mg capsules using cherry syrup. Suspension should be dispensed in amber glass bottles and protected from light.
I.V. use: Add 200 mg to 500 ml of compatible solution, such as normal saline solution or D_5W. Use an infusion pump to administer drug. Don't mix with other drugs; switch to P.O. therapy as soon as possible.
• Discontinue drug if heart block develops, if QRS complex widens by more than 25%, or if QTc interval lengthens by more than 25% above baseline; also notify prescriber.

Patient teaching
• When transferring patient from immediate-release to sustained-release capsules, advise him to take sustained-release capsule 6 hours after last immediate-release capsule was taken.
• Teach patient importance of taking drug on time and exactly as prescribed. This may require use of alarm clock for night doses.
• Advise patient to chew gum or hard candy to relieve dry mouth.
• Teach patient not crush or chew extended release tablets.

Evaluation
• Patient's ECG reveals that arrhythmia has been corrected.
• Patient develops no new arrhythmias as result of therapy.
• Patient and family state understanding of drug therapy.

disulfiram
(digh-SUL-fih-ram)
Antabuse

Pharmacologic class: aldehyde dehydrogenase inhibitor
Therapeutic class: alcohol deterrent
Pregnancy risk category: NR

Indications and dosages
▶ **Adjunct in management of chronic alcoholism.** *Adults:* 250 to 500 mg P.O. as single dose in morning for 1 to 2 weeks. Can be taken in evening if drowsiness occurs. Maintenance dosage is 125 to 500 mg P.O. daily (average dosage 250 mg) until permanent self-control is established. Treatment may continue for months or years.

How supplied
Tablets: 250 mg, 500 mg

Pharmacokinetics
Absorption: absorbed completely from GI tract.
Distribution: drug is highly lipid-soluble and initially localized in adipose tissue.
Metabolism: mostly oxidized in liver.
Excretion: primarily excreted in urine; 5% to 20% eliminated in feces.

Route	Onset	Peak	Duration
P.O.	1-2 hr	Unknown	< 14 days

Pharmacodynamics

Chemical effect: blocks oxidation of ethanol at acetaldehyde stage. Excess acetaldehyde produces highly unpleasant reaction in presence of even small amounts of ethanol.
Therapeutic effect: deters alcohol consumption.

Adverse reactions

CNS: drowsiness, headache, fatigue, delirium, depression, neuritis, peripheral neuritis, polyneuritis, restlessness, and psychotic reactions.
EENT: optic neuritis.
GI: metallic or garlic aftertaste.
GU: impotence.
Skin: acneiform or allergic dermatitis.
Other: ***disulfiram reaction.***

Interactions

Drug-drug. *Alfentanil:* prolonged duration of effect. Monitor patient closely.
Anticoagulants: increased anticoagulant effect. Adjust dosage of anticoagulant.
Bacampicillin: low levels of ethanol and acetaldehyde are produced by bacampicillin metabolism. Monitor patient closely.
CNS depressants: increased CNS depression. Use together cautiously.
Isoniazid: ataxia or marked change in behavior. Don't use concomitantly.
Metronidazole: psychotic reaction. Don't use concomitantly. Wait for 2 weeks following disulfram.
Midazolam: increased plasma levels of midazolam. Use together cautiously.
Paraldehyde: toxic levels of acetaldehyde. Don't use concomitantly.
Phenytoin: increased blood levels of phenytoin. Monitor phenytoin blood levels, and expect prescriber to adjust phenytoin dosages.
Tricyclic antidepressants, especially amitriptyline: transient delirium. Monitor patient closely.
Drug-herb. *Passion flower, pill-bearing spurge, pokeweed, squaw vine, squill, sundew, sweet flag, tormentil, valerian, yarrow:* disulfiram reaction may occur if herb form contains alcohol. Discourage concomitant use.
Drug-lifestyle. *Alcohol use (all sources, including cough syrups, liniments, shaving lotion, back-rub preparations):* may precipitate disulfiram reaction. Don't use concomitantly. Alcohol reaction may occur as long as 2 weeks after a single disulfiram dose; the longer patient remains on drug, the more sensitive he is to alcohol.

Contraindications and precautions

- Contraindicated during alcohol intoxication and within 12 hours of alcohol ingestion. Also contraindicated in patients hypersensitive to disulfiram or thiram derivatives used in pesticides and rubber vulcanization; patients with psychoses, myocardial disease, or coronary occlusion; and patients receiving metronidazole, paraldehyde, alcohol, or alcohol-containing preparations.
- Drug shouldn't be administered to pregnant women.
- Use with extreme caution in patients receiving concurrent phenytoin therapy and in patients with diabetes mellitus, hypothyroidism, seizure disorder, cerebral damage, nephritis, or hepatic cirrhosis or insufficiency.
- Use cautiously in breast-feeding women.
- Safety of drug hasn't been established in children.

NURSING CONSIDERATIONS

Assessment

- Obtain history of patient's alcoholism before therapy.
- Complete physical examination and laboratory studies, including CBC, chemistry panel, and transaminase determination, should precede therapy. Repeat physical examination and laboratory studies regularly, as ordered.
- Monitor effectiveness by assessing patient's abstinence from alcohol.
- Measure serum alcohol level weekly.
- Be alert for adverse reactions and drug interactions. Disulfiram reaction is precipitated by alcohol use, and may include flushing, throbbing headache, dyspnea, nausea, copious vomiting, diaphoresis, thirst, chest pain, palpitations, hyperventilation, hypotension, syncope, anxiety, weakness, blurred vision, and confusion. In severe reactions patient may experience respiratory depression, CV collapse, arrhythmias, MI, acute heart failure, seizures, unconsciousness, and death.

• Mild reactions may occur in sensitive patients with blood alcohol levels of 5 to 10 mg/dl; symptoms are fully developed at 50 mg/dl; unconsciousness typically occurs at 125- to 150-mg/dl level. Reaction may last from 30 minutes to several hours or as long as alcohol remains in blood.
• Evaluate patient's and family's knowledge of drug therapy.

Nursing diagnoses
• Ineffective health maintenance related to alcoholism
• Acute pain related to drug-induced headache
• Deficient knowledge related to drug therapy

Planning and implementation
• Use only under close medical and nursing supervision. Never administer until patient has abstained from alcohol for at least 12 hours. Patient should clearly understand consequences of disulfiram therapy and give permission for its use. Use drug only if patient is cooperative, well motivated, and receiving supportive psychiatric therapy.
• Administration is usually during the day, although drug may be given at night if drowsiness occurs. Establish lowered maintenance dose until permanent self-control is practiced. Keep in mind that treatment may continue for months or years.

Patient teaching
• Caution patient's family that disulfiram should never be given to the patient without his knowledge; severe reaction or death could result if the patient ingests alcohol.
• Warn patient to avoid all sources of alcohol (for example, sauces and cough syrups). Even external application of liniments, shaving lotion, and back-rub preparations may precipitate disulfiram reaction. Tell patient that alcohol reaction may occur as long as 2 weeks after single dose of disulfiram; the longer patient remains on drug, the more sensitive he becomes to alcohol.
• Tell patient to wear or carry medical identification identifying him as a disulfiram user.
• Reassure patient that drug-induced adverse reactions (unrelated to concomitant alcohol use), such as drowsiness, fatigue, impotence, headache, peripheral neuritis, and metallic or garlic taste, subside after about 2 weeks of therapy.

Evaluation
• Patient abstains from alcohol consumption.
• Patient's headache is relieved with mild analgesic therapy.
• Patient and family state understanding of drug therapy.

dobutamine hydrochloride
(doh-BYOO-tuh-meen high-droh-KLOR-ighd)
Dobutrex

Pharmacologic class: adrenergic, $beta_1$ agonist
Therapeutic class: inotropic agent
Pregnancy risk category: B

Indications and dosages
▶ **To increase cardiac output in short-term treatment of cardiac decompensation caused by depressed contractility, such as during refractory heart failure, and as adjunct in cardiac surgery.** *Adults:* 2 to 20 mcg/kg/minute I.V. infusion. Rarely, rates up to 40 mcg/kg/minute may be needed; however, such doses may worsen ischemia.

How supplied
Injection: 12.5 mg/ml in 20-ml vials

Pharmacokinetics
Absorption: not applicable with I.V. administration.
Distribution: widely distributed throughout body.
Metabolism: metabolized by liver.
Excretion: excreted mainly in urine with minor amounts in feces. *Half-life:* about 2 minutes.

Route	Onset	Peak	Duration
I.V.	1-2 min	≤ 10 min	< 5 min after drug stopped

Pharmacodynamics

Chemical effect: directly stimulates $beta_1$ receptors to increase myocardial contractility and stroke volume. At therapeutic dosages, drug decreases peripheral vascular resistance (afterload), reduces ventricular filling pressure (preload), and may facilitate AV node conduction.
Therapeutic effect: increases cardiac output.

Adverse reactions

CNS: headache.
CV: *increased heart rate,* ***hypertension,*** PVCs, angina, nonspecific chest pain, phlebitis, hypotension.
GI: nausea, vomiting.
Musculoskeletal: mild leg cramps or tingling sensation.
Respiratory: shortness of breath, ***asthma attacks.***
Other: ***anaphylaxis.***

Interactions

Drug-drug. *Beta blockers:* may antagonize dobutamine effects. Don't use together.
Bretylium: may potentiate action of vasopressors on adrenergic receptors; arrhythmias may result. Monitor ECG closely.
General anesthetics: greater risk of ventricular arrhythmias. Monitor patient closely.
Tricyclic antidepressants: may potentiate pressor response. Monitor patient closely.
Drug-herb. *Rue:* Increased inotropic potential. Monitor vital signs closely.

Contraindications and precautions

- Contraindicated in patients hypersensitive to drug or its components and in those with idiopathic hypertrophic subaortic stenosis.
- Use cautiously in patients with history of hypertension. Drug may cause exaggerated pressor response.
- Safety of drug hasn't been established in pregnant or breast-feeding women and in children.

NURSING CONSIDERATIONS

Assessment

- Assess patient's condition before therapy and regularly thereafter.
- Continuously monitor ECG, blood pressure, pulmonary capillary wedge pressure, cardiac condition, and urine output.
- Monitor serum electrolyte levels, as ordered. Drug may lower serum potassium level.
- Be alert for adverse reactions and drug interactions.
- Evaluate patient's and family's knowledge of drug therapy.

Nursing diagnoses

- Decreased cardiac output related to underlying condition
- Acute pain related to headache
- Deficient knowledge related to drug therapy

Planning and implementation

- Before starting dobutamine, correct hypovolemia with plasma volume expanders, as ordered.
- Administer cardiac glycoside before dobutamine, as ordered. Because drug increases AV node conduction, patients with atrial fibrillation may develop rapid ventricular rate.
- Administer drug using central venous catheter or large peripheral vein. Titrate infusion according to prescriber's orders and patient's condition. Use infusion pump.
- Dilute concentrate for injection before administration. Compatible solutions include D_5W, half-normal saline solution injection, normal saline solution injection, and lactated Ringer's injection. The contents of one vial (250 mg) diluted with 1,000 ml of solution yield 250 mcg/ml; diluted with 500 ml, 500 mcg/ml; diluted with 250 ml, 1,000 mcg/ml. Concentration shouldn't exceed 5 mg/ml.
- Avoid extravasation; it may cause inflammatory response.

ALERT Don't administer through same I.V. line with other drugs. Drug is incompatible with heparin, hydrocortisone sodium succinate, cefazolin, cefamandole, neutral cephalothin, penicillin, and ethacrynate sodium.

- Don't mix with sodium bicarbonate injection because drug is incompatible with alkaline solutions.
- Keep in mind that I.V. solutions remain stable for 24 hours.
- Oxidation of drug may slightly discolor admixtures containing dobutamine. This

doesn't indicate significant loss of potency, provided drug is used within 24 hours of reconstitution.
- Change I.V. sites regularly to avoid phlebitis.

Patient teaching
- Tell patient to report chest pain, shortness of breath, and headache.

Evaluation
- Patient regains adequate cardiac output exhibited by stable vital signs, normal urine output, and clear mental status.
- Patient's headache is relieved with analgesic administration.
- Patient and family state understanding of drug therapy.

docetaxel
(doks-uh-TAKX-ul)
Taxotere

Pharmacologic class: taxoid antineoplastic
Therapeutic class: antineoplastic
Pregnancy risk category: D

Indications and dosages
▶ **Treatment of patients with locally advanced or metastatic breast cancer who have progressed during anthracycline-based therapy or have relapsed during anthracycline-based adjuvant therapy.** *Adults:* 60 to 100 mg/m^2 I.V. over 1 hour q 3 weeks.
▶ **Locally advanced or metastatic non-small-cell lung cancer after failure of platinum-based chemotherapy.** *Adults:* 75 mg/m^2 I.V. over 1 hour every 3 weeks. Premedicate with dexamethasone 16 mg daily for 3 days, starting 1 day before docetaxel therapy.

How supplied
Injection: 20 mg, 80 mg

Pharmacokinetics
Absorption: not applicable with I.V. administration.
Distribution: 94% is protein-bound.
Metabolism: partly by liver.
Excretion: mainly in feces.

Route	Onset	Peak	Duration
I.V.	Immediate	Unknown	Unknown

Pharmacodynamics
Chemical effect: disrupts the microtubular network essential for mitotic and interphase cellular functions.
Therapeutic effect: inhibits mitosis, producing antineoplastic effect.

Adverse reactions
CNS: *asthenia,* paresthesia, dysesthesia, weakness.
CV: *fluid retention,* hypotension.
GI: *stomatitis, nausea, vomiting, diarrhea.*
Hematologic: *anemia,* **NEUTROPENIA, FEBRILE NEUTROPENIA, MYELOSUPPRESSION, LEUKOPENIA, THROMBOCYTOPENIA,** ***septic and nonseptic death.***
Hepatic: increased liver function test results.
Musculoskeletal: back pain, *myalgia,* arthralgia.
Respiratory: dyspnea.
Skin: *alopecia,* skin eruptions, desquamation, nail pigmentation alterations, nail pain, flushing, rash.
Other: **HYPERSENSITIVITY REACTIONS,** infection, pain, chest tightness, drug fever, chills.

Interactions
Drug-drug. *Agents that are induced, inhibited, or metabolized by cytochrome P-450 3A4 (cyclosporin, ketoconazole, erythromycin, troleandomycin):* may modify docetaxel metabolism when given together. Use cautiously.

Contraindications and precautions
- Contraindicated in patients hypersensitive to drug or to other polysorbate 80–containing drugs and in those with neutrophil counts below 1,500 cells/mm^3.

NURSING CONSIDERATIONS

Assessment
- Premedicate patient with oral corticosteroids.

• Monitor blood count frequently during therapy.
• Evaluate patient's and family's knowledge of drug therapy.

Nursing diagnoses
• Ineffective health maintenance related to neoplastic disease
• Deficient knowledge related to drug therapy

Planning and implementation
• For patients with febrile neutropenia, neutrophils below 500 cells/mm^3 for more than 1 week, severe or cumulative cutaneous reactions, or other grade 3 or 4 nonhematologic toxicities during therapy, docetaxel should be discontinued until toxicity is resolved and then restarted at 55 mg/m^2. For patients who develop grade 3 or higher peripheral neuropathy, docetaxel should be discontinued entirely.
• Dilute drug with diluent supplied before administration. Allow drug and diluent to stand at room temperature for 5 minutes before mixing. After adding diluent contents to vial, rotate vial gently for 15 seconds. Let solution stand for few minutes for foam to dissipate.
• To prepare solution for infusion, withdraw required amount of premixed solution from vial and inject it into 250 ml normal saline solution or D_5W to yield 0.3 to 0.9 mg/ml.
• Wear gloves during drug preparation and administration.

Patient teaching
• Warn patient that alopecia occurs in almost 80% of patients.
• Tell patient to promptly report sore throat, fever, or unusual bruising or bleeding and signs of fluid retention.

Evaluation
• Patient shows positive response to drug.
• Patient and family state understanding of drug therapy.

docusate calcium (dioctyl calcium sulfosuccinate)
(DOK-yoo-sayt KAL-see-um)
DC Softgels†, Pro-Cal-Sof†, Surfak†

docusate potassium (dioctyl potassium sulfosuccinate)
Diocto-K†, Kasof†

docusate sodium (dioctyl sodium sulfosuccinate)
Colace†, Coloxyl ◇, Coloxyl Enema Concentrate ◇, Dialose†, Diocto†, Dioeze†, Disonate†, DOK†, DOS Softgels†, Doxinate†, D-S-S†, Modane Soft†, Pro-Sof†, Regulax SS†, Regulex ♦ †, Regutol†, Therevac Plus†, Therevac-SB†

Pharmacologic class: surfactant
Therapeutic class: emollient laxative
Pregnancy risk category: C

Indications and dosages
▶ **Stool softener.** *Adults and children over age 12:* 50 to 360 mg P.O. daily until bowel movements are normal. Or, give enema (where available). Dilute 1:24 with sterile water before administration, and give 100 to 150 ml (retention enema), 300 to 500 ml (evacuation enema), or 0.5 to 1.5 liters (flushing enema).
Children ages 6 to 12: 40 to 120 mg docusate sodium P.O. daily.
Children ages 3 to 6: 20 to 60 mg docusate sodium P.O. daily.
Children under age 3: 10 to 40 mg docusate sodium P.O. daily.

Higher dosages used for initial therapy. Dosage adjusted to individual response. Usual dosage in children and adults with minimal needs is 50 to 150 mg (docusate calcium) P.O. daily.

How supplied
docusate calcium
Capsules: 50 mg†, 240 mg†
docusate potassium
Capsules: 100 mg†, 240 mg†

docusate sodium
Tablets: 100 mg†
Capsules: 50 mg†, 60 mg†, 100 mg†, 240 mg†, 250 mg†
Oral liquid: 150 mg/15 ml†
Oral solution: 50 mg/ml†
Syrup: 20 mg/5ml*†, 50 mg/15 ml†, 60 mg/15 ml†, 100 mg/30 ml†
Enema concentrate: 18 g/100 ml (must be diluted) ◊

Pharmacokinetics

Absorption: absorbed minimally in duodenum and jejunum.
Distribution: distributed primarily locally, in gut.
Metabolism: none.
Excretion: excreted in feces.

Route	Onset	Peak	Duration
P.O.	Varies	Varies	24-72 hr
P.R.	Unknown	Unknown	Unknown

Pharmacodynamics

Chemical effect: reduces surface tension of interfacing liquid contents of bowel. This detergent activity promotes incorporation of additional liquid into stool, thus forming softer mass.
Therapeutic effect: softens stool.

Adverse reactions

EENT: throat irritation.
GI: bitter taste, mild abdominal cramping, diarrhea, laxative dependence with long-term or excessive use.

Interactions

Drug-drug. *Mineral oil:* may increase mineral oil absorption and cause toxicity and lipoid pneumonia. Separate administration times.

Contraindications and precautions

- Contraindicated in patients hypersensitive to drug and in those with intestinal obstruction, undiagnosed abdominal pain, signs of appendicitis, fecal impaction, or acute surgical abdomen.
- Use cautiously in pregnant women.

NURSING CONSIDERATIONS

Assessment
- Obtain history of patient's bowel patterns before therapy, and reassess regularly thereafter.
- Before giving drug for constipation, determine if patient has adequate fluid intake, exercise, and diet.
- Be alert for adverse reactions and drug interactions.
- Evaluate patient's and family's knowledge of drug therapy.

Nursing diagnoses
- Constipation related to underlying condition
- Diarrhea related to prolonged or excessive use of drug
- Deficient knowledge related to drug therapy

Planning and implementation
P.O. use: Give liquid in milk, fruit juice, or infant formula to mask bitter taste.
P.R. use: Follow manufacturer's directions.
- Drug is laxative of choice for patients who shouldn't strain during defecation, including patients recovering from MI or rectal surgery, for those with rectal or anal disease that makes passage of firm stool difficult, and for those with postpartum constipation.
- Store drug at 59° to 86° F (15° to 30° C), and protect liquid from light.
- Discontinue if abdominal cramping occurs, and notify prescriber; docusate doesn't stimulate intestinal peristaltic movements.

Patient teaching
- Teach patient about dietary sources of bulk, which include bran and other cereals, fresh fruit, and vegetables.
- Instruct patient to use only occasionally and not to use for more than 1 week without prescriber's knowledge.
- Tell patient to discontinue if severe cramping occurs and notify prescriber.

Evaluation
- Patient's constipation is relieved.
- Patient remains free from diarrhea during therapy.

• Patient and family state understanding of drug therapy.

dofetilide

(doh-FET-eh-lighd)
Tikosyn

Pharmacologic class: antiarrhythmic
Therapeutic class: class III antiarrhythmic
Pregnancy risk category: C

Indications and dosages

▶ **Maintenance of normal sinus rhythm in patients with symptomatic atrial fibrillation or atrial flutter of greater than one week's duration who have been converted to normal sinus rhythm; conversion of atrial fibrillation and atrial flutter to normal sinus rhythm.** *Adults:* dosage is individualized and is based on creatinine clearance and QTc interval, which must be determined before first dose (QT interval should be used if heart rate is less than 60 beats/minute). Usual recommended dosage is 500 mcg b.i.d. for patients with creatinine clearance above 60 ml/minute.

How supplied

Distributed only to hospitals and other institutions confirmed to have received applicable dosing and treatment initiation programs. Inpatient and subsequent outpatient discharge and refill prescriptions are filled only upon confirmation that prescriber has received these programs.
Capsules: 125 mcg (0.125 mg), 250 mcg (0.25 mg), 500 mcg (0.5 mg)

Pharmacokinetics

Absorption: bioavailability after oral administration is greater than 90%; plasma levels peak at 2 to 3 hours. Steady-state plasma levels are achieved in 2 to 3 days. Absorption is unaffected by food or antacid.
Distribution: drug is widely distributed throughout the body and has a volume of distribution of 3 L/kg. Plasma protein binding is 60% to 70%.
Metabolism: drug is metabolized to a small extent by the CYP3A4 isoenzyme of the cytochrome P-450 system of the liver.
Excretion: about 80% is excreted in the urine, of which 80% is excreted as unchanged drug with the remaining 20% consisting of inactive or minimally active metabolites.

Route	Onset	Peak	Duration
P.O.	Unknown	2-3 hr	Unknown

Pharmacodynamics

Chemical effect: as a class II antiarrhythmic, dofetilide prolongs repolarization without affecting conduction velocity by blocking the cardiac ion channel carrying potassium current. No effect is seen on sodium channels, alpha-adrenergic receptors, or beta-adrenergic receptors.
Therapeutic effect: maintenance of normal sinus rhythm in patients with symptomatic atrial fibrillation or atrial flutter who have been converted to normal sinus rhythm; conversion of atrial fibrillation and atrial flutter to normal sinus rhythm.

Adverse reactions

CNS: *headache,* dizziness, insomnia, anxiety, migraine, cerebral ischemia, CVA, asthenia, paresthesia, syncope.
CV: ***ventricular fibrillation,*** ventricular tachycardia, ***torsades de pointes,*** AV block, bundle branch block, ***heart block,*** *chest pain,* angina, atrial fibrillation, hypertension, palpitations, ***bradycardia,*** edema, ***cardiac arrest, MI.***
EENT: facial paralysis.
GI: nausea, diarrhea, abdominal pain.
GU: urinary tract infection.
Hepatic: liver damage.
Musculoskeletal: back pain, arthralgia.
Respiratory: respiratory tract infection, dyspnea, increased cough.
Skin: rash, sweating.
Other: flulike syndrome, ***angioedema***, peripheral edema.

Interactions

Drug-drug. *Amiodarone, diltiazem, macrolide antibiotics, nefazadone, norfloxacin, protease inhibitors, quinine, serotonin reuptake inhib-*

itors, zafirlukast: possible increased dofetilide plasma levels. Use with extreme caution.
Cimetidine, ketoconazole, sulfamethozaxole, trimethoprim, verapamil: increased plasma levels of dofetilide. Concomitant use is contraindicated.
Inhibitors of renal cationic secretion (prochlorperazine, megestrol): may increase dofetilide levels. Avoid concomitant use.
Inhibitors of CYP3A4 (macrolide antibiotics, azole antifungals, protease inhibitors, serotonin reuptake inhibitors, amiodarone, cannabinoids, diltiazem, nefazadone, norfloxacin, quinine, zafirlukast): may decrease metabolism and increase dofetilide levels. Use together cautiously.
Triamterene, metformin, amiloride: may increase dofetilide levels. Use cautiously together.
Drug-food. *Grapefruit juice:* possible decreased hepatic metabolism and increased plasma levels. Avoid use together.

Contraindications and precautions

- Dofetilide is contraindicated in patients with congenital or acquired long-QT syndromes. Dofetilide shouldn't be used in patients with baseline QT or QTc interval greater than 440 msec (500 msec in patients with ventricular conduction abnormalities).
- Dofetilide is contraindicated in patients with severe renal impairment (creatinine clearance below 20 ml/min).
- Dofetilide is contraindicated in patients hypersensitive to drug and in those receiving verapamil, cimetidine, trimethoprim (alone or with sulfamethoxazole), or ketoconazole.
- Use cautiously in patients with severe hepatic impairment.

NURSING CONSIDERATIONS

Assessment

- Obtain accurate medication list from patient before starting dofetilide; previous antiarrhythmic therapy should be withdrawn under careful monitoring for a minimum of three plasma half-lives. Dofetilide shouldn't be administered after amiodarone therapy until amiodarone levels are below 0.3 mcg/ml or until amiodarone has been withdrawn for at least 3 months.
- Assess patient's QTc interval, cardiac rhythm, and vital signs before starting medication. Prolongation of the QTc interval requires subsequent dosage adjustments or discontinuation. Continuous ECG monitoring is required for a minimum of 3 days.
- Obtain potassium level before starting therapy and then regularly thereafter. Hypokalemia and hypomagnesemia may occur when giving potassium-depleting diuretics, increasing the risk of torsades de pointes. Potassium levels should be within the normal range before giving dofetilide and maintained in a normal range.
- Monitor patient for prolonged diarrhea, sweating, and vomiting; report them to prescriber because electrolyte imbalance may increase the risk of arrhythmias.
- Patient with creatinine clearance between 20 and 60 ml/minute requires a reduced dosage.
- Monitor renal function and QTc interval every 3 months.
- Evaluate patient's and family's knowledge of drug therapy.

Nursing diagnoses

- Decreased cardiac output related to underlying arrhythmia
- Risk for injury related to drug-induced adverse reactions
- Deficient knowledge related to drug therapy

Planning and implementation

- If patient doesn't convert to normal sinus rhythm within 24 hours after starting dofetilide, electrical conversion should be considered.
- Patient shouldn't be discharged within 12 hours of conversion to normal sinus rhythm.
- If dofetilide must be discontinued to allow administration of other interacting drugs, a washout period of at least 2 days should be observed before starting other drug.

Patient teaching

- Inform the patient to notify prescriber about any change in prescription drugs, OTC medications, or herbal remedies.

• Urge patient to immediately report excessive or prolonged diarrhea, sweating, vomiting, or loss of appetite or thirst to prescriber.
• Inform the patient that dofetilide can be taken without regard to meals or antacids.
• Tell patient not to take drug with grapefruit juice.
• Caution patient not to use OTC Tagamet-HB for ulcers or heartburn. Explain that antacids and such OTC acid reducers as Zantac 75 mg, Pepcid, Axid, and Prevacid are acceptable.
• Instruct woman to notify prescriber about planned, suspected, or known pregnancy.
• Advise patient not to breast-feed while taking dofetilide.
• If patient misses dose, tell him to skip it and wait for the next scheduled dose. Caution against doubling the dose.

Evaluation

• Patient maintains normal sinus rhythm.
• Patient has no injury as a result of drug-induced adverse reactions.
• Patient and family state understanding of drug therapy.

dolasetron mesylate

(doh-LEH-seh-trohn MES-ih layt)
Anzemet

Pharmacologic class: selective serotonin (5-HT_3) receptor antagonist
Therapeutic class: antiemetic
Pregnancy risk category: B

Indications and dosages

▶ **Prevention of nausea and vomiting from cancer chemotherapy.** *Adults:* 100 mg P.O. given as a single dose 1 hour before chemotherapy. Or, 1.8 mg/kg (or a fixed dose of 100 mg) as a single I.V. dose given 30 minutes before chemotherapy.
Children ages 2 to 16: 1.8 mg/kg P.O. 1 hour before chemotherapy. Or, 1.8 mg/kg as single I.V. dose 30 minutes before chemotherapy. Injectable form can be mixed with apple juice and administered P.O. Maximum dose is 100 mg.

▶ **Prevention of postoperative nausea and vomiting.** *Adults:* 100 mg P.O. within 2 hours before surgery. Or, 12.5 mg as single I.V. dose about 15 minutes before cessation of anesthesia.
Children ages 2 to 16: 1.2 mg/kg P.O. given within 2 hours before surgery, up to maximum of 100 mg. Or, 0.35 mg/ kg (up to 12.5 mg) as single I.V. dose about 15 minutes before cessation of anesthesia. Injectable form can be mixed with apple juice and administered P.O.

▶ **Treatment of postoperative nausea and vomiting (I.V. form).** *Adults:* 12.5 mg as a single I.V. dose as soon as nausea or vomiting begins.
Children ages 2 to 16: 0.35 mg/kg, up to maximum dose of 12.5 mg, as a single I.V. dose as soon as nausea or vomiting begins.

How supplied

Tablets: 50 mg, 100 mg
Injection: 20 mg/ml as 12.5 mg/0.625 ml ampule or 100 mg/5 ml vials

Pharmacokinetics

Absorption: rapid for hydrodolasetron, an active metabolite that has an absolute bioavailability of 75%. Absorption of the parent compound is rarely seen.
Distribution: widely distributed with 69% to 77% bound to plasma protein.
Metabolism: dolasetron is metabolized to an active metabolite, hydrodolasetron, by carbonyl reductase. Rarely detected in plasma because of rapid and complete metabolism.
Excretion: about two-thirds of hydrodolasetron is recovered in urine; one-third in feces. *Half-life:* 8 hours.

Route	Onset	Peak	Duration
P.O.	Rapid	1 hr	8 hr
I.V.	Rapid	36 min	7 hr

Pharmacodynamics

Chemical effect: selective serotonin (5-HT_3) receptor antagonist that blocks the action of serotonin, thereby preventing serotonin from stimulating the vomiting reflex.
Therapeutic effect: prevents nausea and vomiting.

Adverse reactions

CNS: *headache*, dizziness, drowsiness, fatigue.
CV: ***arrhythmias, bradycardia,*** ECG changes, hypotension, hypertension, tachycardia.
GI: *diarrhea*, dyspepsia, abdominal pain, constipation, anorexia.
GU: oliguria, urine retention.
Hepatic: elevated liver function test results.
Skin: pruritus, rash.
Other: fever, chills, pain at injection site.

Interactions

Drug-drug. *Drugs that prolong ECG intervals (such as antiarrhythmics):* increased risk of arrhythmia. Monitor patient closely.
Drugs that inhibit P-450 enzymes (such as cimetidine): increased hydrodolasetron levels. Monitor patient for adverse effects.
Drugs that induce P-450 enzymes (such as rifampin): decreased hydrodolasetron levels. Monitor patient for decreased efficacy of drug.

Contraindications and precautions

- Contraindicated in patients hypersensitive to drug.
- Administer cautiously in patients who have or may develop prolonged cardiac conduction intervals, such as those with electrolyte abnormalities, history of arrhythmias, and cumulative high-dose anthracycline therapy.
- Drug isn't recommended for use in children under age 2. Use cautiously in breast-feeding women.

NURSING CONSIDERATIONS

Assessment

- Assess patient for history of nausea and vomiting related to chemotherapy or postoperative recovery.
- Be alert for potential adverse reactions and drug interactions.
- Monitor ECG carefully in patients who have or may develop prolonged cardiac conduction intervals.
- Evaluate patient's and family's knowledge of drug therapy.

Nursing diagnoses

- Imbalanced nutrition: less than body requirements, related to nausea and vomiting
- Risk for injury related to drug-induced adverse CNS reaction
- Deficient knowledge related to drug therapy

Planning and implementation

P.O. use: Injection for P.O. administration is stable in apple juice for 2 hours at room temperature.
I.V. use: Injection can be infused as rapidly as 100 mg/30 seconds or diluted in 50 ml of compatible solution and infused over 15 minutes.
- Discontinue drug and notify prescriber immediately if arrhythmia develops.

Patient teaching
- Tell patient about potential adverse effects.
- Instruct patient not to mix injection in juice for P.O. use until just before dosing.
- Tell patient to report nausea or vomiting.

Evaluation

- Patient has no nausea and vomiting.
- Patient is free from injury.
- Patient and family state understanding of drug therapy

donepezil hydrochloride

(doh-NEH-peh-zil high-droh-KLOR-ighd)
Aricept

Pharmacologic class: reversible inhibitor of acetylcholinesterase
Therapeutic class: psychotherapeutic agent for Alzheimer's disease
Pregnancy risk category: C

Indications and dosages

▶ **Mild to moderate dementia of the Alzheimer's type.** *Adults:* initially, 5 mg P.O. daily h.s. After 4 to 6 weeks, may increase dosage to 10 mg daily.

How supplied

Tablets: 5 mg, 10 mg

Pharmacokinetics

Absorption: well absorbed.
Distribution: 96% plasma protein–bound, mainly to albumin.
Metabolism: extensively metabolized.
Excretion: in urine and feces.

Route	Onset	Peak	Duration
P.O.	Unknown	3-4 hr	Unknown

Pharmacodynamics

Chemical effect: reversibly inhibits acetylcholinesterase in the CNS, thereby increasing the acetylcholine level.
Therapeutic effect: temporarily improves cognitive function in patients with Alzheimer's disease.

Adverse reactions

CNS: *headache, insomnia*, dizziness, depression, abnormal dreams, somnolence, ***seizures,*** tremor, irritability, paresthesia, aggression, vertigo, ataxia, restlessness, abnormal crying, fatigue, nervousness, aphasia.
CV: syncope, chest pain, hypertension, vasodilation, atrial fibrillation, hot flushes, hypotension.
EENT: cataracts, *sore throat,* blurred vision, eye irritation.
GI: *nausea, diarrhea*, vomiting, anorexia, fecal incontinence, GI bleeding, bloating, epigastric pain.
GU: frequent urination.
Hematologic: ecchymosis.
Metabolic: weight decrease.
Musculoskeletal: muscle cramps, arthritis, toothache, bone fracture.
Respiratory: *dyspnea, bronchitis.*
Skin: pruritus, urticaria, diaphoresis.
Other: increased libido, pain, accident, influenza, dehydration.

Interactions

Drug-drug. *Anticholinergics:* may interfere with anticholinergic activity. Monitor patient.
Bethanechol, succinylcholine: additive effects. Monitor patient closely.
Carbamazepine, dexamethasone, phenytoin, phenobarbital, rifampin: may increase rate of donepezil elimination. Monitor patient.
Cholinomimetics, cholinesterase inhibitors: synergistic effect. Monitor patient closely.
Drug-herb. *Jaborandi tree, pill-bearing spurge:* additive effect may occur when combined, and risk of toxicity may be increased. Discourage concomitant use.

Contraindications and precautions

- Contraindicated in patients hypersensitive to drug or to piperidine derivatives.
- Use cautiously in patients with history of ulcer disease, CV disease, asthma or obstructive pulmonary disease, or urinary outflow impairment. Also use cautiously in those currently taking NSAIDs.

NURSING CONSIDERATIONS

Assessment

- Monitor patient for symptoms of active or occult GI bleeding.
- Evaluate patient's and family's knowledge of drug therapy.

Nursing diagnoses

- Risk for injury related to adverse effects of drug
- Deficient knowledge related to drug therapy

Planning and implementation

- Use in pregnancy only if benefit justifies risk to fetus. Tell patient to avoid breast-feeding during therapy.
- Safety and effectiveness in children haven't been established.

Patient teaching

- Explain that drug doesn't alter underlying degenerative disease but can alleviate symptoms.
- Tell caregiver to give drug in the evening, just before bedtime.
- Advise patient and caregiver to immediately report significant adverse effects or changes in overall health status.
- Tell caregiver to inform health-care team that patient is taking drug before patient receives anesthesia.

Evaluation

- Patient remains free from injury.

• Patient and family state understanding of drug therapy.

dopamine hydrochloride

(DOH-puh-meen high-droh-KLOR-ighd)
Intropin, Revimine ♦

Pharmacologic class: adrenergic
Therapeutic class: inotropic, vasopressor
Pregnancy risk category: C

Indications and dosages

▶ **To treat shock and correct hemodynamic imbalances; to improve perfusion to vital organs; to increase cardiac output; to correct hypotension.** *Adults:* initially, 1 to 5 mcg/kg/minute by I.V. infusion. Dosage adjusted to desired hemodynamic or renal response, increased by 1 to 4 mcg/kg/minute at 10- to 30-minute intervals.

How supplied

Injection: 40 mg/ml, 80 mg/ml, 160 mg/ml as concentrate for injection for I.V. infusion; 0.8 mg/ml (200 or 400 mg) in D_5W; 1.6 mg/ml (400 or 800 mg) in D_5W, 3.2 mg/ml (800 mg) in D_5W as parenteral injection for I.V. infusion.

Pharmacokinetics

Absorption: not applicable with I.V. administration.
Distribution: widely distributed throughout body; doesn't cross blood-brain barrier.
Metabolism: metabolized to inactive compounds in liver, kidneys, and plasma.
Excretion: excreted in urine, mainly as its metabolites. *Half-life:* about 9 minutes.

Route	Onset	Peak	Duration
I.V.	≤ 5 min	Unknown	≤ 10 min after drug stopped

Pharmacodynamics

Chemical effect: stimulates dopaminergic, beta-adrenergic, and alpha-adrenergic receptors of sympathetic nervous system.
Therapeutic effect: increases cardiac output and blood pressure.

Adverse reactions

CNS: headache.
CV: ***arrhythmias,*** ectopic beats, tachycardia, anginal pain, palpitations, ***hypotension, bradycardia,*** widening of QRS complex, conduction disturbances, vasoconstriction, hypertension.
GI: nausea, vomiting.
Respiratory: ***asthma attacks,*** dyspnea.
Skin: necrosis, tissue sloughing with extravasation, piloerection.
Other: ***anaphylaxis,*** azotemia.

Interactions

Drug-drug. *Alpha-adrenergic blockers, beta blockers:* may antagonize dopamine effects. Monitor patient closely.
Ergot alkaloids: extreme elevations in blood pressure. Don't use together.
Inhaled anesthetics: increased risk of arrhythmias or hypertension. Monitor patient closely.
MAO inhibitors: may cause hypertensive crisis. Avoid if possible.
Oxytocic drugs: potentiation of pressor effect resulting in severe hypertension. Avoid if possible.
Phenytoin: may lower blood pressure of dopamine-stabilized patients. Monitor patient carefully.
Tricyclic antidepressants: potentiate adverse sympathomimetic effects of dopamine. Monitor patient closely.

Contraindications and precautions

• Contraindicated in patients with uncorrected tachyarrhythmias, pheochromocytoma, or ventricular fibrillation.
• Use cautiously in patients with occlusive vascular disease, cold injuries, diabetic endarteritis, and arterial embolism; in pregnant women; and in those taking MAO inhibitors.
• Safety of drug hasn't been established in breast-feeding women and in children.

NURSING CONSIDERATIONS

Assessment

- Obtain history of patient's underlying condition before therapy.
- During infusion, frequently monitor ECG, blood pressure, cardiac output, central venous pressure, pulmonary capillary wedge pressure, pulse rate, urine output, and color and temperature of limbs.
- Be alert for adverse reactions and drug interactions.
- Be aware that acidosis decreases effectiveness of dopamine.
- After drug is stopped, watch closely for sudden drop in blood pressure.
- Evaluate patient's and family's knowledge of drug therapy.

Nursing diagnoses

- Ineffective tissue perfusion (cerebral, cardiopulmonary, and renal) related to underlying condition
- Risk for injury related to drug-induced adverse reactions
- Deficient knowledge related to drug therapy

Planning and implementation

- Drug isn't used to treat blood or fluid volume deficit. If deficit exists, replace fluid before administering vasopressors, as ordered.
- Use central line or large vein, such as in antecubital fossa, to minimize risk of extravasation.
- Don't mix with alkaline solutions. Use D_5W, normal saline solution, or combination of D_5W and normal saline solution. Mix just before use.
- Don't mix other drugs in I.V. container with dopamine. Don't give alkaline drugs (for example, sodium bicarbonate or phenytoin sodium) through I.V. line containing dopamine.
- Use continuous infusion pump to regulate flow rate.
- Keep in mind that patient response depends on dosage and pharmacologic effect. Dosages of 0.5 to 2 mcg/kg/minute stimulate mainly dopamine receptors and dilate renal vasculature. Dosages of 2 to 10 mcg/kg/minute stimulate beta-adrenergic receptors for positive inotropic effect. Higher dosages also stimulate alpha-adrenergic receptors, causing vasoconstriction and increased blood pressure.
- Most patients are satisfactorily maintained on dosages below 20 mcg/kg/minute.
- Taper dosage slowly to evaluate stability of blood pressure, as ordered.
- Discard after 24 hours or earlier if solution is discolored.
- If disproportionate rise in diastolic pressure (a marked decrease in pulse pressure) is observed in patient receiving dopamine, decrease infusion rate, as ordered, and watch carefully for further evidence of predominant vasoconstrictor activity, unless such effect is desired.
- If extravasation occurs, stop infusion immediately and call prescriber. Extravasation may require treatment by infiltration of area with 5 to 10 mg of phentolamine and 10 to 15 ml of normal saline solution.
- If adverse reactions develop, notify prescriber, who will adjust or discontinue dosage. Also, if urine flow decreases without hypotension, notify prescriber because dosage may need to be reduced.

Patient teaching

- Emphasize importance of reporting discomfort at I.V. site immediately.

Evaluation

- Patient regains adequate cerebral, cardiopulmonary, and renal tissue perfusion.
- Patient doesn't experience injury as result of drug-induced adverse reactions.
- Patient and family state understanding of drug therapy.

doxacurium chloride

(doks-uh-KYOO-ree-um KLOR-ighd)
Nuromax

Pharmacologic class: nondepolarizing neuromuscular blocker
Therapeutic class: skeletal muscle relaxant
Pregnancy risk category: C

Indications and dosages

▶ **To provide skeletal muscle relaxation during surgery as adjunct to general anesthesia.**

Dosage is highly individualized. All times of onset and duration of neuromuscular blockade are averages and considerable individual variation is normal.
Adults: 0.05 mg/kg rapid I.V. produces adequate conditions for endotracheal intubation in 5 minutes in about 90% of patients when used as part of thiopental-narcotic induction technique. Lower doses may require longer delay before intubation is possible. Neuromuscular blockade at this dose lasts for average of 100 minutes.
Children over age 2: initial dose of 0.03 mg/kg I.V. administered during halothane anesthesia produces effective blockade in 7 minutes with duration of 30 minutes. Under same conditions, 0.05 mg/kg produces blockade in 4 minutes with duration of 45 minutes.
▶ **Maintenance of neuromuscular blockade during long procedures.** *Adults and children:* after initial dose of 0.05 mg/kg I.V., maintenance doses of 0.005 to 0.01 mg/kg prolong neuromuscular blockade for an average of 30 minutes. Children usually require more frequent administration of maintenance doses.

How supplied

Injection: 1 mg/ml

Pharmacokinetics

Absorption: not applicable with I.V. administration.
Distribution: plasma protein–binding is about 30% in human plasma.
Metabolism: thought not to be metabolized.
Excretion: eliminated primarily unchanged in urine and bile. *Half-life:* 86 to 123 minutes.

Route	Onset	Peak	Duration
I.V.	≤ 5 min	3-9 min	1-4 hr

Pharmacodynamics

Chemical effect: competes with acetylcholine for receptor sites at motor end plate. Because this action may be antagonized by cholinesterase inhibitors, doxacurium is considered a competitive antagonist.
Therapeutic effect: relaxes skeletal muscles.

Adverse reactions

Respiratory: dyspnea, ***respiratory depression, respiratory insufficiency or apnea.***
Musculoskeletal: prolonged muscle weakness.

Interactions

Drug-drug. *Aminoglycosides (gentamicin, kanamycin, neomycin, streptomycin), bacitracin, colistimethate, colistin, polymyxin B, tetracyclines:* potentiated neuromuscular blockade leading to increased skeletal muscle relaxation and prolongation of effect. Use together cautiously.
Carbamazepine, phenytoin: may prolong time to maximal block or shorten duration of block with neuromuscular blocking agents. Monitor patient closely.
Inhaled anesthetics, quinidine: may enhance activity or prolong action of nondepolarizing neuromuscular blockers. Monitor patient closely.
Magnesium salts: may enhance neuromuscular blockade. Monitor patient for excessive weakness.

Contraindications and precautions

- Contraindicated in patients hypersensitive to drug. Also contraindicated in neonates; drug contains benzyl ethanol, which has been linked to fatalities in neonates.
- Use cautiously, possibly at reduced dosage, in debilitated patients; patients with metastatic cancer, severe electrolyte disturbances, or neuromuscular diseases; and patients in whom neuromuscular blockade may be difficult to initiate or reverse. Patients with myasthenia gravis or myasthenic syndrome (Eaton-Lambert syndrome) are particularly sensitive to effects of nondepolarizing relaxants. Shorter-acting agents are recommended for use in such patients.
- Use cautiously in breast-feeding women.
- Because of lack of data supporting safety, this drug isn't recommended for patients requiring prolonged mechanical ventilation in intensive care unit, before or after administration of nondepolarizing neuromuscular blocking agents, or during cesarean delivery.
- Safety of drug hasn't been established in children under age 2.

NURSING CONSIDERATIONS

Assessment
- Obtain history of patient's underlying condition before therapy.
- Monitor patient continuously throughout drug administration.
- Be alert for adverse reactions and drug interactions.
- Because drug has minimal vagolytic action, watch for bradycardia, which may occur during anesthesia.
- Monitor respirations closely until patient is fully recovered from neuromuscular blockade, as evidenced by tests of muscle strength (hand grip, head lift, and ability to cough).
- Evaluate patient's and family's knowledge of drug therapy.

Nursing diagnoses
- Ineffective health maintenance related to underlying condition
- Impaired spontaneous ventilation related to drug's effects on respiratory muscles
- Deficient knowledge related to drug therapy

Planning and implementation
- To avoid distress to patient, don't administer drug until patient's consciousness is obtunded by general anesthetic. Doxacurium has no effect on consciousness or pain threshold.
- Dosage should be adjusted to ideal body weight in obese patients (patients 30% or more above their ideal weight) to avoid prolonged neuromuscular blockade.
- Use drug only under direct medical supervision by personnel skilled in use of neuromuscular blocking agents and techniques for maintaining patent airway. Don't use unless facilities and equipment for intubation, mechanical ventilation, oxygen therapy, and drug antagonist are within reach.
- Higher initial doses may be needed by patients with severe burns and some patients with severe liver disease. Higher doses (0.8 mg/kg) produce intubating conditions more rapidly (4 minutes), with neuromuscular blockade lasting 160 minutes or longer. Consequently, higher doses should be reserved for long procedures. Administration during steady-state anesthesia with enflurane, halothane, or isoflurane may allow 33% reduction of dose.
- Prepare drug for I.V. use with D_5W, normal saline solution injection, dextrose 5% in normal saline solution injection, lactated Ringer's injection, or dextrose 5% in lactated Ringer's injection.
- When diluted as directed, doxacurium is compatible with alfentanil, fentanyl, and sufentanil.
- Product should be administered immediately after reconstitution. Diluted solutions are stable for 24 hours at room temperature; however, because reconstitution dilutes preservative, risk of contamination increases. Unused solutions should be discarded after 8 hours.
- Acid-base and electrolyte balance may influence actions of nondepolarizing neuromuscular blockers. Alkalosis may counteract paralysis, and acidosis may enhance it.
- Nerve stimulator and train-of-four monitoring are recommended to document antagonism of neuromuscular blockade and recovery of muscle strength. Before attempting pharmacologic reversal with neostigmine, some evidence of spontaneous recovery should be evident.
- Provide respiratory support as needed.
- Administer pain medication regularly if pain is thought to be present; patient may experience pain but not be able to show it.

Patient teaching
- If patient isn't under influence of anesthesia, talk to him and keep him informed of surroundings because drug doesn't affect consciousness. Reassure him that all his vital needs are being met and that he is being monitored constantly.

Evaluation
- Patient shows improvement in underlying condition.
- Patient regains ability to maintain spontaneous ventilation after effects of drug have subsided.
- Patient and family state understanding of drug therapy.

doxapram hydrochloride

(DOKS-uh-prahm high-droh-KLOR-ighd)

Dopram

Pharmacologic class: analeptic
Therapeutic class: CNS and respiratory stimulant
Pregnancy risk category: B

Indications and dosages

▶ **Postanesthesia respiratory stimulation, drug-induced CNS depression, chronic pulmonary disease with acute hypercapnia.** *Adults:* 0.5 to 1 mg/kg of body weight (up to 2 mg/kg in CNS depression) by I.V. injection or infusion. Repeated q 5 minutes, if needed. Maximum, 4 mg/kg, up to 3 g in 1 day.

▶ **COPD.** *Adults:* 1 to 2 mg/minute by I.V. infusion. Maximum, 3 mg/minute for maximum duration of 2 hours.

How supplied

Injection: 20 mg/ml (benzyl alcohol 0.9%)

Pharmacokinetics

Absorption: not applicable with I.V. administration.
Distribution: distributed throughout body.
Metabolism: 99% metabolized by liver.
Excretion: metabolites excreted in urine.

Route	Onset	Peak	Duration
I.V.	20-40 sec	1-2 min	5-12 min

Pharmacodynamics

Chemical effect: not clearly defined; acts either directly on central respiratory centers in medulla or indirectly on chemoreceptors.
Therapeutic effect: stimulates respirations.

Adverse reactions

CNS: ***seizures,*** *headache,* dizziness, apprehension, disorientation, pupillary dilation, bilateral Babinski's signs, paresthesia.
CV: *chest pain and tightness, variations in heart rate, hypertension,* depressed T waves, ***arrhythmias.***
EENT: sneezing, ***laryngospasm.***
GI: nausea, vomiting, diarrhea.
GU: urine retention, bladder stimulation with incontinence.
Respiratory: hiccups, rebound hypoventilation, cough, ***bronchospasm,*** dyspnea.
Musculoskeletal: muscle spasms.
Skin: pruritus, diaphoresis, flushing.
Other: fever.

Interactions

Drug-drug. *MAO inhibitors, sympathomimetics:* potentiate adverse CV effects. Use together cautiously.

Contraindications and precautions

- Contraindicated in patients with seizure disorders; head injury; CV disorders; frank, uncompensated heart failure; severe hypertension; CVA; respiratory failure or incompetence secondary to neuromuscular disorders, muscle paresis, flail chest, obstructed airway, pulmonary embolism, pneumothorax, restrictive respiratory disease, acute bronchial asthma, or extreme dyspnea; or hypoxia not related to hypercapnia.
- Use cautiously in patients with bronchial asthma, severe tachycardia or arrhythmias, cerebral edema or increased CSF pressure, hyperthyroidism, pheochromocytoma, or metabolic disorders. Also use cautiously in pregnant women.
- Safety of drug hasn't been established in breast-feeding women and in children.

NURSING CONSIDERATIONS

Assessment

- Obtain history of patient's underlying condition before therapy.
- Assess blood pressure, heart rate, deep tendon reflexes, and arterial blood gases before giving drug and closely throughout therapy.
- Monitor effectiveness by observing patient for improvement in CNS and respiratory function.
- Be alert for adverse reactions and drug interactions.
- Evaluate patient's (if appropriate) and family's knowledge of drug therapy.

Nursing diagnoses

- Ineffective breathing pattern related to underlying condition
- Risk for trauma related to potential for drug-induced seizure activity
- Deficient knowledge related to drug therapy

Planning and implementation

- Establish adequate airway before administering drug. Prevent patient from aspirating vomitus by placing him on his side. Have suction equipment nearby.
- Administer drug slowly; rapid infusion may cause hemolysis. Doxapram is physically incompatible with strongly alkaline drugs such as thiopental sodium, aminophylline, and sodium bicarbonate.
- Avoid extravasation, which may lead to thrombophlebitis and local skin irritation.
- Drug is used only in surgical or emergency department situations.
- Discontinue drug and notify prescriber if patient shows signs of increased arterial carbon dioxide or oxygen tension or if mechanical ventilation is started.

Patient teaching

- If patient is alert, instruct him to report chest pain or tightness immediately.

Evaluation

- Patient regains normal respiratory pattern.
- Patient has no seizures as result of therapy.
- Patient and family state understanding of drug therapy.

doxazosin mesylate

(doks-AY-zoh-sin MES-ih-layt)
Cardura

Pharmacologic class: alpha-adrenergic blocker
Therapeutic class: antihypertensive
Pregnancy risk category: C

Indications and dosages

▶ **Essential hypertension.** *Adults:* initially, 1 mg P.O. daily. If necessary, increased to 2 mg daily. To minimize adverse reactions, dosage is adjusted slowly (typically increased only q 2 weeks). If necessary, increased to 4 mg daily; then to 8 mg. Maximum, 16 mg daily, but dosage above 4 mg daily increases risk of adverse reactions.

▶ **BPH.** *Adults:* initially, 1 mg P.O. once daily morning or evening; may be increased to 2 mg and, thereafter, to 4 mg and to 8 mg once daily p.r.n. Recommended adjustment interval is 1 to 2 weeks.

How supplied

Tablets: 1 mg, 2 mg, 4 mg, 8 mg

Pharmacokinetics

Absorption: readily absorbed from GI tract.
Distribution: 98% protein-bound.
Metabolism: extensively metabolized in liver.
Excretion: 63% excreted in bile and feces; 9% excreted in urine. *Half-life:* 19 to 22 hours.

Route	Onset	Peak	Duration
P.O.	1-2 hr	5-6 hr	24 hr

Pharmacodynamics

Chemical effect: acts on peripheral vasculature to produce vasodilation.
Therapeutic effect: lowers blood pressure.

Adverse reactions

CNS: *dizziness*, vertigo, *asthenia*, *headache,* somnolence, drowsiness.
CV: *orthostatic hypotension,* hypotension, edema, palpitations, ***arrhythmias,*** tachycardia.
EENT: rhinitis, pharyngitis, abnormal vision.
GI: nausea, vomiting, diarrhea, constipation.
Musculoskeletal: arthralgia, myalgia.
Respiratory: dyspnea.
Skin: rash, pruritus.
Other: pain.

Interactions

Drug-drug. *Clonidine:* clonidine effects may be decreased. Dosage adjustments may be necessary.
Drug-herb. *Butcher's broom:* possible reduction in effects. Discourage concomitant use.

Contraindications and precautions

- Contraindicated in patients hypersensitive to drug and to quinazoline derivatives (including prazosin and terazosin).
- Drug isn't recommended for breast-feeding women because it accumulates in breast milk at levels about 20 times greater than those in maternal plasma.
- Use cautiously in patients with impaired liver function and in pregnant women.
- Safety in children hasn't been established.

NURSING CONSIDERATIONS

Assessment

- Obtain history of patient's blood pressure before therapy, and reassess regularly thereafter.
- Determine effect on standing and supine blood pressure at 2 to 6 hours and 24 hours after administration.
- Be alert for adverse reactions.
- Monitor patient's ECG for arrhythmias.
- Evaluate patient's and family's knowledge of drug therapy.

Nursing diagnoses

- Risk for injury related to presence of hypertension
- Decreased cardiac output related to drug-induced adverse CV reactions
- Deficient knowledge related to drug therapy

Planning and implementation

- Dosage must be increased gradually, with adjustments every 2 weeks for hypertension and every 1 to 2 weeks for benign prostatic hyperplasia.
- If syncope occurs, place patient in recumbent position and treat supportively. A transient hypotensive response isn't considered a contraindication to continued therapy.

Patient teaching

- Advise patient taking doxazosin that he's susceptible to a first-dose effect similar to that produced by other alpha-adrenergic blockers—marked orthostatic hypotension accompanied by dizziness or syncope. Orthostatic hypotension is most common after first dose, but it also can occur when therapy is interrupted or dosages are adjusted.
- Warn patient that dizziness or fainting may occur. Advise patient to refrain from driving and performing other hazardous activities until drug's adverse CNS effects are known.
- Stress importance of regular follow-up visits.

Evaluation

- Patient's blood pressure becomes normal.
- Patient maintains adequate cardiac output throughout therapy.
- Patient and family state understanding of drug therapy.

doxepin hydrochloride

(DOKS-eh-pin high-droh-KLOR-ighd)

Novo-Doxepin ♦, Sinequan, Triadapin ♦

Pharmacologic class: tricyclic antidepressant
Therapeutic class: antidepressant
Pregnancy risk category: C

Indications and dosages

▶ **Depression, anxiety.** *Adults:* initially, 25 to 75 mg P.O. daily in divided doses to maximum of 300 mg daily. Or, entire maintenance dosage may be given once daily with maximum dose of 150 mg P.O.

How supplied

Capsules: 10 mg, 25 mg, 50 mg, 75 mg, 100 mg, 150 mg
Oral concentrate: 10 mg/ml

Pharmacokinetics

Absorption: absorbed rapidly from GI tract.
Distribution: distributed widely in body, including CNS; 90% protein-bound.
Metabolism: metabolized by liver. A significant first-pass effect may explain variability of serum levels in different patients taking same dosage.
Excretion: most of drug excreted in urine.

Route	Onset	Peak	Duration
P.O.	Unknown	≤ 2 hr	Unknown

Pharmacodynamics

Chemical effect: unknown; increases amount of norepinephrine, serotonin, or both in CNS by blocking their reuptake by presynaptic neurons.
Therapeutic effect: relieves depression and anxiety.

Adverse reactions

CNS: *drowsiness, dizziness,* excitation, tremors, weakness, confusion, headache, nervousness, EEG changes, ***seizures,*** extrapyramidal reactions, ataxia, paresthesia, hallucinations.
CV: *orthostatic hypotension, tachycardia, ECG changes,* hypertension.
EENT: *blurred vision,* tinnitus, mydriasis.
GI: *dry mouth, glossitis, constipation,* nausea, vomiting, anorexia.
GU: *urine retention.*
Hematologic: eosinophilia, ***bone marrow depression.***
Skin: rash, urticaria, photosensitivity.
Other: *diaphoresis,* ***hypersensitivity reaction.***

Interactions

Drug-drug. *Barbiturates, CNS depressants:* enhanced CNS depression. Avoid concomitant use.
Cimetidine, fluoxetine, sertraline, methylphenidate: may increase doxepin serum levels. Monitor patient for increased adverse reactions.
Clonidine, epinephrine, norepinephrine: increased hypertensive effect. Use cautiously.
MAO inhibitors: may cause severe excitation, hyperpyrexia, or seizures, usually with high dosage. Avoid concomitant use.
Drug-herb. *St. John's wort, SAMe, yohimbe:* possible elevation of blood serotonin levels. Discourage concurrent use.
Drug-food. *Carbonated beverages, grape juice:* drug is physically incompatible with these beverages. Warn against using together.
Drug-lifestyle. *Alcohol use:* enhanced CNS depression. Discourage concomitant use.
Sun exposure: increased risk of photosensitivity reactions. Discourage unprotected or prolonged exposure to the sun.

Contraindications and precautions

- Contraindicated in patients hypersensitive to drug and in those with glaucoma or a tendency for urine retention.
- Breast-feeding isn't recommended during therapy.
- Safety of drug hasn't been established in pregnant women or in children under age 12.

NURSING CONSIDERATIONS

Assessment

- Assess patient's depression or anxiety before and during therapy.
- Be alert for adverse reactions and drug interactions.
- Evaluate patient's and family's knowledge of drug therapy.

Nursing diagnoses

- Ineffective individual coping related to underlying condition
- Risk for injury related to drug-induced adverse CNS reactions
- Deficient knowledge related to drug therapy

Planning and implementation

- Dosage should be reduced in elderly or debilitated patients, adolescents, and those receiving other drugs (especially anticholinergics).
- Dilute oral concentrate with 120 ml of water, milk, or juice (except grape juice). Don't mix with carbonated beverages because of incompatibility.
- Don't withdraw drug abruptly. Abrupt withdrawal of long-term therapy may cause nausea, headache, and malaise, which don't indicate addiction.
- Because hypertensive episodes have occurred during surgery in patients receiving tricyclic antidepressants, drug should be discontinued gradually several days before surgery.
- If signs of psychosis occur or increase, notify prescriber and expect dosage to be reduced.

Patient teaching

- Tell patient to dilute oral concentrate with 120 ml of water, milk, or juice (orange, grapefruit, tomato, prune, or pineapple). Drug is in-

compatible with carbonated beverages and grape juice.
- Advise patient to take full dose at bedtime, but warn of possible morning orthostatic hypotension.
- Warn patient to avoid hazardous activities that require alertness and good psychomotor coordination until CNS effects of drug are known. Drowsiness and dizziness usually subside after a few weeks.
- Tell patient to avoid alcohol during drug therapy.
- Warn patient not to stop drug therapy suddenly.
- Advise patient to consult prescriber before taking prescription drugs, OTC medications, or herbal remedies.
- Advise patient to use sunblock, wear protective clothing, and avoid prolonged exposure to strong sunlight.

☑ Evaluation

- Patient behavior and communication indicate improvement of depression or anxiety.
- Patient has no injury as result of drug-induced adverse CNS reactions.
- Patient and family state understanding of drug therapy.

doxercalciferol

(dox-er-kal-SIF-eh-rol)
Hectorol

Pharmacologic class: synthetic vitamin D analogue
Therapeutic class: parathyroid hormone antagonist
Pregnancy risk category: B

Indications and dosages

▶ **Reduction of elevated intact parathyroid hormone (PTH) levels in the management of secondary hyperparathyroidism in patients undergoing long-term renal dialysis.** *Adults:* initially, 10 mcg P.O. three times weekly at dialysis. Dosage adjusted as needed to lower intact PTH levels to 150 to 300 pg/ml. Dosage may be increased by 2.5 mcg at 8-week intervals if the intact PTH level isn't decreased by 50% and fails to reach target range. Maximum, 20 mcg P.O. three times weekly. If intact PTH levels fall below 100 pg/ml, drug should be suspended for 1 week and then resumed at a dose that's at least 2.5 mcg lower than the last administered dose.

How supplied

Capsules: 2.5 mcg

Pharmacokinetics

Absorption: absorbed from the GI tract.
Distribution: no information available.
Metabolism: metabolized to its active forms in the liver.
Excretion: major metabolite of doxercalciferol attains peak blood levels at 11 to 12 hours after repeated oral doses. *Elimination half-life:* 32 to 37 hours, with a range of up to 96 hours.

Route	Onset	Peak	Duration
P.O.	Unknown	11-12 hr	Unknown

Pharmacodynamics

Chemical effect: Once activated, doxercalciferol and other biologically active vitamin D metabolites regulate blood calcium levels required for essential body functions. Doxercalciferol acts directly on the parathyroid glands to suppress PTH synthesis and secretion.
Therapeutic effect: reduction of elevated intact PTH levels.

Adverse reactions

CNS: *dizziness, headache, malaise,* sleep disorder.
CV: ***bradycardia****, edema.*
GI: anorexia, dyspepsia, *nausea, vomiting,* constipation.
Metabolic: weight gain.
Musculoskeletal: arthralgia.
Respiratory: *dyspnea.*
Skin: pruritus.
Other: abscess.

Interactions

Drug-drug. *Cholestyramine, mineral oil:* reduced intestinal absorption of doxercalciferol. Avoid concomitant use.
Glutethimide, phenobarbital, and other enzyme inducers; phenytoin and other enzyme

inhibitors: may affect doxercalciferol metabolism. Adjust dosage as directed.
Magnesium-containing antacids: may cause hypermagnesemia. Monitor patient for toxicity.
Calcium-containing or non-aluminum-containing phosphate binders: may cause hypercalcemia or hyperphosphatemia and decrease effectiveness of doxercalciferol. Use cautiously together, and adjust dosage of phosphate binders as directed.
Vitamin D supplements: may cause additive effects and hypercalcemia. Monitor patient for toxicity.

Contraindications and precautions

• Contraindicated in patients with a recent history of hypercalcemia, hyperphosphatemia, or vitamin D toxicity.
• Use cautiously in patients with hepatic insufficiency, and frequently monitor calcium, phosphorus, and intact PTH levels in these patients.

NURSING CONSIDERATIONS

Assessment

• Assess hepatic function before starting therapy.
• Monitor calcium, phosphorus, and intact PTH levels as ordered. Monitor them more frequently in patients with hepatic insufficiency.
• Be alert for adverse reactions and drug interactions.
• Evaluate patient's and family's knowledge about drug therapy.

Nursing diagnoses

• Imbalanced nutrition: less than body requirements related to adverse GI effects
• Risk for injury related to adverse CNS effects
• Deficient knowledge related to drug therapy

Planning and implementation

• Give doxercalciferol with dialysis (about every other day). Dosing must be individualized and based on intact PTH levels, with monitoring of serum calcium and phosphorus levels before doxercalciferol therapy and weekly thereafter.
• If patient has hypercalcemia or hyperphosphatemia, or if the product of serum calcium × serum phosphorus (Ca × P) is greater than 70, immediately stop doxercalciferol, as ordered, until these values decrease.
• Progressive hypercalcemia from vitamin D overdose may require emergency attention. Acute hypercalcemia may worsen arrhythmias and seizures and affects the action of digoxin. Chronic hypercalcemia can lead to vascular and soft-tissue calcification.
• Calcium-based or non-aluminum-containing phosphate binders and a low-phosphate diet are used to control serum phosphorus levels in patients undergoing dialysis. Expect adjustments in doses of doxercalciferol and concurrent therapies such as dietary phosphate binders to sustain PTH suppression and maintain serum calcium and phosphorus levels within acceptable ranges.

Patient teaching

• Inform patient that dosage must be adjusted over several months to achieve satisfactory PTH suppression.
• Tell patient to adhere to a low-phosphorus diet and to follow instructions regarding calcium supplementation.
• Tell patient to obtain prescriber's approval before using OTC drugs, including antacids and vitamin preparations containing calcium or vitamin D.
• Inform patient that early signs and symptoms of hypercalcemia include weakness, headache, somnolence, nausea, vomiting, dry mouth, constipation, muscle pain, bone pain, and metallic taste. Late signs and symptoms include polyuria, polydipsia, anorexia, weight loss, nocturia, conjunctivitis, pancreatitis, photophobia, rhinorrhea, pruritus, hyperthermia, decreased libido, hypertension, and arrhythmias.

Evaluation

• Patient has no nausea and vomiting.
• Patient remains free from injury.
• Patient and family state understanding of drug therapy.

doxorubicin hydrochloride

(doks-oh-ROO-bih-sin high-droh-KLOR-ighd)
Adriamycin ◇, Adriamycin PFS, Adriamycin RDF, Rubex

Pharmacologic class: antineoplastic antibiotic (cell cycle–phase nonspecific)
Therapeutic class: antineoplastic
Pregnancy risk category: D

Indications and dosages

Dosages and indications may vary. Check treatment protocol with prescriber.

▶ **Bladder, breast, lung, ovarian, stomach, testicular, and thyroid cancers; Hodgkin's disease; acute lymphoblastic and myeloblastic leukemia; Wilms' tumor; neuroblastoma; lymphoma; sarcoma.** *Adults:* 60 to 75 mg/m^2 I.V. as single dose q 3 weeks; or 30 mg/m^2 I.V. in single daily dose on days 1 through 3 of 4-week cycle. Alternatively, 20 mg/m^2 I.V. once weekly. Maximum cumulative dosage is 550 mg/m^2.

How supplied

Injection (preservative-free): 2 mg/ml
Powder for injection: 10-mg, 20-mg, 50-mg, 100-mg, 150-mg vials

Pharmacokinetics

Absorption: not applicable with I.V. administration.
Distribution: distributed widely in body tissues; doesn't cross blood-brain barrier.
Metabolism: extensively metabolized by hepatic microsomal enzymes to several metabolites, one of which possesses cytotoxic activity.
Excretion: excreted primarily in bile, minimally in urine. *Half-life:* initial, 30 minutes; terminal, 16½ hours.

Route	Onset	Peak	Duration
I.V.	Unknown	Unknown	Unknown

Pharmacodynamics

Chemical effect: unknown; thought to interfere with DNA-dependent RNA synthesis by intercalation.
Therapeutic effect: hinders or kills certain cancer cells.

Adverse reactions

CV: cardiac depression, seen in such ECG changes as sinus tachycardia, T-wave flattening, ST-segment depression, voltage reduction; ***arrhythmias; irreversible cardiomyopathy.***
EENT: conjunctivitis.
GI: *nausea, vomiting,* diarrhea, *stomatitis,* esophagitis, anorexia.
GU: red urine (transient).
Hematologic: ***leukopenia*** during days 10 through 15, with recovery by day 21; ***thrombocytopenia;*** **MYELOSUPPRESSION.**
Skin: *complete alopecia;* urticaria; facial flushing; *hyperpigmentation of nails, dermal creases, or skin* (especially in previously irradiated areas).
Other: *severe cellulitis or tissue sloughing if drug extravasates,* hyperuricemia, ***anaphylaxis.***

Interactions

Drug-drug. *Calcium channel blockers:* may potentiate cardiotoxic effects. Monitor patient closely.
Digoxin: may decrease serum digoxin levels. Monitor patient closely.
Phenytoin: decreased serum levels of phenytoin. Check levels.
Streptozocin: increased and prolonged blood levels. Dosage may need adjustment.
Drug-herb. *Green tea:* May enhance antitumor effects of doxorubicin. Urge patient to discuss with prescriber before using together.

Contraindications and precautions

- Contraindicated in patients with marked myelosuppression induced by previous treatment with other antitumor drugs or radiotherapy and in those who have received lifetime cumulative dosage of 550 mg/m^2.
- Drug isn't recommended for pregnant or breast-feeding women.
- Safety of drug hasn't been established in children.

NURSING CONSIDERATIONS

Assessment
- Obtain history of patient's neoplastic disorder before therapy, and reassess regularly thereafter.
- Assess ECG before treatment.
- Monitor CBC and liver function tests, as ordered; monitor ECG monthly during therapy.
- Be alert for adverse reactions and drug interactions.
- Evaluate patient's and family's knowledge of drug therapy.

Nursing diagnoses
- Ineffective health maintenance related to presence of neoplastic disease
- Decreased cardiac output related to drug-induced cardiotoxicity
- Deficient knowledge related to drug therapy

Planning and implementation
- Premedicate with antiemetic, as ordered, to reduce nausea.
- Follow facility policy to reduce risks. Preparation and administration of parenteral form create carcinogenic, mutagenic, and teratogenic risks for staff.
- Dosage may need adjustment in elderly patients and those with myelosuppression or impaired cardiac or hepatic function.
- Never give this drug by I.M. or S.C. route.

ALERT Red color of doxorubicin is similar to that of daunorubicin. Take care to avoid confusing these two drugs.

- Reconstitute using preservative-free normal saline solution injection. Add 5 ml to 10-mg vial, 10 ml to 20-mg vial, or 25 ml to 50-mg vial. Shake vial and allow drug to dissolve; final concentration is 2 mg/ml. Give by direct injection into I.V. line of free-flowing compatible I.V. solution containing D_5W or normal saline solution injection.
- Avoid extravasation; don't place I.V. line over joints or in limbs with poor venous or lymphatic drainage.
- If extravasation occurs, stop I.V. infusion immediately, notify prescriber, and apply ice to area for 24 to 48 hours. Monitor area closely because extravasation reaction may be progressive. Early consultation with plastic surgeon may be advisable.
- Precipitate may form if drug is mixed with aminophylline, cephalothin, dexamethasone, fluorouracil, heparin, or hydrocortisone.
- If skin or mucosal contact occurs, immediately wash area with soap and water.
- In case of leak or spill, inactivate drug with 5% sodium hypochlorite solution (household bleach).
- Be prepared to stop drug or slow rate of infusion if tachycardia develops; notify prescriber.
- Stop drug immediately if signs of heart failure develop, and notify prescriber. Heart failure may be prevented by limiting cumulative dosage to 550 mg/m^2 (400 mg/m^2 when patient also receives or has received cyclophosphamide or radiation therapy to cardiac area).
- Alternative dosage schedule (once-weekly dosing) causes a lower risk of cardiomyopathy.
- If vein streaking occurs, slow administration rate. If welts occur, stop administration and notoify prescriber.
- Be prepared to decrease dosage if serum bilirubin level is increased: 50% dosage when bilirubin level is 1.2 to 3 mg/dl; 25% dosage when bilirubin level is greater than 3 mg/dl.
- Refrigerated, reconstituted solution is stable for 48 hours; at room temperature, it's stable for 24 hours.
- Provide adequate hydration; alkalinizing urine or administering allopurinol may prevent or minimize uric acid nephropathy.
- Report adverse reactions to prescriber, and be prepared to provide supportive care to treat such reactions.

ALERT Liposomal doxorubicin and conventional doxorubicin aren't interchangable. Plasma clearance of liposomal form is significantly reduced compared to the conventional form, requiring decreased dosing with liposomal doxorubicin.

Patient teaching
- Warn patient to watch for signs of infection (fever, sore throat, fatigue) and bleeding (easy bruising, nosebleeds, bleeding gums, melena). Have patient take temperature daily.

• Advise patient that orange to red urine for 1 to 2 days is normal and doesn't indicate presence of blood in urine.
• Tell patient that complete alopecia may occur within 3 to 4 weeks. Hair may regrow 2 to 5 months after drug is stopped.
• Instruct patient to report symptoms of heart failure and other cardiac signs and symptoms promptly to prescriber.
• Tell patient to use safety precautions to prevent injury.

Evaluation
• Patient exhibits positive response to therapy, as noted on improved follow-up studies.
• Patient maintains adequate cardiac output throughout therapy.
• Patient and family state understanding of drug therapy.

doxorubicin hydrochloride liposomal
(doks-oh-ROO-bih-sin high-droh-KLOR-ighd li-po-SOE-mal)
Doxil

Pharmacologic class: anthracycline
Therapeutic class: antineoplastic
Pregnancy risk category: D

Indications and dosages
▶ **Metastatic carcinoma of the ovary in patients with disease refractory to paclitaxel- and platinum-based chemotherapy regimens.** *Adults:* 50 mg/m^2 (doxorubicin hydrochloride equivalent) I.V. at an initial infusion rate of 1 mg/minute once every 4 weeks for at least 4 courses. Continue treatment as long as patient doesn't progress, shows no evidence of cardiotoxicity, and continues to tolerate treatment. If no infusion-related adverse events are observed, increase infusion rate to complete administration over 1 hour.
▶ **AIDS-related Kaposi's sarcoma in patients with disease that has progressed with previous combination chemotherapy or in patients who are intolerant to such therapy.** *Adults:* 20 mg/m^2 (doxorubicin hydrochloride equivalent) I.V. over 30 minutes, once every 3 weeks, for as long as patient responds satisfactorily and tolerates treatment.

How supplied
Injection: 2 mg/ml

Pharmacokinetics
Absorption: unknown.
Distribution: distributed mostly to vascular fluid. Plasma protein–binding hasn't been determined; however, plasma protein–binding of doxorubicin is about 70%.
Metabolism: doxorubicinol, the major metabolite of doxorubicin, is detected at very low levels in plasma.
Excretion: plasma elimination is slow and biphasic. *Half-life:* about 5 hours in the first phase, 55 hours in the second phase at doses of 10 to 20 mg/m^2.

Route	Onset	Peak	Duration
I.V.	Unknown	Unknown	Unknown

Pharmacodynamics
Chemical effect: Doxil is doxorubicin hydrochloride encapsulated in liposomes which, because of their small size and persistence in circulation, can penetrate the altered vasculature of tumors. The mechanism of action of doxorubicin hydrochloride is probably related to its ability to bind DNA and inhibit nucleic acid synthesis.
Therapeutic effect: hinders or kills certain cancer cells in patients with ovarian cancer or AIDS-related Kaposi's sarcoma.

Adverse reactions
CNS: *asthenia,* paresthesia, headache, somnolence, dizziness, depression, insomnia, anxiety, malaise, emotional lability, fatigue.
CV: chest pain, hypotension, tachycardia, peripheral edema, cardiomyopathy, ***heart failure, arrhythmias,*** pericardial effusion.
EENT: *mucous membrane disorder,* mouth ulceration, pharyngitis, rhinitis, conjunctivitis, retinitis, optic neuritis.
GI: *nausea, vomiting, constipation, anorexia, diarrhea,* abdominal pain, taste perversion,

dyspepsia, oral candidiasis, enlarged abdomen, esophagitis, dysphagia, *stomatitis,* glossitis.
GU: albuminuria.
Hematologic: ***leukopenia, neutropenia,*** THROMBOCYTOPENIA, ***anemia, increased PT.***
Hepatic: hyperbilirubinemia.
Metabolic: dehydration, weight loss, hypocalcemia, hyperglycemia.
Musculoskeletal: myalgia, back pain.
Respiratory: dyspnea, increased cough, pneumonia.
Skin: *rash, alopecia,* dry skin, pruritus, skin discoloration, skin disorder, exfoliative dermatitis, herpes zoster, sweating, *palmar-plantar erythrodysesthesia,* alopecia.
Other: fever, ***allergic reaction,*** chills, infection, infusion-related reactions.

Contraindications and precautions

- Contraindicated in patients hypersensitive to the conventional form of doxorubicin hydrochloride or any component in the liposomal form. Also, contraindicated in patients with marked myelosuppression or those who have received a lifetime cumulative dosage of 550 mg/m^2 (400 mg/m^2 if patient received radiotherapy to the mediastinal area or concomitant therapy with other cardiotoxic drugs, such as cyclophosphamide). Use in patients with a history of cardiovascular disease only when benefit of drug outweighs risk to patient.
- Use cautiously in patients who have received other anthracyclines. The total dose of doxorubicin hydrochloride should also take into account any previous or concomitant therapy with related compounds, such as daunorubicin. Heart failure and cardiomyopathy may occur after therapy stops.

NURSING CONSIDERATIONS

Assessment

- Obtain an accurate medication list from patient, including previous or current chemotherapeutic drugs.
- Evaluate patient's hepatic function before therapy, and adjust dosage accordingly, as ordered.
- Monitor cardiac function closely by endomyocardial biopsy, echocardiography, or gated radionuclide scans. If results indicate possible cardiac injury, the benefit of continued therapy must be weighed against the risk of myocardial injury.
- Be alert for adverse reactions.
- Evaluate patient's and family's knowledge about drug therapy.

Nursing diagnoses

- Risk for infection related to myelosuppression
- Risk for injury related to drug-induced adverse reactions
- Deficient knowledge related to drug therapy

Planning and implementation

- Patients with impaired hepatic function need a reduced dosage.
- Dosage modifications are recommended for managing adverse reactions, including palmar-plantar erythrodysesthesia, hematologic toxicity, and stomatitis.
- Follow facility procedures for proper handling and disposal of antineoplastic drugs.

ALERT Carefully check label on the I.V. bag before giving drug. Accidental substitution of Doxil for conventional doxorubicin hydrochloride has caused severe adverse effects. Dilute appropriate dose (maximum, 90 mg) in 250 ml of D_5W using aseptic technique. Refrigerate diluted solution at 36° to 46° F (2° to 8° C), and administer within 24 hours.
- Infuse I.V. over 30 to 60 minutes depending on the dose. Don't use with in-line filters.
- Monitor patient carefully during infusion. Acute infusion reactions (flushing, shortness of breath, facial swelling, headache, chills, back pain, tightness in the chest or throat, or hypotension) may occur. These reactions resolve over several hours to a day once the infusion is stopped. The reaction may resolve by slowing the infusion rate.
- Don't give drug by I.M. or S.C. route. Avoid extravasation. If it occurs, stop infusion immediately and restart in another vein. Applying ice over the extravasation site for about 30 minutes may help to alleviate the local reaction.

ALERT Doxil has unique pharmacokinetic properties and shouldn't be substituted on a milligram-per-milligram basis for conventional doxorubicin hydrochloride.

- No drug interactions have been reported; however, Doxil may interact with drugs known to interact with the conventional form of doxorubicin hydrochloride.
- Drug may potentiate the toxicity of other antineoplastic therapies.
- The total dose of doxorubicin hydrochloride should also take into account any previous or concomitant therapy with related compounds, such as daunorubicin. Heart failure and cardiomyopathy may occur after therapy stops.
- Monitor CBC, including platelets, before each dose and frequently throughout therapy. Leukopenia is usually transient. Hematologic toxicity may require dose reduction or suspension or delay of therapy. Persistent severe myelosuppression may result in superinfection or hemorrhage. Patient may need granulocyte colony-stimulating factor (or granulocyte-macrophage colony-stimulating factor) to support blood counts.

Patient teaching
- Tell patient to notify prescriber about symptoms of hand-foot syndrome, such as tingling or burning, redness, flaking, bothersome swelling, small blisters, or small sores on the palms of hands or soles of feet.
- Advise patient to report symptoms of stomatitis, such as painful redness, swelling, or sores in the mouth.
- Advise patient to avoid exposure to people with infections. Tell patient to report fever of 100.5°F or higher.
- Urge patient to report nausea, vomiting, tiredness, weakness, rash, or mild hair loss.
- Advise woman of childbearing age to avoid pregnancy during therapy.

☑ Evaluation
- Patient has no infection.
- Patient has no injury as a result of drug-induced adverse reactions.
- Patient and family state understanding of drug therapy.

doxycycline
(doks-ee-SIGH-kleen)
Doxylin ◇, Monodox, Vibramycin

doxycycline hyclate
Apo-Doxy ♦, Doryx, DoxyCaps, Doxychel Hyclate, Doxycin ♦, Doxy-Tabs, Novo-Doxylin ♦, Periostat, Vibramycin, Vibra-Tabs

doxycycline hydrochloride
Doryx ◇, Vibramycin ◇, Vibramycin IV, Vibra-Tabs 50 ◇

Pharmacologic class: tetracycline
Therapeutic class: antibiotic
Pregnancy risk category: D

Indications and dosages
▶ **Infections caused by sensitive gram-negative and gram-positive organisms, *Chlamydia, Mycoplasma, Rickettsia,* and organisms that cause trachoma and Lyme disease.** *Adults and children weighing more than 45 kg (99 lb):* 100 mg P.O. q 12 hours on first day; then 100 mg P.O. daily. Or, 200 mg I.V. on first day in one or two infusions; then 100 to 200 mg I.V. daily. For severe infections 100 mg P.O. every 12 hours may be used. *Children over age 8 and weighing less than 45 kg:* 4.4 mg/kg P.O. or I.V. daily in divided doses q 12 hours on first day, then 2.2 to 4.4 mg/kg daily.
▶ **Gonorrhea in patients allergic to penicillin.** *Adults:* 100 mg P.O. b.i.d. for 7 days. Or, 300 mg P.O. initially and repeat dose in 1 hour.
▶ **Primary or secondary syphilis in patients allergic to penicillin.** *Adults and children 8 years and older:* 100 mg P.O. b.i.d. for 2 weeks (early detection) or 4 weeks (if more than 1 year's duration).
▶ **Uncomplicated urethral, endocervical, or rectal infection caused by *Chlamydia trachomatis* or *Ureaplasma urealyticum*.** *Adults:* 100 mg P.O. b.i.d. for at least 7 days.
▶ **Prevention of malaria.** *Adults:* 100 mg P.O. daily.

Children over age 8: 2 mg/kg P.O. once daily. Dosage shouldn't exceed adult dose. Therapy should begin 1 to 2 days before travel to malarious area and be continued throughout travel and for 4 weeks thereafter.

How supplied

doxycycline

Tablets: 50 mg ◇, 100 mg ◇
Capsules: 50 mg, 100 mg
Oral suspension: 25 mg/5 ml
Syrup: 50 mg/5 ml

doxycycline hyclate

Tablets: 50 mg, 100 mg
Capsules: 20 mg, 50 mg, 100 mg
Capsules (coated pellets): 100 mg
Injection: 100 mg, 200 mg

doxycycline hydrochloride

Tablets: 50 mg ◇, 100 mg ◇
Capsules: 50 mg ◇, 100 mg ◇, 250 mg ◇
Injection: 100 mg ◇
Powder for injection: 200 mg

Pharmacokinetics

Absorption: 90% to 100% absorbed after P.O. administration; absorption is insignificantly altered by milk or other dairy products.
Distribution: distributed widely in body tissues and fluids. Poor penetration in CSF. Drug is 25% to 93% protein-bound.
Metabolism: insignificantly metabolized; some hepatic degradation occurs.
Excretion: excreted primarily unchanged in urine; some drug is excreted in feces. *Half-life:* 22 to 24 hours after multiple dosing.

Route	Onset	Peak	Duration
P.O.	Unknown	1.5-4 hr	Unknown
I.V.	Immediate	Unknown	Unknown

Pharmacodynamics

Chemical effect: unknown; thought to exert bacteriostatic effect by binding to 30S ribosomal subunit of microorganisms, thus inhibiting protein synthesis.
Therapeutic effect: hinders bacterial growth. Spectrum of activity includes many gram-negative and gram-positive organisms, *Chlamydia, Mycoplasma, Rickettsia,* and spirochetes.

Adverse reactions

CNS: ***intracranial hypertension (pseudotumor cerebri).***
CV: pericarditis, thrombophlebitis.
EENT: glossitis, dysphagia.
GI: anorexia, *epigastric distress, nausea,* vomiting, *diarrhea,* oral candidiasis, enterocolitis, anogenital inflammation.
Hematologic: ***neutropenia,*** eosinophilia, ***thrombocytopenia,*** hemolytic anemia.
Hepatic: elevated liver enzyme levels.
Musculoskeletal: bone growth retardation if used in children under age 8.
Skin: *maculopapular and erythematous rash, photosensitivity, increased pigmentation, urticaria.*
Other: ***hypersensitivity reactions, anaphylaxis,*** superinfection, permanent discoloration of teeth, enamel defects.

Interactions

Drug-drug. *Antacids (including sodium bicarbonate) and laxatives containing aluminum, magnesium, or calcium; antidiarrheals:* decreased antibiotic absorption. Give antibiotic 1 hour before or 2 hours after these drugs.
Ferrous sulfate and other iron products, zinc: decreased antibiotic absorption. Give drug 3 hours after or 2 hours before iron administration.
Methoxyflurane: may cause nephrotoxicity with tetracyclines. Avoid this combination.
Oral anticoagulants: increased anticoagulant effect. Monitor PT and INR, and adjust dosage, as ordered.
Oral contraceptives: decreased contraceptive effectiveness and increased risk of breakthrough bleeding. Recommend nonhormonal form of birth control.
Penicillins: may interfere with bactericidal action of penicillins. Avoid using together.
Carbamazepine, phenobarbital: decreased antibiotic effect. Avoid if possible.
Drug-lifestyle. *Alcohol use:* decreased antibiotic effect. Discourage concomitant use.
Sun exposure: photosensitivity reactions may occur. Urge precautions.

Contraindications and precautions

- Contraindicated in patients hypersensitive to drug or other tetracyclines.

• Avoid use of drug in breast-feeding women.
• Use cautiously in patients with impaired kidney or liver function.
• Use of these drugs during last half of pregnancy and in children under age 8 may cause permanent discoloration of teeth, enamel defects, and bone growth retardation.

NURSING CONSIDERATIONS

Assessment
• Obtain history of patient's infection before therapy, and reassess regularly thereafter.
• Obtain specimen for culture and sensitivity tests before first dose. Therapy may begin pending test results.
• Be alert for adverse reactions and drug interactions.
• Monitor I.V. infusion site for signs of thrombophlebitis, which may occur with I.V. administration.
• Monitor patient's hydration status if adverse GI reactions occur.
• Evaluate patient's and family's knowledge of drug therapy.

Nursing diagnoses
• Infection related to presence of susceptible bacteria
• Risk for deficient fluid volume related to drug-induced adverse GI reactions
• Deficient knowledge related to drug therapy

Planning and implementation
• Check expiration date. Outdated or deteriorated tetracyclines may cause reversible nephrotoxicity (Fanconi's syndrome).
P.O. use: Give drug with milk or food if adverse GI reactions develop.
I.V. use: Reconstitute powder for injection with sterile water for injection. Use 10 ml in 100-mg vial and 20 ml in 200-mg vial. Dilute solution to 100 to 1,000 ml for I.V. infusion. Avoid extravasation. Don't infuse solutions that are more concentrated than 1 mg/ml. Depending on the dose, duration of infusion is typically 1 to 4 hours.
– Don't expose drug to light or heat. Protect it from sunlight during infusion.
– Reconstituted injectable solution is stable for 72 hours if refrigerated.
– Parenteral form may cause false-positive reading of copper sulfate tests (Clinitest). All forms may cause false-negative reading of glucose oxidase reagent (Diastix or Chemstrip uG).
• Notify prescriber of adverse reactions. Some adverse reactions, such as superinfection, may necessitate substitution of another antibiotic.

Patient teaching
• Tell patient to take entire amount of medication exactly as prescribed, even after he feels better.
• Instruct patient to take oral doxycycline with milk or food but not antacids if adverse GI reactions develop. Tell patient to take drug 1 hour or longer before bedtime to prevent irritation from esophageal reflux.
• Tell patient to use sunscreen and avoid strong sunlight during therapy to prevent photosensitivity reactions.
• Stress good oral hygiene.
• Tell patient to check expiration dates and to discard outdated doxycycline because it may become toxic.
• Advise patient taking oral contraceptive to use alternative means of contraception during doxycycline therapy and for 1 week after therapy is discontinued.

Evaluation
• Patient is free from infection.
• Patient maintains adequate hydration throughout therapy.
• Patient and family state understanding of drug therapy.

dronabinol (delta-9-tetrahydrocannabinol)
(droh-NAB-eh-nohl)
Marinol

Pharmacologic class: cannabinoid
Therapeutic class: antiemetic or appetite stimulant

Controlled substance schedule: III
Pregnancy risk category: C

Indications and dosages

▶ **Nausea and vomiting from chemotherapy.** *Adults:* 5 mg/m^2 P.O. 1 to 3 hours before administration of chemotherapy. Then same dose q 2 to 4 hours after chemotherapy for total of four to six doses daily. If needed, dosage increased in increments of 2.5 mg/m^2 to maximum of 15 mg/m^2 per dose.

▶ **Anorexia and weight loss in patients with AIDS.** *Adults:* 2.5 mg P.O. b.i.d. before lunch and dinner, increased p.r.n. to maximum of 20 mg daily.

How supplied

Capsules: 2.5 mg, 5 mg, 10 mg

Pharmacokinetics

Absorption: almost 95% absorbed.
Distribution: distributed rapidly in many tissue sites; 97% to 99% protein-bound.
Metabolism: undergoes extensive metabolism in liver. Metabolite activity is unknown.
Excretion: excreted primarily in feces. *Half-life:* 25 to 35 hours.

Route	Onset	Peak	Duration
P.O.	Unknown	2-4 hr	4-6 hr

Pharmacodynamics

Chemical effect: unknown.
Therapeutic effect: relieves nausea and vomiting caused by chemotherapy and stimulates appetite.

Adverse reactions

CNS: *dizziness, drowsiness, euphoria, ataxia,* depersonalization, disorientation, hallucinations, somnolence, headache, muddled thinking, asthenia, amnesia, confusion, *paranoia.*
CV: tachycardia, orthostatic hypotension, palpitations, vasodilation.
EENT: visual disturbances.
GI: *dry mouth, nausea, vomiting, abdominal pain,* diarrhea.

Interactions

Drug-drug. *CNS depressants, psychotomimetic substances, sedatives:* additive effects. Avoid concomitant use.
Drug-lifestyle. *Alcohol use:* additive effects. Discourage concomitant use.

Contraindications and precautions

- Contraindicated in patients hypersensitive to sesame oil or cannabinoids.
- Drug isn't recommended for breast-feeding women.
- Use cautiously in elderly patients and in those with heart disease, psychiatric illness, or history of drug abuse.
- Safety of drug hasn't been established in children.

NURSING CONSIDERATIONS

Assessment

- Obtain history of patient's underlying condition before therapy.
- Monitor effectiveness by assessing for nausea, vomiting, or weight gain. Drug effects may persist for days after therapy ends.
- Be alert for adverse reactions and drug interactions.
- Monitor patient for dependence. Dronabinol is the principal active substance in *Cannabis sativa* (marijuana). It can produce physical and psychological dependence and has higih potential for abuse.
- Monitor patient's hydration status, weight, and nutritional status regularly.
- Evaluate patient's and family's knowledge of drug therapy.

Nursing diagnoses

- Risk for deficient fluid volume related to nausea and vomiting from chemotherapy
- Disturbed thought processes related to drug-induced adverse CNS reactions
- Deficient knowledge related to drug therapy

Planning and implementation

- Expect drug to be prescribed only for patients who haven't responded satisfactorily to other antiemetics.

• Give drug 1 to 3 hours before chemotherapy starts and again 2 to 4 hours after chemotherapy is administered.

Patient teaching
• Inform patient that drug may cause unusual changes in mood or other adverse behavioral effects.
• Caution patient to avoid hazardous activities until full CNS effects of drug are known.
• Warn family members to make sure patient is supervised by a responsible person during and immediately after treatment.

Evaluation
• Patient maintains adequate hydration.
• Patient regains normal thought processes after effects of drug therapy have dissipated.
• Patient and family state understanding of drug therapy.

E

edetate calcium disodium

(ED-eh-tayt KAL-see-um digh-SOH-dee-um)
Calcium Disodium Versenate, Calcium EDTA

Pharmacologic class: chelating agent
Therapeutic class: heavy metal antagonist
Pregnancy risk category: B

Indications and dosages

▶ **Acute lead encephalopathy or blood lead levels above 70 mcg/dl.** *Adults and children:* 1.5 g/m² I.V. or I.M. daily in divided doses at 12-hour intervals for 3 to 5 days, usually in conjunction with dimercaprol. A second course may be administered in 5 to 7 days.
▶ **Lead poisoning without encephalopathy, or asymptomatic with blood levels below 70 mcg/dl.** *Children:* 1 g/m² I.V. or I.M. daily in divided doses.

How supplied

Injection: 200 mg/ml

Pharmacokinetics

Absorption: well absorbed after I.M. administration.
Distribution: distributed primarily in extracellular fluid.
Metabolism: none.
Excretion: excreted in urine. *Half-life:* 20 minutes to 1½ hours.

Route	Onset	Peak	Duration
I.V., I.M.	1 hr	24-48 hr	Unknown

Pharmacodynamics

Chemical effect: forms stable, soluble complexes with metals, particularly lead.
Therapeutic effect: abolishes effects of lead poisoning.

Adverse reactions

CNS: headache, paresthesia, numbness, fatigue.
CV: ***arrhythmias,*** hypotension.
EENT: sneezing and nasal congestion.
GI: anorexia, nausea, vomiting, excessive thirst.
GU: proteinuria, hematuria, ***nephrotoxicity with renal tubular necrosis leading to fatal nephrosis.***
Metabolic: hypercalcemia.
Musculoskeletal: arthralgia, myalgia.
Other: sudden fever, chills.

Interactions

Drug-drug. *Zinc insulin:* interferes with action of insulin by binding with zinc. Monitor patient closely.
Zinc supplements: decreased effectiveness of edetate calcium disodium and zinc supplements because of chelation. Withhold zinc supplements until therapy is complete.

Contraindications and precautions

• Contraindicated in patients with anuria, hepatitis, or acute renal disease.
• Use with extreme caution in patients with mild renal disease. Expect dosages to be reduced.
• Use cautiously in pregnant women.

NURSING CONSIDERATIONS

Assessment
- Obtain history of patient's underlying condition before therapy.
- Monitor effectiveness by checking serum lead level and observing for decreasing signs and symptoms of lead poisoning.
- Monitor fluid intake and output, urinalysis, BUN, and ECG daily, as ordered.
- Be alert for adverse reactions.
- Observe injection site for local reaction.
- Evaluate patient's and family's knowledge of drug therapy.

Nursing diagnoses
- Risk for injury related to lead poisoning
- Ineffective renal tissue perfusion related to drug-induced fatal nephrosis
- Deficient knowledge related to drug therapy

Planning and implementation
I.V. use: Dilute drug with D_5W or normal saline injection to 2 to 4 mg/ml. Infuse half of daily dose over 1 hour in asymptomatic patients or 2 hours in symptomatic patients. Give rest of infusion at least 6 hours later. Or, give by slow infusion over at least 8 hours.
I.M. use: Add procaine hydrochloride, as ordered, to I.M. solution to minimize pain. Watch for local reactions.
- Because I.V. use may increase intracranial pressure, don't administer by that route to treat lead encephalopathy. Give by I.M. route instead.
- The I.M. route is preferred, especially for children and patients with lead encephalopathy.
- Force fluids to facilitate lead excretion, except in patients with lead encephalopathy.
- To avoid toxicity, use with dimercaprol, as ordered.
- Apply ice or cold compresses to injection site to ease local reaction.

ALERT Don't confuse edetate calcium with edetate disodium, which is used to treat hypercalcemia.

Patient teaching
- Warn patient that some adverse reactions—such as fever, chills, thirst, and nasal congestion—may occur 4 to 8 hours after administration.
- Encourage patient and family to identify and remove source of lead in home.

Evaluation
- Patient sustains no injury as result of lead poisoning.
- Patient has no signs of altered renal tissue perfusion.
- Patient and family state understanding of drug therapy.

edetate disodium
(ED-eh-tayt digh-SOH-dee-um)
EDTA, Disotate, Endrate

Pharmacologic class: chelating agent
Therapeutic class: heavy metal antagonist
Pregnancy risk category: C

Indications and dosages
▶ **Hypercalcemic crisis.** *Adults:* 50 mg/kg by slow I.V. infusion added to 500 ml of D_5W or normal saline solution and given over 3 or more hours. Maximum, 3 g/day.
Children: 40 to 70 mg/kg by slow I.V. infusion, diluted to maximum of 30 mg/ml in D_5W or normal saline solution and given over 3 or more hours. Maximum, 70 mg/kg/day.
▶ **Cardiac glycoside–induced arrhythmias.** *Adults and children:* 15 mg/kg/hour I.V. with maximum of 60 mg/kg daily.

How supplied
Injection: 150 mg/ml

Pharmacokinetics
Absorption: not applicable with I.V. administration.
Distribution: distributed widely throughout body but doesn't enter CSF in significant amounts.
Metabolism: none.
Excretion: excreted in urine.

Route	Onset	Peak	Duration
I.V.	Unknown	Unknown	Unknown

Pharmacodynamics

Chemical effect: chelates with metals, such as calcium, to form stable, soluble complex.
Therapeutic effect: lowers blood calcium level.

Adverse reactions

CNS: circumoral paresthesia, numbness, headache.
CV: hypertension, thrombophlebitis, orthostatic hypotension.
EENT: erythema.
GI: nausea, vomiting, diarrhea, anorexia, abdominal cramps.
Metabolic: ***severe hypocalcemia,*** decreased magnesium level.
GU: nephrotoxicity with urinary urgency, nocturia, dysuria, polyuria, proteinuria, renal insufficiency, ***renal failure, tubular necrosis***.
Skin: dermatitis.
Other: pain at site of infusion.

Interactions

Drug-drug. *Cardiac glycosides:* Sudden drop in serum calcium caused by edate disodium may reverse effects of digitalis. Monitor patient closely.
Insulin: decreased serum glucose and possible chelation of zinc in insulin. Dosage adjustments of insulin may be required.

Contraindications and precautions

- Contraindicated in patients hypersensitive to drug and in those with anuria, known or suspected hypocalcemia, significant renal disease, active or healed tubercular lesions, or a history of seizures or intracranial lesions.
- Use cautiously in patients with limited cardiac reserve, heart failure, or hypokalemia. Also use cautiously in pregnant or breast-feeding women.

NURSING CONSIDERATIONS

Assessment

- Obtain history of patient's calcium level before therapy.
- Monitor effectiveness by obtaining serum calcium level after each dose, as ordered. If used to treat cardiac glycoside–induced arrhythmias, evaluate patient's ECG frequently.
- Monitor kidney function tests frequently, as ordered.
- Be alert for adverse reactions.
- Evaluate patient's and family's knowledge of drug therapy.

Nursing diagnoses

- Risk for injury related to hypercalcemia
- Ineffective protection related to drug-induced hypocalcemia
- Deficient knowledge related to drug therapy

Planning and implementation

ALERT Read label carefully; don't confuse with edetate calcium disodium, which is used for lead toxicity.
- Dilute before use. Avoid rapid I.V. infusion; profound hypocalcemia may occur, leading to tetany, seizures, arrhythmias, and respiratory arrest. Drug isn't recommended for direct or intermittent injection. Avoid extravasation.
- Record I.V. site used, and avoid repeated use of same site, which increases likelihood of thrombophlebitis.
- Keep I.V. calcium available to treat hypocalcemia.
- Keep patient in bed for 15 minutes after infusion to avoid orthostatic hypotension.
- If generalized systemic reactions—fever, chills, back pain, emesis, muscle cramps, urinary urgency—occur 4 to 8 hours after infusion, report them to prescriber. Treatment is usually supportive. Symptoms usually subside within 12 hours.
- Don't use to treat lead toxicity; use edetate calcium disodium instead.
- Other drug treatments for hypercalcemia are safer and more effective than edetate disodium.

Patient teaching

- Instruct patient to report respiratory difficulty, dizziness, and muscle cramping immediately.
- Advise patient to move from sitting or lying position slowly to avoid dizziness.
- Reassure patient that generalized systemic reaction usually subsides within 12 hours.

Evaluation

- Patient sustains no injury as result of hypercalcemia.

• Patient's blood calcium level doesn't fall below normal after edetate disodium therapy.
• Patient and family state understanding of drug therapy.

edrophonium chloride

(ed-roh-FOH-nee-um KLOR-ighd)
Enlon, Reversol, Tensilon

Pharmacologic class: cholinesterase inhibitor
Therapeutic class: cholinergic agonist, diagnostic agent
Pregnancy risk category: NR

Indications and dosages

▶ **As curare antagonist (to reverse nondepolarizing neuromuscular blocking action).** *Adults:* 10 mg I.V. given over 30 to 45 seconds. Dose may be repeated as needed to maximum of 40 mg. Larger dosages may potentiate effect of curare.

▶ **Diagnostic aid in myasthenia gravis (Tensilon test).** *Adults:* 1 to 2 mg I.V. over 15 to 30 seconds; then 8 mg if no response (increase in muscle strength) occurs. Or, 10 mg I.M. If cholinergic reaction occurs, 2 mg I.M. is given 30 minutes later to rule out false-negative response.
Children weighing more than 34 kg (75 lb): 2 mg I.V. If no response within 45 seconds, 1 mg q 45 seconds to maximum of 10 mg. Or, 5 mg I.M.
Children weighing less than 34 kg: 1 mg I.V. If no response within 45 seconds, 1 mg q 45 seconds to maximum of 5 mg. Or, 2 mg I.M. (I.M. route may be used in children because of difficulty with I.V. route.) Expect same reactions as with I.V. test, but they appear after 2- to 10-minute delay.
Infants: 0.5 mg to 1 mg I.M. or S.C.

▶ **To differentiate myasthenic crisis from cholinergic crisis.** *Adults:* 1 mg I.V. If no response in 1 minute, dose is repeated once. Increased muscle strength confirms myasthenic crisis; no increase or exaggerated weakness confirms cholinergic crisis.

How supplied

Injection: 10 mg/ml in 1-ml ampules or in 10-ml or 15-ml vials

Pharmacokinetics

Unknown.

Route	Onset	Peak	Duration
I.V.	30-60 sec	Unknown	5-10 min
I.M.	2-10 min	Unknown	5-30 min

Pharmacodynamics

Chemical effect: inhibits destruction of acetylcholine released from parasympathetic and somatic efferent nerves. Acetylcholine accumulates, promoting increased stimulation of receptor.
Therapeutic effect: reverses nondepolarizing neuromuscular blocker.

Adverse reactions

CNS: ***seizures,*** weakness, dysarthria.
CV: hypotension, ***bradycardia, AV block, cardiac arrest.***
EENT: excessive lacrimation, diplopia, ***laryngospasm,*** miosis, conjunctival hyperemia, dysphagia.
GI: nausea, vomiting, *diarrhea, abdominal cramps,* excessive salivation.
GU: urinary frequency, incontinence.
Musculoskeletal: muscle cramps, muscle fasciculation.
Respiratory: ***respiratory paralysis, bronchospasm,*** increased bronchial secretions.
Skin: diaphoresis.

Interactions

Drug-drug. *Aminoglycosides, anesthetics:* prolonged or enhanced muscle weakness. Monitor patient closely.
Cardiac glycosides: may increase heart's sensitivity to edrophonium. Use together cautiously.
Cholinergics: increased effects. Stop all other cholinergics before giving drug, as ordered.
Corticosteroids, magnesium, procainamide, quinidine: may antagonize cholinergic effects. Observe patient for lack of drug effect.
Drug-herb. *Jaborandi tree, pill-bearing spurge:* Possible additive effect with risk of toxicity. Discourage concomitant use.

Contraindications and precautions

- Contraindicated in patients hypersensitive to anticholinesterases and in those with mechanical obstruction of intestine or urinary tract.
- Use cautiously in patients with bronchial asthma or arrhythmias.
- Safety of drug hasn't been established in pregnant or breast-feeding women.

NURSING CONSIDERATIONS

Assessment

- Obtain history of patient's underlying condition before therapy.
- Monitor effectiveness by evaluating reduction of symptoms of underlying condition. When giving drug to differentiate myasthenic crisis from cholinergic crisis, observe patient's muscle strength closely.
- Be alert for adverse reactions and drug interactions.
- Evaluate patient's and family's knowledge of drug therapy.

Nursing diagnoses

- Ineffective health maintenance related to underlying condition
- Impaired gas exchange related to drug-induced bronchospasm
- Deficient knowledge related to drug therapy

Planning and implementation

- Stop all other cholinergics before giving this drug, as ordered.

I.V. use: For easier parenteral administration, use tuberculin syringe with I.V. needle.

I.M. use: Use I.M. route, as ordered, to give drug to children because of difficulty with I.V. insertion in children.

- Keep atropine injection readily available, and be prepared to give 0.5 to 1 mg S.C. or slow I.V. push, as ordered. Provide respiratory support, as needed.

Patient teaching

- Tell patient to report adverse reactions immediately, especially difficulty breathing.

Evaluation

- Patient shows improvement in underlying condition.
- Patient maintains adequate gas exchange throughout therapy.
- Patient and family state understanding of drug therapy.

efavirenz

(eh-fah-VEER-enz)

Sustiva

Pharmacologic class: nonnucleoside, reverse transcriptase inhibitor
Therapeutic class: antiviral
Pregnancy risk category: C

Indications and dosages

▶ **Treatment of HIV-1 infection.** *Adults:* 600 mg P.O. once daily in combination with a protease inhibitor or nucleoside analogue reverse transcriptase inhibitors.
Children age 3 and older weighing 40 kg (88 lb) or more: 600 mg P.O. once daily in combination with a protease inhibitor or nucleoside analogue reverse transcriptase inhibitors.
Children age 3 and older weighing 10 to under 15 kg (22 to under 33 lb): 200 mg P.O. once daily.
Children weighing 15 to under 20 kg (33 to under 44 lb): 250 mg P.O. once daily.
Children weighing 20 to under 25 kg (44 to under 55 lb): 300 mg P.O. once daily.
Children weighing 25 to under 32.5 kg (55 to under 72 lb): 350 mg P.O. once daily.
Children weighing 32.5 to under 40 kg (72 to under 88 lb): 400 mg P.O. once daily.

Give above doses in combination with protease inhibitor or nucleoside analogue reverse transcriptase inhibitor.

How supplied

Capsules: 50 mg, 100 mg, 200 mg

Pharmacokinetics

Absorption: oral absorption produces peak levels in 3 to 5 hours with steady-state levels in 6 to 10 days.
Distribution: highly bound to human plasma proteins, predominantly albumin.

Metabolism: primarily metabolized by cytochrome P-450 system to metabolites that are inactive against HIV-1.
Excretion: excreted primarily in feces with a small number of metabolites excreted in urine.

Route	Onset	Peak	Duration
P.O.	Unknown	3-5 hr	Unknown

Pharmacodynamics

Chemical effect: a nonnucleoside, reverse transcriptase inhibitor that inhibits the transcription of HIV-1 RNA to DNA, a critical step in the viral replication process.
Therapeutic effect: lowers amount of HIV in the blood (viral load) and increases CD4 lymphocytes.

Adverse reactions

CNS: abnormal dreams or thinking, agitation, amnesia, confusion, depersonalization, depression, *dizziness,* euphoria, fatigue, hallucinations, headache, hypesthesia, impaired concentration, insomnia, somnolence, nervousness.
GI: abdominal pain, anorexia, *diarrhea,* dyspepsia, flatulence, *nausea,* vomiting.
GU: hematuria, renal calculi.
Hepatic: increase in AST, ALT, and total cholesterol levels.
Skin: increased sweating, ***erythema multiforme, Stevens-Johnson syndrome, toxic epidermal necrolysis,*** *rash,* pruritus.
Other: fever.

Interactions

Drug-drug. *Clarithromycin, indinavir:* decreased plasma levels. Alternate therapy or dosage adjustment may be indicated.
Drugs that induce cytochrome P-450 enzyme system (such as phenobarbital, rifampin, rifabutin): increased clearance of efavirenz, resulting in lowered plasma levels. Avoid concomitant use.
Ergot derivatives, midazolam, triazolam: competition for cytochrome P-450 enzyme system may result in inhibited metabolism of these drugs and cause serious or life-threatening adverse events (such as arrhythmias, prolonged sedation, or respiratory depression). Avoid concomitant use.
Estrogens, ritonavir: increased plasma levels. Monitor patient.
Oral contraceptives: potential interaction of efavirenz with oral contraceptive hasn't been determined. Advise use of a reliable method of barrier contraception in addition to oral contraceptives.
Psychoactive drugs: additive CNS effects. Avoid concomitant use.
Saquinavir: plasma saquinavir levels decreased significantly. Don't use with saquinavir as sole protease inhibitor.
Warfarin: plasma levels and effects potentially increased or decreased. Monitor INR.
Drug-food. *High-fat meals:* increased absorption of drug. Instruct patient to maintain a proper low-fat diet.
Drug-lifestyle. *Alcohol use:* enhanced CNS effects. Discourage concomitant use.

Contraindications and precautions

- Contraindicated in patients hypersensitive to drug or its components.
- Use cautiously in patients with hepatic impairment or in those concurrently receiving hepatotoxic drugs.

NURSING CONSIDERATIONS

Assessment

- Monitor liver function test results in patients with history of hepatitis B or C and in those also taking ritonavir.
- Monitor cholesterol levels.
- Children may be more prone to adverse reactions, especially diarrhea, nausea, vomiting, and rash.
- Evaluate patient's and family's knowledge of drug therapy.

Nursing diagnoses

- Risk for infection related to patient's underlying condition
- Risk for impaired skin integrity related to potential adverse effects of drug
- Deficient knowledge related to drug therapy

Planning and implementation

- Drug should be used in combination with other antiretrovirals because resistant viruses emerge rapidly when used alone. Drug should

not be used as monotherapy or added on as a single agent to a failing regimen.
- Combination with ritonavir may cause a higher occurrence of adverse effects (such as dizziness, nausea, paresthesia) and laboratory abnormalities (elevated liver enzyme levels).
- Pregnancy must be ruled out before therapy is started in women of childbearing age.
- Administer drug at bedtime to decrease noticeable CNS adverse effects.

Patient teaching
- Instruct patient to take drug with water, juice, milk, or soda. It may be taken without regard to meals.
- Inform patient about need for scheduled blood tests to monitor liver function and cholesterol levels.
- Tell patient to use reliable method of barrier contraception in addition to oral contraceptives and to notify prescriber immediately if pregnancy is suspected.
- Inform patient that drug doesn't cure HIV infection and that it won't affect the development of opportunistic infections and other complications of HIV disease. Explain that it doesn't reduce the risk of HIV transmission through sexual contact or blood contamination.
- Instruct patient to take drug at same time daily and always in combination with other antiretroviral drugs.
- Tell patient to take drug exactly as prescribed and not to discontinue without medical approval. Also instruct patient to report any adverse reactions.
- Inform patient that rash is most common adverse effect. If it occurs, tell patient to report it immediately because it may be serious in rare cases.
- Instruct patient to report use of other medications.
- Advise patient that dizziness, difficulty sleeping or concentrating, drowsiness, or unusual dreams may occur the first few days of therapy. Reassure patient that these symptoms typically resolve after 2 to 4 weeks and may be less problematic if drug is taken at bedtime.
- Tell patient to avoid alcoholic beverages, driving, or operating machinery until drug's effects are known.

☑ Evaluation
- Patient is free from opportunistic infections.
- Patient's skin integrity is maintained.
- Patient and family state understanding of drug therapy.

enalaprilat
(eh-NAH-leh-prel-at)
Vasotec I.V.

enalapril maleate
Amprace◇, Renitec◇, Vasotec

Pharmacologic class: ACE inhibitor
Therapeutic class: antihypertensive
Pregnancy risk category: C (D in second and third trimesters)

Indications and dosages
▶ **Hypertension.** *Adults:* for patient not taking a diuretic, initially 5 mg P.O. once daily, adjusted according to response. Usual dosage range is 10 to 40 mg daily as single dose or two divided doses. Or, 1.25 mg I.V. over 5 minutes q 6 hours. For patient taking a diuretic, initially 2.5 mg P.O. once daily. Or, 0.625 mg I.V. over 5 minutes, repeated in 1 hour if needed, followed by 1.25 mg I.V. q 6 hours.

▶ **To convert from I.V. to P.O. therapy.** *Adults:* initially, 5 mg P.O. once daily; if patient was receiving 0.625 mg I.V., then 2.5 mg P.O. once daily. Dosage is adjusted to response.

▶ **To convert from P.O. to I.V. therapy.** *Adults:* 1.25 mg I.V. over 5 minutes q 6 hours. Higher amounts haven't shown greater efficacy.

▶ **Heart failure.** *Adults:* Initially, 2.5 mg P.O. once daily. Dosage may be adjusted upward after a few days or weeks according to clinical response. Recommended range is 2.5 to 20 mg twice daily.

▶ **Asymptomatic left ventricular dysfunction.** *Adults:* 2.5 mg P.O. b.i.d., adjusted as tolerated up to target of 20 mg/day in divided doses.

How supplied

Tablets: 2.5 mg, 5 mg, 10 mg, 20 mg
Injection: 1.25 mg/ml

Pharmacokinetics

Absorption: about 60% of P.O. dose absorbed from GI tract.
Distribution: unknown.
Metabolism: metabolized extensively to active metabolite.
Excretion: about 94% excreted in urine and feces as enalaprilat and enalapril. *Half-life:* 12 hours.

Route	Onset	Peak	Duration
P.O.	1 hr	4-6 hr	24 hr
I.V.	15 min	1-4 hr	6 hr

Pharmacodynamics

Chemical effect: unknown; inhibits ACE, which prevents conversion of angiotensin I to angiotensin II, a potent vasoconstrictor. Reduced formation of angiotensin II decreases peripheral arterial resistance, thus decreasing aldosterone secretion.
Therapeutic effect: lowers blood pressure.

Adverse reactions

CNS: *headache, dizziness, fatigue,* vertigo, asthenia, syncope.
CV: *hypotension,* chest pain.
GI: diarrhea, nausea, abdominal pain, vomiting.
GU: decreased renal function (in patients with bilateral renal artery stenosis or heart failure).
Hematologic: ***neutropenia, thrombocytopenia, agranulocytosis.***
Respiratory: *dry, persistent, tickling, nonproductive cough;* dyspnea.
Skin: rash.
Other: ***angioedema.***

Interactions

Drug-drug. *Diuretics:* excessive reduction of blood pressure. Monitor patient.
Insulin, oral antidiabetics: risk of hypoglycemia, especially at start of enalapril therapy. Monitor patient and glucose levels closely.
Lithium: risk of lithium toxicity. Monitor lithium levels.
NSAIDs: may reduce antihypertensive effect. Monitor blood pressure.
Potassium supplements, potassium-sparing diuretics: increased risk of hyperkalemia. Avoid these drugs unless hypokalemic blood levels are confirmed.
Drug-herb. *Licorice:* may cause sodium retention and increase blood pressure, interfering with therapeutic effects of ACE inhibitors. Discourage concomitant use.
Drug-lifestyle. *Alcohol use:* may produce additive hypotensive effect. Discourage concurrent use.
Sunlight: Photosensitivity reaction may occur. Urge precautions.

Contraindications and precautions

- Contraindicated in patients hypersensitive to drug and those with history of angioedema from previous treatment with ACE inhibitor.
- Use with extreme caution and only when absolutely necessary in pregnant women because fetal harm may occur.
- Use cautiously in patients with renal impairment.
- Safety of drug hasn't been established in breast-feeding women and in children.

NURSING CONSIDERATIONS

Assessment

- Obtain history of patient's blood pressure before therapy, and reassess regularly thereafter.
- Monitor CBC with differential counts before therapy, every 2 weeks for first 3 months of therapy, and periodically thereafter.
- Monitor potassium intake and serum potassium level.
- Be alert for adverse reactions and drug interactions.
- Evaluate patient's and family's knowledge of drug therapy.

Nursing diagnoses

- Risk for injury related to presence of hypertension
- Risk for infection related to drug-induced adverse hematologic reactions
- Deficient knowledge related to drug therapy

Planning and implementation

- Patient with renal insufficiency or hyponatremia should start with 2.5 mg P.O. daily, adjusted slowly.

P.O. use: Follow normal protocol.
I.V. use: Inject drug slowly over at least 5 minutes, or dilute in 50 ml of compatible solution and infuse over 15 minutes. Compatible solutions include D_5W, normal saline injection, dextrose 5% in lactated Ringer's injection, and D_5W in normal saline injection.

- First-dose hypotension, following effective management, doesn't negate further, careful dosage adjustment.
- Notify prescriber immediately if CBC becomes abnormal or if evidence of infection arises.
- If angioedema occurs, notify prescriber and stop treatment immediately. Institute appropriate therapy (epinephrine solution 1:1,000 [0.3 to 0.5 ml] S.C.), and take measures to ensure patent airway.

Patient teaching

- Advise patient to report evidence of angioedema, such as breathing difficulty and swelling of face, eyes, lips, or tongue. Angioedema (including laryngeal edema) may occur, especially after first dose.
- Instruct patient to report signs of infection, such as fever and sore throat.
- Advise patient that light-headedness can occur, especially during first few days of therapy. Tell patient to rise slowly to minimize this effect and to report symptoms to prescriber. If patient experiences syncope, he should stop taking drug and call prescriber immediately.
- Tell patient to use caution in hot weather and during exercise. Inadequate fluid intake, vomiting, diarrhea, and excessive perspiration can lead to light-headedness and syncope.
- Advise patient to avoid sodium substitutes; these products may contain potassium, which can cause hyperkalemia in patients taking drug.
- Tell woman to notify prescriber if pregnancy occurs. Drug will need to be discontinued.

Evaluation

- Patient's blood pressure becomes normal.
- Patient's CBC remains normal throughout therapy.
- Patient and family state understanding of drug therapy.

enoxacin

(eh-NOKS-uh-sin)
Penetrex

Pharmacologic class: fluoroquinolone antibacterial
Therapeutic class: antibiotic
Pregnancy risk category: C

Indications and dosages

▶ **Uncomplicated urinary tract infections.** *Adults:* 200 mg P.O. q 12 hours for 7 days.
▶ **Severe or complicated urinary tract infections.** *Adults:* 400 mg P.O. q 12 hours for 14 days.
▶ **Uncomplicated urethral or endocervical gonorrhea.** *Adults:* 400 mg P.O. as single dose. Doxycycline therapy may follow to treat possible coexisting chlamydial infection.

In patients with renal failure with creatinine clearance of 30 ml/minute or less, therapy starts with usual initial dose. Subsequent doses are decreased by 50%.

How supplied

Tablets: 200 mg, 400 mg

Pharmacokinetics

Absorption: absolute oral bioavailability is about 90% after absorption.
Distribution: about 40% bound to plasma proteins.
Metabolism: five metabolites of drug have been identified; they account for 15% to 20% of administered dose.
Excretion: excreted primarily in urine. *Half-life:* 3 to 6 hours.

Route	Onset	Peak	Duration
P.O.	Unknown	1-3 hr	Unknown

Pharmacodynamics

Chemical effect: inhibits bacterial DNA synthesis, mainly by blocking DNA gyrase; bactericidal.

Therapeutic effect: kills susceptible bacteria. Spectrum of activity includes most strains of gram-positive aerobes, such as *Staphylococcus epidermidis* and *Staphylococcus saprophyticus*, and many gram-negative aerobes, such as *Enterobacter cloacae, Escherichia coli, Klebsiella pneumoniae, Neisseria gonorrhoeae, Proteus mirabilis,* and *Pseudomonas aeruginosa.*

Adverse reactions

CNS: headache, restlessness, tremors, lightheadedness, confusion, hallucinations, ***seizures.***

GI: *nausea, diarrhea,* vomiting, abdominal pain or discomfort, oral candidiasis.

GU: crystalluria.

Hemotolic: eosinophilia.

Hepatic: elevated liver enzyme levels.

Respiratory: dyspnea, cough.

Skin: *rash,* photosensitivity, pruritus.

Other: hypersensitivity.

Interactions

Drug-drug. *Aminophylline, cyclosporine, theophylline:* increased levels of these drugs because of decreased metabolism. Use together cautiously.

Antacids containing magnesium hydroxide or aluminum hydroxide, oral iron supplements, sucralfate: decreased enoxacin absorption. Separate administration times by at least 2 hours before or 8 hours after.

Bismuth subsalicylate: bioavailability of enoxacin is decreased when given within 60 minutes of bismuth subsalicylate. Separate administration times.

Digoxin: may increase digoxin serum levels. Monitor patient closely for toxicity.

Drug-food. *Any food:* affects absorption. Give drug on an empty stomach.

Caffeine: increased effect of caffeine. Monitor patient closely.

Contraindications and precautions

- Contraindicated in patients hypersensitive to drug or other fluoroquinolone antibiotics.
- Use cautiously in patients with CNS disorders, such as severe cerebral arteriosclerosis or seizure disorders, and in those at increased risk for seizures. Drug may cause CNS stimulation.
- Use cautiously and with dosage adjustments in patients with impaired kidney or liver function. Also use cautiously in pregnant women.
- Safety of drug hasn't been established in breast-feeding women and in children.

NURSING CONSIDERATIONS

Assessment

- Obtain history of patient's infection before therapy, and reassess regularly thereafter.
- Obtain specimen for culture and sensitivity tests before first dose. Therapy may begin pending test results.
- Have patient being treated for gonorrhea obtain initial serologic test for syphilis before therapy starts. Drug isn't effective in treating syphilis and may mask signs and symptoms of infection. Have patient repeat serologic test in 1 to 3 months.
- Be alert for adverse reactions and drug interactions.
- Monitor patient's hydration status if adverse GI reactions occur.
- Evaluate patient's and family's knowledge of drug therapy.

Nursing diagnoses

- Infection related to presence of susceptible bacteria
- Risk for deficient fluid volume related to drug-induced adverse GI reactions
- Deficient knowledge related to drug therapy

Planning and implementation

- Administer 2 hours after a meal or 2 hours before or after antacids containing magnesium hydroxide or aluminum hydroxide, sucralfate, or products that contain iron (such as vitamins with mineral supplements).

ALERT Don't confuse enoxacin with enoxaparin sodium.

Patient teaching

- Advise patient to avoid overexposure to direct sunlight while taking drug and to use

sunblock and wear protective clothing when outdoors.
• Warn patient not to drink beverages containing caffeine while taking enoxacin. Drug inhibits metabolism of caffeine and can result in toxicity.
• Advise patient to liberally increase fluid intake while taking drug because similar drugs have caused urine microcrystal formation.
• Warn patient to avoid hazardous activities until adverse CNS effects of drug are known.

Evaluation
• Patient is free from infection.
• Patient maintains adequate hydration throughout therapy.
• Patient and family state understanding of drug therapy.

enoxaparin sodium
(eh-NOKS-uh-pah-rin SOH-dee-um)
Lovenox

Pharmacologic class: low-molecular-weight heparin derivative
Therapeutic class: anticoagulant
Pregnancy risk category: B

Indications and dosages
▶ **Prevention of pulmonary embolism and deep vein thrombosis (DVT) after hip or knee replacement surgery.** *Adults:* 30 mg S.C. q 12 hours for 7 to 10 days. Initial dose given 12 to 24 hours after surgery, provided hemostasis has been established. Or, for hip replacement surgery, 40 mg S.C. once daily given initially 12 hours before surgery. May continue with 40 mg S.C. once daily or 30 mg S.C. q 12 hours for 3 weeks.
▶ **Prevention of pulmonary embolism and DVT in patients after abdominal surgery.** *Adults:* 40 mg S.C. once daily for 7 to 10 days with initial dose given 2 hours before surgery.
▶ **Prevention of ischemic complications of unstable angina and non-Q-wave MI, when concurrently administered with aspirin.** *Adults:* 1 mg/kg S.C. q 12 hours for 2 to 8 days together with oral aspirin therapy (100 to 325 mg/day).
▶ **Inpatient treatment of acute DVT with and without pulmonary embolism when administered in conjunction with warfarin sodium.** *Adults:* 1 mg/kg S.C. every 12 hours. Or, 1.5 mg/kg S.C. once daily (at same time every day) for 5 to 7 days until therapeutic oral anticoagulant effect (INR of 2 to 3) has been achieved. Warfarin sodium therapy is usually started within 72 hours of enoxaparin injection.
▶ **Outpatient treatment of acute DVT without pulmonary embolism when administered in conjunction with warfarin sodium.** *Adults:* 1 mg/kg S.C. every 12 hours for 5 to 7 days until therapeutic oral anticoagulant effect (INR of 2 to 3) has been achieved. Warfarin sodium therapy is usually started within 72 hours of enoxaparin injection.

How supplied
Injection: 30 mg/0.3 ml; 40 mg/0.4 ml; 60 mg/0.6 ml; 80 mg/0.8 ml; 100 mg/ml

Pharmacokinetics
Absorption: unknown.
Distribution: unknown.
Metabolism: unknown.
Excretion: unknown. *Half-life:* about 4½ hours after S.C. administration.

Route	Onset	Peak	Duration
S.C.	Unknown	3-5 hr	< 24 hr

Pharmacodynamics
Chemical effect: accelerates formation of antithrombin IIIB–thrombin complex and deactivates thrombin, preventing conversion of fibrinogen to fibrin. Enoxaparin has higher antifactor Xa–antifactor IIa activity ratio.
Therapeutic effect: prevents pulmonary embolism and DVT.

Adverse reactions
CNS: confusion, ***neurologic injury*** (when used with spinal or epidural puncture).
CV: edema, peripheral edema, ***CV toxicity.***
GI: nausea.
Hematologic: ecchymosis, hypochromic anemia, ***thrombocytopenia, hemorrhage,*** bleeding complications.

Skin: irritation, pain, hematoma, or erythema at injection site; *rash; urticaria.*
Other: fever, pain, ***angioedema.***

Interactions

Drug-drug. *Anticoagulants, antiplatelet drugs, NSAIDs:* increased risk of bleeding. Don't use together.
Plicamycin, valproic acid: may cause hypoprothrombinemia and inhibit platelet aggregation. Monitor patient closely.

Contraindications and precautions

- Contraindicated in patients hypersensitive to drug, heparin, or pork products; in those with active major bleeding or thrombocytopenia; and in those who demonstrate antiplatelet antibodies in presence of drug.
- Use with extreme caution, if at all, in patients with postoperative indwelling epidural catheters or patients who have had epidural or spinal anesthesia. Epidural and spinal hematomas have been reported, resulting in long-term or permanent paralysis.
- Use with extreme caution in patients with history of heparin-induced thrombocytopenia.
- Use cautiously in patients with conditions that put them at increased risk for hemorrhage, such as bacterial endocarditis, and in patients with congenital or acquired bleeding disorders, ulcer disease, angiodysplastic GI disease, hemorrhagic CVA, or recent spinal, eye, or brain surgery.
- Use cautiously in pregnant or breast-feeding women.
- Safe use in children hasn't been established.

NURSING CONSIDERATIONS

Assessment

- Obtain history of patient's coagulation parameters before therapy.
- Monitor effectiveness by evaluating patient for signs and symptoms of pulmonary embolism or DVT.
- Monitor platelet counts regularly. Patient with normal coagulation doesn't require regular monitoring of PT, INR, and PTT.
- Frequently monitor neurological status in patients who have had spinal or epidural anesthesia. Alert prescriber immediately if neurological compromise is noted.
- Be alert for adverse reactions and drug interactions.
- Evaluate patient's and family's knowledge of drug therapy.

Nursing diagnoses

- Risk for injury related to risk for pulmonary embolism or DVT after knee or hip replacement surgery
- Ineffective protection related to drug-induced bleeding complications
- Deficient knowledge related to drug therapy

Planning and implementation

ALERT To avoid drug loss, don't expel air bubble from 30- or 40-mg prefilled syringes.
- Never administer drug I.M.
- Don't massage after S.C. injection. Rotate sites and keep accurate record.
- Enoxaparin can't be used interchangeably (unit for unit) with unfractionated heparin or other low-molecular-weight heparins.
- Don't mix enoxaparin with other injections or infusions.
- Avoid excessive I.M. injections of other drugs to prevent or minimize hematomas. If possible, don't give I.M. injections when patient is anticoagulated.
- To treat severe overdose, give protamine sulfate (a heparin antagonist) by slow I.V. infusion at concentration of 1% to equal dosage of enoxaparin injected, as ordered.

ALERT Don't confuse enoxacin with enoxaparin sodium.

Patient teaching
- Instruct patient and family to watch for signs of bleeding and notify prescriber immediately.
- Tell patient to avoid OTC drugs that contain aspirin or other salicylates.

Evaluation

- Patient doesn't develop pulmonary embolism or DVT.
- Patient has no bleeding complications during therapy.
- Patient and family state understanding of drug therapy.

entacapone

(en-TAK-uh-pohn)

Comtan

Pharmacologic class: catechol-O-methyltransferase (COMT) inhibitor
Therapeutic class: antiparkinsonian
Pregnancy risk category: C

Indications and dosages

▶ **Adjunct to levodopa-carbidopa for treatment of idiopathic Parkinson's disease in patients who experience end-of-dose wearing-off.** *Adults:* 200 mg P.O. with each dose of levodopa-carbidopa to maximum of eight times daily. Maximum recommended dosage of entacapone is 1,600 mg daily. Reducing daily levodopa dose or extending the interval between doses may be necessary to optimize patient's response.

How supplied

Tablets: 200 mg

Pharmacokinetics

Absorption: absorption is rapid, with serum levels peaking in about 1 hour. Food doesn't affect absorption.
Distribution: drug is about 98% protein-bound, mainly to albumin, and doesn't distribute widely into tissues.
Metabolism: drug is almost completely metabolized by glucuronidation before elimination. No active metabolites have been identified.
Excretion: about 10% of drug is excreted in urine; the remainder is excreted in bile and feces. *Half-life:* 0.4 to 0.7 hours for first phase and 2.4 hours for second phase.

Route	Onset	Peak	Duration
P.O.	1 hr	1 hr	6 hr

Pharmacodynamics

Chemical effect: entacapone is a reversible inhibitor of peripheral COMT, which is responsible for elimination of various catecholamines, including dopamine. Blocking this pathway when administering levodopa-carbidopa should result in higher serum levels of levodopa, thereby allowing greater dopaminergic stimulation in the CNS and leading to a greater clinical effect in treating parkinsonian symptoms.
Therapeutic effect: control of idiopathic Parkinson's disease signs and symptoms.

Adverse reactions

CNS: *dyskinesia, hyperkinesia,* hypokinesia, dizziness, anxiety, somnolence, agitation, fatigue, asthenia, hallucinations.
GI: *nausea, diarrhea,* abdominal pain, constipation, vomiting, dry mouth, dyspepsia, flatulence, gastritis, taste perversion.
GU: *urine discoloration.*
Hematologic: purpura.
Musculoskeletal: back pain.
Respiratory: dyspnea.
Skin: sweating.
Other: bacterial infection.

Interactions

Drug-drug. *Ampicillin, chloramphenicol, cholestyramine, erythromycin, probenecid:* may block biliary excretion, resulting in higher serum levels of entacapone. Use cautiously.
CNS depressants: additive effect. Use cautiously.
Drugs metabolized by COMT (*bitolterol, dobutamine, dopamine, epinephrine, isoetharine, isoproterenol, norepinephrine*): may cause higher serum levels of these drugs, resulting in increased heart rate, changes in blood pressure, or possibly arrhythmias. Use cautiously.
Nonselective MAO inhibitors (such as phenelzine, tranylcypromine): may inhibit normal catecholamine metabolism. Avoid concomitant use.
Drug-lifestyle. *Alcohol use:* may cause additive CNS effects. Discourage concomitant use.

Contraindications and precautions

- Contraindicated in patients hypersensitive to drug.
- Use cautiously in patients with hepatic impairment, biliary obstruction, or orthostatic hypotension.

NURSING CONSIDERATIONS

Assessment
- Assess hepatic and biliary function before starting therapy.
- Monitor blood pressure closely. Watch for orthostatic hypotension.
- Monitor patient for hallucinations.
- Evaluate patient's and family's knowledge about drug therapy.

Nursing diagnoses
- Impaired physical mobility related to presence of parkinsonism
- Disturbed thought processes related to drug-induced adverse reactions
- Deficient knowledge related to drug therapy

Planning and implementation
- Drug can be given with immediate or sustained-release levodopa-carbidopa and can be taken with or without food.
- Drug should be used only with levodopa-carbidopa; no antiparkinsonian effects will occur when drug is given as monotherapy.
- Levodopa-carbidopa dosage requirements are usually lower when given with entacapone; levodopa-carbidopa dose should be lowered or dosing interval increased, as ordered, to avoid adverse effects.
- Drug may cause or worsen dyskinesia despite reduction of levodopa dosage.
- Watch for the onset of diarrhea. It usually begins 4 to 12 weeks after therapy starts, but may begin as early as first week or as late as many months after therapy starts.
- Rapid withdrawal or abrupt reduction in dose could lead to signs and symptoms of Parkinson's disease; it may also lead to hyperpyrexia and confusion, a symptom complex resembling neuroleptic malignant syndrome. Discontinue drug slowly, as ordered, and monitor patient closely. Adjust other dopaminergic treatments as ordered.
- Observe for urine discoloration.
- Rarely, rhabdomyolysis has occurred with drug use.

Patient teaching
- Instruct patient not to crush or break tablet and to take it at same time as levodopa-carbidopa.
- Warn patient to avoid hazardous activities until CNS effects of drug are known.
- Advise patient to avoid alcohol during treatment.
- Instruct patient to use caution when standing after a prolonged period of sitting or lying down because dizziness may occur. This effect is more common early in therapy.
- Warn patient that hallucinations, increased dyskinesia, nausea, and diarrhea could occur.
- Inform patient that drug may cause urine to turn brownish orange.
- Advise patient to notify prescriber if she is pregnant or breast-feeding or if she plans to become pregnant.

Evaluation
- Patient exhibits improved physical mobility.
- Patient maintains normal thought process.
- Patient and family state understanding of drug therapy.

ephedrine sulfate
(eh-FED-rin SUL-fayt)
Kondon's Nasal†, Pretz-D†

Pharmacologic class: adrenergic
Therapeutic class: bronchodilator, vasopressor (parenteral form), nasal decongestant.
Pregnancy risk category: C

Indications and dosages
▶ **To correct hypotension.** *Adults:* 25 to 50 mg I.M. or S.C. or 10 to 25 mg I.V., p.r.n., to maximum of 150 mg/24 hours.
Children: 3 mg/kg or 100 mg/m^2 S.C. or I.V. daily in four to six divided doses.
▶ **Bronchodilation, nasal decongestion.** *Adults and children age 12 and over:* 25 to 50 mg P.O. q 3 to 4 hours p.r.n. For patient use as a bronchodilator, 12.5 to 25 mg P.O. q 4 hr. Maximum, 150 mg in 24 hours. As a nasal decongestant, 0.5% solution applied topically to nasal mucosa as drops or on nasal pack. Instill no more often than q 4 hours.

Children ages 2 to 12: 2 to 3 mg/kg P.O. daily in four to six divided doses.

How supplied

Tablets: 30 mg ◊
Capsules: 25 mg, 50 mg
Injection: 25 mg/ml, 50 mg/ml
Nasal solution: 0.25%†, 0.5%†, 1%†

Pharmacokinetics

Absorption: rapidly and completely absorbed after P.O., I.M., or S.C. administration; unknown after nasal administration.
Distribution: widely distributed throughout body.
Metabolism: slowly metabolized in liver.
Excretion: excreted unchanged in urine. Rate of excretion depends on urine pH. *Half-life:* 3 to 6 hours.

Route	Onset	Peak	Duration
P.O.	15-60 min	Unknown	3-5 hr
I.V.	≤ 5 min	Unknown	Unknown
I.M.	10-20 min	Unknown	0.5-1 hr
S.C.	Unknown	Unknown	0.5-1 hr
Intranasal	Unknown	Unknown	Unknown

Pharmacodynamics

Chemical effect: stimulates alpha- and beta-adrenergic receptors; direct- and indirect-acting sympathomimetic.
Therapeutic effect: raises blood pressure, causes bronchodilation, and relieves nasal decongestion.

Adverse reactions

CNS: *insomnia, nervousness,* dizziness, headache, muscle weakness, diaphoresis, euphoria, confusion, delirium.
CV: *palpitations,* tachycardia, hypertension, precordial pain.
EENT: dryness of nose and throat.
GI: nausea, vomiting, anorexia.
GU: urine retention, painful urination from visceral sphincter spasm.

Interactions

Drug-drug. *Acetazolamide:* increased serum ephedrine levels. Monitor patient for toxicity.
Alpha-adrenergic blockers: unopposed beta-adrenergic effects, resulting in hypotension. Monitor blood pressure.
Antihypertensives: decreased effects. Monitor blood pressure.
Beta blockers: unopposed alpha-adrenergic effects, resulting in hypertension. Monitor blood pressure.
Cardiac glycosides, general anesthetics (halogenated hydrocarbons): increased risk of ventricular arrhythmias. Monitor patient closely.
Ergot alkaloids: enhanced vasoconstrictor activity. Monitor patient closely.
Guanadrel, guanethidine: enhanced pressor effects of ephedrine. Monitor patient closely.
MAO inhibitors, tricyclic antidepressants: when given with sympathomimetics, may cause severe hypertension (hypertensive crisis). Avoid concomitant use.
Methyldopa, reserpine: may inhibit effects of ephedrine. Use together cautiously.

Contraindications and precautions

- Contraindicated in patients hypersensitive to ephedrine and other sympathomimetic drugs; in those with porphyria, severe coronary artery disease, arrhythmias, angle-closure glaucoma, psychoneurosis, angina pectoris, substantial organic heart disease, or CV disease; and in those taking MAO inhibitors.
- Breast-feeding should be avoided during treatment with ephedrine.
- Use with extreme caution in elderly men and in those with hypertension, hyperthyroidism, nervous or excitable states, diabetes, or prostatic hyperplasia.
- Use cautiously in pregnant women and in children.

NURSING CONSIDERATIONS

Assessment

- Obtain history of patient's underlying condition before therapy, and reassess regularly thereafter.
- Be alert for adverse reactions and drug interactions.
- Evaluate patient's and family's knowledge of drug therapy.

Nursing diagnoses

- Ineffective health maintenance related to underlying condition
- Risk for deficient fluid volume related to drug-induced adverse GI reactions
- Deficient knowledge related to drug therapy

Planning and implementation

- Hypoxia, hypercapnia, and acidosis, which may reduce drug effectiveness or increase adverse reactions, must be identified and corrected before or during ephedrine administration.
- Volume deficit must be corrected before administering vasopressors. This drug isn't a substitute for blood or fluid volume replenishment.
- To prevent insomnia, avoid giving within 2 hours before bedtime.

P.O. use: Follow normal protocol.
I.V. use: Give 10 to 25 mg by I.V. injection slowly; repeat in 5 to 10 minutes, if necessary. Compatible with most common I.V. solutions.
I.M., S.C., and intranasal use: Follow normal protocol.

- Notify prescriber if effectiveness decreases. Effectiveness decreases after 2 to 3 weeks, as tolerance develops. Prescriber may need to increase dosage. Drug isn't addictive.

Patient teaching

- Warn patient not to take OTC drugs that contain ephedrine without consulting prescriber.
- Teach patient how to instill nose drops and caution him not to exceed recommended dosage.
- Advise patient to notify prescriber if effectiveness decreases because dosage may need to be adjusted.
- Instruct patient to notify prescriber if adverse reactions occur.
- Caution patient not to perform hazardous activities if adverse CNS reactions occur.

Evaluation

- Patient exhibits improvement in underlying condition.
- Patient maintains adequate hydration throughout therapy.
- Patient and family state understanding of drug therapy.

epinephrine (adrenaline)

(eh-pih-NEF-rin)

Adrenalin†, Bronkaid Mist†, Bronkaid Mistometer♦, Primatene Mist†

epinephrine bitartrate

AsthmaHaler Mist†, Bronitin Mist†, Bronkaid Mist Suspension†, Medihaler-Epi†, Primatene Mist Suspension†

epinephrine hydrochloride

Adrenalin Chloride†, Ana-Guard, EpiPen Auto-Injector, EpiPen Jr. Auto-Injector, Sus-Phrine

Pharmacologic class: adrenergic
Therapeutic class: bronchodilator, vasopressor, cardiac stimulant, local anesthetic, topical antihemorrhagic
Pregnancy risk category: C

Indications and dosages

▶ **Bronchospasm, hypersensitivity reactions, anaphylaxis.** *Adults:* 0.1 to 0.5 ml of 1:1,000 S.C. or I.M.; repeated q 10 to 15 minutes, p.r.n. Or, 0.1 to 0.25 ml of 1:1,000 (1 to 2.5 ml of commercially available 1:10,000 injection or of 1:10,000 dilution prepared by diluting 1 ml of commercially available 1:1,000 injection with 10 ml of water for injection or normal saline injection) I.V. slowly over 5 to 10 minutes.
Children: 0.01 ml (10 mcg) of 1:1,000/kg S.C.; repeated q 20 minutes to 4 hours, p.r.n. Or, 0.005 ml/kg of 1:200 (Sus-Phrine) S.C.; repeated q 8 to 12 hours, p.r.n.
▶ **Hemostasis.** *Adults:* 1:50,000 to 1:1,000 applied topically.
▶ **Acute asthma attacks.** *Adults and children age 4 and over:* 160 to 250 mcg (metered aerosol), which is equivalent to one inhalation, repeated once if necessary after at least 1 minute; subsequent doses should not be administered for at least 3 hours. Or, 1% (1:100) solution of epinephrine or 2.25% solution of racepinephrine administered by hand-bulb nebulizer as one to three deep inhalations, repeated q 3 hours, p.r.n.

▶ **Prolongation of local anesthetic effect.** *Adults and children:* 1:500,000 to 1:50,000 mixed with local anesthetic.

▶ **Restoration of cardiac rhythm in cardiac arrest.** *Adults:* 0.5 to 1 mg I.V. or into endotracheal tube. Drug may be given intracardiac if no I.V. route or intratracheal route is available. Some clinicians advocate higher dose (up to 5 mg), especially in patients who don't respond to usual I.V. dose. After initial I.V. administration, drug may be infused I.V. at 1 to 4 mcg/minute.
Children: 10 mcg/kg I.V., or 5 to 10 mcg (0.05 to 0.1 ml of 1:10,000)/kg intracardiac.

How supplied

Aerosol inhaler: 160 mcg†, 200 mcg†, 220 mcg†, 250 mcg/metered spray†
Nebulizer inhaler: 0.5%†, 1% (1:100)♦†, 2.25% (racepinephrine)◇†
Injection: 0.01 mg/ml (1:100,000), 0.1 mg/ml (1:10,000), 0.5 mg/ml (1:2,000), 1 mg/ml (1:1,000) parenteral; 5 mg/ml (1:200) parenteral suspension

Pharmacokinetics

Absorption: well absorbed after S.C. or I.M. injection. Rapidly absorbed after inhalation administration.
Distribution: distributed widely throughout body.
Metabolism: metabolized at sympathetic nerve endings, liver, and other tissues to inactive metabolites.
Excretion: excreted in urine, mainly as its metabolites and conjugates.

Route	Onset	Peak	Duration
I.V.	Immediate	≤ 5 min	1-4 hr
I.M.	Varies	Unknown	1-4 hr
S.C.	6-15 min	≤ 30 min	1-4 hr
Inhalation	3-5 min	Unknown	1-3 hr

Pharmacodynamics

Chemical effect: stimulates alpha- and beta-adrenergic receptors in sympathetic nervous system.
Therapeutic effect: relaxes bronchial smooth muscle, causes cardiac stimulation, relieves allergic signs and symptoms, stops local bleeding, and decreases pain sensation.

Adverse reactions

CNS: *nervousness, tremors,* euphoria, anxiety, cold limbs, vertigo, *headache, drowsiness,* diaphoresis, disorientation, agitation, fear, weakness, ***cerebral hemorrhage, CVA,*** increased rigidity and tremors (in patients with Parkinson's disease).
CV: *palpitations,* widened pulse pressure, *hypertension, tachycardia,* ***ventricular fibrillation, shock,*** anginal pain, ECG changes (including decreased T-wave amplitude).
GI: *nausea,* vomiting.
Metabolic: hyperglycemia, glycosuria.
Respiratory: dyspnea.
Skin: urticaria, pain, hemorrhage at injection site.
Other: pallor.

Interactions

Drug-drug. *Alpha-adrenergic blockers:* hypotension from unopposed beta-adrenergic effects. Monitor blood pressure.
Antihistamines, thyroid hormones, tricyclic antidepressants: when given with sympathomimetics, may cause severe adverse cardiac effects. Avoid giving together.
Beta blockers (such as propranolol): vasoconstriction and reflex bradycardia. Monitor patient carefully.
Cardiac glycosides, general anesthetics (halogenated hydrocarbons): increased risk of ventricular arrhythmias. Monitor patient closely.
Doxapram, methylphenidate: enhanced CNS stimulation or pressor effects. Monitor patient closely.
Ergot alkaloids: enhanced vasoconstrictor activity. Monitor patient closely.
Guanadrel, guanethidine: enhanced pressor effects of epinephrine. Monitor patient closely.
Levodopa: enhanced risk of cardiac arrhythmias. Monitor patient closely.
MAO inhibitors: increased risk of hypertensive crisis. Avoid concomitant use.

Contraindications and precautions

- Contraindicated in patients with angle-closure glaucoma, shock (other than anaphylactic shock), organic brain damage, cardiac dilation, arrhythmias, coronary insufficiency, or cerebral arteriosclerosis. Also contraindicated in patients receiving general anesthesia with halogenated hydrocarbons or cyclopropane and in patients in labor (may delay second stage).

- Some commercial products contain sulfites and are contraindicated in patients with sulfite allergies except when epinephrine is being used for treatment of serious allergic reactions or in other emergency situations.
- In conjunction with local anesthetics, epinephrine is contraindicated for use in fingers, toes, ears, nose, or genitalia.
- Breast-feeding should be avoided during drug use.
- Use with extreme caution in patients with long-standing bronchial asthma or emphysema who have developed degenerative heart disease. Also use cautiously in elderly patients and in those with hyperthyroidism, CV disease, hypertension, psychoneurosis, or diabetes, as well as in pregnant women not in labor and in children.

NURSING CONSIDERATIONS

Assessment

- Obtain history of patient's underlying condition before therapy, and reassess regularly thereafter.
- When administering I.V., monitor blood pressure, heart rate, and ECG when therapy starts and frequently thereafter.
- Be alert for adverse reactions and drug interactions.
- Evaluate patient's and family's knowledge of drug therapy.

Nursing diagnoses

- Ineffective health maintenance related to underlying condition
- Decreased cardiac output related to drug-induced adverse CV effects
- Deficient knowledge related to drug therapy

Planning and implementation

- Keep in mind that 1 mg of epinephrine = 1 ml of 1:1,000 or 10 ml of 1:10,000.
- Epinephrine is drug of choice in emergency treatment of acute anaphylactic reactions.
- Discard epinephrine solution after 24 hours or if solution is discolored or contains precipitate. Keep solution in light-resistant container, and don't remove before use.

I.V. use: Don't mix with alkaline solutions. Use D_5W, normal saline injection, lactated Ringer's injection, or combinations of dextrose in sodium chloride. Mix just before use.

I.M. use: Avoid I.M. administration of parenteral suspension into buttocks. Gas gangrene may occur because epinephrine reduces oxygen tension of tissues, encouraging growth of contaminating organisms.

– Massage site after I.M. injection to counteract possible vasoconstriction. Repeated local injection can cause necrosis, resulting from vasoconstriction at injection site.

S.C. use: Follow normal protocol.

Inhalation use: If bronchodilator is administered by inhalation and more than one inhalation is ordered, wait 2 minutes between inhalations. Always administer bronchodilator first and wait 5 minutes before administering the other if more than one type of inhalant is ordered. Remember that the patient shouldn't receive more than 12 bronchodilator inhalations in 24 hours.

- Giving medication on time is extremely important.
- Notify prescriber if adverse reactions develop; he may adjust dosage or discontinue drug. Also notify prescriber if patient's pulse increases by 20% or more when epinephrine is administered.
- If blood pressure rises sharply, rapid-acting vasodilators, such as nitrites or alpha-adrenergic blockers, can be given to counteract marked pressor effect of large doses of epinephrine.
- Epinephrine is destroyed rapidly by oxidizing agents, such as iodine, chromates, nitrates, nitrites, oxygen, and salts of easily reducible metals (such as iron).

Patient teaching

- Tell patient to take drug exactly as prescribed and to take it around the clock.
- Teach patient to perform oral inhalation correctly. Give following instructions for using metered-dose inhaler:

– Clear nasal passages and throat.

– Breathe out, expelling as much air from lungs as possible.
– Place mouthpiece well into mouth and inhale deeply as dose from inhaler is released.
– Hold breath for several seconds, remove mouthpiece, and exhale slowly.
- If more than one inhalation is ordered, tell patient to wait at least 2 minutes before repeating procedure.
- Tell patient who also is using corticosteroid inhaler to use bronchodilator first, then wait about 5 minutes before using corticosteroid. This allows bronchodilator to open air passages for maximum effectiveness.
- Instruct patient who has acute hypersensitivity reactions, such as to bee stings, to self-inject epinephrine at home.
- Tell patient to reduce intake of foods containing caffeine, such as coffee, colas, and chocolates, when taking bronchodilator.
- Instruct patient to contact prescriber immediately if he experiences fluttering of heart, rapid beating of heart, shortness of breath, or chest pain.
- Tell patient not to take any OTC medicines or herbal remedies without medical approval while taking this drug.
- Show patient how to check pulse. Instruct him to check pulse before and after using bronchodilator and to call prescriber if pulse rate increases bymore than 20 beats/minute.

Evaluation
- Patient shows improvement in underlying condition.
- Patient maintains adequate cardiac output throughout therapy.
- Patient and family state understanding of drug therapy.

epinephrine hydrochloride
(eh-pih-NEF-rin high-droh-KLOR-ighd)
Adrenalin Chloride

Pharmacologic class: adrenergic
Therapeutic class: decongestant, topical antihemorrhagic
Pregnancy risk category: NR

Indications and dosages
▶ **Nasal congestion, local superficial bleeding.** *Adults and children:* instill 1 or 2 gtt of solution.

How supplied
Nasal solution: 0.1%

Pharmacokinetics
Unknown.

Route	Onset	Peak	Duration
Nasal	≤ 1 min	Unknown	Unknown

Pharmacodynamics
Chemical effect: causes local vasoconstriction of dilated arterioles, reducing blood flow and nasal congestion.
Therapeutic effect: relieves nasal decongestion and stops local bleeding.

Adverse reactions
CNS: nervousness, excitation.
CV: *tachycardia.*
EENT: rebound nasal congestion, slight sting on application.

Interactions
None significant.

Contraindications and precautions
- Contraindicated in patients hypersensitive to drug.
- Breast-feeding should be avoided during drug therapy.
- Use cautiously in patients with hyperthyroidism, coronary artery disease, hypertension, or diabetes mellitus.
- Also use cautiously in pregnant women and in children.

NURSING CONSIDERATIONS

Assessment
- Obtain history of patient's underlying condition before therapy, and reassess regularly thereafter.
- Monitor effectiveness by noting if patient experiences decreased nasal congestion or cessation of bleeding.
- Be alert for adverse reactions.

• Evaluate patient's and family's knowledge of drug therapy.

Nursing diagnoses

• Ineffective health maintenance related to underlying condition
• Deficient knowledge related to drug therapy

Planning and implementation

• Follow normal protocol for instilling nose drops.

Patient teaching

• Teach patient how to instill nose drops.
• Instruct patient that product should be used by only one person to prevent spread of infection.
• Tell patient not to exceed recommended dosage and to use only when needed.

Evaluation

• Patient shows improvement of underlying condition.
• Patient and family state understanding of drug therapy.

epirubicin hydrochloride

(ep-uh-ROO-bih-sin high-droh-KLOR-ighd)
Ellence

Pharmacologic class: anthracycline
Therapeutic class: antineoplastic
Pregnancy risk category: D

Indications and dosages

▶ **Adjuvant therapy in patients with evidence of axillary node tumor involvement following resection of primary breast cancer.** *Adults:* 100 to120 mg/m^2 I.V. infusion over 3 to 5 minutes via a free-flowing I.V. solution on day 1 of each cycle q 3 to 4 weeks; or divided equally in two doses on days 1 and 8 of each cycle. Maximum cumulative (lifetime) dose is 900 mg/m^2.

Dosage modification after the first cycle is based on toxicity. For patient with platelet count below 50,000/mm^3, absolute neutrophil count (ANC) below 250/mm^3, neutropenic fever, or grade 3 or 4 nonhematologic toxicity, the day 1 dose in subsequent cycles should be reduced to 75% of the day 1 dose given in the current cycle. Day 1 therapy in subsequent cycles should be delayed until platelets are 100,000/mm^3 or above, ANC is 1,500/mm^3 or above, and nonhematologic toxicities recover to grade 1.

For patients receiving divided doses (days 1 and 8), the day 8 dose should be 75% of the day 1 dose if platelet counts are 75,000 to 100,000/mm^3 and ANC is 1,000 to 1,499/mm^3. If day 8 platelet counts are below 75,000/mm^3, ANC is below 1,000/mm^3, or grade 3 or 4 nonhematologic toxicity has occurred, the day 8 dose should be omitted.

How supplied

Injection: 2 mg/ml

Pharmacokinetics

Absorption: drug is a vesicant and must be given I.V.
Distribution: rapidly and widely distributed into tissues. Plasma protein–binding is about 77%, mainly to albumin, and appears to concentrate in RBCs.
Metabolism: extensively and rapidly metabolized by the liver. Several metabolites form with little to no cytotoxic activity.
Excretion: eliminated mostly by biliary excretion and, to a lesser extent, urinary excretion.

Route	Onset	Peak	Duration
I.V.	Unknown	Unknown	Unknown

Pharmacodynamics

Chemical effect: The precise mechanism of epirubicin's cytotoxic effects isn't completely known. It's thought to form a complex with DNA by intercalation between nucleotide base pairs, thereby inhibiting DNA, RNA, and protein synthesis. DNA cleavage occurs, resulting in cytocidal activity. Drug may also interfere with replication and transcription of DNA, and it generates cytotoxic free radicals.
Therapeutic effect: kills certain cancer cells.

Adverse reactions

CNS: *lethargy.*
CV: ***cardiomyopathy, heart failure.***
EENT: *conjunctivitis, keratitis.*

GI: *nausea, vomiting, diarrhea,* anorexia, *mucositis.*
GU: *amenorrhea.*
Hematologic: LEUKOPENIA, NEUTROPENIA, ***febrile neutropenia,*** *anemia,* THROMBOCYTOPENIA.
Skin: *alopecia,* rash, itch, skin changes.
Other: *infection,* fever, *hot flushes, local toxicity.*

Interactions

Drug-drug. *Cytotoxic drugs:* additive toxicities (especially hematologic and GI) may occur. Monitor patient closely.
Calcium channel blockers, other cardioactive compounds: may increase risk of heart failure. Monitor cardiac function closely.
Cimetidine: increased epirubicin level (by 50%) and decreased clearance. Avoid concomitant use.
Radiation therapy: effects may be enhanced. Monitor patient carefully.

Contraindications and precautions

- Contraindicated in patient hypersensitive to this drug, other anthracyclines, or anthracenediones. Also contraindicated in patients with baseline neutrophil counts below 1,500 cells/mm^3, in those with severe myocardial insufficiency or recent MI, in those previously treated with anthracyclines to total cumulative doses, and in those with severe hepatic dysfunction.
- Use cautiously in patients with active or dormant cardiac disease, patients with previous or concomitant radiotherapy to the mediastinal and pericardial area, previous therapy with other anthracyclines or anthracenediones, or concomitant use of other cardiotoxic drugs.

NURSING CONSIDERATIONS

Assessment

- Obtain baseline total bilirubin, AST, creatinine, and CBC (including ANC), and evaluate cardiac function by measuring left ventricular ejection fraction (LVEF) before therapy.
- Monitor LVEF regularly during therapy, and discontinue drug at the first sign of impaired cardiac function. Monitor patient for early signs of cardiac toxicity, including sinus tachycardia, ECG abnormalities, tachyarrhythmias, bradycardia, AV block, and bundle branch block.
- Obtain total and differential WBC, RBC, and platelet counts before and during each cycle of therapy.
- Evaluate patient's and family's knowledge about drug therapy.

Nursing diagnoses

- Risk for injury related to drug-induced adverse reactions
- Risk for infection related to myelosupression
- Deficient knowledge related to drug therapy

Planning and implementation

- Patients with bone marrow dysfunction, hepatic dysfunction, or severe renal dysfunction should receive lower dosages.
- Epirubicin should be given under the supervision of a prescriber experienced in the use of cancer chemotherapy. Pregnant women shouldn't handle this drug.
- Wear protective clothing (goggles, gown, disposable gloves) when handling this drug.
- Drug is a vesicant. Never give I.M. or S.C. Always administer through free-flowing I.V. solution of normal saline solution or D_5W over 3 to 5 minutes.
- Facial flushing and local erythematous streaking along the vein may indicate too-rapid administration.
- Avoid veins over joints or in limbs with compromised venous or lymphatic drainage.
- Immediately stop infusion if burning or stinging occurs, and restart in another vein.
- Don't mix drug with heparin or fluorouracil because precipitation may result.
- Don't mix in same syringe with other drugs.
- Discard unused solution in vial 24 hours after vial penetrated.
- Patients receiving 120 mg/m^2 of epirubicin should also receive prophylactic antibiotic therapy with trimethoprim-sulfamethoxazole or a fluoroquinolone, as ordered.
- Use of antiemetics before epirubicin may be necessary to reduce nausea and vomiting.
- Delayed cardiac toxicity may occur 2 to 3 months after completion of treatment. It causes reduced LVEF, evidence of heart failure (tachycardia, dyspnea, pulmonary edema, de-

pendent edema, hepatomegaly, ascites, pleural effusion, and gallop rhythm). Delayed cardiac toxicity is dependent upon the cumulative dose of epirubicin. Don't exceed a cumulative dose of 900 mg/m^2.

• Monitor serum uric acid, potassium, calcium phosphate, and creatinine immediately after initial chemotherapy administration in patients susceptible to tumor lysis syndrome. Hydration, urine alkalinization, and prophylaxis with allopurinol may prevent hyperuricemia and minimize complications of tumor lysis syndrome.
• The WBC nadir usually occurs 10 to14 days after drug administration and returns to normal by day 21.
• Anthracycline-induced leukemia may occur.
• Administration of drug after previous radiation therapy may induce an inflammatory cell reaction at the site of irradiation.

Patient teaching

• Advise patient to report nausea, vomiting, stomatitis, dehydration, fever, evidence of infection, or symptoms of heart failure (tachycardia, dyspnea, edema) or injection site pain.
• Inform patient of the risk of cardiac damage and treatment-related leukemia with use of drug.
• Women of childbearing age should avoid getting pregnant and men should use effective contraception during treatment.
• Advise women that irreversible amenorrhea or premature menopause may occur.
• Advise patient about probable hair loss. Tell patient that hair regrowth usually occurs 2 to 3 months after therapy is discontinued.
• Advise patient that urine may appear red 1 to 2 days after administration of the drug.

☑ Evaluation

• Patient sustains no injury from drug-induced adverse reactions.
• Patient remains free of infection.
• Patient and family state understanding of drug therapy.

epoetin alfa (erythropoietin)

(ee-POH-eh-tin AL-fah)
Epogen, Eprex♦, Procrit

Pharmacologic class: glycoprotein
Therapeutic class: antianemic
Pregnancy risk category: C

Indications and dosages

▶ **Anemia from reduced production of endogenous erythropoietin caused by end-stage renal disease.** *Adults:* dosage is individualized. Starting dose is 50 to 100 units/kg I.V. three times weekly. (Nondialysis patients with chronic renal failure or patients receiving continuous peritoneal dialysis may receive drug by S.C. injection or I.V.) Dosage reduced when target hematocrit is reached or if hematocrit rises more than 4 points in any 2-week period. Dosage increased if hematocrit doesn't increase by 5 to 6 points after 8 weeks of therapy. Maintenance dosage is individualized.
▶ **Anemia in children with chronic renal failure who are undergoing dialysis.** *Infants and children ages 1 month to 16 years:* 50 units/kg I.V. or S.C. three times weekly. Reduce dosage when target hematocrit is reached or if hematocrit rises more than 4 points in a 2-week period. Increase dosage if hematocrit doesn't rise by 5 to 6 points after 8 weeks of therapy and is below target range. Maintenance dose is highly individualized to maintain hematocrit in target range.
▶ **Adjunct treatment of HIV-infected patients with anemia secondary to zidovudine therapy.** *Adults:* 100 units/kg I.V. or S.C. three times weekly for 8 weeks or until target hemoglobin is reached.
▶ **Anemia secondary to chemotherapy.** *Adults:* 150 units/kg S.C. three times weekly for 8 weeks or until target hemoglobin is reached. Dosage then increased up to 300 units/kg S.C. three times weekly, if needed.

How supplied

Injection: 2,000 units/ml, 3,000 units/ml, 4,000 units/ml, 10,000 units/ml, 20,000 units/ml

Pharmacokinetics

Unknown.

Route	Onset	Peak	Duration
I.V.	1-6 wk	Immediate	Unknown
S.C.	1-6 wk	4-24 hr	Unknown

Pharmacodynamics

Chemical effect: mimics effects of erythropoietin, a naturally occurring hormone produced by the kidneys. Epoetin alfa is one of factors controlling rate of RBC production. It acts on erythroid tissues in bone marrow, stimulating mitotic activity of erythroid progenitor cells and early precursor cells. It functions as a growth factor and as a differentiating factor, enhancing rate of RBC production.
Therapeutic effect: eliminates anemia.

Adverse reactions

CNS: *headache, **seizures,** paresthesia, fatigue,* dizziness, *asthenia.*
CV: increased clotting of arteriovenous grafts, *hypertension, edema.*
GI: *nausea, vomiting, diarrhea.*
Hematologic: iron deficiency, elevated platelet count.
Musculoskeletal: *arthralgia.*
Respiratory: *cough, shortness of breath.*
Skin: *rash, injection site reactions, urticaria.*
Other: *pyrexia.*

Interactions

None significant.

Contraindications and precautions

- Contraindicated in patients with uncontrolled hypertension, hypersensitivity to mammal cell–derived products or albumin (human).
- Use cautiously in pregnant or breast-feeding women.
- Safety of drug hasn't been established in children.

NURSING CONSIDERATIONS

Assessment

- Assess patient's blood count and blood pressure before therapy.
- Assess effectiveness by monitoring blood count results, as ordered. Hematocrit may rise and cause excessive clotting. Watch for evidence of blood clot formation such as shortness of breath, cold, swollen or pulseless limb.
- Patient's response to epoetin alfa depends on amount of endogenous erythropoietin in plasma. Patients with 500 units/L or more usually have transfusion-dependent anemia and will probably not respond to drug. Those with levels below 500 units/L usually respond well.
- Be alert for adverse reactions.
- Monitor blood pressure closely. Up to 80% of patients with chronic renal failure have hypertension. Blood pressure may rise, especially when hematocrit is increasing in early part of therapy.
- After injection (usually within 2 hours), some patients complain of pain or discomfort in their limbs (long bones) and pelvis and of coldness and sweating. Symptoms may persist for up to 12 hours and then disappear.
- Monitor patient's hydration status if adverse GI reactions occur.
- Evaluate patient's and family's knowledge of drug therapy.

Nursing diagnoses

- Ineffective protection related to reduced production of endogenous erythropoietin
- Risk for deficient fluid volume related to drug-induced adverse GI reactions
- Deficient knowledge related to drug therapy

Planning and implementation

I.V. use: Give drug by direct injection without dilution. Solution contains no preservatives. Discard unused portion. Don't mix with other drugs.
S.C. use: Follow normal protocol.
- When used in HIV-infected patient, be prepared to individualize dosage based on response, as ordered. Dosage recommendations are for patients with endogenous erythropoietin levels of 500 units/L or less and cumulative zidovudine doses of 4.2 g/week or less.
- Patient treated with epoetin alfa may need additional heparin to prevent clotting during dialysis.
- Institute diet restrictions or drug therapy to control blood pressure. Reduce dosage in

patient who exhibits rapid rise in hematocrit (more than 4 points in a 2-week period), as ordered, because of risk of hypertension.

Patient teaching
- Advise patient that blood specimens will be drawn weekly for blood counts and that dosage adjustments may be made based on results.
- Warn patient to avoid hazardous activities, such as driving or operating heavy machinery, early in therapy. Excessively rapid rise in hematocrit may increase the risk of seizures.
- Tell patient to notify prescriber if adverse reactions occur.

Evaluation
- Patient's blood count is normal.
- Patient maintains adequate hydration throughout therapy.
- Patient and family state understanding of drug therapy.

eprosartan mesylate
(eh-proh-SAR-ten MEH-sih-layt)
Teveten

Pharmacologic class: angiotensin II receptor antagonist
Therapeutic class: antihypertensive
Pregnancy risk category: C (D in second and third trimesters)

Pharmacodynamics
Chemical effect: Drug is an angiotensin II receptor that blocks vasoconstrictor and aldosterone-secreting effects of angiotensin II by selectively blocking binding of angiotensin II to its receptor sites in many tissues, such as vascular smooth muscle and the adrenal gland.
Therapeutic effect: lowers blood pressure.

Indications and dosages
▶ **Hypertension, alone or with other antihypertensives.** *Adults:* initially, 600 mg P.O. daily. Daily dosage ranges from 400 to 800 mg given as single daily dose or two divided doses.

How supplied
Tablets: 400 mg, 600 mg

Pharmacokinetics
Absorption: absolute bioavailability of single oral dose is about 13%. Plasma levels peak in 1 to 2 hours.
Distribution: plasma protein–binding is about 98%.
Metabolism: no active metabolites.
Excretion: eliminated by biliary and renal excretion, primarily as unchanged drug. Following P.O. administration, about 90% is recovered in feces and about 7% in urine. *Terminal elimination half-life:* typically 5 to 9 hours.

Route	Onset	Peak	Duration
P.O.	1-2 hr	1-3 hr	24 hr

Adverse reactions
CNS: depression, fatigue, headache, dizziness.
CV: chest pain, dependent edema.
EENT: pharyngitis, rhinitis, sinusitis.
GI: abdominal pain, dyspepsia, diarrhea.
GU: urinary tract infection, increased BUN level.
Hematologic: ***neutropenia.***
Metabolic: hypertriglyceridemia.
Musculoskeletal: arthralgia, myalgia.
Respiratory: cough, upper respiratory tract infection, bronchitis.
Other: injury, viral infection.

Interactions
None significant.

Contraindications and precautions
- Contraindicated in patients hypersensitive to drug or its components.
- Use cautiously in patients with an activated renin-angiotensin system, such as volume- or salt-depleted patients, and in patients whose renal function may depend on the activity of the renin-angiotensin-aldosterone system, such as patients with severe heart failure.
- Also use cautiously in patients with renal artery stenosis.

NURSING CONSIDERATIONS

Assessment
- Monitor blood pressure closely during start of treatment. If hypotension occurs, place patient in supine position and, if necessary,

give I.V. infusion of normal saline solution, as ordered.
- Determine patient's fluid balance status and serum sodium level before starting drug therapy.
- Elderly patients have a slightly decreased response to drug.
- Be alert for adverse reactions.
- Evaluate patient's and family's knowledge of drug therapy.

Nursing diagnoses
- Risk for injury related to presence of hypertension
- Risk for infection related to neutropenia
- Deficient knowledge related to drug therapy

Planning and implementation
- Correct hypovolemia and hyponatremia before starting therapy, as ordered, to reduce risk of symptomatic hypotension.
- A transient episode of hypotension doesn't contraindicate continued treatment. Drug may be restarted once patient's blood pressure has stabilized.
- Drug may be used alone or with other antihypertensives, such as diuretics and calcium channel blockers. Maximum blood pressure response may take 2 to 3 weeks.
- Monitor patient for facial or lip swelling because angioedema has occurred with other angiotensin II antagonists.

Patient teaching
- Advise woman of childbearing age to use reliable form of contraception and to notify prescriber immediately if pregnancy is suspected. Drug may need to be discontinued under medical supervision.
- Advise patient to report facial or lip swelling and signs and symptoms of infection, such as fever or sore throat.
- Tell patient to notify prescriber before taking OTC product to treat a dry cough.
- Inform patient that drug may be taken without regard to meals.
- Tell patient to store drug at a controlled room temperature (68° to 77° F [20° to 25° C]).

Evaluation
- Patient's blood pressure is well controlled, and patient remains free of injury.
- WBCs are within normal limits.
- Patient and family state understanding of drug therapy.

eptifibatide
(ep-tih-FY-beh-tide)
Integrilin

Pharmacologic class: glycoprotein IIb/IIIa (GP IIb/IIIa) inhibitor
Therapeutic class: antiplatelet agent
Pregnancy risk category: B

Indications and dosages
▶ **Patients with acute coronary syndrome (unstable angina or non-Q-wave MI), including patients who will be managed medically and those undergoing percutaneous coronary intervention.** *Adults:* I.V. bolus of 180 mcg/kg (maximum dose of 22.6 mg) as soon as possible following diagnosis; then a continuous I.V. infusion of 2 mcg/kg/minute (maximum infusion rate of 15 mg/hour) for up to 72 hours. Infusion rate may be decreased to 0.5 mcg/kg/minute during percutaneous coronary intervention. Infusion should then be continued for another 20 to 24 hours after procedure for up to 96 hours.
▶ **Patients without an acute coronary syndrome who are undergoing percutaneous coronary intervention.** *Adults:* I.V. bolus of 135 mcg/kg given immediately before procedure; then continuous infusion of 0.5 mcg/kg/minute for 20 to 24 hours.

How supplied
Injection: 10-ml (2 mg/ml), 100-ml (0.75 mg/ml) vials

Pharmacokinetics
Absorption: not applicable with I.V. administration.
Distribution: drug is 25% bound to plasma proteins.
Metabolism: not reported. No major metabolites have been detected in human plasma.

Excretion: most of drug is excreted in urine. *Elimination half-life:* 2½ hours.

Route	Onset	Peak	Duration
I.V.	Immediate	Immediate	4-6 hr after end of infusion

Pharmacodynamics

Chemical effect: Drug reversibly binds to the glycoprotein IIb/IIIa (GP IIb/IIIa) receptor on human platelets and inhibits platelet aggregation.
Therapeutic effect: prevent clot formation.

Adverse reactions

CV: hypotension.
GU: hematuria.
Hematologic: *bleeding,* ***thrombocytopenia.***
Other: bleeding at femoral artery access site.

Interactions

Drug-drug. *Clopidogrel, dipyridamole, NSAIDs, oral anticoagulants (warfarin), thrombolytics, ticlopidine:* increased risk of bleeding. Monitor patient closely.
Other inhibitors of platelet receptor IIb/IIIa: potential for serious bleeding. Don't administer together.

Contraindications

- Contraindicated in patients hypersensitive to drug or its ingredients and in those with history of bleeding diathesis, evidence of active abnormal bleeding within previous 30 days, severe hypertension (systolic blood pressure over 200 mm Hg or diastolic blood pressure over 110 mm Hg) not adequately controlled with antihypertensives, major surgery within previous 6 weeks, history of CVA within 30 days, history of hemorrhagic CVA, current or planned use of another parenteral GP IIb/IIIa inhibitor, or platelet count below 100,000/mm³.
- Also, contraindicated in patients whose serum creatinine is 2 mg/dl or higher (for the 180-mcg/kg bolus and 2-mcg/kg/minute infusion) or 4 mg/dl or higher (for the 135-mcg/kg bolus and 0.5-mcg/kg/minute infusion) and in patients who are dependent on renal dialysis.

NURSING CONSIDERATIONS

Assessment

- Obtain history of patient's underlying medical conditions, especially conditions that put patient at increased risk for bleeding.
- Obtain accurate patient weight. Use drug cautiously in patients weighing more than 315 lb (143 kg).
- Perform baseline laboratory tests before start of drug therapy; also determine hematocrit, platelet count, and PT, INR, PTT, hemoglobin, and serum creatinine levels.
- Monitor patient for bleeding.
- Evaluate patient's and family's knowledge about drug therapy.

Nursing diagnoses

- Ineffective cardiopulmonary tissue perfusion related to presence of acute coronary syndrome
- Risk for injury related to increased bleeding tendencies
- Deficient knowledge related to drug therapy

Planning and implementation

- Withdraw bolus dose from 10-ml vial into a syringe and administer by I.V. push over 1 to 2 minutes. Administer I.V. infusion undiluted directly from 100-ml vial using an infusion pump.
- Inspect solution for particulate matter before use. If particles are visible, the sterility is suspect; discard solution.
- Drug may be administered in same I.V. line as alteplase, atropine, dobutamine, heparin, lidocaine, meperidine, metoprolol, midazolam, morphine, nitroglycerin, or verapamil.
- Don't give drug in same I.V. line as furosemide.
- Drug may be administered in same I.V. line with normal saline solution or normal saline and 5% dextrose; main infusion may also contain up to 60 mEq/L of potassium chloride.
- Drug is intended for use with heparin and aspirin.
- Discontinue eptifibatide and heparin and achieve sheath hemostasis by standard compressive techniques at least 4 hours before hospital discharge.

• If patient will undergo coronary artery bypass graft surgery, infusion should be stopped before surgery.
• Minimize use of arterial and venous punctures, I.M. injections, urinary catheters, and nasotracheal and nasogastric tubes.
• When obtaining I.V. access, avoid use of noncompressible sites (such as subclavian or jugular veins).
• If patient's platelet count is below 100,000/mm^3, notify prescriber and discontinue eptifibatide and heparin as ordered.
• Store vials in refrigerator at 36° to 46° F (2° to 8° C). Protect from light until administration.

Patient teaching

• Explain that drug is a blood thinner used to prevent chest pain and heart attack.
• Explain that the risk of serious bleeding is far outweighed by the benefits of drug.
• Instruct patient to report chest discomfort or other adverse events immediately.

☑ Evaluation

• Patient maintains adequate cardiopulmonary tissue perfusion.
• Patient has no life-threatening bleeding episode.
• Patient and family state understanding of drug therapy

ergotamine tartrate

(er-GAH-tuh-meen TAR-trayt)
Cafergot, Ergodryl Mono ◇, Ergomar, Ergostat, Gynergen ♦, Medihaler Ergotamine ♦

Pharmacologic class: ergot alkaloid
Therapeutic class: vasoconstrictor
Pregnancy risk category: X

Indications and dosages

▶ **Vascular or migraine headache.** *Adults:* initially, 2 mg P.O. or S.L.; then 1 to 2 mg P.O. or S.L. q 30 minutes to maximum of 6 mg per attack or 10 mg weekly. For aerosol inhaler, 1 spray (360 mcg) initially, repeated q 5 minutes, p.r.n., to maximum of 6 sprays (2.16 mg) per 24 hours or 15 sprays (5.4 mg) weekly. For suppositories, initially, 2 mg P.R. at onset of attack, repeated in 1 hour, p.r.n. Maximum dosage is two suppositories per attack or five suppositories weekly.

How supplied

Capsules: 1 mg ◇
Tablets: 1 mg ♦
Tablets (sublingual): 2 mg
Aerosol inhaler: 360 mcg/metered spray ♦
Suppositories: 2 mg

Pharmacokinetics

Absorption: rapidly absorbed after inhalation and variably absorbed after P.O. or P.R. administration.
Distribution: widely distributed throughout body.
Metabolism: extensively metabolized in liver.
Excretion: thought to be primarily excreted in feces; 4% excreted in urine.

Route	Onset	Peak	Duration
P.O.	Varies	0.5-3 hr	Varies
P.R., S.L., inhalation	Varies	Unknown	Varies

Pharmacodynamics

Chemical effect: stimulates alpha-adrenergic receptors, causing peripheral vasoconstriction. Drug also inhibits reuptake of norepinephrine, increasing vasoconstrictor activity.
Therapeutic effect: relieves vascular or migraine headache.

Adverse reactions

CV: numbness and tingling in fingers and toes, transient tachycardia or ***bradycardia,*** precordial distress and pain, increased arterial pressure, angina pectoris, peripheral vasoconstriction.
GI: nausea, *vomiting.*
GU: uterine contractions.
Musculoskeletal: weakness in legs, muscle pain in limbs.
Skin: itching, localized edema.

Interactions

Drug-drug. *Erythromycin, other macrolides:* may cause symptoms of ergot toxicity. Vaso-

dilators (nitroprusside, nifedipine, or prazosin) may be ordered to treat such an attack. Monitor patient closely.
Propranolol, other beta blockers: blocked natural pathway for vasodilation in patients receiving ergot alkaloids; may result in excessive vasoconstriction. Watch closely if drugs are used together.

Contraindications and precautions

- Contraindicated in pregnant women and in those with peripheral or occlusive vascular diseases, coronary artery disease, hypertension, hepatic or renal dysfunction, severe pruritus, sepsis, or hypersensitivity to ergot alkaloids.
- Use cautiously in breast-feeding women. Excessive dosage or prolonged administration of drug may inhibit lactation.
- Safety of drug hasn't been established in children.

NURSING CONSIDERATIONS

Assessment
- Obtain history of patient's headache before therapy, and reassess regularly thereafter.
- Be alert for adverse reactions and drug interactions.
- Be alert for ergotamine rebound or increase in frequency and duration of headache, which may occur if drug is discontinued suddenly.
- Evaluate patient's and family's knowledge of drug therapy.

Nursing diagnoses
- Acute pain related to presence of vascular or migraine headache
- Decreased peripheral tissue perfusion related to vasoconstriction
- Deficient knowledge related to drug therapy

Planning and implementation
- Drug is most effective when used during prodromal stage of headache or as soon as possible after onset.
- Avoid prolonged administration; don't exceed recommended dosage.
- Store drug in light-resistant container.

P.O. and Inhalation use: Follow normal protocol.
P.R. use: If suppository softens, chill it in ice-cold water while still in wrapper.
S.L. use: Don't give drug with food or drink while tablets are dissolving.
– S.L. tablets are preferred for use during early stage of attack because of their rapid absorption.

Patient teaching
- Tell patient not to eat, drink, or smoke while S.L. tablet is dissolving.
- Warn patient not to increase dosage without first consulting prescriber.
- Advise patient to avoid prolonged exposure to cold weather whenever possible. Cold may increase adverse reactions to drug.
- Instruct patient receiving long-term therapy to check for and report coldness in limbs or tingling in fingers and toes. Severe vasoconstriction may result in tissue damage.
- Instruct patient on correct use of inhaler.
- Help patient evaluate underlying causes of stress, which may precipitate attacks.

Evaluation
- Patient is free from pain.
- Patient maintains adequate tissue perfusion to limbs throughout therapy.
- Patient and family state understanding of drug therapy.

erythromycin base
(eh-rith-roh-MIGH-sin bays)
Apo-Erythro ♦, EMU-V ◇, E-Mycin, Erybid ♦, ERYC, ERYC-125 ♦, ERYC-250 ♦, Ery-Tab, Erythromid ♦, Erythromycin Base Filmtab, Novo-Rythro ♦, PCE Dispertab

erythromycin estolate
Ilosone, Novo-Rythro ♦

erythromycin ethylsuccinate
Apo-Erythro-ES ♦, E.E.S., EES-400 ◇, EES granules ◇, EryPed, Erythrocin

erythromycin gluceptate
Ilotycin Gluceptate

erythromycin lactobionate

Erythrocin

erythromycin stearate

Apo-Erythro-S ♦, Erythrocin, My-E, Novo-Rythro ♦

Pharmacologic class: erythromycin
Therapeutic class: antibiotic
Pregnancy risk category: B

Indications and dosages

▶ **Acute pelvic inflammatory disease caused by *Neisseria gonorrhoeae.*** *Adults:* 500 mg I.V. (erythromycin gluceptate, lactobionate) q 6 hours for 3 days; then 250 mg (erythromycin base, estolate, stearate) or 400 mg (erythromycin ethylsuccinate) P.O. q 6 hours for 7 days.

▶ **Endocarditis prophylaxis for dental procedures in patients allergic to penicillin.** *Adults:* initially, 800 mg (ethylsuccinate) or 1 g (stearate) P.O. 2 hours before procedure; then 400 mg (ethylsuccinate) or 500 mg (stearate) P.O. 6 hours later.
Children: initially, 20 mg/kg (ethylsuccinate or stearate) P.O. 2 hours before procedure; then one-half initial dose 6 hours later.

▶ **Intestinal amebiasis.** *Adults:* 250 mg (base, estolate, stearate) or 400 mg (ethylsuccinate) P.O. q 6 hours for 10 to 14 days.
Children: 30 to 50 mg/kg (base, estolate, ethylsuccinate, stearate) P.O. daily in divided doses q 6 hours for 10 to 14 days.

▶ **Mild to moderately severe respiratory tract, skin, and soft-tissue infections caused by sensitive group A beta-hemolytic streptococci, *Bordetella pertussis, Corynebacterium diphtheriae, Diplococcus pneumoniae, Listeria monocytogenes, Mycoplasma pneumoniae.*** *Adults:* 250 to 500 mg (erythromycin base, estolate, stearate) P.O. q 6 hours; or 400 to 800 mg (erythromycin ethylsuccinate) P.O. q 6 hours; or 15 to 20 mg/kg I.V. daily as continuous infusion or in divided doses q 6 hours.
Children: 30 to 50 mg/kg (oral erythromycin salts) P.O. daily in divided doses q 6 hours; or 15 to 20 mg/kg I.V. daily in divided doses q 4 to 6 hours.

▶ **Syphilis.** *Adults:* 500 mg (erythromycin base, estolate, stearate) P.O. q.i.d. for 15 days.

▶ **Legionnaires' disease.** *Adults:* 1 to 4 g P.O. or I.V. daily in divided doses for 10 to 21 days.

▶ **Uncomplicated urethral, endocervical, or rectal infections when tetracyclines are contraindicated.** *Adults:* 500 mg (base, estolate, stearate) or 800 mg (ethylsuccinate) P.O. q.i.d. for at least 7 days.

▶ **Urogenital *Chlamydia trachomatis* infections during pregnancy.** *Adults:* 500 mg (base, estolate, stearate) P.O. q.i.d. for at least 7 days, or 250 mg (base, estolate, stearate) or 400 mg (ethylsuccinate) P.O. q.i.d. for at least 14 days.

▶ **Conjunctivitis caused by *C. trachomatis* in neonates.** *Neonates:* 50 mg/kg P.O. daily in four divided doses for at least 2 weeks.

▶ **Pneumonia of infancy caused by *C. trachomatis.*** *Infants:* 50 mg/kg daily in four divided doses for at least 3 weeks.

How supplied

erythromycin base
Tablets (enteric-coated): 250 mg, 333 mg, 500 mg
Tablets (filmtabs): 250 mg, 500 mg
Capsules (enteric-coated pellets): 250 mg, 333 mg

erythromycin estolate
Tablets: 500 mg, 250 mg
Capsules: 250 mg
Oral suspension: 125 mg/5 ml, 250 mg/5 ml

erythromycin ethylsuccinate
Tablets: 400 mg, 600 mg ♦
Tablets (chewable): 200 mg, 400 mg
Oral suspension: 200 mg/5 ml, 400 mg/5 ml, 100 mg/2.5 ml

erythromycin gluceptate
Injection: 1-g vial

erythromycin lactobionate
Injection: 500-mg, 1-g vials

erythromycin stearate
Tablets (film-coated): 250 mg, 500 mg
Oral suspension: 125mg/5ml, 250 mg/5ml

Pharmacokinetics

Absorption: most erythromycin salts are absorbed in duodenum. Because erythromycin base is acid-sensitive, it must be buffered or have enteric coating to prevent destruction by gastric acid. Acid salts and esters (estolate, ethylsuccinate, and stearate) aren't affected by

gastric acidity and, therefore, are well absorbed; they are unaffected or possibly even enhanced by presence of food. Base and stearate preparations should be given on empty stomach.
Distribution: widely distributed in most body tissues and fluids except CSF, where it appears at low levels. About 80% of erythromycin base and 96% of erythromycin estolate are protein-bound.
Metabolism: partially metabolized in liver to inactive metabolites.
Excretion: mainly excreted unchanged in bile; small amount (less than 5%) excreted in urine. *Half-life:* about 1½ hours.

Route	Onset	Peak	Duration
P.O.	Unknown	1-4 hr	Unknown
I.V.	Immediate	Immediate	Unknown

Pharmacodynamics

Chemical effect: inhibits bacterial protein synthesis by binding to 50S subunit of ribosome.
Therapeutic effect: inhibits bacterial growth. Spectrum of activity includes *B. pertussis, C. diphtheriae, Corynebacterium minutissimum, Entamoeba histolytica, Haemophilus influenzae, Legionella pneumophila,* and *M. pneumoniae.* It also may be used to treat infections caused by *C. trachomatis, L. monocytogenes, N. gonorrhoeae, Staphylococcus aureus, Streptococcus pneumoniae, Streptococcus viridans,* and *Treponema pallidum.*

Adverse reactions

CV: ***ventricular arrhythmias,*** *venous irritation or thrombophlebitis* after I.V. injection.
EENT: hearing loss with high I.V. doses.
GI: *abdominal pain and cramping, nausea, vomiting, diarrhea.*
Hepatic: cholestatic jaundice (erythromycin estolate).
Skin: urticaria, rash, eczema.
Other: overgrowth of nonsusceptible bacteria or fungi, ***anaphylaxis,*** fever.

Interactions

Drug-drug. *Carbamazepine:* increased carbamazepine blood levels and increased risk of toxicity. Monitor patient closely.
Clindamycin, lincomycin: may be antagonistic. Don't use together.
Cyclosporine: increased cyclosporine levels. Monitor patient closely.
Digoxin: increased serum digoxin levels. Monitor patient for digoxin toxicity.
Disopyramide: increased disopyramide plasma levels, resulting, in some cases, in arrhythmias and increased QT intervals. Monitor ECG.
Midazolam, triazolam: increased effects of these drugs. Monitor patient closely.
Oral anticoagulants: increased anticoagulant effects. Monitor PT and INR closely.
Theophylline: decreased erythromycin blood level and increased theophylline toxicity. Use together cautiously.
Drug-herb. *Pill-bearing spurge:* May inhibit CYP3A enzymes and alter drug metabolism. Use together cautiously.

Contraindications and precautions

- Contraindicated in patients hypersensitive to drug or other macrolides. Erythromycin estolate is contraindicated in patients with hepatic disease.
- Use other erythromycin salts cautiously in patients with impaired liver function. Also use cautiously in pregnant or breast-feeding women.

NURSING CONSIDERATIONS

Assessment

- Obtain history of patient's infection before therapy, and reassess regularly thereafter.
- Obtain urine specimen for culture and sensitivity tests before first dose. Therapy may begin, pending test results.
- Be alert for adverse reactions and drug interactions.
- Monitor patient's hydration status if adverse GI reactions occur.
- Monitor liver function (increased serum levels of alkaline phosphatase, ALT, AST, and bilirubin may occur). Erythromycin estolate may cause serious hepatotoxicity in adults (reversible cholestatic jaundice). Other erythromycin salts cause hepatotoxicity to lesser degree. Patients who develop hepatotoxicity from estolate may react similarly to treatment with other erythromycin preparations.

• Evaluate patient's and family's knowledge of drug therapy.

Nursing diagnoses

• Infection related to presence of susceptible bacteria
• Risk for deficient fluid volume related to potential for drug-induced adverse GI reactions
• Deficient knowledge related to drug therapy

Planning and implementation

ALERT American Heart Association recommendations no longer include using erythromycins to prevent bacterial endocarditis. However, practitioners who have successfully used the drug as prophalaxis in indivdual patients may continue to do so.
P.O. use: When administering suspension, be sure to note concentration.
– For best absorption, give oral form of drug with full glass of water 1 hour before or 2 hours after meals. Coated tablets may be taken with meals. Tell patient not to drink fruit juice with drug. Chewable erythromycin tablets should not be swallowed whole.
– Coated tablets or encapsulated pellets cause less GI upset; they may be more tolerable in patients who can't tolerate erythromycin.
I.V. use: Reconstitute drug according to manufacturer's directions, and dilute each 250 mg in at least 100 ml of normal saline solution. Infuse over 1 hour.
– Don't administer erythromycin lactobionate with other drugs.
• Drug may falsely elevate urinary catecholamines, 17-hydroxycorticosterone, and 17-ketosteroids.
• Drug may interfere with colorimetric assays, resulting in falsely elevated AST and ALT levels.

Patient teaching

• Instruct patient how to take oral drug.
• Tell patient to take entire amount of drug exactly as prescribed, even after he feels better.
• Instruct patient to notify prescriber if adverse reactions occur, especially nausea, abdominal pain, and fever.

Evaluation

• Patient is free from infection.
• Patient maintains adequate hydration with therapy.
• Patient and family state understanding of drug therapy.

esmolol hydrochloride

(EZ-moh-lohl high-droh-KLOR-ighd)
Brevibloc

Pharmacologic class: beta blocker
Therapeutic class: antiarrhythmic
Pregnancy risk category: C

Indications and dosages

▶ **Supraventricular tachycardia; control of ventricular rate in patients with atrial fibrillation or flutter in perioperative, postoperative, or other emergent circumstances; noncompensatory sinus tachycardia when heart rate requires specific interventions.**
Adults: loading dose is 500 mcg/kg/minute by I.V. infusion over 1 minute, followed by 4-minute maintenance infusion of 50 mcg/kg/minute. If adequate response doesn't occur within 5 minutes, loading dose is repeated and followed by maintenance infusion of 100 mcg/kg/minute for 4 minutes. Loading dose is repeated and maintenance infusion increased in stepwise manner, p.r.n. Maximum maintenance infusion for tachycardia is 200 mcg/kg/minute.
▶ **Management of perioperative and postoperative tachycardia or hypertension.**
Adults: for perioperative treatment, 80 mg (about 1 mg/kg) I.V. bolus over 30 seconds, followed by 150 mcg/kg/minute I.V., if needed. Adjust infusion rate, p.r.n., to maximum of 300 mcg/kg/minute. Postoperative treatment is same as for supraventricular tachycardia, although dosages adequate for control may be as high as 300 mcg/minute.

How supplied

Injection: 10 mg/ml, 250 mg/ml

Pharmacokinetics

Absorption: not applicable with I.V. administration.
Distribution: distributed rapidly throughout plasma; 55% protein-bound.
Metabolism: hydrolyzed rapidly by plasma esterase.
Excretion: excreted by kidneys as metabolites.
Half-life: about 9 minutes.

Route	Onset	Peak	Duration
I.V.	Almost immediate	About 30 min	< 30 min

Pharmacodynamics

Chemical effect: a class II antiarrhythmic, esmolol is an ultrashort-acting selective $beta_1$-adrenergic blocker that decreases heart rate, myocardial contractility, and blood pressure.
Therapeutic effect: restores normal sinus rhythm.

Adverse reactions

CNS: dizziness, somnolence, headache, agitation, fatigue, confusion.
CV: HYPOTENSION, peripheral ischemia.
EENT: nasal congestion.
GI: *nausea,* vomiting.
Respiratory: ***bronchospasm,*** wheezing, dyspnea.
Other: inflammation, induration at infusion site.

Interactions

Drug-drug. *Digoxin:* esmolol may increase serum digoxin levels by 10% to 20%. Monitor serum digoxin levels.
Morphine: may increase esmolol blood levels. Adjust esmolol carefully.
Reserpine, other catecholamine-depleting drugs: may cause additive bradycardia and hypotension. Adjust esmolol carefully.
Succinylcholine: esmolol may prolong neuromuscular blockade. Monitor patient.

Contraindications and precautions

- Contraindicated in patients with sinus bradycardia, heart block greater than first-degree, cardiogenic shock, or overt heart failure.
- Use cautiously in patients with impaired kidney function, diabetes, or bronchospasm. Also use cautiously in pregnant or breast-feeding women.
- Safety of drug hasn't been established in children.

NURSING CONSIDERATIONS

Assessment

- Obtain history of patient's arrhythmias before therapy.
- Monitor ECG and blood pressure continuously during infusion. Up to 50% of patients treated with esmolol develop hypotension. Monitor closely, especially if patient's pretreatment blood pressure was low.
- Be alert for adverse reactions and drug interactions.
- Evaluate patient's and family's knowledge of drug therapy.

Nursing diagnoses

- Decreased cardiac output related to presence of arrhythmias
- Ineffective cerebral tissue perfusion related to drug-induced hypotension
- Deficient knowledge related to drug therapy

Planning and implementation

- Don't give by I.V. push; use infusion-control device. The 10-mg/ml single-dose vial may be used without diluting, but injection concentrate (250 mg/ml) must be diluted to no more than 10 mg/ml before infusion. Remove 20 ml from 500 ml of D_5W, lactated Ringer's solution, half-normal saline solution, or normal saline solution, and add two ampules of esmolol (final concentration 10 mg/ml).
- Hypotension can usually be reversed within 30 minutes by decreasing dose or, if necessary, stopping infusion. Notify prescriber if this becomes necessary.
- Esmolol solutions are incompatible with diazepam, furosemide, sodium bicarbonate, and thiopental sodium.
- When patient's heart rate becomes stable, esmolol will be replaced by a longer-acting antiarrhythmic, such as propranolol, digoxin, or verapamil. A half-hour after first dose of alternative drug is administered, reduce infusion

rate by 50%. Monitor patient response, and if heart rate is controlled for 1 hour after administration of second dose of alternative drug, discontinue esmolol infusion.
- If local reaction develops at infusion site, change to another site. Avoid using butterfly needles.

Patient teaching
- Inform patient of need for continuous ECG, blood pressure, and heart rate monitoring to assess effectiveness of drug and detect adverse reactions.

☑ Evaluation
- Patient regains normal cardiac output with correction of arrhythmias.
- Patient's blood pressure remains normal throughout therapy.
- Patient and family state understanding of drug therapy.

estazolam
(eh-STAZ-uh-lam)
ProSom

Pharmacologic class: benzodiazepine
Therapeutic class: hypnotic
Controlled substance schedule: IV
Pregnancy risk category: X

Indications and dosages
▶ **Insomnia.** *Adults:* 1 mg P.O. h.s. Some patients may need 2 mg.
Elderly patients: 1 mg P.O. h.s. Use higher doses with extreme care. Frail elderly or debilitated patients may take 0.5 mg, but this low dose may be only marginally effective.

How supplied
Tablets: 1 mg, 2 mg

Pharmacokinetics
Absorption: rapidly and completely absorbed through GI tract.
Distribution: 93% protein-bound.
Metabolism: extensively metabolized in liver.
Excretion: metabolites excreted primarily in urine. Less than 5% excreted in urine as unchanged drug; 4% of 2-mg dose excreted in feces. *Half-life:* 10 to 24 hours.

Route	Onset	Peak	Duration
P.O.	Unknown	1-3 hr	Unknown

Pharmacodynamics
Chemical effect: unknown; thought to act on limbic system and thalamus of CNS by binding to specific benzodiazepine receptors.
Therapeutic effect: promotes sleep.

Adverse reactions
CNS: fatigue, dizziness, *daytime drowsiness, somnolence, asthenia, hypokinesia,* headache, abnormal thinking.
GI: dyspepsia, abdominal pain.
Musculoskeletal: back pain, stiffness.

Interactions
Drug-drug. *Cimetidine, disulfiram, isoniazid, oral contraceptives:* may impair metabolism and clearance of benzodiazepines and prolong their plasma half-life. Monitor patient for increased CNS depression.
CNS depressants, including antihistamines, opioid analgesics, and benzodiazepines: increased CNS depression. Avoid concomitant use.
Digoxin, phenytoin: increased serum levels of these drugs, resulting in toxicity. Monitor serum levels closely.
Rifampin: may increase metabolism and clearance and decrease plasma half-life. Watch for decreased effectiveness.
Theophylline: pharmacologic antagonism. Watch for decreased effectiveness.
Drug-herb. *Kava, catnip, lady's slipper, lemon balm, passionflower, sassafras, skullcap, valerian:* sedative effects may be enhanced. Discourage using together.
Drug-lifestyle. *Alcohol use:* increased CNS and respiratory depression. Discourage concomitant use.
Smoking: may increase drug metabolism and clearance and decrease plasma half-life. Monitor patient for decreased effectiveness.

Contraindications and precautions
- Contraindicated during pregnancy and in patients hypersensitive to drug.

• Drug isn't recommended for breast-feeding women.
• Use cautiously in patients with hepatic, renal, or pulmonary disease; depression; or suicidal tendencies.
• Safety of drug hasn't been established in children.

NURSING CONSIDERATIONS

Assessment
• Obtain history of patient's sleep pattern before therapy, and reassess regularly thereafter.
• Monitor liver and kidney function and CBC periodically during long-term therapy, as ordered.
• Be alert for adverse reactions and drug interactions.
• Watch for possible withdrawal symptoms. Patients who receive prolonged treatment with benzodiazepines may experience withdrawal symptoms if drug is discontinued suddenly (possibly after 6 weeks of continuous therapy).
• Evaluate patient's and family's knowledge of drug therapy.

Nursing diagnoses
• Disturbed sleep pattern related to underlying condition
• Risk for trauma related to drug-induced adverse CNS reactions
• Deficient knowledge related to drug therapy

Planning and implementation
• Before leaving bedside, make sure patient has swallowed drug.
• Take precautions to prevent hoarding by depressed, suicidal, or drug-dependent patient or patient who has history of drug abuse.

Patient teaching
• Tell patient not to increase dosage of drug but to inform prescriber if he thinks that drug is no longer effective.
• Caution patient to avoid hazardous activities that require mental alertness or physical coordination. For inpatient (particularly elderly patient), supervise walking and raise side rails.
• Warn patient that additive depressant effects can occur if alcohol is consumed while taking drug or within 24 hours afterward.
• If patient uses an oral contraceptive, recommend an alternate birth control method during therapy because drug may enhance contraceptive hormone metabolism and decrease its effect.

Evaluation
• Patient is able to sleep.
• Patient's safety is maintained.
• Patient and family state understanding of drug therapy.

estradiol (oestradiol)
(eh-struh-DIGH-ol)
Climara, Estrace**, Estrace Vaginal Cream, Estraderm, Vivelle

estradiol cypionate
depGynogen, Depo-Estradiol, Dura-Estrin, E-Cypionate, Estro-Cyp, Estrofem, Estroject-L.A.

estradiol valerate (oestradiol valerate)
Delestrogen, Dioval, Duragen-10, Duragen-20, Duragen-40, Estradiol L.A., Estra-L 20, Estra-L 40, Femogex, Gynogen L.A., Menaval, Primogyn Depot◇, Valergen-10, Valergen-20, Valergen-40

Pharmacologic class: estrogen
Therapeutic class: estrogen replacement, antineoplastic
Pregnancy risk category: X

Indications and dosages
▶ **Vasomotor menopausal symptoms, female hypogonadism, female castration, primary ovarian failure. (Estradiol.)** *Adults:* 1 to 2 mg P.O. daily in cycles of 21 days on and 7 days off or cycles of 5 days on and 2 days off. Or, 1 transdermal system (Estraderm) delivering 0.05 mg/24 hours applied twice weekly. Or, as a system (Vivelle) delivering either 0.05 mg/24 hours or 0.0375 mg/24 hours applied twice weekly. Or, as a system (Climara) delivering 0.05 mg/24 hours or 0.1 mg/24 hours applied once weekly in cycles

of 3 weeks on and 1 week off. **(Cypionate.)** *Adults:* 1 to 5 mg I.M. q 3 to 4 weeks. **(Valerate.)** *Adults:* 10 to 20 mg I.M. q 4 weeks, p.r.n.

▶ **Atrophic vaginitis, kraurosis vulvae. (Estradiol.)** *Adults:* 2 to 4 g intravaginal applications of cream daily for 1 to 2 weeks. When vaginal mucosa is restored, maintenance dosage of 1 g one to three times weekly in cyclic regimen. **(Climara.)** *Adults:* 0.05 mg/24 hours applied weekly in a cyclic regimen. **(Estraderm.)** *Adults:* 0.05 mg/24 hours applied twice weekly in a cyclic regimen. **(Valerate.)** *Adults:* 10 to 20 mg I.M. q 4 weeks, p.r.n.

▶ **Palliative treatment of advanced, inoperable breast cancer. (Estradiol.)** *Men and postmenopausal women:* 10 mg P.O. t.i.d. for 3 months.

▶ **Palliative treatment of advanced inoperable prostate cancer. (Estradiol.)** *Men:* 1 to 2 mg P.O. t.i.d. **(Valerate.)** *Men:* 30 mg I.M. q 1 to 2 weeks.

▶ **Prevention of postmenopausal osteoporosis.** *Women:* place a 6.5 cm^2 (0.025 mg/day) Climera system once weekly on clean, dry skin area of lower abdomen or upper quadrant of buttock; press firmly in place for about 10 seconds, making sure contact is good, especially around the edges.

How supplied

estradiol

Tablets (micronized): 0.5 mg, 1 mg, 2 mg
Transdermal: 0.025 mg/24 hours, 0.0375 mg/24 hours, 0.05 mg/24 hours, 0.075 mg/24 hours, 0.1 mg/24 hours; 4 mg/10 cm^2 (delivers 0.05 mg/24 hours); 6.5 cm^2 (delivers 0.025 mg/day); 8 mg/20 cm^2 (delivers 0.1 mg/24 hours).
Vaginal cream (in nonliquefying base): 0.1 mg/g

estradiol cypionate

Injection (in oil): 5 mg/ml

estradiol valerate

Injection (in oil): 10 mg/ml, 20 mg/ml, 40 mg/ml

Pharmacokinetics

Absorption: after P.O. administration, estradiol and other natural unconjugated estrogens are well absorbed but substantially inactivated by liver. After I.M. administration, absorption begins rapidly and continues for days. Topically applied estradiol is absorbed readily into systemic circulation.
Distribution: distributed throughout body with highest levels in fat. Estradiol and other natural estrogens are about 50% to 80% plasma protein–bound.
Metabolism: metabolized primarily in liver.
Excretion: primarily through kidneys.

Route	Onset	Peak	Duration
All routes	Unknown	Unknown	Unknown

Pharmacodynamics

Chemical effect: increases synthesis of DNA, RNA, and protein in responsive tissues; also reduces release of follicle-stimulating hormone and luteinizing hormone from pituitary gland.
Therapeutic effect: relieves vasomotor menopausal symptoms, provides estrogen replacement, relieves vaginal dryness, and provides palliative action for advanced prostate or breast cancer.

Adverse reactions

CNS: headache, dizziness, chorea, depression, ***seizures.***
CV: thrombophlebitis, ***thromboembolism,*** hypertension, edema.
EENT: worsening of myopia or astigmatism, intolerance of contact lenses.
GI: *nausea,* vomiting, abdominal cramps, bloating, diarrhea, constipation, ***pancreatitis.***
GU: breakthrough bleeding, altered menstrual flow, dysmenorrhea, amenorrhea, ***increased risk of endometrial cancer,*** cervical erosion, altered cervical secretions, enlargement of uterine fibromas, vaginal candidiasis, testicular atrophy, impotence.
Hepatic: cholestatic jaundice, gallbladder disease, ***hepatic adenoma.***
Metabolic: increased appetite, weight changes, hyperglycemia, hypercalcemia.
Skin: melasma, urticaria, erythema nodosum, dermatitis, hair loss.
Other: ***possibility of increased risk of breast cancer,*** breast changes (tenderness, enlargement, secretion), gynecomastia.

Interactions

Drug-drug. *Bromocriptine:* may cause amenorrhea, interfering with bromocriptine effects. Avoid concomitant use.
Carbamazepine, phenobarbital, rifampin: decreased effectiveness of estrogen therapy. Monitor patient closely.
Corticosteroids: possible enhanced effects. Monitor patient closely.
Cyclosporine: increased risk of toxicity. Use together with caution, and frequently monitor cyclosporine levels.
Dantrolene, other hepatotoxic drugs: increased risk of hepatotoxicity. Monitor patient closely.
Oral anticoagulants: dosage adjustments may be necessary. Monitor PT and INR.
Tamoxifen: estrogens may interfere with effectiveness of tamoxifen. Avoid concomitant use.
Drug-food. *Caffeine:* may increase serum caffeine levels. Monitor effects.
Drug-lifestyle. *Smoking:* increased risk of CV effects. If smoking continues, may need alternative therapy.

Contraindications and precautions

- Contraindicated in pregnant or breast-feeding women and in patients with thrombophlebitis, thromboembolic disorders, estrogen-dependent neoplasia, breast or reproductive organ cancer (except for palliative treatment), or undiagnosed abnormal genital bleeding. Also, contraindicated in patients with history of thrombophlebitis or thromboembolic disorders linked to estrogen use (except for palliative treatment of breast and prostate cancer).
- Use cautiously in patients with cerebrovascular or coronary artery disease, asthma, bone diseases, migraine, seizures, or cardiac, hepatic, or renal dysfunction and in women with strong family history of breast cancer or who have breast nodules, fibrocystic disease, or abnormal mammogram findings.
- Drug shouldn't be used in children.

NURSING CONSIDERATIONS

Assessment

- Obtain history of patient's underlying condition before therapy, and reassess regularly thereafter.
- Make sure patient has thorough physical examination before starting estrogen therapy.
- Ask patient about allergies, especially to foods or plants. Estradiol is available as aqueous solution or as solution in peanut oil; estradiol cypionate, as solution in cottonseed oil or vegetable oil; estradiol valerate, as solution in castor oil, sesame oil, or vegetable oil.
- Patient receiving long-term therapy should have yearly examinations. Periodically monitor serum lipid levels, blood pressure, body weight, and liver function, as ordered.
- Evaluate patient's and family's knowledge of drug therapy.

Nursing diagnoses

- Ineffective health maintenance related to underlying condition
- Ineffective tissue perfusion (cerebral, peripheral, pulmonary, or myocardial) related to drug-induced thromboembolism
- Deficient knowledge related to drug therapy

Planning and implementation

P.O. use: Give oral preparations at mealtimes or bedtime (if only one daily dose is required) to minimize nausea.
I.M. use: To give as I.M. injection, make sure drug is well dispersed in solution by rolling vial between palms. Inject deep into large muscle. Rotate injection sites to prevent muscle atrophy. Never give drug I.V.
Intravaginal use: Follow normal protocol.
Transdermal use: Apply transdermal patch to clean, dry, hairless, intact skin on abdomen or buttocks. Don't apply to breasts, waistline, or other areas where clothing can loosen patch. When applying, ensure good contact with skin, especially around edges, and hold in place with palm for about 10 seconds. Rotate application sites.
- In women who take oral estrogen, treatment with Estraderm transdermal patch can begin 1 week after withdrawal of oral therapy, sooner if menopausal symptoms appear before end of week.
- Because of risk of thromboembolism, therapy should be discontinued at least 1 month before procedures that increase risk of prolonged immobilization or thromboembolism, such as knee or hip surgery. Withhold drug

and notify prescriber if you suspect a thromboembolic event.

- Notify pathologist if patient receives estrogen therapy.

ALERT Estrogen preparations aren't interchangeable.

Patient teaching

- Inform patient about package insert that describes adverse effects of estrogen; also, provide verbal explanation.
- Emphasize importance of regular physical examinations. Postmenopausal women who use estrogen replacement for more than 5 years to treat menopausal symptoms may be at increased risk for endometrial carcinoma. This risk is reduced by using cyclic rather than continuous therapy and lowest possible dosages of estrogen. Adding progestins to regimen decreases risk of endometrial hyperplasia; it isn't known if progestins affect risk of endometrial carcinoma. Most studies show no increased risk of breast cancer.
- Teach patient how to use vaginal cream. Patient should wash vaginal area with soap and water before applying. Tell her to apply drug at bedtime or to lie flat for 30 minutes after application to minimize drug loss.
- Warn patient to immediately report abdominal pain; pain, numbness, or stiffness in legs or buttocks; pressure or pain in chest; shortness of breath; severe headaches; visual disturbances, such as blind spots, flashing lights, or blurriness; vaginal bleeding or discharge; breast lumps; swelling of hands or feet; yellow skin or sclera; dark urine; and light-colored stools.
- Explain to patient receiving cyclic therapy for postmenopausal symptoms that, although withdrawal bleeding may occur during week off drug, fertility hasn't been restored. Pregnancy can't occur because patient hasn't ovulated.
- Tell diabetic patient to report elevated blood glucose test results so antidiabetic dosage can be adjusted.
- Teach woman how to perform routine breast self-examination.

☑ Evaluation

- Patient shows improvement in underlying condition.
- Patient has no thromboembolic event during therapy.
- Patient and family state understanding of drug therapy.

estramustine phosphate sodium

(es-truh-MUS-teen FOS-fayt SOE-dee-um)

Emcyt, Estracyt ◇

Pharmacologic class: estrogen, alkylating agent

Therapeutic class: antineoplastic

Pregnancy risk category: NR

Indications and dosages

▶ **Palliative treatment of metastatic or progressive prostate cancer.** *Adults:* 10 to 16 mg/kg P.O. in three to four divided doses. Usual dosage is 14 mg/kg daily. Therapy continued for up to 3 months and, if successful, maintained as long as patient responds.

How supplied

Capsules: 140 mg

Pharmacokinetics

Absorption: about 75% absorbed in GI tract.

Distribution: distributed widely in body tissues.

Metabolism: extensively metabolized in liver.

Excretion: excreted primarily in feces, with small amount excreted in urine. *Half-life:* 20 hours.

Route	Onset	Peak	Duration
P.O.	Unknown	Unknown	Unknown

Pharmacodynamics

Chemical effect: unknown; probably acts by its ability to bind selectively to protein present in human prostate.

Therapeutic effect: hinders prostatic cancer growth.

Adverse reactions

CNS: lethargy, insomnia, headache, anxiety.

CV: ***MI,*** sodium and fluid retention, thrombophlebitis, ***heart failure, CVA,*** hypertension.
GI: *nausea, vomiting,* diarrhea, anorexia, flatulence, GI bleeding, thirst.
Hematologic: ***leukopenia, thrombocytopenia.***
Respiratory: dyspnea, ***pulmonary embolism.***
Skin: rash, pruritus, dry skin, thinning of hair, flushing.
Other: loss of libido, *edema, painful gynecomastia and breast tenderness.*

Interactions

Drug-drug. *Calcium-containing drugs (such as antacids):* impaired estramustine absorption. Don't administer together.
Drug-food. *Calcium-rich foods (milk, dairy products):* impaired estramustine absorption. Don't administer together.
Drug-lifestyle. *Smoking:* Increased risk of CVA, transient ischemic attack, thrombophlebitis, and pulmonary embolism. Urge patient to use cautiously together.

Contraindications and precautions

- Contraindicated in patients hypersensitive to estradiol or nitrogen mustard and in those with active thrombophlebitis or thromboembolic disorders, except when actual tumor mass is cause of thromboembolic phenomenon.
- Use cautiously in patients with history of thrombophlebitis, thromboembolic disorders, and cerebrovascular or coronary artery disease. Monitor weight regularly in these patients. Estramustine may worsen peripheral edema or heart failure.

NURSING CONSIDERATIONS

Assessment

- Obtain history of patient's neoplastic disease before therapy, and reassess regularly thereafter.
- Monitor blood pressure and glucose tolerance periodically throughout therapy. Also monitor CBC and ECG periodically during therapy.
- Be alert for adverse reactions and drug interactions.
- Evaluate patient's and family's knowledge of drug therapy.

Nursing diagnoses

- Ineffective health maintenance related to neoplastic disease
- Risk for injury related to drug-induced adverse reactions
- Deficient knowledge related to drug therapy

Planning and implementation

- Administer drug on empty stomach.
- Patient may continue therapy as long as response is favorable. Some patients have taken drug for more than 3 years.
- Store capsules in refrigerator.
- Each 140-mg capsule contains 12.5 mg of sodium. Limit patient's sodium intake, if not contraindicated, to minimize sodium and fuid retention.

Patient teaching

- Tell patient to take drug on empty stomach (2 hours before or 1 hour after meals) and to avoid taking with milk or dairy products.
- Advise patient and partner to use contraception if woman is of childbearing age.

Evaluation

- Patient shows improvement in health.
- Patient has no injury as result of therapy.
- Patient and family state understanding of drug therapy.

estrogens, conjugated (estrogenic substances, conjugated; oestrogens, conjugated)

(ES-troh-jenz, KAHN-jih-gayt-ed)
C.E.S. ♦, Premarin, Premarin Intravenous

Pharmacologic class: estrogen
Therapeutic class: estrogen replacement, antineoplastic, antiosteoporotic
Pregnancy risk category: X

Indications and dosages

▶ **Abnormal uterine bleeding (hormonal imbalance).** *Women:* 25 mg I.V. or I.M. Repeated in 6 to 12 hours, p.r.n.
▶ **Palliative treatment of breast cancer (at least 5 years after menopause).** *Men and*

postmenopausal women: 10 mg P.O. t.i.d. for 3 months or more.
▶ **Female castration, primary ovarian failure.** *Women:* 1.25 mg P.O. daily in cycles of 3 weeks on and 1 week off.
▶ **Osteoporosis.** *Postmenopausal women:* 0.625 mg P.O. daily in cyclic regimen (3 weeks on, 1 week off).
▶ **Hypogonadism.** *Women:* 2.5 to 7.5 mg P.O. daily in divided doses for 20 consecutive days each month.
▶ **Vasomotor menopausal symptoms.** *Women:* 0.3 to 1.25 mg P.O. daily in cycles of 3 weeks on and 1 week off.
▶ **Atrophic vaginitis, kraurosis vulvae.** *Women:* 2 to 4 g intravaginally once daily on cyclic basis (3 weeks on and 1 week off).
▶ **Palliative treatment of inoperable prostate cancer.** *Men:* 1.25 to 2.5 mg P.O. t.i.d.

How supplied

Tablets: 0.3 mg, 0.625 mg, 0.9 mg, 1.25 mg, 2.5 mg
Injection: 25 mg/5 ml
Vaginal cream: 0.625 mg/g

Pharmacokinetics

Absorption: not well characterized after P.O. or intravaginal administration. After I.M. administration, absorption begins rapidly and continues for days.
Distribution: distributed throughout body with highest levels in fat; about 50% to 80% plasma protein–bound.
Metabolism: metabolized primarily in liver.
Excretion: majority of estrogen elimination occurs through kidneys.

Route	Onset	Peak	Duration
All routes	Unknown	Unknown	Unknown

Pharmacodynamics

Chemical effect: increases synthesis of DNA, RNA, and protein in responsive tissues; also reduces release of follicle-stimulating hormone and luteinizing hormone from pituitary gland.
Therapeutic effect: provides estrogen replacement, relieves vasomotor menopausal symptoms and vaginal dryness, helps prevent severity of osteoporosis, and provides palliative action for prostate and breast cancer.

Adverse reactions

CNS: headache, dizziness, chorea, depression, lethargy, ***seizures.***
CV: thrombophlebitis; ***thromboembolism;*** hypertension; edema; ***increased risk of CVA, pulmonary embolism, and MI.***
EENT: worsening of myopia or astigmatism, intolerance of contact lenses.
GI: *nausea,* vomiting, abdominal cramps, bloating, diarrhea, constipation, anorexia, ***pancreatitis.***
GU: breakthrough bleeding, altered menstrual flow, dysmenorrhea, amenorrhea, ***increased risk of endometrial cancer,*** cervical erosion, altered cervical secretions, enlargement of uterine fibromas, vaginal candidiasis, testicular atrophy, impotence.
Hepatic: gallbladder disease, cholestatic jaundice, ***hepatic adenoma.***
Metabolic: increased appetite, weight changes, hyperglycemia, hypercalcemia.
Skin: melasma, urticaria, erythema nodosum, dermatitis, flushing (with rapid I.V. administration), hirsutism, hair loss.
Other: breast changes (tenderness, enlargement, secretion), ***possibility of increased risk of breast cancer***, gynecomastia.

Interactions

Drug-drug. *Bromocriptine:* may cause amenorrhea, interfering with bromocriptine effects. Avoid concomitant use.
Carbamazepine, phenobarbital, rifampin: decreased estrogen effectiveness. Monitor patient closely.
Corticosteroids: possible enhanced effects. Monitor patient closely.
Cyclosporine: increased risk of toxicity. Use together with caution and frequently monitor cyclosporine levels.
Dantrolene, other hepatotoxic drugs: increased risk of hepatotoxicity. Monitor patient closely.
Oral anticoagulants: dosage adjustments may be necessary. Monitor PT and INR.
Tamoxifen: estrogens may interfere with effectiveness of tamoxifen. Avoid concomitant use.
Drug-food. *Caffeine:* may increase serum caffeine levels. Monitor effects.

Drug-lifestyle. *Smoking:* increased risk of CV effects. If smoking continues, patient may need alternative therapy.

Contraindications and precautions

- Contraindicated in pregnant or breast-feeding women and in patients with thrombophlebitis, thromboembolic disorders, estrogen-dependent neoplasia, breast or reproductive organ cancer (except for palliative treatment), or undiagnosed abnormal genital bleeding.
- Use cautiously in patients with cerebrovascular or coronary artery disease, asthma, bone disease, migraine, seizures, or cardiac, hepatic, or renal dysfunction and in women with family history (mother, grandmother, sister) of breast or genital tract cancer or who have breast nodules, fibrocystic disease, or abnormal mammogram findings.
- Drug shouldn't be used in children.

NURSING CONSIDERATIONS

Assessment

- Obtain history of patient's underlying condition before therapy, and reassess regularly thereafter.
- Make sure patient has thorough physical examination before starting estrogen therapy.
- Patient receiving long-term therapy should have yearly examinations. Periodically monitor serum lipid levels, blood pressure, body weight, and liver function, as ordered.
- Be alert for adverse reactions and drug interactions.
- Evaluate patient's and family's knowledge of drug therapy.

Nursing diagnoses

- Ineffective health maintenance related to underlying condition
- Ineffective tissue perfusion (cerebral, peripheral, pulmonary, or myocardial) related to drug-induced thromboembolism
- Deficient knowledge related to drug therapy

Planning and implementation

P.O. use: Give oral forms at mealtimes or h.s. (if only one daily dose is required) to minimize nausea.
Intravaginal use: Follow normal protocol.
I.V. use: When giving by direct I.V. injection, administer slowly to avoid flushing reaction. Reconstitute powder for injection with diluent provided (sterile water for injection with benzyl alcohol). To facilitate introduction of diluent, withdraw 5 ml of air from vial before adding diluent. Gently agitate to mix drug. Avoid shaking container. Avoid mixing with solutions of acidic pH to prevent incompatibility.
I.M. use: When giving by I.M. injection, inject deep into large muscle. Rotate injection sites to prevent muscle atrophy.

- I.M. or I.V. use is preferred for rapid treatment of dysfunctional uterine bleeding or reduction of surgical bleeding.
- Refrigerate before reconstituting. Agitate gently after adding diluent.
- Because of risk of thromboembolism, therapy should be discontinued at least 1 month before procedures that may cause prolonged immobilization or thromboembolism, such as knee or hip surgery.
- Withhold drug and notify prescriber if thromboembolic event is suspected; be prepared to provide supportive care as indicated.
- Notify pathologist if patient receives estrogen therapy.

ALERT Estrogens aren't interchangeable.

Patient teaching

- Inform patient about package insert that describes adverse effects of estrogen; also, provide verbal explanation.
- Emphasize importance of regular physical examinations. Postmenopausal women who use estrogen replacement for more than 5 years to treat menopausal symptoms may be at increased risk for endometrial carcinoma. This risk is reduced by using cyclic rather than continuous therapy and lowest possible dosages of estrogen. Adding progestins to regimen decreases risk of endometrial hyperplasia; it isn't known if progestins affect risk of endometrial carcinoma. Most studies show no increased risk of breast cancer.
- Teach patient how to use vaginal cream. Patient should wash vaginal area with soap and water before applying. Tell her to apply drug at bedtime or to lie flat for 30 minutes after application to minimize drug loss.

• Explain to patient on cyclic therapy for postmenopausal symptoms that, although withdrawal bleeding may occur during week off drug, fertility hasn't been restored. Pregnancy can't occur because she hasn't ovulated.
• Warn patient to immediately report abdominal pain; pain, numbness, or stiffness in legs or buttocks; pressure or pain in chest; shortness of breath; severe headaches; visual disturbances, such as blind spots, flashing lights, or blurriness; vaginal bleeding or discharge; breast lumps; swelling of hands or feet; yellow skin or sclera; dark urine; and light-colored stools.
• Tell diabetic patient to report elevated blood glucose test results so antidiabetic dosage can be adjusted.
• Teach woman how to perform routine breast self-examination.

✓ Evaluation

• Patient shows improvement in underlying condition.
• Patient has no thromboembolic event during therapy.
• Patient and family state understanding of drug therapy.

estrogens, esterified

(ES-troh-jenz, ES-ter-eh-fighd)
Estratab, Menest, Neo-Estrone ♦

Pharmacologic class: estrogen
Therapeutic class: antineoplastic
Pregnancy risk category: X

Indications and dosages

▶ **Inoperable prostate cancer.** *Men:* 1.25 to 2.5 mg P.O. t.i.d.
▶ **Breast cancer.** *Men and postmenopausal women:* 10 mg P.O. t.i.d. for 3 or more months.
▶ **Female hypogonadism.** *Women:* 2.5 to 7.5 mg P.O. daily in divided doses in cycles of 20 days on, 10 days off.
▶ **Female castration, primary ovarian failure.** *Women:* 2.5 mg P.O. daily to t.i.d. in cycles of 3 weeks on, 1 week off.
▶ **Vasomotor menopausal symptoms.** *Women:* average dosage is 1.25 mg P.O. daily in cycles of 3 weeks on, 1 week off.
▶ **Atrophic vaginitis or urethritis.** *Women:* 0.3 to 1.25 mg P.O. daily in cycles of 3 weeks on, 1 week off.
▶ **Osteoporosis prevention.** *Adults:* initially, 0.3 mg P.O. daily; may be increased to maximum 1.25 mg daily.

How supplied

Tablets: 0.3 mg, 0.625 mg, 1.25 mg, 2.5 mg
Tablets (film-coated): 0.3 mg, 0.625 mg, 1.25 mg, 2.5 mg

Pharmacokinetics

Absorption: well absorbed but substantially inactivated by liver.
Distribution: distributed throughout body with highest levels in fat; about 50% to 80% plasma protein–bound.
Metabolism: metabolized primarily in liver.
Excretion: excreted primarily by kidneys.

Route	Onset	Peak	Duration
P.O.	Unknown	Unknown	Unknown

Pharmacodynamics

Chemical effect: increases synthesis of DNA, RNA, and protein in responsive tissues; also reduces release of follicle-stimulating hormone and luteinizing hormone from pituitary gland.
Therapeutic effect: provides estrogen replacement, hinders prostate and breast cancer cell growth, and relieves vasomotor menopausal symptoms and vaginal dryness.

Adverse reactions

CNS: headache, dizziness, chorea, depression, lethargy, ***seizures.***
CV: thrombophlebitis; ***thromboembolism;*** hypertension; edema; ***increased risk of CVA, pulmonary embolism, and MI.***
EENT: worsening of myopia or astigmatism, intolerance of contact lenses.
GI: *nausea,* vomiting, abdominal cramps, bloating, diarrhea, constipation, anorexia, ***pancreatitis.***
GU: breakthrough bleeding, altered menstrual flow, dysmenorrhea, amenorrhea, ***possibility of***

increased risk of breast cancer, cervical erosion, altered cervical secretions, enlargement of uterine fibromas, vaginal candidiasis, testicular atrophy, impotence.
Hepatic: cholestatic jaundice, ***hepatic adenoma,*** gallbladder disease.
Metabolic: increased appetite, weight changes, hypercalcemia.
Skin: melasma, rash, erythema nodosum, dermatitis, hirsutism, hair loss.
Other: ***increased risk of endometrial cancer,*** gynecomastia, breast changes (tenderness, enlargement, secretion).

Interactions

Drug-drug. *Bromocriptine:* may cause amenorrhea, interfering with bromocriptine effects. Avoid concomitant use.
Carbamazepine, phenobarbital, rifampin: decreased effectiveness of estrogen therapy. Monitor patient closely.
Corticosteroids: possible enhanced effects. Monitor patient closely.
Cyclosporine: increased risk of toxicity. Use together with caution and frequently monitor cyclosporine levels.
Dantrolene, other hepatotoxic drugs: increased risk of hepatotoxicity. Monitor patient closely.
Oral anticoagulants: dosage adjustments may be necessary. Monitor PT and INR.
Tamoxifen: estrogens may interfere with effectiveness of tamoxifen. Avoid concomitant use.
Drug-food. *Caffeine:* may increase serum caffeine levels. Monitor effects.
Drug-lifestyle. *Smoking:* increased risk of CV effects. If smoking continues, patient may need alternative therapy.

Contraindications and precautions

- Contraindicated in pregnant or breast-feeding women and in patients with breast cancer (except metastatic disease), estrogen-dependent neoplasia, active thrombophlebitis or thromboembolic disorders, undiagnosed abnormal genital bleeding, hypersensitivity to drug, or history of thromboembolic disease.
- Use cautiously in patients with history of hypertension, depression, cardiac or renal dysfunction, liver impairment, bone diseases, migraine, seizures, or diabetes mellitus.
- Drug shouldn't be used in children.

NURSING CONSIDERATIONS

Assessment

- Obtain history of patient's underlying condition before therapy, and reassess regularly thereafter.
- Make sure patient has thorough physical examination before starting esterified estrogens therapy.
- Patient receiving long-term therapy should have yearly examinations. Periodically monitor serum lipid levels, blood pressure, body weight, and liver function, as ordered.
- Be alert for adverse reactions and drug interactions.
- Evaluate patient's and family's knowledge of drug therapy.

Nursing diagnoses

- Ineffective health maintenance related to underlying condition
- Ineffective tissue perfusion (cerebral, peripheral, pulmonary, or myocardial) related to drug-induced thromboembolism
- Deficient knowledge related to drug therapy

Planning and implementation

- Give oral forms at mealtimes or bedtime (if only one daily dose is required) to minimize nausea.
- Because of risk of thromboembolism, therapy should be discontinued at least 1 month before procedures that may cause prolonged immobilization or thromboembolism, such as knee or hip surgery.
- Withhold drug and notify prescriber if thromboembolic event is suspected; be prepared to provide supportive care as indicated.
- Notify pathologist if patient receives estrogen therapy.

ALERT Estrogens aren't interchangeable.

Patient teaching

- Inform patient about package insert that describes adverse effects of estrogens; also, provide verbal explanation.
- Emphasize importance of regular physical examinations. Postmenopausal women who use estrogen replacement for more than 5 years to treat menopausal symptoms may be at increased risk for endometrial carcinoma. This

risk is reduced by using cyclic rather than continuous therapy and lowest possible dosages of estrogen. Adding progestins to regimen decreases risk of endometrial hyperplasia; it isn't known if progestins affect risk of endometrial carcinoma. Most studies show no increased risk of breast cancer.

- Explain to patient on cyclic therapy for postmenopausal symptoms that although withdrawal bleeding may occur during week off drug, fertility hasn't been restored. Pregnancy cannot occur because she hasn't ovulated.
- Warn patient to immediately report abdominal pain; pain, numbness, or stiffness in legs or buttocks; pressure or pain in chest; shortness of breath; severe headaches; visual disturbances, such as blind spots, flashing lights, or blurriness; vaginal bleeding or discharge; breast lumps; swelling of hands or feet; yellow skin or sclera; dark urine; and light-colored stools.
- Tell diabetic patient to report elevated blood glucose test results so antidiabetic dosage can be adjusted.
- Teach woman how to perform routine breast self-examination.

☑ Evaluation

- Patient shows improvement in underlying condition.
- Patient has no thromboembolic event during therapy.
- Patient and family state understanding of drug therapy.

estropipate (piperazine estrone sulfate)

(ES-troh-pih-payt)
Ogen, Ortho-Est

Pharmacologic class: estrogen
Therapeutic class: estrogen replacement
Pregnancy risk category: X

Indications and dosages

▶ **Management of moderate to severe vasomotor symptoms, vulvar and vaginal atrophy.** *Women:* 0.75 to 6 mg P.O. daily 3 weeks on, 1 week off, or 2 to 4 g of vaginal cream daily. Typically, dosage given on cyclic, short-term basis.

▶ **Primary ovarian failure, female castration, female hypogonadism.** *Women:* administered on cyclic basis—1.5 to 9 mg P.O. daily for first 3 weeks, followed by rest period of 8 to 10 days. If bleeding doesn't occur by end of rest period, cycle repeated.

▶ **Prevention of osteoporosis.** *Women:* 0.625 mg P.O. daily for 25 days of 31-day cycle. Regimen repeated as necessary.

How supplied

Tablets: 0.75 mg, 1.5 mg, 3 mg, 6 mg
Vaginal cream: 1.5 mg/g (0.15%)

Pharmacokinetics

Absorption: not well characterized after P.O. or intravaginal administration.
Distribution: distributed throughout body with highest levels in fat; about 50% to 80% plasma protein–bound.
Metabolism: metabolized primarily in liver.
Excretion: eliminated primarily by kidneys.

Route	Onset	Peak	Duration
P.O., intravaginal	Unknown	Unknown	Unknown

Pharmacodynamics

Chemical effect: increases synthesis of DNA, RNA, and protein in responsive tissues. Also reduces release of follicle-stimulating hormone and luteinizing hormone from pituitary gland.
Therapeutic effect: provides estrogen replacement, relieves vasomotor menopausal symptoms, and helps reduce severity of osteoporosis.

Adverse reactions

CNS: depression, headache, dizziness, migraine, ***seizures.***
CV: edema; thrombophlebitis; ***increased risk of CVA, pulmonary embolism, thromboembolism, and MI.***
GI: nausea, vomiting, abdominal cramps, bloating.
GU: increased size of uterine fibromas, ***increased risk of endometrial cancer,*** vaginal

candidiasis, cystitis-like syndrome, dysmenorrhea, amenorrhea, breakthrough bleeding.
Hepatic: cholestatic jaundice.
Metabolic: hypercalcemia, weight changes.
Skin: hemorrhagic eruption, erythema nodosum, ***erythema multiforme,*** hirsutism, melasma, hair loss.
Other: ***possibility of increased risk of breast cancer,*** breast engorgement or enlargement, libido changes, aggravation of porphyria.

Interactions

Drug-drug. *Bromocriptine:* may cause amenorrhea, interfering with bromocriptine effects. Avoid concomitant use.
Carbamazepine, phenobarbital, rifampin: decreased effectiveness of estrogen therapy. Monitor patient closely.
Corticosteroids: possible enhanced effects. Monitor patient closely.
Cyclosporine: increased risk of toxicity. Use together with caution and frequently monitor cyclosporine levels.
Dantrolene, other hepatotoxic drugs: increased risk of hepatotoxicity. Monitor patient closely.
Oral anticoagulants: dosage adjustments may be necessary. Monitor PT and INR.
Tamoxifen: estrogens may interfere with effectiveness of tamoxifen. Avoid concomitant use.
Drug-food. *Caffeine:* may increase serum caffeine levels. Monitor effects.
Drug-lifestyle. *Smoking:* increased risk of CV effects. If smoking continues, patient may need alternate therapy.

Contraindications and precautions

- Contraindicated in pregnant or breast-feeding women and in patients with active thrombophlebitis, thromboembolic disorders, estrogen-dependent neoplasia, undiagnosed genital bleeding, or breast, reproductive organ, or genital cancer.
- Use cautiously in patients with cerebrovascular or coronary artery disease, asthma, depression, bone disease, migraine, seizures, or cardiac, hepatic, or renal dysfunction and in women with family history (mother, grandmother, sister) of breast or genital tract cancer or who have breast nodules, fibrocystic disease, or abnormal mammogram findings.
- Drug shouldn't be used in children.

NURSING CONSIDERATIONS

Assessment

- Obtain history of patient's underlying condition before therapy, and reassess regularly thereafter.
- Make sure patient has thorough physical examination before starting estropipate therapy.
- Patient receiving long-term therapy should have yearly examinations. Periodically monitor serum lipid levels, blood pressure, body weight, and liver function, as ordered.
- Be alert for adverse reactions and drug interactions.
- Evaluate patient's and family's knowledge of drug therapy.

Nursing diagnoses

- Ineffective health maintenance related to underlying condition
- Ineffective tissue perfusion (cerebral, peripheral, pulmonary, or myocardial) related to drug-induced thromboembolism
- Deficient knowledge related to drug therapy

Planning and implementation

P.O. use: Give oral forms with meals or at bedtime (if only one daily dose is required) to minimize nausea.
Intravaginal use: Follow normal protocol.
- Because of risk of thromboembolism, therapy should be discontinued at least 1 month before procedures that may cause prolonged immobilization or thromboembolism, such as knee or hip surgery.
- Withhold drug and notify prescriber if thromboembolic event is suspected; be prepared to provide supportive care as indicated.
- Notify pathologist if patient receives this drug.

ALERT Estrogens aren't interchangeable.

Patient teaching

- Inform patient about package insert that describes adverse effects of estrogens; also, provide verbal explanation.
- Emphasize importance of regular physical examinations. Postmenopausal women who use estrogen replacement for more than 5 years to treat menopausal symptoms may be at increased risk for endometrial carcinoma. This

risk is reduced by using cyclic rather than continuous therapy and lowest possible dosages of estrogen. Adding progestins to regimen decreases risk of endometrial hyperplasia; it isn't known if progestins affect risk of endometrial carcinoma. Most studies show no increased risk of breast cancer.
- Teach patient how to use vaginal cream. Patient should wash vaginal area with soap and water before applying. Tell her to use drug at bedtime or to lie flat for 30 minutes after application to minimize drug loss.
- Explain to patient on cyclic therapy for postmenopausal symptoms that, although withdrawal bleeding may occur during week off drug, fertility hasn't been restored. Pregnancy can't occur because she hasn't ovulated.
- Explain to patient being treated for hypogonadism that duration of therapy needed to produce withdrawal bleeding depends on patient's endometrial response to drug. If satisfactory withdrawal bleeding doesn't occur, oral progestin is added to regimen. Explain to patient that despite return of withdrawal bleeding, pregnancy can't occur because she isn't ovulating.
- Warn patient to immediately report abdominal pain; pain, numbness, or stiffness in legs or buttocks; pressure or pain in chest; shortness of breath; severe headaches; visual disturbances, such as blind spots, flashing lights, or blurriness; vaginal bleeding or discharge; breast lumps; swelling of hands or feet; yellow skin or sclera; dark urine; and light-colored stools.
- Tell diabetic patient to report elevated blood glucose test results so antidiabetic dosage can be adjusted.
- Teach woman how to perform routine breast self-examination.

☑ Evaluation
- Patient shows improvement in underlying condition.
- Patient has no thromboembolic event during therapy.
- Patient and family state understanding of drug therapy.

etanercept
(ee-TAN-er-sept)
Enbrel

Pharmacologic class: tumor necrosis factor (TNF) blocker
Therapeutic class: antirheumatic
Pregnancy risk category: B

Indications and dosages
▶ **Reduction in signs and symptoms of moderately to severely active rheumatoid arthritis in patients who demonstrate inadequate response to one or more disease-modifying antirheumatic drugs with methotrexate and who don't respond adequately to methotrexate alone.** *Adults:* 25 mg S.C. twice weekly, 72 to 96 hours apart.
▶ **Reduction in signs and symptoms of moderately to severely active polyarticular-course juvenile rheumatoid arthritis in patients who have had an inadequate response to one or more disease-modifying antirheumatic drugs.** *Children ages 4 to 17:* 0.4 mg/kg (maximum, 25 mg per dose) S.C. twice weekly, 72 to 96 hours apart.

How supplied
Injection: 25 mg single-use vial

Pharmacokinetics
Absorption: serum levels peak in 72 hours.
Distribution: not reported.
Metabolism: not reported.
Excretion: *elimination half-life:* 115 hours.

Route	Onset	Peak	Duration
S.C.	Unknown	72 hr	Unknown

Pharmacodynamics
Chemical effect: Binds specifically to TNF and blocks its action with cell surface TNF receptors, reducing inflammatory and immune responses found in rheumatoid arthritis.
Therapeutic effect: reduces signs and symptoms of rheumatoid arthritis.

Adverse reactions
CNS: asthenia, *headache,* dizziness.

EENT: *rhinitis,* pharyngitis, sinusitis.
GI: abdominal pain, dyspepsia.
Respiratory: *upper respiratory tract infections,* cough, respiratory disorder.
Skin: *injection site reaction,* rash.
Other: *infections,* ***malignancies.***

Interactions

None significant.

NURSING CONSIDERATIONS

Assessment

- Obtain history of patient's underlying condition before therapy, and reassess regularly thereafter.
- Obtain accurate immunization history from parents or guardians of juvenile rheumatoid arthritis patients; if possible, they should be brought up-to-date with all immunizations in compliance with current guidelines before treatment is started.
- Drug isn't recommended for children under age 4.
- Monitor patient for infection.
- Evaluate patient's and family's knowledge about drug therapy.

Nursing diagnoses

- Acute pain related to underlying condition
- Risk for infection related to drug-induced adverse reactions
- Deficient knowledge related to drug therapy

Planning and implementation

- Drug is for S.C. injection only.
- Reconstitute aseptically with 1 ml of supplied sterile bacteriostatic water for injection, USP (0.9% benzyl alcohol). Don't filter reconstituted solution during preparation or administration. Inject diluent slowly into vial. Minimize foaming by gently swirling during dissolution rather than shaking. Dissolution takes less than 5 minutes.
- Visually inspect solution for particulates and discoloration before use. Reconstituted solution should be clear and colorless. Don't use solution if it's discolored, cloudy, or if particulates exist.
- Don't add other drugs or diluents to reconstituted solution.
- Use reconstituted solution as soon as possible; may be refrigerated in vial for up to 6 hours at 36° to 46° F (2° to 8° C).
- Injection sites should be at least 1″ apart; don't use areas where skin is tender, bruised, red, or hard. Recommended sites include the thigh, abdomen, and upper arm. Rotate sites regularly.
- Patient may develop positive antinuclear antibody or positive anti-double-stranded DNA antibodies measured by radioimmunoassay and *Crithidia lucilae* assay.
- Don't give live vaccines during therapy.
- Anti-TNF therapies, including etanercept, may affect defenses against infection. Notify prescriber and discontinue therapy, as ordered, if serious infection occurs.
- Needle cover of diluent syringe contains dry natural rubber (latex) and shouldn't be handled by persons sensitive to latex.

Patient teaching

- If patient will be administering drug, teach mixing and injection techniques, including rotation of injection sites.
- Instruct patient to use puncture-resistant container to dispose of needles and syringes.
- Tell patient that injection site reactions typically occur within first month of therapy and decrease thereafter.
- Urge patient to avoid live vaccines during therapy. Stress importance of alerting prescriber or other health care providers of etanercept use.
- Instruct patient to promptly report evidence of infection to prescriber.
- Advise breast-feeding women to discontinue breast-feeding during drug therapy.

Evaluation

- Patient has decreased pain.
- Patient is free from infection.
- Patient and family state understanding of drug therapy.

ethacrynate sodium
(eth-uh-KRIH-nayt SOH-dee-um)
Sodium Edecrin

ethacrynic acid
Edecril ◇, Edecrin

Pharmacologic class: loop diuretic
Therapeutic class: diuretic
Pregnancy risk category: B

Indications and dosages

▶ **Acute pulmonary edema.** *Adults:* 50 mg or 0.5 to 1 mg/kg I.V. to maximum dose of 100 mg. Usually only one dose is needed; occasionally, second dose may be required.

▶ **Edema.** *Adults:* 50 to 200 mg P.O. daily. Refractory cases may require up to 200 mg b.i.d.
Children: initial dose is 25 mg P.O., increased cautiously in 25-mg increments daily until desired effect is achieved.

How supplied

Tablets: 25 mg, 50 mg
Injection: 50 mg (with 62.5 mg of mannitol and 0.1 mg of thimerosal)

Pharmacokinetics

Absorption: ethacrynic acid is absorbed rapidly from GI tract. Ethacrynate sodium is administered I.V. and doesn't require absorption.
Distribution: unknown.
Metabolism: unknown.
Excretion: unknown.

Route	Onset	Peak	Duration
P.O.	30 min	2 hr	6-8 hr
I.V.	5 min	15-30 min	2 hr

Pharmacodynamics

Chemical effect: inhibits sodium and chloride reabsorption at renal tubules and ascending loop of Henle.
Therapeutic effect: promotes sodium and water excretion.

Adverse reactions

CNS: malaise, confusion, fatigue, vertigo, headache, nervousness.
CV: volume depletion and dehydration, orthostatic hypotension.
EENT: transient deafness (with too-rapid I.V. injection), blurred vision, tinnitus, hearing loss.
GI: cramping, diarrhea, anorexia, nausea, vomiting, *GI bleeding,* ***pancreatitis.***
GU: nocturia, polyuria, frequent urination, oliguria, hematuria.
Hematologic: ***agranulocytosis,*** neutropenia, ***thrombocytopenia,*** azotemia.
Metabolic: asymptomatic hyperuricemia; hypochloremic alkalosis; fluid and electrolyte imbalances, including dilutional hyponatremia, hypokalemia, hypocalcemia, hypomagnesemia; hyperglycemia and impairment of glucose tolerance.
Skin: dermatitis.
Other: rash; fever, chills.

Interactions

Drug-drug. *Aminoglycoside antibiotics:* potentiated ototoxic adverse reactions of both drugs. Use together cautiously.
Antihypertensives: increased risk of hypotension. Use together cautiously.
Cardiac glycosides: increased risk of digoxin toxicity from ethacrynate-induced hypokalemia. Monitor potassium and digoxin levels.
Cisplatin: increased risk of ototoxicity. Avoid concomitant use.
Lithium: decreased lithium clearance, increasing risk of lithium toxicity. Monitor lithium level.
Metolazone: profound diuresis and enhanced electrolyte loss. Use together cautiously.
NSAIDs: decreased diuretic effectiveness. Use together cautiously.
Warfarin: potentiated anticoagulant effect. Use together cautiously.
Drug-herb. *Licorice root:* may contribute to potassium depletion caused by diuretics. Discourage concomitant use.
Drug-lifestyle. *Sun exposure:* Photosensitivity may occur. Discourage prolonged or unprotected exposure to sunlight.

Contraindications and precautions

- Contraindicated in patients hypersensitive to drug, in those with anuria, and in infants.
- Ethacrynic acid isn't recommended for breast-feeding women.
- Use cautiously in patients with electrolyte abnormalities or hepatic impairment. Also, use cautiously in pregnant women.

NURSING CONSIDERATIONS

Assessment

- Obtain history of patient's underlying condition before therapy.
- Monitor effectiveness by regularly checking urine output, weight, peripheral edema, and breath sounds.
- Monitor fluid intake, blood pressure, and serum electrolyte levels.
- Monitor blood uric acid levels, especially in patients with history of gout.
- Be alert for adverse reactions and drug interactions.
- Evaluate patient's and family's knowledge of drug therapy.

Nursing diagnoses

- Excessive fluid volume related to underlying condition
- Impaired urinary elimination related to diuretic therapy
- Deficient knowledge related to drug therapy

Planning and implementation

P.O. use: Give drug with food or milk. P.O. use may cause GI upset.
– To prevent nocturia, give P.O. doses in morning.
I.V. use: Reconstitute vacuum vial with 50 ml of D_5W or normal saline solution. Give slowly through I.V. line of running infusion over several minutes. Discard unused solution after 24 hours. Don't use cloudy or opalescent solutions.
– If more than one I.V. dose is necessary, use new injection site to avoid thrombophlebitis.
– Don't mix with whole blood or its derivatives.

- Don't give S.C. or I.M. because of local pain and irritation.
- Potassium chloride and sodium supplements may be needed.
- Notify prescriber if diarrhea occurs because severe diarrhea may necessitate discontinuing drug.

Patient teaching

- Advise patient to avoid sudden posture changes and to rise slowly to avoid orthostatic hypotension.
- Advise diabetic patient to closely monitor blood glucose levels.
- Teach patient and family to identify and report signs of hypersensitivity or fluid and electrolyte disturbances.
- Teach patient to monitor fluid volume by daily weight and intake and output.
- Tell patient to take oral drug early in day to avoid interruption of sleep by nocturia.

Evaluation

- Patient is free from edema.
- Patient demonstrates adjustment of lifestyle to deal with altered patterns of urinary elimination.
- Patient and family state understanding of drug therapy.

ethambutol hydrochloride

(ee-THAM-byoo-tol high-droh-KLOR-ighd)
Etibi ♦, Myambutol

Pharmacologic class: semisynthetic antitubercular
Therapeutic class: antitubercular agent
Pregnancy risk category: B

Indications and dosages

▶ **Adjunct treatment in pulmonary tuberculosis.** *Adults and children over age 13:* for patients who have not received previous antitubercular therapy, 15 mg/kg P.O. daily in single dose.
Retreatment: 25 mg/kg P.O. daily as single dose for 60 days with at least one other antitubercular drug; then decreased to 15 mg/kg/day as single dose.

How supplied

Tablets: 100 mg, 400 mg

Pharmacokinetics

Absorption: absorbed rapidly from GI tract.
Distribution: distributed widely in body tissues and fluids; 8% to 22% protein-bound.
Metabolism: undergoes partial hepatic metabolism.
Excretion: after 24 hours, about 50% of unchanged drug and 8% to 15% of its metabolites are excreted in urine; 20% to 25% is excreted in feces. *Half-life:* about 3½ hours.

Route	Onset	Peak	Duration
P.O.	Unknown	2-4 hr	Unknown

Pharmacodynamics

Chemical effect: unknown; appears to interfere with synthesis of one or more metabolites of susceptible bacteria, altering cellular metabolism during cell division (bacteriostatic).
Therapeutic effect: hinders bacterial growth. Spectrum of activity includes *Mycobacterium bovis, Mycobacterium marinum, Mycobacterium tuberculosis,* and some strains of *Mycobacterium avium, Mycobacterium fortuitum, Mycobacterium intracellulare,* and *Mycobacterium kansasii.*

Adverse reactions

CNS: malaise, headache, dizziness, confusion, possibly hallucinations, peripheral neuritis.
EENT: dose-related optic neuritis (vision loss and loss of color discrimination, especially red and green).
GI: anorexia, nausea, vomiting, abdominal pain.
GU: elevated uric acid level.
Hematologic: ***thrombocytopenia.***
Hepatic: abnormal liver function test results.
Respiratory: bloody sputum.
Skin: dermatitis, pruritus, ***toxic epidermal necrolysis.***
Other: ***anaphylactoid reactions,*** fever, precipitation of gout.

Interactions

Drug-drug. *Aluminum salts:* may delay and reduce absorption of ethambutol. Separate administrations by several hours.

Contraindications and precautions

- Contraindicated in patients hypersensitive to drug, in patients with optic neuritis, and in children under age 13.
- Use cautiously in patients with impaired kidney function, cataracts, recurrent eye inflammations, gout, and diabetic retinopathy. Also, use cautiously in pregnant or breast-feeding women.

NURSING CONSIDERATIONS

Assessment

- Obtain history of patient's infection before therapy.
- Perform visual acuity and color discrimination tests and obtain AST and ALT levels, as ordered, before therapy.
- Monitor effectiveness by regularly assessing for improvement in patient's condition and evaluating culture and sensitivity test results.
- Monitor AST and ALT levels every 2 to 4 weeks, as ordered, and perform visual acuity and color discrimination tests during treatment.
- Monitor serum uric acid level, as ordered; observe patient for symptoms of gout.
- Be alert for adverse reactions and drug interactions.
- Evaluate patient's and family's knowledge of drug therapy.

Nursing diagnoses

- Infection related to presence of susceptible bacteria
- Disturbed sensory perception (visual) related to drug-induced adverse reactions
- Deficient knowledge related to drug therapy

Planning and implementation

- Anticipate dosage reduction in patient with impaired kidney function.
- Always give ethambutol with other antituberculotics to prevent development of resistant organisms.

Patient teaching

- Reassure patient that visual disturbances will disappear several weeks to months after drug is stopped. Caution patient not to perform haz-

ardous activities if visual disturbances or adverse CNS reactions occur.
- Emphasize need for regular follow-up care.

Evaluation
- Patient is free from infection.
- Patient regains pretreatment visual ability after therapy has stopped.
- Patient and family state understanding of drug therapy.

ethinyl estradiol (ethinyloestradiol)
(ETH-uh-nil es-truh-DIGH-ol)
Estinyl**

Pharmacologic class: estrogen
Therapeutic class: estrogen replacement, antineoplastic
Pregnancy risk category: X

Indications and dosages
▶ **Palliative treatment of metastatic breast cancer (at least 5 years after menopause).** *Women:* 1 mg P.O. t.i.d. for at least 3 months.
▶ **Female hypogonadism.** *Women:* 0.05 mg P.O. once daily to t.i.d. 2 weeks a month, followed by 2 weeks of progesterone therapy; continued for three to six monthly dosing cycles, followed by 2 months off.
▶ **Vasomotor menopausal symptoms.** *Women:* 0.02 to 0.05 mg P.O. daily for cycles of 3 weeks on and 1 week off.
▶ **Palliative treatment of metastatic inoperable prostate cancer.** *Men:* 0.15 to 2 mg P.O. daily.

How supplied
Tablets: 0.02 mg, 0.05 mg, 0.5 mg

Pharmacokinetics
Absorption: well absorbed but substantially inactivated by liver.
Distribution: distributed throughout body with highest levels in fat; about 50% to 80% plasma protein–bound.
Metabolism: metabolized primarily in liver.
Excretion: excreted primarily by kidneys.

Route	Onset	Peak	Duration
P.O.	Unknown	Unknown	Unknown

Pharmacodynamics
Chemical effect: increases synthesis of DNA, RNA, and protein in responsive tissues; also reduces release of follicle-stimulating hormone and luteinizing hormone from pituitary gland.
Therapeutic effect: replaces estrogen, hinders prostate and breast cancer cell growth, and relieves vasomotor menopausal symptoms.

Adverse reactions
CNS: headache, dizziness, chorea, depression, lethargy, ***seizures.***
CV: thrombophlebitis; ***thromboembolism;*** hypertension; edema; ***increased risk of CVA, pulmonary embolism, and MI.***
EENT: worsening of myopia or astigmatism, intolerance to contact lenses.
GI: *nausea,* vomiting, abdominal cramps, bloating, diarrhea, constipation, anorexia.
GU: breakthrough bleeding, altered menstrual flow, dysmenorrhea, amenorrhea, cervical erosion, increased risk of endometrial cancer, altered cervical secretions, enlarged uterine fibromas, vaginal candidiasis; testicular atrophy, impotence.
Hepatic: cholestatic jaundice, gallbladder disease, ***hepatic adenoma.***
Metabolic: hyperglycemia, hypercalcemia, increased appetite, weight changes.
Skin: melasma, urticaria, acne, seborrhea, oily skin, hirsutism or hair loss, erythema nodosum, dermatitis.
Other: ***possibility of increased risk of breast cancer,*** gynecomastia, breast changes (tenderness, enlargement, secretion).

Interactions
Drug-drug. *Bromocriptine:* may cause amenorrhea, interfering with bromocriptine effects. Avoid concomitant use.
Carbamazepine, phenobarbital, rifampin: decreased effectiveness of estrogen therapy. Monitor patient closely.

Corticosteroids: possible enhanced effects. Monitor patient closely.
Cyclosporine: increased risk of toxicity. Use together with caution and frequently monitor cyclosporine levels.
Dantrolene, other hepatotoxic drugs: increased risk of hepatotoxicity. Monitor patient closely.
Oral anticoagulants: dosage adjustments may be necessary. Monitor PT and INR.
Tamoxifen: estrogens may interfere with effectiveness of tamoxifen. Avoid concomitant use.
Drug-food. *Caffeine:* may increase serum caffeine levels. Monitor effects.
Drug-lifestyle. *Smoking:* increased risk of CV effects. If smoking continues, patient may need alternate therapy.

Contraindications and precautions

- Contraindicated in pregnant or breast-feeding women and in patients with thrombophlebitis, thromboembolic disorders, estrogen-dependent neoplasia, breast or reproductive organ cancer (except for palliative treatment), or undiagnosed abnormal genital bleeding.
- Use cautiously in patients with cerebrovascular or coronary artery disease, asthma, depression, bone disease, or cardiac, hepatic, or renal dysfunction and in women with family history (mother, grandmother, sister) of breast or genital tract cancer or who have breast nodules, fibrocystic disease, or abnormal mammogram findings.
- Drug shouldn't be used in children.

NURSING CONSIDERATIONS

Assessment

- Obtain history of patient's underlying condition before therapy, and reassess regularly thereafter.
- Make sure patient has thorough physical examination before starting ethinyl estradiol therapy.
- Patient receiving long-term therapy should have yearly examinations. Periodically monitor serum lipid levels, blood pressure, body weight, and liver function, as ordered.
- Be alert for adverse reactions and drug interactions.
- Evaluate patient's and family's knowledge of drug therapy.

Nursing diagnoses

- Ineffective health maintenance related to underlying condition
- Ineffective tissue perfusion (cerebral, peripheral, pulmonary, or myocardial) related to drug-induced thromboembolism
- Deficient knowledge related to drug therapy

Planning and implementation

- Give oral forms with meals or at bedtime (if only one daily dose is required) to minimize nausea.
- Because of risk of thromboembolism, therapy should be discontinued at least 1 month before procedures that may cause prolonged immobilization or thromboembolism, such as knee or hip surgery.
- Withhold drug and notify prescriber if thromboembolic event is suspected; be prepared to provide supportive care as indicated.
- Notify pathologist if patient receives this drug.

ALERT Estrogen preparations aren't interchangeable.

Patient teaching

- Inform patient about package insert that describes estrogen's adverse effects; also, provide verbal explanation.
- Emphasize importance of regular physical examinations. Postmenopausal women who use estrogen replacement for more than 5 years to treat menopausal symptoms may be at increased risk for endometrial carcinoma. This risk is reduced by using cyclic rather than continuous therapy and lowest possible dosages of estrogen. Adding progestins to regimen decreases risk of endometrial hyperplasia; it isn't known if progestins affect risk of endometrial carcinoma. Most studies show no increased risk of breast cancer.
- Explain to patient on cyclic therapy for postmenopausal symptoms that, although withdrawal bleeding may occur during week off drug, fertility hasn't been restored. Pregnancy can't occur because patient hasn't ovulated.

ALERT Warn patient to immediately report abdominal pain; pain, numbness, or stiffness in legs or buttocks; pressure or pain in chest; shortness of breath; severe headaches; visual disturbances, such as blind spots, flashing lights, or blurriness; vaginal bleeding or discharge; breast lumps; swelling of hands or feet; yellow skin or sclera; dark urine; and light-colored stools.

- Tell diabetic patient to report elevated blood glucose test results so antidiabetic dosage can be adjusted.
- Teach woman how to perform routine breast self-examination.

Evaluation

- Patient shows improvement in underlying condition.
- Patient has no thromboembolic event during therapy.
- Patient and family state understanding of drug therapy.

ethinyl estradiol and desogestrel

(ETH-uh-nil es-truh-DIGH-ol and DAY-so-jest-rul)

monophasic: Desogen, Ortho-Cept

ethinyl estradiol and ethynodiol diacetate

monophasic: Demulen 1/35, Demulen 1/50, Zovia 1/35E, Zovia 1/50E

ethinyl estradiol and levonorgestrel

monophasic: Levlen, Nordette
triphasic: Tri-Levlen, Triphasil

ethinyl estradiol and norethindrone

monophasic: Brevicon, Genora 0.5/35, Genora 1/35, ModiCon, N.E.E. 1/35, Nelova 0.5/35E, Nelova 1/35E, Norethin 1/35E, Norinyl 1+35, Ortho-Novum 1/35, Ovcon-35, Ovcon-50
biphasic: Nelova 10/11, Ortho-Novum 10/11
triphasic: Ortho-Novum 7/7/7, Tri-Norinyl

ethinyl estradiol and norethindrone acetate

monophasic: Loestrin 21 1/20, Loestrin 21 1.5/30

ethinyl estradiol and norgestimate

monophasic: Ortho-Cyclen
triphasic: Ortho Tri-Cyclen

ethinyl estradiol and norgestrel

monophasic: Lo/Ovral, Ovral

ethinyl estradiol, norethindrone acetate, and ferrous fumarate

monophasic: Loestrin Fe 1/20, Loestrin Fe 1.5/30

mestranol and norethindrone

monophasic: Genora 1/50, Nelova 1/50 M, Norethin 1/50 M, Norinyl 1+50, Ortho-Novum 1/50

Pharmacologic class: estrogen with progestin
Therapeutic class: oral contraceptive
Pregnancy risk category: X

Indications and dosages

▶ **Contraception. (Monophasic oral contraceptives.)** *Adults:* 1 tablet P.O. daily, beginning on day 5 of menstrual cycle (first day of menstrual flow is day 1). With 20- and 21-tablet packages, new dosing cycle begins 7 days after last tablet taken. With 28-tablet packages, dosage is 1 tablet daily without interruption; extra tablets are placebos or contain iron. (**Biphasic oral contraceptives.**) *Adults:* 1 color tablet P.O. daily for 10 days; then next color tablet for 11 days. (**Triphasic oral contraceptives.**) *Adults:* 1 tablet P.O. daily in sequence specified by brand.

How supplied

Monophasic oral contraceptives
ethinyl estradiol and desogestrel
Tablets: ethinyl estradiol 30 mcg and desogestrel 0.15 mg (Desogen, Ortho-Cept)

ethinyl estradiol and ethynodiol diacetate
Tablets: ethinyl estradiol 35 mcg and ethynodiol diacetate 1 mg (Demulen 1/35, Zovia 1/35E); ethinyl estradiol 50 mcg and ethynodiol diacetate 1 mg (Demulen 1/50, Zovia 1/50E)
ethinyl estradiol and levonorgestrel
Tablets: ethinyl estradiol 30 mcg and levonorgestrel 0.15 mg (Levlen, Nordette)
ethinyl estradiol and norethindrone
Tablets: ethinyl estradiol 35 mcg and norethindrone 0.4 mg (Ovcon-35); ethinyl estradiol 35 mcg and norethindrone 0.5 mg (Brevicon, Genora 0.5/35, ModiCon, Nelova 0.5/35E); ethinyl estradiol 35 mcg and norethindrone 1 mg (Genora 1/35, N.E.E. 1/35, Nelova 1/35E, Norcept-E 1/35, Norethin 1/35E, Norinyl 1+35, Ortho-Novum 1/35); ethinyl estradiol 50 mcg and norethindrone 1 mg (Ovcon-50)
ethinyl estradiol and norethindrone acetate
Tablets: ethinyl estradiol 20 mcg and norethindrone acetate 1 mg (Loestrin 21 1/20); ethinyl estradiol 30 mcg and norethindrone acetate 1.5 mg (Loestrin 21 1.5/30)
ethinyl estradiol and norgestimate
Tablets: ethinyl estradiol 35 mcg and norgestimate 0.25 mg (Ortho Cyclen)
ethinyl estradiol and norgestrel
Tablets: ethinyl estradiol 30 mcg and norgestrel 0.3 mg (Lo/Ovral); ethinyl estradiol 50 mcg and norgestrel 0.5 mg (Ovral)
ethinyl estradiol, norethindrone acetate, and ferrous fumarate
Tablets: ethinyl estradiol 20 mcg, norethindrone acetate 1 mg, and ferrous fumarate 75 mg (Loestrin Fe 1/20); ethinyl estradiol 30 mcg, norethindrone acetate 1.5 mg, and ferrous fumarate 75 mg (Loestrin Fe 1.5/30
mestranol and norethindrone
Tablets: mestranol 50 mcg and norethindrone 1 mg (Genora 1/50, Nelova 1/50 M, Norethin 1/50 M, Norinyl 1+50, Ortho-Novum 1/50)

Biphasic oral contraceptives
ethinyl estradiol and norethindrone
Tablets: ethinyl estradiol 35 mcg and norethindrone 0.5 mg during phase 1 [10 days]; ethinyl estradiol 35 mcg and norethindrone 1 mg during phase 2 [11 days] (Nelova 10/11, Ortho-Novum 10/11)

Triphasic oral contraceptives
ethinyl estradiol and levonorgestrel
Tablets: (Tri-Levlen, Triphasil) ethinyl estradiol 30 mcg and levonorgestrel 0.05 mg during phase 1 [6 days]; ethinyl estradiol 40 mcg and levonorgestrel 0.075 mg during phase 2 [5 days]; ethinyl estradiol 30 mcg and levonorgestrel 0.125 mg during phase 3 [10 days]
ethinyl estradiol and norethindrone
Tablets: (Tri-Norinyl) ethinyl estradiol 35 mcg and norethindrone 0.5 mg during phase 1 [7 days]; ethinyl estradiol 35 mcg and norethindrone 1 mg during phase 2 [9 days]; ethinyl estradiol 35 mcg and norethindrone 0.5 mg during phase 3 [5 days]; (Ortho-Novum 7/7/7) ethinyl estradiol 35 mcg and norethindrone 0.5 mg during phase 1 [7 days]; ethinyl estradiol 35 mcg and norethindrone 0.75 mg during phase 2 [7 days]; ethinyl estradiol 35 mcg and norethindrone 1 mg during phase 3 [7 days]
ethinyl estradiol and norgestimate
Tablets: (Ortho Tri-Cyclen) ethinyl estradiol 35 mcg and norgestimate 0.18 mg during phase 1 (7 days); ethinyl estradiol 35 mcg and norgestimate 0.215 mg during phase 2 (7 days); ethinyl estradiol 35 mcg and norgestimate 0.25 mg during phase 3 (7 days).

Pharmacokinetics

Absorption: mostly well absorbed.
Distribution: widely distributed and extensively bound to plasma proteins.
Metabolism: metabolized mainly in liver.
Excretion: excreted in urine and feces.

Route	Onset	Peak	Duration
P.O.	Unknown	Varies	Unknown

Pharmacodynamics

Chemical effect: inhibit ovulation through negative feedback mechanism directed at hypothalamus. Estrogen suppresses secretion of follicle-stimulating hormone, blocking follicular development and ovulation. Progestin suppresses secretion of luteinizing hormone so ovulation cannot occur even if follicle develops. Progestin thickens cervical mucus, which interferes with sperm migration, and causes

endometrial changes that prevent implantation of fertilized ovum.
Therapeutic effect: prevent pregnancy and relieve signs and symptoms of endometriosis.

Adverse reactions

CNS: *headache, dizziness,* depression, lethargy, migraine.
CV: ***thromboembolism,*** hypertension, edema, ***pulmonary embolism, CVA.***
EENT: worsening of myopia or astigmatism, intolerance of contact lenses, exophthalmos, diplopia.
GI: granulomatous colitis, *nausea,* vomiting, abdominal cramps, bloating, diarrhea, constipation, anorexia, ***pancreatitis.***
GU: *breakthrough bleeding,* dysmenorrhea, amenorrhea, cervical erosion or abnormal secretions, enlargement of uterine fibromas, vaginal candidiasis.
Hepatic: gallbladder disease, cholestatic jaundice, ***liver tumors.***
Metabolic: changes in appetite, weight gain, hyperglycemia, hypercalcemia.
Skin: rash, acne, ***erythema multiforme.***
Other: breast changes (*tenderness,* enlargement, secretion).

Interactions

Drug-drug. *Bromocriptine:* may cause amenorrhea, interfering with bromocriptine effects. Avoid concomitant use.
Carbamazepine, phenobarbital, phenytoin, rifampin: decreased effectiveness of estrogen therapy. Monitor patient closely.
Corticosteroids: possibly enhanced effects. Monitor patient closely.
Dantrolene, other hepatotoxic drugs: increased risk of hepatotoxicity. Monitor patient closely.
Griseofulvin, penicillins, sulfonamides, tetracyclines: may decrease effectiveness of oral contraceptives. Avoid concomitant use, if possible or use barrier contraception for the duration of concomitant therapy.
Oral anticoagulants: dosage adjustments may be necessary. Monitor PT and INR.
Tamoxifen: estrogens may interfere with effectiveness of tamoxifen. Avoid concomitant use.
Drug-food. *Caffeine:* may increase serum caffeine levels. Monitor effects.
Drug-lifestyle. *Smoking:* increased risk of CV effects. If smoking continues, may need an alternate therapy.

Contraindications and precautions

- Contraindicated in known or suspected pregnancy, in breast-feeding women, and in patients with thromboembolic disorders, cerebrovascular or coronary artery disease, diplopia or ocular lesion arising from ophthalmic vascular disease, classic migraine, MI, known or suspected breast cancer, known or suspected estrogen-dependent neoplasia, benign or malignant liver tumors, active liver disease or history of cholestatic jaundice with pregnancy or prior use of oral contraceptives, or undiagnosed abnormal vaginal bleeding.
- Use cautiously in patients with cardiac, renal, or hepatic insufficiency; hyperlipidemia; hypertension; migraine; seizure disorders; or asthma.
- To avoid later fertility and menstrual problems, hormonal contraception isn't advised for adolescents until after at least 2 years of well-established menstrual cycles and completion of physiologic maturation.

NURSING CONSIDERATIONS

Assessment

- Obtain history of patient's pregnancy status or underlying endometriosis before therapy.
- Monitor effectiveness by determining if pregnancy test is negative or if patient with endometriosis has diminished signs and symptoms.
- Periodically monitor serum lipid levels, blood pressure, body weight, and liver function, as ordered.
- Be alert for adverse reactions and drug interactions.
- Evaluate patient's and family's knowledge of drug therapy.

Nursing diagnoses

- Health-seeking behavior (prevention of pregnancy) related to family planning
- Acute pain related to drug-induced headache
- Deficient knowledge related to drug therapy

Planning and implementation

- Make sure patient has been properly instructed about prescribed oral contraceptive before she takes first dose.

ALERT Make sure patient has negative pregnancy test before drug therapy starts.

- Many laboratory tests are affected by oral contraceptives.
- Stop therapy if patient develops granulomatous colitis, and notify prescriber.
- Drug should be stopped at least 1 week before surgery to decrease risk of thromboembolism. Tell patient to use alternative method of birth control.

Patient teaching

- Tell patient to take tablets at same time each day; nighttime dosing may reduce nausea and headaches.
- Advise patient to use additional method of birth control, such as condoms or diaphragm with spermicide, for first week of first cycle.
- Tell patient that missed doses in midcycle greatly increase likelihood of pregnancy.
- If one tablet is missed, tell patient to take it as soon as remembered or to take two tablets the next day and continue regular schedule. If patient misses 2 consecutive days, instruct her to take two tablets daily for 2 days and then resume normal schedule. Also advise her to use additional method of birth control for 7 days after two missed doses. If she misses three or more doses, tell her to discard remaining tablets in monthly package and to substitute another contraceptive method. If next menstrual period doesn't begin on schedule, warn patient to rule out pregnancy before starting new dosing cycle. If menstrual period begins, have patient start new dosing cycle 7 days after last tablet was taken.
- Warn patient that headache, nausea, dizziness, breast tenderness, spotting, and breakthrough bleeding are common at first. These effects should diminish after three to six dosing cycles (months).
- Instruct patient to weigh herself at least twice weekly and to report sudden weight gain or edema to prescriber.
- Warn patient to avoid exposure to ultraviolet light or prolonged exposure to sunlight.

ALERT Warn patient to immediately report abdominal pain; numbness, stiffness, or pain in legs or buttocks; pressure or pain in chest; shortness of breath; severe headache; visual disturbances, such as blind spots, blurriness, or flashing lights; undiagnosed vaginal bleeding or discharge; two consecutive missed menstrual periods; lumps in breast; swelling of hands or feet; or severe pain in abdomen.

- Advise patient of increased risks associated with simultaneous use of cigarettes and oral contraceptives.
- Teach patient how to perform routine breast self-examination.
- If one menstrual period is missed and tablets have been taken on schedule, tell patient to continue taking them. If two consecutive menstrual periods are missed, tell patient to stop drug and have pregnancy test. Progestins may cause birth defects if taken early in pregnancy.
- Advise patient not to take same drug for longer than 12 months without consulting prescriber. Stress importance of Papanicolaou test and annual gynecologic examination.
- Advise patient to check with prescriber about how soon pregnancy may be attempted after hormonal therapy is stopped. Many prescribers recommend that women not become pregnant within 2 months after stopping drug.
- Warn patient of possible delay in achieving pregnancy when drug is discontinued.
- Tell patient that many prescribers advise women on prolonged therapy (5 years or longer) to stop drug and use other birth control methods. Periodically reassess patient while off hormone therapy.

Evaluation

- Patient doesn't become pregnant.
- Patient obtains relief from drug-induced headache with administration of mild analgesic.
- Patient and family state understanding of drug therapy.

ethosuximide
(eth-oh-SUKS-ih-mighd)
Zarontin

Pharmacologic class: succinimide derivative
Therapeutic class: anticonvulsant
Pregnancy risk category: NR

Indications and dosages

▶ **Absence seizures.** *Adults and children age 6 and older:* 500 mg P.O. daily. Optimal dose is 20 mg/kg/day.
Children ages 3 to 6: 250 mg P.O. daily. Optimal dose is 20 mg/kg/day.

How supplied

Capsules: 250 mg
Syrup: 250 mg/5 ml

Pharmacokinetics

Absorption: absorbed from GI tract.
Distribution: distributed widely throughout body; protein binding is minimal.
Metabolism: metabolized extensively in liver.
Excretion: excreted in urine with small amounts excreted in bile and feces. *Half-life:* about 60 hours.

Route	Onset	Peak	Duration
P.O.	Unknown	3-7 hr	Unknown

Pharmacodynamics

Chemical effect: not well defined; may increase seizure threshold. Reduces paroxysmal spike-and-wave pattern of absence seizures by depressing nerve transmission in motor cortex.
Therapeutic effect: prevents seizures.

Adverse reactions

CNS: *drowsiness, headache, fatigue, dizziness, ataxia, irritability, euphoria, lethargy, depression, psychosis.*
EENT: myopia, tongue swelling, gingival hyperplasia.
GI: *nausea, vomiting, diarrhea, cramps, anorexia, hiccups, epigastric and abdominal pain.*
GU: vaginal bleeding, urinary frequency.
Hematologic: ***leukopenia,*** eosinophilia, ***agranulocytosis, pancytopenia.***
Metabolic: *weight loss.*
Skin: urticaria, pruritic and erythematous rashes, hirsutism.

Interactions

Drug-drug. *Phenytoin:* serum phenytoin levels may be increased. Monitor levels closely.
Drug-lifestyle. *Alcohol use:* increased CNS depression. Discourage concomitant use.

Contraindications and precautions

- Contraindicated in patients hypersensitive to succinimide derivatives.
- Use with extreme caution in patients with hepatic or renal disease.
- Safety of drug hasn't been established in pregnant or breast-feeding women.

NURSING CONSIDERATIONS

Assessment

- Obtain history of patient's seizure disorder before therapy.
- Monitor effectiveness by assessing patient for absence of seizure activity. Drug may increase frequency of generalized tonic-clonic seizures when used alone in patients who have mixed types of seizures.
- Monitor blood levels. Therapeutic blood levels are 40 to 80 mcg/ml.
- Obtain CBC every 3 to 6 months, as ordered.
- Be alert for adverse reactions.
- Evaluate patient's and family's knowledge of drug therapy.

Nursing diagnoses

- Risk for injury related to seizure disorder
- Ineffective protection related to drug-induced blood disorders
- Deficient knowledge related to drug therapy

Planning and implementation

- Ethosuximide is drug of choice for treating absence seizures.
- Give with food to minimize GI distress.

ALERT Never withdraw drug suddenly because doing so could cause absence seizures. Call prescriber immediately if adverse reactions develop.

• Drug may cause positive direct Coombs' test.

Patient teaching
• Advise patient to take drug with food to minimize GI distress.
• Caution patient to avoid hazardous activities that require mental alertness until CNS effects of drug are known.
• Warn patient and parents not to stop drug abruptly and to call prescriber if adverse reactions occur.

Evaluation
• Patient is free from seizure activity.
• Patient maintains normal CBC throughout therapy.
• Patient and family state understanding of drug therapy.

etidronate disodium
(eh-tih-DROH-nayt digh-SOH-dee-um)
Didronel

Pharmacologic class: pyrophosphate analogue
Therapeutic class: antihypercalcemic
Pregnancy risk category: C

Indications and dosages

▶ **Symptomatic Paget's disease of bone (osteitis deformans).** *Adults:* 5 to 10 mg/kg P.O. daily in single dose 2 hours before meal with water or juice. Maximum dosage is 20 mg/kg P.O. daily.
▶ **Heterotopic ossification in spinal cord injuries.** *Adults:* 20 mg/kg P.O. daily for 2 weeks; then 10 mg/kg daily for 10 weeks. Total treatment period is 12 weeks.
▶ **Heterotopic ossification after total hip replacement.** *Adults:* 20 mg/kg P.O. daily for 1 month before total hip replacement and for 3 months afterward.
▶ **Malignancy-related hypercalcemia.** *Adults:* 7.5 mg/kg I.V. daily for 3 consecutive days. Maintenance dosage is 20 mg/kg P.O. daily for 30 days. May be used for maximum of 90 days.

How supplied

Tablets: 200 mg, 400 mg
Injection: 50 mg/ml

Pharmacokinetics

Absorption: absorption after P.O. dose is variable and decreased in presence of food. Absorption may also be dose-related.
Distribution: about half of dose is distributed to bone.
Metabolism: not metabolized.
Excretion: about 50% excreted within 24 hours in urine. *Half-life:* 5 to 7 hours.

Route	Onset	Peak	Duration
P.O., I.V.	Variable	Variable	Variable

Pharmacodynamics

Chemical effect: decreases osteoclastic activity by inhibiting osteocytic osteolysis and decreases mineral release and matrix or collagen breakdown in bone.
Therapeutic effect: slows excessive remodeling of pagetic or heterotropic bone and lowers blood calcium levels in malignant disease.

Adverse reactions

CNS: ***seizures.***
CV: fluid overload.
GI: diarrhea, increased frequency of bowel movements, nausea, constipation, stomatitis (at 20 mg/kg/day).
Hepatic: abnormal hepatic function.
Musculoskeletal: increased or recurrent bone pain, pain at previously asymptomatic sites, increased risk of fracture.
Respiratory: dyspnea.
Other: *elevated serum phosphate level,* fever, ***hypersensitivity reactions.***

Interactions

Drug-drug. *Antacids containing calcium, magnesium, or aluminum; mineral supplements containing calcium, iron, magnesium, or aluminum:* can inhibit absorption. Avoid use within 2 hours of dose.
Drug-food. *Foods containing large amounts of calcium (such as milk, dairy products):* can prevent oral absorption. Avoid use within 2 hours of dose.

Contraindications and precautions

- No known contraindications.
- Use cautiously in pregnant or breast-feeding women and in patients with impaired kidney function.
- Safety of drug hasn't been established in children.

NURSING CONSIDERATIONS

Assessment

- Obtain history of patient's underlying condition before therapy.
- Assess kidney function before therapy and then during therapy, as ordered.
- Monitor effectiveness by evaluating serum alkaline phosphatase level and urinary hydroxyproline excretion; both decrease if therapy is effective.
- Evaluate patient's and family's knowledge of drug therapy.

Nursing diagnoses

- Risk for injury related to underlying bone condition
- Diarrhea related to drug-induced adverse GI reactions
- Deficient knowledge related to drug therapy

Planning and implementation

- Don't give drug longer than 3 months at doses above 10 mg/kg daily. Therapy can be resumed after 3 months, if needed, but shouldn't exceed 6 months.

P.O. use: Don't give drug with food, milk, or antacids; they may reduce absorption.

I.V. use: Dilute daily dose in at least 250 ml of normal saline solution or D_5W, and infuse over at least 2 hours.

– Some patients may receive I.V. etidronate for up to 7 days. However, risk of hypokalemia increases after 3 days of treatment.

- Notify prescriber about elevated serum phosphate level, especially in patients receiving higher doses. However, serum phosphate level usually returns to normal 2 to 4 weeks after drug is discontinued.

Patient teaching

- Stress importance of diet high in calcium and vitamin D.
- Tell patient not to eat for 2 hours after daily dose.
- Tell patient that improvement may not occur for up to 3 months but may continue for months after drug is stopped.

Evaluation

- Patient shows improvement of underlying condition.
- Patient doesn't have severe diarrhea during therapy.
- Patient and family state understanding of drug therapy.

etodolac (ultradol)

(eh-toh-DOH-lak)

Lodine, Lodine XL

Pharmacologic class: NSAID
Therapeutic class: antiarthritic
Pregnancy risk category: C

Indications and dosages

▶ **Acute pain.** *Adults:* 200 to 400 mg P.O. of conventional tablets or capsules q 6 to 8 hours

▶ **Acute or long-term management of osteoarthritis or rheumatoid arthritis.** *Adults:* 600 to 1,000 mg P.O.daily of conventional tablets or capsules in 2 divided doses. For extended-release tablets, usual dosage is 400 to 1,000 mg P.O. once daily.

How supplied

Capsules: 200 mg, 300 mg
Tablets (extended-release): 400 mg, 500 mg, 600 mg
Tablets (film-coated): 400 mg, 500 mg

Pharmacokinetics

Absorption: well absorbed from GI tract.
Distribution: distributed to liver, lungs, heart, and kidneys.
Metabolism: extensively metabolized in liver.
Excretion: excreted in urine primarily as metabolites; 16% is excreted in feces.

Route	Onset	Peak	Duration
P.O.	≤ 30 min	1-2 hr	4-12 hr

Pharmacodynamics

Chemical effect: unknown; may inhibit prostaglandin synthesis.
Therapeutic effect: relieves inflammation and pain.

Adverse reactions

CNS: *asthenia, malaise, dizziness,* depression, drowsiness, nervousness, insomnia, headache.
CV: hypertension, ***heart failure,*** syncope, flushing, palpitations, edema, fluid retention.
EENT: blurred vision, tinnitus, photophobia, dry mouth.
GI: *dyspepsia,* flatulence, abdominal pain, diarrhea, nausea, constipation, gastritis, melena, vomiting, anorexia, peptic ulceration with or without ***GI bleeding*** or ***perforation,*** ulcerative stomatitis, thirst.
GU: dysuria, urinary frequency, ***renal failure.***
Hematologic: hemolytic anemia, ***leukopenia, thrombocytopenia, agranulocytosis.***
Hepatic: ***hepatitis.***
Metabolic: weight gain.
Respiratory: asthma.
Skin: pruritus, rash, photosensitivity, ***Stevens-Johnson syndrome.***
Other: chills, fever.

Interactions

Drug-drug. *Antacids:* may decrease peak levels of drug. Monitor patient for decreased etodolac effect.
Aspirin: reduced protein-binding of etodolac without altering its clearance. Clinical significance unknown. Recommend avoiding concomitant use.
Beta blockers, diuretics: effects may be blunted. Monitor patient closely.
Cyclosporine: impaired elimination and increased risk of nephrotoxicity. Avoid concomitant use.
Digoxin, lithium, methotrexate: etodolac may impair elimination of these drugs, resulting in increased levels and risk of toxicity. Monitor blood levels.
Phenytoin: increased serum levels of phenytoin. Monitor patient and serum levels for toxicity.
Warfarin: etodolac decreases protein-binding of warfarin but doesn't change its clearance. Although no dosage adjustment is necessary, monitor PT and INR closely, and watch for bleeding.
Drug-herb. *Dong quai, feverfew, garlic, ginger, horse chestnut, red clover:* possible increased risk of bleeding. Discourage concomitant use.
St. John's wort: increased risk of photosensitivity. Advise patient to avoid unprotected exposure to sunlight.
Drug-lifestyle. *Alcohol use:* increased chance of adverse effects. Discourage concurrent use.
Sun exposure: photosensitivity reactions may occur. Urge precautions.

Contraindications and precautions

- Contraindicated in patients hypersensitive to drug and in those with history of aspirin- or NSAID-induced asthma, rhinitis, urticaria, or other allergic reactions.
- Use of drug during third trimester of pregnancy isn't recommended.
- Use cautiously in patients with history of GI bleeding, ulceration, and perforation and renal or hepatic impairment. Also use cautiously in pregnant women during first and second trimesters and breast-feeding women.
- Safety of drug hasn't been established in children under age 18.

NURSING CONSIDERATIONS

Assessment

- Obtain history of patient's underlying condition before therapy.
- Monitor effectiveness by evaluating patient for decreased inflammation and pain.
- Be alert for adverse reactions and drug interactions.
- Evaluate patient's and family's knowledge of drug therapy.

Nursing diagnoses

- Acute pain related to underlying condition
- Risk for injury related to drug-induced adverse reactions
- Deficient knowledge related to drug therapy

Planning and implementation

- Give drug with milk or meals to minimize GI discomfort.

• Metabolites of etodolac may cause false-positive test for urinary bilirubin, decreased serum uric acid levels, and borderline elevations of one or more liver function tests.

Patient teaching

• Advise patient that serious GI toxicity, including peptic ulceration and bleeding, can occur as a result of taking NSAIDs, despite absence of GI symptoms. Teach patient evidence of GI bleeding, such as dark tarry stools, generalized weakness, coffee ground emesis, and tell him to contact prescriber immediately if they occur. Also, tell patient to take drug with milk or food.
• Instruct patient to notify prescriber if other adverse reactions occur or of drug doesn't relieve pain.
• Advise patient to use sunblock, wear protective clothing, and avoid prolonged exposure to sunlight to prevent photosensitivity reactions.
• Tell patient not to use drug during last trimester of pregnancy.

☑ Evaluation

• Patient is free from pain.
• Patient has no injury as result of drug-induced adverse reactions.
• Patient and family state understanding of drug therapy.

etoposide (VP-16)

(eh-toh-POH-sighd)
VePesid, Toposar

Pharmacologic class: podophyllotoxin (cell cycle–phase specific, G2 and late S phases)
Therapeutic class: antineoplastic
Pregnancy risk category: D

Indications and dosages

▶ **Testicular cancer.** *Adults:* 50 to 100 mg/m² I.V. on 5 consecutive days q 3 to 4 weeks; or 100 mg/m² on days 1, 3, and 5 q 3 to 4 weeks for 3 to 4 courses of therapy.
▶ **Small-cell carcinoma of lung.** *Adults:* 35 mg/m²/day I.V. for 4 days; or 50 mg/m²/day I.V. for 5 days. P.O. dosage is two times I.V. dose rounded to nearest 50 mg.

How supplied

Capsules: 50 mg
Injection: 20 mg/ml

Pharmacokinetics

Absorption: only moderately absorbed across GI tract after P.O. administration. Bioavailability ranges from 25% to 75%, with average of 50% of dose being absorbed.
Distribution: distributed widely in body tissues; crosses blood-brain barrier to limited and variable extent. Etoposide is about 94% protein-bound.
Metabolism: only small portion of dose is metabolized in liver.
Excretion: excreted primarily in urine as unchanged drug; smaller portion excreted in feces. *Half-life:* initial, 30 minutes to 2 hours; terminal, 5½ to 11 hours.

Route	Onset	Peak	Duration
P.O., I.V.	Unknown	Unknown	Unknown

Pharmacodynamics

Chemical effect: unknown.
Therapeutic effect: inhibits selected cancer cell growth.

Adverse reactions

CNS: peripheral neuropathy.
CV: hypotension.
GI: *nausea, vomiting, anorexia, diarrhea,* abdominal pain, *stomatitis.*
Hematologic: *anemia,* ***myelosuppression*** (dose-limiting), **LEUKOPENIA, THROMBOCYTOPENIA.**
Skin: reversible alopecia.
Other: ***anaphylaxis***, rash.

Interactions

Drug-drug. *Warfarin:* may further prolong PT. Monitor patient and serum levels closely.

Contraindications and precautions

• Contraindicated in patients hypersensitive to drug.
• Drug isn't recommended for use during pregnancy unless absolutely necessary because fetal harm may occur. It also isn't recommended for use in breast-feeding women.

• Use cautiously in patients who have had previous cytotoxic or radiation therapy.
• Safety of drug hasn't been established in children.

NURSING CONSIDERATIONS

Assessment
• Obtain history of patient's underlying condition before therapy.
• Obtain baseline blood pressure before therapy, and monitor blood pressure at 30-minute intervals during infusion.
• Monitor effectiveness by noting results of follow-up diagnostic tests and overall physical status and by regularly checking tumor size and rate of growth through appropriate studies, as ordered. Etoposide has produced complete remission in small-cell lung cancer and testicular cancer.
• Monitor CBC, as ordered. Observe patient for signs of bone marrow suppression.
• Be alert for adverse reactions and drug interactions.
• Evaluate patient's and family's knowledge of drug therapy.

Nursing diagnoses
• Ineffective health maintenance related to presence of neoplastic disease
• Ineffective protection related to drug-induced adverse hematologic reactions
• Deficient knowledge related to drug therapy

Planning and implementation
• Follow facility policy to reduce risks. Preparation and administration of parenteral form create carcinogenic, mutagenic, and teratogenic risks for staff.
P.O. use: Store capsules in refrigerator.
I.V. use: Give drug by slow I.V. infusion (over at least 30 minutes) to prevent severe hypotension. If systolic blood pressure falls below 90 mm Hg, stop infusion and notify prescriber.
– Dilute drug for infusion in either D_5W or normal saline solution to 0.2 or 0.4 mg/ml. Higher concentrations may crystallize.
– Don't administer through membrane-type in-line filter because diluent may dissolve filter.
– Solutions diluted to 0.2 mg/ml are stable 96 hours at room temperature in plastic of glass unprotected from light; solutions diluted to 0.4 mg/ml are stable 48 hours under same conditions.
• Keep diphenhydramine, hydrocortisone, epinephrine, and necessary emergency equipment available to establish airway in case of anaphylaxis.

Patient teaching
• Warn patient to watch for signs of infection and bleeding. Teach patient how to take infection-control and bleeding precautions.
• Tell patient that hair loss is possible but reversible.
• Instruct patient to report discomfort, pain, or burning at I.V. insertion site.

Evaluation
• Patient exhibits positive response to therapy.
• Patient's immune function returns to normal with cessation of therapy.
• Patient and family state understanding of drug therapy.

exemestane
(ecks-eh-MES-tayn)
Aromasin

Pharmacologic class: aromatase inactivator
Therapeutic class: antineoplastic
Pregnancy risk category: D

Indications and dosages
▶ **Advanced breast cancer in postmenopausal women whose disease has progressed following treatment with tamoxifen.** *Adults:* 25 mg P.O. once daily after a meal.

How supplied
Tablets: 25 mg

Pharmacokinetics
Absorption: rapidly absorbed, with about 42% of dose absorbed from the GI tract following P.O. administration. Plasma levels increase by 40% after a high-fat breakfast.
Distribution: extensively distributed in tissues and 90% bound to plasma proteins.

Metabolism: extensively metabolized by the liver. The main liver isoenzyme involved is cytochrome P-450 3A4.
Excretion: excreted equally in urine and feces. Less than 1% is excreted unchanged in urine. *Elimination half-life:* about 24 hours.

Route	Onset	Peak	Duration
P.O.	Unknown	1-2 hr	unknown

Pharmacodynamics

Chemical effect: drug is an irreversible, steroidal aromatase inactivator that acts as a false substrate for the aromatase enzyme, the principal enzyme that converts androgens to estrogens in premenopausal and postmenopausal women. Exemestane is then processed to an intermediate that binds irreversibly to the enzyme's active site, causing inactivation. This effect is known as "suicide inhibition," and results in lower levels of circulating estrogens. Deprivation of estrogen is an effective and selective way to treat estrogen-dependent breast cancer in postmenopausal women.
Therapeutic effect: hinders function of breast cancer cells.

Adverse reactions

CNS: *depression, insomnia, anxiety, fatigue, pain,* dizziness, headache, paresthesia, generalized weakness, asthenia, confusion, hypoesthesia.
CV: hypertension, edema, chest pain.
EENT: sinusitis, rhinitis, pharyngitis.
GI: *nausea,* vomiting, abdominal pain, anorexia, constipation, diarrhea, dyspepsia.
GU: urinary tract infection.
Metabolic: increased appetite.
Musculoskeletal: pathologic fractures, arthralgia, back pain, skeletal pain.
Respiratory: *dyspnea,* bronchitis, coughing, upper respiratory tract infection.
Skin: rash, increased sweating, alopecia, itching.
Other: fever, infection, flulike syndrome, *hot flushes,* lymphedema.

Interactions

Drug-drug. *Drugs that induce CYP3A4:* may decrease exemestane plasma levels. Monitor patient closely for toxicity.

Contraindications and precautions

- Contraindicated in patients hypersensitive to drug or its components.
- Don't administer to premenopausal women or administer concurrently with estrogen-containing drugs.

NURSING CONSIDERATIONS

Assessment

- Assess patient's breast cancer before therapy and regularly thereafter.
- Monitor patient for adverse reactions.
- Monitor patient's hydration status if adverse GI reactions occur.
- Evaluate patient's and family's knowledge about drug therapy.

Nursing diagnoses

- Ineffective health maintenance related to presence of breast cancer
- Risk for impaired physical mobility related to potential adverse musculoskeletal effects
- Deficient knowledge related to drug therapy

Planning and implementation

- Drug should be given only to postmenopausal women.
- Don't administer with estrogen-containing drugs because doing so could interfere with intended action.
- Treatment should continue until tumor progression is evident.

Patient teaching

- Tell patient to take drug after a meal.
- Inform patient that she may need to take drug for a long period of time.
- Advise patient to report adverse effects to prescriber.

Evaluation

- Patient responds well to drug.
- Patient has no musculoskeletal adverse reactions.
- Patient and family state understanding of drug therapy.

F

factor IX complex

(FAK-tor nighn KOM-pleks)
Bebulin VH, BeneFix, Konyne 80, Profilnine Heat-Treated, Proplex T

factor IX (human)

AlphaNine SD, Mononine

Pharmacologic class: blood derivative
Therapeutic class: systemic hemostatic
Pregnancy risk category: C

Indications and dosages

▶ **Factor IX deficiency (hemophilia B or Christmas disease), anticoagulant overdosage.** *Adults and children:* to calculate approximate units of factor IX needed, use following equations.
Human product: 1 U/kg × body weight in kilograms × percentage of desired increase of factor IX level
Recombinant product: 1.2 U/kg × body weight in kilograms × percentage of desired increase of factor IX level
Proplex T: 0.5 U/kg × body weight in kilograms × percentage of desired increase of factor IX level.

Infusion rates vary with product and patient comfort. Dosage is highly individualized, depending on degree of deficiency, level of factor IX desired, patient weight, and severity of bleeding.

How supplied

Injection: vials, with diluent. Units specified on label.

Pharmacokinetics

Absorption: not applicable.
Distribution: equilibration within extravascular space takes 4 to 6 hours.
Metabolism: cleared by plasma.
Excretion: unknown. *Half-life:* about 24 hours.

Route	Onset	Peak	Duration
I.V.	Immediate	10-30 min	Unknown

Pharmacodynamics

Chemical effect: directly replaces deficient clotting factor.
Therapeutic effect: causes clotting.

Adverse reactions

CNS: headache.
CV: ***thromboembolic reactions, MI, disseminated intravascular coagulation, pulmonary embolism,*** changes in blood pressure.
GI: nausea, vomiting.
Skin: urticaria.
Other: *transient fever, chills, flushing, tingling,* ***hypersensitivity reactions (anaphylaxis).***

Interactions

Drug-drug. *Aminocaproic acid:* increased risk of thrombosis. Avoid concomitant use.

Contraindications and precautions

- Contraindicated in patients with hepatic disease in whom there is suspicion of intravascular coagulation or fibrinolysis. Mononine is contraindicated in patients hypersensitive to murine protein.
- Use cautiously in neonates and infants and in pregnant or breast-feeding women.

NURSING CONSIDERATIONS

Assessment

- Assess patient's coagulation studies and bleeding disorder before and after therapy.
- Be alert for adverse reactions and drug interactions.
- Monitor vital signs regularly.
- Evaluate patient's and family's knowledge of drug therapy.

Nursing diagnoses

- Ineffective health maintenance related to underlying disorder
- Ineffective protection related to drug-induced intravascular hemolysis
- Deficient knowledge related to drug therapy

Planning and implementation
- As ordered, give hepatitis B vaccine before factor IX complex.
- Avoid rapid infusion. If tingling sensation, fever, chills, or headache develops, decrease flow rate and notify prescriber.
- Reconstitute with 20 ml of sterile water for injection for each vial of lyophilized drug. Keep refrigerated until ready to use; warm to room temperature before reconstituting. Use within 3 hours of reconstitution. Unstable in solution. Don't shake, refrigerate, or mix solution with other I.V. solutions. Store away from heat.
- Risk of hepatitis must be weighed against risk of not receiving drug. Because of manufacturing process, risk of HIV transmission is extremely low.

Patient teaching
- Explain drug action to patient.
- Tell patient to report adverse reactions promptly.

Evaluation
- Patient is free from bleeding.
- Patient does not experience injury.
- Patient and family state understanding of drug therapy.

famciclovir
(fam-SIGH-kloh-veer)
Famvir

Pharmacologic class: synthetic acyclic guanine derivative
Therapeutic class: antiviral
Pregnancy risk category: B

Indications and dosages
▶ **Acute herpes zoster.** *Adults:* 500 mg P.O. q 8 hours for 7 days.
▶ **Recurrent episodes of genital herpes.** *Adults:* 125 mg P.O. b.i.d. for 5 days. Therapy begins as soon as symptoms occur.
▶ **Treatment of recurrent herpes simplex virus infections in HIV-infected patients.** *Adults:* 500 mg P.O. b.i.d. for 7 days.
▶ **Long-term suppressive therapy of recurrent episodes of genital herpes.** *Adults:* 250 mg P.O. q 12 hours for up to 1 year of therapy.

How supplied
Tablets: 125 mg, 250 mg, 500 mg

Pharmacokinetics
Absorption: absolute bioavailability is 77%.
Distribution: less than 20% is bound to plasma proteins.
Metabolism: extensively metabolized in liver to active drug, penciclovir (98.5%), and other inactive metabolites.
Excretion: primarily in urine.

Route	Onset	Peak	Duration
P.O.	Unknown	$\leq$ 1 hr	Unknown

Pharmacodynamics
Chemical effect: converted to penciclovir, which enters viral cells and inhibits DNA polymerase and viral DNA synthesis.
Therapeutic effect: inhibits viral replication. Spectrum of activity include herpes simplex types 1 and 2 and varicella-zoster viruses.

Adverse reactions
CNS: *headache,* fatigue, dizziness, paresthesia, somnolence.
EENT: pharyngitis, sinusitis.
GI: diarrhea, *nausea,* vomiting, constipation, anorexia, abdominal pain.
Musculoskeletal: back pain, arthralgia.
Skin: pruritus; zoster-related signs, symptoms, and complications.

Interactions
Drug-drug. *Probenecid:* may increase plasma levels of famciclovir. Monitor patient for increased adverse effects.

Contraindications and precautions
- Contraindicated in patients hypersensitive to drug.
- Breast-feeding isn't recommended during drug therapy.
- Use cautiously in patients with renal or hepatic impairment. Dosage adjustment may be

needed. Also use cautiously in pregnant women.
- Safety of drug hasn't been established in children.

NURSING CONSIDERATIONS

Assessment
- Assess patient's viral infection before therapy, and reassess regularly throughout therapy.
- Be alert for adverse reactions and drug interactions.
- Monitor patient's hydration status if adverse GI reactions occur.
- Evaluate patient's and family's knowledge of drug therapy.

Nursing diagnoses
- Infection related to presence of virus susceptible to famciclovir
- Risk for deficient fluid volume related to drug's adverse GI reactions
- Deficient knowledge related to drug therapy

Planning and implementation
- Patients with renal insufficiency need a reduced dosage.
- Drug may be taken without regard to meals.

Patient teaching
- Teach patient how to prevent spread of infection to others.
- Urge patient to recognize and report early symptoms of herpes infection, such as tingling, itching, or pain.

Evaluation
- Patient is free from infection.
- Patient maintains adequate hydration.
- Patient and family state understanding of drug therapy.

famotidine

(fam-OH-tih-deen)
Pepcid, Pepcid AC†, Pepcid RPD, Pepcidine ◇

Pharmacologic class: H_2-receptor antagonist
Therapeutic class: antiulcer agent
Pregnancy risk category: B

Indications and dosages

▶ **Duodenal ulcer (short-term treatment).** *Adults:* For acute therapy, 40 mg P.O. once daily h.s. or 20 mg P.O. b.i.d. Maintenance, 20 mg P.O. once daily h.s.

▶ **Benign gastric ulcer (short-term treatment).** *Adults:* 40 mg P.O. daily h.s. for 8 weeks.

▶ **Pathologic hypersecretory conditions (such as Zollinger-Ellison syndrome).** *Adults:* 20 mg P.O. q 6 hours up to 160 mg q 6 hours.

▶ **Hospitalized patients with intractable ulcerations or hypersecretory conditions or patients who can't take oral medication.** *Adults:* 20 mg I.V. q 12 hours.

▶ **Gastroesophageal reflux disease (GERD).** *Adults:* 20 mg P.O. b.i.d. for up to 6 weeks. For esophagitis caused by GERD, 20 to 40 mg b.i.d. for up to 12 weeks.

▶ **Prevention or treatment of heartburn.** *Adults:* 10 mg (Pepcid AC only) P.O. 1 hour before meals (prevention) or 10 mg (Pepcid AC only) P.O. with water when symptoms occur. Maximum, 20 mg daily. Drug shouldn't be taken daily for more than 2 weeks.

How supplied

Tablets: 10 mg, 20 mg, 40 mg
Tablets, orally disintegrating: 20 mg
Tablets, chewable: 10 mg†
Powder for oral suspension: 40 mg/5 ml after reconstitution
Injection: 10 mg/ml, 20 mg/50 ml (premixed)

Pharmacokinetics

Absorption: when given orally, about 40% to 45% is absorbed.
Distribution: distributed widely to many body tissues.
Metabolism: about 30% to 35% of dose is metabolized by liver.
Excretion: most of drug is excreted unchanged in urine. *Half-life:* 2½ to 3½ hours.

Route	Onset	Peak	Duration
P.O.	≤ 1 hr	1-3 hr	10-12 hr
I.V.	≤ 1 hr	20 min	10-12 hr

Pharmacodynamics

Chemical effect: competitively inhibits action of H_2 at receptor sites of parietal cells, decreasing gastric acid secretion.
Therapeutic effect: decreases gastric acid levels and prevents heartburn.

Adverse reactions

CNS: *headache,* dizziness, vertigo, malaise, paresthesia.
CV: palpitations.
EENT: tinnitus, orbital edema.
GI: diarrhea, constipation, anorexia, taste disorder, dry mouth.
GU: increased BUN and creatinine levels.
Musculoskeletal: musculoskeletal pain.
Skin: acne, dry skin, flushing.
Other: transient irritation at I.V. site, fever.

Interactions

None significant.

Contraindications and precautions

- Contraindicated in patients hypersensitive to drug.
- Use cautiously in pregnant or breast-feeding women.
- Safety of drug hasn't been established in children.

NURSING CONSIDERATIONS

Assessment

- Assess patient's GI disorder before therapy, and reassess regularly throughout therapy.
- Be alert for adverse reactions.
- Evaluate patient's and family's knowledge of drug therapy.

Nursing diagnoses

- Impaired tissue integrity related to underlying GI disorder
- Constipation related to drug's adverse effect on GI tract
- Deficient knowledge related to drug therapy

Planning and implementation

P.O. use: Give drug at bedtime or, if more than one daily dose is ordered, give last dose of day at bedtime.
– Store reconstituted oral suspension below 86° F (30° C). Discard after 30 days.
I.V. use: To prepare I.V. injection, dilute 2 ml (20 mg) drug with compatible I.V. solution to total volume of either 5 or 10 ml, and inject over at least 2 minutes. Compatible solutions include sterile water for injection, normal saline injection, D_5W or $D_{10}W$ injection, 5% sodium bicarbonate injection, and lactated Ringer's injection.
– Or, give by intermittent I.V. infusion. Dilute 20 mg (2 ml) drug in 100 ml of compatible solution and infuse over 15 to 30 minutes. Solution is stable for 48 hours at room temperature after dilution.
– Store I.V. injection in refrigerator at 36° to 46° F (2° to 8° C).
– Change I.V. site if infiltration or signs of phlebitis occur. Apply warm compresses to site.

Patient teaching

- Tell patient to take drug with snack if desired. Remind him that drug is most effective if taken at bedtime. Tell patient taking 20 mg b.i.d. to take one dose at bedtime.
- With prescriber's knowledge, allow patient to take antacids concomitantly, especially at beginning of therapy when pain is severe.
- Urge patient to avoid cigarette smoking because it may increase gastric acid secretion and worsen disease.
- Advise patient not to take drug for more than 8 weeks unless specifically ordered by prescriber. For self-medication prevention or treatment of heartburn, therapy should continue no more than 2 weeks without prescriber's knowledge.

Evaluation

- Patient reports decrease in or relief of GI pain with drug.
- Patient regains normal bowel pattern.
- Patient and family state understanding of drug therapy.

felodipine

(feh-LOH-dih-peen)

Agon ◇, Agon SR ◇, Plendil, Plendil ER ◇, Renedil ◆

Pharmacologic class: calcium channel blocker
Therapeutic class: antihypertensive
Pregnancy risk category: C

Indications and dosages

▶ **Hypertension.** *Adults:* initially, 5 mg P.O. daily. Dosage adjusted based on patient response, usually at no less than 2-week intervals. Usual dosage is 2.5 to 10 mg daily. Maximum recommended dosage is 20 mg daily. *Elderly patients:* 5 mg P.O. daily, adjusted as for adults. Maximum recommended dosage is 10 mg daily.

How supplied

Tablets: 5 mg ◇
Tablets (extended-release): 2.5 mg, 5 mg, 10 mg

Pharmacokinetics

Absorption: almost completely absorbed, but extensive first-pass metabolism reduces absolute bioavailability to about 20%.
Distribution: over 99% bound to plasma proteins.
Metabolism: unknown, although thought to be hepatic.
Excretion: over 70% of dose appears in urine and 10% in feces as metabolites. *Half-life:* 11 to 16 hours.

Route	Onset	Peak	Duration
P.O.	2-5 hr	2.5-5 hr	24 hr

Pharmacodynamics

Chemical effect: unknown; dihydropyridine derivative that prevents entry of calcium ions into vascular smooth-muscle and cardiac cells.
Therapeutic effect: lowers blood pressure.

Adverse reactions

CNS: *headache*, dizziness, paresthesia, asthenia.
CV: *peripheral edema,* chest pain, palpitations.
EENT: rhinorrhea, pharyngitis, gingival hyperplasia.
GI: abdominal pain, nausea, constipation, diarrhea.
Musculoskeletal: muscle cramps, back pain.
Respiratory: upper respiratory infection, cough.
Skin: rash, *flushing.*

Interactions

Drug-drug. *Anticonvulsants:* decreased plasma felodipine level. Avoid concomitant use.
Cimetidine: decreased felodipine clearance. Give lower doses of felodipine.
Metoprolol: may alter pharmacokinetics of metoprolol. No dosage adjustment appears necessary. Monitor patient for adverse effects.
Theophylline: may slightly decrease theophylline levels. Monitor patient's response carefully.
Drug-food. *Grapefruit juice:* increased bioavailability and effect when taken together. Caution patient not to take with grapefruit juice.

Contraindications and precautions

- Contraindicated in patients hypersensitive to drug.
- Breast-feeding isn't recommended during therapy.
- Use cautiously in patients with heart failure, particularly those receiving beta blockers, and in patients with impaired hepatic function because clearance of drug from blood is dependent on liver. Also use cautiously in pregnant women.
- Safety of drug hasn't been established in children.

NURSING CONSIDERATIONS

Assessment

- Assess patient's blood pressure before therapy, and reassess regularly thereafter.
- Be alert for adverse reactions and drug interactions.
- Evaluate patient's and family's knowledge of drug therapy.

Nursing diagnoses

- Risk for injury related to presence of hypertension

- Excessive fluid volume related to drug-induced peripheral edema
- Deficient knowledge related to drug therapy

Planning and implementation

- Drug may be given without regard to food. However, a small study reported more than twofold increase of bioavailability when drug was taken with doubly concentrated grapefruit juice as compared with water or orange juice.

Patient teaching

- Instruct patient to swallow tablets whole and not to crush or chew them.
- Tell patient to take drug even when he feels better; to watch his diet; and to check with prescriber or pharmacist before taking other medications, including OTC medicines and herbal remedies.
- Advise patient to observe good oral hygiene and to see dentist regularly.

Evaluation

- Patient's blood pressure is normal.
- Patient does not develop complications from peripheral edema.
- Patient and family state understanding of drug therapy.

fenofibrate

(feh-noh-FIGH-brayt)
Tricor

Pharmacologic class: fibric acid derivative
Therapeutic class: antilipemic
Pregnancy risk category: C

Indications and dosages

▶ **Adjunct therapy to diet for treatment of patients with very high serum triglyceride levels (type IV and V hyperlipidemia) who are at risk of pancreatitis and who don't respond adequately to a determined dietary effort.** *Adults:* initially, 67 mg P.O. daily. Increase sequentially if necessary following repeat serum triglyceride levels at 4- to 8-week intervals to maximum dose of three capsules daily (201 mg).

▶ **Adjunctive therapy to diet for reducing low-density lipoprotein cholesterol, total cholesterol, triglycerides, and apolipoprotein B in patients with primary hypercholesterolemia or mixed dyslipidemia (Fredrickson types IIa and IIb).** *Adults:* 200 mg P.O. daily.
Elderly patients: initially, 67 mg daily. Increase dose only after evaluation of effects on renal function and lipid levels.

How supplied

Capsules (micronized): 67 mg

Pharmacokinetics

Absorption: well absorbed from GI tract.
Distribution: about 99% bound to plasma proteins.
Metabolism: rapidly hydrolyzed by esterases to active metabolite, fenofibric acid.
Excretion: about 60% excreted in urine mainly as metabolites and 25% in feces. *Half-life:* 20 hours.

Route	Onset	Peak	Duration
P.O.	Unknown	6-8 hr	Unknown

Pharmacodynamics

Chemical effect: exact mechanism unknown. May inhibit triglyceride synthesis, resulting in a decrease in the quantity of very-low-density lipoproteins released into circulation. Drug also may stimulate breakdown of triglyceride-rich protein.
Therapeutic effect: decreases serum triglyceride levels.

Adverse reactions

CNS: dizziness, pain, asthenia, fatigue, paresthesia, insomnia, increased appetite, headache.
CV: ***arrhythmias.***
EENT: eye irritation, eye floaters, earache, conjunctivitis, blurred vision, rhinitis, sinusitis.
GI: dyspepsia, eructation, flatulence, nausea, vomiting, abdominal pain, constipation, diarrhea.
GU: increased BUN and creatinine levels, polyuria, vaginitis.
Hepatic: increased ALT, AST levels.
Musculoskeletal: arthralgia.

Respiratory: cough.
Skin: pruritus, rash.
Other: decreased hemoglobin and uric acid levels, hypersensitivity reaction, *infection,* flu syndrome, decreased libido.

Interactions

Drug-drug. *Bile acid sequestrants:* may bind and inhibit absorption of fenofibrate. Give drug 1 hour before or 4 to 6 hours after bile acid sequestrants.
Coumarin-type anticoagulants: potentiation of anticoagulant effect. Monitor PT and INR closely. Dosage of anticoagulant may need to be reduced.
Cyclosporine, immunosuppressants, nephrotoxic agents: induced renal dysfunction may compromise the elimination of fenofibrate. Use together cautiously.
3-Hydroxy-3-methylglutaryl coenzyme A (HMG-CoA) reductase inhibitors: no data are available on concomitant use with fenofibrate; however, because of risk of myopathy, rhabdomyolysis, and acute renal failure reported with combined use of HMG-CoA reductase inhibitors and gemfibrozil (another fibrate derivative), these drugs shouldn't be given together.
Drug-food. *Any food:* absorption of fenofibrate is increased. Give drug with meals.
Drug-lifestyle. *Alcohol use:* may elevate triglyceride levels. Discourage concomitant use.

Contraindications and precautions

- Contraindicated in patients hypersensitive to drug and in those with gallbladder disease, hepatic dysfunction, primary biliary cirrhosis, severe renal dysfunction, or unexplained persistent liver function abnormalities.
- Use cautiously in patients with history of pancreatitis.
- Safety and efficacy in children haven't been established.

NURSING CONSIDERATIONS

Assessment

- Assess baseline lipid levels and liver function tests before starting therapy and periodically thereafter as ordered.
- Be alert for adverse reactions and drug interactions.
- Evaluate patient's and family's knowledge of drug.

Nursing diagnoses

- Imbalanced nutrition: less than body requirements related to drug-induced adverse GI reactions
- Risk for infection related to adverse drug reactions
- Deficient knowledge related to drug therapy

Planning and implementation

- Patients with severe renal impairment need evaluation of renal function and triglyceride levels before dosage increase.
- Give drug with meals.
- Counsel patient on importance of adhering to triglyceride-lowering diet.

Patient teaching

- Advise patient to promptly report symptoms of unexplained muscle weakness, pain, or tenderness, especially if accompanied by malaise or fever.
- Urge patient to take drug with meals to optimize drug absorption.
- Advise patient to continue weight-control measures, including diet and exercise, and to reduce alcohol intake before starting drug therapy.
- Instruct patient who also takes bile acid resin to take fenofibrate 1 hour before or 4 to 6 hours after bile acid resin.
- Advise breast-feeding patient to discontinue either breast-feeding or drug therapy.

Evaluation

- Patient maintains adequate nutritional intake.
- Patient remains free from infection.
- Patient and family state understanding of drug therapy.

fenoprofen calcium

(fen-uh-PROH-fen KAL-see-um)
Nalfon, Nalfon 200

Pharmacologic class: NSAID
Therapeutic class: nonnarcotic analgesic, anti-inflammatory

Pregnancy risk category: NR

Indications and dosages

▶ **Rheumatoid arthritis and osteoarthritis.** *Adults:* 300 to 600 mg P.O. t.i.d. or q.i.d. Maximum, 3.2 g daily.

▶ **Mild to moderate pain.** *Adults:* 200 mg P.O. q 4 to 6 hours, p.r.n.

How supplied

Tablets: 600 mg
Capsules: 200 mg, 300 mg

Pharmacokinetics

Absorption: absorbed rapidly and completely from GI tract.
Distribution: 99% protein-bound.
Metabolism: metabolized in liver.
Excretion: excreted chiefly in urine with small amount excreted in feces. *Half-life:* 2½ to 3 hours.

Route	Onset	Peak	Duration
P.O.	15-30 min	About 2 hr	4-6 hr

Pharmacodynamics

Chemical effect: unknown; produces anti-inflammatory, analgesic, and antipyretic effects, possibly by inhibiting prostaglandin synthesis.
Therapeutic effect: relieves pain, fever, and inflammation.

Adverse reactions

CNS: *headache,* drowsiness, fatigue, nervousness, asthenia, tremor, confusion, dizziness, *somnolence.*
CV: peripheral edema, palpitations.
EENT: tinnitus, blurred vision, nasopharyngitis, decreased hearing.
GI: *epigastric distress, nausea,* ***GI bleeding,*** vomiting, occult blood loss, peptic ulceration, constipation, anorexia, *dyspepsia,* flatulence.
GU: oliguria, interstitial nephritis, proteinuria, ***reversible renal failure, papillary necrosis,*** cystitis, hematuria.
Hematologic: prolonged bleeding time, anemia, ***aplastic anemia, agranulocytosis, thrombocytopenia, hemorrhage.***
Hepatic: elevated liver enzyme levels, ***hepatitis.***
Respiratory: dyspnea, upper respiratory tract infections.
Skin: *pruritus,* rash, urticaria, increased diaphoresis.
Other: ***anaphylaxis, angioedema.***

Interactions

Drug-drug. *Antacids:* may decrease plasma fenoprofen levels. Dosage adjustment may be necessary.
Aspirin: decreased fenoprofen bioavailability; may increase GI toxicity. Avoid concomitant use.
Corticosteroids: increased risk of adverse GI reactions. Avoid concomitant use.
Diuretics: decreased diuretic effectiveness. Monitor patient closely.
Oral anticoagulants, sulfonylureas: fenoprofen enhances pharmacologic effects of these drugs. Use together cautiously.
Phenobarbital: enhanced fenoprofen metabolism. Monitor patient for lack of fenoprofen effectiveness.
Drug-herb. *Dong quai, feverfew, garlic, ginger, horse chestnut, red clover:* Possible increased risk of bleeding. Discourage concomitant use.
Drug-lifestyle. *Alcohol use:* increased risk of adverse GI reactions. Discourage concomitant use.
Sunlight: May cause photosensitivity. Urge precautions.

Contraindications and precautions

- Contraindicated in patients hypersensitive to drug, in pregnant women, and in patients with significantly impaired kidney function or a history of aspirin- or NSAID-induced asthma, rhinitis, or urticaria.
- Breast-feeding isn't recommended during drug therapy.
- Use cautiously in elderly patients and those with history of serious GI events or peptic ulcer disease, compromised cardiac function, or hypertension.
- Safety of drug hasn't been established in children.

NURSING CONSIDERATIONS

Assessment
- Assess patient's pain or inflammation before and after administration.
- Check renal, hepatic, ocular, and auditory function periodically during long-term therapy.
- Be alert for adverse reactions and drug interactions.
- Evaluate patient's and family's knowledge of drug therapy.

Nursing diagnoses
- Acute pain related to underlying condition
- Risk for injury related to drug-induced adverse reactions
- Deficient knowledge related to drug therapy

Planning and implementation
- Give drug on empty stomach unless adverse GI reactions occur.
- Notify prescriber about abnormalities in renal, hepatic, ocular, or auditory function because drug will need to be discontinued.
- Drug may cause false elevations in free and total serum T_3 levels as measured by Amerlex-T assay. Fenoprofen or its metabolite may cross-react with antibody used in Amerlex-M assay. Limited data suggest that drug may alter free and total T_3 levels determined by Corning method.

Patient teaching
- Tell patient to take drug 30 minutes before or 2 hours after meals. If adverse GI reactions occur, drug may be taken with milk or meals.
- Tell patient that full effect for arthritis may be delayed 2 to 4 weeks.
- Warn patient to avoid hazardous activities that require alertness until adverse CNS effects of drug are known.
- Teach patient signs and symptoms of GI bleeding, and tell him to contact prescriber immediately if they occur. Serious GI toxicity, including peptic ulceration and bleeding, can occur in patients taking NSAIDs despite absence of GI symptoms.

Evaluation
- Patient is free from pain.
- Patient has no injury from adverse reactions.
- Patient and family state understanding of drug therapy.

fentanyl citrate
(FEN-tuh-nihl SIGH-trayt)
Sublimaze

fentanyl transdermal system
Duragesic-25, Duragesic-50, Duragesic-75, Duragesic-100

fentanyl transmucosal
Actiq, Fentanyl Oralet

Pharmacologic class: opioid analgesic
Therapeutic class: analgesic, adjunct to anesthesia, anesthetic
Controlled substance schedule: II
Pregnancy risk category: C

Indications and dosages

▶ **Adjunct to general anesthetic.** *Adults:* for low-dose therapy, 2 mcg/kg I.V. For moderate-dose therapy, 2 to 20 mcg/kg I.V.; then 25 to 100 mcg I.V. or I.M., p.r.n. For high-dose therapy, 20 to 50 mcg/kg I.V.; then 25 mcg to one-half initial loading dose I.V. p.r.n.
Children ages 2 to 12: 2 to 3 mcg/kg I.V. or I.M. during induction and maintenance phases of general anesthesia.
▶ **Adjunct to regional anesthesia.** *Adults:* 50 to 100 mcg I.M. or slow I.V. over 1 to 2 minutes.
▶ **Postoperatively.** *Adults:* 50 to 100 mcg I.M. q 1 to 2 hours, p.r.n.
▶ **Preoperatively.** *Adults:* 50 to 100 mcg I.M. 30 to 60 minutes before surgery. Or, 5 mcg/kg dispensed as Oralet unit, 20 to 40 minutes before desired effects are needed.
Children age 2 or older weighing more than 15 kg (33 lb) and less than 40 kg (44 lb): 5 mcg/kg as an Oralet lozenge. May need a dose 10 to 15 mcg/kg transmucosally.
▶ **Management of chronic pain.** *Adults:* one transdermal system applied to upper torso on area of skin that isn't irritated and hasn't been irradiated. Therapy started with 25-mcg/hour

system; dosage adjusted as needed and tolerated. Each system may be worn 72 hours.
▶ **Breakthrough cancer pain in opioid-tolerant patients (Actiq).** *Adults:* 200 mcg P.O. initially, adjusted based on response. Each dose should be consumed over 15 minutes. An additional lozenge may be taken 30 minutes after start of the previous dose. Don't use more than 2 units per episode of breakthrough pain.

How supplied

Injection: 50 mcg/ml
Transdermal system: patches designed to release 25, 50, 75, or 100 mcg of fentanyl per hour
Transmucosal: 100 mcg, 200 mcg, 300 mcg, 400 mcg, 600 mcg, 800 mcg, 1,200 mcg, 1,600 mcg

Pharmacokinetics

Absorption: varies with transmucosal or transdermal use.
Distribution: distributes and accumulates to adipose tissue and skeletal muscle.
Metabolism: metabolized in liver.
Excretion: excreted in urine. *Half-life:* about 3½ hours after parenteral use, 5 to 15 hours after transmucosal use, 18 hours after transdermal use.

Route	Onset	Peak	Duration
I.V.	1-2 min	3-5 min	0.5-1 hr
I.M.	7-15 min	20-30 min	1-2 hr
Transmucosal	15 min	20-30 min	Unknown
Transdermal	12-24 hr	1-3 days	Varies

Pharmacodynamics

Chemical effect: unknown; binds with opioid receptors in CNS, altering both perception of and emotional response to pain.
Therapeutic effect: relieves pain.

Adverse reactions

CNS: *sedation, somnolence, clouded sensorium, euphoria,* dizziness, headache, *confusion, asthenia,* nervousness, hallucinations, anxiety, depression, ***seizures*** (with large doses).
CV: *hypotension,* hypertension, ***arrhythmias,*** chest pain, ***bradycardia.***
EENT: *dry mouth.*
GI: *nausea, vomiting, constipation,* ileus, abdominal pain.
GU: *urine retention.*
Respiratory: ***respiratory depression,*** hypoventilation, dyspnea, ***apnea.***
Skin: reaction at application site (erythema, papules, edema), *pruritus, diaphoresis.*
Other: physical dependence.

Interactions

Drug-drug. *CNS depressants, general anesthetics, hypnotics, MAO inhibitors, other narcotic analgesics, sedatives, tricyclic antidepressant:* additive effects. Use together with extreme caution. Fentanyl dose should be reduced by one-quarter to one-third. Also, give above drugs in reduced dosages.
Diazepam: CV depression when given with high doses of fentanyl. Monitor patient closely.
Droperidol: hypotension and decreased pulmonary arterial pressure. Monitor patient closely.
Drug-lifestyle. *Alcohol use:* additive effects. Discourage concomitant use.

Contraindications and precautions

• Contraindicated in patients intolerant of drug.
• Use cautiously in elderly or debilitated patients, pregnant or breast-feeding women, and patients with head injury, increased CSF pressure, COPD, decreased respiratory reserve, potentially compromised respirations, hepatic or renal disease, or bradyarrhythmias.
• Safety of drug hasn't been established in children under age 2.

NURSING CONSIDERATIONS

Assessment

• Assess patient's underlying condition before therapy.
• Evaluate degree of pain relief obtained after administration.
• Periodically monitor postoperative vital signs and bladder function. Because drug decreases both rate and depth of respirations,

monitoring of arterial oxygen saturation (SaO_2) may help assess respiratory depression.
• Monitor patient who develops adverse reactions to transdermal system for at least 12 hours after removal. Serum drug levels may take as long as 17 hours to decline by 50%.
• Be alert for adverse reactions and drug interactions.
• Evaluate patient's and family's knowledge of drug therapy.

Nursing diagnoses
• Acute pain related to underlying condition
• Ineffective breathing pattern related to respiratory depression
• Deficient knowledge related to drug therapy

Planning and implementation
• For better analgesic effect, give drug before patient has intense pain.
I.V. use: Only staff trained in giving I.V. anesthetics and managing their adverse effects should give I.V. fentanyl.
– Keep naloxone and resuscitation equipment available when giving drug I.V.
– Drug is commonly used I.V. with droperidol to produce neuroleptanalgesia.
I.M. use: Follow normal protocol.
Transmucosal form: Remove foil overwrap of fentanyl Oralet just before administration.
– Instruct patient to place fentanyl Oralet in mouth and suck (not chew) it.
– Remove fentanyl Oralet unit using handle after it has been consumed, patient shows adequate effect, or patient shows signs of respiratory depression. Place any remaining portion in plastic overwrap and dispose of accordingly for Schedule II drugs.
ALERT Ask patient and caregivers about the presence of children in the home. Actiq lozenges contain enough fentanyl citrate to be fatal to a child.
– Because high doses may cause hypoventilation, transmucosal doses shouldn't exceed 15 mcg/kg (maximum, 400 mcg) in children or 5 mcg/kg (maximum, 400 mcg) in adults.
Transdermal form: Transdermal fentanyl isn't recommended for postoperative pain.
– Dosage equivalency charts are available to calculate fentanyl transdermal dose based on daily morphine intake—for example, for every 90 mg of oral morphine or 15 mg of I.M. morphine per 24 hours, 25 mcg/hour of transdermal fentanyl is needed.
– Dosage adjustments in patient using transdermal system should be made gradually. Reaching steady-state levels of new dosage may take up to 6 days; delay dosage adjustment until after at least two applications.
– High doses can produce muscle rigidity, which can be reversed with neuromuscular blockers; however, patient must be ventilated artificially.
– Immediately report respiratory rate below 12 breaths/minute or decreased respiratory volume or SaO_2.
– When drug is used postoperatively, encourage patient to turn, cough, and deep breathe to prevent atelectasis.
– Most patients have good control of pain for 3 days while wearing transdermal system, but a few may need new application after 48 hours. Because serum fentanyl level rises for first 24 hours after application, analgesic effect can't be evaluated for first day. Make sure patient has adequate supplemental analgesic to prevent breakthrough pain.
– When reducing opioid therapy or switching to different analgesic, transdermal system should be withdrawn gradually. Because fentanyl serum level drops gradually after removal, give half of equianalgesic dose of new analgesic 12 to 18 hours after removal as ordered.

Patient teaching
• Teach patient proper application of transdermal patch. Instruct patient to clip hair at application site, but to avoid razor, which may irritate skin. Tell him to wash area with clear water if necessary, but not with soaps, oils, lotions, alcohol, or other substances that may irritate skin or prevent adhesion. Urge him to dry area completely before application.
• Tell patient to remove transdermal system from package just before applying, to hold in place for 10 to 20 seconds, and to be sure edges of patch adhere to the skin.
• Teach patient to dispose of transdermal patch by folding so adhesive side adheres to itself and then flushing it down toilet.

• If patient needs another patch after 72 hours, tell him to apply it to new site.
• Inform patient that heat from fever or environment may increase transdermal delivery and cause toxicity, which requires dosage adjustment. Instruct patient to notify prescriber if fever occurs or if patient will be spending time in hot climate.
ALERT Strongly warn patient to keep drug safely secured away from children.

Evaluation
• Patient is free from pain.
• Patient maintains adequate ventilation throughout drug therapy.
• Patient and family state understanding of drug therapy.

ferrous fumarate
(FEH-rus FYOO-muh-rayt)
Femiron†, Feostat†, Feostat Drops†, Fumasorb†, Fumerin†, Hemocyte†, Ircon†, Neo-Fer♦†, Nephro-Fer†, (OTC) Novofumar♦,(OTC) Palafer♦, Palafer Pediatric Drops♦, Span-FF†

ferrous gluconate
Fergon†, Fertinic♦, Novoferrogluc♦

ferrous sulfate
Apo-Ferrous Sulfate♦, Feosol*†, Fer-gen-sol†, Fer-In-Sol*†, Fer-Iron Drops†, Fero-Grad♦, Fero-Gradumet†, Ferospace†

ferrous sulfate, dried
Feosol, Ferralyn, Mol-Iron†, Slow-Fe†

Pharmacologic class: oral iron supplement
Therapeutic class: hematinic
Pregnancy risk category: A

Indications and dosages
▶ **Iron deficiency (Fumarate).** *Adults:* 50 to 100 mg elemental iron P.O. t.i.d.
Children: 4 to 6 mg/kg P.O. daily, divided into three doses.
▶ **Iron deficiency (Gluconate).** *Adults:* 325 mg P.O. q.i.d., increased to 650 mg q.i.d. as needed and tolerated.
Children age 2 and older: 3 mg/kg/day P.O. in three to four divided doses.
▶ **Iron deficiency (Sulfate).** *Adults:* 300 mg P.O. b.i.d. to q.i.d. Or, 1 extended-release capsule (160 to 525 mg) P.O. daily to b.i.d.
Children age 2 and older: 3 mg/kg/day P.O. in three or four divided doses.

How supplied
ferrous fumarate
(Each 100 mg provides 33 mg of elemental iron.)
Tablets†: 60 mg, 195 mg, 200 mg, 300 mg, 324 mg, 325 mg, 350 mg
Tablets (chewable): 100 mg†
Capsules (extended-release): 325 mg†
Oral suspension: 100 mg/5 ml†
Drops: 45 mg/0.6 ml†
ferrous gluconate
(Each 100 mg provides 11.6 mg of elemental iron.)
Tablets: 240 mg†, 300 mg†, 320 mg† (contains 37 mg Fe+), 325 mg†
Extended-release tablets: 320 mg†
Capsules: 86 mg†
Elixir: 300 mg/5 ml (contains 35 mg Fe+)*†
ferrous sulfate
(About 20% elemental iron; dried and powdered, it's about 32% elemental iron.)
Tablets: 195 mg†, 300 mg†, 325 mg†; 200 mg (dried)
Tablets (extended-release): 160 mg (dried)†
Capsules: 150 mg†, 159 mg (dried), 190 mg (dried), 250 mg†, 390 mg†
Capsules (extended-release): 150 mg (dried), 159 mg (dried)†, 160 mg (dried), 250 mg (dried), 525 mg†
Elixir: 220 mg/5 ml*†
Syrup: 90 mg/5 ml*†
Solution: 75 mg/0.6 ml
Drops: 75 mg/0.6 ml, 125 mg/ml

Pharmacokinetics
Absorption: absorbed from entire length of GI tract, but primary absorption sites are duodenum and proximal jejunum. Up to 10% of iron absorbed by healthy people; patients with iron-deficiency anemia may absorb up to 60%. Enteric coating and some extended-release formulas have decreased absorption because they're designed to release iron past points of

highest GI absorption. Food may decrease absorption by 33% to 50%.
Distribution: iron is transported through GI mucosal cells directly into blood, where it's bound immediately to carrier protein, transferrin, and transported to bone marrow for incorporation into hemoglobin. Iron is highly protein-bound.
Metabolism: iron is liberated by destruction of hemoglobin, but is conserved and reused by body.
Excretion: healthy people lose only small amounts of iron each day. Men and postmenopausal women lose about 1 mg/day, and premenopausal women about 1.5 mg/day. The loss usually occurs in nails, hair, feces, and urine; trace amounts are lost in bile and sweat.

Route	Onset	Peak	Duration
P.O.	≤ 4 days	7-10 days	2-4 mo

Pharmacodynamics

Chemical effect: provides elemental iron, an essential component in formation of hemoglobin.
Therapeutic effect: relieves iron deficiency.

Adverse reactions

GI: *nausea, epigastric pain, vomiting, constipation,* diarrhea, black stools, anorexia.
Other: suspension and drops may temporarily stain teeth.

Interactions

Drug-drug. *Antacids, cholestyramine resin, fluoroquinolones, levodopa, penicillamine, tetracycline, vitamin E:* decreased iron absorption. Separate doses by 2 to 4 hours.
Chloramphenicol: Increased iron response. Watch patient carefully.
Fluoroquinolones, penicillamine, tetracyclines: Decreased GI absorption, possibly resulting in decreased serum levels or efficacy. Separate doses by 2 to 4 hours.
L-thyroxine: decreased L-thyroxine absorption. Separate doses by at least 2 hours. Monitor thyroid function.
Levodopa, methyldopa: decreased absorption and efficacy of levodopa and methyldopa. Monitor patient for decreased effects of these drugs.
Vitamin C: may increase iron absorption. Beneficial drug interaction.
Drug-food. *Yogurt, cheese, eggs, milk, whole-grain breads, cereals, tea, coffee:* may impair oral iron absorption. Don't administer together.

Contraindications and precautions

- Contraindicated in patients with primary hemochromatosis, hemosiderosis, hemolytic anemia (unless iron deficiency anemia is also present), peptic ulcer disease, regional enteritis, or ulcerative colitis, and in those receiving repeated blood transfusions.
- Use cautiously on long-term basis.

NURSING CONSIDERATIONS

Assessment

- Obtain baseline assessment of patient's iron deficiency before therapy.
- Evaluate hemoglobin and hematocrit levels and reticulocyte counts during therapy, as ordered.
- Be alert for adverse reactions and drug interactions.
- Evaluate patient's and family's knowledge of drug therapy.

Nursing diagnoses

- Fatigue related to iron deficiency
- Constipation related to adverse effect of drug therapy on GI tract
- Deficient knowledge related to drug therapy

Planning and implementation

- Give tablets with juice or water, but not with milk or antacids.
- Dilute liquid forms in juice or water, but not in milk or antacids.
- To avoid staining teeth, give suspension or elixir with straw and place drops at back of throat.
- Don't crush or allow patient to chew extended-release forms.
- GI upset may be related to dose. Between-meal dosing is preferable, but iron can be given with some foods, although absorption may be decreased. Enteric-coated products reduce GI upset but also reduce amount of iron absorbed.

• Oral iron may turn stools black. Although this unabsorbed iron is harmless, it could mask presence of melena.

Patient teaching

ALERT Inform parents that as few as three or four tablets can cause poisoning in children.
• If patient misses dose, tell him to take it as soon as he remembers but not to double-dose.
• Advise patient to avoid certain foods that may impair oral iron absorption, including yogurt, cheese, eggs, milk, whole-grain breads and cereals, tea, and coffee.
• Teach dietary measures for preventing constipation.

Evaluation

• Patient reports fatigue is no longer a problem in daily life.
• Patient states appropriate measures to prevent or relieve constipation.
• Patient and family state understanding of drug therapy.

fexofenadine hydrochloride

(feks-oh-FEN-uh-deen high-droh-KLOR-ighd)
Allegra, Telfast◇

Pharmacologic class: H_1-receptor antagonist
Therapeutic class: antihistamine
Pregnancy risk category: C

Indications and dosagess

▶ **Seasonal allergic rhinitis.** *Adults and children age 12 and older:* 60 mg P.O. b.i.d.
Children ages 6 to 11: 30 mg P.O. b.i.d.
▶ **Chronic idiopathic urticaria.** *Children age 12 and older:* 60 mg P.O. b.i.d.
Children ages 6 to 11: 30 mg P.O. b.i.d.

How supplied

Capsules: 60 mg, 180 mg

Pharmacokinetics

Absorption: drug is rapidly absorbed.
Distribution: plasma protein–binding is 60% to 70%.
Metabolism: not reported.
Excretion: about 80% in feces and 11% in urine. *Half-life:* 14.4 hours.

Route	Onset	Peak	Duration
P.O.	Unknown	3 hr	14 hr

Pharmacodynamics

Chemical effect: principal effects are mediated through a selective inhibition of peripheral H_1-receptors.
Therapeutic effect: relieves symptoms of seasonal allergies.

Adverse reactions

CNS: fatigue, drowsiness.
GI: nausea, dyspepsia.
GU: dysmenorrhea.
Other: viral infection.

Interactions

Drug-drug. *Erythromycin, ketoconazole:* increased fenofenadine levels. Prolonged QT interval has been seen with other antihistamines. Monitor patient closely.

Contraindications and precautions

• Contraindicated in patients hypersensitive to drug or its components.
• Use cautiously in patients with impaired renal function.
• Safety and effectiveness in children under age 6 haven't been established.
• No data exist to demonstrate whether drug appears in breast milk; use caution when giving drug to breast-feeding women.

NURSING CONSIDERATIONS

Assessment

• Assess patient's seasonal allergy symptoms before therapy and thereafter.
• Monitor for adverse reactions.
• Evaluate patient's and family's knowledge of drug therapy.

Nursing diagnoses

• Risk for injury related to fatigue and drowsiness associated with drug
• Ineffective health maintenance related to underlying condition
• Deficient knowledge related to drug therapy

Planning and implementation

- Patient with impaired renal function or currently on dialysis should receive a reduced daily dosage.

Patient teaching

- Advise woman taking drug to avoid breast-feeding.
- Caution patient not to perform hazardous activities if drowsiness occurs as a result of drug use.
- Instruct patient not to exceed prescribed dosage and to take drug only during seasonal allergy symptoms.
- Warn patient to avoid alcohol and hazardous activities that require alertness until CNS effects of drug are known.
- Tell patient that coffee or tea may reduce drowsiness. Suggest sugarless gum, sugarless sour hard candy, or ice chips to relieve dry mouth.

Evaluation

- Patient experiences limited fatigue and drowsiness associated with drug.
- Patient responds well to the drug.
- Patient and family state understanding of drug therapy.

filgrastim (granulocyte colony-stimulating factor; G-CSF)

(fil-GRAH-stem)

Neupogen

Pharmacologic class: biologic response modifier
Therapeutic class: colony-stimulating factor
Pregnancy risk category: C

Indications and dosages

▶ **To decrease risk of infection in patients with nonmyeloid cancers receiving myelosuppressive antineoplastics.** *Adults and children:* 5 mcg/kg/day I.V. or S.C. as single dose. May be increased in increments of 5 mcg/kg for each chemotherapy cycle, depending on duration and severity of nadir of absolute neutrophil count (ANC).

▶ **To decrease risk of infection in patients with nonmyeloid cancers receiving myelosuppressive antineoplastics followed by bone marrow transplant.** *Adults and children:* 10 mcg/kg/day I.V. or S.C. at least 24 hours after cytotoxic chemotherapy and bone marrow infusion. Subsequent dosages adjusted according to neutrophil response.

▶ **Congenital neutropenia.** *Adults:* 6 mcg/kg S.C. b.i.d. Dosage adjusted according to patient's response.

▶ **Idiopathic or cyclic neutropenia.** *Adults:* 5 mcg/kg S.C. daily. Dosage adjusted based on response.

▶ **Peripherial blood progenitor cell collection:** *Adults:* 10 mcg/kg/day S.C. for at least 4 days before first leukapheresis and continuing until the last leukapheresis is completed.

How supplied

Injection: 300 mcg/ml

Pharmacokinetics

Absorption: rapid absorption after S.C. administration.
Distribution: unknown.
Metabolism: unknown.
Excretion: unknown. *Half-life:* about 3½ hours.

Route	Onset	Peak	Duration
I.V.	5-60 min	24 hr	1-7 days
S.C.	5-60 min	2-8 hr	1-7 days

Pharmacodynamics

Chemical effect: glycoprotein that stimulates proliferation and differentiation of hematopoietic cells. Drug is specific for neutrophils.
Therapeutic effect: raises WBC levels.

Adverse reactions

CNS: *fatigue*, headache, weakness.
CV: ***MI, arrhythmias,*** chest pain.
GI: *nausea, vomiting, diarrhea, mucositis*, stomatitis, constipation.
GU: hematuria, proteinuria.
Hematologic: ***thrombocytopenia,*** leukocytosis.
Musculoskeletal: *skeletal pain.*
Respiratory: dyspnea, cough.
Skin: *alopecia*, rash, cutaneous vasculitis.

Other: *fever, **hypersensitivity reactions.***

Interactions

Drug-drug. *Chemotherapy drugs:* rapidly dividing myeloid cells are sensitive to cytotoxic drugs. Don't use filgrastim within 24 hours before or after a chemotherapy dose.

Contraindications and precautions

- Contraindicated in patients hypersensitive to proteins derived from *Escherichia coli* or to drug or its components.
- Use cautiously in pregnant or breast-feeding women.

NURSING CONSIDERATIONS

Assessment

- Assess patient's underlying condition before therapy.
- Obtain baseline CBC and platelet counts before therapy, as ordered.
- Evaluate CBC and platelet count during therapy, as ordered.
- Be alert for adverse reactions and drug interactions.
- Ask patient about skeletal pain.
- Evaluate patient's and family's knowledge of drug therapy.

Nursing diagnoses

- Ineffective protection related to underlying condition or treatment
- Acute pain related to adverse drug effects on skeletal muscle
- Deficient knowledge related to drug therapy

Planning and implementation

I.V. use: Dilute in 50 to 100 ml of D_5W, and give by intermittent infusion over 15 to 60 minutes or continuous infusion over 24 hours. If final concentration will be 2 to 15 mcg/ml, add albumin at 2 mg/ml (0.2%) to minimize binding of drug to plastic containers or tubing.
S.C. use: Follow normal protocol.

- Don't give drug within 24 hours of cytotoxic chemotherapy.
- Once dose is withdrawn, don't reenter vial. Discard unused portion. Vials are for single-dose use and contain no preservatives.
- Give daily for up to 2 weeks or until ANC has returned to 10,000/mm³ after expected chemotherapy-induced neutrophil nadir, as ordered.
- Refrigerate drug at 36° to 46° F (2° to 8° C). Don't freeze; avoid shaking. Store at room temperature for maximum of 6 hours; discard after 6 hours.

Patient teaching

- Teach patient how to give drug and how to dispose of used needles, syringes, drug containers, and unused drug.
- Tell patient to report bruising or spontaneous bleeding, such as frequent nosebleeds.
- Teach patient how to manage skeletal pain.

Evaluation

- Patient's WBC count is normal.
- Patient reports skeletal pain is bearable or relieved with analgesic administration and comfort measures.
- Patient and family state understanding of drug therapy.

finasteride

(fin-ES-teh-righd)

Proscar, Propecia

Pharmacologic class: steroid (synthetic 4-azasteroid) derivative
Therapeutic class: androgen synthesis inhibitor
Pregnancy risk category: X

Indications and dosages

▶ **Symptomatic BPH; reduction of risk for acute urinary retention and need for surgery, including prostatectomy and transurethral resection of prostate (Proscar).** *Adults:* 5 mg P.O. daily

▶ **Male pattern baldness (Propecia).** *Adult men only:* 1 mg P.O. daily.

How supplied

Tablets: 1 mg, 5 mg

Pharmacokinetics

Absorption: not clearly defined, although average bioavailability was 63% in one study.
Distribution: about 90% bound to plasma proteins; crosses blood-brain barrier.
Metabolism: extensively metabolized by liver.
Excretion: 39% of dose is excreted in urine as metabolites; 57% in feces.

Route	Onset	Peak	Duration
P.O.	Unknown	1-2 hr	About 2 wk

Pharmacodynamics

Chemical effect: competitively inhibits steroid 5-reductase, an enzyme responsible for formation of potent androgen 5-dihydrotestosterone (DHT) from testosterone. Because DHT influences development of prostate gland, decreasing levels of this hormone in adult men should relieve symptoms of BPH. In men with male pattern baldness, the balding scalp contains miniaturized hair follicles and increased amounts of DHT. Finasteride decreases scalp and serum DHT concentrations in these men.
Therapeutic effect: relieves symptoms of BPH, reduces hair loss, and promotes hair growth.

Adverse reactions

GU: impotence, decreased volume of ejaculate.
Other: decreased libido.

Interactions

None significant.

Contraindications and precautions

- Contraindicated in patients hypersensitive to drug.
- Drug isn't indicated for use in women or children.

NURSING CONSIDERATIONS

Assessment

- Before therapy, assess patient's BPH, and evaluate him for conditions that could mimic BPH, including hypotonic bladder; prostate cancer, infection, or stricture; or relevant neurologic conditions. Carefully monitor patients with large residual urine volume or severely diminished urine flow. These patients may not be candidates for finasteride therapy.
- Evaluate patient for improvement in BPH symptoms.
- Anticipate periodic digital rectal examinations.
- Be alert for adverse reactions and drug interactions.
- Carefully evaluate sustained increases in serum prostate-specific antigen levels, which could indicate noncompliance.
- Evaluate patient's and family's knowledge of drug therapy.

Nursing diagnoses

- Impaired urinary elimination related to BPH
- Ineffective sexuality patterns related to drug-induced impotence
- Deficient knowledge related to drug therapy

Planning and implementation

- Because it's impossible to identify which patients will respond to finasteride, keep in mind that a minimum of 6 months of therapy may be necessary.

Patient teaching

- Warn woman who is or may become pregnant not to handle crushed or broken tablets because of risk of adverse effects on male fetus.
- Caution man whose sexual partner is or may become pregnant to stop drug or to take precautions to avoid exposing her to his semen.
- Reassure patient that although drug may decrease volume of ejaculate, it doesn't appear to impair normal sexual function. Impotence and decreased libido have occurred in less than 4% of patients.
- Tell patient taking drug for male pattern baldness that he may not notice any effects for 3 months or more.

Evaluation

- Patient's BPH symptoms diminish.
- Patient states appropriate ways to manage sexual dysfunction.
- Patient and family state understanding of drug therapy.

flavoxate hydrochloride
(flah-VOKS-ayt high-droh-KLOR-ighd)
Urispas

Pharmacologic class: flavone derivative
Therapeutic class: urinary tract spasmolytic
Pregnancy risk category: B

Indications and dosages

▶ **Symptomatic relief of dysuria, urinary frequency and urgency, nocturia, incontinence, and suprapubic pain from urologic disorders.** *Adults and children over age 12:* 100 to 200 mg P.O. t.i.d. or q.i.d.

How supplied

Tablets: 100 mg

Pharmacokinetics

Absorption: absorbed well from GI tract.
Distribution: unknown.
Metabolism: unknown.
Excretion: excreted in urine.

Route	Onset	Peak	Duration
P.O.	Unknown	≤ 2 hr	Unknown

Pharmacodynamics

Chemical effect: produces direct spasmolytic effect on smooth muscles of urinary tract and provides some local anesthesia and analgesia.
Therapeutic effect: relieves urinary tract symptoms.

Adverse reactions

CNS: *confusion* (especially in elderly patients), nervousness, dizziness, headache, drowsiness.
CV: tachycardia, palpitations.
EENT: *blurred vision,* disturbed eye accommodation, increased ocular tension.
GI: dry mouth, nausea, vomiting.
GU: dysuria.
Hematologic: eosinophilia, ***leukopenia.***
Skin: urticaria, dermatoses.
Other: fever.

Interactions

Drug-lifestyle. *Exercise, hot weather:* may precipitate heat stroke. Urge precautions to avoid becoming overheated.

Contraindications and precautions

- Contraindicated in patients with pyloric or duodenal obstruction, obstructive intestinal lesions or ileus, achalasia, GI hemorrhage, or obstructive uropathies of lower urinary tract.
- Use cautiously in patients suspected of having glaucoma and in pregnant or breast-feeding women.
- Safety of drug hasn't been established in children age 12 and younger.

NURSING CONSIDERATIONS

Assessment

- Assess patient's urinary function before therapy, and reassess regularly thereafter.
- Check history for other drug use before giving drugs with adverse anticholinergic reactions. Such reactions may be intensified by flavoxate.
- Be alert for adverse reactions.
- Evaluate patient's and family's knowledge of drug therapy.

Nursing diagnoses

- Impaired urinary elimination related to underlying GU disorder
- Risk for injury related to drug-induced adverse reactions
- Deficient knowledge related to drug therapy

Planning and implementation

- Dosage may be reduced if symptoms improve.

Patient teaching

- Warn patient to avoid hazardous activities until CNS effects of drug are known.
- Tell patient to notify prescriber of adverse reactions or persistent symptoms.

Evaluation

- Patient regains normal urinary elimination pattern.
- Patient sustains no injury from adverse reactions.

• Patient and family state understanding of drug therapy.

flecainide acetate
(FLEH-kay-nighd AS-ih-tayt)
Tambocor

Pharmacologic class: benzamide derivative
Therapeutic class: antiarrhythmic
Pregnancy risk category: C

Indications and dosages

▶ **Paroxysmal supraventricular tachycardia; paroxysmal atrial fibrillation or flutter in patients without structural heart disease; life-threatening ventricular arrhythmias, such as sustained ventricular tachycardia.**
Adults: for paroxysmal supraventricular tachycardia, 50 mg P.O. q 12 hours. Increased in increments of 50 mg b.i.d. q 4 days until efficacy is achieved. Maximum, 300 mg daily. In patients with renal impairment (creatinine clearance 35 ml/minute), initial dosage is 100 mg once daily or 50 mg b.i.d. For life-threatening ventricular arrhythmias, 100 mg P.O. q 12 hours. Increase in increments of 50 mg b.i.d. q 4 days until efficacy is achieved. Maximum, 400 mg daily for most patients. Initial dosage for patients with renal failure is 50 mg P.O. q 12 hours. Where available, flecainide may be given to adults by I.V. injection: 2 mg/kg I.V. push over at least 10 minutes; or dilute dose and give as infusion.

How supplied

Tablets: 50 mg, 100 mg, 150 mg
Injection: 10 mg/ml ◊

Pharmacokinetics

Absorption: rapidly and almost completely absorbed from GI tract; bioavailability is 85% to 90%.
Distribution: thought to be well distributed throughout body. Only about 40% binds to plasma proteins.
Metabolism: metabolized in liver to inactive metabolites. About 30% of oral dose escapes metabolism.
Excretion: excreted in urine. *Half-life:* about 20 hours.

Route	Onset	Peak	Duration
P.O.	Unknown	2-3 hr	Unknown
I.V.	Immediate	Immediate	Unknown

Pharmacodynamics

Chemical effect: decreases excitability, conduction velocity, and automaticity as result of slowed atrial, AV node, His-Purkinje system, and intraventricular conduction and causes slight but significant prolongation of refractory periods in these tissues.
Therapeutic effect: restores normal sinus rhythm.

Adverse reactions

CNS: *dizziness, headache,* fatigue, tremor, anxiety, insomnia, depression, malaise, paresthesia, ataxia, vertigo, *light-headedness, syncope*, asthenia.
CV: edema, ***new or worsened arrhythmias,*** chest pain, ***heart failure, cardiac arrest,*** palpitations.
EENT: *blurred vision and other visual disturbances.*
GI: nausea, constipation, abdominal pain, dyspepsia, vomiting, diarrhea, anorexia.
Respiratory: *dyspnea.*
Skin: rash.
Other: flushing, fever.

Interactions

Drug-drug. *Amiodarone, cimetidine:* altered pharmacokinetics. Watch for toxicity.
Cardiac glycosides: may increase plasma digoxin levels by 15% to 25%. Monitor serum digoxin levels and watch for evidence of toxicity.
Disopyramide, verapamil: negative inotropic properties may be additive with flecainide; avoid concurrent administration.
Propranolol, other beta blockers: both flecainide and propranolol plasma levels increase by 20% to 30%. Monitor patient for propranolol and flecainide toxicity.
Urine acidifying and alkalinizing agents: extremes of urine pH may substantially alter excretion of flecainide. Monitor for flecainide toxicity or decreased effectiveness.

Drug-lifestyle. *Smoking:* lowered flecainide levels. Discourage smoking.

Contraindications and precautions

- Contraindicated in patients hypersensitive to drug and in those with cardiogenic shock or second- or third-degree AV block or right bundle branch block related to left hemiblock (in absence of artificial pacemaker).
- Breast-feeding isn't recommended during drug use.
- Use cautiously in patients with heart failure, cardiomyopathy, severe renal or hepatic disease, prolonged QT interval, sick sinus syndrome, or blood dyscrasia. Also use cautiously in pregnant women.
- Safety of drug hasn't been established in children.

NURSING CONSIDERATIONS

Assessment

- Obtain assessment of patient's arrhythmia before therapy.
- Monitor effectiveness by continuous ECG monitoring initially; long-term oral administration requires regular ECG readings.
- Monitor serum flecainide levels, especially in patient with renal failure or heart failure. Therapeutic levels range from 0.2 to 1 mcg/ml. Incidence of adverse effects increases when trough blood levels exceed 1 mcg/ml.
- Monitor serum potassium levels regularly.
- Be alert for adverse reactions and drug interactions.
- Evaluate patient's and family's knowledge of drug therapy.

Nursing diagnoses

- Decreased cardiac output related to underlying arrhythmia
- Ineffective protection related to drug-induced new arrhythmias
- Deficient knowledge related to drug therapy

Planning and implementation

- When used to prevent ventricular arrhythmias, flecainide should be reserved for patient with documented life-threatening arrhythmias.
- If patient has pacemaker, check that pacing threshold was determined 1 week before and after starting therapy because flecainide can alter endocardial pacing thresholds.
- Correct hypokalemia or hyperkalemia as ordered before giving flecainide because these electrolyte disturbances may alter flecainide effect.

P.O. use: Follow normal protocol.

I.V. use: When administering by I.V. push, give over at least 10 minutes. For I.V. infusion, mix only with D_5W.

- Dosage adjustments should be made only once every 3 to 4 days.
- Twice-daily dosing for flecainide enhances patient compliance.
- Because of flecainide's long half-life, its full effect may take 3 to 5 days. Give concomitant I.V. lidocaine as ordered for first several days.
- Keep emergency equipment nearby.
- If ECG disturbances occur, withhold drug, obtain rhythm strip, and notify prescriber immediately.

Patient teaching

- Stress importance of taking oral drug exactly as prescribed.
- Warn patient to avoid hazardous activities that require alertness or good vision if adverse CNS or visual reactions occur.
- Tell patient to limit fluid and sodium intake to minimize heart failure or fluid retention and to weigh himself daily. Urge him to report sudden weight gain promptly.

Evaluation

- Patient regains normal cardiac output with abolishment of underlying arrhythmia after drug therapy.
- Patient does not develop new arrhythmias.
- Patient and family state understanding of drug therapy.

floxuridine

(floks-YOOR-eh-deen)

FUDR

Pharmacologic class: antimetabolite (cell cycle–phase specific, S phase)
Therapeutic class: antineoplastic
Pregnancy risk category: D

Indications and dosages

▶ **GI adenocarcinoma metastatic to liver.** *Adults:* 0.1 to 0.6 mg/kg daily by intra-arterial infusion for 14 to 21 days or until toxicity occurs; or 0.4 to 0.6 mg/kg daily into hepatic artery.

How supplied

Injection: 500-mg vials

Pharmacokinetics

Absorption: not applicable.
Distribution: drug crosses blood-brain barrier to limited extent.
Metabolism: metabolized to fluorouracil in liver.
Excretion: about 60% excreted through lungs as carbon dioxide; small amount excreted by kidneys as unchanged drug and metabolites.

Route	Onset	Peak	Duration
Intra-arterial	Unknown	Unknown	Unknown

Pharmacodynamics

Chemical effect: inhibits DNA synthesis.
Therapeutic effect: hinders growth of GI adenocarcinoma cells that have spread to liver.

Adverse reactions

CNS: malaise, weakness, headache, lethargy, disorientation, confusion, euphoria.
CV: ***myocardial ischemia,*** angina, thrombophlebitis.
EENT: blurred vision, nystagmus, photophobia, epistaxis.
GI: *anorexia, stomatitis, abdominal pain, nausea, vomiting, diarrhea, bleeding, enteritis,* GI ulceration, intrahepatic and extrahepatic biliary sclerosis, acalculous cholecystitis.
Hematologic: ***leukopenia, anemia, thrombocytopenia, agranulocytosis.***
Skin: *erythema,* dermatitis, pruritus, rash, *alopecia,* photosensitivity.
Other: ***anaphylaxis,*** fever.

Interactions

Drug-lifestyle. *Sun exposure:* may increase skin reaction. Urge precautions.

Contraindications and precautions

- Contraindicated in patients with poor nutritional status, bone marrow suppression, or serious infection.
- Drug isn't recommended for pregnant or breast-feeding women.
- Give cautiously after high-dose pelvic radiation therapy or use of alkylating agents and in patients with impaired hepatic or renal function.
- Safety of drug hasn't been established in children.

NURSING CONSIDERATIONS

Assessment

- Assess patient's neoplastic disorder before therapy, and reassess regularly throughout therapy.
- Monitor fluid intake and output, CBC, and renal and hepatic function.
- Be alert for adverse reactions.
- Evaluate patient's and family's knowledge of drug therapy.

Nursing diagnoses

- Ineffective health maintenance related to drug therapy
- Ineffective protection related to immunosuppression
- Deficient knowledge related to drug therapy

Planning and implementation

- Follow facility policy to reduce risks. Preparation and administration of parenteral form create carcinogenic, mutagenic, and teratogenic risks for staff.
- Reconstitute with sterile water for injection. To prepare infusion, dilute in D_5W or normal saline solution.
- Use infusion pump with intra-arterial infusions.
- Check line for bleeding, blockage, displacement, or leakage.
- Refrigerated solution is stable for no more than 2 weeks.
- Use of antacid eases but won't prevent GI distress.
- Notify prescriber immediately about severe adverse skin and GI reactions.

• Discontinue drug and notify prescriber if WBC count falls below 3,500/mm³ or if platelet count falls below 100,000/mm³.

Patient teaching
• Warn patient to watch for signs of infection and bleeding. Teach infection-control and bleeding precautions.
• Advise woman of childbearing age to avoid becoming pregnant during therapy and to consult with prescriber before becoming pregnant.
• Instruct patient to notify prescriber if adverse reactions occur.

Evaluation
• Patient shows positive response to drug therapy.
• Patient develops no infection or bleeding complications.
• Patient and family state understanding of drug therapy.

fluconazole
(floo-KON-uh-zohl)
Diflucan

Pharmacologic class: bis-triazole derivative
Therapeutic class: antifungal
Pregnancy risk category: C

Indications and dosages

▶ **Oropharyngeal and esophageal candidiasis.** *Adults:* 200 mg P.O. or I.V. on first day, followed by 100 mg once daily. Higher doses (up to 400 mg daily) have been used for esophageal disease. Treatment should continue for 2 weeks after symptoms resolve.
Children: 6 mg/kg P.O. or I.V. on first day, followed by 3 mg/kg once daily for at least 2 weeks.
▶ **Vulvovaginal candidiasis.** *Adults:* 150 mg P.O. as a single dose.
▶ **Systemic candidiasis.** *Adults:* 400 mg P.O. or I.V. on first day, followed by 200 mg once daily. Treatment should continue at least 4 weeks or for 2 weeks after symptoms resolve.
Children: 6 to 12 mg/kg/day P.O. or I.V.
▶ **Cryptococcal meningitis.** *Adults:* 400 mg P.O. or I.V. on first day, followed by 200 mg once daily. Higher doses (up to 400 mg daily) may be used. Treatment should continue for 10 to 12 weeks after CSF cultures are negative.
Children: 12 mg/kg/day P.O. or I.V. on first day, followed by 6 mg/kg/daily for 10 to 12 weeks after CSF culture becomes negative.
▶ **Prevention of candidiasis in bone marrow transplant.** *Adults:* 400 mg. P.O. or I.V. once daily. Start prophylaxis several days before anticipated granulocytopenia. Continue therapy for 7 days after neutrophil count rises above 1,000 cells/mm³.
▶ **Suppression of relapse of cryptococcal meningitis in patients with AIDS.** *Adults:* 200 mg P.O. or I.V. daily.
Children: 3 to 6 mg/kg/day P.O.
Patients with renal failure: if creatinine clearance is below 50 ml/minute, dosage is reduced by 50% in patients not receiving dialysis. Patients receiving hemodialysis should receive 100% of usual dose after each session.

How supplied

Tablets: 50 mg, 100 mg, 150 mg, 200 mg
Powder for oral suspension: 10 mg/ml, 40 mg/ml
Injection: 200 mg/100 ml, 400 mg/200 ml

Pharmacokinetics

Absorption: rapid and complete after P.O. administration.
Distribution: well distributed to various sites, including CNS, saliva, sputum, blister fluid, urine, normal skin, nails, and blister skin. Drug is 12% protein-bound.
Metabolism: partially metabolized.
Excretion: primarily excreted by kidneys; over 80% excreted unchanged in urine.

Route	Onset	Peak	Duration
P.O.	Unknown	1-2 hr	Unknown
I.V.	Immediate	Immediate	Unknown

Pharmacodynamics

Chemical effect: inhibits fungal cytochrome P-450, an enzyme responsible for fungal sterol synthesis, and weakens fungal cell walls.
Therapeutic effect: hinders fungal growth. Spectrum of activity includes *Cryptococcus*

neoformans, Candida species (including systemic *C. albicans*), *Aspergillus flavus, Aspergillus fumigatus, Coccidioides immitis,* and *Histoplasma capsulatum.*

Adverse reactions

CNS: headache.
GI: *nausea,* vomiting, abdominal pain, diarrhea.
Hepatic: ***hepatotoxicity***, elevated liver enzyme levels.
Skin: rash, ***Stevens-Johnson syndrome.***
Other: ***anaphylaxis.***

Interactions

Drug-drug. *Cyclosporine, phenytoin:* may increase plasma levels of these drugs. Monitor serum cyclosporine or phenytoin levels.
Isoniazid, phenytoin, rifampin, valproic acid, oral sulfonylureas: increased risk of elevated hepatic transaminases. Monitor patient and serum levels closely.
Oral antidiabetics (tolbutamide, glyburide, glipizide): may increase plasma levels of these drugs. Monitor patient for enhanced hypoglycemic effect.
Rifampin: enhanced fluconazole metabolism. Monitor patient for lack of response.
Theophylline: decreased theophylline clearance. Monitor serum levels.
Warfarin: increased risk of bleeding. Monitor PT and INR.
Zidovudine: zidovudine activity may be increased. Monitor patient closely.
Drug-lifestyle. *Alcohol use:* May increase risk of hepatotoxicity. Discourage concurrent use.

Contraindications and precautions

- Contraindicated in patients hypersensitive to drug.
- Drug isn't recommended for breast-feeding women.
- Although no information exists regarding cross-sensitivity, use cautiously in patients hypersensitive to other antifungal azole compounds. Also, use cautiously in pregnant women.

NURSING CONSIDERATIONS

Assessment

- Assess patient's fungal infection before therapy, and reassess regularly throughout therapy.
- Periodically monitor liver function during prolonged therapy, as ordered. Although adverse hepatic effects are rare, they can be serious.
- Be alert for adverse reactions and drug interactions.
- Monitor patient's hydration status if adverse GI reactions occur.
- Evaluate patient's and family's knowledge of drug therapy.

Nursing diagnoses

- Infection related to presence of susceptible fungi
- Risk for deficient fluid volume related to adverse GI reactions
- Deficient knowledge related to drug therapy

Planning and implementation

P.O. use: Follow normal protocol.
I.V. use: Don't remove protective overwrap from I.V. bags of fluconazole until just before use to ensure product sterility. Plastic container may show some opacity from moisture absorbed during sterilization. This is normal, won't affect drug, and will diminish over time.
– Administer by continuous infusion at no more than 200 mg/hour. Use infusion pump. To prevent air embolism, don't connect in series with other infusions. Don't add any other drugs to solution.
- If patient develops mild rash, monitor him closely. Discontinue drug if lesions progress, and notify prescriber.

Patient teaching

- Urge patient to adhere to regimen and to return for follow-up.
- Tell patient to report adverse reactions to prescriber.

Evaluation

- Patient is free from infection.
- Patient maintains adequate hydration.
- Patient and family state understanding of drug therapy.

flucytosine (5-fluorocytosine, 5-FC)

(floo-SIGH-toh-seen)
Ancobon, Ancotil ◇

Pharmacologic class: fluorinated pyrimidine
Therapeutic class: antifungal
Pregnancy risk category: C

Indications and dosages

▶ **Severe fungal infections caused by susceptible strains of *Candida* (including septicemia, endocarditis, urinary tract and pulmonary infections) and *Cryptococcus* (meningitis, pulmonary infection, and possible urinary tract infections).** *Adults and children weighing more than 50 kg (110 lb):* 50 to 150 mg/kg daily P.O. in divided doses given q 6 hours.
Adults and children weighing less than 50 kg: 1.5 to 4.5 g/m²/day P.O. in four divided doses. Severe infections may require doses up to 250 mg/kg.

How supplied

Capsules: 250 mg, 500 mg

Pharmacokinetics

Absorption: from 75% to 90% of dose is absorbed; food decreases absorption rate.
Distribution: distributed widely into liver, kidneys, spleen, heart, bronchial secretions, joints, peritoneal fluid, and aqueous humor. CSF levels vary from 60% to 100% of serum levels. Drug is 2% to 4% bound to plasma proteins.
Metabolism: only small amounts of drug are metabolized.
Excretion: about 75% to 95% excreted unchanged in urine; less than 10% excreted unchanged in feces. *Half-life:* 2½ to 6 hours.

Route	Onset	Peak	Duration
P.O.	Unknown	1-2 hr	Unknown

Pharmacodynamics

Chemical effect: unknown; appears to penetrate fungal cells, where it's converted to fluorouracil—a known metabolic antagonist—and causes defective protein synthesis.
Therapeutic effect: hinders fungal growth. Spectrum of activity includes some strains of *Cryptococcus* and *Candida.*

Adverse reactions

CNS: dizziness, confusion, headache, vertigo, sedation, fatigue, weakness, hallucinations, psychosis, ataxia, paresthesia, parkinsonism, peripheral neuropathy.
CV: chest pain, ***cardiac arrest.***
EENT: hearing loss.
GI: nausea, vomiting, diarrhea, abdominal pain, dry mouth, duodenal ulcer, ***hemorrhage,*** ulcerative colitis.
GU: azotemia, elevated BUN and creatinine levels, crystalluria, ***renal failure.***
Hematologic: anemia, eosinophilia, ***leukopenia, bone marrow suppression, thrombocytopenia, agranulocytosis, aplastic anemia.***
Hepatic: elevated liver enzyme levels (ALT, AST); elevated serum alkaline phosphatase level, jaundice.
Metabolic: hypoglycemia, hypokalemia.
Respiratory: ***respiratory arrest,*** dyspnea.
Skin: occasional rash, pruritus, urticaria, photosensitivity.

Interactions

Drug-drug. *Amphotericin B:* synergistic effects and possibly enhanced toxicity when used together. Monitor patient.

Contraindications and precautions

- Contraindicated in patients hypersensitive to drug.
- Use with extreme caution in those with impaired hepatic or renal function or bone marrow suppression.
- Use cautiously in pregnant women.

NURSING CONSIDERATIONS

Assessment

- Assess patient's fungal infection before therapy, and reassess regularly throughout therapy.
- Before therapy, obtain hematologic tests and renal and liver function studies. Make sure susceptibility tests showing that organism is flucytosine-sensitive are on chart.

• Monitor blood, liver, and renal function studies frequently; obtain susceptibility tests weekly, as ordered, to monitor drug resistance.
• If possible, regularly perform blood level assays of drug, as ordered, to maintain flucytosine at therapeutic level (25 to 120 mcg/ml). Higher blood levels may be toxic.
• Be alert for adverse reactions and drug interactions.
• Monitor patient's hydration status if adverse GI reactions occur.
• Evaluate patient's and family's knowledge of drug therapy.

Nursing diagnoses
• Infection related to presence of susceptible fungi
• Risk for deficient fluid volume related to adverse GI reactions
• Deficient knowledge related to drug therapy

Planning and implementation
• Give capsules over 15 minutes to reduce adverse GI reactions.

Patient teaching
• Inform patient that therapeutic response may take weeks or months.
• Tell patient how to take capsules.
• Warn patient to avoid hazardous activities requiring mental alertness if adverse CNS reactions occur.

Evaluation
• Patient is free from infection.
• Patient maintains adequate hydration throughout drug therapy.
• Patient and family state understanding of drug therapy.

fludarabine phosphate
(floo-DAR-uh-been FOS-fayt)
Fludara

Pharmacologic class: antimetabolite
Therapeutic class: antineoplastic
Pregnancy risk category: D

Indications and dosages
▶ **B-cell chronic lymphocytic leukemia in patients who either haven't responded or have responded inadequately to at least one standard alkylating agent regimen.** *Adults:* 25 mg/m^2 I.V. over 30 minutes for 5 consecutive days. Cycle repeated q 28 days.

How supplied
Powder for injection: 50 mg

Pharmacokinetics
Absorption: not applicable.
Distribution: unknown.
Metabolism: rapidly dephosphorylated and then phosphorylated intracellularly to its active metabolite.
Excretion: 23% is excreted in urine as unchanged active metabolite. *Half-life:* about 10 hours.

Route	Onset	Peak	Duration
I.V.	7-21 hr	Unknown	Unknown

Pharmacodynamics
Chemical effect: unknown; actions may be multifaceted. After conversion to its active metabolite, fludarabine interferes with DNA synthesis by inhibiting DNA polymerase alpha, ribonucleotide reductase, and DNA primase.
Therapeutic effect: kills susceptible cancer cells.

Adverse reactions
CNS: diaphoresis, *fatigue, malaise, weakness, paresthesia,* headache, peripheral neuropathy, sleep disorder, depression, cerebellar syndrome, ***CVA,*** transient ischemic attack, agitation, *confusion,* ***coma.***
CV: *edema,* angina, phlebitis, ***arrhythmias, heart failure, MI,*** supraventricular tachycardia, deep venous thrombosis, ***aneurysm, hemorrhage.***
EENT: *visual disturbances,* hearing loss, delayed blindness (with high doses), sinusitis, pharyngitis, epistaxis.
GI: *nausea, vomiting, diarrhea,* constipation, *anorexia,* stomatitis, *GI bleeding,* esophagitis, mucositis.
GU: dysuria, *urinary infection,* urinary hesitancy, proteinuria, hematuria, ***renal failure.***

Hematologic: ***hemolytic anemia,*** **MYELOSUPPRESSION.**
Hepatic: ***liver failure,*** cholelithiasis.
Metabolic: hyperglycemia, dehydration, hyperuricemia, hyperphosphatemia.
Musculoskeletal: myalgia.
Respiratory: *cough, pneumonia, dyspnea, upper respiratory infection,* allergic pneumonitis, hemoptysis, hypoxia, bronchitis.
Skin: alopecia, *rash,* pruritus, seborrhea.
Other: *fever, chills,* **INFECTION,** pain, tumor lysis syndrome, ***anaphylaxis.***

Interactions

Drug-drug. *Other myelosuppressants:* increased toxicity. Avoid concomitant use.
Pentostatin: increased risk of pulmonary toxicity. Avoid concomitant administration.

Contraindications and precautions

- Contraindicated in patients hypersensitive to drug or its components.
- Use with extreme caution and only when necessary in pregnant women.
- Use cautiously in patients with renal insufficiency.
- Safety of drug hasn't been established in breast-feeding women and in children.

NURSING CONSIDERATIONS

Assessment

- Assess patient's underlying condition before therapy, and reassess regularly thereafter.
- Careful hematologic monitoring is needed, especially of neutrophil and platelet counts. Bone marrow suppression can be severe.
- Be alert for adverse reactions and drug interactions.
- Evaluate patient's and family's knowledge of drug therapy.

Nursing diagnoses

- Ineffective health maintenance related to presence of leukemia
- Ineffective protection related to drug-induced immunosuppression
- Deficient knowledge related to drug therapy

Planning and implementation

- Follow facility policy to reduce risks. Preparation and administration of parenteral form create mutagenic, teratogenic, and carcinogenic risks for staff.
- To prepare solution, add 2 ml of sterile water for injection to solid cake of drug. Dissolution should occur within 15 seconds; each milliliter will contain 25 mg of drug. Dilute further in 100 or 125 ml of D_5W or normal saline injection. Use within 8 hours of reconstitution.
- Optimal duration of therapy isn't known. Current recommendations suggest three additional cycles after achieving maximal response.
- Store drug in refrigerator at 36° to 46° F (2° to 8° C).

Patient teaching

- Warn patient to watch for evidence of infection and bleeding.
- Advise woman of childbearing age to avoid becoming pregnant during therapy and to consult with prescriber before becoming pregnant.
- Tell patient to notify prescriber if adverse reactions occur.

Evaluation

- Patient shows positive response to fludarabine therapy.
- Patient develops no serious infections or bleeding complications.
- Patient and family state understanding of drug therapy.

fludrocortisone acetate

(floo-droh-KOR-tuh-sohn AS-ih-tayt)
Florinef

Pharmacologic class: mineralocorticoid, glucocorticoid
Therapeutic class: mineralocorticoid replacement therapy
Pregnancy risk category: C

Indications and dosages

▶ **Adrenal insufficiency (partial replacement), adrenogenital syndrome.** *Adults:* 0.1 to 0.2 mg P.O. daily.

How supplied

Tablets: 0.1 mg

Pharmacokinetics

Absorption: absorbed readily from GI tract.
Distribution: distributed to muscle, liver, skin, intestines, and kidneys. It is extensively bound to plasma proteins. Only unbound portion is active.
Metabolism: metabolized in liver to inactive metabolites.
Excretion: excreted in urine; insignificant quantities are excreted in feces. *Half-life:* 18 to 36 hours.

Route	Onset	Peak	Duration
P.O.	Varies	Varies	1-2 days

Pharmacodynamics

Chemical effect: increases sodium reabsorption and potassium and hydrogen secretion at distal convoluted tubule of nephron.
Therapeutic effect: increases sodium levels and decreases potassium and hydrogen levels.

Adverse reactions

CV: *sodium and water retention,* hypertension, cardiac hypertrophy, edema, ***heart failure.***
Metabolic: hypokalemia.
Skin: bruising, diaphoresis, urticaria, allergic rash.

Interactions

Drug-drug. *Barbiturates, phenytoin, rifampin:* increased clearance of fludrocortisone acetate. Monitor patient for effect.
Potassium-depleting drugs (such as thiazide diuretics): enhanced potassium-wasting effects of fludrocortisone. Monitor serum potassium levels.
Drug-food. *Sodium-containing drugs or foods:* may increase blood pressure. Sodium intake may need to be adjusted.

Contraindications and precautions

- Contraindicated in patients hypersensitive to drug and in those with systemic fungal infections.
- Use cautiously in patients with hypothyroidism, cirrhosis, ocular herpes simplex, emotional instability and psychotic tendencies, nonspecific ulcerative colitis, diverticulitis, fresh intestinal anastomoses, active or latent peptic ulcer, renal insufficiency, hypertension, osteoporosis, and myasthenia gravis.
- Long-term use in children may delay growth and maturation.

NURSING CONSIDERATIONS

Assessment

- Assess patient's underlying condition before therapy, and reassess regularly thereafter.
- Monitor patient's blood pressure, weight, and serum electrolyte levels.
- Be alert for adverse reactions and drug interactions.
- Evaluate patient's and family's knowledge of drug therapy.

Nursing diagnoses

- Ineffective health maintenance related to underlying adrenal condition
- Excessive fluid volume related to drug-induced adverse reactions
- Deficient knowledge related to drug therapy

Planning and implementation

- Drug is used with cortisone or hydrocortisone in patients with adrenal insufficiency.
- If hypertension occurs, notify prescriber, who may lower dosage by 50%.
- Potassium supplements may be needed.

Patient teaching

- Tell patient to notify prescriber about worsened symptoms, such as hypotension, weakness, cramping, and palpitations.
- Warn patient that mild peripheral edema is common.

Evaluation

- Patient's health is improved.
- Patient develops no sodium and water retention.
- Patient and family state understanding of drug therapy.

flumazenil
(floo-MAZ-ih-nil)
Romazicon

Pharmacologic class: benzodiazepine antagonist
Therapeutic class: antidote
Pregnancy risk category: C

Indications and dosages

▶ **Complete or partial reversal of sedative effects of benzodiazepines after anesthesia or short diagnostic procedures (conscious sedation).** *Adults:* initially, 0.2 mg I.V. over 15 seconds. If patient doesn't reach desired level of consciousness after 45 seconds, dose is repeated. Repeated at 1-minute intervals until cumulative dose of 1 mg has been given (initial dose plus four more doses), if needed. Most patients respond after 0.6 to 1 mg of drug. In case of resedation, dosage may be repeated after 20 minutes; however, no more than 1 mg should be given at any one time and no more than 3 mg/hour.

▶ **Suspected benzodiazepine overdose.** *Adults:* initially, 0.2 mg I.V. over 15 seconds. If patient doesn't reach desired level of consciousness after 30 seconds, 0.3 mg is given over 30 seconds. If patient still doesn't respond adequately, 0.5 mg is given over 30 seconds; 0.5-mg doses are repeated as needed at 1-minute intervals until cumulative dose of 3 mg has been given. Most patients with benzodiazepine overdose respond to cumulative doses between 1 and 3 mg; rarely, patients who respond partially after 3 mg may need additional doses. No more than 5 mg over 5 minutes should be given initially. Sedation that persists after this dosage is unlikely to be caused by benzodiazepines. In case of resedation, dosage may be repeated after 20 minutes; however, no more than 1 mg should be given at any one time and no more than 3 mg/hour.

How supplied

Injection: 0.1 mg/ml in 5- and 10-ml multiple-dose vials

Pharmacokinetics

Absorption: not applicable.
Distribution: redistributes rapidly; 50% bound to plasma proteins.
Metabolism: metabolized by liver. Ingestion of food during I.V. infusion enhances extraction of drug from plasma, probably by increasing hepatic blood flow.
Excretion: about 90% to 95% appears in urine as metabolites; remainder excreted in feces. *Half-life:* about 54 minutes.

Route	Onset	Peak	Duration
I.V.	Unknown	Unknown	Unknown

Pharmacodynamics

Chemical effect: competitively inhibits actions of benzodiazepines on gamma-aminobutyric acid–benzodiazepine receptor complex.
Therapeutic effect: awakens patient from sedative effects of benzodiazepines.

Adverse reactions

CNS: *dizziness, headache,* ***seizures,*** agitation, emotional lability, tremor, insomnia.
CV: ***arrhythmias,*** cutaneous vasodilation, palpitations.
EENT: *abnormal or blurred vision.*
GI: *nausea, vomiting.*
Respiratory: dyspnea, hyperventilation.
Skin: *diaphoresis.*
Other: *pain at injection site.*

Interactions

Drug-drug. *Antidepressants, drugs that can cause seizures or arrhythmias:* seizures or arrhythmias can develop after effect of benzodiazepine overdose is removed. Use with caution, if at all, in cases of mixed overdose.

Contraindications and precautions

- Contraindicated in patients hypersensitive to drug or benzodiazepines; in patients who show evidence of serious cyclic antidepressant overdose; and in those who received benzodiazepine to treat potentially life-threatening condition (such as status epilepticus).
- Use cautiously in patients at high risk for developing seizures; patients who recently have received multiple doses of parenteral

benzodiazepine; patients displaying signs of seizure activity; patients who may be at risk for unrecognized benzodiazepine dependence, such as intensive care unit patients; patients with head injury; psychiatric or alcohol-dependent patients; and pregnant or breast-feeding women.
• Safety of drug hasn't been established in children.

NURSING CONSIDERATIONS

Assessment
• Assess patient's sedation before therapy.
• Assess patient's level of consciousness frequently.
• Be alert for adverse reactions and drug interactions.
ALERT Monitor patient closely for resedation that may occur after reversal of benzodiazepine effects; flumazenil's duration of action is shorter than that of all benzodiazepines. Monitor patient closely after long-acting benzodiazepines, such as diazepam, or high doses of short-acting benzodiazepines, such as 10 mg of midszolam. In most cases, severe resedation is unlikely in patient who fails to show signs of resedation 2 hours after 1-mg dose of flumazenil.
• Monitor patient's ECG for evidence of arrhythmias.
• Evaluate patient's and family's knowledge of drug therapy.

Nursing diagnoses
• Ineffective protection related to sedated state
• Decreased cardiac output related to drug-induced seizures
• Deficient knowledge related to drug therapy

Planning and implementation
• Give drug by direct injection or dilute with compatible solution. Discard within 24 hours unused drug that has been drawn into syringe or diluted.
• Administer drug into I.V. line in large vein with free-flowing I.V. solution to minimize pain at injection site. Compatible solutions include D_5W, lactated Ringer's injection, and normal saline solution.
• Notify prescriber if arrhythmias or other adverse reactions occur, and be prepared to treat accordingly.

Patient teaching
• Warn patient to avoid hazardous activities within 24 hours of procedure.
• Tell patient to avoid alcohol, CNS depressants, and OTC drugs for 24 hours.
• Give family members important instructions or provide patient with written instructions. Don't expect patient to recall information given in postprocedure period.

Evaluation
• Patient is awake and alert.
• Patient maintains adequate cardiac output.
• Patient and family state understanding of drug therapy.

flunisolide
(floo-NIH-soh-lighd)
AeroBid, AeroBid-M, Bronalide ♦ (oral inhalant), Nasalide, Nasarel, Rhinalar Nasal Mist ◇ (nasal inhalant)

Pharmacologic class: glucocorticoid
Therapeutic class: anti-inflammatory, antiasthmatic
Pregnancy risk category: C

Indications and dosages
▶ **Steroid-dependent asthma (oral inhalant).** *Adults and children age 6 and over:* 2 inhalations (500 mcg) b.i.d. Maximum, 4 inhalations daily, b.i.d.
▶ **Symptoms of seasonal or perennial rhinitis (nasal inhalant).** *Adults:* starting dose is 2 sprays (50 mcg) in each nostril b.i.d. Total, 200 mcg daily. If necessary, dosage may be increased to 2 sprays in each nostril t.i.d. Maximum, 8 sprays in each nostril (400 mcg) daily. *Children ages 6 to 14:* starting dose is 1 spray (25 mcg) in each nostril t.i.d. or 2 sprays (50 mcg) in each nostril b.i.d. Total, 150 to 200 mcg daily. Maximum, 4 sprays in each nostril (200 mcg) daily.

How supplied

Oral inhalant: 250 mcg/metered spray (at least 100 metered inhalations/container)
Nasal inhalant: 25 mcg/metered spray, 200 doses/bottle ◇
Nasal solution: 0.25 mg/ml in pump spray bottle

Pharmacokinetics

Absorption: about 50% of nasally inhaled dose is absorbed systemically. After oral inhalation, about 70% of dose is absorbed from lungs and GI tract. Only about 20% of orally inhaled dose reaches systemic circulation unmetabolized because of extensive metabolism in liver.
Distribution: unknown after intranasal use. After oral inhalation, 10% to 25% of drug is distributed to lungs; remainder is deposited in mouth and swallowed. No evidence exists of tissue storage of drug or its metabolites. When absorbed, it is 50% bound to plasma proteins.
Metabolism: drug that is swallowed undergoes rapid metabolism in liver or GI tract to variety of metabolites, one of which has glucocorticoid activity. Flunisolide and its active metabolite are eventually conjugated in liver to inactive metabolites.
Excretion: unknown for inhalation routes.

Route	Onset	Peak	Duration
Nasal or oral inhalation	1-4 wk	Unknown	Unknown

Pharmacodynamics

Chemical effect: unknown; may stabilize leukocyte lysosomal membranes.
Therapeutic effect: relieves inflammation.

Adverse reactions

CNS: headache, dizziness, irritability, nervousness.
CV: chest pain, edema, palpitations.
EENT: dry mouth, watery eyes, throat irritation, hoarseness, nasopharyngeal fungal infections, *sore throat, nasal congestion, mild and transient nasal burning and stinging,* dryness, sneezing, epistaxis.
GI: *unpleasant taste, nausea, vomiting, upset stomach,* abdominal pain, decreased appetite, *diarrhea.*
Respiratory: *upper respiratory tract infection.*
Skin: pruritus, rash.
Other: *cold symptoms, flu,* fever.

Interactions

None significant.

Contraindications and precautions

- Contraindicated in patients hypersensitive to drug and in those with status asthmaticus or respiratory infection.
- Nasal inhalant shouldn't be used in presence of untreated localized infection involving nasal mucosa.
- Use nasal inhalant cautiously, if at all, in patients with active or quiescent respiratory tract tubercular infections or with untreated fungal, bacterial, or systemic viral or ocular herpes simplex infections. Also use cautiously in patients who recently have had nasal septal ulcers, nasal surgery, or nasal trauma.
- Use cautiously in pregnant or breast-feeding women.
- Safety of drug hasn't been established in children under age 6.

NURSING CONSIDERATIONS

Assessment

- Assess patient's underlying condition before therapy, and reassess regularly thereafter.
- Be alert for adverse reactions and drug interactions.
- Evaluate patient's and family's knowledge of drug therapy.

Nursing diagnoses

- Ineffective health maintenance related to underlying condition
- Impaired tissue integrity related to adverse EENT reactions
- Deficient knowledge related to drug therapy

Planning and implementation

Oral inhalation use: Not recommended in patients with asthma controlled by bronchodila-

tors or other noncorticosteroids alone, or in those with nonasthmatic bronchial diseases.
– Spacer device may help to ensure proper dosage administration.
Nasal inhalation use: Flunisolide isn't effective for acute exacerbations of rhinitis. Decongestants or antihistamines may be needed.
– To instill, shake container before using; have patient blow nose to clear nasal passages; have patient tilt head slightly forward. Insert nozzle into nostril, pointing away from septum. Hold other nostril closed, and then have patient inhale gently and spray. Next, shake container and repeat in other nostril. Clean nosepiece with warm water if it becomes clogged.
- Store drug between 36° and 86° F (2° and 30° C).
- Withdraw drug slowly, as ordered, in patient who has received long-term oral corticosteroid therapy.
- After withdrawal of systemic corticosteroids, patient may need supplemental systemic steroids if he shows evidence of adrenal insufficiency when exposed to trauma, surgery, or infections.

Patient teaching
Oral inhalation
- Warn patient that drug doesn't relieve acute asthma attacks.
- Advise patient to ensure delivery of proper dose by gently warming canister to room temperature before using. Some patients carry canister in pocket to keep it warm.
- Tell patient who also is using bronchodilator to use it several minutes before flunisolide.
- Instruct patient to allow 1 minute to elapse before repeating inhalations and to hold breath for few seconds to enhance drug action.
- Teach patient to keep inhaler clean and unobstructed by washing with warm water and drying thoroughly after use.
- Teach patient to check mucous membranes frequently for signs of fungal infection.
- Advise patient to prevent oral fungal infections by gargling or rinsing mouth with water after each inhaler use. Caution patient not to swallow the water.

Nasal inhalation
- Explain that therapeutic effects of drug, unlike those of decongestants, aren't immediate. Most patients achieve benefit within a few days, but some need 2 to 3 weeks.
- Advise patient to use drug regularly, as prescribed, because its effectiveness depends on regular use.
- Teach patient how to instill drug.
- Warn patient not to exceed recommended dosage to avoid suppression of hypothalamic-pituitary-adrenal function.
- Tell patient to stop drug and notify prescriber if symptoms persist after 3 weeks.

☑ Evaluation
- Patient's health improves.
- Patient maintains upper airway and buccal tissue integrity.
- Patient and family state understanding of drug therapy.

fluorouracil (5-fluorouracil, 5-FU)
(floo-roh-YOOR-uh-sil)
Adrucil, Efudex, Fluoroplex

Pharmacologic class: antimetabolite (cell cycle–phase specific, S phase)
Therapeutic class: antineoplastic
Pregnancy risk category: D

Indications and dosages
▶ **Colon, rectal, breast, stomach, and pancreatic cancers.** *Adults:* 12 mg/kg I.V. daily for 4 days; if no toxicity, give 6 mg/kg on 6th, 8th, 10th, and 12th day; then single weekly maintenance dose of 10 to 15 mg/kg I.V. begun after toxicity (if any) from initial course has subsided. (Dosages recommended based on lean body weight.) Maximum single recommended dose is 800 mg.
▶ **Palliative treatment of advanced colorectal cancer.** *Adults:* 425 mg/m^2 I.V. daily for 5 consecutive days. Given with 20 mg/m^2 of leucovorin I.V. Repeated at 4-week intervals for two additional courses; then repeated at intervals of 4 to 5 weeks if tolerated.
▶ **Multiple actinic (solar) keratoses; superficial basal cell carcinoma.** *Adults:* apply cream or topical solution b.i.d.

How supplied

Injection: 50 mg/ml
Cream: 1%, 5%
Topical solution: 1%, 2%, 5%

Pharmacokinetics

Absorption: unknown for topical forms.
Distribution: distributes widely into all areas of body water and tissues; crosses blood-brain barrier.
Metabolism: small amount converted in tissues to active metabolite with majority of drug degraded in liver.
Excretion: metabolites primarily excreted through lungs as carbon dioxide; small portion excreted in urine as unchanged drug.

Route	Onset	Peak	Duration
I.V., topical	Unknown	Unknown	Unknown

Pharmacodynamics

Chemical effect: inhibits DNA synthesis.
Therapeutic effect: inhibits cell growth of selected cancers.

Adverse reactions

CNS: acute cerebellar syndrome, ataxia, confusion, disorientation, euphoria, headache, nystagmus, *weakness, malaise.*
CV: thrombophlebitis, ***myocardial ischemia,*** angina.
EENT: epistaxis, photophobia, lacrimation, lacrimal duct stenosis, visual changes.
GI: *stomatitis, GI ulcer* (may precede leukopenia), *nausea and vomiting, diarrhea, anorexia,* GI bleeding.
Hematologic: ***leukopenia, thrombocytopenia, agranulocytosis,*** anemia; WBC count nadir 9 to 14 days after first dose; platelet count nadir in 7 to 14 days.
Skin: *reversible alopecia; dermatitis; erythema; scaling; pruritus*; contact dermatitis; nail changes; pigmented palmar creases; erythematous, desquamative rash of hands and feet with long-term use ("hand-foot syndrome"); photosensitivity; *pain, burning,* soreness, suppuration, and swelling with topical use.
Other: ***anaphylaxis.***

Interactions

Drug-drug. *Leucovorin calcium, previous treatment with alkylating agents:* increased fluorouracil toxicity. Use with extreme caution.
Drug-lifestyle. *Sun exposure:* photosensitivity reactions may occur. Urge precautions.

Contraindications and precautions

- Contraindicated in patients hypersensitive to drug and in those with poor nutrition, bone marrow suppression (WBC counts of 5,000/mm^3 or less or platelet counts of 100,000/mm^3 or less), or potentially serious infections and in those who have had major surgery within previous month.
- Drug isn't recommended for pregnant or breast-feeding women.
- Use cautiously after high-dose pelvic radiation therapy and in patients who received alkylating agents or have impaired hepatic or renal function or widespread neoplastic infiltration of bone marrow.
- Safety of drug hasn't been established in children.

NURSING CONSIDERATIONS

Assessment

- Assess patient's condition before therapy, and reassess regularly thereafter.
- Monitor fluid intake and output, CBC, platelet count, and renal and hepatic function tests, as ordered.
- Be alert for adverse reactions and drug interactions.
- Fluorouracil toxicity may be delayed for 1 to 3 weeks.
- Monitor patient receiving topical form for serious adverse reactions. Ingestion and systemic absorption may cause leukopenia, thrombocytopenia, stomatitis, diarrhea, or GI ulceration, bleeding, and hemorrhage. Application to large ulcerated areas may cause systemic toxicity.
- Watch for stomatitis or diarrhea (signs of toxicity).
- Evaluate patient's and family's knowledge of drug therapy.

Nursing diagnoses

- Ineffective health maintenance related to underlying neoplastic condition
- Ineffective protection related to adverse hematologic reactions
- Deficient knowledge related to drug therapy

Planning and implementation

- Follow facility policy to reduce risks. Preparation and administration of parenteral form create carcinogenic, mutagenic, and teratogenic risks for staff.
- Drug sometimes is ordered as 5-fluorouracil or 5-FU. The numeral 5 is part of drug name and shouldn't be confused with dosage units.
- Give antiemetic, as ordered, to reduce nausea before giving parenteral form of drug.

I.V. use: Drug may be given by direct injection without dilution. For I.V. infusion, drug may be diluted with D_5W, sterile water for injection, or normal saline injection. Infuse slowly over 2 to 8 hours.

– Don't use cloudy solution. If crystals form, redissolve by warming.

– Use plastic I.V. containers for giving continuous infusions. Solution is more stable in plastic I.V. bags than in glass bottles.

Topical use: Apply with caution near eyes, nose, and mouth.

– Avoid occlusive dressings because they increase risk of inflammatory reactions in adjacent normal skin.

– Wash hands immediately after handling topical form.

– Expect to use 1% topical concentration on face. Higher concentrations are used for thicker-skinned areas or resistant lesions.

– Expect to use 5% topical strength for superficial basal cell carcinoma confirmed by biopsy.

- Don't refrigerate fluorouracil.
- Use sodium hypochlorite 5% (household bleach) to inactivate drug in event of spill.
- Discontinue drug if diarrhea occurs, and notify prescriber.
- Consider protective isolation if WBC count is less than 2,000/mm^3.

Patient teaching

- Warn patient that alopecia may occur but is reversible.
- Caution patient to avoid prolonged exposure to sunlight or ultraviolet light when topical form is used.
- Tell patient to use sunblock to avoid inflammatory erythematous dermatitis. Long-term use of drug may cause erythematous, desquamative rash of hands and feet. May be treated with pyridoxine (50 to 150 mg P.O. daily) for 5 to 7 days.
- Warn patient that topically treated area may be unsightly during therapy and for several weeks after. Full healing may take 1 or 2 months.

Evaluation

- Patient shows positive response to fluorouracil therapy.
- Patient develops no serious adverse hematologic reactions.
- Patient and family state understanding of drug therapy.

fluoxetine hydrochloride

(floo-OKS-eh-teen high-droh-KLOR-ighd)

Prozac, Prozac-20 ◇

Pharmacologic class: serotonin uptake inhibitor
Therapeutic class: antidepressant
Pregnancy risk category: B

Indications and dosages

▶ **Depression, obsessive-compulsive disorder.** *Adults:* initially, 20 mg P.O. in morning; dosage increased according to patient response. May be given b.i.d. in morning and at noon. Maximum, 80 mg daily.

▶ **Treatment of binge eating and vomiting behaviors in patients with moderate to severe bulimia nervosa.** *Adults:* 60 mg daily P.O. in the morning.

▶ **Treatment of depression in elderly patients.** *Adults age 65 and older:* initially, 20 mg P.O. daily in the morning. Increase dosage based on clinical response. Doses may be given twice daily, in the morning and at noon. Maximum, 80 mg daily. A lower dosage or less frequent dosing should be considered in these patients, especially those with systemic illness and those who take multiple drugs for concomitant illnesses.

How supplied

Tablets: 10 mg
Pulvules: 10 mg, 20 mg, 40 mg
Oral solution: 20 mg/5 ml

Pharmacokinetics

Absorption: well absorbed after P.O. administration.
Distribution: apparently highly protein-bound (about 95%).
Metabolism: metabolized primarily in liver to active metabolites.
Excretion: excreted by kidneys. *Half-life:* 2 to 3 days.

Route	Onset	Peak	Duration
P.O.	1-4 wk	6-8 hr	Unknown

Pharmacodynamics

Chemical effect: unknown; presumed to be linked to inhibition of CNS neuronal uptake of serotonin.
Therapeutic effect: relieves depression and obsessive-compulsive behaviors.

Adverse reactions

CNS: *nervousness, anxiety, insomnia, headache, drowsiness,* fatigue, tremor, dizziness, asthenia.
CV: palpitations, hot flushes.
EENT: nasal congestion, pharyngitis, sinusitis.
GI: *nausea, diarrhea, dry mouth, anorexia,* dyspepsia, constipation, abdominal pain, vomiting, flatulence, increased appetite.
GU: sexual dysfunction.
Metabolic: weight loss.
Musculoskeletal: muscle pain.
Respiratory: cough, upper respiratory infection, respiratory distress.
Skin: rash, pruritus, urticaria.
Other: flulike syndrome, fever.

Interactions

Drug-drug. *Cyproheptadine:* may reverse or decrease pharmacologic effect. Monitor patient closely.
Flecainide, carbamazepine, vinblastine: increased serum levels of these drugs. Monitor serum levels and patient for adverse effects.
Insulin, oral antidiabetics: altered blood glucose levels and possible altered need for antidiabetic. Adjust dosage as ordered.
Lithium, tricyclic antidepressants: risk of increased serum levels. Monitor levels and adjust doses as needed.
Phenytoin: increased plasma phenytoin levels and risk of toxicity. Monitor serum phenytoin levels and adjust dosage as ordered.
Tryptophan: increased toxic reaction with agitation, GI distress, and restlessness. Don't use together.
Warfarin, other highly protein-bound drugs: may increase plasma levels of fluoxetine or other highly protein-bound drugs. Monitor serum levels closely.
Drug-herb. *St. John's wort:* increased risk of serotonin syndrome. Discourage concomitant use.
Drug-lifestyle. *Alcohol use:* increased CNS depression. Discourage concomitant use.

Contraindications and precautions

- Contraindicated in patients hypersensitive to drug and in those taking MAO inhibitors within 14 days of starting therapy.
- Drug isn't recommended for breast-feeding women.
- Use cautiously in patients at high risk for suicide; in those with history of hepatic, renal, or CV disease, diabetes mellitus, or history of seizures; and in pregnant women.
- Safety of drug hasn't been established in children.

NURSING CONSIDERATIONS

Assessment

- Assess patient's condition before therapy, and reassess regularly throughout therapy.
- Be alert for adverse reactions and drug interactions.
- Evaluate patient's and family's knowledge of drug therapy.

Nursing diagnoses

- Ineffective individual coping related to patient's underlying condition

• Disturbed sleep pattern related to drug-induced insomnia
• Deficient knowledge related to drug therapy

Planning and implementation

• Elderly or debilitated patients and patients with renal or hepatic dysfunction may need lower dosages or less frequent dosing.
• Administer drug in morning to prevent insomnia.
• Give antihistamines or topical corticosteroids as ordered to treat rashes or pruritus.

Patient teaching

• Tell patient not to take drug in afternoon because fluoxetine commonly causes nervousness and insomnia.
• Warn patient to avoid hazardous activities that require alertness and psychomotor coordination until CNS effects of drug are known.
• Advise patient to consult prescriber before taking any other prescription or OTC medications.

Evaluation

• Patient behavior and communication indicate improvement of depression with drug therapy.
• Patient has no insomnia with drug use.
• Patient and family state understanding of drug therapy.

fluoxymesterone

(floo-oks-ee-MES-tuh-rohn)
Android-F, Halotestin**

Pharmacologic class: androgen
Therapeutic class: androgen replacement, antineoplastic
Controlled substance schedule: III
Pregnancy risk category: X

Indications and dosages

▶ **Hypogonadism from testicular deficiency.** *Adults:* 5 to 20 mg P.O. daily.
▶ **Delayed puberty.** *Adolescents:* highly individualized; usual range is 2.5 to 10 mg P.O. daily. Don't exceed 20 mg daily. Duration of therapy is 4 to 6 months.
▶ **Palliation of breast cancer in women.** *Adults:* 10 to 40 mg P.O. daily in divided doses. All dosages individualized and reduced to minimum when effect is noted.

How supplied

Tablets: 2 mg, 5 mg, 10 mg

Pharmacokinetics

Absorption: unknown.
Distribution: unknown.
Metabolism: primarily hepatic.
Excretion: unknown.

Route	Onset	Peak	Duration
P.O.	Unknown	Unknown	Unknown

Pharmacodynamics

Chemical effect: stimulates target tissues to develop normally in androgen-deficient men. It also exerts inhibitory, antiestrogenic effects on hormone-responsive breast tumors and metastases.
Therapeutic effect: stimulates puberty, reverses testicular deficiency, and inhibits estrogenic effects on breast tumors and metastases.

Adverse reactions

CNS: headache, anxiety, depression, paresthesia, sleep apnea syndrome.
CV: edema.
GI: nausea.
Hematologic: polycythemia, elevated serum lipid levels, suppression of clotting factors.
Hepatic: reversible jaundice, peliosis hepatis, elevated liver enzyme levels, ***liver cell tumors.***
Metabolic: hypercalcemia.
Skin: hypersensitivity skin reactions.
Other: androgenic effects in women (acne, edema, *weight gain, hirsutism,* hoarseness, clitoral enlargement, *decrease in breast size,* changes in libido, male pattern baldness, *oily skin or hair), hypoestrogenic effects in women (flushing; diaphoresis; vaginitis including itching, dryness, and burning; vaginal bleeding; nervousness; emotional lability; menstrual irregularities);* excessive hormonal effects in men (prepubertal—premature epiphyseal

closure, *acne,* priapism, *growth of body and facial hair,* phallic enlargement; postpubertal—testicular atrophy, oligospermia, decreased ejaculate, impotence, gynecomastia, epididymitis).

Interactions

Drug-drug. *Hepatotoxic drugs:* increased risk of hepatotoxicity. Monitor patient closely.
Insulin, oral antidiabetics: altered dosage requirements. Monitor blood glucose levels in diabetic patients.
Oral anticoagulants: altered dosage requirements. Monitor PT and INR.

Contraindications and precautions

- Contraindicated in patients hypersensitive to drug, in pregnant or breast-feeding women, in males with breast cancer or prostate cancer, and in those with cardiac, hepatic, or renal decompensation.
- Use cautiously in prepubertal males and in patients with BPH and aspirin sensitivity.

NURSING CONSIDERATIONS

Assessment

- Assess patient's underlying condition before therapy and regularly thereafter.
- When given for breast cancer, subjective effects may not occur for about 1 month; objective effects on clinical symptoms may take 3 months.
- Semen evaluation is performed routinely every 3 to 4 months, especially in adolescent males.
- Be alert for adverse reactions and drug interactions.
- Watch for symptoms of jaundice and evaluate hepatic function.
- Monitor male patient for excessive sexual stimulation or priapism.
- Monitor patient for hypercalcemia. Symptoms may be difficult to distinguish from symptoms of condition being treated, unless anticipated and thought of as symptom cluster. Hypercalcemia is particularly likely to occur in patient with metastatic breast cancer and may indicate bone metastases.
- Evaluate patient's and family's knowledge of drug therapy.

Nursing diagnoses

- Sexual dysfunction related to hormonal dysfunction
- Disturbed body image related to adverse androgenic reactions
- Deficient knowledge related to drug therapy

Planning and implementation

- Give drug with food if adverse GI reactions occur.
- Dosage adjustment may reverse hepatic dysfunction. If liver function test results are abnormal, notify prescriber because therapy should be stopped.
- Report signs of virilization or menstrual irregularities to prescriber.

Patient teaching

- Tell patient to take drug with food or meals if GI upset occurs.
- Make sure patient understands importance of using effective nonhormonal contraceptive during therapy.
- Advise woman to wash after intercourse to decrease risk of vaginitis. Instruct her to wear only cotton underwear.
- Tell woman to report menstrual irregularities and to discontinue therapy pending etiologic determination.
- Explain to patient taking drug for palliation of breast cancer that virilization usually occurs. Give emotional support. Tell patient to report androgenic effects. Stopping drug will prevent further changes but will probably not reverse existing effects.

Evaluation

- Patient's underlying condition shows improvement.
- Patient states acceptance of body image changes caused by drug.
- Patient and family state understanding of drug therapy.

fluphenazine decanoate
(floo-FEN-uh-zeen deh-kuh-NOH-ayt)
Modecate ♦ ◇, Modecate Concentrate ♦, Prolixin Decanoate

fluphenazine enanthate
Moditen Enanthate ♦, Prolixin Enanthate

fluphenazine hydrochloride
Anatensol ◇ *, Apo-Fluphenazine ♦, Modecate Concentrate ♦, Moditen HCl ♦, Permitil* **, Permitil Concentrate, Prolixin* **, Prolixin Concentrate* ♦

Pharmacologic class: phenothiazine (piperazine derivative)
Therapeutic class: antipsychotic
Pregnancy risk category: C

Indications and dosages

▶ **Psychotic disorders.** *Adults:* initially, 0.5 to 10 mg hydrochloride P.O. daily in divided doses q 6 to 8 hours; may increase cautiously to 20 mg. Higher doses (50 to 100 mg) have been given. Maintenance, 1 to 5 mg P.O. daily. I.M. doses are one-third to one-half of oral doses. Use lower dosages for elderly patients (1 to 2.5 mg daily). Or, 12.5 to 25 mg of long-acting esters (decanoate or enanthate) I.M. or S.C. q 1 to 6 weeks. Maintenance, 25 to 100 mg, p.r.n.

How supplied

fluphenazine decanoate
Depot injection: 25 mg/ml, 100 mg/ml ♦
fluphenazine enanthate
Depot injection: 25 mg/ml
fluphenazine hydrochloride
Tablets: 1 mg, 2.5 mg, 5 mg, 10 mg
Oral concentrate: 5 mg/ml*
Elixir: 2.5 mg/5 ml*
I.M. injection: 2.5 mg/ml

Pharmacokinetics

Absorption: rate and extent of absorption vary with route of administration; oral tablet absorption is erratic and variable.
Distribution: distributed widely into body. CNS levels are usually higher than those in plasma. Drug is 91% to 99% protein-bound.
Metabolism: metabolized extensively by liver, but no active metabolites are formed.
Excretion: most of drug excreted in urine; some excreted in feces by way of biliary tract.

Route	Onset	Peak	Duration
P.O.	≤ 1 hr	0.5 hr	6-8 hr
I.M., S.C.	1-3 days	Unknown	1-6 wk

Pharmacodynamics

Chemical effect: unknown; may block dopamine receptors in brain.
Therapeutic effect: relieves psychotic signs and symptoms.

Adverse reactions

CNS: *extrapyramidal reactions, tardive dyskinesia,* sedation, pseudoparkinsonism, EEG changes, drowsiness, ***seizures,*** dizziness, ***neuroleptic malignant syndrome.***
CV: orthostatic hypotension, tachycardia, ECG changes.
EENT: *dry mouth,* ocular changes, *blurred vision,* nasal congestion.
GI: *constipation.*
GU: *urine retention,* dark urine, menstrual irregularities, gynecomastia, inhibited ejaculation.
Hematologic: ***leukopenia, agranulocytosis, aplastic anemia,*** eosinophilia, ***hemolytic anemia.***
Hepatic: cholestatic jaundice, abnormal liver function test results.
Metabolic: weight gain, increased appetite.
Skin: *mild photosensitivity,* allergic reactions.

Interactions

Drug-drug. *Antacids:* inhibited absorption of oral phenothiazines. Separate doses by at least 2 hours.
Anticholinergics: increased anticholinergic effects. Avoid concomitant use.
Barbiturates, lithium: may decrease phenothiazine effect. Observe patient.
Centrally acting antihypertensives: decreased antihypertensive effect. Monitor blood pressure.

CNS depressants: increased CNS depression. Avoid concomitant use.
Drug-lifestyle. *Alcohol use:* increased CNS depression. Discourage concomitant use.
Sun exposure: increased risk of photosensitivity. Discourage prolonged or unprotected exposure to sun.

Contraindications and precautions

• Contraindicated in patients hypersensitive to drug and in those with CNS depression, bone marrow suppression, other blood dyscrasia, subcortical damage, liver damage, or coma.
• Use cautiously in elderly or debilitated patients, pregnant or breast-feeding women, and those with pheochromocytoma, severe CV disease (may cause sudden drop in blood pressure), peptic ulcer, exposure to extreme heat or cold (including antipyretic therapy) or phosphorous insecticides, respiratory disorder, hypocalcemia, seizure disorder (may lower seizure threshold), severe reactions to insulin or electroconvulsive therapy, mitral insufficiency, glaucoma, or prostatic hyperplasia. Use parenteral form cautiously in patients with asthma and patients allergic to sulfites.

NURSING CONSIDERATIONS

Assessment

• Assess patient's condition before therapy and regularly thereafter.
• Monitor therapy with weekly bilirubin tests during first month; periodic blood tests (CBC and liver function); and periodic renal function and ophthalmic tests (long-term use).
• Be alert for adverse reactions and drug interactions.
• Monitor patient for tardive dyskinesia, which may occur after prolonged use. It may not appear until months or years later and may disappear spontaneously or persist for life despite discontinuation of drug.
• Evaluate patient's and family's knowledge of drug therapy.

Nursing diagnoses

• Impaired thought processes related to psychosis
• Impaired physical mobility related to extrapyramidal reactions
• Deficient knowledge related to drug therapy

Planning and implementation

ALERT Prolixin concentrate and Permitil concentrate are 10 times more concentrated than Prolixin elixir (5 mg/ml vs. 0.5 mg/ml). Check dosage order carefully.
P.O. use: Dilute liquid concentrate with water, fruit juice (except apple), milk, or semisolid food just before administration.
I.M. and S.C. use: For long-acting forms (decanoate and enanthate), which are oil preparations, use dry needle of at least 21G. Allow 24 to 96 hours for onset of action. Note and report adverse reactions in patient taking these drug forms.
• Oral liquid and parenteral forms can cause contact dermatitis. Wear gloves when preparing solutions, and avoid contact with skin and clothing.
• Protect drug from light. Slight yellowing of injection or concentrate is common and doesn't affect potency. Discard markedly discolored solutions.
• Withhold dose and notify prescriber if patient develops symptoms of blood dyscrasia (fever, sore throat, infection, cellulitis, weakness) or persistent extrapyramidal reactions (longer than a few hours), especially in a pregnant woman or child.
• Acute dystonic reactions may be treated with diphenhydramine.
• Don't withdraw drug abruptly unless severe adverse reactions occur. After abrupt withdrawal of long-term therapy, patient may experience gastritis, nausea, vomiting, dizziness, tremor, feeling of warmth or cold, diaphoresis, tachycardia, headache, and insomnia.

Patient teaching

• Warn patient to avoid activities that require alertness and psychomotor coordination until CNS effects of drug are known.
• Tell patient not to mix concentrate with beverages containing caffeine, tannics (such as tea) or pectinates (such as apple juice).
• Tell patient to avoid alcohol during therapy.
• Advise patient to relieve dry mouth with sugarless gum or hard candy.
• Have patient report urine retention or constipation.

- Tell patient to use sunblock and to wear protective clothing.
- Inform patient that drug may discolor urine.
- Stress importance of not stopping drug suddenly.

☑ Evaluation

- Patient demonstrates decrease in psychotic behavior.
- Patient maintains pretreatment physical mobility.
- Patient and family state understanding of drug therapy.

flurazepam hydrochloride

(floo-RAH-zuh-pam high-droh-KLOR-ighd)
Apo-Flurazepam ♦, Dalmane, Novo-Flupam ♦

Pharmacologic class: benzodiazepine
Therapeutic class: sedative-hypnotic
Controlled substance schedule: IV
Pregnancy risk category: X

Indications and dosages

▶ **Insomnia.** *Adults:* 15 to 30 mg P.O. h.s. Dose repeated once, p.r.n.

How supplied

Capsules: 15 mg, 30 mg

Pharmacokinetics

Absorption: absorbed rapidly through GI tract.
Distribution: distributed widely throughout body; about 97% bound to plasma protein.
Metabolism: metabolized in liver to active metabolite desalkylflurazepam.
Excretion: excreted in urine. Half-life: 50 to 100 hours.

Route	Onset	Peak	Duration
P.O.	Unknown	0.5-1 hr	Unknown

Pharmacodynamics

Chemical effect: unknown; may act on limbic system, thalamus, and hypothalamus of CNS to produce hypnotic effects.
Therapeutic effect: promotes sleep and calmness.

Adverse reactions

CNS: *daytime sedation, dizziness, drowsiness, disturbed coordination,* lethargy, confusion, *headache,* light-headedness, nervousness, hallucinations, staggering, ataxia, disorientation, ***coma.***
GI: nausea, vomiting, heartburn, diarrhea, abdominal pain.
Hepatic: elevated liver enzyme levels.
Other: physical or psychological dependence.

Interactions

Drug-drug. *Cimetidine:* increased sedation. Monitor patient carefully.
CNS depressants, including narcotic analgesics: excessive CNS depression. Use together cautiously.
Digoxin: digoxin serum levels may increase, resulting in toxicity. Monitor patient and digoxin levels closely.
Disulfiram, isoniazid, oral contraceptives: decreased metabolism of benzodiazepines, leading to toxicity. Monitor patient closely.
Phenytoin: increased phenytoin levels. Monitor patient for toxicity.
Rifampin: enhanced metabolism of benzodiazepines. Monitor patient for decreased effectiveness.
Theophylline: antagonist with flurazepam. Monitor patient for decreased effectiveness.
Drug-herb. *Kava, catnip, lady's slipper, lemon balm, passionflower, sassafras, skullcap, valerian:* sedative effects may be enhanced. Discourage concurrent use.
Drug-lifestyle. *Alcohol use:* excessive CNS and respiratory depression. Discourage concurrent use.
Smoking: enhanced metabolism of benzodiazepines. Discourage concomitant use.

Contraindications and precautions

- Contraindicated in patients hypersensitive to drug and in pregnant women.
- Drug isn't recommended for breast-feeding women.
- Use cautiously in patients with impaired hepatic or renal function, chronic pulmonary insufficiency, mental depression, suicidal tendencies, or history of drug abuse.
- Safety of drug hasn't been established in children under age 15.

NURSING CONSIDERATIONS

Assessment
- Assess patient's sleep patterns and CNS status before therapy.
- Evaluate patient's ability to sleep. Drug is more effective on second, third, and fourth nights of use.
- Be alert for adverse reactions and drug interactions.
- Evaluate patient's and family's knowledge of drug therapy.

Nursing diagnoses
- Disturbed sleep pattern related to underlying patient problem
- Risk for trauma related to drug-induced adverse CNS reactions
- Deficient knowledge related to drug therapy

Planning and implementation
- Before leaving bedside, make sure patient has swallowed capsule.

Patient teaching
- Encourage patient to continue drug, even if it doesn't relieve insomnia on first night.
- Warn patient to avoid activities that require alertness or physical coordination. For inpatient, supervise walking and raise bed rails, particularly for elderly patient.
- Advise patient that physical and psychological dependence is possible with long-term use.

Evaluation
- Patient notes drug-induced sleep.
- Patient's safety is maintained.
- Patient and family state understanding of drug therapy.

flurbiprofen
(flur-bih-PROH-fen)

Ansaid, Apo-Flurbiprofen♦, Froben♦, Froben SR♦, Novo-Flurprofen♦, Nu-Flurbiprofen♦

Pharmacologic class: NSAID, phenylalkanoic acid derivative
Therapeutic class: antiarthritic
Pregnancy risk category: B

Indications and dosages
▶ **Rheumatoid arthritis and osteoarthritis.** *Adults:* 200 to 300 mg P.O. daily, divided b.i.d. to q.i.d. Where available, patients maintained on 200 mg daily may switch to one 200-mg extended-release capsule P.O. daily, taken in evening after food.

How supplied
Tablets: 50 mg, 100 mg
Capsules (extended-release)*♦*: 200 mg

Pharmacokinetics
Absorption: well absorbed. Administering with food alters rate, but not extent, of absorption.
Distribution: highly bound to plasma proteins.
Metabolism: metabolized primarily in liver.
Excretion: excreted primarily in urine. *Half-life:* 6½ hours.

Route	Onset	Peak	Duration
P.O.	Unknown	About 2 hr	Unknown

Pharmacodynamics
Chemical effect: unknown; possibly inhibits prostaglandin synthesis.
Therapeutic effect: relieves pain.

Adverse reactions
CNS: *headache,* anxiety, insomnia, increased reflexes, tremors, amnesia, asthenia, drowsiness, malaise, depression, dizziness.
CV: *edema,* ***heart failure,*** hypertension, vasodilation.
EENT: rhinitis, tinnitus, visual changes, epistaxis.
GI: *dyspepsia, diarrhea, abdominal pain, nausea,* constipation, ***bleeding,*** flatulence, vomiting.
GU: *symptoms suggesting urinary tract infection,* hematuria, interstitial nephritis, ***renal failure.***
Hematologic: ***thrombocytopenia, neutropenia,*** anemia, ***aplastic anemia.***
Hepatic: elevated liver enzyme levels, jaundice.
Respiratory: asthma.
Skin: rash, photosensitivity, urticaria.
Other: ***angioedema,*** weight changes.

Interactions

Drug-drug. *Aspirin:* decreased flurbiprofen levels. Concomitant use isn't recommended.
Beta blockers: antihypertensive effect of beta blockers may be impaired. Monitor blood pressure.
Cyclosporine: increased risk of nephrotoxicity. Monitor patient closely.
Diuretics: possible decreased diuretic effect. Monitor patient closely.
Lithium: serum lithium levels may be increased. Monitor levels.
Methotrexate: increased risk of methotrexate toxicity. Monitor patient closely.
Oral anticoagulants: increased bleeding tendency. Monitor patient.
Drug-herb. *Dong quai, feverfew, garlic, ginger, horse chestnut, red clover:* possible increased risk of bleeding. Monitor patient closely.
St. John's wort: increased risk of photosensitivity. Advise patient to avoid unprotected exposure to sunlight.
Drug-lifestyle. *Alcohol use:* increased risk of adverse GI reactions. Discourage concomitant use.
Sun exposure: photosensitivity reactions may occur. Urge precautions.

Contraindications and precautions

- Contraindicated in patients hypersensitive to drug and in those with a history of aspirin- or NSAID-induced asthma, urticaria, or other allergic-type reactions.
- Drug isn't recommended for breast-feeding women or those in the third trimester of pregnancy.
- Use cautiously in patients with history of peptic ulcer disease, hepatic dysfunction, cardiac disease, or other conditions that may cause fluid retention or impaired renal function. Also use cautiously in pregnant women in first and second trimesters.
- Safety of drug hasn't been established in children.

NURSING CONSIDERATIONS

Assessment

- Assess patient's arthritis before therapy and regularly thereafter.
- Patient receiving long-term therapy should have periodic liver function studies, eye examinations, and hematocrit determinations.
- Be alert for adverse reactions and drug interactions.
- Evaluate patient's and family's knowledge of drug therapy.

Nursing diagnoses

- Acute pain related to presence of arthritis
- Diarrhea related to drug-induced adverse effect
- Deficient knowledge related to drug therapy

Planning and implementation

- Elderly or debilitated patient or patient with hepatic or renal dysfunction should be monitored closely and probably should receive reduced dosage.
- Give drug with food, milk, or antacid if GI upset occurs.

Patient teaching

- Tell patient to take drug with food, milk, or antacid if GI upset occurs.
- Tell patient taking extended-release capsule to swallow it whole and not to crush, chew, or break it open.
- Advise patient to avoid hazardous activities that require mental alertness until CNS effects are known.
- Serious GI toxicity, including peptic ulceration and bleeding, can occur in patients taking NSAIDs despite absence of GI symptoms. Teach signs and symptoms of GI bleeding, and tell patient to contact prescriber immediately if they occur.

Evaluation

- Patient is free from pain.
- Patient regains normal bowel pattern.
- Patient and family state understanding of drug therapy.

flutamide

(FLOO-tuh-mighd)
Euflex◆, Eulexin

Pharmacologic class: nonsteroidal antiandrogen
Therapeutic class: antineoplastic
Pregnancy risk category: D

Indications and dosages

▶ **Metastatic prostatic carcinoma (stage D2).** *Adults:* 250 mg P.O. q 8 hours. Used with luteinizing hormone–releasing hormone analogues such as leuprolide acetate.

How supplied

Capsules: 125 mg
Tablets: 250 mg◆

Pharmacokinetics

Absorption: absorbed rapidly and completely.
Distribution: animal studies show drug concentrates in prostate. Drug and its active metabolite are about 95% protein-bound.
Metabolism: over 97% of drug is metabolized rapidly, with at least six metabolites identified.
Excretion: over 95% excreted in urine. *Half-life:* 6 hours.

Route	Onset	Peak	Duration
P.O.	Unknown	2 hr	Unknown

Pharmacodynamics

Chemical effect: inhibits androgen uptake or prevents androgen binding in cell nuclei in target tissues.
Therapeutic effect: hinders prostatic cancer cell activity.

Adverse reactions

CNS: drowsiness, confusion, depression, anxiety, nervousness, paresthesia.
CV: peripheral edema, hypertension.
GI: *diarrhea, nausea, vomiting,* anorexia.
GU: *impotence.*
Hematologic: ***thrombocytopenia, leukopenia,*** anemia, hemolytic anemia.
Hepatic: elevated liver enzyme levels, ***hepatitis,*** encephalopathy.
Skin: rash, photosensitivity.
Other: *hot flushes, loss of libido,* gynecomastia.

Interactions

Drug-drug. *Warfarin:* may increase PT. Monitor patient's PT and INR.
Drug-lifestyle. *Sun exposure:* may cause sensitivity reactions. Warn patient to take appropriate precautions.

Contraindications and precautions

- Contraindicated in patients hypersensitive to drug.
- Drug isn't indicated for female patients.
- Safety of drug hasn't been established in male children.

NURSING CONSIDERATIONS

Assessment

- Assess patient's prostatic cancer before therapy.
- Monitor liver function tests periodically, as ordered.
- Be alert for adverse reactions.
- Monitor hydration status if adverse GI reactions occur.
- Evaluate patient's and family's knowledge of drug therapy.

Nursing diagnoses

- Ineffective health maintenance related to presence of prostatic cancer
- Risk for deficient fluid volume related to adverse GI reactions
- Deficient knowledge related to drug therapy

Planning and implementation

- Drug may be given without regard to meals.
- Give with luteinizing hormone–releasing antagonist (such as leuprolide acetate), as ordered.

Patient teaching

- Make sure patient knows that flutamide must be taken continuously with drug used for medical castration (such as leuprolide acetate) to allow full benefit of therapy. Leuprolide suppresses testosterone production while flutamide inhibits testosterone action at cellular

level. Together they can impair growth of androgen-responsive tumors. Advise patient not to discontinue either drug.
• Tell patient to notify prescriber if adverse reactions occur.

✓ Evaluation
• Patient responds well to drug.
• Patient maintains adequate hydration throughout drug therapy.
• Patient and family state understanding of drug therapy.

fluticasone propionate
(FLU-tih-ka-sohn proh-PIGH-oh-nayt)
Flovent Inhalation Aerosol,
Flovent Rotadisk

Pharmacologic class: corticosteroid
Therapeutic class: topical and inhalation anti-inflammatory
Pregnancy risk category: C

Indications and dosages
▶ **Maintenance treatment of asthma as prevention and for patients who need oral corticosteroid for chronic asthma. (Flovent Inhalation Aerosol.)** *Adults and children age 12 and over:* in those previously taking bronchodilators alone, initially, inhaled dose of 88 mcg b.i.d. to maximum of 440 mcg b.i.d.
Patients previously taking inhaled corticosteroids: initially, inhaled dose of 88 to 220 mcg b.i.d. to maximum of 440 mcg b.i.d.
Patients previously taking oral corticosteroids: inhaled dose of 880 mcg b.i.d. **(Flovent Rotadisk.)** *Adults and adolescents:* in patients previously taking bronchodilators alone, initially, inhaled dose of 100 mcg b.i.d. to maximum of 500 mcg b.i.d.
Patients previously taking inhaled corticosteroids: initially, inhaled dose of 100 to 250 mcg b.i.d. to maximum of 500 mcg b.i.d.
Patients previously taking oral corticosteroids: inhaled dose of 1,000 mcg b.i.d.
Children ages 4 to 11: For patients previously on bronchodilators alone or on inhaled corticosteroids, initially, inhaled dose of 50 mcg b.i.d. to maximum of 100 mcg b.i.d.

How supplied
Oral inhalation aerosol: 44 mcg, 110 mcg, 220 mcg
Oral inhalation powder: 50 mcg, 100 mcg, 250 mcg

Pharmacokinetics
Absorption: rapidly and completely absorbed after P.O. administration.
Distribution: animal studies show drug concentrates in prostate. Drug and its active metabolite are about 95% protein-bound.
Metabolism: rapid, with at least 6 metabolites identified. More than 97% of drug is metabolized within 1 hour of administration.
Excretion: more than 95% of drug is excreted in urine.

Route	Onset	Peak	Duration
Inhalation	24 hr	1-2 wk	Several days

Pharmacodynamics
Chemical effect: synthetic glucocorticoid with potent anti-inflammatory activity inhibits many cell types and mediator production or secretion involved in asthma. These anti-inflammatory actions may contribute to drug's efficacy in asthma.
Therapeutic effect: improves breathing ability.

Adverse reactions
CNS: *headache*, dizziness, migraine, nervousness.
EENT: mouth irritation, *oral candidiasis, pharyngitis,* acute nasopharyngitis, nasal congestion, sinusitis, dysphonia, rhinitis, otitis media, tonsillitis, nasal discharge, earache, laryngitis, epistaxis, sneezing, hoarseness, conjunctivitis, eye irritation.
GI: diarrhea, abdominal pain, viral gastroenteritis, colitis, abdominal discomfort, nausea, vomiting.
GU: dysmenorrhea, candidiasis of vagina, pelvic inflammatory disease, vaginitis, vulvovaginitis, irregular menstrual cycle.
Metabolic: cushingoid features, weight gain.
Musculoskeletal: growth retardation in children, pain in joints, aches and pains, disorder or symptoms of neck sprain or strain, sore muscles.

Respiratory: *upper respiratory tract infection,* bronchitis, chest congestion, dyspnea, irritation from inhalant.
Skin: dermatitis, urticaria.
Other: dental problems, fever, influenza.

Interactions

Drug-drug. *Ketoconazole*: increased mean fluticasone levels. Use care when giving fluticasone with long-term ketoconazole and other known cytochrome P-450 3A4 inhibitors.

Contraindications

- Contraindicated in patients hypersensitive to ingredients of these preparations.
- Also contraindicated in primary treatment of patients with status asthmaticus or other acute episodes of asthma in whom intensive measures are needed.

NURSING CONSIDERATIONS

Assessment

- Obtain history of patient's underlying condition before therapy, and reassess regularly thereafter.
- Because of risk of systemic absorption of inhaled corticosteroids, observe patient carefully for evidence of systemic corticosteroid effects.
- Monitor patient, especially postoperatively or during periods of stress, for evidence of inadequate adrenal response.
- Ask woman if she's breast-feeding; use drug cautiously in these patients.
- Evaluate patient's and family's knowledge of drug therapy.

Nursing diagnoses

- Ineffective breathing pattern related to respiratory condition
- Impaired oral mucous membrane related to potential adverse effect of oral candidiasis
- Deficient knowledge related to drug therapy

Planning and implementation

- For patients starting therapy who are currently receiving oral corticosteroid therapy, reduce prednisone dose to no more than 2.5 mg/day on a weekly basis, beginning after at least 1 week of therapy with fluticasone, as ordered.
- During withdrawal from oral corticosteroids, some patients may have symptoms of systemically active corticosteroid withdrawal, such as joint or muscle pain, lassitude, and depression, despite maintenance or even improvement of respiratory function.
- As with other inhaled asthma drugs, bronchospasm may occur with an immediate increase in wheezing after dosing. If bronchospasm occurs following fluticasone inhalation aerosol, it should be treated immediately with a fast-acting inhaled bronchodilator.
- Some patients on high doses of fluticasone may have an abnormal response to the 6-hour cosyntropin stimulation test.

Patient teaching

- Tell patient that drug isn't intended to relieve acute bronchospasm.
- For proper use of drug and to attain maximum improvement, tell patient to follow carefully the accompanying patient instructions.
- Advise patient to use drug at regular intervals as directed.
- Instruct patient not to increase dosage but to contact prescriber if symptoms don't improve or if condition worsens.
- Instruct patient to contact prescriber immediately when episodes of asthma that aren't responsive to bronchodilators occur during course of treatment with fluticasone. During such episodes, patients may need therapy with oral corticosteroids.
- Warn patient to avoid exposure to chickenpox or measles and, if exposed, to consult prescriber immediately.
- Tell patient to carry or wear medical identification indicating that he may need supplementary corticosteroids during stress or a severe asthma attack.
- During periods of stress or a severe asthma attack, instruct patient who has been withdrawn from systemic corticosteroids to resume oral corticosteroids (in large doses) immediately and to contact prescriber for further instruction. Instruct him to rinse his mouth after inhalation.
- Advise patient to avoid spraying inhalation aerosol into eyes.
- Instruct patient to shake canister well before using inhalation aerosol.

• Advise patient to store fluticasone powder in a dry place.

☑ Evaluation

• Patient has normal breathing pattern.
• Patient doesn't develop oral candidiasis.
• Patient and family state understanding of drug therapy.

fluvastatin sodium

(floo-vuh-STAH-tin SOH-dee-um)

Lescol

Pharmacologic class: hydroxymethylglutaryl-coenzyme A (HMG-CoA) reductase inhibitor
Therapeutic class: cholesterol inhibitor
Pregnancy risk category: X

Indications and dosages

▶ **Reduction of low-density lipoprotein (LDL) and total cholesterol levels in patients with primary hypercholesterolemia (types IIa and IIb) or to slow progression of coronary atherosclerosis in patients with coronary artery disease; treatment of elevated triglyceride and apolipoprotein B levels in patients with primary hypercholesterolemia and mixed dyslipidemia whose response to dietary restriction and other nonpharmacologic measures has been inadequate.** *Adults:* initially, 20 to 40 mg P.O. h.s. Increase dosage as needed to maximum of 80 mg daily (given in divided doses).

How supplied

Capsules: 20 mg, 40 mg

Pharmacokinetics

Absorption: absorbed rapidly and virtually completely (98%) after P.O. administration on empty stomach.
Distribution: more than 98% bound to plasma proteins.
Metabolism: completely metabolized in liver.
Excretion: about 5% excreted in urine, 90% in feces.

Route	Onset	Peak	Duration
P.O.	Unknown	Unknown	Unknown

Pharmacodynamics

Chemical effect: inhibits 3-hydroxy-3-methylglutaryl coenzyme A reductase. This enzyme is early (and rate-limiting) step in synthetic pathway of cholesterol.
Therapeutic effect: lowers blood LDL and cholesterol levels.

Adverse reactions

CNS: headache, fatigue, dizziness, insomnia.
EENT: sinusitis, rhinitis, pharyngitis.
GI: dyspepsia, diarrhea, nausea, vomiting, abdominal pain, constipation, flatulence.
Hematologic: ***thrombocytopenia, leukopenia,*** hemolytic anemia.
Hepatic: increased liver enzyme levels.
Musculoskeletal: arthropathy, muscle pain.
Respiratory: *upper respiratory infection,* cough, bronchitis.
Skin: ***hypersensitivity reactions*** (rash, pruritus).
Other: tooth disorder.

Interactions

Drug-drug. *Cholestyramine, colestipol:* may bind with fluvastatin in GI tract and decrease absorption. Separate administration times by at least 4 hours.
Cimetidine, omeprazole, ranitidine: decreased fluvastatin metabolism. Monitor patient for enhanced effects.
Cyclosporine and other immunosuppressants, erythromycin, gemfibrozil, niacin: possible increased risk of polymyositis and rhabdomyolysis. Avoid concomitant use.
Digoxin: may alter digoxin pharmacokinetics. Monitor serum digoxin levels carefully.
Rifampin: enhanced fluvastatin metabolism and decreased plasma levels. Monitor patient for lack of effect.
Warfarin: increased anticoagulant effect with bleeding. Monitor patient.
Drug-herb. *Red yeast rice:* contains components similar to those of statin drugs, increasing the risk of adverse events or toxicity. Discourage concomitant use.
Drug-lifestyle. *Alcohol use:* increased risk of hepatotoxicity. Discourage concomitant use.

Contraindications and precautions

• Contraindicated in patients hypersensitive to drug, in those with active liver disease or conditions that cause unexplained persistent elevations of serum transaminase levels, in pregnant or breast-feeding women, and in women of childbearing age unless they have no risk of pregnancy.
• Use cautiously in patients with severe renal impairment or with history of liver disease or heavy alcohol use.
• Safety of drug hasn't been established in children under age 18.

NURSING CONSIDERATIONS

Assessment

• Assess patient's blood LDL and cholesterol levels before therapy, and evaluate regularly thereafter.
• Liver function tests should be performed periodically.
• Be alert for adverse reactions and drug interactions.
• Evaluate patient's and family's knowledge of drug therapy.

Nursing diagnoses

• Risk for injury related to elevated LDL and cholesterol blood levels
• Diarrhea related to adverse effect of drug on GI tract
• Deficient knowledge related to drug therapy

Planning and implementation

• Drug should be started only after diet and other nondrug therapies have proven ineffective.
• Give drug at bedtime to enhance effectiveness.
• Maintain standard low-cholesterol diet during therapy.

Patient teaching

• Tell patient that drug may be taken without regard to meals; efficacy is enhanced if taken in evening.
• Teach patient about proper dietary management, weight control, and exercise. Explain their importance in controlling serum lipid levels.
• Warn patient to restrict alcohol consumption.
• Tell patient to inform prescriber of any adverse reactions, particularly muscle aches and pains.
• Tell patient to stop drug and notify prescriber about planned, suspected, or known pregnancy.

Evaluation

• Patient's blood LDL and cholesterol levels are within normal limits.
• Patient maintains normal bowel pattern.
• Patient and family state understanding of drug therapy.

fluvoxamine maleate

(floo-VOKS-uh-meen MAL-ee-ayt)
Luvox

Pharmacologic class: serotonin reuptake inhibitor
Therapeutic class: antidepressant
Pregnancy risk category: C

Indications and dosages

▶ **Obsessive-compulsive disorder.** *Adults:* initially, 50 mg P.O. daily h.s. Increased in 50-mg increments q 4 to 7 days until maximum benefit occurs. Maximum, 300 mg daily. Total daily doses of more than 100 mg should be given in two divided doses.
Children ages 8 to 17: 25 mg P.O. daily h.s. Dose may be increased in 25-mg increments q 4 to 7 days as tolerated until maximum benefit achieved. Maximum, 200 mg daily. Total daily doses exceeding 50 mg should be given in two divided doses.

How supplied

Tablets: 25 mg, 50 mg, 100 mg

Pharmacokinetics

Absorption: unknown.
Distribution: 77% protein-bound.
Metabolism: metabolized in liver.
Excretion: excreted in urine. *Half-life:* 17 hours.

Route	Onset	Peak	Duration
P.O.	Unknown	3-8 hr	Unknown

Pharmacodynamics

Chemical effect: unknown; selectively inhibits neuronal uptake of serotonin, which is thought to reduce obsessive-compulsive disorders.
Therapeutic effect: relieves obsessive-compulsive behavior.

Adverse reactions

CNS: *headache, asthenia, somnolence, insomnia, nervousness,* dizziness, tremor, anxiety, hypertonia, *agitation,* depression, CNS stimulation.
CV: palpitations, vasodilation.
EENT: amblyopia.
GI: *nausea, diarrhea, constipation, dyspepsia,* anorexia, *vomiting,* flatulence, dysphagia, taste perversion, *dry mouth.*
GU: abnormal ejaculation, urinary frequency, impotence, anorgasmia, urine retention.
Respiratory: upper respiratory tract infection, dyspnea, yawning.
Skin: sweating.
Other: decreased libido, flulike syndrome, chills, tooth disorder.

Interactions

Drug-drug. *Benzodiazepines, theophylline, warfarin:* reduced clearance of these drugs by fluvoxamine. Use together cautiously (except for diazepam, which shouldn't be administered together with fluvoxamine). Dosage adjustments may be necessary.
Carbamazepine, clozapine, methadone, metopranolol, propranolol, tricyclic antidepressants: elevated serum levels of these drugs caused by fluvoxamine. Use together cautiously. Monitor patient closely for adverse reactions. Dosage adjustments may be necessary.
Diltiazem: bradycardia may occur. Monitor heart rate.
Lithium, tryptophan: may enhance fluvoxamine effects. Use together cautiously.
MAO inhibitors: may cause severe excitation, hyperpyrexia, myoclonus, delirium, and coma. Avoid concomitant use.
Drug-herb. *St. John's wort:* may cause serotonin syndrome. Discourage concomitant use.
Drug-food. *Caffeine:* decreased caffeine elimination and increased effects. Discourage concurrent use.
Drug-lifestyle. *Smoking:* decreased effectiveness of drug. Advise patient that smoking may decrease effectiveness of drug.

Contraindications and precautions

- Contraindicated in patients hypersensitive to drug or to other phenylpiperazine antidepressants and within 14 days of MAO inhibitor therapy.
- Drug isn't recommended for breast-feeding women.
- Use cautiously in patients with hepatic dysfunction, concomitant conditions that may affect hemodynamic responses or metabolism, or history of mania or seizures. Also use cautiously in pregnant women.
- Safety of drug hasn't been established in children younger than age 8.

NURSING CONSIDERATIONS

Assessment

- Assess patient's condition before therapy, and reassess regularly thereafter. Several weeks of therapy may be needed before positive response occurs.
- Be alert for adverse reactions and drug interactions.
- Evaluate patient's and family's knowledge of drug therapy.

Nursing diagnoses

- Ineffective individual coping related to underlying condition
- Diarrhea related to adverse effect of drug on GI tract
- Deficient knowledge related to drug therapy

Planning and implementation

- At least 14 days should elapse after stopping fluvoxamine before patient starts an MAO inhibitor, and at least 14 days should elapse before patient starts fluvoxamine after MAO inhibitor therapy has stopped.
- Give drug at bedtime.

Patient teaching

- Warn patient to avoid hazardous activities until CNS effects of drug are known.
- Advise patient to avoid alcoholic beverages during drug therapy.

• Alert patient that smoking may decrease effectiveness of drug.
• Instruct woman to notify prescriber about planned, suspected, or known pregnancy.
• Tell patient who develops rash, hives, or related allergic reaction to notify prescriber.
• Inform patient that several weeks of therapy may be needed to obtain full antidepressant effect. Once improvement occurs, advise patient not to stop drug unless directed by prescriber.
• Advise patient to check with prescriber before taking OTC medications or herbal remedies; interactions can occur.

Evaluation

• Patient's obsessive-compulsive behaviors are diminished.
• Patient maintains normal bowel patterns.
• Patient and family state understanding of drug therapy.

folic acid (vitamin B)

(FOH-lek AS-id)

Apo-Folic♦, Folvite, Novo-Folacid♦

Pharmacologic class: folic acid derivative
Therapeutic class: vitamin supplement
Pregnancy risk category: A

Indications and dosages

▶ **To maintain health.** *Neonates and infants to age 6 months:* 25 mcg.
Infants ages 6 months to 1 year: 35 mcg.
Children ages 1 to 3: 50 mcg.
Children ages 4 to 6: 75 mcg.
Children ages 7 to 11: 100 mcg.
Children ages 11 to 14: 150 mcg.
Men age 15 and over: 200 mcg.
Women age 15 and over: 180 mcg.
Pregnant women: 400 mcg.
Breast-feeding women: 280 mcg during first 6 months, 260 mcg during second 6 months.

▶ **Megaloblastic or macrocytic anemia caused by folic acid or other nutritional deficiency, hepatic disease, alcoholism, intestinal obstruction, excessive hemolysis.** *Adults and children over age 4:* 0.4 mg to 1 mg P.O., S.C., or I.M. daily. After anemia caused by folic acid deficiency is corrected, proper diet and supplements are needed to prevent recurrence.
Children under age 4: up to 0.3 mg P.O., S.C., or I.M. daily.
Pregnant and breast-feeding women: 0.8 mg P.O., S.C., or I.M. daily.

▶ **Prevention of megaloblastic anemia in pregnancy and fetal damage.** *Adults:* up to 1 mg P.O., S.C., or I.M. daily throughout pregnancy.

▶ **Nutritional supplement.** *Adults:* 0.1 mg P.O., S.C., or I.M. daily.
Children: 0.05 mg P.O. daily.

▶ **To test folic acid deficiency in patients with megaloblastic anemia without masking pernicious anemia.** *Adults and children:* 0.1 to 0.2 mg P.O. or I.M. for 10 days, with diet low in folate and vitamin B_{12}.

▶ **Tropical sprue.** *Adults:* 3 to 15 mg P.O. daily.

How supplied

Tablets: 0.1 mg†, 0.4 mg†, 0.8 mg†, 1 mg
Injection: 5 mg/ml with 1.5% benzyl alcohol or 10 mg/ml with 1.5% benzyl alcohol and 0.2% EDTA

Pharmacokinetics

Absorption: absorbed rapidly from GI tract, mainly from proximal part of small intestine, when administered orally. Absorption unknown after S.C. or I.M. administration.
Distribution: distributed into all body tissues; liver contains about half of total body folate stores. Folate is concentrated actively in CSF.
Metabolism: metabolized in liver.
Excretion: excess folate is excreted unchanged in urine; small amounts of folic acid have been recovered in feces. About 0.05 mg/day of normal body folate stores is lost by combination of urinary and fecal excretion and oxidative cleavage of molecule.

Route	Onset	Peak	Duration
P.O., S.C., I.M.	Unknown	30-60 min	Unknown

Pharmacodynamics

Chemical effect: stimulates normal erythropoiesis and nucleoprotein synthesis.
Therapeutic effect: nutritional supplement.

Adverse reactions

CNS: general malaise.
GI: bitter taste, anorexia, nausea, flatulence.
Respiratory: ***bronchospasm.***
Skin: allergic reactions (rash, pruritus, erythema).

Interactions

Drug-drug. *Aminosalicylic acid, chloramphenicol, methotrexate, sulfasalazine, trimethoprim:* antagonism of folic acid. Monitor patient for decreased folic acid effect. Use together cautiously.
Anticonvulsants (such as phenobarbital, phenytoin): increased anticonvulsant metabolism and decreased anticonvulsant blood levels. Monitor patient closely.

Contraindications and precautions

- Contraindicated in patients with B_{12} deficiency or undiagnosed anemia.

NURSING CONSIDERATIONS

Assessment

- Assess patient's folic acid deficiency before therapy.
- Evaluate CBC, and assess patient's physical status throughout therapy.
- Be alert for adverse reactions and drug interactions.
- Evaluate patient's and family's knowledge of drug therapy.

Nursing diagnoses

- Imbalanced nutrition: less than body requirements related to presence of folic acid deficiency
- Deficient knowledge related to drug therapy

Planning and implementation

- Patient with small-bowel resection and intestinal malabsorption may need parenteral administration.

P.O. and S.C. use: Follow normal protocol.
I.M. use: Don't mix with other drugs in same syringe for I.M. injections. Follow normal protocol.

- Protect from light and heat; store at room temperature.
- Concurrent folic acid and vitamin B_{12} therapy may be used if supported by diagnosis.
- Make sure patient is getting properly balanced diet.

Patient teaching

- Teach patient proper nutrition to prevent recurrence of anemia.
- Tell patient to report hypersensitivity reactions or breathing difficulty.
- Urge patient to avoid alcohol because it increases folic acid requirements.

Evaluation

- Patient's CBC is normal.
- Patient and family state understanding of drug therapy.

foscarnet sodium (phosphonoformic acid)

(fos-KAR-net SOH-dee-um)
Foscavir

Pharmacologic class: pyrophosphate analogue
Therapeutic class: antiviral
Pregnancy risk category: C

Indications and dosages

▶ **CMV retinitis in patients with AIDS.** *Adults:* initially, in patients with normal renal function, 60 mg/kg I.V. over 1 hour q 8 hours for 2 to 3 weeks, depending on clinical response. Or, 90 mg/kg I.V. q 12 hours over 1.5 to 2 hours for 2 to 3 weeks, depending on clinical response. Follow with maintenance infusion of 90 mg/kg/day I.V. over 2 hours; dose may be increased as needed and tolerated to 120 mg/kg daily if disease progresses.

▶ **Mucocutaneous acyclovir-resistant HSV infections.** *Adults:* 40 mg/kg I.V. infused over at least 1 hour, either q 8 or 12 hours for 2 to 3 weeks or until healed.

How supplied

Injection: 24 mg/ml in 250- and 500-ml bottles

Pharmacokinetics

Absorption: not applicable.
Distribution: unknown.
Metabolism: unknown.
Excretion: about 80% to 90% appears unchanged in urine. *Half-life:* about 3 hours.

Route	Onset	Peak	Duration
I.V.	Immediate	Immediate	Unknown

Pharmacodynamics

Chemical effect: inhibits all known herpes viruses in vitro by blocking pyrophosphate binding site on DNA polymerases and reverse transcriptases.
Therapeutic effect: inhibits herpes virus activity.

Adverse reactions

CNS: *headache,* ***seizures,*** *fatigue, malaise, asthenia, paresthesia, dizziness, hypesthesia, neuropathy,* tremor, ataxia, generalized spasms, dementia, stupor, sensory disturbances, ***meningitis,*** aphasia, abnormal coordination, EEG abnormalities, depression, confusion, anxiety, insomnia, somnolence, nervousness, amnesia, agitation, aggressive reaction.
CV: *hypertension, palpitations, ECG abnormalities, sinus tachycardia,* cerebrovascular disorder, *first-degree AV block, hypotension, flushing,* edema.
EENT: visual disturbances, eye pain, conjunctivitis, sinusitis, pharyngitis, rhinitis.
GI: taste perversion, dry mouth, *nausea, diarrhea, vomiting, abdominal pain, anorexia,* constipation, dysphagia, ***rectal hemorrhage,*** melena, flatulence, ulcerative stomatitis, ***pancreatitis.***
GU: *abnormal renal function, decreased creatinine clearance and increased serum creatinine level, albuminuria, dysuria, polyuria, urethral disorder, urine retention, urinary tract infection,* ***acute renal failure,*** candidiasis.
Hematologic: anemia, granulocytopenia, ***leukopenia, bone marrow suppression, thrombocytopenia,*** platelet abnormalities, thrombocytosis, WBC count abnormalities, lymphadenopathy.
Hepatic: abnormal hepatic function, increased liver enzyme levels.
Metabolic: hypokalemia, hypomagnesemia, hypophosphatemia or hyperphosphatemia, hypocalcemia, hyponatremia.
Musculoskeletal: leg cramps, arthralgia, myalgia.
Respiratory: *cough, dyspnea,* pneumonitis, respiratory insufficiency, pulmonary infiltration, stridor, pneumothorax, ***bronchospasm,*** hemoptysis.
Skin: *rash, increased sweating,* pruritus, skin ulceration, erythematous rash, seborrhea, skin discoloration, facial edema.
Other: *fever,* pain, ***sepsis,*** rigors, inflammation, pain at infusion site, lymphoma-like disorder, sarcoma, back or chest pain, bacterial or fungal infections, abscess, flulike symptoms..

Interactions

Drug-drug. *Nephrotoxic drugs (such as amphotericin B, aminoglycosides):* increased risk of nephrotoxicity. Avoid concomitant use.
Pentamidine: increased risk of nephrotoxicity and severe hypocalcemia. Don't use together.
Zidovudine: possible increased risk or severity of anemia. Monitor blood counts.

Contraindications and precautions

- Contraindicated in patients hypersensitive to drug.
- Use cautiously and in reduced amounts in patients with abnormal renal function, as ordered, because drug will accumulate and toxicity will increase. Because foscarnet is nephrotoxic, it may worsen renal impairment. Some nephrotoxicity occurs in most patients treated with drug.
- Also, use cautiously in pregnant or breast-feeding women.
- Safety of drug hasn't been established in children.

NURSING CONSIDERATIONS

Assessment

- Assess patient's infection before therapy and regularly thereafter.
- Obtain serum electrolyte levels and creatinine clearance before beginning therapy, as ordered.

• Monitor creatinine clearance two to three times weekly during induction and at least once every 1 to 2 weeks during maintenance.
• Because drug can adversely affect potassium, calcium, magnesium, and phosphorus, monitor levels using schedule similar to that established for creatinine clearance.
• Drug may cause dose-related transient decrease in ionized serum calcium, which may not be reflected in laboratory values. Assess for tetany and seizures with abnormal electrolyte levels.
• Monitor patient's hemoglobin and hematocrit levels. Anemia is common (in up to 33% of patients treated with drug). It may be severe enough that patient needs transfusions.
• Be alert for adverse reactions and drug interactions.
• Evaluate patient's and family's knowledge of drug therapy.

Nursing diagnoses
• Infection related to presence of herpesvirus susceptible to drug
• Disturbed sensory perception (tactile) related to drug's adverse effect
• Deficient knowledge related to drug therapy

Planning and implementation
• Use infusion pump to give drug over at least 1 hour. To minimize renal toxicity, ensure adequate hydration before and during infusion.
• Don't exceed recommended dosage, infusion rate, or frequency of administration. All doses must be individualized based on patient's renal function.
• Because drug is highly toxic and toxicity is probably dose-related, use lowest effective maintenance dose.
• Dosage must be adjusted when creatinine clearance is below 1.5 ml/minute/kg. If creatinine clearance falls below 0.4 ml/minute/kg, drug should be discontinued.

Patient teaching
• Advise patient to report circumoral tingling, numbness in limbs, and paresthesia.

Evaluation
• Patient is free from infection.
• Patient has no adverse neurologic reactions.
• Patient and family state understanding of drug therapy.

fosinopril sodium
(foh-SIN-oh-pril SOH-dee-um)
Monopril

Pharmacologic class: ACE inhibitor
Therapeutic class: antihypertensive
Pregnancy risk category: C (D in second and third trimesters)

Indications and dosages
▶ **Hypertension.** *Adults:* initially, 10 mg P.O. daily. Dosage is adjusted based on blood pressure response at peak and trough levels. Usual dosage is 20 to 40 mg, up to 80 mg daily. Dosage is divided if needed.
▶ **Adjunctive therapy for heart failure.** *Adults:* initially, 10 mg P.O. once daily. Dosage should be increased over several weeks to maximum tolerable, but no more than 40 mg P.O. daily.

How supplied
Tablets: 10 mg, 20 mg, 40 mg

Pharmacokinetics
Absorption: absorbed slowly through GI tract, primarily in proximal small intestine.
Distribution: more than 95% protein-bound.
Metabolism: hydrolyzed mainly in liver and gut.
Excretion: 50% excreted in urine; remainder in feces. *Half-life:* 11½ hours.

Route	Onset	Peak	Duration
P.O.	≤ 1 hr	2-6 hr	About 24 hr

Pharmacodynamics
Chemical effect: antihypertensive action not clearly defined. Inhibits ACE, preventing conversion of angiotensin I to angiotensin II, a potent vasoconstrictor. Reduced formation of angiotensin II decreases peripheral arterial resistance, thus decreasing aldosterone secretion.
Therapeutic effect: lowers blood pressure.

Adverse reactions

CNS: headache, dizziness, fatigue, syncope, paresthesia, sleep disturbance, ***CVA.***
CV: chest pain, angina, ***MI,*** rhythm disturbances, palpitations, hypotension, orthostatic hypotension.
EENT: tinnitus, sinusitis.
GI: dry mouth, nausea, vomiting, diarrhea, ***pancreatitis,*** abdominal distention, abdominal pain, constipation.
GU: sexual dysfunction, renal insufficiency.
Hepatic: ***hepatitis.***
Metabolic: gout, hyperkalemia.
Musculoskeletal: arthralgia, musculoskeletal pain, myalgia.
Respiratory: *dry, persistent, tickling, nonproductive cough;* ***bronchospasm.***
Skin: urticaria, rash, photosensitivity, pruritus.
Other: decreased libido, ***angioedema.***

Interactions

Drug-drug. *Antacids:* may impair absorption. Separate administration times by at least 2 hours.
Diuretics, other antihypertensives: risk of excessive hypotension. Diuretic may need to be discontinued or fosinopril dosage lowered.
Lithium: increased serum lithium levels and lithium toxicity. Avoid concomitant use.
Potassium-sparing diuretics, potassium supplements, sodium substitutes containing potassium: risk of hyperkalemia. Monitor serum potassium during concomitant use.
Drug-herb. *Licorice:* may cause sodium retention and increase blood pressure, interfering with therapeutic effect of ACE inhibitor. Discourage concomitant use.
Drug-food. *Salt substitutes containing potassium:* risk of hyperkalemia. Monitor serum potassium closely during concomitant use.
Drug-lifestyle. *Alcohol use:* additive hypotensive effects. Discourage concomitant use.

Contraindications and precautions

- Contraindicated in patients hypersensitive to drug or other ACE inhibitors and in breast-feeding women.
- Use with extreme caution and only when necessary in pregnant women to prevent fetal harm.
- Use cautiously in patients with impaired renal or hepatic function.
- Safety of drug hasn't been established in children.

NURSING CONSIDERATIONS

Assessment

- Assess blood pressure before therapy and regularly thereafter.
- Assess renal and hepatic function before and during therapy.
- Monitor potassium intake and serum potassium level. Diabetic patients, those with impaired renal function, and those receiving drugs that can increase serum potassium may develop hyperkalemia.
- Other ACE inhibitors have been linked to agranulocytosis and neutropenia. Monitor CBC with differential counts before therapy, every 2 weeks for first 3 months of therapy, and periodically thereafter.
- Monitor patient's hydration status if adverse GI reactions occur.
- Evaluate patient's and family's knowledge of drug therapy.

Nursing diagnoses

- Risk for injury related to presence of hypertension
- Risk for deficient fluid volume related to adverse GI reactions
- Deficient knowledge related to drug therapy

Planning and implementation

- Drug may be taken without regard to meals. However, taking drug with food slows absorption of drug.

Patient teaching

- Tell patient to avoid sodium substitutes; they may contain potassium, which increases the risk of hyperkalemia.
- Urge patient to report signs of infection (such as fever and sore throat); easy bruising or bleeding; swelling of tongue, lips, face, eyes, mucous membranes, or limbs; difficulty swallowing or breathing; and hoarseness.
- Tell patient to use caution in hot weather and during exercise. Inadequate fluid intake, vom-

iting, diarrhea, and excessive perspiration can lead to light-headedness and syncope.
• Tell woman to notify prescriber about planned, suspected, or known pregnancy. Drug will probably need to be discontinued.

☑ Evaluation
• Patient's blood pressure is normal.
• Patient maintains adequate hydration throughout drug therapy.
• Patient and family state understanding of drug therapy.

fosphenytoin sodium
(fahs-FEN-eh-toyn SOH-dee-um)
Cerebyx

Pharmacologic class: prodrug of phenytoin
Therapeutic class: anticonvulsant
Pregnancy risk category: D

Indications and dosages
▶ **Status epilepticus.** *Adults:* 15 to 20 mg phenytoin sodium equivalent (PE)/kg I.V. at 100 to 150 mg PE/minute as loading dose; then 4 to 6 mg PE/kg/day I.V. as maintenance dose. (Phenytoin may be used instead of fosphenytoin as maintenance, using the appropriate dose.)
▶ **Prevention and treatment of seizures during neurosurgery (nonemergent loading or maintenance dosing).** *Adults:* loading dose of 10 to 20 mg PE/kg I.M. or I.V. at infusion rate not exceeding 150 mg PE/minute. Maintenance dose is 4 to 6 mg PE/kg/day I.V. or I.M.
▶ **Short-term substitution for oral phenytoin therapy.** *Adults:* same total daily dosage equivalent as oral phenytoin sodium therapy given as a single daily dose I.M. or I.V. at infusion rate not exceeding 150 mg PE/minute. Some patients may need more frequent dosing.

How supplied
Injection: 2 ml (150 mg fosphenytoin sodium equivalent to 100 mg phenytoin sodium), 10 ml (750 mg fosphenytoin sodium equivalent to 500 mg phenytoin sodium)

Pharmacokinetics
Absorption: completely absorbed following I.M. and I.V. use.
Distribution: widely throughout body; 95% plasma protein–bound.
Metabolism: in liver.
Excretion: in urine.

Route	Onset	Peak	Duration
I.V.	Unknown	Immediate	Unknown
I.M.	Unknown	30 min	Unknown

Pharmacodynamics
Chemical effect: because fosphenytoin is a prodrug of phenytoin, its anticonvulsant action is the same. Phenytoin is thought to stabilize neuronal membranes and limit seizure activity.
Therapeutic effect: prevents and controls seizures.

Adverse reactions
CNS: increased or decreased reflexes, speech disorders, dysarthria, asthenia, ***intracranial hypertension***, thinking abnormalities, nervousness, hypesthesia, extrapyramidal syndrome, ***cerebral edema,*** headache, *nystagmus, dizziness, somnolence, ataxia,* stupor, incoordination, paresthesia, tremor, agitation, vertigo.
CV: hypertension, vasodilation, tachycardia, hypotension.
GI: taste perversion, constipation.
Hematologic: ***thrombocytopenia, leukopenia, agranulocytosis, granulocytopenia, pancytopenia.***
Metabolic: hypokalemia, hyperglycemia.
Musculoskeletal: back pain, myasthenia, pelvic pain.
Respiratory: pneumonia.
Skin: ecchymosis, injection site reaction and pain, rash, *pruritus.*
Other: lymphadenopathy, accidental injury, infection, chills.

Interactions
Drug-drug. *Amiodarone, chloramphenicol, chlordiazepoxide, cimetidine, diazepam, dicumarol, disulfiram, estrogens, ethosuximide, fluoxetine,* H_2*-receptor antagonists,*

halothane, isoniazid, methylphenidate, phenothiazines, phenylbutazone, salicylates, succinimides, sulfonamides, tolbutamide, trazodone: may increase plasma phenytoin levels and thus its therapeutic effects. Use together cautiously.
Carbamazepine, reserpine: may decrease plasma phenytoin levels. Monitor patient.
Coumarin, digitoxin, doxycycline, estrogens, furosemide, oral contraceptives, rifampin, quinidine, theophylline, vitamin D: efficacy may be decreased by phenytoin because of increased hepatic metabolism. Monitor patient closely.
Phenobarbital, valproic acid, sodium valproate: may increase or decrease plasma phenytoin levels. Monitor patient.
Tricyclic antidepressants: may lower seizure threshold and require adjustments in phenytoin dosage. Use cautiously.
Drug-lifestyle. *Acute alcohol use:* may increase plasma phenytoin levels and thus its therapeutic effects. Use together cautiously.
Chronic alcohol use: may decrease plasma phenytoin levels. Monitor patient.

Contraindications and precautions

- Contraindicated in patients hypersensitive to drug, its components, phenytoin, or other hydantoins. Also, contraindicated in patients with sinus bradycardia, SA block, second- or third-degree AV block, or Adams-Stokes syndrome.

NURSING CONSIDERATIONS

Assessment
- Don't give drug I.M. for status epilepticus because therapeutic phenytoin levels may not occur as rapidly as with I.V. administration.
- After drug administration, phenytoin levels shouldn't be monitored until about 2 hours after the end of I.V. infusion or 4 hours after I.M. administration.
- Evaluate patient's and family's knowledge of drug therapy.

Nursing diagnoses
- Risk for trauma related to seizures
- Deficient knowledge related to drug therapy

Planning and implementation
- Drug should always be prescribed and dispensed in phenytoin sodium equivalent units (PE). Don't make any adjustments in recommended doses when substituting fosphenytoin for phenytoin, and vice versa.

I.V. use: Before I.V. infusion, dilute drug in D_5W or normal saline solution for injection to a level ranging from 1.5 to 25 mg PE/ml. Don't exceed 150 mg PE/minute.
– Monitor patient's ECG, blood pressure, and respiration throughout period of maximal serum phenytoin levels—about 10 to 20 minutes after end of fosphenytoin infusion.
I.M. use: I.M. use generates systemic phenytoin levels similar to oral phenytoin sodium, allowing essentially interchangeable use.
- Abrupt withdrawal of drug may cause status epilepticus.

ALERT Don't confuse Cerebyx with Celexa or Celebrex.

Patient teaching
- Warn patient that sensory disturbances may occur with I.V. use.
- Instruct patient to immediately report adverse reactions, especially rash.
- Warn patient not to stop drug abruptly or to adjust dosage without consulting prescriber.
- Inform women that breast-feeding isn't recommended.

Evaluation
- Patient is free from seizures.
- Patient and family state understanding of drug therapy.

furosemide (frusemide◆)

(fyoo-ROH-seh-mighd)
Apo-Furosemide◆, Furoside◆, Lasix*, Lasix Special◆, Myrosemide*, Novosemide◆, Uritol◆

Pharmacologic class: loop diuretic
Therapeutic class: diuretic, antihypertensive
Pregnancy risk category: C

Indications and dosages

▶ **Acute pulmonary edema.** *Adults:* 40 mg I.V. injected slowly over 1 to 2 minutes; then 80 mg I.V. in 1 to 1½ hours, if needed.
Infants and children: 1 mg/kg I.M. or I.V. If desired results don't occur after 2 hours, may increase initial dose by 1 mg/kg. Dosing interval should be at least 2 hours.

▶ **Edema.** *Adults:* 20 to 80 mg P.O. daily in a.m., second dose in 6 to 8 hours; carefully adjusted up to 600 mg daily if needed. Or, 20 to 40 mg I.M. or I.V., increased by 20 mg q 2 hours until desired response occurs. Give I.V. dose slowly over 1 to 2 minutes.
Infants and children: 2 mg/kg P.O. daily, increased by 1 to 2 mg/kg in 6 to 8 hours if needed; carefully adjusted up to 6 mg/kg daily if needed.

▶ **Hypertension.** *Adults:* 40 mg P.O. b.i.d. Dosage adjusted according to response.

How supplied

Tablets: 20 mg, 40 mg, 80 mg, 500 mg ♦
Oral solution: 40 mg/5 ml, 10 mg/ml*
Injection: 10 mg/ml

Pharmacokinetics

Absorption: about 60% absorbed from GI tract after P.O. administration; unknown after I.M. use.
Distribution: about 95% plasma protein-bound.
Metabolism: metabolized minimally by liver.
Excretion: about 50% to 80% excreted in urine. *Half-life:* about 30 minutes.

Route	Onset	Peak	Duration
P.O.	20-60 min	1-2 hr	6-8 hr
I.V.	About 5 min	≤ 30 min	2 hr
I.M.	Unknown	Unknown	Unknown

Pharmacodynamics

Chemical effect: inhibits sodium and chloride reabsorption at proximal and distal tubules and ascending loop of Henle.
Therapeutic effect: promotes water and sodium excretion.

Adverse reactions

CNS: vertigo, headache, dizziness, paresthesia, restlessness, weakness.
CV: volume depletion and dehydration, orthostatic hypotension, thrombophlebitis (with I.V. use).
EENT: transient deafness (with too-rapid I.V. injection), blurred or yellow vision.
GI: abdominal discomfort and pain, diarrhea, anorexia, nausea, vomiting, constipation, ***pancreatitis.***
GU: nocturia, polyuria, frequent urination, oliguria.
Hematologic: *agranulocytosis, leukopenia, thrombocytopenia,* azotemia, anemia, ***aplastic anemia.***
Hepatic: *hepatic dysfunction,* increased cholesterol levels.
Metabolic: hypokalemia; hypochloremic alkalosis; asymptomatic hyperuricemia; gout; fluid and electrolyte imbalances, including dilutional hyponatremia, hypocalcemia, and hypomagnesemia; hyperglycemia and glucose intolerance.
Musculoskeletal: muscle spasm.
Skin: dermatitis, purpura, photosensitivity.
Other: fever, transient pain at I.M. injection site.

Interactions

Drug-drug. *Aminoglycoside antibiotics, cisplatin:* potentiated ototoxicity. Use together cautiously.
Amphotericin B, corticosteroids, corticotropin, metolazone: increased risk of hypokalemia. Monitor potassium levels closely.
Antidiabetics: decreased hypoglycemic effects. Monitor blood glucose levels.
Antihypertensives: increased risk of hypotension. Use together cautiously.
Cardiac glycosides, neuromuscular blockers: increased toxicity from furosemide-induced hypokalemia. Monitor potassium levels closely.
Ethacrynic acid: may increase risk of ototoxicity. Don't use concomitantly.
Lithium: decreased lithium excretion, resulting in lithium toxicity. Monitor lithium level.
NSAIDs: inhibited diuretic response. Use together cautiously.
Salicylates: may cause salicylate toxicity. Use together cautiously.

Drug-herb. *Aloe.* Possible increased drug effects. Monitor patient for dehydration.
Licorice: may cause rapid potassium loss. Monitor patient for hypokalemia.
Drug-lifestyle. *Alcohol use:* Additive hypotensive and diuretic effect. Discourage concurrent use.
Sun exposure: photosensitivity reactions may occur. Urge precautions.

Contraindications and precautions

- Contraindicated in patients with anuria or history of hypersensitivity to drug.
- Drug isn't recommended for breast-feeding women.
- Use cautiously in patients with hepatic cirrhosis.
- Use in pregnant women only if benefits outweigh risks.

NURSING CONSIDERATIONS

Assessment

- Assess patient's underlying condition before therapy.
- Monitor weight, peripheral edema, breath sounds, blood pressure, fluid intake and output, and serum electrolyte, blood glucose, BUN, and carbon dioxide levels.
- Monitor blood uric acid, especially if patient has a history of gout.
- Be alert for adverse reactions and drug interactions.
- Evaluate patient's and family's knowledge of drug therapy.

Nursing diagnoses

- Excessive fluid volume related to presence of edema
- Impaired urinary elimination related to diuretic therapy
- Deficient knowledge related to drug therapy

Planning and implementation

P.O. and I.M. use: Administer P.O. and I.M. doses in morning to prevent nocturia. Give second doses in early afternoon.
I.V. use: Give drug by direct injection over 1 to 2 minutes. Or, dilute with D_5W, normal saline solution, or lactated Ringer's solution, and infuse no faster than 4 mg/minute to avoid ototoxicity. Use prepared infusion solution within 24 hours.

- Store tablets in light-resistant container to prevent discoloration. Don't use yellowed injectable preparation.
- Refigerate oral furosemide solution to ensure drug stability.
- Notify prescriber if oliguria or azotemia develops or increases.

Patient teaching

- Advise patient to stand slowly to prevent dizziness, to avoid alcohol, and to minimize strenuous exercise in hot weather.
- Instruct patient to report ringing in ears, severe abdominal pain, or sore throat and fever because they may indicate furosemide toxicity.

ALERT Discourage patient from storing different drugs in same container, because this increases risk of errors. The most popular strengths of furosemide and digoxin are white tablets of similar size.

- Tell patient to check with prescriber before taking OTC medications or herbal remedies.

Evaluation

- Patient is free from edema.
- Patient demonstrates adjustment of lifestyle to cope with altered patterns of urinary elimination.
- Patient and family state understanding of drug therapy.

G

gabapentin

(geh-buh-PEN-tin)
Neurontin

Pharmacologic class: 1-aminomethyl cyclohexoneacetic acid
Therapeutic class: anticonvulsant
Pregnancy risk category: C

Indications and dosages

▶ **Adjunct treatment of partial seizures with and without secondary generalization in adults with epilepsy.** *Adults:* initially 300 mg P.O. h.s. on day 1; then 300 mg P.O. b.i.d. on day 2; then 300 mg P.O. t.i.d. on day 3. Dosage increased as needed and tolerated to 1,800 mg daily in divided doses. Dosages up to 3,600 mg daily have been well tolerated.
Patients with renal failure: if creatinine clearance is over 60 ml/minute, 400 mg P.O. t.i.d.; if creatinine clearance is 30 to 60 ml/minute, 300 mg P.O. b.i.d.; if creatinine clearance is 15 to 30 ml/minute, 300 mg P.O. daily; if creatinine clearance is below 15 ml/minute, 300 mg P.O. every other day. Patients on dialysis should receive loading dose of 300 to 400 mg P.O.; then 200 to 300 mg P.O. after each 4-hour hemodialysis session.

How supplied

Capsules: 100 mg, 300 mg, 400 mg

Pharmacokinetics

Absorption: bioavailability isn't dose proportional but averages about 60%.
Distribution: drug circulates largely unbound to plasma protein.
Metabolism: not appreciably metabolized.
Excretion: excreted by kidneys as unchanged drug. *Half-life:* 5 to 7 hours.

Route	Onset	Peak	Duration
P.O.	Unknown	Unknown	Unknown

Pharmacodynamics

Chemical effect: unknown; although structurally related to gamma-amino butyric acid (GABA), drug doesn't interact with GABA receptors and isn't converted metabolically into GABA or a GABA agonist.
Therapeutic effect: prevents and treats partial seizures.

Adverse reactions

CNS: *somnolence, dizziness, ataxia, fatigue, nystagmus, tremor,* nervousness, dysarthria, amnesia, depression, abnormal thinking, twitching, abnormal coordination.
CV: peripheral edema, vasodilation.
EENT: *diplopia, rhinitis,* pharyngitis, dry throat, *amblyopia.*
GI: nausea, vomiting, dyspepsia, dry mouth, constipation.
GU: impotence.
Hematologic: *leukopenia,* decreased WBC count.
Metabolic: increased appetite, weight gain.
Musculoskeletal: back pain, myalgia, fractures.
Respiratory: cough.
Skin: pruritus, abrasion.
Other: dental abnormalities.

Interactions

Drug-drug. *Antacids:* decreased gabapentin absorption. Separate administration times by at least 2 hours.
Drug-lifestyle. *Alcohol use:* Increased CNS depression. Discourage use.

Contraindications and precautions

- Contraindicated in patients hypersensitive to drug.
- Use cautiously in pregnant women.
- Safety of drug hasn't been established in breast-feeding women or in children younger than age 12.

NURSING CONSIDERATIONS

Assessment

- Assess patient's disorder before therapy and regularly thereafter.
- Routine monitoring of plasma drug levels isn't necessary. Drug doesn't appear to alter plasma levels of other anticonvulsants.
- Be alert for adverse reactions and drug interactions.
- Evaluate patient's and family's knowledge of drug therapy.

Nursing diagnoses

- Risk for trauma related to seizures
- Risk for injury related to drug-induced adverse CNS reactions
- Deficient knowledge related to drug therapy

Planning and implementation

- Give first dose at bedtime to minimize drowsiness, dizziness, fatigue, and ataxia.

ⓢ **ALERT** If gabapentin is discontinued or alternative drug is substituted, do so gradually over at least 1 week as ordered to minimize risk seizures. Don't suddenly withdraw other anticonvulsants in patient starting gabapentin therapy.
- Drug may cause false-positive tests for urine protein when Ames-N-Multistix SG dipstick test is used.
- Take seizure precautions.

Patient teaching
- Tell patient to take drug without regard to meals.
- Warn patient to avoid hazardous activities until CNS effects of drug are known.

Evaluation
- Patient is free from seizures.
- Patient has no injury from adverse CNS reactions.
- Patient and family state understanding of drug therapy.

ganciclovir
(jan-SIGH-kloh-veer)
Cytovene

Pharmacologic class: synthetic nucleoside
Therapeutic class: antiviral
Pregnancy risk category: C

Indications and dosages
▶ **Treatment of CMV retinitis in immunocompromised patients, including those with AIDS.** *Adults:* induction treatment—5 mg/kg I.V. q 12 hours for 14 to 21 days (normal renal function); maintenance treatment—5 mg/kg I.V. daily for 7 days weekly, or 6 mg/kg I.V. daily for 5 days weekly. Or, following induction treatment, 1,000 mg P.O. t.i.d. with food. Dosage is adjusted for patients with impaired renal function and is based on creatinine clearance levels.
▶ **Prevention of CMV disease in transplant recipients at risk for CMV disease.** *Adults:* 5 mg/kg I.V. q 12 hours for 7 to 14 days, followed by 5 mg/kg once daily 7 days weekly or 6 mg/kg once daily 5 days weekly. Alternatively, 1,000 mg P.O. t.i.d. with food. Duration of treatment with I.V. ganciclovir in transplant recipients depends on duration and degree of immunosuppression.
▶ **Prevention of CMV disease in patients with advanced HIV infection at risk for development of CMV disease.** *Adults:* 1,000 mg P.O. t.i.d. with food.

How supplied
Capsules: 250 mg, 500 mg
Injection: 500 mg/vial

Pharmacokinetics
Absorption: poorly absorbed after P.O. administration. Bioavailability is about 5% under fasting conditions.
Distribution: preferentially concentrates in CMV-infected cells; only 2% to 3% protein-bound.
Metabolism: over 90% of drug isn't metabolized.
Excretion: mostly excreted unchanged. *Half-life:* about 3 hours.

Route	Onset	Peak	Duration
P.O.	Unknown	Unknown	Unknown
I.V.	Immediate	Immediate	Unknown

Pharmacodynamics
Chemical effect: unknown; may inhibit viral DNA synthesis of CMV.
Therapeutic effect: inhibits CMV.

Adverse reactions
CNS: altered dreams, confusion, ataxia, dizziness, headache, ***seizures, coma,*** behavioral changes.
CV: ***arrhythmias,*** hypotension, hypertension.
EENT: retinal detachment in CMV retinitis patients.
GI: nausea, vomiting, diarrhea, anorexia.
GU: hematuria, increased serum creatinine levels.
Hematologic: ***thrombocytopenia, agranulocytosis, leukopenia.***
Hepatic: abnormal liver function test results.
Other: inflammation, pain, phlebitis at injection site.

Interactions

Drug-drug. *Cytotoxic drugs:* increased toxic effects, especially hematologic effects and stomatitis. Monitor patient closely.
Imipenem/cilastatin: heightened seizure activity with concomitant use. Monitor patient closely.
Immunosuppressants (such as azathioprine, corticosteroids, cyclosporine): enhanced immune and bone marrow suppression. Use together cautiously.
Probenecid: increased ganciclovir blood levels. Monitor patient closely.
Zidovudine: increased risk of granulocytopenia with concurrent use. Monitor patient closely.

Contraindications and precautions

- Contraindicated in patients hypersensitive to drug and in those with absolute neutrophil count below $500/mm^3$ or platelet count below $25,000/mm^3$.
- Drug not recommended for breast-feeding women.
- Use cautiously and at reduced dosage in patients with renal dysfunction and in pregnant women.
- Safety of drug hasn't been established in children.

NURSING CONSIDERATIONS

Assessment
- Assess patient's condition before therapy and regularly thereafter.
- Obtain neutrophil and platelet counts every 2 days during twice-daily ganciclovir dosing and at least weekly thereafter, as ordered.
- Monitor hydration status if adverse GI reactions occur with oral drug.
- Be alert for adverse reactions and drug interactions.
- Evaluate patient's and family's knowledge of drug therapy.

Nursing diagnoses
- Infection related to CMV retinitis
- Ineffective protection related to adverse hematologic reactions
- Deficient knowledge related to drug therapy

Planning and implementation
P.O. use: Give drug with food.
I.V. use: Reconstitute with 10 ml sterile water for injection. Shake vial to dissolve drug. Further dilute appropriate dose in normal saline, D_5W, Ringer's lactate, or Ringer's solutions (typically 100 ml) and infuse over 1 hour. Faster infusions will cause increased toxicity. Use infusion pump. Don't administer as I.V. bolus. Infusion concentrations greater than 10 mg/ml aren't recommended.
– Use caution when preparing solution, which is alkaline.
- Don't administer drug S.C. or I.M. because severe tissue irritation could result.
- Encourage fluid intake; ganciclovir infusion therapy should be accompanied by adequate hydration.
- Alert prescriber to signs of renal failure because the dosage will need adjustment.

Patient teaching
- Tell patient to take oral form of drug with food.
- Stress importance of drinking adequate fluid throughout therapy.
- Advise patient to report pain or discomfort at I.V. site.
- Instruct patient about infection-control and bleeding precautions.

Evaluation
- Patient is free from infection.
- Patient has no serious adverse hematologic reactions.
- Patient and family state understanding of drug therapy.

ganirelix acetate
(gan-eh-REL-iks AS-ih-tayt)
Antagon

Pharmacologic class: gonadotropin-releasing hormone (Gn-RH) antagonist
Therapeutic class: fertility agent
Pregnancy risk category: X

Indications and dosages

▶ **Inhibition of premature luteinizing hormone (LH) surges in women undergoing medically supervised, controlled ovarian hyperstimulation.** *Adults:* 250 mcg S.C. once daily during early to midfollicular phase of menstrual cycle. Continue daily until enough follicles of sufficient size are confirmed by ultrasound; human chorionic gonadotropin will then be given to induce final maturation of follicles.

How supplied

Injection: 250 mcg/0.5 ml in prefilled syringes

Pharmacokinetics

Absorption: rapidly absorbed after S.C. injection with an average of 91.1% absorbed.
Distribution: 81.9% bound to plasma proteins.
Metabolism: unmetabolized drug is found in urine up to 24 hours after dose. Two metabolites have been detected in feces.
Excretion: primary excretion route is fecal; metabolites can be detected nearly 8 days after a dose.

Route	Onset	Peak	Duration
S.C.	Unknown	1 hr	Unknown

Pharmacodynamics

Chemical effect: Gn-RH, secreted by the pituitary gland, stimulates the synthesis and secretion of gonadotropins LH and follicle-stimulating hormone (FSH). In midcycle, a large increase in Gn-RH leads to a large surge in LH secretion, causing ovulation, a rise in progesterone levels, and a decrease in estradiol levels. Ganirelix blocks pituitary Gn-RH receptors and suppresses LH and, to a smaller degree, FSH secretion. By suppressing LH and FSH secretion in the early-to-mid menstrual cycle, ganirelix stops premature gonadotropin surges that could interfere with medically supervised, controlled ovarian hyperstimulation.
Therapeutic effect: increased fertility.

Adverse reactions

CNS: headache.
GI: abdominal pain, nausea.
GU: vaginal bleeding, gynecologic abdominal pain, ovarian hyperstimulation syndrome, miscarriage.
Skin: injection site reaction.

Interactions

None reported.

Contraindications and precautions

- Contraindicated in patients hypersensitive to ganirelix or its components or to Gn-RH or Gn-RH analogue. Also, contraindicated in pregnant women.
- Use with caution in patients with potential hypersensitivity to Gn-RH and in those with latex allergies because the product packaging contains natural rubber latex.

NURSING CONSIDERATIONS

Assessment

- Before starting treatment, make sure patient isn't pregnant.
- Monitor patient who reports previous potential hypersensitivity to Gn-RH carefully; monitor patient closely after first injection.
- Evaluate patient's and family's knowledge about drug therapy.

Nursing diagnoses

- Disturbed self esteem related to infertility
- Acute pain secondary to drug-induced adverse reactions
- Deficient knowledge related to drug therapy

Planning and implementation

- Only prescribers experienced in infertility treatments should prescribe this drug.
- Natural rubber latex packaging of this product may cause allergic reactions in a hypersensitive patient.
- Increased WBC count and decreased bilirubin levels and hematocrit have been observed in patients receiving ganirelix injections.

Patient teaching

- Tell patient that the correct use of ganirelix injection is extremely important to the success of the fertility treatments. Patient should be able to follow strict administration schedule.

• Teach patient proper technique for S.C. administration of drug.
• Advise patient to use the abdomen or upper thigh for injection and to vary injection site with each dose.
• Advise patient to store drug at room temperature, away from heat and light, and out of children's reach.
• Inform patient to discontinue drug and report suspected or known pregnancy.

Evaluation
• Patient becomes pregnant.
• Patient has no adverse reactions.
• Patient and family state understanding of drug therapy.

gatifloxacin
(ga-tih-FLOCKS-ah-sin)
Tequin

Pharmacologic class: fluoroquinolone antibiotic
Therapeutic class: antibiotic
Pregnancy risk category: C

Indications and dosages

▶ **Acute bacterial exacerbation of chronic bronchitis caused by *Streptococcus pneumoniae, Haemophilus influenzae, Haemophilus parainfluenzae, Moraxella catarrhalis,* or *Staphylococcus aureus*; complicated urinary tract infection caused by *Escherichia coli, Klebsiella pneumoniae,* or *Proteus mirabilis;* acute pyelonephritis caused by *E. coli.*** *Adults:* 400 mg I.V. or P.O. daily for 7 to 10 days.
▶ **Acute sinusitis caused by *S. pneumoniae* or *H. influenzae.*** *Adults:* 400 mg I.V. or P.O. daily for 10 days.
▶ **Community-acquired pneumonia caused by *S. pneumoniae, H. influenzae, H. parainfluenzae, M. catarrhalis, S. aureus, Mycoplasma pneumoniae, Chlamydia pneumoniae,* or *Legionella pneumophila.*** *Adults:* 400 mg I.V. or P.O. daily for 7 to 14 days.
▶ **Uncomplicated urethral gonorrhea in men and cervical gonorrhea or acute uncomplicated rectal infections in women caused by *Neisseria gonorrhoeae.*** *Adults:* 400 mg P.O. as single dose.
▶ **Uncomplicated urinary tract infection caused by *E. coli, K. pneumoniae,* or *P. mirabilis.*** *Adults:* 400 mg I.V. or P.O. as single dose, or 200 mg I.V. or P.O. daily for 3 days.

How supplied

Tablets: 200 mg, 400 mg
Injection: 200 mg/20-ml vial, 400 mg/40-ml vial; 200 mg in 100 ml D_5W, 400 mg in 200 ml D_5W

Pharmacokinetics

Absorption: 96% of gatifloxacin is absorbed after P.O. administration; levels peak in 1 to 2 hours.
Distribution: drug is 20% protein-bound. It's widely distributed into many tissues and fluids.
Metabolism: limited biotransformation.
Excretion: more than 70% excreted unchanged by the kidneys. *Serum half-life:* 7-14 hours.

Route	Onset	Peak	Duration
P.O.	Unknown	1-2 hr	Unknown
I.V.	Unknown	Unknown	Unknown

Pharmacodynamics

Chemical effect: inhibits DNA gyrase and topoisomerase, preventing cell replication and division. It's active against gram-positive and gram-negative organisms, including *S. aureus, S. pneumoniae, E. coli, H. influenzae, H. parainfluenzae, K. pneumoniae, M. catarrhalis, N. gonorrhoeae, P. mirabilis, C. pneumoniae, L. pneumophilia,* and *M. pneumoniae.*
Therapeutic effect: kills susceptible bacteria, including *S. pneumoniae, H. influenzae, H. parainfluenzae, M. catarrhalis, S. aureus, E. coli, K. pneumoniae, P. mirabilis, M. pneumoniae, C. pneumoniae,* and *L. pneumophila.*

Adverse reactions

CNS: headache, dizziness, abnormal dreams, insomnia, paresthesia, tremor, vertigo.
CV: palpitations, chest pain, peripheral edema.
EENT: tinnitus, abnormal vision, pharyngitis.
GI: nausea, diarrhea, abdominal pain, constipation, dyspepsia, oral candidiasis, ***pseudo-***

membranous colitis, glossitis, stomatitis, mouth ulcer, vomiting, disturbed taste.
GU: dysuria, hematuria, vaginitis.
Musculoskeletal: arthralgia, myalgia, back pain.
Respiratory: dyspnea.
Skin: rash, sweating.
Other: ***anaphylaxis***, redness at injection site, chills, fever.

Interactions

Drug-drug. *Antacids containing aluminum or magnesium, didanosine buffered solution tablets or buffered powder, products containing zinc, magnesium, or iron:* decreased gatifloxacin absorption. Give gatifloxacin 4 hours before these products.
Antidiabetics (glyburide, insulin): possible symptomatic hypoglycemia or hyperglycemia. Monitor blood glucose level.
Antipsychotics, cisapride, erythromycin, tricyclic antidepressants: possible prolongation of QTc interval. Use cautiously.
Class IA antiarrhythmics (quinidine, procainamide), class III antiarrhythmics (amiodarone, sotalol): potential for prolongation of QTc interval. Avoid concomitant use.
Digoxin: possible increase in digoxin levels. Watch for signs of digoxin toxicity.
NSAIDs: potential for increased risk of CNS stimulation and seizures. Use together cautiously.
Probenecid: increase in gatifloxacin levels and prolongation of its half-life. Monitor patient closely.
Warfarin: possible enhanced effects of warfarin. Monitor PT and INR.
Drug-lifestyle. *Sun exposure:* photosensitivity reactions may occur. Urge precautions.

Contraindications and precautions

• Contraindicated in patients hypersensitive to fluoroquinolones, patients with prolonged QTc interval, and patients with uncorrected hypokalemia.
• Use cautiously in patients with clinically significant bradycardia, acute myocardial ischemia, known or suspected CNS disorders, or renal insufficiency.

NURSING CONSIDERATIONS

Assessment

• In patient being treated for gonorrhea, test for syphilis at time of diagnosis.
• Monitor kidney function in patient with renal insufficiency.
• Monitor blood glucose in patient with diabetes.
• Monitor patient concurrently on digoxin for evidence of digoxin toxicity.
• Be alert for adverse reactions and drug interactions.
• Evaluate patient's and family's knowledge about drug therapy.

Nursing diagnoses

• Infection related to presence of bacteria susceptible to drug
• Risk for injury related to drug-induced adverse reactions
• Deficient knowledge related to drug therapy

Planning and implementation

• Reduce dosage as directed for patients with creatinine clearance less than 40 ml/min, those on hemodialysis, and those on continuous peritoneal dialysis.
P.O. use: Give gatifloxacin 4 hours before antacids containing aluminum or magnesium, didanosine buffered solution tablets or buffered powder, products containing zinc, magnesium, or iron.
I.V. use: Dilute drug in single-use vials with D_5W or normal saline solution to 2 mg/ml before administration. Diluted solutions are stable 14 days at room temperature or refrigerated. Frozen solutions are stable up to 6 months except for 5% sodium bicarbonate solutions. Thaw at room temperature. After being thawed, solutions are stable 14 days when stored at room temperature or refrigerated. Don't mix with other drugs. Infuse over 60 minutes.
– Discard any unused portion of single-dose vials.
• Discontinue drug and notify prescriber if patient experiences seizures, increased intracranial pressure, psychosis, or CNS stimulation leading to tremors, restlessness, lightheadedness, confusion, hallucinations,

paranoia, depression, nightmares, and insomnia.

- Discontinue drug and notify prescriber about skin rash or other sign of hypersensitivity.
- Discontinue drug and notify prescriber if patient experiences pain, inflammation, or rupture of a tendon.
- Monitor patient for diarrhea because pseudomembranous colitis may occur in patients taking antibiotics.

Patient teaching

- Tell patient to take drug as prescribed and to finish all of the medication even if symptoms disappear.
- Advise patient to take drug 4 hours before products containing aluminum, magnesium, zinc, or iron.
- Advise patient to use sunblock and protective clothing when exposed to excessive sunlight.
- Warn patient to avoid hazardous tasks until adverse CNS effects of drugs are known.
- Advise diabetic patient to monitor blood glucose levels and notify prescriber if hypoglycemia occurs.
- Advise patient to report palpitations, fainting spells, skin rash, hives, difficulty swallowing or breathing, swelling of the lips, tongue, face, tightness in throat, hoarseness, or other symptoms of allergic reaction immediately.
- Advise patient to stop drug, refrain from exercise, and notify prescriber if pain, inflammation, or rupture of a tendon occur.

☑ Evaluation

- Patient is free from infection after drug therapy.
- Patient has no injury as a result of drug-induced adverse reactions.
- Patient and family state understanding of drug therapy.

gemfibrozil
(jem-FIGH-broh-zil)
Lopid

Pharmacologic class: fibric acid derivative
Therapeutic class: antilipemic
Pregnancy risk category: C

Indications and dosages

▶ **Type IV and V hyperlipidemia unresponsive to diet and other drugs; reduction of risk of coronary heart disease in patients with type IIb hyperlipidemia who can't tolerate or who are refractory to treatment with bile acid sequestrants or niacin.** *Adults:* 1,200 mg P.O. daily in two divided doses, 30 minutes before morning and evening meals. If no benefit is seen after 3 months, drug should be discontinued.

How supplied

Tablets: 600 mg
Capsules: 300 mg ♦

Pharmacokinetics

Absorption: well absorbed from GI tract.
Distribution: 95% protein-bound.
Metabolism: metabolized by liver.
Excretion: excreted primarily in urine, with some excretion in feces. *Half-life:* about 1.25 hours. Biological half-life is considerably longer, as a result of enterohepatic circulation and reabsorption in the GI tract.

Route	Onset	Peak	Duration
P.O.	2-5 days	> 4 wk	Unknown

Pharmacodynamics

Chemical effect: inhibits peripheral lipolysis and also reduces triglyceride synthesis in liver.
Therapeutic effect: lowers serum triglyceride levels and raises high-density lipoprotein (HDL) levels.

Adverse reactions

CNS: blurred vision, headache, dizziness.
GI: *abdominal and epigastric pain, diarrhea, nausea,* vomiting, flatulence.
Hematologic: ***anemia, leukopenia, thrombocytopenia.***
Hepatic: bile duct obstruction, elevated liver enzyme levels.
Musculoskeletal: painful limbs.
Skin: rash, dermatitis, pruritus.

Interactions

Drug-drug. *HMG-CoA reductase inhibitors:* myopathy with rhabdomyolysis has been reported. Don't use together.
Oral anticoagulants: gemfibrozil may enhance clinical effects of oral anticoagulants. Monitor patient.

Contraindications and precautions

- Contraindicated in patients hypersensitive to drug and in those with hepatic or severe renal dysfunction (including primary biliary cirrhosis) or gallbladder disease.
- Use cautiously in pregnant women.
- Safety of drug hasn't been established in breast-feeding women or in children.

NURSING CONSIDERATIONS

Assessment

- Assess patient's serum triglyceride and HDL levels before therapy and regularly thereafter.
- Periodic CBCs and liver function tests should be performed during first 12 months of therapy.
- Be alert for adverse reactions and drug interactions.
- Evaluate patient's and family's knowledge of drug therapy.

Nursing diagnoses

- Risk for injury related to elevated blood lipids and cholesterol levels
- Diarrhea related to drug's adverse effect on GI tract
- Deficient knowledge related to drug therapy

Planning and implementation

- Administer drug 30 minutes before breakfast and dinner.
- Make sure patient is following standard low-cholesterol diet.

Patient teaching

- Instruct patient to take drug 30 minutes before breakfast and dinner.
- Teach patient dietary management of serum lipids (restricting total fat and cholesterol intake) and measures to control other cardiac disease risk factors. If appropriate, suggest weight control, exercise, and smoking cessation programs.
- Advise patient to avoid driving or other potentially hazardous activities until drug's CNS effects are known.
- Tell patient to observe bowel movements and to report signs of steatorrhea or bile duct obstruction.

Evaluation

- Patient's blood triglyceride and cholesterol levels are normal.
- Patient regains normal bowel patterns.
- Patient and family state understanding of drug therapy.

gentamicin sulfate

(jen-tuh-MIGH-sin SUL-fayt)

Cidomycin♦, Garamycin, Gentamicin Sulfate ADD-Vantage, Jenamicin

Pharmacologic class: aminoglycoside
Therapeutic class: antibiotic
Pregnancy risk category: D

Indications and dosages

▶ **Serious infections caused by sensitive strains of *Pseudomonas aeruginosa, Escherichia coli, Proteus, Klebsiella, Serratia, Enterobacter, Citrobacter, Staphylococcus.*** *Adults:* 3 mg/kg daily in divided doses I.M. or I.V. infusion q 8 hours (in 50 to 200 ml of normal saline solution or D_5W infused over 30 minutes to 2 hours). For life-threatening infections, patient may receive up to 5 mg/kg daily in three to four divided doses.
Children: 2 to 2.5 mg/kg q 8 hours I.M. or by I.V. infusion.
Neonates over 1 week or infants: 7.5 mg/kg daily in divided doses q 8 hours.
Neonates under 1 week and preterm infants: 2.5 mg/kg I.V. q 12 hours.

▶ **Meningitis.** *Adults:* systemic therapy as above; 4 to 8 mg intrathecally daily also may be used.
Children and infants over age 3 months: systemic therapy as above; 1 to 2 mg intrathecally daily may also be used.

▶ **Endocarditis prophylaxis for GI or GU procedure or surgery.** *Adults:* 1.5 mg/kg I.M.

or I.V. 30 to 60 minutes before procedure or surgery and q 8 hours after, for two doses. Given separately with aqueous penicillin or ampicillin.
Children: 2 mg/kg I.M. or I.V. 30 to 60 minutes before procedure or surgery and q 8 hours after, for two doses. Given separately with aqueous penicillin G or ampicillin G.
▶ **Posthemodialysis to maintain therapeutic blood levels.** *Adults:* 1 to 1.7 mg/kg I.M. or by I.V. infusion after each dialysis.
Children: 2 to 2.5 mg/kg I.M. or by I.V. infusion after each dialysis.

How supplied

Injection: 40 mg/ml (adult), 10 mg/ml (pediatric), 2 mg/ml (intrathecal)
I.V. infusion (premixed): 40 mg, 60 mg, 70 mg, 80 mg, 90 mg, 100 mg, 120 mg, available in normal saline solution

Pharmacokinetics

Absorption: unknown after I.M. administration.
Distribution: distributed widely. CSF penetration is low even in patients with inflamed meninges. Protein-binding is minimal.
Metabolism: not metabolized.
Excretion: excreted primarily in urine; small amounts may be excreted in bile. *Half-life:* 2 to 3 hours.

Route	Onset	Peak	Duration
I.V.	Immediate	30-90 min	Unknown
I.M.	Unknown	30-90 min	Unknown
Intrathecal	Unknown	Unknown	Unknown

Pharmacodynamics

Chemical effect: inhibits protein synthesis by binding to ribosomes.
Therapeutic effect: kills susceptible bacteria (many aerobic gram-negative organisms and some aerobic gram-positive organisms). Drug may act against some aminoglycoside-resistant bacteria.

Adverse reactions

CNS: headache, lethargy, numbness, peripheral neuropathy, ***seizures.***
EENT: *ototoxicity* (tinnitus, vertigo, hearing loss).
GU: *nephrotoxicity* (cells or casts in urine; oliguria; proteinuria; decreased creatinine clearance; increased BUN, nonprotein nitrogen, and serum creatinine levels).
Hematologic: ***thrombocytopenia, leukopenia, agranulocytosis.***
Other: hypersensitivity reactions.

Interactions

Drug-drug. *Acyclovir, amphotericin B, cisplatin, methoxyflurane, other aminoglycosides, vancomycin:* increased ototoxicity and nephrotoxicity. Use together cautiously.
Cephalothin: increased nephrotoxicity. Use together cautiously.
Dimenhydrinate: may mask symptoms of ototoxicity. Use with caution.
General anesthetics, neuromuscular blockers: may potentiate neuromuscular blockade. Monitor patient closely.
Indomethacin: may increase serum peak and trough levels of gentamicin. Monitor serum gentamicin levels.
I.V. loop diuretics (such as furosemide): increased ototoxicity. Use cautiously.
Parenteral penicillins (such as ampicillin, ticarcillin): gentamicin inactivation in vitro. Don't mix together.

Contraindications and precautions

- Contraindicated in patients hypersensitive to drug or other aminoglycosides.
- Use cautiously in patients with impaired renal function or neuromuscular disorders and in neonates, infants, and the elderly.

NURSING CONSIDERATIONS

Assessment

- Assess patient's infection before therapy and regularly thereafter.
- Obtain specimen for culture and sensitivity tests before first dose.
- Evaluate patient's hearing before therapy and regularly thereafter.
- Weigh patient and review baseline renal function studies before therapy and then regularly during therapy.

• Obtain blood for peak drug level 1 hour after I.M. injection and 30 minutes to 1 hour after I.V. infusion; for trough levels, draw blood just before next dose. Don't collect blood in heparinized tube because heparin is incompatible with aminoglycosides.
• Peak blood levels above 12 mcg/ml and trough levels above 2 mcg/ml may increase risk of toxicity.
• Be alert for adverse reactions and drug interactions.
• Evaluate patient's and family's knowledge of drug therapy.

Nursing diagnoses

• Infection related to presence of susceptible bacteria
• Impaired urinary elimination related to nephrotoxicity
• Deficient knowledge related to drug therapy

Planning and implementation

I.V. use: When giving drug by intermittent I.V. infusion, dilute with 50 to 200 ml of D_5W or normal saline injection and infuse over 30 minutes to 2 hours. After infusion, flush line with normal saline solution or D_5W.
I.M. use: Give drug deep into large muscle mass (gluteal or midlateral thigh); rotate injection sites. Don't inject more than 2 g of drug per site.
Intrathecal use: Use preservative-free forms of gentamicin for intrathecal route.
• Hemodialysis (8 hours) removes up to 50% of drug from blood.
• Notify prescriber about signs of decreasing renal function or changes in hearing.
• Therapy usually continues for 7 to 10 days. If no response occurs in 3 to 5 days, therapy may be stopped and new specimens obtained for culture and sensitivity testing.
• Encourage adequate fluid intake; patient should be well hydrated while taking drug to minimize chemical irritation of renal tubules.

Patient teaching

• Instruct patient to notify prescriber about adverse reactions, such as changes in hearing.
• Emphasize importance of drinking at least 2,000 ml of fluids daily, if not contraindicated.

Evaluation

• Patient is free from infection.
• Patient maintains normal renal function throughout drug therapy.
• Patient and family state understanding of drug therapy.

glimepiride

(gligh-MEH-peh-righd)
Amaryl

Pharmacologic class: sulfonylurea
Therapeutic class: antidiabetic
Pregnancy risk category: C

Indications and dosages

▶ **Adjunct to diet and exercise to lower blood glucose in patients with type 2 (non-insulin-dependent) diabetes mellitus whose hyperglycemia can't be managed by diet and exercise alone.** *Adults:* initially, 1 to 2 mg P.O. once daily with first main meal of day. Usual maintenance dosage is 1 to 4 mg P.O. once daily. After reaching 2 mg, dosage increased in increments not exceeding 2 mg q 1 to 2 weeks, based on patient's blood glucose response. Maximum, 8 mg daily.
▶ **Adjunct to insulin therapy in patients with type 2 (non-insulin-dependent) diabetes mellitus whose hyperglycemia can't be managed by diet and exercise in conjunction with oral hypoglycemic agents.** *Adults:* 8 mg P.O. once daily with first main meal of day in combination with low-dose insulin. Adjust insulin upward weekly as needed, based on patient's blood glucose response.

How supplied

Tablets: 1 mg, 2 mg, 4 mg

Pharmacokinetics

Absorption: completely absorbed.
Distribution: 99.5% protein-bound.
Metabolism: completely metabolized.
Excretion: in urine and feces.

Route	Onset	Peak	Duration
P.O.	Within 1 hr	2-3 hr	Unknown

Pharmacodynamics

Chemical effect: stimulates release of insulin from pancreatic beta cells; increases sensitivity of peripheral tissues to insulin.
Therapeutic effect: lowers blood glucose levels.

Adverse reactions

CNS: dizziness, asthenia, headache.
EENT: changes in accommodation.
GI: nausea.
Hematologic: leukopenia, hemolytic anemia, ***agranulocytosis, thrombocytopenia, aplastic anemia, pancytopenia.***
Hepatic: cholestatic jaundice, elevated transaminase levels.
Metabolic: hypoglycemia.
Skin: allergic skin reactions (pruritus, erythema, urticaria, and morbilliform or maculopapular eruptions).

Interactions

Drug-drug. *Beta blockers:* may mask symptoms of hypoglycemia. Monitor glucose levels carefully.
Drugs that produce hyperglycemia, other diuretics: may lead to loss of glucose control. Adjust dosage as ordered.
Insulin: concomitant use may increase potential for hypoglycemia.
NSAIDs, other highly protein-bound drugs: may potentiate hypoglycemic action of sulfonylureas, such as glimepiride.
Drug-herb. *Aloe, bitter melon, bilberry leaf, burdock, dandelion, fenugreek, garlic, ginseng:* improvement in blood glucose control may allow reduction of oral hypoglycemic. Tell patient to discuss herbs with prescriber before use.
Drug-lifestyle. *Alcohol use:* altered glycemic control, most commonly hypoglycemia. May cause disulfiram-like reaction. Discourage concomitant use.

Contraindications and precautions

- Contraindicated in patients hypersensitive to drug and in those with diabetic ketoacidosis.
- Use cautiously in debilitated or malnourished patients and in those with adrenal, pituitary, hepatic, or renal insufficiency.

NURSING CONSIDERATIONS

Assessment

- Monitor fasting blood glucose periodically to determine therapeutic response. Also monitor glycosylated hemoglobin, usually every 3 to 6 months, to more precisely assess long-term glycemic control.
- Evaluate patient's and family's knowledge of drug therapy.

Nursing diagnoses

- Ineffective health maintenance related to hyperglycemia
- Risk for injury related to drug-induced hypoglycemia
- Deficient knowledge related to drug therapy

Planning and implementation

- Oral hypoglycemic drugs have been linked with an increased risk of CV mortality compared with diet alone or with diet and insulin therapy.
- Renally impaired patients should begin therapy with a reduced dosage.
- Don't give drug to breast-feeding women.

Patient teaching

- Tell patient to take drug with first meal of day.
- Stress importance of adhering to diet, weight-reduction, exercise, and personal hygiene programs. Explain to patient and family how to monitor blood glucose levels, and teach them signs, symptoms, and treatment of hyperglycemia and hypoglycemia.
- Advise patient to wear or carry medical identification that describes his condition.
- Advise woman planning pregnancy to consult prescriber before becoming pregnant.
- Instruct patient to avoid alcohol consumption during therapy.

Evaluation

- Patient's blood glucose level is normal.
- Patient recognizes hypoglycemia early and treats it before injury occurs.
- Patient and family state understanding of drug therapy.

glipizide

(GLIGH-peh-zighd)
Glucotrol, Glucotrol XL, Minidiab ◊

Pharmacologic class: sulfonylurea
Therapeutic class: antidiabetic
Pregnancy risk category: C

Indications and dosages

▶ **Adjunct to diet to lower blood glucose level in patients with type 2 (non-insulin-dependent) diabetes mellitus.** *Adults:* initially, 5 mg P.O. daily before breakfast. Elderly patients or those with liver disease may be started on 2.5 mg. Maximum once-daily dosage is 15 mg. Maximum recommended total daily dosage is 40 mg. **(Extended-release tablets.)** *Adults:* 5 mg P.O. daily. Adjust in 5-mg increments q 3 months depending on level of glycemic control. Maximum daily dosage for these tablets is 20 mg.

▶ **To replace insulin therapy.** *Adults:* if insulin dosage is more than 20 units daily, patient is started at usual dosage in addition to 50% of insulin. If insulin dosage is less than 20 units, insulin may be discontinued.

How supplied

Tablets: 5 mg, 10 mg
Tablets (extended-release): 5 mg, 10 mg

Pharmacokinetics

Absorption: absorbed rapidly and completely from GI tract.
Distribution: distributed within extracellular fluid; about 92% to 99% protein-bound.
Metabolism: metabolized by liver to inactive metabolites.
Excretion: primarily in urine; small amounts in feces. *Half-life:* 2 to 4 hours.

Route	Onset	Peak	Duration
P.O.	15-30 min	1-3 hr	10-16 hr

Pharmacodynamics

Chemical effect: may stimulate insulin release from pancreas, reduce glucose output by liver, and increase peripheral sensitivity to insulin.
Therapeutic effect: lowers blood glucose levels.

Adverse reactions

CNS: dizziness.
GI: nausea, vomiting, constipation.
Hematologic: ***agranulocytosis, thrombocytopenia, aplastic anemia.***
Hepatic: cholestatic jaundice.
Metabolic: ***hypoglycemia.***
Skin: rash, pruritus, facial flushing.

Interactions

Drug-drug. *Anabolic steroids, chloramphenicol, clofibrate, guanethidine, MAO inhibitors, phenylbutazone, probenecid, salicylates, sulfonamides:* increased hypoglycemic activity. Monitor blood glucose level.
Beta blockers, clonidine: prolonged hypoglycemic effect and masked symptoms of hypoglycemia. Use together cautiously.
Corticosteroids, glucagon, rifampin, thiazide diuretics: decreased hypoglycemic response. Monitor blood glucose level.
Hydantoins: increased blood levels of hydantoins. Monitor blood levels.
Oral anticoagulants: increased hypoglycemic activity or enhanced anticoagulant effect. Monitor blood glucose levels and PT and INR.
Drug-herb. *Aloe, bitter melon, bilberry leaf, burdock, dandelion, fenugreek, garlic, ginseng:* improvement in blood glucose control may allow reduction of oral hypoglycemic. Tell patient to discuss herbs with prescriber before use.
Drug-lifestyle. *Alcohol use:* altered glycemic control, most commonly hypoglycemia. May also cause disulfiram-like reaction. Discourage concomitant use.

Contraindications and precautions

- Contraindicated in patients hypersensitive to drug and in pregnant or breast-feeding women, and in patients with diabetic ketoacidosis.
- Use cautiously in patients with renal and hepatic disease and in debilitated, malnourished, or elderly patients.
- Safety of drug hasn't been established in children because of the rarity of type 2 diabetes mellitus in this population.

NURSING CONSIDERATIONS

Assessment
- Assess blood glucose level before therapy and regularly thereafter.
- Patient transferring from insulin therapy to oral antidiabetic needs blood glucose monitoring at least three times daily before meals.
- During periods of increased stress, such as from infection, fever, surgery, or trauma, patient may need insulin therapy. Monitor patient closely for hyperglycemia in these situations.
- Be alert for adverse reactions and drug interactions.
- Evaluate patient's and family's knowledge of drug therapy.

Nursing diagnoses
- Ineffective health maintenance related to hyperglycemia
- Risk for injury related to drug-induced hypoglycemia
- Deficient knowledge related to drug therapy

Planning and implementation
- Give drug about 30 minutes before meals.
- Some patients taking drug may attain effective control on once-daily regimen; others show better response with divided dosing.
- Treat hypoglycemic reaction with oral form of rapid-acting carbohydrates if patient can swallow or with glucagon or I.V. glucose if patient can't swallow or is comatose. Follow up treatment with complex carbohydrate snack when patient is awake, and determine cause of reaction.
- Make sure adjunct therapies, such as diet and exercise, are being used appropriately.

Patient teaching
- Instruct patient about nature of disease; importance of following therapeutic regimen; adhering to specific diet, weight reduction, exercise, and personal hygiene programs; and avoiding infection. Explain how and when to monitor blood glucose level, and teach recognition and treatment of hypoglycemia and hyperglycemia.
- Tell patient not to change dosage without prescriber's consent and to report abnormal blood or urine glucose test results.
- Advise patient not to take other medications, including OTC drugs or herbal remedies, without first checking with prescriber.
- Instruct patient to avoid alcohol consumption during drug therapy.
- Advise patient to carry medical identification at all times.

Evaluation
- Patient's blood glucose level is normal with drug therapy.
- Patient doesn't experience hypoglycemia.
- Patient and family state understanding of drug therapy.

glucagon
(GLOO-kuh-gon)

Pharmacologic class: pancreatic hormone
Therapeutic class: antihypoglycemic
Pregnancy risk category: B

Indications and dosages

▶ **Hypoglycemia.** *Adults and children weighing more than 20 kg (44 lb):* 1 mg I.V., I.M., or S.C.
Children weighing 20 kg or less: 0.5 mg I.V., I.M., or S.C.
▶ **Diagnostic aid for radiologic examination.** *Adults:* 0.25 to 2 mg I.V. or I.M. before start of radiologic procedure.

How supplied

Powder for injection: 1 mg (1 unit)/vial, 10 mg (10 units)/vial

Pharmacokinetics

Absorption: unknown.
Distribution: unknown.
Metabolism: drug is degraded extensively by liver, in kidneys and plasma, and at its tissue receptor sites in plasma membranes.
Excretion: excreted by kidneys. *Half-life:* 3 to 10 minutes.

Route	Onset	Peak	Duration
I.V., I.M., S.C.	Almost immediate	≤ 30 min	1-2 hr

Pharmacodynamics

Chemical effect: promotes catalytic depolymerization of hepatic glycogen to glucose.
Therapeutic effect: raises blood glucose level.

Adverse reactions

GI: nausea, vomiting.
Other: ***hypersensitivity reactions.***

Interactions

Drug-drug. *Oral anticoagulants:* anticoagulant effect may be increased. Monitor PT and INR closely.

Contraindications and precautions

- Contraindicated in patients hypersensitive to drug and in those with pheochromocytoma.
- Use cautiously in patients with history of insulinoma or pheochromocytoma.

NURSING CONSIDERATIONS

Assessment

- Assess patient's blood glucose level before therapy and after drug administration.
- Be alert for adverse reactions and drug interactions.
- Monitor patient's hydration status if vomiting occurs.
- Evaluate patient's and family's knowledge of drug therapy.

Nursing diagnoses

- Risk for injury related to patient's hypoglycemia
- Risk for deficient fluid volume related to drug-induced vomiting
- Deficient knowledge related to drug therapy

Planning and implementation

- Reconstitute 1-unit vial with 1 ml of diluent; reconstitute 10-unit vial with 10 ml of diluent. Use only diluent supplied by manufacturer when preparing doses of 2 mg or less. For larger doses, dilute with sterile water for injection.

I.V. use: For I.V. drip infusion, use dextrose solution, which is compatible with glucagon; drug forms precipitate in chloride solutions. Inject directly into vein or into I.V. tubing of free-flowing compatible solution over 2 to 5 minutes. Interrupt primary infusion during glucagon injection if using same I.V. line. May repeat in 15 minutes if necessary. I.V. glucose must be given if patient fails to respond. When patient responds, supplemental carbohydrate needs to be given promptly.

I.M. and S.C. use: Follow normal protocol.

- Arouse patient from coma as quickly as possible and give additional carbohydrates orally to prevent secondary hypoglycemic reactions.
- Notify prescriber that patient's hypoglycemic episode required glucagon use. Be prepared to provide emergency intervention if patient doesn't respond to glucagon administration. Unstable hypoglycemic diabetic patient may not respond to glucagon; give dextrose I.V. instead as ordered.
- Notify prescriber if patient can't retain some form of sugar for 1 hour because of nausea or vomiting.

Patient teaching

- Instruct patient and family in proper drug administration.
- Teach them to recognize hypoglycemia, and tell them to notify prescriber immediately in emergencies.

Evaluation

- Patient's blood glucose level returns to normal.
- Patient remains well hydrated.
- Patient and family state understanding of drug therapy.

glyburide (glibenclamide)

(GLIGH-byoo-righd)

Albert Glyburide♦, Apo-Glyburide♦, DiaBeta**, Euglucon♦, Gen-Glybe♦, Glynase PresTab, Micronase, Novo-Glyburide♦, Nu-Glyburide♦

Pharmacologic class: sulfonylurea
Therapeutic class: antidiabetic
Pregnancy risk category: B

Indications and dosages

▶ **Adjunct to diet to lower blood glucose level in patients with type 2 (non-insulin-dependent) diabetes mellitus.** *Adults:* initially, 1.25 to 5 mg regular tablets P.O. once daily with breakfast. For maintenance, 1.25 to 20 mg daily as single dose or in divided doses. Or initially, 0.75 to 3 mg micronized formulation P.O. daily. For maintenance, 0.75 to 12 mg P.O. daily in single or divided doses.

▶ **To replace insulin therapy.** *Adults:* initially, if insulin dosage is more than 40 units daily, 5 mg regular tablets or 3 mg micronized formulation P.O. once daily in addition to 50% of insulin dosage. If insulin dosage is 20 to 40 units daily, 5 mg regular tablets or 3 mg micronized formulation P.O. once daily with abrupt insulin discontinuation. If insulin dosage is less than 20 units daily, 2.5 to 5 mg regular tablets or 1.5 to 3 mg micronized formulation P.O. once daily with abrupt insulin discontinuation.

How supplied

Tablets: 1.25 mg, 2.5 mg, 5 mg
Tablets (micronized): 1.5 mg, 3 mg, 4.5 mg, 6 mg

Pharmacokinetics

Absorption: absorbed almost completely from GI tract.
Distribution: unknown, although it's 99% protein-bound.
Metabolism: metabolized completely by liver to inactive metabolites.
Excretion: excreted as metabolites in urine and feces in equal proportions. *Half-life:* 10 hours.

Route	Onset	Peak	Duration
P.O.	1-4 hr	2-4 hr	24 hr

Pharmacodynamics

Chemical effect: unknown; may stimulate insulin release from pancreas, reduce glucose output by liver, increase peripheral sensitivity to insulin, and cause mild diuresis.
Therapeutic effect: lowers blood glucose levels.

Adverse reactions

GI: nausea, epigastric fullness, heartburn.
Hematologic: ***agranulocytosis, thrombocytopenia, aplastic anemia.***
Hepatic: cholestatic jaundice.
Metabolic: ***hypoglycemia.***
Skin: rash, pruritus, facial flushing.

Interactions

Drug-drug. *Anabolic steroids, chloramphenicol, clofibrate, guanethidine, MAO inhibitors, phenylbutazone, salicylates, sulfonamides:* increased hypoglycemic activity. Monitor blood glucose level.
Beta blockers, clonidine: prolonged hypoglycemic effect and masked symptoms of hypoglycemia. Use together cautiously.
Corticosteroids, glucagon, rifampin, thiazide diuretics: decreased hypoglycemic response. Monitor blood glucose level.
Hydantoins: increased blood levels of hydantoins. Monitor blood levels.
Oral anticoagulants: increased hypoglycemic activity or enhanced anticoagulant effect. Monitor blood glucose level and PT and INR.
Drug-herb. *Aloe, bitter melon, bilberry leaf, burdock, dandelion, fenugreek, garlic, ginseng:* improvement in blood glucose control may allow reduction of oral hypoglycemic. Tell patient to discuss herbs with prescriber before use.
Drug-lifestyle. *Alcohol use:* altered glycemic control, most commonly hypoglycemia. May also cause disulfiram-like reaction. Discourage concomitant use.

Contraindications and precautions

- Contraindicated in patients hypersensitive to drug, in pregnant or breast-feeding women, in children, and in patients with diabetic ketoacidosis.
- Use cautiously in patients with hepatic or renal impairment and in debilitated, malnourished, or elderly patients.

NURSING CONSIDERATIONS

Assessment

- Assess blood glucose level before therapy and regularly thereafter.
- Patient transferring from insulin therapy to oral antidiabetic needs blood glucose monitoring at least three times daily before meals.
- During periods of increased stress, such as from infection, fever, surgery, or trauma, patient may need insulin therapy. Monitor patient closely for hyperglycemia in these situations.

- Be alert for adverse reactions and drug interactions.
- Evaluate patient's and family's knowledge of drug therapy.

Nursing diagnoses

- Ineffective health maintenance related to hyperglycemia
- Risk for injury related to drug-induced hypoglycemia
- Deficient knowledge related to drug therapy

Planning and implementation

- Micronized glyburide (Glynase PresTab) contains drug in smaller particle size and isn't bioequivalent to regular tablets. Dose for patient who has been taking Micronase or DiaBeta needs adjustment.
- Although most patients take glyburide once daily, patient taking more than 10 mg daily may achieve better results with twice-daily dosage.
- Treat hypoglycemic reaction with oral form of rapid-acting carbohydrates if patient can swallow or with glucagon or I.V. glucose if patient can't swallow or is comatose. Follow up treatment with complex carbohydrate snack when patient is awake, and determine cause of reaction.
- Make sure that adjunct therapy, such as diet and exercise, is being used appropriately.

Patient teaching

- Instruct patient about nature of disease; importance of following therapeutic regimen; adhering to specific diet, weight reduction, exercise, and personal hygiene programs; and avoiding infection. Explain how and when to monitor blood glucose level, and teach recognition and treatment of hypoglycemia and hyperglycemia.
- Tell patient not to change dosage without prescriber's consent and to report abnormal blood or urine glucose test results.
- Advise patient not to take other medications, including OTC drugs and herbal remedies, without first checking with prescriber.
- Instruct patient to avoid alcohol consumption during drug therapy.
- Advise patient to wear or carry medical identification at all times.

Evaluation

- Patient's blood glucose level is normal with drug therapy.
- Patient doesn't experience hypoglycemia.
- Patient and family state understanding of drug therapy.

glycerin

(GLIH-seh-rin)

Fleet Babylax†, Fleet†, Sani-Supp†

Pharmacologic class: trihydric alcohol
Therapeutic class: laxative (osmotic)
Pregnancy risk category: NR

Indications and dosages

▶ **Constipation.** *Adults and children age 6 and over:* 2 to 3 g as rectal suppository or 5 to 15 ml as enema.
Children under age 6: 1 to 1.7 g as rectal suppository; or 2 to 5 ml as enema.

How supplied

Enema (pediatric): 4 ml/applicator†
Suppositories: adult, children, and infant sizes†

Pharmacokinetics

Absorption: suppositories are absorbed poorly.
Distribution: distributed locally.
Metabolism: unknown.
Excretion: excreted in feces.

Route	Onset	Peak	Duration
P.R.	15-60 min	15-60 min	15-60 min

Pharmacodynamics

Chemical effect: hyperosmolar laxative that draws water from tissues into feces to stimulate evacuation.
Therapeutic effect: promotes stool evacuation.

Adverse reactions

GI: *cramping pain,* rectal discomfort, hyperemia of rectal mucosa.

Interactions

None significant.

Contraindications and precautions

- Contraindicated in patients hypersensitive to drug and in those with intestinal obstruction, undiagnosed abdominal pain, vomiting or other signs of appendicitis, fecal impaction, or acute surgical abdomen.

NURSING CONSIDERATIONS

Assessment

- Obtain assessment of patient's constipation before therapy.
- Monitor effectiveness by noting patient's response after drug administration.
- Be alert for adverse GI reactions.
- Evaluate patient's and family's knowledge of drug therapy.

Nursing diagnoses

- Constipation related to interruption of normal pattern of elimination
- Acute pain related to abdominal cramping
- Deficient knowledge related to drug therapy

Planning and implementation

- Drug is used mainly to reestablish proper toilet habits in laxative-dependent patient.
- Drug must be retained for at least 15 minutes; usually acts within 1 hour. Entire suppository need not melt to be effective.
- Notify prescriber if drug isn't effective.

Patient teaching

- Warn patient that abdominal cramping may occur but will subside when bowel is emptied.

Evaluation

- Patient reports return of normal bowel pattern of elimination.
- Patient states that abdominal cramping is transient.
- Patient and family state understanding of drug therapy.

glycopyrrolate

(gligh-koh-PEER-uh-layt)
Robinul, Robinul Forte

Pharmacologic class: anticholinergic
Therapeutic class: antimuscarinic, GI antispasmodic
Pregnancy risk category: B

Indications and dosages

▶ **Blockade of adverse cholinergic effects caused by anticholinesterase agents used to reverse neuromuscular blockade.** *Adults and children:* 0.2 mg I.V. for each 1 mg neostigmine or 5 mg of pyridostigmine. May be given I.V. without dilution or may be added to dextrose injection and given by infusion.

▶ **Preoperatively to diminish secretions and block cardiac vagal reflexes.** *Adults and children age 2 and older:* 0.0044 mg/kg of body weight I.M. 30 to 60 minutes before anesthesia.
Children under age 2: up to 0.0088 mg/kg I.M. 30 to 60 minutes before anesthesia.

▶ **Adjunct therapy in peptic ulcerations and other GI disorders.** *Adults:* 1 to 2 mg P.O. t.i.d. or 0.1 mg I.M. t.i.d. or q.i.d. Dosage must be individualized. Maximum P.O. dosage is 8 mg daily.

How supplied

Tablets: 1 mg, 2 mg
Injection: 0.2 mg/ml

Pharmacokinetics

Absorption: poorly absorbed from GI tract after P.O. use. Rapidly absorbed after I.M. use. Unknown after S.C. use.
Distribution: rapidly distributed; doesn't cross blood-brain barrier or enter CNS.
Metabolism: unknown.
Excretion: small amounts eliminated in urine as unchanged drug and metabolites; most excreted unchanged in feces or bile. *Half-life:* 1.7 hours.

Route	Onset	Peak	Duration
P.O.	Unknown	Unknown	Unknown
I.V.	Unknown	Unknown	3-7 hr
I.M.	15-30 min	30-45 min	3-7 hr
S.C.	15-30 min	Unknown	3-7 hr

Pharmacodynamics

Chemical effect: inhibits cholinergic (muscarinic) actions of acetylcholine on autonomic

effectors innervated by postganglionic cholinergic nerves.
Therapeutic effect: diminishes secretions and GI motility and blocks drug-induced cholinergic effects.

Adverse reactions

CNS: disorientation, irritability, incoherence, weakness, nervousness, drowsiness, dizziness, headache, confusion or excitement.
CV: palpitations, tachycardia, ***paradoxical bradycardia.***
EENT: *dilated pupils, blurred vision,* photophobia, increased intraocular pressure.
GI: abdominal distention, loss of taste, *constipation,* difficulty swallowing, *dry mouth,* nausea, vomiting, epigastric distress.
GU: *urinary hesitancy, urine retention,* impotence.
Respiratory: *bronchial plugging.*
Skin: urticaria, decreased sweating or anhidrosis, other dermal manifestations.
Other: burning at injection site, fever, ***anaphylaxis.***

Interactions

Drug-drug. *Amantadine, antihistamines, antiparkinsons, disopyramide, glutethimide, meperidine, phenothiazines, procainamide, quinidine, tricyclic antidepressants:* additive adverse effects. Avoid concomitant use.
Antacids: decreased absorption of oral anticholinergics. Separate administration times by 2 to 3 hours.
Ketoconazole: anticholinergics may interfere with ketoconazole absorption. Avoid concomitant use.
Methotrimeprazine: anticholinergics may enhance risk of extrapyramidal reactions. Avoid concomitant use.

Contraindications and precautions

- Contraindicated in patients hypersensitive to drug and in those with glaucoma, obstructive uropathy, obstructive disease of GI tract, myasthenia gravis, paralytic ileus, intestinal atony, unstable CV status in acute hemorrhage, severe ulcerative colitis, or toxic megacolon.
- Drug not recommended for breast-feeding women.
- Use cautiously in pregnant women, patients in hot or humid environments (to prevent drug-induced heatstroke), and patients with autonomic neuropathy, hyperthyroidism, coronary artery disease, arrhythmias, heart failure, hypertension, hiatal hernia, hepatic or renal disease, or ulcerative colitis.

NURSING CONSIDERATIONS

Assessment

- Assess patient's condition before therapy and regularly thereafter.
- Be alert for adverse reactions and drug interactions.
- Evaluate patient's and family's knowledge of drug therapy.

Nursing diagnoses

- Ineffective health maintenance related to patient's underlying condition
- Urinary retention related to drug's adverse effect on urinary system
- Deficient knowledge related to drug therapy

Planning and implementation

- Elderly patients typically receive smaller dosages and are more prone to confusion or excitement.

P.O. use: Administer drug 30 minutes to 1 hour before meals.
I.V. use: Give by direct injection without dilution. Or, inject into I.V. line containing free-flowing solution.
– Don't mix with I.V. solution containing sodium bicarbonate or alkaline solutions with pH above 6. Alkaline drugs, such as barbiturates (thiopental, methohexital, secobarbital, pentobarbital), chloramphenicol, dexamethasone, dimenhydrinate, diazepam, methylprednisolone, and pentazocine, are incompatible with glycopyrrolate.
I.M. and S.C. use: Follow normal protocol.

- Check all dosages carefully; slight overdose can lead to toxicity.
- Notify prescriber of urine retention; be prepared to catheterize patient.

Patient teaching

- Warn patient to avoid activities that require alertness until drug's CNS effects are known.

• Advise patient to report signs of urinary hesitancy or urine retention.

Evaluation
• Patient responds well to drug.
• Patient regains normal voiding pattern.
• Patient and family state understanding of drug therapy.

gonadorelin acetate
(goh-nah-doh-REH-lin AS-ih-tayt)
Lutrepulse

Pharmacologic class: gonadotropin-releasing hormone (Gn-RH)
Therapeutic class: fertility agent
Pregnancy risk category: B

Indications and dosages
▶ **Induction of ovulation in women with primary hypothalamic amenorrhea.** *Adults:* 5 mcg I.V. q 90 minutes for 21 days. If no response follows three treatment intervals, increase dosage as ordered.

How supplied
Injection: 0.8 mg/10 ml, 3.2 mg/10 ml vials; supplied as kit with I.V. supplies and ambulatory infusion pump

Pharmacokinetics
Absorption: not applicable.
Distribution: has low plasma volume of distribution and high rate of clearance from plasma.
Metabolism: rapidly metabolized.
Excretion: excreted primarily in urine. *Half-life:* initial, 2 to 10 minutes; terminal, 10 to 40 minutes.

Route	Onset	Peak	Duration
I.V.	Unknown	Unknown	Unknown

Pharmacodynamics
Chemical effect: mimics action of Gn-RH, which results in synthesis and release of luteinizing hormone (LH) from anterior pituitary gland. LH then acts on reproductive organs to regulate hormone synthesis.
Therapeutic effect: induces ovulation.

Adverse reactions
GU: multiple pregnancy, ovarian hyperstimulation.
Skin: hematoma, local infection, inflammation, mild phlebitis.

Interactions
Drug-drug. *Ovary-stimulating drugs:* additive effects. Avoid concomitant use.

Contraindications and precautions
• Contraindicated in patients hypersensitive to drug, in women with conditions that could be complicated by pregnancy (such as prolactinoma), in those who are anovulatory from any cause other than hypothalamic disorder, and in those with ovarian cysts.
• Safety of drug hasn't been established in adolescent girls.

NURSING CONSIDERATIONS

Assessment
• Assess patient's underlying condition before therapy.
• Monitor effectiveness by making sure patient has regular pelvic examinations, midluteal phase serum progesterone determinations, and pelvic ultrasound on days 7 and 14 after establishment of baseline scan.
• Closely monitor patient response; this is critical to ensure adequate ovarian stimulation without hyperstimulation (sudden ovarian enlargement, ascites, or pleural effusion).
• Be alert for adverse reactions.
• Inspect I.V. site at each visit, noting signs of infection.
• Evaluate patient's and family's knowledge of drug therapy.

Nursing diagnoses
• Sexual dysfunction related to underlying condition
• Risk for infection related to prolonged need for I.V. site
• Deficient knowledge related to drug therapy

Planning and implementation
• To mimic naturally occurring hormone, administer gonadorelin in pulsatile fashion with available ambulatory infusion pump. Set pulse

period at 1 minute (infuse drug over 1 minute) and pulse interval at 90 minutes.

- To administer 2.5 mcg/pulse, reconstitute 0.8-mg vial with 8 ml of supplied diluent and set pump to deliver 25 microliters/pulse. To administer 5 mcg/pulse, use same dosage strength and dilution but set pump to deliver 50 microliters/pulse.
- Some patients may need higher I.V. doses. To give 10 mcg/pulse, reconstitute 3.2-mg vial with 8 ml of supplied diluent and set pump to deliver 25 microliters/pulse. To give 20 mcg/pulse, use same dosage strength and dilution but set pump to deliver 50 microliters/pulse.
- Cannula and I.V. site should be changed every 48 hours.

Patient teaching

- Inform patient that multiple pregnancy is possible. (It happens about 12% of the time.) Close monitoring of dosage plus ovarian ultrasonography to monitor drug response is necessary.
- Instruct patient about proper aseptic technique and care of I.V. site. Cannula and I.V. site should be changed every 48 hours. Written instructions are available for patients.
- Teach patient to recognize and report hypersensitivity reactions (hives, wheezing, difficulty breathing); anaphylaxis has been reported with similar drugs.
- Advise patient to report signs of infection, hematoma, inflammation, or phlebitis at injection site, as well as severe abdominal pain, bloating, swelling of hands or feet, nausea, vomiting, diarrhea, substantial weight gain, or shortness of breath.
- Encourage patient to adhere to monitoring schedule required by therapy. Regular pelvic examinations, midluteal phase serum progesterone determinations, and multiple ovarian ultrasound scans are needed.

✔ Evaluation

- Patient ovulates during therapy.
- Patient is free from infection.
- Patient and family state understanding of drug therapy.

goserelin acetate

(GOH-seh-reh-lin AS-ih-tayt)
Zoladex, Zoladex 3-Month

Pharmacologic class: synthetic decapeptide
Therapeutic class: luteinizing hormone-releasing hormone (LH-RH; Gn-RH) analogue
Pregnancy risk category: X

Indications and dosages

▶ **Palliative treatment of advanced carcinoma of prostate; endometriosis and advanced breast carcinoma.** *Adults:* 1 implant S.C. q 28 days into upper abdominal wall for 6 months. For endometriosis, maximum duration of therapy is 6 months.

▶ **Palliative treatment of advanced carcinoma of the prostate.** *Adult men:* 1 (10.8 mg) implant S.C. q 12 weeks into upper abdominal wall.

▶ **Endometrial thinning before endometrial ablation for dysfunctional uterine bleeding.** *Adults:* one or two 3.6-mg implants S.C. into upper abdominal wall. Each implant should be given 4 weeks apart.

How supplied

Implants: 3.6 mg, 10.8 mg

Pharmacokinetics

Absorption: slowly absorbed from implant site.
Distribution: unknown.
Metabolism: unknown.
Excretion: route unknown. *Half-life:* about 4.2 hours.

Route	Onset	Peak	Duration
S.C.	2-4 wk	12-15 days	Throughout therapy

Pharmacodynamics

Chemical effect: LH-RH analogue that acts on pituitary to decrease release of follicle-stimulating hormone and LH, resulting in dramatically lowered serum levels of sex hormones.
Therapeutic effect: decreases effects of sex hormones on tumor growth in prostate gland and tissue growth in uterus.

Adverse reactions

CNS: lethargy, pain (worsened in first 30 days), dizziness, insomnia, anxiety, depression, headache, chills, emotional lability.
CV: edema, ***heart failure, arrhythmias, CVA,*** hypertension, ***MI,*** peripheral vascular disorder, chest pain.
GI: nausea, vomiting, diarrhea, constipation, ulcer.
GU: *impotence, sexual dysfunction, lower urinary tract symptoms,* renal insufficiency, urinary obstruction, urinary tract infection, amenorrhea, vaginal dryness.
Hematologic: anemia.
Metabolic: gout, hyperglycemia, weight increase.
Musculoskeletal: loss of bone mineral density (in women).
Respiratory: COPD, upper respiratory tract infection.
Skin: rash, diaphoresis.
Other: *hot flushes,* breast swelling and tenderness, changes in breast size, fever.

Interactions

None reported.

Contraindications and precautions

- Contraindicated in pregnant or breast-feeding women and in patients hypersensitive to LH-RH, LH-RH agonist analogues, or goserelin acetate.
- The 10.8-mg implant is contraindicated for use in women.
- Use cautiously in patients with risk factors for osteoporosis, such as family history of osteoporosis, chronic alcohol or tobacco abuse, or use of drugs that affect bone density.
- Drug should not be used in children.

NURSING CONSIDERATIONS

Assessment

- Assess patient's condition before therapy and regularly thereafter.
- Before giving drug to female patient, rule out pregnancy.
- When used for prostate cancer, LH-RH analogues such as goserelin may initially worsen symptoms because drug initially increases testosterone serum levels. Some patients may have increased bone pain. Rarely, disease (spinal cord compression or ureteral obstruction) has worsened.
- Be alert for adverse reactions.
- Evaluate patient's and family's knowledge of drug therapy.

Nursing diagnoses

- Ineffective health maintenance related to underlying condition
- Acute pain related to drug's adverse effect
- Deficient knowledge related to drug therapy

Planning and implementation

- Drug should be given under supervision of prescriber.
- Administer drug into upper abdominal wall using aseptic technique. After cleaning area with alcohol swab (and injecting local anesthetic), stretch patient's skin with one hand while grasping barrel of syringe with the other. Insert needle into S.C. fat; then change direction of needle so that it parallels abdominal wall. Needle should then be pushed in until hub touches patient's skin and then withdrawn about 1 cm (this creates gap for drug to be injected) before depressing plunger completely.
- To avoid need for new syringe and injection site, don't aspirate after inserting needle.
- Implant comes in preloaded syringe. If package is damaged, don't use syringe. Make sure drug is visible in translucent chamber.
- After implantation, area requires bandage after needle is withdrawn.
- Be prepared to schedule patient for ultrasound to locate goserelin implants if they require removal.
- Notify prescriber of adverse reactions and provide supportive care as indicated and ordered.

Patient teaching

- Advise patient to report every 28 days for new implant. A delay of a couple of days is permissible.
- Tell woman to use nonhormonal form of contraception during treatment. Caution her about significant risks to fetus should pregnancy occur.

• Tell patient to call prescriber if menstruation persists or breakthrough bleeding occurs. Menstruation should stop during treatment.
• After therapy ends, inform patient that she may experience delayed return of menses. Persistent amenorrhea is rare.
• Warn patient that pain may occur.

Evaluation

• Patient responds well to drug.
• Patient has no pain.
• Patient and family state understanding of drug therapy.

granisetron hydrochloride

(grah-NEEZ-eh-trohn high-droh-KLOR-ighd)
Kytril

Pharmacologic class: selective 5-hydroxytryptamine (5-HT_3) receptor antagonist
Therapeutic class: antiemetic, antinauseant
Pregnancy risk category: B

Indications and dosages

▶ **Prevention of nausea and vomiting caused by emetogenic cancer chemotherapy.** *Adults and children ages 2 to 16:* 10 mcg/kg I.V. infused over 5 minutes. Begin infusion within 30 minutes before chemotherapy starts. Or, 1 mg P.O. up to 1 hour before chemotherapy. Dosage repeated 12 hours later.

▶ **Prevention of nausea and vomiting from radiation, including total body irradiation and fractionated abdominal radiation.** *Adults:* 2 mg P.O. once daily within 1 hour of radiation.

How supplied

Tablets: 1 mg
Injection: 1 mg/ml

Pharmacokinetics

Absorption: unknown after P.O. administration.
Distribution: distributed freely between plasma and RBCs; plasma protein–binding about 65%.
Metabolism: metabolized by liver.
Excretion: excreted in urine and feces.

Route	Onset	Peak	Duration
P.O., I.V.	Unknown	Unknown	Unknown

Pharmacodynamics

Chemical effect: located in CNS at area postrema (chemoreceptor trigger zone) and in peripheral nervous system on nerve terminals of vagus nerve. Drug's blocking action may occur at both sites.
Therapeutic effect: prevents nausea and vomiting from chemotherapy.

Adverse reactions

CNS: *headache, asthenia,* somnolence.
CV: hypertension.
GI: taste disorder, diarrhea, constipation.
Hematologic: ***thrombocytopenia.***
Other: fever.

Interactions

Drug-herb. *Horehound:* May enhance serotonergic effects. Discourage use.

Contraindications and precautions

• Contraindicated in patients hypersensitive to drug.
• Use cautiously in pregnant or breast-feeding women.

NURSING CONSIDERATIONS

Assessment

• Assess patient's chemotherapy and GI reactions before therapy.
• Monitor patient for nausea and vomiting.
• Be alert for adverse reactions.
• Monitor hydration status if drug is ineffective or diarrhea occurs.
• Evaluate patient's and family's knowledge of drug therapy.

Nursing diagnoses

• Risk for deficient fluid volume related to nausea and vomiting
• Acute pain related to drug-induced headache
• Deficient knowledge related to drug therapy

Planning and implementation

P.O. use: Give drug 1 hour before chemotherapy; repeat in 12 hours.

I.V. use: Dilute drug with normal saline injection or D_5W to 20 to 50 ml. Infuse over 5 minutes beginning within 30 minutes before chemotherapy starts, and only on day(s) chemotherapy is given. Diluted solutions are stable for 24 hours at room temperature.

– Don't mix with other drugs; compatibility data are limited.

- Alert prescriber if patient experiences nausea or vomiting.

Patient teaching

- Tell patient to notify prescriber if adverse drug reactions occur.

Evaluation

- Patient has no nausea or vomiting with chemotherapy.
- Patient's headache is relieved with mild analgesic.
- Patient and family state understanding of drug therapy.

griseofulvin microsize

(gris-ee-oh-FUHL-vin MIGH-kroh-sighz)

Fulcin ◇, Fulvicin-U/F, Grifulvin V*, Grisactin, Grisovin ◇, Grisovin-FP

griseofulvin ultramicrosize

Fulvicin P/G, Grisactin Ultra, Gris-PEG

Pharmacologic class: *Penicillium* antibiotic
Therapeutic class: antifungal
Pregnancy risk category: C

Indications and dosages

▶ **Ringworm infection of skin, hair, nails (tinea corporis, tinea capitis) when caused by *Trichophyton, Microsporum,* or *Epidermophyton.*** *Adults:* 500 mg (microsize) P.O. daily in single or divided doses. Severe infections may require up to 1 g daily. Or, 330 to 375 mg ultramicrosize daily in single or divided doses.

▶ **Tinea pedis and tinea unguium.** *Adults:* 0.75 to 1 g (microsize) P.O. daily. Or, 660 to 750 mg ultramicrosize P.O. daily in divided doses.

Children: 11 mg/kg/day (microsize) P.O. Or, 7.3 mg/kg/day (ultramicrosize).

How supplied

griseofulvin microsize

Tablets: 250 mg, 500 mg
Capsules: 250 mg
Oral suspension: 125 mg/5 ml*

griseofulvin ultramicrosize

Tablets: 125 mg, 165 mg, 250 mg, 330 mg

Pharmacokinetics

Absorption: absorbed primarily in duodenum; varies among patients. Ultramicrosize preparations are absorbed almost completely; microsize absorption ranges from 25% to 70% and may be increased by giving with high-fat meal.
Distribution: drug concentrates in skin, hair, nails, fat, liver, and skeletal muscle; tightly bound to new keratin.
Metabolism: metabolized in liver.
Excretion: about 50% excreted in urine, 33% in feces, less than 1% unchanged in urine; also excreted in perspiration. *Half-life:* 9 to 24 hours.

Route	Onset	Peak	Duration
P.O.	Unknown	4-8 hr	Unknown

Pharmacodynamics

Chemical effect: arrests fungal cell activity by disrupting its mitotic spindle structure.
Therapeutic effect: inhibits fungal cell growth. Spectrum of activity includes *Trichophyton, Microsporum,* and *Epidermophyton.*

Adverse reactions

CNS: headache, transient decrease in hearing, fatigue with large doses, occasional mental confusion, impaired performance of routine activities, psychotic symptoms, dizziness, insomnia.
GI: oral thrush, nausea, vomiting, excessive thirst, flatulence, diarrhea, ***bleeding.***
Hematologic: leukopenia, ***agranulocytosis***, porphyria.
Hepatic: ***hepatic toxicity.***
Skin: rash, urticaria, photosensitivity, ***toxic epidermal necrolysis.***

Other: estrogen-like effects in children, hypersensitivity reactions (rash, ***angioedema,*** serum sickness–like reactions), lupuslike syndrome or worsening of existing lupus erythematosus.

Interactions

Drug-drug. *Coumarin anticoagulants:* decreased effectiveness. Monitor PT and INR when used concurrently.
Cyclosporine: cyclosporine levels may be reduced, resulting in decreased pharmacologic effects. Avoid concomitant use.
Oral contraceptives: decreased effectiveness. Suggest alternate methods of contraception.
Phenobarbital: decreased griseofulvin blood levels as a result of decreased absorption or increased metabolism. Avoid using together or administer griseofulvin t.i.d.
Drug-food. *High-fat meals:* increased absorption. Administer together.
Drug-lifestyle. *Alcohol use:* may cause tachycardia, diaphoresis, and flushing. Discourage concomitant use.
Sunlight: Photosensitivity may occur. Urge precautions.

Contraindications and precautions

• Contraindicated in patients hypersensitive to drug and in those with porphyria or hepatocellular failure.
• Also contraindicated in pregnant women or women who intend to become pregnant during therapy.
• Use cautiously in penicillin-sensitive patients because griseofulvin is penicillin derivative.
• Safety of drug hasn't been established in breast-feeding women.

NURSING CONSIDERATIONS

Assessment

• Assess patient's fungal infection before therapy.
• Monitor for improvement of signs and symptoms and for laboratory confirmation of complete eradication of organism.
• Assess hematologic, renal, and hepatic function periodically during prolonged therapy, as ordered.
• Be alert for adverse reactions and drug interactions.
• Evaluate patient's and family's knowledge of drug therapy.

Nursing diagnoses

• Infection related to presence of susceptible fungi
• Ineffective protection related to drug-induced granulocytopenia
• Deficient knowledge related to drug therapy

Planning and implementation

• Because of potential toxicity, drug is used only when topical treatment fails to arrest mycotic disease.
• Obtain laboratory tests as ordered to confirm diagnosis of infecting organism. Continue drug until clinical and laboratory examinations confirm complete eradication.
• Because griseofulvin ultramicrosize is dispersed in polyethylene glycol, it's absorbed more rapidly and completely than microsize preparations and is effective at one-half to two-thirds the usual griseofulvin dose.
• Give after high-fat meal to enhance absorption and minimize GI distress.
• Keep in mind that effective treatment of tinea pedis may require concomitant use of topical agent.
• Notify prescriber immediately of granulocytopenia or agranulocytosis, which requires discontinuation of drug.

Patient teaching

• Advise patient that prolonged treatment may be needed to control infection and prevent relapse, even if symptoms abate in first few days. Tell him to keep skin clean and dry and to maintain good hygiene.
• Instruct woman not to become pregnant while on drug therapy.
• Caution patient to avoid intense sunlight.
• Instruct patient to avoid alcohol consumption during therapy.
• Instruct patient to take drug after high-fat meal.
• Warn patient to avoid hazardous activities that require alertness if adverse CNS reactions occur.

Evaluation

• Patient's infection is alleviated.

- Patient's CBC remains within normal limits.
- Patient and family state understanding of drug therapy.

guaifenesin (glyceryl guaiacolate)

(gwah-FEH-nih-sin)

Anti-Tuss*†, Balminil Expectorant♦†, Breonesin†, Gee-Gee†, GG-Cen*†, Glyate*†, Glycotuss†, Glytuss†, Guiatuss*†, Halotussin *, Humibid L.A., Hytuss†, Hytuss-2X†, Naldecon Senior EX†, Resyl♦†, Robitussin*†, Scot-Tussin Expectorant*†

Pharmacologic class: propanediol derivative
Therapeutic class: expectorant
Pregnancy risk category: C

Indications and dosages

▶ **Expectorant.** *Adults and children age 12 and over:* 200 to 400 mg P.O. q 4 hours, or 600 to 1,200 mg extended-release capsules q 12 hours. Maximum, 2,400 mg daily.
Children ages 6 to 12: 100 to 200 mg P.O. q 4 hours. Maximum, 1,200 mg daily.
Children ages 2 to 6: 50 to 100 mg P.O. q 4 hours. Maximum, 600 mg daily.

How supplied

Tablets: 100 mg†, 200 mg†
Tablets (extended-release): 600 mg
Capsules: 200 mg†
Capsules (extended-release): 300 mg
Solution: 100 mg/ml*†, 200 mg/5 ml*†

Pharmacokinetics

Unknown.

Route	Onset	Peak	Duration
P.O.	Unknown	Unknown	Unknown

Pharmacodynamics

Chemical effect: increases production of respiratory tract fluids to help liquefy and reduce viscosity of tenacious secretions.
Therapeutic effect: thins respiratory secretions for easier removal.

Adverse reactions

CNS: drowsiness.
GI: stomach pain, diarrhea, vomiting, nausea (with large doses).
Skin: rash.

Interactions

None significant

Contraindications and precautions

- Contraindicated in patients hypersensitive to drug.
- Use cautiously in pregnant women.
- Safety of drug hasn't been established in breast-feeding women.

NURSING CONSIDERATIONS

Assessment

- Assess patient's sputum production before and after giving drug.
- Be alert for adverse reactions and drug interactions.
- Monitor patient's hydration status if adverse GI reactions occur.
- Evaluate patient's and family's knowledge of drug therapy.

Nursing diagnoses

- Ineffective airway clearance related to underlying condition
- Risk for deficient fluid volume related to adverse GI reactions
- Deficient knowledge related to drug therapy

Planning and implementation

- Give drug with a full glass of water.
- Drug may interfere with laboratory tests for 5-hydroxyindoleacetic acid and vanillylmandelic acid.

Patient teaching

- Inform patient that persistent cough may indicate a serious condition. Tell him to contact prescriber if cough lasts longer than 1 week, recurs frequently, or accompanies a high fever, rash, or severe headache.
- Advise patient to take each dose with a full glass of water before and after dose; increasing fluid intake may prove beneficial.

• Encourage patient to perform deep-breathing exercises.

Evaluation
• Patient's lungs are clear and respiratory secretions are normal.
• Patient maintains adequate hydration.
• Patient and family state understanding of drug therapy.

guanabenz acetate
(GWAH-nuh-benz AS-ih-tayt)
Wytensin

Pharmacologic class: centrally acting antiadrenergic
Therapeutic class: antihypertensive
Pregnancy risk category: C

Indications and dosages
▶ **Hypertension.** *Adults:* initially, 2 to 4 mg P.O. b.i.d. Dosage increased in increments of 4 to 8 mg/day q 1 to 2 weeks. Maximum daily dosage is 32 mg b.i.d. To ensure overnight blood pressure control, give last dose h.s.

How supplied
Tablets: 4 mg, 8 mg

Pharmacokinetics
Absorption: 70% to 80% absorbed from GI tract.
Distribution: appears to be distributed widely into body; about 90% protein-bound.
Metabolism: metabolized extensively in liver.
Excretion: excreted primarily in urine, remainder in feces. *Half-life:* about 6 hours.

Route	Onset	Peak	Duration
P.O.	≤ 1 hr	2-5 hr	About 12 hr

Pharmacodynamics
Chemical effect: unknown; may be from central alpha-adrenergic stimulation, which results in decreased sympathetic outflow to heart, kidneys, and peripheral vasculature.
Therapeutic effect: lowers blood pressure.

Adverse reactions
CNS: *drowsiness, sedation, dizziness,* weakness, headache, ataxia, depression.
CV: *rebound hypertension.*
GI: *dry mouth.*
GU: sexual dysfunction.

Interactions
Drug-drug. *CNS depressants:* may cause increased sedation. Use together cautiously.
MAO inhibitors, tricyclic antidepressants: may decrease antihypertensive effect. Monitor patient closely.
Drug-lifestyle. *Alcohol use.* May enhance CNS effect. Discourage use.

Contraindications and precautions
• Contraindicated in patients hypersensitive to drug.
• Drug not recommended for breast-feeding women.
• Use cautiously in patients with severe coronary insufficiency, recent MI, cerebrovascular disease, or severe hepatic or renal failure. Also use cautiously in elderly patients and pregnant women.
• Safety of drug hasn't been established in children.

NURSING CONSIDERATIONS

Assessment
• Assess blood pressure before therapy and regularly thereafter.
• Be alert for adverse reactions and drug interactions.
• Evaluate patient's and family's knowledge of drug therapy.

Nursing diagnoses
• Risk for injury related to presence of hypertension
• Risk for trauma related to drug-induced adverse reactions
• Deficient knowledge related to drug therapy

Planning and implementation
• Give last dose of day just before sleep to help ensure adequate blood pressure control.
• Don't stop drug abruptly because rebound hypertension may occur.

• Thiazide diuretics may be used concomitantly to treat hypertension.

Patient teaching

• Caution patient that stopping drug abruptly may cause rebound hypertension.
• Advise patient to avoid hazardous tasks that require alertness until CNS effects of drug are known.
• Inform patient that orthostatic hypotension can be minimized by rising slowly and avoiding sudden position changes. Dry mouth can be relieved with chewing gum, sour hard candy, or ice chips.
• Warn patient that tolerance to alcohol or other CNS depressants may be diminished.

Evaluation

• Patient's blood pressure is within normal limits.
• Patient doesn't experience trauma from adverse reactions.
• Patient and family state understanding of drug therapy.

guanfacine hydrochloride

(GWAHN-fuh-seen high-droh-KLOR-ighd)

Tenex

Pharmacologic class: centrally acting antiadrenergic
Therapeutic class: antihypertensive
Pregnancy risk category: B

Indications and dosages

▶ **Hypertension.** *Adults:* initially, 1 mg P.O. daily h.s. May be increased to 2 mg P.O. h.s. after 3 to 4 weeks, as needed. May be further increased to 3 mg P.O. h.s. after another 3 to 4 weeks, as needed. Average is 1 to 3 mg daily.

How supplied

Tablets: 1 mg, 2 mg

Pharmacokinetics

Absorption: absorbed well and completely; about 80% bioavailable.
Distribution: thought to be highly distributed; about 70% protein-bound.
Metabolism: metabolized in liver.
Excretion: excreted in urine. *Half-life:* about 17 hours.

Route	Onset	Peak	Duration
P.O.	Unknown	1-4 hr	24 hr

Pharmacodynamics

Chemical effect: unknown; may inhibit central vasomotor center, decreasing sympathetic outflow to heart, kidneys, and peripheral vasculature.
Therapeutic effect: lowers blood pressure.

Adverse reactions

CNS: *drowsiness, dizziness,* fatigue, headache, insomnia.
CV: ***bradycardia***, orthostatic hypotension, rebound hypertension.
GI: *constipation,* diarrhea, nausea, *dry mouth.*
Skin: dermatitis, pruritus.

Interactions

Drug-drug. *CNS depressants:* potential for increased sedation. Avoid concomitant use.
Drug-lifestyle. *Alcohol use.* May enhance CNS effect. Discourage use.

Contraindications and precautions

• Contraindicated in patients hypersensitive to drug.
• Use cautiously in patients with severe coronary insufficiency, cerebrovascular disease, recent MI, or chronic renal or hepatic insufficiency, and in pregnant women.
• Safety of drug hasn't been established in breast-feeding women or in children.

NURSING CONSIDERATIONS

Assessment

• Assess blood pressure before therapy and regularly thereafter.
• Be alert for adverse reactions. Incidence and severity increase with higher dosages.
• Evaluate patient's and family's knowledge of drug therapy.

Nursing diagnoses
- Risk for injury related to presence of hypertension
- Constipation related to adverse effects on GI tract
- Deficient knowledge related to drug therapy

Planning and implementation
- Give daily dosage at bedtime to minimize daytime drowsiness.
- Drug may be used alone or with diuretic.

Patient teaching
- Tell patient not to stop therapy abruptly. Rebound hypertension is less common than with similar drugs but may occur.
- Advise patient to avoid activities that require alertness until response to drug is known.
- Instruct patient to check with prescriber before taking other OTC medications.

Evaluation
- Patient's blood pressure is normal.
- Patient's bowel pattern is normal.
- Patient and family state understanding of drug therapy.

H

haloperidol
(hal-oh-PER-uh-dol)
Apo-Haloperidol ♦, Haldol**, Novo-Peridol ♦, Peridol ♦, PMS Haloperidol, Serenace ◇

haloperidol decanoate
Haldol Decanoate, Haldol LA ♦

haloperidol lactate
Haldol

Pharmacologic class: butyrophenone
Therapeutic class: antipsychotic
Pregnancy risk category: C

Indications and dosagess
▶ **Psychotic disorders.** *Adults and children age 12 and older:* dosage varies for each patient. Initial range, 0.5 to 5 mg P.O. b.i.d. or t.i.d. Or, 2 to 5 mg I.M. q 4 to 8 hours, although q-1-hour administration may be needed until control is obtained. Maximum, 100 mg P.O. daily.
Children ages 3 to 12: 0.05 to 0.15 mg/kg/day P.O. given b.i.d. or t.i.d. Severely disturbed children may need higher doses.
▶ **Chronically psychotic patients who need prolonged therapy.** *Adults:* 50 to 100 mg I.M. decanoate q 4 weeks.
▶ **Nonpsychotic behavior disorders.** *Children ages 3 to 12:* 0.05 to 0.075 mg/kg/day P.O. b.i.d. or t.i.d. Maximum, 6 mg daily.
▶ **Tourette syndrome.** *Adults:* 0.5 to 5 mg P.O. b.i.d., t.i.d., or p.r.n.
Children ages 3 to 12: 0.05 to 0.075 mg/kg/day P.O. b.i.d. or t.i.d.

How supplied
haloperidol
Tablets: 0.5 mg, 1 mg, 2 mg, 5 mg, 10 mg, 20 mg
haloperidol decanoate
Injection: 50 mg/ml, 100 mg/ml
haloperidol lactate
Oral concentrate: 2 mg/ml
Injection: 5 mg/ml

Pharmacokinetics
Absorption: about 60% of P.O. dose absorbed; about 70% of I.M. dose absorbed within 30 minutes.
Distribution: distributed widely, with high levels in adipose tissue; 91% to 99% protein-bound.
Metabolism: metabolized extensively by liver.
Excretion: about 40% excreted in urine within 5 days; about 15% excreted in feces by way of biliary tract. *Half-life:* P.O., 24 hours; I.M., 21 hours.

Route	Onset	Peak	Duration
P.O.	Unknown	3-6 hr	Unknown
I.M.	Unknown	10-20 min	Unknown (lactate); 3-9 days (decanoate)

Pharmacodynamics

Chemical effect: may block postsynaptic dopamine receptors in brain.
Therapeutic effect: decreases psychotic behaviors.

Adverse reactions

CNS: *severe extrapyramidal reactions, tardive dyskinesia,* sedation, ***seizures, neuroleptic malignant syndrome.***
CV: CV effects.
EENT: *blurred vision.*
GU: urine retention, menstrual irregularities.
Hematologic: transient leukopenia and leukocytosis.
Hepatic: altered liver function test results, jaundice.
Skin: rash.
Other: gynecomastia.

Interactions

Drug-drug. *Carbamazepine:* may decrease haloperidol serum levels. Monitor patient.
CNS depressants: increased CNS depression. Avoid concomitant use.
Fluoxetine: possibility of severe extrapyramidal reaction when administered with haloperidol. Avoid concomitant use.
Lithium: lethargy and confusion with high doses. Monitor patient.
Methyldopa: symptoms of dementia or psychosis. Monitor patient.
Phenytoin: serum haloperidol levels may be decreased. Monitor patient.
Drug-herb. *Nutmeg:* possible loss of symptom control or interference with therapy for psychiatric illness. Discourage concomitant use.
Drug-lifestyle. *Alcohol use:* increased CNS depression. Discourage concomitant use.

Contraindications and precautions

- Contraindicated in patients hypersensitive to drug or in those with parkinsonism, coma, or CNS depression.
- Drug isn't recommended for breast-feeding women.
- Safety of drug hasn't been established in pregnant women.
- Use cautiously in elderly or debilitated patients; patients who take anticonvulsants, anticoagulants, antiparkinsonians, or lithium; and patients with history of seizures or EEG abnormalities, severe CV disorders, allergies, glaucoma, or urine retention.

NURSING CONSIDERATIONS

Assessment

- Assess patient's disorder before therapy and regularly thereafter.
- Be alert for adverse reactions and drug interactions.
- Monitor patient for tardive dyskinesia. It may occur after prolonged use. It may not appear until months or years later and may disappear spontaneously or persist for life despite discontinuation of drug.
- Evaluate patient's and family's knowledge of drug therapy.

Nursing diagnoses

- Disturbed thought processes related to underlying condition
- Impaired physical mobility related to extrapyramidal effects
- Deficient knowledge related to drug therapy

Planning and implementation

P.O. use: Follow normal protocol.
I.M. use: Give drug by deep I.M. injection in gluteal region using a 21G needle. Maximum volume of injection should not exceed 3 ml.

- Elderly patient usually requires lower initial doses and more gradual dosage adjustment.
- Don't administer decanoate I.V.
- When changing from tablets to injection, patient should be given 10 to 15 times oral dose once monthly (maximum, 100 mg).
- Protect drug from light. Slight yellowing of injection or concentrate is common; doesn't affect potency. Discard markedly discolored solutions.
- Don't stop drug abruptly unless required by severe adverse reactions.
- Acute dystonic reactions may be treated with diphenhydramine.

Patient teaching

- Warn patient to avoid activities that require alertness and psychomotor coordination until CNS effects of drug are known.

• Tell patient to avoid alcohol while taking drug.
• Tell patient to relieve dry mouth with sugarless gum or hard candy.
• Instruct patient to take drug exactly as prescribed and not to double doses to compensate for missed ones.

Evaluation

• Patient demonstrates decreased psychotic behavior.
• Patient maintains physical mobility.
• Patient and family state understanding of drug therapy.

heparin sodium

(HEH-puh-rin SOH-dee-um)

Hepalean ♦, Heparin Leo ♦, Heparin Lock Flush Solution (with Tubex), Hep-Lock, Liquaemin Sodium, Uniparin ◊

Pharmacologic class: anticoagulant
Therapeutic class: anticoagulant
Pregnancy risk category: C

Indications and dosages

Heparin dosing is highly individualized, depending upon disease state, age, and renal and hepatic status.

▶ **Deep vein thrombosis, pulmonary embolism.** *Adults:* initially, 10,000 units I.V. push; then adjusted according to PTT and given I.V. q 4 to 6 hours (5,000 to 10,000 units). Or, 5,000 units I.V. bolus; then 20,000 to 40,000 units in 24 hours by I.V. infusion pump. Hourly rate adjusted 4 to 6 hours after bolus dose according to PTT.
Children: initially, 50 units/kg I.V. drip. Maintenance dosage is 100 units/kg I.V. drip q 4 hours. Constant infusion: 20,000 units/m^2 daily. Dosages adjusted according to PTT.

▶ **Embolism prevention.** *Adults:* 5,000 units S.C. q 8 to 12 hours. In surgical patients, first dose given 2 hours before procedure; followed with 5,000 units S.C. q 8 to 12 hours for 5 to 7 days or until patient is fully ambulatory.

▶ **Open-heart surgery.** *Adults:* (total body perfusion) 150 to 400 units/kg continuous I.V infusion.

▶ **Disseminated intravascular coagulation.** *Adults:* 50 to 100 units/kg I.V. q 4 hours as a single injection or constant infusion. Discontinue if no improvement in 4 to 8 hours.
Children: 25 to 50 units/kg I.V. q 4 hours, as a single injection or constant infusion. Discontinue if no improvement in 4 to 8 hours.

▶ **Maintaining patency of I.V. indwelling catheters.** *Adults:* 10 to 100 units I.V. flush. Use sufficient volume to fill device. Not intended for therapeutic use.

How supplied

Products are derived from beef lung or porcine intestinal mucosa.

heparin sodium

Carpuject: 5,000 units/ml
Disposable syringes: 1,000 units/ml, 2,500 units/ml, 5,000 units/ml, 7,500 units/ml, 10,000 units/ml, 15,000 units/ml, 20,000 units/ml, 40,000 units/ml
Premixed I.V. solutions: 1,000 units in 500 ml of normal saline solution; 2,000 units in 1,000 ml of normal saline solution; 12,500 units in 250 ml of half-normal saline solution; 25,000 units in 250 ml of half-normal saline solution; 25,000 units in 500 ml of half-normal saline solution; 10,000 units in 100 ml of D_5W; 12,500 units in 250 ml of D_5W; 25,000 units in 250 ml of D_5W; 25,000 units in 500 ml of D_5W; 20,000 units in 500 ml of D_5W
Unit-dose ampules: 1,000 units/ml, 5,000 units/ml, 10,000 units/ml
Vials: 1,000 units/ml, 2,500 units/ml, 5,000 units/ml, 7,500 units/ml, 10,000 units/ml, 15,000 units/ml, 20,000 units/ml, 40,000 units/ml

heparin sodium flush

Disposable syringes: 10 units/ml, 100 units/ml
Vials: 10 units/ml, 100 units/ml

Pharmacokinetics

Absorption: absorbed after S.C. administration.
Distribution: extensively bound to lipoprotein, globulins, and fibrinogen.
Metabolism: thought to be removed by reticuloendothelial system, with some metabolism occurring in liver.
Excretion: small amount excreted in urine as unchanged drug. *Half-life:* 1 to 2 hours. Half-

life is dose-dependent and nonlinear and may be disproportionately prolonged at higher doses.

Route	Onset	Peak	Duration
I.V.	Immediate	Unknown	Unknown
S.C.	20-60 min	2-4 hr	Unknown

Pharmacodynamics

Chemical effect: accelerates formation of antithrombin III–thrombin complex and deactivates thrombin, preventing conversion of fibrinogen to fibrin.
Therapeutic effect: decreases ability of blood to clot.

Adverse reactions

Hematologic: ***hemorrhage*** (with excessive dosage), *overly prolonged clotting time,* ***thrombocytopenia.***
Skin: irritation, mild pain, hematoma, ulceration, cutaneous or subcutaneous necrosis.
Other: ***white clot syndrome; hypersensitivity reactions,*** including chills, fever, pruritus, rhinitis, burning of feet, conjunctivitis, lacrimation, arthralgia, urticaria, ***anaphylaxis.***

Interactions

Drug-drug. *Oral anticoagulants:* increased additive anticoagulation. Monitor PT, INR, and PTT.
Salicylates, other antiplatelet drugs: increased anticoagulant effect. Don't use together.
Thrombolytics: increased risk of hemorrhage. Monitor patient closely.
Drug-herb. *Dong quai, feverfew, garlic, ginger, horse chestnut, motherwort, red clover:* possible increased risk of bleeding. Monitor patient closely for bleeding if he has been using these herbal products.

Contraindications and precautions

- Contraindicated in patients hypersensitive to drug.
- Conditionally contraindicated in patients with active bleeding; blood dyscrasia; bleeding tendencies, such as hemophilia, thrombocytopenia, or hepatic disease with hypoprothrombinemia; suspected intracranial hemorrhage; suppurative thrombophlebitis; inaccessible ulcerative lesions (especially of GI tract) and open ulcerative wounds; extensive denudation of skin; ascorbic acid deficiency and other conditions causing increased capillary permeability; subacute bacterial endocarditis; shock; advanced renal disease; threatened abortion; severe hypertension. Also conditionally contraindicated during or after brain, eye, or spinal cord surgery; during spinal tap or spinal anesthesia and during continuous tube drainage of stomach or small intestine. Although heparin is clearly hazardous in these conditions, risk versus benefits must be evaluated.
- Use cautiously during menses; immediately postpartum; in patients with mild hepatic or renal disease, alcoholism, or occupations with risk of physical injury; and in patients with history of allergies, asthma, or GI ulcerations.
- When patient needs anticoagulation during pregnancy, most clinicians use heparin.

NURSING CONSIDERATIONS

Assessment

- Assess patient's underlying condition before therapy.
- Draw blood to establish baseline coagulation values before therapy.
- Monitor effectiveness by measuring PTT carefully and regularly. Anticoagulation present when PTT values are 1½ to 2 times control values.
- During intermittent I.V. therapy, always draw blood 30 minutes before next dose to avoid falsely elevated PTT. Blood for PTT may be drawn 8 hours after start of continuous I.V. heparin therapy. Blood for PTT should never be drawn from I.V. tubing of heparin infusion or from infused vein; falsely elevated PTT will result. Always draw blood from opposite arm.
- Be alert for adverse reactions and drug interactions.
- Monitor platelet counts regularly. Thrombocytopenia caused by heparin may be associated with a type of arterial thrombosis known as white clot syndrome.
- Concentrated heparin solutions (greater than 100 units/ml) can irritate blood vessels.
- Evaluate patient's and family's knowledge of drug therapy.

Nursing diagnoses

- Risk for injury related to potential for thrombosis or emboli development from underlying condition
- Ineffective protection related to increased bleeding risks
- Deficient knowledge related to drug therapy

Planning and implementation

- Check order and vial carefully. Heparin comes in various concentrations.

I.V. use: Give drug I.V. using infusion pump to provide maximum safety because of long-term effect and irregular absorption when given S.C. Check constant I.V. infusions regularly, even when pumps are in good working order, to prevent giving too much or too little.
– Never piggyback other drugs into infusion line while heparin infusion is running. Many antibiotics and other drugs deactivate heparin. Never mix any drug with heparin in syringe when bolus therapy is used.
ALERT Don't skip dose or "catch up" with I.V. containing heparin. If I.V. is out, restart it as soon as possible, and reschedule bolus dose immediately.
S.C. use: Give low-dose injections sequentially between iliac crests in lower abdomen deep into S.C. fat. Inject drug slowly. Leave needle in place for 10 seconds after injection; then withdraw. Don't massage after S.C. injection, and watch for bleeding at injection site. Alternate sites every 12 hours—right for morning, left for evening.

- Drug requirements are higher in early phases of thrombogenic diseases and febrile states; lower when patient's condition stabilizes.
- Elderly patients should usually start at lower doses.
- Place notice above patient's bed to inform I.V. team or laboratory staff to apply pressure dressings after taking blood.
- Take bleeding precautions.
- To minimize the risk of hematoma, avoid excessive I.M. injection of other drugs. If possible, don't give I.M. injections at all.
- To treat severe heparin calcium or heparin sodium overdose, use protamine sulfate, a heparin antagonist, as ordered. Dosage is based on dose of heparin, its route of administration, and time elapsed since it was given. As a general rule, 1 to 1.5 units of protamine/100 units of heparin are given if only a few minutes have elapsed; 0.5 to 0.75 mg protamine/100 units heparin if 30 to 60 minutes have elapsed; and 0.25 to 0.375 mg protamine/100 units heparin if 2 hours or more have elapsed.
- Abrupt withdrawal may cause increased coagulability, and heparin therapy is usually followed by oral anticoagulants for prophylaxis.

Patient teaching

- Instruct patient and family to watch for signs of bleeding and to notify prescriber immediately if they occur.
- Tell patient to avoid OTC medications containing aspirin, other salicylates, including components of some herbal remedies, and drugs that may interact with heparin.

Evaluation

- Patient's PTT is reflective of goal of heparin therapy.
- Patient has no injury from bleeding.
- Patient and family state understanding of drug therapy.

hepatitis B immune globulin, human

(hep-uh-TIGH-tus bee ih-MYOON GLOH-byoo-lin, HYOO-mun)
H-BIG

Pharmacologic class: immune serum
Therapeutic class: hepatitis B prophylaxis
Pregnancy risk category: C

Indications and dosages

▶ **Hepatitis B exposure in high-risk patients.** *Adults and children:* 0.06 ml/kg I.M. within 7 days after exposure (preferably within first 24 hours). Dosage repeated 28 days after exposure if patient refuses hepatitis B vaccine. *Neonates born to patients who test positive for hepatitis B surface antigen (HBsAg):* 0.5 ml I.M. within 12 hours of birth.

How supplied

Injection: 1-ml, 4-ml, 5-ml vials

Pharmacokinetics

Absorption: absorbed slowly after I.M. injection.
Distribution: unknown.
Metabolism: unknown.
Excretion: unknown. *Half-life:* antibodies to HBsAg, 21 days.

Route	Onset	Peak	Duration
I.M.	1-6 days	3-11 days	≥ 2 mo

Pharmacodynamics

Chemical effect: provides passive immunity to hepatitis B.
Therapeutic effect: prevents hepatitis B.

Adverse reactions

Skin: urticaria; *pain, tenderness* at injection site.
Other: ***anaphylaxis, angioedema.***

Interactions

Drug-drug. *Live-virus vaccines:* may interfere with response to live-virus vaccines. Defer routine immunization for 3 months.

Contraindications and precautions

- Contraindicated in patients with history of anaphylactic reactions to immune serum.
- Use cautiously in pregnant women.
- No data exist to demonstrate whether drug appears in breast milk.

NURSING CONSIDERATIONS

Assessment

- Assess patient's allergies and reaction to immunizations before therapy.
- Monitor effectiveness by checking patient's antibody titers.
- Be alert for anaphylaxis.
- Evaluate patient's and family's knowledge of drug therapy.

Nursing diagnoses

- Ineffective protection related to lack of immunity to hepatitis B
- Deficient knowledge related to drug therapy

Planning and implementation

- Inject drug into anterolateral aspect of thigh or deltoid muscle in older children and adults; inject into anterolateral aspect of thigh for neonates and children under age 3.
- Make sure epinephrine 1:1,000 is available in case anaphylaxis occurs.
- For postexposure prophylaxis (for example, needle stick, direct contact), drug is usually given with hepatitis B vaccine.

Patient teaching

- Instruct patient to report respiratory difficulty immediately.

Evaluation

- Patient exhibits passive immunity to hepatitis B.
- Patient and family state understanding of drug therapy.

hetastarch

(HET-uh-starch)
Hespan

Pharmacologic class: amylopectin derivative
Therapeutic class: plasma volume expander
Pregnancy risk category: C

Indications and dosages

▶ **Plasma expander.** *Adults:* 500 to 1,000 ml I.V., depending on amount of blood lost and resulting hemoconcentration. Total dosage usually not to exceed 1,500 ml daily. Up to 20 ml/kg hourly may be used in hemorrhagic shock.

How supplied

Injection: 500 ml (6 g/100 ml in normal saline solution)

Pharmacokinetics

Absorption: not applicable.
Distribution: distributed in blood plasma.
Metabolism: hetastarch molecules larger than 50,000 molecular weight are slowly enzymatically degraded to molecules that can be excreted.

*Liquid form contains alcohol. **May contain tartrazine. ♦ Canada ◊ Australia †OTC

Excretion: 40% of hetastarch molecules smaller than 50,000 molecular weight are excreted in urine within 24 hours. Hetastarch molecules that are not hydroxyethylated are slowly degraded to glucose. *Half-life:* 17 to 48 days.

Route	Onset	Peak	Duration
I.V.	Immediate	Immediate	Unknown

Pharmacodynamics

Chemical effect: expands plasma volume.
Therapeutic effect: reverses fluid volume deficit.

Adverse reactions

CNS: headaches.
CV: peripheral edema of legs.
EENT: periorbital edema.
GI: nausea, vomiting.
Respiratory: wheezing.
Skin: urticaria.
Other: mild fever, ***hypersensitivity reactions.***

Interactions

None significant.

Contraindications and precautions

- Contraindicated in patients with severe bleeding disorders, severe heart failure, and renal failure with oliguria and anuria.
- Women receiving hetastarch should temporarily stop breast-feeding.
- Use cautiously in pregnant women.
- Safety of drug hasn't been established in children.

NURSING CONSIDERATIONS

Assessment

- Assess patient's underlying condition before therapy.
- Check for improvement in underlying condition. Assess vital signs and cardiopulmonary status.
- To avoid circulatory overload, monitor patient with impaired renal function carefully.
- Monitor CBC, total leukocyte and platelet counts, leukocyte differential count, hemoglobin, hematocrit, PT, INR, PTT, and electrolyte, BUN, and creatinine levels.
- Be alert for adverse reactions.
- Evaluate patient's and family's knowledge of drug therapy.

Nursing diagnoses

- Deficient fluid volume related to underlying condition
- Ineffective health maintenance related to hypersensitivity reaction
- Deficient knowledge related to drug therapy

Planning and implementation

- Hetastarch isn't a substitute for blood or plasma.
- During continuous-flow centrifugation, leukapheresis ratio is usually 1 part hetastarch to 8 parts venous whole blood.
- Discard partially used bottles.
- Discontinue drug if allergic or sensitivity reaction occurs, and notify prescriber. If necessary, administer antihistamine as ordered.

Patient teaching

- Inform patient about need for drug.
- Tell patient to report difficulty breathing.

Evaluation

- Patient regains normal fluid volume after drug therapy.
- Patient doesn't develop hypersensitivity reaction to drug.
- Patient and family state understanding of drug therapy.

hyaluronidase

(high-el-yoo-RON-ih-dayz)
Wydase

Pharmacologic class: protein enzyme
Therapeutic class: adjunct to increase absorption and dispersion of injected drugs
Pregnancy risk category: C

Indications and dosages

▶ **Adjunct to increase absorption and dispersion of other injected drugs.** *Adults and children:* 150 units added to solution containing other drug.

▶ **Hypodermoclysis.** *Adults and children over age 3:* 150 units injected S.C. before clysis or injected into clysis tubing near needle for each 1,000 ml clysis solution.
▶ **Excretory urography when contrast medium is given S.C.** *Adults and children:* with patient in prone position, 75 units S.C. over each scapula, followed by injection of contrast medium at same sites.

How supplied

Injection: 150 units/vial, 1,500 units/vial; 150 units/ml in 1-ml, 10-ml vials

Pharmacokinetics

Unknown.

Route	Onset	Peak	Duration
S.C.	Unknown	Unknown	Unknown

Pharmacodynamics

Chemical effect: hydrolyzes hyaluronic acid, promoting diffusion of fluids in tissues.
Therapeutic effect: increases fluid diffusion.

Adverse reactions

Skin: rash, urticaria, irritation.

Interactions

Drug-drug. *Local anesthetics:* increased risk of toxic local reaction. Use together cautiously.

Contraindications and precautions

- Contraindicated in patients hypersensitive to drug.
- Use cautiously in pregnant women.
- Distribution of drug into human breast milk isn't known.

NURSING CONSIDERATIONS

Assessment

- Assess patient's condition before therapy and regularly thereafter.
- Perform skin test for sensitivity, as ordered. Avoid injecting into diseased areas to prevent the spread of infection, and observe injection site for local reactions.
- Be alert for adverse reactions and drug interactions.
- Evaluate patient's and family's knowledge of drug therapy.

Nursing diagnoses

- Ineffective health maintenance related to underlying condition
- Deficient knowledge related to drug therapy

Planning and implementation

- Don't inject into acutely inflamed or cancerous areas.
- Drug isn't recommended for I.V. use.
- For child, add 15 units to each 100 ml of solution. Drip rate of solution to which hyaluronidase was added shouldn't exceed 2 ml/minute.
- Don't add to solutions containing epinephrine and heparin. Hyaluronidase is incompatible with these drugs.
- In patients with hypodermoclysis, be prepared to adjust dosage, rate of injection, and type of solution based on patient response.
- Protect drug from heat. Don't use cloudy or discolored solution.
- Avoid getting solution in eyes; if it does, flush with water at once.

Patient teaching

- Instruct patient to report skin reactions.

Evaluation

- Patient shows improved health.
- Patient and family state understanding of drug therapy.

hydralazine hydrochloride

(high-DRAL-uh-zeen high-droh-KLOR-ighd)
Alphapress ◇, Apresoline**, Novo-Hylazin ♦

Pharmacologic class: peripheral vasodilator
Therapeutic class: antihypertensive
Pregnancy risk category: C

Indications and dosages

▶ **Essential hypertension (orally, alone, or in combination with other antihypertensives); severe essential hypertension (parenterally, to lower blood pressure quickly).** *Adults:* **(P.O.)** initially, 10 mg P.O. q.i.d.; gradually increased to 50 mg q.i.d., as needed. Maximum recommended dosage is 200 mg daily, but some patients may need 300 to 400 mg daily. **(I.V.)** 10 to 20 mg given slowly and repeated as necessary. Switch to P.O. antihypertensives as soon as possible. **(I.M.)** 10 to 50 mg, repeated as necessary. Switch to P.O. form as soon as possible.

How supplied

Tablets: 10 mg, 25 mg, 50 mg, 100 mg
Injection: 20 mg/ml

Pharmacokinetics

Absorption: absorbed rapidly from GI tract. Food enhances absorption. Degree of absorption is unknown after I.M. administration.
Distribution: distributed widely throughout body; about 88% to 90% protein-bound.
Metabolism: metabolized extensively in GI mucosa and liver.
Excretion: excreted primarily in urine; about 10% of P.O. dose is excreted in feces. *Half-life:* 3 to 7 hours.

Route	Onset	Peak	Duration
P.O.	20-30 min	1-2 hr	3-8 hr
I.V.	≤ 5 min	15-30 min	3-8 hr
I.M.	Unknown	Unknown	3-8 hr

Pharmacodynamics

Chemical effect: unknown. A direct-acting vasodilator, its predominant effect relaxes arteriolar smooth muscle.
Therapeutic effect: lowers blood pressure.

Adverse reactions

CNS: peripheral neuritis, *headache,* dizziness.
CV: orthostatic hypotension, tachycardia, arrhythmias, angina, palpitations, sodium retention.
GI: nausea, vomiting, diarrhea, anorexia.
Hematologic: ***neutropenia, leukopenia, agranulocytopenia.***
Metabolic: *weight gain.*
Skin: rash.
Other: *lupuslike syndrome* (especially with high doses).

Interactions

Drug-drug. *Diazoxide, MAO inhibitors:* may cause severe hypotension. Use together cautiously.
Indomethacin: may decrease hydralazine effects. Monitor patient.
Metoprolol, propranolol (beta blockers): serum levels of either drug may be increased. Avoid concurrent use.

Contraindications and precautions

- Contraindicated in patients hypersensitive to drug and in those with coronary artery disease or mitral valvular rheumatic heart disease.
- Use cautiously in patients with suspected cardiac disease, CVA, or severe renal impairment and in those taking other antihypertensives. Also use cautiously in pregnant women.
- Safety of drug hasn't been established in breast-feeding women or in children.

NURSING CONSIDERATIONS

Assessment

- Assess blood pressure before therapy and regularly thereafter.
- Monitor CBC, lupus erythematosus cell preparation, and antinuclear antibody titer determination during long-term therapy, as ordered.
- Be alert for adverse reactions and drug interactions.
- Evaluate patient's and family's knowledge of drug therapy.

Nursing diagnoses

- Risk for injury related to presence of hypertension
- Excessive fluid volume related to sodium retention
- Deficient knowledge related to drug therapy

Planning and implementation

P.O. use: Give drug with meals to increase absorption.
I.V. use: Give drug slowly, and repeat as necessary, usually every 4 to 6 hours.
– Hydralazine changes color in most infusion solutions, but the change doesn't indicate loss of potency.

– Drug is compatible with normal saline solution, Ringer's and lactated Ringer's solutions, and several other common I.V. solutions. Drug may react with dextrose. Manufacturer doesn't recommend mixing drug in infusion solutions. Check with pharmacist for additional compatibility information.
I.M. use: Follow normal protocol.

- Some clinicians combine hydralazine therapy with diuretics and beta blockers to decrease sodium retention and tachycardia and to prevent angina.
- Compliance may be improved by giving drug twice daily. Check with prescriber.

Patient teaching

- Instruct patient to take oral form with meals to increase absorption.
- Inform patient that orthostatic hypotension can be minimized by rising slowly and avoiding sudden position changes.
- Tell patient not to stop drug suddenly but to call prescriber if unpleasant adverse reactions occur.
- Tell patient to limit sodium intake.

☑ Evaluation

- Patient's blood pressure is normal.
- Fluid retention doesn't develop.
- Patient and family state understanding of drug therapy.

hydrochlorothiazide

(high-droh-klor-oh-THIGH-uh-zighd)

Apo-Hydro ♦, Dichlotride ◇, Diuchlor H ♦, Esidrix, Ezide, Hydro-chlor, Hydro-D, HydroDIURIL, Hydro-Par, Microzide, Neo-Codema ♦, Novo-Hydrazide ♦, Oretic, Urozide ♦

Pharmacologic class: thiazide diuretic
Therapeutic class: diuretic, antihypertensive
Pregnancy risk category: D

Indications and dosages

▶ **Edema.** *Adults:* 25 to 100 mg P.O. daily or intermittently.

▶ **Hypertension.** *Adults:* 12.5 to 50 mg P.O. daily as single dose. Daily dosage may be gradually increased until desired effect is achieved, adverse reactions are intolerable, or maximum dose of 50 mg daily is reached.
Children ages 2 to 12: 37.5 to 100 mg P.O. daily in two divided doses.
Children ages 6 months to 2 years: 12.5 to 37.5 mg P.O. daily in two divided doses.
Infants under age 6 months: up to 3.3 mg/kg P.O. daily in two divided doses.

How supplied

Tablets: 25 mg, 50 mg, 100 mg
Oral solution: 10 mg/ml, 50 mg/5 ml, 100 mg/ml
Capsules: 12.5 mg

Pharmacokinetics

Absorption: absorbed from GI tract. Rate and extent of absorption vary with different forms of drug.
Distribution: unknown.
Metabolism: none.
Excretion: excreted unchanged in urine.

Route	Onset	Peak	Duration
P.O.	2 hr	4-6 hr	6-12 hr

Pharmacodynamics

Chemical effect: increases sodium and water excretion by inhibiting sodium and chloride reabsorption in nephron's distal segment.
Therapeutic effect: promotes sodium and water excretion and lowers blood pressure.

Adverse reactions

CV: volume depletion and dehydration, orthostatic hypotension.
GI: anorexia, nausea, ***pancreatitis.***
GU: nocturia, polyuria, frequent urination, ***renal failure.***
Hematologic: ***aplastic anemia, agranulocytosis, leukopenia, thrombocytopenia.***
Hepatic: hepatic encephalopathy.
Metabolic: hypokalemia; asymptomatic hyperuricemia; hyperglycemia and impairment of glucose tolerance; fluid and electrolyte imbalances, including dilutional hyponatremia and hypochloremia, metabolic alkalosis, hypercalcemia; gout.
Skin: dermatitis, photosensitivity, rash.

Other: ***anaphylactic reactions,*** hypersensitivity reactions such as pneumonitis and vasculitis.

Interactions

Drug-drug. *Antidiabetics:* decreased effectiveness of hypoglycemics; dosage adjustments may be needed. Monitor blood glucose levels.
Antihypertensives: additive antihypertensive effect. Use together cautiously.
Barbiturates, opiates: increased orthostatic hypotensive effect. Monitor patient closely.
Cardiac glycosides: increased risk of digitalis toxicity from hydrochlorothiazide-induced hypokalemia. Monitor potassium and cardiac glycoside levels.
Cholestyramine, colestipol: decreased intestinal absorption of thiazides. Separate doses.
Diazoxide: increased antihypertensive, hyperglycemic, and hyperuricemic effects. Use together cautiously.
Lithium: decreased lithium excretion, increasing risk of lithium toxicity. Monitor lithium level.
NSAIDs: increased risk of NSAID-induced renal failure. Monitor patient closely.
Drug-herb. *Licorice root:* may contribute to the potassium depletion caused by thiazides. Discourage concomitant use.
Drug-lifestyle. *Alcohol use:* increased orthostatic hypotensive effect. Discourage concomitant use.
Sun exposure: increased sensitivity to sun. Urge appropriate precautions during sun exposure.

Contraindications and precautions

- Contraindicated in patients with anuria and in patients hypersensitive to other thiazides or sulfonamide derivatives.
- Drug isn't recommended for pregnant women because fetal harm may occur.
- Use cautiously in patients with severe renal disease, impaired hepatic function, and progressive hepatic disease.
- Safety of drug hasn't been established for breast-feeding women.

NURSING CONSIDERATIONS

Assessment

- Assess patient's edema or blood pressure before starting therapy.
- Monitor effectiveness by regularly checking blood pressure, urine output, and weight. In patient with hypertension, therapeutic response may be delayed several days.
- Monitor serum electrolyte levels.
- Monitor serum creatinine and BUN levels regularly. Drug isn't as effective if these levels are more than twice normal.
- Monitor blood uric acid levels, especially in patient with history of gout.
- Be alert for adverse reactions and drug interactions.
- Evaluate patient's and family's knowledge of drug therapy.

Nursing diagnoses

- Ineffective health maintenance related to presence of edema or hypertension
- Impaired urinary elimination related to diuretic effect of drug
- Deficient knowledge related to drug therapy

Planning and implementation

- Give drug in morning to prevent nocturia. Give it with food if nausea occurs.
- Drug may be used with potassium-sparing diuretic to prevent potassium loss.

Patient teaching

- Advise patient to take drug with food to minimize GI upset.
- Caution patient to avoid sudden posture changes and to rise slowly to avoid orthostatic hypotension.
- Instruct patient to avoid alcohol consumption during drug therapy.
- Advise patient to use sunblock to prevent photosensitivity reactions.
- Tell patient to check with prescriber before taking OTC medications or herbal remedies.

Evaluation

- Patient's blood pressure is normal, and no edema is present.

• Patient demonstrates adjustment of lifestyle to deal with altered patterns of urinary elimination.
• Patient and family state understanding of drug therapy.

hydrocortisone
(high-droh-KOR-tuh-sohn)
Cortef, Cortenema, Hydrocortone

hydrocortisone acetate
Cortifoam, Hydrocortone Acetate

hydrocortisone cypionate
Cortef
hydrocortisone sodium phosphate
Hydrocortone Phosphate

hydrocortisone sodium succinate
A-hydroCort, Solu-Cortef

Pharmacologic class: glucocorticoid, mineralocorticoid
Therapeutic class: adrenocorticoid replacement
Pregnancy risk category: NR

Indications and dosages

▶ **Severe inflammation, adrenal insufficiency.** *Adults:* 5 to 30 mg P.O. b.i.d., t.i.d., or q.i.d. (as much as 80 mg q.i.d. may be given in acute situations). Or, initially, 100 to 500 mg succinate I.M. or I.V., and then 50 to 100 mg I.M., as indicated. Or, 15 to 240 mg phosphate I.V., I.M., or S.C. q 12 hours. Or, 10 to 75 mg acetate into joints or soft tissue. Dosage varies with size of joint. Local anesthetics commonly are injected with dose.
▶ **Shock.** *Adults:* initially, 50 mg/kg succinate I.V. repeated in 4 hours. Repeat dosage q 24 hours, p.r.n. Or, 0.5 to 2 g I.V. q 2 to 6 hours, p.r.n.
Children: 0.16 to 1 mg/kg or 6 to 30 mg/m^2 phosphate I.M. or succinate I.M. or I.V. daily or b.i.d.
▶ **Adjunct for ulcerative colitis and proctitis.** *Adults:* 1 enema (100 mg) P.R. nightly for 21 days.

How supplied

hydrocortisone
Tablets: 5 mg, 10 mg, 20 mg
Enema: 100 mg/60 ml
hydrocortisone acetate
Injection: 25 mg/ml*, 50 mg/ml* suspension
Enema: 10% aerosol foam (provides 90 mg/application)
Suppositories: 25 mg
hydrocortisone cypionate
Oral suspension: 10 mg/5 ml
hydrocortisone sodium phosphate
Injection: 50 mg/ml solution
hydrocortisone sodium succinate
Injection: 100 mg/vial*, 250 mg/vial*, 500 mg/vial*, 1,000 mg/vial*

Pharmacokinetics

Absorption: absorbed rapidly after P.O. use. Variable absorption after I.M. or intra-articular injection. Unknown after rectal use.
Distribution: distributed to muscle, liver, skin, intestines, and kidneys. Drug is bound extensively to plasma proteins. Only unbound portion is active.
Metabolism: metabolized in liver.
Excretion: inactive metabolites and small amounts of unmetabolized drug excreted in urine; insignificant quantities excreted in feces. *Half-life:* 8 to 12 hours.

Route	Onset	Peak	Duration
All routes	Varies	Varies	Varies

Pharmacodynamics

Chemical effect: not clearly defined; decreases inflammation, mainly by stabilizing leukocyte lysosomal membranes; suppresses immune response; stimulates bone marrow; and influences nutrient metabolism.
Therapeutic effect: reduces inflammation, suppresses immune function, raises adrenocorticoid hormonal levels.

Adverse reactions

Most adverse reactions are dose- or duration-dependent.
CNS: *euphoria, insomnia,* psychotic behavior, pseudotumor cerebri, ***seizures.***

CV: ***heart failure,*** hypertension, edema, ***arrhythmias, thromboembolism.***
EENT: cataracts, glaucoma.
GI: *peptic ulceration,* GI irritation, increased appetite, ***pancreatitis.***
Metabolic: possible hypokalemia, hyperglycemia, and carbohydrate intolerance.
Musculoskeletal: muscle weakness, growth suppression in children, osteoporosis.
Skin: hirsutism, delayed wound healing, acne, various skin eruptions, easy bruising.
Other: susceptibility to infections, ***acute adrenal insufficiency with increased stress (infection, surgery, or trauma) or abrupt withdrawal after long-term therapy.***

Interactions

Drug-drug. *Aspirin, indomethacin, other NSAIDs:* increased risk of GI distress and bleeding. Give together cautiously.
Barbiturates, phenytoin, rifampin: decreased corticosteroid effect. Increase corticosteroid dosage, as ordered.
Live-attenuated virus vaccines, other toxoids and vaccines: decreased antibody response and increased risk of neurologic complications. Avoid concomitant use.
Oral anticoagulants: altered dosage requirements. Monitor PT and INR closely.
Potassium-depleting drugs (such as thiazide diuretics): enhanced potassium-wasting effects of hydrocortisone. Monitor potassium levels.
Skin-test antigens: decreased response. Defer skin testing until therapy is completed.
Drug-lifestyle. *Alcohol use:* Increased risk of GI effects. Discourage use.

Contraindications and precautions

- Contraindicated in patients allergic to drug or its components, in those with systemic fungal infections, and in premature infants (succinate).
- Drug use isn't recommended in high doses for breast-feeding women.
- Use with extreme caution in patients with recent MI.
- Use cautiously in pregnant women and in patients with GI ulcer, renal disease, hypertension, osteoporosis, diabetes mellitus, hypothyroidism, cirrhosis, diverticulitis, nonspecific ulcerative colitis, recent intestinal anastomoses, thromboembolic disorders, seizures, myasthenia gravis, heart failure, tuberculosis, ocular herpes simplex, emotional instability, and psychotic tendencies.
- Long-term use in children may delay growth and maturation.

NURSING CONSIDERATIONS

Assessment

- Assess patient's condition before therapy and regularly thereafter.
- Monitor patient's weight, blood pressure, and serum electrolyte levels.
- Monitor patient for stress. Fever, trauma, surgery, and emotional problems may increase adrenal insufficiency.
- Periodic measurement of growth and development may be needed during high-dose or prolonged therapy in child.
- Be alert for adverse reactions and drug interactions.
- Evaluate patient's and family's knowledge of drug therapy.

Nursing diagnoses

- Ineffective health maintenance related to underlying condition
- Ineffective protection related to immunosuppression
- Deficient knowledge related to drug therapy

Planning and implementation

- For better results and less toxicity, give once-daily dose in morning.

P.O. use: Give P.O. dose with food when possible.
I.V. use: Don't use acetate or suspension form for I.V. use. When administering as direct injection, inject directly into vein or I.V. line containing free-flowing compatible solution over 30 seconds to several minutes. When administering as intermittent or continuous infusion, dilute solution according to manufacturer's instructions and give over prescribed duration. If used for continuous infusion, change solution every 24 hours.

– Hydrocortisone sodium phosphate may be added directly to D_5W or normal saline solution for I.V. administration.
– Reconstitute hydrocortisone sodium succinate with bacteriostatic water or bacteriostatic sodium chloride solution before adding to I.V. solutions. When giving by direct I.V. injection, inject over at least 30 seconds. For infusion, dilute with D_5W, normal saline solution, or D_5W in normal saline solution to 1 mg/ml or less.
I.M. use: Give I.M. injection deep into gluteal muscle. Rotate injection sites to prevent muscle atrophy.
P.R. use: Enema may produce the same systemic effects as other forms of hydrocortisone. If therapy must exceed 21 days, discontinue gradually by reducing administration to every other night for 2 or 3 weeks, as ordered.
• Avoid S.C. injection because atrophy and sterile abscesses may occur.
ALERT Don't confuse Solu-Cortef with Solu-Medrol (methylprednisolone sodium succinate).
• Injectable forms aren't used for alternate-day therapy.
• High-dose therapy usually doesn't continue beyond 48 hours.
• Always adjust to lowest effective dose, and gradually reduce dosage after long-term therapy, as ordered.
• Administer potassium supplements, as ordered.
• Notify prescriber if evidence of adrenal insufficiency appears. Dosage may need to be increased.
• Notify prescriber about adverse reactions. Provide supportive care as indicated and ordered.

Patient teaching
• Teach patient signs of early adrenal insufficiency: fatigue, muscle weakness, joint pain, fever, anorexia, nausea, dyspnea, dizziness, and fainting.
• Instruct patient to carry or wear medical identification that identifies need for supplemental systemic glucocorticoids during stress.
ALERT Tell patient not to discontinue drug abruptly or without prescriber's consent. Abrupt withdrawal may lead to rebound inflammation, fatigue, weakness, arthralgia, fever, dizziness, lethargy, depression, fainting, orthostatic hypotension, dyspnea, anorexia, and hypoglycemia. After prolonged use, sudden withdrawal may be fatal.
• Warn patient receiving long-term therapy about cushingoid symptoms, and tell him to report sudden weight gain or swelling to prescriber. Also, advise him to consider exercise or physical therapy, to ask his prescriber about vitamin D or calcium supplements, and to have periodic ophthalmic examinations.
• Caution patient about easy bruising.

☑ Evaluation
• Patient's condition improves.
• Serious complications related to drug-induced immunosuppression don't develop.
• Patient and family state understanding of drug therapy.

hydromorphone hydrochloride (dihydromorphinone hydrochloride)
(high-droh-MOR-fohn high-droh-KLOR-ighd)
Dilaudid, Dilaudid-HP, HydroStat

Pharmacologic class: opioid
Therapeutic class: analgesic, antitussive
Controlled substance schedule: II
Pregnancy risk category: C

Indications and dosages
▶ **Moderate to severe pain.** *Adults:* 2 to 4 mg P.O. q 4 to 6 hours, p.r.n. Or, 1 to 2 mg I.M., S.C., or I.V. (slowly over at least 2 to 3 minutes) q 4 to 6 hours p.r.n. Or, 3 mg rectal suppository q 6 to 8 hours p.r.n.
▶ **Cough.** *Adults:* 1 mg P.O. q 3 to 4 hours p.r.n.
Children ages 6 to 12: 0.5 mg P.O. q 3 to 4 hours p.r.n.

How supplied
Tablets: 1 mg, 2 mg, 3 mg, 4 mg, 8 mg
Injection: 1 mg/ml, 2 mg/ml, 4 mg/ml, 10 mg/ml
Injection (lyophilized powder): 250 mg/vial

Suppositories: 3 mg
Syrup: 1 mg/5 ml
Liquid: 5 mg/5 ml

Pharmacokinetics

Absorption: well absorbed after oral, rectal, or parenteral administration.
Distribution: unknown.
Metabolism: metabolized primarily in liver.
Excretion: excreted primarily in urine. *Half-life:* 2.6 to 4 hours.

Route	Onset	Peak	Duration
P.O.	30 min	1.5-2 hr	4-5 hr
I.V.	10-15 min	15-30 min	2-3 hr
I.M.	15 min	30-60 min	4-5 hr
S.C.	15 min	30-90 min	4 hr
P.R.	Unknown	Unknown	4 hr

Pharmacodynamics

Chemical effect: binds with opioid receptors in CNS, altering perception of and emotional response to pain. Suppresses cough reflex by direct action on cough center in medulla.
Therapeutic effect: relieves pain and cough.

Adverse reactions

CNS: *sedation, somnolence, clouded sensorium,* dizziness, *euphoria,* ***seizures.***
CV: hypotension, ***bradycardia.***
EENT: blurred vision, diplopia, nystagmus.
GI: nausea, vomiting, constipation, ileus.
GU: urine retention.
Respiratory: ***respiratory depression, bronchospasm.***
Other: induration with repeated S.C. injections, physical dependence.

Interactions

Drug-drug. *CNS depressants, general anesthetics, hypnotics, MAO inhibitors, other narcotic analgesics, sedatives, tranquilizers, tricyclic antidepressants:* additive effects. Use together with extreme caution. Reduce hydromorphone dose and monitor patient response.
Drug-lifestyle. *Alcohol use:* additive effects. Discourage concomitant use.

Contraindications and precautions

- Contraindicated in patients hypersensitive to drug, in patients with intracranial lesions from increased intracranial pressure, and whenever ventilator function is depressed, as in status asthmaticus, COPD, cor pulmonale, emphysema, or kyphoscoliosis.
- Use with extreme caution in patients with hepatic or renal disease, hypothyroidism, Addison's disease, prostatic hypertrophy, or urethral stricture.
- Use with caution in elderly or debilitated patients and in pregnant or breast-feeding women.

NURSING CONSIDERATIONS

Assessment

- Assess patient's pain or cough before and after drug administration.
- Respiratory depression and hypotension can occur with I.V. administration. Monitor respiratory and circulatory status constantly.
- Drug may worsen or mask gallbladder pain.
- Drug is a commonly abused narcotic.
- Be alert for adverse reactions and drug interactions.
- Evaluate patient's and family's knowledge of drug therapy.

Nursing diagnoses

- Acute pain related to underlying condition
- Ineffective breathing pattern related to respiratory depression
- Deficient knowledge related to drug therapy

Planning and implementation

- For better analgesic effect, give drug before patient has intense pain.
- Dilaudid-HP, a highly concentrated form (10 mg/ml), may be given in smaller volumes to prevent discomfort caused by large-volume I.M. or S.C. injections. Check dosage carefully.

P.O., I.M., and P.R. use: Follow normal protocol.
I.V. use: Give drug by direct injection over no less than 2 minutes. For infusion, drug may be mixed in D_5W, normal saline, D_5W in normal

saline, D_5W in half-normal saline, or Ringer's or lactated Ringer's solutions.
S.C. use: Rotate injection sites to avoid induration with S.C. injection.
- Keep resuscitation equipment and narcotic antagonist (naloxone) available.
- Postoperatively, encourage patient to turn, cough, and deep-breathe to avoid atelectasis.

Patient teaching
- Caution ambulatory patient about getting out of bed or walking. Warn outpatient to avoid activities that require mental alertness until CNS effects of drug are known.
- Suggest measures to prevent constipation during maintenance therapy.
- Encourage patient to ask for drug before pain becomes severe.
- Tell patient or family caregiver to notify health care professional if patient's respiratory rate decreases.
- Instruct patient to avoid alcohol consumption during drug therapy.

☑ Evaluation
- Patient is free from pain.
- Patient maintains adequate breathing patterns.
- Patient and family state understanding of drug therapy.

hydroxychloroquine sulfate

(high-droks-ee-KLOR-oh-kwin SUL-fayt)
Plaquenil

Pharmacologic class: 4-aminoquinoline
Therapeutic class: antimalarial, anti-inflammatory
Pregnancy risk category: NR

Indications and dosages

▶ **Suppressive prophylaxis of malaria attacks caused by *Plasmodium vivax, P. malariae, P. ovale,* and susceptible strains of *P. falciparum.*** *Adults and children:* for suppression—5 mg (base)/kg P.O. (maximum, 310 mg) weekly on same day of week (starting 2 weeks before entering and continuing 8 weeks after leaving endemic area). If not started before exposure, initial dose is doubled (620 mg for adults, 10 mg/kg for children) in two divided doses P.O. 6 hours apart.

▶ **Acute malarial attacks.** *Adults:* initially, 800 mg (sulfate) P.O.; then 400 mg (sulfate) after 6 to 8 hours; then 400 mg (sulfate) daily for 2 days (total 2 g sulfate salt).
Children: initial dose, 10 mg base/kg (up to 620 mg base); second dose, 5 mg base/kg (up to 310 mg base) 6 hours after first dose; third dose, 5 mg base/kg 18 hours after second dose; fourth dose, 5 mg base/kg 24 hours after third dose.

▶ **Lupus erythematosus (chronic discoid and systemic).** *Adults:* 400 mg (sulfate) P.O. daily or b.i.d., continued for several weeks or months, depending on response. Prolonged maintenance dosage—200 to 400 mg (sulfate) daily.

▶ **Rheumatoid arthritis.** *Adults:* initially, 400 to 600 mg (sulfate) P.O. daily. When response occurs (usually in 4 to 12 weeks), dosage is halved.

How supplied

Tablets: 200 mg (155-mg base)

Pharmacokinetics

Absorption: absorbed readily and almost completely.
Distribution: concentrates in liver, spleen, kidneys, heart, and brain and is strongly bound in melanin-containing cells. Drug is bound to plasma proteins.
Metabolism: metabolized by liver.
Excretion: most excreted unchanged in urine.
Half-life: 32 to 50 days.

Route	Onset	Peak	Duration
P.O.	Unknown	2-4.5 hr	Unknown

Pharmacodynamics

Chemical effect: unknown; may bind to and alter properties of DNA in susceptible organisms.
Therapeutic effect: prevents or hinders growth of *P. malariae, P. ovale, P. vivax,* and *P. falciparum.* Also relieves inflammation.

Adverse reactions

CNS: irritability, nightmares, ataxia, ***seizures***, psychic stimulation, toxic psychosis, vertigo, nystagmus, lassitude, fatigue, dizziness, hypoactive deep tendon reflexes.
EENT: visual disturbances (blurred vision; difficulty in focusing; reversible corneal changes; typically irreversible, sometimes progressive or delayed retinal changes, such as narrowing of arterioles; macular lesions; pallor of optic disk; optic atrophy; visual field defects; patchy retinal pigmentation, commonly leading to blindness), ototoxicity (irreversible nerve deafness, tinnitus, labyrinthitis).
GI: anorexia, abdominal cramps, diarrhea, nausea, vomiting.
Hematologic: ***agranulocytosis, leukopenia, thrombocytopenia, aplastic anemia; hemolysis*** (in patients with G6PD deficiency).
Metabolic: weight loss.
Musculskeletal: skeletal muscle weakness.
Skin: pruritus, lichen planus eruptions, skin and mucosal pigmentary changes, pleomorphic skin eruptions, alopecia, bleaching of hair.

Interactions

Drug-drug. *Aluminum and magnesium salts, kaolin:* decreased GI absorption. Separate administration times.
Cimetidine: decreased hepatic metabolism of hydroxychloroquine. Monitor patient for toxicity.

Contraindications and precautions

- Contraindicated in patients hypersensitive to drug, in children who need long-term therapy, and in patients with retinal or visual field changes or porphyria.
- Use with extreme caution in patients with severe GI, neurologic, or blood disorders.
- Use cautiously in patients with hepatic disease or alcoholism because drug concentrates in liver. Also, use cautiously in those with G6PD deficiency or psoriasis because drug may worsen these conditions. Also, use cautiously in pregnant women.
- Safety of drug hasn't been established in breast-feeding women.

NURSING CONSIDERATIONS

Assessment

- Assess patient's condition before therapy and regularly thereafter.
- Make sure baseline and periodic ophthalmic examinations are performed. Check periodically for ocular muscle weakness after long-term use.
- Obtain audiometric examinations before, during, and after therapy, especially if long-term.
- Monitor CBCs and liver function studies periodically during long-term therapy, as ordered.
- Assess patient for overdose, which can quickly lead to toxic symptoms: headache, drowsiness, visual disturbances, CV collapse, and seizures, followed by cardiopulmonary arrest. Children are extremely susceptible to toxicity; long-term treatment should be avoided.
- Be alert for adverse reactions and drug interactions.
- Evaluate patient's and family's knowledge of drug therapy.

Nursing diagnoses

- Infection related to susceptible organisms
- Disturbed sensory perception (visual and auditory) related to adverse reactions to drug
- Deficient knowledge related to drug therapy

Planning and implementation

- Give drug right before or after meals on same day of each week.
- Notify prescriber immediately about severe blood disorder that can't be attributed to disease under treatment. Blood reaction may require discontinuation.

Patient teaching

- Advise patient to take drug immediately before or after meals on same day each week to enhance compliance for prophylaxis.
- Warn patient to avoid hazardous activities if adverse CNS or visual disturbances occur.
- Tell patient to promptly report visual or auditory changes.

Evaluation
- Patient is free from infection.
- Patient maintains normal visual and auditory function.
- Patient and family state understanding of drug therapy.

hydroxyurea
(high-droks-ee-yoo-REE-uh)
Hydrea**

Pharmacologic class: antimetabolite (cell cycle–phase specific, S phase)
Therapeutic class: antineoplastic
Pregnancy risk category: D

Indications and dosages
▶ **Melanoma; resistant chronic myelocytic leukemia; recurrent, metastatic, or inoperable ovarian cancer; head and neck cancers.** *Adults:* 80 mg/kg P.O. as single dose q 3 days; or 20 to 30 mg/kg P.O. as single daily dose.
▶ **Reduction of frequency of painful crises and need for transfusions in adult sickle-cell anemia patients with recurrent moderate-to-severe painful crises.** *Adults:* 15 mg/kg P.O. once daily. If blood counts are in acceptable range, dosage may be increased by 5 mg/kg/day q 12 weeks until maximum tolerated dosage or 35 mg/kg/day has been reached. If blood counts are considered toxic, withhold drug until hematologic recovery occurs. Resume treatment after reducing dose by 2.5 mg/kg/day. Every 12 weeks, drug may then be adjusted up or down in 2.5-mg/kg/day increments until patient is at stable, nontoxic dose for 24 weeks.

How supplied
Capsules: 500 mg

Pharmacokinetics
Absorption: well absorbed. Serum levels are higher with a large, single dose than with divided doses.
Distribution: crosses blood-brain barrier.
Metabolism: about 50% of dose is degraded in liver.
Excretion: 50% of drug excreted in urine as unchanged drug; metabolites excreted through lungs as carbon dioxide and in urine as urea.
Half-life: 3 to 4 hours.

Route	Onset	Peak	Duration
P.O.	Unknown	2 hr	Unknown

Pharmacodynamics
Chemical effect: unknown; thought to inhibit DNA synthesis.
Therapeutic effect: hinders growth of certain cancer cells.

Adverse reactions
CNS: drowsiness, hallucinations, ***seizures.***
GI: anorexia, nausea, vomiting, diarrhea, stomatitis.
GU: increased BUN and serum creatinine levels.
Hematologic: ***leukopenia, thrombocytopenia,*** anemia, *megaloblastosis,* ***bone marrow suppression*** (dose-limiting and dose-related, with rapid recovery).
Metabolic: hyperuricemia.
Skin: rash, pruritus.

Interactions
Drug-drug. *Cytotoxic drugs, radiation therapy:* enhanced toxicity of hydroxyurea. Use together cautiously.

Contraindications and precautions
- Contraindicated in patients hypersensitive to drug and in those with marked bone marrow depression.
- Drug use isn't recommended in pregnant or breast-feeding women.
- Use cautiously in patients with renal dysfunction.
- Safety of drug hasn't been established in children.

NURSING CONSIDERATIONS

Assessment
- Assess patient's condition before therapy and regularly thereafter.
- Measure CBC, BUN, uric acid, and serum creatinine levels, as ordered.

• Auditory and visual hallucinations and hematologic toxicity increase with decreased renal function.
• Concomitant radiation therapy may increase risk or severity of GI distress or stomatitis.
• Be alert for adverse reactions and drug interactions.
• Evaluate patient's and family's knowledge of drug therapy.

Nursing diagnoses
• Ineffective health maintenance related to presence of neoplastic disease
• Ineffective protection related to adverse hematologic reactions
• Deficient knowledge related to drug therapy

Planning and implementation
• Keep patient hydrated.
• Dosage modification may be needed after chemotherapy or radiation therapy.
• Bone marrow suppression is dose-limited and dose-related with rapid recovery.

Patient teaching
• If patient can't swallow capsules, tell him to empty contents into water and take immediately.
• Warn patient to watch for signs of infection (fever, sore throat, fatigue) and bleeding (easy bruising, nosebleeds, bleeding gums, melena). Instruct patient to take infection-control and bleeding precautions. Tell patient to take temperature daily.
• Advise woman of childbearing age to avoid becoming pregnant during therapy and to consult with prescriber before becoming pregnant.

Evaluation
• Patient responds well to drug therapy.
• Serious infections or bleeding complications don't develop.
• Patient and family state understanding of drug therapy.

hydroxyzine embonate ◇
(high-DROKS-ih-zeen EM-boh-nayt)
Atarax

hydroxyzine hydrochloride
Apo-Hydroxyzine ♦, Atarax*, Evista, Hyzine-50, Multipax ♦, Novo-Hydroxyzin ♦, Vistaril, Vistazine 50

hydroxyzine pamoate
Vistaril

Pharmacologic class: antihistamine (piperazine derivative)
Therapeutic class: antianxiety, sedative, antipruritic, antiemetic, antispasmodic
Pregnancy risk category: NR

Indications and dosages
▶ **Anxiety.** *Adults:* 50 to 100 mg P.O. q.i.d.
Children age 6 and over: 50 to 100 mg P.O. daily in divided doses.
Children under age 6: 50 mg P.O. daily in divided doses.
▶ **Preoperative and postoperative adjunct therapy.** *Adults:* 25 to 100 mg I.M. q 4 to 6 hours.
Children: 1.1 mg/kg I.M. q 4 to 6 hours.
▶ **Pruritus from allergies.** *Adults:* 25 mg P.O. t.i.d. or q.i.d.
Children age 6 and over: 50 to 100 mg P.O. daily in divided doses.
Children under age 6: 50 mg P.O. daily in divided doses.
▶ **Psychiatric and emotional emergencies, including acute alcoholism.** *Adults:* 50 to 100 mg I.M. q 4 to 6 hours, p.r.n.
▶ **Nausea and vomiting (excluding nausea and vomiting of pregnancy).** *Adults:* 25 to 100 mg I.M.
Children: 1.1 mg/kg I.M.
▶ **Prepartum and postpartum adjunct therapy.** *Adults:* 25 to 100 mg I.M.

How supplied
hydroxyzine embonate ◇
Capsules: 25 mg, 50 mg
hydroxyzine hydrochloride
Tablets: 10 mg, 25 mg, 50 mg, 100 mg

Capsules: 10 mg♦ ◊, 25 mg♦ ◊, 50 mg♦ ◊
Syrup: 10 mg/5 ml
Injection: 25 mg/ml, 50 mg/ml
hydroxyzine pamoate
Capsules: 25 mg, 50 mg, 100 mg
Oral suspension: 25 mg/5 ml

Pharmacokinetics

Absorption: absorbed rapidly and completely after P.O. administration. Unknown for I.M. administration.
Distribution: unknown.
Metabolism: metabolized almost completely in liver.
Excretion: metabolites excreted primarily in urine; small amounts of drug and metabolites excreted in feces. *Half-life:* 3 hours.

Route	Onset	Peak	Duration
P.O.	15-30 min	About 2 hr	4-6 hr
I.M.	Unknown	Unknown	4-6 hr

Pharmacodynamics

Chemical effect: unknown; may suppress activity in key regions of subcortical area of CNS.
Therapeutic effect: relieves anxiety and itching, promotes calmness, and alleviates nausea and vomiting.

Adverse reactions

CNS: *drowsiness,* involuntary motor activity.
GI: *dry mouth.*
Other: marked discomfort at I.M. injection site, ***hypersensitivity reactions*** (wheezing, dyspnea, chest tightness).

Interactions

Drug-drug. *MAO inhibitors*: Enhanced anticholinergic effects. Use cautiously together.
CNS depressants: increased CNS depression. Avoid concomitant use.
Drug-lifestyle. *Alcohol use:* increased CNS depression. Discourage concomitant use.
Sunlight: Photosensitivity may occur. Urge precautions.

Contraindications and precautions

• Contraindicated in early pregnancy and in patients hypersensitive to drug.
• Safety of drug hasn't been established in breast-feeding women.

NURSING CONSIDERATIONS

Assessment
• Assess patient's condition before therapy and regularly thereafter.
• Be alert for adverse reactions and drug interactions.
• Evaluate patient's and family's knowledge of drug therapy.

Nursing diagnoses
• Ineffective health maintenance related to underlying condition
• Risk for injury related to adverse CNS reactions
• Deficient knowledge related to drug therapy

Planning and implementation
• Dosage should be reduced in elderly or debilitated patients.
P.O. use: Follow normal protocol.
I.M. use: Parenteral form (hydroxyzine hydrochloride) for I.M. use only; never administer drug I.V. Z-track injection method is preferred.
– Aspirate I.M. injection carefully to prevent inadvertent intravascular injection. Inject deep into large muscle mass.
• Drug may cause false elevations of urine 17-hydroxycorticosteroids, depending on test method used.

Patient teaching
• Warn patient to avoid hazardous activities until CNS effects of drug are known.
• Tell patient to avoid alcohol during drug therapy.
• Suggest sugarless hard candy or gum to relieve dry mouth.

Evaluation
• Patient exhibits improved health.
• Patient doesn't experience injury.
• Patient and family state understanding of drug therapy.

I-J

ibuprofen

(igh-byoo-PROH-fen)

ACT-3 ◇, Advil†, Apo-Ibuprofen ♦, Bayer Select Pain Relief Formula Caplets, Brufen ◇, Children's Advil, Children's Motrin, Excedrin IB Caplets†, Excedrin-IB Tablets†, Genpril Caplets†, Genpril Tablets†, Haltran†, Ibuprin†, Ibuprohm Caplets†, Ibuprohm Tablets†, Ibu-Tab†, Menadol, Medipren Caplets†, Midol IB, Motrin, Motrin IB Caplets†, Motrin IB Tablets†, Novo-Profen ♦, Nuprin Caplets†, Nuprin Tablets†, Nurofen ◇, Pamprin-IB, Pedia Profen, Rafen ◇, Rufen, Saleto-200, Trendar†

Pharmacologic class: NSAID
Therapeutic class: nonnarcotic analgesic, antipyretic, anti-inflammatory
Pregnancy risk category: NR

Indications and dosages

▶ **Rheumatoid or osteoarthritis, arthritis.** *Adults:* 300 to 800 mg P.O. t.i.d. or q.i.d. not to exceed 3.2 g/day.
▶ **Mild to moderate pain, dysmenorrhea.** *Adults:* 400 mg P.O. q 4 to 6 hours, p.r.n.
▶ **Fever.** *Adults and children over age 12:* 200 to 400 mg P.O. q 4 to 6 hours, p.r.n. Don't exceed 1.2 g/day or give longer than 3 days. *Children ages 6 months to 12 years:* if fever is below 102.5° F (39.2° C), recommended dose is 5 mg/kg P.O. q 6 to 8 hours, p.r.n. Treat higher fevers with 10 mg/kg P.O. q 6 to 8 hours p.r.n., to maximum dose of 40 mg/kg daily.

How supplied

Tablets: 200 mg†, 300 mg, 400 mg, 600 mg, 800 mg
Tablets (chewable): 50 mg, 100 mg
Caplets: 100 mg, 200 mg†
Oral suspension: 100 mg/5 ml
Oral drops: 40 mg/ml

Pharmacokinetics

Absorption: absorbed rapidly and completely from GI tract when administered orally.
Distribution: highly protein-bound.
Metabolism: undergoes biotransformation in liver.
Excretion: excreted mainly in urine, with some biliary excretion. *Half-life:* 2 to 4 hours.

Route	Onset	Peak	Duration
P.O.	≤ 30 min	2-4 hr	≥ 4 hr

Pharmacodynamics

Chemical effect: unknown; produces anti-inflammatory, analgesic, and antipyretic effects, possibly by inhibiting prostaglandin synthesis.
Therapeutic effect: relieves pain, fever, and inflammation.

Adverse reactions

CNS: *headache, drowsiness, dizziness,* cognitive dysfunction, aseptic meningitis.
CV: *peripheral edema,* edema, hypertension, ***heart failure.***
EENT: visual disturbances, *tinnitus.*
GI: *epigastric distress, nausea, occult blood loss, peptic ulceration.*
GU: reversible renal failure.
Hematologic: prolonged bleeding time, anemia, ***neutropenia, pancytopenia, thrombocytopenia, aplastic anemia, leukopenia, agranulocytosis.***
Hepatic: elevated liver enzyme levels.
Respiratory: ***bronchospasm.***
Skin: pruritus, rash, urticaria, photosensitivity, ***Stevens-Johnson syndrome.***

Interactions

Drug-drug. *Antihypertensives, furosemide, thiazide diuretics:* ibuprofen may decrease effectiveness of diuretics or antihypertensives. Monitor patient.
Aspirin: may decrease serum ibuprofen levels. Avoid concomitant use.
Aspirin, corticosteroids: increased risk of adverse GI reactions. Avoid concomitant use.
Cyclosporine: nephrotoxicity of both drugs may be increased. Avoid concomitant use.
Digoxin, hydantoins: may increase serum levels of these drugs. Monitor levels closely.

Lithium, oral anticoagulants: may increase plasma levels or effects of these drugs. Monitor patient for toxicity.
Methotrexate: risk of methotrexate toxicity may be increased. Monitor patient closely.
Probenecid: probenecid may increase concentration and toxicity of NSAIDs. Monitor patient for signs of toxicity.
Drug-herb. *Dong quai, feverfew, garlic, ginger, horse chestnut, red clover:* possible increased risk of bleeding. Monitor patient closely.
St. John's wort: increased risk of photosensitivity. Advise patient to avoid unprotected exposure to sunlight.
Drug-lifestyle. *Alcohol use:* increased risk of adverse GI reactions. Discourage concomitant use.
Sun exposure: may cause photosensitivity reactions. Advise appropriate precautions.

Contraindications and precautions

- Contraindicated in patients hypersensitive to drug and in those with syndrome of nasal polyps, angioedema, and bronchospastic reactivity to aspirin or other NSAIDs.
- Drug isn't recommended for pregnant or breast-feeding women.
- Use cautiously in patients with GI disorders, history of peptic ulcer disease, hepatic or renal disease, cardiac decompensation, hypertension, or intrinsic coagulation defects.

NURSING CONSIDERATIONS

Assessment
- Obtain assessment of patient's underlying condition before drug therapy.
- Assess patient for relief from pain, fever, or inflammation. Full effects in arthritis may take 2 to 4 weeks.
- Check renal and hepatic function periodically in long-term therapy.
- Be alert for adverse reactions and drug interactions.
- Evaluate patient's and family's knowledge of drug therapy.

ALERT Don't confuse Trendar with Trandate.

Nursing diagnoses
- Chronic pain related to underlying condition
- Risk for injury related to drug-induced adverse reactions
- Deficient knowledge related to drug therapy

Planning and implementation
- Give with meals or milk to reduce adverse GI reactions.
- Notify prescriber if drug is ineffective.
- Stop drug if renal or hepatic abnormalities occur, and notify prescriber.

Patient teaching
- Tell patient to take drug with meals or milk to reduce adverse GI reactions.

ALERT Tell patient not to exceed 1.2 g daily, not to give drug to children under age 12, and not to take drug for extended periods without consulting prescriber.
- Caution patient that use with aspirin, alcohol, or corticosteroids may increase risk of adverse GI reactions.
- Serious GI toxicity, including peptic ulceration and bleeding, can occur in patients taking NSAIDs despite absence of GI symptoms. Teach patient to recognize and report signs and symptoms of GI bleeding.
- Instruct patient to avoid alcohol during drug therapy.
- Instruct patient to use sunblock, wear protective clothing, and avoid prolonged exposure to the sun.

Evaluation
- Patient is free from pain.
- Patient doesn't experience injury from adverse reactions.
- Patient and family state understanding of drug therapy.

ibutilide fumarate
(igh-BYOO-tih-lighd FYOO-muh-rayt)
Corvert

Pharmacologic class: ibutilide derivative
Therapeutic class: supraventricular antiarrhythmic
Pregnancy risk category: C

Indications and dosages

▶ **Rapid conversion of recent atrial fibrillation or atrial flutter to sinus rhythm.** *Adults weighing 60 kg (132 lb) or more:* 1 mg I.V. infused over 10 minutes.
Adults weighing less than 60 kg: 0.01 mg/kg I.V. infused over 10 minutes.
Note: Stop infusion if arrhythmia stops or if patient develops sustained or nonsustained ventricular tachycardia or marked prolongation of QT interval. If arrhythmia doesn't stop within 10 minutes after infusion ends, a second 10-minute infusion of equal strength may be administered.

How supplied

Injection: 0.1 mg/ml

Pharmacokinetics

Absorption: not applicable.
Distribution: highly distributed; about 40% protein-bound.
Metabolism: not clearly defined.
Excretion: excreted in urine and feces. *Half-life:* averages about 6 hours.

Route	Onset	Peak	Duration
I.V.	Unknown	Unknown	Unknown

Pharmacodynamics

Chemical effect: prolongs action potential in isolated cardiac myocyte and increases atrial and ventricular refractoriness; has predominantly class III properties.
Therapeutic effect: restores normal sinus rhythm.

Adverse reactions

CNS: headache.
CV: ventricular extrasystoles, nonsustained ventricular tachycardia, hypotension, bundle branch block, ***sustained polymorphic ventricular tachycardia,*** AV block, hypertension, QT interval prolongation, ***bradycardia,*** palpitations, tachycardia.
GI: nausea.

Interactions

Drug-drug. *Class Ia antiarrhythmics (such as disopyramide, procainamide, quinidine), other class III drugs (such as amiodarone, sotalol):* increased risk of prolonged refractoriness. Avoid concomitant administration.
Digoxin: supraventricular arrhythmias may mask cardiotoxicity from excessive digoxin levels. Use cautiously.
H_1-receptor antagonist antihistamines, phenothiazines, tetracyclic antidepressants, tricyclic antidepressants, other drugs that prolong QT interval: increased risk for proarrhythmia. Monitor patient closely.

Contraindications and precautions

- Contraindicated in patients hypersensitive to drug or its components.
- Drug isn't recommended for use in patients with history of polymorphic ventricular tachycardia, such as torsades de pointes, or in breast-feeding women.
- Use cautiously in pregnant women and in patients with hepatic or renal dysfunction (usually, no dosage adjustments are necessary).
- Safety of drug hasn't been established in breast-feeding women and in children.

NURSING CONSIDERATIONS

Assessment

- Assess patient's arrhythmia before therapy.

ALERT Monitor ECG continuously during therapy and for at least 4 hours afterward (or until QT interval returns to baseline) because drug can induce or worsen ventricular arrhythmias. Longer monitoring is required if ECG shows arrhythmic activity.

- Be alert for adverse reactions and drug interactions.
- Evaluate patient's and family's knowledge of drug therapy.

Nursing diagnoses

- Decreased cardiac output related to arrhythmia
- Risk for injury related to life-threatening arrhythmia
- Deficient knowledge related to drug therapy

Planning and implementation

- Drug should be administered only by skilled personnel, with proper equipment and facilities available during and after administration,

such as cardiac monitoring, intracardiac pacing, cardioverter/defibrillator, and medication for treatment of sustained ventricular tachycardia.
• Hypokalemia and hypomagnesemia should be corrected before therapy to reduce risk of proarrhythmia.
• Drug may be administered undiluted or diluted in 50 ml of diluent. It may be added to normal saline solution for injection or D_5W injection before infusion. Contents of one 10-ml vial (0.1 mg/ml) may be added to a 50-ml infusion bag to form admixture of about 0.017 mg/ml ibutilide fumarate. Use strict aseptic technique. Drug is compatible with polyvinyl chloride plastic bags and polyolefin bags.
• Admixtures with approved diluents are chemically and physically stable for 24 hours at room temperature or 48 hours if refrigerated.
• Inspect parenteral drugs for particles and discoloration before administration.

Patient teaching
• Tell patient to report adverse reactions promptly.
• Instruct him to report discomfort at injection site.

Evaluation
• Patient regains normal sinus rhythm.
• Life-threatening arrhythmia doesn't develop.
• Patient and family state understanding of drug therapy.

idarubicin hydrochloride
(igh-duh-ROO-bih-sin high-droh-KLOR-ighd)
Idamycin, Idamycin PFS

Pharmacologic class: antibiotic antineoplastic
Therapeutic class: antineoplastic
Pregnancy risk category: D

Indications and dosages
Dosages and indications vary. Check current literature for recommended protocol.
▶ **Acute myeloid leukemia, including French-American-British classifications M1 through M7, in combination with other approved antileukemic drugs.** *Adults:* 12 mg/m²/day for 3 days by slow I.V. injection (over 10 to 15 minutes) in combination with 100 mg/m²/day of cytarabine for 7 days by continuous I.V. infusion or cytarabine as 25-mg/m² bolus followed by 200 mg/m²/day for 5 days by continuous infusion. A second course may be administered if needed. If patient develops severe mucositis, administration is delayed until recovery is complete, and dosage may be reduced by 25%. Dosage also should be reduced in patients with hepatic or renal impairment. Idarubicin shouldn't be given if bilirubin level is above 5 mg/dl.

How supplied
Powder for injection: 1 mg/ml available in 5-, 10-, or 20-mg vials

Pharmacokinetics
Absorption: not applicable.
Distribution: drug is highly lipophilic and tissue-bound (97%), with highest levels in nucleated blood and bone marrow cells.
Metabolism: extensive extrahepatic metabolism is indicated. Metabolite has cytotoxic activity.
Excretion: primarily biliary excretion, minimally by renal excretion. *Half-life:* 20 to 22 hours.

Route	Onset	Peak	Duration
I.V.	Unknown	≤ 3 min	Unknown

Pharmacodynamics
Chemical effect: may inhibit nucleic acid synthesis by intercalation; interacts with enzyme topoisomerase II.
Therapeutic effect: hinders growth of susceptible cancer cells.

Adverse reactions
CNS: headache, changed mental status, peripheral neuropathy, ***seizures.***
CV: ***heart failure,*** atrial fibrillation, chest pain, ***MI,*** asymptomatic decline in left ventricular ejection fraction, ***myocardial insufficiency, arrhythmias,*** **HEMORRHAGE,** ***myocardial toxicity.***
GI: *nausea, vomiting,* cramps, diarrhea, *mucositis,* ***severe enterocolitis with perforation.***

GU: decreased renal function.
Hematologic: ***myelosuppression.***
Hepatic: changes in hepatic function.
Metabolic: hyperuricemia.
Skin: alopecia, rash, urticaria, bullous erythrodermatous rash on palms and soles, urticaria at injection site, erythema at previously irradiated sites, tissue necrosis at injection site if extravasation occurs.
Other: INFECTION, fever, ***hypersensitivity reactions.***

Interactions

Drug-drug. *Alkaline solutions, heparin:* incompatible. Idarubicin shouldn't be mixed with other drugs unless specific compatibility data are available.

Contraindications and precautions

- No known contraindications. Drug isn't recommended for pregnant or breast-feeding women.
- Use with extreme caution in patients with bone marrow suppression induced by previous drug therapy or radiotherapy and in patients with impaired hepatic or renal function.
- Safety of drug hasn't been established in children.

NURSING CONSIDERATIONS

Assessment

- Assess patient's condition before therapy and regularly thereafter.
- Assess patient for systemic infection, which should be controlled before therapy begins.
- Monitor CBC and hepatic and renal function test results frequently, as ordered.
- Be alert for adverse reactions and drug interactions, especially signs of heart failure.
- Evaluate patient's and family's knowledge of drug therapy.

Nursing diagnoses

- Ineffective health maintenance related to presence of underlying condition
- Ineffective protection related to adverse hematologic reactions
- Deficient knowledge related to drug therapy

Planning and implementation

- Follow facility policy to reduce risks. Preparation and administration of parenteral form are linked to carcinogenic, mutagenic, and teratogenic risks for personnel.
- Take appropriate preventive measures (including adequate hydration) before starting treatment.

ALERT Don't confuse idarubicin with daunorubicin.

- Reconstitute to final concentration of 1 mg/ml using unpreserved normal saline solution for injection. Add 5 ml to 5-mg vial or 10 ml to 10-mg vial. Don't use bacteriostatic saline solution. Vial is under negative pressure.
- Administer over 10 to 15 minutes into free-flowing I.V. infusion of normal saline solution or 5% dextrose solution that is running into large vein.

ALERT Never give drug by I.M. or S.C. route.

- Reconstituted solutions are stable for 72 hours at 59°to 86°F (15°to 30°C); 7 days if refrigerated. Label unused solutions with CHEMOTHERAPY HAZARD label.
- Hyperuricemia may result from rapid lysis of leukemic cells. Allopurinol may be ordered.
- If extravasation occurs, discontinue infusion immediately, elevate limb, and notify prescriber. Treat with intermittent ice packs—30 minutes immediately and then 30 minutes four times daily for 4 days.

Patient teaching

- Teach patient to recognize and report signs of extravasation, infection, bleeding, and heart failure, such as shortness of breath and leg swelling.
- Advise patient that red urine for several days is normal and doesn't indicate blood in urine.
- Advise women of childbearing age to use a reliable contraceptive during therapy and to consult with prescriber before becoming pregnant.

Evaluation

- Patient responds well to drug.
- Serious adverse hematologic reactions don't develop.
- Patient and family state understanding of drug therapy.

ifosfamide

(igh-FOHS-fuh-mighd)
IFEX

Pharmacologic class: alkylating agent (cell cycle–phase nonspecific)
Therapeutic class: antineoplastic
Pregnancy risk category: D

Indications and dosages

▶ **Testicular cancer.** *Adults:* 1.2 g/m²/day I.V. for 5 consecutive days. Repeated q 3 weeks or after patient recovers from hematologic toxicity.

How supplied

Injection: 1 g (supplied with 200-mg ampule of mesna), 2 g, 3 g (supplied with 400-mg ampule of mesna)

Pharmacokinetics

Exhibits dose-dependent pharmacokinetics.
Absorption: not applicable.
Distribution: drug crosses blood-brain barrier but its metabolites don't; therefore, alkylating activity doesn't occur in CSF.
Metabolism: about 50% of dose is metabolized in liver.
Excretion: excreted primarily in urine. *Half-life:* about 14 hours.

Route	Onset	Peak	Duration
I.V.	Unknown	Unknown	Unknown

Pharmacodynamics

Chemical effect: cross-links strands of cellular DNA and interferes with RNA transcription, causing growth imbalance that leads to cell death.
Therapeutic effect: kills testicular cancer cells.

Adverse reactions

CNS: *lethargy, somnolence, confusion, depressive psychosis,* ***coma, seizures,*** ataxia.
GI: *nausea, vomiting.*
GU: *hemorrhagic cystitis* (dose-limiting, occurring in up to 50% of patients), *hematuria,* ***nephrotoxicity.***
Hematologic: *leukopenia, thrombocytopenia,* ***myelosuppression.***
Hepatic: elevated liver enzyme levels.
Skin: *alopecia.*

Interactions

Drug-drug. *Allopurinol:* may produce excessive ifosfamide effect by prolonging half-life. Monitor patient for enhanced toxicity.
Anticoagulants, aspirin: increased risk of bleeding. Avoid concomitant use.
Barbiturates, chloral hydrate, phenytoin: may increase ifosfamide toxicity by inducing hepatic enzymes that hasten formation of toxic metabolites. Monitor patient closely.
Corticosteroids: may inhibit hepatic enzymes, reducing ifosfamide's effect. Monitor patient for enhanced ifosfamide toxicity if concurrent corticosteroid dosage is abruptly reduced or discontinued.
Myelosuppressants: enhanced hematologic toxicity. Dosage adjustment may be necessary.

Contraindications and precautions

- Contraindicated in patients hypersensitive to drug and in those with severely depressed bone marrow function.
- Off-label use not recommended in pregnant or breast-feeding women.
- Use cautiously in patients with renal impairment or compromised bone marrow from leukopenia, granulocytopenia, extensive bone marrow metastases, previous radiation therapy, or previous therapy with cytotoxic drugs.
- Safety of drug hasn't been established in children.

NURSING CONSIDERATIONS

Assessment

- Assess patient's condition before therapy and regularly thereafter.
- Obtain urinalysis before each dose. If microscopic hematuria is present, patient should be evaluated for hemorrhagic cystitis. Dosage adjustments of mesna—a protecting agent given with ifosfamide—may be necessary.
- Monitor CBC and renal and liver function tests, as ordered.
- Be alert for adverse reactions and drug interactions.

• Assess patient for mental status changes; dosage may need to be decreased.
• Evaluate patient's and family's knowledge of drug therapy.

Nursing diagnoses

• Ineffective health maintenance related to presence of cancer
• Ineffective protection related to adverse CNS and hematologic reactions
• Deficient knowledge related to drug therapy

Planning and implementation

• Administer antiemetics, as ordered, before giving ifosfamide to decrease nausea.
• As ordered, administer ifosfamide with protecting agent (mesna) to prevent hemorrhagic cystitis. Mesna must be given with or before ifosfamide to prevent cystitis. Adequate fluid intake (2 L/day, either P.O. or I.V.) is essential.
• Follow facility policy to reduce risks. Preparation and administration of parenteral form are linked to carcinogenic, mutagenic, and teratogenic risks for personnel.
ALERT Don't confuse ifosfamide with cyclophosphamine.
• Reconstitute each gram of drug with 20 ml of diluent to yield 50 mg/ml. Use sterile water for injection or bacteriostatic water for injection. Solutions may be further diluted with sterile water, dextrose 2.5% or 5% in water, half-normal or normal saline solution for injection, D_5W and normal saline solution for injection, or lactated Ringer's injection.
• Infuse each dose over at least 30 minutes.
• Ifosfamide and mesna are physically compatible and may be mixed in same I.V. solution.
• Reconstituted solution is stable for 1 week at room temperature or 6 weeks refrigerated. However, use solution within 6 hours if drug was reconstituted with unpreserved sterile water.
• Don't give drug at bedtime; infrequent voiding during night may increase risk of cystitis. If cystitis develops, discontinue drug and notify prescriber.
• Bladder irrigation with normal saline solution may decrease possibility of cystitis.
• Institute infection-control and bleeding precautions.

Patient teaching

• Tell patient to void frequently to minimize contact of drug and its metabolites with bladder mucosa.
• Warn patient to watch for evidence of infection (fever, sore throat, fatigue), CNS effects (sommolence and dizziness), and bleeding (easy bruising, nosebleeds, bleeding gums, melena). Teach patient about infection-control and bleeding precautions, and tell him to report adverse effects. Tell him to take his temperature daily.
• Instruct patient to avoid OTC medications that contain aspirin.
• Stress importance of adequate fluid intake during therapy. Explain that it may help prevent hemorrhagic cystitis.
• Warn patient that hyperpigmentation may occur.

Evaluation

• Patient responds well to drug.
• Serious infections and CNS and bleeding complications don't develop.
• Patient and family state understanding of drug therapy.

imipenem and cilastatin sodium

(im-ih-PEN-em and sigh-luh-STAT-in SO-dee-um)
Primaxin IM, Primaxin IV

Pharmacologic class: carbapenem (thienamycin class); beta-lactam antibiotic
Therapeutic class: antibiotic
Pregnancy risk category: C

Indications and dosages

▶ **Mild to moderate lower respiratory tract, skin, skin-structure, and gynecologic infections.** *Adults weighing at least 70 kg (154 lb):* 500 to 750 mg I.M. q 12 hours. Or, 250 to 500 mg I.V. q 6 hours. Maximum I.V. dosage is 50 mg/kg/day or 4 g/day, whichever is less. *Children age 3 months and older:* 15 to 25 mg/kg I.V. q 6 hours. Maximum dosage for fully susceptible organisms is 2 g/day and for moderately susceptible organisms, 4 g/day (based on adult studies).

Infants ages 4 weeks to 3 months and weighing at least 1.5 kg (3.3 lb): 25 mg/kg I.V. q 6 hours.
Neonates ages 1 to 4 weeks and weighing at least 1.5 kg: 25 mg/kg I.V. q 8 hours.
Neonates less than 1 week old and weighing at least 1.5 kg: 25 mg/kg I.V. q 12 hours.

▶ **Mild to moderate intra-abdominal infections.** *Adults:* 750 mg I.M. q 12 hours.
Children age 3 months and older: 15 to 25 mg/kg I.V. q 6 hours. Maximum dosage for fully susceptible organisms is 2 g/day and for moderately susceptible organisms, 4 g/day (based on adult studies).
Infants ages 4 weeks to 3 months and weighing at least 1.5 kg (3.3 lb): 25 mg/kg I.V. q 6 hours.
Neonates ages 1 to 4 weeks and weighing at least 1.5 kg: 25 mg/kg I.V. q 8 hours.
Neonates less than 1 week old and weighing at least 1.5 kg: 25 mg/kg I.V. q 12 hours.

▶ **Serious infections of lower respiratory and urinary tracts, intra-abdominal and gynecologic infections, bacterial septicemia, bone and joint infections, skin and soft-tissue infections, and endocarditis.** *Adults weighing at least 70 kg (154 lb):* 500 mg I.V. q 6 hours or 1 g q 6 to 8 hours by I.V. infusion. Maximum dosage is 50 mg/kg/day or 4 g/day, whichever is less.

▶ **Infections (other than CNS infections) in children.** *Children age 3 months and older:* 15 to 25 mg/kg I.V. q 6 hours. Maximum dosage for fully susceptible organisms is 2 g/day and for moderately susceptible organisms, 4 g/day (based on adult studies).
Infants ages 4 weeks to 3 months and weighing at least 1.5 kg (3.3 lb): 25 mg/kg I.V. q 6 hours.
Neonates ages 1 to 4 weeks and weighing at least 1.5 kg: 25 mg/kg I.V. q 8 hours.
Neonates less than 1 week old and weighing at least 1.5 kg: 25 mg/kg I.V. q 12 hours.

How supplied

Powder for I.M. injection: 500-mg, 750-mg vials
Powder for I.V. injection: 250 mg, 500 mg

Pharmacokinetics

Absorption: imipenem is about 75% bioavailable and cilastatin is about 95% bioavailable after I.M. use.
Distribution: distributed rapidly and widely. About 20% of imipenem is protein-bound; 40% of cilastatin is protein-bound.
Metabolism: imipenem is metabolized by kidney dehydropeptidase I, resulting in low urine levels. Cilastatin inhibits this enzyme, thereby reducing imipenem metabolism.
Excretion: about 70% excreted unchanged by kidneys. *Half-life:* 1 hour after I.V. dose; 2 to 3 hours after I.M. dose.

Route	Onset	Peak	Duration
I.V.	Unknown	Immediate	Unknown
I.M.	Unknown	1-2 hr	Unknown

Pharmacodynamics

Chemical effect: imipenem is bactericidal and inhibits bacterial cell wall synthesis. Cilastatin inhibits enzymatic breakdown of imipenem in kidneys, making it effective in urinary tract.
Therapeutic effect: kills susceptible organisms. Spectrum of activity includes many gram-positive, gram-negative, and anaerobic bacteria, including *Staphylococcus* and *Streptococcus* species, *Escherichia coli, Klebsiella, Proteus, Enterobacter* species, *Pseudomonas aeruginosa,* and *Bacteroides* species, including *B. fragilis.*

Adverse reactions

CNS: ***seizures,*** dizziness, somnolence.
CV: hypotension, thrombophlebitis.
GI: nausea, vomiting, diarrhea, *pseudomembranous colitis.*
Hepatic: transient increases in liver enzyme levels.
Skin: rash, urticaria, pruritus.
Other: ***hypersensitivity reactions (anaphylaxis),*** pain at injection site, fever.

Interactions

Drug-drug. *Beta-lactam antibiotics:* possible in vitro antagonism. Avoid concomitant use.
Cyclosporine: adverse CNS effects of both drugs may be increased, possibly because of additive or synergistic toxicity. Avoid concomitant use.

Ganciclovir: may cause seizures. Avoid concomitant use.
Probenecid: increased serum cilastatin levels. Avoid concomitant use.

Contraindications and precautions

- Contraindicated in patients hypersensitive to drug.
- Use cautiously in pregnant or breast-feeding women, in patients allergic to penicillins or cephalosporins, and in those with history of seizure disorders, especially if they also have compromised renal function.
- I.M. safety and efficacy in children under age 12 haven't been established.
- I.V. use isn't recommended in children with CNS infections because of risk of seizures; also not recommended in children weighing less than 30 kg (66 lb) with impaired renal function because no data are available.

NURSING CONSIDERATIONS

Assessment

- Assess patient's infection before therapy and regularly thereafter.
- Obtain urine specimen for culture and sensitivity tests before first dose. Therapy may begin pending results.
- Be alert for adverse reactions and drug interactions.
- Monitor patient's hydration status if adverse GI reactions occur.
- Evaluate patient's and family's knowledge of drug therapy.

Nursing diagnoses

- Infection related to presence of susceptible organisms
- Risk for deficient fluid volume related to adverse GI reactions
- Deficient knowledge related to drug therapy

Planning and implementation

I.V. use: Don't administer drug by direct I.V. bolus injection. Give 250- or 500-mg dose by I.V. infusion over 20 to 30 minutes. Infuse each 1-g dose over 40 to 60 minutes. If nausea occurs, slow infusion.
– When reconstituting powder, shake until solution is clear. Solutions may range from colorless to yellow, and variations of color within this range don't affect drug's potency. After reconstitution, solution is stable for 10 hours at room temperature and for 48 hours when refrigerated.
I.M. use: Follow normal protocol. Reconstitute vials for I.M. injection with 1% lidocaine hydrochloride (without epinephrine) as directed.
- Patients with impaired renal function or who weigh less than 70 kg (154 lb) may need lower dose or longer intervals between doses.

ALERT If seizures develop and persist despite anticonvulsants, notify prescriber, who may discontinue drug.

Patient teaching

- Instruct patient to report adverse reactions because supportive therapy may be needed.
- Warn patient about pain at injection site.

Evaluation

- Patient is free from infection.
- Patient maintains adequate hydration throughout therapy.
- Patient and family state understanding of drug therapy.

imipramine hydrochloride

(ih-MIP-ruh-meen high-droh-KLOR-ighd)
Apo-Imipramine♦, Impril♦, Melipramine◇, Norfranil, Novopramine♦, Tipramine, Tofranil**

imipramine pamoate

Tofranil-PM**

Pharmacologic class: dibenzazepine tricyclic antidepressant
Therapeutic class: antidepressant
Pregnancy risk category: D

Indications and dosages

▶ **Depression.** *Adults:* 75 to 100 mg P.O. or I.M. daily in divided doses, increased in 25- to 50-mg increments to maximum dosage. Or, 25 mg P.O. daily, increased in 25-mg increments every other day. Or, entire dosage may be given h.s. Maximum dosage is 200 mg/day for outpatients, 300 mg/day for inpatients, 100 mg/day for elderly patients.

▶ **Childhood enuresis.** *Children age 6 and older:* 25 mg P.O. 1 hour before bedtime. If no response within 1 week, dosage may be increased to 50 mg nightly for children under age 12 or 75 mg nightly for children age 12 and older. Maximum dosage shouldn't exceed 2.5 mg/kg/day.

How supplied

imipramine hydrochloride
Tablets: 10 mg, 25 mg, 50 mg
Injection: 12.5 mg/ml
imipramine pamoate
Capsules: 75 mg, 100 mg, 125 mg, 150 mg

Pharmacokinetics

Absorption: absorbed rapidly from GI tract after P.O. use and rapidly from muscle tissue after I.M. use.
Distribution: distributed widely into body, including CNS. Drug is 90% protein-bound.
Metabolism: metabolized by liver. A significant first-pass effect may explain variability of serum levels in different patients taking same dose.
Excretion: most of drug is excreted in urine.

Route	Onset	Peak	Duration
P.O.	Unknown	1-2 hr	Unknown
I.M.	Unknown	30 min	Unknown

Pharmacodynamics

Chemical effect: increases amount of norepinephrine, serotonin, or both in CNS by blocking their reuptake by presynaptic neurons.
Therapeutic effect: relieves depression and childhood enuresis (hydrochloride form).

Adverse reactions

CNS: *drowsiness, dizziness,* excitation, tremors, weakness, confusion, headache, nervousness, EEG changes, ***seizures,*** extrapyramidal reactions.
CV: *orthostatic hypotension, tachycardia, ECG changes,* hypertension, ***MI, CVA, arrhythmias, heart block.***
EENT: *blurred vision,* tinnitus, mydriasis.
GI: *dry mouth, constipation,* nausea, vomiting, anorexia, paralytic ileus.
GU: *urine retention,* impotence, testicular swelling.
Metabolic: hypoglycemia, hyperglycemia.
Skin: rash, urticaria, *diaphoresis,* photosensitivity.
Other: ***hypersensitivity reactions,*** gynecomastia, galactorrhea and breast enlargement, altered libido, SIADH.

Interactions

Drug-drug. *Barbiturates, CNS depressants:* enhanced CNS depression. Avoid concomitant use.
Cimetidine, methylphenidate: may increase imipramine serum levels. Monitor patient for adverse reactions.
Clonidine, epinephrine, norepinephrine: increased hypertensive effect. Use cautiously.
Fluoxetine: may increase the pharmacologic and toxic effects of tricyclic antidepressants; symptoms may persist several weeks after fluoxetine therapy stops. Monitor symptoms closely.
MAO inhibitors: may cause hyperpyretic crisis, severe seizures, and death. Avoid concomitant use.
Drug-herb. *SAMe, St. John's wort, yohimbe:* may elevate serotonin levels. Discourage concomitant use.
Drug-lifestyle. *Alcohol use:* enhanced CNS depression. Discourage concomitant use.
Smoking: may lower plasma imipramine levels. Monitor patient for lack of effect.
Sun exposure: increased risk of photosensitivity. Recommend appropriate precautions.

Contraindications and precautions

- Contraindicated in patients hypersensitive to drug, patients receiving MAO inhibitors, and patients in acute recovery phase of MI.
- Drug isn't recommended for use in pregnant or breast-feeding women.
- Use with extreme caution in patients at risk for suicide; patients with history of urine retention or angle-closure glaucoma, increased intraocular pressure, CV disease, impaired hepatic function, hyperthyroidism, seizure disorder, or impaired renal function; and patients receiving thyroid medications. Injectable form contains sulfites, which may cause allergic reactions in hypersensitive patients.

• Safety of drug hasn't been established for treating depression in children.

NURSING CONSIDERATIONS

Assessment
• Assess patient's condition before therapy and regularly thereafter.
• Be alert for adverse reactions and drug interactions.
• Evaluate patient's and family's knowledge of drug therapy.

Nursing diagnoses
• Ineffective individual coping related to depression
• Deficient knowledge related to drug therapy

Planning and implementation
• Dosage should be reduced in elderly or debilitated patients, adolescents, and patients with aggravated psychotic symptoms.

ALERT Don't confuse imipramine with desipramine.

P.O. use: Although doses have been administered up to four times daily, patients may receive entire daily dosage at one time because of drug's long action.

I.M. use: Follow normal protocol.

• Don't withdraw drug abruptly.
• Drug causes high risk of orthostatic hypotension. Check sitting and standing blood pressures after initial dose.
• Because of hypertensive episodes during surgery in patients receiving tricyclic antidepressants, drug should be gradually discontinued several days before surgery. After abrupt withdrawal of long-term therapy, patient may experience nausea, headache, and malaise. These symptoms don't indicate addiction.
• If signs of psychosis occur or increase, notify prescriber and expect to reduce dosage.

Patient teaching
• Advise patient to take full dose at bedtime but warn about possible morning orthostatic hypotension.
• Suggest taking drug with food or milk if it causes stomach upset.
• Suggest relieving dry mouth with sugarless chewing gum or hard candy. Encourage good dental prophylaxis because persistent dry mouth may increase the risk of dental caries.
• Tell patient to avoid alcohol and smoking during drug therapy.
• Warn patient to avoid hazardous activities until CNS effects of drug are known.
• Warn patient not to stop taking drug suddenly.
• Advise patient to consult prescriber before taking other prescription drugs, OTC medications, or herbal remedies.
• Advise patient to use sunblock, wear protective clothing, and avoid prolonged exposure to sunlight to prevent photosensitivity reactions.

Evaluation
• Patient behavior and communication show diminished depression.
• Patient and family state understanding of drug therapy.

immune globulin intramuscular (gamma globulin, IG, IGIM)
(ih-MYOON GLOB-yoo-lin in-truh-MUS-kyoo-ler)
BayGam

immune globulin intravenous (IGIV)
Gamimune N, Gammagard S/D, Gammar-P IV, Iveegam, Polygam S/D, Sandoglobulin, Venoglobulin-I, Venoglobulin-S

Pharmacologic class: immune serum
Therapeutic class: immune serum
Pregnancy risk category: C

Indications and dosages
▶ **Primary humoral immunodeficiency (IGIV).** *Adults and children:*
Gamimune N—100 to 200 mg/kg I.V. monthly, at 0.01 to 0.02 ml/kg/minute for 30 minutes. If no discomfort, rate can slowly be increased to a maximum of 0.08 ml/kg/minute.
Gammagard S/D—200 to 400 mg/kg I.V.; then monthly doses of 100 mg/kg. Start infusion at 0.5 ml/kg/hour and increase to maximum of

4 ml/kg/hour. Dose is related to patient response.
Gammar-P IV—200 to 400 mg/kg I.V. every 3 to 4 weeks. Infuse at 0.01 ml/kg/minute and increase to 0.02 ml/kg/minute after 15 to 30 minutes if no problems occur. Maximum infusion rate is 0.06 ml/kg/minute.
Iveegam—200 ml/kg I.V. monthly. May increase dose to maximum of 800 mg/kg or give more frequently to produce desired effect. Infusion rate is 1 to 2 ml/minute for 5% solution.
Polygam S/D—200 to 400 mg/kg I.V. at 0.5 ml/kg/hour, increasing to a maximum of 4 ml/kg/hour. Subsequent dose is 100 mg/kg I.V. monthly.
Sandoglobulin—200 mg/kg I.V. monthly. Start with 0.5 to 1 ml/minute of 3% solution; gradually increase dose to 2.5 ml/minute after 15 to 30 minutes.
Venoglobulin-I—200 mg/kg I.V. monthly at 0.01 to 0.02 ml/kg/minute for 30 minutes; increase to 0.04 ml/kg/minute or more if no adverse reaction occurs. Dose may be increased to 300 to 400 mg/kg and given more often than once monthly if needed and tolerated.
Venoglobulin-S—200 mg/kg I.V. monthly. Dose may be increased to 300 to 400 mg/kg and given more often than once monthly if IgG levels aren't adequate. Infuse at 0.01 to 0.02 ml/kg/minute for 30 minutes; if tolerated, increase 5% solutions to 0.04 ml/kg/minute and 10% solutions to 0.05 ml/kg/minute.
▶ **Idiopathic thrombocytopenic purpura (IGIV).** *Adults and children*:
Gamimune N—400 mg/kg 5% solution I.V. for 5 days; or 1,000 mg/kg 10% solution I.V. for 1 to 2 days with maintenance dose of 10% solution at 400 to 1,000 mg/kg I.V. single infusion to maintain 30,000/mm^3 platelet count.
Gammagard S/D or Polygam S/D—1,000 mg/kg I.V. as a single dose. Give up to three doses on alternate days if required.
Sandoglobulin—0.4 mg/kg I.V. for 2 to 5 consecutive days.
Venoglobulin-S—maximum of 2,000 mg/kg I.V. over 5 days or less. Maintenance dose is 1,000 mg/kg administered as needed.
▶ **Bone marrow transplant (IGIV).** *Adults over age 20:*
Gamimune N—500 mg/kg 5% or 10% solution I.V. on days 7 and 2 pretransplantation; then weekly until 90 days posttransplantation.
▶ **B-cell chronic lymphocytic leukemia (IGIV).** *Adults:*
Gammagard S/D or Polygam S/D—400 mg/kg I.V. every 3 to 4 weeks.
▶ **Pediatric HIV infection (IGIV).** *Children:*
Gamimune N—400 mg/kg I.V. every 28 days, at 0.01 to 0.02 ml/kg/minute for 30 minutes; increase to maximum of 0.08 ml/kg/minute.
▶ **Kawasaki Syndrome (IGIV).** *Adults:*
Iveegam—400 mg/kg/day I.V. over 2 hours for 4 consecutive days, or a single dose of 2,000 mg/kg I.V. over 10 to 12 hours. Start within 10 days of disease onset. Treat concurrently with aspirin (80 to 100 mg/kg/day P.O. through day 14; then 3 to 10 mg/kg/day for 5 weeks).
▶ **Hepatitis A exposure (IGIM).** *Adults and children:* 0.02 ml/kg I.M. as soon as possible after exposure. Up to 0.01 ml/kg may be administered for prolonged or intense exposure.
▶ **Measles exposure (IGIM).** *Adults and children:* 0.025 ml/kg I.M. within 6 days after exposure.
▶ **Measles postexposure prophylaxis (IGIM).** *Children:* 0.5 ml/kg I.M. (maximum, 15 ml) within 6 days after exposure.
▶ **Chickenpox exposure (IGIM).** *Adults and children:* 0.6 to 1.2 ml/kg I.M. as soon as exposed.
▶ **Rubella exposure in first trimester of pregnancy (IGIM).** *Women:* 0.55 ml/kg I.M. as soon as possible postexposure (within 72 hours).

How supplied

IGIM
Injection: 2-ml, 10-ml vials

IGIV
Injection: 5% and 10% in 10-ml, 50-ml, 100-ml, 250-ml vials (Gamimune N); 5% in 2.5-g, 5-g, 10-g vials; 5%, 10% in 5-g, 10-g, 20-g vials (Venoglobulin-S)
Powder for injection: 50 mg protein/ml in 2.5-g, 5-g, 10-g vials (Gammagard S/D); 1-gm, 2.5-g, 5-g vials (Gammar-P IV); 500-mg and 1-g, 2.5-g, 5-g vials (Iveegam); 2.5-g, 5-g, 10-g vials (Polygam S/D); 1-g, 3-g, 6-g, 12-g vials (Sandoglobulin); 500-mg, 2.5-g, 5-g, 10-g vials (Venoglobulin-I)

Pharmacokinetics

Absorption: absorbed slowly after I.M. administration.
Distribution: distributed evenly between intravascular and extravascular spaces.
Metabolism: unknown.
Excretion: unknown. *Half-life:* 21 to 24 days in immunocompetent patients.

Route	Onset	Peak	Duration
I.V.	Immediate	Immediate	Unknown
I.M.	Unknown	2-5 days	Unknown

Pharmacodynamics

Chemical effect: provides passive immunity by increasing antibody titer. The primary component is IgG.
Therapeutic effect: helps prevent infections.

Adverse reactions

CNS: headache, malaise.
GI: nausea, vomiting.
GU: nephrotic syndrome.
Musculoskeletal: muscle stiffness at injection site.
Skin: urticaria, erythema.
Other: pain, ***anaphylaxis,*** fever.

Interactions

Drug-drug. *Live-virus vaccines:* antibodies in the vaccine may interfere with drug therapy. Don't give within 3 months after giving immune globulin.

Contraindications and precautions

- Contraindicated in patients hypersensitive to drug.
- Use cautiously in pregnant or breast-feeding women.
- I.M. administration contraindicated in patients with severe thrombocytopenia or other coagulation disorders that contraindicate I.M. administration.

NURSING CONSIDERATIONS

Assessment

- Obtain history of allergies and reaction to immunizations.
- Observe patient for signs of anaphylaxis immediately after injection.
- Inspect injection site for local reactions.
- Monitor effectiveness by checking antibody titers after administration.
- Be alert for adverse reactions and drug interactions.
- Evaluate patient's and family's knowledge of drug therapy.

Nursing diagnoses

- Ineffective protection related to lack of or decreased immunity
- Ineffective breathing pattern related to anaphylaxis
- Deficient knowledge related to drug therapy

Planning and implementation

I.V. use: I.V. products aren't interchangeable. Gammagard requires a filter, which is supplied by manufacturer.
- Most adverse effects are related to rapid infusion rate. Infuse slowly.

ALERT Don't confuse Sandoglobulin with Sandimmune or Sandostatin.

I.M. use: When giving I.M., use gluteal region. Doses over 10 ml should be divided and injected into several muscle sites to reduce local pain and discomfort.
- Immune globulin shouldn't be given for prophylaxis against hepatitis A if 6 weeks or more have elapsed since exposure or since clinical illness has begun.
- Make sure epinephrine 1:1,000 is available in case of anaphylaxis.

ALERT I.V. and I.M. products aren't interchangeable.

Patient teaching

- Instruct patient to report respiratory difficulty immediately.
- Tell patient that local reactions may occur at injection site. Instruct patient to notify prescriber promptly if adverse reaction persists or becomes severe.

Evaluation

- Patient exhibits increased passive immunity.
- Patient shows no signs of anaphylaxis.
- Patient and family state understanding of drug therapy.

indapamide

(in-DAP-uh-mighd)
Lozide ♦, Lozol, Natrilix ◇

Pharmacologic class: thiazide-like diuretic
Therapeutic class: diuretic, antihypertensive
Pregnancy risk category: B

Indications and dosages

Edema. *Adults:* initially, 2.5 mg P.O. daily in morning. Increased to 5 mg daily after 1 week, if needed.
Hypertension. *Adults:* initially, 1.25 mg P.O. daily in morning. Increased to 2.5 mg daily after 4 weeks, if needed. Increased to 5 mg daily after 4 more weeks, if needed.

How supplied

Tablets: 1.25 mg, 2.5 mg

Pharmacokinetics

Absorption: absorbed completely from GI tract.
Distribution: distributed widely into body tissues because of its lipophilicity; 71% to 79% plasma protein–bound.
Metabolism: undergoes significant hepatic metabolism.
Excretion: primarily excreted in urine; smaller amounts excreted in feces. *Half-life:* about 14 hours.

Route	Onset	Peak	Duration
P.O.	1-2 hr	≤ 2 hr	≤ 36 hr

Pharmacodynamics

Chemical effect: unknown; probably inhibits sodium reabsorption in distal segment of nephron. Also has direct vasodilating effect, possibly from calcium channel–blocking action.
Therapeutic effect: promotes water and sodium excretion and lowers blood pressure.

Adverse reactions

CNS: headache, irritability, nervousness, dizziness, light-headedness, weakness.
CV: volume depletion and dehydration, orthostatic hypotension.
GI: nausea, ***pancreatitis.***
GU: nocturia, polyuria, frequent urination.
Metabolic: anorexia, hypokalemia; asymptomatic hyperuricemia; fluid and electrolyte imbalances, including metabolic alkalosis and dilutional hyponatremia and hypochloremia; gout.
Musculoskeletal: muscle cramps and spasms.
Skin: dermatitis, photosensitivity, rash.

Interactions

Drug-drug. *Cardiac glycosides:* increased risk of digoxin toxicity from indapamide-induced hypokalemia. Monitor potassium and digoxin levels.
Diazoxide: increased antihypertensive, hyperglycemic, and hyperuricemic effects. Use together cautiously.
NSAIDs: increased risk of NSAID-induced renal failure. Monitor patient for signs of renal failure.

Contraindications and precautions

- Contraindicated in patients hypersensitive to other sulfonamide-derived drugs and in those with anuria.
- Use cautiously in patients with severe renal disease, impaired hepatic function, and progressive hepatic disease.
- Use cautiously in pregnant women.
- Safety of drug hasn't been established in breast-feeding women or in children.

NURSING CONSIDERATIONS

Assessment

- Assess patient's underlying condition before therapy.
- Monitor effectiveness by assessing fluid intake and output, weight, and blood pressure. In hypertensive patient, therapeutic response may be delayed several days.
- Monitor serum electrolytes and blood glucose.
- Monitor serum creatinine and BUN levels regularly. Drug isn't as effective if these levels are more than twice normal.
- Monitor blood uric acid levels, especially if patient has history of gout.
- Be alert for adverse reactions and drug interactions.

• Evaluate patient's and family's knowledge of drug therapy.

Nursing diagnoses
• Risk for injury related to presence of hypertension
• Excessive fluid volume related to presence of edema
• Deficient knowledge related to drug therapy

Planning and implementation
• To prevent nocturia, give drug in morning.
• Drug may be used with potassium-sparing diuretic to prevent potassium loss.

Patient teaching
• Advise patient to avoid sudden postural changes and to rise slowly to avoid orthostatic hypotension.
• Advise patient to use sunblock to prevent photosensitivity reactions.
• Teach patient to monitor fluid volume by recording daily weight and intake and output.
• Tell patient to avoid high-sodium foods and to choose high-potassium foods.
• Advise patient to take drug early in day to avoid nocturia.

Evaluation
• Patient's blood pressure is normal.
• Patient is free from edema.
• Patient and family state understanding of drug therapy.

indinavir sulfate
(in-DIH-nuh-veer SUL-fayt)
Crixivan

Pharmacologic class: protease inhibitor
Therapeutic class: antiviral
Pregnancy risk category: C

Indications and dosages
▶ **Treatment of patients with HIV infection when antiretroviral therapy is warranted.**
Adults: 800 mg P.O. q 8 hours. Dosage reduced to 600 mg P.O. q 8 hours in mild to moderate hepatic insufficiency resulting from cirrhosis.

How supplied
Capsules: 200 mg, 400 mg

Pharmacokinetics
Absorption: rapidly absorbed.
Distribution: 60% bound to plasma proteins.
Metabolism: metabolized by liver and kidneys.
Excretion: excreted in urine.

Route	Onset	Peak	Duration
P.O.	Unknown	< 1 hr	1-8 hr

Pharmacodynamics
Chemical effect: binds to protease active sites and inhibits their activity.
Therapeutic effect: prevents cleavage of viral polyproteins, resulting in formation of immature, noninfectious viral particles.

Adverse reactions
CNS: headache, insomnia, dizziness, malaise, somnolence, asthenia, fatigue.
GI: abdominal pain, *nausea,* diarrhea, vomiting, acid regurgitation, anorexia, dry mouth, taste perversion.
GU: nephrolithiasis.
Hematologic: decreased hemoglobin or neutrophil count.
Hepatic: *hyperbilirubinemia;* elevated ALT, AST, and serum amylase levels.
Musculoskeletal: flank pain, back pain.

Interactions
Drug-drug. *Didanosine:* possible degradation of didanosine. If given with indinavir, administer at least 1 hour apart on an empty stomach.
Ketoconazole: increases plasma indinavir levels. Reduce indinavir dosage as directed.
Midazolam, triazolam: possible inhibited metabolism of these drugs. Don't administer concurrently.
Rifabutin: increased plasma levels of indinavir. Reduce dosage of rifabutin by 50% if administered together.
Rifampin: markedly diminishes plasma indinavir levels. Avoid concomitant use.
Drug-herb. *St. John's wort:* substantially reduces drug levels and may cause loss of therapeutic effects. Discourage concomitant use.

Drug-food. *Any food*: substantially decreases absorption of oral indinavir. Give drug on an empty stomach.

Contraindications and precautions

• Contraindicated in patients hypersensitive to drug.
• Use cautiously in patients with hepatic insufficiency resulting from cirrhosis.

NURSING CONSIDERATIONS

Assessment
• Monitor adverse reactions and drug interactions.
• Evaluate patient's and family's knowledge of drug therapy.

Nursing diagnoses
• Infection related to presence of virus
• Risk for deficient fluid volume related to effect on kidneys
• Deficient knowledge related to drug therapy

Planning and implementation
• Patient should maintain adequate hydration (at least 48 oz or 1.5 L of fluids every 24 hours while taking indinavir).

Patient teaching
• Instruct patient to use barrier protection during sexual intercourse.
• Advise patient that if a dose is missed, he should take the next dose at regular, scheduled time and not double the dose.
• Instruct patient to take drug on an empty stomach with water 1 hour before or 2 hours after a meal.
• Instruct patient to store capsules in the original container and to keep the desiccant in the bottle.
• Instruct patient to drink at least 48 oz (or 1.5 L) of fluid daily.
• Advise HIV-positive woman to avoid breastfeeding to prevent transmitting virus to infant.
• Instruct patient to report evidence of nephrolithiasis (flank pain, hematuria) or diabetes (increased thirst, polyuria) promptly.

Evaluation
• Patient's health improves and signs and symptoms of underlying condition diminish with use of drug.
• Patient maintains adequate hydration.
• Patient and family state understanding of drug therapy.

indomethacin

(in-doh-METH-uh-sin)
Apo-Indomethacin♦, Arthrexin◇, Indocid♦ ◇, Indocid SR♦, Indocin, Indocin SR, Novo-Methacin♦

indomethacin sodium trihydrate

Apo-Indomethacin♦, Indocid PDA♦, Indocin I.V., Novo-Methacin♦

Pharmacologic class: NSAID
Therapeutic class: nonnarcotic analgesic, antipyretic, anti-inflammatory
Pregnancy risk category: NR

Indications and dosages

▶ **Moderate to severe rheumatoid arthritis or osteoarthritis, ankylosing spondylitis.** *Adults:* 25 mg P.O. b.i.d. or t.i.d. with food or antacids, increased by 25 mg or 50 mg daily q 7 days up to 200 mg daily. Or, 50 mg P.R. q.i.d. Or, 75 mg sustained-release capsules P.O. to start, in morning or h.s., followed, if necessary, by another 75 mg b.i.d.

▶ **Acute gouty arthritis.** *Adults:* 50 mg P.O. t.i.d. Dose reduced as soon as possible; then discontinued. Don't use sustained-release capsules for this condition.

▶ **Acute painful shoulders (bursitis or tendinitis).** *Adults:* 75 to 150 mg P.O. daily b.i.d. or t.i.d. with food or antacids for 7 to 14 days.

▶ **To close hemodynamically significant patent ductus arteriosus in premature infants (I.V. form).** *Neonates less than 48 hours old:* 0.2 mg/kg I.V. followed by two doses of 0.1 mg/kg at 12- to 24-hour intervals.
Neonates ages 2 to 7 days: 0.2 mg/kg I.V. followed by two doses of 0.2 mg/kg at 12- to 24-hour intervals.

Neonates over age 7 days: 0.2 mg/kg I.V. followed by two doses of 0.25 mg/kg at 12- to 24-hour intervals.

How supplied

indomethacin
Capsules: 25 mg, 50 mg
Capsules (sustained-release): 75 mg
Oral suspension: 25 mg/5 ml
Suppositories: 50 mg

indomethacin sodium trihydrate
Injection: 1-mg vials

Pharmacokinetics

Absorption: absorbed rapidly and completely from GI tract after P.O. and P.R. administration.
Distribution: highly protein-bound.
Metabolism: metabolized in liver.
Excretion: excreted mainly in urine, with some biliary excretion.

Route	Onset	Peak	Duration
P.O.	0.5 hr	1-4 hr	4-6 hr
I.V.	Immediate	Immediate	Unknown
P.R.	2-4 hr	Unknown	4-6 hr

Pharmacodynamics

Chemical effect: unknown; produces anti-inflammatory, analgesic, and antipyretic effects, possibly by inhibiting prostaglandin synthesis.
Therapeutic effect: relieves pain, fever, and inflammation.

Adverse reactions

P.O. and P.R. form
CNS: *headache, dizziness,* depression, drowsiness, confusion, peripheral neuropathy, ***seizures,*** psychic disturbances, syncope, *vertigo.*
CV: hypertension, *edema,* ***heart failure.***
EENT: blurred vision, corneal and retinal damage, hearing loss, tinnitus.
GI: *nausea, vomiting,* anorexia, *diarrhea, peptic ulceration,* ***GI bleeding, pancreatitis.***
GU: hematuria, ***acute renal failure.***
Hematologic: ***hemolytic anemia, aplastic anemia, agranulocytosis,*** leukopenia, ***thrombocytopenic purpura,*** iron-deficiency anemia.
Hepatic: elevated liver enzyme levels.
Metabolic: hyperkalemia.
Skin: pruritus, urticaria, ***Stevens-Johnson syndrome.***
Other: hypersensitivity (rash, respiratory distress, ***anaphylaxis, angioedema***).

I.V. form
GI: ***bleeding,*** vomiting.
GU: ***renal dysfunction, azotemia.***
Hematologic: decreased platelet aggregation.
Metabolic: ***hyponatremia, hyperkalemia, hypoglycemia.***
Other: hypersensitivity reactions (rash, respiratory distress, ***anaphylaxis, angioedema***).

Interactions

Drug-drug. *Aminoglycosides, cyclosporine, methotrexate:* indomethacin may enhance toxicity of these drugs. Avoid concomitant use.
Antihypertensives: reduced antihypertensive effect. Monitor blood pressure closely.
Aspirin: decreased blood levels of indomethacin. Avoid concomitant use.
Corticosteroids: increased risk of GI toxicity. Don't use together.
Diflunisal, probenecid: decreased indomethacin excretion; watch for increased adverse reactions to indomethacin.
Digoxin: indomethacin may prolong half-life of digoxin. Use together cautiously.
Dipyridamole: enhanced fluid retention. Avoid concomitant use.
Furosemide, thiazide diuretics: impaired response to both drugs. Avoid using with indomethacin if possible.
Lithium: increased plasma lithium levels. Monitor patient for toxicity.
Triamterene: possible nephrotoxicity. Monitor patient closely.
Drug-herb. *Dong quai, feverfew, garlic, ginger, horse chestnut, red clover:* possible increased risk of bleeding. Monitor patient closely.
St. John's wort: increased risk of photosensitivity. Advise patient to avoid unprotected exposure to sunlight.
Senna: blocked laxative effects. Discourage concomitant use.
Drug-lifestyle. *Alcohol use:* increased risk of GI toxicity. Discourage concomitant use.

Contraindications and precautions

- Contraindicated in patients hypersensitive to drug; in those with history of aspirin- or NSAID-induced asthma, rhinitis, or urticaria; and in pregnant or breast-feeding women. Also contraindicated in infants with untreated infection, active bleeding, coagulation defects, thrombocytopenia, congenital heart disease (in whom patency of ductus arteriosus is necessary for satisfactory pulmonary or systemic blood flow), necrotizing enterocolitis, or impaired renal function. Suppositories contraindicated in patients with history of proctitis or recent rectal bleeding.
- Because of its high risk of adverse effects during prolonged use, indomethacin shouldn't be used routinely as analgesic or antipyretic.
- Drug isn't recommended for use in pregnant or breast-feeding women.
- Use cautiously in elderly patients and in those with epilepsy, parkinsonism, hepatic or renal disease, CV disease, infection, mental illness or depression, or history of GI disease.

NURSING CONSIDERATIONS

Assessment

- Assess patient's condition before therapy and regularly thereafter.
- Monitor patient carefully for bleeding and for reduced urine output during I.V. use.
- Be alert for adverse reactions and drug interactions.
- Evaluate patient's and family's knowledge of drug therapy.

Nursing diagnoses

- Chronic pain related to underlying condition
- Risk for injury related to adverse reactions
- Deficient knowledge related to drug therapy

Planning and implementation

P.O. use: Administer drug with food, milk, or antacid if GI upset occurs.

I.V. use: Reconstitute powder for injection with sterile water for injection or normal saline solution. For each 1-mg vial, add 1 ml of diluent to yield 1 mg/ml; add 2 ml of diluent to yield 0.5 mg/ml. Give by direct injection over 5 to 10 seconds.

ALERT Use only preservative-free diluents to prepare I.V. injection. Never use diluents containing benzyl alcohol because it has been linked to fatal gasping syndrome in neonates. Because injection contains no preservatives, reconstitute immediately before administration and discard unused solution.

- Don't administer second or third scheduled I.V. dose if patient has anuria or marked oliguria; instead, notify prescriber.

P.R. use: Follow normal protocol.

- If ductus arteriosus reopens, second course of one to three doses may be given. If ineffective, surgery may be necessary.
- Discontinue drug and notify prescriber if patient has bleeding or reduced urine output.
- Drug may enhance hypothalamic-pituitary-adrenal axis response to dexamethasone suppression test.
- Notify prescriber if drug is ineffective.

Patient teaching

- Tell patient to take oral form of drug with food, milk, or antacid if GI upset occurs.
- Alert patient that use of oral form with aspirin, alcohol, or corticosteroids may increase risk of adverse GI reactions.
- Teach patient to recognize and urge him to report signs and symptoms of GI bleeding. Serious GI toxicity, including peptic ulceration and bleeding, can occur in patients taking oral NSAIDs despite absence of GI symptoms.
- Instruct patient to avoid alcohol consumption during drug therapy.
- Tell patient to notify prescriber immediately about visual or hearing changes. Patient receiving long-term oral therapy should have regular eye examinations, hearing tests, CBC, and renal function tests to detect toxicity.
- Advise patient to avoid hazardous activities if adverse CNS reactions occur.

Evaluation

- Patient is free from pain.
- Patient doesn't experience injury from adverse reactions.
- Patient and family state understanding of drug therapy.

infliximab
(in-FLIX-i-mab)
Remicade

Pharmacologic class: monoclonal antibody
Therapeutic class: anti-inflammatory
Pregnancy risk category: C

Indications and dosages

▶ **Reduction of signs and symptoms in patients with moderately to severely active Crohn's disease and inadequate response to conventional therapy.** *Adults:* 5 mg/kg single I.V. infusion over at least 2 hours.

▶ **Reduction in number of draining enterocutaneous fistulas in patients with fistulizing Crohn's disease.** *Adults:* 5 mg/kg I.V. infused over at least 2 hours. Additional doses of 5 mg/kg should be given 2 and 6 weeks after initial infusion.

▶ **Reduction in signs and symptoms of rheumatoid arthritis in patients who have had inadequate response to methotrexate alone.** *Adults:* 3 mg/kg I.V. infused over at least 2 hours, followed by additional 3-mg/kg doses 2 and 6 weeks after first infusion; then every 8 weeks thereafter. Give with methotrexate.

How supplied

Injection: 100-mg vial

Pharmacokinetics

Absorption: absorption is incomplete.
Distribution: not reported.
Metabolism: not reported.
Excretion: not reported. *Terminal half-life:* 9½ days.

Route	Onset	Peak	Duration
I.V.	Unknown	Unknown	Unknown

Pharmacodynamics

Chemical effect: a monoclonal antibody that binds to human tumor necrosis factor (TNF)-alpha to neutralize its activity and inhibit its binding with receptors, thereby reducing the infiltration of inflammatory cells and production of TNF-alpha in inflamed areas of the intestine.
Therapeutic effect: relieves inflammation in the GI tract.

Adverse reactions

CNS: *headache, fatigue,* dizziness, malaise, insomnia.
CV: hypertension, peripheral edema, hypotension, tachycardia, chest pain, flushing.
EENT: pharyngitis, rhinitis, sinusitis, conjunctivitis.
GI: *nausea, abdominal pain,* vomiting, constipation, dyspepsia, flatulence, intestinal obstruction, mouth pain, ulcerative stomatitis.
GU: dysuria, increased micturition frequency.
Hematologic: anemia, ecchymosis, hematoma.
Hepatic: elevated liver enzyme levels.
Musculoskeletal: myalgia, arthralgia, arthritis, back pain.
Respiratory: *upper respiratory tract infections,* bronchitis, coughing, dyspnea, allergic reaction.
Skin: rash, pruritus, candidiasis, acne, alopecia, eczema, erythema, erythematous rash, maculopapular rash, papular rash, dry skin, increased sweating, urticaria.
Other: *fever,* chills, pain, flu syndrome, hot flushes, abscess, toothache.

Interactions

None significant.

Contraindications and precautions

- Contraindicated in patients hypersensitive to murine proteins or other components of drug.
- Use drug cautiously in elderly patients.

NURSING CONSIDERATIONS

Assessment

- Obtain history of patient's underlying condition before therapy, and reassess regularly thereafter.
- Observe patient for infusion-related reactions, including fever, chills, pruritus, urticaria, dyspnea, hypotension, hypertension, and chest pain, during and for 2 hours after administration.
- Monitor liver function.

• Observe patient for development of lymphomas and infection. Patients with chronic Crohn's disease and long-term exposure to immunosuppressants are more likely to develop lymphomas and infections.
• Drug may affect normal immune responses. Monitor patient for development of autoimmune antibodies and lupus-like syndrome; drug should be discontinued, as ordered. Expect symptoms to resolve.
• Evaluate patient's and family's knowledge of drug therapy.

Nursing diagnoses
• Chronic pain related to inflammation of the GI tract
• Imbalanced nutrition: Less than body requirements related to underlying medical condition
• Deficient knowledge related to drug therapy

Planning and implementation
I.V. use: Drug is incompatible with plasticized polyvinyl chloride equipment or devices; prepare only in glass infusion bottles or polypropylene or polyolefin infusion bags. Administer through polyethylene-lined administration sets with an in-line, sterile, nonpyrogenic, low-protein-binding filter (pore size of 1.2 mm or less).
• Vials don't contain antibacterial preservatives; use reconstituted drug immediately. Reconstitute with 10 ml sterile solution for injection using syringe with 21G or smaller needle. Don't shake; gently swirl to dissolve powder. Solution should be colorless to light yellow and opalescent; it may contain a few translucent particles. Don't use if you see other particles or discoloration.
• Dilute total volume of reconstituted drug to 250 ml with normal saline solution for injection. Infusion concentration range is 0.4 to 4 mg/ml. Infusion should begin within 3 hours of preparation and must last at least 2 hours.
• Don't infuse drug in same I.V. line with other drugs.
• If an infusion reaction occurs, discontinue drug, notify prescriber, and be prepared to give acetaminophen, antihistamines, corticosteroids, and epinephrine, as ordered.

Patient teaching
• Tell patient about infusion reaction symptoms, and instruct him to report them.
• Inform patient of postinfusion adverse effects, and tell him to report them promptly.
• Tell breast-feeding woman to stop breast-feeding if drug is to be administered.

Evaluation
• Patient is free from pain.
• Patient maintains adequate nutrition.
• Patient and family state understanding of drug therapy.

insulin glargine (rDNA) injection
IN-suh-lin GLAR-gene (rDNA) in-JEK-shun
Lantus

Pharmacologic class: pancreatic hormone
Therapeutic class: antidiabetic
Pregnancy risk category: C

Indications and dosages
▶ **Management of type 1 diabetes mellitus in patients who need basal (long-acting) insulin for the control of hyperglycemia.** *Adults and children:* for patients taking once-daily NPH or ultralente human insulin, start drug at the same dose as the current insulin dose. For patients taking twice-daily NPH human insulin, start drug at a dose that is 20% less than the current daily dose of insulin. Adjust dose based on patient response.
▶ **Management of type 2 diabetes mellitus in patients previously treated with oral antidiabetics.** *Adults:* 10 IU S.C. once daily h.s. Adjust as needed to total daily dose of 2 IU to 100 IU S.C. h.s.

How supplied
Injection: 100 units/ml

Pharmacokinetics
Absorption: slower, more prolonged absorption than NPH insulin and a relatively constant level over 24 hours with no pronounced peak in comparison to NPH insulin. After injection into S.C. tissue, the acidic solution is neutralized, leading to formation of microprecipi-

tates. From these microprecipitates, small amounts of insulin glargine are slowly released.
Distribution: unknown.
Metabolism: partly metabolized to form two active metabolites with in vitro activity similar to that of insulin.
Excretion: unknown.

Route	Onset	Peak	Duration
S.C.	Slow	None	10.8-24 hr

Pharmacodynamics

Chemical effect: increases glucose transport across muscle and fat cell membranes to reduce blood glucose level. Promotes conversion of glucose to its storage form, glycogen. Triggers amino acid uptake and conversion to protein in muscle cells and inhibits protein degradation. Stimulates triglyceride formation and inhibits release of free fatty acids from adipose tissue. Stimulates lipoprotein lipase activity, which converts circulating lipoproteins to fatty acids.
Therapeutic effect: lowers blood glucose levels.

Adverse reactions

Metabolic: hypoglycemia.
Skin: lipodystrophy, pruritus, rash.
Other: allergic reactions, pain at injection site.

Interactions

Drug-drug: *ACE inhibitors, disopyramide, fibrates, fluoxetine, MAO inhibitors, octreotide, oral antidiabetics, propoxyphene, salicylates, sulfonamide antibiotics:* may cause hypoglycemia and increased insulin effect. Monitor blood glucose. Insulin glargine dosage may need adjustment.
Beta blockers, clonidine: may mask signs of hypoglycemia and may either potentiate or weaken the blood glucose–lowering effect of insulin. Monitor blood glucose carefully. Insulin glargine dosage may need adjustment.
Corticosteroids, danazol, diuretics, estrogens, isoniazid, phenothiazines (prochlorperazine, promethazine), progestins (oral contraceptives), sympathomimetics (albuterol, epinephrine, terbutaline), thyroid hormones: may reduce the blood glucose–lowering effect of insulin. Monitor blood glucose. Insulin glargine dosage may need adjustment.
Guanethidine, reserpine: may mask signs of hypoglycemia. Avoid concurrent use if possible. Monitor blood glucose carefully.
Lithium: may either potentiate or weaken the blood glucose–lowering effect of insulin. Monitor blood glucose. Insulin glargine dosage may need adjustment.
Pentamidine: may cause hypoglycemia, which may be followed by hyperglycemia. Avoid concurrent use, if possible.
Drug-herb. *Aloe, bitter melon, bilberry leaf, burdock, dandelion, fenugreek, garlic, ginseng:* concomitant use may improve blood glucose control and allow a reduced antidiabetic dosage. Tell patient to discuss the use of herbal remedies with prescriber before use.
Licorice root: may increase dosage requirements of insulin. Advise against concurrent use.
Drug-lifestyle. *Alcohol use, emotional stress, exercise:* may potentiate or weaken the blood glucose–lowering effect of insulin. Monitor blood glucose. Dosage adjustments of insulin glargine may be required.

Contraindications and precautions

- Contraindicated in patients hypersensitive to insulin glargine or its excipients. Don't use drug during episodes of hypoglycemia.
- Use cautiously in patients with renal or hepatic impairment, and adjust dosage as directed.

NURSING CONSIDERATIONS

Assessment

- Obtain history of patient's underlying condition before therapy, and reassess regularly thereafter. As with any insulin, the desired blood glucose levels and the doses and timing of antidiabetic medication must be determined individually.
- Monitor blood glucose levels closely.
- Monitor patient for hypoglycemia. Early symptoms may be different or less pronounced in patients with longstanding diabetes, diabetic nerve disease, or intensified diabetes control.
- Evaluate patient's and family's knowledge of drug therapy.

Nursing diagnoses

- Ineffective health maintenance related to hyperglycemia
- Risk for injury related to drug-induced hypoglycemia
- Deficient knowledge related to drug therapy

Planning and implementation

- Drug isn't intended for I.V. use. Its prolonged duration of activity depends on injection into the S.C. space.
- Because of its prolonged duration, insulin glargine isn't the insulin of choice for diabetic ketoacidosis.
- The rate of absorption, onset, and duration of action may be affected by exercise and other circumstances such as illness and emotional stress.
- Don't dilute drug or mix it with any other insulin or solution.
- As with any insulin therapy, lipodystrophy may occur at injection site and delay insulin absorption. Rotate injection sites to reduce lipodystrophy.

Patient teaching

- Teach patient proper blood glucose monitoring techniques and proper diabetes management.
- Teach diabetic patient signs and symptoms of hypoglycemia, such as fatigue, weakness, confusion, headache, and pale skin.
- Advise patient to treat mild episodes of hypoglycemia with oral glucose tablets. Encourage patient to always carry glucose tablets in case of a hypoglycemic episode.
- Teach patient the importance of maintaining a diabetic diet. Explain that adjustments in drug dosage, meal patterns, and exercise may be needed to regulate blood glucose.
- Any change of insulin should be made cautiously and only under medical supervision. Changes in insulin strength, manufacturer, type (regular, NPH, insulin analogs), species (animal, human), or method of manufacture (rDNA versus animal source), may necessitate a dosage change. Concomitant oral antidiabetic treatment may need to be adjusted.
- Tell patient to consult prescriber before using OTC medications.
- Advise patient not to dilute or mix any other insulin or solution with insulin glargine. If the solution is cloudy, tell patient to discard the vial.
- Instruct patient to store insulin glargine vials and cartridges in the refrigerator.

Evaluation

- Patient's blood glucose level is normal.
- Patient doesn't experience hypoglycemic reactions.
- Patient and family state understanding of drug therapy.

insulins

(IN-suh-linz)

insulin analog injection

Humalog

insulin injection (regular insulin, crystalline zinc insulin)

Actrapid HM ◊, Actrapid HM Penfill ◊, Actrapid MC ◊, Actrapid MC Penfill ◊, Humulin R†, Hypurin Neutral ◊, Insulin 2 Neutral ◊, Novolin R†, Novolin R PenFill†, Pork Regular Iletin II†, Regular (Concentrated) Iletin II, Regular Iletin I†, Regular Purified Pork Insulin†, Velosulin Human ◊, Velosulin Insuject ◊

insulin zinc suspension (lente)

Humulin L†, Lente Iletin II†, Lente Insulin†, Lente MC ◊, Lente Purified Pork Insulin†, Monotard HM ◊, Monotard MC ◊, Novolin L†

insulin zinc suspension, extended (ultralente)

Humulin U†, Ultralente Insulin†, Ultratard HM ◊, Ultratard MC ◊

insulin zinc suspension, prompt (semilente)

Semilente MC ◊

isophane insulin suspension (neutral protamine Hagedorn insulin, NPH)

Humulin N†, Humulin NPH◇, Hypurin Isophane◇, Insulatard◇, Insulatard Human◆, Isotard MC◇, Novolin N†, Novolin N PenFill†, NPH Insulin†, NPH Purified Pork†, Pork NPH Iletin II†, Protaphane HM◇, Protaphane HM Penfill◇, Protaphane MC◇

isophane insulin suspension with insulin injection

Actraphane HM◇, Actraphane HM Penfill◇, Actraphane MC◇, Humulin 50/50†, Humulin 70/30†, Novolin 70/30, Novolin 70/30 PenFill†

protamine zinc suspension (PZI)

Protamine Zinc Insulin MC◇

Pharmacologic class: pancreatic hormone
Therapeutic class: antidiabetic
Pregnancy risk category: NR

Indications and dosages

▶ **Diabetic ketoacidosis. (Regular insulin.)** *Adults:* 0.15 units/kg as I.V. bolus, followed by 0.1 units/kg/hour by continuous infusion. Continue infusion until blood glucose level drops to 250 mg/dl; then start S.C. insulin with dosage and interval adjusted according to patient's blood glucose levels. Or, 50 to 100 units I.V. and 50 to 100 units S.C. immediately; then additional doses q 1 to 2 hours based on blood glucose levels.
Children: 0.1 unit/kg as I.V. bolus; then 0.1 unit/kg hourly by continuous infusion until blood glucose level drops to 250 mg/dl; then start S.C. insulin. Or, 0.5 to 1 unit/kg in two divided doses, one I.V. and the other S.C., followed by 0.5 to 1 unit/kg I.V. q 1 to 2 hours based on blood glucose levels.

▶ **Type 1 diabetes mellitus (insulin-dependent), adjunct to type 2 diabetes mellitus (non-insulin-dependent) inadequately controlled by diet and oral antidiabetics.** *Adults and children:* therapeutic regimen is adjusted based on patient's blood glucose levels.

▶ **Control of hyperglycemia with longer-acting insulin in patients with type 1 diabetes mellitus and with sulfonylureas in patients with type 2 diabetes mellitus (insulin lispro rDNA origin, Humalog).** *Adults and children over age 3:* Dosage varies and must be determined by a prescriber familiar with patient's metabolic needs, eating habits, and other lifestyle variables. Inject S.C. up to 15 minutes before or immediately after a meal.

How supplied

insulin injection
Injection (human): 100 units/ml (Actrapid HM◇, Humulin R†, Novolin R†, Humalog [lispro], Velosulin Human◇); 100 units/ml in 1.5-ml cartridge system† (Actrapid HM Penfill◇, Novolin R PenFill†)
Injection (from pork): 100 units/ml†
Injection (purified beef): 100 units/ml (Hypurin Neutral◇, Insulin 2◇)
Injection (purified pork): 100 units/ml (Actrapid MC◇, Pork Regular Iletin II†, Regular Purified Pork Insulin†); 100 units/ml in 1.5-ml cartridge system◇ (Actrapid MC Penfill◇); 100 units/ml in 2-ml cartridge system◇; 500 units/ml (Regular [Concentrated] Iletin II)

insulin zinc suspension, prompt
Injection (purified pork): 100 units/ml† (Semilente MC◇)

isophane insulin suspension
Injection (from beef): 100 units/ml† (NPH Insulin†)
Injection (human, recombinant): 100 units/ml (Humulin N†, Humulin NPH◇, Insulatard Human◆, Novolin N†, Protaphane HM◇); 100 units/ml in 1.5-ml cartridge system (Protaphane HM PenFill◇, Novolin N PenFill†)
Injection (purified beef): 100 units/ml (Hypurin Isophane◇, Isotard MC◇)
Injection (purified pork): 100 units/ml (Insulatard◇, NPH Purified Pork†, Pork NPH Iletin II, Protaphane MC◇)

isophane insulin suspension 50% with insulin injection 50%
Injection (human): 100 units/ml (Humulin 50/50†)

isophane insulin suspension 70% with insulin injection 30%
Injection (human): 100 units/ml (Actraphane HM ◇, Humulin 70/30†, Novolin 70/30†); 100 units/ml in 1.5-ml cartridge system (Actraphane HM Penfill ◇, Novolin 70/30 PenFill†)
Injection (purified pork): 100 units/ml (Actraphane MC ◇)
insulin zinc suspension
Injection (from beef): 100 units/ml (Lente Insulin†, Lente MC ◇)
Injection (purified beef): 100 units/ml (Lente MC ◇)
Injection (purified pork): 100 units/ml (Lente Iletin II†, Monotard MC ◇, Lente Purified Pork Insulin†)
Injection (human): 100 units/ml† (Humulin L†, Monotard HM ◇, Novolin L†)
protamine zinc suspension
Injection (purified pork): Protamine Zinc Insulin MC ◇
insulin zinc suspension, extended
Injection (from beef): 100 units/ml† (Ultralente Insulin†)
Injection (human): 100 units/ml (Ultratard HM ◇, Humulin U†)
Injection (purified pork): 100 units/ml ◇ (Ultratard MC ◇)

Pharmacokinetics

Absorption: highly variable after S.C. administration depending on insulin type and injection site.
Distribution: distributed widely throughout body.
Metabolism: some is bound and inactivated by peripheral tissues, but most appears to be degraded in liver and kidneys.
Excretion: filtered by renal glomeruli; undergoes some tubular reabsorption. *Half-life:* about 9 minutes after I.V. administration.

Route	Onset	Peak	Duration
I.V.	≤ 0.5 hr	0.25-0.5 hr	0.5-1 hr
S.C.	0.25-8 hr	2-30 hr	5-36 hr

Pharmacodynamics

Chemical effect: increases glucose transport across muscle and fat cell membranes to reduce blood glucose level. Promotes conversion of glucose to its storage form, glycogen; triggers amino acid uptake and conversion to protein in muscle cells and inhibits protein degradation; stimulates triglyceride formation and inhibits release of free fatty acids from adipose tissue; and stimulates lipoprotein lipase activity, which converts circulating lipoproteins to fatty acids.
Therapeutic effect: lowers blood glucose levels.

Adverse reactions

Metabolic: ***hypoglycemia,*** hyperglycemia (rebound, or Somogyi, effect).
Skin: urticaria, itching, swelling, redness, stinging, warmth at injection site.
Other: *lipoatrophy, lipohypertrophy,* ***hypersensitivity reactions, anaphylaxis,*** rash.

Interactions

Drug-drug. *AIDS antivirals, corticosteroids, dextrothyroxine, epinephrine, thiazide diuretics:* diminished insulin response. Monitor patient for hyperglycemia.
Anabolic steroids, beta blockers, clofibrate, fenfluramine, guanethidine, MAO inhibitors, salicylates, tetracycline: prolonged hypoglycemic effect. Monitor blood glucose level carefully.
Diazoxide, phenytoin (high doses): may inhibit endogenous insulin secretion and may cause hypoglycemia in patients with diabetes. Carefully adjust insulin dosage.
Oral contraceptives: may decrease glucose tolerance in diabetic patients. Monitor blood glucose levels and adjust insulin dosage carefully.
Drug-herb. *Basil, bay, bee pollen, burdock, ginseng, glucomannion, horehound, marshmallow, myrrh, sage:* May affect glycemic control. Monitor blood glucose carefully.
Drug-lifestyle. *Alcohol use:* hypoglycemic effect. Discourage concomitant use.
Marijuana use: may increase serum glucose levels. Discourage concomitant use.
Smoking: may increase glucose levels and decrease response to insulin. Encourage smoking cessation.

Contraindications and precautions

- No known contraindications.

• Insulin is drug of choice to treat diabetes in pregnant and breast-feeding women.

NURSING CONSIDERATIONS

Assessment

• Assess patient's blood glucose level before therapy and regularly thereafter. Monitor levels more frequently if patient is under stress, unstable, pregnant, recently diagnosed, or taking medications that can interact with insulin.
• Monitor patient's hemoglobin A1c level regularly, as ordered.
• Monitor urine ketone levels when blood glucose levels are elevated.
• Be alert for adverse reactions and drug interactions.
• Monitor injection sites for local reactions.
• Evaluate patient's and family's knowledge of drug therapy.

Nursing diagnoses

• Ineffective health maintenance related to hyperglycemia
• Risk for injury related to drug-induced hypoglycemia
• Deficient knowledge related to drug therapy

Planning and implementation

ALERT Regular insulin is used in patients with circulatory collapse, diabetic ketoacidosis, or hyperkalemia. Don't use regular insulin concentrated (500 units/ml) I.V. Don't use intermediate- or long-acting insulins for coma or other emergency that needs rapid drug action.
ALERT Dosage is always expressed in USP units. Use only syringes calibrated for particular concentration of insulin administered. U-500 insulin must be administered with U-100 syringe because no syringes are made for this strength.
• Insulin resistance may develop and large insulin doses are needed to control symptoms of diabetes in these patients. U-500 insulin is available as Regular (Concentrated) Iletin II for such patients. Although not normally stocked in every pharmacy, it's readily available. Give hospital pharmacy sufficient notice before needing to refill in-house prescription. Never store U-500 insulin in same area with other insulin preparations because of danger of severe overdose if given accidentally to other patients.
• To mix insulin suspension, swirl vial gently or rotate between palms or between palm and thigh. Don't shake vigorously because doing so causes bubbling and air in syringe.
• Humalog insulin has a rapid onset of action and should be given within 15 minutes before meals.
• Lente, semilente, and ultralente insulins may be mixed in any proportion.
• Regular insulin may be mixed with NPH or lente insulins in any proportion.
• Switching from separate injections to prepared mixture may alter patient response. Whenever NPH or lente is mixed with regular insulin in same syringe, give immediately to avoid loss of potency.
• Don't use insulin that has changed color or become clumped or granular.
• Check expiration date on vial before using.
S.C. use: Usual administration route is S.C. Pinch fold of skin with fingers starting at least 3″ apart, and insert needle at 45- to 90-degree angle.
• Press but don't rub site after injection. Rotate and chart injection sites to avoid overuse of one area. Diabetic patients may achieve better control if injection sites are rotated within same anatomic region.
I.V. use: Use only regular insulin. Inject directly at ordered rate into vein, through intermittent infusion device, or into port close to I.V. access site. Intermittent infusion isn't recommended. If given by continuous infusion, infuse drug diluted in normal saline solution at prescribed rate.
• Ketosis-prone type I, severely ill, and newly diagnosed diabetic patients with very high blood glucose levels may require hospitalization and I.V. treatment with regular fast-acting insulin.
• Store drug in cool area. Refrigeration is desirable but not essential except for concentrated regular insulin.
• Notify prescriber of sudden changes in blood glucose levels, dangerously high or low levels, or ketosis.

• Be prepared to provide supportive measures if patient develops diabetic ketoacidosis or hyperglycemic hyperosmolar nonketotic coma.
• Treat hypoglycemic reaction with oral form of rapid-acting glucose if patient can swallow or with glucagon or I.V. glucose if patient can't be roused. Follow with complex carbohydrate snack when patient is awake, and determine cause of reaction.
• Make sure patient is following appropriate diet and exercise programs. Expect to adjust insulin dosage when other aspects of regimen are altered.
• Discuss with prescriber how to deal with noncompliance.
• Treat lipoatrophy or lipohypertrophy according to prescribed protocol.

Patient teaching
• Tell patient that insulin relieves symptoms but doesn't cure disease.
• Inform patient about nature of disease; importance of following therapeutic regimen; adherence to specific diet, weight reduction, exercise, and personal hygiene programs; and ways of avoiding infection. Review timing of injections and eating, and explain that meals must not be skipped.
• Stress that accuracy of measurement is very important, especially with concentrated regular insulin. Aids, such as magnifying sleeve or dose magnifier, may improve accuracy. Instruct patient and family how to measure and administer insulin.
• Advise patient not to alter order of mixing insulins or change model or brand of syringe or needle.
• Tell patient that blood glucose monitoring and urine ketone tests are essential guides to dosage and success of therapy. Stress the importance of recognizing hypoglycemic symptoms because insulin-induced hypoglycemia is hazardous and may cause brain damage if prolonged; most adverse effects are self-limiting and temporary.
• Teach patient about proper use of equipment for monitoring blood glucose levels.
• Instruct patient to avoid alcohol consumption during drug therapy.
• Advise patient not to smoke within 30 minutes after insulin injection. Smoking decreases absorption.
• Tell patient that marijuana use may increase insulin requirements.
• Advise patient to wear or carry medical identification at all times, to carry ample insulin supply and syringes on trips, to have carbohydrates (lump of sugar or candy) on hand for emergencies, and to note time zone changes for dose scheduling when traveling.

☑ Evaluation
• Patient's blood glucose level is normal.
• Patient sustains no injury from drug-induced hypoglycemia.
• Patient and family state understanding of drug therapy.

interferon alfa-2a, recombinant (rIFN-A)
(in-ter-FEER-on AL-fuh too-ay ree-COM-bih-nent)
Roferon-A

interferon alfa-2b, recombinant (IFN-alpha 2)
Intron-A

Pharmacologic class: biological response modifier
Therapeutic class: antineoplastic
Pregnancy risk category: C

Indications and dosages
▶ **Hairy-cell leukemia. Alfa-2a.** *Adults:* for induction, 3 million units S.C. or I.M. daily for 16 to 24 weeks. For maintenance, 3 million units S.C. or I.M. three times weekly.
Alfa-2b. *Adults:* 2 million units/m^2 I.M. or S.C., three times weekly for up to 6 months.
▶ **AIDS-related Kaposi's sarcoma. Alfa-2a.** *Adults:* for induction, 36 million units S.C. or I.M. daily for 10 to 12 weeks. For maintenance, 36 million units S.C. or I.M. three times weekly.

Alfa-2b. *Adults:* 30 million units/m² S.C. or I.M. three times weekly.

▶ **Condylomata acuminata (genital or venereal warts). Alfa-2b.** *Adults:* 1 million units/lesion intralesionally three times weekly for 3 weeks.

▶ **Chronic hepatitis B. Alfa-2b.** *Adults:* 30 to 35 million units weekly I.M. or S.C., administered either as 5 million units daily or 10 million units three times weekly, for 16 weeks. *Children age 1 and older*: 3 million IU/m² S.C. three times weekly for first week, increased to 6 million IU/m² S.C. three times weekly (maximum of 10 million IU three times weekly) for total of 16 to 24 weeks

▶ **Chronic hepatitis C. Alfa-2a and alfa-2b.** *Adults:* 3 million units I.M. or S.C. three times weekly.

▶ **Chronic myelogenous leukemia (chronic phase Ph positive). Alfa-2a.** *Adults:* initial dose of 9 million units daily administered S.C. or I.M. Optimal maintenance dosage and duration of therapy haven't been determined. See package insert for specific recommendations.

▶ **Malignant melanoma. Alfa-2b.** *Adults:* initial dose of 20 million IU/m² I.V. on 5 consecutive days weekly for 4 weeks. Maintenance dosage is 10 million IU/m² S.C. three times weekly for 48 weeks.

How supplied

alfa-2a

Injection: 3 million IU/vial, 6 million IU/ml, 9 million IU/ml, 18 and 36 million IU/multiple-dose vial

Sterile powder for injection: 18 million IU/vial

alfa-2b

Injection: 3 million IU/vial with diluent, 5 million IU/vial with diluent, 10 million IU/vial with diluent, 18 million IU/vial with diluent, 25 million IU/vial with diluent, 50 million IU/vial with diluent

Pharmacokinetics

Absorption: more than 80% absorbed after I.M. or S.C. injection.

Distribution: not applicable.

Metabolism: drug appears to be metabolized in liver and kidney.

Excretion: reabsorbed from glomerular filtrate with minor biliary elimination.

Route	Onset	Peak	Duration
I.M.	Unknown	3.8 hr	Unknown
S.C.	Unknown	7.3 hr	Unknown
Intra-lesional	Unknown	Unknown	Unknown

Pharmacodynamics

Chemical effect: unknown; appears to involve direct antiproliferative action against tumor cells or viral cells to inhibit replication and modulation of host immune response by enhancing phagocytic activity of macrophages and by augmenting specific cytotoxicity of lymphocytes for target cells.

Therapeutic effect: inhibits growth of certain tumor cells and viral cells.

Adverse reactions

CNS: *dizziness,* confusion, paresthesia, numbness, lethargy, depression, nervousness, difficulty in thinking or concentrating, insomnia, sedation, apathy, anxiety, irritability, fatigue, vertigo, gait disturbances, poor coordination.

CV: hypotension, chest pain, ***arrhythmias,*** palpitations, syncope, ***heart failure,*** hypertension, edema, ***MI.***

EENT: excessive salivation, visual disturbances, dry or inflamed oropharynx, rhinorrhea, sinusitis, conjunctivitis, earache, eye irritation, rhinitis.

GI: *anorexia, nausea, diarrhea,* vomiting, abdominal fullness, abdominal pain, flatulence, constipation, hypermotility, gastric distress, dysgeusia.

GU: transient impotence.

Hematologic: ***leukopenia, mild thrombocytopenia.***

Hepatic: ***hepatitis.***

Respiratory: coughing, dyspnea, tachypnea, cyanosis.

Skin: *rash,* dryness, *pruritus,* partial alopecia, diaphoresis, urticaria, flushing.

Other: flu syndrome (fever, fatigue, myalgia, headache, chills, arthralgia), hot flushes.

Interactions

Drug-drug. *Aminophylline, theophylline:* may reduce theophylline clearance. Monitor serum levels.
Cardiotoxic, hematotoxic, or neurotoxic drugs: effects of previously or concurrently administered drugs may be increased by interferons. Monitor patient closely.
CNS depressants: enhanced CNS effects. Avoid concomitant use.
Interleukin-2: increased risk of renal failure from interleukin-2. Monitor patient closely.
Live-virus vaccines: increased risk of adverse reactions and decreased antibody response. Don't use together.
Zidovudine: possible synergistic adverse effects between alfa-2b and zidovudine. Carefully monitor WBC count.
Drug-lifestyle. *Alcohol use:* increased risk of GI bleeding. Discourage concomitant use.

Contraindications and precautions

- Contraindicated in patients hypersensitive to drug or to mouse immunoglobulin.
- Drug isn't recommended for breast-feeding women.
- Use cautiously in patients with severe hepatic or renal function impairment, seizure disorders, compromised CNS function, cardiac disease, or myelosuppression. Also use cautiously in pregnant women.
- Safety of drug hasn't been established in children.

NURSING CONSIDERATIONS

Assessment

- Assess patient's condition before therapy and regularly thereafter.
- Obtain allergy history. Drug contains phenol as preservative and serum albumin as stabilizer.
- At beginning of therapy, assess for flulike symptoms, which tend to diminish with continued therapy.
- Monitor blood studies, as ordered. Interferons may decrease hemoglobin, hematocrit, WBC count, platelet count, and neutrophil count; increase PT and PTT; and increase serum levels of AST, ALT, LD, alkaline phosphatase, calcium, phosphorus, and fasting glucose. All of these effects are dose-related and reversible. Recovery occurs within several days or weeks after withdrawal.
- Be alert for adverse reactions and drug interactions.
- Evaluate patient's and family's knowledge of drug therapy.

Nursing diagnoses

- Ineffective health maintenance related to underlying condition
- Risk for injury related to drug-induced adverse CNS reactions
- Deficient knowledge related to drug therapy

Planning and implementation

- Premedicate patient with acetaminophen to minimize flulike symptoms.
- Administer drug at bedtime to minimize daytime drowsiness.
- Make sure patient is well hydrated, especially during initial stages of treatment.

ALERT Different brands of interferon may not be equivalent and may require different dosage.

I.M. use: Follow normal protocol.
S.C. use: Use S.C. administration route in patients whose platelet count is below 50,000/mm^3.
Intralesional use: When administering interferon alfa-2b for condylomata acuminata, use only 10 million-IU vial because dilution of other strengths required for intralesional use results in hypertonic solution. Don't reconstitute 10 million-IU vial with more than 1 ml of diluent. Use tuberculin or similar syringe and 25G to 30G needle. Don't inject too deeply beneath lesion or too superficially. As many as five lesions can be treated at one time. To ease discomfort, administer drug in evening with acetaminophen.

- Refrigerate drug.
- Notify prescriber of severe adverse reactions, which may require dosage reduction or discontinuation.
- Use with blood dyscrasia–causing drugs, bone marrow suppressants, or radiation therapy may increase bone marrow suppression. Dosage reduction may be needed.

Patient teaching

- Advise patient that laboratory tests will be performed before and periodically during therapy. Tests include CBC with differential, platelet count, blood chemistry and electrolyte studies, liver function tests, and, if patient has cardiac disorder or advanced stages of cancer, ECGs.
- Instruct patient in proper oral hygiene during treatment because bone marrow–suppressant effects of interferon may lead to microbial infection, delayed healing, and gingival bleeding. This drug also may decrease salivary flow.
- Emphasize need to follow prescriber's instructions about taking and recording temperature. Explain how and when to take acetaminophen.
- Advise patient to check with prescriber for instructions after missing dose.
- Tell patient that drug may cause temporary hair loss; explain that it should grow back when therapy ends.
- Teach patient how to prepare and administer drug and how to dispose of used needles, syringes, containers, and unused drug. Give him a copy of information for patients included with product, and make sure he understands it. Also provide information on drug stability.
- Warn patient not to receive any immunization without prescriber's approval and to avoid contact with people who have taken oral polio vaccine. Concurrent use with live-virus vaccine may potentiate replication of vaccine virus, increase adverse reactions, and decrease patient's antibody response. Patients are at increased risk for infection during therapy.
- Instruct patient to avoid alcohol during drug therapy.
- Advise patient to report signs of depression.

☑ Evaluation

- Patient shows improved health.
- Patient sustains no injury from adverse CNS reactions.
- Patient and family state understanding of drug therapy.

interferon beta-1b, recombinant

(in-ter-FEER-on BAY-tuh wun bee ree-COM-bih-nent)

Betaseron

Pharmacologic class: biological response modifier

Therapeutic class: antiviral, immunoregulator

Pregnancy risk category: C

Indications and dosages

▶ **To reduce frequency of exacerbations in patients with relapsing-remitting multiple sclerosis.** *Adults:* 8 million IU (0.25 mg) S.C. every other day.

How supplied

Powder for injection: 9.6 million IU (0.3 mg)

Pharmacokinetics

Unknown.

Route	Onset	Peak	Duration
S.C.	Unknown	1-8 hr	Unknown

Pharmacodynamics

Chemical effect: attaches to membrane receptors and causes cellular changes, including increased protein synthesis.

Therapeutic effect: decreases exacerbations in multiple sclerosis.

Adverse reactions

CNS: depression, anxiety, emotional lability, depersonalization, *malaise,* ***suicidal tendencies,*** confusion, somnolence, ***seizures,*** headache, dizziness.

CV: ***hemorrhage.***

EENT: laryngitis.

GI: *nausea, diarrhea, constipation.*

GU: *menstrual disorders (bleeding or spotting, early or delayed menses, decreased days of menstrual flow, menorrhagia).*

Hematologic: *decreased WBC and absolute neutrophil counts.*

Hepatic: elevated ALT levels, elevated bilirubin levels.

Respiratory: dyspnea.

Other: *flulike symptoms (fever, chills, myalgia, diaphoresis);* breast pain; *pelvic pain; lymphadenopathy;* ***hypersensitivity reaction;*** *inflammation, pain, and necrosis* at injection site.

Interactions

None significant.

Contraindications and precautions

- Contraindicated in patients hypersensitive to interferon beta or human albumin.
- Drug isn't recommended for pregnant or breast-feeding women. No data exist to demonstrate whether drug appears in breast milk.
- Use cautiously in women of childbearing age.
- Safety of drug hasn't been established in children.

NURSING CONSIDERATIONS

Assessment

- Obtain assessment of patient's underlying condition before therapy.
- Monitor frequency of exacerbations after drug therapy begins.
- Monitor WBC counts, platelet counts, and blood chemistries, including liver function tests.
- Be alert for adverse reactions.
- Monitor patient for depression and suicidal ideation.
- Evaluate patient's and family's knowledge of drug therapy.

Nursing diagnoses

- Ineffective health maintenance related to exacerbations of multiple sclerosis
- Risk for injury related to drug-induced adverse CNS reactions
- Deficient knowledge related to drug therapy

Planning and implementation

- Premedicate patient with acetaminophen, as ordered, to minimize flulike symptoms.
- To reconstitute, inject 1.2 ml of supplied diluent (0.54% saline solution for injection) into vial and gently swirl to dissolve drug. Don't shake. Reconstituted solution will contain 8 million IU (0.25 mg)/ml. Discard vials that contain particles or discolored solution.
- Inject immediately after preparation.
- Rotate injection sites to minimize local reactions.

Patient teaching

- Warn woman of childbearing age about dangers to fetus. Tell her to notify prescriber promptly if she becomes pregnant during therapy.
- Teach patient how to give S.C. injections, including solution preparation, use of aseptic technique, rotation of injection sites, and equipment disposal. Periodically reevaluate patient's technique.
- Advise patient to take drug at bedtime to minimize mild flulike symptoms.
- Advise patient to report thoughts of depression or suicidal ideation.

Evaluation

- Patient exhibits decreased frequency of exacerbations.
- Patient sustains no injury from adverse CNS reactions.
- Patient and family state understanding of drug therapy.

interferon gamma-1b

(in-ter-FEER-on GAH-muh wun bee)

Actimmune

Pharmacologic class: biological response modifier
Therapeutic class: antineoplastic
Pregnancy risk category: C

Indications and dosages

▶ **Chronic granulomatous disease; to delay disease progression in patients with severe, malignant osteopetrosis.** *Patients with body surface area greater than 0.5 m²:* 50 mcg/m² (1 million IU/m²) S.C. three times weekly in the deltoid or anterior thigh.

Patients with body surface area 0.5 m² or less: 1.5 mcg/kg S.C. three times weekly in the deltoid muscle or anterior thigh.

How supplied

Injection: 100 mcg (3 million units)/vial

Pharmacokinetics

Absorption: about 90% absorbed after S.C. administration.
Distribution: unknown.
Metabolism: unknown.
Excretion: unknown. *Half-life:* 6 hours.

Route	Onset	Peak	Duration
S.C.	Unknown	≤ 7 hr	Unknown

Pharmacodynamics

Chemical effect: acts as interleukin-type lymphokine. Drug has potent phagocyte-activating properties and enhances oxidative metabolism of tissue macrophages.
Therapeutic effect: promotes phagocyte activity.

Adverse reactions

CNS: *fatigue, decreased mental status, gait disturbance.*
GI: *nausea, vomiting, diarrhea.*
Hematologic: ***neutropenia, thrombocytopenia.***
Hepatic: elevated liver enzyme levels.
Skin: erythema and tenderness at injection site, rash.
Other: flulike syndrome.

Interactions

Drug-drug. *Myelosuppressive drugs:* possible additive myelosuppression. Monitor patient closely.
Zidovudine: increased plasma zidovudine levels. Adjust dosages as directed.

Contraindications and precautions

- Contraindicated in patients hypersensitive to drug or to genetically engineered products derived from *Escherichia coli.*
- Drug isn't recommended for use in breast-feeding women.
- Use cautiously in pregnant women and in patients with cardiac disease, compromised CNS function, or seizure disorders.
- Safety of drug hasn't been established in children under age 18.

NURSING CONSIDERATIONS

Assessment

- Assess patient's condition before therapy and regularly thereafter.
- Be alert for adverse reactions and drug interactions. Symptoms of flu syndrome include headache, fever, chills, myalgia, and arthralgia.
- Monitor patient's hydration status if adverse GI reactions occur.
- Evaluate patient's and family's knowledge of drug therapy.

Nursing diagnoses

- Ineffective health maintenance related to underlying condition
- Risk for fluid volume deficit related to adverse GI reactions
- Deficient knowledge related to drug therapy

Planning and implementation

- Premedicate with acetaminophen to minimize symptoms at beginning of therapy. Flu-like symptoms tend to diminish with continued therapy.
- Discard unused portion. Each vial is for single-dose use and doesn't contain preservative.
- Give drug at bedtime to reduce discomfort from flulike symptoms.
- Refrigerate drug immediately. Vials must be stored at 36° to 46° F (2° to 8° C); don't freeze. Don't shake vial; avoid excessive agitation. Discard vials that have been left at room temperature for more than 12 hours.

Patient teaching

- Teach patient how to administer drug and how to dispose of used needles, syringes, containers, and unused drug. Give him a copy of patient information included with product, and make sure he understands it.
- Instruct patient to notify prescriber if adverse reactions occur.

Evaluation

- Patient responds well to drug.
- Patient maintains adequate hydration.
- Patient and family state understanding of drug therapy.

ipecac syrup
(IH-pih-kak SIH-rup)

Pharmacologic class: alkaloid emetic
Therapeutic class: emetic
Pregnancy risk category: C

Indications and dosages

▶ **To induce vomiting in poisoning.** *Adults and children age 12 and older:* 30 ml P.O., followed by 200 to 300 ml of water.
Children ages 1 to 12: 15 ml P.O., followed by about 200 ml of water or milk.
Children ages 6 months to 1 year: 5 ml P.O., followed by 100 to 200 ml of water or milk. If necessary, repeat dose once after 20 minutes.

How supplied

Syrup: 70 mg powdered ipecac/ml (contains glycerin 10% and alcohol 1% to 2.5%)†**

Pharmacokinetics

Absorption: absorbed in significant amounts mainly when it doesn't produce emesis.
Distribution: unknown.
Metabolism: unknown.
Excretion: slowly excreted in urine.

Route	Onset	Peak	Duration
P.O.	20-30 min	Unknown	20-25 min

Pharmacodynamics

Chemical effect: acts locally on gastric mucosa and centrally on the chemoreceptor trigger zone.
Therapeutic effect: induces vomiting.

Adverse reactions

CNS: depression.
CV: ***arrhythmias, bradycardia,*** hypotension, atrial fibrillation, ***fatal myocarditis*** (after excessive dose).
GI: diarrhea.

Interactions

Drug-drug. *Activated charcoal:* neutralized emetic effect. Don't give together; may give activated charcoal after patient vomits.

Contraindications and precautions

- Contraindicated in semicomatose or unconscious patients and in those with severe inebriation, seizures, shock, or loss of gag reflex. Don't use if patient has ingested strychnine, corrosives (such as alkalies and strong acids), or petroleum distillates.

NURSING CONSIDERATIONS

Assessment

- Assess patient to determine substance ingested before starting therapy.
- Monitor effectiveness by observing patient for vomiting. Ipecac syrup usually induces vomiting in 20 to 30 minutes. In antiemetic toxicity, ipecac syrup is usually effective if less than 1 hour has passed since ingestion of antiemetic.
- No systemic toxicity occurs with doses of 30 ml or less.
- Monitor blood pressure, ECG, and fluid and electrolyte balance.
- Be alert for adverse reactions and drug interactions.
- Evaluate patient's and family's knowledge of drug therapy.

Nursing diagnoses

- Ineffective health maintenance related to ingestion of poisonous substance
- Decreased cardiac output related to adverse cardiac reactions
- Deficient knowledge related to drug therapy

Planning and implementation

ALERT Unless advised otherwise by poison control center, don't give ipecac syrup after patient ingests petroleum distillates (for example, kerosene, gasoline) or volatile oils; retching and vomiting may cause aspiration and lead to bronchospasm, pulmonary edema, or aspiration pneumonitis. Vegetable oil will delay absorption of these substances. Don't give ipecac syrup after patient ingests caustic substances, such as lye; additional injury to esophagus and mediastinum can occur.

ALERT Clearly indicate ipecac *syrup,* not single word "ipecac," to avoid confusion with fluidextract, which is 14 times more concentrated

and, if inadvertently used instead of syrup, may cause death.
- Follow dose with 200 to 300 ml of water.
- If two doses don't induce vomiting, be prepared to perform gastric lavage.
- Position patient on side to prevent aspiration of vomitus. Have airway and suction equipment nearby.

Patient teaching
- Recommend that parents keep 1 oz (30 ml) of syrup available in home for use in emergency when child reaches age 1.
- Advise parent or guardian to consult prescriber or poison control center before administering to child.

Evaluation
- Patient regains health after elimination of poisonous substance.
- Patient's cardiac output remains adequate.
- Patient and family state understanding of drug therapy.

ipratropium bromide
(ip-ruh-TROH-pee-um BROH-mighd)
Atrovent

Pharmacologic class: anticholinergic
Therapeutic class: bronchodilator
Pregnancy risk category: B

Indications and dosages

▶ **Bronchospasm caused by COPD.** *Adults and children over age 12:* 1 to 2 inhalations q.i.d. Additional inhalations may be needed. However, total inhalations shouldn't exceed 12 in 24 hours. Or, use inhalation solution, giving up to 500 mcg q 6 to 8 hours via oral nebulizer.
Children ages 5 to 12: 125 to 250 mcg nebulizer solution dissolved in normal saline solution and administered by nebulizer q 4 to 6 hours.

▶ **Rhinorrhea linked to allergic and nonallergic perennial rhinitis (0.03% nasal spray).** *Adults and children age 6 and older:* 2 sprays (42 mcg) in each nostril b.i.d. or t.i.d (total dosage 168 to 252 mcg/day).

▶ **Rhinorrhea caused by the common cold (0.06% nasal spray).** *Adults and children age 12 and over:* 2 sprays (84 mcg) per nostril t.i.d. or q.i.d. (total dosage 504 to 672 mcg/day).
Children ages 5 to 11: 2 sprays (84 mcg) per nostril t.i.d. (total dosage 504 mcg/day).
Infants and children under age 5: 25 mcg/kg t.i.d. by nebulizer.

How supplied

Inhaler: each metered dose supplies 18 mcg
Solution for inhalation: 0.02% (500 mcg vial)
Solution for nebulizer: 0.025% (250 mcg/ml)◊, 0.02% (200 mcg/ml)
Nasal spray: 0.03% (21 mcg), 0.06% (42 mcg)

Pharmacokinetics

Absorption: drug isn't readily absorbed into systemic circulation.
Distribution: not applicable.
Metabolism: small amount that is absorbed is metabolized in liver.
Excretion: absorbed drug excreted in urine and bile; remainder excreted unchanged in feces. *Half-life:* about 2 hours.

Route	Onset	Peak	Duration
Inhalation	5-15 min	1-2 hr	3-6 hr

Pharmacodynamics

Chemical effect: inhibits vagally mediated reflexes by antagonizing acetylcholine.
Therapeutic effect: relieves bronchospasms and symptoms of seasonal allergic rhinitis.

Adverse reactions

CNS: nervousness, dizziness, headache.
CV: palpitations.
EENT: blurred vision, epistaxis.
GI: nausea, GI distress, dry mouth.
Respiratory: cough, *upper respiratory tract infection, bronchitis,* ***bronchospasm.***
Skin: rash.

Interactions

Drug-drug. *Anticholinergics:* increased anticholinergic effects. Avoid concomitant use.
Cromolyn sodium: will form precipitate if mixed in same nebulizer. Don't use together.

Drug-herb. *Jaborandi tree, pill-bearing spurge:* decreased drug effects. Use cautiously.

Contraindications and precautions

ALERT Contraindicated in patients hypersensitive to drug or to atropine or its derivatives and in those hypersensitive to soyalecithin or related food products such as soybeans and peanuts.

- Use cautiously in pregnant women, breast-feeding patients, and patients with angle-closure glaucoma, prostatic hyperplasia, or bladder-neck obstruction.
- Safety of drug hasn't been established in children under age 6 for rhinorrhea linked to allergic and non-allergic perennial rhinitis.
- Safety and efficacy of use beyond 4 days for rhinorrhea from the common cold haven't been established.

NURSING CONSIDERATIONS

Assessment

- Assess patient's condition before and after drug administration; monitor peak expiratory flow.
- Be alert for adverse reactions and drug interactions.
- Evaluate patient's and family's knowledge of drug therapy.

Nursing diagnoses

- Ineffective breathing pattern related to patient's underlying condition
- Acute pain related to drug-induced headache
- Deficient knowledge related to drug therapy

Planning and implementation

ALERT Don't confuse Atrovent with Alupent.

- Drug isn't effective for treating acute episodes of bronchospasm when rapid response is needed.
- Total inhalations shouldn't exceed 12 in 24 hours, and total nasal sprays shouldn't exceed eight in each nostril in 24 hours.
- If more than one inhalation is ordered, 2 minutes should elapse between inhalations. If more than one type of inhalant is ordered, always give bronchodilator first and wait 5 minutes before giving the other.
- Give medication on time to ensure maximal effect.
- Notify prescriber if drug fails to relieve bronchospasms.

Patient teaching

- Warn patient that drug isn't effective for treating acute episodes of bronchospasm where rapid response is required.
- Give patient these instructions for using metered-dose inhaler: Clear nasal passages and throat. Breathe out, expelling as much air from lungs as possible. Place mouthpiece well into mouth and inhale deeply as you release dose from inhaler. Hold breath for several seconds, remove mouthpiece, and exhale slowly.
- Tell patient to avoid accidentally spraying into eyes. Temporary blurring of vision may result.
- If more than one inhalation is ordered, tell patient to wait at least 2 minutes before repeating procedure.
- If patient also uses a corticosteroid inhaler, tell him to use ipratropium first, and then wait about 5 minutes before using the corticosteroid. This process allows bronchodilator to open air passages for maximum effectiveness of the corticosteroid.
- Tell patient to take a missed dose as soon as remembered, unless it's almost time for next dose. In that case, tell him to skip the missed dose. Advise against doubling the dose.

Evaluation

- Patient's bronchospasms are relieved.
- Patient and family state understanding of drug therapy.

irbesartan

(ir-buh-SAR-tun)

Avapro

Pharmacologic class: angiotensin II receptor antagonist
Therapeutic class: antihypertensive
Pregnancy risk category: C (D in second and third trimesters)

Indications and dosages

▶ **Hypertension.** *Adults:* initially, 150 mg P.O. daily, increased to a maximum of 300 mg daily if necessary.

How supplied

Tablets: 75 mg, 150 mg, 300 mg

Pharmacokinetics

Absorption: rapid and complete with an average absolute bioavailability of 60% to 80%.
Distribution: widely distributed into body tissues; 90% bound to plasma proteins.
Metabolism: metabolized primarily by conjugation and oxidation.
Excretion: excreted by biliary and renal routes. About 20% is recovered in urine and the rest in feces. *Half-life:* 11 to 15 hours.

Route	Onset	Peak	Duration
P.O.	Unknown	1.5-2 hr	24 hr

Pharmacodynamics

Chemical effect: inhibits the vasoconstricting and aldosterone-secreting effects of angiotensin II by selectively blocking binding of angiotension II to receptor sites in many tissues.
Therapeutic effect: lowers blood pressure.

Adverse reactions

CNS: fatigue, anxiety, dizziness, headache.
CV: chest pain, edema, tachycardia.
EENT: pharyngitis, rhinitis, sinus abnormality.
GI: diarrhea, dyspepsia, abdominal pain, nausea, vomiting.
GU: urinary tract infection.
Musculoskeletal: musculoskeletal trauma or pain.
Respiratory: upper respiratory tract infection.
Skin: rash.

Interactions

None reported.

Contraindications and precautions

- Contraindicated in patients hypersensitive to drug or its components.
- Use during pregnancy can cause fetal injury or death. When pregnancy is detected, drug should be discontinued as soon as possible.
- Use cautiously in volume- or salt-depleted patients and in patients with impaired renal function or renal artery stenosis.

NURSING CONSIDERATIONS

Assessment

- Monitor patient's blood pressure regularly.
- Monitor patient's electrolytes, and assess patient for volume or salt depletion before starting drug therapy.
- Make sure woman of childbearing age is using effective birth control before starting this drug because of danger to fetus.
- Evaluate patient's and family's knowledge of drug therapy.

Nursing diagnoses

- Risk for hypotension in volume- or salt-depleted patients
- Risk of injury related to the presence of hypertension
- Deficient knowledge related to drug therapy

Planning and implementation

- Drug may be administered with a diuretic or other antihypertensive if necessary to control blood pressure.
- If patient becomes hypotensive, place in a supine position and give an I.V. infusion of normal saline solution, as ordered.

Patient teaching

- Warn woman of childbearing age about consequences of exposing fetus to drug. Tell her to call prescriber immediately if pregnancy is suspected.
- Tell patient that drug may be taken once daily with or without food.
- Instruct patient to avoid driving and hazardous activities until CNS effects of drug are known.

Evaluation

- Patient doesn't experience hypotension as a result of volume or salt depletion.
- Patient's blood pressure remains within normal limits and no injury is suffered as a result of drug therapy.
- Patient and family state understanding of drug therapy.

iron dextran

(IGH-ern DEKS-tran)

DexFerrum, Dexiron ♦, InFeD

Pharmacologic class: parenteral iron supplement
Therapeutic class: hematinic
Pregnancy risk category: C

Indications and dosages

▶ **Iron-deficiency anemia.** Dosage is individualized and based on patient's weight and hemoglobin level. One ml iron dextran provides 50 mg elemental iron. An I.M. or I.V. test dose is required before administration.
Adults and children: For I.M. use, 0.5-ml test dose injected by Z-track method. If no reactions occur, maximum daily doses are 0.5 ml (25 mg) for infants weighing less than 5 kg (11 lb), 1 ml (50 mg) for children weighing less than 10 kg (22 lb), and 2 ml (100 mg) for heavier children and adults. For I.V. use, 0.5-ml test dose injected over 30 seconds. If no reactions occur in 1 hour, remainder of therapeutic dose is given I.V. Therapeutic dose repeated I.V. daily. Maximum single dose 100 mg. Give slowly (1 ml/minute).

How supplied

Injection: 50 mg elemental iron/ml

Pharmacokinetics

Absorption: I.M. doses are absorbed in two stages: 60% after 3 days and up to 90% by 3 weeks. Remainder is absorbed over several months or longer.
Distribution: during first 3 days, local inflammation facilitates passage of drug into lymphatic system; drug is then ingested by macrophages, which enter lymph and blood.
Metabolism: drug is cleared from plasma by reticuloendothelial cells of liver, spleen, and bone marrow.
Excretion: trace amounts excreted in urine, bile, and feces. *Half-life:* 6 hours.

Route	Onset	Peak	Duration
I.V., I.M.	72 hr	Unknown	3-4 wk

Pharmacodynamics

Chemical effect: provides elemental iron, a component of hemoglobin.
Therapeutic effect: increases levels of plasma iron, an essential component of hemoglobin.

Adverse reactions

CNS: headache, transitory paresthesia, arthralgia, myalgia, dizziness, malaise, syncope.
CV: chest pain, chest tightness, shock, hypertension, arrhythmias, *hypotensive reaction, peripheral vascular flushing with overly rapid I.V. administration, tachycardia.*
GI: nausea, vomiting, metallic taste, transient loss of taste, abdominal pain, diarrhea.
Respiratory: ***bronchospasm.***
Skin: rash, urticaria, *brown discoloration* at I.M. injection site.
Other: *soreness, inflammation, and local phlebitis* at I.V. injection site; sterile abscess; necrosis; atrophy; fibrosis; ***anaphylaxis;*** delayed sensitivity reactions.

Interactions

None significant.

Contraindications and precautions

- Contraindicated in patients hypersensitive to drug and in those with acute infectious renal disease or anemia disorders (except iron-deficiency anemia).
- Use with extreme caution in patients who have serious hepatic impairment, rheumatoid arthritis, and other inflammatory diseases.
- Use cautiously in patients with history of significant allergies or asthma.

NURSING CONSIDERATIONS

Assessment

- Assess patient's iron deficiency before therapy.
- Monitor effectiveness by evaluating hemoglobin level, hematocrit, and reticulocyte count, and monitor patient's health status.
- Be alert for adverse reactions and drug interactions.
- Observe patient for delayed reactions (1 to 2 days), which may include arthralgia, backache, chills, dizziness, headache, malaise, fever, myalgia, nausea, and vomiting.

- Evaluate patient's and family's knowledge of drug therapy.

Nursing diagnoses

- Ineffective health maintenance related to iron deficiency
- Risk for injury related to potential drug-induced anaphylaxis
- Deficient knowledge related to drug therapy

Planning and implementation

- Don't administer iron dextran with oral iron preparations.
- I.M. or I.V. injections of iron are recommended only for patients for whom oral administration is impossible or ineffective.

I.V. use: Check facility policy before administering I.V.

ALERT I.M. or I.V. test dose is required.

- Use I.V. when patient has insufficient muscle mass for deep I.M. injection, impaired absorption from muscle as a result of stasis or edema, possibility of uncontrolled I.M. bleeding from trauma (as may occur in hemophilia), or massive and prolonged parenteral therapy (as may be needed in chronic substantial blood loss).
- When I.V. dose is complete, flush vein with 10 ml of normal saline solution. The patient should rest 15 to 30 minutes after I.V. administration.

I.M. use: Use a 19G or 20G needle that's 2 to 3 inches long inject drug deep into upper outer quadrant of buttock—never into arm or other exposed area. Use Z-track method to avoid leakage into S.C. tissue and staining of skin.

- Minimize skin staining by using separate needle to withdraw drug from its container.
- Keep epinephrine and resuscitation equipment readily available to treat anaphylaxis.

Patient teaching

- Warn patient to avoid OTC vitamins that contain iron.
- Teach patient to recognize and report symptoms of reaction or toxicity.

Evaluation

- Patient's hemoglobin, hematocrit, and reticulocyte counts are normal.
- Patient doesn't experience anaphylaxis.
- Patient and family state understanding of drug therapy.

isoniazid (isonicotinic acid hydride INH)

(igh-soh-NIGH-uh-sid)

Isotamine♦, Laniazid, Nydrazid**, PMS Isoniazid♦

Pharmacologic class: isonicotinic acid hydrazine
Therapeutic class: antituberculotic
Pregnancy risk category: C

Indications and dosages

▶ **Actively growing tubercle bacilli.** *Adults:* 5 mg/kg P.O. or I.M. daily in single dose, maximum 300 mg/day, continued for 6 months to 2 years.

Infants and children: 10 mg/kg P.O. or I.M. daily in single dose, maximum 300 mg/day, continued for 18 months to 2 years. Concomitant administration of at least one other antituberculotic is recommended.

▶ **Prevention of tubercle bacilli in those closely exposed to tuberculosis or those with positive skin tests whose chest X-rays and bacteriologic studies are consistent with nonprogressive tuberculosis.** *Adults:* 300 mg P.O. daily in single dose, for 6 months to 1 year.

Infants and children: 10 mg/kg P.O. daily in single dose. Maximum 300 mg/day, for 1 year.

How supplied

Tablets: 50 mg, 100 mg, 300 mg
Oral solution: 50 mg/5 ml
Injection: 100 mg/ml

Pharmacokinetics

Absorption: completely and rapidly absorbed from GI tract after P.O. administration. Also absorbed readily after I.M. injection.
Distribution: distributed widely into body tissues and fluids.
Metabolism: metabolized primarily in liver. Rate of metabolism varies individually; fast acetylators metabolize drug five times as rap-

idly as others. About 50% of blacks and whites are slow acetylators, whereas more than 80% of Chinese, Japanese, and Eskimos are fast acetylators.
Excretion: excreted primarily in urine; some drug excreted in saliva, sputum, feces, and breast milk. *Half-life:* 1 to 4 hours.

Route	Onset	Peak	Duration
P.O., I.M.	Unknown	1-2 hr	Unknown

Pharmacodynamics

Chemical effect: appears to inhibit cell wall biosynthesis by interfering with lipid and DNA synthesis.
Therapeutic effect: kills susceptible bacteria, such as *Mycobacterium tuberculosis, M. bovis,* and some strains of *M. kansasii.*

Adverse reactions

CNS: *peripheral neuropathy* (especially in patients who are malnourished, alcoholic, diabetic, or slow acetylators), usually preceded by paresthesia of hands and feet; psychosis; ***seizures.***
GI: nausea, vomiting, epigastric distress, constipation, dry mouth.
Hematologic: ***agranulocytosis,*** hemolytic anemia, ***aplastic anemia,*** eosinophilia, leukopenia, neutropenia, ***thrombocytopenia,*** methemoglobinemia, pyridoxine-responsive hypochromic anemia.
Hepatic: ***hepatitis*** (occasionally severe and sometimes fatal, especially in elderly patients).
Metabolic: hyperglycemia, metabolic acidosis.
Other: rheumatic syndrome and lupus-like syndrome, ***hypersensitivity reactions*** (fever, rash, lymphadenopathy, vasculitis), irritation at I.M. injection site.

Interactions

Drug-drug. *Acetaminophen:* increased hepatotoxic effects of acetaminophen. Don't administer together.
Aluminum-containing antacids and laxatives: may decrease rate and amount of isoniazid absorbed. Give isoniazid at least 1 hour before antacid or laxative.
Carbamazepine: increased risk of isoniazid hepatotoxicity. Use together cautiously.
Carbamazepine, phenytoin: increased plasma levels of these anticonvulsants. Monitor patient closely.
Corticosteroids: may decrease therapeutic effect of isoniazid. Monitor patient's need for larger isoniazid dose.
Cyclosporine: possible increased adverse CNS effects of cyclosporine. Monitor patient closely.
Disulfiram: may cause neurologic symptoms, including changes in behavior and coordination. Avoid concomitant use.
Ketoconazole: decreased ketoconazole levels. Monitor patient closely.
Oral anticoagulants: possible increased anticoagulant activity. Monitor patient for signs of bleeding.
Rifampin: increased risk of hepatotoxicity. Monitor patient closely.
Theophylline: increased serum theophylline levels. Monitor serum levels closely, and adjust theophylline dosage as directed.
Drug-food. *Foods containing tyramine:* may cause hypertensive crisis. Tell patients to avoid such foods or eat them in small quantities.
Drug-lifestyle. *Alcohol use:* may increase risk of isoniazid-related hepatitis. Discourage concomitant use.

Contraindications and precautions

- Contraindicated in patients with acute hepatic disease or isoniazid-related liver damage.
- Use cautiously in patients with chronic non-isoniazid-related liver disease, seizure disorders (especially in those taking phenytoin), severe renal impairment, or chronic alcoholism. Also use cautiously in elderly patients and in pregnant or breast-feeding women.

NURSING CONSIDERATIONS

Assessment

- Assess patient's infection before therapy.
- Monitor patient for improvement, and evaluate culture and sensitivity tests.
- Be alert for adverse reactions and drug interactions.
- Monitor hepatic function closely for changes.
- Monitor patient for paresthesia of hands and feet, which usually precedes peripheral neuropathy, especially in patients who are mal-

nourished, alcoholic, diabetic, or slow acetylators.

• Evaluate patient's and family's knowledge of drug therapy.

Nursing diagnoses

• Infection related to presence of susceptible bacteria

• Disturbed sensory perception (tactile) related to drug-induced peripheral neuropathy

• Deficient knowledge related to drug therapy

Planning and implementation

P.O. use: Give drug 1 hour before or 2 hours after meals to avoid decreased absorption.

I.M. use: Follow normal protocol. Switch to P.O. form as soon as possible.

• Always give isoniazid with other antituberculotics to prevent development of resistant organisms.

• Administer pyridoxine, as ordered, to prevent peripheral neuropathy, especially in malnourished patients.

Patient teaching

• Tell patient to take drug as prescribed; warn against stopping drug without prescriber's consent.

• Advise patient to take with food if GI irritation occurs.

• Instruct patient to avoid alcohol during drug therapy.

• Instruct patient to avoid certain foods (fish, such as skipjack and tuna, and tyramine-containing products, such as aged cheese, beer, and chocolate) because drug has some MAO inhibitor activity.

• Tell patient to notify prescriber immediately if symptoms of liver impairment occur (loss of appetite, fatigue, malaise, jaundice, dark urine).

• Urge patient to comply with treatment, which may take months or years.

Evaluation

• Patient is free from infection.

• Patient maintains normal peripheral nervous system function.

• Patient and family state understanding of drug therapy.

isoproterenol (isoprenaline)

(igh-soh-proh-TEER-uh-nol)

Isuprel

isoproterenol hydrochloride

Isuprel, Isuprel Mistometer, Norisodrine

isoproterenol sulfate

Medihaler-Iso

Pharmacologic class: adrenergic
Therapeutic class: bronchodilator, cardiac stimulant
Pregnancy risk category: C

Indications and dosages

▶ **Bronchospasm.** *Adults and children:* for acute dyspneic episodes, one inhalation of sulfate form initially. Repeated if needed after 2 to 5 minutes. Maintenance dosage is one to two inhalations four to six times daily. Repeated once more 10 minutes after second dose. No more than three doses should be given for each attack.

▶ **Bronchospasm in COPD.** Administered by IPPB or for nebulization by compressed air or oxygen.

Adults: 2 ml of 0.125% or 2.5 ml of 0.1% solution (prepared by diluting 0.5 ml of 0.5% solution to 2 or 2.5 ml or by diluting 0.25 ml of 1% solution to 2 or 2.5 ml with water or half-normal or normal saline solution) up to five times daily.

Children: 2 ml of 0.125% solution or 2.5 ml of 0.1% solution up to five times daily.

▶ **Heart block and ventricular arrhythmias.** *Adults:* (hydrochloride) initially, 0.02 to 0.06 mg I.V. Subsequent doses 0.01 to 0.2 mg I.V. or 5 mcg/minute I.V. Or, 0.2 mg I.M. initially; then 0.02 to 1 mg, p.r.n.

Children: (hydrochloride) half of initial adult dose.

▶ **Shock.** *Adults and children:* (hydrochloride) 0.5 to 5 mcg/minute by continuous I.V. infusion. Usual concentration is 1 mg (5 ml) in 500 ml D_5W. Infusion rate adjusted according to heart rate, CVP, blood pressure, and urine flow.

How supplied

isoproterenol
Nebulizer inhaler: 0.25%, 0.5%, 1%
isoproterenol hydrochloride
Aerosol inhaler: 131 mcg/metered spray
Injection: 20 mcg/ml, 200 mcg/ml
Solution for inhalation: 0.5%, 1%
isoproterenol sulfate
Aerosol inhaler: 80 mcg/metered spray

Pharmacokinetics

Absorption: variable and often unreliable after S.L. administration. Rapid after P.O. inhalation.
Distribution: distributed widely throughout body.
Metabolism: metabolized by conjugation in GI tract and by enzymatic reduction in liver, lungs, and other tissues.
Excretion: excreted primarily in urine.

Route	Onset	Peak	Duration
Inhalation	2-5 min	Unknown	0.5-2 hr
I.V.	Immediate	Unknown	< 1 hr

Pharmacodynamics

Chemical effect: relaxes bronchial smooth muscle by acting on beta$_2$-adrenergic receptors. As cardiac stimulant, acts on beta$_1$-adrenergic receptors in heart.
Therapeutic effect: relieves bronchospasms and heart block and restores normal sinus rhythm after ventricular arrhythmia.

Adverse reactions

CNS: *headache,* mild tremor, weakness, dizziness, nervousness, insomnia, ***Stokes-Adams seizures.***
CV: *palpitations, tachycardia, angina,* ***cardiac arrest,*** *blood pressure that rises and then falls,* ***arrhythmias.***
GI: nausea, vomiting.
Metabolic: hyperglycemia.
Respiratory: ***bronchospasm.***
Skin: diaphoresis, flushing of face.

Interactions

Drug-drug. *Epinephrine, other sympathomimetics:* increased risk of arrhythmias. Avoid concomitant use.
Propranolol, other beta blockers: blocked bronchodilating effect of isoproterenol. Monitor patient carefully if used together.

Contraindications and precautions

- Contraindicated in patients with tachycardia caused by digitalis intoxication, in those with arrhythmias (other than those that may respond to treatment with isoproterenol), and in those with angina pectoris.
- Use cautiously in elderly patients; in patients with renal or CV disease, coronary insufficiency, diabetes, hyperthyroidism, or history of sensitivity to sympathomimetic amines; in pregnant or breast-feeding women; and in children.

NURSING CONSIDERATIONS

Assessment

- Assess patient's underlying condition before therapy.
- Monitor cardiopulmonary status frequently.
- Be alert for adverse reactions and drug interactions.
- This drug may aggravate ventilation and perfusion abnormalities; even while ease of breathing is improved, arterial oxygen tension may fall paradoxically.
- Evaluate patient's and family's knowledge of drug therapy.

Nursing diagnoses

- Ineffective health maintenance related to underlying condition
- Risk for injury related to drug-induced adverse reactions
- Deficient knowledge related to drug therapy

Planning and implementation

- Drug doesn't treat blood or fluid volume deficit. Volume deficit should be corrected before administering vasopressors.
- Don't use injection or inhalation solution if it's discolored or contains precipitate.

I.V. use: Give drug by direct injection or I.V. infusion. For infusion, drug may be diluted with most common I.V. solutions. However, don't use with sodium bicarbonate injection; drug decomposes rapidly in alkaline solutions.

ALERT If heart rate exceeds 110 beats/minute with I.V. infusion, notify prescriber. Doses sufficient to increase heart rate to more than 130 beats/minute may induce ventricular arrhythmias.
• When administering I.V. isoproterenol to treat shock, closely monitor blood pressure, CVP, ECG, arterial blood gas measurements, and urine output. Carefully adjust infusion rate according to these measurements, as ordered. Use continuous infusion pump to regulate flow rate.
ALERT Don't confuse Isuprel with Ismelin or Isordil.
Inhalation use: If drug is administered by inhalation with oxygen, make sure oxygen concentration won't suppress respiratory drive.
• Follow same instructions for metered powder nebulizer, although deep inhalation isn't necessary.
• Notify prescriber if adverse reactions occur. Dosage adjustment or discontinuation of drug may be required.
• Stop drug immediately if precordial distress or anginal pain occurs.

Patient teaching
• Give patient the following instructions for using metered-dose inhaler: Clear nasal passages and throat. Breathe out, expelling as much air from lungs as possible. Place mouthpiece well into mouth and inhale deeply as you release dose from inhaler. Hold breath for several seconds, remove mouthpiece, and exhale slowly.
• If more than one inhalation is ordered, tell patient to wait at least 2 minutes before repeating procedure.
• If patient also uses a corticosteroid inhaler, tell him to use bronchodilator first, and then wait about 5 minutes before using corticosteroid. This process allows bronchodilator to open air passages for maximum effectiveness of the corticosteroid.
• Warn patient using oral inhalant that this drug may turn sputum and saliva pink.
• Tell patient to stop drug and notify prescriber about chest tightness or dyspnea.
• Warn patient against overuse of drug. Tell him that tolerance can develop.
• Tell patient to reduce caffeine intake during drug therapy.

Evaluation
• Patient exhibits improved health.
• Patient doesn't experience injury from adverse reactions.
• Patient and family state understanding of drug therapy.

isosorbide dinitrate
(igh-soh-SOR-bighd digh-NIGH-trayt)
Apo-ISDN♦, Cedocard SR♦, Coronex♦, Dilatrate-SR, Isordil, Isotrate, Sorbitrate

isosorbide mononitrate
IMDUR, ISMO, Monoket

Pharmacologic class: nitrate
Therapeutic class: antianginal, vasodilator
Pregnancy risk category: C

Indications and dosages
▶ **Acute angina (S.L. and chewable tablets of isosorbide dinitrate only), prophylaxis in situations likely to cause angina.** *Adults:* **S.L. form.** 2.5 to 5 mg under tongue for prompt relief of angina, repeated q 5 to 10 minutes (maximum of three doses for each 30-minute period). For prophylaxis, 2.5 to 10 mg q 2 to 3 hours. **Chewable form.** 5 to 10 mg, p.r.n., for acute attack or q 2 to 3 hours for prophylaxis, but only after initial test dose of 5 mg to determine risk of severe hypotension. **P.O. form (isosorbide dinitrate).** 30 mg P.O. t.i.d. or q.i.d. for prophylaxis only (use smallest effective dose); 40 mg P.O. (sustained-release form) q 6 to 12 hours. **P.O. form (isosorbide mononitrate).** for prophylaxis only, 20 mg P.O. b.i.d. with doses 7 hours apart and first dose upon awakening. For sustained-release form, 30 to 60 mg P.O. once daily on arising; after several days, dosage may be increased to 120 mg once daily; rarely, 240 mg may be required.

How supplied
isosorbide dinitrate
Tablets: 5 mg, 10 mg, 20 mg, 30 mg, 40 mg

Tablets (chewable): 5 mg, 10 mg
Tablets (S.L.): 2.5 mg, 5 mg, 10 mg
Tablets (sustained-release): 40 mg
Capsules: 40 mg
Capsules (sustained-release): 40 mg
isosorbide mononitrate
Tablets: 10 mg, 20 mg
Tablets (extended-release): 30 mg, 60 mg, 120 mg

Pharmacokinetics

Absorption: dinitrate is well absorbed from GI tract but undergoes first-pass metabolism, resulting in bioavailability of about 50% (depending on dosage form used). Mononitrate is also absorbed well, with almost 100% bioavailability.
Distribution: distributed widely throughout body.
Metabolism: metabolized in liver to active metabolites.
Excretion: excreted in urine. *Half-life:* dinitrate P.O., 5 to 6 hours; S.L., 2 hours; mononitrate, about 5 hours.

Route	Onset	Peak	Duration
P.O.	2-60 min	2-60 min	1-12 hr
S.L.	2-5 min	2-5 min	1-2 hr

Pharmacodynamics

Chemical effect: may reduce cardiac oxygen demand by decreasing left ventricular end-diastolic pressure (preload) and, to a lesser extent, systemic vascular resistance (afterload). Drug also may increase blood flow through collateral coronary vessels. Most isosorbide dinitrate activity is attributed to its active metabolite, isosorbide mononitrate.
Therapeutic effect: relieves angina.

Adverse reactions

CNS: *headache, sometimes with throbbing; dizziness;* weakness.
CV: orthostatic hypotension, tachycardia, palpitations, ankle edema, fainting.
GI: nausea, vomiting.
Skin: cutaneous vasodilation, *flushing.*
Other: ***hypersensitivity reactions,*** S.L. burning.

Interactions

Drug-drug. *Antihypertensives:* possibly increased hypotensive effects. Monitor patient closely during initial therapy.
Sildenafil: may increase hyotensive effects. Avoid concomitant use.
Drug-lifestyle. *Alcohol use:* may increase hypotension. Discourage concomitant use.

Contraindications and precautions

- Contraindicated in patients hypersensitive to nitrates, in those with idiosyncratic reactions to them, and in those with severe hypotension, shock, or acute MI with low left ventricular filling pressure.
- Use cautiously in pregnant and breast-feeding women and in patients with blood volume depletion (such as that resulting from diuretic therapy) or mild hypotension.
- Safety of drug hasn't been established in children.

NURSING CONSIDERATIONS

Assessment

- Assess patient's angina before therapy and regularly thereafter.
- Monitor blood pressure, heart rate and rhythm, and intensity and duration of drug response.
- Be alert for adverse reactions and drug interactions.
- Evaluate patient's and family's knowledge of drug therapy.

Nursing diagnoses

- Acute pain related to angina
- Risk for injury related to drug-induced adverse reactions
- Deficient knowledge related to drug therapy

Planning and implementation

ALERT Don't confuse Isordil with Isuprel or Inderal.

- To prevent development of tolerance, a nitrate-free interval of 8 to 12 hours per day has been recommended. The dosage regimen for isosorbide mononitrate (one tablet upon awakening with second dose in 7 hours, or one extended-release tablet daily) is intended to minimize

nitrate tolerance by providing substantial nitrate-free interval.
P.O. use: Administer drug on empty stomach, either 30 minutes before or 1 to 2 hours after meals, and have patient swallow tablets whole. Have patient chew chewable tablets thoroughly before swallowing.
S.L. use: Administer drug at first sign of angina. Have patient wet tablet with saliva, place it under his tongue until completely absorbed, and sit down and rest. Dose may be repeated every 10 to 15 minutes for maximum of three doses.
- Don't discontinue drug abruptly because coronary vasospasm may occur.
- Notify prescriber immediately if patient's pain doesn't subside.

Patient teaching
- Caution patient to take drug regularly, as prescribed, and to keep it accessible at all times.

ALERT Advise patient that abrupt discontinuation causes coronary vasospasm.
- Tell patient to take S.L. tablet at first sign of attack. Explain that tablet should be wet with saliva and placed under tongue until completely absorbed, and that patient should sit down and rest until pain subsides. Tell patient that dose may be repeated every 10 to 15 minutes for maximum of three doses. If drug doesn't provide relief, medical help should be obtained promptly.
- Tell patient who complains of tingling sensation with drug placed S.L. to try holding tablet in buccal pouch.

ALERT Warn patient not to confuse S.L. form with P.O. form.
- Teach patient taking P.O. form to take tablet on empty stomach, either 30 minutes before or 1 to 2 hours after meals and to swallow tablet whole or chew chewable tablet thoroughly before swallowing.
- Tell patient to minimize orthostatic hypotension by changing to upright position slowly. Tell him to go up and down stairs carefully and to lie down at first sign of dizziness.
- Instruct patient to avoid alcohol consumption during drug therapy.
- Tell patient to store drug in cool place, in tightly closed container, away from light.

Evaluation
- Patient is free from pain.
- Patient doesn't experience injury from adverse reactions.
- Patient and family state understanding of drug therapy.

isotretinoin
(igh-soh-TREH-tih-noyn)
Accutane, Accutane Roche ♦, Roaccutane ◇

Pharmacologic class: retinoic acid derivative
Therapeutic class: antiacne
Pregnancy risk category: X

Indications and dosages
▶ **Severe recalcitrant nodular acne unresponsive to conventional therapy.** *Adults and adolescents:* 0.5 to 2 mg/kg P.O. daily in two divided doses for 15 to 20 weeks.

How supplied
Capsules: 10 mg, 20 mg, 40 mg

Pharmacokinetics
Absorption: absorbed rapidly from GI tract.
Distribution: distributed widely in body; 99.9% protein-bound, primarily to albumin.
Metabolism: metabolized in liver and possibly in gut wall.
Excretion: unknown.

Route	Onset	Peak	Duration
P.O.	Unknown	About 3 hr	Unknown

Pharmacodynamics
Chemical effect: unknown; thought to normalize keratinization, reversibly decrease size of sebaceous glands, and alter composition of sebum to less viscous form that is less likely to cause follicular plugging.
Therapeutic effect: improves skin integrity.

Adverse reactions
CNS: headache, fatigue, *pseudotumor cerebri* (benign intracranial hypertension).
EENT: *conjunctivitis,* corneal deposits, dry eyes, visual disturbances.

GI: nonspecific GI symptoms, gum bleeding and inflammation, nausea, vomiting.
Hematologic: anemia, elevated platelet count.
Hepatic: elevated AST, ALT, and alkaline phosphatase levels.
Metabolic: *hypertriglyceridemia,* hyperglycemia.
Musculoskeletal: *musculoskeletal pain (skeletal hyperostosis).*
Skin: *cheilosis, rash, dry skin,* peeling of palms and toes, skin infection, thinning of hair, photosensitivity.

Interactions

Drug-drug. *Carbamazepine:* reduced plasma carbamazepine levels. Monitor patient for loss of therapeutic effects.
Tetracyclines: increased risk of pseudotumor cerebri. Avoid concomitant use.
Vitamin A, products that contain vitamin A: increased toxic effects of isotretinoin. Don't use together without prescriber's permission.
Drug-food. *Any food:* enhanced absorption of drug. Take drug with food.
Drug-lifestyle. *Alcohol use:* increased risk of hypertriglyceridemia. Discourage concomitant use.
Sun exposure: increased photosensitivity reactions. Advise patient to use sunscreen and wear protective clothing.

Contraindications and precautions

- Contraindicated in women of childbearing age unless patient has had negative serum pregnancy test within 2 weeks before beginning therapy, will begin drug therapy on second or third day of next menstrual period, and will comply with stringent contraceptive measures for 1 month before therapy, during therapy, and at least 1 month after therapy.

ALERT Severe fetal abnormalities may occur if drug is used during pregnancy.

- Also contraindicated in patients hypersensitive to parabens, which are used as preservatives.
- Drug isn't recommended for breast-feeding women.
- Safety of drug hasn't been established in children under age 12.

NURSING CONSIDERATIONS

Assessment

- Assess patient's skin before therapy and regularly thereafter.
- Obtain baseline serum lipid studies and liver function tests before therapy, as ordered. Monitor these values at regular intervals until response to drug is established (usually about 4 weeks).
- Monitor blood glucose levels and CK levels in patients who engage in vigorous physical activity.
- Be alert for adverse reactions and drug interactions.
- Most adverse reactions appear to be dose-related, occurring at dosages greater than 1 mg/kg daily. They're usually reversible when therapy is discontinued or dosage reduced.
- Evaluate patient's and family's knowledge of drug therapy.

Nursing diagnoses

- Impaired skin integrity related to underlying skin condition
- Impaired tissue integrity related to adverse reactions
- Deficient knowledge related to drug therapy

Planning and implementation

- Anticipate second course of therapy, if needed, to start at least 8 weeks after completion of first course because improvement may continue after withdrawal of drug.
- Give drug with meals or shortly thereafter to enhance absorption.

ALERT Patient who experiences headache, nausea, vomiting, or visual disturbances should be screened for papilledema. Signs and symptoms of pseudotumor cerebri require immediate discontinuation of therapy and prompt neurologic intervention.

Patient teaching

- Advise patient to take drug with milk, meals, or shortly after meals to ensure adequate absorption.
- Tell patient to immediately report visual disturbances and bone, muscle, or joint pain.
- Warn patient that contact lenses may feel uncomfortable during drug therapy.

• Warn patient against using abrasives, medicated soaps and cleansers, acne preparations containing peeling agents, and topical alcohol preparations (including cosmetics, aftershave, cologne) because these agents cause cumulative irritation or excessive drying of skin.
• Instruct patient to avoid alcohol during drug therapy.
• Tell patient to avoid prolonged exposure to sun, to use sunblock, and to wear protective clothing.
ALERT Advise patient not to donate blood during or for 30 days after therapy; severe fetal abnormalities may occur if a pregnant woman receives blood containing isotretinoin.
• Advise women of childbearing age to use two reliable forms of contraception simultaneously for 1 month before, during, and 1 month after treatment.

Evaluation

• Patient has improved skin condition.
• Patient is free from conjunctivitis, corneal deposits, and dry eyes.
• Patient and family state understanding of drug therapy.

isradipine

(is-RAH-deh-peen)
DynaCirc

Pharmacologic class: calcium channel blocker
Therapeutic class: antihypertensive
Pregnancy risk category: C

Indications and dosages

▶ **Essential hypertension.** *Adults:* initially, 2.5 mg P.O. b.i.d., alone or with thiazide diuretic. Dosage increased gradually. If response is inadequate after first 2 to 4 weeks, dosage increased by 5 mg daily at 2- to 4-week intervals to maximum of 20 mg daily.

How supplied

Capsules: 2.5 mg, 5 mg

Pharmacokinetics

Absorption: 90% to 95% absorbed after P.O. administration.
Distribution: 95% is bound to plasma protein.
Metabolism: completely metabolized before elimination with extensive first-pass metabolism.
Excretion: 60% to 65% of drug excreted in urine; 25% to 30% in feces. *Half-life:* about 8 hours.

Route	Onset	Peak	Duration
P.O.	≤ 20 min	≤ 1.5 hr	12 hr

Pharmacodynamics

Chemical effect: inhibits calcium ion influx across cardiac and smooth-muscle cells and may decrease arteriolar resistance and blood pressure.
Therapeutic effect: lowers blood pressure.

Adverse reactions

CNS: dizziness.
CV: edema, flushing, palpitations, tachycardia, orthostatic hypotension.
GI: nausea, diarrhea.
GU: frequent urination.
Respiratory: dyspnea.
Skin: rash.

Interactions

Drug-drug. *Cimetidine:* increases isradipine levels. Monitor patient for increased effects.
Fentanyl anesthesia: severe hypotension has been reported with concomitant use of beta blocker and calcium channel blocker. Avoid concomitant use.
Rifampin: reduced isradipine effects. Monitor patient closely.

Contraindications and precautions

• Contraindicated in patients hypersensitive to drug.
• Use cautiously in pregnant and breastfeeding women and in patients with heart failure, especially those who take beta blockers.
• Safety of drug hasn't been established in children.
ALERT Don't confuse DynaCirc with Dynacin.

NURSING CONSIDERATIONS

Assessment
- Assess blood pressure before therapy and regularly thereafter.
- Be alert for adverse reactions and drug interactions.
- Monitor patient's hydration status if adverse GI reactions occur.
- Evaluate patient's and family's knowledge of drug therapy.

Nursing diagnoses
- Risk for injury related to presence of hypertension
- Risk for deficient fluid volume related to adverse GI reactions
- Deficient knowledge related to drug therapy

Planning and implementation
- Drug may be given without regard to meals. However, giving drug with food slows its absorption.
- Before surgery, inform anesthesiologist that patient is taking calcium channel blocker.

Patient teaching
- Explain that patient may note increased need to void because drug has some diuretic activity.
- Instruct patient to notify prescriber of adverse reactions or significant changes in blood pressure.

Evaluation
- Patient's blood pressure is normal.
- Patient maintains normal hydration.
- Patient and family state understanding of drug therapy.

itraconazole
(ih-truh-KAHN-uh-zohl)
Sporanox

Pharmacologic class: synthetic triazole
Therapeutic class: antifungal
Pregnancy risk category: C

Indications and dosages

▶ **Pulmonary and extrapulmonary blastomycosis; histoplasmosis.** *Adults (capsules):* 200 mg P.O. daily. Dosage may be increased as needed and tolerated in 100-mg increments to maximum of 400 mg daily. Amounts that exceed 200 mg daily should be divided into two doses. Treatment should continue for at least 3 months. In life-threatening illness, loading dose of 200 mg t.i.d. is administered for 3 days. Or, administer 200 mg by I.V. infusion over 1 hour twice daily for four doses; then 200 mg I.V. once daily.

▶ **Aspergillosis.** *Adults (capsules):* 200 to 400 mg P.O. daily. Or, administer 200 mg by I.V. infusion over 1 hour twice daily for four doses; then decrease to 200 mg I.V. once daily for up to 14 days.

▶ **Onychomycosis for toenails with or without fingernail involvement.** *Adults (capsules):* 200 mg P.O. once daily for 12 weeks.

▶ **Onychomycosis for fingernails.** *Adults (capsules):* two treatment phases each consisting of 200 mg P.O. b.i.d. for 1 week. Phases are separated by a 3-week period without drug.

▶ **Esophageal candidiasis.** *Adults (oral solution):* 100 mg to 200 mg swished in mouth vigorously and swallowed daily for a minimum of 3 weeks.

▶ **Oropharyngeal candidiasis.** *Adults (oral solution):* 200 mg swished in mouth vigorously and swallowed daily for 1 to 2 weeks. For patients unresponsive to fluconazole tablets, give 100 mg swished in mouth vigorously and swallowed twice daily for 2 to 4 weeks.

How supplied

Capsules: 100 mg
Injection: 10 mg/ml
Oral solution: 10 mg/ml

Pharmacokinetics

Absorption: P.O. bioavailability is maximal when taken with food. Absolute P.O. bioavailability is 55%.
Distribution: plasma protein–binding of itraconazole is 99.8%; that of its metabolite, hydroxyitraconazole, 99.5%.

Metabolism: extensively metabolized by liver into large number of metabolites, including hydroxyitraconazole, the major metabolite.
Excretion: excreted in feces and urine.

Route	Onset	Peak	Duration
P.O.	Unknown	Unknown	Unknown

Pharmacodynamics

Chemical effect: interferes with fungal cell wall synthesis by inhibiting formation of ergosterol and increasing cell wall permeability.
Therapeutic effect: hinders fungal activity. Spectrum of activity includes *Aspergillus* species and *Blastomyces dermatitidis.*

Adverse reactions

CNS: fatigue, malaise.
CV: edema.
GI: nausea, vomiting, diarrhea, abdominal pain, anorexia.
Skin: rash, pruritus.
Other: fever.

Interactions

Drug-drug. *Antacids, H_2-receptor antagonists, phenytoin, rifampin:* possible decreased plasma itraconazole levels. Avoid concomitant use.
Cyclosporine, digoxin: possible increased plasma levels of these drugs. Monitor plasma levels closely.
Isoniazid: may decrease plasma itraconazole levels. Monitor patient closely.
Oral anticoagulants: possible enhanced anticoagulant effects. Monitor PT and INR closely.
Oral antidiabetics: similar antifungals have caused hypoglycemia. Monitor blood glucose levels.

Contraindications and precautions

- Contraindicated in patients hypersensitive to drug; in those receiving astemizole, cisapride, oral triazolam, or oral midazolam; and in breast-feeding women (drug appears in breast milk).
- Use cautiously in patients with hypochlorhydria (they may not absorb drug as readily as patients with normal gastric acidity), in HIV-infected patients (hypochlorhydria can accompany HIV infection), and in pregnant women.
- Safety of drug hasn't been established in children.
- Don't use injection in patients with a creatinine clearance less than 30 ml/minute.

NURSING CONSIDERATIONS

Assessment

- Assess patient's infection before therapy and regularly thereafter.
- Monitor liver and renal function test results.
- Be alert for adverse reactions and drug interactions.
- Evaluate patient's and family's knowledge of drug therapy.

Nursing diagnoses

- Infection related to presence of susceptible fungi
- Risk for deficient fluid volume related to adverse reactions
- Deficient knowledge related to drug therapy

Planning and implementation

- Administer capsules with food. Don't administer oral solution with food.

ALERT Oral solution and capsules aren't interchangeable.

- Report signs and symptoms of liver disease and abnormal liver test results.

I.V. use: Dilute in normal saline solution for injection. Add dose to 50-ml I.V. bag of normal saline solution. Infuse over 60 minutes, using an infusion set with a filter. Flush I.V. line with 15 to 20 ml of normal saline solution after each infusion. Compatibility with other drugs is unknown.
P.O. use: Instruct patient to swish solution vigorously in the mouth (10 ml at a time) for several seconds and then swallow.

Patient teaching

- Teach patient to recognize and report signs and symptoms of liver disease (anorexia, dark urine, pale stools, unusual fatigue, or jaundice).
- Tell patient to take capsules with food to ensure maximal absorption.

Evaluation

- Patient is free from infection.

Photoguide to tablets and capsules

This photoguide provides full-color photographs of some of the most commonly prescribed tablets and capsules in the United States. Shown in actual size, the drugs are organized alphabetically by trade or generic name for quick reference.

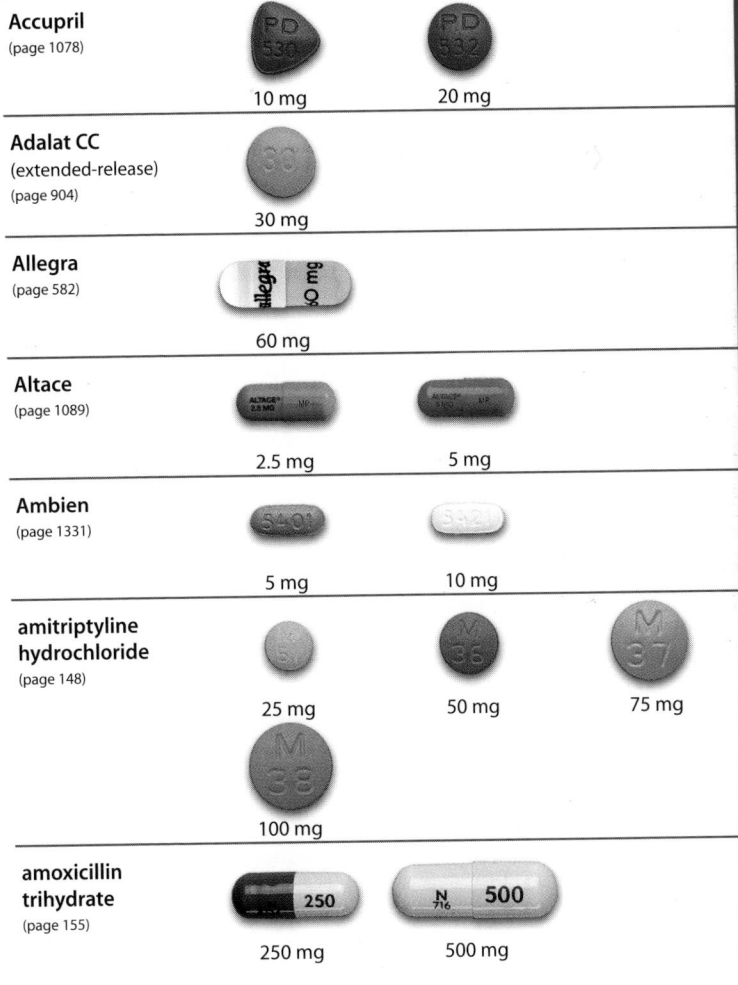

Accupril
(page 1078)

10 mg | 20 mg

Adalat CC
(extended-release)
(page 904)

30 mg

Allegra
(page 582)

60 mg

Altace
(page 1089)

2.5 mg | 5 mg

Ambien
(page 1331)

5 mg | 10 mg

amitriptyline hydrochloride
(page 148)

25 mg | 50 mg | 75 mg

100 mg

amoxicillin trihydrate
(page 155)

250 mg | 500 mg

Amoxil
(page 155)

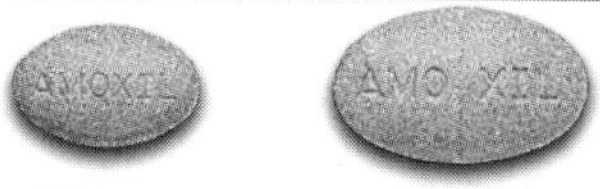

125 mg (chewable) | 250 mg (chewable)

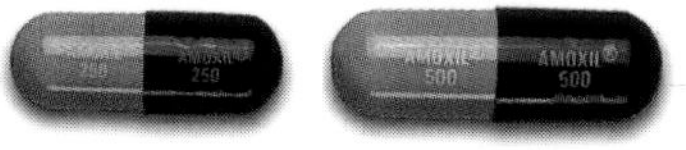

250 mg | 500 mg

atenolol
(page 183)

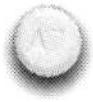

25 mg

Ativan
(page 769)

0.5 mg | 1 mg

Augmentin
(page 153)

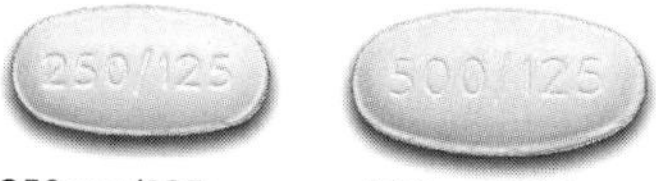

250 mg/125 mg | 500 mg/125 mg

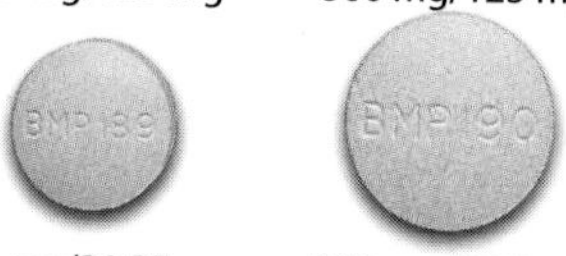

125 mg/31.25 mg (chewable) | 250 mg/62.5 mg (chewable)

Axid
(page 914)

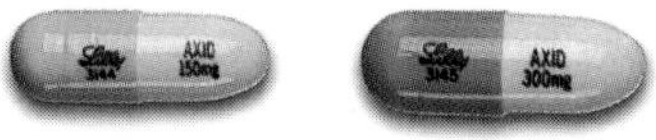

150 mg | 300 mg

Biaxin
(page 356)

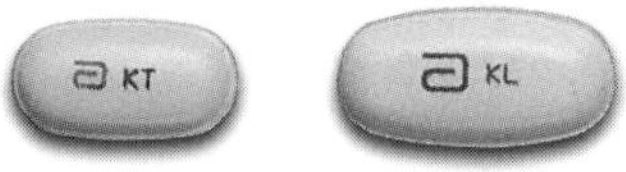

250 mg | 500 mg

Bumex
(page 243)

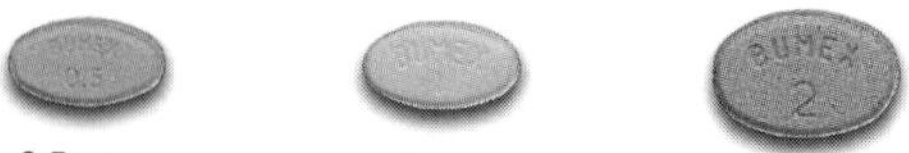

0.5 mg | 1 mg | 2 mg

BuSpar
(page 247)

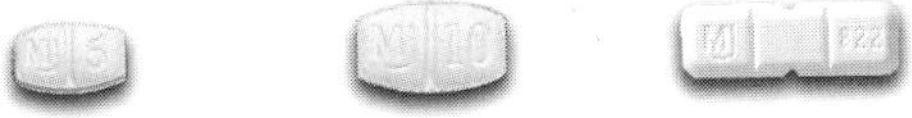

5 mg | 10 mg | 15 mg

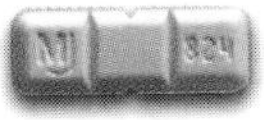

30 mg

Calan
(page 1303)

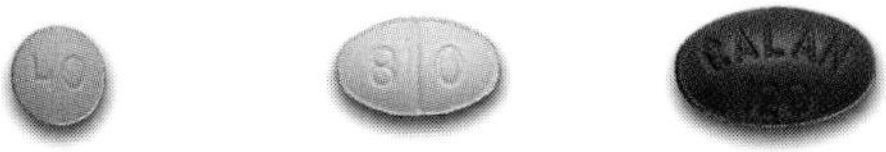

40 mg | 80 mg | 120 mg

Capoten
(page 268)

12.5 mg | 25 mg

Carafate
(page 1174)

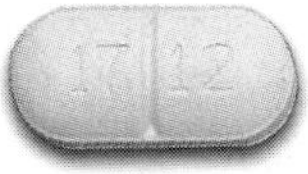

1 g

Cardizem
(page 463)

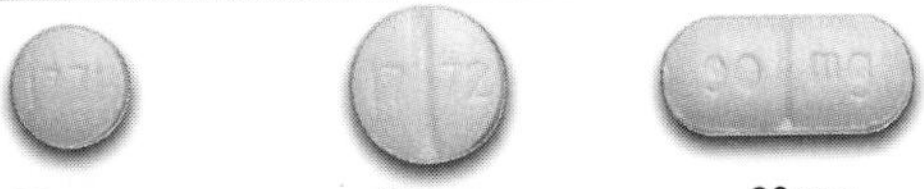

30 mg | 60 mg | 90 mg

Cardizem CD
(extended-release)
(page 463)

120 mg | 180 mg | 240 mg

Cardura
(page 494)

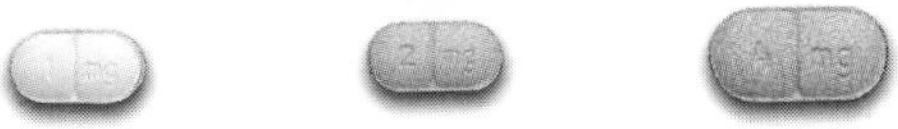

1 mg | 2 mg | 4 mg

Ceclor
(page 285)

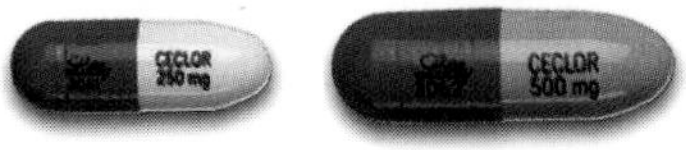

250 mg | 500 mg

Ceftin
(page 313)

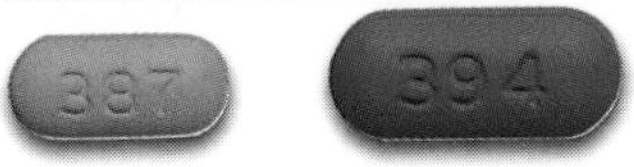

250 mg | 500 mg

Cefzil
(page 305)

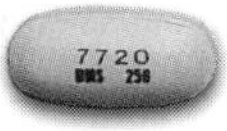

250 mg

Celebrex
(page 315)

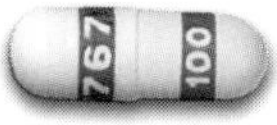

100 mg

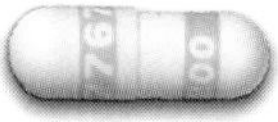
200 mg

Celexa
(page 353)

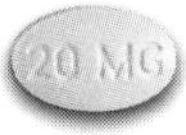

20 mg

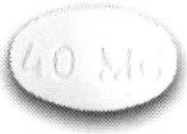
40 mg

cephalexin
(page 317)

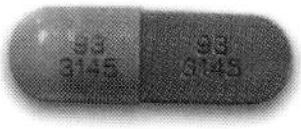
250 mg

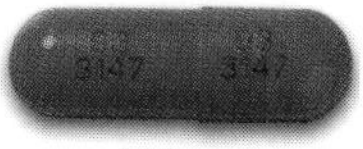
500 mg

cimetidine
(page 346)

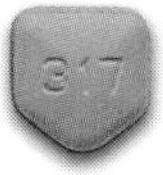

300 mg

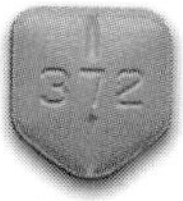

400 mg

Cipro
(page 349)

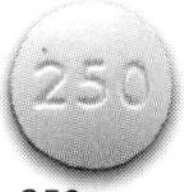

250 mg

500 mg

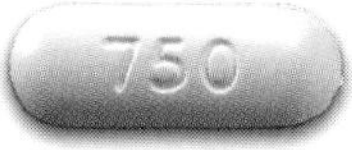

750 mg

Claritin
(page 768)

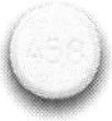
10 mg

Compazine
(page 1051)

5 mg

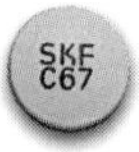

10 mg

Cordarone
(page 146)

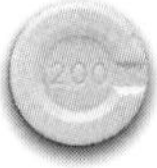
200 mg

Coreg
(page 281)

3.125 mg

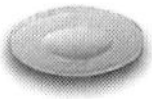
6.25 mg

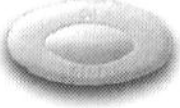
12.5 mg

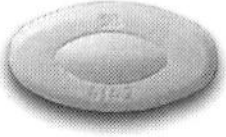
25 mg

Coumadin
(page 1317)

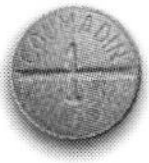
1 mg

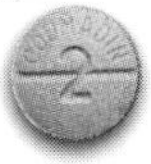
2 mg

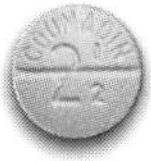
2.5 mg

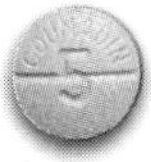
5 mg

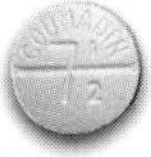
7.5 mg

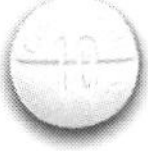
10 mg

Cozaar
(page 771)

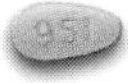
25 mg

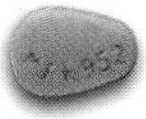
50 mg

cyclobenzaprine hydrochloride
(page 394)

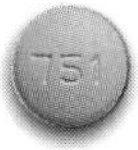

10 mg

Daypro
(page 940)

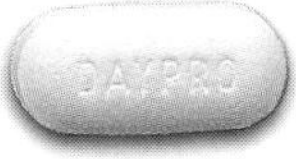

600 mg

Deltasone
(page 1042)

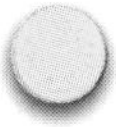
2.5 mg

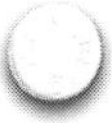
5 mg

10 mg

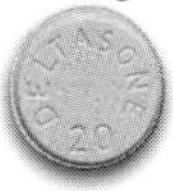

20 mg

Depakote
(page 1292)

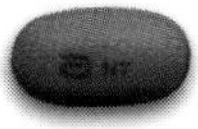
125 mg

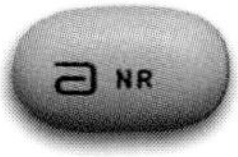

250 mg

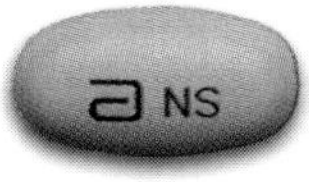

500 mg

Depakote Sprinkle
(delayed-release)
(page 1292)

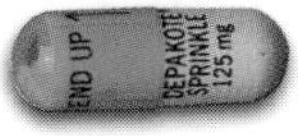

125 mg

DiaBeta
(page 638)

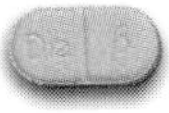
1.25 mg

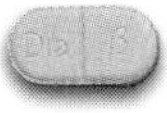
2.5 mg

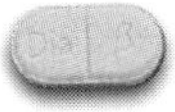
5 mg

Diflucan
(page 590)

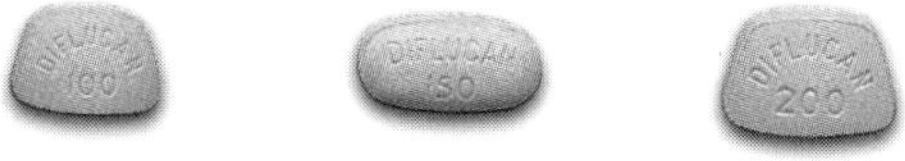

100 mg | 150 mg | 200 mg

Dilacor XR
(page 463)

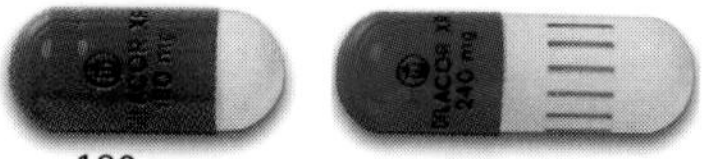

180 mg | 240 mg

Dilantin Infatabs
(page 1002)

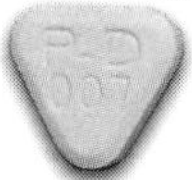

50 mg

Dilantin Kapseals
(page 1002)

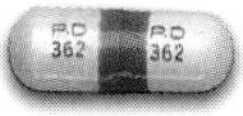

100 mg

doxepin hydrochloride
(page 495)

75 mg

Duricef
(page 287)

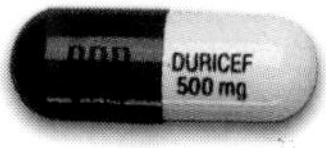

500 mg

E.E.S.
(page 534)

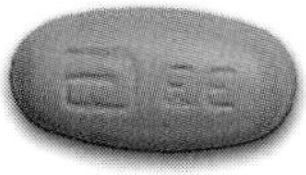

400 mg

Effexor
(page 1301)

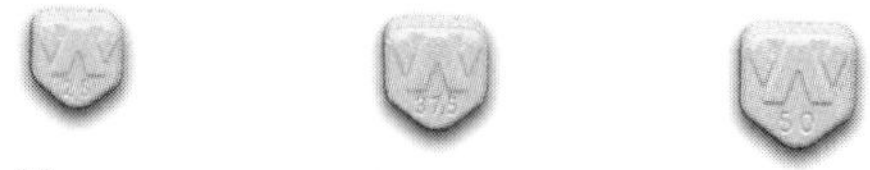

25 mg | 37.5 mg | 50 mg

75 mg | 100 mg

Ery-Tab
(delayed-release)
(page 534)

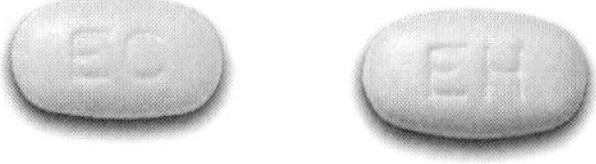

250 mg | 333 mg

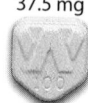

Erythrocin Stearate Filmtab
(page 534)

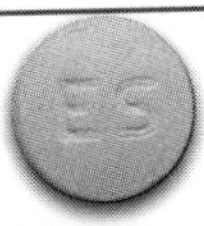

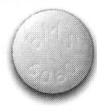

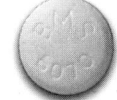

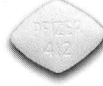

250 mg

Erythromycin Base Filmtab
(page 534)

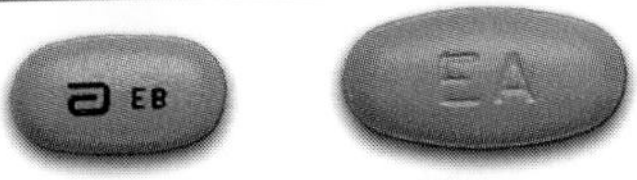

250 mg | 500 mg

Estrace
(page 540)

1 mg | 2 mg

Evista
(page 670)

60 mg

Floxin
(page 926)

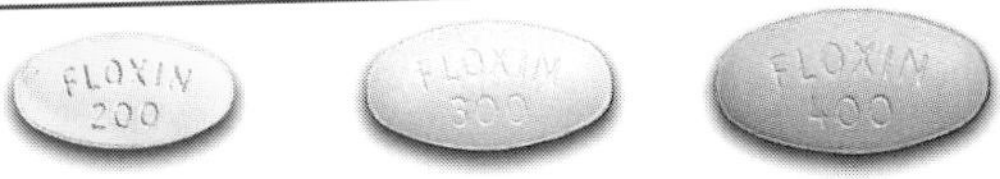

200 mg | 300 mg | 400 mg

Fosamax
(page 119)

10 mg | 40 mg

furosemide
(page 622)

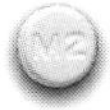

20 mg

glipizide
(page 636)

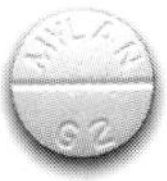

10 mg

Glucophage
(page 812)

500 mg | 850 mg

Glucotrol
(page 636)

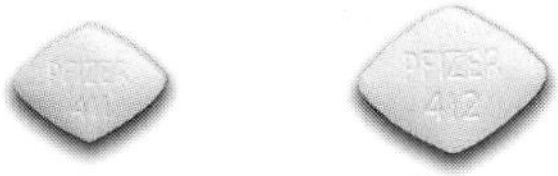

5 mg | 10 mg

Glucotrol XL
(page 636)

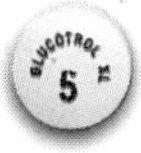

5 mg

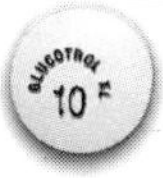

10 mg

Glynase Prestab
(page 638)

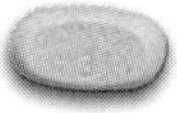
3 mg

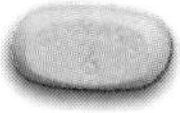
6 mg

Hytrin
(page 1201)

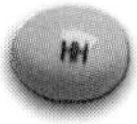
1 mg

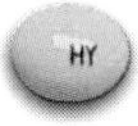

2 mg

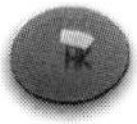
5 mg

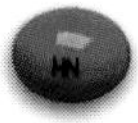
10 mg

Inderal
(page 1061)

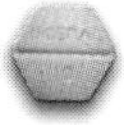
10 mg

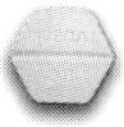
20 mg

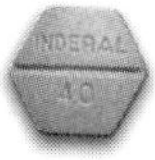

40 mg

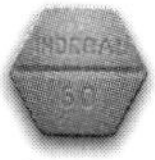
60 mg

K-Dur
(page 1029)

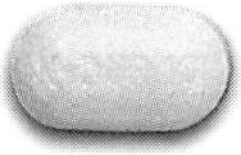
10 mEq

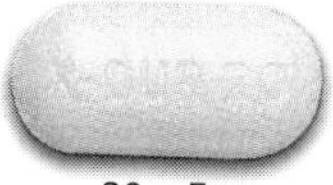
20 mEq

Klonopin
(page 367)

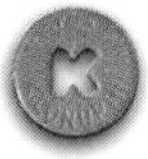
0.5 mg

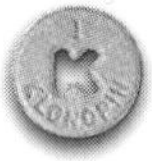
1 mg

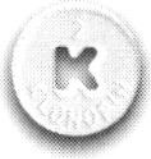
2 mg

Lanoxin
(page 455)

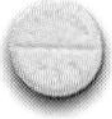
0.125 mg

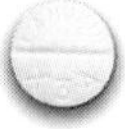
0.25 mg

Lasix
(page 622)

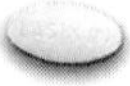
20 mg

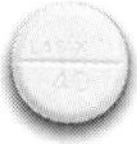
40 mg

Levaquin
(page 747)

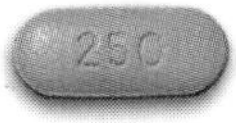

250 mg

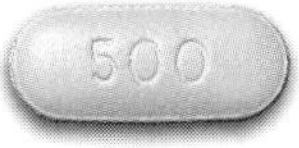

500 mg

Levoxyl
(page 750)

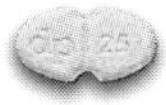
25 mcg

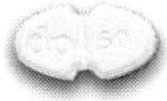
50 mcg

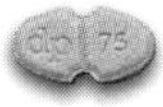
75 mcg

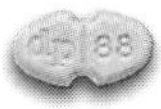
88 mcg

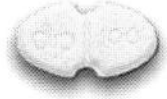
100 mcg

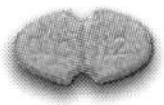
112 mcg

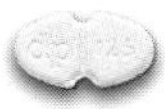
125 mcg

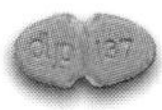
137 mcg

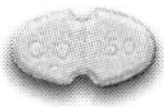
150 mcg

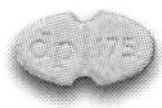
175 mcg

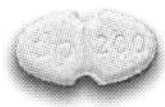
200 mcg

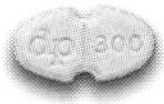
300 mcg

Lipitor
(page 184)

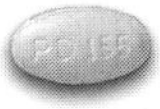
10 mg

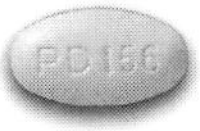
20 mg

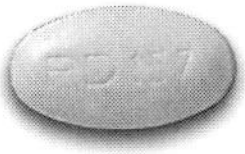
40 mg

Lodine
(page 564)

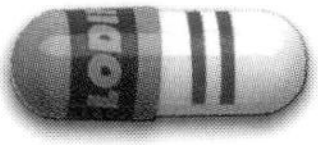
200 mg

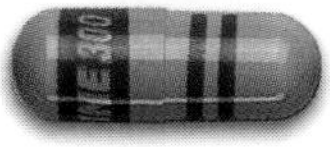
300 mg

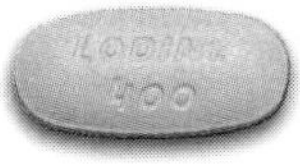
400 mg

Lopid
(page 631)

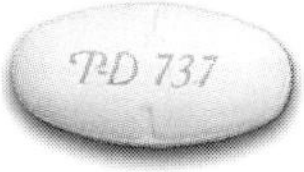

600 mg

Lorabid
(page 766)

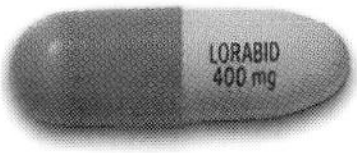

400 mg

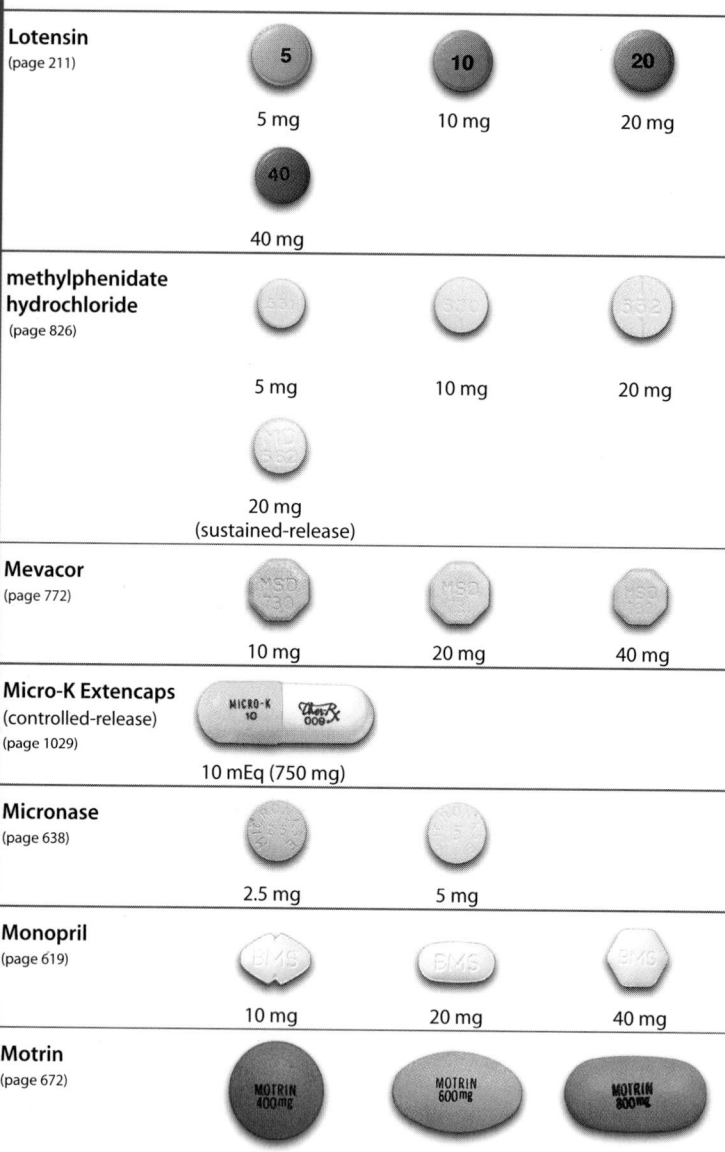

Lotensin
(page 211)

5 mg

10 mg

20 mg

40 mg

methylphenidate hydrochloride
(page 826)

5 mg

10 mg

20 mg

20 mg
(sustained-release)

Mevacor
(page 772)

10 mg

20 mg

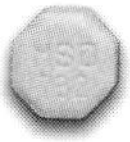
40 mg

Micro-K Extencaps
(controlled-release)
(page 1029)

10 mEq (750 mg)

Micronase
(page 638)

2.5 mg

5 mg

Monopril
(page 619)

10 mg

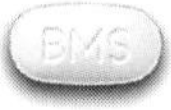
20 mg

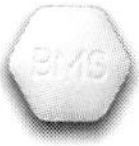
40 mg

Motrin
(page 672)

400 mg

600 mg

800 mg

Naprosyn
(page 885)

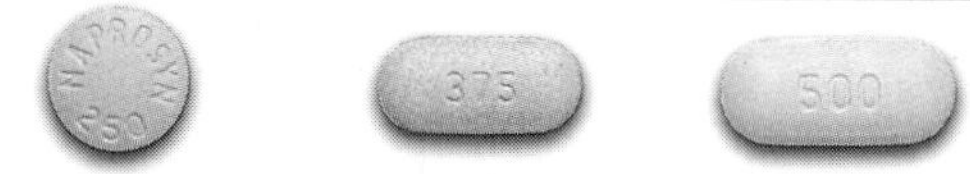

250 mg | 375 mg | 500 mg

naproxen
(page 885)

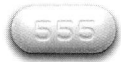

375 mg | 500 mg

Neurontin
(page 624)

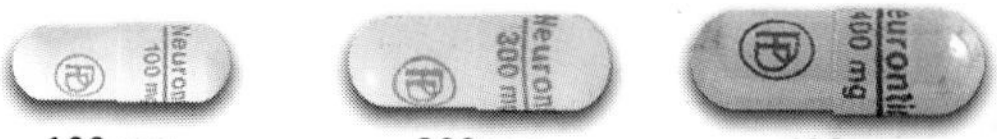

100 mg | 300 mg | 400 mg

Nitrostat
(page 910)

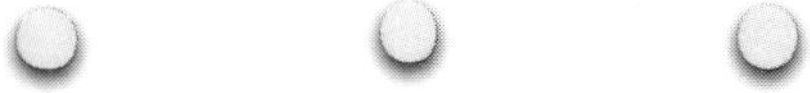

0.3 mg | 0.4 mg | 0.6 mg

Nolvadex
(page 1192)

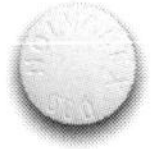

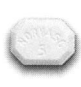

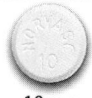

10 mg

nortriptyline hydrochloride
(page 921)

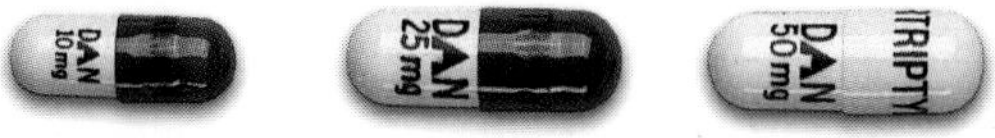

10 mg | 25 mg | 50 mg

Norvasc
(page 150)

5 mg | 10 mg

Oruvail
(page 721)

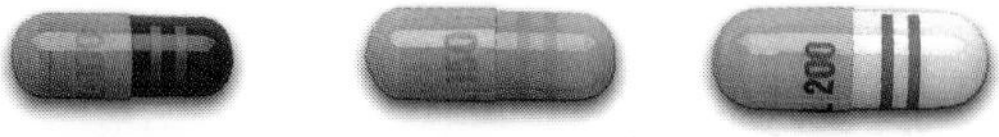

100 mg | 150 mg | 200 mg

Pamelor
(page 921)

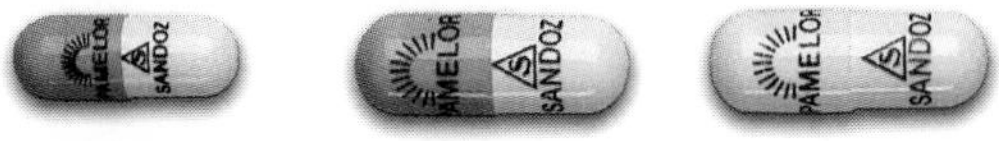

10 mg | 25 mg | 50 mg

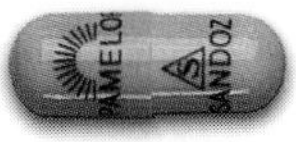

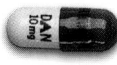

75 mg

Paxil
(page 964)

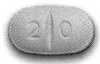

20 mg | 30 mg

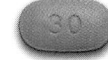

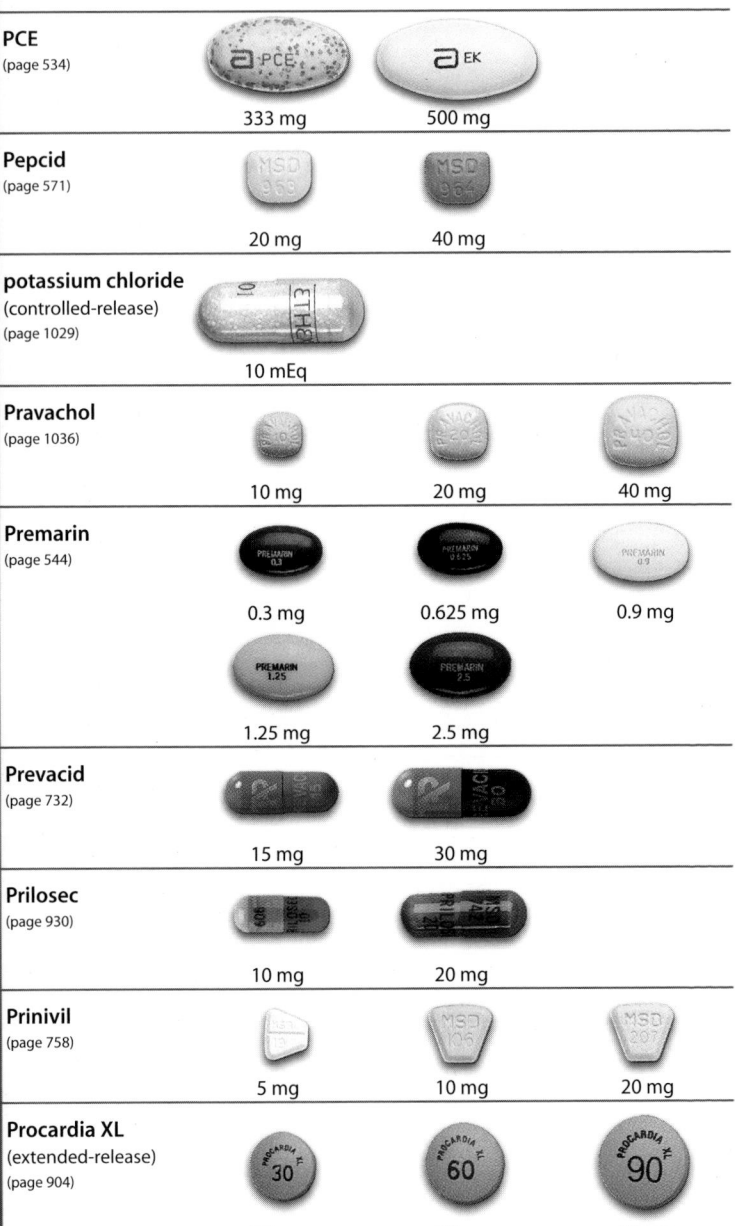

PCE
(page 534)

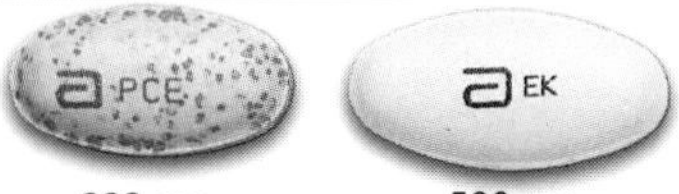

333 mg | 500 mg

Pepcid
(page 571)

20 mg | 40 mg

potassium chloride
(controlled-release)
(page 1029)

10 mEq

Pravachol
(page 1036)

10 mg | 20 mg | 40 mg

Premarin
(page 544)

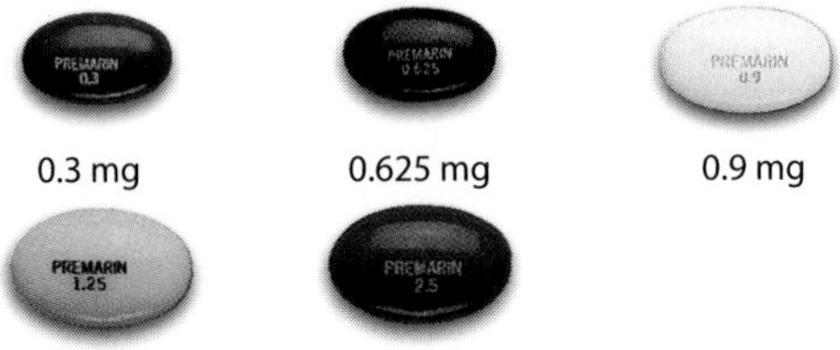

0.3 mg | 0.625 mg | 0.9 mg

1.25 mg | 2.5 mg

Prevacid
(page 732)

15 mg | 30 mg

Prilosec
(page 930)

10 mg | 20 mg

Prinivil
(page 758)

5 mg | 10 mg | 20 mg

Procardia XL
(extended-release)
(page 904)

30 mg | 60 mg | 90 mg

Provera
(page 791)

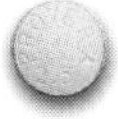
2.5 mg

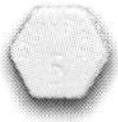
5 mg

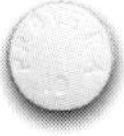
10 mg

Prozac
(page 601)

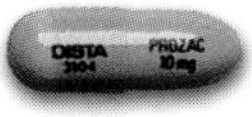

10 mg

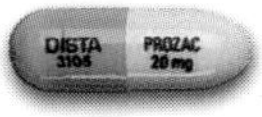

20 mg

Relafen
(page 873)

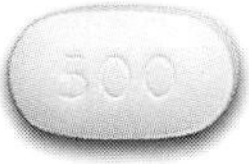

500 mg

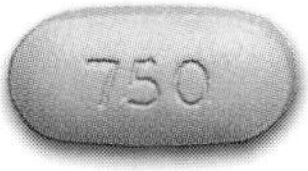

750 mg

Risperdal
(page 1110)

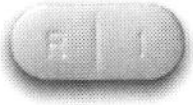

1 mg

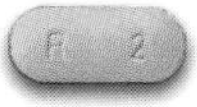

2 mg

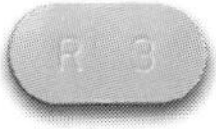

3 mg

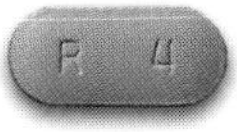

4 mg

Serzone
(page 890)

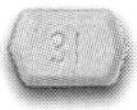

50 mg

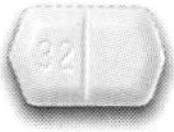

100 mg

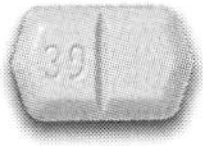

150 mg

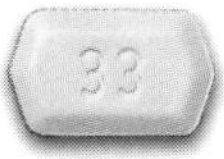

200 mg

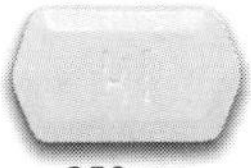
250 mg

Sinemet
(page 272)

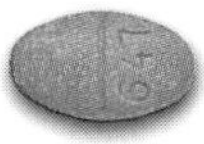
10 mg/100 mg

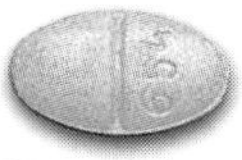
25 mg/250 mg

Sinemet CR
(extended-release)
(page 272)

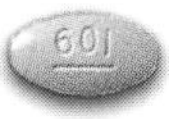

25 mg/100 mg

Singulair
(page 863)

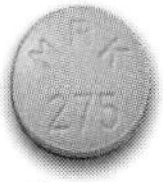

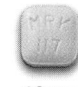

5 mg

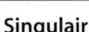

10 mg

Sumycin
(page 1210)

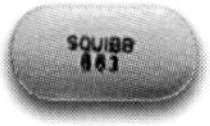

250 mg

Tagamet
(page 346)

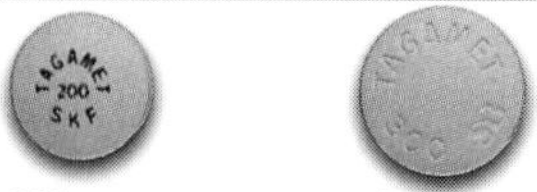

200 mg | 300 mg

Tenormin
(page 183)

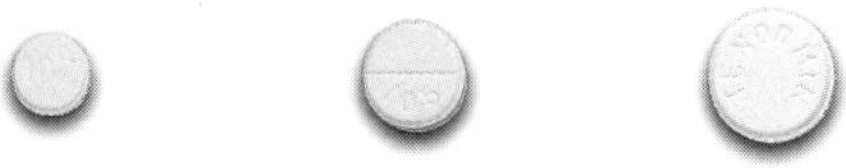

25 mg | 50 mg | 100 mg

Theo-Dur
(extended-release)
(page 1212)

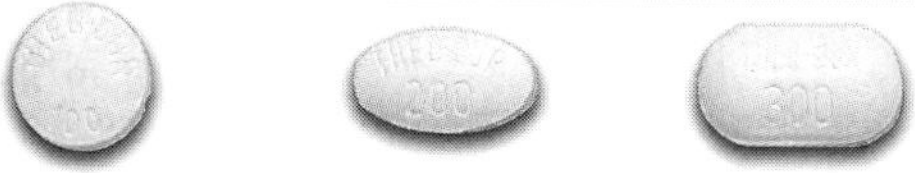

100 mg | 200 mg | 300 mg

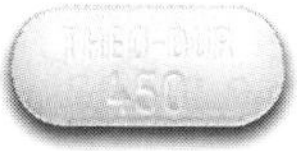

450 mg

Ticlid
(page 1230)

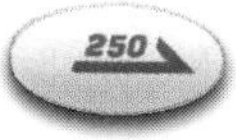

250 mg

Toprol-XL
(page 834)

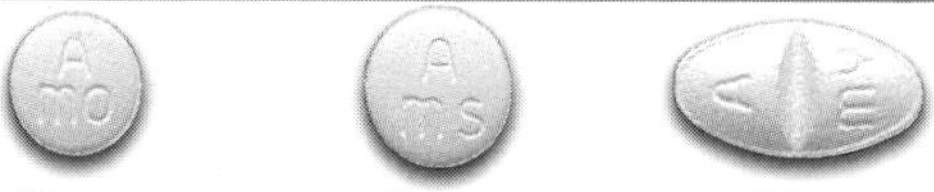

50 mg | 100 mg | 200 mg

Toradol
(page 723)

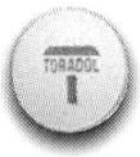

10 mg

Trental
(page 987)

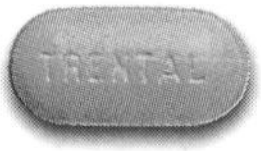

400 mg

Trimox
(page 155)

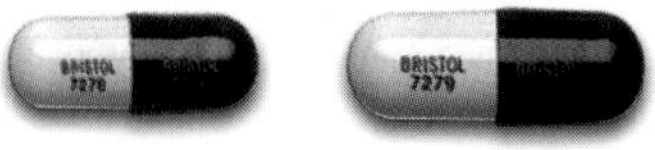

250 mg | 500 mg

Ultram
(page 1254)

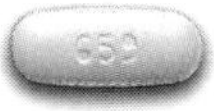

50 mg

Valium
(page 443)

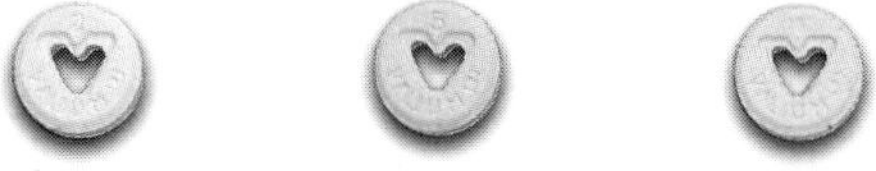

2 mg | 5 mg | 10 mg

Vasotec
(page 513)

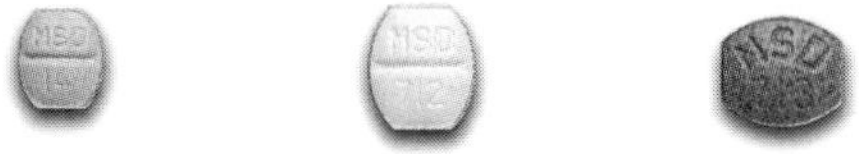

2.5 mg | 5 mg | 10 mg

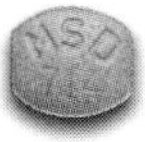

20 mg

Veetids
(page 978)

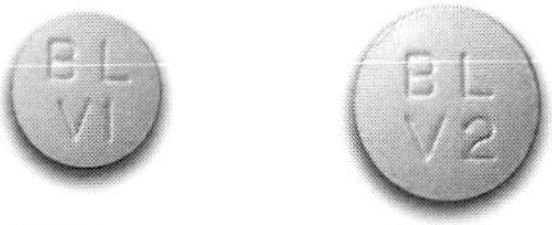

250 mg | 500 mg

verapamil hydrochloride
(extended-release)
(page 1303)

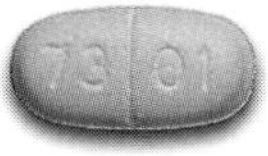

180 mg

Verelan
(extended-release)
(page 1303)

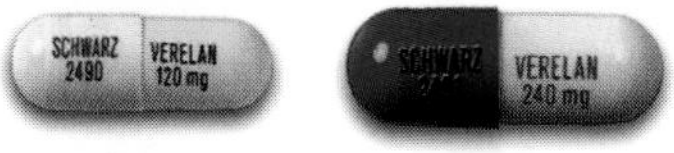

120 mg | 240 mg

Viagra
(page 1140)

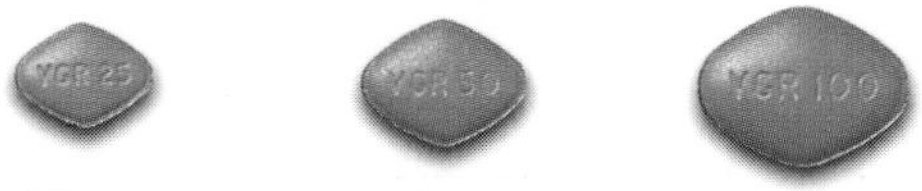

25 mg | 50 mg | 100 mg

Vioxx
(page 1118)

12.5 mg | 25 mg

Wellbutrin
(page 246)

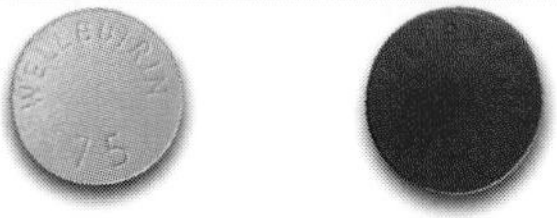

75 mg | 100 mg

Wellbutrin SR
(page 246)

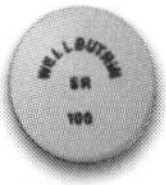
100 mg

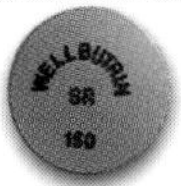

150 mg

Xanax
(page 125)

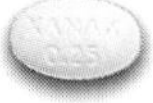
0.25 mg

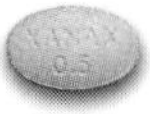
0.5 mg

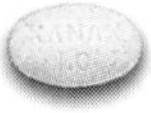
1 mg

Zantac
(page 1091)

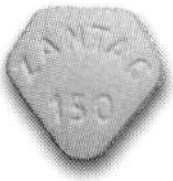

150 mg

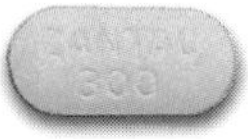
300 mg

Zestril
(page 758)

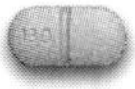
5 mg

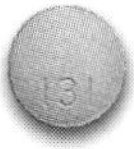

10 mg

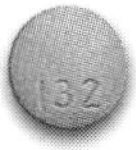

20 mg

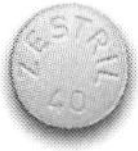

40 mg

Zithromax
(page 197)

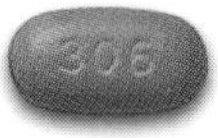

250 mg

Zocor
(page 1143)

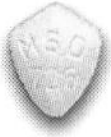
5 mg

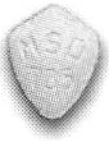
10 mg

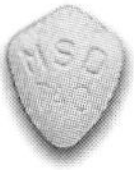
20 mg

Zoloft
(page 1135)

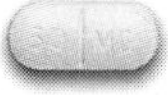
50 mg

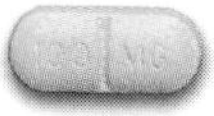
100 mg

Zovirax
(page 110)

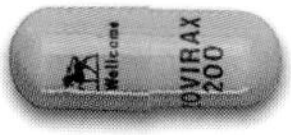

200 mg

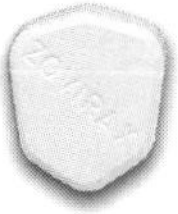
400 mg

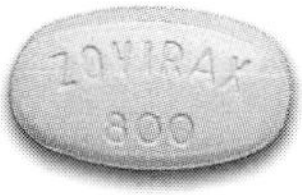

800 mg

• Patient maintains adequate fluid balance.
• Patient and family state understanding of drug therapy.

K

kaolin and pectin mixtures
(KAY-oh-lin and PEK-tin MIX-cherz)
Kaodene Non-Narcotic †, Kaolin w/Pectin†, Kao-Spen, Kapectolin†, K-C†, K-P†

Pharmacologic class: absorbent
Therapeutic class: antidiarrheal
Pregnancy risk category: NR

Indications and dosages
▶ **Mild, nonspecific diarrhea. Regular-strength suspension.** *Adults:* 60 to 120 ml P.O. after each bowel movement.
Children over age 12: 60 ml P.O. after each bowel movement.
Children ages 6 to 12: 30 to 60 ml P.O. after each bowel movement.
Children ages 3 to 6: 15 to 30 ml P.O. after each bowel movement.
Liquid. *Adults:* 45 ml P.O. 1 to 3 times daily or after each loose bowel movement.
Children ages 6 to 12: 22.5 ml P.O.
Children ages 3 to 6: 15 ml P.O.

How supplied
Oral suspension: 5.2 g kaolin and 260 mg pectin per 30 ml† (Kao-Spen, K-C†,), 90 g kaolin and 2 g pectin per 30ml† (Kapectolin†, Kaolin w/Pectin†)
Liquid: 3.9 g Kaolin and 194.4 mg pectin per 30 ml with bismuth subsalicylate (Kaodene)

Pharmacokinetics
Absorption: none.
Distribution: none.
Metabolism: none.
Excretion: excreted in feces.

Route	Onset	Peak	Duration
P.O.	Unknown	Unknown	Unknown

Pharmacodynamics
Chemical effect: decreases fluid content of stool, although total water loss seems to remain the same.
Therapeutic effect: alleviates diarrhea.

Adverse reactions
GI: constipation; drug absorption of nutrients, other drugs, and enzymes; fecal impaction or ulceration (in infants and elderly or debilitated patients after long-term use).

Interactions
Drug-drug. *Oral drugs:* decreased drug absorption. Separate administration times by 2 to 3 hours or more.

Contraindications and precautions
• No known contraindications.
• Use cautiously in pregnant women.

NURSING CONSIDERATIONS

Assessment
• Assess patient's bowel patterns before and after therapy.
• Be alert for adverse GI reactions and drug interactions.
• Evaluate patient's and family's knowledge of drug therapy.

Nursing diagnoses
• Diarrhea related to underlying condition
• Constipation related to long-term use of drug
• Deficient knowledge related to drug therapy

Planning and implementation
• Read label carefully. Check dosage and strength.
• Administer dose after each loose bowel movement.
• Don't use in place of specific therapy for underlying cause of diarrhea.

Patient teaching
• Warn patient not to use drug to replace therapy for underlying cause.
• Advise patient not to use drug for more than 2 days.

✓ Evaluation

- Patient reports decrease in or absence of loose stools.
- Patient doesn't have constipation.
- Patient and family state understanding of drug therapy.

ketoconazole

(kee-toh-KAHN-uh-zohl)
Nizoral

Pharmacologic class: imidazole derivative
Therapeutic class: antifungal
Pregnancy risk category: C

Indications and dosages

▶ **Systemic candidiasis, chronic mucocandidiasis, oral thrush, candiduria, coccidioidomycosis, histoplasmosis, chromomycosis, and paracoccidioidomycosis; severe cutaneous dermatophyte infection resistant to therapy with topical or oral griseofulvin.**
Adults and children weighing more than 40 kg (88 lb): initially, 200 mg P.O. daily in single dose. Dosage may be increased to 400 mg once daily in patients who don't respond to lower dosage.
Children age 2 and older: 3.3 to 6.6 mg/kg P.O. daily as single dose.

How supplied

Tablets: 200 mg

Pharmacokinetics

Absorption: decreased by raised gastric pH and may be increased in extent and consistency by food.
Distribution: distributed into bile, saliva, cerumen, synovial fluid, and sebum. Penetration into CSF is erratic and probably minimal. Drug is 84% to 99% bound to plasma proteins.
Metabolism: metabolized in liver.
Excretion: primarily in feces, with smaller amount excreted in urine. *Half-life:* 8 hours.

Route	Onset	Peak	Duration
P.O.	Unknown	1-2 hr	Unknown

Pharmacodynamics

Chemical effect: inhibits purine transport and DNA, RNA, and protein synthesis; increases cell wall permeability, making fungus more susceptible to osmotic pressure.
Therapeutic effect: kills susceptible fungi or hinders growth. Spectrum of activity includes most pathogenic fungi.

Adverse reactions

CNS: headache, nervousness, dizziness, ***suicidal tendencies.***
GI: *nausea, vomiting,* abdominal pain, diarrhea, constipation.
Hematologic: ***thrombocytopenia.***
Hepatic: elevated liver enzyme levels, ***hepatotoxicity.***
Skin: itching.
Other: gynecomastia with tenderness.

Interactions

Drug-drug. *Antacids, anticholinergics, H_2-receptor antagonists:* decreased ketoconazole absorption. Wait at least 2 hours after ketoconazole dose before giving these drugs.
Corticosteroids: corticosteroid bioavailability may be increased and clearance may be decreased, possibly resulting in toxicity. Monitor patient closely.
Cyclosporine, methylprednisolone, tacrolimus: increased serum levels of these drugs. Adjust their dosages as directed, and monitor their levels closely.
Isoniazid, rifampin: increased ketoconazole metabolism. Monitor patient for decreased antifungal effect.
Oral anticoagulants: anticoagulant response may be enhanced. Monitor PT and INR.
Oral midazolam, triazolam: elevated plasma levels of these drugs, which may potentiate or prolong sedative or hypnotic effects. Avoid concomitant use.

Contraindications and precautions

- Contraindicated in patients hypersensitive to drug and in those taking oral midazolam or triazolam.
- Breast-feeding women should use other feeding methods during therapy.

• Use cautiously in patients with hepatic disease, in those taking other hepatotoxic drugs, and in pregnant women.

NURSING CONSIDERATIONS

Assessment

• Assess patient's infection before therapy and regularly thereafter.
• Evaluate laboratory studies for eradication of fungi.
• Be alert for adverse reactions and drug interactions.
• Monitor patient's hydration status if adverse GI reactions occur.
• Evaluate patient's and family's knowledge of drug therapy.

Nursing diagnoses

• Infection related to presence of susceptible fungi
• Risk for deficient fluid volume related to adverse GI reactions
• Deficient knowledge related to drug therapy

Planning and implementation

• Because of risk of serious hepatotoxicity, drug shouldn't be used for less serious conditions, such as fungus infections of skin or nails.
• To minimize nausea, divide daily amount into two doses. Also, giving drug with meals helps to decrease nausea.
• Have patient dissolve each tablet in 4 ml aqueous solution of 0.2 N hydrochloric acid and sip mixture through straw to avoid contact with teeth. Have patient drink full glass (8 oz) of water afterward.

Patient teaching

• Instruct patient with achlorhydria to dissolve each tablet in 4 ml aqueous solution of 0.2 N hydrochloric acid, sip mixture through a straw (to avoid contact with teeth), and drink a glass of water after the dose because ketoconazole requires gastric acidity for dissolution and absorption.
• Make sure patient understands that treatment should continue until all clinical and laboratory tests indicate that active fungal infection has subsided. If drug is discontinued too soon, infection will recur. Minimum treatment for candidiasis is 7 to 14 days; for other systemic fungal infections, 6 months; for resistant dermatophyte infections, at least 4 weeks.
• Reassure patient that nausea will subside.

Evaluation

• Patient is free from infection.
• Patient maintains adequate hydration.
• Patient and family state understanding of drug therapy.

ketoprofen

(kee-toh-PROH-fen)
Actron caplets†, Apo-Keto♦, Apo-Keto-E♦, Novo-Keto-EC♦, Orudis, Orudis E♦, Orudis KT†, Orudis SR♦ ◇, Oruvail, Rhodis♦, Rhodis-EC♦

Pharmacologic class: NSAID
Therapeutic class: nonnarcotic analgesic, antipyretic, anti-inflammatory
Pregnancy risk category: B

Indications and dosages

▶ **Rheumatoid arthritis and osteoarthritis.** *Adults:* 75 mg t.i.d., 50 mg q.i.d., or 200 mg as sustained-release tablet once daily. Maximum, 300 mg/day. Or, where suppository is available, 100 mg P.R. b.i.d. or one suppository h.s. (with ketoprofen P.O. during day).
▶ **Mild to moderate pain; dysmenorrhea.** *Adults:* 25 to 50 mg P.O. q 6 to 8 hours, p.r.n.
▶ **Minor aches and pain or fever.** *Adults:* 12.5 mg with full glass of water q 4 to 6 hours. Don't exceed 25 mg in 4 hours or 75 mg in 24 hours. Don't give to children under age 16 unless directed by prescriber.

How supplied

Tablets: 12.5 mg†**
Tablets (sustained-release): 200 mg♦
Tablets (enteric-coated): 50 mg♦, 100 mg♦
Capsules (extended-release): 100 mg, 150 mg, 200 mg
Capsules: 25 mg, 50 mg, 75 mg
Suppositories: 100 mg♦

Pharmacokinetics

Absorption: absorbed rapidly and completely from GI tract.
Distribution: highly protein-bound.
Metabolism: metabolized extensively in liver.
Excretion: excreted in urine.

Route	Onset	Peak	Duration
P.O., P.R.	1-2 hr	0.5-2 hr	3-4 hr

Pharmacodynamics

Chemical effect: may inhibit prostaglandin synthesis.
Therapeutic effect: relieves pain, fever, and inflammation.

Adverse reactions

CNS: *headache,* dizziness, *CNS excitation* or depression.
EENT: tinnitus, visual disturbances, ***laryngeal edema.***
GI: *nausea, abdominal pain, diarrhea, constipation, flatulence,* ***peptic ulceration,*** anorexia, vomiting, stomatitis.
GU: ***nephrotoxicity,*** *elevated BUN level.*
Hematologic: prolonged bleeding time, *thrombocytopenia, agranulocytosis.*
Hepatic: elevated liver enzyme levels.
Respiratory: dyspnea, ***bronchospasm.***
Skin: rash, photosensitivity, ***exfoliative dermatitis.***

Interactions

Drug-drug. *Anticoagulants:* may increase anticoagulant effect. Monitor PT and INR.
Aspirin: increased risk of adverse GI reactions and increased ketoprofen levels. Avoid concomitant use.
Corticosteroids: increased risk of adverse GI reactions. Avoid concomitant use.
Hydrochlorothiazide, other diuretics: decreased diuretic effectiveness. Monitor patient for lack of effect.
Lithium, methotrexate: increased levels of these drugs, leading to toxicity. Monitor levels closely.
Oral anticoagulants: increased risk of bleeding. Monitor patient closely.
Probenecid: increased plasma ketoprofen levels. Avoid concomitant use.
Drug-herb. *Dong quai, feverfew, garlic, ginger, horse chestnut, red clover:* possible increased risk of bleeding. Monitor patient closely.
St. John's wort: increased risk of photosensitivity. Advise patient to avoid unprotected exposure to sunlight.
Drug-lifestyle. *Alcohol use:* increased risk of GI toxicity. Discourage concomitant use.
Sun exposure: may cause photosensitivity reactions. Recommend appropriate precautions.

Contraindications and precautions

- Contraindicated in patients hypersensitive to drug and in those with a history of aspirin- or NSAID-induced asthma, urticaria, or other allergic reactions.
- Avoid use of drug during third trimester of pregnancy. Drug isn't recommended for breast-feeding women.
- Use cautiously in patients with history of peptic ulcer disease, renal dysfunction, hypertension, heart failure, or fluid retention.
- Safety of drug hasn't been established in children.
- Don't give drug to children under age 16 unless directed by prescriber.

NURSING CONSIDERATIONS

Assessment

- Assess patient's pain before and after drug administration. Full effect may not occur for 2 to 4 weeks.
- Check renal and hepatic function every 6 months or as directed during long-term therapy.
- Be alert for adverse reactions and drug interactions.
- Monitor patient's hydration status if adverse GI reactions occur.
- Evaluate patient's and family's knowledge of drug therapy.

Nursing diagnoses

- Chronic pain related to underlying condition
- Risk for deficient fluid volume related to adverse GI reactions
- Deficient knowledge related to drug therapy

Planning and implementation

P.O. use: Sustained-release form isn't recommended for patients in acute pain.
- Administer drug on empty stomach unless GI upset occurs.

P.R. use: Follow normal protocol.
- Inform laboratory personnel that patient is taking ketoprofen. Drug may interfere with some laboratory determinations of blood glucose and serum iron levels, depending on testing method used.

Patient teaching
- Tell patient to take drug 30 minutes before or 2 hours after meals. If adverse GI reactions occur, patient may take drug with milk or meals.
- Tell patient that full therapeutic effect may be delayed for 2 to 4 weeks.
- Instruct patient to report adverse visual or auditory reactions immediately.
- Teach patient to recognize and immediately report evidence of GI bleeding. Also, explain that serious GI toxicity, including peptic ulceration and bleeding, can occur in patients taking NSAIDs despite an absence of GI symptoms.
- Alert patient that concomitant use with aspirin, alcohol, or corticosteroids may increase risk of adverse GI reactions.
- Advise patient to use sunblock, wear protective clothing, and avoid prolonged exposure to sunlight. Explain that drug may cause photosensitivity reactions.

Evaluation
- Patient is free from pain.
- Patient maintains normal hydration status.
- Patient and family state understanding of drug therapy.

ketorolac tromethamine
(KEE-toh-roh-lak troh-METH-uh-meen)
Toradol

Pharmacologic class: NSAID
Therapeutic class: analgesic
Pregnancy risk category: C

Indications and dosages

▶ **Short-term management of pain.** *Adults under age 65:* dosage based on patient response. Initially, 60 mg I.M. or 30 mg I.V. as single dose or doses of 30 mg I.M. or I.V. q 6 hours. Maximum, 120 mg daily. To switch to P.O. dosing, initially give 20 mg P.O., and then 10 mg P.O. q 4 to 6 hours, p.r.n., up to 40 mg daily.
Adults age 65 or older, renally impaired patients, and those weighing less than 50 kg (110 lb): initially, 30 mg I.M. or 15 mg I.V. as single dose or doses of 15 mg I.M. or I.V. q 6 hours. Maximum, 60 mg daily. To switch to P.O. dosing, 10 mg P.O. q 4 to 6 hours, p.r.n., up to 40 mg daily. Maximum combined use of drug not to exceed 5 days.

How supplied

Tablets: 10 mg
Injection: 15 mg/ml, 30 mg/ml

Pharmacokinetics

Absorption: completely absorbed after I.M. use. After P.O. use, food delays absorption but doesn't decrease total amount absorbed.
Distribution: more than 99.9% protein-bound.
Metabolism: metabolized mainly in liver.
Excretion: more than 90% excreted in urine, with the remainder excreted in feces. *Half-life:* 3.8 to 6.3 hours.

Route	Onset	Peak	Duration
P.O.	30-60 min	30-60 min	6-8 hr
I.V.	Immediate	Immediate	8 hr
I.M.	≤ 10 min	30-60 min	6-8 hr

Pharmacodynamics

Chemical effect: unknown; may inhibit prostaglandin synthesis.
Therapeutic effect: relieves pain.

Adverse reactions

CNS: drowsiness, sedation, dizziness, headache, sweating.
CV: edema, hypertension, palpitations, arrhythmias.
GI: *nausea, dyspepsia, GI pain,* diarrhea, ***peptic ulceration.***
GU: ***acute renal failure.***

Hematologic: decreased platelet adhesion, purpura, ***thrombocytopenia.***
Metabolic: hyperkalemia.
Respiratory: ***bronchospasm.***
Other: pain at injection site.

Interactions

Drug-drug. *Antihypertensives, diuretics:* decreased effectiveness of these drugs. Monitor reactions closely.
Lithium: increased lithium levels. Monitor levels closely.
Methotrexate: decreased methotrexate clearance and increased toxicity. Don't use together.
Salicylates, warfarin: ketorolac may increase levels of free (unbound) salicylates or warfarin in blood. Clinical significance is unknown.
Drug-herb. *Dong quai, feverfew, garlic, ginger, horse chestnut, red clover:* possible increased risk of bleeding. Monitor patient closely.
St. John's wort: increased risk of photosensitivity. Advise patient to avoid unprotected exposure to sunlight.

Contraindications and precautions

- Contraindicated in patients hypersensitive to drug and in those with a history of syndrome of nasal polyps, angioedema, bronchospastic reactivity, or allergic reactions to aspirin or other NSAIDs.
- Also contraindicated in patients currently receiving aspirin or other NSAIDs, in those with advanced renal impairment, and in those at risk for renal failure as a result of volume depletion.
- Contraindicated in patients with a high risk of bleeding and in those with suspected or confirmed cerebrovascular bleeding, hemorrhage diathesis, and incomplete hemostasis.
- Contraindicated for intrathecal or epidural administration because of its alcohol content.
- Use cautiously in women patients, women giving birth, patients in the perioperative period; and patients with hepatic or renal impairment, history of serious GI events or peptic ulcer disease, cardiac decompensation, hypertension, or coagulation disorders.
- Use cautiously in breast-feeding patients. Trace amounts of drug have been detected in breast milk.
- Safety of drug hasn't been established in children.

NURSING CONSIDERATIONS

Assessment
- Assess patient's pain before and after drug administration.
- Be alert for adverse reactions and drug interactions.
- Evaluate patient's and family's knowledge of drug therapy.

Nursing diagnoses
- Acute pain related to underlying condition
- Risk for injury related to drug-induced adverse CNS reactions
- Deficient knowledge related to drug therapy

Planning and implementation
P.O. use: When switching from injectable to P.O. form, don't exceed 120 mg of drug (including maximum of 40 mg P.O.) on day of transition.
I.V. use: Give I.V. bolus over at least 15 seconds.
I.M. use: Administration by I.M. route may cause pain at injection site. Apply pressure to site for 15 to 30 seconds after injection to minimize local effects.
- Notify prescriber if pain persists or worsens.

Patient teaching
- Teach patient to recognize and immediately report signs and symptoms of GI bleeding. Also explain that serious GI toxicity, including peptic ulceration and bleeding, can occur in patient taking oral NSAIDs despite an absence of GI symptoms.
- Advise patient to report persistent or worsening pain.
- Explain that drug is intended only for short-term use.

Evaluation
- Patient is free from pain.
- Patient sustains no injury from adverse reactions.
- Patient and family state understanding of drug therapy.

L

labetalol hydrochloride

(lah-BAY-tuh-lol high-droh-KLOR-ighd)
Normodyne, Presolol ◇, Trandate

Pharmacologic class: alpha-adrenergic and beta blocker
Therapeutic class: antihypertensive
Pregnancy risk category: C

Indications and dosages

▶ **Hypertension.** *Adults:* 100 mg P.O. b.i.d. with or without diuretic. If needed, increase dosage to 200 mg b.i.d. after 2 days as directed. Further increases may be made q 2 to 3 days until optimum response is reached. Usual maintenance dosage is 200 to 400 mg b.i.d.

▶ **Severe hypertension, hypertensive emergencies.** *Adults:* 200 mg diluted in 160 ml of D_5W, infused at 2 mg/minute until satisfactory response is obtained; then infusion stopped. Dose may be repeated q 6 to 12 hours. Or, administered by repeated I.V. injection: initially, 20 mg I.V. slowly over 2 minutes. Then repeat injections of 40 to 80 mg q 10 minutes until maximum dosage of 300 mg is reached, p.r.n.

How supplied

Tablets: 100 mg, 200 mg, 300 mg
Injection: 5 mg/ml

Pharmacokinetics

Absorption: 90% to 100% absorbed with P.O. administration; however, drug undergoes extensive first-pass metabolism in liver and only about 25% of P.O. dose reaches systemic circulation unchanged.
Distribution: distributed widely throughout body; about 50% protein-bound.
Metabolism: drug administered P.O. metabolized extensively in liver and, possibly, GI mucosa.
Excretion: about 5% excreted unchanged in urine; remainder excreted as metabolites in urine and feces. *Half-life:* about 5½ hours after I.V. dose; 6 to 8 hours after P.O. dose.

Route	Onset	Peak	Duration
P.O.	≤ 20 min	2-4 hr	8-12 hr
I.V.	≤ 2-5 min	5 min	2-4 hr

Pharmacodynamics

Chemical effect: unknown; may be related to reduced peripheral vascular resistance as result of alpha-adrenergic blockade.
Therapeutic effect: lowers blood pressure.

Adverse reactions

CNS: vivid dreams, fatigue, headache, transient scalp tingling.
CV: *orthostatic hypotension and dizziness,* peripheral vascular disease, ***bradycardia, ventricular arrhythmias.***
EENT: nasal stuffiness.
GI: nausea, vomiting, diarrhea.
GU: sexual dysfunction, urine retention.
Respiratory: increased airway resistance.
Skin: rash.

Interactions

Drug-drug. *Cimetidine:* may enhance labetalol's effect. Give together cautiously.
Halothane: additive hypotensive effect. Monitor blood pressure.
Insulin, oral antidiabetics: can alter dosage requirements in previously stabilized diabetic patients. Observe patient carefully.

Contraindications and precautions

- Contraindicated in patients hypersensitive to drug and in those with bronchial asthma, overt cardiac failure, greater than first-degree heart block, cardiogenic shock, severe bradycardia, and other conditions linked to severe and prolonged hypotension.
- Use cautiously in pregnant or breast-feeding women and in patients with heart failure, hepatic failure, chronic bronchitis, emphysema, peripheral vascular disease, or pheochromocytoma.
- Safety of drug hasn't been established in children.

NURSING CONSIDERATIONS

Assessment
- Obtain history of patient's hypertension before therapy.
- Monitor blood pressure frequently. Drug masks common signs of shock.
- When administered I.V. for hypertensive emergencies, labetalol produces rapid, predictable fall in blood pressure within 5 to 10 minutes.
- Be alert for adverse reactions and drug interactions.
- Evaluate patient's and family's knowledge of drug therapy.

Nursing diagnoses
- Ineffective health maintenance related to presence of hypertension
- Risk for trauma related to drug-induced hypotension
- Deficient knowledge related to drug therapy

Planning and implementation
ALERT Don't confuse Trandate with Tridrate.
P.O. use: If dizziness occurs, ask prescriber if patient may take dose at bedtime or take smaller doses t.i.d. to help minimize this reaction.
I.V. use: Administer diluted infusion with infusion-control device. Monitor blood pressure q 5 minutes for 30 minutes, then q 30 minutes for 2 hours, then hourly for 6 hours. Patient should remain in supine position for 3 hours after infusion. For I.V. injection, blood pressure should be monitored immediately before and 5 to 10 minutes after injection.
ALERT Sodium bicarbonate injection is incompatible with I.V. labetalol.

Patient teaching
- Tell patient that abrupt discontinuation of therapy can exacerbate angina and precipitate MI.
- Inform patient that dizziness can be minimized by rising slowly and avoiding sudden position changes.

Evaluation
- Patient's blood pressure is normal.
- Patient doesn't experience trauma caused by drug-induced hypotension.
- Patient and family state understanding of drug therapy.

lactulose
(LAK-tyoo-lohs)
Cephulac, Cholac, Chronulac, Constilac, Constulose, Duphalac, Enulose, Evalose, Heptalac, Lac-Dol ◇

Pharmacologic class: disaccharide
Therapeutic class: laxative
Pregnancy risk category: B

Indications and dosages
▶ **Constipation.** *Adults:* 10 to 20 g (15 to 30 ml) P.O. daily.
▶ **Prevention and treatment of hepatic encephalopathy, including hepatic precoma and coma in patients with severe hepatic disease.** *Adults:* initially, 20 to 30 g (30 to 45 ml) P.O. t.i.d. or q.i.d. until two or three soft stools are produced daily. Usual dosage is 30 to 50 g daily t.i.d. Or, 200 g (300 ml) diluted with 700 ml of water or saline solution and administered as retention enema q 4 to 6 hours, p.r.n.

How supplied
Syrup: 10 g/15 ml

Pharmacokinetics
Absorption: absorbed minimally.
Distribution: distributed locally, primarily in colon.
Metabolism: metabolized by colonic bacteria (absorbed portion isn't metabolized).
Excretion: most excreted in feces; absorbed portion excreted in urine.

Route	Onset	Peak	Duration
P.O.	24-48 hr	Varies	Varies
P.R.	Unknown	Unknown	Unknown

Pharmacodynamics
Chemical effect: produces osmotic effect in colon. Resulting distention promotes peristalsis. Lactulose also decreases blood ammonia, probably as result of bacterial degradation, which lowers pH of colon contents.

Therapeutic effect: relieves constipation.

Adverse reactions

GI: *abdominal cramps, belching, diarrhea, distention, flatulence.*
Metabolic: hypernatremia.

Interactions

Drug-drug. *Antacids, antibiotics, orally administered neomycin:* decreased effectiveness of lactulose. Avoid concomitant use.

Contraindications and precautions

- Contraindicated in patients on low-galactose diet.
- Use cautiously in patients with diabetes mellitus.

NURSING CONSIDERATIONS

Assessment

- Assess patient's condition before therapy and regularly thereafter, including mental status if patient has hepatic encephalopathy.
- Monitor serum sodium levels.
- Be alert for adverse reactions and drug interactions.
- Evaluate patient's and family's knowledge of drug therapy.

Nursing diagnoses

- Constipation related to underlying condition
- Deficient knowledge related to drug therapy

Planning and implementation

ALERT Don't confuse lactulose with lactose.

- Be prepared to replace fluid loss.
- Store drug at room temperature, preferably below 86° F (30° C). Don't freeze.
- To minimize sweet taste, dilute with water or fruit juice or give with food.
- If enema isn't retained for at least 30 minutes, be prepared to repeat dose.

Patient teaching

- Advise patient to dilute drug with juice or water or to take it with food to improve taste.
- Inform patient of adverse reactions and tell him to notify prescriber if reactions become bothersome or if diarrhea occurs.

Evaluation

- Patient's constipation is relieved.
- Patient and family state understanding of drug therapy.

lamivudine

(la-MI-vyoo-deen)
Epivir, Epivir-HBV

Pharmacologic class: synthetic nucleoside analogue
Therapeutic class: antiviral
Pregnancy risk category: C

Indications and dosages

▶ **HIV infection concomitantly with zidovudine.** *Adults weighing 50 kg (110 lb) or more and children age 12 and older:* 150 mg P.O. b.i.d.
Adults weighing less than 50 kg: 2 mg/kg P.O. b.i.d.
Children ages 3 months to 12 years: 4 mg/kg P.O. b.i.d. Maximum dose is 150 mg b.i.d.
▶ **Treatment of chronic hepatitis B with evidence of hepatitis B viral replication and active liver inflammation.** *Adults:* 100 mg P.O. once daily. Safety and effectiveness of treatment beyond 1 year haven't been established; optimum duration of treatment isn't known. If lamivudine is given to patients with HBV and HIV, higher dosage indicated for HIV therapy should be used as part of an appropriate combination regimen.

How supplied

Tablets: 100 mg, 150 mg
Oral solution: 5 mg/ml, 10 mg/ml

Pharmacokinetics

Absorption: rapidly absorbed after P.O. administration in HIV-infected patients.
Distribution: believed to distribute into extravascular spaces. Volume of distribution is independent of dose and doesn't correlate with body weight. Less than 36% is bound to plasma proteins.
Metabolism: drug has a minor route of elimination. The only known metabolite is the trans-sulfoxide metabolite.

Excretion: drug is primarily eliminated unchanged in urine. *Mean elimination half-life:* 5 to 7 hours.

Route	Onset	Peak	Duration
P.O.	Unknown	1-3 hr	Unknown

Pharmacodynamics

Chemical effect: A synthetic nucleoside analogue that inhibits HIV reverse transcription via viral DNA chain termination. RNA- and DNA-dependent DNA polymerase activities are also inhibited.

Therapeutic effect: reduces the symptoms linked to HIV infection.

Adverse reactions

Adverse reactions pertain to the combination therapy of lamivudine and zidovudine.

CNS: *headache, fatigue, neuropathy, malaise, dizziness, insomnia, sleep disorders,* depressive disorders.

GI: *nausea, diarrhea, vomiting, anorexia,* abdominal pain, abdominal cramps, dyspepsia, ***pancreatitis.***

EENT: *nasal symptoms.*

Hematologic: ***neutropenia,*** anemia, ***thrombocytopenia.***

Hepatic: elevated liver enzyme and bilirubin levels.

Musculoskeletal: *musculoskeletal pain,* myalgia, arthralgia.

Respiratory: *cough.*

Skin: rash.

Other: *fever, chills.*

Interactions

Drug-drug. *Trimethoprim/sulfamethoxazole:* decreased lamivudine clearance and possible increased blood levels. Monitor patient closely.

Zidovudine: increased serum zidovudine level. Monitor patient closely.

Contraindications and precautions

- Contraindicated in patients hypersensitive to drug. Drug should be used with extreme caution, if at all, in children with history of pancreatitis or other significant risk factors for development of pancreatitis. Women infected with HIV and those taking lamivudine shouldn't breast-feed.

NURSING CONSIDERATIONS

Assessment

- Obtain history of patient's underlying condition before therapy, and reassess regularly thereafter.
- Patients should be tested for HIV before and during treatment because formulation and dosage of lamivudine in Epivir-HBV aren't appropriate for those dually infected with hepatitis B virus and HIV.
- Monitor renal function before and during therapy.
- Monitor serum amylase level.
- Monitor patient's CBC, platelet count, and renal and liver function studies, as ordered. Report abnormalities.
- Evaluate patient's and family's knowledge of drug therapy.

Nursing diagnoses

- Risk for infection related to the presence of HIV
- Risk for injury related to drug-induced CNS adverse reactions
- Deficient knowledge related to drug therapy

Planning and implementation

- Patients with renal insufficiency need a dosage adjustment.
- If lamivudine is given to patients with hepatitis B virus and HIV, the higher dosage indicated for HIV therapy should be used as part of an appropriate combination regimen.
- Administer drug with zidovudine. It's not currently indicated for use alone unless for chronic hepatitis B virus infection.
- Safety and effectiveness of treatment with Epivir-HBV beyond 1 year haven't been established; optimum duration of treatment isn't known.
- Stop lamivudine treatment immediately and notify prescriber if clinical signs, symptoms, or laboratory abnormalities suggest pancreatitis.
- An Antiretroviral Pregnancy Registry has been established to monitor maternal-fetal outcomes of pregnant women exposed to lamivu-

dine. To register a pregnant patient, the prescriber can call 1-800-258-4263.

Patient teaching

• Inform patient that long-term effects of lamivudine are unknown.
• Stress importance of taking lamivudine exactly as prescribed.
• Teach parents the signs and symptoms of pancreatitis. Advise them to report signs and symptoms immediately.

☑ Evaluation

• Patient responds well to drug therapy.
• Patient sustains no injury as a result of drug-induced CNS adverse reactions.
• Patient and family state understanding of drug therapy.

lamivudine/zidovudine

(la-MI-vyoo-deen/zye-DOE-vyoo-deen)
Combivir

Pharmacologic class: reverse transcriptase inhibitor
Therapeutic class: antiretroviral
Pregnancy risk category: C

Indications and dosages

▶ **Treatment of HIV infection.** *Adults and children age 12 and older weighing more than 50 kg (110 lb):* one tablet P.O. b.i.d.

How supplied

Tablets: 150 mg lamivudine and 300 mg zidovudine

Pharmacokinetics

Absorption: both drugs are rapidly absorbed after P.O. administration, with bioavailability of 86% and 64%, respectively.
Distribution: both drugs are extensively distributed with low protein-binding.
Metabolism: only about 5% of lamivudine is metabolized; zidovudine is primarily (74%) metabolized in the liver.
Excretion: lamivudine is primarily eliminated unchanged in the urine. Zidovudine and its major metabolite are primarily eliminated in the urine. Elimination half-lives of lamivudine and zidovudine are 5 to 7 hours and ½ to 3 hours, respectively. Renal excretion is a principal route of elimination, and dosage adjustments are necessary in patients with compromised renal function making this fixed ratio combination unsuitable. Hemodialysis and peritoneal dialysis have negligible effect on the removal of zidovudine, but removal of its metabolite, GZDV, is enhanced. The effect of dialysis on lamivudine is unknown.

Route	Onset	Peak	Duration
P.O.	Unknown	Unknown	Unknown

Pharmacodynamics

Chemical effect: inhibits reverse transcriptase via DNA chain termination. Both drugs are also weak inhibitors of DNA polymerase. Together, they have synergistic antiretroviral activity. Combination therapy with lamivudine and zidovudine is targeted at suppressing or delaying the emergence of resistant strains that can occur with retroviral monotherapy because dual resistance requires multiple mutations.
Therapeutic effect: reduces the symptoms of HIV infection.

Adverse reactions

CNS: *headache, malaise, fatigue, insomnia, dizziness, neuropathy,* depression.
EENT: *nasal signs and symptoms.*
GI: *nausea, diarrhea, vomiting, anorexia,* abdominal pain, abdominal cramps, dyspepsia.
Hematologic: ***neutropenia,*** anemia.
Hepatic: increased ALT, AST, and amylase levels.
Musculoskeletal: *musculoskeletal pain,* myalgia, arthralgia.
Respiratory: *cough.*
Skin: rash.
Other: *fever, chills.*

Interactions

Drug-drug. *Ganciclovir, interferon-alpha, other bone marrow suppressive or cytotoxic drugs:* may increase zidovudine's hematologic toxicity. Monitor patient.

Contraindications and precautions

• Contraindicated in patients hypersensitive to drug or its components and in those who need dosage adjustments, such as children under age 12, those weighing less than 50 kg, and those with creatinine clearance below 50 ml/minute. Also contraindicated in patients experiencing dose-limiting adverse effects. Women infected with HIV and those taking Combivir shouldn't breast-feed.

NURSING CONSIDERATIONS

Assessment

• Obtain history of patient's underlying condition before therapy, and reassess regularly thereafter.
• Watch for bone marrow toxicity with frequent blood counts, particularly in patients with advanced HIV infection.
• Monitor patient for signs of lactic acidosis or hepatotoxicity (abdominal pain, jaundice) and notify the prescriber.
• Assess patient's fine motor skills and peripheral sensation for evidence of peripheral neuropathies.
• Evaluate patient's and family's knowledge of drug therapy.

Nursing diagnoses

• Risk for infection related to the presence of HIV
• Disturbed sensory perception (tactile) related to drug-induced peripheral neuropathy
• Deficient knowledge related to drug therapy

Planning and implementation

• This drug combination may be inappropriate for patients with compromised renal function.
• Use drug cautiously in patients with bone marrow suppression as evidenced by granulocyte count below 1,000 cells/mm^3 or hemoglobin level below 9.5 g/dl.
• An Antiretroviral Pregnancy Registry has been established to monitor maternal-fetal outcomes of pregnant women exposed to Combivir. To register a pregnant patient, prescriber can call 1-800-258-4263.

Patient teaching

• Advise patient that therapy with lamivudine and zidovudine won't cure HIV infection and that he may continue to experience illness, including opportunistic infections.
• Warn patient that HIV transmission can still occur with drug therapy.
• Educate patient about using barrier contraception when engaging in sexual activities to prevent disease transmission.
• Teach patient signs and symptoms of neutropenia and anemia (fever, chills, infection, fatigue) and instruct him to report such occurrences.
• Tell patient to have blood counts followed closely while on drug, especially if he has advanced disease.
• Advise patient to consult prescriber or pharmacist before taking other drugs.
• Warn patient to report abdominal pain immediately.
• Instruct patient to report signs and symptoms of myopathy or myositis (muscle inflammation, pain, weakness, decrease in muscle size).
• Stress importance of taking combination drug therapy exactly as prescribed to reduce the development of resistance.
• Tell patient he may take combination with or without food.
• Inform women that breast-feeding is contraindicated in HIV infection and during drug therapy.

Evaluation

• Patient responds well to drug.
• Patient doesn't develop peripheral neuropathy.
• Patient and family state understanding of drug therapy.

lamotrigine

(lah-MOH-trigh-jeen)
Lamictal

Pharmacologic class: phenytriazine
Therapeutic class: anticonvulsant
Pregnancy risk category: C

Indications and dosages

▶ **Adjunct therapy in treatment of partial seizures caused by epilepsy.** *Adults and children over age 16:* 50 mg P.O. daily for 2 weeks, followed by 100 mg daily in two divided doses for 2 weeks. Usual maintenance dosage is 300 to 500 mg P.O. daily in two divided doses. For patients also taking valproic acid, 25 mg P.O. every other day for 2 weeks, followed by 25 mg P.O. daily for 2 weeks. Thereafter, maximum 150 mg P.O. daily in divided doses.

▶ **Adjunctive treatment for Lennox-Gaustaut Syndrome.** *Adults and children over age 12:* for patients receiving an antiepileptic drug regimen with valproic acid, 25 mg P.O. every other day for 2 weeks; then 25 mg P.O. daily for 2 weeks. Thereafter, usual maintenance dosage is 100 to 400 mg P.O. daily in one or two divided doses. For patients taking enzyme-inducing antiepileptics but not valproic acid, 50 mg P.O. daily for 2 weeks; then 100 mg P.O. daily in two divided doses for 2 weeks. Thereafter, usual maintenance dosage is 300 to 500 mg P.O. daily in divided doses.

Children ages 2 to 12 weighing more than 17 kg (37 lb): for patients receiving antiepileptic drug regimen with valproic acid, 0.15mg/kg/day P.O. in one or two doses (rounded down to nearest 5 mg) for 2 weeks. If calculated daily dose of lamotrigine is 2.5 to 5 mg, 5 mg of lamotrigine should be taken on alternate days; then 0.3 mg/kg/day P.O. in one or two doses rounded down to nearest 5 mg for 2 weeks. Thereafter, usual maintenance dosage is 1 to 5 mg/kg/day (maximum 200 mg/day in one dose or two divided doses). For patients receiving an antiepileptic drug regimen without valproic acid, 0.6 mg/kg/day P.O. in two divided doses rounded down to nearest 5 mg for 2 weeks; then 1.2 mg/kg/day P.O. in divided doses rounded down to nearest 5 mg for 2 weeks. Thereafter, usual maintenance dosage is 5 to 15 mg/kg/day (maximum 400 mg/day in divided doses).

How supplied

Tablets: 25 mg, 100 mg, 150 mg, 200 mg
Tablets (chewable dispersible): 5 mg, 25 mg

Pharmacokinetics

Absorption: rapidly and completely absorbed after P.O. administration with negligible first-pass metabolism.
Distribution: 55% protein-bound.
Metabolism: predominantly by glucuronic acid conjugation.
Excretion: excreted primarily in urine. *Half-life:* 14.4 to 70.3 hours, depending on dosage schedule and use of other anticonvulsants.

Route	Onset	Peak	Duration
P.O.	Unknown	1.4-4.8 hr	Unknown

Pharmacodynamics

Chemical effect: unknown; may inhibit release of glutamate and aspartate, excitatory neurotransmitters in the brain, through action at sodium channels.
Therapeutic effect: prevents partial seizure activity.

Adverse reactions

CNS: *dizziness, headache, ataxia, somnolence,* incoordination, insomnia, tremors, depression, anxiety, ***seizures,*** irritability, speech disorder, decreased memory, aggravated reaction, concentration disturbance, sleep disorder, emotional lability, vertigo, malaise, mind racing, ***suicide attempts.***
CV: palpitations.
EENT: *diplopia, blurred vision,* vision abnormality, nystagmus, rhinitis, pharyngitis.
GI: *nausea, vomiting,* diarrhea, dyspepsia, abdominal pain, constipation, anorexia, dry mouth.
GU: dysmenorrhea, vaginitis, amenorrhea.
Musculoskeletal: dysarthria, muscle spasm, neck pain.
Respiratory: cough, dyspnea.
Skin: ***Stevens-Johnson syndrome, toxic epidermal necrolysis,*** *rash,* pruritus, hot flushes, alopecia, acne.
Other: flu syndrome, fever, infection, chills, tooth disorder.

Interactions

Drug-drug. *Acetaminophen*: serum lamotrigine levels may be reduced, decreasing therapeutic effects. Monitor patient.

Carbamazepine, phenobarbital, phenytoin, primidone: decreased steady-state levels of lamotrigine. Monitor patient closely.
Folate inhibitors (such as co-trimoxazole, methotrexate): may have additive effect because lamotrigine inhibits dihydrofolate reductase, an enzyme involved in folic acid synthesis. Monitor patient closely.
Valproic acid: decreases lamotrigine clearance, which increases steady-state levels. Monitor patient closely for toxicity.
Drug-lifestyle. *Sun exposure:* photosensitivity reactions may occur. Urge precautions.

Contraindications and precautions

- Contraindicated in patients hypersensitive to drug and in children under age 16.
- Use of drug in breast-feeding women isn't recommended.
- Use cautiously in patients with renal, hepatic, or cardiac impairment and in pregnant women.

NURSING CONSIDERATIONS

Assessment

- Obtain history of patient's seizure disorder before therapy.
- Evaluate patient for reduction in frequency and duration of seizures after therapy begins. Check adjunct anticonvulsant's serum levels periodically, as ordered.
- Evaluate patient's and family's knowledge of drug therapy.

Nursing diagnoses

- Risk for trauma related to seizures
- Risk for impaired skin integrity related to dermatologic reactions
- Deficient knowledge related to drug therapy

Planning and implementation

- Dosage should be lowered if drug is added to multidrug regimen that includes valproic acid.
- Lowered maintenance dosage should be used in patients with severe renal impairment.
- Don't stop drug abruptly because doing so increases the risk of seizures. Instead, drug should be tapered over at least 2 weeks.

ALERT Rash may be life-threatening. Stop drug and notify prescriber at first sign of rash, unless it isn't drug-related.

Patient teaching

- Inform patient that lamotrigine may cause rash. Combination therapy with valproic acid and lamotrigine may be more likely to cause serious rash. Tell patient to report rash or signs or symptoms of hypersensitivity promptly because they could be serious enough to warrant discontinuation of drug.
- Instruct patient to avoid prolonged exposure to the sun, use sunblock, and wear protective clothing.
- Warn patient not to engage in hazardous activity until CNS effects of drug are known.

Evaluation

- Patient is seizure-free.
- Drug-induced skin impairment doesn't develop.
- Patient and family state understanding of drug therapy.

lansoprazole

(lan-soh-PRAY-zohl)
Prevacid

Pharmacologic class: substituted benzimidazole
Therapeutic class: antiulcer agent
Pregnancy risk category: B

Indications and dosages

▶ **Short-term treatment of active duodenal ulcer.** *Adults:* 15 mg P.O. daily before meals for 4 weeks.
▶ **Maintenance of healed duodenal ulcers.** *Adults:* 15 mg P.O. once daily.
▶ **Short-term treatment of erosive esophagitis.** *Adults:* 30 mg P.O. daily before meals for up to 8 weeks. If healing doesn't occur, additional 8 weeks of therapy may be given. Maintenance dosage for healing is 15 mg P.O. daily.
▶ **Short-term treatment of active benign gastric ulcer.** *Adults:* 30 mg P.O. once daily for up to 8 weeks.

▶ ***Helicobacter pylori* eradication to reduce risk of duodenal ulcer recurrence. Triple therapy.** *Adults:* 30 mg P.O. lansoprazole with 500 mg P.O. clarithromycin and 1 g P.O. amoxicillin, each given q 12 hours for 14 days. **Dual therapy.** *Adults:* 30 mg P.O. lansoprazole with 1 g P.O. amoxicillin, each given q 8 hours for 14 days.

▶ **Long-term treatment of pathologic hypersecretory conditions, including Zollinger-Ellison syndrome.** *Adults:* initially, 60 mg P.O. once daily. Dosage increased as needed. If more than 120 mg/day, give in divided doses.

▶ **Short-term treatment of symptomatic gastroesophageal reflux disease (GERD).** *Adults:* 15 mg P.O. daily for up to 8 weeks.

How supplied

Capsules (delayed-release): 15 mg, 30 mg

Pharmacokinetics

Absorption: absorbed rapidly.
Distribution: 97% bound to plasma proteins.
Metabolism: metabolized extensively in liver.
Excretion: excreted mainly in feces, minimally in urine. *Half-life:* less than 2 hours.

Route	Onset	Peak	Duration
P.O.	Unknown	1.7 hr	> 24 hr

Pharmacodynamics

Chemical effect: inhibits activity of proton pump and binds to hydrogen or potassium adenosine triphosphatase, located at secretory surface of gastric parietal cells.
Therapeutic effect: decreases gastric acid formation.

Adverse reactions

GI: diarrhea, nausea, abdominal pain.

Interactions

Drug-drug. *Ampicillin esters, digoxin, iron salts, ketoconazole:* lansoprazole may interfere with absorption. Monitor patient closely.
Sucralfate: delays lansoprazole absorption. Give lansoprazole at least 30 minutes before sucralfate.
Theophylline: theophylline clearance may increase slightly. Use together cautiously. Dosage adjustment of theophylline may be necessary when lansoprazole is started or stopped.
Drug-herb. *Male fern:* male fern is inactivated in alkaline environments. Discourage concomitant use.
St. John's wort: increased risk of photosensitivity. Advise patient to avoid unprotected exposure to sunlight.

Contraindications and precautions

- Contraindicated in patients hypersensitive to drug.
- Drug isn't recommended for breast-feeding women.
- Use cautiously in pregnant women.
- Safety of drug hasn't been established in children.

NURSING CONSIDERATIONS

Assessment

- Assess patient's condition before therapy and regularly thereafter.
- Be alert for adverse reactions and drug interactions.
- Evaluate patient's and family's knowledge of drug therapy.

Nursing diagnoses

- Impaired tissue integrity related to underlying condition
- Ineffective health maintenance related to drug-induced adverse reactions
- Deficient knowledge related to drug therapy

Planning and implementation

- Give drug on empty stomach.
- Dosage adjustment may be necessary for patients with severe liver disease.
- Drug shouldn't be used as maintenance therapy for patient with duodenal ulcer or erosive esophagitis.
- Notify prescriber if adverse reactions occur, and be prepared to provide supportive care.

Patient teaching

- Instruct patient to take drug before eating. Tell the patient who has trouble swallowing capsules to open and sprinkle contents over

applesauce, and to swallow immediately. The contents shouldn't be chewed or crushed.
- Instruct patient to notify prescriber if adverse reactions occur.

☑ Evaluation
- Patient regains normal GI tissue integrity.
- Patient doesn't experience serious adverse reactions.
- Patient and family state understanding of drug therapy.

leflunomide
(leh-FLOO-noh-mighd)
Arava

Pharmacologic class: pyrimidine synthesis inhibitor
Therapeutic class: immunomodulatory agent
Pregnancy risk category: X

Indications and dosages

▶ **Treatment of active rheumatoid arthritis to reduce signs and symptoms and to retard structural damage as evidenced by X-ray erosions and joint space narrowing.** *Adults:* 100 mg P.O. q 24 hours for 3 days followed by 20 mg (maximum daily dosage) P.O. q 24 hours. Dosage may be decreased to 10 mg daily if higher dosage isn't well-tolerated.

How supplied

Tablets: 10 mg, 20 mg, 100 mg

Pharmacokinetics

Absorption: 80% of dose is absorbed following P.O. administration.
Distribution: extensively bound to albumin; has low volume of distribution.
Metabolism: primary route of metabolism hasn't been identified.
Excretion: excreted renally as well as by direct biliary elimination; 43% excreted in urine, 48% eliminated in feces.

Route	Onset	Peak	Duration
P.O.	Unknown	6-12 hr	Unknown

Pharmacodynamics

Chemical effect: inhibits dihydroorotate dehydrogenase, an enzyme involved in pyrimidine synthesis, and has antiproliferative activity and anti-inflammatory effects.
Therapeutic effect: reduces pain and inflammation related to rheumatoid arthritis.

Adverse reactions

CNS: asthenia, dizziness, headache, paresthesia, malaise, migraine, sleep disorder, vertigo, neuritis, anxiety, depression, insomnia, neuralgia.
CV: angina pectoris, *hypertension,* chest pain, peripheral edema, palpitations, tachycardia, vasculitis, vasodilation, varicose veins.
EENT: pharyngitis, rhinitis, sinusitis, epistaxis, enlarged salivary gland, blurred vision, cataract, conjunctivitis, eye disorder.
GI: mouth ulcer, oral candidiasis, stomatitis, dry mouth, anorexia, *diarrhea,* dyspepsia, gastroenteritis, nausea, abdominal pain, vomiting, cholelithiasis, colitis, constipation, esophagitis, flatulence, gastritis, melena, gingivitis, taste perversion.
GU: urinary tract infection, albuminuria, cystitis, dysuria, hematuria, menstrual disorder, pelvic pain, vaginal candidiasis, prostate disorder, urinary frequency.
Hematologic: anemia, hyperlipidemia.
Hepatic: elevated liver enzyme levels.
Metabolic: weight loss, diabetes mellitus, hyperglycemia, hyperthyroidism, hypokalemia.
Musculoskeletal: arthrosis, back pain, bursitis, muscle cramps, myalgia, bone necrosis, bone pain, arthralgia, leg cramps, joint disorder, neck pain, synovitis, tendon rupture, tenosynovitis.
Respiratory: bronchitis, increased cough, pneumonia, *respiratory infection,* asthma, dyspnea, lung disorder.
Skin: *alopecia,* eczema, pruritus, *rash,* dry skin, acne, contact dermatitis, fungal dermatitis, hair discoloration, hematoma, nail disorder, skin nodule, subcutaneous nodule, maculopapular rash, skin disorder, skin discoloration, skin ulcer, increased sweating, ecchymosis.

Other: allergic reaction, flu syndrome, fever, injury or accident, pain, abscess, cyst, hernia, increased CK, tooth disorder, herpes simplex, herpes zoster.

Interactions

Drug-drug. *Cholestyramine, charcoal:* decreased plasma leflunomide levels. Sometimes used for this effect in overdose.
Methotrexate, other hepatotoxic drugs: increased risk of hepatotoxicity. Monitor liver enzyme levels, as ordered.
NSAIDs (diclofenac, ibuprofen): increased NSAID levels. Clinical significance is unknown.
Rifampin: increased active leflunomide metabolite level. Use together cautiously.
Tolbutamide: increased tolbutamide levels. Clinical significance is unknown.

Contraindications and precautions

- Contraindicated in patients hypersensitive to drug or its components, in women who are or may become pregnant, and in women who are breast-feeding.
- Drug isn't recommended for patients with hepatic insufficiency, hepatitis B or C, severe immunodeficiency, bone marrow dysplasia, or severe uncontrolled infections.
- Vaccination with live vaccines isn't recommended. Long half-life of drug should be considered when contemplating administration of a live vaccine after stopping drug treatment.
- Drug isn't recommended for children under age 18 and men attempting to father children.
- Use cautiously in patients with renal insufficiency.
- Some immunosuppression drugs, including leflunomide, cause an increased risk of malignancy, particularly lymphoproliferative disorders.

NURSING CONSIDERATIONS

Assessment

- Assess patient's condition before therapy and regularly thereafter.
- Be alert for adverse reactions and drug interactions.
- Monitor liver enzymes (ALT and AST) before starting therapy and monthly thereafter until stable. Frequency of monitoring can then be decreased based on clinical situation.
- Evaluate patient's and family's knowledge of drug therapy.

Nursing diagnoses

- Ineffective health maintenance related to underlying disease.
- Deficient knowledge related to drug therapy.

Planning and implementation

ALERT Drug can cause fetal harm when given to pregnant women. Discontinue drug in women planning to become pregnant, and notify prescriber.

- Drug should be discontinued in man who plans to father a child. Tell patient to follow recommended leflunomide removal protocol (cholestyramine 8 g P.O. t.i.d. for 11 days).

Patient teaching

- Explain need for and frequency of required blood test monitoring.
- Instruct patient to use contraceptive measures during drug therapy and until drug is no longer active.
- Advise patient to notify prescriber immediately if pregnancy is suspected.
- Advise breast-feeding patient to discontinue breast-feeding during drug therapy.
- Inform patient that aspirin, other NSAIDs, and low-dose corticosteroids may be continued during treatment; however, combined use of drug with antimalarials, I.M. or P.O. gold, penicillamine, azathioprine, or methotrexate hasn't been adequately studied.

Evaluation

- Patient has improvement in symptoms of rheumatoid arthritis.
- Patient and family state understanding of drug therapy.

leucovorin calcium (citrovorum factor, folinic acid)

(loo-koh-VOR-in KAL-see-um)
Wellcovorin

Pharmacologic class: formyl derivative (active reduced form of folic acid)
Therapeutic class: vitamin, antidote
Pregnancy risk category: C

Indications and dosages

▶ **Overdose of folic acid antagonist.** *Adults and children:* P.O., I.M., or I.V. dose equivalent to weight of antagonist given.

▶ **Rescue after high methotrexate dose in treatment of cancer.** *Adults and children:* 10 mg/m^2 P.O., I.M., or I.V. q 6 hours until methotrexate level falls below 5×10^{-8} M.

▶ **Megaloblastic anemia caused by congenital enzyme deficiency.** *Adults and children:* 3 to 6 mg I.M. daily; then 1 mg P.O. or I.M. daily for life.

▶ **Folate-deficient megaloblastic anemia.** *Adults and children:* up to 1 mg P.O. or I.M daily. Duration of treatment depends on hematologic response.

▶ **Treatment of hematologic toxicity caused by pyrimethamine or trimethoprim therapy.** *Adults and children:* 5 to 15 mg P.O. or I.M. daily.

▶ **Palliative treatment of advanced colorectal carcinoma.** *Adults:* 20 mg/m^2 I.V., followed by fluorouracil, for 5 consecutive days. Repeated q 4 weeks for two additional courses; then q 4 to 5 weeks, if tolerated.

How supplied

Tablets: 5 mg, 10 mg, 15 mg, 25 mg
Injection: 1-ml ampule (3 mg/ml with 0.9% benzyl alcohol)
Powder for injection: 50 mg/vial, 100 mg/vial, 350 mg/vial

Pharmacokinetics

Absorption: absorbed rapidly after P.O. administration.
Distribution: distributed throughout body; liver contains about one-half of total body folate stores.
Metabolism: metabolized in liver.
Excretion: excreted by kidneys. *Half-life:* 6.2 hours.

Route	Onset	Peak	Duration
P.O.	20-30 min	2-3 hr	3-6 hr
I.V.	5 min	10 min	3-6 hr
I.M.	10-20 min	< 1 hr	3-6 hr

Pharmacodynamics

Chemical effect: readily converts to other folic acid derivatives.
Therapeutic effect: raises folic acid level in body.

Adverse reactions

Respiratory: ***bronchospasm.***
Skin: hypersensitivity reactions (rash, pruritus, erythema).

Interactions

Drug-drug. *Anticonvulsants:* may decrease anticonvulsant effectiveness. Monitor patient closely.
Fluorouracil: may enhance fluorouracil toxicity. Avoid concomitant use.
Methotrexate: may decrease efficacy of intrathecal methotrexate. Avoid concomitant use.

Contraindications and precautions

- Contraindicated in patients with pernicious anemia and other megaloblastic anemias caused by lack of vitamin B_{12}.

NURSING CONSIDERATIONS

Assessment

- Assess patient's condition before therapy and regularly thereafter.
- Monitor serum creatinine level daily to detect renal dysfunction.
- Be alert for adverse reactions and drug interactions.
- Monitor patient for rash, wheezing, pruritus, and urticaria, which can be signs of drug allergy.
- Evaluate patient's and family's knowledge of drug therapy.

Nursing diagnoses
- Ineffective health maintenance related to underlying conditions
- Deficient knowledge related to drug therapy

Planning and implementation
ALERT Don't confuse leucovorin (folinic acid) with folic acid.
P.O. and I.M. use: Follow normal protocol.
I.V. use: When using powder for injection, reconstitute 50-mg vial with 5 ml, 100-mg vial with 10 ml, or 350-mg vial with 17 ml of sterile water or bacteriostatic water for injection. When doses are greater than 10 mg/m^2, don't use diluents containing benzyl alcohol.
ALERT Don't exceed 160 mg/minute when giving by direct injection.
- To avoid confusion, don't refer to leucovorin as folinic acid.
- Follow leucovorin rescue schedule and protocol closely to maximize therapeutic response.
- Don't give simultaneously with systemic methotrexate.
- Protect drug from light and heat, especially reconstituted parenteral forms.

Patient teaching
- Tell patient reason for drug use.

Evaluation
- Patient's condition improves.
- Patient and family state understanding of drug therapy.

leuprolide acetate
(loo-PROH-lighd AS-ih-tayt)
Leupron for Pediatric use, Lucrin ◇, Lupron, Lupron Depot, Lupron Depot-Ped, Lupron Depot-3 Month, Lupron Depot-4 Month

Pharmacologic class: gonadotropin-releasing hormone
Therapeutic class: antineoplastic, luteinizing hormone-releasing hormone analogue
Pregnancy risk category: X

Indications and dosages
▶ **Advanced prostate cancer.** *Adults:* 1 mg S.C. daily. Or, 7.5 mg I.M. (depot injection) monthly. Or, 22.5 mg I.M. q 3 months (84 days). Or, 30 mg I.M. q 4 months (4 weeks, depot).
▶ **Endometriosis.** *Adults:* 3.75 mg I.M. (depot injection only) as single injection once monthly for up to 6 months.
▶ **Central precocious puberty.** *Children:* initially, 0.3 mg/kg (minimum 7.5 mg) I.M. (depot injection only) as single injection q 4 weeks. Dosage may be increased in increments of 3.75 mg q 4 weeks, if needed. Or, (injection form) 50 mcg/kg/day S.C. If total downregulation isn't achieved, adjust dosage upward by 10 mcg/kg/day. This becomes the maintenance dosage. Therapy should be discontinued before girl reaches age 11 and before boy reaches age 12.

How supplied
Injection: 5 mg/ml in 2.8-ml multiple-dose vial
Depot injection:
Lupron Depot—3.75 mg, 7.5 mg
Lupron Depot-Ped—7.5 mg, 11.25 mg, 15 mg
Lupron Depot-3 month—11.25 mg, 22.5 mg
Lupron Depot-4 month—30 mg

Pharmacokinetics
Absorption: after S.C. administration, drug is rapidly and completely absorbed; unknown for I.M. use.
Distribution: unknown; about 7% to 15% bound to plasma proteins.
Metabolism: unknown.
Excretion: unknown. *Half-life:* 3 hours.

Route	Onset	Peak	Duration
I.M., S.C.	Unknown	1-2 mo	1-3 mo

Pharmacodynamics
Chemical effect: initially stimulates but then inhibits release of follicle-stimulating hormone and luteinizing hormone, resulting in testosterone suppression.
Therapeutic effect: hinders prostatic cancer cell growth and eases signs and symptoms of endometriosis.

Adverse reactions
CNS: dizziness, depression, headache.
CV: ***arrhythmias,*** angina, ***MI,*** peripheral edema.

GI: nausea, vomiting.
GU: impotence.
Hepatic: elevated liver enzyme levels.
Musculoskeletal: transient bone pain (during first week of treatment).
Respiratory: ***pulmonary embolism.***
Skin: skin reactions at injection site.
Other: *hot flushes,* decreased libido, gynecomastia.

Interactions

None significant.

Contraindications and precautions

- Contraindicated in patients hypersensitive to drug or other gonadotropin-releasing hormone analogues, in pregnant or breast-feeding women, and in women with undiagnosed vaginal bleeding.
- Use cautiously in patients hypersensitive to benzyl alcohol.
- The 30-mg depot formulation is contraindicated in women.

NURSING CONSIDERATIONS

Assessment

- Assess patient's condition before therapy and regularly thereafter.
- Be alert for adverse reactions.
- Evaluate patient's and family's knowledge of drug therapy.

Nursing diagnoses

- Ineffective health maintenance related to underlying condition
- Disturbed thought processes related to drug-induced depression
- Deficient knowledge related to drug therapy

Planning and implementation

- Never administer drug by I.V. injection.

I.M. use: Once-monthly depot injection should be administered under medical supervision. Use supplied diluent to reconstitute drug (extra diluent is provided and should be discarded).

– Draw 1 ml into syringe with 22G needle. (When preparing Lupron Depot-3 Month 22.5 mg, use a 23G or larger needle.) Withdraw 1.5 ml from ampule for the 3-month formulation.

– Inject into vial; then shake well. Suspension will appear milky.

– Although suspension is stable for 24 hours after reconstitution, it contains no bacteriostatic agent. Use immediately.

- When using prefilled dual-chamber syringes, prepare for injection by screwing white plunger into end stopper until stopper begins to turn. Remove and discard tab around base of needle. Hold syringe upright and release diluent by slowly pushing plunger until first stopper is at blue line in middle of barrel. Gently shake syringe to form a uniform milky suspension. If particles adhere to stopper, tap syringe against finger. Remove needle guard and advance plunger to expel air from syringe. Inject entire contents I.M. as for a normal injection.

S.C. use: Follow normal protocol.

- Leuprolide is nonsurgical alternative to orchiectomy for prostate cancer.
- A fractional dose of drug formulated to give q 3 months isn't equivalent to same dose of once-monthly formulation.

Patient teaching

- Before starting therapy in child for central precocious puberty, make sure parents understand importance of continuous therapy.
- Carefully instruct patient who will administer S.C. injection about proper administration techniques, and advise him to use only syringes provided by manufacturer.
- Advise patient that if another syringe must be substituted, a low-dose insulin syringe (U-100, 0.5 ml) is acceptable.
- Advise patient to store drug at room temperature, protected from light and heat.
- Reassure patient with history of undesirable effects from other endocrine therapies that leuprolide is much easier to tolerate. Tell patient that adverse effects are transient and will disappear after about 1 week.
- Warn patient that worsening of prostate cancer symptoms may occur when therapy starts.

Evaluation

- Patient exhibits improvement in underlying condition.

• Patient demonstrates pretreatment thought processes.
• Patient and family state understanding of drug therapy.

levalbuterol hydrochloride

(leev-al-BYOO-teh-rohl high-droh-KLOR-ighd)
Xopenex

Pharmacologic class: $beta_2$ agonist
Therapeutic class: bronchodilator
Pregnancy risk category: C

Indications and dosages

▶ **To prevent or treat bronchospasm in patients with reversible obstructive airway disease.** *Adults and adolescents age 12 and older:* 0.63 mg administered t.i.d. every 6 to 8 hours by P.O. inhalation via a nebulizer. Patients with more severe asthma who don't respond adequately to 0.63-mg doses may benefit from 1.25 mg t.i.d.

How supplied

Solution for inhalation: 0.63 mg or 1.25 mg in 3-ml vials

Pharmacokinetics

Absorption: some levalbuterol is absorbed following P.O. inhalation.
Distribution: unknown.
Metabolism: unknown.
Excretion: unknown.

Route	Onset	Peak	Duration
Inhalation	10-17 min	90 min	5-8 hr

Pharmacodynamics

Chemical effect: Levalbuterol activates $beta_2$ receptors on airway smooth muscle, which causes smooth muscle from trachea to terminal bronchioles to relax, thereby relieving bronchospasm and reducing airway resistance. Drug also inhibits the release of mediators from mast cells in the airway.
Therapeutic effect: improves ventilation.

Adverse reactions

CNS: dizziness, migraine, nervousness, tremor, anxiety.
CV: tachycardia.
EENT: *rhinitis*, sinusitis, turbinate edema.
GI: dyspepsia.
Musculoskeletal: leg cramps.
Respiratory: increased cough.
Other: flu syndrome, accidental injury, pain, *viral infection.*

Interactions

Drug-drug. *Beta blockers:* blocked pulmonary effect of the drug and, possibly, severe bronchospasm. Don't use together, if possible. If concomitant use is necessary, a cardioselective beta blocker could be considered but should be administered with caution.
Digoxin: decreased digoxin levels (up to 22%). Monitor serum digoxin levels, and watch for loss of therapeutic effect.
Epinephrine, short-acting sympathomimetic aerosol bronchodilators: increased adverse adrenergic effects. To avoid serious CV effects, additional adrenergics should be used with caution.
Loop or thiazide diuretics: increased risk of ECG changes and hypokalemia. Use together cautiously.
MAO inhibitors, tricyclic antidepressants: potentiated action of levalbuterol on the vascular system. Use extreme caution when administering these drugs within 2 weeks of each other.

Contraindications and precautions

• Contraindicated in patients hypersensitive to levalbuterol or racemic albuterol.
• Use cautiously in patients with CV disorders, especially coronary insufficiency, hypertension, and arrhythmias. Also use cautiously in patients with seizure disorders, hyperthyroidism, or diabetes mellitus and in patients who are unusually responsive to sympathomimetic amines.

NURSING CONSIDERATIONS

Assessment

• Obtain history of patient's underlying condition before therapy, and reassess regularly thereafter.

• Make sure that patient has a thorough physical examination before starting drug therapy.
• Be alert for adverse reactions and drug interactions.
• Evaluate patient's and family's knowledge of drug therapy.

Nursing diagnoses
• Impaired gas exchange related to underlying respiratory condition
• Risk for injury related to drug-induced adverse reactions
• Deficient knowledge related to drug therapy

Planning and implementation
• Like other inhaled beta agonists, levalbuterol can produce paradoxical bronchospasm, which may be life-threatening. If this occurs, discontinue levalbuterol immediately and start alternative therapy, as directed.
• Like other beta agonists, levalbuterol can produce significant CV effects in some patients. Although such effects are uncommon at recommended doses, drug may be discontinued if they occur.
• Compatibility, efficacy, and safety of levalbuterol when mixed with other drugs in a nebulizer haven't been established.

Patient teaching
• Warn patient to stop drug and notify prescriber if drug causes breathing to worsen.
• Urge patient not to increase the dosage or frequency without consulting prescriber.
• Tell patient to seek medical attention immediately if levalbuterol becomes less effective, if signs and symptoms worsen, or if drug is needed more often than usual.
• Tell patient that the effects of levalbuterol may last up to 8 hours.
• Urge patient to use other inhalations and antiasthma drugs only as directed while taking levalbuterol.
• Inform patient that common adverse reactions include palpitations, rapid heart rate, headache, dizziness, tremor, and nervousness.
• Caution woman to notify prescriber if she becomes pregnant or intends to breast-feed.
• Tell patient to keep unopened vials in foil pouch. Once the foil pouch is opened, the vials should be used within 2 weeks. Inform patient that vials removed from the pouch, if not used immediately, should be protected from light and heat and used within 1 week.
• Teach patient to correctly administer drug by oral inhalation via a nebulizer.
• Tell patient to breathe as calmly, deeply, and evenly as possible until no more mist is formed in the nebulizer reservoir (5 to 15 minutes). At this point, the treatment is finished.

Evaluation
• Patient's respiratory status improves.
• Patient doesn't experience injury from adverse reactions caused by drug.
• Patient and family state understanding of drug therapy.

levamisole hydrochloride
(lee-VUH-mee-sohl high-droh-KLOR-ighd)
Ergamisol

Pharmacologic class: immunomodulator
Therapeutic class: antineoplastic
Pregnancy risk category: C

Indications and dosages
▶ **Adjuvant treatment of Dukes' stage C colon cancer (with fluorouracil) after surgical resection.** *Adults:* 50 mg P.O. q 8 hours for 3 days. Therapy begun no sooner than 7 days and no later than 30 days after surgery, provided that patient is out of hospital, walking, and maintaining normal P.O. nutrition; has well-healed wounds; and has recovered from any postoperative complications. Fluorouracil (450 mg/m^2/day I.V.) is given for 5 days with 3-day course of levamisole starting 21 to 34 days after surgery. Maintenance dosage is 50 mg P.O. q 8 hours for 3 days q 2 weeks for 1 year. Given in conjunction with fluorouracil maintenance therapy (450 mg/m^2/day by rapid I.V. push, once a week beginning 28 days after initial 5-day course) for 1 year.

How supplied
Tablets: 50 mg (base)

Pharmacokinetics
Absorption: rapidly absorbed from GI tract.

Distribution: unknown.
Metabolism: extensively metabolized by liver.
Excretion: excreted primarily in urine, with some excretion in feces. *Half-life:* 3 to 4 hours.

Route	Onset	Peak	Duration
P.O.	Unknown	1.5-2 hr	Unknown

Pharmacodynamics

Chemical effect: unknown; appears to restore depressed immune function and may potentiate actions of monocytes and macrophages and enhance T-cell responses.
Therapeutic effect: increases immune response.

Adverse reactions

CNS: *dizziness, headache, paresthesia, somnolence, depression, nervousness, insomnia, anxiety, fatigue.*
CV: chest pain, edema.
EENT: blurred vision, conjunctivitis, *altered sense of smell.*
GI: *stomatitis, nausea, diarrhea, vomiting, anorexia, abdominal pain, constipation, flatulence, dyspepsia, altered taste.*
Hematologic: ***agranulocytosis, leukopenia, thrombocytopenia.***
Hepatic: hyperbilirubinemia.
Musculoskeletal: *arthralgia, myalgia.*
Skin: *dermatitis,* ***exfoliative dermatitis,*** pruritus, urticaria, *alopecia.*
Other: rigors, *infection, fever.*

Interactions

Drug-drug. *Phenytoin:* plasma phenytoin levels may be elevated when administered with levamisole and fluorouracil. Monitor phenytoin plasma levels.
Drug-lifestyle. *Alcohol use:* may precipitate disulfiram-like reaction. Discourage concomitant use.

Contraindications and precautions

- Contraindicated in patients hypersensitive to drug.
- Use cautiously in pregnant women.
- Safety of drug in breast-feeding women and in children hasn't been established.

NURSING CONSIDERATIONS

Assessment

- Assess patient's condition before therapy and regularly thereafter.
- Obtain baseline CBC with differential, platelet count, electrolyte levels, and liver function studies, as ordered, immediately before starting therapy.
- Obtain CBC with differential and platelet count at weekly intervals, as ordered, before treatment with fluorouracil. Obtain electrolyte levels and liver function studies every 3 months for 1 year, as ordered.
- Be alert for adverse reactions and drug interactions.
- Evaluate patient's and family's knowledge of drug therapy.

Nursing diagnoses

- Ineffective health maintenance related to underlying condition
- Ineffective immune protection related to adverse hematologic reactions
- Deficient knowledge related to drug therapy

Planning and implementation

- If levamisole therapy begins 7 to 20 days after surgery, fluorouracil should be started with second course of levamisole therapy. It should begin no sooner than 21 days and no later than 35 days after surgery. If levamisole is deferred until 21 to 30 days after surgery, fluorouracil therapy should begin with first course of levamisole.

ALERT Dosage modifications are based on hematologic parameters. If WBC count is between 2,500/mm³ and 3,500/mm³, don't give fluorouracil until WBC count is above 3,500/mm³. When fluorouracil is restarted, reduce dosage by 20%, as directed. If WBC count stays below 2,500/mm³ for more than 10 days after fluorouracil is withdrawn, discontinue levamisole. If platelet count is below 100,000/mm³, therapy with both fluorouracil and levamisole should be discontinued and the prescriber notified.

- Don't exceed recommended doses. Higher doses increase the risk of agranulocytosis.
- Promptly report development of stomatitis or diarrhea. If either occurs during initial course

of fluorouracil therapy, drug is discontinued and weekly fluorouracil therapy starts 28 days after start of initial course. If stomatitis or diarrhea develops during weekly doses of fluorouracil, fluorouracil therapy is deferred until these symptoms subside. Then fluorouracil therapy is started at reduced dosages (decreased by 20%).

Patient teaching

- Instruct patient to report stomatitis, diarrhea, or flulike symptoms, such as fever and chills.
- Advise patient to use soft toothbrush and electric razor to avoid trauma and excessive bleeding.
- Instruct patient to avoid alcohol consumption during drug therapy.
- Tell patient to avoid exposure to people with infection.

☑ Evaluation

- Patient responds well to therapy.
- Patient regains normal hematologic parameters.
- Patient and family state understanding of drug therapy.

levetiracetam

(leev-ah-tah-RACE-ah-tam)
Keppra

Pharmacologic class: anticonvulsant
Therapeutic class: anticonvulsant
Pregnancy risk category: C

Indications and dosages

▶ Adjunctive therapy for partial seizures. *Adults:* initially, 500 mg b.i.d. Dosage can be increased by 500 mg b.i.d., as needed, for seizure control at 2-week intervals to maximum dosage of 1,500 mg b.i.d.

How supplied

Tablets: 250 mg, 500 mg, 750 mg

Pharmacokinetics

Absorption: rapidly absorbed in the GI tract. Serum levels peak in about 1 hour. Although drug can be taken with food, time to reach peak levels is delayed by about 1.5 hours and serum levels are slightly lower. Serum levels reach steady-state in about 2 days.
Distribution: protein binding is minimal.
Metabolism: no active metabolites. Drug isn't metabolized through the cytochrome P-450 system.
Excretion: about 66% of drug is eliminated unchanged by glomerular filtration and tubular reabsorption. *Elimination half-life:* about 7 hours in patients with normal renal function.

Route	Onset	Peak	Duration
P.O.	1 hr	1 hr	12 hr

Pharmacodynamics

Chemical effect: unknown. Thought to inhibit kindling activity in hippocampus, thus preventing simultaneous neuronal firing that leads to seizure activity.
Therapeutic effect: prevents seizure activity.

Adverse reactions

CNS: *asthenia, headache, somnolence,* dizziness, depression, vertigo, paresthesia, nervousness, hostility, emotional lability, ataxia, amnesia, anxiety.
EENT: diplopia, pharyngitis, rhinitis, sinusitis.
GI: anorexia.
Hematologic: ***leukopenia, neutropenia.***
Musculoskeletal: pain.
Respiratory: cough, infection.

Interactions

Drug-drug. *Antihistamines, benzodiazepines, narcotics, tricyclic antidepressants, other drugs that cause drowsiness:* Concomitant use may lead to severe sedation.
Carbamazepine, clozapine, and other drugs known to cause leukopenia or neutropenia: may increase the risk of infection. Monitor patient closely.
Drug-lifestyle. *Alcohol:* increased risk of severe sedation. Discourage concurrent use.

Contraindications and precautions

- Contraindicated in patients hypersensitive to drug. Use cautiously in immunocompromised patients and in those with poor renal function.

NURSING CONSIDERATIONS

Assessment
- Obtain history of patient's underlying condition before therapy, and reassess regularly thereafter.
- Assess renal function before therapy starts.
- Monitor patient closely for such adverse reactions as dizziness, which may lead to falls.
- Evaluate patient's and family's knowledge of drug therapy.

Nursing diagnoses
- Risk for trauma related to seizures
- Risk for infection related to leukopenia and neutropenia
- Deficient knowledge related to drug therapy

Planning and implementation
- Patients with renal insufficiency need dosage adjustment.

P.O. use: Drug can be taken with or without food.
- Use drug only with other anticonvulsants; not recommended for monotherapy.
- Leukopenia and neutropenia have been reported with drug use. Use cautiously in immunocompromised patients (such as those with cancer or HIV infection).
- Seizures can occur if drug is stopped abruptly. Tapering is recommended.

Patient teaching
- Warn patient to use extra care when rising to a sitting or standing position to avoid dizziness and falling.
- Advise patient to call prescriber and not to stop drug suddenly if adverse reactions occur.
- Tell patient to take with other prescribed seizure drugs.
- Inform patient that drug can be taken with or without food.

Evaluation
- Patient is free from seizure activity.
- Patient doesn't develop infection.
- Patient and family state understanding of drug therapy.

levocarnitine (L-carnitine)
(lee-voh-KAR-nuh-teen)
Carnitor, L-Carnitine, VitaCarn

Pharmacologic class: amino acid derivative
Therapeutic class: nutritional supplement
Pregnancy risk category: B

Indications and dosages

▶ **Primary and secondary systemic carnitine deficiency.** All dosages based on clinical response. Higher dosages may be given.
Adults: 990 mg P.O. b.i.d. or t.i.d. Or, 10 to 30 ml (1 to 3 g) of oral liquid daily.
Children: 50 to 100 mg/kg/day P.O. in divided doses. Maximum, 3 g/day.
▶ **Acute and long-term treatment of secondary carnitine deficiency.** *Adults:* 50 mg/kg/day, divided and given I.V. slowly over 2 to 3 minutes q 3 to 4 hours.

How supplied

Tablets: 330 mg
Capsules: 250 mg
Oral liquid: 100 mg/ml
Injection: 1 g/5 ml

Pharmacokinetics

Absorption: unknown after P.O. administration.
Distribution: not bound to plasma proteins or albumin.
Metabolism: major metabolites are trimethylamine *N*-oxide and gamma butyrobetaine.
Excretion: excreted mainly in urine; small amount excreted in feces.

Route	Onset	Peak	Duration
P.O., I.V.	Unknown	Unknown	Unknown

Pharmacodynamics

Chemical effect: facilitates transport of fatty acids (used to produce energy) into cellular mitochondria.
Therapeutic effect: relieves signs and symptoms of carnitine deficiency.

Adverse reactions

GI: *nausea, vomiting, cramps, diarrhea.*

Other: body odor.

Interactions

Drug-drug. *L-carnitine (sold as vitamin B_T):* inhibition of levocarnitine and possible deficiency. Avoid concomitant use.
Valproic acid: increases levocarnitine requirement. Adjust dosage as ordered.
Drug-lifestyle. *Any food:* decreased GI upset. Give with food.

Contraindications and precautions

- No known contraindications.
- Drug isn't recommended for use in breast-feeding women.
- Use cautiously in pregnant women.

NURSING CONSIDERATIONS

Assessment

- Obtain history of patient's underlying condition before therapy.
- Monitor blood chemistry and plasma drug levels periodically, as ordered, as well as vital signs and patient's overall condition.
- Monitor patient's tolerance during first week of therapy and after increasing dosage, as ordered.
- Be alert for adverse reactions and drug interactions.
- Monitor patient's hydration status if adverse GI reactions occur.
- Evaluate patient's and family's knowledge of drug therapy.

Nursing diagnoses

- Fatigue related to levocarnitine deficiency
- Risk for deficient fluid volume related to drug-induced adverse GI reactions
- Deficient knowledge related to drug therapy

Planning and implementation

P.O. use: Give enteral liquid alone or dissolve in drinks or liquid food.
- Space doses evenly every 3 to 4 hours, and give drug with or after meals, if possible.
- Don't refrigerate solution.

I.V. use: Administer drug slowly over 2 to 3 minutes.

Patient teaching

- Tell patient to consume oral liquid slowly to minimize GI distress. If GI intolerance persists, dosage may have to be reduced.
- Instruct patient to dissolve drug in drink or liquid food or take with meals to reduce GI upset.
- Warn patient to avoid "vitamin B_T" in health food stores because it interacts with drug and renders it ineffective.
- Caution patient not to share drug with others. Some people have used it to improve athletic performance.

Evaluation

- Patient's energy level is increased.
- Patient maintains adequate hydration throughout therapy.
- Patient and family state understanding of drug therapy.

levodopa

(lee-voh-DOH-puh)
Dopar, Larodopa

Pharmacologic class: precursor of dopamine
Therapeutic class: antiparkinsonian
Pregnancy risk category: C

Indications and dosages

▶ **Idiopathic parkinsonism, postencephalitic parkinsonism, and symptomatic parkinsonism after carbon monoxide or manganese intoxication or with cerebral arteriosclerosis.** *Adults and children over age 12:* initially, 0.5 to 1 g P.O. daily divided into two or more doses with food; increased by no more than 0.75 g daily q 3 to 7 days until usual optimal daily dosage of 3 to 6 g is reached. Maximum 8 g daily. Dosage carefully adjusted to patient requirements, tolerance, and response. Higher dosage requires close supervision.

How supplied

Tablets: 100 mg, 250 mg, 500 mg
Capsules: 100 mg, 250 mg, 500 mg

Pharmacokinetics

Absorption: absorbed rapidly from small intestine by active amino acid transport system, with 30% to 50% reaching general circulation.
Distribution: distributed widely to most body tissues but not to CNS, which receives less than 1% of dose because of extensive metabolism in periphery.
Metabolism: 95% of levodopa is converted to dopamine in lumen of stomach and intestines and on first pass through liver.
Excretion: excreted primarily in urine. *Half-life:* 1 to 3 hours.

Route	Onset	Peak	Duration
P.O.	3 wk-6 mo	1-3 hr	About 5 hr but varies greatly

Pharmacodynamics

Chemical effect: unknown; may be decarboxylated to dopamine, countering dopamine depletion in extrapyramidal centers.
Therapeutic effect: relieves signs and symptoms of parkinsonism.

Adverse reactions

CNS: *aggressive behavior, abnormal movements (choreiform, dystonic, dyskinetic), involuntary grimacing and head movements, myoclonic body jerks,* ***seizures,*** *ataxia, tremors, muscle twitching, bradykinetic episodes, psychiatric disturbance, memory loss, mood changes, nervousness, anxiety, disturbing dreams, euphoria, malaise, fatigue, severe depression,* ***suicidal tendencies,*** *dementia, delirium, hallucinations* (may necessitate reduction or withdrawal of drug).
CV: *orthostatic hypotension,* cardiac irregularities, flushing, hypertension, phlebitis.
EENT: blepharospasm, blurred vision, diplopia, mydriasis or miosis, widening of palpebral fissures, activation of latent Horner's syndrome, oculogyric crises, nasal discharge.
GI: dry mouth, excessive salivation, bitter taste, *nausea, vomiting, anorexia,* constipation, flatulence, diarrhea, epigastric pain.
GU: urinary frequency, urine retention, incontinence, darkened urine, priapism.
Hematologic: ***hemolytic anemia, leukopenia, agranulocytosis.***
Hepatic: ***hepatotoxicity.***
Metabolic: weight loss.
Respiratory: hyperventilation, hiccups.
Other: dark perspiration, excessive and inappropriate sexual behavior.

Interactions

Drug-drug. *Antacids:* increased levodopa absorption. Administer antacids 1 hour after levodopa.
Anticholinergics: increased gastric deactivation and decreased intestinal absorption of levodopa. Avoid concomitant use.
Benzodiazepine: levodopa's therapeutic value may be attenuated. Monitor patient closely.
Furazolidone, MAO inhibitors, procarbazine: risk of severe hypertension. Avoid concomitant use.
Inhaled halogen anesthetics, sympathomimetics: increased risk of arrhythmias. Monitor patient closely.
Metoclopramide: accelerated gastric emptying of levodopa. Give metoclopramide 1 hour after levodopa.
Papaverine, phenothiazines and other antipsychotics, phenytoin, rauwolfia alkaloids: decreased levodopa effect. Use together cautiously.
Pyridoxine: reversal of antiparkinsonian effects. Check vitamin preparations and nutritional supplements for pyridoxine (vitamin B_6) content. Don't give together.
Tricyclic antidepressants: delayed absorption and decreased bioavailability of levodopa. Hypertensive episodes have occurred. Monitor patient closely.
Drug-herb. *Kava:* may interfere with drug and with natural dopamine, worsening symptoms of Parkinson's disease. Discourage concomitant use.
Rauwolfia: decreased effectiveness of levodopa. Discourage concomitant use.
Drug-food. *Foods high in protein:* decreased levodopa absorption. Don't give with high-protein foods.

Contraindications and precautions

• Contraindicated in patients hypersensitive to drug, in those who have taken an MAO inhibitor within 14 days, and in those with acute

angle-closure glaucoma, melanoma, or undiagnosed skin lesions.
• Drug shouldn't be used in breast-feeding women.
• Use cautiously in pregnant women and in patients with severe CV, renal, hepatic, or pulmonary disorders; peptic ulcer; psychiatric illness; MI with residual arrhythmias; bronchial asthma; emphysema; or endocrine disease.
• Safety of drug hasn't been established in children age 12 and younger.

NURSING CONSIDERATIONS

Assessment
• Assess patient's condition before therapy and regularly thereafter.
• Observe and monitor vital signs, especially during dosage adjustments.
• Patient receiving long-term therapy should be tested regularly for diabetes and acromegaly; periodically monitor kidney, liver, and hematopoietic function, as ordered.
• Be alert for adverse reactions and drug interactions.
• Evaluate patient's and family's knowledge of drug therapy.

Nursing diagnoses
• Impaired physical mobility related to presence of parkinsonism
• Disturbed thought processes related to drug-induced adverse reactions
• Deficient knowledge related to drug therapy

Planning and implementation
• To minimize GI upset, give drug with food. However, keep in mind that high-protein meals can impair absorption and reduce effectiveness.
• Patient who must undergo surgery should continue levodopa as long as oral intake is permitted, usually until 6 to 24 hours before surgery. Drug should be resumed as soon as patient can take oral medication.
• Protect drug from heat, light, and moisture. If preparation darkens, it has lost potency and should be discarded.
• Report significant changes in vital signs.

ALERT Muscle twitching and eyelid twitching may be early signs of drug overdose; report immediately.
• Prescriber-supervised period of drug discontinuance (called a drug holiday) may reestablish effectiveness of lower dosage regimen.
• Coombs' test occasionally becomes positive during extended use. Expect elevated uric acid levels with colorimetric method but not with urate oxidase.
• Alkaline phosphatase, AST, ALT, LD, bilirubin, BUN, and protein-bound iodine levels show transient elevations in patient receiving levodopa; WBC count, hemoglobin, and hematocrit show occasional reductions.
• False-positive tests for urine glucose can occur with reagents that use copper sulfate; false-negative results can occur with tests that use glucose enzymatic methods. Levodopa also interferes with tests for urine ketones and urine phenylketonuria, falsely elevates urine catecholamine levels, and may falsely decrease urine vanillylmandelic acid levels.

Patient teaching
• Advise patient to take drug with food but not with high-protein meals. If patient has trouble swallowing pills, tell him or family member to crush tablets and mix with applesauce or baby food.
• Warn patient and family not to increase dosage without prescriber's orders.
• Warn patient about possible dizziness and light-headedness, especially at start of therapy. Tell patient to change positions slowly and dangle legs before getting out of bed. Elastic stockings may help control this reaction.
• Advise patient and family that multivitamin preparations, fortified cereals, and certain OTC medications may contain pyridoxine (vitamin B_6), which can block effects of levodopa.
• Warn patient about risk of arrhythmias if he uses cocaine with drug.

Evaluation
• Patient has improved physical mobility.
• Patient maintains normal thought process.
• Patient and family state understanding of drug therapy.

levofloxacin

(lee-voe-FLOX-a-sin)
Levaquin

Pharmacologic class: fluorinated carboxyquinolone
Therapeutic class: broad spectrum antibacterial
Pregnancy risk category: C

Indications and dosages

▶ **Acute maxillary sinusitis caused by susceptible strains of *Streptococcus pneumoniae, Moraxella catarrhalis,* or *Haemophilus influenzae.*** *Adults age 18 and older:* 500 mg P.O. or I.V. daily for 10 to 14 days.

▶ **Acute bacterial exacerbation of chronic bronchitis caused by *Staphylococcus aureus, S. pneumoniae, M. catarrhalis,* or *H. influenzae* or *parainfluenzae.*** *Adults age 18 and older:* 500 mg P.O. or I.V. daily for 7 days.

▶ **Community-acquired pneumonia caused by *S. aureus, S. pneumoniae, M. catarrhalis, H. influenzae, H. parainfluenzae, Klebsiella pneumoniae, Chlamydia pneumoniae, Legionella pneumophila,* or *Mycoplasma pneumoniae*.** *Adults age 18 and older:* 500 mg P.O. or I.V. daily for 7 to 14 days.

▶ **Mild to moderate skin and skin-structure infections caused by *S. aureus* or *S. pyogenes.*** *Adults age 18 and older:* 500 mg P.O. or I.V. daily for 7 to 10 days.

▶ **Mild to moderate uncomplicated urinary tract infection caused by *Escherichia coli, K. pneumoniae,* or *Staphylococcus saprophyticus*.** *Adults age 18 and older:* 250 mg P.O. daily for 3 days.

▶ **Mild to moderate urinary tract infections caused by *Enterococcus faecalis, Enterobacter cloacae, E. coli, K. pneumoniae, Proteus mirabilis,* or *Pseudomonas aeruginosa.*** *Adults age 18 and older:* 250 mg P.O. or I.V. daily for 10 days.

▶ **Mild to moderate acute pyelonephritis caused by *E. coli.*** *Adults age 18 and older:* 250 mg P.O. or I.V. daily for 10 days.

▶ **Community-acquired pneumonia caused by penicillin-resistant *Streptococcus pneumoniae.*** *Adults age 18 and older:* 500 mg P.O. or I.V. infusion over 60 minutes once daily for 7 to 14 days.

How supplied

Tablets: 250 mg, 500 mg
Single-use vials: 500 mg
Infusion (premixed): 250 mg in 50 ml D_5W, 500 mg in 100 ml D_5W

Pharmacokinetics

Absorption: plasma level after I.V. administration is comparable to that observed for equivalent P.O. doses (on a mg-per-mg basis). Therefore, P.O. and I.V. routes can be considered interchangeable. Plasma levels peak within 1 to 2 hours after P.O. dosing. Steady state occurs within 48 hours on a 500 mg/day regimen.
Distribution: mean volume of distribution ranges from 89 to 112 L after single and multiple 500-mg doses, indicating widespread distribution into body tissues. Drug also penetrates well into lung tissues; levels are generally two to five times higher than plasma levels.
Metabolism: drug undergoes limited metabolism. The only identified metabolites are the desmethyl and N-oxide metabolites, which have little relevant pharmacologic activity.
Excretion: primarily excreted unchanged in the urine. *Mean terminal half-life:* about 6 to 8 hours.

Route	Onset	Peak	Duration
P.O., I.V.	Unknown	1-2 hr	Unknown

Pharmacodynamics

Chemical effect: inhibits bacterial DNA gyrase and prevents DNA replication, transcription, repair, and recombination in susceptible bacteria.
Therapeutic effect: kills susceptible bacteria. Spectrum of activity includes *S. pneumoniae, M. catarrhalis, H. influenzae, H. parainfluenzae, S. aureus, S. pyogenes, K. pneumoniae, C. pneumoniae, L. pneumophila, M. pneumoniae, E. coli, K. pneumoniae, S. saprophyticus, E. faecalis, E. cloacae,* and *P. aeruginosa.*

Adverse reactions

CNS: headache, insomnia, dizziness, encephalopathy, paresthesia, ***seizures.***
CV: chest pain, palpitations, vasodilation, abnormal ECG.
GI: nausea, diarrhea, constipation, vomiting, abdominal pain, dyspepsia, flatulence, pseudomembranous colitis.
GU: vaginitis.
Hematologic: eosinophilia, hemolytic anemia, lymphopenia.
Metabolic: hypoglycemia.
Musculoskeletal: back pain, tendon rupture.
Respiratory: allergic pneumonitis.
Skin: rash, photosensitivity, pruritus, erythema multiforme, ***Stevens-Johnson syndrome.***
Other: pain, hypersensitivity reactions, ***anaphylaxis, multisystem organ failure.***

Interactions

Drug-drug. *Aluminum- or magnesium-containing antacids, iron salts, products containing zinc, sucralfate:* may interfere with GI absorption of levofloxacin. Administer at least 2 hours apart.
Antidiabetics: may alter blood glucose levels. Monitor them closely.
NSAIDs: may increase CNS stimulation. Monitor patient for seizure activity.
Theophylline: decreased theophylline clearance with some fluoroquinolones. Monitor theophylline levels.
Warfarin and derivatives: increased effect of oral anticoagulant with some fluoroquinolones. Monitor PT and INR.
Drug-lifestyle. *Sun exposure:* possible photosensitivity reactions. Urge patient to take precautions.

Contraindications and precautions

- Contraindicated in patients hypersensitive to drug, its components, or other fluoroquinolones.

NURSING CONSIDERATIONS

Assessment

- Obtain specimen for culture and sensitivity tests before starting therapy and as needed to detect bacterial resistance.
- Obtain history of seizure disorders or other CNS diseases, such as cerebral arteriosclerosis, before therapy starts.
- Monitor blood glucose and renal, hepatic, and hematopoietic blood studies, as ordered.
- Evaluate patient's and family's knowledge of drug therapy.

Nursing diagnoses

- Risk for infection related to presence of bacteria susceptible to drug
- Risk for deficient fluid volume related to drug-induced adverse GI reactions
- Deficient knowledge related to drug therapy

Planning and implementation

P.O. use: Give dose with plenty of fluids. Antacids, sucralfate, and products containing iron or zinc should be avoided for at least 2 hours before and after each dose.
I.V. use: Levofloxacin injection should be administered only by I.V. infusion.
– Dilute drug in single-use vials, according to manufacturer's instructions, with D_5W or normal saline solution for injection to a final concentration of 5 mg/ml.
– Reconstituted solution should be clear, slightly yellow, and free of particulates. It's stable 72 hours at room temperature, 14 days when refrigerated in plastic containers, and 6 months when frozen. Thaw at room temperature or in refrigerator.
– Don't mix with other drugs. Infuse over 60 minutes.
- Acute hypersensitivity reactions may require treatment with epinephrine, oxygen, I.V. fluids, antihistamines, corticosteroids, pressor amines, and airway management.
- If patient has symptoms of excessive CNS stimulation (restlessness, tremor, confusion, hallucinations), stop drug and notify prescriber. Take seizure precautions.
- Patients with creatinine clearence below 50 ml/minute need a dosage adjustment.
- Most antibacterial drugs can cause pseudomembranous colitis. Notify prescriber if diarrhea occurs. Drug may be discontinued.

Patient teaching

- Tell patient to take drug as prescribed, even if symptoms resolve.

• Advise patient to take drug with plenty of fluids and to avoid antacids, sucralfate, and products containing iron or zinc for at least 2 hours before and after each dose.
• Warn patient to avoid hazardous tasks until adverse CNS effects of drug are known.
• Advise patient to avoid excessive sunlight, use sunblock, and wear protective clothing when outdoors.
• Instruct patient to stop drug and notify prescriber if rash or other signs or symptoms of hypersensitivity develop.
• Tell patient to notify prescriber if he experiences pain or inflammation; tendon rupture can occur with drug.
• Instruct diabetic patient to monitor blood glucose levels and notify prescriber if a hypoglycemic reaction occurs.
• Instruct patient to notify prescriber about loose stools or diarrhea.

☑ Evaluation

• Patient is free from infection after drug therapy.
• Patient maintains adequate hydration throughout drug therapy.
• Patient and family state understanding of drug therapy.

levonorgestrel

(lee-voh-nor-JES-trel)
Norplant System

Pharmacologic class: progestin
Therapeutic class: contraceptive
Pregnancy risk category: X

Indications and dosages

▶ **Prevention of pregnancy.** *Women:* six capsules implanted subdermally in midportion of upper arm, about 8 cm above elbow crease, during first 7 days after menses starts. Capsules are placed fanlike, 15 degrees apart (total of 75 degrees). Contraceptive effect lasts for 5 years.

How supplied

Implants: 36 mg/capsule; each kit contains six capsules

Pharmacokinetics

Absorption: 100% bioavailable.
Distribution: bound by circulating protein sex hormone–binding globulin (SHBG).
Metabolism: metabolized by liver.
Excretion: metabolites excreted in urine.

Route	Onset	Peak	Duration
Subdermal	≤ 24 hr	≤ 24 hr	5 yr

Pharmacodynamics

Chemical effect: slowly releases synthetic progestin levonorgestrel into bloodstream. How progestins provide contraception isn't understood, but they alter mucus covering the cervix, prevent implantation of ovum and, in some patients, prevent ovulation.
Therapeutic effect: prevents pregnancy.

Adverse reactions

CNS: headache, nervousness, dizziness.
GI: nausea, *abdominal discomfort,* appetite change.
GU: *amenorrhea, prolonged bleeding, spotting, irregular onset of bleeding, frequent onset of bleeding, scanty bleeding, cervicitis, vaginitis, leukorrhea.*
Metabolic: weight gain.
Musculoskeletal: *musculoskeletal pain.*
Skin: dermatitis; acne; hirsutism; hypertrichosis; scalp hair loss; infection, transient pain, or itching at implant site.
Other: adnexal enlargement, mastalgia, *removal difficulty, breast discharge.*

Interactions

Drug-drug. *Carbamazepine, phenytoin, rifampin:* may reduce contraceptive efficacy of levonorgestrel implants. Avoid concomitant use.
Drug-food. *Caffeine:* may increase serum caffeine levels. Monitor effects.
Drug-lifestyle. *Smoking:* increased risk of adverse CV effects. Advise patient to stop smoking.

Contraindications and precautions

• Contraindicated in patients with active thrombophlebitis or thromboembolic disorders, undiagnosed abnormal genital bleeding, acute liver disease, malignant or benign liver

tumors, known or suspected breast cancer, or known or suspected pregnancy.
- Use cautiously in patients with hyperlipidemia or history of depression and in diabetic or prediabetic patients.
- Little is known about effects of drug in breast-feeding women.

NURSING CONSIDERATIONS

Assessment
- Obtain pregnancy test before therapy, and retest if pregnancy is suspected.
- Closely monitor patient with condition that may be aggravated by fluid retention because steroid hormones may cause fluid retention.
- Be alert for adverse reactions and drug interactions.
- Evaluate patient's and family's knowledge of drug therapy.

Nursing diagnoses
- Health-seeking behavior related to desire to prevent pregnancy
- Chronic pain related to drug-induced adverse reactions
- Deficient knowledge related to drug therapy

Planning and implementation
- During insertion, pay special attention to asepsis and correct placement of capsules; use careful technique to minimize tissue trauma.
- Laboratory tests may show decreased SHBG and T_4 levels and increased T_3 uptake.
- Expect implants to be removed if active thrombophlebitis or thromboembolic disease develops or if patient will be immobilized for a long time.
- If jaundice develops, expect implants to be removed because steroid hormone metabolism is impaired in patients with liver failure.
- Although retinal thrombosis after use of oral contraceptives has been reported, no similar incidents have been documented after use of implant system. However, patients with sudden, unexplained vision problems, including contact lense wearers in whom vision or lens tolerance changes, should be immediately evaluated by an ophthalmologist.

Patient teaching

ALERT Tell patient to report to prescriber immediately if implant capsule falls out. Efficacy may be impaired.
- Warn patient that missed menstrual periods aren't accurate indicators of early pregnancy because drug may induce amenorrhea. Advise patient that 6 weeks or more of amenorrhea (after pattern of regular menstrual periods) could indicate pregnancy. If pregnancy is confirmed, implants must be removed.
- Encourage regular (at least annual) physical examinations.
- Inform patient that most patients develop variations in menstrual bleeding patterns, including irregular bleeding, prolonged bleeding, spotting, and amenorrhea. These irregularities usually diminish over time.
- Instruct patient to avoid caffeine consumption and smoking while on drug therapy.

Evaluation
- Patient doesn't become pregnant.
- Patient is free from pain.
- Patient and family state understanding of drug therapy.

levothyroxine sodium (T_4, L-thyroxine sodium)

(lee-voh-thigh-ROKS-een SOH-dee-um)

Eltroxin, Levo-T, Levothroid, Levoxine, Levoxyl, Oroxine ◊, Synthroid**

Pharmacologic class: thyroid hormone
Therapeutic class: thyroid hormone replacement
Pregnancy risk category: A

Indications and dosages

▶ **Cretinism.** *Children under age 1:* initially, 0.025 to 0.05 mg P.O. daily, increased to 0.05 mg P.O. in 4 to 6 weeks, as needed.

▶ **Myxedema coma.** *Adults:* 300 to 500 mcg I.V.; if no response in 24 hours, give an additional 100 to 300 mcg I.V. in 48 hours, followed by parenteral maintenance dosage of 50 to 200 mcg I.V. daily. Patient should be switched to P.O. maintenance as soon as possible.

▶ **Thyroid hormone replacement.** *Adults age 65 and younger:* initially, 0.025 to 0.05 mg P.O. daily, increased by 0.025 mg P.O. q 2 to 4 weeks until desired response occurs. Maintenance dosage is 0.1 to 0.2 mg P.O. daily. May administer I.V. or I.M. when P.O. ingestion is precluded for long periods. Dosage adjustment may be necessary.
Adults over age 65: 0.0125 to 0.025 mg P.O. daily. Increased by 0.0125 to 0.025 mg at 3- to 8-week intervals, depending on response.
Children: initially, 0.025 to 0.075 mg (children younger than age 1) or 3 to 5 mcg/kg (children age 1 and older) P.O. daily, gradually increased by 0.025 to 0.05 mg q 2 to 4 weeks until desired response occurs.

How supplied

Tablets: 0.025 mg, 0.05 mg, 0.075 mg, 0.088 mg, 0.1 mg, 0.112 mg, 0.125 mg, 0.137 mg, 0.15 mg, 0.175 mg, 0.2 mg, 0.3 mg
Injection: 200 mcg/vial, 500 mcg/vial

Pharmacokinetics

Absorption: well absorbed from GI tract after P.O. administration.
Distribution: distributed widely; 99% protein-bound.
Metabolism: metabolized in peripheral tissues, primarily in liver, kidneys, and intestines.
Excretion: 20% to 40% excreted in feces.
Half-life: 6 to 7 days.

Route	Onset	Peak	Duration
P.O., I.V., I.M.	24 hr	3-4 wk	1-3 wk

Pharmacodynamics

Chemical effect: not fully defined; stimulates metabolism by accelerating cellular oxidation.
Therapeutic effect: raises thyroid hormone levels in body.

Adverse reactions

Adverse reactions to thyroid hormones are extensions of their pharmacologic properties and reflect patient sensitivity to them.
CNS: headache, *nervousness, insomnia, tremors.*
CV: *tachycardia, palpitations,* ***arrhythmias,*** angina pectoris, hypertension, ***cardiac arrest.***
GI: appetite change, nausea, diarrhea.
GU: menstrual irregularities.
Metabolic: weight loss.
Musculoskeletal: leg cramps.
Skin: diaphoresis.
Other: heat intolerance, fever.

Interactions

Drug-drug. *Cholestyramine, colestipol:* impaired levothyroxine absorption. Separate doses by 4 to 5 hours.
Insulin, oral antidiabetics: altered serum glucose levels. Monitor blood glucose levels. Dosage adjustments may be necessary.
I.V. phenytoin: free thyroid released. Monitor patient for tachycardia.
Oral anticoagulants: altered PT. Monitor PT and INR. Dosage adjustments may be necessary.
Sympathomimetics (such as epinephrine): increased risk of coronary insufficiency. Monitor patient closely.

Contraindications and precautions

- Contraindicated in patients hypersensitive to drug and in patients with acute MI uncomplicated by hypothyroidism, untreated thyrotoxicosis, or uncorrected adrenal insufficiency.
- Use with extreme caution in elderly patients and those with angina pectoris, hypertension, other CV disorders, renal insufficiency, or ischemia.
- Rapid replacement in patients with arteriosclerosis may precipitate angina, coronary occlusion, or CVA. Use cautiously in these patients.
- Use cautiously in breast-feeding women and in patients with diabetes mellitus, diabetes insipidus, or myxedema.

NURSING CONSIDERATIONS

Assessment

- Assess patient's condition before therapy and regularly thereafter. Normal serum levels of T_4 should occur within 24 hours, followed by threefold increase in serum T_3 in 3 days.
- Be alert for adverse reactions and drug interactions.

• In patients with coronary artery disease who must receive thyroid hormone, watch carefully for possible coronary insufficiency.
• Evaluate patient's and family's knowledge of drug therapy.

Nursing diagnoses

• Ineffective health maintenance related to presence of hypothyroidism
• Risk for injury related to drug-induced adverse reactions
• Deficient knowledge related to drug therapy

Planning and implementation

ALERT Don't confuse mg with mcg dosage (1 mg = 1,000 mcg).
• Thyroid hormone replacement requirements are about 25% lower in patients over age 60 than in young adults.
• Patients with adult hypothyroidism are unusually sensitive to thyroid hormone. Patient should be started at lowest dosage and adjusted to higher dosage until reaching a euthyroid state based on symptoms and laboratory data.
P.O. use: When changing from levothyroxine to liothyronine, levothyroxine should be stopped and liothyronine begun. Dosage increased in small increments after residual effects of levothyroxine disappear. When changing from liothyronine to levothyroxine, levothyroxine is started several days before withdrawing liothyronine to avoid relapse.
I.V. use: Prepare I.V. dose immediately before injection. Don't mix with other solutions. Inject into vein over 1 to 2 minutes.
I.M. use: Follow normal protocol.
• Thyroid hormones alter thyroid function test results. Patients taking levothyroxine who need radioactive iodine uptake studies must discontinue drug 4 weeks before test.
• Patients taking a prescribed anticoagulant with thyroid hormones usually need a reduced anticoagulant dosage.
ALERT Don't confuse levothyroxine sodium with liothyronine sodium.

Patient teaching

• Stress importance of compliance. Tell patient to take thyroid hormones at same time each day, preferably before breakfast, to maintain constant hormone levels. Suggest morning dosage to prevent insomnia.
• Warn patient (especially elderly patient) to notify prescriber at once of chest pain, palpitations, sweating, nervousness, shortness of breath, or other signs of overdose or aggravated CV disease.
• Advise patient who has achieved stable response not to change brands.
• Tell patient to report unusual bleeding and bruising.

Evaluation

• Patient's thyroid hormone levels are normal.
• Patient doesn't experience injury.
• Patient and family state understanding of drug therapy.

lidocaine hydrochloride (lignocaine hydrochloride)

(LIGH-doh-kayn high-droh-KLOR-ighd)
LidoPen Auto-Injector, Xylocaine, Xylocard ♦ ◇

Pharmacologic class: amide derivative
Therapeutic class: ventricular antiarrhythmic
Pregnancy risk category: B

Indications and dosages

▶ **Ventricular arrhythmias resulting from MI, cardiac manipulation, or cardiac glycosides.** *Adults:* 50 to 100 mg (1 to 1.5 mg/kg) by I.V. bolus at 25 to 50 mg/minute. Elderly patients or patients weighing less than 50 kg (110 lb) and those with heart failure or hepatic disease receive half the normal dose. Bolus dose is repeated q 3 to 5 minutes until arrhythmias subside or adverse reactions develop. Don't exceed 300-mg total bolus during 1-hour period. Simultaneously, constant infusion of 20 to 50 mcg/kg/minute (1 to 4 mg/minute) is begun. If single bolus has been given, smaller bolus dose may be repeated 5 to 10 minutes after start of infusion to maintain therapeutic serum level. After 24 hours of continuous infusion, rate is decreased by one-half. Or, 200 to 300 mg I.M., followed by second I.M. dose 60 to 90 minutes later, if needed.

Children: 1 mg/kg by I.V. bolus, followed by infusion of 20 to 50 mcg/kg/minute.

How supplied

Injection for I.M. use: 300 mg/3 ml automatic injection device
Injection for direct I.V. use: 1% (10 mg/ml), 2% (20 mg/ml)
Injection for I.V. admixtures: 4% (40 mg/ml), 10% (100 mg/ml), 20% (200 mg/ml)
Infusion (premixed): 0.2% (2 mg/ml), 0.4% (4 mg/ml), 0.8% (8 mg/ml)

Pharmacokinetics

Absorption: nearly complete after I.M. administration.
Distribution: distributed widely, especially to adipose tissue.
Metabolism: most of drug metabolized in liver to two active metabolites.
Excretion: less than 10% excreted in urine unchanged. *Half-life:* 15 minutes to 2 hours (may be prolonged in patients with heart failure or hepatic disease).

Route	Onset	Peak	Duration
I.V. (no bolus)	Immediate	30-60 min	10-20 min
I.M.	5-15 min	10 min	2 hr

Pharmacodynamics

Chemical effect: decreases depolarization, automaticity, and excitability in ventricles during diastolic phase by direct action on tissues.
Therapeutic effect: abolishes ventricular arrhythmias.

Adverse reactions

CNS: *confusion, tremors,* lethargy, somnolence, *stupor, restlessness,* slurred speech, euphoria, depression, *light-headedness,* paresthesia, muscle twitching, ***seizures.***
CV: *hypotension,* ***bradycardia, new or worsened arrhythmias, cardiac arrest.***
EENT: *tinnitus, blurred or double vision.*
Respiratory: ***respiratory arrest.***
Skin: diaphoresis.
Other: ***anaphylaxis,*** soreness at injection site, cold sensation, ***status asthmaticus.***

Interactions

Drug-drug. *Beta blockers, cimetidine:* decreased lidocaine metabolism. Monitor patient for toxicity.
Phenytoin, procainamide, propranolol, quinidine: additive cardiac depressant effects. Monitor patient.
Succinylcholine: possible prolonged neuromuscular blockage. Monitor patient for increased effects.
Tocainide: increased risk of adverse reactions. Avoid concomitant use.
Drug-herb. *Pareira:* may add to or potentiate neuromuscular blockade. Avoid concomitant use.
Drug-lifestyle. *Smoking:* may increase lidocaine metabolism. Monitor patient closely.

Contraindications and precautions

- Contraindicated in patients hypersensitive to amide-type local anesthetics and in those with Adams-Stokes syndrome, Wolff-Parkinson-White syndrome, or severe degrees of SA, AV, or intraventricular block in absence of artificial pacemaker.
- Use cautiously in patients with complete or second-degree heart block or sinus bradycardia, in elderly patients, in those with heart failure or renal or hepatic disease, and in those weighing less than 50 kg. These patients require reduced dosage.
- Safety of drug hasn't been established in children and in breast-feeding women.

NURSING CONSIDERATIONS

Assessment

- Assess patient's condition before therapy and regularly thereafter.
- Patient receiving infusion must be on cardiac monitor and be attended at all times.
- Monitor patient's response, especially ECG, blood pressure, and serum electrolyte, BUN, and creatinine levels, as ordered.
- Check for therapeutic serum levels (2 to 5 mcg/ml) as ordered.
- Be alert for adverse reactions and drug interactions.

ALERT Monitor patient for toxicity. Seizures may be first clinical sign. Severe reactions

usually are preceded by somnolence, confusion, and paresthesia.
• Evaluate patient's and family's knowledge of drug therapy.

Nursing diagnoses
• Decreased cardiac output related to presence of ventricular arrhythmia
• Disturbed thought processes related to adverse CNS reactions
• Deficient knowledge related to drug therapy

Planning and implementation
I.V. use: Use infusion-control device to administer infusion precisely. Don't exceed 4 mg/minute; faster rate greatly increases risk of toxicity.
ALERT Don't give concentrated lidocaine solutions (4%, 10%, 20%) by direct I.V. injection. Lidocaine injections containing 40, 100, or 200 mg/ml are for the preparation of I.V. infusion solutions and must be diluted before use.
I.M. use: Give I.M. injections only in deltoid muscle.
• Remind prescriber to test isoenzymes if I.M. route is prescribed in patients with suspected MI. This is necessary because patients who received I.M. lidocaine show sevenfold increase in serum CK level. Such an increase originates in skeletal muscle, not cardiac muscle.
• If signs of toxicity (such as dizziness) occur, stop drug at once and notify prescriber. Continued infusion could lead to seizures and coma. Give oxygen by way of nasal cannula, if not contraindicated. Keep oxygen and cardiopulmonary resuscitation equipment available.
• Discontinue drug and notify prescriber if arrhythmias worsen or if ECG changes, such as widening QRS complex or substantially prolonged PR interval, are evident.

Patient teaching
• Explain purpose of drug.
• Tell patient or caregiver to report adverse reactions.
• Instruct patient to avoid smoking during drug therapy.

Evaluation
• Patient's cardiac output returns to normal with abolishment of ventricular arrhythmia.
• Patient maintains normal thought processes throughout therapy.
• Patient and family state understanding of drug therapy.

linezolid
(linn-AYE-zoe-lid)
Zyvox

Pharmacologic class: oxazolidinone
Therapeutic class: antibiotic
Pregnancy risk category: C

Indications and dosages
▶ **Vancomycin-resistant *Enterococcus faecium* infections, including cases with concurrent bacteremia.** *Adults:* 600 mg I.V. or P.O. (tablets or suspension) q 12 hours for 14 to 28 days.
▶ **Nosocomial pneumonia caused by *Staphylococcus aureus* (methicillin-susceptible [MSSA] and methicillin-resistant [MRSA] strains) or penicillin-susceptible strains of *Streptococcus pneumonia*.** *Adults:* 600 mg I.V. or P.O. (tablets or suspension) q 12 hours for 10 to 14 days.
▶ **Complicated skin and skin-structure infections caused by *S. aureus* (MSSA and MSRA), *Streptococcus pyogenes*, or *Streptococcus agalactiae*.** *Adults:* 600 mg I.V. or P.O. (tablets or suspension) q 12 hours for 10 to 14 days.
▶ **Uncomplicated skin and skin-structure infections caused by *S. aureus* (MSSA) or *S. pyogenes*.** *Adults:* 400 mg P.O. (tablets or suspension) q 12 hours for 10 to 14 days.
▶ **Community-acquired pneumonia caused by *S. pneumoniae* (penicillin-susceptible strains), including case with concurrent bacteremia, or *S. aureus* (MSSA).** *Adults:* 600 mg I.V. or P.O. (tablets or suspension) q 12 hours for 10 to 14 days.

How supplied:
Tablets: 400 mg, 600 mg

Powder for oral suspension: 100 mg/5 ml when constituted
Injection: 2 mg/ml

Pharmacokinetics

Absorption: rapid and complete after P.O. dose. Levels peak in 1 to 2 hours. Bioavailability is about 100%.
Distribution: distributed readily into well-perfused tissues. Protein-binding is about 31%.
Metabolism: undergoes oxidative metabolism to two inactive metabolites. Linezolid doesn't appear to be metabolized by the cytochrome P-450 oxidative system.
Excretion: at steady-state, about 30% of an administered dose appears in urine as linezolid and about 50% as metabolites. Linezolid undergoes significant renal tubular reabsorption, such that renal clearance is low. Non-renal clearance accounts for about 65% of the total clearance.

Route	Onset	Peak	Duration
P.O			
tablet	Unknown	1 hr	4.7-5.4 hr
suspension	Unknown	1 hr	4.6 hr
I.V.	Unknown	0.5 hr	4.8 hr

Pharmacodynamics

Chemical effect: bacteriostatic against enterococci and staphylococci. Bactericidal against most strains of streptococci. Linezolid is active against methicillin-susceptible and resistant strains of *S. aureus* and penicillin-susceptible strains of *S. pneumoniae.* It's also active against *S. pyogenes,* and *S. algatactiae.* Linezolid exerts antimicrobial effects by interfering with bacterial protein synthesis. It binds to the 23S ribosomal DNA on the bacterial 50S ribosomal subunit. This action prevents formation of a functional 70S ribosomal subunit, thereby blocking the translation step of bacterial protein synthesis.
Therapeutic effect: hinders or kills susceptible bacteria.

Adverse reactions

CNS: headache, insomnia, dizziness.
GI: diarrhea, nausea, vomiting, constipation, elevated amylase, elevated lipase, altered taste, tongue discoloration, oral candidiasis.
GU: elevated BUN, vaginal candidiasis.
Hematologic: anemia, ***leukopenia, neutropenia, thrombocytopenia.***
Hepatic: elevated liver enzyme levels.
Skin: rash.
Other: fever, fungal infection.

Interactions

Drug-drug. *Adrenergics such as dopamine, epinephrine, and pseudoephedrine:* increased risk of hypertension. Monitor blood pressure and heart rate. Start continuous infusions of dopamine and epinephrine at lower doses, and adjust to response.
Serotoninergic drugs: increased risk of serotonin syndrome (confusion, delirium, restlessness, tremors, blushing, diaphoresis, hyperpyrexia). If these symptoms occur, consider stopping serotoninergic drug as directed.
Drug-food: *Foods and beverages high in tyramine, such as aged cheese, tap beer, red wine, air-dried meat, soy sauce, sauerkraut:* increased blood pressure. Tyramine content of meals shouldn't exceed 100 mg.

Contraindications and precautions

- Contraindicated in patients hypersensitive to linezolid or any inactive components of the formulation.

NURSING CONSIDERATIONS

Assessment

- Obtain history of patient's underlying condition before therapy, and reassess regularly thereafter.
- Obtain specimen for culture and sensitivity tests before starting linezolid therapy. Sensitivity results should be used to guide subsequent therapy.
- Monitor platelet count in patients with increased risk of bleeding, patients with thrombocytopenia, patients receiving drugs that may cause thrombocytopenia, and patients receiving linezolid for more than 14 days.
- Monitor patient for persistent diarrhea; consider pseudomembranous colitis.

• Evaluate patient's and family's knowledge of drug therapy.

Nursing diagnoses

• Infection related to susceptible bacteria
• Risk for injury related to drug-induced adverse reactions
• Deficient knowledge related to drug therapy

Planning and implementation

• Because inappropriate use of antibiotics may lead to resistant organisms, careful consideration should be given to alternative drugs before starting linezolid therapy, especially in the outpatient setting.

P.O. use: Reconstitute suspension according to manufacturer's instructions. Store at room temperature and use within 21 days.

I.V. use: Inspect for particulate matter and leaks.

– Infuse over 30 to 120 minutes. Don't infuse linezolid in a series connection.

– Don't inject additives into the infusion bag. Administer other I.V. medications separately or in a separate I.V. line to avoid physical incompatibilities. If a single I.V. line is used, flush the line with a compatible solution before and after linezolid infusion.

– Linezolid is compatible with the following I.V. solutions: D_5W, USP; normal saline solution for injection, USP; and lactated Ringer's injection, USP.

– Drugs known to be incompatible with linezolid include amphotericin B, ceftriaxone sodium, chlorpromazine hydrochloride, diazepam, erythromycin lactobionate, pentamidine isothionate, phenytoin sodium, and trimethoprim-sulfamethoxazole.

• Store drug at room temperature in its protective overwrap. The solution may turn yellow over time, but this doesn't indicate a change in potency.

• No dosage adjustment is needed when switching from I.V. to P.O. dosage forms.

• Safety and efficacy of linezolid therapy for longer than 28 days haven't been studied.

Patient teaching

• Inform patient that tablets and oral suspension may be taken with or without meals.

• Stress the importance of completing the entire course of therapy, even if the patient feels better.

• Teach patient to alert prescriber if he has hypertension, is taking cough or cold preparations, or is being treated with selective serotonin-reuptake inhibitors or other antidepressants.

• Inform patient with phenylketonuria that each 5 ml of linezolid oral suspension contains 20 mg of phenylalanine. Linezolid tablets and injection don't contain phenylalanine.

Evaluation

• Patient is free from infection.
• Patient doesn't experience injury as a result of drug-induced adverse reactions.
• Patient and family state understanding of drug therapy.

liothyronine sodium (T_3)

(lee-oh-THIGH-roh-neen SOH-dee-um)

Cytomel, Tertroxin ◇, Triostat

Pharmacologic class: thyroid hormone
Therapeutic class: thyroid hormone replacement
Pregnancy risk category: A

Indications and dosages

▶ **Congenital hypothyroidism.** *Children:* 5 mcg P.O. daily with a 5-mcg increase q 3 to 4 days until desired response is achieved.

▶ **Myxedema.** *Adults:* initially, 5 mcg P.O. daily, increased by 5 to 10 mcg q 1 to 2 weeks until daily dose reaches 25 mcg. Then, increased by 12.5 to 25 mcg daily q 1 to 2 weeks. Maintenance dose is 50 to 100 mcg daily.

▶ **Myxedema coma, precoma.** *Adults:* initially, 10 to 20 mcg I.V. for patients with known or suspected CV disease; 25 to 50 mcg I.V. for those not known to have CV disease. Subsequent dosages are based on patient's condition and response.

▶ **Nontoxic goiter.** *Adults:* initially, 5 mcg P.O. daily; may increase by 5 to 10 mcg daily q 1 to 2 weeks until daily dose reaches 25 mcg. Then, increase by 12.5 to 25 mcg daily q 1 to 2 weeks. Usual maintenance dose is 75 mcg daily.

▶ **Thyroid hormone replacement.** *Adults:* initially, 25 mcg P.O. daily, increased by 12.5 to 25 mcg q 1 to 2 weeks until satisfactory response is achieved. Usual maintenance dose is 25 to 75 mcg daily.

▶ **T_3 suppression test to differentiate hyperthyroidism from euthyroidism.** *Adults:* 75 to 100 mcg P.O. daily for 7 days.

How supplied

Tablets: 5 mcg, 25 mcg, 50 mcg
Injection: 10 mcg/ml

Pharmacokinetics

Absorption: 95% absorbed from GI tract.
Distribution: highly protein-bound.
Metabolism: unknown.
Excretion: unknown. *Half-life:* 1 to 2 days.

Route	Onset	Peak	Duration
P.O.	Unknown	2-3 days	About 3 days
I.V.	Unknown	Unknown	Unknown

Pharmacodynamics

Chemical effect: not clearly defined; enhances oxygen consumption by most body tissues and increases basal metabolic rate and metabolism of carbohydrates, lipids, and proteins.
Therapeutic effect: raises thyroid hormone levels in body.

Adverse reactions

Adverse reactions to thyroid hormones are extensions of their pharmacologic properties and reflect patient sensitivity to them.
CNS: irritability, *nervousness, insomnia, tremors,* headache.
CV: *tachycardia,* ***arrhythmias,*** angina pectoris, increased blood pressure, ***cardiac arrest.***
GI: diarrhea, abdominal cramps, vomiting.
GU: menstrual irregularities.
Metabolic: weight loss.
Musculoskeletal: accelerated bone maturation in infants and children.
Skin: diaphoresis.
Other: heat intolerance.

Interactions

Drug-drug. *Cholestyramine, colestipol:* impaired liothyronine absorption. Separate doses by 4 to 5 hours.
Insulin, oral antidiabetics: initial thyroid replacement therapy may increase insulin or oral hypoglycemic requirements. Monitor blood glucose levels. Dosage adjustments may be necessary.
I.V. phenytoin: free thyroid released. Monitor patient for tachycardia.
Oral anticoagulants: altered PT. Monitor PT and INR. Dosage adjustments may be necessary.
Sympathomimetics (such as epinephrine): increased risk of coronary insufficiency. Monitor patient closely.

Contraindications and precautions

- Contraindicated in patients hypersensitive to drug and in those with untreated thyrotoxicosis, uncorrected adrenal insufficiency, and acute MI uncomplicated by hypothyroidism.
- Use with extreme caution in elderly patients and those with angina pectoris, hypertension, other CV disorders, renal insufficiency, or ischemia.
- Rapid replacement in patients with arteriosclerosis may precipitate angina, coronary occlusion, or CVA. Use cautiously in these patients.
- Use cautiously in breast-feeding women and patients with diabetes mellitus, diabetes insipidus, or myxedema.

NURSING CONSIDERATIONS

Assessment

- Assess patient's condition before therapy and regularly thereafter.
- Monitor pulse rate and blood pressure.
- Observe patient with coronary artery disease for coronary insufficiency.
- Be alert for adverse reactions and drug interactions.
- Evaluate patient's and family's knowledge of drug therapy.

Nursing diagnoses

- Ineffective health maintenance related to underlying thyroid condition

- Disturbed sleep pattern related to drug-induced insomnia
- Deficient knowledge related to drug therapy

Planning and implementation

ALERT Don't confuse liothyronine with levothyroxine.

- Levothyroxine is usually preferred for thyroid hormone replacement therapy. Liothyronine may be used when rapid onset or rapidly reversible agent is desirable or in patients with impaired peripheral conversion of levothyroxine to liothyronine.
- In most patients, regulation of liothyronine dosage is difficult.

P.O. use: Give drug at same time every day, preferably in the morning to prevent insomnia.
I.V. use: Repeat doses should be given more than 4 hours but less than 12 hours apart. Don't give I.M. or S.C.

- Thyroid hormone replacement requirements are about 25% lower in patients over age 60 than in young adults.
- When changing from levothyroxine to liothyronine, levothyroxine should be stopped and liothyronine begun at low dosage and increased in small increments after residual effects of levothyroxine have disappeared. When changing from liothyronine to levothyroxine, levothyroxine is started several days before withdrawing liothyronine to avoid relapse.
- Thyroid hormones alter thyroid function tests. Patient taking liothyronine who needs radioactive iodine uptake studies must discontinue drug 7 to 10 days before test.
- Patient who takes thyroid hormone and prescribed anticoagulant usually needs decreased anticoagulant dosage.

Patient teaching

- Stress importance of compliance. Tell patient to take thyroid hormones at same time each day, preferably before breakfast, to maintain constant hormone levels and prevent insomnia.
- Advise patient who has achieved stable response not to change brands to avoid problems with bioequivalence.
- Warn patient (especially elderly patient) to notify prescriber at once if chest pain, palpitations, sweating, nervousness, or other signs of overdose occur or if signs of aggravated CV disease (chest pain, dyspnea, and tachycardia) develop.
- Tell patient to report unusual bleeding and bruising.

Evaluation

- Patient's thyroid hormone levels are normal.
- Patient doesn't have insomnia.
- Patient and family state understanding of drug therapy.

lisinopril

(ligh-SIN-uh-pril)
Prinivil, Zestril

Pharmacologic class: ACE inhibitor
Therapeutic class: antihypertensive
Pregnancy risk category: C (D in second and third trimesters)

Indications and dosages

▶ **Hypertension.** *Adults:* initially, 10 mg P.O. daily. If patient also takes a diuretic, reduce initial dosage to 5 mg P.O. daily. Most patients are well controlled on 20 to 40 mg daily as single dose.

▶ **Treatment adjunct in heart failure (with diuretics and cardiac glycosides).** *Adults:* initially, 5 mg P.O. daily. Usual effective dosage range is 5 to 20 mg daily as single dose. In patients with hyponatremia (serum sodium below 130 mEq/L) or serum creatinine above 3 mg/dl, start with 2.5 mg P.O. once daily.

▶ **Treatment of hemodynamically stable patients within 24 hours of acute MI to improve survival.** *Adults*: initially, 5 mg P.O. Then 5 mg P.O. after 24 hours, 10 mg P.O. after 48 hours, and 10 mg P.O. once daily for 6 weeks. Patients with systolic blood pressure of 120 mm Hg or less at start of therapy or during first 3 days after an infarct should receive reduced dosage of 2.5 mg P.O.

How supplied

Tablets: 2.5 mg, 5 mg, 10 mg, 20 mg, 40 mg

Pharmacokinetics

Absorption: variable.
Distribution: distributed widely in tissues, although only minimal amount enters brain. Plasma protein–binding appears insignificant.
Metabolism: not metabolized.
Excretion: excreted unchanged in urine. *Half-life:* 12 hours.

Route	Onset	Peak	Duration
P.O.	1 hr	7 hr	24 hr

Pharmacodynamics

Chemical effect: unknown; may result primarily from suppression of renin-angiotensin-aldosterone system.
Therapeutic effect: lowers blood pressure.

Adverse reactions

CNS: *dizziness, headache, fatigue,* depression, somnolence, paresthesia.
CV: hypotension, *orthostatic hypotension,* chest pain.
EENT: *nasal congestion.*
GI: *diarrhea,* nausea, dyspepsia, dysgeusia.
GU: impotence.
Hematologic: neutropenia, ***agranulocytopenia.***
Metabolic: hyperkalemia.
Musculoskeletal: *muscle cramps.*
Respiratory: *dry, persistent, tickling, nonproductive cough.*
Skin: rash.
Other: ***angioedema, anaphylaxis,*** decreased libido.

Interactions

Drug-drug. *Capsaicin:* may cause or worsen coughing caused by ACE inhibitors. Monitor patient closely.
Diuretics: excessive hypotension. Monitor blood pressure.
Indomethacin: attenuated hypotensive effect. Monitor blood pressure.
Insulin, oral antidiabetics: risk of hypoglycemia, especially when starting lisinopril. Monitor patient closely.
Lithium: increased serum lithium levels. Monitor patient for toxicity.
Potassium-sparing diuretics, potassium supplements: hyperkalemia. Monitor potassium level.
Thiazide diuretics: attenuation of potassium loss caused by thiazide diuretics. Discontinue diuretics 2 to 3 days before lisinopril therapy or reduce lisinopril dosage to 5 mg P.O. once daily, as ordered.
Drug-herb. *Licorice:* can cause sodium retention and increase blood pressure, interfering with the therapeutic effects of ACE inhibitors. Discourage concomitant use.
Drug-food. *Potassium-containing salt substitutes*: possible hyperkalemia. Monitor patient closely.

Contraindications and precautions

- Contraindicated in patients hypersensitive to ACE inhibitors, in those with a history of angioedema from previous treatment with an ACE inhibitor, and in pregnant women.
- Use cautiously in patients with impaired kidney function; adjust dosage as directed. Also use cautiously in patients at risk for hyperkalemia (those with renal insufficiency or diabetes or who use drugs that raise potassium level) and in breast-feeding women.
- Safety of drug hasn't been established in children.

NURSING CONSIDERATIONS

Assessment

- Assess patient's condition before therapy and regularly thereafter. Beneficial effects of drug may require several weeks of therapy.
- Monitor WBC with differential counts before therapy, every 2 weeks for first 3 months of therapy, and periodically thereafter.
- Be alert for adverse reactions and drug interactions.
- Evaluate patient's and family's knowledge of drug therapy.

Nursing diagnoses

- Risk for injury related to presence of hypertension
- Decreased cardiac output related to drug-induced hypotension
- Deficient knowledge related to drug therapy

Planning and implementation

ALERT Don't confuse lisinopril with fosinopril or Lioresal. Don't confuse Prinivil with Proventil or Prilosec. Don't confuse Zestril with Zostrix.

- If drug doesn't control blood pressure, diuretics may be added.

Patient teaching

- Advise patient to report signs or symptoms of angioedema (including laryngeal edema), such as breathing difficulty or swelling of face, eyes, lips, or tongue.
- Tell patient that light-headedness may occur, especially during first few days of therapy. Tell him to rise slowly to minimize this effect and to report symptoms to prescriber. If syncope occurs, tell patient to stop taking drug and call prescriber immediately.
- Tell patient not to discontinue drug suddenly but to call prescriber if adverse reactions occur.
- Advise patient to report signs of infection, such as fever and sore throat.
- Tell women to notify prescriber if pregnancy occurs. Drug will need to be discontinued.

Evaluation

- Patient's blood pressure is within normal limits.
- Patient maintains adequate cardiac output throughout therapy.
- Patient and family state understanding of drug therapy.

lithium carbonate

(LITH-ee-um KAR-buh-nayt)

Carbolith ♦, Duralith ♦, Eskalith, Eskalith CR, Lithane**, Lithicarb ◇, Lithizine ♦, Lithobid, Lithonate, Lithotabs

lithium citrate

Cibalith-S*

Pharmacologic class: alkali metal
Therapeutic class: antimanic agent
Pregnancy risk category: D

Indications and dosages

▶ **Prevention or control of mania.** *Adults:* 300 to 600 mg P.O. up to q.i.d., increasing on basis of blood levels to achieve optimal dosage, usually 1,800 mg/day. Recommended therapeutic lithium blood levels: 1 to 1.5 mEq/L for acute mania; 0.6 to 1.2 mEq/L for maintenance therapy; and 2 mEq/L as maximum dosage.

How supplied

lithium carbonate
Tablets: 300 mg (300 mg = 8.12 mEq lithium)
Tablets (controlled-release): 300 mg, 450 mg
Capsules: 150 mg, 300 mg, 600 mg
lithium citrate
Syrup (sugarless): 8 mEq (of lithium) per 5 ml (8 mEq lithium = 300 mg of lithium carbonate)

Pharmacokinetics

Absorption: rate and extent vary with dosage form; absorption is complete within 8 hours of P.O. use.
Distribution: distributed widely; levels in thyroid gland, bone, and brain exceed serum levels.
Metabolism: not metabolized.
Excretion: 95% excreted unchanged in urine. *Half-life:* 18 hours (adolescents) to 36 hours (elderly).

Route	Onset	Peak	Duration
P.O.	1-3 wk	0.5-3 hr	Unknown

Pharmacodynamics

Chemical effect: unknown; probably alters chemical transmitters in CNS, possibly by interfering with ionic pump mechanisms in brain cells, and may compete with sodium ions.
Therapeutic effect: prevents or controls mania.

Adverse reactions

CNS: tremors, drowsiness, headache, confusion, restlessness, dizziness, psychomotor retardation, stupor, lethargy, ***coma,*** blackouts, ***epileptiform seizures,*** EEG changes, worsened organic mental syndrome, impaired speech, ataxia, weakness, incoordination.
CV: *reversible ECG changes,* ***arrhythmias,*** hypotension.

EENT: tinnitus, blurred vision.
GI: dry mouth, metallic taste, nausea, vomiting, anorexia, diarrhea, thirst, abdominal pain, flatulence, indigestion.
GU: polyuria, glycosuria, ***renal toxicity*** with long-term use, decreased creatinine clearance, albuminuria.
Hematologic: *leukocytosis with leukocyte count of 14,000 to 18,000/mm³* (reversible).
Metabolic: transient hyperglycemia, goiter, hypothyroidism (lowered T_3, T_4, and protein-bound iodine but elevated ^{131}I [radioactive iodine] uptake), hyponatremia.
Skin: pruritus, rash, diminished or absent sensation, drying and thinning of hair, psoriasis, acne, alopecia.
Other: ankle and wrist edema.

Interactions

Drug-drug. *Aminophylline, sodium bicarbonate, urine alkalinizers:* increased lithium excretion. Avoid salt loads and monitor lithium levels.
Carbamazepine, indomethacin, methyldopa, piroxicam, probenecid: increased effect of lithium. Monitor patient for lithium toxicity.
Diuretics: increased reabsorption of lithium by kidneys with possible toxic effect. Use with extreme caution, and monitor lithium and electrolyte levels (especially sodium).
Fluoxetine: increased lithium serum levels. Monitor patient for toxicity.
Neuroleptics: may cause encephalopathy. Watch for signs and symptoms (lethargy, tremors, extrapyramidal symptoms), and stop drug if they occur.
Neuromuscular blockers: may cause prolonged paralysis or weakness. Monitor patient closely.
Thyroid hormones: may induce hypothyroidism. Monitor thyroid function.
Drug-herb. *Parsley:* may promote or produce serotonin syndrome. Discourage concomitant use.

Contraindications and precautions

- Contraindicated if therapy can't be closely monitored.
- Drug shouldn't be used in pregnant or breast-feeding women.
- Drug isn't recommended for use in children under age 12.
- Use with extreme caution in patients receiving neuroleptics, neuromuscular blockers, or diuretics; in elderly or debilitated patients; and in patients with thyroid disease, seizure disorder, renal or CV disease, severe debilitation or dehydration, or sodium depletion.

NURSING CONSIDERATIONS

Assessment

- Assess patient's condition before therapy and regularly thereafter. Expect delay of 1 to 3 weeks before drug's beneficial effects are noticed.
- Monitor baseline ECG, thyroid and kidney studies, and electrolyte levels, as ordered. Monitor lithium blood levels 8 to 12 hours after first dose, usually before morning dose, two or three times weekly in first month, then weekly to monthly during maintenance therapy.
- With blood levels of lithium below 1.5 mEq/L, adverse reactions usually remain mild.
- Check urine-specific gravity and report level below 1.005, which may indicate diabetes insipidus.
- Lithium may alter glucose tolerance in diabetic patient. Monitor blood glucose level closely.
- Perform outpatient follow-up of thyroid and kidney function every 6 to 12 months. Palpate thyroid to check for enlargement.
- Be alert for adverse reactions and drug interactions.
- Evaluate patient's and family's knowledge of drug therapy.

Nursing diagnoses

- Disturbed thought processes related to presence of manic disorder
- Ineffective health maintenance related to drug-induced endocrine dysfunction
- Deficient knowledge related to drug therapy

Planning and implementation

ALERT Don't confuse Lithobid with Levbid, Lithonate with Lithostat, or Lithotabs with Lithobid or Lithostat.

• Determination of lithium blood levels is crucial to safe use of drug. Drug shouldn't be used in patients who can't have blood level checked regularly.
• Give with plenty of water and after meals to minimize GI reactions.
• Before leaving bedside, make sure patient has swallowed medication.
• Notify prescriber if patient's behavior hasn't improved in 3 weeks or if it worsens.

Patient teaching
• Tell patient to take drug with plenty of water and after meals to minimize GI upset.
• Explain that lithium has narrow therapeutic margin of safety. A blood level that is even slightly high can be dangerous.
• Warn patient and family to watch for signs of toxicity (diarrhea, vomiting, tremors, drowsiness, muscle weakness, ataxia) and to expect transient nausea, polyuria, thirst, and discomfort during first few days. Tell patient to withhold one dose and call prescriber if toxic symptoms appear but not to stop drug abruptly.
• Warn patient to avoid activities that require alertness and good psychomotor coordination until CNS effects of drug are known.
• Tell patient not to switch brands or take other prescription or OTC drugs without prescriber's approval.
• Advise patient to wear or carry medical identification.

Evaluation
• Patient exhibits improved behavior and thought processes.
• Patient maintains normal endocrine function throughout therapy.
• Patient and family state understanding of drug therapy.

lomefloxacin hydrochloride
(loh-muh-FLOKS-uh-sin high-droh-KLOR-ighd)
Maxaquin

Pharmacologic class: fluoroquinolone
Therapeutic class: broad-spectrum antibiotic
Pregnancy risk category: C

Indications and dosages
▶ **Acute bacterial exacerbations of chronic bronchitis caused by *Haemophilus influenzae* or *Moraxella catarrhalis*.** *Adults:* 400 mg P.O. daily for 10 days.
▶ **Uncomplicated urinary tract infections (cystitis) caused by *Escherichia coli, Klebsiella pneumoniae, Proteus mirabilis,* or *Staphylococcus saprophyticus*.** *Adults:* 400 mg P.O. daily for 10 days.
▶ **Complicated urinary tract infections caused by *E. coli, K. pneumoniae, P. mirabilis,* or *Pseudomonas aeruginosa*; possibly effective against infections caused by *Citrobacter diversus* or *Enterobacter cloacae*.** *Adults:* 400 mg P.O. daily for 14 days.
▶ **Prevention of infections after transurethral surgical procedures.** *Adults:* 400 mg P.O. as single dose 2 to 6 hours before surgery. Patients with creatinine clearance of 10 to 40 ml/minute should receive loading dose of 400 mg P.O. on first day, followed by 200 mg daily for duration of therapy. Hemodialysis removes negligible amounts of drug.

How supplied
Tablets (film-coated): 400 mg

Pharmacokinetics
Absorption: absorbed rapidly from GI tract; absolute bioavailability is 95% to 98%. Food impairs absorption by reducing total amount absorbed and slowing absorption rate.
Distribution: 10% bound to plasma proteins.
Metabolism: metabolized in liver.
Excretion: most of drug excreted in urine; about 10% excreted in feces. *Half-life:* 8 hours.

Route	Onset	Peak	Duration
P.O.	Unknown	1.5 hr	Unknown

Pharmacodynamics
Chemical effect: inhibits bacterial DNA gyrase, an enzyme necessary for bacterial replication (bactericidal).
Therapeutic effect: inhibits bacterial growth. Spectrum of activity includes *E. coli, H. influenzae, K. pneumoniae, M. catarrhalis, P.*

mirabilis, P. aeruginosa, S. saprophyticus, and possibly *C. diversus* or *E. cloacae.*

Adverse reactions

CNS: *dizziness, headache,* abnormal dreams, fatigue, malaise, asthenia, agitation, anxiety, confusion, depersonalization, depression, insomnia, nervousness, somnolence, ***seizures, coma,*** hyperkinesia, tremors, vertigo, paresthesia.
CV: flushing, hypotension, hypertension, edema, syncope, arrhythmia, tachycardia, ***bradycardia***, extrasystoles, cyanosis, angina pectoris, ***MI, cardiac failure, pulmonary embolisms,*** cerebrovascular disorder, ***cardiomyopathy,*** phlebitis.
EENT: epistaxis, abnormal vision, conjunctivitis, eye pain, earache, tinnitus.
GI: taste perversion, *diarrhea, nausea,* anorexia, increased appetite, tongue discoloration, dry mouth, abdominal pain, dyspepsia, vomiting, flatulence, constipation, inflammation, dysphagia, bleeding.
GU: dysuria, hematuria, anuria, epididymitis, orchitis, vaginal candidiasis, perineal pain, intermenstrual bleeding, leukorrhea, vaginitis.
Hematologic: thrombocythemia, ***thrombocytopenia,*** lymphadenopathy, increased fibrinolysis.
Hepatic: elevated liver enzyme levels.
Metabolic: hypoglycemia, gout.
Musculoskeletal: leg cramps, back pain, arthralgia, myalgia.
Respiratory: cough, dyspnea, chest pain, ***bronchospasm,*** respiratory disorder, infection, increased sputum, stridor.
Skin: pruritus, skin disorder, diaphoresis, skin exfoliation, eczema, rash, urticaria, *photosensitivity.*
Other: ***anaphylaxis,*** thirst, chills, allergic reaction, facial edema, flulike symptoms, decreased heat tolerance.

Interactions

Drug-drug. *Antacids, didanosine, iron salts, sucralfate, zinc salts:* impaired absorption after binding with lomefloxacin in GI tract. Give at least 4 hours before or 2 hours after dose.
Antineoplastic drugs: fluoroquinolone serum levels may be decreased. Monitor patient.
Cimetidine: increased half-life of other fluoroquinolones when administered to patient taking cimetidine; lomefloxacin hasn't been tested. Monitor patient for toxicity.
Cyclosporine, warfarin: increased effects on serum levels when combined with other fluoroquinolones; lomefloxacin hasn't been tested. Monitor patient for toxicity.
Probenecid: decreased excretion of lomefloxacin. Monitor patient for toxicity.
Drug-herb. *St. John's wort:* increased risk of photosensitivity. Advise patient to avoid unprotected exposure to sunlight.
Drug-lifestyle. *Sun exposure:* photosensitivity reactions may occur. Advise patient to take precautions.

Contraindications and precautions

- Contraindicated in patients hypersensitive to drug or other fluoroquinolones.
- Drug isn't recommended for use in breastfeeding women.
- Use cautiously in patients with known or suspected CNS disorders that may predispose them to seizures, such as seizure disorder or cerebral arteriosclerosis.
- Safety of drug hasn't been established in children.

NURSING CONSIDERATIONS

Assessment

- Assess patient's infection before therapy and regularly thereafter.
- Obtain specimen for culture and sensitivity tests before first dose. Therapy may begin pending test results.
- Be alert for adverse reactions and drug interactions.
- Monitor patient's hydration status if adverse GI reactions occur.
- Evaluate patient's and family's knowledge of drug therapy.

Nursing diagnoses

- Infection related to presence of susceptible bacteria
- Risk for deficient fluid volume related to drug-induced adverse GI reactions
- Deficient knowledge related to drug therapy

Planning and implementation
- Administer drug on empty stomach.
- Prolonged use may result in overgrowth of organisms resistant to lomefloxacin.

Patient teaching
- Advise patient that hypersensitivity reactions may occur even after first dose. If rash or other allergic reaction occurs, tell patient to stop taking drug and notify prescriber.
- Warn patient to refrain from driving and performing other hazardous tasks until CNS effects of drug are known. Drug may cause dizziness or light-headedness.
- Advise patient to wear protective clothing, use sunblock, and avoid prolonged exposure to sunlight during treatment and for a few days after therapy ends. If sunburn occurs, tell him to call prescriber promptly.

Evaluation
- Patient is free from infection.
- Patient maintains adequate hydration throughout therapy.
- Patient and family state understanding of drug therapy.

lomustine (CCNU)
(loh-MUH-steen)
CeeNU

Pharmacologic class: alkylating agent, nitrosourea (cell cycle–phase nonspecific)
Therapeutic class: antineoplastic
Pregnancy risk category: D

Indications and dosages
▶ **Brain tumor, Hodgkin's disease.** *Adults and children:* 100 to 130 mg/m² P.O. as single dose q 6 weeks. Dosage reduced according to degree of bone marrow suppression. Repeat doses shouldn't be given until WBC count is more than 4,000/mm³ and platelet count is more than 100,000/mm³.

How supplied
Capsules: 10 mg, 40 mg, 100 mg, dose pack (two 10-mg, two 40-mg, two 100-mg capsules)

Pharmacokinetics
Absorption: absorbed rapidly and well across GI tract after P.O. use.
Distribution: distributed widely in body tissues and crosses blood-brain barrier to significant extent.
Metabolism: metabolized rapidly and extensively in liver.
Excretion: metabolites excreted primarily in urine with smaller amounts excreted in feces and through lungs. *Half-life:* 1 to 2 days.

Route	Onset	Peak	Duration
P.O.	Unknown	Unknown	Unknown

Pharmacodynamics
Chemical effect: cross-links strands of cellular DNA and interferes with RNA transcription.
Therapeutic effect: kills selected cancer cells.

Adverse reactions
GI: *nausea, vomiting* (beginning within 4 to 5 hours), stomatitis.
GU: ***nephrotoxicity,*** progressive azotemia, ***renal failure.***
Hematologic: anemia, leukopenia (delayed up to 6 weeks, lasting 1 to 2 weeks), ***thrombocytopenia*** (delayed up to 4 weeks, lasting 1 to 2 weeks), ***bone marrow suppression*** (delayed up to 6 weeks).
Hepatic: ***hepatotoxicity.***
Respiratory: ***pulmonary fibrosis.***
Other: ***secondary malignant disease.***

Interactions
Drug-drug. *Anticoagulants, aspirin:* increased bleeding risk. Avoid concomitant use.

Contraindications and precautions
- Contraindicated in patients hypersensitive to drug.
- Drug isn't recommended for use in pregnant or breast-feeding women.
- Use cautiously in patients with decreased platelet, WBC, or RBC count and in those receiving other myelosuppressant drugs.

NURSING CONSIDERATIONS

Assessment
- Assess patient's condition before therapy and regularly thereafter.
- Monitor CBC weekly, as ordered; bone marrow toxicity is delayed.
- Periodically monitor liver function tests, as ordered.
- Be alert for adverse reactions and drug interactions.
- Evaluate patient's and family's knowledge of drug therapy.

Nursing diagnoses
- Ineffective health maintenance related to presence of neoplastic disease
- Ineffective protection related to adverse hematologic reactions
- Deficient knowledge related to drug therapy

Planning and implementation
- To avoid nausea, give antiemetic before giving drug, as ordered.
- Give 2 to 4 hours after meals; drug is better absorbed if taken on empty stomach.
- Drug administration is repeated only when CBC results reveal safe hematologic parameters.
- Institute infection-control and bleeding precautions.

Patient teaching
- Warn patient to watch for signs of infection (fever, sore throat, fatigue) and bleeding (easy bruising, nosebleeds, bleeding gums, melena) and to take temperature daily.
- Instruct patient to avoid OTC products containing aspirin.
- Advise woman of childbearing age to avoid becoming pregnant during therapy and to consult with prescriber before becoming pregnant.

Evaluation
- Patient responds well to therapy.
- Patient regains normal hematologic function.
- Patient and family state understanding of drug therapy.

loperamide
(loh-PEH-ruh-mighd)

Imodium, Imodium A-D†, Kaopectate II Caplets†, Maalox Anti-Diarrheal Caplets†, Neo-Diaral†, Pepto Diarrhea Control†

Pharmacologic class: piperidine derivative
Therapeutic class: antidiarrheal
Pregnancy risk category: B

Indications and dosages

▶ **Acute, nonspecific diarrhea.** *Adults and children over age 12:* initially, 4 mg P.O.; then 2 mg after each unformed stool. Maximum dosage is 16 mg daily.
Children ages 8 to 12: 10 ml (2 mg) t.i.d. P.O. on first day. Subsequent doses of 5 ml (1 mg)/10 kg (22 lb) of body weight may be given after each unformed stool. Maximum dosage is 6 mg daily.
Children ages 6 to 8: 10 ml (2 mg) P.O. b.i.d. on first day. Report persistent diarrhea.
Children ages 2 to 6: 5 ml (1 mg) P.O. t.i.d. on first day. Report persistent diarrhea.

▶ **Chronic diarrhea.** *Adults:* initially, 4 mg P.O.; then 2 mg after each unformed stool until diarrhea subsides. Dosage adjusted to individual response.

▶ **Acute diarrhea including traveler's diarrhea (OTC).** *Adults:* 4 mg after first loose bowel movement followed by 2 mg after each subsequent loose bowel movement; maximum 8 mg/day for 2 days.

How supplied

Tablets: 2 mg†
Capsules: 2 mg
Oral liquid*: 1 mg/5 ml†, 1 mg/ml†

Pharmacokinetics

Absorption: absorbed poorly from GI tract.
Distribution: unknown.
Metabolism: metabolized in liver.
Excretion: excreted primarily in feces; less than 2% excreted in urine. *Half-life:* 9.1 to 14.4 hours.

Route	Onset	Peak	Duration
P.O.	Unknown	2.5-5 hr	24 hr

Pharmacodynamics

Chemical effect: inhibits peristaltic activity, prolonging transit of intestinal contents.
Therapeutic effect: relieves diarrhea.

Adverse reactions

CNS: drowsiness, fatigue, dizziness.
GI: dry mouth; abdominal pain, distention, or discomfort; *constipation;* nausea; vomiting.
Skin: rash, hypersensitivity reactions.

Interactions

None significant.

Contraindications and precautions

- Contraindicated in patients hypersensitive to drug, in children younger than age 2, and in patients in whom constipation must be avoided.
- Use cautiously in patients with hepatic disease and in pregnant or breast-feeding women.
- OTC form is contraindicated in patients with bloody diarrhea and those with fever over 101° F (38° C).

NURSING CONSIDERATIONS

Assessment

- Assess patient's diarrhea before therapy and regularly thereafter.
- Be alert for adverse reactions.

ALERT Monitor children closely for CNS effects because they may be more sensitive than adults to such effects.

- Monitor patient's hydration status if adverse GI reactions occur.
- Evaluate patient's and family's knowledge of drug therapy.

Nursing diagnoses

- Diarrhea related to underlying condition
- Risk for deficient fluid volume related to drug-induced adverse GI reactions
- Deficient knowledge related to drug therapy

Planning and implementation

ALERT Don't confuse Imodium with Ionamin.

- Notify prescriber if acute abdominal signs occur or drug is ineffective.
- If drug is given by nasogastric tube, flush tube to clear it and ensure drug's passage to stomach.

ALERT Oral liquids are available in different concentrations. Check dosage carefully. For children, consider an oral liquid product that doesn't contain alcohol.

Patient teaching

- Advise patient not to exceed recommended dosage.
- Tell patient with acute diarrhea to discontinue drug and seek medical attention if no improvement occurs within 48 hours; for chronic diarrhea, tell him to notify prescriber and discontinue drug if no improvement occurs after giving 16 mg daily for at least 10 days.
- Advise patient to stop taking drug and to notify prescriber immediately if abdominal distention or other symptoms develop in acute colitis.

Evaluation

- Patient's diarrhea is relieved.
- Patient maintains adequate hydration throughout therapy.
- Patient and family state understanding of drug therapy.

loracarbef

(loh-ruh-KAR-bef)
Lorabid

Pharmacologic class: synthetic beta-lactam antibiotic of carbacephem class
Therapeutic class: antibiotic
Pregnancy risk category: B

Indications and dosages

▶ **Secondary bacterial infections of acute bronchitis.** *Adults:* 200 to 400 g P.O. q 12 hours for 7 days.
▶ **Acute bacterial exacerbations of chronic bronchitis.** *Adults:* 400 mg P.O. q 12 hours for 7 days.
▶ **Pneumonia.** *Adults:* 400 mg P.O. q 12 hours for 14 days.
▶ **Pharyngitis, sinusitis, tonsillitis.** *Adults:* 200 to 400 mg P.O. q 12 hours for 10 days.

Children: 15 mg/kg P.O. daily in divided doses q 12 hours for 10 days.

▶ **Acute otitis media.** *Children:* 30 mg/kg (oral suspension) P.O. daily in divided doses q 12 hours for 10 days.

▶ **Uncomplicated skin and skin-structure infections.** *Adults:* 200 mg P.O. q 12 hours for 7 days.

▶ **Impetigo.** *Children:* 15 mg/kg P.O. daily in divided doses q 12 hours for 7 days.

▶ **Uncomplicated cystitis.** *Adults:* 200 mg P.O. daily for 7 days.

▶ **Uncomplicated pyelonephritis.** *Adults:* 400 mg P.O. q 12 hours for 14 days. Patients with creatinine clearance of 50 ml/minute or more don't need dose and interval changes. Patients with creatinine clearance of 10 to 49 ml/minute should receive half of usual dose at same interval. Patients with creatinine clearance below 10 ml/minute should receive usual dose q 3 to 5 days. Hemodialysis patients require another dose after dialysis.

How supplied

Pulvules: 200 mg, 400 mg
Powder for oral suspension: 100 mg/5 ml, 200 mg/5 ml in 50-ml, 75-ml and 100-ml bottles

Pharmacokinetics

Absorption: about 90% absorbed from GI tract. Absorption of suspension is greater than that of capsule.
Distribution: about 25% of circulating drug is bound to plasma proteins.
Metabolism: doesn't appear to be metabolized.
Excretion: excreted primarily in urine. *Half-life:* about 1 hour.

Route	Onset	Peak	Duration
P.O.	Unknown	0.5-1 hr	Unknown

Pharmacodynamics

Chemical effect: inhibits cell-wall synthesis, promoting osmotic instability; usually bactericidal.
Therapeutic effect: kills susceptible bacteria. Spectrum of activity includes gram-positive aerobes, such as *Staphylococcus aureus* and *saprophyticus, Streptococcus pneumoniae* and *pyogenes;* and gram-negative aerobes, such as *Escherichia coli, Haemophilus influenzae*, and *Moraxella catarrhalis.*

Adverse reactions

CNS: headache, somnolence, nervousness, insomnia, dizziness.
CV: vasodilation.
GI: diarrhea, nausea, vomiting, abdominal pain, anorexia, pseudomembranous colitis.
GU: vaginal candidiasis, elevated BUN and creatinine levels.
Hematologic: ***transient thrombocytopenia, leukopenia,*** eosinophilia.
Hepatic: transient elevations in AST, ALT, and alkaline phosphatase levels.
Skin: rash, urticaria, pruritus, ***erythema multiforme.***
Other: hypersensitivity reactions, ***anaphylaxis.***

Interactions

Drug-drug. *Probenecid:* decreased loracarbef excretion, causing increased plasma levels. Monitor patient for toxicity.
Drug-food. *Any food:* decreased absorption. Give drug 1 hour before or 2 hours after meals.

Contraindications and precautions

- Contraindicated in patients hypersensitive to drug or other cephalosporins and in patients with diarrhea caused by pseudomembranous colitis.
- Use cautiously in pregnant or breast-feeding women.
- Safety and efficacy haven't been established in infants under age 6 months.

NURSING CONSIDERATIONS

Assessment

- Assess patient's infection before therapy and regularly thereafter.
- Obtain specimen for culture and sensitivity tests before giving first dose. Therapy may begin pending test results.
- Be alert for adverse reactions and drug interactions.

ALERT Watch for seizures. Beta-lactam antibiotics may trigger seizures in susceptible

patients, especially when given without dosage modification to those with renal impairment.
• Monitor patient's hydration status if adverse GI reactions occur.
• Evaluate patient's and family's knowledge of drug therapy.

Nursing diagnoses
• Infection related to presence of susceptible bacteria
• Risk for deficient fluid volume related to drug-induced adverse GI reactions
• Deficient knowledge related to drug therapy

Planning and implementation
ALERT Don't confuse Lorabid with Lortab.
• To reconstitute powder for oral suspension, add 30 ml of water in two portions to 50-ml bottle or 60 ml of water in two portions to 100-ml bottle. Shake after each addition.
• After reconstitution, store oral suspension for 14 days at constant room temperature (59° to 86° F [15° to 30° C]).
• If seizures occur, stop drug and tell prescriber. Give anticonvulsants, as ordered.
• Between 40% and 75% of patients receiving cephalosporins show false-positive direct Coombs' test; only some indicate hemolytic anemia.

Patient teaching
• Tell patient to take drug on an empty stomach, at least 1 hour before or 2 hours after meals.
• Tell patient to shake suspension well before measuring dose.
• Tell patient to take drug exactly as prescribed.
• Instruct patient to discard unused portion after 14 days.

Evaluation
• Patient is free from infection.
• Patient maintains adequate hydration throughout therapy.
• Patient and family state understanding of drug therapy.

loratadine
(loo-RAH-tuh-deen)
Claratyne ◇, Claritin, Claritin Reditabs, Claritin Syrup

Pharmacologic class: tricyclic antihistamine
Therapeutic class: antihistamine
Pregnancy risk category: B

Indications and dosages
▶ **Symptomatic treatment of seasonal allergic rhinitis.** *Adults and children age 12 and over:* 10 mg P.O. daily.
Children ages 6 to 11: 10 mg (10 ml) once daily.

How supplied
Tablets: 10 mg
Tablets (rapidly disintegrating): 10 mg
Syrup: 1 mg/ml

Pharmacokinetics
Absorption: readily absorbed. Food may delay peak plasma levels by 1 hour.
Distribution: doesn't readily cross blood-brain barrier; about 97% bound to plasma protein.
Metabolism: extensively metabolized, although specific enzyme systems responsible for metabolism haven't been identified.
Excretion: about 80% distributed equally between urine and feces. *Half-life:* 8.4 hours.

Route	Onset	Peak	Duration
P.O.	1 hr	4-6 hr	24 hr

Pharmacodynamics
Chemical effect: blocks effects of histamine at H_1-receptor sites. Loratadine is a nonsedating antihistamine; its chemical structure prevents entry into CNS.
Therapeutic effect: relieves allergy symptoms.

Adverse reactions
CNS: headache, somnolence, fatigue.
GI: dry mouth.

Interactions
Drug-drug. *Erythromycin:* increased plasma loratadine levels. Monitor patient closely.

Drug-lifestyle. *Alcohol use:* increased CNS depression. Urge caution.
Sun exposure: photosensitivity reactions may occur. Tell patient to take precautions.

Contraindications and precautions

- Contraindicated in patients hypersensitive to drug.
- Drug isn't recommended for use in breast-feeding women.
- Use in pregnant women only when absolutely necessary.
- Use cautiously in patients with hepatic impairment.
- Safety of drug hasn't been established in children younger than age 6.

NURSING CONSIDERATIONS

Assessment

- Assess patient's condition before therapy and regularly thereafter.
- Be alert for adverse reactions and drug interactions.
- Evaluate patient's and family's knowledge of drug therapy.

Nursing diagnoses

- Ineffective health maintenance related to underlying allergy condition
- Fatigue related to drug's adverse effect
- Deficient knowledge related to drug therapy

Planning and implementation

- Dosage for patients with hepatic failure or renal insufficiency should be reduced.
- Give drug on empty stomach.
- Notify prescriber if drug is ineffective.

Patient teaching

- Tell patient to take drug at least 2 hours after meal, to avoid eating for at least 1 hour after taking drug, and to take drug only once daily.
- Advise patient taking Claritin Reditabs to place tablet on the tongue, where it disintegrates within a few seconds. It can be swallowed with or without water.
- Tell patient to contact prescriber if symptoms persist or worsen.
- Advise patient to stop taking drug 4 days before allergy skin tests to preserve accuracy of tests.
- Instruct patient to avoid prolonged exposure to the sun and to wear sunblock and protective clothing during drug therapy.
- Tell patient to avoid alcohol and driving or other activities that require alertness until CNS effects of drug are known.
- Review patient's coping strategies for fatigue.

Evaluation

- Patient states that allergy symptoms are relieved.
- Patient describes coping strategies for fatigue.
- Patient and family state understanding of drug therapy.

lorazepam

(loo-RAZ-eh-pam)

Apo-Lorazepam ♦, Ativan, Lorazepam Intensol, Novo-Lorazem ♦, Nu-Loraz ♦

Pharmacologic class: benzodiazepine
Therapeutic class: antianxiety agent, sedative-hypnotic
Controlled substance schedule: IV
Pregnancy risk category: NR

Indications and dosages

▶ **Anxiety.** *Adults:* 2 to 6 mg P.O. daily in divided doses. Maximum, 10 mg daily.

▶ **Insomnia caused by anxiety.** *Adults:* 2 to 4 mg P.O. h.s.

▶ **Premedication before operative procedure.** *Adults:* 0.05 mg/kg I.M. 2 hours before procedure. Total dosage shouldn't exceed 4 mg. Or, 2 mg total or 0.044 mg/kg I.V., whichever is smaller. Larger doses up to 0.05 mg/kg I.V. (to total of 4 mg) may be required.

How supplied

Tablets: 0.5 mg, 1 mg, 2 mg
Tablets (S.L.): 0.5 mg ♦, 1 mg ♦, 2 mg ♦
Oral solution (concentrated): 2 mg/ml
Injection: 2 mg/ml, 4 mg/ml

Pharmacokinetics

Absorption: well absorbed through GI tract after P.O. administration; unknown after I.M. administration.
Distribution: distributed widely throughout body; about 85% protein-bound.
Metabolism: metabolized in liver.
Excretion: excreted in urine. *Half-life:* 10 to 20 hours.

Route	Onset	Peak	Duration
P.O.	1 hr	2 hr	12-24 hr
I.V.	1-5 min	1-1.5 hr	6-8 hr
I.M.	15-30 min	1-1.5 hr	6-8 hr

Pharmacodynamics

Chemical effect: unknown; probably stimulates gamma-aminobutyric receptors in ascending reticular activating system.
Therapeutic effect: relieves anxiety and promotes calmness and sleep.

Adverse reactions

CNS: *drowsiness, lethargy, hangover,* fainting, anterograde amnesia, restlessness, psychosis.
CV: transient hypotension.
EENT: visual disturbances.
GI: dry mouth, abdominal discomfort.
GU: incontinence, urine retention.
Other: ***acute withdrawal syndrome*** (after sudden discontinuation in physically dependent people).

Interactions

Drug-drug. *CNS depressants:* increased CNS depression. Avoid concomitant use.
Digoxin: may increase serum digoxin levels, increasing toxicity. Monitor patient closely.
Drug-herb. *Catnip, kava, lady's slipper, lemon balm, passion flower, sassafras, skullcap, valerian:* sedative effects may be enhanced. Discourage using together.
Drug-lifestyle. *Alcohol use:* increased CNS depression. Discourage concomitant use.
Smoking: decreased benzodiazepine effectiveness. Monitor patient closely.

Contraindications and precautions

- Contraindicated in patients hypersensitive to drug, other benzodiazepines, or vehicle used in parenteral dosage form; also contraindicated in patients with acute angle-closure glaucoma.
- Avoid use in pregnant women, especially during first trimester, and in breast-feeding women.
- Use cautiously in patients with pulmonary, renal, or hepatic impairment. Also use cautiously in elderly, acutely ill, or debilitated patients.
- Safety of drug hasn't been established in children.

NURSING CONSIDERATIONS

Assessment

- Assess patient's condition before therapy and regularly thereafter.

ALERT Check respirations before each I.V. dose and every 5 to 15 minutes thereafter until respiratory status is stable.

- Monitor liver, kidney, and hematopoietic function studies periodically in patient receiving repeated or prolonged therapy, as ordered.
- Be alert for adverse reactions and drug interactions.
- Evaluate patient's and family's knowledge of drug therapy.

Nursing diagnoses

- Anxiety related to underlying condition
- Risk for injury related to drug-induced adverse CNS effects
- Deficient knowledge related to drug therapy

Planning and implementation

ALERT Don't confuse lorazepam with alprazolam.

- Reduce dosage in elderly or debilitated patient. Preoperative I.V. dose shouldn't exceed 2 mg in patients older than age 50.

P.O. use: Follow normal protocol.
I.V. use: Give drug slowly, at no more than 2 mg/minute. Dilute with equal volume of sterile water for injection, normal saline solution for injection, or D_5W injection.
I.M. use: Inject drug deep into muscle mass. Don't dilute.

- Have emergency resuscitation equipment and oxygen available.
- Refrigerate parenteral form to prolong shelf life.

• Possibility of abuse and addiction exists. Don't withdraw drug abruptly after long-term use; withdrawal symptoms may occur.

Patient teaching
• Warn patient to avoid hazardous activities until CNS effects of drug are known.
• Tell patient to avoid alcohol and smoking during drug therapy.
• As premedication before surgery, lorazepam provides substantial preoperative amnesia. Patient teaching requires extra care to ensure adequate recall. Provide written materials or inform family member, if possible.

Evaluation
• Patient is less anxious.
• Patient doesn't experience injury as result of adverse CNS reactions.
• Patient and family state understanding of drug therapy.

losartan potassium
(loh-SAR-tan poh-TAH-see-um)
Cozaar

Pharmacologic class: angiotensin II receptor antagonist
Therapeutic class: antihypertensive
Pregnancy risk category: C (D in second and third trimesters)

Indications and dosages
▶ **Hypertension.** *Adults:* initially, 25 to 50 mg P.O. daily. Maximum daily dosage is 100 mg in one or two divided doses.

How supplied
Tablets: 25 mg, 50 mg

Pharmacokinetics
Absorption: absorbed well and undergoes extensive first-pass metabolism; systemic bioavailability of drug is about 33%.
Distribution: highly bound to plasma proteins.
Metabolism: cytochrome P-450 2C9 and 3A4 are involved in biotransformation of losartan to its metabolites.
Excretion: excreted primarily in feces with smaller amount excreted in urine. *Half-life:* about 2 hours.

Route	Onset	Peak	Duration
P.O.	Unknown	1-4 hr	Unknown

Pharmacodynamics
Chemical effect: inhibits vasoconstricting and aldosterone-secreting effects of angiotensin II by selectively blocking binding of angiotensin II to receptor sites in many tissues, including vascular smooth muscle and adrenal glands.
Therapeutic effect: lowers blood pressure.

Adverse reactions
CNS: dizziness, insomnia.
EENT: nasal congestion, sinus disorder, sinusitis.
GI: diarrhea, dyspepsia.
Musculoskeletal: muscle cramps, myalgia, back or leg pain.
Respiratory: cough, upper respiratory tract infection.

Interactions
Drug-drug. *Potassium-sparing diuretics, potassium supplements:* possible hyperkalemia. Monitor patient closely.
Drug-herb. *Red yeast rice:* contains components similar to those of statin drugs, increasing the risk of adverse events or toxicity. Discourage concomitant use.
Drug-food: *Salt substitutes containing potassium:* risk of hyperkalemia. Monitor patient closely.

Contraindications and precautions
• Contraindicated in patients hypersensitive to drug.
• Breast-feeding isn't recommended during drug therapy.
• Drug should be used in pregnant women only when absolutely necessary. It acts directly on renin-angiotensin system and can cause fetal and neonatal morbidity and death. These problems haven't been detected when exposure has been limited to first trimester.
• Use cautiously in patients with impaired kidney or liver function.

• Safety of drug hasn't been established in children.

NURSING CONSIDERATIONS

Assessment

• Assess patient's blood pressure before therapy and regularly thereafter. When drug is used alone, its effect on blood pressure is notably less in black patients than in those of other races.
• Regularly assess patient's kidney function (by way of serum creatinine and BUN levels), as ordered. Patients with severe heart failure whose kidney function depends on angiotensin-aldosterone system have experienced acute renal failure during ACE inhibitor therapy. Manufacturer states that losartan would be expected to do the same. Closely monitor patient, especially during first few weeks of therapy.
• Be alert for adverse reactions.
• Monitor for symptomatic hypotension in patient taking a diuretic.
• Evaluate patient's and family's knowledge of drug therapy.

Nursing diagnoses

• Risk for injury related to presence of hypertension
• Disturbed sleep pattern related to drug-induced insomnia
• Deficient knowledge related to drug therapy

Planning and implementation

ALERT Don't confuse Cozaar with Zocor.
• Lowest dosage (25 mg) should be used initially in patients with impaired liver function and in those with volume depletion (such as those receiving diuretics).
• Drug can be used alone or with other antihypertensives.
• If antihypertensive effect measured by serum trough level of drug using once-daily dosing is inadequate, a twice-daily regimen using same total daily dosage or an increase in dosage may give better response.
• Administer once-daily dosing in morning to prevent insomnia.
• If pregnancy is suspected, notify prescriber because drug should probably be discontinued.

Patient teaching
• Tell patient to avoid sodium substitutes; these products may contain potassium, which can cause hyperkalemia in patients taking losartan.
• Inform woman of childbearing age about consequences of second- and third-trimester exposure to losartan, and instruct her to notify prescriber immediately if pregnancy occurs or is suspected.

Evaluation

• Patient's blood pressure is normal.
• Patient states that insomnia hasn't occurred.
• Patient and family state understanding of drug therapy.

lovastatin (mevinolin)

(loh-vuh-STAH-tin)
Mevacor

Pharmacologic class: lactone
Therapeutic class: cholesterol-lowering agent
Pregnancy risk category: X

Indications and dosages

▶ **Primary prevention of coronary heart disease in patients without symptomatic CV disease, average to moderately elevated total cholesterol and low-density lipoprotein (LDL) cholesterol levels, and below average high-density lipoprotein cholesterol levels; reduction of LDL and total cholesterol levels in patients with primary hypercholesterolemia (types IIa and IIb), to slow the progression of coronary atherosclerosis with coronary artery disease.** *Adults:* initially, 20 mg P.O. once daily with evening meal. Recommended dosage range is 10 to 80 mg daily in one or two divided doses. For patients receiving immunosuppressants, initially 10 mg P.O. daily; maximum, 20 mg daily.

How supplied

Tablets: 10 mg, 20 mg, 40 mg

Pharmacokinetics

Absorption: about 30% absorbed. Administration with food improves plasma levels of total inhibitors by about 30%.
Distribution: less than 5% of dose reaches systemic circulation because of extensive first-pass hepatic extraction; liver is principal site of action. Drug and its principal metabolite are more than 95% bound to plasma proteins.
Metabolism: metabolized in liver.
Excretion: about 80% excreted in feces, about 10% in urine. *Half-life:* 3 hours.

Route	Onset	Peak	Duration
P.O.	Unknown	2-6 hr	4-6 wk

Pharmacodynamics

Chemical effect: inhibits 3-hydroxy-3-methylglutaryl coenzyme A reductase. This enzyme is an early (and rate-limiting) step in synthetic pathway of cholesterol.
Therapeutic effect: lowers LDL and total cholesterol levels.

Adverse reactions

CNS: headache, dizziness, peripheral neuropathy.
EENT: blurred vision.
GI: constipation, diarrhea, dyspepsia, flatulence, abdominal pain or cramps, heartburn, dysgeusia, nausea.
Hepatic: elevated serum transaminase levels, abnormal liver function test results.
Musculoskeletal: muscle cramps, myalgia, myositis, ***rhabdomyolysis.***
Skin: rash, pruritus.

Interactions

Drug-drug. *Bile acid sequestrants*: decreased lovastatin bioavailability. Administer separately.
Cyclosporine or other immunosuppressants, erythromycin, gemfibrozil, niacin: increased risk of polymyositis and rhabdomyolysis. Monitor patient closely.
Digoxin: slight elevation in digoxin levels is possible. Monitor patient.
Isradipine: increased clearance of lovastatin and its metabolites via increased hepatic blood flow. Monitor patient for loss of therapeutic effect.
Itraconazole: may increase HMG-COA reductase inhibitor levels about 20-fold. Temporarily interrupt HMG-COA reductase inhibitor if patient needs systemic azole antifungal.
Oral anticoagulants: lovastatin may enhance oral anticoagulant effects. Monitor patient closely.
Drug-herb. *Red yeast rice:* contains components similar to those of statin drugs, increasing the risk of adverse events or toxicity. Discourage concomitant use.
Drug-lifestyle. *Alcohol use:* increased risk of hepatotoxicity. Discourage concomitant use.

Contraindications and precautions

- Contraindicated in patients hypersensitive to drug, in those with active liver disease or conditions linked to unexplained persistent elevations of serum transaminase levels, in pregnant or breast-feeding women, and in women of childbearing age unless they have no risk of pregnancy.
- Use cautiously in patients who consume substantial quantities of alcohol or have history of liver disease.
- Safety of drug hasn't been established in children.

NURSING CONSIDERATIONS

Assessment

- Obtain history of patient's lipoprotein and cholesterol levels before therapy, and reassess regularly thereafter.
- Liver function tests should be performed at start of therapy and periodically thereafter.
- Be alert for adverse reactions and drug interactions.
- Evaluate patient's and family's knowledge of drug therapy.

Nursing diagnoses

- Risk for injury related to underlying condition
- Pain related to drug-induced adverse musculoskeletal reactions
- Deficient knowledge related to drug therapy

Planning and implementation

- Drug therapy should begin only after diet and other nonpharmacologic therapies have

proven ineffective. Patient should follow a standard low-cholesterol diet during therapy.
• Administer drug with evening meal; absorption is enhanced and cholesterol biosynthesis is greater in evening.
ALERT Don't confuse lovastatin with Lotensin, Leustatin, or Livostin. Don't confuse Mevacor with Mivacron.

Patient teaching
• Instruct patient to take drug with evening meal.
• Teach patient dietary management of serum lipids (restricting total fat and cholesterol intake) and measures to control other cardiac disease risk factors. If appropriate, recommend weight control, exercise, and smoking cessation programs.
• Advise patient to have periodic eye examinations.
• Tell patient to store drug at room temperature in light-resistant container.
• Instruct patient to avoid alcohol consumption during drug therapy.
ALERT Inform woman that drug is contraindicated during pregnancy. Tell her to notify prescriber immediately if she becomes pregnant.

Evaluation
• Patient's LDL and cholesterol levels are within normal limits.
• Patient doesn't experience musculoskeletal pain.
• Patient and family state understanding of drug therapy.

loxapine hydrochloride
(LOKS-uh-peen high-droh-KLOR-ighd)
Loxapac♦, Loxitane C, Loxitane IM

loxapine succinate
Loxapac♦, Loxitane

Pharmacologic class: dibenzoxazepine
Therapeutic class: antipsychotic
Pregnancy risk category: NR

Indications and dosages
▶ **Psychotic disorders.** *Adults:* 10 mg P.O. b.i.d. to q.i.d., rapidly increasing to 60 to 100 mg P.O. daily for most patients (dosage varies from patient to patient); or 12.5 to 50 mg I.M. q 4 to 6 hours or longer, both dose and interval depending on patient response. Maximum dosage is 250 mg daily.

How supplied
loxapine hydrochloride
Oral concentrate: 25 mg/ml
Injection: 50 mg/ml
loxapine succinate
Capsules: 5 mg, 10 mg, 25 mg, 50 mg
Tablets: 5 mg♦, 10 mg♦, 25 mg♦, 50 mg♦

Pharmacokinetics
Absorption: absorbed rapidly and completely from GI tract.
Distribution: distributed widely in body; 91% to 99% protein-bound.
Metabolism: metabolized extensively by liver.
Excretion: most of drug excreted as metabolites in urine; some excreted in feces. *Half-life:* P.O. form, 3 to 4 hours; I.M. form, 12 hours.

Route	Onset	Peak	Duration
P.O.	30 min	1.5-3 hr	≤ 2 hr
I.M.	30 min	1.5-3 hr	≤ 12 hr

Pharmacodynamics
Chemical effect: unknown; probably blocks postsynaptic dopamine receptors in brain.
Therapeutic effect: relieves psychotic symptoms.

Adverse reactions
CNS: *extrapyramidal reactions, sedation, tardive dyskinesia,* ***seizures,*** pseudoparkinsonism, EEG changes, dizziness, ***neuroleptic malignant syndrome.***
CV: *orthostatic hypotension,* tachycardia, ECG changes.
EENT: *blurred vision.*
GI: *dry mouth, constipation.*
GU: *urine retention,* dark urine, menstrual irregularities.
Hematologic: ***leukopenia, agranulocytosis, thrombocytopenia.***

Metabolic: weight gain, increased appetite.
Skin: *mild photosensitivity,* allergic reactions.
Other: gynecomastia.

Interactions

Drug-drug. *CNS depressants:* increased CNS depression. Avoid concomitant use.
Drug-lifestyle. *Alcohol use:* increased CNS depression. Discourage concomitant use.

Contraindications and precautions

• Contraindicated in patients hypersensitive to dibenzoxazepines and in patients experiencing coma, severe CNS depression, or drug-induced depression.
• Drug isn't recommended for use in breast-feeding women.
• Use with extreme caution in those with seizure disorder, CV disorder, glaucoma, or history of urine retention.
• Safety of drug hasn't been established in children and in pregnant women.

NURSING CONSIDERATIONS

Assessment

• Assess patient's condition before therapy and regularly thereafter.
• Assess blood pressure before therapy and monitor regularly.
• Be alert for adverse reactions and drug interactions.
• Monitor patient for tardive dyskinesia. It may occur after prolonged use. It may not appear until months or years later and may disappear spontaneously or persist for life despite discontinuation of drug.
• Evaluate patient's and family's knowledge of drug therapy.

Nursing diagnoses

• Disturbed thought processes related to underlying psychotic condition
• Impaired physical mobility related to drug-induced extrapyramidal symptoms
• Deficient knowledge related to drug therapy

Planning and implementation

P.O. use: Dilute liquid concentrate with orange or grapefruit juice just before giving.
I.M. use: Follow normal protocol.
• Acute dystonic reactions may be treated with diphenhydramine.

Patient teaching

• Warn patient to avoid activities that require alertness and psychomotor coordination until CNS effects of drug are known.
• Tell patient to avoid alcohol consumption.
• Advise patient to get up slowly to avoid orthostatic hypotension.
• Tell patient to relieve dry mouth with sugarless gum or hard candy.
• Tell patient that periodic eye examinations are recommended.

Evaluation

• Patient's psychotic behavior declines.
• Patient maintains physical mobility throughout therapy.
• Patient and family state understanding of drug therapy.

Lyme disease vaccine (recombinant OspA)

(LIGHM dih-ZEEZ vak-SEEN)
LYMErix

Pharmacologic class: bacterial vaccine
Therapeutic class: Lyme disease prophylaxis
Pregnancy risk category: C

Indications and dosages

▶ **Active immunization against Lyme disease.** *Adolescents and adults ages 15 to 70:* 30 mcg I.M. in deltoid region; repeat dose at 1 and 12 months after first dose. Administration of second and third doses should take place several weeks before onset of *Borrelia burgdorferi* transmission season, which varies regionally.

How supplied

Injection: 30 mcg/0.5 ml single-dose vials and prefilled syringes

Pharmacokinetics

No information available.

Route	Onset	Peak	Duration
I.M.	Unknown	Unknown	Unknown

Pharmacodynamics

Chemical effect: Vaccine stimulates specific antibodies directed against *B. burgdorferi,* the bacterial spirochete that causes Lyme disease. The Lyme disease vaccine contains lipoprotein OspA, an outer-surface protein of *B. burgdorferi,* which, following administration, stimulates formation of anti-OspA antibodies that have bactericidal activity against *B. burgdorferi.*
Therapeutic effect: provides active immunization against Lyme disease.

Adverse reactions

CNS: *headache, fatigue,* dizziness, depression, hypoesthesia, paresthesia.
EENT: pharyngitis, rhinitis, sinusitis.
GI: diarrhea, nausea.
Musculoskeletal: *arthralgia,* back pain, achiness, myalgia, arthritis, arthrosis, stiffness, tendinitis.
Respiratory: bronchitis, cough, upper respiratory tract infection.
Skin: *rash*; contact dermatitis; *injection site reaction, pain, redness, soreness, swelling.*
Other: chills or rigors, fever, viral infection, flulike symptoms.

Interactions

None reported.

Contraindications and precautions

- Contraindicated in patients hypersensitive to vaccine or its components. Don't administer vaccine to patients outside the indicated age range or to those with treatment-resistant Lyme arthritis (antibiotic refractory) or moderate to severe febrile illness. Lyme disease vaccine shouldn't be given to patients receiving anticoagulants unless potential benefit outweighs risk.
- Use cautiously in immunosuppressed patients or in those receiving immunosuppressive therapy because the expected immune response may not occur. For patients receiving immunosuppressive therapy, consider deferring vaccination for 3 months after therapy ends.
- Also use cautiously in patients who may be allergic to the natural rubber packaging for the prefilled syringe. Note that the packaging for the vial doesn't contain rubber.
- Use cautiously in breast-feeding women because it's unknown whether the vaccine appears in breast milk.

NURSING CONSIDERATIONS

Assessment

- Assess patient for appropriateness of receiving vaccine. Immunization against Lyme disease is appropriate in people who live in, work in, travel to, or pursue recreational activities in *B. burgdorferi*–infected grassy or wooded areas.
- Assess patient for immunosupression risk factors before starting immunization series. For patients receiving immunosuppressive therapy, consider deferring vaccination until 3 months after therapy ends.
- Before immunization, review patient's history for possible vaccine sensitivity, allergies, previous vaccination-related adverse reactions, and occurrence of any adverse event–related signs and symptoms. Epinephrine injection and other drugs appropriate for controlling immediate allergic reactions must be readily available.
- Evaluate patient's and family's knowledge about drug therapy.

Nursing diagnoses

- Risk for injury if patient contracts Lyme disease
- Chronic pain related to drug-induced adverse reactions
- Deficient knowledge related to drug therapy

Planning and implementation

- Refrigerate vaccine between 36° and 46° F (2° and 8° C). Don't freeze; discard if product has been frozen.
- Shake well before use. Inspect for particulates or discoloration before administering. With thorough agitation, the Lyme disease vaccine is a turbid, white suspension. Discard if it appears otherwise.

• Use vaccine as supplied, without diluting or reconstituting. Give the full, recommended dose. Any vaccine remaining in a single-dose vial should be discarded. Lyme disease vaccine should be given I.M. in the deltoid region. Don't administer I.V., I.D., or S.C.
• Patients with a history of Lyme disease may benefit from vaccination because previous infection with *B. burgdorferi* may not provide protective immunity.
• Vaccine is a preventive measure, not a treatment for Lyme disease.
• No information is available on the immune response to the Lyme disease vaccine when administered with other vaccines. When vaccine must be given with other vaccines, each should be given with a different syringe and at a different injection site.
• Immunization with Lyme disease vaccine may cause a false-positive enzyme-linked immunosorbent assay (ELISA) result for *B. burgdorferi* in the absence of infection. Therefore, it's important to perform Western blot testing if the ELISA test is positive or equivocal in vaccinated patients who are being evaluated for suspected Lyme disease.
• Register pregnant women who receive the Lyme disease vaccine by calling GlaxoSmithKline at 1-800-366-8900.

Patient teaching
• Inform patient that this vaccine prevents and doesn't treat Lyme disease.
• Inform patient that Lyme disease vaccine may not protect everyone.
• Inform patient of the benefits and risks of immunization with the vaccine and of the importance of completing all three vaccinations several weeks before the start of the *B. burgdorferi* season in his geographic area.
• Urge patient to report any adverse signs and symptoms that may have occurred after the previous dose when he returns for the next dose in the series.
• Tell patient to notify prescriber if he takes an anticoagulant, such as warfarin, heparin, or aspirin.
• Inform patient that, besides getting the Lyme disease vaccine, he can help prevent tick-borne diseases by wearing long-sleeved shirts and long pants, tucking pants into socks, treating clothing with tick repellent, and checking for and removing attached ticks after returning from endemic areas.
• Show patient the proper way to remove a tick—with fine-pointed tweezers, being careful to not squash the tick before removal.
• Tell patient that Lyme disease vaccine may cause a false-positive test result for *B. burgdorferi* infection. Advise patient to inform prescriber that he has received Lyme disease vaccine because it may affect laboratory testing for diagnosing Lyme disease.

☑ Evaluation
• Patient doesn't develop Lyme disease.
• Patient remains free from adverse reactions.
• Patient and family state understanding of drug therapy.

lymphocyte immune globulin (antithymocyte globulin [equine], ATG), (LIG)
(LIM-foh-sight ih-MYOON GLOH-byoo-lin)
Atgam

Pharmacologic class: immunoglobulin
Therapeutic class: immunosuppressant
Pregnancy risk category: C

Indications and dosages
▶ **Prevention of acute renal allograft rejection.** *Adults and children:* 15 mg/kg I.V. daily for 14 days, followed by alternate-day dosing for 14 days. First dose should be given within 24 hours of transplantation.
▶ **Treatment of acute renal allograft rejection.** *Adults and children:* 10 to 15 mg/kg I.V. daily for 14 days, followed by alternate-day dosing for 14 days. Therapy should start when rejection is diagnosed.
▶ **Aplastic anemia.** *Adults:* 10 to 20 mg/kg I.V. daily for 8 to 14 days. Additional alternate-day therapy up to total of 21 doses can be administered.

How supplied
Injection: 50 mg of equine IgG/ml in 5-ml ampules

Pharmacokinetics

Absorption: not applicable.
Distribution: unknown.
Metabolism: unknown.
Excretion: about 1% excreted in urine, principally as unchanged drug. *Half-life:* about 6 days.

Route	Onset	Peak	Duration
I.V.	Unknown	5 days	Unknown

Pharmacodynamics

Chemical effect: unknown; inhibits cell-mediated immune responses by either altering T-cell function or eliminating antigen-reactive T cells.
Therapeutic effect: prevents or relieves signs and symptoms of renal allograft rejection; also relieves signs and symptoms of aplastic anemia.

Adverse reactions

CNS: malaise, ***seizures,*** headache.
CV: *hypotension, chest pain,* thrombophlebitis, tachycardia, edema, iliac vein obstruction, renal artery stenosis.
EENT: ***laryngospasm.***
GI: *nausea, vomiting,* diarrhea, hiccups, epigastric pain, abdominal distention, stomatitis.
Hematologic: ***leukopenia, thrombocytopenia,*** hemolysis, ***aplastic anemia.***
Hepatic: elevated liver enzyme levels.
Metabolic: hyperglycemia.
Musculoskeletal: arthralgia.
Respiratory: *dyspnea,* ***pulmonary edema.***
Skin: rash.
Other: febrile reactions, serum sickness, ***anaphylaxis,*** infection, night sweats, lymphadenopathy.

Interactions

Drug-drug. *Muromonab-CD3:* increased risk of infection. Monitor patient closely.

Contraindications and precautions

- Contraindicated in patients hypersensitive to drug. An intradermal skin test is recommended at least 1 hour before first dose. Marked local swelling or erythema larger than 10 mm indicates increased risk of severe systemic reaction, such as anaphylaxis. Severe reactions to skin test, such as hypotension, tachycardia, dyspnea, generalized rash, or anaphylaxis, usually preclude further administration.
- Drug isn't recommended for use in breast-feeding women.
- Use cautiously in pregnant women. Also use cautiously in patients receiving additional immunosuppressive therapy (such as corticosteroids and azathioprine) because of increased potential for infection.

NURSING CONSIDERATIONS

Assessment

- Assess patient's condition before therapy and regularly thereafter.
- Be alert for adverse reactions and drug interactions.
- Evaluate patient's and family's knowledge of drug therapy.

Nursing diagnoses

- Ineffective health maintenance related to underlying condition
- Ineffective immune protection related to adverse hematologic reactions
- Deficient knowledge related to drug therapy

Planning and implementation

I.V. use: Dilute concentrated drug before administration. Dilute required dose in 250 to 1,000 ml of half-normal or normal saline solution for injection. Final concentration of drug shouldn't exceed 1 mg/ml.
– When adding ATG to infusion solution, make sure container is inverted so drug doesn't contact air inside container. Gently rotate or swirl container to mix contents; don't shake because this may cause excessive foaming or denature drug protein.
– Infuse with in-line filter with pore size of 0.2 to 1 micron over no less than 4 hours (most facilities specify 4 to 8 hours). ATG solutions must be filtered during administration; filters with pore sizes of 0.2 to 5 microns have been used.
– Don't use solutions that are more than 12 hours old, including actual infusion time.
- Don't dilute ATG concentrate with dextrose solutions or solutions with low salt concentration because precipitate may form. The pro-

teins in ATG can be denatured by air. ATG is unstable in acidic solutions.
• Refrigerate drug at 35° to 47° F (2° to 8° C). Don't freeze. ATG concentrate is heat-sensitive.

Patient teaching
• Warn patient that fever is likely. Instruct him to report adverse drug effects.
• Instruct patient to take infection-control and bleeding precautions.

Evaluation
• Patient responds well to therapy.
• Patient doesn't experience serious adverse hematologic reactions.
• Patient and family state understanding of drug therapy.

M

magaldrate (aluminum-magnesium complex)
(muh-GAL-drayt)
Isopan†, Riopan†

Pharmacologic class: aluminum-magnesium salt
Therapeutic class: antacid
Pregnancy risk category: NR

Indications and dosages
▶ **Antacid.** *Adults:* 540 to 1,080 mg (5 to 10 ml) of suspension or liquid P.O. with water between meals and h.s.

How supplied
Liquid, oral suspension: 540 mg/5 ml†

Pharmacokinetics
Absorption: may be absorbed systemically, posing risk to patient with renal failure. Absorption is unrelated to mechanism of action.
Distribution: primarily local.
Metabolism: none.
Excretion: excreted in feces.

Route	Onset	Peak	Duration
P.O.	≤ 20 min	Unknown (fasting); 3 hr (non-fasting)	20-60 min

Pharmacodynamics
Chemical effect: reduces total acid load in GI tract, elevates gastric pH to reduce pepsin activity, strengthens gastric mucosal barrier, and increases esophageal sphincter tone.
Therapeutic effect: soothes stomach upset.

Adverse reactions
GI: mild constipation or diarrhea.

Interactions
Drug-drug. *Allopurinol, antibiotics (including fluoroquinolones and tetracyclines), diflunisal, digoxin, iron, isoniazid, penicillamine, phenothiazines, quinidine:* decreased pharmacologic effect possible because of impaired absorption. Separate administration times.
Enteric-coated drugs: may release prematurely in stomach. Separate doses by at least 1 hour.

Contraindications and precautions
• Contraindicated in patients with severe renal disease. Drug isn't typically used in patients with renal failure to help control hypophosphatemia because it contains magnesium, which may accummulate.
• Use cautiously in patients with mild renal impairment and in pregnant or breast-feeding women.

NURSING CONSIDERATIONS

Assessment
• Assess patient's condition before therapy and regularly thereafter.
• Record amount and consistency of stools.
• Monitor serum magnesium level in patient with mild renal impairment. Symptomatic hypermagnesemia usually occurs only in severe renal failure.
• Be alert for adverse reactions and drug interactions.
• Evaluate patient's and family's knowledge of drug therapy.

Nursing diagnoses
• Chronic pain related to gastric hyperacidity
• Diarrhea related to drug-induced adverse GI reactions
• Deficient knowledge related to drug therapy

Planning and implementation
• Shake suspension well. Give with water to facilitate passage.
• When giving through nasogastric tube, make sure tube is placed properly and is patent. After instilling drug, flush tube with water to ensure passage to stomach and to clear tube.
• Drug has very low sodium content and is acceptable for patient on restricted sodium intake.

Patient teaching
• Advise patient not to take drug indiscriminately or to switch antacids without prescriber's advice.

Evaluation
• Patient states that pain is relieved.
• Patient maintains normal bowel patterns throughout therapy.
• Patient and family state understanding of drug therapy.

magnesium chloride
(mag-NEE-see-um KLOR-ighd)
Slow-Mag†

magnesium sulfate

Pharmacologic class: magnesium salt
Therapeutic class: anticonvulsant, electrolyte supplement, antiarrhythmic
Pregnancy risk category: D

Indications and dosages
▶ **Mild hypomagnesemia.** *Adults:* 1 g I.M. q 6 hours for four doses, depending on serum magnesium level.
▶ **Severe hypomagnesemia (serum magnesium level 0.8 mEq/L or less with symptoms).** *Adults:* 5 g I.V. in 1 L of solution over 3 hours. Subsequent doses depend on serum magnesium level.
▶ **Magnesium supplementation.** *Adults:* 2 tablets magnesium chloride P.O. daily.
▶ **Magnesium supplementation in total parenteral nutrition (TPN).** *Adults:* 4 to 24 mEq I.V. daily added to TPN solution. *Infants:* 2 to 10 mEq I.V. daily added to TPN solution. Each 2 ml of 50% solution contains 1 g, or 8.12 mEq, magnesium sulfate.
▶ **Hypomagnesemic seizures.** *Adults:* 1 to 2 g of 10% solution I.V. over 15 minutes; then 1 g I.M. q 4 to 6 hours, based on patient's response and serum magnesium level.
▶ **Seizures caused by hypomagnesemia in acute nephritis.** *Children:* 0.2 ml/kg of 50% solution I.M. q 4 to 6 hours, p.r.n., or 100 mg/kg of 10% solution I.V. very slowly. Adjust dosage according to serum magnesium level and seizure response.
▶ **Paroxysmal atrial tachycardia unresponsive to other treatments.** *Adults:* 3 to 4 g I.V. of 10% solution over 30 seconds with close monitoring of ECG.

How supplied
magnesium chloride
Tablets (delayed-release): 64 mg
Injectable solutions: 20% in 50-ml vials
magnesium sulfate
Injectable solutions: 10%, 12.5%, 50% in 2-ml, 5-ml, 10-ml, 20-ml, and 30-ml ampules, vials, and prefilled syringes

Pharmacokinetics
Absorption: 35% to 40% of P.O. dose is absorbed through GI tract. High-fat diets may interfere with absorption.
Distribution: about 30% of magnesium is bound intracellularly to proteins and energy-rich phosphates.
Metabolism: unknown.
Excretion: parenteral dose excreted primarily in urine; P.O. dose excreted in urine and feces.

Route	Onset	Peak	Duration
P.O.	Unknown	4 hr	4-6 hr
I.V., I.M.	Unknown	Unknown	4-6 hr

Pharmacodynamics
Chemical effect: replaces and maintains magnesium levels; as anticonvulsant, reduces mus-

cle contractions by interfering with release of acetylcholine at myoneural junction.
Therapeutic effect: raises magnesium levels, alleviates seizure activity, and restores normal sinus rhythm.

Adverse reactions

CNS: *weak or absent deep tendon reflexes,* flaccid paralysis, hypothermia, drowsiness, perioral paresthesia, twitching carpopedal spasm, tetany, ***seizures.***
CV: slow, weak pulse; ***arrhythmias;*** *hypotension;* ***circulatory collapse.***
Metabolic: hypocalcemia.
Respiratory: ***respiratory paralysis.***
Skin: diaphoresis, flushing.

Interactions

Drug-drug. *Cardiac glycosides:* possible serious cardiac conduction changes. Administer with extreme caution.
Neuromuscular blockers: possible increased neuromuscular blockage. Use cautiously.
Nitrofurantoin, penicillamine, tetracyclines: decreased bioavailability with oral magnesium supplements. Separate administration times by 2 to 3 hours.

Contraindications and precautions

- Contraindicated in patients with myocardial damage or heart block and in women who are actively progressing in labor.
- Use parenteral magnesium with extreme caution in patients with impaired kidney function.

NURSING CONSIDERATIONS

Assessment

- Assess patient's condition before therapy and regularly thereafter.
- When administering I.V. for severe hypomagnesemia, watch for respiratory depression and signs of heart block. Respirations should be more than 16 breaths/minute before dose is given.
- Check serum magnesium level after repeated doses.
- Monitor patient's fluid intake and output. Output should be 100 ml or more during 4-hour period before dose.
- Be alert for adverse reactions and drug interactions.
- Evaluate patient's and family's knowledge of drug therapy.

Nursing diagnoses

- Ineffective health maintenance related to underlying condition
- Risk for injury related to drug-induced adverse reactions
- Deficient knowledge related to drug therapy

Planning and implementation

P.O. use: Follow normal protocol.
I.V. use: Inject I.V. bolus dose slowly, using infusion pump for continuous infusion if available, to avoid respiratory or cardiac arrest. Infusion shouldn't exceed 150 mg/minute. Rapid drip causes feeling of heat.
ALERT When giving I.V. for severe hypomagnesemia, watch for respiratory depression and signs and symptoms of heart block. Respirations should be more than 16 breaths/minute before dose is given.
- Magnesium sulfate may form precipitate when mixed with solutions containing arsenates, barium, calcium, clindamycin, ethanol, heavy metals, hydrocortisone sodium succinate, phosphates, polymyxin B sulfate, procaine, salicylates, or tartrates. Drug is also incompatible with alkalis, including carbonates and bicarbonates.

I.M. use: Undiluted 50% solutions may be administered to adults by deep I.M. injection. When administering to children, dilute solutions to 20% or less.
- Keep I.V. calcium available to reverse magnesium intoxication.
- Test knee-jerk and patellar reflexes before each additional dose. If absent, notify prescriber and don't give magnesium until reflexes return; otherwise, patient may develop temporary respiratory failure and need cardiopulmonary resuscitation or I.V. administration of calcium.

Patient teaching

- Instruct patient receiving parenteral drug to report adverse reactions immediately.

• Review oral administration schedule with patient. Tell him not to take more than prescribed.

☑ Evaluation

• Patient has positive response to drug administration.
• Patient sustains no injury from adverse reactions.
• Patient and family state understanding of drug therapy.

magnesium citrate (citrate of magnesia)

(mag-NEE-see-um SIH-trayt)
Citroma†, Citro-Mag♦

magnesium hydroxide (milk of magnesia)

Milk of Magnesia†, Milk of Magnesia Concentrate†, Phillips' Milk of Magnesia†, Concentrated Phillips' Milk of Magnesia†

magnesium sulfate (epsom salts)

Pharmacologic class: magnesium salt
Therapeutic class: saline laxative
Pregnancy risk category: NR

Indications and dosages

▶ **Constipation; to evacuate bowel before surgery. Magnesium citrate.** *Adults and children age 12 and older:* 11 to 25 g P.O. daily as single dose or divided.
Children ages 6 to 11: 5.5 to 12.5 g P.O. daily as single dose or divided.
Children ages 2 to 5: 2.7 to 6.25 g P.O. daily as single dose or divided.
Magnesium hydroxide. *Adults and children age 12 and older:* 2.4 to 4.8 g (30 to 60 ml) P.O. daily as single dose or divided.
Children ages 6 to 11: 1.2 to 2.4 g (15 to 30 ml) P.O. daily as single dose or divided.
Children ages 2 to 5: 0.4 to 1.2 g (5 to 15 ml) P.O. daily as single dose or divided.
Magnesium sulfate. *Adults and children age 12 and older:* 10 to 30 g P.O. daily as single dose or divided.
Children ages 6 to 11: 5 to 10 g P.O. daily as single dose or divided.
Children ages 2 to 5: 2.5 to 5 g P.O. daily as single dose or divided.
▶ **As antacid. Magnesium hydroxide.** *Adults:* 5 to 15 ml P.O. t.i.d. or q.i.d.

How supplied

magnesium citrate
Oral solution: about 168 mEq magnesium/240 ml†
magnesium hydroxide
Oral suspension: 7% to 8.5% (about 80 mEq magnesium/30 ml)†
magnesium sulfate
Granules: about 40 mEq magnesium/5 g†

Pharmacokinetics

Absorption: about 15% to 30% may be absorbed systemically (posing risk to patients with renal failure).
Distribution: unknown.
Metabolism: unknown.
Excretion: unabsorbed drug excreted in feces; absorbed drug excreted rapidly in urine.

Route	Onset	Peak	Duration
P.O.	0.5-3 hr	Varies	Varies

Pharmacodynamics

Chemical effect: reduces total acid load in GI tract, elevates gastric pH to reduce pepsin activity, strengthens gastric mucosal barrier, and increases esophageal sphincter tone.
Therapeutic effect: soothes stomach upset, relieves constipation, and raises serum magnesium level.

Adverse reactions

GI: *abdominal cramping, nausea, diarrhea,* laxative dependence with long-term or excessive use.
Metabolic: fluid and electrolyte disturbances.

Interactions

Drug-drug. *Oral drugs:* impaired absorption. Separate administration times.

Contraindications and precautions

- Contraindicated in patients with abdominal pain, nausea, vomiting, other symptoms of appendicitis or acute surgical abdomen, myocardial damage, heart block, fecal impaction, rectal fissures, intestinal obstruction or perforation, or renal disease, and in women during labor and delivery.
- Use cautiously in patients with rectal bleeding and in pregnant or breast-feeding women.

NURSING CONSIDERATIONS

Assessment

- Assess patient's condition before therapy and regularly thereafter.
- Before giving for constipation, determine whether patient has adequate fluid intake, exercise, and diet.

ALERT Monitor serum electrolyte levels, as ordered, during prolonged use. Magnesium may accumulate in patient with renal insufficiency.

- Be alert for adverse reactions and drug interactions.
- Evaluate patient's and family's knowledge of drug therapy.

Nursing diagnoses

- Constipation related to underlying condition
- Diarrhea related to therapy
- Deficient knowledge related to drug therapy

Planning and implementation

- Time drug administration so that it doesn't interfere with scheduled activities or sleep.
- Chill magnesium citrate before use to improve its palatability.
- Shake suspension well. Give with large amount of water when used as laxative. When administering through nasogastric tube, make sure tube is placed properly and is patent. After instilling drug, flush tube with water to ensure passage to stomach and maintain tube patency.
- Drug is for short-term therapy.
- Magnesium sulfate is more potent than other saline laxatives.

Patient teaching

- Teach patient about dietary sources of bulk, such as bran and other cereals, fresh fruit, and vegetables.
- Warn patient that frequent or prolonged use may cause dependence.

Evaluation

- Patient's constipation is relieved.
- Diarrhea doesn't develop.
- Patient and family state understanding of drug therapy.

magnesium oxide

(mag-NEE-see-um OKS-ighd)

Mag-Ox 400†, Maox†, Uro-Mag†

Pharmacologic class: magnesium salt
Therapeutic class: antacid, laxative
Pregnancy risk category: NR

Indications and dosages

▶ **Antacid.** *Adults:* 140 mg P.O. with water or milk after meals and h.s.

▶ **Laxative.** *Adults:* 4 g P.O. with water or milk, usually h.s.

▶ **Oral replacement therapy in mild hypomagnesemia.** *Adults:* 400 to 840 mg P.O. daily. Monitor serum magnesium response.

How supplied

Tablets: 400 mg†, 420 mg†
Capsules: 140 mg†

Pharmacokinetics

Absorption: small amount absorbed from GI tract.
Distribution: unknown.
Metabolism: none.
Excretion: unabsorbed drug excreted in feces; absorbed drug excreted in urine.

Route	Onset	Peak	Duration
P.O.	20 min	Unknown	20-60 min (fasting); 3 hr (non-fasting)

Pharmacodynamics

Chemical effect: reduces total acid load in GI tract, elevates gastric pH to reduce pepsin activity, strengthens gastric mucosal barrier, and increases esophageal sphincter tone.
Therapeutic effect: soothes stomach upset, relieves constipation, and raises serum magnesium level.

Adverse reactions

GI: *diarrhea,* nausea, abdominal pain.
Metabolic: hypermagnesemia.

Interactions

Drug-drug. *Allopurinol, antibiotics (including fluoroquinolones and tetracyclines), diflunisal, digoxin, iron, isoniazid, penicillamine, phenothiazines, quinidine:* decreased pharmacologic effect, possibly because of impaired absorption. Separate administration times.
Enteric-coated drugs: may release prematurely in stomach. Separate doses by at least 1 hour.

Contraindications and precautions

- Contraindicated in patients with severe renal disease.
- Use cautiously in patients with mild renal impairment and in pregnant or breast-feeding women.

NURSING CONSIDERATIONS

Assessment

- Assess patient's condition before therapy and regularly thereafter.

ALERT Monitor serum magnesium level. With prolonged use and renal impairment, watch for symptoms of hypermagnesemia (hypotension, nausea, vomiting, depressed reflexes, respiratory depression, and coma).

- Be alert for adverse reactions and drug interactions.
- Evaluate patient's and family's knowledge of drug therapy.

Nursing diagnoses

- Ineffective health maintenance related to underlying condition
- Risk for injury related to potential for hypermagnesemia
- Deficient knowledge related to drug therapy

Planning and implementation

- When using as laxative, don't give other oral drugs 1 to 2 hours before or after treatment.
- If diarrhea occurs, be prepared to suggest alternative preparation.

Patient teaching

- Advise patient not to take drug indiscriminately or to switch antacids without prescriber's advice.

Evaluation

- Patient responds well to therapy.
- Patient maintains normal serum magnesium level throughout therapy.
- Patient and family state understanding of drug therapy.

magnesium sulfate

(mag-NEE-see-um SUL-fayt)

Pharmacologic class: mineral, electrolyte
Therapeutic class: anticonvulsant
Pregnancy risk category: A

Indications and dosages

▶ **Prevention or control of seizures in preeclampsia or eclampsia.** *Women:* initially, 4 g I.V. in 250 ml of D_5W and 4 to 5 g deep I.M. each buttock; then 4 g deep I.M. into alternate buttock q 4 hours, p.r.n. Or, 4 g I.V. loading dose, followed by 1 to 2 g hourly as I.V. infusion.
▶ **Hypomagnesemia.** *Adults:* 1 g I.M. q 6 hours for four doses for mild deficiency; up to 250 mg/kg I.M. over 4-hour period for severe deficiency.
▶ **Seizures, hypertension, and encephalopathy linked to acute nephritis in children.** *Children:* 0.2 ml/kg of 50% solution I.M. q 4 to 6 hours, p.r.n. For severe symptoms, 100 to 200 mg/kg I.V. very slowly over 1 hour with one-half of dose administered in first 15 to 20 minutes. Dosage adjusted according to serum magnesium level and seizure response.
▶ **Management of paroxysmal atrial tachycardia.** *Adults:* 3 to 4 g I.V. over 30 seconds.

▶ **Management of life-threatening ventricular arrhythmias, such as sustained ventricular tachycardia or torsades de pointes.**
Adults: 2 to 6 g I.V. over several minutes, followed by continuous infusion of 3 to 20 mg/minute for 5 to 48 hours. Dosage and duration of therapy based on patient response and serum magnesium level.

How supplied

Injection: 4%, 8%, 10%, 12.5%, 25%, 50%
Injection solution: 1% in D_5W, 2% in D_5W

Pharmacokinetics

Absorption: unknown after I.M.use.
Distribution: distributed throughout body.
Metabolism: none.
Excretion: excreted unchanged in urine.

Route	Onset	Peak	Duration
I.V.	1-2 min	Almost immediate	About 30 min
I.M.	1 hr	Unknown	3-4 hr

Pharmacodynamics

Chemical effect: may decrease acetylcholine released by nerve impulses, but anticonvulsant mechanism is unknown.
Therapeutic effect: prevents or controls seizures, raises serum magnesium levels, stops paroxysmal atrial tachycardia, and alleviates selected symptoms of acute nephritis in children.

Adverse reactions

CNS: drowsiness, *depressed reflexes,* flaccid paralysis, hypothermia.
CV: *hypotension, flushing,* ***circulatory collapse,*** depressed cardiac function, ***heart block.***
Metabolic: hypocalcemia.
Respiratory: ***respiratory paralysis.***
Skin: diaphoresis.

Interactions

Drug-drug. *Anesthetics, CNS depressants:* may cause additive CNS depression. Use together cautiously.
Cardiac glycosides: concomitant use may exacerbate arrhythmias. Use together cautiously.
Neuromuscular blockers: may increase neuromuscular blockade. Use together cautiously.

Contraindications and precautions

- Parenteral administration contraindicated in patients with heart block or myocardial damage.
- Drug isn't recommended for use in breast-feeding women.
- Use cautiously in patients with impaired kidney function and in women who are in labor.

NURSING CONSIDERATIONS

Assessment

- Assess patient's condition before therapy and regularly thereafter.
- Monitor vital signs every 15 minutes when giving drug I.V.

ALERT Watch for respiratory depression and signs of heart block. Respirations should be about 16 breaths/minute before each dose.

- Monitor fluid intake and output. Output should be 100 ml or more in 4-hour period before each dose.
- Be alert for adverse reactions and drug interactions.
- Check serum magnesium level after repeated doses. Disappearance of knee-jerk and patellar reflexes is sign of pending magnesium toxicity. Signs of hypermagnesemia begin to appear at serum levels of 4 mEq/L.
- Observe neonate for signs of magnesium toxicity, including neuromuscular or respiratory depression, when giving I.V. form to toxemic mother within 24 hours before delivery.
- Evaluate patient's and family's knowledge of drug therapy.

Nursing diagnoses

- Ineffective health maintenance related to underlying condition
- Risk for injury related to drug-induced adverse reactions
- Deficient knowledge related to drug therapy

Planning and implementation

ALERT Don't confuse magnesium sulfate with magnese sulfate.
I.V. use: If necessary, dilute to maximum concentration of 20%. Drug is compatible with D_5W.
– Infuse no faster than 150 mg/minute (1.5 ml/minute of 10% solution or 0.75 ml/minute of

20% solution). Rapid drip induces uncomfortable feeling of heat.
I.M. use: Follow normal protocol.
- Keep I.V. calcium gluconate available to reverse magnesium intoxication; use cautiously in patients undergoing digitalization because of danger of arrhythmias.
- If used to treat seizures, institute appropriate seizure precautions.

Patient teaching
- Stress importance of reporting adverse reactions immediately.

Evaluation
- Patient responds well to therapy.
- Patient doesn't experience injury.
- Patient and family state understanding of drug therapy.

mannitol
(MAN-ih-tol)
Osmitrol

Pharmacologic class: osmotic diuretic
Therapeutic class: diuretic, diagnostic and nephrotic treatment agent, treatment of drug intoxication, reduction of intracranial or intraocular pressure
Pregnancy risk category: C

Indications and dosages

▶ **Test dose for marked oliguria or suspected inadequate kidney function.** *Adults and children over age 12:* 200 mg/kg or 12.5 g as 15% or 20% I.V. solution over 3 to 5 minutes. Response is adequate if 30 to 50 ml of urine/hour is excreted over 2 to 3 hours. If response is inadequate, second test dose is given. If still no response after second dose, drug should be discontinued.
▶ **Oliguria.** *Adults and children over age 12:* 100 g I.V. as 15% to 20% solution over 90 minutes to several hours.
▶ **Prevention of oliguria or acute renal failure.** *Adults and children over age 12:* 50 to 100 g I.V. of concentrated solution, followed by 5% to 10% solution. Exact concentration determined by fluid requirements.
▶ **Edema; ascites caused by renal, hepatic, or cardiac failure.** *Adults and children over age 12:* 100 g I.V. as 10% to 20% solution over 2 to 6 hours.
▶ **Reduction of intraocular or intracranial pressure.** *Adults and children over age 12:* 1.5 to 2 g/kg as 15% to 25% I.V. solution over 30 to 60 minutes.
▶ **Diuresis in drug intoxication.** *Adults and children over age 12:* 25-g loading dose followed by an infusion maintaining 100- to 500-ml urine output/hour and positive fluid balance.
▶ **Irrigating solution during transurethral resection of prostate.** *Adults:* 2.5% solution, p.r.n.

How supplied

Injection: 5%, 10%, 15%, 20%, 25%

Pharmacokinetics

Absorption: not applicable.
Distribution: remains in extracellular compartment; doesn't cross blood-brain barrier.
Metabolism: metabolized minimally to glycogen in liver.
Excretion: excreted in urine. *Half-life:* about 100 minutes.

Route	Onset	Peak	Duration
I.V.	30-60 min	≤ 1 hr	6-8 hr

Pharmacodynamics

Chemical effect: increases osmotic pressure of glomerular filtrate, inhibiting tubular reabsorption of water and electrolytes. This elevates blood plasma osmolality, enhancing water flow into extracellular fluid.
Therapeutic effect: increases water excretion, decreases intracranial or intraocular pressure, prevents or treats kidney dysfunction, and alleviates drug intoxication.

Adverse reactions

CNS: headache, confusion, ***seizures.***
CV: transient expansion of plasma volume during infusion, causing circulatory overload and ***heart failure;*** tachycardia; angina-like chest pain.
EENT: blurred vision, rhinitis.
GI: thirst, nausea, vomiting, *diarrhea.*

GU: urine retention.
Metabolic: fluid and electrolyte imbalance, water intoxication, cellular dehydration.

Interactions

Drug-drug. *Lithium:* increased urinary excretion of lithium. Monitor patient closely.

Contraindications and precautions

- Contraindicated in patients hypersensitive to drug and in those with anuria, severe pulmonary congestion, frank pulmonary edema, severe heart failure, severe dehydration, metabolic edema, progressive renal disease or dysfunction, or active intracranial bleeding except during craniotomy.
- Drug isn't recommended for use in breast-feeding women.
- Use cautiously in pregnant women.

NURSING CONSIDERATIONS

Assessment

- Assess patient's condition before therapy and regularly thereafter.
- Monitor vital signs, central venous pressure, and fluid intake and output hourly. Insert urethral catheter in comatose or incontinent patient because therapy is based on strict evaluation of fluid intake and output. In patient with urethral catheter, use hourly urometer collection bag to facilitate accurate evaluation.
- Monitor weight, kidney function, and serum and urine sodium and potassium levels daily.
- Be alert for adverse reactions and drug interactions.
- Evaluate patient's and family's knowledge of drug therapy.

Nursing diagnoses

- Ineffective health maintenance related to underlying condition
- Risk for deficient fluid volume related to drug-induced adverse GI reactions
- Deficient knowledge related to drug therapy

Planning and implementation

- To redissolve crystallized solution (occurs at low temperatures or in concentrations greater than 15%), warm bottle in hot water bath and shake vigorously. Cool to body temperature before giving. Don't use solution with undissolved crystals.
- Give as intermittent or continuous infusion at prescribed rate, using in-line filter and infusion pump. Direct injection isn't recommended. Check I.V. line patency at infusion site before and during administration.
- Avoid infiltration; if it occurs, observe for inflammation, edema, and necrosis.
- For maximum intraocular pressure reduction before surgery, give 1 to 1½ hours preoperatively, as ordered.
- When used as irrigating solution for prostate surgery, concentrations of 3.5% or greater are needed to avoid hemolysis.
- Notify prescriber immediately if oliguria increases or adverse reactions occur.

Patient teaching

- Tell patient he may feel thirsty or have a dry mouth, and emphasize the importance of drinking only amount of fluid provided.
- Instruct patient to immediately report pain in chest, back, or legs or shortness of breath.

Evaluation

- Patient responds well to mannitol.
- Patient maintains adequate hydration throughout therapy.
- Patient and family state understanding of drug therapy.

mebendazole

(meh-BEN-duh-zohl)
Vermox

Pharmacologic class: benzimidazole
Therapeutic class: anthelmintic
Pregnancy risk category: C

Indications and dosages

▶ **Pinworm.** *Adults and children over age 2:* 100 mg P.O. as single dose. If infection persists 3 weeks later, treatment is repeated.
▶ **Roundworm, whipworm, hookworm.** *Adults and children over age 2:* 100 mg P.O. b.i.d. for 3 days. If infection persists 3 weeks later, treatment is repeated.

How supplied

Tablets (chewable): 100 mg
Oral suspension: 100 mg/5 ml ◊

Pharmacokinetics

Absorption: about 5% to 10% of dose is absorbed; varies widely among patients.
Distribution: highly bound to plasma proteins.
Metabolism: metabolized to inactive metabolites.
Excretion: mostly excreted in feces; 2% to 10% excreted in urine. *Half-life:* 3 to 9 hours.

Route	Onset	Peak	Duration
P.O.	Unknown	2-5 hr	Varies

Pharmacodynamics

Chemical effect: selectively and irreversibly inhibits uptake of glucose and other nutrients in susceptible helminths.
Therapeutic effect: kills helminth infestation.

Adverse reactions

GI: transient abdominal pain, diarrhea.

Interactions

Drug-drug. *Carbamazepine, hydantoins:* may reduce plasma levels of mebendazole, possibly decreasing its therapeutic effect. Monitor patient.
Cimetidine: increased mebendazole levels. Monitor patient closely.

Contraindications and precautions

- Contraindicated in patients hypersensitive to drug.
- Use cautiously in pregnant women.
- Safety of drug hasn't been established in breast-feeding women.

NURSING CONSIDERATIONS

Assessment

- Assess patient's condition before therapy and regularly thereafter.
- Be alert for adverse reactions and drug interactions.
- Evaluate patient's and family's knowledge of drug therapy.

Nursing diagnoses

- Infection related to presence of helminths
- Diarrhea related to drug-induced adverse GI reactions
- Deficient knowledge related to drug therapy

Planning and implementation

- Tablets may be chewed, swallowed whole, or crushed and mixed with food.
- Administer drug to all family members, as prescribed, to decrease risk of spreading infection.
- No dietary restrictions, laxatives, or enemas are necessary.

Patient teaching

- Teach patient about personal hygiene, especially good hand-washing technique. To avoid reinfection, teach patient to wash perianal area daily, to change undergarments and bedclothes daily, and to wash hands and clean fingernails before meals and after bowel movements.
- Advise patient not to prepare food for others.

Evaluation

- Patient is free from infestation.
- Patient's bowel pattern returns to normal after therapy is stopped.
- Patient and family state understanding of drug therapy.

mechlorethamine hydrochloride (nitrogen mustard)

(meh-klor-ETH-uh-meen high-droh-KLOR-ighd)
Mustargen

Pharmacologic class: alkylating agent (cell cycle–phase nonspecific)
Therapeutic class: antineoplastic
Pregnancy risk category: D

Indications and dosages

▶ **Polycythemia vera, chronic lymphocytic leukemia, chronic myelocytic leukemia, malignant effusions (pericardial, peritoneal, pleural), mycosis fungoides, Hodgkin's disease, lymphosarcoma, bronchogenic cancer.** *Adults:* 0.4 mg/kg or 10 mg/m^2 I.V. as single dose or in divided doses of 0.1 to 0.2 mg/kg/day on 2 to 4 successive days q 3 to 6 weeks. Given through running I.V. infusion. Subsequent courses given when patient has recovered hematologically from previous course (usually 3 to 6 weeks).

▶ **Malignant effusions.** *Adults:* 0.2 to 0.4 mg/kg intracavitarily.

How supplied

Injection: 10-mg vials

Pharmacokinetics

Absorption: after intracavitary administration, drug is absorbed incompletely, probably from deactivation by body fluids in cavity.
Distribution: doesn't cross blood-brain barrier.
Metabolism: converted rapidly to its active form, which reacts quickly with various cellular components before being deactivated.
Excretion: metabolites excreted in urine.

Route	Onset	Peak	Duration
I.V., intracavitary	Rapid	Unknown	Unknown

Pharmacodynamics

Chemical effect: cross-links strands of cellular DNA and interferes with RNA transcription, causing imbalance of growth that leads to cell death.
Therapeutic effect: kills certain cancer cells.

Adverse reactions

CNS: headache, weakness, drowsiness, vertigo.
CV: *thrombophlebitis.*
EENT: tinnitus, hearing loss with high doses.
GI: *metallic taste, nausea, vomiting, anorexia.*
Hematologic: ***thrombocytopenia, agranulocytosis,*** lymphocytopenia, myelosuppression that peaks in 4 to 10 days and lasts 10 to 21 days, mild anemia that begins in 2 to 3 weeks.
Metabolic: hyperuricemia.
Skin: *alopecia,* rash, sloughing, severe irritation if drug extravasates or touches skin.
Other: precipitation of herpes zoster, ***anaphylaxis, secondary malignant disease.***

Interactions

Drug-drug. *Anticoagulants, aspirin:* increased risk of bleeding. Avoid concomitant use.

Contraindications and precautions

- Contraindicated in patients hypersensitive to drug and in those with infectious diseases.
- Drug isn't recommended for use in pregnant or breast-feeding women.
- Use cautiously in patients with severe anemia or depressed neutrophil or platelet count and in those who have recently undergone radiation therapy or chemotherapy.
- Safety of drug hasn't been established in children.

NURSING CONSIDERATIONS

Assessment

- Assess patient's condition before therapy and regularly thereafter.
- Monitor CBC and platelet counts regularly, as ordered.
- Monitor serum uric acid level, as ordered.
- Be alert for adverse reactions and drug interactions.
- Neurotoxicity increases with dose and patient age.
- Evaluate patient's and family's knowledge of drug therapy.

Nursing diagnoses

- Ineffective health maintenance related to presence of neoplastic disease
- Ineffective immune protection related to adverse hematologic reactions
- Deficient knowledge related to drug therapy

Planning and implementation

- Follow facility policy to reduce risks. Preparation and administration of parenteral form are linked to carcinogenic, mutagenic, and teratogenic risks for personnel.

I.V. use: Reconstitute drug using 10 ml of sterile water for injection or normal saline solution injection. Resulting solution contains 1 mg/ml of mechlorethamine.
– Give by direct injection into vein or into I.V. line containing free-flowing solution.

ALERT Make sure I.V. solution doesn't extravasate because mechlorethamine is a potent vesicant. If it does, apply cold compresses and infiltrate area with isotonic sodium thiosulfate, as ordered.

Intracavitary use: When given intracavitarily for sclerosing effect, dilute with up to 100 ml of normal saline solution for injection. Turn patient from side to side every 15 minutes to 1 hour to distribute drug.
- Prepare immediately before infusion. Solution is very unstable. Use within 15 minutes, and discard unused solution.
- Don't use solutions that are discolored or contain particulates. Don't use vials that appear to contain droplets of water.
- Dispose of equipment used in drug preparation and administration properly and according to facility policy. Neutralize unused solution with equal volume of 5% sodium bicarbonate and 5% sodium thiosulfate.
- To prevent hyperuricemia with resulting uric acid nephropathy, patient should be adequately hydrated.

Patient teaching
- Warn patient to watch for signs of infection (fever, sore throat, fatigue) and bleeding (easy bruising, nosebleeds, bleeding gums, melena). Have patient take temperature daily.
- Instruct patient to avoid OTC products that contain aspirin.
- Advise woman of childbearing age to avoid becoming pregnant during therapy and to consult with prescriber before becoming pregnant.

☑ Evaluation
- Patient responds positively to drug.
- Patient regains normal hematologic parameters.
- Patient and family state understanding of drug therapy.

meclizine hydrochloride (meclozine hydrochloride)

(MEK-lih-zeen high-droh-KLOR-ighd)
Ancolan ◇, Antivert, Antivert/25†, Antivert/50, Bonamine ♦, Bonine†, Dizmiss†, Meni-D, Vergon†

Pharmacologic class: piperazine-derivative antihistamine
Therapeutic class: antiemetic, antivertigo agent
Pregnancy risk category: B

Indications and dosages

▶ **Vertigo.** *Adults:* 25 to 100 mg P.O. daily in divided doses. Dosage varies with patient response.
▶ **Motion sickness.** *Adults:* 25 to 50 mg P.O. 1 hour before travel, repeated daily for duration of journey.

How supplied

Tablets: 12.5 mg, 25 mg†, 50 mg
Tablets (chewable): 25 mg†
Capsules: 15 mg, 25 mg, 30 mg

Pharmacokinetics

Absorption: unknown.
Distribution: well distributed throughout body.
Metabolism: unknown, although thought to metabolize in liver.
Excretion: excreted unchanged in feces; metabolites found in urine. *Half-life:* about 6 hours.

Route	Onset	Peak	Duration
P.O.	About 1 hr	Unknown	8-24 hr

Pharmacodynamics

Chemical effect: unknown; may affect neural pathways originating in labyrinth to inhibit nausea and vomiting.
Therapeutic effect: relieves vertigo and nausea.

Adverse reactions

CNS: *drowsiness,* fatigue.
EENT: blurred vision.
GI: dry mouth.

Interactions

Drug-drug. *CNS depressants:* increased drowsiness. Use together cautiously.

Contraindications and precautions

- Contraindicated in patients hypersensitive to drug.

• Use cautiously in breast-feeding women and in patients with asthma, glaucoma, or prostatic hyperplasia.
• Safety of drug hasn't been established in children and in pregnant women.

NURSING CONSIDERATIONS

Assessment
• Assess patient's condition before therapy and regularly thereafter.
• Be alert for adverse reactions and drug interactions.
• Evaluate patient's and family's knowledge of drug therapy.

Nursing diagnoses
• Risk for injury related to vertigo
• Risk for deficient fluid volume related to motion sickness
• Deficient knowledge related to drug therapy

Planning and implementation
• If used to prevent motion sickness, drug should be taken 1 hour before travel.
• Don't discontinue abruptly after long-term therapy because paradoxical reactions or sudden reversal of improved state may occur.

Patient teaching
• Advise patient to refrain from driving and performing other hazardous activities that require alertness until CNS effects of drug are known.
• Teach patient how to take drug.
• Stress importance of not stopping drug abruptly if used long-term.
• Advise patient not to use alcohol while taking this drug and to consult a prescriber before taking drug if already taking sedatives or tranquilizers.

Evaluation
• Patient states that vertigo is relieved.
• Patient states that motion sickness doesn't occur.
• Patient and family state understanding of drug therapy.

medroxyprogesterone acetate
(med-roks-ee-proh-JES-ter-ohn AS-ih-tayt)
Amen, Cycrin, Depo-Provera, Provera

Pharmacologic class: progestin
Therapeutic class: progestin antineoplastic
Pregnancy risk category: X

Indications and dosages
▶ **Abnormal uterine bleeding caused by hormonal imbalance.** *Women:* 5 to 10 mg P.O. daily for 5 to 10 days beginning on day 16 of menstrual cycle. If patient also has received estrogen, 10 mg P.O. daily for 10 days beginning on day 16 of cycle.
▶ **Secondary amenorrhea.** *Women:* 5 to 10 mg P.O. daily for 5 to 10 days.
▶ **Endometrial or renal carcinoma.** *Women:* 400 to 1,000 mg I.M. weekly.
▶ **Contraception in women.** *Women:* 150 mg I.M. once q 3 months.

How supplied
Tablets: 2.5 mg, 5 mg, 10 mg
Injection (suspension): 150 mg/ml, 400 mg/ml

Pharmacokinetics
Absorption: slow after I.M. use; unknown for P.O. use.
Distribution: unknown.
Metabolism: primarily in liver; not well characterized.
Excretion: primarily in urine; not well characterized.

Route	Onset	Peak	Duration
P.O., I.M.	Unknown	Unknown	Unknown

Pharmacodynamics
Chemical effect: suppresses ovulation, possibly by inhibiting pituitary gonadotropin secretion, and forms thick cervical mucus.
Therapeutic effect: stops abnormal uterine bleeding, reverses secondary amenorrhea, prevents pregnancy, and hinders cancer cell growth.

Adverse reactions

CNS: dizziness, migraine, lethargy, depression.
CV: hypertension, thrombophlebitis, ***pulmonary embolism,*** edema, ***thromboembolism, CVA.***
GI: nausea, vomiting, abdominal cramps.
GU: breakthrough bleeding, dysmenorrhea, amenorrhea, cervical erosion, abnormal secretions, uterine fibromas, vaginal candidiasis.
Hepatic: cholestatic jaundice.
Metabolic: hyperglycemia.
Skin: melasma, rash, pain, induration, sterile abscesses.
Other: breast tenderness, enlargement, or secretion; decreased libido.

Interactions

Drug-drug. *Aminoglutethimide, rifampin:* decreased progestin effects. Monitor patient for diminished therapeutic response. Tell patient to use nonhormonal contraceptive during therapy with these drugs.
Bromocriptine: may cause amenorrhea, interfering with bromocriptine's effects. Avoid concomitant use.
Drug-food. *Caffeine:* may increase serum caffeine levels. Monitor patient for effect.
Drug-lifestyle. *Smoking:* increased risk of adverse CV effects. If smoking continues, may need alternative therapy.

Contraindications and precautions

- Contraindicated in patients hypersensitive to drug, in pregnant women, and in those with active thromboembolic disorders, breast cancer, undiagnosed abnormal vaginal bleeding, missed abortion, hepatic dysfunction, or a history of thromboembolic disorders, cerebrovascular disease, or apoplexy. Tablets are also contraindicated in patients with liver dysfunction or known or suspected cancer of genital organs.
- Drug isn't recommended for use in breast-feeding women.
- Use cautiously in patients with diabetes mellitus, seizure disorder, migraine, cardiac or renal disease, asthma, or depression.

NURSING CONSIDERATIONS

Assessment

- Assess patient's condition before therapy and regularly thereafter.
- Be alert for adverse reactions and drug interactions.
- Monitor injection sites for evidence of sterile abscess.
- Evaluate patient's and family's knowledge of drug therapy.

Nursing diagnoses

- Ineffective health maintenance related to underlying condition
- Excessive fluid volume related to drug-induced edema
- Deficient knowledge related to drug therapy

Planning and implementation

P.O. use: Follow normal protocol.
I.M. use: Rotate injection sites to prevent muscle atrophy.

Patient teaching

- Have patient read package insert explaining possible adverse effects of progestins before administering first dose; then provide verbal explanation.
- Instruct patient to avoid caffeine and smoking during drug therapy.

ALERT Tell patient to report unusual symptoms immediately and to stop drug and notify prescriber if visual disturbance or migraine occurs.

- Teach woman how to perform routine monthly breast self-examination.
- Warn patient that I.M. injection may be painful.

Evaluation

- Patient responds well to drug therapy.
- Patient doesn't develop fluid excess throughout drug therapy.
- Patient and family state understanding of drug therapy.

mefloquine hydrochloride

(MEF-loh-kwin high-droh-KLOR-ighd)
Lariam

Pharmacologic class: quinine derivative
Therapeutic class: antimalarial
Pregnancy risk category: C

Indications and dosages

▶ **Acute malaria infections caused by mefloquine-sensitive strains of *Plasmodium falciparum* and *P. vivax*.** *Adults:* 1,250 mg P.O. as single dose. Patients with *P. vivax* infections should receive primaquine or other 8-aminoquinolones to avoid relapse after treatment of initial infection.

▶ **Malaria prophylaxis.** *Adults:* 250 mg P.O. once weekly. Prophylaxis should start 1 week before entering endemic area and continue for 4 weeks after return.

How supplied

Tablets: 250 mg

Pharmacokinetics

Absorption: well absorbed.
Distribution: concentrated in RBCs; about 98% protein-bound.
Metabolism: metabolized by liver.
Excretion: excreted primarily by liver; small amounts found in urine. *Half-life:* about 21 days.

Route	Onset	Peak	Duration
P.O.	Unknown	7-24 hr	Unknown

Pharmacodynamics

Chemical effect: unknown; may be related to its ability to form complexes with hemin.
Therapeutic effect: kills malaria-causing organisms. Spectrum of activity includes all human types of malaria, including chloroquine-resistant malaria and strains of *P. falciparum* and *P. vivax*.

Adverse reactions

CNS: dizziness, fatigue, syncope, headache, ***seizures.***
CV: extrasystoles.
EENT: tinnitus.
GI: loss of appetite, vomiting, *nausea,* loose stools, diarrhea, GI discomfort.
Skin: rash.
Other: fever, chills.

Interactions

Drug-drug. *Beta blockers, quinidine, quinine:* ECG abnormalities and cardiac arrest may occur. Avoid concomitant use.
Chloroquine, quinine: increased risk of seizures. Monitor patient.
Halofantrine: risk of fatal prolongation of QTC interval. Don't use together.
Valproic acid: decreased valproic acid blood levels and loss of seizure control at start of mefloquine therapy. Check anticonvulsant blood levels.

Contraindications and precautions

- Contraindicated in patients hypersensitive to mefloquine or related compounds.
- Use cautiously in patients with cardiac disease or seizure disorders and in pregnant or breast-feeding women.
- Safety of drug hasn't been established in children.

NURSING CONSIDERATIONS

Assessment

- Assess patient's condition before therapy and regularly thereafter.
- Monitor liver function tests periodically, as ordered.
- Be alert for adverse reactions and drug interactions.
- Monitor patient's hydration status if adverse GI reactions occur.
- Evaluate patient's and family's knowledge of drug therapy.

Nursing diagnoses

- Infection related to presence of malaria organisms
- Risk of deficient fluid volume related to drug-induced adverse reactions
- Deficient knowledge related to drug therapy

Planning and implementation
- Because health risks from concomitant administration of quinine and mefloquine are great, drug therapy shouldn't begin less than 12 hours after last dose of quinine or quinidine.
- Patients with infections caused by *P. vivax* are at high risk for relapse because drug doesn't eliminate hepatic phase (exoerythrocytic parasites). Follow-up therapy with primaquine is advisable.
- Give drug with food and full glass of water to minimize adverse GI reactions.

Patient teaching
- Advise patient to take drug on same day of week when using it for prophylaxis.
- Advise patient to use caution when performing hazardous activities that require alertness and coordination because dizziness, disturbed sense of balance, and neuropsychiatric reactions may occur.
- Instruct patient taking mefloquine prophylaxis to discontinue drug and notify prescriber if he notices signs or symptoms of impending toxicity, such as unexplained anxiety, depression, confusion, or restlessness.
- Recommend to patient undergoing long-term therapy that he have periodic ophthalmologic examinations.

Evaluation
- Patient is free from infection.
- Patient maintains adequate hydration throughout therapy.
- Patient and family state understanding of drug therapy.

megestrol acetate
(meh-JES-trol AS-ih-tayt)
Megace, Megostat◇

Pharmacologic class: progestin
Therapeutic class: antineoplastic
Pregnancy risk category: D

Indications and dosages
▶ **Breast cancer.** *Adults:* 40 mg P.O. q.i.d.
▶ **Endometrial cancer.** *Adults:* 40 to 320 mg P.O. daily in divided doses.
▶ **Treatment of anorexia, cachexia, or unexplained significant weight loss in patients with AIDS.** *Adults:* 800 mg P.O. (oral suspension) daily in divided doses; 100 to 400 mg for AIDS-related cachexia.

How supplied
Tablets: 20 mg, 40 mg
Oral suspension: 40 mg/ml

Pharmacokinetics
Absorption: well absorbed across GI tract.
Distribution: appears to be stored in fatty tissue; highly bound to plasma proteins.
Metabolism: completely metabolized in liver.
Excretion: excreted in urine.

Route	Onset	Peak	Duration
P.O.	Unknown	Unknown	Unknown

Pharmacodynamics
Chemical effect: changes tumor's hormonal environment and alters neoplastic process. Mechanism of appetite stimulation is unknown.
Therapeutic effect: hinders cancer cell growth and increases appetite.

Adverse reactions
CV: hypertension, thrombophlebitis, ***heart failure.***
GI: nausea, vomiting.
GU: breakthrough menstrual bleeding.
Metabolic: weight gain, increased appetite.
Musculoskeletal: carpal tunnel syndrome.
Respiratory: ***pulmonary embolism.***
Skin: alopecia, hirsutism.
Other: breast tenderness.

Interactions
None significant.

Contraindications and precautions
- Contraindicated in patients hypersensitive to drug and in pregnant women.
- Drug isn't recommended for use in breast-feeding women.
- Use cautiously in patients with history of thrombophlebitis.

• Safety of drug hasn't been established in children.

NURSING CONSIDERATIONS

Assessment
• Assess patient's condition before therapy and regularly thereafter.
• Be alert for adverse reactions.
• Monitor patient's hydration status if adverse GI reactions occur.
• Evaluate patient's and family's knowledge of drug therapy.

Nursing diagnoses
• Ineffective health maintenance related to underlying condition
• Risk for deficient fluid volume related to drug-induced adverse GI reactions
• Deficient knowledge related to drug therapy

Planning and implementation
• Two months is adequate trial when treating cancer.

Patient teaching
• Inform patient that therapeutic response isn't immediate.
• Advise breast-feeding woman to discontinue breast-feeding during therapy because of possible infant toxicity.

Evaluation
• Patient responds well to therapy.
• Patient maintains adequate hydration throughout therapy.
• Patient and family state understanding of drug therapy.

meloxicam
(mell-OX-ih-kam)
Mobic

Pharmacologic class: enolic acid NSAID
Therapeutic class: anti-inflammatory, analgesic
Pregnancy risk category: C

Indications and dosages
▶ **Relief of signs and symptoms of osteoarthritis.** *Adults:* 7.5 mg P.O. once daily. May increase to maximum of 15 mg daily, p.r.n.

How supplied
Tablets: 7.5 mg

Pharmacokinetics
Absorption: bioavailability after P.O. administration is 89% and doesn't appear to be affected by food or antacids. Steady-state conditions are reached after 5 days of daily administration.
Distribution: 99.4% bound to human plasma proteins.
Metabolism: almost completely metabolized to pharmacologically inactive metabolites.
Excretion: excreted in both urine and feces, primarily as metabolites. *Elimination half-life:* 15 to 20 hours.

Route	Onset	Peak	Duration
P.O.	Unknown	Unknown	Unknown

Pharmacodynamics
Chemical effect: mechanism of action of meloxicam may be related to prostaglandin (cyclooxygenase) synthetase inhibition.
Therapeutic effect: relief of signs and symptoms of osteoarthritis.

Adverse reactions
CNS: dizziness, headache, insomnia, fatigue, ***seizures,*** paresthesia, tremor, vertigo, anxiety, confusion, depression, nervousness, somnolence, malaise, syncope.
CV: ***arrhythmias,*** palpitations, tachycardia, angina, ***heart failure,*** hypertension, hypotension, ***MI,*** edema.
EENT: pharyngitis, abnormal vision, conjunctivitis, tinnitus.
GI: abdominal pain, diarrhea, dyspepsia, flatulence, nausea, constipation, colitis, dry mouth, duodenal ulcer, esophagitis, gastric ulcer, gastritis, GI reflux, ***hemorrhage***, ***pancreatitis,*** vomiting, increased appetite, taste perversion.
GU: albuminuria, elevated BUN and creatinine levels, hematuria, urinary frequency, ***renal failure,*** urinary tract infection.

Hematologic: anemia, ***leukopenia,*** purpura, ***thrombocytopenia.***
Hepatic: elevated liver enzyme levels, bilirubinemia, ***hepatitis.***
Metabolic: dehydration, weight changes.
Musculoskeletal: arthralgia, back pain.
Respiratory: upper respiratory tract infection, asthma, ***bronchospasm,*** dyspnea, cough.
Skin: rash, pruritus, alopecia, bullous eruption, photosensitivity, sweating, urticaria.
Other: accidental injury, allergic reaction, fever, ***angioedema,*** flulike symptoms.

Interactions

Drug-drug. *ACE inhibitors:* diminished antihypertensive effects. Monitor patient's blood pressure.
Aspirin: increased risk of adverse effects. Avoid concomitant use.
Furosemide, thiazide diuretics: NSAIDs can reduce sodium excretion linked to diuretics, leading to sodium retention. Monitor patient for edema and increased blood pressure.
Lithium: increased lithium levels. Monitor plasma lithium levels closely during treatment.
Warfarin: increased PT or INR and increased risk of bleeding complications. Monitor PT and INR, and check for signs and symptoms of bleeding.
Drug-herb. *Dong quai, feverfew, garlic, ginger, horse chestnut, red clover:* possible increased risk of bleeding. Monitor patient closely.
St. John's wort: increased risk of photosensitivity. Advise patient to avoid unprotected exposure to sunlight.
Drug-lifestyle. *Smoking:* increased risk of GI irritation and bleeding. Monitor patient for bleeding.
Alcohol: increased risk of GI irritation and bleeding. Monitor patient for bleeding.

Contraindications and precautions

- Contraindicated in patients hypersensitive to meloxicam and in those who have experienced asthma, urticaria, or allergic-type reactions after taking aspirin or other NSAIDs. Avoid use in late pregnancy.
- Use with extreme caution in patients with a history of ulcers or GI bleeding. Use cautiously in patients with dehydration, anemia, hepatic disease, renal disease, hypertension, fluid retention, heart failure, and asthma. Also use cautiously in elderly and debilitated patients because of increased risk of fatal GI bleeding.

NURSING CONSIDERATIONS

Assessment

- Obtain accurate history of drug allergies; meloxicam can produce allergic-like reactions in patients hypersensitive to aspirin and other NSAIDs.
- Assess patient for increased risk of GI bleeding. Risk factors include history of ulcers or GI bleeding, treatment with corticosteroids or anticoagulants, longer duration of NSAID treatment, smoking, alcoholism, older age, and poor overall health.
- Monitor patient for signs and symptoms of overt and occult bleeding.
- Monitor patient for fluid retention; closely monitor patients who have hypertension, edema, or heart failure.
- Monitor liver function.
- Evaluate patient's and family's knowledge of drug therapy.

Nursing diagnoses

- Chronic pain related to underlying condition
- Risk for injury related to drug-induced adverse reactions
- Deficient knowledge related to drug therapy

Planning and implementation

- Drug may be taken with food to avoid GI upset.
- Rehydrate patients who are dehydrated before starting treatment with meloxicam.
- If patient develops evidence of liver disease (eosinophilia, rash, etc.), drug should be discontinued, as directed.

Patient teaching

- Tell patient to notify prescriber about history of allergic reactions to aspirin or other NSAIDs before starting therapy.
- Teach patient to report signs and symptoms of GI ulcerations and bleeding, such as vomit-

ing blood, blood in stool, and black, tarry stools.
• Instruct patient to report skin rash, weight gain, or edema.
• Advise patient to report warning signs of hepatotoxicity (nausea, fatigue, lethargy, pruritus, jaundice, right upper quadrant tenderness, and flulike symptoms).
• Warn patient with a history of asthma that it may recur while taking meloxicam and that he should stop taking the drug and notify prescriber if it does.
• Tell woman to notify prescriber if she becomes pregnant or is planning to become pregnant while taking this drug.
• Inform patient that it may take several days before consistent pain relief is achieved.

☑ Evaluation
• Patient is free from pain.
• Patient sustains no injury as a result of drug-induced adverse reactions.
• Patient and family state understanding of drug therapy.

melphalan (L-phenylalanine mustard)
(MEL-feh-len)
Alkeran

Pharmacologic class: alkylating agent (cell cycle–phase nonspecific)
Therapeutic class: antineoplastic
Pregnancy risk category: C

Indications and dosages
▶ **Multiple myeloma.** *Adults:* 6 mg P.O. daily for 2 to 3 weeks; then drug stopped for up to 4 weeks or until WBC and platelet counts begin to rise again; maintenance dosage of 2 mg daily then given.
Alternative therapy: 0.15 mg/kg P.O. daily for 7 days at 2- to 6-week intervals. Or, 0.25 mg/kg P.O. daily for 4 days, repeated q 4 to 6 weeks. Or, administered I.V. to patients who can't tolerate oral therapy: 16 mg/m^2 given by infusion over 15 to 20 minutes q 2 weeks for four doses. After patient has recovered from toxicity, drug given q 4 weeks.
▶ **Nonresectable advanced ovarian cancer.** *Adults:* 0.2 mg/kg P.O. daily for 5 days. Repeated q 4 to 6 weeks, depending on bone marrow recovery.

How supplied
Tablets (scored): 2 mg
Injection: 50 mg

Pharmacokinetics
Absorption: incomplete and variable from GI tract.
Distribution: distributed rapidly and widely in total body water; initially 50% to 60% bound to plasma proteins and increases to 80% to 90% over time.
Metabolism: extensively deactivated by hydrolysis.
Excretion: excreted primarily in urine. *Half-life:* 2 hours.

Route	Onset	Peak	Duration
P.O., I.V.	Unknown	Unknown	Unknown

Pharmacodynamics
Chemical effect: cross-links strands of cellular DNA and interferes with RNA transcription.
Therapeutic effect: kills certain cancer cells.

Adverse reactions
Hematologic: ***thrombocytopenia, leukopenia, bone marrow suppression.***
Hepatic: ***hepatotoxicity.***
Respiratory: ***pneumonitis, pulmonary fibrosis.***
Skin: dermatitis, pruritus, rash, alopecia.
Other: ***anaphylaxis, hypersensitivity reactions.***

Interactions
Drug-drug. *Anticoagulants, aspirin:* increased risk of bleeding. Avoid concomitant use.
Antigout agents: decreased effectiveness. Dosage adjustments may be necessary.
Bone marrow suppressants: additive toxicity. Monitor patient closely.
Carmustine: carmustine lung toxicity threshold may be reduced. Monitor patient closely.

Cisplatin: cisplatin may affect melphalan kinetics by inducing renal dysfunction and subsequently altering melphalan clearance. Monitor patient closely.
Cyclosporine: increased toxicity of cyclosporine, particularly nephrotoxicity. Use cautiously together.
Interferon alpha: serum melphalan levels may be decreased. Monitor serum levels closely.
Nalidixic acid: risk of severe hemorrhagic necrotic enterocolitis may increase in children. Monitor patient closely.
Vaccines: decreased effectiveness of killed-virus vaccines and increased risk of toxicity from live-virus vaccines. Postpone routine immunization for at least 3 months after last dose of melphalan.
Drug-food. *Any food:* decreased absorption of oral drug. Separate administration times.

Contraindications and precautions

- Contraindicated in patients hypersensitive to drug and in those whose disease is resistant to drug. Patients hypersensitive to chlorambucil may have cross-sensitivity to melphalan.
- Drug isn't recommended for pregnant or breast-feeding women.
- Drug isn't recommended for patients with severe leukopenia, thrombocytopenia, anemia, or chronic lymphocytic leukemia.
- Safety of drug hasn't been established in children.

NURSING CONSIDERATIONS

Assessment

- Assess patient's condition before therapy and regularly thereafter.
- Monitor serum uric acid level and CBC, as ordered.
- Be alert for adverse reactions and drug interactions.
- Evaluate patient's and family's knowledge of drug therapy.

Nursing diagnoses

- Ineffective health maintenance related to presence of neoplastic disease
- Ineffective immune protection related to adverse hematologic reactions
- Deficient knowledge related to drug therapy

Planning and implementation

- Follow facility policy to reduce risks. Preparation and administration of parenteral form are linked to carcinogenic, mutagenic, and teratogenic risks for personnel.
- Dosage may need to be reduced in patient with renal impairment.
- Melphalan is drug of choice in combination with prednisone in patients with multiple myeloma.

ALERT Don't confuse melphalan with Mephyton.
P.O. use: Give drug on empty stomach.
I.V. use: Because drug isn't stable in solution, reconstitute immediately before administering with 10 ml of sterile diluent supplied by manufacturer. Shake vigorously until solution is clear. Resulting solution contains 5 mg of melphalan per ml.
– Immediately dilute required dose in normal saline solution for injection. Final concentration shouldn't exceed 0.45 mg/ml.
– Give by I.V. infusion over 15 to 20 minutes.
– Administer promptly after diluting; reconstituted product begins to degrade within 30 minutes. After final dilution, nearly 1% of drug degrades every 10 minutes.
– Don't refrigerate reconstituted product because precipitate will form.

Patient teaching

- Tell patient to take oral drug on empty stomach.
- Warn patient to watch for signs of infection (fever, sore throat, fatigue) and bleeding (easy bruising, nosebleeds, bleeding gums, melena). Have patient take temperature daily.
- Instruct patient to avoid OTC products that contain aspirin.
- Advise woman of childbearing age to avoid becoming pregnant during therapy and to consult with prescriber before becoming pregnant.

Evaluation

- Patient responds well to therapy.
- Patient regains normal hematologic function when therapy is completed.

• Patient and family state understanding of drug therapy.

menotropins
(meh-noh-TROH-pins)
Humegon, Pergonal, Repronex

Pharmacologic class: gonadotropin
Therapeutic class: ovulation stimulant, spermatogenesis stimulant
Pregnancy risk category: X

Indications and dosages

▶ **Anovulation.** *Women:* 75 IU each of follicle-stimulating hormone (FSH) and luteinizing hormone (LH) I.M. daily for 7 to 12 days, followed by 5,000 to 10,000 USP units of human chorionic gonadotropin (HCG) I.M. 1 day after last dose of menotropins. Repeated for one to three menstrual cycles until ovulation occurs.

▶ **Infertility with ovulation.** *Women:* 75 IU each of FSH and LH I.M. daily for 7 to 12 days, followed by 5,000 to 10,000 USP units of HCG I.M. 1 day after last dose of menotropins. Repeated for two menstrual cycles and then increased to 150 IU each of FSH and LH daily for 7 to 12 days, followed by 5,000 to 10,000 USP units of HCG I.M. 1 day after last dose of menotropins. Repeated for two menstrual cycles.

▶ **Infertility in men.** *Men:* Treatment with HCG of 5,000 USP units three times a week for 4 to 6 months; then 75 IU each of FSH and LH I.M. three times weekly (given with 2,000 USP units of HCG twice weekly) for at least 4 months. If spermatogenesis doesn't increase, dosage increased to 150 IU each of FSH and LH three times weekly (dosage of HCG remains unchanged).

How supplied

Injection: 75 IU of LH and 75 IU of FSH activity/ampule; 150 IU of LH and 150 IU of FSH activity/ampule

Pharmacokinetics

Absorption: unknown.
Distribution: unknown.
Metabolism: unknown.
Excretion: excreted in urine.

Route	Onset	Peak	Duration
I.M.	9-12 days	Unknown	Unknown

Pharmacodynamics

Chemical effect: when given to women who haven't had primary ovarian failure, mimics FSH in inducing follicular growth and LH in aiding follicular maturation.
Therapeutic effect: stimulates ovulation and fertility.

Adverse reactions

CV: ***CVA,*** tachycardia.
GI: nausea, vomiting, diarrhea.
GU: *ovarian enlargement with pain and abdominal distention,* multiple births, ovarian hyperstimulation syndrome (sudden ovarian enlargement, ascites, or pleural effusion).
Hematologic: hemoconcentration with fluid loss into abdomen.
Respiratory: ***atelectasis, acute respiratory distress syndrome, pulmonary embolism, pulmonary infarction, arterial occlusion.***
Other: fever, *gynecomastia,* ***hypersensitivity reactions, anaphylaxis.***

Interactions

None significant.

Contraindications and precautions

• Contraindicated in patients hypersensitive to drug; in women with primary ovarian failure, uncontrolled thyroid or adrenal dysfunction, pituitary tumor, abnormal uterine bleeding, uterine fibromas, or ovarian cysts or enlargement; in pregnant women; and in men with normal pituitary function, primary testicular failure, or infertility disorders other than hypogonadotropic hypogonadism.
• Drug shouldn't be used in breast-feeding women or children.

NURSING CONSIDERATIONS

Assessment
• Assess patient's condition before therapy and regularly thereafter.
• Be alert for adverse reactions.

• Evaluate patient's and family's knowledge of drug therapy.

Nursing diagnoses

• Sexual dysfunction related to underlying disorder
• Risk for deficient fluid volume related to drug-induced adverse reactions
• Deficient knowledge related to drug therapy

Planning and implementation

• Monitor patient closely to ensure adequate ovarian stimulation.
• Reconstitute with 1 to 2 ml of sterile normal saline solution. Use immediately.
• Rotate injection sites.

Patient teaching

• Discuss risk of multiple births.
• In infertility, encourage daily intercourse from day before HCG is given until ovulation occurs.
• Tell patient that pregnancy usually occurs 4 to 6 weeks after therapy.
• Instruct patient to immediately report severe abdominal pain, bloating, swelling of hands or feet, nausea, vomiting, diarrhea, substantial weight gain, or shortness of breath.

Evaluation

• Patient or partner becomes pregnant.
• Patient maintains adequate hydration throughout therapy.
• Patient and family state understanding of drug therapy.

meperidine hydrochloride (pethidine hydrochloride)

(meh-PER-uh-deen high-droh-KLOR-ighd)
Demerol

Pharmacologic class: opioid
Therapeutic class: analgesic, adjunct to anesthesia
Controlled substance schedule: II
Pregnancy risk category: C

Indications and dosages

▶ **Moderate to severe pain.** *Adults:* 50 to 150 mg P.O., I.M., or S.C. q 3 to 4 hours, p.r.n. Or, 15 to 35 mg/hour by continuous I.V. infusion.
Children: 1.1 to 1.76 mg/kg P.O., I.M., or S.C. q 3 to 4 hours. Maximum dosage is 100 mg q 4 hours, p.r.n.
▶ **Preoperatively.** *Adults:* 50 to 100 mg I.M., I.V., or S.C. 30 to 90 minutes before surgery.
Children: 1 to 2.2 mg/kg I.M., I.V., or S.C. up to adult dose 30 to 90 minutes before surgery.
▶ **Adjunct to anesthesia.** *Adults:* Repeated slow I.V. injections of fractional doses (i.e., 10 mg/ml). Or, continuous I.V. infusion of more dilute solution (1 mg/ml) adjusted to needs of patient.
▶ **Obstetric analgesia.** *Adults:* 50 to 100 mg I.M. or S.C. when pain becomes regular, repeated at 1- to 3-hour intervals.

How supplied

Tablets: 50 mg, 100 mg
Syrup: 50 mg/5 ml
Injection: 10 mg/ml, 25 mg/ml, 50 mg/ml, 75 mg/ml, 100 mg/ml

Pharmacokinetics

Absorption: unknown.
Distribution: distributed widely throughout body.
Metabolism: metabolized primarily by hydrolysis in liver.
Excretion: excreted primarily in urine. Excretion enhanced by acidifying urine. *Half-life:* 2.4 to 4 hours.

Route	Onset	Peak	Duration
P.O.	15 min	60-90 min	2-4 hr
I.V.	1 min	5-7 min	2-4 hr
I.M., S.C.	10-15 min	30-50 min	2-4 hr

Pharmacodynamics

Chemical effect: binds with opioid receptors in CNS, altering both perception of and emotional response to pain through unknown mechanism.
Therapeutic effect: relieves pain.

Adverse reactions

CNS: *sedation, somnolence, clouded sensorium, euphoria,* paradoxical excitement, tremors, dizziness, ***seizures.***
CV: *hypotension,* ***bradycardia,*** tachycardia, ***cardiac arrest, shock.***
GI: *nausea, vomiting, constipation,* ileus.
GU: *urine retention.*
Musculoskeletal: muscle twitching.
Respiratory: ***respiratory depression, respiratory arrest.***
Skin: pain at injection site, local tissue irritation and induration (after S.C. injection), phlebitis (after I.V. use).
Other: physical dependence.

Interactions

Drug-drug. *CNS depressants, general anesthetics, hypnotics, other narcotic analgesics, phenothiazines, sedatives, tricyclic antidepressants:* possible respiratory depression, hypotension, profound sedation, or coma. Use together with extreme caution. Reduce meperidine dosage as directed.
MAO inhibitors: increased CNS excitation or depression that can be severe or fatal. Don't use together.
Phenytoin: decreased serum levels of meperidine. Monitor patient for decreased analgesia.
Drug-herb. *Parsley:* may promote or produce serotonin syndrome. Discourage concomitant use.
Drug-lifestyle. *Alcohol use:* additive effects. Urge caution.

Contraindications and precautions

- Contraindicated in patients hypersensitive to drug and in those who have received MAO inhibitors within 14 days.
- Use with extreme caution in elderly patients, debilitated patients, and patients with increased intracranial pressure, head injury, asthma, other respiratory conditions, supraventricular tachycardias, seizures, acute abdominal conditions, hepatic or renal disease, hypothyroidism, Addison's disease, urethral stricture, or prostatic hyperplasia.
- Use cautiously in pregnant or breast-feeding women.

NURSING CONSIDERATIONS

Assessment

- Assess patient's pain before therapy and regularly thereafter.
- Be alert for adverse reactions and drug interactions.
- Meperidine and its active metabolite normeperidine accumulate in body. Monitor patient for increased toxic effect, especially in patient with impaired renal function.
- Monitor respirations of neonate exposed to drug during labor.
- Monitor patient for withdrawal symptoms if drug is discontinued abruptly after long-term use.
- Evaluate patient's and family's knowledge of drug therapy.

Nursing diagnoses

- Acute pain related to underlying condition
- Risk for injury related to drug-induced adverse reactions
- Deficient knowledge related to drug therapy

Planning and implementation

- Drug may be used in some patients who are allergic to morphine.
- Because meperidine toxicity often appears after several days of treatment, it isn't recommended for treatment of chronic pain.
- Keep resuscitation equipment and naloxone available.
- Don't give drug if respirations are below 12 breaths/minute, if respiratory rate or depth is decreased, or if change in pupils is noted.

P.O. use: P.O. dose is less than half as effective as parenteral dose. Give I.M., if possible. When changing from parenteral to P.O. route, dosage should be increased.
– Syrup has local anesthetic effect. Give with full glass of water.
I.V. use: Give slowly by direct I.V. injection or slow continuous I.V. infusion. Drug is compatible with most I.V. solutions, including D_5W, normal saline solution, and Ringer's or lactated Ringer's solutions.
– Drug is incompatible with aminophylline, barbiturates, heparin, morphine sulfate, phenytoin, sodium bicarbonate, or sulfonamides.
I.M. use: Follow normal protocol.

S.C. use: S.C. injection isn't recommended because it's painful.
ALERT Don't confuse Demerol with Demulen, Dymelor, or Temaril.

Patient teaching
- Warn outpatient to avoid hazardous activities until CNS effects of drug are known.
- Instruct patient to avoid alcohol consumption during drug therapy.
- Teach patient to manage adverse reactions, such as constipation.
- Tell family members to withhold drug and notify prescriber if patient's respiratory rate decreases.

Evaluation
- Patient is free from pain.
- Patient doesn't experience injury.
- Patient and family state understanding of drug therapy.

meprobamate
(meh-PROH-bah-mayt)
Apo-Meprobamate◆, Equanil**, 'Miltown'-200, 'Miltown'-400, 'Miltown'-600, Neuramate, Probate, Trancot

Pharmacologic class: carbamate
Therapeutic class: antianxiety agent
Controlled substance schedule: IV
Pregnancy risk category: D

Indications and dosages
▶ **Anxiety.** *Adults:* 1.2 to 1.6 g P.O. daily in three or four equally divided doses. Maximum dosage is 2.4 g daily. Or, 400 to 800 mg sustained-release capsule P.O. b.i.d.
Children ages 6 to 12: 100 to 200 mg P.O. b.i.d. or t.i.d. Or, 200 mg sustained-release capsule P.O. b.i.d. Drug isn't recommended for children younger than age 6.

How supplied
Tablets: 200 mg, 400 mg, 600 mg

Pharmacokinetics
Absorption: well absorbed from GI tract.
Distribution: distributed throughout body; 20% protein-bound.
Metabolism: metabolized rapidly in liver.
Excretion: excreted in urine. *Half-life:* about 10 hours.

Route	Onset	Peak	Duration
P.O.	Unknown	Unknown	Unknown

Pharmacodynamics
Chemical effect: unknown; appears to act at multiple sites in CNS.
Therapeutic effect: relieves anxiety.

Adverse reactions
CNS: *drowsiness,* ataxia, dizziness, slurred speech, headache, vertigo, ***seizures.***
CV: palpitations, tachycardia, hypotension, ***arrhythmias.***
GI: anorexia, nausea, vomiting, diarrhea, stomatitis.
Hematologic: ***aplastic anemia, thrombocytopenia, leukopenia, agranulocytosis.***
Skin: pruritus, urticaria, erythematous maculopapular rash.
Other: ***hypersensitivity reactions.***

Interactions
Drug-drug. *CNS depressants:* increased CNS depression. Avoid concomitant use.
Drug-lifestyle. *Alcohol use:* increased CNS depression. Discourage concomitant use.

Contraindications and precautions
- Contraindicated in patients hypersensitive to drug or related compounds (such as carisoprodol, mebutamate, tybamate, and carbromal) and in patents with porphyria.
- Drug should be avoided in pregnant women, especially during first trimester, and in breast-feeding women.
- Use cautiously in patients with impaired liver or kidney function, seizure disorders, or suicidal tendencies.

NURSING CONSIDERATIONS

Assessment
- Assess patient's anxiety before therapy and regularly thereafter.

• Periodically monitor CBC and kidney and liver function tests in patient receiving high doses, as ordered.
• Be alert for adverse reactions and drug interactions.
• Evaluate patient's and family's knowledge of drug therapy.

Nursing diagnoses
• Anxiety related to underlying condition
• Risk for injury related to drug-induced adverse CNS reactions
• Deficient knowledge related to drug therapy

Planning and implementation
• Dosage should be reduced in elderly or debilitated patient.
• Give drug with meals to reduce GI distress.
• Possibility of abuse and addiction exists with long-term use. Withdraw drug gradually over 2 weeks to avoid withdrawal symptoms.
• Drug may interfere with certain laboratory tests for urinary 17-ketogenic steroids and 17-hydroxycorticosteroids.
ALERT Don't confuse Miltown with Milontin.
ALERT After abrupt withdrawal of long-term therapy, severe generalized tonic-clonic seizures may occur.

Patient teaching
• Tell patient to take drug with food.
• Warn patient to avoid hazardous activities until CNS effects of drug are known.
• Tell patient to avoid alcohol.
• Tell patient to report signs of hematologic toxicity, such as bruising or bleeding, fever, or sore throat.

Evaluation
• Patient states that he is less anxious.
• Patient doesn't experience injury from adverse CNS reactions.
• Patient and family state understanding of drug therapy.

mercaptopurine (6-mercaptopurine, 6-MP)
(mer-cap-toh-PYOO-reen)
Purinethol

Pharmacologic class: antimetabolite (cell cycle–phase specific, S phase)
Therapeutic class: antineoplastic
Pregnancy risk category: D

Indications and dosages
Dosage and indications may vary.
▶ **Acute lymphoblastic leukemia in children, acute myeloblastic leukemia, chronic myelocytic leukemia.** *Adults:* 2.5 mg/kg P.O. daily as single dose, up to 5 mg/kg/day. Maintenance dosage is 1.5 to 2.5 mg/kg/day. *Children age 5 and over:* 2.5 mg/kg P.O. daily. Maintenance dosage is 1.5 to 2.5 mg/kg/day.

How supplied
Tablets (scored): 50 mg

Pharmacokinetics
Absorption: incomplete and variable; about 50% of dose is absorbed.
Distribution: distributed widely in total body water.
Metabolism: extensively metabolized in liver.
Excretion: excreted in urine.

Route	Onset	Peak	Duration
P.O.	Unknown	Unknown	Unknown

Pharmacodynamics
Chemical effect: inhibits RNA and DNA synthesis.
Therapeutic effect: inhibits growth of certain cancer cells.

Adverse reactions
GI: *nausea, vomiting, anorexia,* painful oral ulcers.
Hematologic: ***leukopenia, thrombocytopenia,*** *anemia* (may persist several days after drug is stopped).
Hepatic: biliary stasis, *jaundice,* ***hepatotoxicity.***

Metabolic: hyperuricemia.
Skin: rash, hyperpigmentation.

Interactions

Drug-drug. *Allopurinol:* slowed inactivation of mercaptopurine. Decrease mercaptopurine to one-fourth or one-third normal dose, as directed.
Hepatotoxic drugs: may enhance hepatotoxicity of mercaptopurine. Monitor patient closely.
Nondepolarizing neuromuscular blockers: antagonized muscle relaxant effect. Notify anesthesiologist that patient is receiving drug.
Warfarin: antagonized anticoagulant effect. Monitor PT and INR.

Contraindications and precautions

- Contraindicated in patients whose disease has resisted drug.
- Drug isn't recommended for use in pregnant or breast-feeding women.

NURSING CONSIDERATIONS

Assessment

- Assess patient's condition before therapy and regularly thereafter.
- Monitor blood count and serum transaminase, alkaline phosphatase, and bilirubin levels weekly during induction and monthly during maintenance, as ordered.
- Observe for signs of bleeding and infection.
- Monitor fluid intake and output and serum uric acid levels, as ordered.
- Be alert for adverse reactions and drug interactions. Adverse GI reactions are less common in children.

ALERT Watch for jaundice, clay-colored stools, and frothy, dark urine. Hepatic dysfunction is reversible when drug is stopped. If hepatic tenderness occurs, stop drug and notify prescriber.

- Evaluate patient's and family's knowledge of drug therapy.

Nursing diagnoses

- Ineffective health maintenance related to presence of leukemia
- Ineffective immune protection related to drug-induced adverse hematologic reactions
- Deficient knowledge related to drug therapy

Planning and implementation

- Dosage modifications may be required after chemotherapy or radiation therapy and in patient with depressed neutrophil or platelet count or impaired liver or kidney function.

ALERT Sometimes drug is ordered as 6-mercaptopurine or 6-MP. The numeral 6 is part of drug name and doesn't signify number of dosage units. To prevent confusion, avoid the use of these designations.

- Drug regimen must continue despite nausea and vomiting. Notify prescriber if adverse GI reactions occur, and obtain order for antiemetic.
- Encourage adequate fluid intake (3 L daily).
- If allopurinol is ordered, use cautiously.
- Discontinue drug if hepatic tenderness occurs and notify prescriber.

Patient teaching

- Tell patient to notify prescriber if vomiting occurs shortly after taking dose because antiemetic will be needed so drug therapy can continue.
- Warn patient to watch for signs of infection (fever, sore throat, fatigue) and bleeding (easy bruising, nosebleeds, bleeding gums, melena). Have patient take his temperature daily.
- Advise woman of childbearing age to avoid becoming pregnant during therapy and to consult with prescriber before becoming pregnant.

Evaluation

- Patient responds well to therapy.
- Patient doesn't develop serious ill effects when hematologic studies are abnormal.
- Patient and family state understanding of drug therapy.

meropenem
(mer-oh-PEN-em)
Merrem I.V.

Pharmacologic class: synthetic broad-spectrum carbapenem antibiotic

Therapeutic class: antibiotic
Pregnancy risk category: B

Indications and dosages

▶ **Complicated appendicitis and peritonitis caused by viridans group streptococci, *Escherichia coli, Klebsiella pneumoniae, Pseudomonas aeruginosa, Bacteroides fragilis, Bacteroides thetaiotaomicron,* and *Peptostreptococcus* species; bacterial meningitis (children only) caused by *Streptococcus pneumoniae, Haemophilus influenzae,* and *Neisseria meningitidis.*** *Adults:* 1 g I.V. q 8 hours over 15 to 30 minutes as I.V. infusion or over 3 to 5 minutes as I.V. bolus injection (5 to 20 ml).
Children weighing more than 50 kg (110 lb): 1 g I.V. q 8 hours for intra-abdominal infections and 2 g I.V. q 8 hours for meningitis.
Children age 3 months and older: 20 mg/kg (intra-abdominal infection) or 40 mg/kg (bacterial meningitis) q 8 hours over 15 to 30 minutes as I.V. infusion or over 3 to 5 minutes as I.V. bolus injection (5 to 20 ml). Maximum dosage is 2 g I.V. q 8 hours.

How supplied

Powder for injection: 500 mg/15 ml, 500 mg/20 ml, 500 mg/100 ml, 1 g/15 ml, 1 g/30 ml, 1 g/100 ml

Pharmacokinetics

Absorption: penetrates into most body fluids and tissues including CSF.
Distribution: plasma protein–binding is 2%.
Metabolism: in kidneys.
Excretion: excreted in urine.

Route	Onset	Peak	Duration
I.V.	Unknown	Within 1 hr	Unknown

Pharmacodynamics

Chemical effect: readily penetrates the cell wall of most gram-positive and gram-negative bacteria to reach penicillin binding protein targets, where it inhibits cell wall synthesis.
Therapeutic effect: bactericidal.

Adverse reactions

CNS: ***seizures,*** headache.
CV: phlebitis, thrombophlebitis at injection site.
GI: diarrhea, nausea, vomiting, constipation, oral candidiasis, glossitis.
GU: increased creatinine or BUN levels, presence of RBCs in urine.
Hematologic: increased or decreased platelet count, increased eosinophil count, decreased hemoglobin or hematocrit, decreased WBC count.
Hepatic: increased levels of ALT, AST, alkaline phosphatase, LD, and bilirubin.
Respiratory: ***apnea.***
Skin: rash, pruritus.
Other: ***hypersensitivity reaction, anaphylaxis,*** inflammation.

Interactions

Drug-drug. *Probenecid:* inhibited renal excretion of meropenem. Concomitant administration isn't recommended.

Contraindications and precautions

- Contraindicated in patients hypersensitive to drug, its components, or other drugs in same class. Also contraindicated in those who have had anaphylactic reactions to beta-lactams.

NURSING CONSIDERATIONS

Assessment

- Obtain specimen for culture and sensitivity tests before giving first dose.

ALERT Serious and occasionally fatal hypersensitivity reactions have been reported in patients receiving therapy with beta-lactams. Before starting therapy, determine whether previous hypersensitivity reactions have occurred to penicillins, cephalosporins, other beta-lactams, or other allergens.

- Monitor patient for signs and symptoms of superinfection.
- Periodically assess organ system functions, as ordered, during prolonged therapy.
- Evaluate patient's and family's knowledge of drug therapy.

Nursing diagnoses

- Infection related to bacteria
- Risk for deficient fluid volume related to effect on kidneys

• Deficient knowledge related to drug therapy

Planning and implementation

• For I.V. bolus administration, add 10 ml of sterile water for injection to 500-mg/20-ml vial or add 20 ml to 1-g/30-ml vial.
• For I.V. infusion, reconstitute infusion vials (500 mg/100 ml and 1 g/100 ml) with compatible infusion fluid. Or, reconstitute an injection vial, add resulting solution to an I.V. container, and further dilute with appropriate infusion fluid.
• Dosages need to be adjusted for patients with renal insufficiency or renal failure or with creatinine clearance below 51 ml/minute.
• Follow manufacturer's guidelines closely when using ADD-Vantage vials.

Patient teaching
• Advise breast-feeding patient of risk of drug transmission to infant.
• Instruct patient to report adverse reactions.

Evaluation

• Patient is free from infection.
• Patient maintains adequate hydration.
• Patient and family state understanding of drug therapy.

mesalamine

(mez-AL-uh-meen)
Asacol, Pentasa, Rowasa

Pharmacologic class: salicylate
Therapeutic class: anti-inflammatory
Pregnancy risk category: B

Indications and dosages

▶ **Active mild to moderate distal ulcerative colitis, proctitis, proctosigmoiditis.** *Adults:* 800 mg P.O. (tablets) t.i.d. for total dose of 2.4 g/day for 6 weeks; 1 g P.O. (capsules) q.i.d. for total dose of 4 g up to 8 weeks; 500 mg P.R. (suppository) b.i.d. retained for 1 to 3 hours or longer, or 4 g as retention enema once daily (preferably h.s.) retained overnight (for about 8 hours). Usual course of therapy for P.R. form is 3 to 6 weeks.

How supplied

Tablets (delayed-release): 400 mg
Capsules (controlled-release): 250 mg
Rectal suspension: 4 g/60 ml
Suppositories: 500 mg

Pharmacokinetics

Absorption: poorly absorbed with P.R. administration; P.O. tablets and capsules are made to have delayed absorption from GI tract.
Distribution: not clearly defined.
Metabolism: undergoes acetylation, but whether this takes place at colonic or systemic sites is unknown.
Excretion: P.O. form primarily excreted in urine; most of P.R. form excreted in feces.
Half-life: mesalamine, 30 to 75 minutes; acetylated metabolite, about 5 to 10 hours.

Route	Onset	Peak	Duration
P.O., P.R.	Unknown	3-12 hr	Unknown

Pharmacodynamics

Chemical effect: unknown; probably acts topically by inhibiting prostaglandin production in colon.
Therapeutic effect: relieves inflammation in lower GI tract.

Adverse reactions

CNS: headache, dizziness, fatigue, malaise.
GI: abdominal pain, cramps, discomfort, flatulence, diarrhea, rectal pain, bloating, nausea, *pancolitis.*
Respiratory: wheezing.
Skin: pruritus, rash, urticaria, hair loss.
Other: ***anaphylaxis,*** fever.

Interactions

None significant.

Contraindications and precautions

• Contraindicated in patients hypersensitive to drug, its components, or salicylates.
• Drug isn't recommended for use in breast-feeding women.
• Use cautiously in patients with renal impairment. Nephrotoxic potential from absorbed mesalamine exists. Also use cautiously in pregnant women.

NURSING CONSIDERATIONS

Assessment
- Assess patient's condition before therapy and regularly thereafter.
- Monitor periodic kidney function studies in patient on long-term therapy, as ordered.
- Because it contains potassium metabisulfite, drug may cause hypersensitivity reactions in patient sensitive to sulfites.
- Be alert for adverse reactions.
- Evaluate patient's and family's knowledge of drug therapy.

Nursing diagnoses
- Impaired tissue integrity related to underlying condition
- Acute pain related to drug-induced adverse GI reactions
- Deficient knowledge related to drug therapy

Planning and implementation
ALERT Don't confuse Asacol with Os-Cal.

P.O. use: Patient should swallow tablets and capsules whole and not crush or chew them.

P.R. use: For maximum effectiveness, have patient retain suppository as long as possible (1 to 3 hours). When giving suspension, shake bottle before application.

Patient teaching
- Teach patient how to take oral form or administer rectal form, and instruct him to carefully follow instructions supplied with medication.
- Instruct patient to discontinue drug if he experiences fever or rash. Patient intolerant of sulfasalazine may also be hypersensitive to mesalamine.

Evaluation
- Patient reports relief from GI symptoms.
- Patient states that no new pain is experienced during therapy.
- Patient and family state understanding of drug therapy.

mesna
(MEZ-nah)
MESNEX

Pharmacologic class: thiol derivative
Therapeutic class: uroprotectant
Pregnancy risk category: B

Indications and dosages
▶ **Prophylaxis of hemorrhagic cystitis in patients receiving ifosfamide.** *Adults:* dosage varies with amount of ifosfamide administered. Usual dosage is 240 mg/m^2 as I.V. bolus with ifosfamide. Dosage repeated at 4 hours and 8 hours after ifosfamide given.

How supplied
Injection: 100 mg/ml

Pharmacokinetics
Absorption: not applicable.
Distribution: remains in vascular compartment; isn't distributed through tissues.
Metabolism: rapidly metabolized to mesna disulfide, its only metabolite.
Excretion: excreted in urine. *Half-life:* mesna, 1 ¼ hour; mesna disulfide, 1 hour.

Route	Onset	Peak	Duration
I.V.	Unknown	Unknown	Unknown

Pharmacodynamics
Chemical effect: prevents ifosfamide-induced hemorrhagic cystitis by reacting with urotoxic ifosfamide metabolites.
Therapeutic effect: prevents ifosfamide from adversely affecting bladder tissue.

Adverse reactions
GI: soft stools, nausea, vomiting, diarrhea, dysgeusia.

Interactions
None significant.

Contraindications and precautions
- Contraindicated in patients hypersensitive to mesna or thiol-containing compounds.
- Use cautiously in pregnant women.

• Safety of drug hasn't been established in children and in breast-feeding women.

NURSING CONSIDERATIONS

Assessment

• Assess patient's condition before therapy and regularly thereafter.
• Up to 6% of patients may not respond to drug's protective effects.
• Monitor urine samples daily in patient receiving mesna for hematuria.
• Be alert for adverse reactions.
• Monitor patient's hydration status if adverse GI reactions occur.
• Evaluate patient's and family's knowledge of drug therapy.

Nursing diagnoses

• Risk for deficient fluid volume related to drug-induced adverse GI reactions
• Deficient knowledge related to drug therapy

Planning and implementation

• Because mesna is used with ifosfamide and other chemotherapeutic drugs, it's difficult to determine adverse reactions attributable solely to mesna.
• Mesna isn't effective in preventing hematuria from other causes (such as thrombocytopenia).
• Although formulated to prevent hemorrhagic cystitis from ifosfamide, drug won't protect against other toxicities linked to ifosfamide.
• Mesna may interfere with diagnostic tests for urine ketones.
• Prepare I.V. solution by diluting commercially available ampules with D_5W, D_5W and normal saline solution for injection, normal saline solution for injection, or lactated Ringer's solution to obtain final solution of 20 mg/ml of mesna.
• Refrigerate diluted solutions after preparation, and use within 6 hours. Diluted solutions are stable for 24 hours at room temperature.
• After opening ampule, discard any unused drug because it decomposes quickly into inactive compound.
• Don't mix mesna I.V. with cisplatin because they're incompatible.

Patient teaching

• Instruct patient to report hematuria immediately and to notify prescriber about adverse GI reactions.

Evaluation

• Patient maintains adequate hydration throughout therapy.
• Patient and family state understanding of drug therapy.

mesoridazine besylate

(mes-oh-RID-eh-zeen BES-eh-layt)
Serentil*, Serentil Concentrate

Pharmacologic class: phenothiazine (piperidine derivative)
Therapeutic class: antipsychotic
Pregnancy risk category: NR

Indications and dosages

▶ **Alcoholism.** *Adults and children over age 12:* 25 mg P.O. b.i.d. up to maximum of 200 mg daily.
▶ **Behavioral problems related to chronic organic mental syndrome.** *Adults and children over age 12:* 25 mg P.O. t.i.d. up to maximum of 300 mg daily.
▶ **Psychoneurotic manifestations (anxiety).** *Adults and children over age 12:* 10 mg P.O. t.i.d. up to maximum of 150 mg daily.
▶ **Schizophrenia.** *Adults and children over age 12:* initially, 50 mg P.O. t.i.d. up to 400 mg/day. Or, 25 mg I.M. repeated in 30 to 60 minutes, p.r.n., up to 200 mg daily.

How supplied

Tablets: 10 mg, 25 mg, 50 mg, 100 mg
Oral concentrate: 25 mg/ml*
Injection: 25 mg/ml

Pharmacokinetics

Absorption: erratic and variable with P.O. use; unknown with I.M. use.
Distribution: distributed widely in body; 91% to 99% protein-bound.
Metabolism: metabolized extensively by liver.

Excretion: excreted primarily in urine with some excretion in feces by way of biliary tract.

Route	Onset	Peak	Duration
P.O., I.M.	Up to several wk	Unknown	Unknown

Pharmacodynamics

Chemical effect: unknown. A piperidine phenothiazine and major sulfoxide metabolite of thioridazine, mesoridazine may block postsynaptic dopamine receptors in brain.
Therapeutic effect: relieves psychotic and alcoholic signs and symptoms.

Adverse reactions

CNS: extrapyramidal reactions, *tardive dyskinesia, sedation,* EEG changes, dizziness, ***neuroleptic malignant syndrome.***
CV: *orthostatic hypotension,* tachycardia, ECG changes.
EENT: *ocular changes, blurred vision,* retinitis pigmentosa.
GI: *dry mouth, constipation.*
GU: *urine retention,* dark urine, menstrual irregularities, inhibited ejaculation.
Hematologic: ***leukopenia, agranulocytosis,*** hyperprolactinemia, ***aplastic anemia, thrombocytopenia.***
Hepatic: cholestatic jaundice, abnormal liver function test results.
Metabolic: weight gain, increased appetite.
Skin: *mild photosensitivity,* allergic reactions, pain at I.M. injection site, sterile abscess.
Other: gynecomastia.

Interactions

Drug-drug. *Antacids:* inhibited absorption of oral phenothiazines. Separate doses by at least 2 hours.
Anticholinergics: may increase anticholinergic effects. Use together cautiously.
Barbiturates: may decrease phenothiazine effect. Observe patient.
CNS depressants: increased CNS depression. Use together cautiously.
Lithium, phenothiazine: possible disorientation, unconsciousness, and extrapyramidal symptoms. Use cautiously.
Metrizamide: increased risk of seizures. Monitor patient closely.
Drug-herb. *Dong quai, St. John's wort:* increased risk of photosensitivity. Advise patient to avoid unprotected exposure to sunlight.
Kava: increased risk or severity of dystonic reactions. Discourage concomitant use.
Yohimbe: phenothiazines may increase the risk of toxicity. Discourage concomitant use.
Drug-lifestyle. *Alcohol use:* increased CNS depression. Discourage concomitant use.
Sun exposure: increased photosensitivity reactions. Urge patient to take precautions.

Contraindications and precautions

- Contraindicated in patients hypersensitive to drug and in those experiencing severe CNS depression or coma.
- Drug isn't recommended for use in breastfeeding women.
- Use cautiously in pregnant women.
- Safety of drug hasn't been established in children younger than age 12.

NURSING CONSIDERATIONS

Assessment

- Assess patient's condition before therapy and regularly thereafter.
- Obtain baseline measures of blood pressure before starting therapy and monitor regularly. Watch for orthostatic hypotension, especially with parenteral administration.
- Monitor therapy with weekly bilirubin tests during first month, periodic blood tests (CBC and liver function), and ophthalmologic tests (long-term use), as ordered.
- Be alert for adverse reactions and drug interactions.
- Monitor patient for tardive dyskinesia. It may occur after prolonged use, although it may not appear until months or years later and may disappear spontaneously or persist for life, despite discontinuation of drug.

ALERT Watch for symptoms of neuroleptic malignant syndrome (extrapyramidal effects, hyperthermia, autonomic disturbance), which is rare but can be fatal.

- Evaluate patient's and family's knowledge of drug therapy.

Nursing diagnoses

- Disturbed thought processes related to underlying condition
- Constipation related to drug-induced adverse GI reactions
- Deficient knowledge related to drug therapy

Planning and implementation

ALERT Don't confuse Serentil with Serevent or Aventyl.

- Oral liquid and parenteral forms may cause contact dermatitis. Wear gloves when preparing solutions, and avoid contact with skin and clothing.

P.O. use: P.O. therapy should replace parenteral therapy as soon as possible. When P.O. concentrate solution is used, dilute dose with water, orange juice, or grape juice just before administration.

I.M. use: Administer drug deep in upper outer quadrant of buttocks. Massage slowly afterward to prevent sterile abscess. Injection may sting.

- Protect drug from light. Slight yellowing of injection or concentrate is common; this doesn't affect potency. Discard markedly discolored solutions.
- Withhold dose and notify prescriber if jaundice, symptoms of blood dyscrasia (fever, sore throat, infection, cellulitis, weakness), or persistent extrapyramidal reactions (longer than a few hours) develop, especially in pregnant woman or in children.
- Acute dystonic reactions may be treated with diphenhydramine.
- Don't discontinue drug abruptly unless severe adverse reactions occur. After abrupt withdrawal of long-term therapy, patient may experience gastritis, nausea, vomiting, dizziness, tremors, feeling of warmth or cold, diaphoresis, tachycardia, headache, and insomnia.

Patient teaching

- Warn patient to avoid activities that require alertness and psychomotor coordination until CNS effects of drug are known.
- Advise patient to change positions slowly.
- Tell patient to avoid alcohol during drug therapy.
- Have patient report urine retention or constipation.
- Tell patient that drug may discolor urine.
- Advise patient to relieve dry mouth with sugarless gum or hard candy.
- Tell patient to avoid prolonged exposure to the sun, use sunblock, and wear protective clothing to avoid photosensitivity reactions.

Evaluation

- Patient exhibits improved behavior.
- Patient maintains normal bowel pattern.
- Patient and family state understanding of drug therapy.

metaproterenol sulfate

(met-uh-proh-TER-eh-nul SUL-fayt)

Alupent, Arm-a-Med Metaproterenol, Dey-Lute Metaproterenol

Pharmacologic class: adrenergic
Therapeutic class: bronchodilator
Pregnancy risk category: C

Indications and dosages

▶ **Acute episodes of bronchial asthma.** *Adults and children:* 2 to 3 inhalations. Don't repeat inhalations more often than q 3 to 4 hours. Maximum 12 inhalations daily.

▶ **Bronchial asthma and reversible bronchospasm.** *Adults:* 20 mg P.O. q 6 to 8 hours. *Children over age 9 or weighing more than 27 kg (60 lb):* 20 mg P.O. q 6 to 8 hours. *Children ages 6 to 9 or weighing less than 27 kg:* 10 mg P.O. q 6 to 8 hours.

Or, by way of IPPB or nebulizer. *Adults and children age 12 and older:* by IPPB, 0.2 to 0.3 ml of 5% solution diluted in 2.5 ml of normal saline solution or 2.5 ml of commercially available 0.4% or 0.6% solution q 4 hours, p.r.n. By hand-bulb nebulizer, 10 inhalations of an undiluted 5% solution.

Children ages 6 to 12: 0.1 to 0.2 ml of 5% solution diluted in normal saline solution to final volume of 3 ml q 4 hours, p.r.n.

How supplied

Tablets: 10 mg, 20 mg
Syrup: 10 mg/5 ml

Aerosol inhaler: 0.65 mg/metered spray
Nebulizer inhaler: 0.4%, 0.6%, 5% solution

Pharmacokinetics

Absorption: well absorbed.
Distribution: widely distributed.
Metabolism: extensively metabolized on first pass through liver.
Excretion: excreted in urine.

Route	Onset	Peak	Duration
P.O.	1 min	≤ 1 hr	1-4 hr
Inhalation	15 min	≤ 1 hr	2-6 hr
Nebulization	5-30 min	≤ 1 hr	2-6 hr

Pharmacodynamics

Chemical effect: relaxes bronchial smooth muscle by acting on $beta_2$-adrenergic receptors.
Therapeutic effect: improves breathing.

Adverse reactions

CNS: nervousness, weakness, drowsiness, tremors.
CV: tachycardia, hypertension, palpitations, ***cardiac arrest.***
GI: vomiting, nausea, bad taste.
Respiratory: ***paradoxical bronchiolar constriction.***

Interactions

Drug-drug. *Levodopa:* risk of arrhythmias. Avoid concomitant use.
Propranolol, other beta blockers: blocked bronchodilating effect of metaproterenol. Monitor patient.

Contraindications and precautions

- Contraindicated in patients hypersensitive to drug or its ingredients, in those receiving cyclopropane or halogenated hydrocarbon general anesthetics, and in those with tachycardia or arrhythmias caused by tachycardia, peripheral or mesenteric vascular thrombosis, or profound hypoxia or hypercapnia.
- Use cautiously in patients with hypertension, hyperthyroidism, heart disease, diabetes, or cirrhosis; in those who are receiving cardiac glycosides; and in pregnant or breast-feeding women.

NURSING CONSIDERATIONS

Assessment

- Assess patient's condition before therapy and regularly thereafter.
- Be alert for adverse reactions and drug interactions.
- Monitor patient's hydration status if adverse GI reactions occur.
- Evaluate patient's and family's knowledge of drug therapy.

Nursing diagnoses

- Impaired gas exchange related to underlying respiratory condition
- Risk for deficient fluid volume related to drug-induced adverse GI reactions
- Deficient knowledge related to drug therapy

Planning and implementation

ALERT Don't confuse metaproterenol with metoprolol or metipranolol. Don't confuse Alupent with Atrovent.

- Patient may use tablets and aerosol concomitantly. Watch for toxicity.

P.O. and oral inhalation use: Follow normal protocol.
Aerosol nebulization use: Solution can be given by IPPB with drug diluted in normal saline solution or by hand-bulb nebulizer at full strength.

Patient teaching

- Give patient the following instructions for using metered-dose inhaler: Clear nasal passages and throat. Breathe out, expelling as much air from lungs as possible.Place mouthpiece well into mouth and inhale deeply as you release a dose from inhaler. Hold breath for several seconds, remove mouthpiece, and exhale slowly. Allow 2 minutes between inhalations.
- Instruct patient to store drug in light-resistant container.
- Advise patient that metaproterenol inhalations should precede corticosteroid inhalations (when prescribed) by 10 to 15 minutes to maximize effectiveness of corticosteroid therapy.
- Tell patient using corticosteroid inhaler to use bronchodilator first, and then wait 5 min-

utes before using corticosteroid. This allows bronchodilator to open air passages for maximum effectiveness of corticosteroid.
• If more than one inhalation of metaproterenol is ordered, tell patient to wait at least 2 minutes before repeating procedure.
• Warn patient to discontinue immediately and notify prescriber if paradoxical bronchospasm occurs.
• If no response is derived from dosage, tell patient to notify prescriber or request dosage adjustments.

✓ Evaluation
• Patient's status improves.
• Patient maintains adequate hydration.
• Patient and family state understanding of drug therapy.

metformin hydrochloride
(met-FOR-min high-droh-KLOR-ighd)
Glucophage

Pharmacologic class: biguanide
Therapeutic class: antidiabetic
Pregnancy risk category: B

Indications and dosages
▶ **Adjunct to diet to lower blood glucose level in patients with type 2 (non-insulin-dependent) diabetes mellitus.** *Adults:* initially, 500 mg P.O. b.i.d. with morning and evening meals, or 850 mg P.O. once daily with morning meal. When 500-mg dose form is used, dosage increased 500 mg weekly to maximum of 2,500 mg P.O. daily, as necessary. When 850-mg dose form is used, dosage increased 850 mg every other week to maximum of 2,550 mg P.O. daily, as necessary.

How supplied
Tablets: 500 mg, 850 mg

Pharmacokinetics
Absorption: absorbed from GI tract, with food decreasing extent of absorption as well as slightly delaying absorption.
Distribution: only negligibly bound to plasma proteins in contrast to sulfonylureas, which are more than 90% protein-bound.
Metabolism: not metabolized.
Excretion: excreted unchanged in urine. *Half-life:* about 6.2 hours.

Route	Onset	Peak	Duration
P.O.	Unknown	Unknown	Unknown

Pharmacodynamics
Chemical effect: decreases hepatic glucose production and intestinal absorption of glucose and improves insulin sensitivity (increases peripheral glucose uptake and utilization).
Therapeutic effect: lowers blood glucose levels.

Adverse reactions
GI: diarrhea, nausea, vomiting, abdominal bloating, flatulence, anorexia, unpleasant or metallic taste.
Hematologic: megaloblastic anemia.
Metabolic: ***lactic acidosis.***
Skin: rash, dermatitis.

Interactions
Drug-drug. *Calcium channel blockers, corticosteroids, estrogens, isoniazid, nicotinic acid, oral contraceptives, phenothiazines, phenytoin, sympathomimetics, thiazide and other diuretics, thyroid agents:* may produce hyperglycemia. Monitor patient's glycemic control. Metformin dosage may need to be increased.
Cationic drugs (such as amiloride, cimetidine, digoxin, morphine, procainamide, quinidine, quinine, ranitidine, triamterene, trimethoprim, vancomycin): may compete for common renal tubular transport systems, which may increase plasma metformin levels. Monitor patient's blood glucose level.
Iodinated contrast material: parenteral contrast studies with iodinated materials have been linked to lactic acidosis leading to acute renal failure. Withhold metformin on or before the day of the study, and resume after 48 hours, provided renal function is within normal limits.
Nifedipine: increased metformin levels. Monitor patient. Metformin dosage may need to be decreased.

Drug-herb. *Aloe, bilberry leaf, bitter melon, burdock, dandelion, fenugreek, garlic, ginseng:* improved blood glucose control may allow reduction of antidiabetic. Tell patient to discuss use of herbal remedies with prescriber before therapy.
Drug-lifestyle. *Alcohol use:* potentiated drug effects. Discourage concomitant use.

Contraindications and precautions

• Contraindicated in patients hypersensitive to drug and in those with renal disease or metabolic acidosis. Drug should be temporarily withheld in patients undergoing radiologic studies involving parenteral administration of iodinated contrast materials; use of such products may result in acute renal dysfunction. Drug also should be stopped if patient enters hypoxic state. Metformin should be avoided in patients with hepatic disease.
• Drug isn't recommended for use in breast-feeding women.
• Use cautiously in elderly, debilitated, or malnourished patients and those with adrenal or pituitary insufficiency because of increased risk of hypoglycemia.
• Safety hasn't been established in pregnant women and in children.

NURSING CONSIDERATIONS

Assessment

• Assess patient's blood glucose level before therapy and regularly thereafter.
• Before beginning therapy, assess patient's kidney function, and then reassess at least annually. If renal impairment is detected, expect prescriber to switch to different antidiabetic agent.
• Monitor patient's hematologic status for megaloblastic anemia. Patients with inadequate vitamin B_{12} or calcium intake or absorption seem predisposed to developing subnormal vitamin B_{12} levels when taking metformin. They should have serum vitamin B_{12} level determinations every 2 to 3 years.
• Be alert for adverse reactions and drug interactions.
• Monitor patient closely during times of increased stress, such as infection, fever, surgery, or trauma; insulin therapy may be required.
• Risk of metformin-induced lactic acidosis is very low. Cases have been reported primarily in diabetic patients with significant renal insufficiency; with other medical or surgical problems; and with multiple, concomitant drug regimens. The risk of lactic acidosis increases with the degree of renal impairment and patient's age.
• Evaluate patient's and family's knowledge of drug therapy.

Nursing diagnoses

• Ineffective health maintenance related to presence of hyperglycemia
• Risk for deficient fluid volume related to drug-induced adverse GI reactions
• Deficient knowledge related to drug therapy

Planning and implementation

• When switching from standard oral antidiabetic (except chlorpropamide) to metformin, no transition period usually is necessary. When switching patient from chlorpropamide to metformin, use care during first 2 weeks of metformin therapy because prolonged retention of chlorpropamide increases risk of hypoglycemia during this time.
• Notify prescriber if blood glucose level rises despite therapy.
• If patient hasn't responded to 4 weeks of therapy using maximum dosage, prescriber may add oral sulfonylurea while continuing metformin at maximum dosage. If patient still doesn't respond after several months, prescriber may stop both drugs and start insulin therapy.
ALERT Stop drug immediately and notify prescriber if patient develops conditions linked to hypoxemia or dehydration because of risk of lactic acidosis.
• Metformin therapy may be temporarily suspended for surgical procedure (except minor procedures not related to restricted intake of food and fluids) and not restarted until patient's oral intake has resumed and kidney function is normal.

Patient teaching

- Tell patient to take once-daily dose with breakfast and twice-daily dose with breakfast and dinner.
- Instruct patient to stop drug and tell prescriber about unexplained hyperventilation, myalgia, malaise, unusual somnolence, or other symptoms of early lactic acidosis.
- Warn patient to minimize alcohol consumption while taking drug.

ALERT Teach patient about diabetes and the importance of following therapeutic regimen; adhering to diet, weight reduction, exercise, and hygiene programs; and avoiding infection. Explain how and when to monitor blood glucose level and how to differentiate between hypoglycemia and hyperglycemia.

- Tell patient not to change dosage without prescriber's consent. Encourage patient to report abnormal blood glucose test results.
- Advise patient not to take other medication, including OTC drugs, without checking with prescriber.
- Instruct patient to wear or carry medical identification.

Evaluation

- Patient's blood glucose level is normal.
- Patient maintains adequate hydration throughout therapy.
- Patient and family state understanding of drug therapy.

methadone hydrochloride

(METH-eh-dohn high-droh-KLOR-ighd)

Dolophine, Methadose, Physeptone ◇

Pharmacologic class: opioid
Therapeutic class: analgesic, narcotic detoxification adjunct
Controlled substance schedule: II
Pregnancy risk category: C

Indications and dosages

▶ **Severe pain.** *Adults:* 2.5 to 10 mg P.O., I.M., or S.C. q 3 to 4 hours, p.r.n.

▶ **Narcotic withdrawal syndrome.** *Adults:* 15 to 20 mg P.O. daily (highly individualized). Maintenance dosage is 20 to 120 mg P.O. daily. Dosage adjusted as needed. Daily dosages greater than 120 mg require state and federal approval.

How supplied

Tablets: 5 mg, 10 mg
Dispersible tablets (for methadone maintenance therapy): 40 mg
Oral solution: 5 mg/5 ml, 10 mg/5 ml, 10 mg/ml (concentrate)
Injection: 10 mg/ml

Pharmacokinetics

Absorption: well absorbed from GI tract; unknown for I.M. route.
Distribution: highly bound to tissue protein.
Metabolism: metabolized primarily in liver.
Excretion: excreted primarily in urine; metabolites excreted in feces. *Half-life:* 15 to 25 hours.

Route	Onset	Peak	Duration
P.O.	30-60 min	1.5-2 hr	4-6 hr
I.M.	10-20 min	1-2 hr	4-5 hr
S.C.	Unknown	Unknown	Unknown

Pharmacodynamics

Chemical effect: binds with opioid receptors at many sites in CNS, altering both perception of and emotional response to pain through unknown mechanism.
Therapeutic effect: relieves pain and symptoms of opioid withdrawal.

Adverse reactions

CNS: *sedation, somnolence, clouded sensorium, euphoria,* dizziness, chorea, ***seizures.***
CV: *hypotension,* ***bradycardia, shock, cardiac arrest.***
EENT: visual disturbances.
GI: *nausea, vomiting, constipation,* ileus.
GU: *urine retention.*
Respiratory: ***respiratory depression, respiratory arrest.***
Skin: pain at injection site, tissue irritation, induration after S.C. injection, diaphoresis.
Other: decreased libido, physical dependence.

Interactions

Drug-drug. *Ammonium chloride and other urine acidifiers, phenytoin:* may reduce methadone effect. Monitor patient for decreased pain control.
CNS depressants, general anesthetics, hypnotics, MAO inhibitors, sedatives, tranquilizers, tricyclic antidepressants: possible respiratory depression, hypotension, profound sedation, or coma. Use together cautiously. Monitor patient.
Rifampin: withdrawal symptoms; reduced blood levels of methadone. Use together cautiously.
Drug-lifestyle. *Alcohol use:* additive effects. Advise caution.

Contraindications and precautions

- Contraindicated in patients hypersensitive to drug.
- Use with extreme caution in patients with acute abdominal conditions, severe hepatic or renal impairment, hypothyroidism, Addison's disease, prostatic hyperplasia, urethral stricture, head injury, increased intracranial pressure, asthma, or other respiratory conditions.
- Use cautiously in elderly or debilitated patients and in pregnant or breast-feeding women.
- Safety of drug hasn't been established in children.

NURSING CONSIDERATIONS

Assessment

- Assess patient's pain or opioid dependence before and during therapy.
- Monitor patient closely because drug has cumulative effect; marked sedation can occur after repeated doses.
- Be alert for adverse reactions and drug interactions.
- Evaluate patient's and family's knowledge of drug therapy.

Nursing diagnoses

- Chronic pain related to underlying condition
- Ineffective individual coping related to opioid dependence
- Deficient knowledge related to drug therapy

Planning and implementation

P.O. use: Liquid form is legally required in maintenance programs. Dissolve tablets in 120 ml of orange juice or powdered citrus drink.
– P.O. dose is one-half as potent as injected dose.
I.M. and S.C. use: For parenteral use, I.M. injection is preferred. Rotate injection sites.
- Around-the-clock regimen is needed to manage severe, chronic pain.
- When drug is used as adjunct in treating narcotic addiction, withdrawal usually is delayed and mild.

Patient teaching

- Caution patient about getting out of bed or walking. Warn outpatient to avoid hazardous activities until drug's CNS effects are known.
- Instruct patient to avoid alcohol consumption during drug therapy.

Evaluation

- Patient is free from pain.
- Patient doesn't exhibit opioid withdrawal symptoms.
- Patient and family state understanding of drug therapy.

methamphetamine hydrochloride

(meth-am-FET-uh-meen high-droh-KLOR-ighd)
Desoxyn, Desoxyn Gradumet

Pharmacologic class: amphetamine
Therapeutic class: CNS stimulant, short-term adjunct anorexigenic, sympathomimetic amine
Controlled substance schedule: II
Pregnancy risk category: C

Indications and dosages

▶ **Attention deficit hyperactivity disorder.** *Children age 6 and older:* initially, 5 mg P.O. once daily or b.i.d., with 5-mg increments weekly, p.r.n. Usual effective dosage is 20 to 25 mg daily.
▶ **Short-term adjunct in exogenous obesity.** *Adults:* 2.5 to 5 mg P.O. b.i.d. to t.i.d. 30 minutes before meals. Or, 10- or 15-mg long-acting tablet daily before breakfast.

How supplied

Tablets: 5 mg
Tablets (extended release): 5 mg, 10 mg, 15 mg**

Pharmacokinetics

Absorption: rapidly absorbed from GI tract.
Distribution: widely distributed.
Metabolism: metabolized in liver to at least seven metabolites.
Excretion: excreted in urine. *Half-life:* 4 to 5 hours.

Route	Onset	Peak	Duration
P.O.	Unknown	Unknown	≤ 24 hr

Pharmacodynamics

Chemical effect: unknown; probably promotes nerve impulse transmission by releasing stored norepinephrine from nerve terminals in brain. Main sites of activity appear to be cerebral cortex and reticular activating system. In hyperkinetic children, drug has paradoxical calming effect.
Therapeutic effect: promotes calmness in children with attention deficit disorder and causes weight loss.

Adverse reactions

CNS: *nervousness, insomnia,* irritability, *talkativeness,* dizziness, headache, hyperexcitability, tremors.
CV: hypertension, hypotension, *tachycardia, palpitations,* ***arrhythmias.***
EENT: blurred vision, mydriasis.
GI: metallic taste, dry mouth, nausea, vomiting, abdominal cramps, diarrhea, constipation, anorexia.
GU: impotence.
Skin: urticaria.
Other: altered libido.

Interactions

Drug-drug. *Acetazolamide, antacids, sodium bicarbonate:* increased renal reabsorption. Monitor patient for enhanced effects.
Ammonium chloride, ascorbic acid: decreased serum levels and increased renal excretion of methamphetamine. Monitor patient for decreased methamphetamine effects.
Guanethidine: amphetamines may decrease the antihypertensive effectiveness of guanethidine. Monitor blood pressure.
Haloperidol, phenothiazines, tricyclic antidepressants: increased CNS effects. Avoid concomitant use.
Insulin, oral antidiabetics: may decrease antidiabetic requirement. Monitor blood glucose levels.
MAO inhibitors: severe hypertension; possible hypertensive crisis. Don't use together or within 14 days of MAO inhibitor therapy.
Drug-herb. *Melatonin:* enhanced monoaminergic effects of methamphetamine; may worsen insomnia. Discourage concomitant use.
Drug-food. *Caffeine-containing beverages:* may increase amphetamine and related amine effects. Discourage concomitant use.

Contraindications and precautions

- Contraindicated in patients hypersensitive to sympathomimetic amines; patients with idiosyncratic reactions to sympathomimetic amines; patients with moderate to severe hypertension, hyperthyroidism, symptomatic CV disease, advanced arteriosclerosis, glaucoma, or history of drug abuse; patients who have taken an MAO inhibitor within 14 days; and agitated patients.
- Don't use in pregnant women.
- Use cautiously in patients who are elderly, debilitated, asthenic, or psychopathic or who have history of suicidal or homicidal tendencies.
- Safety of drug hasn't been established in breast-feeding women.

NURSING CONSIDERATIONS

Assessment

- Assess patient's condition before therapy and regularly thereafter.
- Be alert for adverse reactions and drug interactions.
- Evaluate patient's and family's knowledge of drug therapy.

Nursing diagnoses

- Ineffective health maintenance related to underlying condition

• Disturbed sleep pattern related to drug-induced insomnia
• Deficient knowledge related to drug therapy

Planning and implementation

ALERT Don't confuse Desoxyn with digitoxin or digoxin.
• Drug isn't the first-line treatment for obesity. Use as anorexigenic is prohibited in some states.
• When used for obesity, be sure patient is on weight-reduction program.
• If tolerance to anorexigenic effect develops, notify prescriber because drug will need to be discontinued.

Patient teaching
• Warn patient of high potential for abuse. Advise him that drug shouldn't be used to prevent fatigue.
• Tell patient not to crush long-acting tablets.
• Advise patient to take last dose of drug at least 6 hours before bedtime.
• Warn patient to avoid activities that require alertness or good coordination until CNS effects are known.
• Tell patient to avoid caffeine during drug therapy.
• Instruct patient to report signs of excessive stimulation.

Evaluation

• Patient exhibits positive response to methamphetamine therapy.
• Patient doesn't experience insomnia.
• Patient and family state understanding of drug therapy.

methimazole

(meth-IH-muh-zohl)
Tapazole

Pharmacologic class: thyroid hormone antagonist
Therapeutic class: antihyperthyroid agent
Pregnancy risk category: D

Indications and dosages

▶ **Hyperthyroidism.** *Adults:* if mild, 15 mg P.O. daily. If moderately severe, 30 to 40 mg daily. If severe, 60 mg daily. Daily dose divided into three doses at 8-hour intervals. Maintenance dosage is 5 to 15 mg daily.
Children: 0.4 mg/kg P.O. daily in divided doses q 8 hours. Maintenance dosage is 0.2 mg/kg daily in divided doses q 8 hours.

How supplied

Tablets: 5 mg, 10 mg

Pharmacokinetics

Absorption: absorbed rapidly from GI tract.
Distribution: concentrated in thyroid and isn't protein-bound.
Metabolism: undergoes hepatic metabolism.
Excretion: excreted primarily in urine. *Half-life:* 5 to 13 hours.

Route	Onset	Peak	Duration
P.O.	≤ 5 days	0.5-1 hr	Unknown

Pharmacodynamics

Chemical effect: inhibits oxidation of iodine in thyroid gland, blocking iodine's ability to combine with tyrosine to form T_4. Also may prevent coupling of monoiodotyrosine and diiodotyrosine to form T_4 and T_3.
Therapeutic effect: reduces thyroid hormone level.

Adverse reactions

CNS: headache, drowsiness, vertigo.
GI: diarrhea, nausea, vomiting, salivary gland enlargement, loss of taste.
Hematologic: ***agranulocytosis,*** leukopenia, ***thrombocytopenia, aplastic anemia.***
Hepatic: jaundice, hepatic dysfunction.
Metabolic: hypothyroidism.
Musculoskeletal: arthralgia, myalgia.
Skin: rash, urticaria, skin discoloration.
Other: drug-induced fever, lymphadenopathy.

Interactions

Drug-drug. *Anticoagulants:* enhanced effects from anti-vitamin K activity attributed to drug. Monitor PT and INR as indicated.

Contraindications and precautions

• Contraindicated in patients hypersensitive to drug.
• Drug isn't recommended for breast-feeding women.
• Use with extreme caution in pregnant women.

NURSING CONSIDERATIONS

Assessment

• Assess patient's thyroid condition before therapy and regularly thereafter.
• Monitor thyroid function studies.
• Monitor CBC and liver function periodically, as ordered.
ALERT Dosages higher than 30 mg/day increase risk of agranulocytosis. Patients over age 40 may have an increased risk of developing drug-induced agranulocytosis.
• Be alert for adverse reactions.
• Evaluate patient's and family's knowledge of drug therapy.

Nursing diagnoses

• Ineffective health maintenance related to presence of hyperthyroidism
• Ineffective immune protection related to drug-induced adverse hematologic reactions
• Deficient knowledge related to drug therapy

Planning and implementation

ALERT Don't confuse methimazole with mebendazole or methazolamide.
• Pregnant women may need less drug as pregnancy progresses. Thyroid hormone may be added. Drug may be stopped during last weeks of pregnancy.
• Notify prescriber about signs and symptoms of hypothyroidism because dosage may need to be adjusted.
ALERT Stop drug and notify prescriber if severe rash occurs or cervical lymph nodes become enlarged.

Patient teaching

• Tell patient to take drug with meals.
• Warn patient to immediately report fever, sore throat, or mouth sores (signs of agranulocytosis); skin eruptions (sign of hypersensitivity); and anorexia, pruritus, right upper quadrant pain, and yellow skin or sclera (signs of hepatic dysfunction).
• Tell patient to ask prescriber about using iodized salt and eating shellfish.
• Warn patient against taking OTC cough medications; many contain iodine.
• Instruct patient to store drug in light-resistant container.

Evaluation

• Patient has normal thyroid hormone level.
• Patient maintains normal hematologic parameters throughout therapy.
• Patient and family state understanding of drug therapy.

methocarbamol

(meth-oh-KAR-buh-mol)
Carbacot, Robaxin, Robaxin-750, Skelex

Pharmacologic class: carbamate derivative of guaifenesin
Therapeutic class: skeletal muscle relaxant
Pregnancy risk category: NR

Indications and dosages

▶ **As adjunct in acute, painful musculoskeletal conditions.** *Adults:* 1.5 g P.O. q.i.d. for 2 to 3 days; then 1 g P.O. q.i.d., or not more than 500 mg (5 ml) I.M. into each buttock. Repeated q 8 hours, p.r.n. Or 1 to 3 g daily (10 to 30 ml) I.V. directly into vein at 3 ml/minute, or 10 ml may be added to no more than 250 ml of D_5W or normal saline solution. Maximum dosage is 3 g daily I.M. or I.V. for 3 consecutive days.
▶ **Supportive therapy in tetanus management.** *Adults:* 1 to 2 g by direct I.V. or 1 to 3 g as infusion q 6 hours.
Children: 15 mg/kg I.V. q 6 hours.

How supplied

Tablets: 500 mg, 750 mg
Injection: 100 mg/ml

Pharmacokinetics

Absorption: rapidly and completely absorbed from GI tract after P.O. administration; unknown after I.M. administration.

Distribution: widely distributed throughout body.
Metabolism: extensively metabolized in liver.
Excretion: excreted primarily in urine. *Half-life:* 0.9 to 2.2 hours.

Route	Onset	Peak	Duration
P.O.	≤ 0.5 hr	≤ 2 hr	Unknown
I.V.	Immediate	Immediate	Unknown
I.M.	Unknown	Unknown	Unknown

Pharmacodynamics

Chemical effect: unknown; probably modifies central perception of pain without modifying pain reflexes.
Therapeutic effect: relieves skeletal muscle pain.

Adverse reactions

CNS: drowsiness, dizziness, light-headedness, headache, syncope, mild muscle incoordination with I.M. or I.V. use, ***seizures*** with I.V. use.
CV: hypotension, ***bradycardia*** with I.M. or I.V. use, thrombophlebitis.
GI: nausea, anorexia, GI upset, metallic taste.
GU: hematuria with I.V. use, discoloration of urine.
Hematologic: hemolysis, decreased hemoglobin level with I.V. use.
Skin: urticaria, pruritus, rash.
Other: extravasation with I.V. use, fever, flushing, ***anaphylaxis*** with I.M. or I.V. use.

Interactions

Drug-drug. *CNS depressants:* increased CNS depression. Avoid concomitant use.
Drug-lifestyle. *Alcohol use:* increased CNS depression. Discourage concomitant use.

Contraindications and precautions

- Contraindicated in patients hypersensitive to drug and in those with impaired kidney function or seizure disorder (injectable form).
- Drug isn't recommended for use in breast-feeding women.
- Use cautiously in pregnant women.

NURSING CONSIDERATIONS

Assessment

- Assess patient's condition before therapy and regularly thereafter.
- Watch for orthostatic hypotension, especially with parenteral route.
- Monitor CBC periodically during prolonged therapy.
- Be alert for adverse reactions and drug interactions.
- Monitor patient's hydration status if adverse GI reactions occur.
- Evaluate patient's and family's knowledge of drug therapy.

Nursing diagnoses

- Acute pain related to underlying musculoskeletal condition
- Risk for deficient fluid volume related to drug-induced adverse GI reactions
- Deficient knowledge related to drug therapy

Planning and implementation

ALERT Don't confuse methocarbamol with mephobarbital.
P.O. use: Give tablets with meals or milk.
– Prepare liquid by crushing tablets into water or saline solution. Give through nasogastric tube.
I.V. use: Dilute 10 ml of drug in no more than 250 ml of D_5W or normal saline solution injection. Infuse slowly; maximum rate is 300 mg (3 ml)/minute.
– Drug irritates veins; may cause phlebitis and fainting and aggravate seizures if injected rapidly. Keep patient supine during infusion and for 15 minutes afterward. Drug is an irritant; avoid extravasation.
I.M. use: Give drug I.M. deep into upper outer quadrant of buttocks, with maximum of 5 ml in each buttock.
- Don't give drug S.C.
- In tetanus, methocarbamol is used with tetanus antitoxin, penicillin, tracheotomy, and aggressive supportive care. Long course of I.V. methocarbamol therapy is required.
- Have epinephrine, antihistamines, and corticosteroids available.

• Drug may interfere with urine tests to determine 5-hydroxyindoleacetic acid and vanillylmandelic acid levels.

Patient teaching

• Advise patient to get up slowly after parenteral administration.

• Tell patient that urine may turn green, black, or brown.

• Advise patient to follow prescriber's orders regarding physical activity.

• Warn patient to avoid activities that require alertness until drug's CNS effects are known.

• Tell patient not to combine drug with alcohol or other CNS depressants. Instruct patient to avoid alcohol consumption during drug therapy.

☑ Evaluation

• Patient is free from pain.

• Patient maintains adequate hydration throughout therapy.

• Patient and family state understanding of drug therapy.

methotrexate (amethopterin, MTX)

(meth-oh-TREKS-ayt)

Rheumatrex

methotrexate sodium

Methotrexate LPF, Rheumatrex Dose Pack

Pharmacologic class: antimetabolite (cell cycle–phase specific, S phase)
Therapeutic class: antineoplastic
Pregnancy risk category: X

Indications and dosages

▶ **Trophoblastic tumors (choriocarcinoma, hydatidiform mole).** *Adults:* 15 to 30 mg P.O. or I.M. daily for 5 days. Repeated after 1 or more weeks, based on response or toxicity.

▶ **Acute lymphoblastic and lymphatic leukemia.** *Adults and children:* 3.3 mg/m^2/day P.O. or I.M. for 4 to 6 weeks or until remission occurs; then 20 to 30 mg/m^2 P.O. or I.M. twice weekly.

▶ **Meningeal leukemia.** *Adults and children:* 12 mg/m^2 intrathecally or an empirical dose of 15 mg q 2 to 5 days and repeat until cell count of CSF returns to normal, then give one additional dose.

▶ **Burkitt's lymphoma (stage I or stage II).** *Adults:* 10 to 25 mg P.O. daily for 4 to 8 days with 1-week rest intervals.

▶ **Lymphosarcoma (stage III).** *Adults:* 0.625 to 2.5 mg/kg daily P.O., I.M., or I.V.

▶ **Osteosarcoma.** *Adults:* initially, 12 g/m^2 I.V. as 4-hour infusion. Subsequent doses 12 to 15 g/m^2 I.V. as 4-hour infusion given weeks 4, 5, 6, 7, 11, 12, 15, 16, 29, 30, 44, and 45 after surgery. Given with leucovorin, 15 mg P.O. q 6 hours for 10 doses after start of methotrexate infusion.

▶ **Mycosis fungoides.** *Adults:* 2.5 to 10 mg P.O. daily, or 50 mg I.M. weekly, or 25 mg I.M. twice weekly.

▶ **Psoriasis.** *Adults:* 10 to 25 mg P.O., I.M., or I.V. as single weekly dose.

▶ **Rheumatoid arthritis.** *Adults:* initially, 7.5 mg P.O. weekly, either in single dose or divided as 2.5 mg P.O. q 12 hours for three doses once a week. Dosage may be gradually increased to maximum of 20 mg weekly.

How supplied

Tablets (scored): 2.5 mg
Injection: 20-mg, 25-mg, 50-mg, 100-mg, 250-mg, 1-g vials, lyophilized powder, preservative-free; 25-mg/ml vials, preservative-free solution; 2.5-mg/ml, 25-mg/ml vials, lyophilized powder, preserved

Pharmacokinetics

Absorption: P.O. absorption appears to be dose-related; smaller doses are almost completely absorbed, whereas absorption of larger doses is incomplete and variable. I.M. doses are absorbed completely.
Distribution: distributed widely throughout body with highest levels in kidneys, gallbladder, spleen, liver, and skin; about 50% bound to plasma protein.
Metabolism: metabolized only slightly in liver.
Excretion: excreted primarily in urine. *Half-life:* 4 hours. *Terminal half-life:* about 3 to 10 hours for patients receiving low-dose antineo-

plastic therapy (below 30 mg/m^2). For patients receiving high doses, the terminal half-life is 8 to 15 hours.

Route	Onset	Peak	Duration
P.O.	Unknown	1-2 hr	Unknown
I.V., intrathecal	Unknown	Immediate	Unknown
I.M.	Unknown	0.5-1 hr	Unknown

Pharmacodynamics

Chemical effect: prevents reduction of folic acid to tetrahydrofolate by binding to dihydrofolate reductase.
Therapeutic effect: kills certain cancer cells and reduces inflammation.

Adverse reactions

CNS: ***arachnoiditis*** (within hours of intrathecal use), subacute neurotoxicity (may begin few weeks later), demyelination, ***leukoencephalopathy.***
EENT: pharyngitis.
GI: *stomatitis, diarrhea,* enteritis, ***intestinal perforation,*** *nausea, vomiting.*
GU: nephropathy, *tubular necrosis,* ***renal failure.***
Hematologic: WBC and platelet count nadirs occurring on day 7, ***anemia, leukopenia, thrombocytopenia.***
Hepatic: ***acute toxicity, chronic toxicity,*** cirrhosis, ***hepatic fibrosis.***
Metabolic: hyperuricemia.
Musculoskeletal: osteoporosis in children with long-term use.
Respiratory: ***pulmonary fibrosis, pulmonary interstitial infiltrates,*** pneumonitis.
Skin: *urticaria,* pruritus, alopecia, hyperpigmentation, psoriatic lesions, rash, photosensitivity.
Other: ***sudden death.***

Interactions

Drug-drug. *Digoxin:* may decrease serum digoxin levels. Monitor patient closely.
Folic acid derivatives: antagonized methotrexate effect. Monitor patient.
NSAIDs, phenylbutazone, probenecid, salicylates, sulfonamides: increased methotrexate toxicity. Don't use together.
Phenytoin: may decrease serum phenytoin levels. Monitor patient.
Procarbazine: may increase hepatotoxicity of methotrexate. Monitor liver function closely.
Vaccines: immunizations may be ineffective; risk of disseminated infection with live-virus vaccines. Consult with prescriber about safe time to administer vaccine.
Drug-lifestyle. *Alcohol use:* may increase hepatotoxicity. Discourage concomitant use.
Sun exposure: photosensitivity reactions may occur. Urge precautions.

Contraindications and precautions

- Contraindicated in patients hypersensitive to drug; in pregnant or breast-feeding women; and in those with psoriasis or rheumatoid arthritis who also have alcoholism, alcoholic liver, chronic liver disease, immunodeficiency syndromes, or blood dyscrasias.
- Use cautiously and at modified dosage in patients with impaired liver or kidney function, bone marrow suppression, aplasia, leukopenia, thrombocytopenia, or anemia. Also use cautiously in patients with infection, peptic ulceration, or ulcerative colitis and in very young, elderly, or debilitated patients.

NURSING CONSIDERATIONS

Assessment

- Assess patient's condition before therapy and regularly thereafter.
- Perform baseline pulmonary function tests and repeat periodically.
- Monitor fluid intake and output daily.
- Monitor serum uric acid level.
- Watch for increases in AST, ALT, and alkaline phosphatase levels—signs of hepatic dysfunction.
- Monitor CBC regularly, as ordered.
- Be alert for adverse reactions and drug interactions.
- Evaluate patient's and family's knowledge of drug therapy.

Nursing diagnoses

- Ineffective health maintenance related to underlying condition

- Ineffective immune protection related to drug-induced adverse hematologic reactions
- Deficient knowledge related to drug therapy

Planning and implementation

- Follow facility policy to reduce risks. Preparation and administration of parenteral forms are linked to carcinogenic, mutagenic, and teratogenic risks.

P.O. and I.M. use: Follow normal protocol.
I.V. use: Give undiluted by direct injection. Or, dilute with up to 25 ml of normal saline solution injection (for Folex) or 2 to 10 ml of sterile water for injection, normal saline solution injection, or bacteriostatic water for injection containing parabens or benzyl alcohol (for Mexate).
Intrathecal use: Use only 20-, 50-, or 100-mg vials of powder with no preservatives. Reconstitute immediately before using with preservative-free normal saline solution injection. Dilute to maximum of 1 mg/ml. Use only new vials of drug and diluent.

- Reconstitute solutions without preservatives immediately before use, and discard unused drug.
- CSF volume depends on age, not body surface area (BSA). Using BSA for dosing when treating meningeal leukemia has resulted in low CSF methotrexate level in children and high level and neurotoxicity in adults. Or, a dosing regimen based on age may be used. Elderly patients may require a reduced dosage because CSF volume and turnover may decrease with age.
- Have patient drink 2 to 3 L of fluids daily.

ALERT Alkalinize urine, as ordered, by giving sodium bicarbonate tablets to prevent precipitation of drug, especially with high doses. Maintain urine pH at more than 6.5. Reduce dosage, as ordered, if BUN level reaches 20 to 30 mg/dl or creatinine level reaches 1.2 to 2 mg/dl. Report BUN level over 30 mg/dl or creatinine level over 2 mg/dl, and stop use of drug.

- Rash, redness, or ulcerations in mouth or adverse pulmonary reactions may signal serious complications. Therapy may be discontinued if ulcerative stomatitis or other severe adverse GI reaction occurs or if pulmonary toxicity is detected.
- Leucovorin rescue necessary with high-dose (greater than 100 mg) protocols. This technique works against systemic toxicity but doesn't interfere with tumor cells' absorption of methotrexate.

Patient teaching

- Teach and encourage diligent mouth care to reduce risk of superinfection in mouth.
- Warn patient to avoid prolonged exposure to the sun, wear protective clothing, and use highly protective sunblock.
- Tell patient to continue leucovorin rescue despite severe nausea and vomiting and to tell prescriber. Parenteral leucovorin therapy may be needed.
- Warn patient to avoid becoming pregnant during and immediately after therapy because of risk of abortion or congenital anomalies.
- Instruct patient to avoid alcohol consumption during drug therapy.

Evaluation

- Patient exhibits positive response to drug therapy.
- Patient doesn't experience serious complications when hematologic parameters are depressed during therapy.
- Patient and family state understanding of drug therapy.

methylcellulose

(meth-il-SEL-yoo-lohs)
Citrucel†, Citrucel Sugar Free†

Pharmacologic class: adsorbent
Therapeutic class: bulk-forming laxative
Pregnancy risk category: NR

Indications and dosages

▶ **Chronic constipation.** *Adults:* 1 to 3 heaping tablespoons in 8 oz (240 ml) cold water daily to t.i.d. Usual dosage up to 6 g daily (3 tablespoons).
Children ages 6 to 12: 1 to 1½ level tablespoons in 4 oz (120 ml) cold water daily to t.i.d. Usual dosage up to 3 g daily (1½ tablespoons).

How supplied

Powder: 2 g/heaping tablespoon†

Pharmacokinetics

Absorption: not absorbed.
Distribution: distributed locally, in intestine.
Metabolism: none.
Excretion: excreted in feces.

Route	Onset	Peak	Duration
P.O.	12-24 hr	≤ 3 days	Varies

Pharmacodynamics

Chemical effect: absorbs water and expands to increase bulk and moisture content of stool, which encourages peristalsis and bowel movement.
Therapeutic effect: relieves constipation.

Adverse reactions

GI: *nausea,* vomiting, and diarrhea with excessive use; esophageal, gastric, small intestinal, or colonic strictures when drug is chewed or taken in dry form; *abdominal cramps,* especially in severe constipation; laxative dependence with long-term or excessive use.

Interactions

None significant.

Contraindications and precautions

- Contraindicated in patients with abdominal pain, nausea, vomiting, or other symptoms of appendicitis or acute surgical abdomen and in those with intestinal obstruction or ulceration, disabling adhesions, or difficulty swallowing.
- Use cautiously in pregnant or breast-feeding women.

NURSING CONSIDERATIONS

Assessment

- Assess patient's constipation before therapy and regularly thereafter.
- Before giving drug for constipation, determine whether patient has adequate fluid intake, exercise, and diet.
- Be alert for adverse reactions.
- Monitor patient's hydration status if adverse GI reactions occur.
- Evaluate patient's and family's knowledge of drug therapy.

Nursing diagnoses

- Constipation related to underlying condition
- Risk for deficient fluid volume related to drug-induced adverse GI reactions
- Deficient knowledge related to drug therapy

Planning and implementation

ALERT Don't confuse Citrucel with Citracal.

- Drug is especially useful in debilitated patients and in those with postpartum constipation, irritable bowel syndrome, diverticulitis, or colostomies. Drug is also used to treat laxative abuse and to empty colon before barium enema.

Patient teaching

- Tell patient to take drug with at least 8 oz of pleasant-tasting liquid.
- Teach patient about dietary sources of bulk, such as bran and other cereals, fresh fruit, and vegetables.

Evaluation

- Patient's constipation is relieved.
- Patient maintains adequate hydration throughout therapy.
- Patient and family state understanding of drug therapy.

methyldopa

(meth-il-DOH-puh)

Aldomet, Apo-Methyldopa ♦, Dopamet ♦, Hydopa ◊, Novomedopa ♦, Nu-Medopa ♦

methyldopate hydrochloride

Aldomet

Pharmacologic class: centrally acting antiadrenergic agent
Therapeutic class: antihypertensive
Pregnancy risk category: B (P.O.), C (I.V.)

Indications and dosages

▶ **Hypertension, hypertensive crisis.** *Adults:* **P.O.** initially, 250 mg P.O. b.i.d. to t.i.d. in first 48 hours. Then increased as needed q 2 days. Entire daily dose may be given in evening or

h.s. Adjust dosages, as needed, if other antihypertensives are added to or deleted from therapy. Maintenance dosage is 500 mg to 2 g daily in two to four divided doses. Maximum recommended daily dose is 3 g.
Adults: **I.V.** 250 to 500 mg q 6 hours, diluted in D_5W and given over 30 to 60 minutes. Maximum dosage is 1 g q 6 hours. Switch to P.O. antihypertensives as soon as possible.
Children: initially, 10 mg/kg P.O. daily in two to four divided doses. Or, 20 to 40 mg/kg I.V. daily in four divided doses. Increase dosage at least q 2 days until desired response occurs. Maximum 65 mg/kg, 2 g/m^2, or 3 g daily, whichever is least.

How supplied

methyldopa
Tablets: 125 mg, 250 mg, 500 mg
Oral suspension: 250 mg/5 ml
methyldopate hydrochloride
Injection: 250 mg/5 ml

Pharmacokinetics

Absorption: absorbed partially from GI tract after P.O. administration.
Distribution: distributed throughout body; bound weakly to plasma proteins.
Metabolism: metabolized extensively in liver and intestinal cells.
Excretion: absorbed drug excreted in urine; unabsorbed drug excreted in feces. *Half-life:* about 2 hours.

Route	Onset	Peak	Duration
P.O.	Unknown	4-6 hr	12-48 hr
I.V.	Unknown	4-6 hr	10-16 hr

Pharmacodynamics

Chemical effect: unknown; thought to involve inhibition of central vasomotor centers, thereby decreasing sympathetic outflow to heart, kidneys, and peripheral vasculature.
Therapeutic effect: lowers blood pressure.

Adverse reactions

CNS: *sedation,* headache, asthenia, weakness, dizziness, *decreased mental acuity,* involuntary choreoathetoid movements, psychic disturbances, depression, nightmares.
CV: ***bradycardia,*** *orthostatic hypotension,* aggravated angina, ***myocarditis,*** *edema.*
EENT: *nasal congestion.*
GI: nausea, vomiting, diarrhea, ***pancreatitis,*** *dry mouth.*
GU: impotence.
Hematologic: ***hemolytic anemia,*** reversible agranulocytosis, ***thrombocytopenia.***
Hepatic: ***hepatic necrosis.***
Metabolic: *weight gain.*
Skin: rash.
Other: gynecomastia, galactorrhea, *drug-induced fever.*

Interactions

Drug-drug. *Amphetamines, norepinephrine, phenothiazines, tricyclic antidepressants:* possible hypertensive effects. Monitor patient carefully.
Barbiturates: may reduce the action of methyldopa. Monitor patient.
Levodopa: additive hypotensive effects may increase adverse CNS reactions. Monitor patient closely.
Lithium: may increase lithium levels. Monitor patient for increased lithium levels.
Drug-herb. *Capsicum:* may reduce antihypertensive effectiveness. Avoid concomitant use.

Contraindications and precautions

- Contraindicated in patients hypersensitive to drug and in those with active hepatic disease (such as acute hepatitis) or active cirrhosis. Also contraindicated if previous methyldopa therapy has been linked to liver disorders.
- Use cautiously in patients with history of impaired liver function and in breast-feeding women.

NURSING CONSIDERATIONS

Assessment

- Assess patient's blood pressure before therapy and regularly thereafter.
- Monitor CBC with differential counts before therapy, every 2 weeks for first 3 months of therapy, and periodically thereafter.
- Monitor patient's Coombs' test results. In patient who has received this drug for several months, positive reaction to direct Coombs' test indicates hemolytic anemia.

• Be alert for adverse reactions and drug interactions.
• Evaluate patient's and family's knowledge of drug therapy.

Nursing diagnoses

• Ineffective health maintenance related to presence of hypertension
• Risk for injury related to drug-induced adverse CNS reactions
• Deficient knowledge related to drug therapy

Planning and implementation

ALERT Don't confuse Aldomet with Aldoril or Anzemet.
P.O. use: Follow normal protocol.
I.V. use: Report involuntary choreoathetoid movements; drug may be stopped.
• After dialysis, notify prescriber if hypertension occurs; patient may need extra dose of methyldopa.
• Patient who needs blood transfusions should have direct and indirect Coombs' tests to prevent crossmatching problems.

Patient teaching

• Advise patient to report signs of infection, such as fever and sore throat.
• Tell patient to report adverse reactions but not to stop taking drug.
• Tell patient to check his weight daily and to report weight gain over 5 lb (2.27 kg). Diuretics can relieve sodium and water retention.
• Warn patient that drug may impair mental alertness, particularly at start of therapy. Once-daily dosage at bedtime minimizes daytime drowsiness.
• Tell patient to rise slowly and avoid sudden position changes.
• Tell patient that dry mouth can be relieved with ice chips or sugarless gum or hard candy.
• Advise patient that urine may turn dark in bleached toilet bowls.

Evaluation

• Patient's blood pressure is normal.
• Patient doesn't experience injury as result of drug-induced adverse CNS reactions.
• Patient and family state understanding of drug therapy.

methylergonovine maleate

(meth-il-er-goh-NOH-veen MAL-ee-ayt)
Methergine

Pharmacologic class: ergot alkaloid
Therapeutic class: oxytocic
Pregnancy risk category: C

Indications and dosages

▶ **Prevention and treatment of postpartum hemorrhage caused by uterine atony or subinvolution.** *Women:* 0.2 mg I.M. q 2 to 4 hours. For excessive uterine bleeding or other emergencies, 0.2 mg I.V. over 1 minute while blood pressure and uterine contractions are monitored. After initial I.M. or I.V. dose, 0.2 to 0.4 mg P.O. q 6 to 12 hours for 2 to 7 days. Dosage is decreased if patient develops severe cramping.

How supplied

Tablets: 0.2 mg
Injection: 0.2 mg/ml

Pharmacokinetics

Absorption: absorption is rapid, with 60% of P.O. dose appearing in blood; unknown after I.M. administration.
Distribution: rapidly distributed in tissues.
Metabolism: extensive first-pass metabolism precedes hepatic metabolism.
Excretion: excreted primarily in feces with small amount in urine.

Route	Onset	Peak	Duration
P.O.	5-10 min	30 min	≥ 3 hr
I.V.	Immediate	Unknown	45 min
I.M.	2-5 min	Unknown	≥ 3 hr

Pharmacodynamics

Chemical effect: increases motor activity of uterus by direct stimulation.
Therapeutic effect: prevents or stops postpartum hemorrhage.

Adverse reactions

CNS: dizziness, headache, ***seizures, CVA*** with I.V. use.

CV: hypertension, transient chest pain, palpitations, peripheral vasoconstriction, gangrene, thrombophlebitis.
EENT: tinnitus.
GI: *nausea, vomiting.*
GU: ***uterine tetany.***
Respiratory: dyspnea.
Skin: diaphoresis.
Other: ***hypersensitivity reactions.***

Interactions

Drug-drug. *Dopamine, I.V. oxytocin, regional anesthetics, vasoconstrictors:* excessive vasoconstriction. Use together cautiously.

Contraindications and precautions

- Contraindicated in pregnant women and in patients with hypertension, toxemia, or sensitivity to ergot preparations.
- Drug isn't recommended for use in breast-feeding women.
- Use cautiously in patients with sepsis, obliterative vascular disease, or hepatic or renal disease. Also use cautiously during last stage of labor.
- Drug isn't indicated for use in children.

NURSING CONSIDERATIONS

Assessment

- Assess patient's condition before therapy and regularly thereafter.
- Monitor blood pressure, pulse rate, and uterine response; report sudden change in vital signs, frequent periods of uterine relaxation, and character and amount of vaginal bleeding.
- Monitor contractions, which may continue 3 hours or more after P.O. or I.M. administration.
- Be alert for adverse reactions and drug interactions.
- Monitor patient's hydration status if adverse GI reactions occur.
- Evaluate patient's and family's knowledge of drug therapy.

Nursing diagnoses

- Decreased cardiac output related to postpartum hemorrhage
- Risk for deficient fluid volume related to drug therapy
- Deficient knowledge related to drug therapy

Planning and implementation

P.O. and I.M. use: Follow normal protocol.
I.V. use: Drug shouldn't routinely be given I.V. because of risk of severe hypertension and CVA. If it must be given I.V., give slowly over 1 minute with careful blood pressure monitoring. I.V. dose may be diluted to 5 ml with normal saline solution.
– Store in tightly closed, light-resistant container. Discard solution if discolored.
– Store I.V. solutions below 46.4° F (8° C). Daily stock may be kept at room temperature for 60 to 90 days.

Patient teaching

- Advise patient to report adverse reactions promptly.

Evaluation

- Patient's bleeding stops.
- Patient maintains adequate hydration throughout therapy.
- Patient and family state understanding of drug therapy.

methylphenidate hydrochloride

(meth-il-FEN-ih-dayt high-droh-KLOR-ighd)
Concerta, Methylin, Methylin ER, PMS-Methylphenidate ♦, Ritalin, Ritalin-SR

Pharmacologic class: piperidine CNS stimulant
Therapeutic class: CNS stimulant (analeptic)
Controlled substance schedule: II
Pregnancy risk category: NR (C for Concerta)

Indications and dosages

▶ **Attention deficit hyperactivity disorder (ADHD). Ritalin, Methylin.** *Children age 6 and older:* initial dose, 5 mg P.O. daily before breakfast and lunch, increased by 5- to 10-mg increments weekly, p.r.n., until an optimum daily dose of 2 mg/kg is reached. Not to exceed 60 mg daily.

▶ **ADHD. Concerta.** *Children age 6 and older not currently taking methylphenidate:* initially, 18 mg P.O. once daily in the morning. *Children age 6 and older currently taking methylphenidate:* if previous methylphenidate dosage is 5 mg b.i.d. or t.i.d. or 20 mg sustained-release, give 18 mg P.O. q morning. If previous methylphenidate dosage is 10 mg b.i.d. or t.i.d. or 40 mg sustained-release, give 36 mg P.O. q morning. If previous methylphenidate dosage is 15 mg b.i.d. or t.i.d. or 60 mg sustained release, give 54 mg P.O. q morning. Adjust dosages in 18-mg increments weekly, p.r.n. Maximum dosage is 54 mg/day.

▶ **Narcolepsy. Ritalin, Methylin.** *Adults:* 10 mg P.O. b.i.d. or t.i.d. 30 to 45 minutes before meals. Dosage varies with patient needs.

How supplied

Tablets: 5 mg, 10 mg, 20 mg
Tablets (sustained-release): 20 mg
Tablets (extended-release): 10 mg, 18 mg, 20 mg, 36 mg

Pharmacokinetics

Absorption: absorbed rapidly and completely.
Distribution: unknown.
Metabolism: metabolized by liver.
Excretion: excreted in urine.

Route	Onset	Peak	Duration
P.O.	Unknown	2-5 hr	Unknown

Pharmacodynamics

Chemical effect: unknown; probably promotes nerve impulse transmission by releasing stored norepinephrine from nerve terminals in brain. Main site of activity appears to be cerebral cortex and reticular activating system. In hyperkinetic children, drug has paradoxical calming effect.
Therapeutic effect: promotes calmness and prevents sleep.

Adverse reactions

CNS: *nervousness, insomnia,* Tourette syndrome, dizziness, headache, akathisia, dyskinesia, ***seizures.***
CV: *palpitations,* angina, *tachycardia,* changes in blood pressure and pulse rate.
EENT: dry throat, pharyngitis and sinusitis (Concerta).
GI: vomiting; nausea, abdominal pain, and anorexia (Concerta).
Hematologic: ***thrombocytopenia,*** thrombocytopenic purpura, ***leukopenia.***
Metabolic: weight loss.
Musculoskeletal: delayed growth.
Respiratory: upper respiratory tract infection (Concerta), cough.
Skin: rash, urticaria, ***exfoliative dermatitis, erythema multiforme.***

Interactions

Drug-drug. *Centrally acting antihypertensives:* decreased antihypertensive effect. Monitor blood pressure.
MAO inhibitors: severe hypertension; possible hypertensive crisis. Don't use together or within 14 days of MAO inhibitor therapy.
Tricyclic antidepressants: increased plasma levels of these drugs. Avoid concomitant use.
Drug-food. *Caffeine:* may increase amphetamine and related amine effects. Discourage concomitant use.

Contraindications and precautions

- Contraindicated in patients hypersensitive to drug and in those with glaucoma, motor tics, family history or diagnosis of Tourette syndrome, or history of marked anxiety, tension, or agitation.
- Use cautiously in pregnant or breast-feeding women and in patients with hypertension, history of drug abuse, seizures, or EEG abnormalities.
- Drug isn't recommended for use in children younger than age 6.

NURSING CONSIDERATIONS

Assessment

- Assess patient's condition before therapy and regularly thereafter.
- Drug may precipitate Tourette syndrome in children. Monitor effects, especially at start of therapy.
- Observe patient for signs of excessive stimulation. Monitor blood pressure.
- Monitor results of periodic CBC, differential, and platelet counts with long-term use.

- Monitor height and weight in child receiving prolonged therapy. Drug may delay growth, but child will attain normal height when drug is stopped.
- Monitor patient for tolerance or psychological dependence.
- Be alert for adverse reactions and drug interactions.
- Evaluate patient's and family's knowledge of drug therapy.

Nursing diagnoses
- Ineffective health maintenance related to underlying condition
- Disturbed sleep pattern related to drug-induced insomnia
- Deficient knowledge related to drug therapy

Planning and implementation
- This is drug of choice for ADHD. It's usually discontinued after puberty.
- Drug shouldn't be used to prevent fatigue.
- Give at least 6 hours before bedtime to prevent insomnia. Give after meals to reduce appetite suppression.
- Ritalin SR tablets have a duration of about 8 hours and may be used in place of regular tablets when 8-hour dosage of SR tablets corresponds to the adjusted dosage of the regular tablets.

ALERT Don't confuse Ritalin with Rifadin.

Patient teaching
- Tell patient to swallow Ritalin SR and Concerta tablets whole and not to chew or crush them.
- Caution patient to avoid activities that require alertness until CNS effects of drug are known.
- Tell patient to avoid caffeine.
- Advise patient with seizure disorder to notify prescriber if seizure occurs.
- Inform patient that he will need more rest as drug effects wear off.
- Warn patient that the shell of the Concerta tablet may appear in the stool.

Evaluation
- Patient responds positively to drug therapy.
- Patient doesn't experience insomnia during therapy.
- Patient and family state understanding of drug therapy.

methylprednisolone
(meth-il-pred-NIS-uh-lohn)
Medrol**, Meprolone

methylprednisolone acetate
depMedalone 40, depMedalone 80, Depoject-40, Depoject-80, Depo-Medrol, Depopred-40, Depopred-80, Depo-Predate 40, Depo-Predate 80, Duralone-40, Duralone-80, M-Prednisol-40, M-Prednisol-80, Medralone 40, Medralone 80

methylprednisolone sodium succinate
A-methaPred, Solu-Medrol

Pharmacologic class: glucocorticoid
Therapeutic class: anti-inflammatory, immunosuppressant
Pregnancy risk category: NR

Indications and dosages
▶ **Severe inflammation or immunosuppression. Methylprednisolone.** *Adults:* 2 to 60 mg P.O. daily in four divided doses.
Methylprednisolone acetate. *Adults:* 10 to 80 mg I.M. daily, or 4 to 80 mg into joint or soft tissue, p.r.n.
Methylprednisolone succinate. *Adults:* 10 to 250 mg I.M. or I.V. q 4 hours.
Children: 0.03 to 0.2 mg/kg or 1 to 6.25 mg/m^2 I.M. or I.V. daily in divided doses.

▶ **Shock. Methylprednisolone succinate.** *Adults:* 100 to 250 mg I.V. at 2- to 6-hour intervals. Or, 30 mg/kg I.V. initially, repeated q 4 to 6 hours, p.r.n. Continue therapy for 2 to 3 days or until patient is stable.

How supplied
methylprednisolone
Tablets: 2 mg, 4 mg, 8 mg, 16 mg, 24 mg, 32 mg

methylprednisolone acetate
Injection (suspension): 20 mg/ml, 40 mg/ml, 80 mg/ml
methylprednisolone sodium succinate
Injection: 40 mg/vial, 125 mg/vial, 500 mg/vial, 1,000 mg/vial, 2,000 mg/vial

Pharmacokinetics

Absorption: absorbed readily after P.O. administration; unknown after I.M. administration.
Distribution: distributed rapidly to muscle, liver, skin, intestines, and kidneys.
Metabolism: metabolized in liver.
Excretion: excreted primarily in urine; insignificant amount excreted in feces. *Half-life:* 18 to 36 hours.

Route	Onset	Peak	Duration
P.O.	Rapid	1-2 hr	30-36 hr
I.V.	Immediate	Immediate	Unknown
I.M.	6-48 hr	4-8 days	1-4 wk

Pharmacodynamics

Chemical effect: not clear; decreases inflammation, mainly by stabilizing leukocyte lysosomal membranes. Drug also suppresses immune response, stimulates bone marrow, and influences protein, fat, and carbohydrate metabolism.
Therapeutic effect: relieves inflammation and suppresses immune system function.

Adverse reactions

Most adverse reactions are dose- or duration-dependent.
CNS: *euphoria, insomnia,* psychotic behavior, pseudotumor cerebri.
CV: ***heart failure,*** hypertension, edema, ***thromboembolism, fatal arrest or circulatory collapse*** after rapid administration of large I.V. doses.
EENT: cataracts, glaucoma.
GI: ***peptic ulceration,*** GI irritation, increased appetite, ***pancreatitis.***
Metabolic: hypokalemia, hyperglycemia, and carbohydrate intolerance.
Musculoskeletal: muscle weakness, osteoporosis, growth suppression in children.
Skin: hirsutism, delayed wound healing, acne, various skin eruptions.
Other: susceptibility to infections, ***acute adrenal insufficiency*** with increased stress (infection, surgery, or trauma) or abrupt withdrawal after long-term therapy.

Interactions

Drug-drug. *Aspirin, indomethacin, other NSAIDs:* increased risk of GI distress and bleeding. Give together cautiously.
Barbiturates, phenytoin, rifampin: decreased corticosteroid effect. Increase corticosteroid dosage, as ordered.
Oral anticoagulants: altered dosage requirements. Monitor PT closely.
Potassium-depleting drugs (such as thiazide diuretics): enhanced potassium-wasting effects. Monitor serum potassium level.
Skin-test antigens: decreased response. Defer skin testing until therapy is completed.
Toxoids, vaccines: decreased antibody response and increased risk of neurologic complications. Avoid concomitant use.

Contraindications and precautions

- Contraindicated in patients allergic to drug or its components, in those with systemic fungal infections, and in premature infants (acetate and succinate).
- Use cautiously in pregnant women and in patients with GI ulceration or renal disease, hypertension, osteoporosis, diabetes mellitus, hypothyroidism, cirrhosis, diverticulitis, nonspecific ulcerative colitis, recent intestinal anastomoses, thromboembolic disorders, seizures, myasthenia gravis, heart failure, tuberculosis, ocular herpes simplex, emotional instability, or psychotic tendencies.
- Drug isn't recommended for breast-feeding women.

NURSING CONSIDERATIONS

Assessment

- Assess patient's condition before therapy and regularly thereafter.
- Watch for enhanced response in patient with hypothyroidism or cirrhosis.
- Monitor patient's weight, blood pressure, serum electrolyte levels (especially glucose),

and sleep patterns. Euphoria may initially interfere with sleep, but patient typically adjusts to drug after 1 to 3 weeks.
- Be alert for adverse reactions and drug interactions.
- Evaluate patient's and family's knowledge of drug therapy.

Nursing diagnoses
- Ineffective health maintenance related to underlying condition
- Risk for injury related to drug-induced adverse reactions
- Deficient knowledge related to drug therapy

Planning and implementation
- Drug may be used for alternate-day therapy.
- For better results and less risk of toxicity, give once-daily dose in morning.

P.O. use: Give P.O. dose with food when possible. Critically ill patients may need concomitant antacid or H_2-receptor antagonist therapy.
I.V. use: Give only methylprednisolone sodium succinate by I.V. route, never the acetate form. Reconstitute according to manufacturer's directions using supplied diluent or bacteriostatic water for injection with benzyl alcohol.
– For direct injection, inject diluted drug into vein or I.V. line containing free-flowing compatible solution over at least 1 minute. For treatment of shock, give massive doses over at least 10 minutes to prevent arrhythmias and circulatory collapse.
– When giving as intermittent or continuous infusion, dilute solution according to manufacturer's instructions and give over prescribed duration.
– If used for continuous infusion, change solution every 24 hours.
– Compatible solutions include D_5W, normal saline solution, and D_5W in normal saline solution.
I.M. use: Give I.M. injection deep into gluteal muscle.
– Dermal atrophy may occur with large doses of acetate salt. Use multiple small injections rather than single large dose and rotate injection sites.
- Avoid S.C. injection because atrophy and sterile abscesses may occur.

ALERT Don't confuse Solu-Medrol with Solu-Cortef (hydrocortisone sodium succinate) or methylprednisolone with medroxyprogesterone.
ALERT Manufacturers of Solu-Medrol state that drug should not be given intrathecally because severe adverse reactions have been reported.
- Don't use acetate salt when immediate onset of action is needed.
- Discard reconstituted solutions after 48 hours.
- Always adjust to lowest effective dose, as ordered.
- Administer potassium supplements, as needed.
- Gradually reduce drug dosage after long-term therapy, as ordered. Abrupt withdrawal may cause inflammation, fatigue, weakness, arthralgia, fever, dizziness, lethargy, depression, fainting, orthostatic hypotension, dyspnea, anorexia, and hypoglycemia. After prolonged use, sudden withdrawal may be fatal.

Patient teaching
- Tell patient not to discontinue drug abruptly or without prescriber's consent.
- Teach patient signs of early adrenal insufficiency: fatigue, muscle weakness, joint pain, fever, anorexia, nausea, dyspnea, dizziness, and fainting.
- Instruct patient to wear or carry medical identification.
- Warn patient receiving long-term therapy about cushingoid symptoms, and tell him to report sudden weight gain or swelling. Suggest exercise or physical therapy, and advise him to ask prescriber about vitamin D or calcium supplements.

Evaluation
- Patient responds positively to drug therapy.
- Patient sustains no injury from adverse reactions.
- Patient and family state understanding of drug therapy.

metoclopramide hydrochloride

(met-oh-KLOH-preh-mighd high-droh-KLOR-ighd)

Apo-Metoclop ♦, Clopra, Maxeran ♦, Maxolon, Octamide, Octamide PFS, Pramin ◇, Reclomide, Reglan

Pharmacologic class: para-aminobenzoic acid derivative
Therapeutic class: antiemetic, GI stimulant
Pregnancy risk category: B

Indications and dosages

▶ **Prevention or reduction of nausea and vomiting induced by cisplatin and other chemotherapeutic agents.** *Adults:* 1 to 2 mg/kg I.V. 30 minutes before chemotherapy; then repeated q 2 hours for two doses; then q 3 hours for three doses.

▶ **Prevention or reduction of postoperative nausea and vomiting.** *Adults:* 10 to 20 mg I.M. near end of surgical procedure, repeated q 4 to 6 hours, p.r.n.

▶ **To facilitate small-bowel intubation and aid in radiologic examinations.** *Adults and children over age 14:* 10 mg (2 ml) I.V. as single dose over 1 to 2 minutes.
Children ages 6 to 14: 2.5 to 5 mg I.V. (0.5 to 1 ml).
Children under age 6: 0.1 mg/kg I.V.

▶ **Delayed gastric emptying caused by diabetic gastroparesis.** *Adults:* 10 mg P.O. for mild symptoms, slow I.V. for severe symptoms 30 minutes before meals and h.s. for 2 to 8 weeks, depending on response.

▶ **Gastroesophageal reflux disease.** *Adults:* 10 to 15 mg P.O. q.i.d., p.r.n., 30 minutes before meals and h.s.

How supplied

Tablets: 5 mg, 10 mg
Syrup: 5 mg/5 ml
Injection: 5 mg/ml

Pharmacokinetics

Absorption: after P.O. dose, absorbed rapidly and completely from GI tract; after I.M. dose, about 74% to 96% bioavailable.
Distribution: distributed to most body tissues and fluids, including brain.
Metabolism: not metabolized extensively; small amount metabolized in liver.
Excretion: excreted in urine and feces. *Half-life:* 4 to 6 hours.

Route	Onset	Peak	Duration
P.O.	30-60 min	1-2 hr	1-2 hr
I.V.	1-3 min	Unknown	1-2 hr
I.M.	10-15 min	Unknown	1-2 hr

Pharmacodynamics

Chemical effect: stimulates motility of upper GI tract by increasing lower esophageal sphincter tone and blocks dopamine receptors at chemoreceptor trigger zone.
Therapeutic effect: prevents or minimizes nausea and vomiting from chemotherapy or surgery. Also reduces gag reflex in small-bowel intubation and radiologic examinations, improves gastric emptying when diabetic gastroparesis is present, and reduces gastric reflux.

Adverse reactions

CNS: *restlessness, anxiety, drowsiness,* fatigue, *lassitude,* insomnia, ***suicide ideation, seizures,*** headache, dizziness, extrapyramidal symptoms, tardive dyskinesia, dystonic reactions, sedation.
CV: transient hypertension.
GI: nausea, bowel disturbances.
Hematologic: ***agranulocytosis, neutropenia.***
Skin: rash.
Other: fever, prolactin secretion, loss of libido.

Interactions

Drug-drug. *Anticholinergics, opioid analgesics:* antagonized GI motility effects of metoclopramide. Use together cautiously.
Butyrophenones, phenothiazines: increased risk of extrapyramidal effects. Monitor patient closely.
CNS depressants: additive CNS depression. Avoid concomitant use.
Drug-lifestyle. *Alcohol use:* additive CNS depression. Discourage concomitant use.

Contraindications and precautions

- Contraindicated in patients hypersensitive to drug, in those for whom stimulation of GI motility might be dangerous (such as those with hemorrhage), and in those with pheochromocytoma or seizure disorder.
- Use cautiously in pregnant women, breast-feeding women, and patients with a history of depression, Parkinson's disease, or hypertension.
- Safety and effectiveness haven't been established for therapy that lasts longer than 12 weeks.

NURSING CONSIDERATIONS

Assessment

- Assess patient's condition before therapy and regularly thereafter.
- Monitor blood pressure frequently in patient receiving I.V. form of drug.
- Be alert for adverse reactions and drug interactions.
- Evaluate patient's and family's knowledge of drug therapy.

Nursing diagnoses

- Risk for deficient fluid volume related to nausea and vomiting
- Risk for injury related to drug-induced adverse CNS reactions
- Deficient knowledge related to drug therapy

Planning and implementation

P.O. use: Follow normal protocol. Dilute P.O. concentrate just before administration in water, juice, or carbonated beverage. Semisolid food such as applesauce or pudding also may be used.

I.V. use: Give doses of 10 mg or less by direct injection over 1 to 2 minutes.

– Dilute doses larger than 10 mg in 50 ml of compatible diluent and infuse over at least 15 minutes.

– Protection from light is unnecessary if infusion mixture is given within 24 hours.

– Drug is compatible with D_5W, normal saline solution injection, and D_5W in half-normal saline solution.

ALERT Diphenhydramine 25 mg I.V. counteracts extrapyramidal effects caused by high drug doses.

I.M. use: Commercially available preparation may be used for I.M. injection without further dilution.

Patient teaching

- Instruct patient to avoid alcohol consumption during drug therapy.
- Advise patient to avoid activities requiring alertness for 2 hours after taking each dose.

Evaluation

- Patient responds positively to drug and doesn't develop fluid volume deficit.
- Patient doesn't experience injury from adverse reactions.
- Patient and family state understanding of drug therapy.

metolazone

(meh-TOH-luh-zohn)

Mykrox, Zaroxolyn**

Pharmacologic class: quinazoline derivative (thiazide-like) diuretic

Therapeutic class: diuretic, antihypertensive

Pregnancy risk category: B

Indications and dosages

▶ **Edema in heart failure or renal disease.** *Adults:* 5 to 20 mg (extended) P.O. daily.

▶ **Hypertension.** *Adults:* 2.5 to 5 mg (extended) P.O. daily. Maintenance dosage determined by patient's blood pressure. Or, 0.5 mg (prompt) P.O. once daily in morning, increased to 1 mg P.O. daily, p.r.n. If response is inadequate, another antihypertensive is added.

How supplied

Tablets (extended): 2.5 mg, 5 mg, 10 mg

Tablets (prompt): 0.5 mg

Pharmacokinetics

Absorption: about 65% absorbed in healthy people; in cardiac patients, absorption falls to 40%. Rate and extent vary among preparations.

Distribution: 50% to 70% erythrocyte-bound; 33% protein-bound.
Metabolism: insignificant.
Excretion: 70% to 95% excreted unchanged in urine. *Half-life:* about 14 hours.

Route	Onset	Peak	Duration
P.O.	1 hr	2-8 hr	12-24 hr

Pharmacodynamics

Chemical effect: increases sodium and water excretion by inhibiting sodium reabsorption in cortical diluting site of ascending loop of Henle.
Therapeutic effect: promotes water and sodium elimination and lowers blood pressure.

Adverse reactions

CNS: dizziness, headache, fatigue.
CV: volume depletion and dehydration, orthostatic hypotension.
GI: anorexia, nausea, ***pancreatitis.***
GU: nocturia, polyuria, frequent urination.
Hematologic: ***aplastic anemia, agranulocytosis, leukopenia, thrombocytopenia.***
Hepatic: hepatic encephalopathy.
Metabolic: asymptomatic hyperuricemia; hyperglycemia and glucose tolerance impairment; fluid and electrolyte imbalances, including hypokalemia, metabolic alkalosis, hypercalcemia, and dilutional hyponatremia and hypochloremia.
Musculoskeletal: gout, muscle cramps, swelling.
Skin: dermatitis, photosensitivity, rash.
Other: ***hypersensitivity reactions.***

Interactions

Drug-drug. *Barbiturates, opioids:* increased orthostatic hypotensive effect. Monitor patient closely.
Cardiac glycosides: increased risk of digitalis toxicity from metolazone-induced hypokalemia. Monitor potassium and digitalis levels.
Cholestyramine, colestipol: decreased intestinal absorption of thiazides. Separate doses.
Diazoxide: increased antihypertensive, hyperglycemic, and hyperuricemic effects. Use together cautiously.
Lithium: decreased lithium clearance, increasing risk of lithium toxicity. Monitor lithium level.
NSAIDs: increased risk of NSAID-induced renal failure. Monitor patient for signs of renal failure.
Drug-lifestyle. *Alcohol use:* increased orthostatic hypotensive effect. Discourage concomitant use.
Sun exposure: photosensitivity reactions may occur. Urge patient to take precautions.

Contraindications and precautions

- Contraindicated in patients hypersensitive to thiazides or other sulfonamide-derived drugs and in patients with anuria or hepatic coma or precoma.
- Drug isn't recommended for pregnant women.
- Use cautiously in patients with impaired kidney or liver function.
- Safety of drug hasn't been established in breast-feeding women and in children.

NURSING CONSIDERATIONS

Assessment

- Assess patient's condition before therapy and regularly thereafter. In hypertensive patients, therapeutic response may be delayed several days.
- Unlike thiazide diuretics, drug is effective in patient with decreased kidney function.
- Monitor fluid intake and output, weight, blood pressure, and serum electrolyte levels.
- Monitor blood uric acid levels, especially in patient with history of gout.
- Be alert for adverse reactions and drug interactions.
- Evaluate patient's and family's knowledge of drug therapy.

Nursing diagnoses

- Excessive fluid volume related to presence of edema
- Risk for injury related to presence of hypertension
- Deficient knowledge related to drug therapy

Planning and implementation

ALERT Don't confuse Zaroxolyn with Zarontin or Metolazone with Metoprolol.
- Give drug in morning to prevent nocturia.

• Mykrox (prompt) tablets are more rapidly and completely absorbed than other brands mimicking oral solution. Don't interchange Mykrox with Zaroxolyn (extended) tablets.
• Drug may be used with potassium-sparing diuretic to prevent potassium loss.
• Drug is used as adjunct in furosemide-resistant edema.

Patient teaching
• Advise patient to avoid sudden posture changes and to rise slowly to avoid orthostatic hypotension.
• Advise patient to wear protective clothing, avoid prolonged exposure to sun, and use sunblock to prevent photosensitivity reactions.
• Instruct patient to avoid alcohol consumption during drug therapy.

☑ Evaluation
• Patient doesn't have edema.
• Patient's blood pressure is normal.
• Patient and family state understanding of drug therapy.

metoprolol succinate
(meh-TOH-pruh-lol SUHK-seh-nayt)
Toprol-XL

metoprolol tartrate
(meh-TOH-pruh-lol TAR-trayt)
Apo-Metoprolol ♦, Apo-Metoprolol (Type L) ♦, Betaloc ♦ ◇, Betaloc Durules ♦, Lopresor ♦, Lopresor SR ♦, Lopressor, Minax ◇, Novometoprol ♦, Nu-Metop ♦

Pharmacologic class: beta blocker
Therapeutic class: antihypertensive, adjunct treatment of acute MI
Pregnancy risk category: C

Indications and dosages
▶ **Hypertension. Metoprolol succinate.** *Adults:* initially, 100 to 150 mg (extended-release tablets) P.O. once daily. Dosage is adjusted as needed and tolerated at intervals of not less than 1 week to maximum of 400 mg daily.
Metoprolol tartrate. *Adults:* 100 mg P.O. daily in single or divided doses; usual maintenance dosage is 100 to 450 mg daily.
▶ **Early intervention in acute MI. Metoprolol tartrate.** *Adults:* 2.5 to 5 mg I.V. push q 2 to 5 minutes to a total of 15 mg within 15 minutes. Then, 15 minutes after last dose, 25 to 50 mg P.O. q 6 hours for 48 hours. Maintenance dosage is 100 mg P.O. b.i.d.
▶ **Angina pectoris. Metoprolol succinate.** *Adults:* initially, 100 mg (extended-release tablets) P.O. daily as single dose. Dosage increased at weekly intervals until adequate response or pronounced decrease in heart rate is seen. Daily dosage beyond 400 mg hasn't been studied.
Metoprolol tartrate. *Adults:* 100 mg P.O. in two divided doses. Dosage increased at weekly intervals until adequate response or pronounced decrease in heart rate is seen. Maintenance dosage is 100 to 400 mg/day.

How supplied
metoprolol succinate
Tablets (extended-release): 50 mg, 100 mg, 200 mg
metoprolol tartrate
Tablets: 50 mg, 100 mg
Tablets (extended-release): 100 mg ♦, 200 mg ♦
Injection: 1 mg/ml in 5-ml ampules

Pharmacokinetics
Absorption: absorbed rapidly and almost completely from GI tract with P.O. administration; food enhances absorption.
Distribution: distributed widely throughout body; about 12% protein-bound.
Metabolism: metabolized in liver.
Excretion: about 95% excreted in urine. *Half-life:* 3 to 7 hours.

Route	Onset	Peak	Duration
P.O.	≤ 15 min	1-12 hr	6-24 hr
I.V.	≤ 5 min	20 min	5-8 hr

Pharmacodynamics
Chemical effect: unknown for antihypertensive action. Drug decreases myocardial con-

tractility, heart rate, and cardiac output; lowers blood pressure; reduces myocardial oxygen consumption; and depresses renin secretion. ***Therapeutic effect:*** reduces blood pressure and angina and helps to prevent myocardial tissue damage.

Adverse reactions

CNS: fatigue, lethargy, dizziness.
CV: ***bradycardia,*** *hypotension,* ***heart failure, AV block,*** peripheral vascular disease.
GI: nausea, vomiting, diarrhea.
Metabolic: arthralgia.
Respiratory: dyspnea, ***bronchospasm.***
Skin: rash.
Other: fever.

Interactions

Drug-drug. *Barbiturates, rifampin:* increased metabolism of metoprolol. Monitor patient for decreased effect.
Cardiac glycosides, diltiazem, verapamil: excessive bradycardia and increased depressant effect on myocardium. Use together cautiously.
Chlorpromazine, cimetidine, verapamil: decreased hepatic clearance. Monitor patient for increased beta-blocking effect.
Hydralazine: serum levels and, hence, pharmacologic effects of beta blockers and hydralazine may be enhanced. Monitor patient closely.
Indomethacin: decreased antihypertensive effect. Monitor blood pressure and adjust dosage.
Insulin, oral antidiabetics: altered dosage requirements in previously stabilized diabetic patient. Observe patient carefully.
MAO inhibitors: bradycardia may develop during concurrent use. Monitor ECG and patient closely.
Drug-food. *Any food:* may increase absorption. Give together.

Contraindications and precautions

- Contraindicated in patients hypersensitive to drug or other beta blockers and in those with sinus bradycardia, heart block greater than first-degree, cardiogenic shock, or overt cardiac failure when used to treat hypertension or angina. When used to treat MI, drug is also contraindicated in patients with heart rate below 45 beats/minute, second- or third-degree heart block, PR interval of 0.24 second or more with first-degree heart block, systolic blood pressure under 100 mm Hg, or moderate to severe cardiac failure.
- Drug isn't recommended for breast-feeding women.
- Use cautiously in pregnant patients and patients with heart failure, diabetes, or respiratory or hepatic disease.
- Safety of drug hasn't been established in children.

NURSING CONSIDERATIONS

Assessment

- Assess patient's condition before therapy and regularly thereafter.
- Monitor blood pressure frequently. Drug masks common signs of shock.
- Be alert for adverse reactions and drug interactions.
- Evaluate patient's and family's knowledge of drug therapy.

Nursing diagnoses

- Ineffective health maintenance related to underlying disorder
- Risk for injury related to drug-induced adverse CNS reactions
- Deficient knowledge related to drug therapy

Planning and implementation

- Always check patient's apical pulse rate before giving drug. If it's slower than 60 beats/minute, withhold drug and call prescriber immediately.

P.O. use: Give drug with meals because food may increase absorption.
I.V. use: Give drug undiluted and by direct injection.
– Although mixing with other drugs should be avoided, studies have shown that metoprolol is compatible with meperidine hydrochloride or morphine sulfate or with alteplase infusions at Y-site connection.
– Store drug at room temperature and protect from light. Discard solution if discolored or contains particulates.
ALERT Don't confuse metoprolol with metaproterenol or metolazone.

Patient teaching

- Tell patient that abrupt discontinuation of therapy can worsen angina and precipitate MI. Withdraw drug gradually over 1 to 2 weeks.
- Instruct patient to take oral form of drug with meals to enhance absorption.
- Advise patient to report adverse reactions to prescriber.
- Warn patient to avoid performing hazardous activities until CNS effects of drug are known.

☑ Evaluation

- Patient responds well to therapy.
- Patient doesn't experience injury from adverse CNS reactions.
- Patient and family state understanding of drug therapy.

metronidazole

(met-roh-NIGH-duh-zohl)

Apo-Metronidazole ♦, Flagyl, Flagyl ER, Flagyl 375, Metric 21, Metrogyl ◇, Metrozine ◇, Novonidazol ♦, Protostat, Trikacide ♦

metronidazole hydrochloride

Flagyl I.V. RTU, Metro I.V., Novonidazol ♦

Pharmacologic class: nitroimidazole
Therapeutic class: antibacterial, antiprotozoal, amebicide
Pregnancy risk category: B

Indications and dosages

▶ **Amebic hepatic abscess.** *Adults:* 500 to 750 mg P.O. t.i.d. for 5 to 10 days.
Children: 35 to 50 mg/kg daily (in three doses) for 10 days.

▶ **Intestinal amebiasis.** *Adults:* 750 mg P.O. t.i.d. for 5 to 10 days.
Children: 35 to 50 mg/kg daily (in three doses) for 10 days. Therapy followed with P.O. iodoquinol.

▶ **Trichomoniasis.** *Adults:* 375 mg P.O. b.i.d. for 7 days or 2 g P.O. in single dose (may give 2-g dose in two 1-g doses on same day); 4 to 6 weeks should elapse between courses of therapy.
Children: 5 mg/kg dose P.O. t.i.d. for 7 days.

▶ **Refractory trichomoniasis.** *Adults:* 500 mg P.O. b.i.d. for 10 days.

▶ **Bacterial infections caused by anaerobic microorganisms.** *Adults:* loading dose is 15 mg/kg I.V. infused over 1 hour (about 1 g for 70-kg [154-lb] adult). Maintenance dosage is 7.5 mg/kg I.V. or P.O. q 6 hours (about 500 mg for 70-kg adult). First maintenance dose should be given 6 hours after loading dose. Maximum, 4 g daily.

▶ **Prevention of postoperative infection in contaminated or potentially contaminated colorectal surgery.** *Adults:* 15 mg/kg I.V. infused over 30 to 60 minutes and completed about 1 hour before surgery. Then, 7.5 mg/kg I.V. infused over 30 to 60 minutes at 6 and 12 hours after initial dose.

How supplied

Capsules: 375 mg
Tablets: 200 mg ◇, 250 mg, 400 mg ◇, 500 mg
Tablets (extended release): 750 mg
Oral suspension (benzoyl metronidazole): 200 mg/5 ml ◇
Injection: 500 mg/100 ml
Powder for injection: 500-mg single-dose vials

Pharmacokinetics

Absorption: about 80% of P.O. dose absorbed; food delays peak levels to about 2 hours.
Distribution: distributed in most body tissues and fluids; less than 20% bound to plasma proteins.
Metabolism: metabolized to active metabolite and to other metabolites.
Excretion: excreted primarily in urine; 6% to 15% in feces. *Half-life:* 6 to 8 hours (may be longer in patients with impaired liver function).

Route	Onset	Peak	Duration
P.O.	Unknown	1-2 hr	Unknown
I.V.	Immediate	Immediate	Unknown

Pharmacodynamics

Chemical effect: direct-acting trichomonacide and amebicide that works at both intestinal and extraintestinal sites.

Therapeutic effect: hinders growth of selected organisms. Spectrum of activity includes most anaerobic bacteria and protozoa, including *Bacteroides fragilis, Bacteroides melaninogenicus, Balantidium coli, Clostridium, Entamoeba histolytica, Fusobacterium, Giardia lamblia, Peptococcus, Peptostreptococcus, Trichomonas vaginalis,* and *Veillonella.*

Adverse reactions

CNS: vertigo, headache, ataxia, incoordination, confusion, irritability, depression, restlessness, weakness, fatigue, drowsiness, insomnia, sensory neuropathy, paresthesia of limbs, psychic stimulation, ***seizures,*** neuropathy.
CV: flattened T wave, edema.
GI: abdominal cramping, stomatitis, *nausea, vomiting, anorexia,* diarrhea, constipation, proctitis, dry mouth, metallic taste.
GU: darkened urine, polyuria, dysuria, pyuria, incontinence, cystitis, dyspareunia, dry vagina and vulva, sense of pelvic pressure.
Hematologic: transient leukopenia, ***neutropenia.***
Skin: pruritus, flushing, rash.
Other: decreased libido; gynecomastia; overgrowth of nonsusceptible organisms, especially *Candida* (glossitis, furry tongue); fever; thrombophlebitis after I.V. infusion.

Interactions

Drug-drug. *Cimetidine:* increased risk of metronidazole toxicity because of inhibited hepatic metabolism. Monitor patient.
Disulfiram: acute psychoses and confusional states. Don't use together.
Lithium: increased lithium levels, possibly resulting in toxicity. Monitor serum lithium levels closely.
Oral anticoagulants: increased anticoagulant effects. Monitor patient.
Phenobarbital, phenytoin: decreased metronidazole effectiveness because of increased hepatic clearance. Monitor patient closely.
Drug-lifestyle. *Alcohol use:* disulfiram-like reaction (nausea, vomiting, headache, cramps, flushing). Discourage concurrent use.

Contraindications and precautions

- Contraindicated in patients hypersensitive to drug or other nitroimidazole derivatives.
- Drug isn't recommended for breast-feeding women.
- Use cautiously in patients receiving hepatotoxic drugs and in patients with history of blood dyscrasia or CNS disorder, retinal or visual field changes, hepatic disease, or alcoholism.

NURSING CONSIDERATIONS

Assessment

- Assess patient's infection before therapy and regularly thereafter.
- Watch carefully for edema, especially in patients also receiving corticosteroids, because Flagyl I.V. RTU may cause sodium retention.
- Record number and character of stools when used in amebiasis.
- Be alert for adverse reactions and drug interactions.
- Evaluate patient's and family's understanding of drug therapy.

Nursing diagnoses

- Infection related to presence of susceptible organisms
- Risk for deficient fluid volume related to drug-induced adverse GI reactions
- Deficient knowledge related to drug therapy

Planning and implementation

- Metronidazole should be used only after *T. vaginalis* has been confirmed by wet smear or culture or *E. histolytica* has been identified. Asymptomatic sexual partners of patients being treated for *T. vaginalis* infection should be treated simultaneously to avoid reinfection.
- For trichomoniasis during pregnancy, 7-day regimen is preferred over 2-g single-dose regimen.

P.O. use: Give drug with meals to minimize GI distress.
I.V. use: No preparation is necessary for RTU form.
– To prepare lyophilized vials of metronidazole, add 4.4 ml of sterile water for injection, bacteriostatic water for injection, sterile normal saline solution injection, or bacteriostatic normal saline solution injection. Reconstituted drug contains 100 mg/ml.

– Add contents of vial to 100 ml of D_5W, lactated Ringer's injection, or normal saline solution for final concentration of 5 mg/ml.
– Resulting highly acidic solution must be neutralized before administering. Carefully add 5 mEq of sodium bicarbonate for each 500 mg of metronidazole. Carbon dioxide will form and may need to be vented.
ALERT Infuse drug over at least 1 hour. Don't give I.V. push.
– Don't refrigerate neutralized diluted solution. Precipitation may occur. If Flagyl I.V. RTU is refrigerated, crystals may form. These will disappear after solution is gently warmed to room temperature.

Patient teaching
- Tell patient to avoid alcohol or alcohol-containing medications during therapy and for at least 48 hours after therapy is completed.
- Tell patient that metallic taste and dark or red-brown urine may occur.
- Instruct patient to take oral form with meals to minimize reactions.
- Instruct patient in proper hygiene.

Evaluation
- Patient is free from infection.
- Patient maintains adequate hydration throughout therapy.
- Patient and family state understanding of drug therapy.

mexiletine hydrochloride
(MEKS-il-eh-teen high-droh-KLOR-ighd)
Mexitil

Pharmacologic class: lidocaine analogue, sodium channel antagonist
Therapeutic class: ventricular antiarrhythmic
Pregnancy risk category: C

Indications and dosages
▶ **Refractory life-threatening ventricular arrhythmias, including ventricular tachycardia and PVCs.** *Adults:* 200 to 400 mg P.O., followed by 200 mg q 8 hours. Dose increased q 2 to 3 days to 400 mg q 8 hours if satisfactory control isn't obtained. Patients who respond well to q-12-hour schedule may be given up to 450 mg q 12 hours. Maximum daily dosage is 1,200 mg.
I.V. ◇ *Adults:* loading dose is 100 to 250 mg I.V. at 25 mg/minute. Then prepare infusion solution of 250 mg of mexiletine in 500 ml of D_5W, and administer first 120 ml (60 mg) over 1 hour. If response is inadequate, give another bolus of 200 mg over 10 to 20 minutes. Maintenance dosage is 0.5 mg/minute (1 ml/minute of prepared solution).

How supplied
Capsules: 50 mg ◇, 100 mg ♦, 150 mg, 200 mg, 250 mg
Injection: 250 mg/10 ml ◇

Pharmacokinetics
Absorption: about 90% absorbed from GI tract after P.O. use.
Distribution: distributed widely throughout body. Distribution volume declines in patients with liver disease, resulting in toxic serum drug levels with usual doses. About 50% to 60% of circulating drug is bound to plasma proteins.
Metabolism: most of drug metabolized in liver.
Excretion: excreted in urine. *Half-life:* 10 to 12 hours.

Route	Onset	Peak	Duration
P.O.	0.5-2 hr	2-3 hr	Unknown
I.V.	Immediate	Immediate	Unknown

Pharmacodynamics
Chemical effect: class Ib antiarrhythmic that blocks fast sodium channel in cardiac tissues, especially Purkinje network, without involvement of autonomic nervous system. Drug reduces rate of rise and amplitude of action potential and decreases automaticity in Purkinje fibers. It also shortens action potential and, to a lesser extent, decreases effective refractory period in Purkinje fibers.
Therapeutic effect: abolishes ventricular arrhythmias.

Adverse reactions

CNS: *tremors, dizziness,* blurred vision, ataxia, diplopia, confusion, nystagmus, nervousness, headache.
CV: hypotension, ***bradycardia,*** widened QRS complex, ***arrhythmias,*** palpitations, chest pain.
GI: nausea, vomiting.
Skin: rash.

Interactions

Drug-drug. *Antacids, atropine, narcotics:* slowed mexiletine absorption. Monitor patient.
Cimetidine: increased or decreased mexiletine blood levels. Monitor patient carefully.
Methylxanthines (such as caffeine, theophylline): reduced clearance of methylxanthines, possibly resulting in toxicity. Monitor patient.
Metoclopramide: mexiletine absorption may be accelerated. Monitor patient for toxicity.
Phenobarbital, phenytoin, rifampin, urine acidifiers: decreased mexiletine blood levels. Monitor patient.
Urine alkalinizers: increased mexiletine blood levels. Monitor patient.

Contraindications and precautions

- Contraindicated in patients with cardiogenic shock or second- or third-degree AV block in absence of artificial pacemaker.
- Drug isn't recommended for breast-feeding women.
- Use cautiously in pregnant patients and in patients with first-degree heart block, ventricular pacemaker, sinus node dysfunction, intraventricular conduction disturbances, hypotension, severe heart failure, or seizure disorder.
- Safety of drug hasn't been established in children.

NURSING CONSIDERATIONS

Assessment

- Assess patient's condition until arrhythmia is abolished.
- Monitor drug levels, as ordered. Therapeutic levels range from 0.75 to 2 mcg/ml.
- Be alert for adverse reactions and drug interactions.
- Monitor patient for toxicity. An early sign is tremors, usually fine tremor of hands. This progresses to dizziness and later to ataxia and nystagmus as drug's blood level increases. Ask patient about these symptoms.
- Monitor patient's hydration status if adverse GI reactions occur.
- Evaluate patient's and family's knowledge of drug therapy.

Nursing diagnoses

- Decreased cardiac output related to presence of ventricular arrhythmia
- Risk for deficient fluid volume related to drug-induced adverse GI reactions
- Deficient knowledge related to drug therapy

Planning and implementation

P.O. use: Give with meals or antacids to lessen GI distress.
I.V. use: Mexiletine injection is compatible with normal saline solution, D_5W, 5% sodium bicarbonate, 1/6 M sodium lactate, and 10% fructose (levulose).
– When changing from lidocaine to mexiletine, stop lidocaine infusion when first mexiletine dose is given. Keep infusion line open, however, until arrhythmia is controlled.
- If patient appears to be good candidate for every-12-hour therapy, notify prescriber. Twice-daily dosage enhances compliance.
- Notify prescriber of significant change in blood pressure and heart rate and rhythm.

Patient teaching

- Instruct patient taking oral form of drug to take it with food.
- Instruct patient to report adverse reactions.

Evaluation

- Patient regains normal cardiac output.
- Patient maintains adequate hydration throughout therapy.
- Patient and family state understanding of drug therapy.

mezlocillin sodium

(mez-loh-SIL-in SOH-dee-um)
Mezlin

Pharmacologic class: extended-spectrum penicillin, acyclaminopenicillin
Therapeutic class: antibiotic
Pregnancy risk category: B

Indications and dosages

▶ **Systemic infections caused by susceptible strains of gram-positive and especially gram-negative organisms (including *Proteus* and *Pseudomonas aeruginosa*).** *Adults:* 200 to 300 mg/kg daily I.V. or I.M. in four to six divided doses. Usual dosage is 3 g q 4 hours or 4 g q 6 hours. For serious infections, up to 24 g daily may be given.
Children ages 1 month to 12 years: 50 mg/kg q 4 hours I.V. or I.M.
Neonates weighing over 2,000 g (4.4 lb) and older than age 1 week: 75 mg/kg I.V. q 6 hours (300 mg/kg/day).
Neonates weighing over 2,000 g and age 1 week or less: 75 mg/kg I.V. q 12 hours (150 mg/kg/day).
Neonates weighing 2,000 g or less and older than age 1 week: 75 mg/kg I.V. q 8 hours (225 mg/kg/day).
Neonates weighing 2,000 g or less and age 1 week or less: 75 mg/kg I.V. q 12 hours (150 mg/kg/day).

How supplied

Injection: 1 g, 2 g, 3 g, 4 g,

Pharmacokinetics

Absorption: unknown after I.M. use.
Distribution: distributed widely; 16% to 42% protein-bound.
Metabolism: metabolized partially.
Excretion: excreted primarily in urine; up to 30% of dose excreted in bile. *Half-life:* 45 to 90 minutes.

Route	Onset	Peak	Duration
I.V.	Immediate	Immediate	Unknown
I.M.	Unknown	45-90 min	Unknown

Pharmacodynamics

Chemical effect: inhibits cell wall synthesis during microorganism multiplication; bacteria resist mezlocillin by producing penicillinases—enzymes that hydrolyze mezlocillin. Mezlocillin resists these enzymes.
Therapeutic effect: kills susceptible bacteria. Spectrum of activity includes many gram-negative bacilli, many gram-positive and gram-negative aerobic cocci, and some gram-positive bacilli.

Adverse reactions

CNS: neuromuscular irritability, ***seizures.***
GI: nausea, diarrhea.
Hematologic: ***bleeding, neutropenia, thrombocytopenia,*** eosinophilia, ***leukopenia,*** hemolytic anemia.
Metabolic: *hypokalemia.*
Skin: rash, pruritus.
Other: ***hypersensitivity reactions,*** overgrowth of nonsusceptible organisms, pain at injection site, vein irritation, phlebitis.

Interactions

Drug-drug. *Aminoglycoside antibiotics (such as gentamicin, tobramycin):* chemically incompatible. Don't mix in I.V. solution. Give 1 hour apart, especially in patients with renal insufficiency.
Anticoagulants: large I.V. doses of penicillins can increase bleeding risk of anticoagulants by prolonging bleeding time. Monitor patient.
Probenecid: increased blood levels of mezlocillin. Probenecid may be used for this purpose.
Vecuronium: may prolong neuromuscular blockage of vecuronium. Use with caution.

Contraindications and precautions

- Contraindicated in patients hypersensitive to drug or other penicillins.
- Use cautiously in pregnant women; patients with other drug allergies, especially to cephalosporins (possible cross-sensitivity); and patients with bleeding tendencies, uremia, or hypokalemia.
- Safety of drug hasn't been established in breast-feeding women.

NURSING CONSIDERATIONS

Assessment
- Assess patient's infection before therapy and regularly thereafter.
- Before giving, ask patient about any allergic reactions to penicillin. A negative history of penicillin allergy is no guarantee against future reaction.
- Obtain specimen for culture and sensitivity tests before giving first dose. Therapy may begin pending results.
- Check CBC and platelet counts frequently, as ordered. Drug may cause thrombocytopenia.
- Monitor serum potassium level.
- Be alert for adverse reactions and drug interactions.
- Monitor patient's hydration status if adverse GI reactions occur.
- Evaluate patient's and family's knowledge of drug therapy.

Nursing diagnoses
- Infection related to presence of susceptible bacteria
- Risk of deficient fluid volume related to drug-induced adverse GI reactions
- Deficient knowledge related to drug therapy

Planning and implementation
I.V. use: Reconstitute vial with at least 10 ml/g of drug using sterile water for injection, D_5W, or normal saline solution injection.
– Solutions not exceeding 10% concentration may be given by direct injection over 3 to 5 minutes.
– Or, dilute in 50 to 100 ml of I.V. solution and give by intermittent infusion over 30 minutes.
– Give I.V. intermittently to prevent vein irritation. Change site every 48 hours.
I.M. use: Don't give more than 2 g per injection. Inject slowly (12 to 15 seconds), deep into body of large muscle.
- Drug is almost always used with another antibiotic, such as gentamicin.
- Give drug at least 1 hour before bacteriostatic antibiotics.

ALERT Institute seizure precautions. Patient with high serum drug levels may have seizures.
- Dosage should be altered in patients with impaired kidney function.
- Drug may interfere with positive direct antiglobulin (Coombs') test results and with certain tests for serum and urine proteins; tests that use bromphenol blue (Albustix, Albutest) aren't affected.

ALERT Don't confuse mezlocillin with methicillin.

Patient teaching
- Advise patient to promptly report adverse reactions.

Evaluation
- Patient is free from infection.
- Patient maintains adequate hydration throughout therapy.
- Patient and family state understanding of drug therapy.

midazolam hydrochloride
(MID-ayz-oh-lam high-droh-KLOR-ighd)
Hypnovel ◇, Versed, Versed Syrup

Pharmacologic class: benzodiazepine
Therapeutic class: preoperative sedative, agent for conscious sedation, adjunct for induction of general anesthesia
Controlled substance schedule: IV
Pregnancy risk category: D

Indications and dosages
▶ **Preoperative sedation (to induce sleepiness or drowsiness and relieve apprehension).** *Adults under age 60:* 0.07 mg to 0.08 mg/kg I.M. about 1 hour before surgery.
▶ **Conscious sedation before short diagnostic or endoscopic procedures.** *Adults under age 60:* initially, small dose not to exceed 2.5 mg I.V. administered slowly; repeated in 2 minutes if needed in small increments of initial dose over at least 2 minutes to achieve desired effect. Total dose of up to 5 mg may be given.
Adults age 60 and over: 1.5 mg or less over at least 2 minutes. If additional adjustment is needed, give at no more than 1 mg over 2 min-

utes. Total doses exceeding 3.5 mg aren't usually necessary.

▶ **Induction of general anesthesia.** *Adults under age 55:* 0.3 to 0.35 mg/kg I.V. over 20 to 30 seconds if patient hasn't received preanesthesia medication, or 0.15 to 0.35 mg/kg I.V. over 20 to 30 seconds if patient has received preanesthesia medication. Additional increments of 25% of initial dose may be needed to complete induction.
Adults age 55 and over: 0.3 mg/kg I.V. over 20 to 30 seconds if patient hasn't received premedication, or 0.2 mg/kg I.V. over 20 to 30 seconds if patient has received sedation or narcotic premedication. Additional increments of 25% of initial dose may be needed to complete induction.

▶ **To induce sleepiness and amnesia and to relieve apprehension before anesthesia or before or during procedures in children.** *Children:* 0.1 to 0.15 mg/kg I.M. Doses up to 0.5 mg/kg can be used for more anxious patients.
Children ages 6 months to 5 years: 0.05 to 0.1 mg/kg I.V. over 2 to 3 minutes. Additional doses may be given in small increments after 2 to 3 minutes. Total dose of up to 0.6 mg/kg (not to exceed 6 mg) may be given.
Children ages 6 to 12: 0.025 to 0.05 mg/kg I.V. over 2 to 3 minutes. Additional doses may be given in small increments after 2 to 3 minutes. Total dose of up to 0.4 mg/kg (not to exceed 10 mg) may be given.
Infants and children ages 6 months to 5 years and less cooperative patients: 0.25 to 1 mg/kg P.O. as a single dose, not to exceed 20 mg.
Children ages 6 to 16 and cooperative patients: 0.25 to 0.5 mg/kg P.O. as a single dose, up to 20 mg.

▶ **Continuous infusion for sedation of intubated patients in the critical care setting:** *Adults:* initially 0.01 to 0.05 mg/kg may be given I.V. over several minutes, repeated at 10- to 15-minute intervals, until adequate sedation is achieved. For maintenance of sedation, usual initial infusion rate is 0.02 to 0.1 mg/kg/hour. Higher loading dose or infusion rates may be needed in some patients. Use the lowest effective rate.
Children: initially, 0.05 to 0.2 mg/kg may be given I.V. over at least 2 to 3 minutes; then continuous infusion at 0.06 to 0.12 mg/kg/hour. Increase or decrease infusion to maintain desired effect.
Neonates over 32 weeks gestational age: initially 0.06 mg/kg/hr. Adjust rate, p.r.n., using lowest possible rate.
Neonates under 32 weeks gestational age: initially 0.03 mg/kg/hr. Adjust rate, p.r.n., using lowest possible rate.

How supplied

Injection: 1 mg/ml, 5 mg/ml
Syrup: 2 mg/ml

Pharmacokinetics

Absorption: absorption after I.M. use appears to be 80% to 100%.
Distribution: drug has large volume of distribution; about 97% protein-bound.
Metabolism: metabolized in liver.
Excretion: excreted in urine. *Half-life:* 2 to 6 hours.

Route	Onset	Peak	Duration
I.V.	1.5-5 min	Rapid	2-6 hr
I.M.	≤ 15 min	15-60 min	2-6 hr

Pharmacodynamics

Chemical effect: unknown; thought to depress CNS at limbic and subcortical levels of brain by potentiating effects of gamma-aminobutyric acid.
Therapeutic effect: promotes calmness and sleep.

Adverse reactions

CNS: headache, oversedation, involuntary movements, combativeness, amnesia.
CV: variations in blood pressure ***(hypotension)*** and pulse rate, ***cardiac arrest.***
GI: *nausea,* vomiting, *hiccups.*
Respiratory: *decreased respiratory rate,* APNEA.
Skin: pain, tenderness at injection site.

Interactions

Drug-drug. *CNS depressants:* may increase risk of apnea. Avoid concomitant use.
Indinavir, ritonavir: possible prolonged or severe sedation and respiratory depression. Monitor patient closely.

Oral contraceptives: may prolong benzodiazepine half-life. Monitor patient closely.
Verapamil: effects of benzodiazepine may be increased. Monitor patient closely.
Drug-lifestyle. *Alcohol use:* may increase risk of apnea. Discourage concurrent use.

Contraindications and precautions

- Contraindicated in patients hypersensitive to drug and in those with acute angle-closure glaucoma, shock, coma, or acute alcohol intoxication.
- Drug isn't recommended for use in pregnant women.
- Use cautiously in patients with uncompensated acute illness, in elderly or debilitated patients, and in breast-feeding women.

NURSING CONSIDERATIONS

Assessment

- Assess patient's condition before therapy and regularly thereafter.
- Monitor blood pressure, heart rate and rhythm, respirations, airway integrity, and arterial oxygen saturation during procedure, especially in patients premedicated with narcotics.
- Be alert for adverse reactions and drug interactions.
- Evaluate patient's and family's knowledge of drug therapy.

Nursing diagnoses

- Anxiety related to surgery
- Ineffective breathing pattern related to drug's effect on respiratory system
- Deficient knowledge related to drug therapy

Planning and implementation

- Before administering drug, have oxygen and resuscitation equipment available in case of severe respiratory depression. Excessive dosage or rapid infusion has been linked to respiratory arrest, particularly in elderly or debilitated patients.
- Midazolam may be mixed in same syringe with morphine sulfate, meperidine, atropine sulfate, or scopolamine.

I.V. use: Administer drug slowly over at least 2 minutes, and wait at least 2 minutes when adjusting doses to effect.
– Take care to avoid extravasation.
I.M. use: Administer drug deep into large muscle mass.
ALERT Don't confuse Versed with Vepesid.

Patient teaching

- Drug's beneficial amnesic effect diminishes recall of perioperative events. This effect requires extra caution when teaching patients. Written information, family member instruction, and follow-up contact may be required to ensure that patient has adequate information.
- Instruct patient to avoid alcohol consumption during drug therapy.

Evaluation

- Patient exhibits calmness.
- Patient maintains adequate breathing pattern throughout therapy.
- Patient and family state understanding of drug therapy.

miglitol
(MIG-lih-tall)
Glyset

Pharmacologic class: alpha-glucosidase inhibitor
Therapeutic class: antidiabetic
Pregnancy risk category: B

Indications and dosages

▶ **Monotherapy as an adjunct to diet to improve glycemic control in patients with type 2 diabetes mellitus whose hyperglycemia can't be managed with diet alone, or in combination with a sulfonylurea when diet plus either miglitol or sulfonylurea alone yield inadequate glycemic control.** *Adults:* 25 mg P.O. t.i.d. at the start (with the first bite) of each main meal; may be increased after 4 to 8 weeks to a maintenance dosage of 50 mg P.O. t.i.d. The dosage may then be further increased after three months, based on glycosylated hemoglobin level, to maximum of 100 mg P.O. t.i.d.

How supplied

Tablets: 25 mg, 50 mg, 100 mg

Pharmacokinetics

Absorption: saturable absorption at high doses. A 25-mg dose of miglitol is completely absorbed, whereas a dose of 100 mg is only 50% to 70% absorbed; levels peak 2 to 3 hours after P.O. dose.
Distribution: distributed primarily into the extracellular fluid. Protein-binding is negligible (less than 4 %).
Metabolism: not metabolized.
Excretion: primarily renal excretion. More than 95% of a dose appears in urine as unchanged drug. *Half-life:* about 2 hours.

Route	Onset	Peak	Duration
P.O.	Unknown	2-3 hr	Unknown

Pharmacodynamics

Chemical effect: lowers blood glucose through reversible inhibition of alpha-glucosidases in the brush border of the small intestine. Alpha-glucosidases are responsible for the conversion of oligosaccharides and disaccharides to glucose. Inhibition of these enzymes results in delayed glucose absorption and a lowering of postprandial hyperglycemia. In contrast to sulfonylureas, miglitol has no effect on insulin secretion.
Therapeutic effect: lowers blood glucose.

Adverse reactions

GI: abdominal pain, diarrhea, flatulence.
Skin: rash.
Other: decreased serum iron levels.

Interactions

Drug-drug. *Digoxin, propranolol, ranitidine:* may decrease the bioavailability of these drugs. Monitor patient for loss of efficacy, and adjust dosages as directed.
Intestinal absorbents (such as charcoal) and digestive enzyme preparations (such as amylase, pancreatin): may reduce the effectiveness of miglitol. Avoid concomitant use.
Drug-herb. *Aloe, bilberry leaf, bitter melon, burdock, dandelion, fenugreek, garlic, ginseng:* concomitant use may improve blood glucose control, allowing reduced antidiabetic dosage. Advise patient to discuss the use of herbal remedies with prescriber before therapy.

Contraindications and precautions

- Drug is contraindicated in patients hypersensitive to drug or its components. Also contraindicated in patients with diabetic ketoacidosis, inflammatory bowel disease, colonic ulceration, or partial intestinal obstruction; patients predisposed to intestinal obstruction or those with chronic intestinal diseases related to disorders of digestion or absorption; and patients with conditions that may deteriorate as a result of increased gas formation in the intestine.
- Drug isn't recommended for patients with significant renal dysfunction (serum creatinine less than 2 mg/dL). Use cautiously in patients also receiving insulin or oral sulfonylureas.

NURSING CONSIDERATIONS

Assessment

- Obtain history of patient's underlying condition before therapy, and reassess regularly thereafter.
- Monitor blood glucose regularly, especially during situations of increased stress, such as infection, fever, surgery, and trauma.
- Check glycosylated hemoglobin every three months, as ordered, to monitor long-term glycemic control.
- Evaluate patient's and family's knowledge about drug therapy.

Nursing diagnoses

- Ineffective health maintenance related to hyperglycemia
- Risk for injury related to drug-induced hypoglycemia
- Deficient knowledge related to drug therapy

Planning and implementation

P.O. use: Miglitol should be given with the first bite of each main meal.
- In patients also receiving insulin or oral sulfonylureas, miglitol may increase the hypoglycemic potential of insulin or sulfonylureas. Dosage adjustments of these drugs may be

needed, as ordered. Monitor these patients for an increased frequency of hypoglycemia.
- Management of type 2 diabetes should include diet control, exercise program, and regular testing of urine and blood glucose.
- Treat mild to moderate hypoglycemia with a form of dextrose such as glucose tablets or gel. Severe hypoglycemia may require I.V. glucose or glucagon.

Patient teaching
- Instruct patient about the importance of adhering to prescriber's diet, weight reduction, and exercise instructions and to have blood glucose and glycosylated hemoglobin tested regularly.
- Inform patient that treatment with miglitol relieves symptoms but doesn't cure diabetes.
- Teach patient to recognize the signs and symptoms of hyperglycemia and hypoglycemia.
- Instruct patient to treat hypoglycemia with glucose tablets and to have a source of glucose readily available when miglitol is taken with a sulfonylurea or insulin.
- Advise patient to seek medical advice promptly during periods of stress such as fever, trauma, infection, or surgery because medication requirements may change.
- Instruct patient to take miglitol three times a day with the first bite of each main meal.
- Show patient how and when to monitor glucose levels.
- Advise patient that adverse GI effects are most common during the first few weeks of therapy and should improve over time.
- Urge patient to wear or carry medical identification at all times.

☑ Evaluation
- Patient's blood glucose level is normal.
- Patient sustains no injury from drug-induced hypoglycemia.
- Patient and family state understanding of drug therapy.

milrinone lactate
(MIL-rih-nohn LAK-tayt)
Primacor

Pharmacologic class: bipyridine phosphodiesterase inhibitor
Therapeutic class: inotropic vasodilator
Pregnancy risk category: C

Indications and dosages
▶ **Short-term treatment of heart failure.** *Adults:* loading dose is 50 mcg/kg I.V., given slowly over 10 minutes, followed by continuous I.V. infusion of 0.375 to 0.75 mcg/kg/minute. Adjust infusion dose based on clinical and hemodynamic responses, as ordered.
Patients with creatinine clearance of 50 ml/minute or less: dosage is adjusted to maximum clinical effect, not to exceed 1.13 mg/kg/day.

How supplied
Injection: 1 mg/ml
Premixed injection: 200 mcg/ml in 100 ml D_5W injection; 200 mcg/ml in 200 ml D_5W injection.

Pharmacokinetics
Absorption: not applicable.
Distribution: about 70% bound to plasma protein.
Metabolism: about 12% metabolized to glucuronide metabolite.
Excretion: about 83% excreted unchanged in urine. *Half-life:* 2.3 to 2.7 hours.

Route	Onset	Peak	Duration
I.V.	5-15 min	1-2 hr	3-6 hr

Pharmacodynamics
Chemical effect: produces inotropic action by increasing cellular levels of cAMP; produces vasodilation by relaxing vascular smooth muscle.
Therapeutic effect: relieves acute signs and symptoms of heart failure.

Adverse reactions
CNS: headache.

CV: VENTRICULAR ARRHYTHMIAS, *ventricular ectopic activity,* nonsustained ventricular tachycardia, ***sustained ventricular tachycardia, ventricular fibrillation.***

Interactions

None reported.

Contraindications and precautions

- Contraindicated in patients hypersensitive to drug.
- Drug isn't recommended for patients with severe aortic or pulmonic valvular disease in place of surgical correction of obstruction or for patients in acute phase of MI.
- Use cautiously in patients with atrial flutter or fibrillation because drug slightly shortens AV node conduction time and may increase ventricular response rate. Also use cautiously in pregnant or breast-feeding women.
- Safety of drug hasn't been established in children.

NURSING CONSIDERATIONS

Assessment

- Assess patient's heart failure before therapy and regularly thereafter.
- Monitor fluid and electrolyte status, blood pressure, heart rate, and kidney function during therapy.
- Monitor patient's ECG continuously during therapy.
- Be alert for adverse reactions.
- Evaluate patient's and family's knowledge of drug therapy.

Nursing diagnoses

- Impaired gas exchange related to presence of heart failure
- Decreased cardiac output related to drug-induced cardiac arrhythmias
- Deficient knowledge related to drug therapy

Planning and implementation

- Milrinone typically is given with digoxin and diuretics.
- Inotropics may aggravate outflow tract obstruction in hypertrophic subaortic stenosis.
- Prepare I.V. infusion solution using half-normal or normal saline solution or D_5W. Prepare 100-mcg/ml solution by adding 180 ml of diluent per 20-mg (20-ml) vial, 150-mcg/ml solution by adding 113 ml of diluent per 20-mg (20-ml) vial, and 200-mcg/ml solution by adding 80 ml of diluent per 20-mg (20-ml) vial.

ALERT Improvement of cardiac output may result in enhanced urine output. Expect dosage reduction in diuretic therapy as heart failure improves. Potassium loss may predispose patient to digitalis toxicity.

- Excessive decrease in blood pressure requires discontinuation or slower infusion.

ALERT Administering furosemide into an I.V. line containing milrinone causes precipitate to form.

Patient teaching

- Tell patient to report headache; mild analgesic can be given for relief.

Evaluation

- Patient exhibits adequate gas exchange as heart failure is resolved.
- Drug-induced arrhythmias don't develop during therapy.
- Patient and family state understanding of drug therapy.

mineral oil (liquid petrolatum)

(MIN-er-ul OYL)

Fleet Enema Mineral Oil†, Kondremul†, Kondremul Plain†, Lansoyl♦, Liqui-Doss†, Milkinol†, Petrogalar Plain†

Pharmacologic class: lubricant oil
Therapeutic class: laxative
Pregnancy risk category: C

Indications and dosages

▶ **Constipation, preparation for bowel studies or surgery.** *Adults and children age 12 and older:* 5 to 45 ml P.O. h.s. Or, 120 ml P.R. (as enema).
Children ages 6 to 12: 5 to 15 ml P.O. h.s. Or, 30 to 60 ml P.R. (as enema).
Children ages 2 to 6: 30 to 60 ml P.R. (as enema).

How supplied

Emulsion: 50%†
Oral liquid: in pints, quarts, gallons†
Enema: 120 ml†, 133 ml†

Pharmacokinetics

Absorption: absorbed minimally except for emulsified drug form, which has significant absorption.
Distribution: distributed locally, primarily in colon.
Metabolism: none.
Excretion: excreted in feces.

Route	Onset	Peak	Duration
P.O., P.R.	6-8 hr	Varies	Varies

Pharmacodynamics

Chemical effect: increases water retention in stool by creating barrier between colon wall and feces that prevents colonic reabsorption of fecal water.
Therapeutic effect: relieves constipation.

Adverse reactions

GI: *nausea,* vomiting, decreased absorption of nutrients and fat-soluble vitamins, anal pruritus, diarrhea with excessive use, *abdominal cramps* (especially in severe constipation), slowed healing after hemorrhoidectomy.
Respiratory: ***lipid pneumonia.***
Other: laxative dependence with long-term or excessive use.

Interactions

Drug-drug. *Docusate salts:* may increase mineral oil absorption and cause lipid pneumonia. Separate administration times.
Fat-soluble vitamins (A, D, E, and K): possible decreased absorption after prolonged administration. Monitor patient for deficiencies.

Contraindications and precautions

- Contraindicated in patients with abdominal pain, nausea, vomiting, or other symptoms of appendicitis or acute surgical abdomen and in those with fecal impaction or intestinal obstruction or perforation.
- Use cautiously in young children; in pregnant or breast-feeding women; in elderly or debilitated patients because of susceptibility to lipid pneumonia through aspiration, absorption, and transport from intestinal mucosa; and in patients with rectal bleeding.

NURSING CONSIDERATIONS

Assessment

- Assess patient's condition before therapy and regularly thereafter.
- Before giving drug for constipation, determine whether patient has adequate fluid intake, exercise, and diet.
- Be alert for adverse reactions and drug interactions.
- Evaluate patient's and family's knowledge of drug therapy.

Nursing diagnoses

- Constipation related to underlying condition
- Risk for deficient fluid volume related to drug-induced adverse GI reactions
- Deficient knowledge related to drug therapy

Planning and implementation

P.O. use: Give drug on empty stomach.
– Give drug with fruit juice or carbonated drink to disguise taste.
P.R. use: Follow normal protocol.

Patient teaching

- Advise patient to take drug only at bedtime and not to take for more than 1 week.
- Warn patient of possible rectal leakage from excessive dosages.
- Teach patient about dietary sources of bulk, such as bran and cereals, fresh fruit, and vegetables.

Evaluation

- Patient regains normal bowel pattern.
- Patient maintains adequate hydration throughout therapy.
- Patient and family state understanding of drug therapy.

minocycline hydrochloride

(migh-noh-SIGH-kleen high-droh-KLOR-ighd)
Apo-Minocycline ◇, Dynacin, Minocin*, Minocin IV, Minomycin ◇, Minomycin IV ◇, Vectrin

Pharmacologic class: tetracycline
Therapeutic class: antibiotic
Pregnancy risk category: D

Indications and dosages

▶ **Infections caused by sensitive gram-negative and gram-positive organisms, trachoma, amebiasis.** *Adults:* 200 mg I.V.; then 100 mg I.V. q 12 hours. Maximum 400 mg/day. Or, 200 mg P.O. initially; then 100 mg P.O. q 12 hours. Some clinicians use 100 or 200 mg P.O. initially, followed by 50 mg q.i.d.
Children over age 8: initially, 4 mg/kg P.O. or I.V., followed by 2 mg/kg P.O. q 12 hours. Given I.V. in 500- to 1,000-ml solution without calcium over 6 hours.

▶ **Gonorrhea in patients sensitive to penicillin.** *Adults:* initially, 200 mg P.O.; then 100 mg q 12 hours for at least 4 days.

▶ **Syphilis in patients sensitive to penicillin.** *Adults:* initially, 200 mg P.O.; then 100 mg q 12 hours for 10 to 15 days.

▶ **Meningococcal carrier state.** *Adults:* 100 mg P.O. q 12 hours for 5 days.

▶ **Uncomplicated urethral, endocervical, or rectal infection caused by *Chlamydia trachomatis* or *Ureaplasma urealyticum*.** Adults: 100 mg P.O. b.i.d. for at least 7 days.

▶ **Uncomplicated gonococcal urethritis in men.** *Adults:* 100 mg P.O. b.i.d. for 5 days.

How supplied

Tablets (film-coated): 50 mg, 100 mg
Capsules: 50 mg, 100 mg
Oral suspension: 50 mg/5 ml
Injection: 100 mg

Pharmacokinetics

Absorption: 90% to 100% absorbed after P.O. administration.
Distribution: distributed widely in body tissues and fluids, including synovial, pleural, prostatic, and seminal fluids; bronchial secretions; saliva; and aqueous humor. CSF penetration is poor. Drug is 70% to 80% protein-bound.
Metabolism: metabolized partially.
Excretion: excreted primarily unchanged in liver. *Half-life:* 11 to 26 hours.

Route	Onset	Peak	Duration
P.O.	Unknown	1-4 hr	Unknown
I.V.	Immediate	Immediate	Unknown

Pharmacodynamics

Chemical effect: unknown; may exert bacteriostatic effect by binding to ribosomal subunit of microorganisms, inhibiting protein synthesis.
Therapeutic effect: hinders bacterial cell growth. Spectrum of activity includes many gram-negative and gram-positive organisms, *Chlamydia, Mycoplasma, Rickettsia,* and spirochetes.

Adverse reactions

CNS: *light-headedness or dizziness from vestibular toxicity,* ***intracranial hypertension (pseudotumor cerebri).***
CV: pericarditis, *thrombophlebitis.*
EENT: dysphagia, glossitis.
GI: *anorexia,* epigastric distress, oral candidiasis, *nausea,* vomiting, *diarrhea,* enterocolitis, inflammatory lesions in anogenital region.
GU: increased BUN level.
Hematologic: ***neutropenia,*** eosinophilia, ***thrombocytopenia.***
Hepatic: elevated liver enzyme levels.
Musculoskeletal: and bone growth retardation if used in children under age 8; superinfection.
Skin: *maculopapular and erythematous rashes, photosensitivity, increased pigmentation, urticaria.*
Other: permanent discoloration of teeth, enamel defects, hypersensitivity reactions (***anaphylaxis***).

Interactions

Drug-drug. *Antacids (including sodium bicarbonate) and laxatives containing aluminum, magnesium, or calcium; antidiarrheals:* de-

creased antibiotic absorption. Give antibiotic 1 hour before or 2 hours after these drugs.
Ferrous sulfate, other iron products, zinc: decreased antibiotic absorption. Give drug 3 hours after or 2 hours before iron.
Methoxyflurane: may cause nephrotoxicity with tetracyclines. Monitor patient carefully.
Oral anticoagulants: increased anticoagulant effect. Monitor PT and INR and adjust dosage, as ordered.
Oral contraceptives: decreased contraceptive effectiveness and increased risk of breakthrough bleeding. Recommend nonhormonal form of birth control.
Penicillins: may interfere with bactericidal action of penicillins. Avoid using together.
Drug-lifestyle. *Sun exposure:* photosensitivity reactions may occur. Urge precautions.

Contraindications and precautions

- Contraindicated in patients hypersensitive to drug or other tetracyclines.
- Drug isn't recommended for breast-feeding women.
- Use cautiously in patients with impaired kidney or liver function. Use of this drug during last half of pregnancy and in children under age 8 may cause permanent discoloration of teeth, enamel defects, and bone growth retardation.

NURSING CONSIDERATIONS

Assessment

- Assess patient's infection before therapy and regularly thereafter.
- Obtain specimen for culture and sensitivity tests before giving first dose. Therapy may begin pending results.
- Be alert for adverse reactions and drug interactions.
- Monitor patient's hydration status if adverse GI reactions occur.
- Evaluate patient's and family's knowledge of drug therapy.

Nursing diagnoses

- Infection related to presence of susceptible bacteria
- Risk for deficient fluid volume related to drug-induced adverse reactions
- Deficient knowledge related to drug therapy

Planning and implementation

ALERT Don't confuse minocin with niacin and mithracin.
ALERT Check expiration date. Outdated or deteriorated tetracyclines have been linked to reversible nephrotoxicity (Fanconi's syndrome).
- Don't expose these drugs to light or heat. Keep cap tightly closed.

P.O. use: Follow normal protocol.
I.V. use: Reconstitute 100 mg of powder with 5 ml of sterile water for injection, with further dilution of 500 to 1,000 ml for I.V. infusion. Solution is stable for 24 hours at room temperature.
– Thrombophlebitis may develop with I.V. administration of drug. Avoid extravasation. Switch to P.O. form as soon as possible.
- Drug may cause tooth discoloration in children and young adults. Inform prescriber if brown pigmentation occurs.
- Parenteral form may cause false-positive reading of copper sulfate tests (Clinitest). All forms may cause false-negative reading of glucose enzymatic tests (Diastix).

Patient teaching

- Inform patient that drug may be taken with food, and instruct him to take drug exactly as prescribed.
- Instruct patient to take oral form of drug with full glass of water, and to avoid taking it within 1 hour of bedtime to avoid esophagitis.
- Warn patient to avoid hazardous tasks until adverse CNS effects of drug are known.
- Warn patient to avoid direct sunlight and ultraviolet light, to use a sunblock, and wear protective clothing.
- Advise patient using oral contraceptives that another form of birth control should be used. Also inform her that she may experience breakthrough bleeding.

Evaluation

- Patient is free from infection.
- Patient maintains adequate hydration throughout therapy.
- Patient and family state understanding of drug therapy.

minoxidil

(migh-NOKS-uh-dil)
Loniten

Pharmacologic class: peripheral vasodilator
Therapeutic class: antihypertensive
Pregnancy risk category: C

Indications and dosages

▶ **Severe hypertension.** *Adults:* initially, 5 mg P.O. as single dose. Effective dosage range is usually 10 to 40 mg daily. Maximum dosage is 100 mg daily.
Children under age 12: 0.2 mg/kg P.O. (maximum 5 mg) as single daily dose. Effective dosage range usually is 0.25 to 1 mg/kg daily. Maximum dosage is 50 mg.

How supplied

Tablets: 2.5 mg, 10 mg, 25 mg ◊

Pharmacokinetics

Absorption: absorbed rapidly from GI tract.
Distribution: distributed widely in body tissues; not bound to plasma proteins.
Metabolism: about 90% metabolized.
Excretion: excreted primarily in urine. *Half-life:* 4.2 hours.

Route	Onset	Peak	Duration
P.O.	About 30 min	≤ 1 hr	2-5 days

Pharmacodynamics

Chemical effect: unknown; produces direct arteriolar vasodilation.
Therapeutic effect: lowers blood pressure.

Adverse reactions

CV: *edema, tachycardia, pericardial effusion and tamponade,* ***heart failure,*** ECG changes.
Metabolic: weight gain.
Skin: *hypertrichosis* (elongation, thickening, and enhanced pigmentation of fine body hair), rash, ***Stevens-Johnson syndrome.***
Other: breast tenderness.

Interactions

Drug-drug. *Guanethidine:* severe orthostatic hypotension. Advise patient to stand up slowly.

Contraindications and precautions

- Contraindicated in patients hypersensitive to drug and in those with pheochromocytoma.
- Drug isn't recommended for breast-feeding women.
- Use cautiously in pregnant women and in patients with impaired kidney function or recent acute MI.

NURSING CONSIDERATIONS

Assessment

- Obtain history of patient's blood pressure and pulse rate before therapy and reassess regularly thereafter.
- Be alert for adverse reactions and drug interactions.
- Monitor fluid intake and output and check for weight gain and edema.
- Evaluate patient's and family's knowledge of drug therapy.

Nursing diagnoses

- Risk for injury related to presence of hypertension
- Excessive fluid volume related to drug-induced edema
- Deficient knowledge related to drug therapy

Planning and implementation

ALERT Don't confuse Loniten with Lotensin.
- Drug is removed by hemodialysis. Administer dose after dialysis.
- Drug usually is prescribed with a beta blocker to control tachycardia and a diuretic to counteract fluid retention.
- Notify prescriber if blood pressure changes significantly or pulse rate rises more than 20 beats/minute from baseline.

Patient teaching

- Make sure patient reads package insert describing drug's adverse reactions. Provide verbal explanation.

• Teach patient how to take his own pulse and instruct him to report increases over 20 beats/minute to prescriber.
• Tell patient not to suddenly stop taking drug but to call prescriber if unpleasant adverse effects occur.
• Tell patient to weigh himself at least weekly and to report weight gain of more than 5 lb (2.27 kg).
• Inform patient that excessive hair growth commonly occurs within 3 to 6 weeks of beginning treatment. Unwanted hair can be removed by depilatory cream or by shaving. Assure patient that extra hair will disappear within 1 to 6 months of stopping minoxidil. Advise him not to discontinue drug without prescriber's approval.

Evaluation
• Patient's blood pressure is normal.
• Patient exhibits no evidence of edema throughout therapy.
• Patient and family state understanding of drug therapy.

mirtazapine
(mir-TAH-zuh-peen)
Remeron

Pharmacologic class: piperazinoazepine group of compounds
Therapeutic class: antidepressant
Pregnancy risk category: C

Indications and dosages
▶ **Depression.** *Adults:* initially, 15 mg P.O. h.s. Maintenance dosage is 15 to 45 mg daily. Adjust dosage at intervals of at least 1 to 2 weeks.

How supplied
Tablets: 15 mg, 30 mg

Pharmacokinetics
Absorption: rapidly absorbed.
Distribution: 85% bound to plasma proteins.
Metabolism: extensively metabolized in liver.
Excretion: mainly excreted in urine; some in feces. *Mean elimination half-life:* about 20 to 40 hours.

Route	Onset	Peak	Duration
P.O.	Unknown	Within 2 hr	Unknown

Pharmacodynamics
Chemical effect: enhances central noradrenergic and serotonergic activity; potent antagonist of histamine receptors.
Therapeutic effect: relieves depression.

Adverse reactions
CNS: somnolence, dizziness, asthenia, abnormal dreams, abnormal thinking, tremors, confusion.
CV: edema, peripheral edema.
GI: nausea, increased appetite, dry mouth, constipation.
GU: urinary frequency.
Metabolic: weight gain.
Musculoskeletal: back pain, myalgia.
Respiratory: dyspnea.
Other: flu syndrome.

Interactions
Drug-drug. *Diazepam, other CNS depressants:* possible additive CNS effects. Avoid concomitant use.
MAO inhibitors: potentially serious, sometimes fatal reactions. Don't use drug within 14 days of an MAO inhibitor.
Drug-lifestyle. *Alcohol use:* possible additive CNS effects. Discourage concomitant use.

Contraindications and precautions
• Contraindicated in patients hypersensitive to drug.
• Use cautiously in patients with CV or cerebrovascular disease, seizure disorders, suicidal ideations, impaired hepatic or renal function, or history of mania or hypomania.
• Coadministration with MAO inhibitors is contraindicated.

NURSING CONSIDERATIONS

Assessment
• Stop drug and monitor patient closely if he develops a sore throat, fever, stomatitis, or

other signs of infection together with a low WBC count.
- Evaluate patient's and family's knowledge of drug therapy.

Nursing diagnoses
- Disturbed thought processes related to adverse effects
- Risk for injury related to sedation and orthostatic hypotension
- Deficient knowledge related to drug therapy

Planning and implementation
- Use cautiously when administering drug to breast-feeding women.

Patient teaching
- Warn patient to avoid hazardous activities if somnolence occurs.
- Tell patient to report signs and symptoms of infection or flulike symptoms.
- Advise patient to avoid alcohol or other CNS depressants.
- Stress importance of compliance with therapy.
- Instruct patient not to take other drugs without prescriber's approval.
- Tell woman to notify prescriber if she suspects pregnancy or if she is breast-feeding.

Evaluation
- Patient regains normal thought processes.
- Patient sustains no injury from adverse reactions.
- Patient and family state understanding of drug therapy.

misoprostol
(mee-SOH-pruh-stol)
Cytotec

Pharmacologic class: prostaglandin E_1 analogue
Therapeutic class: gastric mucosal protectant
Pregnancy risk category: X

Indications and dosages
▶ **Prevention of NSAID-induced gastric ulcer in elderly or debilitated patients at high risk for complications from gastric ulcer and in patients with history of NSAID-induced ulcer.** *Adults:* 200 mcg P.O. q.i.d. with food. If dosage isn't tolerated, decreased to 100 mcg P.O. q.i.d.

How supplied
Tablets: 100 mcg, 200 mcg

Pharmacokinetics
Absorption: absorbed rapidly from GI tract.
Distribution: highly bound to plasma proteins.
Metabolism: rapidly de-esterified to misoprostol acid, the biologically active metabolite.
Excretion: about 15% excreted in feces; balance excreted in urine. *Half-life:* 20 to 40 minutes.

Route	Onset	Peak	Duration
P.O.	30 min	10-15 min	About 3 hr

Pharmacodynamics
Chemical effect: replaces gastric prostaglandins depleted by NSAID therapy. Misoprostol also decreases basal and stimulated gastric acid secretion and may increase gastric mucus and bicarbonate production.
Therapeutic effect: protects gastric mucosa from ulcerating.

Adverse reactions
CNS: headache.
GI: *diarrhea, abdominal pain,* nausea, flatulence, dyspepsia, vomiting, constipation.
GU: hypermenorrhea, dysmenorrhea, spotting, cramps, menstrual disorders.

Interactions
Drug-drug. *Antacids:* reduced plasma levels of misoprostol. Not considered significant.

Contraindications and precautions
- Contraindicated in pregnant or breast-feeding women and in patients with history of allergy to prostaglandins.

NURSING CONSIDERATIONS

Assessment
- Obtain history of patient's GI condition before therapy.

• In woman of childbearing age, make sure that negative pregnancy test is obtained within 2 weeks before therapy begins.
• Be alert for adverse reactions and drug interactions.
• Evaluate patient's and family's knowledge of drug therapy.

Nursing diagnoses

• Risk for injury related to potential for gastric ulceration
• Acute pain related to headache
• Deficient knowledge related to drug therapy

Planning and implementation

• Drug shouldn't be routinely administered to women of childbearing age unless they are at high risk for development of ulcers or complications from NSAID-induced ulcers.
ALERT Take special precautions to prevent use of drug during pregnancy. Make sure patient is fully aware of dangers of misoprostol to fetus and that she receives both verbal and written warnings regarding these dangers. Also make sure patient can comply with effective contraceptive means.

Patient teaching

• Instruct patient not to share drug. Remind her that drug may cause miscarriage, usually with life-threatening bleeding.
• Advise her not to begin therapy until second or third day of next normal menstrual period.

Evaluation

• Patient remains free from signs and symptoms of gastric ulceration.
• Patient states that drug-induced headache doesn't occur.
• Patient and family state understanding of drug therapy.

mitomycin (mitomycin-C)

(might-oh-MIGH-sin)
Mutamycin

Pharmacologic class: antineoplastic antibiotic (cell cycle–phase nonspecific)
Therapeutic class: antineoplastic
Pregnancy risk category: NR

Indications and dosages

Dosage and indications may vary. Check protocol with prescriber.
▶ **Pancreatic and stomach cancers.** *Adults:* 20 mg/m^2 I.V. as single dose. Cycle repeated after 6 to 8 weeks, with dosage adjusted if needed based on nadir WBC and platelet counts.

How supplied

Injection: 5-mg, 20-mg, 40-mg vials

Pharmacokinetics

Absorption: not applicable with I.V. administration.
Distribution: distributed widely in body tissues; doesn't cross blood-brain barrier.
Metabolism: metabolized by hepatic microsomal enzymes and deactivated in kidneys, spleen, brain, and heart.
Excretion: excreted primarily in urine; small portion excreted in bile and feces. *Half-life:* about 50 minutes.

Route	Onset	Peak	Duration
I.V.	Unknown	Unknown	Unknown

Pharmacodynamics

Chemical effect: acts like alkylating agent, cross-linking strands of DNA. This causes imbalance of cell growth, leading to cell death.
Therapeutic effect: kills certain cancer cells.

Adverse reactions

GI: *nausea, vomiting,* anorexia, stomatitis.
Hematologic: THROMBOCYTOPENIA, LEUKOPENIA (may be delayed up to 8 weeks and be cumulative with successive doses), ***microangiopathic hemolytic anemia.***
Respiratory: ***interstitial pneumonitis.***
Skin: desquamation, induration, pruritus, and *pain* at injection site; ***septicemia,*** cellulitis, ulceration, and sloughing with extravasation; *reversible alopecia;* purple coloration of nail beds.

Interactions

Drug-drug. *Vinca alkaloids:* may cause acute respiratory distress. Avoid concomitant use.

Contraindications and precautions

- Contraindicated in patients hypersensitive to drug and in those with thrombocytopenia, coagulation disorder, or increased bleeding tendency from other causes.
- Drug isn't recommended for pregnant or breast-feeding women.
- Safety of drug hasn't been established in children.

NURSING CONSIDERATIONS

Assessment

- Assess patient's condition before therapy and regularly thereafter.
- Obtain CBC and blood studies, as ordered.
- Monitor kidney function tests, as ordered.
- Be alert for adverse reactions and drug interactions.
- Evaluate patient's and family's knowledge of drug therapy.

Nursing diagnoses

- Ineffective health maintenance related to presence of neoplastic disease
- Ineffective protection related to adverse hematologic reactions
- Deficient knowledge related to drug therapy

Planning and implementation

ALERT Don't confuse mitomycin with mithramycin.

- Follow facility policy to reduce risks. Preparation and administration of parenteral form are related to mutagenic, teratogenic, and carcinogenic risks to personnel.
- Using sterile water for injection, reconstitute 5-mg vials with 10 ml, 20-mg vials with 40 ml, and 40-mg vials with 80 ml.
- For infusion, dilute with normal saline solution injection, D_5W, or sodium lactate for injection. After dilution, drug is stable at room temperature for 3 hours in D_5W, 12 hours in normal saline solution injection, and 24 hours in sodium lactate for injection.
- Avoid extravasation. If it occurs, stop infusion immediately and notify prescriber because of potential for severe ulceration and necrosis.
- Never administer drug I.M. or S.C.

Patient teaching

- Instruct patient to watch for signs of infection and bleeding and to take temperature daily.
- Warn patient that alopecia may occur but assure him that it's reversible.
- Tell patient to report adverse reactions to prescriber promptly.

Evaluation

- Patient responds well to therapy.
- Patient doesn't develop serious complications.
- Patient and family state understanding of drug therapy.

mitotane (o,p′-DDD)

(MIGH-toh-tayn)

Lysodren

Pharmacologic class: chlorophenothane (DDT) analogue
Therapeutic class: antineoplastic
Pregnancy risk category: C

Indications and dosages

▶ **Inoperable adrenocortical cancer.** *Adults:* initially, 2 to 6 g P.O. daily in divided doses t.i.d. or q.i.d.; increased to 9 to 10 g P.O. daily in divided doses t.i.d. or q.i.d. Dosage is adjusted until maximum tolerated dosage is achieved (varies from 2 to 19 g/day but is usually 8 to 10 g/day).

How supplied

Tablets (scored): 500 mg

Pharmacokinetics

Absorption: 35% to 40% absorbed across GI tract.
Distribution: widely distributed in body tissue; fatty tissue is primary storage site. Slow release of drug from fatty tissue into plasma occurs after drug is discontinued.

Metabolism: metabolized in liver and other tissue.
Excretion: excreted in urine and bile. *Half-life:* 18 to 159 days.

Route	Onset	Peak	Duration
P.O.	2-3 days (steroid); ≤ 6 mo (tumor)	3-5 hr	Unknown

Pharmacodynamics

Chemical effect: unknown; thought to selectively destroy adrenocortical tissue and hinder extra-adrenal metabolism of cortisol.
Therapeutic effect: hinders adrenocortical cancer cell growth.

Adverse reactions

CNS: *depression, somnolence, lethargy, vertigo,* brain damage and dysfunction in long-term high-dose therapy.
CV: hypertension.
EENT: visual disturbances.
GI: *severe nausea, vomiting,* diarrhea, anorexia.
GU: hemorrhagic cystitis.
Skin: dermatitis, maculopapular rash.
Other: hypouricemia, increased serum cholesterol level, adrenal insufficiency.

Interactions

Drug-drug. *Corticosteroids:* corticosteroid metabolism may be altered; higher corticosteroid doses may be needed.
Warfarin: increased metabolism, which may require higher warfarin doses. Monitor PT and INR closely.

Contraindications and precautions

- Contraindicated in patients hypersensitive to drug and in those who are in shock or who have suffered trauma.
- Drug isn't recommended for breast-feeding women.
- Use cautiously in patients with hepatic disease and in pregnant women.
- Safety of drug hasn't been established in children.

NURSING CONSIDERATIONS

Assessment

- Obtain history of patient's adrenocortical cancer before therapy.
- Monitor effectiveness according to reduction in pain, weakness, and anorexia.
- Assess and record behavioral and neurologic signs daily throughout therapy. Prolonged therapy has been linked to significant neurologic impairment.
- Be alert for adverse reactions.
- Monitor patient's hydration status if adverse GI reactions occur.
- Evaluate patient's and family's knowledge of drug therapy.

Nursing diagnoses

- Ineffective health maintenance related to presence of neoplastic disease
- Risk for deficient fluid volume related to drug-induced adverse GI reactions
- Deficient knowledge related to drug therapy

Planning and implementation

- Give antiemetic before mitotane, as ordered.
- Be prepared to reduce dosage if adverse GI or skin reactions are severe.
- Use of corticosteroids may avoid acute adrenocorticoid insufficiency and is usually required. Glucocorticoid dosage should be increased in periods of stress, such as infection or trauma, as ordered.
- Drug is distributed mostly to body fat. Obese patients may need higher dosage and have longer-lasting adverse reactions.
- Adequate therapeutic trial is at least 3 months, but treatment can continue if clinical benefits are observed.
- Monitor PT and INR on patient receiving mitotane and warfarin concurrently.

Patient teaching

- Warn patient to avoid activities that require alertness and good motor coordination until CNS effects of drug are known.
- Tell patient to report adverse reactions promptly.
- For patient also receiving warfarin, instruct him to watch for and report signs of bleeding.

Evaluation
- Patient responds well to therapy.
- Patient maintains adequate hydration throughout therapy.
- Patient and family state understanding of drug therapy.

mitoxantrone hydrochloride
(migh-toh-ZAN-trohn high-droh-KLOR-ighd)
Novantrone

Pharmacologic class: antibiotic antineoplastic
Therapeutic class: antineoplastic
Pregnancy risk category: D

Indications and dosages
▶ **Combination initial therapy for acute nonlymphocytic leukemia.** *Adults:* induction begins with 12 mg/m² I.V. daily on days 1 through 3, in combination with 100 mg/m² daily of cytarabine on days 1 through 7. A second induction may be given if response isn't adequate. Maintenance therapy: 12 mg/m² on days 1 and 2, in combination with cytarabine on days 1 through 5.

How supplied
Injection: 2 mg/ml in 10-ml, 12.5-ml, 15-ml vials

Pharmacokinetics
Absorption: not applicable.
Distribution: 78% plasma protein–bound.
Metabolism: metabolized by liver.
Excretion: excreted by way of renal and hepatobiliary systems. *Half-life:* 5.8 days.

Route	Onset	Peak	Duration
I.V.	Unknown	Unknown	Unknown

Pharmacodynamics
Chemical effect: not fully understood; probably cell cycle–nonspecific. Drug reacts with DNA, producing cytotoxic effect.
Therapeutic effect: hinders susceptible cancer cell growth.

Adverse reactions
CNS: ***seizures,*** headache.
CV: ***heart failure, arrhythmias,*** tachycardia.
EENT: conjunctivitis.
GI: *bleeding, abdominal pain, diarrhea, nausea, mucositis, vomiting, stomatitis.*
GU: uric acid nephropathy, ***renal failure.***
Hematologic: ***myelosuppression.***
Hepatic: jaundice.
Metabolic: hyperuricemia.
Respiratory: dyspnea, cough.
Skin: petechiae, ecchymoses, alopecia.

Interactions
None significant.

Contraindications and precautions
- Contraindicated in patients hypersensitive to drug.
- Drug isn't recommended for pregnant or breast-feeding women.
- Use cautiously in patients previously exposed to anthracyclines or other cardiotoxic drugs.
- Safety of drug hasn't been established in children.

NURSING CONSIDERATIONS

Assessment
- Assess patient's condition before therapy and regularly thereafter.
- Monitor hematologic and laboratory chemistry parameters, as ordered.
- Left ventricular ejection fraction should be monitored.
- Be alert for adverse reactions and drug interactions.
- Evaluate patient's and family's knowledge of drug therapy.

Nursing diagnoses
- Ineffective health maintenance related to presence of leukemia
- Ineffective immune protection related to drug-induced myelosuppression
- Deficient knowledge related to drug therapy

Planning and implementation
- Patients with significant myelosuppression shouldn't receive drug unless benefits outweigh risks.

• Follow facility policy to minimize risks. Preparation and administration of parenteral form are linked to mutagenic, teratogenic, and carcinogenic risks to personnel.
• Dilute dose (available as aqueous solution of 2 mg/ml in volumes of 10, 12.5, and 15 ml) in at least 50 ml of normal saline solution injection or D_5W injection. Administer drug by direct injection into free-flowing I.V. line of normal saline solution or D_5W injection over at least 3 minutes. Don't mix with other drugs. Heparin is physically incompatible. Don't mix.
• Although drug isn't a vesicant, discontinue infusion immediately and notify prescriber if it extravasates.
• Be prepared to give allopurinol, as ordered. Uric acid nephropathy can be avoided by adequately hydrating patient before and during therapy.
• If severe nonhematologic toxicity occurs during first course of therapy, second course should be delayed until patient recovers.
• Store undiluted solution at room temperature. Once diluted, mixture is stable for 7 days at room temperature.

Patient teaching
• Inform patient that urine may appear blue-green within 24 hours after administration and that some bluish discoloration of sclera may occur. These effects aren't harmful.
• Teach patient infection-control and bleeding precautions. Tell him to watch for and report signs of bleeding and infection.
• Advise woman of childbearing age to avoid pregnancy during therapy and to consult prescriber before becoming pregnant.

☑ Evaluation
• Patient responds well to therapy.
• Patient develops no serious complications from drug-induced myelosuppression.
• Patient and family state understanding of drug therapy.

mivacurium chloride
(migh-vuh-KYOO-ree-um KLOR-ighd)
Mivacron

Pharmacologic class: nondepolarizing neuromuscular blocker
Therapeutic class: skeletal muscle relaxant
Pregnancy risk category: C

Indications and dosages
▶ **Adjunct to general anesthesia, to facilitate endotracheal intubation, and to relax skeletal muscles during surgery or mechanical ventilation.** *Adults:* dosage is highly individualized. Usually, 0.15 mg/kg I.V. push over 5 to 15 seconds provides adequate muscle relaxation within 135 seconds for endotracheal intubation. Supplemental doses of 0.1 mg/kg I.V. q 15 minutes is usually sufficient to maintain muscle relaxation. Or, maintain neuromuscular blockade with continuous infusion of 4 mcg/kg/minute begun simultaneously with initial dose, or 9 to 10 mcg/kg/minute started after evidence of spontaneous recovery caused by initial dose. When used with isoflurane or enflurane anesthesia, dosage usually is reduced about 35% to 40%.
Children ages 2 to 12: 0.2 mg/kg I.V. push given over 5 to 15 seconds. Neuromuscular blockade is usually evident in less than 2 minutes. Maintenance doses are generally required more frequently in children. Or, neuromuscular blockade maintained with continuous I.V. infusion adjusted to effect. Most children respond to 5 to 31 mcg/kg/minute (average 14 mcg/kg/minute).

How supplied
Injection: 2 mg/ml in 5-ml and 10-ml vials
Infusion: 0.5 mg/ml in 50 ml of D_5W

Pharmacokinetics
Absorption: not applicable.
Distribution: not extensively distributed to tissues.
Metabolism: rapidly hydrolyzed by plasma pseudocholinesterase to inactive components.
Excretion: metabolites excreted in urine and bile. *Half-life: cis-trans* and *trans-trans* iso-

mers, less than 2.3 minutes; *cis-cis* isomer, 55 minutes.

Route	Onset	Peak	Duration
I.V.	1-2 min	2-5 min	20-35 min

Pharmacodynamics

Chemical effect: competes with acetylcholine for receptor sites at motor end plate. Because this action may be antagonized by cholinesterase inhibitors, drug is considered a competitive antagonist. Drug is mixture of three stereoisomers, each with neuromuscular blocking activity.
Therapeutic effect: relaxes skeletal muscles.

Adverse reactions

CNS: dizziness.
CV: *flushing,* hypotension, tachycardia, ***bradycardia, arrhythmias,*** phlebitis.
Musculoskeletal: prolonged muscle weakness, muscle spasms.
Respiratory: ***bronchospasm,*** wheezing, ***respiratory insufficiency or apnea.***
Skin: rash, urticaria, erythema.

Interactions

Drug-drug. *Alkaline solutions (such as barbiturate solutions):* physically incompatible; precipitate may form. Don't administer through same I.V. line.
Aminoglycosides (gentamicin, kanamycin, neomycin, streptomycin), bacitracin, colistimethate, colistin, polymyxin B sulfate, tetracycline: potentiated neuromuscular blockade, leading to increased skeletal muscle relaxation and prolonged effect. Use together cautiously.
Carbamazepine, phenytoin: may prolong time to maximal blockade or shorten duration of neuromuscular blockers. Monitor patient.
Inhaled anesthetics (especially enflurane, isoflurane), magnesium salts, quinidine: may enhance activity or prolong action of nondepolarizing neuromuscular blockers. Monitor patient for excessive weakness.

Contraindications and precautions

- Contraindicated in patients hypersensitive to drug.
- Use very cautiously, if at all, in patients who are homozygous for atypical plasma pseudocholinesterase gene. Drug is metabolized to inactive compounds by plasma pseudocholinesterase.
- Use cautiously in patients with significant CV disease, in those who may be adversely affected by release of histamine (such as asthmatic patients), and in pregnant or breast-feeding women.
- Also use cautiously, possibly at reduced dosage, in debilitated patients; in patients with metastatic cancer, severe electrolyte disturbances, or neuromuscular diseases; and in those in whom potentiation or difficulty in reversal of neuromuscular blockade is anticipated. Patients with myasthenia gravis or myasthenic syndrome (Eaton-Lambert syndrome) are particularly sensitive to effects of nondepolarizing relaxants.

NURSING CONSIDERATIONS

Assessment

- Assess patient's need for drug before therapy and regularly thereafter.
- Monitor respiratory rate closely until patient is fully recovered from neuromuscular blockade, as evidenced by tests of muscle strength (hand grip, head lift, and ability to cough).
- Be alert for adverse reactions and drug interactions.
- Evaluate patient's and family's knowledge of drug therapy.

Nursing diagnoses

- Ineffective breathing pattern related to drug's effect on respiratory muscle
- Deficient knowledge related to drug therapy

Planning and implementation

ALERT Don't confuse Mivacron with Mazicon or Mevacor.
ALERT Administer only under direct medical supervision of clinician skilled in use of neuromuscular blockers and techniques for maintaining airway. Don't use unless emergency equipment for respiratory support and antagonist are within reach.
- To avoid patient distress, don't administer until patient's consciousness is obtunded by

general anesthetic because drug has no effect on consciousness or pain threshold.
- Administer test dose to assess patient's sensitivity to drug. Patients with severe burns develop resistance to nondepolarizing neuromuscular blockers; however, they also may have reduced plasma pseudocholinesterase activity.
- Drug may be given by direct injection over 5 to 15 seconds.
- Prepare drug for I.V. use with D_5W, normal saline solution injection, D_5W in normal saline solution injection, lactated Ringer's injection, or D_5W in lactated Ringer's injection. Diluted solutions are stable for 24 hours at room temperature.
- When diluted as directed, drug is compatible with alfentanil, fentanyl, sufentanil, droperidol, and midazolam.
- For drug available as premixed infusion in D_5W, remove protective outer wrap, and then check container for minor leaks by squeezing bag before administering. Don't add other drugs to container, and don't use container in series connections.
- Nerve stimulator and train-of-four monitoring are recommended to document antagonism of neuromuscular blockade and recovery of muscle strength. Before attempting reversal with neostigmine or edrophonium, some signs of spontaneous recovery should be evident.
- Experimental evidence suggests that acid-base and electrolyte balances may influence actions of nondepolarizing neuromuscular blockers. Alkalosis may counteract paralysis; acidosis may enhance it.
- Dosage should be adjusted to ideal body weight in obese patients (patients 30% or more above their ideal weight) to avoid prolonged neuromuscular blockade.
- Duration of effect is increased about 150% in patients with end-stage renal disease and 300% in patients with hepatic dysfunction.
- Like other neuromuscular blockers, dosage requirements for children are higher on mg/kg basis than those for adults. Onset and recovery of neuromuscular blockade occur more rapidly in children.

Patient teaching
- Describe use of drug to patient and family, and answer their questions.

☑ Evaluation
- Patient maintains adequate ventilation with or without assistance.
- Patient and family state understanding of drug therapy.

modafinil
(moh-DAF-ih-nil)
Provigil

Pharmacologic class: nonamphetamine CNS stimulant
Therapeutic class: analeptic
Controlled substance schedule: IV
Pregnancy risk category: C

Indications and dosages
▶ **Improvement of wakefulness in patients with excessive daytime sleepiness caused by narcolepsy.** *Adults:* 200 mg P.O. daily, given as a single dose in the morning. In patients with severe hepatic impairment, 100 mg P.O. daily, given as a single dose in the morning.

How supplied
Tablets: 100 mg, 200 mg

Pharmacokinetics
Absorption: rapid, with plasma levels peaking in 2 to 4 hours.
Distribution: well distributed in body tissue. About 60% binds to plasma protein, primarily albumin.
Metabolism: about 90% of drug is metabolized in the liver, with subsequent renal elimination of the metabolites.
Excretion: less than 10% is excreted from the kidneys as unchanged drug.

Route	Onset	Peak	Duration
P.O.	Unknown	2-4 hr	Unknown

Pharmacodynamics
Chemical effect: unknown. It has wake-promoting actions similar to those of sympathomimetics, including amphetamines, but it's structurally distinct from amphetamines and doesn't appear to alter the release of either

dopamine or norepinephrine to produce CNS stimulation.
Therapeutic effect: improved daytime wakefulness.

Adverse reactions

CNS: *headache,* nervousness, dizziness, depression, anxiety, cataplexy, insomnia, paresthesia, dyskinesia, hypertonia, confusion, amnesia, emotional lability, ataxia, tremor.
CV: hypotension, hypertension, vasodilation, ***arrhythmias,*** syncope, chest pain.
EENT: *rhinitis,* pharyngitis, epistaxis, amblyopia, abnormal vision.
GI: *nausea,* diarrhea, dry mouth, mouth ulcer, gingivitis, thirst, anorexia, vomiting.
GU: abnormal urine, urine retention, abnormal ejaculation, albuminuria.
Hematologic: eosinophilia.
Hepatic: abnormal liver function.
Metabolic: hyperglycemia.
Musculoskeletal: neck pain, rigid neck, joint disorder.
Respiratory: lung disorder, dyspnea, asthma.
Skin: herpes simplex, dry skin.
Other: chills, fever.

Interactions

Drug-drug. *Carbamazepine, phenobarbital, rifampin, other inducers of CYP3A4; itraconazole, ketoconazole, other inhibitors of CYP3A4:* altered modafinil levels. Monitor patient closely.
Cyclosporine, theophylline: reduced serum levels of these drugs. Use together cautiously.
Diazepam, phenytoin, propranolol, other drugs metabolized by CYP2C19: modafinil is a reversible inhibitor of cytochrome P-450 isoenzyme CYP2C19, and thus may increase serum levels of drugs that this enzyme metabolizes. Use together cautiously. Adjust dosage as necessary.
Hormonal contraceptives: reduced serum levels of these drugs, resulting in reduced contraceptive effectiveness. Recommend additional or alternative contraceptive method during modafinil therapy and for 1 month afterward.
Methylphenidate: delayed modafinil absorption. Separate administration times.
Phenytoin, warfarin: concentration-dependent inhibition of CYP2C9 activity and increased serum levels of phenytoin and warfarin. Monitor patient closely for signs of toxicity.
Tricyclic antidepressants (such as clomipramine, desipramine): increased tricyclic antidepressant levels. Reduce dosage of these drugs, as directed.

Contraindications and precautions

- Contraindicated in patients hypersensitive to modafinil. Don't use in patients with a history of left ventricular hypertrophy or ischemic ECG changes, chest pain, arrhythmias, or other signs or symptoms of mitral valve prolapse caused by CNS stimulant use.
- Use cautiously in patients with recent MI or unstable angina and in those with history of psychosis.
- Use cautiously and at reduced dosage in patients with severe hepatic impairment, with or without cirrhosis.
- Also use cautiously in patients concurrently treated with MAO inhibitors.

NURSING CONSIDERATIONS

Assessment
- Obtain history of patient's underlying condition before therapy, and reassess regularly thereafter.
- Assess patient's renal function before starting drug therapy.
- Monitor hypertensive patients on modafinil therapy closely.
- Evaluate patient's and family's knowledge about drug therapy.

Nursing diagnoses
- Disturbed sleep pattern related to drug-induced insomnia
- Risk for injury related to drug-induced CNS adverse effects
- Deficient knowledge related to drug therapy

Planning and implementation
- Food has no effect on overall bioavailability, but it may delay modafinil absorption by 1 hour.
- Although single, daily, 400-mg doses have been well tolerated, no consistent evidence exists that this dosage provides additional benefit beyond the 200-mg dose.

Patient teaching

- Modafinil may impair judgment. Advise patient to be careful while driving or performing other activities that require alertness until full effects of drug are known.
- Instruct patient not to take other prescription or OTC drugs without consulting prescriber because of possible drug interactions.
- Advise patient to avoid alcohol while taking modafinil.
- Tell patient to notify prescriber if he develops a rash, hives, or a related allergic reaction.
- Caution woman that concurrent use of hormonal contraceptives (including depot or implantable contraceptives) with modafinil tablets may increase the risk of pregnancy. Recommend an alternative or additional method of contraception during modafinil therapy and for 1 month afterward.
- Advise woman to notify prescriber if she becomes pregnant or intends to become pregnant during therapy.
- Tell woman to notify prescriber if she's breast-feeding.

✓ Evaluation

- Patient develops and maintains normal sleep-wake patterns.
- Patient has no adverse CNS effects.
- Patient and family state understanding of drug therapy.

moexipril hydrochloride

(moh-EKS-eh-pril high-droh-KLOR-ighd)

Univasc

Pharmacologic class: ACE inhibitor
Therapeutic class: antihypertensive
Pregnancy risk category: C (D in second and third trimesters)

Indications and dosages

▶ **Hypertension.** *Adults:* 7.5 mg P.O. once daily before meals (3.75 mg for patients receiving diuretics). Inadequate response may lead to increased dose or divided dosing. Recommended dosage is 7.5 to 30 mg daily, in one or two divided doses 1 hour before meals. Subsequent adjustments made based on patient response.

How supplied

Tablets: 7.5 mg, 15 mg

Pharmacokinetics

Absorption: incompletely absorbed from GI tract, with bioavailability of about 13%. Food significantly decreases bioavailability.
Distribution: about 50% protein-bound.
Metabolism: metabolized extensively to the active metabolite moexiprilat.
Excretion: excreted primarily in feces, with small amount in urine. *Half-life:* 2 to 9 hours.

Route	Onset	Peak	Duration
P.O.	1 hr	3-6 hr	24 hr

Pharmacodynamics

Chemical effect: unknown; thought to result mainly from suppression of renin-angiotensin-aldosterone system. Inhibits ACE, thereby inhibiting production of angiotensin II (a potent vasoconstrictor and stimulator of aldosterone secretion). Other mechanisms also may be involved.
Therapeutic effect: lowers blood pressure.

Adverse reactions

CNS: *dizziness,* headache, fatigue.
CV: peripheral edema, hypotension, orthostatic hypotension, chest pain, flushing.
EENT: pharyngitis, rhinitis, sinusitis.
GI: diarrhea, dyspepsia, nausea.
GU: urinary frequency.
Hematologic: neutropenia.
Metabolic: hyperkalemia.
Musculoskeletal: myalgia.
Respiratory: *persistent, nonproductive cough,* upper respiratory tract infection.
Skin: rash.
Other: ***anaphylaxis, angioedema,*** flu syndrome, pain.

Interactions

Drug-drug. *Antacids:* bioavailability of ACE inhibitors may be decreased. Give drug on an empty stomach.

Digoxin: increased plasma digoxin levels. Monitor digoxin levels and patient closely.
Diuretics: risk of excessive hypotension. Monitor blood pressure closely.
Indomethacin: reduced hypotensive effects of ACE inhibitors. Avoid concomitant use.
Lithium: increased serum lithium levels and lithium toxicity. Use together cautiously. Monitor serum lithium levels frequently.
Potassium-sparing diuretics, potassium supplements: risk of hyperkalemia. Monitor serum potassium level closely.
Drug-herb. *Capsaicin:* may cause or worsen coughing linked to ACE inhibitor treatment. Advise against concomitant use.
Drug-food. *Salt substitutes that contain potassium:* risk of hyperkalemia. Monitor serum potassium level closely.

Contraindications and precautions

- Contraindicated in patients hypersensitive to drug and in those with history of angioedema with previous treatment with ACE inhibitor.
- Drug isn't recommended for pregnant women.
- Use cautiously in breast-feeding women and in patients with impaired kidney function, heart failure, or renal artery stenosis.
- Safety of drug hasn't been established in children.

NURSING CONSIDERATIONS

Assessment

- Assess patient's blood pressure before therapy.
- Measure blood pressure at trough (just before dose) to verify adequate control. Drug is less effective in reducing trough blood pressure in blacks than in nonblacks.
- Monitor patient for hypotension.
- Assess kidney function before therapy and periodically thereafter. Monitor serum potassium level, as ordered.
- Other ACE inhibitors have been linked to agranulocytosis and neutropenia. Monitor CBC with differential counts before therapy, especially in patient who has collagen-vascular disease with impaired kidney function.
- Be alert for adverse reactions and interactions.
- Evaluate patient's and family's knowledge of drug therapy.

Nursing diagnoses

- Risk for injury related to presence of hypertension
- Disturbed sleep pattern related to cough
- Deficient knowledge related to drug therapy

Planning and implementation

- Excessive hypotension can occur when drug is given with diuretics. If possible, diuretic therapy should be discontinued 2 to 3 days before starting moexipril to decrease potential for excessive hypotensive response. If moexipril doesn't adequately control blood pressure, prescriber may reinstitute diuretic with care.
- Angioedema involving tongue, glottis, or larynx may be fatal because of airway obstruction. Be prepared with appropriate therapy, such as epinephrine and equipment to ensure a patent airway.
- Notify prescriber if drug-induced cough interferes with patient's ability to sleep.

Patient teaching

- Instruct patient to take drug on an empty stomach; high-fat meals can impair absorption.
- Tell patient to avoid salt substitutes; these products may contain potassium, which can cause hyperkalemia.
- Advise patient to rise slowly to minimize light-headedness. If syncope occurs, tell him to stop drug and call prescriber immediately.
- Urge patient to use caution in hot weather and during exercise. Inadequate fluid intake, vomiting, diarrhea, and excessive perspiration can lead to light-headedness and syncope.
- Advise patient to report signs of infection, such as fever and sore throat; easy bruising or bleeding; swelling of tongue, lips, face, eyes, mucous membranes, or limbs; difficulty swallowing or breathing; and hoarseness.
- Tell woman to notify prescriber if pregnancy occurs.

Evaluation
- Patient's blood pressure is normal.
- Patient states that sleep disturbance doesn't occur.
- Patient and family state understanding of drug therapy.

montelukast sodium
(mon-tih-LOO-kist SOH-dee-um)
Singulair

Pharmacologic class: leukotriene receptor antagonist
Therapeutic class: antiasthmatic
Pregnancy risk category: B

Indications and dosages
▶ **Prevention and long-term treatment of asthma.** *Adults and children age 15 and older:* 10 mg P.O. once daily in evening.
Children ages 6 to 14: 5-mg chewable tablet P.O. once daily in evening.
Children ages 2 to 5: 4-mg chewable tablet P.O. once daily in the evening.

How supplied
Tablets (film-coated): 10 mg
Tablets (chewable): 4 mg, 5 mg

Pharmacokinetics
Absorption: rapid with an oral bioavailability of 64%.
Distribution: over 99% bound to plasma proteins.
Metabolism: extensively metabolized by cytochrome P-450 isoenzymes.
Excretion: about 86% is recovered in the feces, indicating montelukast and its metabolites are excreted almost exclusively via the bile.
Half-life: 2.7 to 5.5 hours.

Route	Onset	Peak	Duration
P.O.			
coated	Unknown	3-4 hr	Unknown
chewable	Unknown	2-2.5 hr	Unknown

Pharmacodynamics
Chemical effect: inhibits airway cysteinyl leukotriene ($CysLT_1$) receptors. Binds with high affinity and selectivity to the $CysLT_1$ receptor, and inhibits physiologic action of the cysteinyl leukotriene LTD_4. This receptor inhibition reduces early- and late-phase bronchoconstriction caused by antigen challenge.
Therapeutic effect: improves breathing.

Adverse reactions
CNS: *headache,* dizziness, fatigue, asthenia.
EENT: nasal congestion.
GI: dyspepsia, infectious gastroenteritis, abdominal pain.
GU: pyuria.
Hepatic: increased ALT and AST levels.
Respiratory: cough.
Skin: rash.
Other: fever, trauma, influenza, dental pain.

Interactions
Drug-drug. *Phenobarbital, rifampin:* may decrease bioavailability of montelukast via induction of hepatic metabolism. Monitor patient closely.

Contraindications and precautions
- Contraindicated in patients hypersensitive to drug or its components and in patients with acute asthmatic attacks or status asthmaticus.
- Use cautiously and with appropriate monitoring when systemic corticosteroid dosages are reduced.
- Safety and efficacy for patients under age 6 haven't been established.

NURSING CONSIDERATIONS

Assessment
- Assess patient's underlying condition and monitor drug's effectiveness.
- Monitor patient for adverse reactions and drug interactions.
- Evaluate patient's and family's knowledge of drug therapy.

Nursing diagnoses
- Impaired gas exchange related to asthma
- Activity intolerance related to asthma
- Deficient knowledge related to drug therapy

Planning and implementation

- Don't abruptly substitute drug for inhaled or oral corticosteroids.
- Drug isn't indicated for patients with acute asthmatic attacks or status asthmaticus. Also not indicated as monotherapy for managing exercise-induced bronchospasm. Appropriate rescue drug should be continued for acute exacerbations.
- Give drug daily and not on as-needed basis.

Patient teaching

- Advise patient to take drug daily, even if asymptomatic, and to contact prescriber if asthma isn't well controlled.
- Warn patient not to reduce or stop taking other prescribed antiasthma drugs without prescriber's approval.
- Warn patient that drug isn't beneficial in acute asthma attacks, or in exercise-induced bronchospasm and advise him to keep appropriate rescue medications available.
- Advise patient with known aspirin sensitivity to continue to avoid using aspirin and NSAIDs.
- Advise patient with phenylketonuria that chewable tablet contains phenylalanine.

Evaluation

- Patient's respiratory signs and symptoms improve.
- Patient can perform normal activities of daily living.
- Patient and family state understanding of drug therapy.

moricizine hydrochloride

(MOR-ih-sigh-zeen high-droh-KLOR-ighd)
Ethmozine

Pharmacologic class: sodium channel blocker
Therapeutic class: antiarrhythmic
Pregnancy risk category: B

Indications and dosages

▶ **Life-threatening ventricular arrhythmias.** *Adults:* individualized dosage is based on clinical response and patient tolerance. Therapy should begin in hospital. Most patients respond to 600 to 900 mg P.O. daily in divided doses q 8 hours. Daily dosage increased within this range q 3 days by 150 mg until desired clinical effect is achieved.
Patients with hepatic or renal impairment: 600 mg or less P.O. daily.

How supplied

Tablets: 200 mg, 250 mg, 300 mg

Pharmacokinetics

Absorption: absorbed from GI tract. Administration within 30 minutes of mealtime delays absorption and lowers peak plasma levels but has no effect on extent of absorption.
Distribution: 95% protein-bound.
Metabolism: undergoes significant first-pass metabolism. At least 26 metabolites have been found; none represent more than 1% of a dose. Drug induces its own metabolism.
Excretion: 50% excreted in feces; 39% excreted in urine; some recycled through enterohepatic circulation. *Half-life:* 1½ to 3½ hours.

Route	Onset	Peak	Duration
P.O.	≤ 2 hr	0.5-2 hr	10-24 hr

Pharmacodynamics

Chemical effect: class I antiarrhythmic that reduces fast inward current carried by sodium ions across myocardial cell membranes. Moricizine has potent local anesthetic activity and membrane-stabilizing effect.
Therapeutic effect: alleviates ventricular arrhythmias.

Adverse reactions

CNS: *dizziness, headache, fatigue,* anxiety, hypoesthesia, asthenia, nervousness, paresthesia, sleep disorders.
CV: ***proarrhythmic events (ventricular tachycardia, PVCs, supraventricular arrhythmias),*** *ECG abnormalities (including conduction defects, sinus pause, junctional rhythm, or AV block),* ***heart failure,*** *palpitations,* ***cardiac death,*** *chest pain.*
EENT: blurred vision.
GI: *nausea, vomiting, abdominal pain, dyspepsia, diarrhea, dry mouth.*

GU: urine retention, urinary frequency, dysuria.
Musculoskeletal: pain.
Respiratory: dyspnea.
Skin: diaphoresis, rash.
Other: drug-induced fever.

Interactions

Drug-drug. *Cimetidine:* increased plasma levels and decreased clearance of moricizine. Begin moricizine therapy at low dosage (not more than 600 mg daily) and monitor plasma levels and therapeutic effect closely.
Digoxin, propranolol: additive prolongation of PR interval. Monitor patient closely.
Theophylline: increased clearance and reduced plasma levels of theophylline. Monitor plasma levels and therapeutic response; adjust theophylline dosage as ordered.

Contraindications and precautions

- Contraindicated in patients hypersensitive to drug, in patients with second- or third-degree AV block or right bundle-branch heart block when linked to left hemiblock (bifascicular block) unless artificial pacemaker is present, and in patients with cardiogenic shock.
- Drug isn't recommended for breast-feeding women.
- Use with extreme caution in patients with sick sinus syndrome because drug may cause sinus bradycardia or sinus arrest. Also use with extreme caution in patients with coronary artery disease and left ventricular dysfunction because these patients may be at risk for sudden death when treated with drug.
- Administer cautiously to patients with hepatic or renal impairment and to pregnant women.
- Safety of drug hasn't been established in children.

NURSING CONSIDERATIONS

Assessment

- Assess patient's condition before therapy and regularly thereafter.
- Be alert for adverse reactions and drug interactions.
- Evaluate patient's and family's knowledge of drug therapy.

Nursing diagnoses

- Decreased cardiac output related to presence of ventricular arrhythmia
- Risk for injury related to drug-induced adverse reactions
- Deficient knowledge related to drug therapy

Planning and implementation

ALERT Don't confuse Ethmozine with Erythrocin.

- When substituting moricizine for another antiarrhythmic, previous drug should be withdrawn for one or two of drug's half-lives before moricizine is started. Patients with tendency to develop life-threatening arrhythmias after drug withdrawal should be hospitalized during withdrawal of therapy and adjustment to moricizine. Guidelines that prescribers use for starting moricizine therapy are as follows:
  - disopyramide, 6 to 12 hours after last dose.
  - mexiletine, 8 to 12 hours after last dose.
  - procainamide, 3 to 6 hours after last dose.
  - propafenone, 8 to 12 hours after last dose.
  - quinidine, 6 to 12 hours after last dose.
  - tocainide, 8 to 12 hours after last dose.
- Determine electrolyte status and correct imbalances before therapy, as ordered. Hypokalemia, hyperkalemia, and hypomagnesemia may alter effects of drug.

Patient teaching

- Tell patient to report adverse reactions promptly.

Evaluation

- Patient regains normal cardiac output with alleviation of ventricular arrhythmia.
- Patient sustains no injury from adverse reactions.
- Patient and family state understanding of drug therapy.

morphine hydrochloride
(MOR-feen high-droh-KLOR-ighd)
Morphitec ♦, M.O.S. ♦, M.O.S.-SR ♦

morphine sulfate
Astramorph PF, DMS Concentrate, Duramorph, Duramorph PF, Epimorph ♦, Infumorph 200, Infumorph 500, Kadian, Morphine H.P. ♦, MS Contin, MSIR, Oramorph SR, RMS Uniserts, Roxanol, Roxanol 100, Roxanol Rescudose, Roxanol SR, Roxanol UD, Statex ♦

morphine tartrate ◇
Pharmacologic class: opioid
Therapeutic class: narcotic analgesic
Controlled substance schedule: II
Pregnancy risk category: C

Indications and dosages
▶ **Severe pain.** *Adults:* 10 mg S.C. or I.M. Or, 2.5 to 15 mg I.V. q 4 hours, p.r.n. Or, 10 to 30 mg P.O. Or, 10 to 20 mg P.R. q 4 hours, p.r.n. When given by continuous I.V. infusion, loading dose of' 15 mg I.V. may be followed by continuous infusion of 0.8 to 10 mg/hour. Or, 30 mg controlled-release tablets P.O. q 8 to 12 hours may be administered. As epidural injection, 5 mg by epidural catheter. If adequate pain relief not obtained within 1 hour, additional doses of 1 to 2 mg are given at intervals sufficient to assess efficacy. Maximum total epidural dosage shouldn't exceed 10 mg. *Children:* 0.1 to 0.2 mg/kg S.C. q 4 hours. Maximum single dose is 15 mg.

How supplied
morphine hydrochloride
Tablets: 10 mg ♦, 20 mg ♦, 40 mg ♦, 60 mg ♦
Tablets (extended-release): 30 mg ♦, 60 mg ♦
Oral solution ♦: 1 mg/ml, 5 mg/ml, 10 mg/ml, 20 mg/ml, 50 mg/ml
Syrup: 1 mg/ml ♦, 5 mg/ml ♦, 10 mg/ml ♦, 20 mg/ml ♦, 50 mg/ml ♦
Suppositories: 10 mg ♦, 20 mg ♦, 30 mg ♦

morphine sulfate
Capsules (sustained release): 20 mg, 50 mg, 100 mg
Tablets: 15 mg, 30 mg
Tablets (extended-release): 15 mg, 30 mg, 60 mg, 100 mg, 200 mg
Soluble tablets: 10 mg, 15 mg, 30 mg
Oral solution: 10 mg/5 ml, 20 mg/5 ml, 20 mg/ml (concentrate)
Oral solution (concentrated): 20 mg/ml, 30 mg/1.5 ml, 100 mg/5 ml
Syrup: 1 mg/ml, 5 mg/ml
Injection (with preservative): 500 mcg/ml, 1 mg/ml, 2 mg/ml, 3 mg/ml, 4 mg/ml, 5 mg/ml, 8 mg/ml, 10 mg/ml, 15 mg/ml, 25 mg/ml, 50 mg/ml
Injection (without preservative): 500 mcg/ml, 1 mg/ml, 10 mg/ml, 25 mg/ml
Suppositories: 5 mg, 10 mg, 20 mg, 30 mg

morphine tartrate
Injection: 80 mg/ml ◇

Pharmacokinetics
Absorption: absorbed variably from GI tract when administered P.O.; unknown for other routes.
Distribution: distributed widely throughout body.
Metabolism: metabolized primarily in liver.
Excretion: excreted in urine and bile. *Half-life:* 2 to 3 hours.

Route	Onset	Peak	Duration
P.O.	1 hr	1-2 hr	4-12 hr
I.V.	< 5 min	20 min	4-5 hr
I.M.	10-30 min	30-60 min	4-5 hr
S.C.	10-30 min	50-90 min	4-5 hr
P.R.	20-60 min	20-60 min	4-5 hr
Epidural	15-60 min	15-60 min	24 hr
Intrathecal	15-60 min	Unknown	24 hr

Pharmacodynamics
Chemical effect: binds with opioid receptors in CNS, altering both perception of and emotional response to pain through unknown mechanism.
Therapeutic effect: relieves pain.

Adverse reactions

CNS: *sedation, somnolence, clouded sensorium, euphoria,* ***seizures*** (with large doses), dizziness, *nightmares* (with long-acting oral forms).
CV: *hypotension,* ***bradycardia, shock, cardiac arrest.***
GI: *nausea, vomiting, constipation,* ileus.
GU: *urine retention.*
Hematologic: ***thrombocytopenia.***
Respiratory: ***respiratory depression, respiratory arrest.***
Skin: pruritus and flushing with epidural administration.
Other: *physical dependence.*

Interactions

Drug-drug. *CNS depressants, general anesthetics, hypnotics, MAO inhibitors, other narcotic analgesics, sedatives, tranquilizers, tricyclic antidepressants:* possible respiratory depression, hypotension, profound sedation, or coma. Use together with extreme caution. Reduce morphine dosage and monitor patient response.
Drug-lifestyle. *Alcohol use:* additive effects. Urge caution.

Contraindications and precautions

- Contraindicated in patients hypersensitive to drug and in those with conditions that preclude I.V. administration of opioids (acute bronchial asthma or upper airway obstruction).
- Use with extreme caution in elderly and debilitated patients and in patients with head injury, increased intracranial pressure, seizures, chronic pulmonary disease, prostatic hyperplasia, severe hepatic or renal disease, acute abdominal conditions, hypothyroidism, Addison's disease, or urethral stricture.
- Use cautiously in pregnant women.
- Breast-feeding women should wait 2 to 3 hours after last dose before breast-feeding to avoid sedation in infant.

NURSING CONSIDERATIONS

Assessment

- Assess patient's pain before therapy and regularly thereafter.
- Morphine may worsen or mask gallbladder pain.
- Monitor patient for respiratory depression after administration. When given epidurally, monitor for up to 24 hours after injection. Check respiratory rate and depth every 30 to 60 minutes for 24 hours.
- Be alert for adverse reactions and drug interactions.
- Evaluate patient's and family's knowledge of drug therapy.

Nursing diagnoses

- Acute pain related to underlying condition
- Ineffective breathing pattern related to drug's depressive effect on respiratory system
- Deficient knowledge related to drug therapy

Planning and implementation

ALERT Don't confuse morphine with hydromorphone.
- Morphine is drug of choice in relieving pain of MI. It may cause transient decrease in blood pressure.
- Keep narcotic antagonist and resuscitation equipment available.
- An around-the-clock regimen best manages severe, chronic pain.
- Withhold dose and notify prescriber if respiratory rate is below 12 breaths/minute.
- Because constipation is often severe with maintenance dosage, make sure prescriber has ordered stool softener or other laxative.

P.O. use: Solutions of various concentrations are available as well as intensified P.O. solution (20 mg/ml). Carefully note strength administered.
– Don't crush or break extended-release tablets.
– If S.L. administration is ordered, measure solution with tuberculin syringe. Administer dose a few drops at a time to allow maximal S.L. absorption and minimize swallowing.
I.V. use: When given by direct injection, 2.5 to 15 mg may be diluted in 4 or 5 ml of sterile water for injection and given over 4 to 5 minutes.

– Or, drug may be mixed with D_5W to yield 0.1 to 1 mg/ml and administered by continuous infusion device.
– Morphine sulfate is compatible with most common I.V. solutions.
I.M. and S.C. use: Follow normal protocol.
P.R. use: Refrigeration of rectal suppository isn't necessary.
– In some patients, P.R. and P.O. absorption may not be equivalent.
Epidural and intrathecal use: Preservative-free preparations are available for epidural or intrathecal administration.

Patient teaching
- Caution patient about getting out of bed or walking. Warn outpatient not to drive or perform other potentially hazardous activities until full CNS effects of drug are known.
- Tell patient to report continued pain.
- Instruct patient to avoid alcohol consumption during drug therapy.

☑ Evaluation
- Patient states that pain is relieved.
- Patient maintains adequate breathing patterns throughout therapy.
- Patient and family state understanding of drug therapy.

moxifloxacin hydrochloride
(mox-ih-FLOX-uh-sin high-droh-CLOR-ighd)
Avelox

Pharmacologic class: fluoroquinolone
Therapeutic class: antibiotic
Pregnancy risk category: C

Indications and dosages
▶ **Acute bacterial sinusitis caused by *Streptococcus pneumoniae, Haemophilus influenzae,* or *Moraxella catarrhalis.*** *Adults:* 400 mg P.O. once daily for 10 days.
▶ **Acute bacterial exacerbation of chronic bronchitis caused by *S. pneumoniae, H. influenzae, H. parainfluenzae, Klebsiella pneumoniae, Staphylococcus aureus,* or *M. catarrhalis.*** *Adults:* 400 mg P.O. once daily for 5 days.
▶ **Mild to moderate community-acquired pneumonia caused by *S. pneumoniae, H. influenzae, Mycoplasma pneumoniae, Chlamydia pneumoniae,* or *M. catarrhalis.*** *Adults:* 400 mg P.O. once daily for 10 days.

How supplied
Tablets (film-coated): 400 mg

Pharmacokinetics
Absorption: well absorbed after P.O. administration, with an absolute bioavailability of about 90%. Plasma levels peak in 1 to 3 hours. Steady-state is reached after 3 days on a 400 mg once daily dose.
Distribution: widely distributed with a distribution volume of 1.7 to 2.7 L/kg. Plasma protein–binding is about 50%. Penetrates well into nasal and bronchial secretions, sinus mucosa, and saliva.
Metabolism: drug is metabolized to inactive glucuronide and sulfate conjugates. About 14% of dose is converted to the glucuronide metabolite. Sulfate metabolite accounts for about 38% of the dose.
Excretion: about 45% of dose is excreted unchanged, about 20% in urine and 25% in feces. Sulfate metabolite is eliminated mainly in feces; glucuronide metabolite undergoes renal excretion. *Half-life:* about 12 hours.

Route	Onset	Peak	Duration
P.O.	Unknown	1-3 hr	Unknown

Pharmacodynamics
Chemical effect: inhibits the activity of topoisomerase I (DNA gyrase) and topoisomerase IV in susceptible bacteria. These enzymes are necessary for bacterial DNA replication, transcription, repair, and recombination.
Therapeutic effect: kills susceptible bacteria, including *S. pneumoniae, H. influenzae, H. parainfluenzae, K. pneumoniae, S. aureus, M. pneumoniae, C. pneumoniae,* and *M. catarrhalis.*

Adverse reactions
CNS: dizziness, headache.
GI: abdominal pain, diarrhea, dyspepsia, nausea, vomiting, taste perversion.

Hematologic: thrombocythemia, ***thrombocytopenia,*** eosinophilia, ***leukopenia,*** altered PT.
Hepatic: abnormal liver function test results.
Metabolic: hyperglycemia, hyperlipidemia, increased amylase.

Interactions

Drug-drug. *Antacids; didanosine; metal cations, such as aluminum, magnesium, iron, zinc; multivitamins; sucralfate:* metal cations chelate with moxifloxacin, resulting in decreased absorption and lower serum levels. Administer drug at least 4 hours before or 8 hours after drugs containing metal cations.
Class IA (quinidine, procainamide) or Class III (amiodarone, sotalol) antiarrhythmics: possible enhanced adverse CV effects. Avoid concurrent use.
Drugs known to prolong the QT interval, such as erythromycin, antipsychotics, and tricyclic antidepressants: may have an additive effect when combined with these drugs. Avoid concomitant use.
NSAIDs: may increase risk of CNS stimulation and seizures. Don't use together.
Drug-lifestyle. *Sun exposure:* although photosensitivity hasn't occurred with moxifloxacin, it has been reported with other fluoroquinolones. Discourage excessive sun exposure.

Contraindications and precautions

- Contraindicated in patients hypersensitive to drug, its components, or other fluoroquinolones.
- Safety and efficacy hasn't been documented in children, adolescents (less than 18 years of age), pregnant women, and breast-feeding women.
- Use cautiously in patients with known or suspected CNS disorders and in patients with risk factors that may predispose to seizures or lower the seizure threshold. Use cautiously in patients with prolonged QT interval or uncorrected hypokalemia.

NURSING CONSIDERATIONS

Assessment

- Obtain history of patient's underlying condition before therapy, and reassess regularly thereafter.
- Obtain specimen for culture and sensitivity tests before first dose. Therapy may begin pending culture results.
- Monitor for hypersensitivity reactions, CNS toxicities including seizures, QT interval prolongation, pseudomembranous colitis, phototoxicity, and tendon rupture.
- Evaluate patient's and family's knowledge about drug therapy.

Nursing diagnoses

- Infection related to presence of bacteria susceptible to drug
- Risk for injury related to drug-induced adverse reactions
- Deficient knowledge related to drug therapy

Planning and implementation

- Correct hypokalemia before starting therapy, as directed.
- Drug may be given without regard to meals. Administer at same time to provide consistent absorption.
- Provide liberal fluid intake.
- Give moxifloxacin 4 hours before or 8 hours after antacids, sucralfate, and products containing iron or zinc.
- The most common adverse reactions are nausea, vomiting, stomach pain, diarrhea, dizziness, and headache.
- Monitor patient for seizures and other adverse CNS reactions linked to fluoroquinolones including dizziness, confusion, tremors, hallucinations, depression, and, rarely, suicidal thoughts or acts. These may occur after the initial dose. Notify prescriber and discontinue moxifloxacin; institute appropriate therapy if any of these reactions occur.
- Store drug at controlled room temperature.

Patient teaching

- Instruct patient to take drug once daily, at the same time each day.
- Tell patient to finish the entire course of therapy, even if symptoms resolve.
- Advise the patient to drink plenty of fluids and to take moxifloxacin 4 hours before or 8 hours after antacids, sucralfate, and products containing iron and zinc.

• Most common adverse reactions are nausea, vomiting, stomach pain, diarrhea, dizziness, and headache.
• Tell patient to avoid hazardous activities, such as driving or operating machinery, until effects of drug are known.
• Instruct patient to contact prescriber if he experiences allergic reaction, palpitations, fainting, persistent diarrhea, severe sunburn, injury to a muscle tendon, or seizures.

Evaluation
• Patient is free from infection after drug therapy.
• Patient sustains no injury as a result of drug-induced adverse reactions.
• Patient and family state understanding of drug therapy.

muromonab-CD3
(myoo-roh-MOH-nab see dee three)
Orthoclone OKT3

Pharmacologic class: monoclonal antibody
Therapeutic class: immunosuppressive
Pregnancy risk category: C

Indications and dosages
▶ **Acute allograft rejection in kidney transplant patients; steroid-resistant hepatic or cardiac allograft rejection.** *Adults:* 5 mg I.V. bolus once daily for 10 to 14 days.

How supplied
Injection: 1 mg/ml in 5-ml ampules

Pharmacokinetics
Absorption: not applicable.
Distribution: unknown.
Metabolism: unknown.
Excretion: unknown.

Route	Onset	Peak	Duration
I.V.	Almost immediately	Unknown	1 wk after drug stopped

Pharmacodynamics
Chemical effect: IgG antibody that reacts in T-lymphocyte membrane with a molecule (CD3) needed for antigen recognition. This drug depletes blood of CD3-positive T cells, which leads to restoration of allograft function and reversal of rejection.
Therapeutic effect: halts acute allograft rejection in kidney transplantation.

Adverse reactions
CNS: *tremors,* headache, ***seizures, encephalopathy, aseptic meningitis, cerebral edema.***
CV: *chest pain,* tachycardia, ***cardiac arrest, shock, heart failure.***
GI: *nausea, vomiting,* diarrhea.
Respiratory: ***severe pulmonary edema, adult respiratory distress syndrome,*** *dyspnea.*
Other: *fever, chills,* INFECTION, ***anaphylaxis, cytokine release syndrome, risk of neoplasia.***

Interactions
Drug-drug. *Immunosuppressants:* increased risk of infection. Monitor patient closely.
Indomethacin: increased muromonab-CD3 levels with CNS effects. Encephalopathy has occurred. Monitor patient closely.
Live-virus vaccines: may increase replication and effects of vaccine. Postpone vaccination when possible and consult prescriber.

Contraindications and precautions
• Contraindicated in pregnant or breast-feeding women and in patients hypersensitive to drug or to other products of murine origin. Also contraindicated in patients who have antimouse antibody titers of 1:1,000 or more; who have fluid overload, as evidenced by chest X-ray or weight gain greater than 3% within week before treatment; and who have history of or predisposition to seizures.
• Safety of drug hasn't been established in children.

NURSING CONSIDERATIONS

Assessment
• Assess patient's condition before therapy and regularly thereafter.

• Obtain chest X-ray within 24 hours before drug treatment, as ordered.
• Assess patient for signs of fluid overload before treatment.
• Be alert for adverse reactions and drug interactions.
• Monitor patient's hydration status if adverse GI reactions occur.
• Evaluate patient's and family's knowledge of drug therapy.

Nursing diagnoses
• Risk for injury related to presence of acute allograft rejection
• Risk for deficient fluid volume related to drug-induced adverse GI reactions
• Deficient knowledge related to drug therapy

Planning and implementation
• Treatment should begin in facility equipped and staffed for cardiopulmonary resuscitation where patient can be monitored closely.
• Most adverse reactions develop within 30 minutes to 6 hours after first dose.
• Administer antipyretic, as ordered, before giving drug to help lower risk of expected pyrexia and chills. Corticosteroids also may be administered, as ordered, before first injection to help decrease risk of adverse reactions. Methylprednisolone sodium succinate (1 mg/kg) preinjection followed by hydrocortisone sodium succinate (100 mg) 30 minutes postinjection may alleviate severity of first-dose reaction.
• Muromonab-CD3 is a monoclonal antibody. Patients develop antibodies to it that can lead to loss of effectiveness and more severe adverse reactions if second course of therapy is attempted. Therefore, experts believe that this drug should be used for only one course of treatment.

Patient teaching
• Inform patient of expected adverse reactions, and reassure him that they will lessen as treatment progresses.

Evaluation
• Patient shows no signs of organ rejection.
• Patient maintains adequate hydration.
• Patient and family state understanding of drug therapy.

mycophenolate mofetil
(migh-koh-FEN-oh-layt MOH-feh-til)
CellCept

mycophenolate mofetil hydrochloride
CellCept Intravenous

Pharmacologic class: mycophenolic acid derivative
Therapeutic class: immunosuppressant
Pregnancy risk category: C

Indications and dosages
▶ **Prevention of organ rejection in patients receiving allogeneic renal transplant.**
Adults: 1 g P.O. or I.V. b.i.d., with corticosteroids and cyclosporine (begun within 72 hours after transplantation).
▶ **Prevention of organ rejection in patients receiving allogeneic cardiac transplant.**
Adults: 1.5 g P.O. or I.V. b.i.d. with cyclosporine and corticosteroids.

How supplied
mycophenolate mofetil
Capsules: 250 mg
Tablets: 500 mg
mycophenolate mofetil hydrochloride
Injection: 500 mg/vial

Pharmacokinetics
Absorption: absorbed from GI tract.
Distribution: 97% bound to plasma proteins.
Metabolism: undergoes complete presystemic metabolism to mycophenolic acid.
Excretion: excreted primarily in urine, with small amount in feces. *Half-life:* about 18 hours.

Route	Onset	Peak	Duration
P.O.	Unknown	Unknown	Unknown
I.V.	Unknown	Unknown	10-17 hr

Pharmacodynamics

Chemical effect: inhibits proliferative responses of T- and B-lymphocytes, suppresses antibody formation by B-lymphocytes, and may inhibit recruitment of leukocytes into sites of inflammation and graft rejection.
Therapeutic effect: prevents organ rejection.

Adverse reactions

CNS: *tremor,* insomnia, dizziness, *headache.*
CV: *chest pain, hypertension, edema,* peripheral edema.
EENT: pharyngitis.
GI: *diarrhea, constipation, nausea, dyspepsia, vomiting, oral candidiasis, abdominal pain,* **HEMORRHAGE.**
GU: urinary tract infection, hematuria, kidney tubular necrosis.
Hematologic: anemia, ***leukopenia***, **THROMBOCYTOPENIA,** hypochromic anemia, leukocytosis.
Metabolic: *hypercholesteremia, hypophosphatemia, hypokalemia,* hyperkalemia, hyperglycemia.
Musckuloskeletal: *back pain.*
Respiratory: *dyspnea, cough,* infection, bronchitis, pneumonia.
Skin: *acne,* rash.
Other: *pain, fever, infection,* ***sepsis,*** *asthenia.*

Interactions

Drug-drug. *Acyclovir, ganciclovir, other drugs known to undergo tubular secretion:* increased risk of toxicity for both drugs. Monitor patient closely.
Antacids with magnesium and aluminum hydroxides: decreased absorption of mycophenolate mofetil. Separate administration times.
Azathioprine: hasn't been clinically studied. Avoid concurrent use.
Cholestyramine: may interfere with enterohepatic recirculation, reducing mycophenolate bioavailability. Don't administer concurrently.
Oral contraceptives: may affect efficacy of oral contraceptives. Advise patient to use barrier birth control methods.

Contraindications and precautions

- Contraindicated in patients hypersensitive to drug, mycophenolic acid, or other components of product and in pregnant (unless benefits outweigh risks) or breast-feeding women.
- Use cautiously in patients with GI disorders.
- Safety of drug hasn't been established in children.

NURSING CONSIDERATIONS

Assessment

- Obtain history of patient's kidney transplant.
- Monitor CBC regularly, as ordered.
- Be alert for adverse reactions and drug interactions.
- Evaluate patient's and family's knowledge of drug therapy.

Nursing diagnoses

- Ineffective health maintenance related to need for kidney transplant
- Ineffective immune protection related to drug-induced immunsupression
- Deficient knowledge related to drug therapy

Planning and implementation

P.O. use: Give drug on an empty stomach.
ALERT Because of potential teratogenic effects, don't open or crush capsules. Avoid inhaling powder in capsules or letting it contact skin or mucous membranes. If contact occurs, wash skin thoroughly with soap and water and rinse eyes with plain water.
I.V. use: CellCept Intravenous must be reconstituted and diluted to 6 mg/ml using D_5W injection.
ALERT Never administer drug by rapid or bolus I.V. injection. Give infusion over at least 2 hours.
- In patients with severe chronic renal impairment (GFR less than 25 ml/minute) outside the immediate posttransplant period, avoid use of doses above 1 g b.i.d.
- Notify prescriber if neutropenia occurs.

Patient teaching

- Warn patient not to open or crush capsule but to swallow it whole on an empty stomach.
- Stress importance of not interrupting therapy without consulting prescriber.
- Inform woman that a pregnancy test should be done 1 week before therapy. Advise her to use effective contraception until at least 6

weeks after therapy stops, even if she has a history of infertility (unless she has had a hysterectomy). Tell her to use two forms of contraception simultaneously unless abstinence is the chosen method. If pregnancy occurs despite these measures, have patient contact prescriber immediately.

✔ Evaluation

- Patient shows no signs and symptoms of organ rejection.
- Neutropenia doesn't develop.
- Patient and family state understanding of drug therapy.

N

nabumetone

(nuh-BYOO-meh-tohn)
Relafen

Pharmacologic class: NSAID
Therapeutic class: antiarthritic
Pregnancy risk category: C

Indications and dosages

▶ **Rheumatoid arthritis, osteoarthritis.**
Adults: initially, 1,000 mg P.O. daily as single dose or in divided doses b.i.d. Maximum, 2,000 mg daily.

How supplied

Tablets: 500 mg, 750 mg

Pharmacokinetics

Absorption: well absorbed from GI tract. Administration with food increases absorption rate and peak levels of principal metabolite but doesn't change total drug absorbed.
Distribution: over 99% of metabolite is bound to plasma proteins.
Metabolism: metabolized to inactive metabolites in liver.
Excretion: metabolites excreted primarily in urine; about 9% appears in feces. *Half-life:* about 24 hours.

Route	Onset	Peak	Duration
P.O.	Unknown	2-4 hr	Unknown

Pharmacodynamics

Chemical effect: unknown; may inhibit prostaglandin synthesis.
Therapeutic effect: relieves pain.

Adverse reactions

CNS: *dizziness, headache,* fatigue, increased sweating, insomnia, nervousness, somnolence.
CV: vasculitis, *edema.*
EENT: *tinnitus.*
GI: *diarrhea, dyspepsia, abdominal pain, constipation, flatulence, nausea,* dry mouth, gastritis, stomatitis, vomiting, ***bleeding,*** ulceration.
Respiratory: dyspnea, pneumonitis.
Skin: *pruritus, rash.*

Interactions

Drug-drug. *Diuretics:* NSAIDs may decrease diuretic effectiveness. Monitor patient closely.
Drugs highly bound to plasma proteins (such as warfarin): increased risk of adverse effects from displacement of drug by nabumetone. Use together cautiously.
Drug-herb. *Dong quai, feverfew, garlic, ginger, horse chestnut, red clover:* possible increased risk of bleeding. Discourage concomitant use.
St. John's wort: increased risk of photosensitivity. Advise patient to avoid unprotected exposure to sunlight.
Drug-food. *Any food:* increases the rate of absorption. Give together.
Drug-lifestyle. *Alcohol use:* increased risk of additive GI toxicity. Discourage concomitant use.

Contraindications and precautions

- Contraindicated in patients hypersensitive to drug and patients with history of aspirin- or NSAID-induced asthma, urticaria, or other allergic reactions.
- Drug isn't recommended for use during third trimester of pregnancy or in breast-feeding women.
- Use cautiously in patients with renal or hepatic impairment, peptic ulcer disease, and

heart failure, hypertension, or other conditions that may predispose patient to fluid retention.
• Use cautiously in elderly patients.
• Safety of drug hasn't been established in children.

NURSING CONSIDERATIONS

Assessment
• Assess patient's arthritis before therapy and regularly thereafter.
• During long-term therapy, periodically monitor renal and liver function, CBC, and hematocrit as ordered; assess these patients for evidence of GI bleeding.
• Watch for fluid retention, especially among patients with heart failure and hypertension.
• Be alert for adverse reactions and drug interactions.
• Evaluate patient's and family's knowledge of drug therapy.

Nursing diagnoses
• Chronic pain related to arthritic condition
• Impaired tissue integrity related to adverse drug effect on GI mucosa
• Deficient knowledge related to drug therapy

Planning and implementation
• Administer drug with food to enhance time of absorption.
• Notify prescriber about adverse reactions.

Patient teaching
• Instruct patient to take drug with food, milk, or antacids for best absorption.
• Advise patient to limit alcohol intake because of additive GI toxicity.
• Teach patient to recognize and report signs and symptoms of GI bleeding.

Evaluation
• Patient is free from pain.
• Patient's GI tissue integrity is maintained throughout drug therapy.
• Patient and family state understanding of drug therapy.

nadolol
(nay-DOH-lol)
Corgard, Syn-Nadolol ♦

Pharmacologic class: beta blocker
Therapeutic class: antihypertensive, antianginal
Pregnancy risk category: C

Indications and dosages
▶ **Angina pectoris.** *Adults:* initially, 40 mg P.O. once daily. Increased in 40- to 80-mg increments q 3 to 7 days until optimum response occurs. Usual maintenance dosage is 40 to 240 mg daily.
▶ **Hypertension.** *Adults:* initially, 20 to 40 mg P.O. once daily. Increased in 40- to 80-mg increments/day q 2 to 14 days until optimum response occurs. Usual maintenance dosage is 40 to 320 mg daily (in rare cases, 640 mg).

How supplied
Tablets: 20 mg, 40 mg, 80 mg, 120 mg, 160 mg

Pharmacokinetics
Absorption: 30% to 40% of dose is absorbed from GI tract.
Distribution: distributed throughout body; about 30% protein-bound.
Metabolism: none.
Excretion: most excreted unchanged in urine; remainder in feces. *Half-life:* about 20 hours.

Route	Onset	Peak	Duration
P.O.	Unknown	2-4 hr	Unknown

Pharmacodynamics
Chemical effect: reduces cardiac oxygen demand by blocking catecholamine-induced increases in heart rate, blood pressure, and myocardial contraction. Depresses renin secretion.
Therapeutic effect: lowers blood pressure and relieves angina.

Adverse reactions
CNS: fatigue, lethargy, dizziness.

CV: ***bradycardia,*** *hypotension,* ***heart failure,*** peripheral vascular disease.
GI: nausea, vomiting, diarrhea, constipation.
Respiratory: *increased airway resistance.*
Skin: rash.
Other: fever.

Interactions

Drug-drug. *Antihypertensives:* enhanced antihypertensive effect. Monitor patient.
Cardiac glycosides: excessive bradycardia and additive effects on AV conduction. Use together cautiously.
Epinephrine: severe vasoconstriction and reflex bradycardia. Monitor patient closely.
Insulin, oral antidiabetics: can alter dosage requirements in diabetic patients. Monitor patient.
NSAIDs: decreased antihypertensive effect. Monitor blood pressure and adjust dosage.

Contraindications and precautions

- Contraindicated in patients with bronchial asthma, sinus bradycardia, greater than first-degree heart block, and cardiogenic shock.
- Drug isn't recommended for breast-feeding women.
- Use cautiously in patients undergoing major surgery involving general anesthesia and in those with heart failure, chronic bronchitis, emphysema, renal or hepatic impairment, or diabetes.
- Safety of drug hasn't been established in children.

NURSING CONSIDERATIONS

Assessment

- Assess patient's condition before therapy and regularly thereafter.
- Drug masks common signs of shock and hyperthyroidism.
- Be alert for adverse reactions and drug interactions.
- Evaluate patient's and family's knowledge of drug therapy.

Nursing diagnoses

- Risk for injury related to presence of hypertension
- Acute pain related to angina
- Deficient knowledge related to drug therapy

Planning and implementation

- Always check apical pulse before giving drug. If slower than 60 beats/minute, withhold drug and notify prescriber.
- If patient develops severe hypotension, give vasopressor, as prescribed.

ALERT Reduce dosage gradually over 1 to 2 weeks. Abrupt discontinuation can worsen angina and MI.

Patient teaching

- Explain importance of taking drug as prescribed, even when feeling well. Caution patient not to stop drug suddenly.

Evaluation

- Patient's blood pressure is normal.
- Patient reports reduced angina.
- Patient and family state understanding of drug therapy.

nafcillin sodium

(naf-SIL-in SOH-dee-um)
Nafcil, Nallpen, Unipen

Pharmacologic class: penicillinase-resistant penicillin
Therapeutic class: antibiotic
Pregnancy risk category: B

Indications and dosages

▶ **Systemic infections caused by penicillinase-producing staphylococci.**
Adults: 2 to 4 g P.O. daily, divided into doses given q 6 hours. Or, 2 to 12 g I.M. or I.V. daily in divided doses q 4 to 6 hours.
Children older than age 1 month: 50 mg/kg P.O. daily, divided into doses given q 6 hours. Or, 50 to 100 mg/kg I.M. or I.V. daily in divided doses q 6 hours for mild to moderate infections. For severe infections, 100 to 200 mg/kg/day I.M. or I.V. in equally divided doses q 4 to 6 hours.

How supplied

Tablets: 500 mg
Capsules: 250 mg

Oral solution: 250 mg/5 ml (after reconstitution)
Injection: 500 mg, 1 g, 2 g
I.V. infusion piggyback: 1 g, 2 g

Pharmacokinetics

Absorption: absorbed erratically and poorly from GI tract after P.O. administration; unknown after I.M. administration.
Distribution: distributed widely. CSF penetration is poor but enhanced by meningeal inflammation. Drug is 70% to 90% protein-bound.
Metabolism: metabolized primarily in liver; undergoes enterohepatic circulation.
Excretion: excreted primarily in bile; 25% to 30% is excreted in urine unchanged. *Half-life:* 30 to 90 minutes.

Route	Onset	Peak	Duration
P.O.	Unknown	0.5-2 hr	Unknown
I.V.	Immediate	Immediate	Unknown
I.M.	Unknown	30-60 min	Unknown

Pharmacodynamics

Chemical effect: inhibits cell wall synthesis during microorganism multiplication; bacteria resist penicillins by producing penicillinases—enzymes that hydrolyze penicillins. Nafcillin resists these enzymes.
Therapeutic effect: kills susceptible bacteria, such as penicillinase-producing staphylococci, and some gram-positive aerobic and anaerobic bacilli.

Adverse reactions

GI: *nausea,* vomiting, diarrhea.
Hematologic: ***transient leukopenia, neutropenia, granulocytopenia, thrombocytopenia*** (with high doses).
Other: hypersensitivity reactions (chills, fever, rash, pruritus, urticaria, ***anaphylaxis***), vein irritation, thrombophlebitis.

Interactions

Drug-drug. *Aminoglycosides:* synergistic effect. Monitor patient closely.
Probenecid: increased blood levels of nafcillin. Probenecid may be used for this purpose.
Rifampin: dose-dependent antagonism. Monitor patient closely.
Warfarin: increased risk of bleeding when used with I.V. nafcillin. Monitor patient for bleeding.

Contraindications and precautions

- Contraindicated in patients hypersensitive to drug or other penicillins.
- Use cautiously in patients with GI distress and those with other drug allergies, especially to cephalosporins.
- Also use cautiously in pregnant or breast-feeding women.

NURSING CONSIDERATIONS

Assessment

- Assess patient's infection before therapy and regularly thereafter.
- Before giving drug, ask patient about allergic reactions to penicillin. Remember that negative history of penicillin allergy is no guarantee against future allergic reaction.
- Obtain specimen for culture and sensitivity tests before giving first dose. Therapy may begin pending results.
- Be alert for adverse reactions and drug interactions.
- Monitor patient's hydration status if adverse GI reactions occur.
- Evaluate patient's and family's knowledge of drug therapy.

Nursing diagnoses

- Infection related to susceptible bacteria
- Risk for deficient fluid volume related to drug-induced adverse GI reactions
- Deficient knowledge related to drug therapy

Planning and implementation

- Give drug at least 1 hour before bacteriostatic antibiotics.
- Drug may falsely elevate urine or serum proteins or cause false-positive results in certain tests for them.

P.O. use: Give drug 1 to 2 hours before or 2 to 3 hours after meals. Oral drug may cause GI disturbances. Food may interfere with absorption.

I.V. use: Reconstitute piggyback containers according to manufacturer's instructions. Reconstitute 500-mg, 1-g, or 2-g vials using sterile water for injection, D_5W, or normal saline solution for injection. Add 1.7 ml for each 500 mg of drug.
– Or, dilute with 15 to 30 ml of sterile water for injection or half-normal or normal saline solution for injection, and give by direct injection into vein or into tubing of free-flowing I.V. solution over 5 to 10 minutes.
– Or, dilute drug to 2 to 40 mg/ml and give by intermittent I.V. infusion over 30 to 60 minutes.
– Avoid continuous I.V. infusions to prevent vein irritation. Change site every 48 hours.
ALERT Aminoglycosides are chemically and physically incompatible with drug; don't mix together in same I.V. solution.
I.M. use: Follow normal protocol.

Patient teaching
- Tell patient to take entire quantity of drug exactly as prescribed, even after he feels better.
- Tell patient to call prescriber if rash, fever, or chills develop.

Evaluation
- Patient is free from infection.
- Patient maintains adequate hydration throughout drug therapy.
- Patient and family state understanding of drug therapy.

nalbuphine hydrochloride
(NAL-byoo-feen high-droh-KLOR-ighd)
Nubain

Pharmacologic class: narcotic agonist-antagonist, opioid partial agonist
Therapeutic class: analgesic; adjunct to anesthesia
Pregnancy risk category: B

Indications and dosages
▶ **Moderate to severe pain.** *Adults:* for average (70 kg [154 lb]) person, give 10 to 20 mg I.V., I.M., or S.C., q 3 to 6 hours, p.r.n. Maximum daily dosage is 160 mg.
▶ **Adjunct to balanced anesthesia.** *Adults:* 0.3 mg/kg to 3 mg/kg I.V. over 10 to 15 minutes, followed by maintenance doses of 0.25 to 0.5 mg/kg in single I.V. doses p.r.n.

How supplied
Injection: 10 mg/ml, 20 mg/ml

Pharmacokinetics
Absorption: unknown for S.C. and I.M. administration.
Distribution: not appreciably bound to plasma proteins.
Metabolism: metabolized in liver.
Excretion: excreted in urine and bile. *Half-life:* 5 hours.

Route	Onset	Peak	Duration
I.V.	2-3 min	≤ 30 min	3-4 hr
I.M.	≤ 15 min	≤ 60 min	3-6 hr
S.C.	≤ 15 min	Unknown	3-6 hr

Pharmacodynamics
Chemical effect: binds with opioid receptors in CNS, altering pain perception and response to pain by unknown mechanism.
Therapeutic effect: relieves pain and enhances anesthesia.

Adverse reactions
CNS: *headache, sedation, dizziness, vertigo,* nervousness, depression, restlessness, crying, euphoria, hostility, unusual dreams, confusion, hallucinations, speech difficulty, delusions.
CV: hypertension, hypotension, tachycardia, ***bradycardia***.
EENT: blurred vision.
GI: cramps, dyspepsia, bitter taste, *dry mouth, nausea, vomiting,* constipation.
GU: urinary urgency.
Respiratory: ***respiratory depression, pulmonary edema.***
Skin: itching; burning; urticaria; *sweaty, clammy feeling.*

Interactions

Drug-drug. *CNS depressants, general anesthetics, hypnotics, MAO inhibitors, sedatives, tranquilizers, tricyclic antidepressants:* possible respiratory depression, hypertension, profound sedation, or coma. Use together cautiously, and monitor patient's response.
Narcotic analgesics: possible decreased analgesic effect and withdrawal symptoms. Avoid concomitant use.
Drug-lifestyle: *Alcohol use:* possible respiratory depression, hypertension, profound sedation, or coma. Discourage concomitant use.

Contraindications and precautions

- Contraindicated in patients hypersensitive to drug.
- Use cautiously in pregnant or breast-feeding women, substance abusers, and in those with emotional instability, head injury, increased intracranial pressure, impaired ventilation, MI accompanied by nausea and vomiting, upcoming biliary surgery, and hepatic or renal disease.

NURSING CONSIDERATIONS

Assessment

- Assess patient's pain or anesthetic requirement before therapy and regularly thereafter.
- Observe for signs of withdrawal in patient receiving long-term opioid therapy.
- Monitor patient closely for respiratory depression.
- Be alert for adverse reactions and drug interactions.
- Evaluate patient's and family's knowledge of drug therapy.

Nursing diagnoses

- Acute pain related to condition
- Disturbed thought processes related to drug's effect on CNS
- Deficient knowledge related to drug therapy

Planning and implementation

- Psychological and physical dependence may occur with prolonged use.
- Drug acts as a narcotic antagonist and may precipitate withdrawal syndrome. For patients receiving long-term opioid therapy, start with 25% of usual dose, as directed.
- Make sure stool softener or other laxative is ordered for severe constipation.
- Withhold dose and notify prescriber if patient's respirations are shallow or rate is below 12 breaths/minute.
- Respiratory depression can be reversed with naloxone. Keep resuscitation equipment available, particularly when administering I.V.

I.V. use: Inject slowly over at least 2 minutes into vein or into I.V. line containing compatible, free-flowing I.V. solution, such as D_5W, normal saline solution, or lactated Ringer's solution.
I.M. and S.C use: Follow normal protocol.
ALERT Don't confuse Nubain with Navane.

Patient teaching

- Caution ambulatory patient about getting out of bed or walking. Warn outpatient to avoid hazardous activities until CNS effects of drug are known.

Evaluation

- Patient is free from pain.
- Patient maintains normal thought processes throughout therapy.
- Patient and family state understanding of drug therapy.

nalidixic acid

(nal-uh-DIK-sik AS-id)
NegGram

Pharmacologic class: fluoroquinolone antibiotic
Therapeutic class: urinary tract anti-infective
Pregnancy risk category: B (safe use in first trimester unknown)

Indications and dosages

▶ **Acute and chronic urinary tract infections caused by susceptible gram-negative organisms (*Proteus, Klebsiella, Enterobacter,* and *Escherichia coli*).** *Adults:* 1 g P.O. q.i.d. for 7 to 14 days; 2 g daily for long-term use.

Children over age 3 months: 55 mg/kg P.O. daily divided q.i.d. for 7 to 14 days; 33 mg/kg divided q.i.d. for long-term use.

How supplied

Tablets: 250 mg, 500 mg, 1 g
Oral suspension: 250 mg/5 ml

Pharmacokinetics

Absorption: well absorbed from GI tract.
Distribution: concentrates in renal tissue and seminal fluid; doesn't penetrate prostatic tissue and only minimal amounts appear in CSF. Drug is highly protein-bound.
Metabolism: metabolized in liver.
Excretion: 13% of metabolites and 2% to 3% of unchanged drug are excreted by kidneys.
Half-life: 1 to 2½ hours.

Route	Onset	Peak	Duration
P.O.	Unknown	1-4 hr	Unknown

Pharmacodynamics

Chemical effect: inhibits microbial DNA synthesis by bacterial DNA gyrase.
Therapeutic effect: kills susceptible bacteria, including most gram-negative organisms except *Pseudomonas*.

Adverse reactions

CNS: weakness, headache, dizziness, vertigo, ***seizures,*** malaise, confusion, hallucinations, drowsiness, ***increased intracranial pressure*** and ***bulging fontanelles*** in infants and children.
EENT: light sensitivity, color perception changes, diplopia, blurred vision.
GI: *abdominal pain, nausea, vomiting,* diarrhea.
Hematologic: eosinophilia, ***leukopenia, thrombocytopenia.***
Skin: pruritus, photosensitivity, urticaria, rash.
Other: ***angioedema,*** fever, chills.

Interactions

Drug-drug. *Oral anticoagulants:* increased anticoagulant effect. Monitor patient for bleeding.
Drug-lifestyle. *Sun exposure:* photosensitivity reactions may occur. Urge patient to take precautions.

Contraindications and precautions

- Contraindicated in patients hypersensitive to drug, in infants under age 3 months, and in patients with seizure disorders.
- Use with extreme caution in prepubertal children because drug has caused cartilage erosion.
- Use cautiously in pregnant women, breast-feeding women, and patients with impaired hepatic or renal function, severe cerebral arteriosclerosis, or pulmonary disease (because of increased respiratory depression).

NURSING CONSIDERATIONS

Assessment

- Assess patient's infection before therapy and regularly thereafter. Resistant bacteria may emerge within first 48 hours of therapy.
- Obtain specimen for culture and sensitivity tests before starting therapy and repeat p.r.n. Therapy may begin pending results.
- Monitor CBC and renal and liver function studies during long-term therapy, as ordered.
- Be alert for adverse reactions and drug interactions.
- Monitor patient's hydration status if adverse GI reactions occur.
- Evaluate patient's and family's knowledge of drug therapy.

Nursing diagnoses

- Infection related to susceptible bacteria
- Risk for deficient fluid volume related to drug-induced adverse GI reactions
- Deficient knowledge related to drug therapy

Planning and implementation

- Drug may cause false-positive Clinitest reaction. Use Diastix to monitor urine glucose. Also gives false elevations in urine vanillylmandelic acid and 17-ketosteroids. Tests should be repeated after therapy is complete.

Patient teaching

- Tell patient to avoid undue exposure to sunlight because of photosensitivity. Patient may continue to be photosensitive for as long as 3 months after therapy ends.

• Tell patient to report visual disturbances; these usually disappear with reduced dose.
• Teach patient to take with food and drink fluids liberally.

Evaluation

• Patient is free from infection.
• Patient maintains adequate hydration throughout drug therapy.
• Patient and family state understanding of drug therapy.

naloxone hydrochloride

(nal-OKS-ohn high-droh-KLOR-ighd)
Narcan

Pharmacologic class: narcotic (opioid) antagonist
Therapeutic class: narcotic antagonist
Pregnancy risk category: B

Indications and dosages

▶ **Known or suspected narcotic-induced respiratory depression, including that caused by pentazocine and propoxyphene.** *Adults:* 0.4 to 2 mg I.V., I.M, or S.C. Repeated q 2 to 3 minutes, p.r.n. If no response is observed after 10 mg has been administered, diagnosis of narcotic-induced toxicity should be questioned.

▶ **Postoperative narcotic depression.** *Adults:* 0.1 to 0.2 mg I.V. q 2 to 3 minutes, p.r.n.
Children: 0.005 to 0.01 mg/kg dose I.V. Repeated q 2 to 3 minutes, p.r.n.
Neonates (asphyxia neonatorum): 0.01 mg/kg I.V. into umbilical vein. May be repeated q 2 to 3 minutes for three doses.

How supplied

Injection: 0.02 mg/ml, 0.4 mg/ml, 1 mg/ml

Pharmacokinetics

Absorption: unknown after I.M. or S.C. administration.
Distribution: rapidly distributed into body tissues and fluids.
Metabolism: rapidly metabolized in liver.
Excretion: excreted in urine. *Half-life:* 60 to 90 minutes in adults, 3 hours in neonates.

Route	Onset	Peak	Duration
I.V.	1-2 min	Unknown	Varies
I.M., S.C.	2-5 min	Unknown	Varies

Pharmacodynamics

Chemical effect: unknown; may displace narcotic analgesics from their receptors (competitive antagonism). Has no pharmacologic activity of its own.
Therapeutic effect: reverses opioid effects.

Adverse reactions

CNS: tremors, ***seizures.***
CV: tachycardia and hypertension with high doses, ***ventricular fibrillation.***
GI: nausea and vomiting with high doses.
Respiratory: ***pulmonary edema.***
Other: withdrawal symptoms in narcotic-dependent patients with higher-than-recommended doses.

Interactions

None significant.

Contraindications and precautions

• Contraindicated in patients hypersensitive to drug.
• Use cautiously in pregnant women and in patients with cardiac irritability and opioid addiction. Abrupt reversal of opioid-induced CNS depression may cause nausea, vomiting, diaphoresis, tachycardia, CNS excitement, and increased blood pressure.
• Safety of drug hasn't been established in breast-feeding women.

NURSING CONSIDERATIONS

Assessment

• Assess patient's opioid use before therapy.
• Assess effectiveness of drug regularly throughout therapy.
• Duration of narcotic may exceed that of naloxone, causing relapse into respiratory depression. Monitor patient's respiratory depth and rate.

• Patients who receive naloxone to reverse opioid-induced respiratory depression may develop tachypnea.
• Monitor patient's hydration status if adverse GI reactions occur.
• Evaluate patient's and family's knowledge of drug therapy.

Nursing diagnoses
• Ineffective health maintenance related to opioid use
• Risk for deficient fluid volume related to drug-induced adverse GI reactions
• Deficient knowledge related to drug therapy

Planning and implementation
ALERT Drug is effective only in reversing respiratory depression caused by opioids. Flumazenil should be used to treat respiratory depression caused by diazepam or other benzodiazepines.
• Provide oxygen, ventilation, and other resuscitation measures if patient has severe respiratory depression.
I.V. use: Be prepared to give continuous I.V. infusion to control adverse effects of epidural morphine.
– To make neonatal concentration (0.02 mg/ml), adult concentration (0.4 mg) may be diluted by mixing 0.5 ml with 9.5 ml of sterile water or saline solution for injection.
I.M. and S.C. use: Follow normal protocol.
ALERT Don't confuse naloxone with naltrexone.

Patient teaching
• Instruct patient and family to report adverse reactions.

Evaluation
• Patient responds well to drug.
• Patient maintains adequate hydration.
• Patient and family state understanding of drug therapy.

naltrexone hydrochloride
(nal-TREKS-ohn high-droh-KLOR-ighd)
ReVia

Pharmacologic class: narcotic (opioid) antagonist
Therapeutic class: narcotic detoxification adjunct
Pregnancy risk category: C

Indications and dosages
▶ **Adjunct for maintenance of opioid-free state in detoxified patients.** *Adults:* initially, 25 mg P.O. If no withdrawal signs occur within 1 hour, additional 25 mg is given. Once patient receives 50 mg q 24 hours, flexible maintenance schedule may be used.
▶ **Treatment of alcohol dependence.** *Adults:* 50 mg P.O. once daily.

How supplied
Tablets: 50 mg

Pharmacokinetics
Absorption: well absorbed from GI tract.
Distribution: widely distributed throughout body but varies considerably. Drug is about 21% to 28% protein-bound.
Metabolism: undergoes extensive first-pass hepatic metabolism. Its major metabolite may be pure antagonist and contribute to its efficacy. Drug and metabolites may undergo enterohepatic recirculation.
Excretion: excreted mainly by kidneys. *Half-life:* about 4 hours.

Route	Onset	Peak	Duration
P.O.	15-30 min	> 12 hr	About 24 hr

Pharmacodynamics
Chemical effect: unknown; may reversibly block subjective effects of I.V. opioids by occupying opioid receptors in brain.
Therapeutic effect: helps prevent opioid dependence and treats alcohol dependence.

Adverse reactions
CNS: *insomnia, anxiety, nervousness, headache,* depression, ***suicide ideation.***

GI: *nausea, vomiting,* anorexia, *abdominal pain.*
Hepatic: ***hepatotoxicity.***
Musculoskeletal: *muscle and joint pain.*

Interactions

Drug-drug. *Thioridazine:* increased somnolence and lethargy. Monitor patient closely.

Contraindications and precautions

• Contraindicated in patients hypersensitive to drug; in those who are receiving opioid analgesics, have a positive urine screen for opioids, or are opioid dependent; in those who have acute opioid withdrawal; and in those with acute hepatitis or liver failure.
• Use cautiously in pregnant women and in patients with mild hepatic disease or history of recent hepatic disease.
• Safety of drug hasn't been established in breast-feeding women.

NURSING CONSIDERATIONS

Assessment

• Assess patient's opioid or alcohol dependence before therapy.
• Monitor effectiveness of drug.
• Evaluate patient's and family's knowledge of drug therapy.

Nursing diagnoses

• Health-seeking behavior related to desire to remain free from opioid dependence
• Disturbed sleep pattern related to drug-induced insomnia
• Deficient knowledge related to drug therapy

Planning and implementation

ALERT Treatment for opioid dependency should begin after patient receives naloxone challenge, a provocative test of opioid dependency. If signs of opioid withdrawal persist after challenge, don't give naltrexone.
• Patient must be completely free from opioids before taking naltrexone or severe withdrawal symptoms may occur. Patient who has been addicted to short-acting opioids, such as heroin and meperidine, must wait at least 7 days after last opioid dose before starting naltrexone. Patient who has been addicted to longer-acting opioids, such as methadone, should wait at least 10 days.
• In emergency, expect patient receiving naltrexone to be given an opioid analgesic, but in a higher dose than usual to surmount naltrexone's effect. Respiratory depression caused by opioid analgesic may be longer and deeper.
• For patient with opioid dependence who isn't expected to comply, use flexible maintenance regimen: 100 mg on Monday and Wednesday, 150 mg on Friday, as ordered.
• Use naltrexone only as part of comprehensive rehabilitation program.
ALERT Don't confuse naloxone and naltrexone.

Patient teaching

• Advise patient to wear or carry medical identification. Warn him to tell medical personnel that he takes naltrexone.
• Give patient names of nonopioid drugs he can continue to take for pain, diarrhea, or cough.

Evaluation

• Patient maintains opioid-free state.
• Patient reports no insomnia.
• Patient and family state understanding of drug therapy.

nandrolone decanoate

(NAN-druh-lohn deh-kuh-NOH-ayt)
Androlone-D, Deca-Durabolin, Hybolin Decanoate, Kabolin, Neo-Durabolic

nandrolone phenpropionate

Durabolin, Hybolin Improved

Pharmacologic class: anabolic steroid
Therapeutic class: erythropoietic and anabolic (nandrolone decanoate), antineoplastic (nandrolone phenpropionate)
Controlled substance schedule: III
Pregnancy risk category: X

Indications and dosages

▶ **Severe debility or disease states, refractory anemias. Nandrolone decanoate.** *Adults:* 50 to 100 mg/week I.M. for women;

100 to 200 mg I.M. at weekly intervals for men. Therapy should be intermittent.
Children ages 2 to 13: 25 to 50 mg I.M. q 3 to 4 weeks.
▶ **Control of metastatic breast cancer.**
Nandrolone phenpropionate. *Adults:* 50 to 100 mg I.M. weekly.

How supplied

nandrolone decanoate
Injection (in oil): 50 mg/ml, 100 mg/ml, 200 mg/ml
nandrolone phenpropionate
Injection (in oil): 25 mg/ml, 50 mg/ml

Pharmacokinetics

Absorption: nandrolone decanoate is slowly released from I.M. depot. Nandrolone phenpropionate's absorption is unknown.
Distribution: unknown.
Metabolism: nandrolone decanoate is hydrolyzed to free nandrolone by plasma esterase and metabolized in liver. Nandrolone phenpropionate is metabolized in liver.
Excretion: excreted in urine. *Half-life:* 6 to 8 days for nandrolone decanoate; unknown for nandrolone phenpropionate.

Route	Onset	Peak	Duration
I.M.	Unknown	3-6 days (decanoate); 1-2 days (phenpropionate)	Unknown

Pharmacodynamics

Chemical effect: promotes tissue building, reverses catabolism, and stimulates erythropoiesis.
Therapeutic effect: promotes tissue building and RBC growth (decanoate); hinders growth of breast cancer cells (phenpropionate).

Adverse reactions

CV: edema.
GI: gastroenteritis, nausea, vomiting, diarrhea, change in appetite.
GU: bladder irritability.
Hematologic: ***thrombocytopenia,*** elevated serum lipid levels.
Hepatic: reversible jaundice, peliosis hepatis, elevated liver enzyme levels, ***liver cell tumors.***
Metabolic: hypercalcemia.
Musculoskeletal: muscle cramps or spasms.
Skin: pain, induration at injection site.
Other: androgenic effects in women (acne, edema, *weight gain, hirsutism,* hoarseness, clitoral enlargement, *decreased breast size,* altered libido, male-pattern baldness, *oily skin or hair*), hypoestrogenic effects in women (flushing, diaphoresis, vaginitis, vaginal bleeding, nervousness, emotional lability, menstrual irregularities), excessive hormonal effects in prepubertal men (premature epiphyseal closure, *acne,* priapism, *growth of body and facial hair,* phallic enlargement), excessive hormonal effects in postpubertal men (testicular atrophy, oligospermia, decreased ejaculatory volume, impotence, gynecomastia, epididymitis).

Interactions

Drug-drug. *Hepatotoxic drugs:* increased risk of hepatotoxicity. Monitor patient closely.
Insulin, oral antidiabetics: altered antidiabetic dosage requirements. Monitor blood glucose levels in diabetic patients.
Oral anticoagulants: altered anticoagulant dosage requirements. Monitor PT and INR.

Contraindications and precautions

• Contraindicated in patient hypersensitive to anabolic steroids, in men with breast or prostate cancer, in patients with nephrosis, in patients experiencing the nephrotic phase of nephritis, in women with breast cancer and hypercalcemia, and in pregnant or breast-feeding women.
• Use cautiously in patients with diabetes; cardiac, renal, or hepatic disease; epilepsy; or migraine or other conditions that may be aggravated by fluid retention.

NURSING CONSIDERATIONS

Assessment

• Assess patient's condition before therapy and regularly thereafter.
• Make sure that pregnancy test is negative for woman of childbearing age before therapy starts.

• In child, X-rays of wrist bones should be taken before treatment to assess bone maturation. During treatment, bone maturation may proceed rapidly; periodically review X-ray results to monitor it.
• Closely observe boy under age 7 for precocious development of male sexual characteristics.
• Semen evaluation is routinely performed every 3 to 4 months, especially in adolescent male.
• Evaluate hepatic function, as ordered.
• Watch for symptoms of hypoglycemia in diabetic patient. Check blood glucose levels regularly because antidiabetic dosage may need to be adjusted.
• Check quantitative urine and serum calcium levels.
• Be alert for adverse reactions and drug interactions.
• Evaluate patient's and family's knowledge of drug therapy.
• Check weight regularly and assess for fluid retention.

Nursing diagnoses

• Ineffective health maintenance related to underlying condition
• Disturbed body image related to adverse androgenic reactions
• Deficient knowledge related to drug therapy

Planning and implementation

• Inject I.M. drug deeply, preferably into upper outer quadrant of gluteal muscle in adults. Rotate injection sites to prevent muscle atrophy.
• Notify prescriber immediately about signs of virilization; they may be irreversible despite stopping therapy promptly.
• Dosage adjustment may reverse jaundice. If liver function test results are abnormal, therapy should be stopped.
• Drug-induced edema usually can be controlled with sodium restrictions or diuretics.
• When used to promote erythropoiesis, make sure patient has adequate daily iron intake.
• Anabolic steroids may alter results of laboratory studies performed during therapy and for 2 to 3 weeks after therapy ends.

Patient teaching

• Make sure patient understands importance of using effective nonhormonal contraceptive during therapy.
• Advise washing after intercourse to decrease risk of vaginitis. Instruct patient to wear only cotton underwear.
• Tell woman to report menstrual irregularities and to stop therapy until the cause of irregularity has been determined.
• Instruct patient to report sudden weight gain.

Evaluation

• Patient responds well to therapy.
• Patient states acceptance of body image changes.
• Patient and family state understanding of drug therapy.

naphazoline hydrochloride

(naf-AZ-oh-leen high-droh-KLOR-ighd)
Privine†

Pharmacologic class: sympathomimetic
Therapeutic class: decongestant, vasoconstrictor
Pregnancy risk category: NR

Indications and dosages

▶ **Nasal congestion.** *Adults and children age 12 and older:* 1 or 2 gtt or sprays in each nostril q 3 to 4 hours.
Children ages 6 to 12: 1 to 2 gtt or sprays in each nostril q 3 to 6 hours, p.r.n. Not to be used longer than 3 to 5 days.

How supplied

Nasal drops: 0.05% solution
Nasal spray: 0.05% solution

Pharmacokinetics

Unknown.

Route	Onset	Peak	Duration
Intranasal	≤ 10 min	Unknown	2-6 hr

Pharmacodynamics

Chemical effect: causes local vasoconstriction of dilated arterioles, reducing blood flow.

Therapeutic effect: relieves nasal congestion.

Adverse reactions

CNS: marked sedation.
EENT: rebound nasal congestion with excessive or long-term use, sneezing, stinging, mucosal dryness.
Other: systemic effects in children after excessive or long-term use.

Interactions

None significant.

Contraindications and precautions

- Contraindicated in patients hypersensitive to drug.
- Drug isn't recommended for breast-feeding women.
- Use cautiously in pregnant women and in patients with hyperthyroidism, heart disease, hypertension, or diabetes mellitus.

NURSING CONSIDERATIONS

Assessment
- Assess patient's condition before therapy and regularly thereafter.
- Be alert for adverse reactions.
- Evaluate patient's and family's knowledge of drug therapy.

Nursing diagnoses
- Ineffective health maintenance related to nasal congestion
- Impaired tissue integrity related to drug's adverse effect on nasal tissue
- Deficient knowledge related to drug therapy

Planning and implementation
- To instill nasal drops, have patient tilt head back as far as possible; instill drops; then have patient lean head forward while inhaling. Repeat procedure for other nostril.
- To instill nasal spray, hold spray container and patient's head upright; then spray. Don't shake container.

Patient teaching
- Teach patient how to use drug.
- Explain that product should be used by only one person to prevent spread of infection.
- Warn patient not to exceed recommended dosage.
- Tell patient to contact prescriber if nasal congestion persists after 5 days.

Evaluation
- Patient's congestion is relieved.
- Patient's nasal tissue doesn't dry or crack.
- Patient and family state understanding of drug therapy.

naproxen
(nuh-PROK-sin)
Apo-Naproxen♦, Naprosyn, Naprosyn-E♦, Naprosyn SR♦ ◇, Naxen♦ ◇, Novo-Naprox♦, Nu-Naprox♦

naproxen sodium
Aleve†, Anaprox, Anaprox DS, Apo-Napro-Na♦, Novo-Naprox Sodium♦, Synflex♦

Pharmacologic class: NSAID
Therapeutic class: nonnarcotic analgesic, antipyretic, anti-inflammatory
Pregnancy risk category: B

Indications and dosages

▶ **Rheumatoid arthritis, osteoarthritis, ankylosing spondylitis.** *Adults:* 250 to 500 mg naproxen P.O. b.i.d. Or, 275 to 550 mg naproxen sodium P.O. b.i.d. Or, where suppository is available, 500 mg P.R. h.s. with naproxen P.O. during day. Maximum dosage is 1,500 mg daily.

▶ **Juvenile arthritis.** *Children:* 10 mg/kg naproxen P.O. in two divided doses.

▶ **Acute gout.** *Adults:* 750 mg naproxen P.O., followed by 250 mg q 8 hours until attack subsides. Or, 825 mg naproxen sodium initially; then 275 mg q 8 hours until attack subsides.

▶ **Mild to moderate pain, primary dysmenorrhea, acute tendinitis and bursitis.** *Adults:* 500 mg naproxen P.O., followed by 250 mg q 6 to 8 hours p.r.n. Or, 550 mg naproxen sodium P.O. initially; then 275 mg P.O. q 6 to 8 hours p.r.n.

How supplied

naproxen
Tablets: 250 mg, 375 mg, 500 mg
Tablets (extended-release) ♦***:*** 750 mg, 1,000 mg
Oral suspension: 125 mg/5 ml
Suppositories: 500 mg ◊
naproxen sodium
275 mg naproxen sodium = 250 mg naproxen
Tablets (film-coated): 220 mg, 275 mg, 550 mg

Pharmacokinetics

Absorption: absorbed rapidly and completely from GI tract.
Distribution: highly protein-bound.
Metabolism: metabolized in liver.
Excretion: excreted in urine. *Half-life:* 1.3 hours.

Route	Onset	Peak	Duration
P.O.	≤ 1 hr	1-4 hr	About 7 hr
P.R.	Unknown	Unknown	Unknown

Pharmacodynamics

Chemical effect: unknown; produces anti-inflammatory, analgesic, and antipyretic effects, possibly by inhibiting prostaglandin synthesis.
Therapeutic effect: relieves pain, fever, and inflammation.

Adverse reactions

CNS: *headache, drowsiness, dizziness,* tinnitus, cognitive dysfunction, aseptic meningitis.
CV: *peripheral edema,* palpitations, digital vasculitis.
EENT: visual disturbances, *tinnitus.*
GI: *epigastric distress, occult blood loss, nausea,* ***peptic ulceration.***
GU: nephrotoxicity.
Hematologic: prolonged bleeding time, ***agranulocytosis, thrombocytopenia, neutropenia.***
Hepatic: elevated liver enzyme levels.
Metabolic: ***hyperkalemia.***
Respiratory: dyspnea.
Skin: *pruritus, rash,* urticaria.

Interactions

Drug-drug. *Antihypertensives, diuretics:* decreased effect of these drugs. Monitor patient.
Aspirin, corticosteroids: increased risk of adverse GI reactions. Use cautiously.
Methotrexate: increased risk of toxicity. Monitor patient closely.
Oral anticoagulants, sulfonylureas, drugs that are highly protein-bound: increased risk of toxicity. Monitor patient closely.
Probenecid: decreased elimination of naproxen. Monitor patient for toxicity.
Drug-herb. *Dong quai, feverfew, garlic, ginger, horse chestnut, red clover:* possible increased risk of bleeding. Discourage concomitant use.
St. John's wort: increased risk of photosensitivity. Advise patient to avoid unprotected exposure to sunlight.
Drug-lifestyle. *Alcohol use:* increased risk of adverse GI reactions. Discourage concomitant use.

Contraindications and precautions

- Contraindicated in patients hypersensitive to drug, breast-feeding patients, patients in the last trimester of pregnancy, and patients with asthma, rhinitis, or nasal polyps.
- Use cautiously in elderly patients and in those with renal disease, CV disease, GI disorders, hepatic disease, or peptic ulcer disease.

NURSING CONSIDERATIONS

Assessment

- Assess patient's condition before therapy and regularly thereafter.
- Monitor CBC and renal and hepatic function every 4 to 6 months or as ordered during long-term therapy.
- NSAIDs may mask signs and symptoms of infection.
- Monitor patient's hydration status if adverse GI reactions occur.
- Evaluate patient's and family's knowledge of drug therapy.

Nursing diagnoses

- Acute pain related to condition
- Risk for deficient fluid volume related to drug-induced adverse GI reactions

• Deficient knowledge related to drug therapy

Planning and implementation

• Inform laboratory personnel that patient is taking naproxen. Drug may interfere with urinary assays of 5-hydroxyindoleacetic acid and may falsely elevate urine 17-ketosteroid concentrations.

P.O. use: Give drug with food or milk to minimize GI upset.

– Tell patient to take a full glass of water or other liquid with each dose.

P.R. use: Not commercially available in the United States.

– Don't use in patients with inflammatory lesion of the rectum or anus.

Patient teaching

• Tell patient taking prescription doses of naproxen for arthritis that full therapeutic effect may take 2 to 4 weeks.

ALERT Warn patient against taking naproxen and naproxen sodium at the same time.

• Teach patient to recognize and report evidence of GI bleeding. Serious GI toxicity, including peptic ulceration and bleeding, can occur in patients taking NSAIDs despite absence of GI symptoms.

• Caution patient that concomitant use with aspirin, alcohol, or corticosteroids may increase risk of adverse GI reactions.

• Advise patient to have periodic eye examinations.

Evaluation

• Patient is free from pain.

• Patient maintains adequate hydration.

• Patient and family state understanding of drug therapy.

naratriptan hydrochloride

(nah-rah-TRIP-tin high-droh-KLOR-ighd)

Amerge

Pharmacologic class: selective 5-hydroxytryptamine$_1$ (5-HT$_1$) receptor subtype agonist

Therapeutic class: antimigraine agent

Pregnancy risk category: C

Indications and dosages

▶ **Treatment of acute migraine headaches with or without aura.** *Adults:* 1 or 2.5 mg P.O. as a single dose. If headache returns or responds only partially, dose may be repeated after 4 hours, for maximum dose of 5 mg in 24 hours.

How supplied

Tablets: 1 mg, 2.5 mg

Pharmacokinetics

Absorption: well absorbed with a bioavailability of 70%.

Distribution: about 28% to 31% plasma protein–bound.

Metabolism: metabolized to a number of inactive metabolites by wide range of cytochrome P-450 isoenzymes.

Excretion: primarily excreted in urine with 50% of dose recovered unchanged and 30% as metabolites. *Half-life:* 6 hours.

Route	Onset	Peak	Duration
P.O.	Unknown	2-3 hr	Unknown

Pharmacodynamics

Chemical effect: thought to activate receptors in intracranial blood vessels leading to vasoconstriction and relief of migraine headache; activation of receptors on sensory nerve endings in trigeminal system may inhibit proinflammatory neuropeptide release.

Therapeutic effect: relieves migraine pain.

Adverse reactions

CNS: paresthesias, dizziness, drowsiness, malaise, fatigue, vertigo, syncope.

CV: palpitations, increased blood pressure, ***tachyarrhythmias, abnormal ECG changes (PR and QTc interval prolongation, ST/T wave abnormalities, PVCs, atrial flutter or fibrillation), coronary vasospasm.***

EENT: ear, nose, and throat infections; photophobia.

GI: nausea, hyposalivation, vomiting.

Other: warm or cold temperature sensations; pressure, tightness, and heaviness sensations.

Interactions

Drug-drug. *Ergot-containing or ergot-type drugs (methysergide, dihydroergotamine), other 5-HT_1 agonists:* prolonged vasospastic reactions. Don't give within 24 hours of naratriptan.
Oral contraceptives: slightly higher naratriptan levels. Monitor patient.
Selective serotonin reuptake inhibitors (fluoxetine, fluvoxamine, paroxetine, sertraline): may cause weakness, hyperreflexia, and incoordination. Monitor patient.
Drug-lifestyle. *Smoking:* increased naratriptan clearance. Discourage concomitant use.

Contraindications and precautions

- Contraindicated in patients hypersensitive to drug or its components; elderly patients; patients who have received ergot-containing, ergot-type, or other 5-HT_1 agonists in the previous 24 hours; patients with history, symptoms, or signs of cardiac ischemia, cerebrovascular disease, or peripheral vascular disease; and patients with significant underlying CV disease, a history of uncontrolled hypertension, severe renal impairment (creatinine clearance below 15 ml/minute), or severe hepatic impairment (Child-Pugh grade C).
- Unless a CV evaluation has determined that patient is free from cardiac disease, use cautiously in patients with risk factors for coronary artery disease, such as hypertension, hypercholesterolemia, obesity, diabetes, a strong family history of coronary artery disease, surgical or physiologic menopause (women), age over 40 (men), and smoking. For patients with cardiac risk factors but a satisfactory CV evaluation, give first dose in a medical facility and consider ECG monitoring.

NURSING CONSIDERATIONS

Assessment

- Assess baseline cardiac function before starting therapy. Perform periodic cardiac reevaluation in patients who develop risk factors for coronary artery disease.
- Monitor renal and liver function test results before starting drug therapy, and report abnormalities.
- Evaluate patient's and family's knowledge of drug therapy.

Nursing diagnoses

- Acute pain related to presence of migraine headache
- Risk for injury related to drug-induced adverse CV reactions
- Deficient knowledge related to drug therapy

Planning and implementation

- Administer drug once a definite diagnosis of migraine has been established. Drug isn't intended for preventing migraine headaches or treating hemiplegic headaches, basilar migraines, or cluster headaches.
- Withhold drug and notify prescriber if patient has pain or tightness in chest or throat, arrhythmias, or increased blood pressure.

ALERT Patients with mild to moderate renal or hepatic impairment receive a reduced starting dose. Don't exceed 2.5 mg in a 24-hour period in these patients.

- Don't give drug to patients with history of coronary artery disease, hypertension, arrhythmias, or risk factors for coronary artery disease because drug may cause coronary vasospasm and hypertension.
- For patients with cardiac risk factors who have had a satisfactory cardiac evaluation, administer first dose while monitoring ECG. Keep emergency equipment readily available.
- Safety and effectiveness haven't been established for cluster headaches or for treating more than four migraine headaches in a 30-day period.

Patient teaching

- Instruct patient to take drug only as prescribed.
- Tell patient that drug is intended to relieve migraine headaches, not prevent them.
- Instruct patient to take dose soon after headache starts. If no response occurs to first tablet, tell patient to seek medical approval before taking second tablet. If prescriber approves a second dose, patient may take a second tablet, but no sooner than 4 hours after first tablet. Warn patient not to exceed two tablets in 24 hours.

- Instruct patient not to use drug if she is or could be pregnant.
- Teach patient to alert prescriber about bothersome adverse effects or risk factors for coronary artery disease.
- Instruct patient to read the patient instructions before taking drug.

Evaluation
- Patient has relief of migraine headache.
- Patient has no pain or tightness in chest or throat, arrhythmias, or increase in blood pressure.
- Patient and family state understanding of drug therapy.

nedocromil sodium
(nee-DOK-roh-mil SOH-dee-um)
Tilade

Pharmacologic class: pyranoquinoline
Therapeutic class: anti-inflammatory respiratory inhalant
Pregnancy risk category: B

Indications and dosages
▶ **Maintenance in mild to moderate reversible obstructive airway disease.** *Adults and children age 12 and over:* 2 inhalations q.i.d., preferably at regular intervals.

How supplied
Inhalation aerosol: 1.75 mg/activation

Pharmacokinetics
Absorption: 2% to 3% of drug swallowed after inhalation is absorbed. From 6% to 9% of drug deposited in lungs is absorbed.
Distribution: distributed only to plasma. About 89% reversibly bound to plasma proteins when plasma levels are 0.5 to 50 mcg/ml.
Metabolism: not metabolized.
Excretion: rapidly excreted unchanged in bile and urine. *Half-life:* about 1½ to 3¼ hours.

Route	Onset	Peak	Duration
Inhalation	2 days-4 wk	5-90 min	6-12 hr

Pharmacodynamics
Chemical effect: reduces inflammatory changes in airway by blocking release of inflammatory mediators from mast cells, eosinophils, monocytes, neutrophils, macrophages, and other immune cells.
Therapeutic effect: improves gas exchange.

Adverse reactions
CNS: headache.
EENT: rhinitis.
GI: nausea, vomiting, *unpleasant taste*.
Respiratory: upper respiratory tract infection, ***bronchospasm.***

Interactions
None significant.

Contraindications and precautions
- Contraindicated in patients hypersensitive to drug or its components and in those experiencing acute asthmatic attack or acute bronchospasm.
- Use cautiously in pregnant or breast-feeding women.
- Safety of drug hasn't been established in children under age 12.

NURSING CONSIDERATIONS

Assessment
- Assess patient's condition before therapy and regularly thereafter.
- Be alert for adverse reactions.
- Evaluate patient's and family's knowledge of drug therapy.

Nursing diagnoses
- Impaired gas exchange related to respiratory condition
- Acute pain related to drug-induced headache
- Deficient knowledge related to drug therapy

Planning and implementation
- Dosage may be reduced to two inhalations t.i.d., as ordered, and then b.i.d. after several weeks, when patient's asthma is under control.
- Administer regularly, even during symptom-free periods, to achieve maximum benefit in maintenance therapy.

• Administer mild analgesic, as ordered, for drug-induced headache.
ALERT Don't confuse Ticlid with Tilade.

Patient teaching
• Warn patient that drug can't replace bronchodilators during acute asthmatic attack.
• Tell patient that drug is adjunct to regular bronchodilator regimen and may reduce need for corticosteroids or bronchodilators.
• Explain that regular use yields the best results. Most patients report benefits after 1 week; some need longer treatment.
• Advise patient that use of an aerochamber may enhance drug delivery to the lungs.
• Teach patient how to use inhaler. Instruct him to shake canister and invert it just before use.
• Advise patient to clean inhaler at least twice weekly and to remove canister before rinsing inhaler in hot, running water. Tell patient to let inhaler air dry overnight.

✓ Evaluation
• Patient demonstrates adequate gas exchange with drug therapy.
• Patient is free from drug-induced headache.
• Patient and family state understanding of drug therapy.

nefazodone hydrochloride
(nef-AZ-oh-dohn high-droh-KLOR-ighd)
Serzone

Pharmacologic class: synthetically derived phenylpiperazine
Therapeutic class: antidepressant
Pregnancy risk category: C

Indications and dosages
▶ **Depression.** *Adults:* initially, 200 mg/day P.O. in two divided doses. Dosage increased in increments of 100 to 200 mg/day at intervals of no less than 1 week, as indicated. Usual dosage range is 300 to 600 mg/day.

How supplied
Tablets: 100 mg, 150 mg, 200 mg, 250 mg

Pharmacokinetics
Absorption: rapidly and completely absorbed with low, variable absolute bioavailability (about 20%).
Distribution: widely distributed in body tissues, including CNS. Drug is extensively bound to plasma proteins.
Metabolism: extensively metabolized.
Excretion: excreted in urine. *Half-life:* 2 to 4 hours.

Route	Onset	Peak	Duration
P.O.	Unknown	About 1 hr	Unknown

Pharmacodynamics
Chemical effect: not precisely defined. Drug inhibits neuronal uptake of serotonin ($5\text{-}HT_2$) and norepinephrine; it also occupies serotonin and $alpha_1$-adrenergic receptors in CNS.
Therapeutic effect: relieves depression.

Adverse reactions
CNS: headache, *somnolence, dizziness, asthenia,* insomnia, *light-headedness, confusion,* memory impairment, paresthesia, abnormal dreams, decreased concentration, ataxia, incoordination, psychomotor retardation, tremor, hypertonia.
CV: vasodilation, orthostatic hypotension, hypotension, peripheral edema.
EENT: *blurred vision, abnormal vision,* pharyngitis, tinnitus, visual field defect.
GI: *dry mouth, nausea, constipation,* dyspepsia, diarrhea, increased appetite, vomiting, taste perversion.
GU: urinary frequency, urinary tract infection, urine retention, vaginitis.
Musculoskeletal: neck rigidity, arthralgia.
Respiratory: cough.
Skin: pruritus, rash.
Other: infection, flu syndrome, chills, fever, thirst, breast pain.

Interactions
Drug-drug. *Alprazolam, triazolam:* increased effects of these drugs. Either avoid concurrent use or give greatly reduced dosage of alprazolam and triazolam.
Calcium channel blockers and HMG-CoA reductase inhibitors: may increase levels of

these drugs. Dosage adjustment may be needed.
CNS-active drugs: may alter CNS activity. Use together cautiously.
Digoxin: may increase digoxin level. Use together cautiously, and monitor digoxin levels.
MAO inhibitors: may cause severe excitation, hyperpyrexia, seizures, delirium, or coma. Avoid concomitant use.
Other drugs highly bound to plasma proteins: may increase adverse reactions. Monitor patient closely.
Drug-lifestyle. *Alcohol use:* enhanced CNS depression. Discourage concomitant use.

Contraindications and precautions

- Contraindicated in patients hypersensitive to drug or other phenylpiperazine antidepressants and within 14 days of MAO inhibitor therapy.
- Use cautiously in patients with CV or cerebrovascular disease that could be worsened by hypotension (such as history of MI, angina, or CVA) and conditions that predispose to hypotension (such as dehydration, hypovolemia, and treatment with antihypertensives).
- Also use cautiously in patients with history of mania and in pregnant or breast-feeding women.
- Safety of drug hasn't been established in children under age 18.

NURSING CONSIDERATIONS

Assessment
- Assess patient's depression before therapy and regularly thereafter.
- Record mood changes. Monitor patient for suicidal tendencies.
- Be alert for adverse reactions and drug interactions.
- Evaluate patient's and family's knowledge of drug therapy.

Nursing diagnoses
- Disturbed thought processes related to depression
- Risk for injury related to drug-induced adverse CNS reactions
- Deficient knowledge related to drug therapy

Planning and implementation
- Allow at least 1 week after stopping drug before patient starts an MAO inhibitor. Allow at least 14 days after stopping an MAO inhibitor before patient starts drug.

Patient teaching
- Warn patient not to engage in hazardous activity until CNS effects of drug are known.

ALERT Instruct man with prolonged or inappropriate erections to stop drug at once and call prescriber.
- Instruct woman to call prescriber if she becomes pregnant or intends to become pregnant during therapy.
- Instruct patient not to drink alcoholic beverages during drug therapy.
- Tell patient who develops rash, hives, or related allergic reaction to notify prescriber.
- Inform patient that several weeks of therapy may be needed to obtain full antidepressant effect. Once improvement occurs, tell patient not to stop drug until directed by prescriber.
- Urge patient to notify prescriber before taking any OTC medications.

Evaluation
- Patient exhibits improved behavior.
- Patient sustains no injuries from drug-induced adverse CNS reactions.
- Patient and family state understanding of drug therapy.

nelfinavir mesylate
(nel-FIN-uh-veer MES-ih-layt)
Viracept

Pharmacologic class: HIV protease inhibitor
Therapeutic class: antiviral
Pregnancy risk category: B

Indications and dosages

▶ **Treatment of HIV infection when antiretroviral therapy is warranted.** *Adults:* 750 mg P.O. t.i.d. with meals or light snacks. *Children ages 2 to 13:* 20 to 30 mg/kg/dose P.O. t.i.d. with meals or light snacks; not to exceed 750 mg t.i.d. Recommended children's dose given t.i.d. is shown below.

Body weight (kg)	Level 1-g scoops	Level teaspoons	Tablets
7 to < 8.5	4	1	-
8.5 to < 10.5	5	1.25	-
10.5 to < 12	6	1.5	-
12 to < 14	7	1.75	-
14 to < 16	8	2	-
16 to < 18	9	2.25	-
18 to < 23	10	2.5	2
> 23	15	3.75	3

How supplied

Tablets: 250 mg
Powder: 50 mg/g powder

Pharmacokinetics

Absorption: not reported; plasma levels peak higher when drug is taken with food.
Distribution: more than 98% bound to plasma protein.
Metabolism: metabolized primarily by cytochrome P-450 3A (CYP3A).
Excretion: excreted mainly in feces. *Half-life:* 3½ to 5 hours.

Route	Onset	Peak	Duration
P.O.	Unknown	2-4 hr	Unknown

Pharmacodynamics

Chemical effect: inhibition of protease enzyme prevents cleavage of the viral polyprotein.
Therapeutic effect: production of immature, noninfectious virus.

Adverse reactions

CNS: asthenia, anxiety, depression, dizziness, emotional lability, hyperkinesia, insomnia, migraine, malaise, headache, paresthesia, ***seizures,*** sleep disorders, somnolence, ***suicide ideation.***
EENT: iritis, eye disorder, pharyngitis, rhinitis, sinusitis.
GI: abdominal pain, nausea, *diarrhea,* flatulence, anorexia, dyspepsia, epigastric pain, GI bleeding, ***pancreatitis,*** mouth ulceration, vomiting.
GU: sexual dysfunction, renal calculus, urine abnormality.
Hematologic: anemia, ***leukopenia, thrombocytopenia.***
Hepatic: ***hepatitis,*** elevated liver function test results.
Metabolic: dehydration, hyperglycemia, hyperlipidemia, hyperuricemia, hypoglycemia, increased amylase and creatinine phosphokinase levels.
Musculoskeletal: back pain, arthralgia, arthritis, cramps, myalgia, myasthenia, myopathy.
Respiratory: dyspnea.
Skin: rash, dermatitis, folliculitis, fungal dermatitis, pruritus, diaphoresis, urticaria.
Other: ***allergic reactions***, fever.

Interactions

Drug-drug. *Amiodarone, ergot derivatives, midazolam, quinidine, triazolam:* nelfinavir may produce large increases in plasma levels of these drugs, which may increase risk for serious or life-threatening adverse events. Don't administer concurrently.
HIV protease inhibitors (indinavir, ritonavir): may increase plasma nelfinavir levels. Monitor serum levels carefully.
Carbamazepine, phenobarbital, phenytoin: may reduce effectiveness of nelfinavir by decreasing plasma nelfinavir levels. Monitor patient.
Oral contraceptives (ethinyl estradiol, norethindrone): nelfinavir may decrease plasma contraceptive levels. Suggest alternate or additional contraceptive measures during nelfinavir therapy.
Rifabutin: increased rifabutin plasma levels. Expect dosage of rifabutin to be reduced by half.
Rifampin: decreased nelfinavir plasma levels. Don't use together.
Drug-herb. *St. John's wort:* substantially reduces blood levels of drug, which may cause loss of therapeutic effects. Discourage concomitant use.

Contraindications and precautions

- Contraindicated in patients hypersensitive to drug or its components.
- Use cautiously in patients with hepatic dysfunction or hemophilia type A and B.

NURSING CONSIDERATIONS

Assessment
- Obtain baseline assessment of patient's condition, and reassess regularly thereafter to monitor drug effectiveness.
- Monitor liver function test results.
- Assess patient for increased bleeding tendencies, especially if he has hemophilia type A or B.
- Monitor patient for excessive diarrhea, and treat as directed.
- Evaluate patient's and family's knowledge of drug therapy.

Nursing diagnoses
- Risk for injury related to adverse GI effects of drug
- Risk for impaired skin integrity secondary to drug adverse effects
- Deficient knowledge related to drug therapy

Planning and implementation
- Administer oral powder in children unable to take tablets. May mix oral powder with small amount of water, milk, formula, soy formula, soy milk, or dietary supplements. Tell patient to consume entire contents.
- Don't reconstitute drug with water in its original container.
- Use reconstituted powder within 6 hours.
- Mixing with acidic foods or juice isn't recommended because of the bitter taste.

ALERT Don't confuse nelfinavir with nevirapine.

Patient teaching
- Advise patient to take drug with food.
- Inform patient that drug doesn't cure HIV infection.
- Tell patient that long-term effects of drug are unknown and that there are no data to support assumption that drug reduces risk of HIV transmission to others.
- Advise patient to take drug daily as prescribed and not to alter dose or stop drug without medical approval.
- Tell patient that diarrhea is most common adverse effect and it can be controlled with loperamide if necessary.
- If patient misses a dose, tell him to take it as soon as possible and then return to his normal schedule. If a dose is skipped, advise patient not to double the dose.
- Instruct patient taking oral contraceptives to use alternate or additional contraceptive measures while taking nelfinavir.
- Advise patient not to breast-feed to avoid transmitting virus to infant.
- Warn patient with phenylketonuria that powder contains 11.2 mg phenylalanine per gram.
- Advise patient to report use of other prescribed or OTC drugs because of possible drug interactions.

Evaluation
- Patient has no adverse GI reactions.
- Skin integrity remains intact.
- Patient and family state understanding of drug therapy.

neomycin sulfate
(nee-oh-MIGH-sin SUL-fayt)

Mycifradin, Neo-fradin, Neo-Tabs

Pharmacologic class: aminoglycoside
Therapeutic class: antibiotic
Pregnancy risk category: D

Indications and dosages

▶ **Infectious diarrhea caused by enteropathogenic *Escherichia coli*.** *Adults:* 50 mg/kg daily P.O. in four divided doses for 2 to 3 days.
Children: 50 to 100 mg/kg daily P.O. divided q 4 to 6 hours for 2 to 3 days.

▶ **Suppression of intestinal bacteria preoperatively.** *Adults:* 1 g P.O. q hour for four doses; then 1 g q 4 hours for balance of 24 hours. A saline cathartic should precede therapy.
Children: 40 to 100 mg/kg daily P.O. divided q 4 to 6 hours. First dose should follow saline cathartic.

▶ **Adjunct treatment in hepatic coma.** *Adults:* 1 to 3 g P.O. q.i.d. for 5 to 6 days. Or, 200 ml of 1% solution or 100 ml of 2% solution as enema retained for 20 to 60 minutes q 6 hours.

How supplied

Tablets: 500 mg
Oral solution: 125 mg/5 ml

Pharmacokinetics

Absorption: absorbed poorly (about 3%), although absorption is enhanced in patients with impaired GI motility or mucosal intestinal ulcerations.
Distribution: distributed locally in GI tract.
Metabolism: not metabolized.
Excretion: excreted primarily unchanged in feces. *Half-life:* 2 to 3 hours.

Route	Onset	Peak	Duration
P.O.	Unknown	1-4 hr	About 8 hr

Pharmacodynamics

Chemical effect: inhibits protein synthesis by binding directly to 30S ribosomal subunit.
Therapeutic effect: kills susceptible bacteria, such as many aerobic gram-negative organisms and some aerobic gram-positive organisms. Inhibits ammonia-forming bacteria in GI tract, reducing ammonia and improving neurologic status of patients with hepatic encephalopathy.

Adverse reactions

CNS: headache, lethargy.
EENT: *ototoxicity.*
GI: nausea, vomiting.
GU: ***nephrotoxicity*** (cells or casts in urine, oliguria, proteinuria, decreased creatinine clearance, increased BUN and serum creatinine levels).
Skin: rash, urticaria.
Other: ***hypersensitivity reactions***.

Interactions

Drug-drug. *Acyclovir, amphotericin B, cisplatin, methoxyflurane, other aminoglycosides, vancomycin:* increased nephrotoxicity. Use together cautiously.
Cephalothin: increased nephrotoxicity. Use together cautiously.
Digoxin: decreased digoxin absorption. Monitor patient for loss of therapeutic effect.
Dimenhydrinate: may mask symptoms of ototoxicity. Use cautiously.
I.V. loop diuretics (such as furosemide): increased risk of ototoxicity. Use cautiously.
Oral anticoagulants: inhibited vitamin K–producing bacteria; may potentiate anticoagulant effect. Monitor patient for bleeding.

Contraindications and precautions

- Contraindicated in patients hypersensitive to other aminoglycosides and in those with intestinal obstruction.
- Use cautiously in elderly patients and in those with impaired renal function, neuromuscular disorders, or ulcerative bowel lesions.
- Safety of drug hasn't been established in breast-feeding women.

NURSING CONSIDERATIONS

Assessment

- Assess patient's condition before therapy and regularly thereafter.
- Evaluate patient's hearing before therapy and regularly thereafter.
- Monitor renal function (output, specific gravity, urinalysis, BUN and creatinine levels, and creatinine clearance).
- Be alert for adverse reactions and drug interactions.
- Monitor patient's hydration status if adverse GI reactions occur.
- Evaluate patient's and family's knowledge of drug therapy.

Nursing diagnoses

- Infection related to organisms
- Risk for deficient fluid volume related to drug-induced adverse GI reactions
- Deficient knowledge related to drug therapy

Planning and implementation

- Drug is nonabsorbable at recommended dosage. More than 4 g/day may be systemically absorbed and lead to nephrotoxicity.
- Make sure patient is well hydrated while taking drug to minimize chemical irritation of renal tubules.
- For preoperative disinfection, provide low-residue diet and cathartic immediately before oral administration of drug, as ordered.

ALERT Never administer drug parenterally.

• In adjunct treatment of hepatic coma, decrease patient's dietary protein and assess neurologic status frequently during therapy.
• The ototoxic and nephrotoxic properties of neomycin limit its usefulness.
• Drug is available in combination with polymyxin B as urinary bladder irrigant.
• Notify prescriber about signs of decreasing renal function or complaints of tinnitus, vertigo, or hearing loss. Deafness may begin several weeks after drug is stopped.

Patient teaching
• Instruct patient to report adverse reactions, especially hearing loss or change in urinary elimination.
• Emphasize the need to drink 2 L of fluid each day.
• Tell patient to alert prescriber if infection worsens or doesn't improve.

☑ Evaluation
• Patient is free from infection.
• Patient maintains adequate hydration throughout drug therapy.
• Patient and family state understanding of drug therapy.

neostigmine bromide
(nee-oh-STIG-meen BROH-mighd)
Prostigmin

neostigmine methylsulfate
Prostigmin

Pharmacologic class: cholinesterase inhibitor
Therapeutic class: muscle stimulant
Pregnancy risk category: C

Indications and dosages
▶ **Treatment of myasthenia gravis.** *Adults:* 15 to 30 mg P.O. t.i.d. (range, 15 to 375 mg daily). Or, 0.5 mg S.C. or I.M.
Children: 7.5 to 15 mg P.O. t.i.d. or q.i.d. Subsequent dosages must be highly individualized, depending on response and tolerance of adverse effects. Therapy may be required day and night.

▶ **Diagnosis of myasthenia gravis.** *Adults:* 0.022 mg/kg I.M. 30 minutes after 0.011 mg/kg I.M. of atropine sulfate.
Children: 0.025 to 0.04 mg/kg. I.M. after 0.011 mg/kg atropine sulfate S.C.

▶ **Postoperative abdominal distention and bladder atony.** *Adults:* 0.25 to 0.5 mg I.M. or S.C. q 4 to 6 hours for 2 to 3 days.

▶ **Antidote for nondepolarizing neuromuscular blockers.** *Adults:* 0.5 to 2 mg I.V. slowly. Repeat p.r.n. to total of 5 mg. Before antidote dose, 0.6 to 1.2 mg atropine sulfate is given I.V.
Note: 1:1,000 solution of injectable solution contains 1 mg/ml; 1:2,000 solution contains 0.5 mg/ml.

How supplied
neostigmine bromide
Tablets: 15 mg
neostigmine methylsulfate
Injection: 0.25 mg/ml, 0.5 mg/ml, 1 mg/ml

Pharmacokinetics
Absorption: poorly absorbed (1% to 2%) from GI tract after P.O. administration. Unknown after S.C. or I.M. administration.
Distribution: about 15% to 25% of dose binds to plasma proteins.
Metabolism: hydrolyzed by cholinesterases and metabolized by microsomal liver enzymes.
Excretion: about 80% of drug excreted in urine.

Route	Onset	Peak	Duration
P.O.	45-75 min	1-2 hr	2-4 hr
I.V.	4-8 min	1-2 hr	2-4 hr
I.M.	20-30 min	1-2 hr	2-4 hr
S.C.	Unknown	1-2 hr	2-4 hr

Pharmacodynamics
Chemical effect: inhibits destruction of acetylcholine released from parasympathetic and somatic efferent nerves. Acetylcholine accumulates, promoting increased stimulation of receptor.
Therapeutic effect: stimulates muscle contraction.

Adverse reactions

CNS: dizziness, headache, mental confusion, jitters.
CV: ***bradycardia***, hypotension, ***cardiac arrest.***
EENT: blurred vision, lacrimation, miosis.
GI: *nausea, vomiting, diarrhea, abdominal cramps,* excessive salivation.
GU: urinary frequency.
Musculoskeletal: *muscle cramps,* muscle weakness, muscle fasciculations.
Respiratory: ***depressed respiratory drive, bronchospasm, bronchoconstriction, respiratory arrest.***
Skin: rash (with bromide), diaphoresis.
Other: hypersensitivity reactions ***(anaphylaxis).***

Interactions

Drug-drug. *Aminoglycosides, anticholinergics, atropine, corticosteroids, magnesium sulfate, procainamide, quinidine:* may reverse cholinergic effects. Observe patient for lack of drug effect.

Contraindications and precautions

- Contraindicated in patients hypersensitive to cholinergics or bromide and in those with peritonitis or mechanical obstruction of intestine or urinary tract.
- Use cautiously in patients with bronchial asthma, bradycardia, seizure disorders, recent coronary occlusion, vagotonia, hyperthyroidism, arrhythmias, or peptic ulcer.

NURSING CONSIDERATIONS

Assessment

- Assess patient's condition before therapy.
- Monitor patient's response after each dose. Watch closely for improvement in strength, vision, and ptosis 45 to 60 minutes after each dose. Show patient how to record variations in muscle strength.
- Monitor vital signs frequently.
- Evaluate patient's and family's knowledge of drug therapy.

Nursing diagnoses

- Impaired physical mobility related to condition
- Diarrhea related to drug's adverse effect on GI tract
- Deficient knowledge related to drug therapy

Planning and implementation

- Stop all other cholinergics before giving drug, as ordered.
- In myasthenia gravis, schedule doses before fatigue. For example, if patient has dysphagia, schedule dose 30 minutes before each meal.
- Be prepared to give atropine injection, as ordered; provide respiratory support as needed.
- When drug is used to prevent abdominal distention and GI distress, prescriber may order a rectal tube to help passage of gas.

ALERT Although drug is commonly used to reverse effects of nondepolarizing neuromuscular blockers in patients who have undergone surgery, be aware that it may worsen blockade produced by succinylcholine.

- Patient may develop resistance to drug.

P.O. use: Give drug with food or milk.
– If appropriate, obtain order for hospitalized patient to have bedside supply of tablets. A patient with long-standing disease may insist on self-administration.
I.V. use: Give drug at slow, controlled rate of no more than 1 mg/minute in adults and 0.5 mg/minute in children.
I.M. and S.C. use: Follow normal protocol.

- I.M. neostigmine may be used instead of edrophonium to diagnose myasthenia gravis. May be preferable to edrophonium when limb weakness is only symptom.

Patient teaching

- Tell patient to take drug with food or milk to reduce GI distress.
- When using for myasthenia gravis, explain that drug will relieve ptosis, double vision, difficulty chewing and swallowing, and trunk and limb weakness. Stress need to take drug exactly as ordered. Explain that it may have to be taken for life.
- Advise patient to wear or carry medical identification indicating that he has myasthenia gravis.

Evaluation

- Patient performs activities of daily living without assistance.
- Patient has normal bowel patterns.
- Patient and family state understanding of drug therapy.

nevirapine

(neh-VEER-uh-peen)
Viramune

Pharmacologic class: nonnucleoside reverse transcriptase inhibitor
Therapeutic class: antiviral
Pregnancy risk category: C

Indications and dosages

▶ **Adjunct treatment in patients with HIV-1 infection who have experienced clinical or immunologic deterioration.** *Adults:* 200 mg P.O. daily for first 14 days, followed by 200 mg P.O. b.i.d., in combination with nucleoside analogue antiretroviral drugs.
▶ **Adjunct treatment in children infected with HIV-1.** *Children age 8 and older:* 4 mg/kg P.O. once daily for first 14 days, followed by 4 mg/kg P.O. twice daily thereafter. Maximum 400 mg daily.
Children ages 2 months to 8 years: 4 mg/kg P.O. once daily for first 14 days, followed by 7 mg/kg P.O. twice daily thereafter. Maximum 400 mg daily.

How supplied

Tablets: 200 mg
Oral suspension: 50 mg/5 ml

Pharmacokinetics

Absorption: readily absorbed.
Distribution: widely distributed.
Metabolism: metabolized by liver.
Excretion: excreted in urine and feces.

Route	Onset	Peak	Duration
P.O.	Unknown	4 hr	Unknown

Pharmacodynamics

Chemical effect: binds to reverse transcriptase and blocks RNA-dependent and DNA-dependent DNA polymerase activities.
Therapeutic effect: may inhibit replication of HIV-1.

Adverse reactions

CNS: *headache,* paresthesia.
GI: *nausea,* diarrhea, abdominal pain, ulcerative stomatitis.
Hematologic: ***decreased neutrophil count,*** decreased hemoglobin.
Hepatic: ***hepatitis;*** increased ALT, AST, GGT, and total bilirubin levels.
Musculoskeletal: myalgia.
Skin: rash, blistering, ***Stevens-Johnson syndrome.***
Other: *fever.*

Interactions

Drug-drug. *Drugs extensively metabolized by P-450 CYP3A:* may lower plasma levels of these drugs. Adjust dosage as directed.
Oral contraceptives, other hormonal contraceptives, protease inhibitors: may decrease plasma levels of these drugs. Don't use together.
Rifabutin, rifampin: more data needed to assess whether dosage adjustments are needed. Monitor patient closely with concomitant use.

Contraindications and precautions

- Contraindicated in patients hypersensitive to drug.
- Use cautiously in patients with impaired renal and hepatic function.

NURSING CONSIDERATIONS

Assessment

- Obtain clinical chemistry tests, including liver and renal function tests, before and during therapy, as ordered.
- Monitor patient for blistering, oral lesions, conjunctivitis, muscle or joint aches, or general malaise. Be especially alert for severe rash or rash accompanied by fever. Report such signs and symptoms to prescriber.

Nursing diagnoses
- Infection related to presence of virus
- Deficient knowledge related to drug therapy

Planning and implementation
- Drug should be used with at least one other antiretroviral.
- Drug appears in breast milk.

ALERT Don't confuse nelfinavir with nevirapine.

Patient teaching
- Inform patient that drug doesn't cure HIV infection and that he can still develop illnesses linked to advanced HIV infection. Explain that drug doesn't reduce the risk of HIV transmission.
- Instruct patient to report rash at once and to stop drug if rash develops.
- Tell patient not to use other drugs unless approved by prescriber.
- Advise woman of childbearing age to avoid use of hormonal contraceptive methods during therapy.
- Tell patient to stop breast-feeding during therapy to reduce risk of postnatal HIV transmission.
- If therapy is interrupted for more than 7 days, instruct patient to resume it as if for the first time.

Evaluation
- Patient shows no signs of worsening condition.
- Patient and family state understanding of drug therapy.

niacin (vitamin B_3, nicotinic acid)
(NIGH-uh-sin)

Niac, Niacin TR Tablets, Niacor, Niaspan, Nico-400, Nicobid†, Nicolar**, Nicotinex, Slo-Niacin

niacinamide (nicotinamide)†

Pharmacologic class: B-complex vitamin
Therapeutic class: vitamin B_3, antilipemic, peripheral vasodilator
Pregnancy risk category: C

Indications and dosages
▶ **RDA.** *Neonates and infants to age 6 months:* 5 mg.
Infants ages 6 months to 1 year: 6 mg.
Children ages 1 to 3: 9 mg.
Children ages 4 to 6: 12 mg.
Children ages 7 to 10: 13 mg.
Men ages 11 to 14: 17 mg.
Men ages 15 to 18: 20 mg.
Men ages 19 to 50: 19 mg.
Men age 51 and over: 15 mg.
Women ages 11 to 50: 15 mg.
Women age 51 and over: 13 mg.
Pregnant women: 17 mg.
Breast-feeding women: 20 mg.

▶ **Pellagra.** *Adults:* 300 to 500 mg P.O., S.C., I.M., or I.V. infusion daily in divided doses, depending on severity of niacin deficiency.
Children: up to 300 mg P.O. or 100 mg I.V. daily, depending on severity of niacin deficiency. After symptoms subside, advise adequate nutrition and RDA supplements to prevent recurrence.

▶ **Hartnup disease.** *Adults:* 50 to 200 mg P.O. daily.

▶ **Niacin deficiency.** *Adults:* up to 100 mg P.O. daily.

▶ **Hyperlipidemias, especially with hypercholesterolemia.** *Adults:* 1 to 2 g P.O. t.i.d. with meals, increased at intervals to 6 g daily, or 375 mg to 2000 mg P.O. daily h.s (Niaspan extended-release tablets).

How supplied
niacin
Tablets: 25 mg†, 50 mg†, 100 mg†, 250 mg†, 500 mg
Tablets (timed-release): 150 mg†, 250 mg†, 500 mg†, 750 mg†
Tablets (extended-release): 375 mg, 500 mg, 750 mg, 1 g
Capsules (timed-release): 125 mg†, 250 mg†, 300 mg†, 400 mg†, 500 mg, 1000 mg
Elixir: 50 mg/5 ml†
Injection: 100 mg/ml in 30-ml vials

niacinamide
Tablets: 50 mg†, 100 mg†, 125 mg†, 250 mg†, 500 mg†

Pharmacokinetics

Absorption: absorbed rapidly from GI tract. Absorption unknown after S.C. or I.M. administration.
Distribution: niacin coenzymes are distributed widely in body tissues.
Metabolism: metabolized by liver to active metabolites.
Excretion: excreted in urine. *Half-life:* about 45 minutes.

Route	Onset	Peak	Duration
P.O.	Unknown	45 min	Unknown
I.V., I.M., S.C.	Unknown	Unknown	Unknown

Pharmacodynamics

Chemical effect: niacin and niacinamide stimulate lipid metabolism, tissue respiration, and glycogenolysis; niacin decreases synthesis of low-density lipoproteins and inhibits lipolysis in adipose tissue.
Therapeutic effect: restores normal levels of vitamin B_3, lowers triglyceride and cholesterol levels, and dilates peripheral blood vessels.

Adverse reactions

CNS: dizziness, transient headache.
CV: *excessive peripheral vasodilation,* ***arrhythmias.***
GI: *nausea, vomiting, diarrhea,* possible activation of peptic ulceration, epigastric or substernal pain.
Hepatic: ***hepatic dysfunction.***
Metabolic: hyperglycemia, hyperuricemia.
Skin: *flushing,* pruritus, dryness, tingling.

Interactions

Drug-drug. *Antihypertensives:* potential orthostatic hypotension. Use together cautiously; also warn patient about orthostatic hypotension.

Contraindications and precautions

- Contraindicated in patients hypersensitive to drug and in those with hepatic dysfunction, active peptic ulcers, severe hypotension, or arterial hemorrhage.
- Use cautiously in patients with gallbladder disease, diabetes mellitus, or coronary artery disease and in patients with history of liver disease, peptic ulcer, allergy, or gout.

NURSING CONSIDSERATIONS

Assessment

- Assess patient's condition before therapy and regularly thereafter.
- Monitor hepatic function and blood glucose, as ordered.
- Be alert for adverse reactions and drug interactions.
- Monitor patient's hydration status if adverse GI reactions occur.
- Evaluate patient's and family's knowledge of drug therapy.

Nursing diagnoses

- Imbalanced nutrition: less than body requirements related to decreased intake of vitamin B_3
- Risk for deficient fluid volume related to drug-induced adverse GI reactions
- Deficient knowledge related to drug therapy

Planning and implementation

- Administer aspirin (325 mg P.O. 30 minutes before niacin dose) as ordered to help reduce flushing.
- Timed-release niacin or niacinamide may prevent excessive flushing that occurs with large doses. However, timed-release niacin has been linked to hepatic dysfunction, even at doses as low as 1 g/day.

P.O. use: Give drug with meals to minimize GI adverse effects.
I.V. use: Give drug by slow I.V. (no more than 2 mg/minute).
I.M. and S.C. use: Follow normal protocol.

Patient teaching

- Explain that flushing sensation is harmless.
- To decrease flushing, advise patient to take drug with a low-fat snack and to avoid taking it after alcohol, hot beverages, hot or spicy foods, a hot shower, or exercise.
- Stress that drug is a potent medication that may cause serious adverse effects. Explain importance of adhering to therapeutic regimen.

• Advise patient against self-medicating for hyperlipidemia.

Evaluation

• Patient's vitamin B_3 levels are normal.
• Patient maintains adequate hydration throughout drug therapy.
• Patient and family state understanding of drug therapy.

nicardipine hydrochloride

(nigh-KAR-dih-peen high-droh-KLOR-ighd)
Cardene, Cardene I.V., Cardene SR

Pharmacologic class: calcium channel blocker
Therapeutic class: antianginal, antihypertensive
Pregnancy risk category: C

Indications and dosages

▶ **Chronic stable angina (alone or with other antianginals).** *Adults:* initially, 20 mg P.O. t.i.d. (immediate-release only). Dosage titrated based on response q 3 days. Usual dosage range is 20 to 40 mg t.i.d.
▶ **Hypertension.** *Adults:* initially, 20 to 40 mg P.O. t.i.d. (immediate-release) or 30 to 60 mg b.i.d. (sustained-release). Dosage increased based on response. Or, for patients unable to take oral nicardipine, 50 ml/hour (5 mg/hour) I.V. infusion initially, increased by 25 ml/hour (2.5 mg/hour) q 15 minutes up to 150 ml/hour (15 mg/hour).

How supplied

Capsules (immediate-release): 20 mg, 30 mg
Capsules (sustained-release): 30 mg, 45 mg, 60 mg
Injection: 2.5 mg/ml

Pharmacokinetics

Absorption: completely absorbed after P.O. administration; may be decreased if drug is taken with food.
Distribution: extensively (over 95%) bound to plasma proteins.
Metabolism: absolute bioavailability of about 35%; extensively metabolized in liver.
Excretion: about 60% excreted in urine, 35% in bile. *Half-life:* 2 to 4 hours.

Route	Onset	Peak	Duration
P.O.	< 20 min	0.5-4 hr	6-12 hr
I.V.	Immediate	Within min	Rapid decline after infusion ends

Pharmacodynamics

Chemical effect: inhibits calcium ion influx across cardiac and smooth-muscle cells, decreasing myocardial contractility and oxygen demand. Also dilates coronary arteries and arterioles.
Therapeutic effect: lowers blood pressure and relieves angina.

Adverse reactions

CNS: *dizziness, light-headedness, headache, paresthesia, drowsiness, asthenia.*
CV: *peripheral edema, palpitations,* angina, tachycardia.
GI: nausea, abdominal discomfort, dry mouth.
Skin: rash, *flushing*.

Interactions

Drug-drug. *Antihypertensives:* enhanced antihypertensive effect. Monitor patient.
Beta blockers: may increase cardiac depressant effects. Monitor patient.
Cimetidine: may decrease metabolism of calcium channel blockers. Monitor patient for toxicity.
Cyclosporine: nicardipine may increase plasma cyclosporine levels. Monitor serum levels closely.
Theophylline: pharmacologic effects of theophylline may be enhanced. Monitor patient.

Contraindications and precautions

• Contraindicated in patients hypersensitive to drug and in those with advanced aortic stenosis.
• Drug use isn't recommended for breast-feeding women.

• Use cautiously in pregnant women and in patients with cardiac conduction disturbances, hypotension, heart failure, and impaired hepatic or renal function.
• Safety of drug hasn't been established in children.

NURSING CONSIDERATIONS

Assessment
• Assess patient's condition before therapy and regularly thereafter.
• Measure blood pressure frequently during initial therapy. Maximum blood pressure response occurs about 1 hour after immediate-release form and 2 to 4 hours after sustained-release form. Check for orthostatic hypotension. Because blood pressure may vary widely based on blood level of drug, assess adequacy of antihypertensive effect 8 hours after dosing.
• Be alert for adverse reactions and drug interactions.
• Evaluate patient's and family's knowledge of drug therapy.

Nursing diagnoses
• Risk for injury related to hypertension
• Acute pain related to angina
• Deficient knowledge related to drug therapy

Planning and implementation
P.O. use: When switching to oral nicardipine, administer first dose of t.i.d. regimen 1 hour before stopping infusion. If using an oral drug other than nicardipine, start therapy after stopping infusion.
I.V. use: Dilute with compatible solution before administration.
– Administer by slow I.V. infusion at 0.1 mg/ml.
– Closely monitor blood pressure during infusion.
– Titrate rate, as ordered, if hypotension or tachycardia occurs.
– Change peripherial infusion site every 12 hours to minimize risk of venous irritation. Adjust infusion rate if hypotension or tachycardia occurs, as ordered.
ALERT Don't confuse nicardipine with nifedipine or nimodipine.

Patient teaching
• Advise patient to report chest pain immediately. Some patients may experience increased frequency, severity, or duration of chest pain at start of therapy or during dosage adjustments.
• Stress need to take drug exactly as prescribed even when feeling well.
• Instruct patient how to minimize orthostatic hypotension.

Evaluation
• Patient's blood pressure is normal.
• Patient's anginal attacks are less frequent and less severe.
• Patient and family state understanding of drug therapy.

nicotine polacrilex
(NIH-koh-teen poh-luh-KRIGH-leks)
Nicorette†, Nicorette DS

Pharmacologic class: nicotinic agonist
Therapeutic class: smoking cessation aid
Pregnancy risk category: X

Indications and dosages
▶ **Relief of nicotine withdrawal symptoms in patients undergoing smoking cessation.**
Adults: initially, one 2-mg square (4-mg square if highly dependent). Patient should chew one piece of gum slowly and intermittently for 30 minutes whenever the urge to smoke occurs. Most patients need 9 to 12 pieces of gum daily during first month. With 4-mg squares, maximum dosage is 20 pieces daily. With 2-mg squares, maximum dosage is 30 pieces daily.

How supplied
***Chewing gum*†:** 2 mg/square, 4 mg/square

Pharmacokinetics
Absorption: nicotine is bound to ion-exchange resin and is released only during chewing. Blood level depends on vigor of gum chewing.
Distribution: not clearly defined.

Metabolism: metabolized by liver and somewhat by kidney and lung.
Excretion: excreted in urine. Excretion increased with acidic urine and high urine output. *Half-life:* 1 to 2 hours.

Route	Onset	Peak	Duration
P.O.	Unknown	15-30 min	Unknown

Pharmacodynamics

Chemical effect: provides nicotine, which stimulates nicotinic acetylcholine receptors in CNS, neuromuscular junction, autonomic ganglia, and adrenal medulla.
Therapeutic effect: blocks nicotine withdrawal symptoms.

Adverse reactions

CNS: dizziness, light-headedness.
CV: ***atrial fibrillation***.
EENT: sore throat, jaw muscle ache (from chewing).
GI: nausea, vomiting, indigestion.
Other: hiccups.

Interactions

Drug-drug. *Beta blockers, methylxanthines, propoxyphene, propranolol:* decreased metabolism of these drugs, increasing therapeutic effects. Dosages may need to be adjusted.
Drug-lifestyle. *Smoking:* reduced effectiveness of drug. Warn patient to avoid smoking while taking drug.

Contraindications and precautions

- Contraindicated in pregnant women, nonsmokers, and patients with recent MI, life-threatening arrhythmias, severe or worsening angina pectoris, or active temporomandibular joint disease.
- Drug isn't recommended for children or breast-feeding women.
- Use cautiously in patients with hyperthyroidism, pheochromocytoma, insulin-dependent diabetes, peptic ulcer disease, history of esophagitis, oral or pharyngeal inflammation, or dental conditions that could be worsened by chewing gum.

NURSING CONSIDERATIONS

Assessment

- Assess patient's smoking history before therapy.
- Evaluate effectiveness of drug by assessing patient for nicotine withdrawal signs and symptoms.
- Be alert for adverse reactions and drug interactions.
- Evaluate patient's and family's knowledge of drug therapy.

Nursing diagnoses

- Ineffective health maintenance related to smoking
- Risk for injury related to drug-induced adverse CNS reactions
- Deficient knowledge related to drug therapy

Planning and implementation

- Smokers most likely to benefit from nicotine gum are those with high "physical" nicotine dependence—those who smoke more than 15 cigarettes daily, prefer high-nicotine brands, usually inhale the smoke, smoke their first cigarette within 30 minutes of arising, find the first morning cigarette the hardest to give up, smoke most frequently in the morning, find it difficult to refrain from smoking in places where it's forbidden, or smoke even when ill and confined to bed.

Patient teaching

ALERT Instruct patient to chew gum slowly and intermittently (chew several times, and then place between cheek and gum) for about 30 minutes to promote slow, even absorption. Fast chewing tends to produce more adverse reactions.

- Make sure patient reads and understands instruction sheet included in package.
- Emphasize importance of withdrawing gum gradually.
- Tell patient that successful abstainers will begin to gradually withdraw gum usage after 3 months. Use of gum for longer than 6 months isn't recommended. For gradual withdrawal, tell patient to cut gum in halves or quarters and mix with other sugarless gum.

☑ Evaluation

- Patient has no nicotine withdrawal symptoms.
- Patient sustains no injuries from drug-induced CNS reactions.
- Patient and family state understanding of drug therapy.

nicotine transdermal system

(NIH-koh-teen trans-DER-mul SIS-tum)
Habitrol†, Nicoderm, Nicotrol†, ProStep

Pharmacologic class: nicotinic cholinergic agonist
Therapeutic class: smoking cessation aid
Pregnancy risk category: D

Indications and dosages

▶ **Relief of nicotine withdrawal symptoms in patients undergoing smoking cessation.** *Adults:* initially, one transdermal system, delivering largest available nicotine dosage in its dosage series, applied once daily in morning to nonhairy part of body and removed before retiring. After 4 to 12 weeks (depending on brand) dosage tapered to next largest available dosage in series followed in 2 to 4 weeks by lowest dosage in series. Drug is then stopped in 2 to 4 weeks.

How supplied

Habitrol—21 mg/day, 14 mg/day, 7 mg/day
Nicoderm—21 mg/day, 14 mg/day, 7 mg/day
Nicotrol—15 mg/16 hours, 10 mg/16 hours, 5 mg/16 hours
ProStep—22 mg/day, 11 mg/day

Pharmacokinetics

Absorption: rapidly absorbed.
Distribution: plasma protein–binding of drug is below 5%.
Metabolism: metabolized by liver, kidney, and lung.
Excretion: excreted primarily in urine as metabolites; about 10% excreted unchanged. With high urine flow rates or acidified urine, up to 30% can be excreted unchanged. *Half-life:* 1 to 2 hours.

Route	Onset	Peak	Duration
Trans-dermal	Unknown	3-9 hr	Varies

Pharmacodynamics

Chemical effect: provides nicotine, which stimulates nicotinic acetylcholine receptors in CNS, neuromuscular junction, autonomic ganglia, and adrenal medulla.
Therapeutic effect: blocks nicotine withdrawal symptoms.

Adverse reactions

CNS: somnolence, dizziness, *headache, insomnia.*
EENT: pharyngitis, sinusitis.
GI: abdominal pain, constipation, dyspepsia, nausea.
GU: dysmenorrhea.
Musculoskeletal: back pain, myalgia.
Skin: *local or systemic erythema, pruritus or burning* at application site, cutaneous hypersensitivity, rash, diaphoresis.

Interactions

Drug-drug. *Acetaminophen, imipramine, oxazepam, pentazocine, propranolol, theophylline:* may decrease induction of hepatic enzymes that help metabolize certain drugs. Dosage may be reduced.
Adrenergic agonists (such as isoproterenol, phenylephrine), adrenergic antagonists (such as labetalol, prazosin): may alter circulating catecholamines. Dosage may need adjustment according to smoking status.
Insulin: may increase amount of S.C. insulin absorbed. Insulin dosage may be reduced.
Drug-herb. *Blue cohosh:* Increases effects of nicotine. Discourage concomitant use.
Drug-lifestyle. *Caffeine:* may decrease induction of hepatic enzymes that help metabolize certain drugs. Dosage may be reduced.

Contraindications and precautions

- Contraindicated in patients hypersensitive to nicotine or components of transdermal system,

in nonsmokers, and in patients with recent MI, life-threatening arrhythmias, or severe or worsening angina pectoris.
• Drug isn't recommended for pregnant women, breast-feeding women, or children.
• Use cautiously in patients with hyperthyroidism, pheochromocytoma, hypertension, insulin-dependent diabetes, or peptic ulcer disease.

NURSING CONSIDERATIONS

Assessment
• Assess patient's smoking history before therapy.
• Evaluate effectiveness of drug by assessing patient for nicotine withdrawal signs and symptoms.
• Be alert for adverse reactions and drug interactions.
• Evaluate patient's and family's knowledge of drug therapy.

Nursing diagnoses
• Ineffective health maintenance related to smoking
• Risk for injury related to drug-induced adverse CNS reactions
• Deficient knowledge related to drug therapy

Planning and implementation
• Exposure of health care workers to nicotine in transdermal systems probably is minimal; however, avoid unnecessary contact. Wash hands with water alone because soap can enhance absorption.
ALERT Don't confuse Nicoderm with Nitro-Derm.

Patient teaching
• Discourage use of transdermal system for more than 3 months. Prolonged nicotine consumption by any route can be habit-forming.
• Warn patient not to smoke. If he smokes while using system, serious adverse effects may occur because peak serum nicotine levels will be much higher than those achieved by smoking alone.
• Make sure patient reads and understands information dispensed with drug.
• Advise patient to apply patch promptly because nicotine can evaporate from transdermal system once it's removed from protective packaging. Patch shouldn't be altered in any way (folded or cut) before application.
• Urge patient not to store at temperatures above 86° F (30° C).
• Teach patient to fold patch in half after removal, bringing adhesive sides together. If system comes in protective pouch, tell patient to place used patch in it. Explain that careful disposal prevents accidental poisoning of children or pets.
• Tell patient with persistent or severe local skin reactions or generalized rash to immediately stop use of patch and contact prescriber.
• Explain that patient who can't stop cigarette smoking during first 4 weeks of therapy probably won't benefit from continued use of drug. Unsuccessful patient may benefit from counseling to identify factors that led to treatment failure. Encourage patient to minimize or eliminate factors contributing to treatment failure and to try again after a while.

Evaluation
• Patient has no nicotine withdrawal symptoms.
• Patient sustains no injuries from drug-induced adverse CNS reactions.
• Patient and family state understanding of drug therapy.

nifedipine
(nigh-FEH-duh-peen)
Adalat, Adalat CC, Adalat P.A.♦, Nu-Nifed♦, Procardia, Procardia XL

Pharmacologic class: calcium channel blocker
Therapeutic class: antianginal
Pregnancy risk category: C

Indications and dosages
▶ **Vasospastic angina (also called Prinzmetal's [variant] angina) and classic chronic stable angina pectoris.** *Adults:* starting dose is 10 mg P.O. t.i.d. Usual effective dosage range is 10 to 20 mg t.i.d. Some patients may

need up to 30 mg q.i.d. Maximum daily dose is 180 mg (capsules).

▶ **Hypertension.** *Adults:* 30 or 60 mg P.O. (extended-release form) once daily. Adjusted over 7- to 14-day period. Maximum 120 mg daily.

How supplied

Tablets (extended-release): 30 mg, 60 mg, 90 mg
Capsules: 10 mg, 20 mg

Pharmacokinetics

Absorption: about 90% of drug is absorbed rapidly from GI tract; however, only about 65% to 70% of drug reaches systemic circulation because of significant first-pass effect in liver.
Distribution: about 92% to 98% of circulating drug is bound to plasma proteins.
Metabolism: metabolized in liver.
Excretion: excreted in urine and feces as inactive metabolites. *Half-life:* 2 to 5 hours.

Route	Onset	Peak	Duration
P.O.	20 min	0.5-2 hr	4-24 hr

Pharmacodynamics

Chemical effect: unknown; may inhibit calcium ion influx across cardiac and smooth-muscle cells, decreasing myocardial contractility and oxygen demand. Also may dilate coronary arteries and arterioles.
Therapeutic effect: reduces blood pressure and prevents angina.

Adverse reactions

CNS: *dizziness, light-headedness, headache,* weakness, syncope.
CV: peripheral edema, hypotension, palpitations, heart failure, pulmonary edema, ***MI.***
EENT: nasal congestion.
GI: nausea, heartburn, diarrhea.
Metabolic: ***hypokalemia.***
Musculoskeletal: muscle cramps.
Respiratory: dyspnea.
Skin: rash, *flushing,* pruritus.

Interactions

Drug-drug. *Cimetidine, ranitidine:* decreased nifedipine metabolism. Monitor patient closely.
Propranolol, other beta blockers: may cause hypotension and heart failure. Use together cautiously.
Drug-food. *Grapefruit juice:* increased bioavailability. Discourage concurrent use because effects vary.

Contraindications and precautions

- Contraindicated in patients hypersensitive to drug and in pregnant or breast-feeding women.
- Use cautiously in elderly patients and in those with heart failure or hypotension.
- Use extended-release tablets cautiously in patients with severe GI narrowing because obstructive symptoms may occur.
- Safety of drug hasn't been established in children.

NURSING CONSIDERATIONS

Assessment

- Assess patient's condition before therapy and regularly thereafter.
- Monitor blood pressure regularly, especially if patient also takes a beta blocker or an antihypertensive.
- Monitor serum potassium level regularly, as ordered.
- Be alert for adverse reactions and drug interactions.
- Evaluate patient's and family's knowledge of drug therapy.

Nursing diagnoses

- Risk for injury related to presence of hypertension
- Pain related to angina
- Deficient knowledge related to drug therapy

Planning and implementation

- When rapid response to drug is desired, instruct patient to bite and swallow capsule. If he can't chew capsules, liquid can be withdrawn by puncturing capsule with needle and squeezing contents into mouth. When using these methods, continuous blood pressure and ECG monitoring is recommended.

• Despite widespread S.L. use of nifedipine capsules, avoid this route of administration. Peak serum levels are lower and it takes longer for levels to peak than when capsules are bitten and swallowed.
• S.L. nitroglycerin may be taken as needed for acute angina.
• Although rebound effect hasn't been observed when drug is stopped, dosage should still be reduced slowly under prescriber's supervision.
ALERT Don't confuse nifedipine with nicardipine or nimodipine.

Patient teaching
• If patient is kept on nitrate therapy while nifedipine dosage is being adjusted, urge continued compliance.
• Warn patient that angina may worsen when therapy starts or dosage increases. Reassure him that this is temporary.
• Instruct patient to swallow extended-release tablets without breaking, crushing, or chewing them.
• Advise patient who takes extended-release form of drug that the wax-matrix "ghost" of tablet may be passed in stool.
• Warn patient not to switch brands. Procardia XL and Adalat CC aren't equivalent because of their differing pharmacokinetics.
• Tell patient to protect capsules from direct light and moisture and to store them at room temperature.

Evaluation
• Patient's blood pressure is normal.
• Patient's angina is less frequent and severe.
• Patient and family state understanding of drug therapy.

nimodipine
(nigh-MOH-dih-peen)
Nimotop

Pharmacologic class: calcium channel blocker
Therapeutic class: cerebral vasodilator
Pregnancy risk category: C

Indications and dosages
▶ **Reduction of neurologic deficits after subarachnoid hemorrhage from ruptured congenital aneurysm.** *Adults:* 60 mg P.O. q 4 hours for 21 days. Therapy begun within 96 hours after subarachnoid hemorrhage. In patients with hepatic failure, 30 mg P.O. q 4 hours for 21 days.

How supplied
Capsules: 30 mg

Pharmacokinetics
Absorption: well absorbed from GI tract, but bioavailability is 3% to 30%.
Distribution: drug is more than 95% protein-bound.
Metabolism: extensively metabolized in liver. Drug and metabolites undergo enterohepatic recycling.
Excretion: excreted mainly in feces; less than 1% in urine. *Half-life:* 8 to 9 hours.

Route	Onset	Peak	Duration
P.O.	Unknown	≤ 1 hr	Unknown

Pharmacodynamics
Chemical effect: inhibits calcium ion influx across cardiac and smooth-muscle cells, decreasing myocardial contractility and oxygen demand. Also dilates coronary and cerebral arteries and arterioles.
Therapeutic effect: improves neurologic deficits in selected patients.

Adverse reactions
CNS: headache.
CV: decreased blood pressure, flushing, edema.
GI: nausea, diarrhea, abdominal discomfort.
Musculoskeletal: muscle cramps.
Respiratory: dyspnea.
Skin: dermatitis, rash.

Interactions
Drug-drug. *Antihypertensives:* possible enhanced hypotensive effect. Monitor patient. *Calcium channel blockers:* possible enhanced CV effects. Monitor patient.

Contraindications and precautions

- No known contraindications.
- Drug isn't recommended for pregnant or breast-feeding women.
- Use cautiously in patients with hepatic failure.
- Safety of drug hasn't been established in children.

NURSING CONSIDERATIONS

Assessment

- Assess patient's condition before therapy and regularly thereafter.
- Monitor blood pressure and heart rate, especially at start of therapy.
- Evaluate patient's and family's knowledge of drug therapy.

Nursing diagnoses

- Ineffective health maintenance related to underlying condition
- Acute pain related to drug-induced headache
- Deficient knowledge related to drug therapy

Planning and implementation

- Nimodipine should be reserved for patients who are in good neurologic condition (for example, Hunt and Hess grades I to II).

ALERT Don't confuse nimodipine with nicardipine or nifedipine.

Patient teaching

- Inform patient and family that nimodipine therapy is required for 21 days.
- Tell patient to take mild analgesic if headache develops.
- Instruct patient to avoid sudden position changes, which may cause dizziness and orthostatic hypotension.

Evaluation

- Patient responds well to therapy.
- Patient is free from pain.
- Patient and family state understanding of drug therapy.

nisoldipine

(nigh-SOHL-dih-peen)

Sular

Pharmacologic class: calcium channel blocker
Therapeutic class: antihypertensive
Pregnancy risk category: C

Indications and dosages

▶ **Hypertension.** *Adults:* initially, 20 mg (10 mg if patient is over age 65 or has liver dysfunction) P.O. once daily; then increased by 10 mg/week or at longer intervals, as indicated. Usual maintenance dosage is 20 to 40 mg once daily. Dosages above 60 mg daily aren't recommended.

How supplied

Extended-release tablets: 10 mg, 20 mg, 30 mg, 40 mg

Pharmacokinetics

Absorption: well absorbed from GI tract; high-fat foods significantly affect release of drug from coat-core form.
Distribution: about 99% protein-bound.
Metabolism: extensively metabolized, with five major metabolites identified.
Excretion: excreted in urine. *Half-life:* 7 to 12 hours.

Route	Onset	Peak	Duration
P.O.	Unknown	6-12 hr	Unknown

Pharmacodynamics

Chemical effect: prevents entry of calcium ions into vascular smooth-muscle cells, causing dilation of arterioles, which decreases peripheral vascular resistance.
Therapeutic effect: lowers blood pressure.

Adverse reactions

CNS: *headache,* dizziness.
CV: vasodilation, palpitations, chest pain, *peripheral edema.*
EENT: sinusitis, pharyngitis.
GI: nausea.
Skin: rash.

Interactions

Drug-drug. *Cimetidine:* increases bioavailability and peak levels of nisoldipine. Monitor patient.
Quinidine: decreases bioavailability, but not peak levels, of nisoldipine. Monitor patient.
Drug-food. *Grapefruit juice:* increased bioavailability and peak levels of drug. Discourage concurrent use.
High-fat meal: increased peak drug levels. Discourage high-fat meals.

Contraindications and precautions

- Contraindicated in patients hypersensitive to dihydropyridine calcium channel blockers.
- Use cautiously in pregnant women and in patients with severe hepatic impairment, heart failure, or compromised ventricular function, and particularly in those taking beta blockers.
- Drug shouldn't be used by breast-feeding women.

NURSING CONSIDERATIONS

Assessment

- Assess patient's blood pressure before therapy and monitor regularly thereafter, especially during dosage adjustment.
- Monitor patient carefully. Some patients, especially those with severe obstructive coronary artery disease, have developed increased frequency, duration, or severity of angina or acute MI when starting calcium channel blocker therapy or increasing dosage.
- Be alert for adverse reactions and interactions.
- Evaluate patient's and family's knowledge of drug therapy.

Nursing diagnoses

- Risk for injury related to hypertension
- Excessive fluid volume related to edema
- Deficient knowledge related to drug therapy

Planning and implementation

- Don't give drug with a high-fat meal or grapefruit products.

Patient teaching

- Tell patient to take drug as prescribed.
- Instruct patient to swallow tablet whole and not to chew, divide, or crush it.

Evaluation

- Patient's blood pressure is normal.
- Patient doesn't exhibit signs of edema.
- Patient and family state understanding of drug therapy.

nitrofurantoin macrocrystals

(nigh-troh-fyoo-RAN-toyn MAH-kroh-kris-tuls)
Macrodantin

nitrofurantoin microcrystals

Apo-Nitrofurantoin ♦, Furadantin, Furalan, Macrodantin

Pharmacologic class: nitrofuran
Therapeutic class: urinary tract anti-infective
Pregnancy risk category: B

Indications and dosages

▶ **Urinary tract infection caused by susceptible *Escherichia coli, Staphylococcus aureus,* enterococci, and certain strains of *Klebsiella, Proteus,* and *Enterobacter.*** *Adults and children over age 12:* 50 to 100 mg P.O. q.i.d. with milk or meals.
Children ages 1 month to 12 years: 5 to 7 mg/kg P.O. daily, divided q.i.d.

▶ **Long-term suppression therapy.** *Adults:* 50 to 100 mg P.O. daily h.s.
Children: 1 to 2 mg/kg P.O. daily h.s.

How supplied

nitrofurantoin macrocrystals
Capsules: 25 mg, 50 mg, 100 mg
nitrofurantoin microcrystals
Tablets: 50 mg, 100 mg
Capsules: 50 mg, 100 mg
Oral suspension: 25 mg/5 ml

Pharmacokinetics

Absorption: well absorbed from GI tract. Food aids drug's dissolution and speeds absorption. Macrocrystal form has slower dissolution and absorption.
Distribution: drug crosses into bile; 60% binds to plasma proteins.

Metabolism: metabolized partially in liver.
Excretion: about 30% to 50% of dose is eliminated in urine. *Half-life:* ¼ to 1 hour.

Route	Onset	Peak	Duration
P.O.	Unknown	Unknown	Unknown

Pharmacodynamics

Chemical effect: unknown; may interfere with bacterial enzyme systems and cell wall formation.
Therapeutic effect: hinders growth of many common gram-positive and gram-negative urinary pathogens including *E. coli, S. aureus,* enterococci, and certain strains of *Klebsiella* and *Enterobacter.*

Adverse reactions

CNS: ***peripheral neuropathy,*** headache, dizziness, drowsiness, *ascending polyneuropathy with high doses or renal impairment.*
GI: *anorexia, nausea, vomiting,* abdominal pain, *diarrhea.*
Hematologic: ***hemolysis in patients with G6PD deficiency*** (reversed after stopping drug), ***agranulocytosis, thrombocytopenia.***
Hepatic: ***hepatitis, hepatic necrosis.***
Respiratory: asthmatic attacks in patients with history of asthma, pulmonary sensitivity (cough, chest pains, fever, chills, dyspnea).
Skin: maculopapular, erythematous, or eczematous eruption; pruritus; urticaria; ***exfoliative dermatitis; Stevens-Johnson syndrome.***
Other: hypersensitivity reactions, ***anaphylaxis,*** transient alopecia, drug fever, overgrowth of nonsusceptible organisms in urinary tract.

Interactions

Drug-drug. *Magnesium-containing antacids:* decreased nitrofurantoin absorption. Separate ingestion by 1 hour.
Nalidixic acid, norfloxacin: possible decreased effectiveness. Avoid using together.
Probenecid, sulfinpyrazone: increased blood levels and decreased urine levels. May result in increased toxicity and lack of therapeutic effect. Don't use together.
Drug-food. *Any food:* increased absorption. Give drug with food.

Contraindications and precautions

- Contraindicated in children age 1 month and under and in patients with moderate to severe renal impairment (creatinine clearance less than 60 ml/minute), anuria, or oliguria.
- Use cautiously in pregnant or breast-feeding women and in patients with renal impairment, anemia, diabetes mellitus, electrolyte abnormalities, vitamin B deficiency, debilitating disease, or G6PD deficiency.

NURSING CONSIDERATIONS

Assessment

- Assess patient's infection before therapy and regularly thereafter.
- Obtain urine specimen for culture and sensitivity tests before starting therapy, and repeat p.r.n. Therapy may begin pending results.
- Monitor fluid intake and output. May turn urine brown or darker.
- Monitor CBC and pulmonary status regularly.
- Be alert for adverse reactions and drug interactions.
- Monitor patient's hydration status if adverse GI reactions occur.
- Evaluate patient's and family's knowledge of drug therapy.

Nursing diagnoses

- Infection related to susceptible bacteria
- Risk for deficient fluid volume related to drug-induced adverse GI reactions
- Deficient knowledge related to drug therapy

Planning and implementation

- Drug has no effect in blood or tissue outside urinary tract.

ALERT Hypersensitivity may develop during long-term therapy.

- Dual-release capsules (25 mg nitrofurantoin macrocrystals combined with 75 mg nitrofurantoin monohydrate) enable twice-daily dosing.
- Continue treatment for 3 days after urine specimens become sterile.
- Some patients may experience fewer adverse GI effects with nitrofurantoin macrocrystals.

• Store drug in amber container. Avoid metals other than stainless steel or aluminum to avoid precipitate formation.
• Drug may cause false-positive results with urine glucose test using copper sulfate reduction method (Clinitest) but not with glucose oxidase tests (Diastix).

Patient teaching
• Tell patient to take drug with food or milk to minimize GI distress.
• Teach patient how to measure intake and output. Warn him that drug will turn urine brown or darker.
• Instruct patient how to store drug.

Evaluation
• Patient is free from infection.
• Patient maintains adequate hydration throughout drug therapy.
• Patient and family state understanding of drug therapy.

nitroglycerin (glyceryl trinitrate)
(nigh-troh-GLIH-suh-rin)
Anginine ◇, Deponit, GTN-Pohl ◇, Minitran, Nitradisc ◇, Nitro-Bid, Nitro-Bid IV, Nitrocine, Nitrodisc, Nitro-Dur, Nitrogard, Nitroglyn, Nitroject, Nitrol, Nitrolingual, Nitrong, Nitrostat, Transderm-Nitro, Transiderm-Nitro ◇, Tridil

Pharmacologic class: nitrate
Therapeutic class: antianginal, vasodilator
Pregnancy risk category: C

Indications and dosages
▶ **Prophylaxis against chronic anginal attacks.** *Adults:* 2.5 mg or 2.6 mg (sustained-release capsule) q 8 to 12 hours. Or, 2% ointment: Start with ½ inch of ointment and increase by ½-inch increments until headache occurs; then decrease to previous dose. Range of dosage with ointment is ½ to 5 inches. Usual dose is 1 to 2 inches. Or, transdermal disc or pad (Nitrodisc, Nitro-Dur, or Transderm-Nitro): 0.2 to 0.4 mg/hour once daily.
▶ **Acute angina pectoris; to prevent or minimize anginal attacks when taken immediately before stressful events.** *Adults:* 1 S.L. tablet (gr 1/400, 1/200, 1/150, 1/100) dissolved under tongue or in buccal pouch as soon as angina begins. Repeat q 5 minutes, if needed, for 15 minutes. Or, using Nitrolingual spray, 1 or 2 sprays into mouth, preferably onto or under tongue. Repeat q 3 to 5 minutes if needed, to maximum of three doses in 15-minute period. Or, 1 to 3 mg transmucosally q 3 to 5 hours during waking hours.
▶ **Hypertension related to surgery; heart failure linked to MI; angina pectoris in acute situations; to produce controlled hypotension during surgery (by I.V. infusion).** *Adults:* initial infusion rate is 5 mcg/minute. Increased as needed by 5 mcg/minute q 3 to 5 minutes until response occurs. If 20-mcg/minute rate doesn't produce response, dosage is increased by as much as 20 mcg/minute q 3 to 5 minutes. Up to 100 mcg/minute may be needed.

How supplied
Tablets (buccal): 1 mg, 2 mg, 3 mg
Tablets (S.L.): 0.15 mg (gr 1/400), 0.3 mg (gr 1/200), 0.4 mg (gr 1/150), 0.6 mg (gr 1/100)
Tablets (sustained-release): 2.6 mg, 6.5 mg, 9 mg
Capsules (sustained-release): 2.5 mg, 6.5 mg, 9 mg, 13 mg
Aerosol (translingual): 0.4 mg metered spray
Topical: 2% ointment
Transdermal: 2.5 mg/24 hours, 5 mg/24 hours, 7.5 mg/24 hours, 10 mg/24 hours, 15 mg/24 hours
I.V.: 0.5 mg/ml, 0.8 mg/ml, 5 mg/ml
I.V. premixed solutions in dextrose: 100 mcg/ml, 200 mcg/ml, 400 mcg/ml

Pharmacokinetics
Absorption: well absorbed from GI tract. However, because it undergoes first-pass metabolism in liver, drug is incompletely absorbed into systemic circulation. For S.L. form, absorption from oral mucosa is relatively complete. For topical or transdermal form, well absorbed. Data not reported for other forms.
Distribution: distributed widely; about 60% of circulating drug is bound to plasma proteins.
Metabolism: metabolized in liver.

Excretion: metabolites excreted in urine. *Half-life:* about 1 to 4 minutes.

Route	Onset	Peak	Duration
P.O.	20-45 min	Unknown	8-12 hr
I.V.	Immediate	Immediate	3-5 min
Buccal	3 min	Unknown	5 hr
Ointment	30 min	Unknown	4-8 hr
S.L.	1-3 min	Unknown	30-60 min
Trans-dermal	30 min	Unknown	≤ 24 hr
Trans-lingual	2-4 min	Unknown	30-60 min

Pharmacodynamics

Chemical effect: reduces cardiac oxygen demand by decreasing left ventricular end-diastolic pressure (preload) and, to a lesser extent, systemic vascular resistance (afterload). Also increases blood flow through collateral coronary vessels.
Therapeutic effect: prevents or relieves acute angina, lowers blood pressure, and helps minimize heart failure caused by MI.

Adverse reactions

CNS: *headache, sometimes with throbbing; dizziness;* weakness.
CV: *orthostatic hypotension, tachycardia, flushing, palpitations,* fainting.
EENT: sublingual burning.
GI: nausea, vomiting.
Skin: cutaneous vasodilation, contact dermatitis (patch), rash.
Other: ***hypersensitivity reactions***.

Interactions

Drug-drug. *Antihypertensives:* may enhance hypotensive effect. Monitor patient closely.
Drug-lifestyle. *Alcohol use:* may increase hypotension. Advise patient to avoid alcohol during therapy.

Contraindications and precautions

- Contraindicated in patients hypersensitive to nitrates and in those with early MI (S.L. nitroglycerin), severe anemia, increased intracranial pressure, angle-closure glaucoma, orthostatic hypotension, and allergy to adhesives (transdermal form).
- I.V. nitroglycerin is contraindicated in patients with cardiac tamponade, restrictive cardiomyopathy, constrictive pericarditis, or hypersensitivity to I.V. form.
- Use cautiously in patients with hypotension or volume depletion and in pregnant or breast-feeding women.
- Safety of drug hasn't been established in children.

NURSING CONSIDERATIONS

Assessment

- Assess patient's condition before therapy and regularly thereafter.
- Monitor vital signs and drug response. Be particularly aware of blood pressure. Excessive hypotension may worsen MI.
- Be alert for adverse reactions and drug interactions.
- Evaluate patient's and family's knowledge of drug therapy.

Nursing diagnoses

- Pain related to angina
- Risk for injury related to drug-induced adverse reactions
- Deficient knowledge related to drug therapy

Planning and implementation

P.O. use: Give tablets on empty stomach, either 30 minutes before or 1 to 2 hours after meals.
– Tell patient to swallow tablets whole and not to chew them.
I.V. use: Dilute drug with D_5W or normal saline solution for injection. Concentration shouldn't exceed 400 mcg/ml.
– Administer with infusion control device and titrate to desired response.
– Mix in glass bottles and avoid I.V. filters because drug binds to plastic. Regular polyvinyl chloride tubing can bind up to 80% of drug, making it necessary to infuse higher dosages. A special nonabsorbent (non-polyvinyl chloride) tubing is available from manufacturer.
– Always use same type of infusion set when changing I.V. lines.
– When changing concentration of nitroglycerin infusion, flush I.V. administration set with

15 to 20 ml of new concentration before use. This will clear line of old drug solution.
Buccal use: Tell patient to place transmucosal tablet between lip and gum above incisors, or between cheek and gum.
– Tablets shouldn't be swallowed or chewed.
Topical use: To apply ointment, measure prescribed amount on application paper; then place paper on any nonhairy area. Don't rub in. Cover with plastic film to aid absorption and protect clothing.
– If using Tape-Surrounded Appli-Ruler (TSAR) system, keep TSAR on skin to protect patient's clothing and to make sure that ointment remains in place.
– Remove excess ointment from previous site before applying next dose. Avoid getting ointment on your fingers.
S.L. use: Administer tablet at first sign of attack. The tablet should be wet with patient's saliva and placed under tongue until completely absorbed. Patient should sit down and rest until pain subsides.
– Dose may be repeated every 10 to 15 minutes for up to three doses. If drug doesn't provide relief, medical help should be obtained promptly.
– Patient who complains of tingling sensation with S.L. form may try holding tablet in buccal pouch.
Transdermal use: Apply transdermal dosage forms to any nonhairy area except distal parts of arms or legs. Absorption won't be maximal from distal sites.
ALERT Remove transdermal patch before defibrillation. Because of aluminum backing on patch, electric current may cause patch to explode.
– When stopping transdermal treatment of angina, gradually reduce dose and frequency of application over 4 to 6 weeks, as ordered.
Translingual use: When administering translingual aerosol form, make sure patient doesn't inhale spray. Release it onto or under tongue, and have patient wait about 10 seconds or so before swallowing.
• Notify prescriber immediately if nitroglycerin is ineffective; keep patient at rest.
• Drug may cause headache, especially at start of therapy. Dosage may need to be reduced temporarily, but tolerance usually develops. Treat headache with aspirin or acetaminophen.
• Minimize drug tolerance with 10- to 12-hour daily nitrate-free interval. For example, remove transdermal system in early evening and apply a new system the next morning. Or omit last daily dose of buccal, sustained-release, or ointment form. Check with prescriber for alterations in dosage regimen if tolerance is suspected.
ALERT Don't confuse Nitro-Bid with Nicobid or nitroglycerin with nitroprusside.

Patient teaching
• Teach patient how to use form of drug prescribed.
• Caution patient to take drug regularly, as prescribed, and to have it accessible at all times.
• Tell patient that stopping drug abruptly causes coronary vasospasm.
• Inform patient that an additional dose may be taken before anticipated stress or at bedtime if angina is nocturnal.
• Instruct patient to use caution when wearing transdermal patch near microwave oven. Leaking radiation may heat metallic backing of patch and cause burns.
• Advise patient to avoid alcohol during drug therapy.
• Tell patient to change to upright position slowly. Advise him to go up and down stairs carefully and to lie down at first sign of dizziness.
• Urge patient to store drug in cool, dark place in tightly closed container. To ensure freshness, tell him to replace S.L. tablets every 3 months and to remove cotton because it absorbs drug.
• Tell patient to store S.L. tablets in original container or other container specifically approved for this use and to carry container in jacket pocket or purse, not in a pocket close to body.

Evaluation
• Patient reports pain relief.
• Patient doesn't experience injury from adverse reactions.
• Patient and family state understanding of drug therapy.

nitroprusside sodium

(nigh-troh-PRUS-ighd SOH-dee-um)
Nipride ♦, Nitropress

Pharmacologic class: vasodilator
Therapeutic class: antihypertensive
Pregnancy risk category: C

Indications and dosages

▶ **To lower blood pressure quickly in hypertensive emergencies; to produce controlled hypotension during anesthesia; to reduce preload and afterload in cardiac pump failure or cardiogenic shock (may be used with or without dopamine).** *Adults:* 50-mg vial diluted with 2 to 3 ml of D_5W and then added to 250, 500, or 1,000 ml of D_5W. Infused at 0.3 to 10 mcg/kg/minute. Average dose is 3 mcg/kg/minute. Maximum infusion rate is 10 mcg/kg/minute. Patients taking other antihypertensives are extremely sensitive to nitroprusside. Dosage is adjusted accordingly.

How supplied

Injection: 50 mg/vial in 2-ml, 5-ml vials

Pharmacokinetics

Absorption: not applicable.
Distribution: unknown.
Metabolism: metabolized rapidly in erythrocytes and tissues to cyanide radical and then converted to thiocyanate in liver.
Excretion: excreted primarily as metabolites in urine. *Half-life:* 2 minutes.

Route	Onset	Peak	Duration
I.V.	Almost immediate	1-2 min	10 min

Pharmacodynamics

Chemical effect: relaxes arteriolar and venous smooth muscle.
Therapeutic effect: lowers blood pressure and reduces preload and afterload.

Adverse reactions

The following adverse reactions usually indicate overdose.

CNS: *headache, dizziness,* ataxia, loss of consciousness, ***coma, increased intracranial pressure,*** weak pulse, absent reflexes, dilated pupils, *restlessness, muscle twitching.*
CV: distant heart sounds, palpitations, ***bradycardia***, tachycardia, hypotension.
GI: vomiting, nausea, abdominal pain.
Metabolic: ***acidosis.***
Respiratory: dyspnea, shallow breathing.
Skin: pink color, *diaphoresis.*
Other: ***thiocyanate toxicity, methemoglobinemia, cyanide toxicity.***

Interactions

Drug-drug. *Antihypertensives:* may cause sensitivity to nitroprusside. Adjust dosage as ordered.
Ganglionic blockers, general anesthetics, negative inotropics, other antihypertensives: additive effects. Monitor blood pressure closely.

Contraindications and precautions

- Contraindicated in patients hypersensitive to drug and in those with compensatory hypertension (as in arteriovenous shunt or coarctation of aorta), inadequate cerebral circulation, congenital optic atrophy, or tobacco-induced amblyopia.
- Use with extreme caution in patients with increased intracranial pressure.
- Use cautiously in pregnant women and in patients with hypothyroidism, hepatic or renal disease, hyponatremia, or low vitamin B_{12} level.
- Safety of drug hasn't been established in breast-feeding women and in children.

NURSING CONSIDERATIONS

Assessment

- Assess patient's condition before therapy.
- Obtain baseline vital signs before giving drug, and find out what parameters prescriber wants to achieve.

ALERT Excessive doses or rapid infusion (more than 15 mcg/kg/minute) can cause cyanide toxicity; therefore, check serum thiocyanate levels every 72 hours. Levels above 100 mcg/ml may cause toxicity. Watch for profound hypotension, metabolic acidosis,

dyspnea, headache, loss of consciousness, ataxia, and vomiting.
- Be alert for adverse reactions and drug interactions.
- Evaluate patient's (if appropriate) and family's knowledge of drug therapy.

Nursing diagnoses
- Risk for injury related to hypertension
- Decreased cardiac output related to heart failure
- Deficient knowledge related to drug therapy

Planning and implementation
- Keep patient in supine position when starting therapy or adjusting dosage.
- Don't use bacteriostatic water for injection or sterile saline solution for reconstitution.
- Because drug is sensitive to light, wrap I.V. solution in foil; it's not necessary to wrap tubing. Fresh solution should have faint brownish tint. Discard drug after 24 hours.
- Infuse with infusion pump. Drug is best given by piggyback through peripheral line with no other medication. Don't adjust rate of main I.V. line while drug is being infused. Even small bolus of nitroprusside can cause severe hypotension.
- Check blood pressure every 5 minutes at start of infusion and every 15 minutes thereafter. If severe hypotension occurs, stop infusion. Effects of drug quickly reverse. Notify prescriber. If possible, start arterial pressure line. Adjust flow to specified level.
- If cyanide toxicity occurs, stop drug immediately and notify prescriber.

ALERT Don't confuse nitroprusside with nitroglycerin.

Patient teaching
- Advise patient, if alert, to report adverse reactions or discomfort at the I.V. site immediately.

Evaluation
- Patient's blood pressure is normal.
- Patient has normal cardiac output.
- Patient and family state understanding of drug therapy.

nizatidine
(nigh-ZAT-ih-deen)
Axid, Tazac ◇

Pharmacologic class: histamine$_2$ (H_2)-receptor antagonist
Therapeutic class: antiulcer drug
Pregnancy risk category: B

Indications and dosages
▶ **Active duodenal ulcer.** *Adults:* 300 mg P.O. daily h.s. Or, 150 mg P.O. b.i.d.
▶ **Maintenance therapy for duodenal ulcer.** *Adults:* 150 mg P.O. daily h.s.
▶ **Benign gastric ulcer.** *Adults:* 150 mg P.O. b.i.d. or 300 mg h.s. for 8 weeks.
▶ **Gastroesophageal reflux disease.** *Adults:* 150 mg P.O. b.i.d.
Patients with impaired renal function: if creatinine clearance is 20 to 50 ml/minute, 150 mg P.O. daily for treatment of active duodenal ulcer or 150 mg every other day for maintenance therapy. If creatinine clearance is below 20 ml/minute, 150 mg P.O. every other day for treatment or 150 mg every third day for maintenance.

How supplied
Capsules: 75 mg†, 150 mg, 300 mg

Pharmacokinetics
Absorption: well absorbed (greater than 90%) from GI tract. Absorption may be slightly enhanced by food and slightly impaired by antacids.
Distribution: about 35% of drug is bound to plasma proteins.
Metabolism: unknown, but may undergo hepatic metabolism.
Excretion: more than 90% excreted in urine; less than 6% in feces. *Half-life:* 1 to 2 hours.

Route	Onset	Peak	Duration
P.O.	≤ 30 min	0.5-3 hr	≤ 12 hr

Pharmacodynamics
Chemical effect: competitively inhibits action of H_2 at receptor sites of parietal cells.

Therapeutic effect: decreases gastric acid secretion.

Adverse reactions

CNS: *somnolence.*
CV: ***arrhythmias.***
Hematologic: ***thrombocytopenia.***
Hepatic: liver damage.
Metabolic: hyperuricemia.
Skin: *diaphoresis,* rash, urticaria, ***exfoliative dermatitis.***
Other: fever.

Interactions

Drug-drug. *Aspirin:* possibly elevated serum salicylate levels (with high doses). Monitor patient for salicylate toxicity.
Drug-food. *Tomato-based, mixed-vegetable juices:* may decrease drug potency. Monitor diet.

Contraindications and precautions

- Contraindicated in patients hypersensitive to H_2-receptor antagonists.
- Use cautiously in patients with impaired renal function and in pregnant or breast-feeding women.
- Safety of drug hasn't been established in children.

NURSING CONSIDERATIONS

Assessment
- Assess patient's condition before therapy and regularly thereafter.
- Be alert for adverse reactions and drug interactions.
- Evaluate patient's and family's knowledge of drug therapy.
- Assess patient for abdominal pain. Note presence of blood in emesis, stool or gastric aspirate.

Nursing diagnoses
- Impaired tissue integrity related to ulceration of GI mucosa
- Decreased cardiac output related to drug-induced arrhythmias
- Deficient knowledge related to drug therapy

Planning and implementation
- If necessary, open capsules and mix contents with apple juice. However, drug loses some potency when combined with tomato-based, mixed-vegetable juices.
- False-positive test results for urobilinogen may occur.

Patient teaching
- Urge patient to avoid cigarette smoking because it may increase gastric acid secretion and worsen disease.
- Have patient report blood in stool or emesis.
- Warn patient to take drug as directed, even after pain subsides, to allow for adequate healing.

Evaluation
- Patient reports pain relief.
- Patient maintains normal cardiac output throughout drug therapy.
- Patient and family state understanding of drug therapy.

norepinephrine bitartrate (levarterenol bitartrate, noradrenaline acid tartrate)

(nor-ep-ih-NEF-rin bigh-TAR-trayt)
Levophed

Pharmacologic class: adrenergic (direct acting)
Therapeutic class: vasopressor
Pregnancy risk category: C

Indications and dosages

▶ **To restore blood pressure in acute hypotensive states.** *Adults:* initially, 8 to 12 mcg/minute by I.V. infusion, adjusted to maintain normal blood pressure. Average maintenance dosage is 2 to 4 mcg/minute.
Children: 2 mcg/m^2/minute by I.V. infusion; dosage adjusted based on patient response.
▶ **Severe hypotension during cardiac arrest.** *Children:* initial I.V. infusion rate is 0.1 mcg/kg/minute. Rate adjusted based on response.

How supplied

Injection: 1 mg/ml

Pharmacokinetics

Absorption: not applicable.
Distribution: drug localizes in sympathetic nerve tissues.
Metabolism: metabolized in liver and other tissues to inactive compounds.
Excretion: excreted in urine. *Half-life:* about 1 minute.

Route	Onset	Peak	Duration
I.V.	Immediate	Immediate	1-2 min

Pharmacodynamics

Chemical effect: stimulates alpha- and $beta_1$-adrenergic receptors in sympathetic nervous system.
Therapeutic effect: raises blood pressure.

Adverse reactions

CNS: *headache,* anxiety, weakness, dizziness, tremor, restlessness, insomnia.
CV: ***bradycardia, severe hypertension,*** marked increase in peripheral resistance, decreased cardiac output, ***arrhythmias.***
GU: decreased urine output.
Metabolic: ***metabolic acidosis***, hyperglycemia, increased glycogenolysis.
Respiratory: respiratory difficulties, ***asthmatic episodes.***
Other: fever, irritation with extravasation, swelling and enlargement of thyroid, ***anaphylaxis.***

Interactions

Drug-drug. *Alpha-adrenergic blockers:* may antagonize drug effects. Monitor patient.
Antihistamines, ergot alkaloids, guanethidine, methyldopa: use with sympathomimetics may cause severe hypertension. Don't give together.
Inhaled anesthetics: increased risk of arrhythmias. Monitor ECG closely.
MAO inhibitors: increased risk of hypertensive crisis. Monitor patient closely.
Tricyclic antidepressants: increased vasopressor effect. Don't give together.

Contraindications and precautions

- Contraindicated in pregnant or breast-feeding women, patients receiving cyclopropane or halothane anesthesia, and patients with mesenteric or peripheral vascular thrombosis, profound hypoxia, hypercapnia, or hypotension caused by blood volume deficits.
- Use with extreme caution in patients receiving MAO inhibitors, tricyclic antidepressants, and certain antihistamines.
- Use cautiously in patients with sulfite sensitivity.

NURSING CONSIDERATIONS

Assessment

- Assess patient's condition before therapy.
- During infusion, frequently monitor ECG, cardiac output, central venous pressure, pulmonary capillary wedge pressure, pulse rate, urine output, and color and temperature of limbs. Also, check blood pressure every 2 minutes until stabilized; then check every 5 minutes.
- Be alert for adverse reactions and drug interactions.
- Monitor vital signs closely when therapy ends. Watch for sudden drop in blood pressure.
- Evaluate patient's and family's knowledge of drug therapy.

Nursing diagnoses

- Decreased cardiac output related to hypotension
- Risk for injury related to drug-induced adverse reactions
- Deficient knowledge related to drug therapy

Planning and implementation

- Drug isn't a substitute for blood or fluid volume deficit. If deficit exists, replace fluid before giving vasopressors.
- Use central venous catheter or large vein, such as in antecubital fossa, to minimize risk of extravasation. Administer in dextrose 5% in normal saline solution for injection; normal saline solution for injection alone isn't recommended. Use continuous infusion pump to regulate flow rate and piggyback setup so I.V. line remains open if norepinephrine is stopped.

• Titrate infusion rate according to assessment findings and prescriber's guidelines. In previously hypertensive patients, blood pressure should be raised no higher than 40 mm Hg below previous systolic pressure.
• Never leave patient unattended during infusion.
• Check site frequently for extravasation. If it occurs, stop infusion immediately and call prescriber. As directed, counteract effect by infiltrating area with 5 to 10 mg phentolamine and 10 to 15 ml of normal saline solution. Also check for blanching along course of infused vein; may progress to superficial sloughing.
• If prolonged I.V. therapy is needed, change injection site frequently.
• Keep emergency drugs on hand to reverse effects of norepinephrine: atropine for reflex bradycardia, phentolamine for vasopressor effects, and propranolol for arrhythmias.
• Report decreased urine output to prescriber immediately.
• When stopping drug, gradually slow infusion rate, as ordered, and report sudden drop in blood pressure.
• Drug solutions deteriorate after 24 hours.
• Protect drug from light. Discard discolored solutions or solutions that contain precipitate.

Patient teaching
• Tell patient to immediately report discomfort at infusion site or difficulty breathing.

☑ Evaluation
• Patient has normal cardiac output.
• Patient sustains no injuries from drug-induced adverse reactions.
• Patient and family state understanding of drug therapy.

norethindrone
(nor-ETH-in-drohn)
Micronor, Nor-Q.D.

norethindrone acetate
Aygestin, Norlutate

Pharmacologic class: progestin
Therapeutic class: contraceptive
Pregnancy risk category: X

Indications and dosages
▶ **Amenorrhea, abnormal uterine bleeding. Norethindrone acetate.** *Adults:* 2.5 to 10 mg P.O. daily on days 5 to 25 of menstrual cycle.
▶ **Endometriosis. Norethindrone acetate.** *Adults:* 5 mg P.O. daily for 14 days; then increased by 2.5 mg daily q 2 weeks up to 15 mg daily.
▶ **Contraception in women. Norethindrone.** *Adults:* initially, 0.35 mg P.O. on first day of menstruation; then 0.35 mg daily.

How supplied
norethindrone
Tablets: 0.35 mg, 0.5 mg
norethindrone acetate
Tablets: 5 mg

Pharmacokinetics
Absorption: well absorbed from GI tract.
Distribution: distributed widely; about 80% protein-bound.
Metabolism: metabolized primarily in liver; it undergoes extensive first-pass metabolism.
Excretion: excreted primarily in feces. *Half-life:* 5 to 14 hours.

Route	Onset	Peak	Duration
P.O.	Unknown	Unknown	Unknown

Pharmacodynamics
Chemical effect: suppresses ovulation, possibly by inhibiting pituitary gonadotropin secretion, and forms thick cervical mucus.
Therapeutic effect: prevents pregnancy and relieves symptoms of endometriosis, amenorrhea, and abnormal uterine bleeding.

Adverse reactions
CNS: dizziness, migraine, lethargy, depression.
CV: hypertension, thrombophlebitis, ***pulmonary embolism, thromboembolism, CVA,*** edema.
GI: nausea, vomiting, abdominal cramps.
GU: breakthrough bleeding, dysmenorrhea, amenorrhea, cervical erosion, abnormal secretions, uterine fibromas, vaginal candidiasis.
Hepatic: cholestatic jaundice.

Metabolic: hyperglycemia.
Skin: melasma, rash.
Other: decreased libido; breast tenderness, enlargement, or secretion.

Interactions

Drug-drug. *Barbiturates, carbamazepine, rifampin:* decreased progestin effects. Monitor patient for lack of effect.
Bromocriptine: may cause amenorrhea, thus interfering with bromocriptine effects. Avoid concomitant use.
Drug-food. *Caffeine:* may increase serum caffeine level. Monitor patient for caffeine effects.
Drug-lifestyle. *Smoking:* increased risk of CV effects. If smoking continues, may need alternative therapy.

Contraindications and precautions

- Contraindicated in pregnant patients; patients hypersensitive to drug; patients with thromboembolic disorders, cerebral apoplexy, or a history of these conditions; and patients with breast cancer, undiagnosed abnormal vaginal bleeding, severe hepatic disease, or missed abortion.
- Drug use isn't recommended for breast-feeding women.
- Use cautiously in patients with diabetes mellitus, seizure disorder, migraine, cardiac or renal disease, asthma, and depression.
- Safety of drug hasn't been established in children.

NURSING CONSIDERATIONS

Assessment

- Assess patient's condition before therapy and regularly thereafter.
- Be alert for adverse reactions and drug interactions.
- Evaluate patient's and family's knowledge of drug therapy.
- Monitor blood pressure and edema.

Nursing diagnoses

- Ineffective health maintenance related to underlying condition
- Excessive fluid volume related to drug-induced edema
- Deficient knowledge related to drug therapy

Planning and implementation

ALERT Norethindrone acetate is twice as potent as norethindrone. It shouldn't be used for contraception.
- Don't use drug as test for pregnancy; norethindrone may cause birth defects and masculinization of female fetus.
- Preliminary estrogen treatment is usually needed by patients with menstrual disorders.
- Withhold drug and notify prescriber if visual disturbance, migraine, or headache occurs or if pulmonary emboli are suspected; provide supportive care.

Patient teaching
- Make sure patient reads package insert explaining adverse effects of progestin before taking first dose. Also, provide verbal explanation.
- Instruct patient to report unusual symptoms immediately. Tell her to stop drug and call prescriber if visual disturbance or migraine occurs.
- Teach patient how to perform routine monthly breast self-examination.
- Warn patient that edema and weight gain are likely. Advise her to restrict sodium intake.

Evaluation

- Patient responds well to therapy.
- Patient's drug-induced edema is minimized with sodium restriction.
- Patient and family state understanding of drug therapy.

norfloxacin

(nor-FLOKS-uh-sin)
Noroxin

Pharmacologic class: fluoroquinolone
Therapeutic class: broad-spectrum antibiotic
Pregnancy risk category: C

Indications and dosages

▶ **Complicated or uncomplicated urinary tract infections caused by susceptible strains of *Escherichia coli, Klebsiella, Enter-***

***obacter, Proteus, Pseudomonas aeruginosa, Citrobacter, Staphylococcus aureus, Staphylococcus epidermidis,* and group D streptococci.** *Adults:* for uncomplicated infections, 400 mg P.O. b.i.d. for 7 to 10 days. For complicated infections, 400 mg b.i.d. for 10 to 21 days.

▶ **Cystitis caused by *E. coli, K. pneumoniae,* or *Proteus mirabilis.*** *Adults:* 400 mg P.O. b.i.d. for 3 days.

▶ **Acute, uncomplicated gonorrhea.** *Adults:* 800 mg P.O. as single dose, followed by doxycycline therapy to treat coexisting chlamydial infection. Adults with creatinine clearance of 30 ml/minute or less should receive 400 mg once daily.

How supplied

Tablets: 400 mg

Pharmacokinetics

Absorption: about 30% to 40% absorbed from GI tract (as dose increases, percentage of absorbed drug decreases). Food may reduce absorption.
Distribution: distributed into renal tissue, liver, gallbladder, prostatic fluid, testicles, seminal fluid, bile, and sputum. From 10% to 15% binds to plasma proteins.
Metabolism: unknown.
Excretion: most systemically absorbed drug is excreted by kidneys, with about 30% appearing in bile. *Half-life:* 3 to 4 hours.

Route	Onset	Peak	Duration
P.O.	Unknown	1-2 hr	Unknown

Pharmacodynamics

Chemical effect: inhibits bacterial DNA synthesis, mainly by blocking DNA gyrase.
Therapeutic effect: kills certain bacteria, such as most aerobic gram-positive and gram-negative urinary pathogens, including *P. aeruginosa.*

Adverse reactions

CNS: fatigue, somnolence, headache, dizziness, ***seizures.***
GI: nausea, constipation, flatulence, heartburn, dry mouth.
GU: increased serum creatinine and BUN levels, crystalluria.
Hematologic: eosinophilia.
Hepatic: transient elevation of AST and ALT levels.
Musculoskeletal: arthralgia, arthritis, myalgia, joint swelling.
Skin: rash, photosensitivity.
Other: ***hypersensitivity reactions (rash, anaphylactoid reactions),*** fever.

Interactions

Drug-drug. *Antacids, iron products, sucralfate:* may hinder absorption. Separate administration times by 2 hours.
Cyclosporine: increased serum cyclosporine levels. Monitor serum levels.
Nitrofurantoin: decreased norfloxacin effectiveness. Don't use together.
Oral anticoagulants: increased anticoagulant effect. Monitor patient closely.
Probenecid: may increase serum levels of norfloxacin by decreasing its excretion. Monitor patient for toxicity.
Theophylline: possible impaired theophylline metabolism, resulting in increased plasma levels and risk of toxicity. Monitor patient closely.
Drug-lifestyle. *Sunlight:* May cause photosensitivity reaction. Urge patient to take precautions.

Contraindications and precautions

- Contraindicated in children and in patients hypersensitive to fluoroquinolones.
- Use cautiously in pregnant women and patients with conditions that may predispose them to seizure disorders, such as cerebral arteriosclerosis.
- Safety of drug hasn't been established in breast-feeding women or in children who are under age 18.

NURSING CONSIDERATIONS

Assessment

- Assess patient's infection before therapy and regularly thereafter.
- Obtain culture and sensitivity tests before starting therapy, and repeat as needed throughout therapy.

• Be alert for adverse reactions and drug interactions.
• Evaluate patient's and family's knowledge of drug therapy.

Nursing diagnoses
• Infection related to bacteria
• Risk for injury related to drug-induced adverse CNS reactions
• Deficient knowledge related to drug therapy

Planning and implementation
• Give drug on empty stomach.
• Make sure patient is well hydrated before and during therapy to avoid crystalluria.

Patient teaching
• Urge patient to take drug 1 hour before or 2 hours after meals to promote absorption.
• Warn patient not to exceed recommended dosage and to drink several glasses of water throughout day to maintain hydration and adequate urine output.
• Caution patient to avoid hazardous activities until CNS effects of drug are known.

Evaluation
• Patient is free from infection.
• Patient has no injuries from drug-induced adverse CNS reactions.
• Patient and family state understanding of drug therapy.

norgestrel
(nor-JES-trel)
Ovrette**

Pharmacologic class: progestin
Therapeutic class: contraceptive
Pregnancy risk category: X

Indications and dosages
▶ **Contraception.** *Women:* 0.075 mg P.O. daily.

How supplied
Tablets: 0.075 mg

Pharmacokinetics
Absorption: well absorbed.
Distribution: unknown.
Metabolism: unknown.
Excretion: unknown.

Route	Onset	Peak	Duration
P.O.	Unknown	Unknown	Unknown

Pharmacodynamics
Chemical effect: unknown; may suppress ovulation, possibly by inhibiting pituitary gonadotropin secretion, and forms thick cervical mucus.
Therapeutic effect: prevents pregnancy.

Adverse reactions
CNS: cerebral thrombosis or hemorrhage, migraine headache, lethargy, depression.
CV: hypertension, thrombophlebitis, ***pulmonary embolism, thromboembolism, CVA,*** edema.
GI: nausea, vomiting, abdominal cramps, gallbladder disease.
GU: *breakthrough bleeding, altered menstrual flow,* dysmenorrhea, spotting, amenorrhea, cervical erosion, vaginal candidiasis.
Hepatic: cholestatic jaundice.
Skin: melasma, rash.
Other: breast tenderness, enlargement, or secretion.

Interactions
Drug-drug. *Barbiturates, carbamazepine, rifampin:* decreased progestin effects. Monitor patient for reduced response.
Bromocriptine: may cause amenorrhea, interfering with bromocriptine's effects. Avoid concomitant use.
Drug-food. *Caffeine:* may increase serum caffeine levels. Monitor patient for caffeine effects.
Drug-lifestyle. *Smoking:* increased risk of CV effects. Patient who continues to smoke may need a different therapy.

Contraindications and precautions
• Contraindicated in pregnant or breast-feeding women; patients hypersensitive to drug; patients with thromboembolic disorders, cerebral apoplexy, or a history of these condi-

tions; and patients with breast cancer, undiagnosed abnormal vaginal bleeding, severe hepatic disease, or missed abortion.

- Use cautiously in patients with diabetes mellitus, seizure disorder, migraine, cardiac disease, renal disease, asthma, or depression.
- Safety of drug hasn't been established in children.

NURSING CONSIDERATIONS

Assessment

- Assess patient's pregnancy status before therapy and regularly thereafter. Failure rate of progestin-only contraceptive is about three times higher than that of combination contraceptives.
- Be alert for adverse reactions and drug interactions.
- Evaluate patient's and family's knowledge of drug therapy.

Nursing diagnoses

- Health-seeking behavior related to request for contraceptive
- Excessive fluid volume related to drug-induced edema
- Deficient knowledge related to drug therapy

Planning and implementation

- Norgestrel is a progestin-only oral contraceptive known as the minipill.
- Make sure pregnancy test is negative before starting therapy.

Patient teaching

- Make sure patient reads package insert explaining adverse effects of progestins before taking first dose. Also, provide verbal explanation.
- Tell patient to take pill at same time every day, even if menstruating.
- Inform patient that risk of pregnancy increases with each tablet missed. Tell patient who misses one tablet to take it as soon as remembered and then to take next tablet at regular time. Advise patient who misses two tablets to take one as soon as remembered and then take next regular dose at usual time and to use a nonhormonal method of contraception along with norgestrel until 14 tablets have been taken. Tell patient who misses three or more tablets to stop drug and use a nonhormonal method of contraception until after menses. If menstrual period doesn't occur within 45 days, tell her to test for pregnancy.
- Advise patient about increased risk of serious adverse CV reactions caused by heavy cigarette smoking.
- Instruct patient to immediately report excessive bleeding, bleeding between menstrual cycles, breast pain or tenderness, vaginal discharge, or swelling of hands or feet.
- Tell patient to report unusual symptoms immediately and to stop drug and call prescriber if she has visual disturbance, migraine, or numbness or tingling in limbs.
- Teach patient how to perform routine breast self-examination.

Evaluation

- Patient doesn't become pregnant.
- Patient develops minimal edema.
- Patient and family state understanding of drug therapy.

nortriptyline hydrochloride

(nor-TRIP-teh-leen high-droh-KLOR-ighd)
Allegron ◇, Aventyl*, Pamelor*

Pharmacologic class: tricyclic antidepressant
Therapeutic class: antidepressant
Pregnancy risk category: NR

Indications and dosages

▶ **Depression.** *Adults:* 25 mg P.O. t.i.d. or q.i.d., gradually increased to maximum of 150 mg daily. Or, entire dosage may be given h.s.

How supplied

Tablets: 10 mg ◇, 25 mg ◇
Capsules: 10 mg, 25 mg, 50 mg, 75 mg
Oral solution: 10 mg/5 ml*

Pharmacokinetics

Absorption: absorbed rapidly.
Distribution: distributed widely into body, including CNS. Drug is 95% protein-bound.

Metabolism: metabolized by liver; significant first-pass effect may account for variability of serum levels in different patients taking same dosage.
Excretion: most excreted in urine; some in feces. *Half-life:* 18 to 24 hours.

Route	Onset	Peak	Duration
P.O.	Unknown	7-8.5 hr	Unknown

Pharmacodynamics

Chemical effect: unknown; increases amount of norepinephrine, serotonin, or both in CNS by blocking their reuptake by presynaptic neurons.
Therapeutic effect: relieves depression.

Adverse reactions

CNS: *drowsiness, dizziness,* excitation, ***seizures,*** tremor, weakness, confusion, headache, nervousness, EEG changes, extrapyramidal reactions.
CV: *tachycardia,* ECG changes, hypertension, ***heart block, CVA, MI.***
EENT: *blurred vision,* tinnitus, mydriasis.
GI: dry mouth, *constipation,* nausea, vomiting, anorexia, paralytic ileus.
GU: urine retention.
Hematologic: bone marrow depression, eosinophilia, ***agranulocytosis, thrombocytopenia.***
Skin: diaphoresis, rash, urticaria, photosensitivity.
Other: ***hypersensitivity reaction.***

Interactions

Drug-drug. *Barbiturates, CNS depressants:* enhanced CNS depression. Avoid concomitant use.
Cimetidine, methylphenidate: may increase serum nortriptyline levels. Monitor patient for adverse reactions.
Clonidine, epinephrine, norepinephrine: increased hypertensive effect. Use together cautiously.
MAO inhibitors: may cause severe excitation, hyperpyrexia, or seizures. Use together cautiously.
Drug-herb. *SAMe, St. John's wort, yohimbe:* use with some tricyclic antidepressants may increase serotonin levels. Discourage concomitant use.
Drug-lifestyle. *Alcohol use:* enhanced CNS depression. Discourage concomitant use.
Smoking: may lower plasma nortriptyline levels. Monitor patient for lack of drug effect.
Sun exposure: increased risk of photosensitivity reaction. Urge patient to take precautions.

Contraindications and precautions

- Contraindicated in patients hypersensitive to drug, patients in acute recovery phase after MI, and patients who took an MAO inhibitor within 14 days.
- Drug isn't recommended for pregnant women, breast-feeding women, or children.
- Use with extreme caution in patients taking thyroid drugs and in patients with glaucoma, suicidal tendency, history of urine retention or seizures, CV disease, or hyperthyroidism.

NURSING CONSIDERATIONS

Assessment

- Assess patient's depression before therapy and regularly thereafter.
- Be alert for adverse reactions and drug interactions.
- Evaluate patient's and family's knowledge of drug therapy.

Nursing diagnoses

- Disturbed thought processes related to depression
- Risk for injury related to drug-induced adverse CNS reactions
- Deficient knowledge related to drug therapy

Planning and implementation

- Dosage should be reduced in elderly or debilitated patient.
- Don't withdraw drug abruptly. After abrupt withdrawal of long-term therapy, patient may experience nausea, headache, and malaise.
- Because hypertensive episodes have occurred during surgery in patients receiving tricyclic antidepressants, drug should be gradually stopped several days before surgery.
- If signs of psychosis occur or increase, expect to reduce dosage.

ALERT Don't confuse nortriptyline with amitriptyline.

Patient teaching

- Whenever possible, advise patient to take full dose at bedtime to reduce risk of orthostatic hypotension.
- Warn patient to avoid hazardous activities until CNS effects of drug are known. Drowsiness and dizziness usually subside after a few weeks.
- Tell patient to avoid alcohol during drug therapy.
- Warn patient not to stop drug suddenly.
- Advise patient to consult prescriber before taking other prescription or OTC drugs.
- Advise patient to use sunblock, wear protective clothing, and avoid prolonged exposure to sunlight.

Evaluation

- Patient's depression improves.
- Patient experiences no injuries due to drug-induced adverse CNS reactions.
- Patient and family state understanding of drug therapy.

nystatin

(nigh-STAT-in)

Mycostatin*, Nadostine♦, Nilstat, Nystex*

Pharmacologic class: polyene macrolide
Therapeutic class: antifungal
Pregnancy risk category: C

Indications and dosages

▶ **GI tract infections.** *Adults:* 500,000 to 1 million units as tablets P.O. t.i.d.

▶ **Oral, vaginal, and intestinal infections caused by *Candida albicans* and other *Candida* species.** *Adults:* 500,000 to 1 million units suspension P.O. t.i.d. for oral candidiasis. *Children and infants over age 3 months:* 250,000 to 500,000 units suspension P.O. q.i.d. *Neonates and premature infants:* 100,000 units suspension P.O. q.i.d.

▶ **Vaginal infections.** *Adults:* 100,000 units, as vaginal tablets, inserted high into vagina, daily or b.i.d. for 14 days.

How supplied

Tablets: 500,000 units
Oral suspension: 100,000 units/ml
Vaginal suppositories: 100,000 units

Pharmacokinetics

Absorption: not absorbed from GI tract, intact skin, or mucous membranes.
Distribution: none.
Metabolism: none.
Excretion: oral form excreted almost entirely unchanged in feces.

Route	Onset	Peak	Duration
P.O., topical	Unknown	Unknown	Unknown

Pharmacodynamics

Chemical effect: unknown; probably acts by binding to sterols in fungal cell membrane, altering cell permeability and allowing leakage of intracellular components.
Therapeutic effect: kills susceptible yeasts and fungi.

Adverse reactions

GI: transient nausea, vomiting, diarrhea (with large oral dosage).

Interactions

None significant.

Contraindications and precautions

- Contraindicated in patients hypersensitive to drug.
- Safety of drug hasn't been established in breast-feeding women.

NURSING CONSIDERATIONS

Assessment

- Assess patient's infection before therapy and regularly thereafter.
- Be alert for adverse reactions.
- Monitor patient's hydration status if adverse GI reactions occur.
- Evaluate patient's and family's knowledge of drug therapy.

Nursing diagnoses

- Infection related to organisms

• Risk for deficient fluid volume related to drug-induced adverse GI reactions
• Deficient knowledge related to drug therapy

Planning and implementation

• Drug isn't effective against systemic infections.
P.O. use: When treating oral candidiasis (thrush), clean food debris from patient's mouth and have patient hold suspension in mouth for several minutes before swallowing.
– When treating an infant, swab medication on oral mucosa.
– Immunosuppressed patients with oral candidiasis are sometimes instructed by prescriber to suck on vaginal tablets (100,000 units) because doing so provides prolonged contact with oral mucosa.
Vaginal use: Pregnant patients can use vaginal tablets up to 6 weeks before term to treat infection that may cause thrush in neonates.

Patient teaching

• Advise patient to take drug for at least 2 days after symptoms disappear to prevent reinfection. Consult prescriber for duration of therapy.
• Instruct patient to continue therapy during menstruation.
• Instruct patient in oral hygiene techniques. Poorly fitting dentures and overuse of mouthwash may alter oral flora and promote infection.
• Explain that predisposing factors for vaginal infection include use of antibiotics, oral contraceptives, and corticosteroids; diabetes; reinfection by sexual partner; and tight-fitting panty hose. Encourage patient to wear cotton (not synthetic) underpants.
• Teach patient about hygiene for affected areas, including wiping perineal area from front to back.
• Advise patient to report redness, swelling, or irritation.

Evaluation

• Patient is free from infection.
• Patient maintains adequate hydration throughout drug therapy.
• Patient and family state understanding of drug therapy.

O

octreotide acetate

(ok-TREE-oh-tighd AS-ih-tayt)
Sandostatin, Sandostatin LAR Depot

Pharmacologic class: synthetic octapeptide
Therapeutic class: somatotropic hormone
Pregnancy risk category: B

Indications and dosages

▶ **Flushing and diarrhea caused by carcinoid tumors.** *Adults:* 0.1 to 0.6 mg daily S.C. in two to four divided doses for first 2 weeks (usual daily dosage is 0.3 mg). Subsequent dosage based on response. Patients currently on Sandostatin can switch to Sandostatin LAR Depot 20 mg I.M. to gluteal area q 4 weeks for 2 months.
▶ **Watery diarrhea caused by vasoactive intestinal polypeptide secreting tumors (VIPomas).** *Adults:* 0.2 to 0.3 mg daily S.C. in two to four divided doses for first 2 weeks of therapy. Subsequent dosage based on individual response; typically doesn't exceed 0.45 mg daily. Patients currently on Sandostatin can switch to Sandostatin LAR Depot 20 mg I.M. to gluteal area q 4 weeks for 2 months.
▶ **Acromegaly.** *Adults:* initially, 50 mcg S.C. t.i.d.; then adjusted according to somatomedin C levels q 2 weeks. Patients currently on Sandostatin can switch to Sandostatin LAR Depot 20 mg I.M. to gluteal area q 4 weeks for 3 months.

How supplied

Injection: 0.05-mg, 0.1-mg, 0.5-mg ampules; 0.2-mg/ml, 1-mg/ml multidose vials
Depot: 10 mg/5 ml, 20 mg/5 ml, 30 mg/5 ml

Pharmacokinetics

Absorption: absorbed rapidly and completely after S.C. injection.
Distribution: distributed to plasma, where it binds to serum lipoprotein and albumin.
Metabolism: not clearly defined.

Excretion: about 35% of drug appears unchanged in urine. *Half-life:* about 1½ hours.

Route	Onset	Peak	Duration
S.C., I.M.	≤ 30 min	30-60 min	12 hr-6 wk

Pharmacodynamics

Chemical effect: mimics action of naturally occurring somatostatin.
Therapeutic effect: relieves flushing and diarrhea caused by certain tumors, and treats acromegaly.

Adverse reactions

CNS: dizziness, headache, light-headedness, fatigue.
CV: ***arrhythmias, bradycardia.***
GI: *nausea, diarrhea, abdominal pain or discomfort,* loose stools, vomiting, fat malabsorption, gallbladder abnormalities.
Metabolic: hyperglycemia, hypoglycemia, hypothyroidism.
Skin: flushing, edema, wheal, erythema and pain at injection site.
Other: pain, burning at S.C. injection site.

Interactions

Drug-drug. *Cyclosporine:* may decrease plasma cyclosporine levels. Monitor patient.

Contraindications and precautions

- Contraindicated in patients hypersensitive to drug or its components.
- Use cautiously in pregnant women.
- Safety of drug hasn't been established in breast-feeding women and in children.

NURSING CONSIDERATIONS

Assessment

- Assess patient's condition before therapy and regularly thereafter.
- Monitor baseline thyroid function tests as ordered.
- Monitor somatomedin C levels every 2 weeks as ordered. Dosage is adjusted based on this level.
- Monitor laboratory tests periodically, such as thyroid function tests, urine 5-hydroxyindoleacetic acid, plasma serotonin, plasma substance P (for carcinoid tumors), and plasma vasoactive intestinal peptide (for VIPomas).
- Monitor fluid and electrolyte status.
- Be alert for adverse reactions and drug interactions.
- Evaluate patient's and family's knowledge of drug therapy.

Nursing diagnoses

- Diarrhea related to condition
- Fatigue related to drug-induced adverse CNS reaction
- Deficient knowledge related to drug therapy

Planning and implementation

- Give drug in divided doses for first 2 weeks of therapy; subsequent daily dosage depends on patient's response.
- Read drug labels carefully, and check dosage and strength.

ALERT For LAR Depot injection, administer only by I.M. route. Don't give I.V. or S.C. Avoid deltoid muscle because of possible discomfort at site.

- Drug therapy may alter fluid and electrolyte balance and may require adjustment of other drugs.

Patient teaching

- Tell patient to report signs of gallbladder disease such as abdominal discomfort. Drug may be linked to development of cholelithiasis.
- Instruct patient that laboratory tests are needed during therapy.
- Advise diabetic patient to monitor blood glucose levels closely. Antidiabetics may need dosage adjustment.

Evaluation

- Patient's bowel pattern is normal.
- Patient uses energy-saving measures to combat fatigue.
- Patient and family state understanding of drug therapy.

ofloxacin

(oh-FLOKS-eh-sin)
Floxin

Pharmacologic class: fluoroquinolone
Therapeutic class: antibiotic
Pregnancy risk category: C

Indications and dosages

▶ **Lower respiratory tract infections caused by susceptible strains of *Haemophilus influenzae* or *Streptococcus pneumoniae.*** *Adults:* 400 mg I.V. or P.O. q 12 hours for 10 days.

▶ **Cervicitis or urethritis caused by *Chlamydia trachomatis* or *Neisseria gonorrhoeae.*** *Adults:* 300 mg I.V. or P.O. q 12 hours for 7 days.

▶ **Acute, uncomplicated gonorrhea.** *Adults:* 400 mg I.V. or P.O. as single dose.

▶ **Mild to moderate skin and skin-structure infections caused by susceptible strains of *Staphylococcus aureus, Staphylococcus epidermidis, Streptococcus pyogenes,* or *Proteus mirabilis.*** *Adults:* 400 mg I.V. or P.O. q 12 hours for 10 days.

▶ **Cystitis caused by *Escherichia coli* or *Klebsiella pneumoniae.*** *Adults:* 200 mg I.V. or P.O. q 12 hours for 3 days.

▶ **Urinary tract infections caused by susceptible strains of *Citrobacter diversus, Enterobacter aerogenes, E. coli, P. mirabilis,* or *Pseudomonas aeruginosa.*** *Adults:* 200 mg I.V. or P.O. q 12 hours for 7 days. Complicated infections may need 10 days of therapy.

▶ **Prostatitis caused by *E. coli.*** *Adults:* 300 mg I.V. or P.O. q 12 hours for 6 weeks. If creatinine clearance is 10 to 50 ml/minute, decrease dosage interval to once q 24 hours. If clearance is below 10 ml/minute, give half recommended dose q 24 hours.

How supplied

Tablets: 200 mg, 300 mg, 400 mg
Injection: 20 mg/ml, 40 mg/ml; 4 mg/ml premixed in D_5W

Pharmacokinetics

Absorption: well absorbed after P.O. administration.
Distribution: widely distributed to body tissues and fluids.
Metabolism: pyridobenzoxazine ring decreases extent of metabolism in liver.
Excretion: 70% to 80% of drug is excreted unchanged in urine; less than 5% in feces.

Route	Onset	Peak	Duration
P.O.	Unknown	1-2 hr	Unknown
I.V.	Almost immediate	Immediate	Unknown

Pharmacodynamics

Chemical effect: unknown; may inhibit bacterial DNA gyrase and prevent DNA replication in susceptible bacteria.
Therapeutic effect: kills susceptible aerobic gram-positive and gram-negative organisms.

Adverse reactions

CNS: headache, dizziness, fatigue, lethargy, malaise, drowsiness, sleep disorders, nervousness, light-headedness, insomnia, ***seizures.***
CV: chest pain.
EENT: visual disturbances.
GI: nausea, anorexia, abdominal pain or discomfort, diarrhea, vomiting, dry mouth, flatulence, dysgeusia.
GU: vaginitis, vaginal discharge, genital pruritus.
Hematologic: eosinophilia.
Hepatic: elevated liver enzyme levels.
Musculoskeletal: trunk pain, transient arthralgia, myalgia.
Skin: rash, pruritus, photosensitivity.
Other: hypersensitivity reactions, ***anaphylactoid reaction,*** fever.

Interactions

Drug-drug. *Antacids that contain aluminum or magnesium hydroxide, iron salts, sucralfate, products containing zinc:* may interfere with GI absorption of ofloxacin. Separate administration by at least 2 hours.
Antineoplastics: may lower serum fluoroquinolone levels. Monitor patient for lack of effect.

Oral anticoagulants: increased effect. Monitor patient for bleeding and altered PT and INR.
Theophylline: decreased theophylline clearance with some fluoroquinolones. Monitor theophylline levels.
Drug-food. *Any food:* decreased absorption. Give drug on an empty stomach.
Drug-lifestyle. *Sun exposure:* photosensitivity reactions may occur. Urge precautions.

Contraindications and precautions

- Contraindicated in patients hypersensitive to drug or other fluoroquinolones.
- Use cautiously in pregnant women and in patients with renal impairment, history of seizures, or other CNS diseases such as cerebral arteriosclerosis.
- Safety of drug hasn't been established in breast-feeding women and in children.

NURSING CONSIDERATIONS

Assessment

- Assess patient's infection before therapy and regularly thereafter.
- Monitor regular blood studies and hepatic and renal function tests during prolonged therapy, as ordered.
- Patient treated for gonorrhea should have serologic test for syphilis. Drug isn't effective against syphilis, and treatment of gonorrhea may mask or delay symptoms of syphilis.
- Be alert for adverse reactions and drug interactions.
- Monitor patient's hydration status if adverse GI reactions occur.
- Evaluate patient's and family's knowledge of drug therapy.

Nursing diagnoses

- Infection related to presence of bacteria
- Risk for deficient fluid volume related to drug-induced adverse GI reactions
- Deficient knowledge related to drug therapy

Planning and implementation

P.O. use: Administer drug on empty stomach.
I.V. use: Dilute concentrate for injection before use. Single-use vials containing 20 or 40 mg/ml must be diluted to maximum of 4 mg/ml using compatible I.V. solution, such as D_5W, normal saline solution for injection, D_5W in normal saline solution for injection, or sterile water for injection. Infuse over at least 1 hour.
– Because compatibility with other drugs isn't known, don't mix ofloxacin with other drugs. If giving infusion at Y-site, discontinue other solution during infusion.
– If patient experiences restlessness, tremor, confusion, or hallucinations, stop medication and notify prescriber. Take seizure precautions.

Patient teaching

- Advise patient to take drug with plenty of fluids but not with meals. Also, tell patient to avoid antacids, sucralfate, and products containing iron or zinc for at least 2 hours before and after each dose.
- Advise patient to take full dose of antibiotic as directed.
- Warn patient to avoid hazardous tasks until CNS effects of drug are known.
- Advise patient to use sunblock and protective clothing to avoid photosensitivity reactions.
- Tell patient to stop drug and notify prescriber if rash or other signs of hypersensitivity reactions develop.

Evaluation

- Patient is free from infection.
- Patient maintains adequate hydration throughout drug therapy.
- Patient and family state understanding of drug therapy.

olanzapine

(oh-LAN-za-peen)
Zyprexa

Pharmacologic class: thienobenzodiazepine derivative
Therapeutic class: antipsychotic
Pregnancy risk category: C

Indications and dosages

▶ **Psychotic disorders.** *Adults:* initially, 5 to 10 mg P.O. once daily. Dosage adjustments should be limited to 5-mg daily increments and occur no more often than weekly. Most patients respond to 10 mg/day. Don't exceed 20 mg/day.

▶ **Short-term treatment of acute manic episodes with bipolar I disorder.** *Adults:* Initially, 10 to 15 mg P.O. daily. Adjust dosage as needed by increments of 5 mg daily at intervals of 24 hours or more. Maximum dose is 20 mg P.O. daily. Duration of treatment is 3 to 4 weeks.

Give 5 mg as initial dose if patient is debilitated, predisposed to hypotension, or pharmacologically sensitive to drug. Also give 5 mg initially if patient's metabolism is altered by smoking status, sex, or age.

How supplied

Tablets: 5 mg, 7.5 mg, 10 mg

Pharmacokinetics

Absorption: levels peak about 6 hours after P.O. dose. Food doesn't affect rate or extent of absorption. About 40% of dose is limited by first-pass metabolism.

Distribution: distributes extensively throughout the body, with a volume of distribution of about 1,000 L. Drug is about 93% protein-bound, primarily to albumin and alpha$_1$-acid glycoprotein.

Metabolism: metabolized by direct glucuronidation and cytochrome P-450–mediated oxidation.

Excretion: about 57% of drug appears in urine and 30% in feces as metabolites. Only 7% of dose is recovered in urine unchanged. *Elimination half-life:* 21 to 54 hours.

Route	Onset	Peak	Duration
P.O.	Unknown	6 hr	Unknown

Pharmacodynamics

Chemical effect: unknown. Binds to dopamine and serotonin receptors; may antagonize adrenergic, cholinergic, and histaminergic receptors.

Therapeutic effect: relieves signs and symptoms of psychoses.

Adverse reactions

CNS: *somnolence, agitation, insomnia, headache, nervousness, hostility,* parkinsonism, *dizziness,* anxiety, personality disorder, akathisia, hypertonia, tremor, amnesia, articulation impairment, euphoria, stuttering, tardive dyskinesia.

CV: orthostatic hypotension, tachycardia, chest pain, hypotension, edema.

EENT: amblyopia, blepharitis, corneal lesion, *rhinitis,* pharyngitis.

GI: constipation, dry mouth, abdominal pain, increased appetite, increased salivation, nausea, vomiting, thirst.

GU: premenstrual syndrome, hematuria, metrorrhagia, urinary incontinence, urinary tract infection.

Hematologic: asymptomatic increases in eosinophil count.

Hepatic: asymptomatic increases in AST, ALT, and GGT levels.

Metabolic: weight gain or loss, fever, asymptomatic increases in CK and serum prolactin levels.

Musculoskeletal: joint pain, limb pain, back pain, neck rigidity, twitching.

Respiratory: increased cough, dyspnea.

Skin: vesiculobullous rash.

Interactions

Drug-drug. *Antihypertensives:* may potentiate hypotensive effects. Monitor blood pressure closely.

Carbamazepine, omeprazole, rifampin: increased olanzapine clearance. Monitor patient.

Diazepam: increased CNS effects. Monitor patient closely.

Dopamine agonists, levodopa: antagonized activity of these drugs. Monitor patient.

Drug-herb. *Nutmeg:* may reduce effectiveness of or interfere with drug therapy. Discourage concomitant use.

Drug-lifestyle. *Alcohol use:* increased CNS effects. Discourage concomitant use.

Contraindications

- Contraindicated in patients hypersensitive to drug.
- Use cautiously in patients with heart disease, cerebrovascular disease, conditions that predispose patient to hypotension, history of seizures or conditions that might lower the seizure threshold, or hepatic impairment.
- Also use cautiously in elderly patients, those with a history of paralytic ileus, and those at

risk for aspiration pneumonia, prostatic hyperplasia, or angle-closure glaucoma.

NURSING CONSIDERATIONS

Assessment
- Obtain history of patient's underlying condition before therapy, and reassess regularly thereafter.
- Obtain baseline and periodic liver function tests, as ordered.
- Monitor patient for signs of neuroleptic malignant syndrome (hyperpyrexia, muscle rigidity, altered mental status, autonomic instability), which is rare but commonly fatal. Drug should be stopped immediately and patient monitored and treated as needed.
- Monitor patient for tardive dyskinesia, which may occur after prolonged use. It may not appear until months or years later, and it may disappear spontaneously or persist for life despite discontinuation of drug.
- Evaluate patient's and family's knowledge about drug therapy.

Nursing diagnoses
- Disturbed thought processes related to underlying condition
- Risk for injury related to drug-induced adverse CNS reactions
- Deficient knowledge related to drug therapy

Planning and implementation
- Therapy starts at 5 mg/dose, as directed, in patients who are debilitated, predisposed to hypotension, pharmacologically sensitive to drug, or affected by altered metabolism caused by smoking status, sex, or age.

ALERT Don't confuse olanzapine with olsalazine or Zyprexa with Zyrtec.

- Drug should be given to pregnant woman only if benefit justifies risk to fetus. Women taking drug shouldn't breast-feed.

Patient teaching
- Tell patient to avoid hazardous tasks until adverse CNS effects of drug are known.
- Warn patient against exposure to extreme heat; drug may impair body's ability to reduce core temperature.
- Tell patient to avoid alcohol during therapy.
- Tell patient to rise slowly to avoid effects of orthostatic hypotension.
- Instruct patient to relieve dry mouth with ice chips or sugarless candy or gum.
- Advise woman to notify prescriber if she becomes pregnant or intends to become pregnant during drug therapy. Advise her not to breastfeed during therapy.

Evaluation
- Patient's behavior and communication show improved thought processes.
- Patient sustains no injury from adverse CNS reactions.
- Patient and family state understanding of drug therapy.

olsalazine sodium
(olh-SAL-uh-zeen SOH-dee-um)
Dipentum

Pharmacologic class: salicylate
Therapeutic class: anti-inflammatory
Pregnancy risk category: C

Indications and dosages
▶ **Maintenance of remission of ulcerative colitis in patients intolerant of sulfasalazine.** *Adults:* 500 mg P.O. b.i.d. with meals.

How supplied
Capsules: 250 mg

Pharmacokinetics
Absorption: about 2.4% of single dose is absorbed.
Distribution: liberated mesalamine is absorbed slowly from colon, resulting in very high local levels.
Metabolism: 0.1% is metabolized in liver; remainder reaches colon, where it's rapidly converted to mesalamine by colonic bacteria.
Excretion: about 80% excreted in feces; less than 1% in urine. *Half-life:* of two metabolites, 0.9 hours to 7 days.

Route	Onset	Peak	Duration
P.O.	Unknown	1 hr	Unknown

Pharmacodynamics

Chemical effect: unknown; converts to 5-aminosalicylic acid (5-ASA or mesalamine) in colon, where it has local anti-inflammatory effect.
Therapeutic effect: prevents flare-up of ulcerative colitis.

Adverse reactions

CNS: headache, depression, vertigo, dizziness.
GI: *diarrhea,* nausea, abdominal pain, heartburn.
Musculoskeletal: arthralgia.
Skin: rash, itching.

Interactions

Drug-drug. *Anticoagulants, coumarin derivatives:* prolonged PT and INR. Monitor patient closely.
Drug-food. *Any food:* decreased GI irritation. Give drug with food.

Contraindications and precautions

- Contraindicated in patients hypersensitive to salicylates.
- Use cautiously in pregnant women, breast-feeding women, and patients with renal disease. Renal tubular damage may result from absorbed mesalamine or its metabolites.
- Safety of drug hasn't been established in children.

NURSING CONSIDERATIONS

Assessment
- Assess patient's condition before therapy and regularly thereafter.
- Monitor BUN and creatinine levels and urinalysis in patient with renal disease, as ordered.
- Be alert for adverse reactions.
- Evaluate patient's and family's knowledge of drug therapy.

Nursing diagnoses
- Impaired tissue integrity related to ulcerative colitis
- Diarrhea related to drug's adverse effect on GI tract
- Deficient knowledge related to drug therapy

Planning and implementation
- Give drug with food in evenly divided doses.
- Report diarrhea to prescriber. Although diarrhea appears dose-related, it's difficult to distinguish from worsening of disease symptoms. Worsening of disease has been noted with similar drugs.

Patient teaching
- Teach patient to take drug in evenly divided doses and with food to minimize adverse GI reactions.
- Urge patient to notify prescriber about adverse reactions, especially diarrhea or increased pain.

Evaluation
- Patient has no evidence of ulcerative colitis.
- Patient is free from diarrhea.
- Patient and family state understanding of drug therapy.

omeprazole

(oh-MEH-pruh-zohl)
Losec ◆ ◇, Prilosec

Pharmacologic class: substituted benzimidazole
Therapeutic class: gastric acid suppressant.
Pregnancy risk category: C

Indications and dosages

▶ **Erosive esophagitis; symptomatic, poorly responsive gastroesophageal reflux disease (GERD).** *Adults:* 20 mg P.O. daily for 4 to 8 weeks. (Patients with GERD should have failed therapy with H_2-receptor antagonist.)
▶ **Pathologic hypersecretory conditions (such as Zollinger-Ellison syndrome).** *Adults:* initially, 60 mg P.O. daily, adjusted according to patient response. If daily amount exceeds 80 mg, give in divided doses. Dosages up to 120 mg t.i.d. have been given. Continue therapy as long as clinically indicated.
▶ **Duodenal ulcer (short-term treatment).** *Adults:* 20 mg P.O. daily for 4 to 8 weeks.
▶ **Gastric ulcer.** *Adults:* 40 mg P.O. daily for 4 to 8 weeks

▶ ***Helicobacter pylori* eradication to reduce risk of duodenal ulcer recurrence; triple therapy with omeprazole, clarithromycin, amoxicillin.** *Adults:* 20 mg P.O. with clarithromycin 500 mg P.O. and amoxicillin 1,000 mg P.O., each given b.i.d. for 10 days. For patients with an ulcer present when therapy starts, another 18 days of omeprazole 20 mg P.O. once daily is recommended.

How supplied

Capsules (delayed-release): 20 mg

Pharmacokinetics

Absorption: absorbed rapidly after drug leaves stomach. However, bioavailability is about 40% because of instability in gastric acid as well as substantial first-pass effect. Bioavailability increases slightly with repeated dosing.
Distribution: protein-binding is about 95%.
Metabolism: metabolized primarily in liver.
Excretion: excreted primarily in urine. *Half-life:* 30 to 60 minutes.

Route	Onset	Peak	Duration
P.O.	≤ 1 hr	2 hr	≥ 3 days

Pharmacodynamics

Chemical effect: inhibits activity of acid (proton) pump and binds to hydrogen-potassium adenosine triphosphatase on secretory surface of gastric parietal cells to block formation of gastric acid.
Therapeutic effect: relieves symptoms caused by excessive gastric acid.

Adverse reactions

CNS: headache, dizziness.
GI: diarrhea, abdominal pain, nausea, vomiting, constipation, flatulence.
Musculoskeletal: back pain.
Respiratory: cough.
Skin: rash.

Interactions

Drug-drug. *Ampicillin esters, iron derivatives, ketoconazole:* these drugs may have poor bioavailability because optimal absorption requires low gastric pH. Administer separately.
Diazepam, phenytoin, warfarin: decreased hepatic clearance, possibly leading to increased serum levels. Monitor patient closely.
Drug-herb. *Male fern:* herb is inactivated in alkaline environments. Discourage concomitant use.
Pennyroyal: may change the rate at which toxic metabolites of pennyroyal form. Discourage concomitant use.

Contraindications and precautions

- Contraindicated in patients hypersensitive to drug or its components.
- Use cautiously in pregnant or breast-feeding women.
- Safety of drug hasn't been established in children.

NURSING CONSIDERATIONS

Assessment

- Assess patient's condition before therapy and regularly thereafter.
- Be alert for adverse reactions and drug interactions.
- Monitor patient's hydration status if adverse GI reactions occur.
- Evaluate patient's and family's knowledge of drug therapy.

Nursing diagnoses

- Impaired tissue integrity related to upper gastric disorder
- Risk for deficient fluid volume related to drug-induced adverse GI reactions
- Deficient knowledge related to drug therapy

Planning and implementation

- Give drug 30 minutes before meals.
- Dosage adjustments aren't needed for patients with renal or hepatic impairment.

ALERT Don't confuse Prilosec with Prozac, Prilocaine, or Prinivil.

Patient teaching

- Explain importance of taking drug exactly as prescribed.
- Tell patient to swallow capsules whole and not to open or crush.

Evaluation
- Patient responds well to therapy.
- Patient maintains adequate hydration throughout drug therapy.
- Patient and family state understanding of drug therapy.

ondansetron hydrochloride
(on-DAN-seh-tron high-droh-KLOR-ighd)
Zofran

Pharmacologic class: serotonin (5-HT_3) receptor antagonist
Therapeutic class: antiemetic
Pregnancy risk category: B

Indications and dosages
▶ **Prevention of nausea and vomiting caused by emetogenic chemotherapy.** *Adults and children age 12 and over:* 8 mg P.O. 30 minutes before start of chemotherapy. Follow with 8 mg P.O. 4 and 8 hours after first dose. Then follow with 8 mg q 8 hours for 1 to 2 days. Or, administer single dose of 32 mg by I.V. infusion over 15 minutes beginning 30 minutes before chemotherapy; or three divided doses of 0.15 mg/kg I.V. (first dose given 30 minutes before chemotherapy; subsequent doses given 4 and 8 hours after first dose). Infuse drug over 15 minutes.
Children ages 4 to 12: 4 mg P.O. 30 minutes before start of chemotherapy. Follow with 4 mg P.O. 4 and 8 hours after first dose. Then follow with 4 mg q 8 hours for 1 to 2 days. Or, three doses of 0.15 mg/kg I.V. Give first dose 30 minutes before chemotherapy; give subsequent doses 4 and 8 hours after first dose. Infuse drug over 15 minutes.
▶ **Prevention of postoperative nausea and vomiting.** *Adults:* 4 mg I.V. (undiluted) over 2 to 5 minutes.

How supplied
Tablets: 4 mg, 8 mg
Injection: 2 mg/ml, 4 mg/ml

Pharmacokinetics
Absorption: absorption is variable with P.O. administration; bioavailability is 50% to 60%.
Distribution: 70% to 76% is plasma protein–bound.
Metabolism: extensively metabolized.
Excretion: primarily excreted in urine. *Half-life:* 4 hours.

Route	Onset	Peak	Duration
P.O., I.V.	Unknown	Unknown	Unknown

Pharmacodynamics
Chemical effect: blocking action may take place in CNS at area postrema (chemoreceptor trigger zone) and in peripheral nervous system on terminals of vagus nerve.
Therapeutic effect: prevents nausea and vomiting from emetogenic chemotherapy or surgery.

Adverse reactions
CNS: headache.
GI: diarrhea, constipation.
Hepatic: transient elevations in AST and ALT levels.
Skin: rash.

Interactions
Drug-drug. *Drugs that alter hepatic drug-metabolizing enzymes (such as cimetidine, phenobarbital):* may alter pharmacokinetics of ondansetron. No dosage adjustment appears necessary.
Drug-herb. *Horehound:* May enhance serotonergic effects. Discourage concomitant use.

Contraindications and precautions
- Contraindicated in patients hypersensitive to drug.
- Use cautiously in patients with liver failure and in pregnant or breast-feeding women.

NURSING CONSIDERATIONS

Assessment
- Assess patient's condition before therapy and regularly thereafter.
- Be alert for adverse reactions and drug interactions.
- Evaluate patient's and family's knowledge of drug therapy.

Nursing diagnoses
- Risk for deficient fluid volume related to nausea and vomiting
- Pain related to drug-induced headache
- Deficient knowledge related to drug therapy

Planning and implementation
P.O. use: Follow normal protocol.
I.V. use: Dilute drug in 50 ml of D_5W injection or normal saline solution for injection before administration.
– Infuse drug over 15 minutes.
Drug is stable for up to 48 hours after dilution in 5% dextrose in normal saline solution for injection, 5% dextrose in half-normal saline solution for injection, and 3% saline solution for injection.
ALERT Don't confuse Zofran with Zantac or Zosyn.

Patient teaching
- Instruct patient when to take drug.
- Tell patient to report adverse reactions.
- Advise patient to report any discomfort at I.V. site.

Evaluation
- Patient maintains adequate hydration.
- Patient reports no headache.
- Patient and family state understanding of drug therapy.

opium tincture*
(OH-pee-um TINK-shur)

opium tincture, camphorated* (paregoric)

Pharmacologic class: opium
Therapeutic class: antidiarrheal
Controlled substance schedule: II (III for opium tincture, camphorated)
Pregnancy risk category: NR

Indications and dosages
▶ **Acute, nonspecific diarrhea. Opium tincture.** *Adults:* 0.6 ml (range 0.3 to 1 ml) P.O. q.i.d. Maximum dosage is 6 ml daily.
Camphorated opium tincture. *Adults:* 5 to 10 ml once daily, b.i.d., t.i.d., or q.i.d. until diarrhea subsides.
Children: 0.25 to 0.5 ml/kg P.O. once daily, b.i.d., t.i.d., or q.i.d. until diarrhea subsides.

How supplied
opium tincture
Oral solution: equivalent to morphine 10 mg/ml*
opium tincture, camphorated
Oral solution: each 5 ml contains morphine, 2 mg; anise oil, 0.2 ml; benzoic acid, 20 mg; camphor, 20 mg; glycerin, 0.2 ml; and ethanol to make 5 ml*

Pharmacokinetics
Absorption: absorbed variably.
Distribution: distributed widely in body.
Metabolism: metabolized in liver.
Excretion: excreted in urine.

Route	Onset	Peak	Duration
P.O.	Unknown	Unknown	Unknown

Pharmacodynamics
Chemical effect: increases smooth-muscle tone in GI tract, inhibits motility and propulsion, and diminishes secretions.
Therapeutic effect: relieves diarrhea.

Adverse reactions
CNS: dizziness, light-headedness.
GI: nausea, vomiting.
Other: physical dependence after long-term use.

Interactions
None significant.

Contraindications and precautions
- Contraindicated in patients with acute diarrhea resulting from poisoning until toxic material is removed from GI tract. Also contraindicated in patients with diarrhea caused by organisms that penetrate intestinal mucosa.
- Use cautiously in patients with asthma, prostatic hyperplasia, hepatic disease, or opioid dependence.
- Safety of drug hasn't been established in pregnant or breast-feeding women.

NURSING CONSIDERATIONS

Assessment
- Assess patient's condition before therapy and regularly thereafter.
- Be alert for adverse reactions.
- Monitor patient's hydration status throughout drug therapy.
- Evaluate patient's and family's knowledge of drug therapy.

Nursing diagnoses
- Diarrhea related to GI disorder
- Risk for deficient fluid volume related to diarrhea and drug-induced adverse GI reactions
- Deficient knowledge related to drug therapy

Planning and implementation
ALERT Read label carefully. Opium content of opium tincture is 25 times greater than that of camphorated opium tincture. Camphorated opium tincture is more dilute, and teaspoonful doses are easier to measure than dropper quantities of opium tincture.
- Mix drug with water to form a milky fluid.
- Store drug in tightly capped, light-resistant container.
- For overdose, use narcotic antagonist naloxone, as ordered, to reverse respiratory depression.

Patient teaching
- Advise patient against using drug for more than 2 days; risk of dependence increases with long-term use.
- Encourage proper storage to keep drug out of children's hands.

Evaluation
- Patient's diarrhea ceases.
- Patient maintains adequate hydration.
- Patient and family state understanding of drug.

orlistat
(OR-lih-stat)
Xenical

Pharmacologic class: lipase inhibitor
Therapeutic class: antiobesity drug
Pregnancy risk category: B

Indications and dosages
▶ **Management of obesity, including weight loss and weight maintenance in conjunction with a reduced-calorie diet; reduction of risk of weight regain after weight loss.**
Adults: 120 mg P.O. t.i.d. with each main meal containing fat (during or up to 1 hour after the meal).

How supplied
Capsules: 120 mg

Pharmacokinetics
Absorption: systemic exposure to orlistat is minimal because only a small amount of drug is absorbed.
Distribution: more than 99% of drug binds to plasma proteins. Lipoproteins and albumin are major binding proteins.
Metabolism: drug is primarily metabolized in GI wall.
Excretion: most unabsorbed drug is excreted in feces.

Route	Onset	Peak	Duration
P.O.	Unknown	Unknown	Unknown

Pharmacodynamics
Chemical effect: a reversible inhibitor of lipases, orlistat bonds with the active site of gastric and pancreatic lipases. These inactivated enzymes are thus unavailable to hydrolyze dietary fat, in the form of triglycerides, into absorbable free fatty acids and monoglycerides. Because the undigested triglycerides aren't absorbed, the resulting caloric deficit may help with weight control. The recommended dosage of 120 mg t.i.d. inhibits dietary fat absorption by about 30%.
Therapeutic effect: weight loss and weight maintenance.

Adverse reactions

CNS: *headache,* dizziness, fatigue, sleep disorder, anxiety, depression.
CV: pedal edema.
EENT: otitis.
GI: *oily spotting, flatus with discharge, fecal urgency, fatty or oily stool, oily evacuation, increased defecation, abdominal pain,* fecal incontinence, nausea, infectious diarrhea, rectal pain, vomiting.
GU: menstrual irregularity, vaginitis, urinary tract infection.
Musculoskeletal: *back pain,* leg pain, arthritis, myalgia, joint disorder, tendinitis.
Respiratory: *influenza, upper respiratory tract infection,* lower respiratory tract infection.
Skin: rash, dry skin.
Other: tooth and gingival disorders.

Interactions

Drug-drug. *Fat-soluble vitamins such as vitamin E, beta-carotene:* decreased vitamin absorption. Separate administration times by 2 hours.
Pravastatin: slightly increased pravastatin levels and additive lipid-lowering effects of drug. Monitor patient.
Warfarin: possible change in coagulation parameters. Monitor INR.

Contraindications and precautions

- Contraindicated in patients hypersensitive to orlistat or any component of the drug and in patients with chronic malabsorption syndrome or cholestasis.
- Use cautiously in patients with a history of hyperoxaluria or calcium oxalate nephrolithiasis.
- Use cautiously in patients with a risk of anorexia nervosa or bulimia.
- Use cautiously in patients receiving cyclosporine therapy because of possible changes in cyclosporine absorption related to variations in diet.

NURSING CONSIDERATIONS

Assessment

- Obtain history of patient's underlying condition before therapy, and reassess regularly thereafter.
- Screen patient for anorexia nervosa or bulimia; as with any weight-loss drug, orlistat carries a risk of misuse in certain patient populations.
- Organic causes of obesity, such as hypothyroidism, must be ruled out before patient starts orlistat therapy.
- In diabetic patients, monitor serum glucose frequently during weight loss. Dosage of oral antidiabetic or insulin may need to be reduced.
- Evaluate patient's and family's knowledge about drug therapy.

Nursing diagnoses

- Imbalanced nutrition: More than body requirements related to obesity
- Disturbed body image related to obesity
- Deficient knowledge related to drug therapy

Planning and implementation

- Drug is recommended for patients with an initial body mass index of 30 kg/m^2 or more (27 kg/m^2 or more if patient has other risk factors, such as hypertension, diabetes, or dyslipidemia).
- It's unknown whether orlistat is safe and effective to use longer than 2 years.
- Tell patient to follow dietary guidelines. GI effects may increase when patient takes orlistat with high-fat foods—specifically, when more than 30% of total daily calories come from fat.
- Orlistat reduces absorption of some fat-soluble vitamins and beta-carotene.

Patient teaching

- Advise patient to follow a nutritionally balanced, reduced-calorie diet that derives only 30% of its calories from fat. Daily intake of fat, carbohydrate, and protein should be distributed over three main meals. If a meal is occasionally missed or contains no fat, tell patient that the orlistat dose can be omitted.
- To ensure adequate nutrition, advise patient to take a daily multivitamin supplement that contains fat-soluble vitamins at least 2 hours before or after taking orlistat, such as at bedtime.
- Tell patient with diabetes that weight loss may improve glycemic control, so the dosage

of his oral antidiabetic or insulin may need to be reduced.

• Tell woman to inform prescriber if she is pregnant, plans to become pregnant, or is breast-feeding.

Evaluation

• Patient reaches and maintains a stable weight.

• Patient and family state understanding of drug therapy.

orphenadrine citrate

(or-FEN-uh-dreen SIH-trayt)

Banflex, Flexoject, Flexon, Myolin, Norflex, Orphenate

Pharmacologic class: diphenhydramine analogue
Therapeutic class: skeletal muscle relaxant
Pregnancy risk category: C

Indications and dosages

▶ **Adjunct in painful, acute musculoskeletal conditions.** *Adults:* 100 mg P.O. b.i.d., or 60 mg I.V. or I.M. q 12 hours, p.r.n. For maintenance therapy, P.O. doses begin 12 hours after last parenteral dose.

How supplied

Tablets: 100 mg
Tablets (extended-release): 100 mg
Injection: 30 mg/ml

Pharmacokinetics

Absorption: rapidly absorbed from GI tract after P.O. administration. Unknown for I.M. administration.
Distribution: widely distributed throughout body.
Metabolism: biotransformed in liver. Metabolized almost completely to at least eight metabolites.
Excretion: excreted in urine, mainly as metabolites. *Half-life:* about 14 hours.

Route	Onset	Peak	Duration
P.O.	≤ 1 hr (regular); 6-8 hr (extended-release)	≤ 2 hr	Unknown
I.V.	Immediate	Immediate	Unknown
I.M.	≤ 5 min	≤ 30 min	Unknown

Pharmacodynamics

Chemical effect: unknown; appears to modify central perception of pain without modifying pain reflexes. Blocks interneuronal activity in descending reticular activating system and in spinal cord.
Therapeutic effect: relaxes skeletal muscles.

Adverse reactions

CNS: disorientation, restlessness, irritability, weakness, *drowsiness,* headache, dizziness, hallucinations, insomnia.
CV: palpitations, tachycardia.
EENT: dilated pupils, blurred vision, difficulty swallowing, increased intraocular pressure.
GI: constipation, *dry mouth,* nausea, vomiting, paralytic ileus, epigastric distress.
GU: urinary hesitancy, urine retention.
Hematologic: ***aplastic anemia.***
Other: ***anaphylaxis.***

Interactions

Drug-drug. *CNS depressants, propoxyphene:* increased CNS depression. Avoid concomitant use.
Drug-lifestyle. *Alcohol use:* increased CNS depression. Discourage concomitant use.

Contraindications and precautions

• Contraindicated in patients hypersensitive to drug and in those with glaucoma; prostatic hyperplasia; pyloric, duodenal, or bladder-neck obstruction; myasthenia gravis; or peptic ulceration.

• Use cautiously in pregnant women, elderly or debilitated patients, and those with tachycardia, cardiac disease, arrhythmias, or sulfite sensitivity.

• Safety of drug hasn't been established in children and in breast-feeding women.

NURSING CONSIDERATIONS

Assessment

- Assess patient's condition before therapy and regularly thereafter.
- When giving drug I.V., assess for paradoxical initial bradycardia; it usually disappears in 2 minutes.
- Monitor CBC, hepatic function, and urinalysis as directed if patient receives long-term therapy.
- Monitor vital signs carefully.
- Be alert for adverse reactions and drug interactions.
- Evaluate patient's and family's knowledge of drug therapy.

Nursing diagnoses

- Chronic pain related to condition
- Risk for injury related to drug-induced adverse CNS reactions
- Deficient knowledge related to drug therapy

Planning and implementation

ALERT Check all dosages; slight overdose can lead to toxicity. Early evidence includes excessive dry mouth, dilated pupils, blurred vision, skin flushing, and fever.

P.O. and I.M. use: Follow normal protocol.

I.V. use: Inject drug over about 5 minutes with patient supine. After 5 to 10 minutes, help patient sit up.

Patient teaching

- Tell patient to report urinary hesitancy and urine retention. Instruct him to void before taking drug.
- Advise patient to relieve dry mouth with sugarless gum or hard candy.
- Warn patient to avoid tasks that require alertness until CNS effects of drug are known.
- Advise patient to avoid alcohol or other CNS depressants during drug therapy.

Evaluation

- Patient is free from pain.
- Patient sustains no injury from adverse CNS reactions.
- Patient and family state understanding of drug therapy.

oseltamivir phosphate

(ah-sul-TAM-ih-veer FOS-fayt)

Tamiflu

Pharmacologic class: neuraminidase inhibitor
Therapeutic class: antiviral
Pregnancy risk category: C

Indications and dosages

▶ **Uncomplicated, acute illness from influenza in patients who have been symptomatic for 2 days or less.** *Adults:* 75 mg P.O. b.i.d. for 5 days. For patients with creatinine clearance less than 30 ml/minute, reduce dosage to 75 mg P.O. once daily for 5 days.

How supplied

Capsules: 75 mg

Pharmacokinetics

Absorption: well absorbed after P.O. administration. More than 75% of administered dose reaches systemic circulation as oseltamivir carboxylate.

Distribution: serum protein–binding for oseltamivir is 42%; 3% for oseltamivir carboxylate.

Metabolism: extensively metabolized by hepatic esterases to its active component, oseltamivir carboxylate.

Excretion: oseltamivir carboxylate is almost entirely eliminated in urine via glomerular filtration and tubular secretion. Less than 20% of orally administered dose is eliminated in feces.

Route	Onset	Peak	Duration
P.O.	Unknown	Unknown	Unknown

Pharmacodynamics

Chemical effect: oseltamivir carboxylate, the active form of oseltamivir, inhibits the enzyme neuraminidase in influenza virus particles. This action is thought to inhibit viral replication, possibly by interfering with viral particle aggregation and release from the host cell.

Therapeutic effect: lessens the symptoms of influenza.

Adverse reactions

CNS: dizziness, insomnia, headache, vertigo, fatigue.
GI: abdominal pain, diarrhea, nausea, vomiting.
Respiratory: bronchitis, cough.

Interactions

None significant.

Contraindications

- Contraindicated in patients hypersensitive to drug or its components.

NURSING CONSIDERATIONS

Assessment

- Obtain complete medical history before treatment.
- Evaluate renal function before giving drug, as directed.
- Ask woman if she's breast-feeding. Use drug only if potential benefits outweigh risks to infant.
- Evaluate patient's and family's knowledge of drug therapy.

Nursing diagnoses

- Infection related to influenza virus
- Imbalanced nutrition: Less than body requirements related to drug's adverse GI effects
- Deficient knowledge related to drug therapy

Planning and implementation

- Drug is used to treat symptoms, not to prevent influenza. Drug isn't a replacement for the annual influenza vaccination.
- There's no evidence to support use of drug in treating viral infections other than influenza virus types A and B.
- Drug may be given with meals to decrease adverse GI effects.
- Safety and efficacy of repeated treatment courses haven't been established.
- Store at controlled room temperature (59° to 86° F [15° to 30° C]).

Patient teaching

- Tell patient to take drug within 2 days of start of symptoms.
- Inform patient that drug is used to treat symptoms, not to prevent influenza. Urge patient to continue receiving an annual influenza vaccination.

Evaluation

- Patient recovers from influenza.
- Patient has no adverse GI effects.
- Patient and family state understanding of drug therapy.

oxacillin sodium

(oks-uh-SIL-in SOH-dee-um)
Bactocill, Prostaphlin

Pharmacologic class: penicillinase-resistant penicillin
Therapeutic class: antibiotic
Pregnancy risk category: B

Indications and dosages

▶ **Systemic infections caused by penicillinase-producing staphylococci.**
Adults and children weighing more than 40 kg (88 lb): 500 mg P.O. q 4 to 6 hours. Or, 1 to 12 g I.M. or I.V. daily, in divided doses q 4 to 6 hours.
Children weighing 40 kg or less: 50 to 100 mg/kg P.O. daily, in divided doses q 6 hours. Or, 50 to 200 mg/kg I.M. or I.V. daily, in divided doses q 4 to 6 hours.

How supplied

Capsules: 250 mg, 500 mg
Oral solution: 250 mg/5 ml (after reconstitution)
Injection: 250 mg, 500 mg, 1 g, 2 g, 4 g
I.V. infusion: 1 g, 2 g, 4 g

Pharmacokinetics

Absorption: absorbed rapidly but incompletely from GI tract after P.O. administration; food decreases absorption. Absorption unknown after I.M. administration.
Distribution: distributed widely. CSF penetration is poor but enhanced by meningeal inflammation. Drug is 89% to 94% protein-bound.
Metabolism: metabolized partially.

Excretion: excreted primarily in urine; small amount in bile. *Half-life:* 30 to 60 minutes.

Route	Onset	Peak	Duration
P.O.	Unknown	0.5-2 hr	Unknown
I.V.	Immediate	Immediate	Unknown
I.M.	Unknown	≤ 30 min	Unknown

Pharmacodynamics

Chemical effect: inhibits cell wall synthesis during microorganism multiplication. Bacteria resist penicillins by producing penicillinases (enzymes that convert penicillins to inactive penicilloic acid); oxacillin resists these enzymes.
Therapeutic effect: kills susceptible bacteria, such as penicillinase-producing staphylococci and a few gram-positive aerobic and anaerobic bacilli.

Adverse reactions

CNS: neuropathy, neuromuscular irritability, ***seizures.***
GI: oral lesions.
GU: interstitial nephritis, transient hematuria, proteinuria.
Hematologic: ***agranulocytopenia, thrombocytopenia,*** eosinophilia, ***hemolytic anemia, transient neutropenia.***
Hepatic: hepatitis, elevated liver enzyme levels.
Other: hypersensitivity reactions (fever, chills, rash, urticaria, ***anaphylaxis***), overgrowth of nonsusceptible organisms, *thrombophlebitis.*

Interactions

Drug-drug. *Aminoglycosides:* possible synergistic effect. Monitor patient closely.
Probenecid: increased blood levels of oxacillin and other penicillins. Probenecid may be used for this purpose.
Rifampin: possible antagonism. Monitor patient for loss of therapeutic effect.

Contraindications and precautions

• Contraindicated in patients hypersensitive to drug or other penicillins.
• Use cautiously in patients with other drug allergies, especially to cephalosporins; in premature neonates; in infants; and in breast-feeding or pregnant women.

NURSING CONSIDERATIONS

Assessment

• Assess patient's infection before therapy and regularly thereafter.
• Before giving drug, ask about allergic reactions to penicillin. However, negative history of allergy is no guarantee against future allergic reaction.
• Obtain specimen for culture and sensitivity tests before giving first dose. Therapy may begin pending results.
• Monitor CBC and platelet count as ordered.
• Monitor periodic liver function studies; watch for elevated AST and ALT levels.
• Be alert for adverse reactions and drug interactions.
• Evaluate patient's and family's knowledge of drug therapy.

Nursing diagnoses

• Infection related to presence of bacteria
• Ineffective protection related to drug-induced adverse hematologic reactions
• Deficient knowledge related to drug therapy

Planning and implementation

I.M. use: Follow normal protocol.
P.O. use: Give drug 1 to 2 hours before or 2 to 3 hours after meals. When given orally, drug may cause GI disturbances. Food may interfere with absorption.
I.V. use: For direct I.V. injection, reconstitute vials with sterile water for injection or normal saline solution for injection. Use 5 ml of diluent for 250- or 500-mg vial, 10 ml of diluent for 1-g vial, 20 ml of diluent for 2-g vial, or 40 ml of diluent for 4-g vial.
– When solution is clear, withdraw ordered dose and inject slowly over 10 minutes.
– When giving by piggyback injection, reconstitute 1-g piggyback vial with 20 to 100 ml of diluent; reconstitute 2-g vial with 19 to 99 ml of diluent.
– For intermittent infusion, further dilute drug to 5 to 40 mg/ml.

ALERT Aminoglycosides are chemically and physically incompatible with drug; don't mix in same I.V. solution.
– To prevent vein irritation, avoid continuous infusions. Change site every 48 hours.
- Don't give I.V. or I.M. unless ordered and infection is severe or patient can't take P.O. dose.
- Give drug at least 1 hour before bacteriostatic antibiotics.
- Drug may falsely elevate urine or serum proteins or cause false-positive results in certain tests of these substances.
- Notify prescriber about abnormal laboratory test results, and be prepared to provide supportive care.

Patient teaching
- Instruct patient to take drug exactly as prescribed, even if he feels better.
- Tell patient to take oral drug on empty stomach.
- Tell patient to call prescriber if he develops rash, fever, or chills.

Evaluation
- Patient is free from infection.
- Patient has no adverse hematologic reactions.
- Patient and family state understanding of drug therapy.

oxaprozin
(oks-uh-PROH-zin)
Daypro

Pharmacologic class: NSAID
Therapeutic class: nonnarcotic analgesic, antipyretic, anti-inflammatory
Pregnancy risk category: C

Indications and dosages
▶ **Osteoarthritis, rheumatoid arthritis.** *Adults:* initially, 1,200 mg P.O. daily. Then, individualized to smallest effective dosage to minimize adverse reactions. Smaller patients or those with mild symptoms may need only 600 mg daily. Maximum is 1,800 mg or 26 mg/kg, whichever is lower, in divided doses.

How supplied
Caplets: 600 mg

Pharmacokinetics
Absorption: high oral bioavailability (95%); food may reduce rate but not extent of absorption.
Distribution: about 99.9% protein-bound.
Metabolism: metabolized in liver.
Excretion: metabolites are excreted in urine (65%) and feces (35%). *Half-life:* 5 hours.

Route	Onset	Peak	Duration
P.O.	Unknown	3-5 hr	Unknown

Pharmacodynamics
Chemical effect: unknown; may inhibit prostaglandin synthesis.
Therapeutic effect: relieves pain, fever, and inflammation.

Adverse reactions
CNS: depression, sedation, somnolence, confusion, sleep disturbances.
EENT: tinnitus, visual disturbances.
GI: *nausea, dyspepsia, diarrhea, constipation,* abdominal pain or distress, anorexia, flatulence, vomiting, ***hemorrhage.***
GU: dysuria, ***renal insufficiency,*** urinary frequency.
Hepatic: elevated liver enzyme levels.
Skin: *rash,* photosensitivity.

Interactions
Drug-drug. *Antihypertensives, diuretics:* decreased effect. Monitor patient closely and adjust dosage as ordered.
Aspirin: oxaprozin displaces salicylates from plasma protein–binding sites, increasing risk of salicylate toxicity. Avoid concomitant use.
Aspirin, corticosteroids: increased risk of adverse GI reactions. Avoid concomitant use.
Methotrexate: increased risk of methotrexate toxicity. Avoid concomitant use.
Oral anticoagulants: increased risk of bleeding. Use together cautiously.
Drug-herb. *Dong quai, feverfew, garlic, ginger, horse chestnut, red clover:* possible

increased risk of bleeding. Discourage concomitant use.
St. John's wort: increased risk of photosensitivity. Advise patient to avoid unprotected exposure to sunlight.
Drug-lifestyle. *Alcohol use:* increased risk of adverse GI reactions. Discourage concomitant use.
Sun exposure: photosensitivity reactions may occur. Urge precautions.

Contraindications and precautions

- Contraindicated in patients hypersensitive to drug and in those with syndrome of nasal polyps, angioedema, and bronchospastic reactivity to aspirin or other NSAIDs.
- Use cautiously in pregnant or breast-feeding women and in those with history of peptic ulcer disease, hepatic or renal dysfunction, hypertension, CV disease, or conditions that predispose to fluid retention.
- Safety of drug has not been established in children.

NURSING CONSIDERATIONS

Assessment

- Assess patient's condition before therapy and regularly thereafter.
- Monitor liver function test results periodically during long-term therapy, and closely monitor patient with abnormal test results. Liver function values may be elevated. These abnormal findings may persist, worsen, or resolve with continued therapy. Rarely, patient may progress to severe hepatic dysfunction.
- Be alert for adverse reactions and drug interactions.
- Evaluate patient's and family's knowledge of drug therapy.

Nursing diagnoses

- Chronic pain related to condition
- Impaired tissue integrity related to adverse GI effects of drug
- Deficient knowledge related to drug therapy

Planning and implementation

- Administer drug on empty stomach unless adverse GI reactions occur.

ALERT Don't confuse oxaprozin with oxazepam.

- Notify prescriber immediately about adverse reactions, especially GI symptoms.

Patient teaching

- To minimize adverse GI effects, tell patient to take drug with milk or meals.
- Explain that full therapeutic effects may be delayed for 2 to 4 weeks.
- Tell patient to report adverse visual or auditory reactions immediately.
- Teach patient to recognize and promptly report signs and symptoms of GI bleeding.
- Advise patient to use sunscreen, wear protective clothing, and avoid prolonged exposure to sunlight.
- Warn patient to avoid hazardous activities until CNS effects of drug are known.

Evaluation

- Patient is free from pain.
- Patient maintains GI tissue integrity.
- Patient and family state understanding of drug therapy.

oxazepam

(oks-AZ-ih-pam)
Alepam ◇, Apo-Oxazepam ♦, Murelax ◇, Novoxapam ♦, Serax**, Serepax ◇

Pharmacologic class: benzodiazepine
Therapeutic class: antianxiety, sedative-hypnotic
Controlled substance schedule: IV
Pregnancy risk category: D

Indications and dosages

▶ **Alcohol withdrawal.** *Adults:* 15 to 30 mg P.O. t.i.d. or q.i.d.
▶ **Severe anxiety.** *Adults:* 15 to 30 mg P.O. t.i.d. or q.i.d.
▶ **Mild to moderate anxiety.** *Adults:* 10 to 15 mg P.O. t.i.d. or q.i.d.

How supplied

Tablets: 10 mg, 15 mg, 30 mg
Capsules: 10 mg, 15 mg, 30 mg

Pharmacokinetics

Absorption: well absorbed.
Distribution: distributed widely throughout body. Drug is 85% to 95% protein-bound.
Metabolism: metabolized in liver.
Excretion: metabolites are excreted in urine.
Half-life: 5 to 13 hours.

Route	Onset	Peak	Duration
P.O.	Unknown	About 3 hr	Unknown

Pharmacodynamics

Chemical effect: unknown; believed to stimulate gamma-aminobutyric receptors in ascending reticular activating system.
Therapeutic effect: relieves anxiety and promotes calmness.

Adverse reactions

CNS: drowsiness, lethargy, hangover, fainting, *mental status changes.*
CV: transient hypotension.
GI: nausea, vomiting, abdominal discomfort.
Hepatic: ***hepatic dysfunction.***
Other: falls.

Interactions

Drug-drug. *Cimetidine, CNS depressants:* increased CNS depression. Avoid concomitant use.
Digoxin: may increase serum digoxin levels, increasing toxicity. Monitor levels closely
Drug-herb. *Catnip, kava, lady's slipper, lemon balm, passion flower, sassafras, skullcap, valerian:* sedative effects may be enhanced. Discourage concomitant use.
Drug-lifestyle. *Alcohol use:* increased CNS depression. Discourage concomitant use.
Smoking: increased benzodiazepine clearance. Monitor patient for lack of drug effect.

Contraindications and precautions

- Contraindicated in patients hypersensitive to drug.
- Avoid use of drug in pregnant or breast-feeding women.
- Use cautiously in elderly patients, in those with history of drug abuse, and in those for whom a drop in blood pressure could lead to cardiac problems.
- Safety of drug hasn't been established in children.

NURSING CONSIDERATIONS

Assessment

- Assess patient's condition before therapy and regularly thereafter.
- Monitor liver, renal, and hematopoietic function studies periodically in patient receiving repeated or prolonged therapy, as ordered.
- Be alert for adverse reactions and drug interactions.
- Evaluate patient's and family's knowledge of drug therapy.

Nursing diagnoses

- Disturbed thought processes related to condition
- Risk for injury related to drug-induced adverse CNS reactions
- Deficient knowledge related to drug therapy

Planning and implementation

- Expect to reduce dosage in elderly or debilitated patient.

ALERT Don't confuse oxazepam with oxaprozin.

- Possibility of abuse and addiction exists. Don't stop drug abruptly; withdrawal symptoms may occur.

Patient teaching

- Warn patient to avoid hazardous activities until CNS effects of drug are known.
- Tell patient to avoid alcohol during drug therapy.
- Warn patient not to stop drug abruptly; withdrawal signs may occur.

Evaluation

- Patient has less anxiety.
- Patient sustains no injury as result of drug therapy.
- Patient and family state understanding of drug therapy.

oxcarbazepine

(ox-car-BAY-zah-peen)
Trileptal

Pharmacologic class: carboxamide derivative
Therapeutic class: antiepileptic
Pregnancy risk category: C

Indications and dosages

▶ **Adjunctive therapy for partial seizures in patients with epilepsy.** *Adults:* initially, 300 mg P.O. b.i.d. Increased by maximum of 600 mg/day (300 mg P.O. b.i.d.) at weekly intervals. Recommended daily dose is 1,200 mg P.O., divided b.i.d.
Children ages 4 to 16: initially, 8 to 10 mg/kg/day P.O. divided b.i.d., not to exceed 600 mg/day. Target maintenance dosage depends on patient weight and should be divided b.i.d. If patient weighs 20 to 29 kg (44 to 64 lb), target maintenance dosage is 900 mg/day. If 29.1 to 39 kg (64 to 86 lb), target maintenance dosage is 1,200 mg/day. If more than 39 kg, target maintenance dosage is 1,800 mg/day. Target dosage should be achieved over 2 weeks.
▶ **Conversion to monotherapy for treatment of partial seizures in patients with epilepsy.** *Adults:* initially, 300 mg P.O. b.i.d. with simultaneous reduction in dosage of concomitant antiepileptic. Increased by a maximum of 600 mg/day at weekly intervals over 2 to 4 weeks. Recommended daily dose is 2,400 mg P.O., divided b.i.d. Concomitant antiepileptics should be completely withdrawn over 3 to 6 weeks.
▶ **Start of monotherapy for treatment of partial seizures in patients with epilepsy.** *Adults:* initially, 300 mg P.O. b.i.d. Increased by 300 mg/day every third day to a daily dose of 1,200 mg divided b.i.d.

Note: For adults with creatinine clearance less than 30 ml/minute, therapy starts at 150 mg P.O. b.i.d. (one-half the usual starting dose) and increases slowly to achieve desired clinical response.

How supplied

Tablets (film-coated): 150 mg, 300 mg, 600 mg

Pharmacokinetics

Absorption: completely absorbed following P.O. administration.
Distribution: about 40% of 10-monohydroxy metabolite (MHD) is bound to serum proteins, mostly to albumin.
Metabolism: rapidly metabolized in the liver to MHD, which is primarily responsible for pharmacologic effects. Minor amounts (4% of dose) are oxidized to pharmacologically inactive 10,11-dihydroxy metabolite (DHD).
Excretion: oxcarbazepine and its metabolites are mainly excreted by the kidneys. More than 95% of dose appears in urine, with less than 1% as unchanged oxcarbazepine. Fecal excretion accounts for less than 4% of dose. *Half-life:* about 2 hours for parent compound, about 9 hours for MHD. Children under age 8 have about 30% to 40% increased clearance of drug.

Route	Onset	Peak	Duration
P.O.	Unknown	Variable	Unknown

Pharmacodynamics

Chemical effect: activity is primarily in response to MHD. Antiseizure activity of oxcarbazepine and MHD is thought to result from blockade of voltage-sensitive sodium channels, which causes stabilization of hyperexcited neural membranes, inhibition of repetitive neuronal firing, and reduction of propagation of synaptic impulses. This activity is thought to prevent seizure spread in the brain. Anticonvulsant effects also may stem from increased potassium conductance and modulation of high-voltage activated calcium channels.
Therapeutic effect: control of partial seizures.

Adverse reactions

CNS: *fatigue*, asthenia, feeling abnormal, *headache, dizziness, somnolence, ataxia, abnormal gait*, insomnia, *tremor*, nervousness, agitation, abnormal coordination, speech disorder, confusion, anxiety, amnesia, ***aggravated seizures,*** hypoesthesia, emotional lability, impaired concentration, *vertigo.*
CV: hypotension, edema, chest pain.

EENT: *nystagmus, diplopia, abnormal vision,* abnormal accommodation, rhinitis, sinusitis, pharyngitis, epistaxis.
GI: *nausea, vomiting, abdominal pain,* diarrhea, dyspepsia, constipation, gastritis, anorexia, dry mouth, rectal hemorrhage, taste perversion, thirst.
GU: urinary tract infection, urinary frequency, vaginitis.
Metabolic: hyponatremia, weight gain, decreased thyroxine level.
Musculoskeletal: muscle weakness, back pain.
Respiratory: *upper respiratory tract infection,* coughing, bronchitis, chest infection.
Skin: acne, purpura, rash, bruising, increased sweating.
Other: fever, ***allergy***, hot flushes, lymphadenopathy, toothache.

Interactions

Drug-drug. *Carbamazepine, valproic acid, verapamil:* decreased serum levels of the active metabolite of oxcarbazepine. Monitor patient and serum levels closely.
Felodipine: decreased felodipine level. Monitor patient closely.
Hormonal contraceptives: decreased plasma levels of ethinylestradiol and levonorgestrel, which reduce contraceptive effect. Women of childbearing age should use other forms of contraception.
Phenobarbital: decreased serum levels of the active metabolite of oxcarbazepine and increased phenobarbital level. Monitor patient closely.
Phenytoin: decreased serum levels of the active metabolite of oxcarbazepine. May increase phenytoin level in adults receiving high doses of oxcarbazepine. Monitor phenytoin levels closely when starting therapy in these patients.
Drug-lifestyle. *Alcohol use:* increased CNS depression. Discourage concomitant use.

Contraindications and precautions

- Contraindicated in patients hypersensitive to oxcarbazepine or its components.
- Use cautiously in patients who have had hypersensitivity reactions to carbamazepine.

NURSING CONSIDERATIONS

Assessment

- Question patient about history of hypersensitivity reaction to carbamazepine because 25% to 30% of affected patients may develop hypersensitivity to oxcarbazepine. Discontinue drug immediately if signs or symptoms of hypersensitivity occur.
- Obtain history of patient's underlying condition before therapy, and reassess regularly thereafter.
- Monitor patient for evidence of hyponatremia, including nausea, malaise, headache, lethargy, confusion, and decreased sensation.
- Evaluate patient's and family's knowledge of drug therapy.

Nursing diagnoses

- Risk for trauma related to seizures
- Risk for injury related to drug-induced adverse reactions
- Deficient knowledge related to drug therapy

Planning and implementation

- Withdraw drug gradually to minimize risk of increased seizure frequency.
- Correct hyponatremia as needed and ordered.

ALERT Oxcarbazepine has been linked to several adverse neurologic events, including psychomotor slowing, difficulty with concentration, speech or language problems, somnolence, fatigue, and abnormal coordination (including ataxia and gait disturbances).

Patient teaching

- Advise patient to tell prescriber if he has ever had a hypersensitivity reaction to carbamazepine.
- Tell patient that drug may be taken with or without food.
- Caution patient to avoid hazardous activities until effects of drug are known.
- Caution patient to avoid alcohol while taking drug.
- Advise patient not to interrupt therapy without consulting prescriber.

• Advise patient to report signs and symptoms of hyponatremia, such as nausea, malaise, headache, lethargy, or confusion.
• Advise women using oral contraceptives for birth control to use another form of birth control while taking drug.

☑ Evaluation
• Patient has no seizures.
• Patient sustains no injury from drug-induced adverse reactions.
• Patient and family state understanding of drug therapy.

oxybutynin chloride
(oks-ee-BYOO-tih-nin KLOR-ighd)
Ditropan, Ditropan XL

Pharmacologic class: synthetic tertiary amine
Therapeutic class: antispasmodic
Pregnancy risk category: B

Indications and dosages
▶ **Antispasmodic for uninhibited or reflex neurogenic bladder.** *Adults:* 5 mg P.O. b.i.d. to t.i.d., up to 5 mg q.i.d.
Children over age 5: 5 mg P.O. b.i.d., up to 5 mg t.i.d.
▶ **Treatment of overactive bladder.**
Ditropan XL. *Adults:* initially, 5 mg P.O. once daily. Dosage adjustments may be made weekly in 5-mg increments, as needed, to a maximum of 30 mg P.O. daily.

How supplied
Tablets: 5 mg
Tablets (extended-release): 5 mg, 10 mg, 15 mg
Syrup: 5 mg/5 ml

Pharmacokinetics
Absorption: absorbed rapidly.
Distribution: unknown.
Metabolism: metabolized by liver.
Excretion: excreted primarily in urine.

Route	Onset	Peak	Duration
P.O.	30-60 min	3-4 hr	6-10 hr

Pharmacodynamics
Chemical effect: produces direct spasmolytic effect and antimuscarinic (atropine-like) effect on smooth muscles of urinary tract, increasing bladder capacity and providing some local anesthesia and mild analgesia.
Therapeutic effect: relieves bladder spasms.

Adverse reactions
CNS: *drowsiness,* dizziness, insomnia, restlessness, impaired alertness.
CV: palpitations, tachycardia.
EENT: *transient blurred vision,* mydriasis, cycloplegia.
GI: nausea, vomiting, *constipation,* bloated feeling, *dry mouth.*
GU: impotence, urinary hesitancy, urine retention.
Skin: decreased diaphoresis, rash, urticaria, allergic reactions.
Other: fever, suppressed lactation, flushing.

Interactions
Drug-drug. *Anticholinergics:* increased anticholinergic effects. Use together cautiously.
Atenolol, digoxin: increased levels of these drugs. Monitor patient closely.
CNS depressants: increased CNS effects. Use cautiously.
Haloperidol, levodopa: decreased levels of these drugs. Monitor patient closely.
Drug-lifestyle: *Alcohol use:* increased CNS effects. Discourage concomitant use.
Exercise, hot weather: may precipitate heatstroke. Urge caution.

Contraindications and precautions
• Contraindicated in patients hypersensitive to drug, elderly or debilitated patients with intestinal atony, hemorrhaging patients with unstable CV status, and patients with myasthenia gravis, GI obstruction, glaucoma, adynamic ileus, megacolon, severe colitis, ulcerative colitis with megacolon, or obstructive uropathy.
• Use cautiously in pregnant or breast-feeding women, elderly patients, and those with autonomic neuropathy, reflux esophagitis, or hepatic or renal disease.

NURSING CONSIDERATIONS

Assessment
- Assess patient's bladder condition before therapy.
- Before giving drug, prescriber will most likely confirm neurogenic bladder by cystometry and rule out partial intestinal obstruction in patients with diarrhea, especially those with colostomy or ileostomy.
- Prepare patient for periodic cystometry to evaluate response to therapy.
- Watch elderly patients for confusion and mental status changes.
- Be alert for adverse reactions.
- Drug may aggravate symptoms of hyperthyroidism, coronary artery disease, heart failure, arrhythmias, tachycardia, hypertension, or prostatic hyperplasia.
- Evaluate patient's and family's knowledge of drug therapy.

Nursing diagnoses
- Acute pain related to bladder spasms
- Risk for injury related to drug-induced adverse CNS reactions
- Deficient knowledge related to drug therapy

Planning and implementation
- If patient has a urinary tract infection, give antibiotics as directed.
- To minimize tendency toward tolerance, be prepared to stop therapy periodically to determine whether patient can get along without it.

ALERT Don't confuse Ditropan with diazepam or Dithranol.

Patient teaching
- Warn patient to avoid hazardous activities until CNS effects of drug are known.
- Tell patient to avoid alcohol during drug therapy.
- Caution patient that taking drug in hot weather raises the risk of fever or heatstroke.
- Advise patient to store drug in tightly closed containers at 59° to 86° F (15° to 30° C).

Evaluation
- Patient is free from bladder pain.
- Patient sustains no injuries from drug-induced adverse CNS reactions.
- Patient and family state understanding of drug therapy.

oxycodone hydrochloride
(oks-ee-KOH-dohn high-droh-KLOR-ighd)
Endone ◇, Oxycontin, OxyFAST, OxyIR, Roxicodone, Roxicodone Intensol, Supeudol ♦

oxycodone pectinate
Proladone ◇

Pharmacologic class: opioid
Therapeutic class: analgesic
Controlled substance schedule: II
Pregnancy risk category: C

Indications and dosages
▶ **Moderate to severe pain.** *Adults:* 5 mg P.O. q 6 hours, p.r.n. Or, 10 to 40 mg P.R., p.r.n., t.i.d., or q.i.d. Or, 10 mg q 12 hours (extended-release tablets) if patient isn't presently taking opiates. If patient is taking a conventional opiate preparation, extended-release dosing is dependent upon the amount being taken.

How supplied
oxycodone hydrochloride
Tablets: 5 mg
Tablets (extended-release): 10 mg, 20 mg, 40 mg, 80 mg
Capsules: 5 mg
Oral solution: 5 mg/5 ml, 20 mg/ml (concentrate)
Suppositories: 10 mg, 20 mg
oxycodone pectinate
Suppositories: 30 mg ◇

Pharmacokinetics
Absorption: unknown.
Distribution: unknown.
Metabolism: metabolized in liver.
Excretion: excreted primarily in urine. *Half-life:* 2 to 3 hours.

Route	Onset	Peak	Duration
P.O.	10-15 min	≤ 1 hr	3-6 hr
P.R.	Unknown	Unknown	Unknown

Pharmacodynamics

Chemical effect: binds with opioid receptors in CNS, altering response to pain via unknown mechanism.
Therapeutic effect: relieves pain.

Adverse reactions

CNS: *sedation, somnolence, clouded sensorium, euphoria,* dizziness.
CV: *hypotension,* ***bradycardia.***
GI: nausea, vomiting, constipation, ileus.
GU: urine retention.
Respiratory: ***respiratory depression.***
Other: physical dependence.

Interactions

Drug-drug. *Anticoagulants:* oxycodone products containing aspirin may increase anticoagulant effect. Monitor PT and INR. Use together cautiously.
CNS depressants, general anesthetics, hypnotics, MAO inhibitors, other narcotic analgesics, sedatives, tranquilizers, tricyclic antidepressants: additive effects. Use together with extreme caution. Reduce oxycodone dose as directed, and monitor patient response.
Drug-lifestyle. *Alcohol use:* increased CNS depression. Discourage concomitant use.

Contraindications and precautions

- Contraindicated in patients hypersensitive to drug
- Use with extreme caution in elderly or debilitated patients and those with head injury, increased intracranial pressure, seizures, asthma, COPD, prostatic hyperplasia, severe hepatic or renal disease, acute abdominal conditions, urethral stricture, hypothyroidism, Addison's disease, or arrhythmias.
- Use cautiously in pregnant or breast-feeding women.

NURSING CONSIDERATIONS

Assessment

- Assess patient's pain before and after drug administration.
- Monitor circulatory and respiratory status.
- Be alert for adverse reactions and drug interactions.
- Evaluate patient's and family's knowledge of drug therapy.

Nursing diagnoses

- Acute pain related to condition
- Ineffective breathing pattern related to drug-induced respiratory depression
- Deficient knowledge related to drug therapy

Planning and implementation

P.O. use: Give drug with food or milk to avoid GI upset.
P.R. use: Not commercially available in the United States.
- For best results, give drug before patient has intense pain.
- Single-agent oxycodone solution and tablets are especially good for patient who shouldn't take aspirin or acetaminophen.

ALERT Withhold dose and notify prescriber if respirations are shallow or rate falls below 12 breaths/minute.

Patient teaching

- Instruct patient to take drug with food or milk to minimize GI upset.
- Tell patient to ask for drug before pain becomes intense.
- Tell patient not to chew or crush OxyIR or extended-release forms.
- Caution ambulatory patient about getting out of bed or walking. Warn outpatient to avoid hazardous activities until CNS effects of drug are known.

Evaluation

- Patient is free from pain.
- Patient's respiratory rate and pattern remain within normal limits.
- Patient and family state understanding of drug therapy.

oxymetazoline hydrochloride

(oks-ee-met-AHZ-oh-leen high-droh-KLOR-ighd)

Afrin†, Afrin Children's Strength Nose Drops†, Allerest 12 Hour Nasal†, Chlorphed-LA†, Dristan Long Lasting†, Drixine Nasal◇, Duramist Plus†, Duration†, 4-Way Long-Acting Nasal, Genasal Spray†, Neo-Synephrine 12 Hour†, Nostrilla†, NTZ Long Acting Nasal†, Sinarest 12 Hour†, Sinex Long-Acting†, Twice-A-Day Nasal†

Pharmacologic class: sympathomimetic
Therapeutic class: decongestant, vasoconstrictor
Pregnancy risk category: NR

Indications and dosages

▶ **Nasal congestion.** *Adults and children age 6 and older:* 2 to 3 gtt or sprays of 0.05% solution in each nostril b.i.d.
Children ages 2 to 6: 2 to 3 gtt of 0.025% solution in each nostril b.i.d. Don't use for more than 5 days.

How supplied

Nasal solution: 0.025%, 0.05%

Pharmacokinetics

Unknown.

Route	Onset	Peak	Duration
Intranasal	5-10 min	≤ 6 hr	< 12 hr

Pharmacodynamics

Chemical effect: may cause local vasoconstriction of dilated arterioles, reducing blood flow and nasal congestion.
Therapeutic effect: relieves nasal congestion.

Adverse reactions

CNS: headache, *restlessness, anxiety,* dizziness, insomnia, possible sedation.
CV: palpitations, ***CV collapse,*** hypertension.
EENT: rebound nasal congestion or irritation with excessive or long-term use, dry nose and throat, increased nasal discharge, stinging, sneezing.
Other: systemic effects in children with excessive or long-term use.

Interactions

None significant.

Contraindications and precautions

- Contraindicated in patients hypersensitive to drug.
- Use cautiously in pregnant patients, breast-feeding patients, elderly patients, and patients with hyperthyroidism, cardiac disease, hypertension, or diabetes mellitus.

NURSING CONSIDERATIONS

Assessment

- Assess patient's congestion before therapy and regularly thereafter.
- Be alert for adverse reactions.
- Evaluate patient's and family's knowledge of drug therapy.

Nursing diagnoses

- Ineffective health maintenance related to nasal congestion
- Risk for injury related to drug-induced adverse CNS reactions
- Deficient knowledge related to drug therapy

Planning and implementation

- When giving drug, have patient hold head upright while you insert nozzle and then sniff the spray briskly.

Patient teaching

- Teach patient how to use drug.
- Inform patient that product should be used by only one person to prevent spread of infection.
- Tell patient not to exceed recommended dosage and to use only when needed.
- Warn patient that excessive use may cause bradycardia, hypotension, dizziness, and weakness.

Evaluation

- Patient's nasal congestion is relieved.

• Patient sustains no injuries from drug-induced adverse CNS reactions.
• Patient and family state understanding of drug therapy.

oxymorphone hydrochloride

(oks-ee-MOR-fohn high-droh-KLOR-ighd)
Numorphan, Numorphan HP

Pharmacologic class: opioid
Therapeutic class: analgesic
Controlled substance schedule: II
Pregnancy risk category: C

Indications and dosages

▶ **Moderate to severe pain.** *Adults:* 1 to 1.5 mg I.M. or S.C. q 4 to 6 hours, p.r.n. Or, 0.5 mg I.V. q 4 to 6 hours, p.r.n. Or, 5 mg P.R. q 4 to 6 hours, p.r.n.

How supplied

Injection: 1 mg/ml, 1.5 mg/ml
Suppositories: 5 mg

Pharmacokinetics

Absorption: well absorbed.
Distribution: widely distributed.
Metabolism: metabolized primarily in liver.
Excretion: excreted primarily in urine.

Route	Onset	Peak	Duration
I.V.	5-10 min	15-30 min	3-4 hr
I.M.	10-15 min	30-90 min	3-6 hr
S.C.	10-20 min	60-90 min	3-6 hr
P.R.	15-30 min	About 2 hr	3-6 hr

Pharmacodynamics

Chemical effect: binds with opioid receptors in CNS, altering response to pain via unknown mechanism.
Therapeutic effect: relieves pain.

Adverse reactions

CNS: *sedation, somnolence, clouded sensorium, euphoria,* dizziness, ***seizures*** with large doses.
CV: *hypotension,* ***bradycardia.***
GI: *nausea, vomiting, constipation,* ileus.
GU: urine retention.
Respiratory: ***respiratory depression.***
Other: physical dependence.

Interactions

Drug-drug. *CNS depressants, general anesthetics, MAO inhibitors, tricyclic antidepressants:* additive effects. Use together with extreme caution.
Drug-lifestyle. *Alcohol use:* additive effects. Discourage concomitant use.

Contraindications and precautions

• Contraindicated in patients hypersensitive to drug and in children under age 18.
• Use with extreme caution in elderly or debilitated patients and in those with head injury, increased intracranial pressure, seizures, asthma, COPD, acute abdominal conditions, prostatic hyperplasia, severe hepatic or renal disease, urethral stricture, respiratory depression, hypothyroidism, Addison's disease, or arrhythmias.
• Use cautiously in pregnant or breast-feeding women.

NURSING CONSIDERATIONS

Assessment

• Assess patient's pain before and after drug administration.
• Be alert for adverse reactions and drug interactions.
• Evaluate patient's and family's knowledge of drug therapy.

Nursing diagnoses

• Acute pain related to condition
• Ineffective breathing pattern related to drug-induced respiratory depression
• Deficient knowledge related to drug therapy

Planning and implementation

• Keep narcotic antagonist (naloxone) and resuscitation equipment available.
• Don't give drug for mild to moderate pain.
• Drug may worsen gallbladder pain.
• Give drug before patient has intense pain.

• Withhold dose and notify prescriber if respirations decrease or rate is below 12 breaths/minute.
• Dependence can develop with long-term use.
• Administering laxatives may help avoid or relieve constipation.
I.V. use: Give drug by direct I.V. injection. If needed, dilute in normal saline solution.
– Keep patient supine during administration to minimize hypotension.
I.M., S.C., and P.R. use: Follow normal protocol.
ALERT Don't confuse oxymorphone with oxymetholone.

Patient teaching
• Instruct patient to take drug before pain becomes intense.
• Caution ambulatory patient about getting out of bed or walking. Warn outpatient to avoid hazardous activities until CNS effects of drug are known.
• Tell patient to refrigerate suppositories.
• Caution patient or family to report a decreased respiratory rate.

Evaluation
• Patient is free from pain.
• Patient's respiratory status is within normal limits.
• Patient and family state understanding of drug therapy.

oxytocin, synthetic injection
(oks-ih-TOH-sin, sin-THET-ik in-JEK-shun)
Oxytocin, Pitocin, Syntocinon

Pharmacologic class: exogenous hormone
Therapeutic class: oxytocic, lactation stimulant
Pregnancy risk category: C

Indications and dosages
▶ **Induction or stimulation of labor.** *Adults:* initially, 1 ml (10 units) ampule in 1,000 ml of dextrose 5% injection or normal saline solution I.V. infused at 1 to 2 milliunits/minute. Rate increased in increments of no more than 1 to 2 milliunits/minute at 15- to 30-minute intervals until normal contraction pattern is established. Rate decreased when labor is firmly established. Maximum dose is 20 milliunits/minute.
▶ **Reduction of postpartum bleeding after expulsion of placenta.** *Adults:* 10 to 40 units added to 1,000 ml of D_5W or normal saline solution infused at rate necessary to control bleeding, usually 20 to 40 milliunits/minute. Also, 1 ml (10 units) can be given I.M. after delivery of placenta.
▶ **Incomplete or inevitable abortion.** *Adults:* 10 units of oxytocin I.V. in 500 ml of normal saline solution or dextrose 5% in normal saline solution. Infuse at 20 to 40 gtt/minute.

How supplied
Injection: 10 units/ml in ampule or vial

Pharmacokinetics
Absorption: unknown after I.M. administration.
Distribution: distributed through extracellular fluid.
Metabolism: metabolized rapidly in kidneys and liver. In early pregnancy, a circulating enzyme, oxytocinase, can inactivate drug.
Excretion: small amounts excreted in urine. *Half-life:* 3 to 5 minutes.

Route	Onset	Peak	Duration
I.V.	Immediate	Unknown	1 hr
I.M.	3-5 min	Unknown	2-3 hr

Pharmacodynamics
Chemical effect: causes potent and selective stimulation of uterine and mammary gland smooth muscle.
Therapeutic effect: induces labor and milk ejection and reduces postpartum bleeding.

Adverse reactions
Maternal
CNS: ***subarachnoid hemorrhage*** from hypertension, ***seizures, coma*** from water intoxication.
CV: ***hypertension;*** increased heart rate, systemic venous return, and cardiac output; ***arrhythmias.***

GI: nausea, vomiting.
GU: tetanic uterine contractions, ***abruptio placentae, impaired uterine blood flow,*** pelvic hematoma, ***increased uterine motility.***
Hematologic: afibrinogenemia (may be related to postpartum bleeding).
Other: hypersensitivity reactions, ***anaphylaxis.***

Fetal

CV: ***bradycardia***, tachycardia, ***PVCs.***
Hematologic: hyperbilirubinemia.
Respiratory: ***anoxia, asphyxia.***

Interactions

Drug-drug. *Cyclopropane anesthetics:* less pronounced bradycardia and hypotension. Use together cautiously.
Thiopental anesthetics: possible delayed induction. Use together cautiously.
Vasoconstrictors: severe hypertension if oxytocin given within 3 or 4 hours of vasoconstrictor in patients receiving caudal block anesthetic. Avoid concomitant use.

Contraindications and precautions

- Contraindicated in cephalopelvic disproportion or delivery that requires conversion, as in transverse lie; in fetal distress when delivery isn't imminent; in prematurity; in other obstetric emergencies; and in severe toxemia, hypertonic uterine patterns, total placenta previa, or vasoprevia. Also contraindicated in patients hypersensitive to drug.
- Use with extreme caution during first and second stages of labor because cervical laceration, uterine rupture, and maternal and fetal death have been reported.
- Use with extreme caution, if at all, in patients with invasive cervical carcinoma and patients with history of cervical or uterine surgery, grand multiparity, uterine sepsis, traumatic delivery, or overdistended uterus.

NURSING CONSIDERATIONS

Assessment

- Assess patient's condition before therapy and regularly thereafter.
- Monitor and record uterine contractions, heart rate, blood pressure, intrauterine pressure, fetal heart rate, and blood loss every 15 minutes.
- Be alert for adverse reactions and drug interactions.
- Monitor fluid intake and output. Antidiuretic effect may lead to fluid overload, seizures, and coma.
- Evaluate patient's and family's knowledge of drug therapy.

Nursing diagnoses

- Risk for deficient fluid volume related to postpartum bleeding
- Excessive fluid volume related to drug-induced antidiuretic effect
- Deficient knowledge related to drug therapy

Planning and implementation

- Drug is used to induce or reinforce labor only when pelvis is known to be adequate, vaginal delivery is indicated, fetal maturity is assured, and fetal position is favorable. Should be used only in hospital where critical care facilities and experienced clinician are immediately available.

I.V. use: Don't give drug by I.V. bolus injection. Administer only by infusion.
– Give by piggyback infusion so drug can be stopped without interrupting I.V. line.
– Use an infusion pump.
I.M. use: Drug isn't recommended for routine I.M. use. However, 10 units may be given I.M. after delivery of placenta to control postpartum uterine bleeding.

- Never give oxytocin simultaneously by more than one route.
- Have magnesium sulfate (20% solution) available for relaxation of myometrium.
- If contractions are less than 2 minutes apart, if they're above 50 mm Hg, or if they last 90 seconds or longer, stop infusion, turn patient on her side, and notify prescriber.

ALERT Don't confuse Pitocin with Pitressin.

Patient teaching

- Instruct patient to report unusual feelings or adverse effects at once.

Evaluation

- Patient maintains adequate fluid balance with drug therapy.
- Patient shows no signs of edema.
- Patient and family state understanding of drug therapy.

P

paclitaxel

(pak-lih-TAK-sil)
Taxol

Pharmacologic class: novel antimicrotubule
Therapeutic class: antineoplastic
Pregnancy risk category: D

Indications and dosages

▶ **Metastatic ovarian cancer after failure of first-line or subsequent chemotherapy.** *Adults:* 135 mg/m^2 or 175 mg/m^2 I.V. over 3 hours q 3 weeks.

▶ **Breast cancer after failure of combination chemotherapy for metastatic disease or relapse within 6 months of adjuvant chemotherapy.** *Adults:* 175 mg/m^2 I.V. over 3 hours q 3 weeks.

▶ **Non-small cell lung cancer.** *Adults:* 135 mg/m^2 I.V. over 24 hours followed by 75 mg/m^2 cisplatin q 3 weeks.

▶ **AIDS-related Kaposi's sarcoma.** *Adults:* 135 mg/m^2 I.V. over 3 hours q 3 weeks or 100 mg/m^2 I.V. over 3 hours q 2 weeks.

▶ **Adjuvant treatment of node-positive breast cancer.** *Adults:* 175 mg/m^2 I.V. over 3 hours q 3 weeks for four courses given sequentially to doxorubicin-containing combination chemotherapy.

How supplied

Injection: 30 mg/5 ml

Pharmacokinetics

Absorption: not applicable.
Distribution: about 89% to 98% of drug is bound to serum proteins.
Metabolism: may be metabolized in liver.
Excretion: unknown.

Route	Onset	Peak	Duration
I.V.	Unknown	Unknown	Unknown

Pharmacodynamics

Chemical effect: prevents depolymerization of cellular microtubules, thus inhibiting normal reorganization of microtubule network necessary for mitosis and other vital cellular functions.
Therapeutic effect: hinders ovarian and breast cancer cell activity.

Adverse reactions

CNS: ***peripheral neuropathy.***
CV: ***bradycardia,*** *hypotension, abnormal ECG.*
GI: *nausea, vomiting, diarrhea, mucositis.*
Hematologic: **NEUTROPENIA, LEUKOPENIA, THROMBOCYTOPENIA,** *anemia, bleeding.*
Hepatic: elevated liver enzyme levels.
Musculoskeletal: *myalgia, arthralgia.*
Skin: alopecia, phlebitis, cellulitis at injection site.
Other: hypersensitivity reactions ***(anaphylaxis).***

Interactions

Drug-drug. *Cisplatin:* possible additive myelosuppressive effects. Use together cautiously.
Cyclosporine, dexamethasone, diazepam, estradiol, etoposide, ketoconazole, quinidine, retinoic acid, teniposide, testosterone, verapamil, vincristine: inhibited paclitaxel metabolism. Use together cautiously.
Doxorubicin: possible increase in levels of doxorubicin and its metabolites. Dose adjustments may be needed.

Contraindications and precautions

- Contraindicated in patients hypersensitive to drug or polyoxyethylated castor oil, a vehicle used in drug solution, and in patients with baseline neutrophil counts below 1,500/mm^3.
- Drug use isn't recommended for pregnant or breast-feeding women.

• Use cautiously in patients who have received radiation therapy; they may have more frequent or severe myelosuppression.
• Safety of drug hasn't been established in children.

NURSING CONSIDERATIONS

Assessment
• Assess patient's condition before therapy and regularly thereafter.
• Continuously monitor patient for first 30 minutes of infusion. Monitor closely throughout infusion.
• Monitor blood counts and liver function test results frequently during therapy.
• Be alert for adverse reactions and drug interactions.
• Evaluate patient's and family's knowledge of drug therapy.

Nursing diagnoses
• Ineffective health maintenance related to cancer
• Ineffective protection related to drug-induced adverse hematologic reactions
• Deficient knowledge related to drug therapy

Planning and implementation
• To reduce severe hypersensitivity, expect to pretreat patient with corticosteroids, such as dexamethasone, and antihistamines, as ordered. H_1-receptor antagonists, such as diphenhydramine, and H_2-receptor antagonists, such as cimetidine or ranitidine, may be used.
• Follow facility protocol for safe handling, preparation, and use of chemotherapy drugs. Preparation and administration of parenteral form are linked to carcinogenic, mutagenic, and teratogenic risks for personnel. Mark all waste materials with CHEMOTHERAPY HAZARD labels.
• Dilute concentrate to 0.3 to 1.2 mg/ml before infusion. Compatible solutions include normal saline solution for injection, D_5W, dextrose 5% in normal saline solution for injection, and dextrose 5% in Ringer's lactate injection. Diluted solutions are stable for 27 hours at room temperature.
• Prepare and store infusion solutions in glass containers. Undiluted concentrate shouldn't come in contact with polyvinylchloride I.V. bags or tubing. Store diluted solution in glass or polypropylene bottles, or use polypropylene or polyolefin bags. Administer through polyethylene-lined administration sets, and use in-line 0.22-micron filter.
• Take care to avoid extravasation.
ALERT Don't confuse paclitaxel with paroxetine or Taxol with Paxil.

Patient teaching
• Warn patient to watch for signs of bleeding and infection.
• Teach patient symptoms of peripheral neuropathy, such as tingling, burning, or numbness in limbs, and urge her to report them immediately. Although mild symptoms are common, severe symptoms occur infrequently. Dosage reduction may be necessary.
• Warn patient that alopecia occurs in up to 82% of patients.
• Advise woman of childbearing age to avoid pregnancy during therapy. Also recommend consulting with prescriber before becoming pregnant.

Evaluation
• Patient responds well to therapy.
• Patient develops no serious complications from drug-induced adverse hematologic reactions.
• Patient and family state understanding of drug therapy.

palivizumab
(pal-i-VI-zu-mab)
Synagis

Pharmacologic class: recombinant monoclonal antibody $IgG1_k$
Therapeutic class: RSV prophylactic
Pregnancy risk category: C

Indications and dosages
▶**Prevention of serious lower respiratory tract disease caused by RSV in children at high risk.** *Children:* 15 mg/kg I.M. monthly

throughout RSV season, with first administration before RSV season.

How supplied

Injection: 100 mg vial

Pharmacokinetics

Absorption: unknown.
Distribution: unknown.
Metabolism: unknown.
Excretion: unknown. *Half-life:* about 18 days.

Route	Onset	Peak	Duration
I.M.	Unknown	Unknown	Unknown

Pharmacodynamics

Chemical effect: has neutralizing and fusion-inhibitory activity against RSV, which inhibits RSV replication.
Therapeutic effect: prevents RSV infection in high-risk children.

Adverse reactions

CNS: nervousness, pain.
EENT: *otitis media, rhinitis*, pharyngitis, sinusitis, conjunctivitis.
GI: diarrhea, vomiting, gastroenteritis, oral candidiasis.
Hematologic: anemia.
Hepatic: liver function abnormality (increased ALT and AST levels).
Respiratory: *upper respiratory tract infection,* cough, wheeze, bronchiolitis, ***apnea,*** pneumonia, bronchitis, ***asthma***, croup, dyspnea.
Skin: *rash,* fungal dermatitis, eczema, seborrhea.
Other: hernia, failure to thrive, injection site reaction, viral infection, flu syndrome.

Interactions

None significant.

Contraindications and precautions

- Contraindicated in children hypersensitive to drug or its components.
- Use cautiously in patients with thrombocytopenia or other coagulation disorders.

NURSING CONSIDERATIONS

Assessment

- Obtain accurate medical history before giving drug; ask if child has any coagulation disorders or liver dysfunction.
- Be alert for adverse reactions.
- Evaluate patient's and family's knowledge about drug therapy.

Nursing diagnoses

- Risk for infection related to RSV infection
- Risk for injury related to drug-induced adverse reactions
- Deficient knowledge related to drug therapy

Planning and implementation

- To reconstitute, slowly add 1 ml of sterile water for injection into a 100-mg vial. Gently swirl vial for 30 seconds to avoid foaming; don't shake. Let reconstituted solution stand at room temperature for 20 minutes. Give within 6 hours of reconstitution.
- Administer drug in anterolateral aspect of thigh. Don't use gluteal muscle routinely as an injection site because of risk of damage to sciatic nerve. Injection volumes over 1 ml should be divided.
- Patients should receive monthly doses throughout RSV season, even if RSV infection develops. In the northern hemisphere, RSV season typically lasts from November to April.
- Anaphylactoid reactions haven't been observed after drug administration, but they can occur after administration of proteins. If anaphylaxis or severe allergic reaction occurs, notify prescriber, administer epinephrine (1:1,000) as ordered, and provide supportive care as needed.

Patient teaching

- Explain to parent or caregiver that drug is used to prevent RSV and not to treat it.
- Advise parent that monthly injections are recommended throughout RSV season.
- Advise parent to report adverse reactions immediately or any unusual bruising, bleeding, or weakness.

☑ Evaluation

- Patient doesn't develop RSV infection.
- Patient sustains no injury from drug-induced adverse reactions.
- Patient and family state understanding of drug therapy.

pamidronate disodium
(pam-ih-DROH-nayt digh-SOH-dee-um)
Aredia

Pharmacologic class: bisphosphonate, pyrophosphate analogue
Therapeutic class: antihypercalcemic
Pregnancy risk category: C

Indications and dosages

▶ **Moderate to severe hypercalcemia related to cancer (with or without bone metastases).** *Adults:* dosage depends on severity of hypercalcemia. Serum calcium levels are corrected for serum albumin as follows:

$$\text{Corrected serum calcium (CCa) (in mg/dl)} = \text{serum calcium (in mg/dl)} + 0.8\,(4 - \text{serum albumin (in g/dl)})$$

Patients with moderate hypercalcemia (CCa levels of 12 to 13.5 mg/dl) may receive 60 to 90 mg by I.V. infusion; 60-mg dose given over at least 4 hours, 90-mg dose infused over 24 hours. Those with severe hypercalcemia (CCa levels over 13.5 mg/dl) may receive 90 mg by I.V. infusion over 24 hours. At least 7 days should elapse before retreatment to allow full response to initial dose.

▶ **Moderate to severe Paget's disease.** *Adults:* 30 mg I.V. as 4-hour infusion on 3 consecutive days for total dose of 90 mg. Cycle repeated, p.r.n.

How supplied

Injection: 30 mg/vial, 60 mg/vial, 90 mg/vial

Pharmacokinetics

Absorption: not applicable.
Distribution: about 50% to 60% of dose is rapidly taken up by bone; drug is also taken up by kidneys, liver, spleen, teeth, and tracheal cartilage.
Metabolism: none.
Excretion: excreted by kidneys. *Half-life:* alpha, 1½ hours; beta, 27¼ hours.

Route	Onset	Peak	Duration
I.V.	Unknown	Unknown	Unknown

Pharmacodynamics

Chemical effect: inhibits bone resorption. Adsorbs to hydroxyapatite crystals in bone and may directly block calcium phosphate dissolution.
Therapeutic effect: lowers blood calcium levels.

Adverse reactions

CNS: ***seizures.***
CV: *fluid overload, hypertension,* ***atrial fibrillation.***
GI: *abdominal pain, anorexia, constipation, nausea, vomiting,* ***GI hemorrhage.***
GU: *urinary tract infection.*
Hematologic: ***leukopenia, thrombocytopenia,*** *anemia.*
Metabolism: hypophosphatemia, hypokalemia, hypomagnesemia, hypocalcemia.
Musckuloskeletal: bone pain.
Other: fever, pain.

Interactions

None significant.

Contraindications and precautions

- Contraindicated in patients hypersensitive to drug or to other biphosphonates, such as etidronate.
- Use with extreme caution in patients with renal impairment.
- Use cautiously in pregnant or breast-feeding women.
- Safety of drug hasn't been established in children.

NURSING CONSIDERATIONS

Assessment

- Assess patient's condition before therapy and regularly thereafter.
- Assess hydration before treatment.

• Closely monitor serum electrolytes, creatinine level, CBC and differential, hematocrit, and hemoglobin level, as ordered.
• Carefully monitor patient with anemia, leukopenia, or thrombocytopenia during first 2 weeks of therapy.
• Monitor patient's temperature. Fever is most likely 24 to 48 hours after therapy.
• Be alert for adverse reactions and drug interactions.
• Evaluate patient's and family's knowledge of drug therapy.

Nursing diagnoses

• Ineffective health maintenance related to hypercalcemia
• Risk for injury related to drug-induced hypocalcemia
• Deficient knowledge related to drug therapy

Planning and implementation

• Use drug only after patient has been vigorously hydrated with saline solution. In patients with mild to moderate hypercalcemia, hydration alone may be sufficient.
• Reconstitute vial with 10 ml of sterile water for injection. After drug is dissolved, add to 1,000 ml of half-normal or normal saline solution injection or D_5W. Don't mix with infusion solutions that contain calcium, such as Ringer's injection or lactated Ringer's injection. Inspect for precipitate before administering.
• Give drug only by I.V. infusion. Animals have developed nephropathy when drug is given as bolus.
• Short-term administration of calcium may be needed if patient has severe hypocalcemia.
• Solution is stable for 24 hours at room temperature.

Patient teaching

• Instruct patient to report unusual signs or symptoms at once.
• Inform patient of need for frequent tests to monitor effectiveness of drug and detect adverse reactions.

Evaluation

• Patient's blood calcium level returns to normal.
• Patient doesn't develop hypocalcemia during drug therapy.
• Patient and family state understanding of drug therapy.

pancreatin

(pan-kree-AH-tin)

Creon Capsules, Creon 10, Creon 20, Digepepsin Tablets, Dizymes Tablets†, Donnazyme, Entozyme, 8X Pancreatin 900 mg†, 4X Pancreatin 600 mg†, Hi-Vegi-Lip Tablets†, Pancrezyme 4X Tablets†

Pharmacologic class: pancreatic enzyme
Therapeutic class: digestant
Pregnancy risk category: C

Indications and dosages

▶ **Exocrine pancreatic secretion insufficiency; digestive aid in diseases related to deficiency of pancreatic enzymes, such as cystic fibrosis.** *Adults and children:* dosage varies with condition being treated. Usual initial dosage is 8,000 to 24,000 units of lipase activity before or with each meal or snack. Total daily dose also may be given in divided doses at 1- to 2-hour intervals throughout day.

How supplied

Creon
Capsules: 300 mg pancreatin, 8,000 units lipase, 13,000 units protease, and 30,000 units amylase
Creon 10
Capsules: 10,000 units lipase, 37,500 units protease, and 33,200 units amylase
Creon 20
Capsules: 20,000 units lipase, 75,000 units protease, and 66,400 units amylase
Digepepsin
Tablets: 300 mg pancreatin
Dizymes
Tablets (enteric-coated): 250 mg pancreatin, 6,750 units lipase, 41,250 units protease, and 43,750 units amylase†

Donnazyme
Tablets: 500 mg pancreatin, 1,000 units lipase, 12,500 units protease, and 12,500 units amylase
Entozyme
Tablets: 500 mg pancreatin, 600 units lipase, 7,500 units protease, and 7,500 units amylase
8X Pancreatin 900 mg
Tablets (enteric-coated): 7,200 mg pancreatin, 22,500 units lipase, 180,000 units protease, and 180,000 units amylase†
4X Pancreatin 600 mg
Tablets (enteric-coated): 2,400 mg pancreatin, 12,000 units lipase, 60,000 units protease, and 60,000 units amylase†
Hi-Vegi-Lip
Tablets (enteric-coated): 2,400 mg pancreatin, 4,800 units lipase, 60,000 units protease, and 60,000 units amylase†
Pancrezyme 4X
Tablets (enteric-coated): 2,400 mg pancreatin, 12,000 units lipase, 60,000 units protease, and 60,000 units amylase†

Pharmacokinetics

Absorption: not absorbed; it acts locally in GI tract.
Distribution: none.
Metabolism: none.
Excretion: excreted in feces.

Route	Onset	Peak	Duration
P.O.	Unknown	1-2 hr	Unknown

Pharmacodynamics

Chemical effect: replaces endogenous exocrine pancreatic enzymes.
Therapeutic effect: aids digestion of starches, fats, and proteins.

Adverse reactions

GI: nausea, diarrhea with high doses.
Metabolic: hyperuricuria with high doses.

Interactions

Drug-drug. *Antacids:* may negate effects of pancreatin. Avoid concomitant use.

Contraindications and precautions

- Contraindicated in patients hypersensitive to drug or to pork protein or enzymes and in those with acute pancreatitis or acute exacerbation of chronic pancreatitis.
- Use cautiously in pregnant or breast-feeding women.

NURSING CONSIDERATIONS

Assessment

- Assess patient's condition before therapy and regularly thereafter. Decreased number of bowel movements and improved stool consistency indicate effective therapy.
- Monitor patient's diet to ensure proper balance of fat, protein, and starch intake to avoid indigestion. Dosage varies according to degree of maldigestion and malabsorption, amount of fat in diet, and enzyme activity of drug.
- Evaluate patient's and family's knowledge of drug therapy.

Nursing diagnoses

- Imbalanced nutrition: less than body requirements related to condition
- Noncompliance related to long-term therapy
- Deficient knowledge related to drug therapy

Planning and implementation

- USP standards dictate that each milligram of bovine or porcine pancreatin contain lipase 2 units, protease 25 units, and amylase 25 units.

ALERT Drug isn't effective in GI disorders unrelated to pancreatic enzyme deficiency.

- Enteric coating on some products may reduce availability of enzyme in upper portion of jejunum.

Patient teaching

- Tell patient not to crush or chew enteric-coated dosage forms. Capsules containing enteric-coated microspheres may be opened and contents sprinkled on small quantity of soft food, such as applesauce. Follow with a glass of water or juice.
- Tell patient to store in airtight containers at room temperature.

Evaluation

- Patient maintains normal digestion of fats, carbohydrates, and proteins.

• Patient complies with prescribed drug regimen.
• Patient and family state understanding of drug therapy.

pancrelipase
(pan-krih-LIGH-pays)
Cotazym Capsules, Cotazym-S Capsules, Creon 5 Delayed-Release Minimicrospheres Capsules, Creon 10 Delayed-Release Minimicrospheres Capsules, Creon 20 Delayed-Release Minimicrospheres Capsules, Ilozyme Tablets, Ku-Zyme HP Capsules, Pancrease Capsules, Pancrease MT 4, Pancrease MT 10, Pancrease MT 16, Pancrelipase Capsules, Protilase Capsules, Ultrase MT 12, Ultrase MT 20, Viokase Powder, Viokase Tablets, Zymase Capsules

Pharmacologic class: pancreatic enzyme
Therapeutic class: digestant
Pregnancy risk category: C

Indications and dosages

▶ **Exocrine pancreatic secretion insufficiency, cystic fibrosis in adults and children, steatorrhea and other disorders of fat metabolism secondary to insufficient pancreatic enzymes.** *Adults and children:* dosage adjusted to patient's response. Usual initial dosage is 4,000 to 33,000 units of lipase activity with each meal or snack.

How supplied

Cotazym
Capsules: 8,000 units lipase, 30,000 units protease, 30,000 units amylase, and 25 mg calcium carbonate
Cotazym-S
Capsules (enteric-coated spheres): 5,000 units lipase, 20,000 units protease, and 20,000 units amylase
Creon 5
Capsules (delayed-release minimicrospheres): 5,000 units lipase, 18,750 units protease, 16,600 units amylase
Creon 10
Capsules (delayed-release minimicrospheres): 10,000 units lipase, 37,500 units protease, 33,200 units amylase
Creon 20
Capsules (delayed-release minimicrospheres): 20,000 units lipase, 75,000 units protease, 66,400 units amylase
Ilozyme
Tablets: 11,000 units lipase, 30,000 units protease, and 30,000 units amylase
Ku-Zyme HP
Capsules: 8,000 units lipase, 30,000 units protease, and 30,000 units amylase
Pancrease
Capsules (enteric-coated microspheres): 4,000 units lipase, 25,000 units protease, and 20,000 units amylase
Pancrease MT 4
Capsules (enteric-coated microtablets): 4,000 units lipase, 12,000 units protease, and 12,000 units amylase
Pancrease MT 10
Capsules (enteric-coated microtablets): 10,000 units lipase, 30,000 units protease, and 30,000 units amylase
Pancrease MT 16
Capsules (enteric-coated microtablets): 16,000 units lipase, 48,000 units protease, and 48,000 units amylase
Pancrelipase
Capsules (enteric-coated pellets): 4,000 units lipase, 25,000 units protease, and 20,000 units amylase
Protilase
Capsules (enteric-coated spheres): 4,000 units lipase, 25,000 units protease, and 20,000 units amylase
Ultrase MT 12
Capsules (delayed-release): 12,000 units lipase, 39,000 units protease, and 39,000 units amylase
Ultrase MT 20
Capsules: 20,000 units lipase, 65,000 units protease, and 65,000 units amylase
Viokase
Tablets: 8,000 units lipase, 30,000 units protease, 30,000 units amylase
Powder: 16,800 units lipase, 70,000 units protease, and 70,000 units amylase per 0.7 g powder

Zymase
Capsules (enteric-coated spheres):
12,000 units lipase, 24,000 units protease, and 24,000 units amylase

Pharmacokinetics

Absorption: not absorbed; it acts locally in GI tract.
Distribution: none.
Metabolism: none.
Excretion: excreted in feces.

Route	Onset	Peak	Duration
P.O.	Varies	Varies	Varies

Pharmacodynamics

Chemical effect: replaces endogenous exocrine pancreatic enzymes.
Therapeutic effect: aids digestion of starches, fats, and proteins.

Adverse reactions

GI: *nausea,* cramping, diarrhea with large doses.

Interactions

Drug-drug. *Antacids:* may destroy enteric coating and enhance degradation of pancrelipase. Avoid concomitant use.

Contraindications and precautions

- Contraindicated in patients hypersensitive to drug or pork protein or enzymes and in those with acute pancreatitis or acute exacerbation of chronic pancreatitis.
- Use cautiously in pregnant or breast-feeding women.

NURSING CONSIDERATIONS

Assessment

- Assess patient's condition before therapy and regularly thereafter. Decreased number of bowel movements and improved stool consistency indicate effective therapy.
- Monitor patient's diet to ensure proper balance of fat, protein, and starch intake to avoid indigestion. Dosage varies according to degree of maldigestion and malabsorption, amount of fat in diet, and enzyme activity of drug.
- Be alert for adverse reactions and drug interactions.
- Evaluate patient's and family's knowledge of drug therapy.

Nursing diagnoses

- Imbalanced nutrition: less than body requirements related to condition
- Noncompliance related to long-term therapy
- Deficient knowledge related to drug therapy

Planning and implementation

- For infant, mix powder with applesauce and give with meals. Avoid contact with or inhalation of powder; it may be irritating. Older child may take capsules with food.
- Enteric coating on some products may reduce availability of enzyme in upper portion of jejunum.

ALERT Drug isn't effective in GI disorders unrelated to pancreatic enzyme deficiency.

Patient teaching

- Advise patient not to crush or chew enteric-coated dosage forms.
- Tell patient to store in airtight containers at room temperature.

Evaluation

- Patient maintains normal digestion of fats, carbohydrates, and proteins.
- Patient complies with prescribed drug regimen.
- Patient and family state understanding of drug therapy.

pancuronium bromide
(pan-kyoo-ROH-nee-um BROH-mighd)
Pavulon

Pharmacologic class: nondepolarizing neuromuscular blocker
Therapeutic class: skeletal muscle relaxant
Pregnancy risk category: C

Indications and dosages

▶ **Adjunct to anesthesia to induce skeletal muscle relaxation; to facilitate intubation;**

to lessen muscle contractions in pharmacologically or electrically induced seizures; to assist with mechanical ventilation. Dosage depends on anesthetic used, individual needs, and response. Dosages are representative and must be adjusted.
Adults and children age 1 month and over: initially, 0.04 to 0.1 mg/kg I.V.; then 0.01 mg/kg q 25 to 60 minutes.
Neonates up to age 1 month: individualized.

How supplied

Injection: 1 mg/ml, 2 mg/ml

Pharmacokinetics

Absorption: not applicable.
Distribution: drug has very low protein-binding regardless of dose.
Metabolism: unknown.
Excretion: excreted mainly in urine; some biliary excretion. *Half-life:* About 2 hours.

Route	Onset	Peak	Duration
I.V.	30-45 sec	3-4.5 min	35-45 min

Pharmacodynamics

Chemical effect: prevents acetylcholine from binding to receptors on muscle end plate, thus blocking depolarization.
Therapeutic effect: relaxes skeletal muscles.

Adverse reactions

CV: tachycardia, increased blood pressure.
EENT: excessive salivation.
Musculoskeletal: residual muscle weakness.
Respiratory: ***prolonged, dose-related respiratory insufficiency or apnea;*** wheezing.
Skin: transient rashes, excessive diaphoresis.
Other: burning sensation, ***allergic or idiosyncratic hypersensitivity reactions.***

Interactions

Drug-drug. *Aminoglycoside antibiotics, including amikacin, gentamicin, kanamycin, neomycin, streptomycin; clindamycin; general anesthetics; polymyxin antibiotics, such as polymyxin B sulfate, colistin, and polymyxin B sulfate; quinidine:* potentiated neuromuscular blockade, leading to increased skeletal muscle relaxation and prolonged effect. Use cautiously during surgical and postoperative periods.
Lithium, opioid analgesics: potentiated neuromuscular blockade, leading to increased skeletal muscle relaxation and possible respiratory paralysis. Use with extreme caution, and reduce pancuronium dosage as directed.
Succinylcholine: increased intensity and duration of blockade. Allow succinylcholine effects to subside before giving pancuronium.

Contraindications and precautions

- Contraindicated in patients hypersensitive to bromides, in those with tachycardia, and in those for whom even a minor increase in heart rate is undesirable.
- Use cautiously in elderly or debilitated patients and in those with respiratory depression, myasthenia gravis, myasthenic syndrome of lung cancer, bronchogenic carcinoma, dehydration, thyroid disorders, collagen diseases, porphyria, electrolyte disturbances, hyperthermia, toxemic states, or renal, hepatic, or pulmonary impairment. Use large doses cautiously in pregnant women undergoing cesarean section and in breast-feeding women.

NURSING CONSIDERATIONS

Assessment

- Assess patient's condition before therapy and regularly thereafter.
- Monitor baseline electrolyte determinations (electrolyte imbalance can potentiate neuromuscular effects) and vital signs.
- Measure fluid intake and output; renal dysfunction may prolong duration of action because 25% of drug is unchanged before excretion.
- Nerve stimulator and train-of-four monitoring are recommended to confirm antagonism of neuromuscular blockade and recovery of muscle strength. Before attempting pharmacologic reversal with neostigmine, you should see some evidence of spontaneous recovery.
- Monitor respirations closely until patient fully recovers from neuromuscular blockade, as evidenced by tests of muscle strength (hand grip, head lift, and ability to cough).

• Be alert for adverse reactions and drug interactions.
• Evaluate patient's and family's knowledge of drug therapy.

Nursing diagnoses
• Ineffective health maintenance related to condition
• Ineffective breathing pattern related to drug's effect on respiratory muscles
• Deficient knowledge related to drug therapy

Planning and implementation
• Administer sedatives or general anesthetics before neuromuscular blockers, as ordered. Neuromuscular blockers don't obtund consciousness or alter pain threshold. Give analgesics for pain, as ordered.
• Pancuronium should be used only by personnel skilled in airway management.
• Mix drug only with fresh solutions; precipitates will form if alkaline solutions such as barbiturate solutions are used.
• Allow succinylcholine effects to subside before giving pancuronium, as ordered.
• Store drug in refrigerator. Don't store in plastic containers or syringes, although plastic syringes may be used for administration.
• Have emergency respiratory support equipment (endotracheal equipment, ventilator, oxygen, atropine, edrophonium, epinephrine, and neostigmine) immediately available.
• Once spontaneous recovery starts, drug-induced neuromuscular blockade may be reversed with anticholinesterase drug (such as neostigmine or edrophonium). Usually administered with an anticholinergic such as atropine.
ALERT Don't confuse pancuronium with pipercuronium or Pavulon with Peptavlon.

Patient teaching
• Explain all events to patient because he can still hear.
• Reassure patient that he'll be monitored at all times and that pain medication will be provided, if appropriate.
• Tell patient that he may feel burning sensation at injection site.

Evaluation
• Patient's condition improves.
• Patient maintains adequate ventilation with mechanical assistance.
• Patient and family state understanding of drug therapy.

papaverine hydrochloride
(puh-PAV-eh-reen high-droh-KLOR-ighd)
Cerespan, Genabid, Pavabid, Pavabid HP, Pavabid Plateau Caps, Pavacels, Pavagen, Pavarine, Pavased, Pavatym, Paverolan

Pharmacologic class: benzylisoquinoline derivative, opioid alkaloid
Therapeutic class: peripheral vasodilator
Pregnancy risk category: C

Indications and dosages
▶ **Relief of cerebral and peripheral ischemia from arterial spasm and myocardial ischemia; treatment of coronary occlusion and certain cerebral angiospastic states.** *Adults:* 100 to 300 mg P.O. three to five times daily. Or, 150- to 300-mg timed-release preparations q 8 to 12 hours. Or, 30 to 120 mg I.M. or I.V. slowly over 1 to 2 minutes q 3 hours, as indicated.

How supplied
Tablets: 60 mg, 100 mg, 200 mg, 300 mg
Tablets (timed-release): 200 mg
Capsules (timed-release): 150 mg
Injection: 30 mg/ml, 32.5 mg/ml♦

Pharmacokinetics
Absorption: 54% of P.O. drug is bioavailable; sustained-release forms are sometimes absorbed poorly and erratically. Absorption unknown after I.M. administration.
Distribution: drug tends to localize in adipose tissue and in liver; remainder is distributed throughout body. About 90% of drug is protein-bound.
Metabolism: metabolized by liver.
Excretion: excreted in urine as metabolites.

Route	Onset	Peak	Duration
P.O.	Rapid	1-2 hr	12 hr (timed-release); unknown (regular)
I.V.	Unknown	Unknown	Unknown
I.M.	Unknown	Unknown	Unknown

Pharmacodynamics

Chemical effect: has direct, nonspecific relaxant effect on vascular, cardiac, and other smooth muscle.
Therapeutic effect: relieves vascular spasms.

Adverse reactions

CNS: *headache,* depression, malaise.
CV: *increased heart rate, increased blood pressure* (parenteral use), depressed AV and intraventricular conduction, hypotension, ***arrhythmias.***
GI: constipation, dry mouth, *nausea.*
Hepatic: ***hepatitis, cirrhosis.***
Respiratory: increased depth of respiration, ***apnea.***
Skin: *diaphoresis.*
Other: *flushing.*

Interactions

Drug-drug. *Levodopa:* papaverine may interfere with therapeutic effects of levodopa in patients with Parkinson's disease. Monitor patient closely.

Contraindications and precautions

• I.V. use is contraindicated in patients with Parkinson's disease or complete AV block.
• Use cautiously in patients with glaucoma and in pregnant women.
• Safety of drug hasn't been established in breast-feeding women and in children.

NURSING CONSIDERATIONS

Assessment

• Assess patient's condition before therapy and regularly thereafter.
• Monitor blood pressure and heart rate and rhythm, especially in patient with cardiac disease.
• Be alert for adverse reactions and drug interactions.
• Monitor for adverse hepatic reactions during long-term therapy.
• Evaluate patient's and family's knowledge of drug therapy.

Nursing diagnoses

• Ineffective tissue perfusion (cerebral, cardiopulmonary, peripheral, GI) related to vascular spasms
• Constipation related to drug's effect on GI tract
• Deficient knowledge related to drug therapy

Planning and implementation

P.O. and I.M. use: Follow normal protocol.
I.V. use: Give drug by direct injection over 1 to 2 minutes to minimize risk of serious adverse reactions. Don't add to lactated Ringer's injection because precipitate forms.
• Drug is most effective when given early in course of disorder.
ALERT FDA has announced that drug may not be effective for diseases indicated.
• Hold dose and notify prescriber at once if vital signs change.

Patient teaching

• Tell patient to take drug regularly; long-term therapy is required.
• Advise patient to avoid hazardous activities until CNS effects of drug are known.
• Instruct patient to avoid sudden position changes.

Evaluation

• Patient maintains adequate tissue perfusion.
• Patient states measures used to prevent constipation.
• Patient and family state understanding of drug therapy.

paricalcitol

(pair-ee-KAL-sih-tohl)
Zemplar

Pharmacologic class: vitamin D analog
Therapeutic class: hyperparathyroidism agent

Pregnancy risk category: C

Indications and dosages

Prevention and treatment of secondary hyperparathyroidism caused by chronic renal failure. *Adults:* 0.04 to 0.1 mcg/kg (2.8 to 7 mcg) I.V. no more often than every other day during dialysis. Doses as high as 0.24 mcg/kg (16.8 mcg) have been safely administered. If satisfactory response isn't observed, dosage may be increased by 2 to 4 mcg at 2- to 4-week intervals.

How supplied

Injection: 5 mcg/ml

Pharmacokinetics

Absorption: not applicable.
Distribution: unknown.
Metabolism: unknown.
Excretion: eliminated primarily by hepatobiliary excretion, 74% in feces and 16% in urine. *Half-life:* about 15 hours.

Route	Onset	Peak	Duration
I.V.	Immediate	Unknown	15 hr

Pharmacodynamics

Chemical effect: synthetic vitamin D analogue that reduces parathyroid hormone (PTH) levels.
Therapeutic effect: reduced PTH levels in patients with chronic renal failure.

Adverse reactions

CNS: light-headedness, malaise.
CV: edema, palpitations.
GI: dry mouth, GI bleeding, *nausea*, vomiting.
Hepatic: reduced serum total alkaline phosphatase level.
Respiratory: pneumonia.
Other: chills, fever, flu syndrome, ***sepsis.***

Interactions

None significant.

Contraindications and precautions

- Contraindicated in patients hypersensitive to drug or its ingredients and in those with evidence of vitamin D toxicity or hypercalcemia.
- Use cautiously in patients taking digitalis compounds. Patients taking digoxin are at greater risk for digitalis toxicity during therapy because of risk of hypercalcemia.

NURSING CONSIDERATIONS

Assessment

- Obtain history of patient's underlying condition before therapy, and reassess regularly thereafter.
- Watch for ECG abnormalities.
- Monitor patient for symptoms of hypercalcemia, such as fatigue, muscle weakness, anorexia, depression, nausea, and constipation. Immediately notify prescriber if you suspect hypercalcemia.
- Monitor serum calcium and phosphorus levels twice weekly when dosage is being adjusted, and then monitor monthly. Measure PTH level every 3 months during therapy, as directed.
- Evaluate patient's and family's knowledge about drug therapy.

Nursing diagnoses

- Risk for injury related to drug-induced hypercalcemia
- Imbalanced nutrition: less than body requirements related to drug-induced GI adverse effects
- Deficient knowledge related to drug therapy

Planning and implementation

- Drug is only administered as an I.V. bolus. Discard unused portion.
- Inspect drug for particulates and discoloration before use.

ALERT As PTH level decreases, paricalcitol dose may need to be decreased, as ordered. Acute paricalcitol overdose may cause hypercalcemia, which may require emergency attention.

- In patients with chronic renal failure, appropriate types of phosphate-binding compounds may be needed to control serum phosphorus levels, but excessive use of aluminum-containing compounds should be avoided.
- Store drug at controlled room temperature (59° to 86° F [15° to 30° C]).

Patient teaching

- Stress importance of adhering to a dietary regimen of calcium supplementation and phosphorus restriction during drug therapy.
- Caution against use of phosphate or vitamin D–related compounds during drug therapy.
- Explain need for frequent laboratory tests.
- Instruct patient with chronic renal failure to take phosphate-binding compounds as prescribed but to avoid excessive use of aluminum-containing compounds. Alert patient to early symptoms of hypercalcemia and vitamin D intoxication, such as weakness, headache, somnolence, nausea, vomiting, dry mouth, constipation, muscle pain, bone pain, and metallic taste.
- Instruct patient to promptly report adverse reactions.
- Remind patient taking digoxin to watch for signs and symptoms of digitalis toxicity.

☑ Evaluation

- Patient doesn't experience hypercalcemia.
- Patient doesn't experience adverse GI effects.
- Patient and family state understanding of drug therapy.

paroxetine hydrochloride

(par-OKS-eh-teen high-droh-KLOR-ighd)
Paxil

Pharmacologic class: selective serotonin reuptake inhibitor (SSRI)
Therapeutic class: antidepressant
Pregnancy risk category: B

Indications and dosages

▶ **Depression.** *Adults:* initially, 20 mg P.O. daily, preferably in morning, as directed. Increased by 10 mg/day at weekly intervals, to maximum of 50 mg daily, if necessary.

▶ **Obsessive-compulsive disorder.** *Adults:* initially, 20 mg P.O. daily, preferably in morning, as directed. Increased by 10 mg/day at weekly intervals to target of 40 mg/day. Maximum, 60 mg/day.

▶ **Panic disorder.** *Adults:* initially, 10 mg P.O. daily. Increased by 10-mg increments at no less than weekly intervals to maximum of 60 mg/day.

▶ **Social anxiety disorder.** *Adults:* initially, 20 mg P.O. daily, usually in the morning. Maintain lowest effective dosage, and periodically assess patient to determine need for continued treatment. Maximum, 60 mg/day.
Elderly or debilitated patients; patients with severe hepatic or renal disease: initially, 10 mg P.O. daily, preferably in morning, as directed. If patient doesn't respond after full antidepressant effect has occurred, increased by 10-mg/day increments at weekly intervals to maximum of 40 mg/day.

How supplied

Tablets: 20 mg, 30 mg

Pharmacokinetics

Absorption: completely absorbed.
Distribution: distributed throughout body, including CNS; only 1% remains in plasma. About 93% to 95% bound to plasma protein.
Metabolism: about 36% metabolized in liver.
Excretion: about 64% excreted in urine. *Half-life:* about 24 hours.

Route	Onset	Peak	Duration
P.O.	1-4 wk	2-8 hr	Unknown

Pharmacodynamics

Chemical effect: unknown; presumed to be linked to inhibition of CNS neuronal uptake of serotonin.
Therapeutic effect: relieves depression.

Adverse reactions

CNS: asthenia, blurred vision, somnolence, dizziness, insomnia, tremor, nervousness, anxiety, paresthesia, confusion.
CV: palpitations, vasodilation, orthostatic hypotension.
EENT: lump or tightness in throat, dysgeusia.
GI: *dry mouth, nausea, constipation, diarrhea, decreased appetite,* taste perversion, increased appetite, flatulence, vomiting, dyspepsia, increased appetite.
GU: ejaculatory disturbances, male genital disorders (including anorgasmy, erectile difficulties, delayed ejaculation or orgasm, impotence, and sexual dysfunction), urinary fre-

quency, other urinary disorder, female genital disorder (including anorgasmy, difficulty with orgasm).
Metabolic: hyponatremia.
Musculoskeletal: myopathy, myalgia, myasthenia.
Skin: *diaphoresis,* rash.
Other: decreased libido, yawning.

Interactions

Drug-drug. *Cimetidine:* decreased hepatic metabolism of paroxetine, leading to risk of toxicity. Dosage adjustments may be necessary.
Digoxin: may decrease digoxin levels. Monitor levels closely.
MAO inhibitors: may increase risk of serious, sometimes fatal, adverse reactions. Avoid concomitant use.
Phenobarbital, phenytoin: may alter pharmacokinetics of both drugs. Dosage adjustments may be needed.
Procyclidine: may increase procyclidine levels. Monitor patient for excessive anticholinergic effects.
Tryptophan: may increase risk of adverse reactions, such as nausea and dizziness. Avoid concomitant use.
Warfarin: increased risk of bleeding. Use concomitantly with caution.
Drug-herb. *St. John's wort:* May result in sedative-hypnotic intoxication with concurrent ingestion of the herb. Discourage using together.
Drug-lifestyle. *Alcohol use:* may alter psychomotor function. Discourage concomitant use.

Contraindications and precautions

- Contraindicated in patients taking MAO inhibitors.
- Use cautiously in pregnant or breast-feeding women; patients with a history of seizures or mania; patients with severe, concomitant systemic illness; and patients at risk for volume depletion.
- Safety of drug hasn't been established in children.

NURSING CONSIDERATIONS

Assessment

- Assess patient's depression before therapy and regularly thereafter.
- Be alert for adverse reactions and drug interactions.
- Evaluate patient's and family's knowledge of drug therapy.

Nursing diagnoses

- Disturbed thought processes related to depression
- Risk for injury related to drug-induced adverse CNS reactions
- Deficient knowledge related to drug therapy

Planning and implementation

- Don't administer drug with, or within 14 days of discontinuing, MAO inhibitor therapy. Allow at least 2 weeks after stopping paroxetine before starting an MAO inhibitor, as ordered.
- If signs of psychosis occur or increase, expect to reduce dosage.

ALERT Don't confuse paroxetine with paclitaxel or Paxil with Taxol.

Patient teaching

- Warn patient to avoid hazardous activities until CNS effects of drug are known.
- Tell patient that he may notice improvement in 1 to 4 weeks but that he must continue with prescribed regimen to obtain continued benefits.
- Tell patient to abstain from alcohol during drug therapy.

ALERT If patient wishes to switch from an SSRI to St. John's wort, tell him to wait a few weeks for the SSRI to fully leave his system before starting the herb. The exact time required will depend on which SSRI he takes.

Evaluation

- Patient's depression improves.
- Patient sustains no injuries because of drug-induced adverse CNS reactions.
- Patient and family state understanding of drug therapy.

pegaspargase (PEG-L-asparaginase)

(peg-AHS-per-jays)
Oncaspar

Pharmacologic class: modified version of enzyme L-asparaginase
Therapeutic class: antineoplastic
Pregnancy risk category: C

Indications and dosages

▶ **Acute lymphoblastic leukemia (ALL) in patients who need L-asparaginase but have developed hypersensitivity to native forms of L-asparaginase.** *Adults and children with body surface area of at least 0.6 m²:* 2,500 IU/m² I.M. or I.V. q 14 days. *Children with body surface area less than 0.6 m²:* 82.5 IU/kg I.M. or I.V. q 14 days.

How supplied

Injection: 750 IU/ml

Pharmacokinetics

Unknown.

Route	Onset	Peak	Duration
I.V., I.M.	Unknown	Unknown	Unknown

Pharmacodynamics

Chemical effect: exerts cytotoxic effect by inactivating amino acid asparagine. Asparagine is required by tumor cells to synthesize proteins. Because tumor cells can't synthesize their own asparagine, protein synthesis and, eventually, synthesis of DNA and RNA are inhibited.
Therapeutic effect: kills selected leukemic cells.

Adverse reactions

CNS: ***seizures,*** headache, paresthesia, ***status epilepticus,*** somnolence, coma, mental status changes, dizziness, emotional lability, mood changes, parkinsonism, confusion, disorientation, fatigue, malaise.
CV: hypotension, tachycardia, chest pain, subacute bacterial endocarditis, hypertension, edema.
EENT: epistaxis.
GI: nausea, vomiting, abdominal pain, anorexia, diarrhea, constipation, indigestion, flatulence, GI pain, mucositis, ***pancreatitis (sometimes fulminant and fatal),*** increased serum amylase and lipase levels, colitis, mouth tenderness.
GU: increased BUN level, increased creatinine level, increased urinary frequency, hematuria, severe hemorrhagic cystitis, renal dysfunction, ***renal failure.***
Hematologic: ***thrombosis, leukopenia, pancytopenia, agranulocytosis, thrombocytopenia,*** prolonged PT and PTT, decreased antithrombin III, ***disseminated intravascular coagulation,*** decreased fibrinogen, hemolytic anemia, increased thromboplastin, easy bruising, ecchymosis, ***hemorrhage*** (may be fatal).
Hepatic: jaundice, bilirubinemia, increased ALT and AST, ascites, hypoalbuminemia, fatty changes in liver, ***liver failure.***
Metabolic: hyperuricemia, hyponatremia, uric acid nephropathy, hypoproteinemia, proteinuria, weight loss, metabolic acidosis, increased blood ammonia level, hyperglycemia, hypoglycemia.
Musculoskeletal: arthralgia, myalgia, musculoskeletal pain, joint stiffness, cramps.
Respiratory: cough, ***severe bronchospasm,*** upper respiratory tract infection.
Skin: itching, alopecia, fever blister, purpura, white hands, urticaria, fungal changes, nail whiteness and ridging, erythema simplex, petechial rash, nighttime sweating.
Other: ***hypersensitivity reactions, including anaphylaxis,*** pain, fever, chills, peripheral edema; infection; ***sepsis; septic shock;*** injection pain or reaction; localized edema.

Interactions

Drug-drug. *Aspirin, dipyridamole, heparin, NSAIDs, warfarin:* imbalances in coagulation factors may occur, predisposing patient to bleeding or thrombosis. Use together cautiously.
Methotrexate: may interfere with action of methotrexate, which requires cell replication for its lethal effect. Monitor patient for decreased effectiveness.

Protein-bound drugs: serum protein depletion may increase toxicity of other drugs that bind to proteins. Monitor patient for toxicity. May interfere with enzymatic detoxification of other drugs, particularly in liver. Administer concomitantly with caution.

Contraindications and precautions

• Contraindicated in patients with pancreatitis or history of pancreatitis; in those who have had significant hemorrhagic events with previous L-asparaginase therapy; and in those with previous serious allergic reactions, such as generalized urticaria, bronchospasm, laryngeal edema, hypotension, or other unacceptable adverse reactions to pegaspargase.
• Drug isn't recommended for pregnant or breast-feeding women.
• Use cautiously in patients with liver dysfunction.

NURSING CONSIDERATIONS

Assessment

• Assess patient's condition before therapy and regularly thereafter.
• Monitor patient closely for hypersensitivity reactions, including life-threatening anaphylaxis, which may occur during therapy, especially in patient hypersensitive to other forms of L-asparaginase.
• Monitor patient's peripheral blood count and bone marrow, as ordered. A drop in circulating lymphoblasts is often noted after therapy begins. This may be accompanied by marked rise in serum uric acid levels.
• Monitor serum amylase levels, as ordered, to detect early evidence of pancreatitis. Monitor patient's blood glucose during therapy because hyperglycemia may occur.
• Monitor patient for liver dysfunction when pegaspargase is used with hepatotoxic chemotherapeutic agents.
• Drug may affect a number of plasma proteins; therefore, monitor fibrinogen, PT, and PTT. Question prescriber if not ordered.
• Be alert for adverse reactions and drug interactions.
• Evaluate patient's and family's knowledge of drug therapy.

Nursing diagnoses

• Ineffective health maintenance related to leukemia
• Ineffective protection related to drug-induced adverse hematologic reactions
• Deficient knowledge related to drug therapy

Planning and implementation

• Drug should be used as sole induction agent only in unusual situation when combined regimen that uses other chemotherapeutic drugs is inappropriate because of toxicity, because patient is refractory to other therapy, or because of other specific patient-related factors.
• Don't use drug that has been frozen. Although drug may not look different, its activity is destroyed by freezing. Obtain new dose from pharmacist.
• Avoid excessive agitation; don't shake. Keep refrigerated at 36° to 46° F (2° to 8° C). Don't use if cloudy, precipitated, or stored at room temperature for more than 48 hours. Discard unused portions. Use only one dose per vial; don't reenter vial. Don't save unused drug for later use.
• Hydrate patient before treatment. Hyperuricemia may result from rapid lysis of leukemic cells. Allopurinol may be ordered.
I.V. use: Give drug over 1 to 2 hours in 100 ml of normal saline solution or D_5W through infusion that is already running.
I.M. use: I.M. route is preferred over I.V. route because of its lower risk of hepatotoxicity, coagulopathy, and GI and renal disorders.
• Limit volume administered at single injection site to 2 ml. If volume is larger than 2 ml, use multiple injection sites.
• Keep patient under observation for 1 hour and keep resuscitation equipment (such as epinephrine, oxygen, and I.V. steroids) within reach to treat anaphylaxis. Moderate to life-threatening hypersensitivity reactions require discontinuation of drug.
• Handle and administer solution with care. Gloves are recommended. Avoid inhalation of vapors and contact with skin or mucous membranes, especially in eyes. If contact occurs, wash with copious amounts of water for at least 15 minutes.

Patient teaching

• Inform patient about hypersensitivity reactions and importance of alerting staff at once if they occur.
• Instruct patient not to take other drugs, including OTC preparations, until approved by prescriber. Concomitant use may increase risk of bleeding or may increase toxicity of other drugs.
• Instruct patient to report signs and symptoms of infection (fever, chills, and malaise) to prescriber because drug may suppress immune system.

Evaluation

• Patient responds well to therapy.
• Patient develops no serious complications caused by drug-induced adverse hematologic reactions.
• Patient and family state understanding of drug therapy.

pemoline

(PEH-moh-leen)

Cylert, Cylert Chewable

Pharmacologic class: oxazolidinedione derivative
Therapeutic class: analeptic
Controlled substance schedule: IV
Pregnancy risk category: B

Indications and dosages

▶ **Attention deficit hyperactivity disorder (ADHD).** *Children age 6 and older:* initially, 37.5 mg P.O. in morning. Increased by 18.75 mg/day q week, as necessary. Effective dosage range is 56.25 to 75 mg daily. Maximum dosage is 112.5 mg daily.

How supplied

Tablets: 18.75 mg, 37.5 mg, 75 mg
Tablets (chewable): 37.5 mg

Pharmacokinetics

Absorption: well absorbed.
Distribution: distribution is unknown. Drug is 50% protein-bound.
Metabolism: metabolized in liver.
Excretion: excreted in urine. *Half-life:* 12 hours.

Route	Onset	Peak	Duration
P.O.	Unknown	2-4 hr	Unknown

Pharmacodynamics

Chemical effect: may promote nerve impulse transmission by releasing stored norepinephrine from nerve terminals in brain, mainly in cerebral cortex and reticular activating system.
Therapeutic effect: promotes calmness in children with ADHD.

Adverse reactions

CNS: *insomnia,* malaise, dyskinetic movements, irritability, fatigue, mild depression, dizziness, headache, drowsiness, hallucinations, nervousness, ***seizures,*** *Tourette syndrome,* psychosis.
CV: *tachycardia.*
GI: anorexia, abdominal pain, nausea, diarrhea.
Hematologic: ***aplastic anemia.***
Hepatic: elevated liver enzyme levels, hepatitis, jaundice, ***hepatic failure.***
Skin: rash.

Interactions

Drug-drug. *Insulin, oral antidiabetics:* may decrease antidiabetic requirement. Monitor blood glucose levels.

Contraindications and precautions

• Contraindicated in patients hypersensitive to drug, in those who have idiosyncratic reactions to drug, and in those with hepatic dysfunction.
• Because of risk of hepatic failure, drug shouldn't be considered as first-line therapy.
• Use cautiously in patients with impaired renal function.

NURSING CONSIDERATIONS

Assessment

• Assess patient's condition, including liver function test results, before and during therapy.

• May precipitate Tourette syndrome in child. Monitor patient closely, especially at start of therapy.
• Monitor patient for blood or hepatic function changes and growth suppression.
• Drug should be stopped if significant hepatic dysfunction occurs.
• Drug may produce similar adverse reactions to amphetamines or methylphenidate, including lowered seizure threshold. Has potential for abuse and dependence.
• Evaluate patient's and family's knowledge of drug therapy.

Nursing diagnoses
• Risk for injury related to ADHD
• Disturbed sleep pattern related to drug-induced insomnia
• Deficient knowledge related to drug therapy

Planning and implementation
• Give drug at least 6 hours before bedtime.
ALERT Don't confuse pemoline with pelamine.

Patient teaching
• Warn patient and parent to avoid hazardous activities until effects of drug are known.
• Tell patient to report insomnia and other adverse effects.

Evaluation
• Patient shows less hyperactivity.
• Patient can sleep without difficulty throughout drug therapy.
• Patient and family state understanding of drug therapy.

penbutolol sulfate
(pen-BYOO-toh-lol SUL-fayt)
Levatol

Pharmacologic class: beta blocker
Therapeutic class: antihypertensive
Pregnancy risk category: C

Indications and dosages
▶ **Mild to moderate hypertension.** *Adults:* 20 mg P.O. once daily. May increase up to 80 mg/day. Full effect of drug may not be seen for 2 weeks. Usually given with other antihypertensives, such as thiazide diuretics.

How supplied
Tablets: 20 mg

Pharmacokinetics
Absorption: almost completely absorbed from GI tract.
Distribution: 80% to 98% of drug is bound to plasma proteins.
Metabolism: metabolized by liver.
Excretion: most metabolites excreted in urine. *Half-life:* 5 hours.

Route	Onset	Peak	Duration
P.O.	≤ 1 hr	1.5-3 hr	≤ 24 hr

Pharmacodynamics
Chemical effect: unknown.
Therapeutic effect: lowers blood pressure.

Adverse reactions
CNS: *dizziness,* vertigo, headache, fatigue, sleep disturbances.
CV: ***bradycardia,*** chest pain, ***heart failure.***
GI: gastric pain, flatulence, nausea, constipation, heartburn, vomiting, taste alteration, dry mouth.
GU: impotence, nocturia, urine retention.
Metabolic: hyperglycemia, hypoglycemia.
Respiratory: respiratory distress, shortness of breath.
Skin: pallor, flushing, rash.
Other: hypersensitivity reactions, decreased libido.

Interactions
Drug-drug. *Clonidine:* may cause paradoxical hypertension. May enhance rebound hypertension when clonidine is withdrawn. Monitor blood pressure closely.
Digoxin, diltiazem, verapamil: may cause additive depression of AV node conduction. Monitor patient closely.
Insulin, oral antidiabetics: hypoglycemic response to these drugs may be altered. Monitor patient closely.

NSAIDs: may decrease antihypertensive effects. Monitor patient.
Prazosin, terazosin: "first-dose" orthostatic hypotension may be enhanced. Monitor patient closely.
Sympathomimetics, including dobutamine, dopamine, isoproterenol, norepinephrine: decreased hypotensive response. Monitor patient.
Theophylline: may decrease bronchodilator effect. Monitor patient.

Contraindications and precautions

- Contraindicated in patients hypersensitive to drug or other beta blockers and in patients with sinus bradycardia, cardiogenic shock, overt cardiac failure, greater than first-degree heart block, or chronic bronchitis.
- Use cautiously in pregnant women, breast-feeding women, patients with heart failure controlled by drug therapy, and patients with a history of bronchospastic disease. Also use cautiously in diabetic patients because drug may mask signs and symptoms of hypoglycemia.
- Safety of drug hasn't been established in children.

NURSING CONSIDERATIONS

Assessment
- Assess patient's condition before therapy and regularly thereafter.
- Monitor ECG and heart rate and rhythm frequently.
- Be alert for adverse reactions and drug interactions.
- Evaluate patient's and family's knowledge of drug therapy.

Nursing diagnoses
- Risk for injury related to hypertension
- Ineffective tissue perfusion (cerebral, cardiopulmonary, peripheral) related to drug-induced adverse reactions
- Deficient knowledge related to drug therapy

Planning and implementation
- Always check patient's apical pulse before giving drug. If you detect extremes in pulse rates, withhold drug and call prescriber immediately.
- Don't stop therapy abruptly; sudden withdrawal of other beta blockers may precipitate angina and MI.
- To slowly discontinue drug, taper dosage over 1 to 2 weeks, especially in patient with ischemic heart disease. If symptoms of angina develop, notify prescriber immediately because drug should be immediately reinstituted, at least temporarily, and supportive care may be needed to control patient's unstable angina.

Patient teaching
- Tell patient to avoid abrupt discontinuation of therapy.
- Teach patient signs and symptoms of heart failure (edema and pulmonary congestion). Advise him to contact prescriber if these symptoms occur.
- Teach patient how to take his pulse and tell him to contact prescriber if pulse is slower than usual. Also tell him to report other adverse reactions.

Evaluation
- Patient's blood pressure is normal.
- Patient maintains adequate tissue perfusion.
- Patient and family state understanding of drug therapy.

penicillamine
(pen-ih-SIL-uh-meen)
Cuprimine, Depen

Pharmacologic class: chelating agent
Therapeutic class: heavy metal antagonist, antirheumatic
Pregnancy risk category: NR

Indications and dosages

▶ **Wilson's disease.** *Adults and children:* 250 mg P.O. q.i.d. 30 to 60 minutes before meals. Dosage adjusted to achieve urinary copper excretion of 0.5 to 1 mg/day.
▶ **Cystinuria.** *Adults:* 250 mg to 1 g P.O. q.i.d. before meals. Dosage adjusted to

achieve urinary cystine excretion of less than 100 mg daily when renal calculi are present or 100 to 200 mg daily when no calculi are present. Maximum dosage is 4 g/day.
Children: 30 mg/kg P.O. daily divided q.i.d. before meals. Dosage adjusted to achieve urinary cystine excretion of less than 100 mg daily when renal calculi are present or 100 to 200 mg daily when no calculi are present.
▶ **Rheumatoid arthritis.** *Adults:* initially, 125 to 250 mg P.O. daily, with increases of 125 to 250 mg q 1 to 3 months, if necessary. Maximum dosage is 1.5 g/day.

How supplied

Tablets (scored): 250 mg
Capsules: 125 mg, 250 mg

Pharmacokinetics

Absorption: well absorbed from GI tract.
Distribution: limited data available.
Metabolism: uncomplexed penicillamine is metabolized in liver to inactive disulfides.
Excretion: only small amount of penicillamine excreted unchanged; after 24 hours, 50% of drug excreted in urine, 20% in feces, and 30% is unaccounted for.

Route	Onset	Peak	Duration
P.O.	Unknown	1 hr	Unknown

Pharmacodynamics

Chemical effect: chelates heavy metals and may inhibit collagen formation; unknown for rheumatoid arthritis.
Therapeutic effect: chelates copper in Wilson's disease, combines with cystine to form complex more soluble than cystine alone, and relieves symptoms of rheumatoid arthritis.

Adverse reactions

EENT: tinnitus, *optic neuritis.*
GI: *anorexia, epigastric pain, nausea, vomiting, diarrhea, loss of taste or altered taste perception, stomatitis.*
GU: nephrotic syndrome, glomerulonephritis, proteinuria, hematuria.
Hematologic: ***leukopenia,*** *eosinophilia,* ***thrombocytopenia,*** *monocytosis,* ***agranulocytopenia, aplastic anemia,*** elevated sedimentation rate, lupuslike syndrome.
Hepatic: ***hepatotoxicity.***
Musculoskeletal: *arthralgia.*
Respiratory: *pneumonitis.*
Skin: alopecia; friability, especially at pressure spots; wrinkling; erythema; urticaria; ecchymoses.
Other: myasthenia gravis syndrome with long-term use, ***allergic reactions,*** *lymphadenopathy.*

Interactions

Drug-drug. *Antacids, oral iron:* decreased effectiveness of D-penicillamine. Give at least 2 hours apart.
Antimalaria drugs, cytotoxic drugs: increased risk of toxicity. Avoid combination.
Digoxin: may decrease digoxin effect. Dosage adjustment may be required.
Drug-food. *Any food:* delayed absorption of drug. Administer drug 1 hour before or 3 hours after meals.

Contraindications and precautions

- Contraindicated in patients with previous penicillamine-related aplastic anemia or granulocytosis, patients with rheumatoid arthritis and renal insufficiency, and pregnant patients except those with Wilson's disease.
- Use with extreme caution, if at all, in patients hypersensitive to penicillin.
- Safety of drug hasn't been established in breast-feeding women.

NURSING CONSIDERATIONS

Assessment

- Obtain history of patient's underlying condition before therapy.
- Monitor effectiveness by evaluating patient's urinary copper or cysteine excretion or improvement in rheumatoid arthritis.
- Monitor CBC and kidney and liver function every 2 weeks for first 6 months, and then monthly, as ordered.
- Monitor urinalysis regularly for protein loss.

• Check patient's range of motion and joint mobility.
• Be alert for adverse reactions and drug interactions.
• Evaluate patient's and family's knowledge of drug therapy.

Nursing diagnoses
• Impaired physical mobility related to Wilson's disease
• Impaired urinary elimination related to drug-induced renal dysfunction
• Deficient knowledge related to drug therapy

Planning and implementation
• Give dose on empty stomach to facilitate absorption, preferably 1 hour before or 3 hours after meals.
• Patient should receive supplemental pyridoxine daily.
• If patient has a skin reaction, give antihistamines, as prescribed. Handle patient carefully to avoid skin damage.
ALERT Report rash and fever (important signs of toxicity) to prescriber immediately.
• Withhold drug and notify prescriber if WBC count falls below 3,500/mm³ or platelet count falls below 100,000/mm³. A progressive decline in platelet or WBC count in three successive blood tests may necessitate temporary cessation of therapy, even if such counts are within normal limits.

Patient teaching
• Tell patient that therapeutic effect may be delayed up to 3 months in treatment of rheumatoid arthritis.
• Tell patient to maintain adequate fluid intake, especially at night.
• Advise patient to report early signs of granulocytopenia: fever, sore throat, chills, bruising, and prolonged bleeding time.
• Reassure patient that taste impairment usually resolves in 6 weeks without change in dosage.

Evaluation
• Patient reports increase in physical mobility.
• Patient maintains normal urinary elimination pattern.
• Patient and family state understanding of drug therapy.

penicillin G benzathine (benzylpenicillin benzathine)
(pen-ih-SIL-in gee BENZ-uh-theen)
Bicillin L-A, Permapen

Pharmacologic class: natural penicillin
Therapeutic class: antibiotic
Pregnancy risk category: B

Indications and dosages
▶ **Congenital syphilis.** *Children under age 2:* 50,000 units/kg I.M. as single dose.
▶ **Group A streptococcal upper respiratory tract infections.** *Adults:* 1.2 million units I.M. as single injection.
Children weighing more than 27 kg (59 lb): 900,000 units I.M. as single injection.
Children weighing less than 27 kg (59 lb): 300,000 to 600,000 units I.M. as single injection.
▶ **Prophylaxis of poststreptococcal rheumatic fever.** *Adults and children:* 1.2 million units I.M. once monthly or 600,000 units twice monthly.
▶ **Syphilis of less than 1 year's duration.** *Adults:* 2.4 million units I.M. as single dose.
▶ **Syphilis of more than 1 year's duration.** *Adults:* 2.4 million units I.M. weekly for 3 successive weeks.

How supplied
Injection: 300,000 units/ml, 600,000 units/ml

Pharmacokinetics
Absorption: absorbed slowly from I.M. injection site.
Distribution: distributed widely into synovial, pleural, pericardial, and ascitic fluids; bile; and liver, skin, lungs, kidneys, muscle, intestines, tonsils, maxillary sinuses, saliva, and erythrocytes. CSF penetration is poor but enhanced in patients with inflamed meninges. Drug is 45% to 68% protein-bound.
Metabolism: between 16% and 30% of drug is metabolized to inactive compounds.

Excretion: excreted primarily in urine. *Half-life:* 30 to 60 minutes.

Route	Onset	Peak	Duration
I.M.	Unknown	13-24 hr	1-4 wk

Pharmacodynamics

Chemical effect: inhibits cell wall synthesis during microorganism multiplication; bacteria resist penicillins by producing penicillinases, enzymes that convert penicillins to inactive penicilloic acid. Penicillin G benzathine resists these enzymes.
Therapeutic effect: kills susceptible bacteria, such as most non-penicillinase–producing strains of gram-positive and gram-negative aerobic cocci; spirochetes; and some gram-positive aerobic and anaerobic bacilli.

Adverse reactions

CNS: neuropathy, ***seizures.***
Hematologic: eosinophilia, hemolytic anemia, ***thrombocytopenia, leukopenia.***
Other: hypersensitivity reactions (maculopapular and ***exfoliative dermatitis,*** chills, fever, edema, ***anaphylaxis***), pain, sterile abscess at injection site.

Interactions

Drug-drug. *Colestipol:* decreased serum levels of penicillin G benzathine. Give penicillin 1 hour before or 4 hours after colestipol.
Probenecid: increased blood levels of penicillin. Probenecid may be used for this purpose.

Contraindications and precautions

- Contraindicated in patients hypersensitive to drug or other penicillins.
- Use cautiously in pregnant women and patients with other drug allergies, especially to cephalosporins.
- Drug appears in breast milk; use in breast-feeding women may sensitize infant to penicillin and cause some adverse effects.

NURSING CONSIDERATIONS

Assessment

- Assess patient's infection before therapy and regularly thereafter.
- Before giving drug, ask patient about allergic reactions to penicillin. However, negative history of penicillin allergy is no guarantee against future allergic reaction.
- Obtain specimen for culture and sensitivity tests before giving first dose. Therapy may begin pending results.
- Be alert for adverse reactions and drug interactions.
- Observe patient closely. Large doses and prolonged therapy raise the risk of bacterial or fungal superinfection, especially in elderly, debilitated, or immunosuppressed patients.
- Evaluate patient's and family's knowledge of drug therapy.

Nursing diagnoses

- Infection related to presence of bacteria
- Ineffective protection related to risk of hypersensitivity reactions to drug
- Deficient knowledge related to drug therapy

Planning and implementation

- Shake drug well before injection.
- Never give drug I.V.; doing so has caused cardiac arrest and death.
- Inject deep into upper outer quadrant of buttocks in adult; in midlateral thigh in infant and young child. Avoid injection into or near major nerves or blood vessels to prevent neurovascular damage.
- Give drug at least 1 hour before bacteriostatic antibiotics.
- Drug's extremely slow absorption makes allergic reactions difficult to treat. Stop drug immediately if patient develops signs of anaphylactic shock (rapidly developing dyspnea and hypotension). Notify prescriber and prepare for immediate treatment with epinephrine, corticosteroids, antihistamines, and other resuscitative measures as indicated.

ALERT Be aware of the various preparations of penicillin. They aren't interchangable.

Patient teaching

- Tell patient to call prescriber if rash, fever, or chills develop.
- Warn patient that injection may be painful but that ice applied to site may ease discomfort.

☑ **Evaluation**

- Patient is free from infection.
- Patient shows no signs of allergy.
- Patient and family state understanding of drug therapy.

penicillin G potassium (benzylpenicillin potassium)

(pen-ih-SIL-in gee poh-TAH-see-um)
Megacillin ♦, Pfizerpen

Pharmacologic class: natural penicillin
Therapeutic class: antibiotic
Pregnancy risk category: B

Indications and dosages

▶ **Moderate to severe systemic infections.** *Adults:* 500,000 units P.O. q 6 to 8 hours; 12 to 24 million units I.M. or I.V. daily in divided doses q 4 hours.
Children: 25,000 to 90,000 units/kg/day P.O. in three to six divided doses; or 25,000 to 300,000 units/kg I.M. or I.V. daily in divided doses q 4 hours.

How supplied

Tablets: 500,000 units ♦
Oral suspension: 250,000 units ♦, 500,000 units ♦
Injection: 1 million units, 5 million units, 10 million units, 20 million units

Pharmacokinetics

Absorption: only 15% to 30% of P.O. dose is absorbed; remainder is hydrolyzed by gastric secretions. Food in stomach reduces rate and extent of absorption. Absorbed rapidly from I.M. injection site.
Distribution: distributed widely into synovial, pleural, pericardial, and ascitic fluids; bile; and liver, skin, lungs, kidneys, muscle, intestines, tonsils, maxillary sinuses, saliva, and erythrocytes. CSF penetration is poor but is enhanced in patients with inflamed meninges. Drug is 45% to 68% protein-bound.
Metabolism: hepatic metabolism accounts for less than 30% of biotransformation of penicillin.
Excretion: excreted primarily in urine. *Half-life:* 30 to 60 minutes.

Route	Onset	Peak	Duration
P.O.	Unknown	0.5-1 hr	Unknown
I.V.	Immediate	Immediate	Unknown
I.M.	Unknown	15-30 min	Unknown

Pharmacodynamics

Chemical effect: inhibits cell wall synthesis during microorganism multiplication; bacteria resist penicillins by producing penicillinases, enzymes that convert penicillins to inactive penicilloic acid. Penicillin G potassium resists these enzymes.
Therapeutic effect: kills susceptible bacteria, such as most nonpenicillinase-producing strains of gram-positive and gram-negative aerobic cocci; spirochetes; and certain gram-positive aerobic and anaerobic bacilli.

Adverse reactions

CNS: neuropathy, ***seizures.***
Hematologic: hemolytic anemia, ***thrombocytopenia, leukopenia.***
Metabolic: severe potassium poisoning with high doses (hyperreflexia, ***seizures, coma***).
Other: hypersensitivity reactions (rash, urticaria, maculopapular eruptions, ***exfoliative dermatitis,*** chills, fever, edema, ***anaphylaxis***), overgrowth of nonsusceptible organisms, thrombophlebitis, pain at injection site.

Interactions

Drug-drug. *Colestipol:* decreased serum levels of penicillin G potassium. Give penicillin 1 hour before or 4 hours after colestipol.
Potassium-sparing diuretics: possible increased risk of hyperkalemia. Don't use together.
Probenecid: increased blood levels of penicillin. Probenecid may be used for this purpose.

Contraindications and precautions

- Contraindicated in patients hypersensitive to drug or other penicillins.
- Use cautiously in pregnant women and patients with other drug allergies, especially to cephalosporins.

• Drug appears in breast milk; use in breast-feeding women may sensitize infant to penicillin and cause some adverse effects.

NURSING CONSIDERATIONS

Assessment
• Assess patient's infection before therapy and regularly thereafter.
• Before giving, ask patient about any allergic reactions to penicillin. However, negative history of penicillin allergy is no guarantee against future allergic reaction.
• Obtain specimen for culture and sensitivity tests before first dose. Therapy may begin pending results.
• Be alert for adverse reactions and drug interactions.
• Observe patient closely. Large doses and prolonged therapy raise the risk of bacterial or fungal superinfection, especially in elderly, debilitated, or immunosuppressed patients.
• Evaluate patient's and family's knowledge of drug therapy.

Nursing diagnoses
• Infection related to presence of bacteria
• Ineffective protection related to risk of hypersensitivity reactions to drug
• Deficient knowledge related to drug therapy

Planning and implementation
• Reconstitute vials with sterile water for injection, D_5W, or normal saline solution for injection. Volume of diluent varies with manufacturer.
• Give drug at least 1 hour before bacteriostatic antibiotics.
ALERT Be aware of the various preparations of penicillin. They aren't interchangable.
• Monitor blood levels in patients taking large doses. High levels may lead to seizures. Take precautions.
P.O. use: Give drug 1 to 2 hours before or 2 to 3 hours after meals. Drug may cause GI disturbances. Food may interfere with absorption.
I.V. use: Use continuous I.V. infusion when large doses are required (10 million units or more). Otherwise, give via intermittent I.V. infusion over 1 to 2 hours.
– Aminoglycosides are physically and chemically incompatible with drug. Administer separately.
I.M. use: Administer drug deep into large muscle; may be painful.

Patient teaching
• Tell patient to take drug exactly as prescribed, even after he feels better.
• Warn patient never to use leftover penicillin for a new illness or to share penicillin with family and friends.
• Tell patient to call prescriber if rash, fever, or chills develop.
• Warn patient that I.M. injection may be painful but that ice applied to site may ease discomfort.

Evaluation
• Patient is free from infection.
• Patient shows no signs of allergy.
• Patient and family state understanding of drug therapy.

penicillin G procaine (benzylpenicillin procaine)
(pen-ih-SIL-in gee PROH-kayn)
Ayercillin♦, Crysticillin 300 AS, Pfizerpen-AS, Wycillin

Pharmacologic class: natural penicillin
Therapeutic class: antibiotic
Pregnancy risk category: B

Indications and dosages
▶ **Moderate to severe systemic infections.** *Adults:* 600,000 to 1.2 million units I.M. daily in single dose.
Children over age 1 month: 25,000 to 50,000 units/kg I.M. daily in single dose.
▶ **Uncomplicated gonorrhea.** *Adults and children over age 12:* 1 g probenecid; after 30 minutes, 4.8 million units of penicillin G procaine I.M., divided between two injection sites.
▶ **Pneumococcal pneumonia.** *Adults and children over age 12:* 600,000 units to 1.2 million units I.M. daily for 7 to 10 days.

How supplied

Injection: 300,000 units/ml, 500,000 units/ml, 600,000 units/ml

Pharmacokinetics

Absorption: absorbed slowly.
Distribution: distributed widely into synovial, pleural, pericardial, and ascitic fluids; bile; and liver, skin, lungs, kidneys, muscle, intestines, tonsils, maxillary sinuses, saliva, and erythrocytes. CSF penetration usually poor, but enhanced in patients with inflamed meninges. Drug is 45% to 68% protein-bound.
Metabolism: from 16% to 30% metabolized to inactive compounds.
Excretion: excreted primarily in urine. *Half-life:* 30 to 60 minutes.

Route	Onset	Peak	Duration
I.M.	Unknown	1-4 hr	1-2 days

Pharmacodynamics

Chemical effect: inhibits cell wall synthesis during microorganism multiplication; bacteria resist penicillins by producing penicillinases, enzymes that convert penicillins to inactive penicilloic acid. Penicillin G procaine resists these enzymes.
Therapeutic effect: kills susceptible bacteria, such as most nonpenicillinase-producing strains of gram-positive and gram-negative aerobic cocci, spirochetes, and some gram-positive aerobic and anaerobic bacilli.

Adverse reactions

CNS: ***seizures.***
Hematologic: ***thrombocytopenia,*** hemolytic anemia, ***leukopenia.***
Musculoskeletal: arthralgia.
Other: hypersensitivity reactions (rash, urticaria, chills, fever, edema, prostration, ***anaphylaxis***), overgrowth of nonsusceptible organisms.

Interactions

Drug-drug. *Colestipol:* decreased serum levels of penicillin G procaine. Give penicillin 1 hour before or 4 hours after colestipol.
Probenecid: increased blood levels of penicillin. Probenecid may be used for this purpose.

Contraindications and precautions

- Contraindicated in patients hypersensitive to drug or other penicillins.
- Use cautiously in pregnant women and in patients with other drug allergies, especially to cephalosporins.
- Drug appears in breast milk; use in breast-feeding women may sensitize infant to penicillin and cause some adverse effects.

NURSING CONSIDERATIONS

Assessment

- Assess patient's infection before therapy and regularly thereafter.
- Before giving, ask patient about allergic reactions to penicillin. However, negative history of penicillin allergy is no guarantee against future allergic reaction.
- Obtain specimen for culture and sensitivity tests before giving first dose. Therapy may begin pending results.
- Be alert for adverse reactions and drug interactions.
- Observe patient closely. Large doses and prolonged therapy raise the risk of bacterial or fungal superinfection, especially in elderly, debilitated, or immunosuppressed patients.
- Evaluate patient's and family's knowledge of drug therapy.

Nursing diagnoses

- Infection related to presence of bacteria
- Ineffective protection related to risk of hypersensitivity reactions to drug
- Deficient knowledge related to drug therapy

Planning and implementation

- Shake drug well before injection.
- Never give I.V.; doing so has caused cardiac arrest and death.
- Inject deep into upper outer quadrant of buttocks in adults; in midlateral thigh in infants and small children. Avoid injection into or near major nerves or blood vessels to prevent neurovascular damage.
- Give penicillin G procaine at least 1 hour before bacteriostatic antibiotics.
- Drug's extremely slow absorption makes allergic reactions difficult to treat. Stop drug immediately if patient develops signs of

anaphylactic shock (rapidly developing dyspnea and hypotension). Notify prescriber and prepare for immediate treatment with epinephrine, corticosteroids, antihistamines, and other resuscitative measures as indicated.

ALERT Be aware of the various preparations of penicillin. They aren't interchangable.

Patient teaching

- Tell patient to call prescriber if rash, fever, or chills develop.
- Warn patient that injection may be painful but that ice applied to site may ease discomfort.

Evaluation

- Patient is free from infection.
- Patient shows no signs of allergy.
- Patient and family state understanding of drug therapy.

penicillin G sodium (benzylpenicillin sodium)

(pen-ih-SIL-in gee SOH-dee-um)

Crystapen ♦

Pharmacologic class: natural penicillin
Therapeutic class: antibiotic
Pregnancy risk category: B

Indications and dosages

▶ **Moderate to severe systemic infections.** *Adults:* 12 to 24 million units daily I.M. or I.V. in divided doses q 4 to 6 hours.
Children: 25,000 to 300,000 units/kg daily I.M. or I.V. in divided doses q 4 to 6 hours.

▶ **Endocarditis prophylaxis for dental surgery.** *Adults and children weighing more than 27 kg (59 lb):* 2 million units I.V. or I.M. 30 to 60 minutes before procedure; then 1 million units 6 hours later.

How supplied

Injection: 5 million-units vial

Pharmacokinetics

Absorption: absorbed rapidly from I.M. injection site.
Distribution: distributed widely into synovial, pleural, pericardial, and ascitic fluids; bile; and liver, skin, lungs, kidneys, muscle, intestines, tonsils, maxillary sinuses, saliva, and erythrocytes. CSF penetration is poor but is enhanced in patients with inflamed meninges. Drug is 45% to 68% protein-bound.
Metabolism: between 16% and 30% of drug is metabolized to inactive compounds.
Excretion: excreted primarily in urine. *Half-life:* 30 to 60 minutes.

Route	Onset	Peak	Duration
I.V.	Immediate	Immediate	Unknown
I.M.	Unknown	15-30 min	Unknown

Pharmacodynamics

Chemical effect: inhibits cell wall synthesis during microorganism multiplication; bacteria resist penicillins by producing penicillinases, enzymes that convert penicillins to inactive penicilloic acid.Penicillin G sodium resists these enzymes.
Therapeutic effect: kills susceptible bacteria, such as most non-penicillinase-producing strains of gram-positive and gram-negative aerobic cocci, spirochetes, and some gram-positive aerobic and anaerobic bacilli.

Adverse reactions

CNS: neuropathy, ***seizures.***
Hematologic: hemolytic anemia, ***leukopenia, thrombocytopenia.***
Musculoskeletal: arthralgia.
Other: hypersensitivity reactions (***exfoliative dermatitis,*** urticaria, ***anaphylaxis***), overgrowth of nonsusceptible organisms, vein irritation, thrombophlebitis, pain at injection site.

Interactions

Drug-drug. *Colestipol:* decreased serum levels of penicillin G sodium. Give penicillin 1 hour before or 4 hours after colestipol.
Probenecid: increased blood levels of penicillin. Probenecid may be used for this purpose.

Contraindications and precautions

- Contraindicated in patients hypersensitive to drug or other penicillins.

• Use cautiously in pregnant women and patients with other drug allergies, especially to cephalosporins.
• Drug appears in breast milk; use in breast-feeding women may sensitize infant to penicillin and cause some adverse effects.

NURSING CONSIDERATIONS

Assessment
• Assess patient's infection before therapy and regularly thereafter.
• Before giving, ask patient about allergic reactions to penicillin. However, negative history of penicillin allergy is no guarantee against future allergic reaction.
• Obtain specimen for culture and sensitivity tests before first dose. Therapy may begin pending results.
• Be alert for adverse reactions and drug interactions.
• Observe patient closely. Large doses and prolonged therapy raise the risk of bacterial or fungal superinfection, especially in elderly, debilitated, or immunosuppressed patients.
• Evaluate patient's and family's knowledge of drug therapy.

Nursing diagnoses
• Infection related to presence of bacteria
• Ineffective protection related to risk of hypersensitivity reactions to drug
• Deficient knowledge related to drug therapy

Planning and implementation
I.V. use: Reconstitute vials with sterile water for injection, normal saline solution for injection, or D_5W. Volume of diluent varies with manufacturer and concentration needed.
– For patient receiving 10 million units of drug or more daily, dilute in 1 to 2 liters of compatible solution and administer over 24 hours. Otherwise, give by intermittent I.V. infusion: Dilute drug in 50 to 100 ml and give over 1 to 2 hours q 4 to 6 hours.
– In neonate or child, give divided doses usually over 15 to 30 minutes.
– Aminoglycosides are physically and chemically incompatible with drug. Administer separately.

I.M. use: Give drug deep in upper outer quadrant of buttocks in adult; in midlateral thigh in young child. Don't massage injection site. Avoid injection near major nerves or blood vessels to prevent neurovascular damage.

ALERT Don't give by S.C. route.
• Give penicillin G sodium at least 1 hour before bacteriostatic antibiotics.

ALERT Be aware of the various preparations of penicillin. They aren't interchangable.
• Monitor blood levels in patients taking large doses. High levels may lead to seizures. Take precautions.

Patient teaching
• Tell patient to report discomfort at I.V. site
• Warn patient that I.M. injection may be painful but that ice applied to site may ease discomfort.

Evaluation
• Patient is free from infection.
• Patient shows no signs of allergy.
• Patient and family state understanding of drug therapy.

penicillin V (phenoxymethylpenicillin)
(pen-ih-SIL-in VEE)

penicillin V potassium (phenoxymethylpenicillin potassium)
Abbocillin VK◇, Apo-Pen-VK◇, Beepen-VK, Betapen-VK, Cilicaine VK◇, Ledercillin VK, Nadopen-V-200♦, Nadopen-V 400♦, Nadopen-V♦, Novo-Pen-VK♦, Nu-Pen VK♦, Pen Vee, Pen Vee K, PVF K♦, PVK◇, V-Cillin K, Veetids**

Pharmacologic class: natural penicillin
Therapeutic class: antibiotic
Pregnancy risk category: B

Indications and dosages
▶ **Mild to moderate systemic infections.** *Adults:* 125 to 500 mg (200,000 to 800,000 units) P.O. q 6 hours.

Children: 15 to 50 mg/kg (25,000 to 90,000 units/kg) P.O. daily, in divided doses q 6 to 8 hours.

▶ **Endocarditis prophylaxis for dental surgery.** *Adults:* 2 g P.O. 30 to 60 minutes before procedure; then 500 mg P.O. q 6 hours for eight doses.

Children weighing less than 30 kg (66 lb): half of adult dose.

How supplied

penicillin V

Tablets: 250 mg, 500 mg

Oral suspension: 125 mg/5 ml, 250 mg/5 ml (after reconstitution)

penicillin V potassium

Tablets: 125 mg, 250 mg, 500 mg

Tablets (film-coated): 250 mg, 500 mg

Capsules: 250 mg ◊

Oral suspension: 125 mg/5 ml, 250 mg/5 ml (after reconstitution)

Pharmacokinetics

Absorption: about 60% to 75% absorbed from GI tract.

Distribution: distributed widely into synovial, pleural, pericardial, and ascitic fluids; bile; and liver, skin, lungs, kidneys, muscle, intestines, tonsils, maxillary sinuses, saliva, and erythrocytes. CSF penetration is poor but is enhanced in patients with inflamed meninges. It's 75% to 89% protein-bound.

Metabolism: between 35% and 70% metabolized to inactive compounds.

Excretion: excreted primarily in urine. *Half-life:* 30 minutes.

Route	Onset	Peak	Duration
P.O.	Unknown	30-60 min	Unknown

Pharmacodynamics

Chemical effect: inhibits cell wall synthesis during microorganism multiplication; bacteria resist penicillins by producing penicillinases. Penicillin V resists those enzymes.

Therapeutic effect: kills susceptible bacteria, such as most nonpenicillinase-producing strains of gram-positive and gram-negative aerobic cocci, spirochetes, and some gram-positive aerobic and anaerobic bacilli.

Adverse reactions

CNS: neuropathy.

GI: *epigastric distress,* vomiting, diarrhea, *nausea.*

Hematologic: eosinophilia, hemolytic anemia, ***leukopenia, thrombocytopenia.***

Other: hypersensitivity reactions (rash, urticaria, chills, fever, edema, ***anaphylaxis***), overgrowth of nonsusceptible organisms.

Interactions

Drug-drug. *Oral contraceptives containing estrogen:* decreased effectiveness of oral contraceptive. Monitor patient for breakthrough bleeding.

Probenecid: increased blood levels of penicillin. Probenecid may be used for this purpose.

Contraindications and precautions

- Contraindicated in patients hypersensitive to drug or other penicillins.
- Use cautiously in pregnant women and patients with other drug allergies, especially to cephalosporins.
- Drug appears in breast milk; use in breast-feeding women may sensitize infant to penicillin and cause some adverse effects.

NURSING CONSIDERATIONS

Assessment

- Assess patient's infection before therapy and regularly thereafter.
- Before giving drug, ask patient about any allergic reactions to penicillin. However, negative history of penicillin allergy is no guarantee against future allergic reaction.
- Obtain specimen for culture and sensitivity tests before giving first dose. Therapy may begin pending results.
- As ordered, periodically assess renal and hematopoietic function in patient receiving long-term therapy.
- Be alert for adverse reactions and drug interactions.
- Observe patient closely. Large doses and prolonged therapy raise the risk of bacterial or fungal superinfection, especially in elderly, debilitated, or immunosuppressed patients.

• Evaluate patient's and family's knowledge of drug therapy.

Nursing diagnoses

• Infection related to presence of bacteria
• Ineffective protection related to risk of hypersensitivity reactions to drug
• Deficient knowledge related to drug therapy

Planning and implementation

• Give drug at least 1 hour before bacteriostatic antibiotics.
• American Heart Association considers amoxicillin the preferred drug for endocarditis prophylaxis because GI absorption is better and serum levels are sustained longer. Penicillin V is considered an alternative choice.
ALERT Be aware of the various preparations of penicillin. They aren't interchangable.

Patient teaching

• Tell patient to take drug exactly as prescribed, even after he feels better.
• Tell patient that drug may be taken without regard to meals. However, if GI disturbances occur, drug may be taken with meals.
• Warn patient never to use leftover penicillin V for new illness or to share penicillin with family and friends.
• Tell patient to call prescriber if rash, fever, or chills develop.

Evaluation

• Patient is free from infection.
• Patient shows no signs of allergy.
• Patient and family state understanding of drug therapy.

pentamidine isethionate

(pen-TAM-eh-deen ighs-eh-THIGH-oh-nayt)
NebuPent, Pentacarinat, Pentam 300, Pneumopent

Pharmacologic class: diamidine derivative
Therapeutic class: antiprotozoal
Pregnancy risk category: C

Indications and dosages

▶ ***Pneumocystis carinii* pneumonia.** *Adults and children:* 4 mg/kg I.V. or I.M. once daily for 14 to 21 days.
▶ **Prevention of *P. carinii* pneumonia in high-risk patients.** *Adults:* 300 mg by inhalation (using Respirgard II nebulizer) once q 4 weeks.

How supplied

Injection: 300-mg vial
Aerosol: 300-mg vial

Pharmacokinetics

Absorption: absorption is limited after aerosol administration. Unknown after I.M. administration.
Distribution: drug appears to be extensively tissue-bound. CNS penetration is poor. Extent of plasma protein–binding is unknown.
Metabolism: unknown.
Excretion: excreted unchanged in urine. *Half-life:* varies according to route of administration: 9 to 13¼ hours for I.M., about 6½ hours for I.V., and unknown for aerosol.

Route	Onset	Peak	Duration
I.V.	Unknown	Immediate	Unknown
I.M.	Unknown	0.5-1 hr	Unknown
Aerosol	Unknown	Unknown	Unknown

Pharmacodynamics

Chemical effect: interferes with organism's biosynthesis of DNA, RNA, phospholipids, and proteins.
Therapeutic effect: hinders growth of susceptible organisms, such as *P. carinii* and *Trypanosoma.*

Adverse reactions

CNS: confusion, hallucinations.
CV: ***hypotension,*** tachycardia.
GI: nausea, anorexia, metallic taste.
GU: *elevated serum creatinine levels,* renal toxicity, ***acute renal failure.***
Hematologic: ***leukopenia, thrombocytopenia, anemia.***
Hepatic: elevated liver enzyme levels.

Metabolic: ***hypoglycemia,*** hyperglycemia, hypocalcemia.
Respiratory: cough, ***bronchospasm.***
Skin: rash, facial flushing, pruritus, ***Stevens-Johnson syndrome.***
Other: fever, *sterile abscess, pain and induration* at injection site.

Interactions

Drug-drug. *Aminoglycosides, amphotericin B, capreomycin, cisplatin, colistin, methoxyflurane, polymyxin B, vancomycin:* increased risk of nephrotoxicity. Monitor patient closely.

Contraindications and precautions

- Contraindicated in patients with history of anaphylactic reaction to drug.
- Drug isn't recommended for breast-feeding women.
- Use cautiously in pregnant women and patients with hypertension, hypotension, hypoglycemia, hypocalcemia, leukopenia, thrombocytopenia, anemia, or hepatic or renal dysfunction.

NURSING CONSIDERATIONS

Assessment

- Assess patient's infection before therapy and regularly thereafter.
- Monitor blood glucose, serum calcium, serum creatinine, and BUN levels daily. After parenteral administration, blood glucose level may decrease initially; hypoglycemia may be severe in 5% to 10% of patients. This may be followed by hyperglycemia and insulin-dependent diabetes mellitus, which may be permanent.
- Closely monitor blood pressure during I.V. administration.
- Be alert for adverse reactions and drug interactions.
- Evaluate patient's and family's knowledge of drug therapy.

Nursing diagnoses

- Infection related to presence of organisms
- Risk for injury related to drug-induced adverse CNS reactions
- Deficient knowledge related to drug therapy

Planning and implementation

I.V. use: Reconstitute drug with 3 ml of sterile water for injection; then dilute in 50 to 250 ml of D_5W. Inject over at least 1 hour.
– To minimize hypotension, infuse drug slowly with patient lying down.
I.M. use: Reconstitute drug with 3 ml of sterile water for solution containing 100 mg/ml; administer deeply. Expect pain and induration.

- In patient with AIDS, pentamidine may produce less severe adverse reactions than co-trimoxazole, the alternative treatment, and may be treatment of choice.

Aerosol use: Administer aerosol form only by Respirgard II nebulizer manufactured by Marquest. Dosage recommendations are based on particle size and delivery rate of this device.
– To use aerosol, mix contents of one vial in 6 ml of sterile water for injection. Don't use normal saline solution; it will cause precipitation. Don't mix with other drugs.
– Don't use low-pressure (below 20 psi) compressors. The flow rate should be 5 to 7 liters/minute from 40- to 50-psi air or oxygen source.

Patient teaching

- Instruct patient to use aerosol device until chamber is empty, which may take up to 45 minutes.
- Warn patient that I.M. injection is painful. However, application of warm soaks is helpful.
- Stress need to report light-headedness or signs and symptoms of hypoglycemia immediately.

Evaluation

- Patient is free from infection.
- Patient sustains no injuries because of drug-induced adverse CNS reactions.
- Patient and family state understanding of drug therapy.

pentazocine hydrochloride
(pen-TAZ-oh-seen high-droh-KLOR-ighd)
Fortral ♦ ◇, Talwin

pentazocine hydrochloride and naloxone hydrochloride
Talwin NX

pentazocine lactate
Fortral ◇, Talwin

Pharmacologic class: narcotic agonist-antagonist, opioid partial agonist
Therapeutic class: analgesic, adjunct to anesthesia
Controlled substance schedule: IV
Pregnancy risk category: NR

Indications and dosages

▶ **Moderate to severe pain.** *Adults:* 50 to 100 mg P.O. q 3 to 4 hours, p.r.n. Maximum oral dosage is 600 mg/day. Or, 30 mg I.M., I.V., or S.C. q 3 to 4 hours, p.r.n. Maximum parenteral dosage is 360 mg/day. Single doses above 30 mg I.V. or 60 mg I.M. or S.C. aren't recommended.

▶ **Labor.** *Adults:* 30 mg I.M. or 20 mg I.V. q 2 to 3 hours when contractions become regular.

How supplied

pentazocine hydrochloride
Tablets: 25 mg ◇, 50 mg ♦ ◇
pentazocine hydrochloride and naloxone hydrochloride
Tablets: 50 mg pentazocine hydrochloride and 500 mcg naloxone hydrochloride
pentazocine lactate
Injection: 30 mg/ml

Pharmacokinetics

Absorption: well absorbed after P.O. or parenteral administration, although P.O. form undergoes first-pass metabolism in liver and less than 20% of dose reaches systemic circulation unchanged. Bioavailability is increased in patients with hepatic dysfunction; patients with cirrhosis absorb 60% to 70% of drug.
Distribution: appears to be widely distributed throughout body.
Metabolism: metabolized in liver. Metabolism may be prolonged in patients with impaired hepatic function.
Excretion: excreted primarily in urine, with very small amounts excreted in feces. *Half-life:* 2 to 3 hours.

Route	Onset	Peak	Duration
P.O.	15-30 min	60-90 min	2-3 hr
I.V.	2-3 min	15-30 min	2-3 hr
I.M., S.C.	15-20 min	30-60 min	2-3 hr

Pharmacodynamics

Chemical effect: binds with opioid receptors at many sites in CNS, altering pain response by unknown mechanism.
Therapeutic effect: relieves pain.

Adverse reactions

CNS: *sedation,* visual disturbances, hallucinations, drowsiness, *dizziness, light-headedness,* confusion, *euphoria,* headache, psychotomimetic effects.
CV: hypotension, ***shock.***
EENT: dry mouth, dysgeusia.
GI: *nausea, vomiting,* constipation.
GU: urine retention.
Respiratory: ***respiratory depression.***
Skin: induration, nodules, sloughing, and sclerosis of injection site.
Other: hypersensitivity reactions ***(anaphylaxis),*** physical and psychological dependence.

Interactions

Drug-drug. *CNS depressants:* additive effects. Use together cautiously.
Narcotic analgesics: possible decreased analgesic effect. Avoid concomitant use.
Drug-lifestyle. *Alcohol use:* additive effects. Discourage concomitant use.
Smoking: may increase requirements for pentazocine. Monitor drug's effectiveness.

Contraindications and precautions

- Contraindicated in patients hypersensitive to drug or its components.
- Drug isn't recommended for children under age 12.

• Use cautiously in pregnant or breast-feeding women and in patients with hepatic or renal disease, acute MI, head injury, increased intracranial pressure, or respiratory depression.

NURSING CONSIDERATIONS

Assessment
• Assess patient's pain before and after drug administration.
• Monitor vital signs closely, especially respirations.
• Be alert for adverse reactions and drug interactions.
• Evaluate patient's and family's knowledge of drug therapy.

Nursing diagnoses
• Acute pain related to condition
• Ineffective breathing pattern related to drug-induced respiratory depression
• Deficient knowledge related to drug therapy

Planning and implementation
P.O. use: Talwin NX, the oral pentazocine available in the U.S., contains the narcotic antagonist naloxone, which prevents illicit I.V. use.
I.V. use: Give drug by direct I.V. injection. Administer slowly. Don't mix in same syringe with aminophylline, barbiturates, or other alkaline substances.
I.M. and S.C. use: Rotate injection sites to minimize tissue irritation. If possible, avoid giving by S.C. route.
• Drug has narcotic antagonist properties. May precipitate withdrawal syndrome in narcotic-dependent patient.
• Dependence may occur with prolonged use.
ALERT Hold drug and notify prescriber if respiratory rate drops significantly. Have naloxone readily available to reverse respiratory depression.
• Drug may interfere with certain laboratory tests for urinary 17-hydroxycorticosteroids.

Patient teaching
• Caution ambulatory patient about getting out of bed or walking. Warn outpatient to avoid hazardous activities until CNS effects of drug are known.
• Warn patient about the risk of dependence.

Evaluation
• Patient is free from pain.
• Patient maintains respiratory rate and pattern within normal limits.
• Patient and family state understanding of drug therapy.

pentobarbital (pentobarbitone)
(pen-toh-BAR-beh-tol)
Nembutal* **

pentobarbital sodium
Carbrital ◇, Nembutal Sodium*, Nova Rectal ♦, Novopentobarb ♦

Pharmacologic class: barbiturate
Therapeutic class: anticonvulsant, sedative-hypnotic
Controlled substance schedule: II
Pregnancy risk category: D

Indications and dosages
▶ **Sedation.** *Adults:* 20 to 40 mg P.O. b.i.d., t.i.d., or q.i.d.
Children: 2 to 6 mg/kg daily P.O. or P.R. in three divided doses. Maximum daily dosage is 100 mg.
▶ **Hypnotic.** *Adults:* 100 to 200 mg P.O. h.s. or 150 to 200 mg I.M. Or, initially, 100 mg I.V. with additional small doses, to a total of 500 mg. Or, 120 or 200 mg P.R.
Children: 2 to 6 mg/kg I.M. Maximum dosage is 100 mg. P.R. doses are 30 mg for patients ages 2 months to 1 year, 30 or 60 mg for patients ages 1 to 4 years, 60 mg for patients ages 5 to 12 years, and 60 or 120 mg for patients ages 12 to 14 years.
▶ **Preoperative sedation.** *Adults:* 150 to 200 mg I.M.
Children age 10 or older: 5 mg/kg P.O. or I.M.
Children younger than age 10: 5 mg/kg P.R.

How supplied
pentobarbital
Elixir: 18.2 mg/5 ml
pentobarbital sodium
Capsules: 50 mg, 100 mg

Injection: 50 mg/ml
Suppositories: 30 mg, 60 mg, 120 mg, 200 mg

Pharmacokinetics

Absorption: absorbed rapidly after P.O. or P.R. administration. Unknown after I.M. administration.
Distribution: distributed widely throughout body. About 35% to 45% of drug is protein-bound.
Metabolism: metabolized in liver.
Excretion: 99% of drug is excreted in urine. *Half-life:* 35 to 50 hours.

Route	Onset	Peak	Duration
P.O.	≤ 15 min	30-60 min	1-4 hr
I.V.	Immediate	Immediate	15 min
I.M.	10-25 min	Unknown	Unknown
P.R.	≤ 15 min	Unknown	1-4 hr

Pharmacodynamics

Chemical effect: unknown; may interfere with transmission of impulses from thalamus to cortex of brain.
Therapeutic effect: promotes sleep and calmness.

Adverse reactions

CNS: *drowsiness, lethargy, hangover,* paradoxical excitement in elderly patients.
GI: nausea, vomiting.
Hematologic: worsening of porphyria.
Respiratory: ***respiratory depression.***
Skin: rash, urticaria, ***Stevens-Johnson syndrome.***
Other: ***angioedema.***

Interactions

Drug-drug. *Corticosteroids, doxycycline, estrogens and oral contraceptives, oral anticoagulants:* pentobarbital may enhance metabolism of these drugs. Monitor patient for decreased effect.
CNS depressants, including narcotic analgesics: excessive CNS and respiratory depression. Use together cautiously.
Griseofulvin: decreased absorption of griseofulvin. Separate administration times.
MAO inhibitors: inhibited barbiturate metabolism and possible prolonged CNS depression. Reduce barbiturate dosage.
Rifampin: may decrease barbiturate levels. Monitor patient for decreased effect.
Drug-lifestyle. *Alcohol use:* excessive CNS and respiratory depression. Discourage concomitant use.

Contraindications and precautions

- Contraindicated in patients with porphyria or hypersensitivity to barbiturates.
- Drug isn't recommended for pregnant or breast-feeding women.
- Use cautiously in elderly or debilitated patients and in those with acute or chronic pain, depression, suicidal tendencies, history of drug abuse, or hepatic impairment.

NURSING CONSIDERATIONS

Assessment

- Assess patient's condition before therapy and regularly thereafter.
- Assess mental status before therapy, and give reduced doses, as ordered. Elderly patients are more sensitive to adverse CNS effects of drug.
- Inspect patient's skin. Skin eruptions may precede life-threatening reactions to barbiturate therapy.
- Be alert for adverse reactions and drug interactions.
- Evaluate patient's and family's knowledge of drug therapy.

Nursing diagnoses

- Disturbed sleep pattern related to condition
- Risk for injury related to drug-induced adverse CNS reactions
- Deficient knowledge related to drug therapy

Planning and implementation

P.O. use: Follow normal protocol.
I.V. use: I.V. use of barbiturates may cause severe respiratory depression, laryngospasm, or hypotension. Have emergency resuscitation equipment available.
– To minimize deterioration, use I.V injection solution within 30 minutes after opening container. Don't use cloudy solution.

– Reserve I.V. injection for emergency treatment, which should be given under close supervision. Give slowly (50 mg/minute or less).
– Parenteral solution is alkaline. Local tissue reactions and injection site pain have followed I.V. use. Avoid extravasation. Assess patency of I.V. site before and during administration.
– Don't mix with other drugs in syringe or in I.V. solutions or lines.
I.M. use: Give I.M. injection deeply. Superficial injection may cause pain, sterile abscess, and sloughing.
P.R. use: To ensure accurate dosage, don't divide suppositories.
• Stop drug and notify prescriber if skin reactions occur. In some patients, high fever, stomatitis, headache, or rhinitis may precede skin reactions.
• Pentobarbital has no analgesic effect and may cause restlessness or delirium in patient with pain.
• Long-term use isn't recommended; drug loses its efficacy in promoting sleep after 14 days of continued use. Long-term high dosage may cause dependence and may lead to withdrawal symptoms if drug is suddenly discontinued. Withdraw barbiturates gradually.
ALERT Don't confuse pentobarbital with phenobarbital.

Patient teaching
• Warn patient about performing activities that require alertness or physical coordination. For inpatient, particularly elderly patient, supervise walking and raise bed rails.
• Inform patient that morning hangover is common after hypnotic dose, which suppresses REM sleep. Patient may experience increased dreaming after therapy stops.
• Tell patient who uses oral contraceptives that she should consider a different birth control methods because drug may decrease contraceptive effect.

Evaluation
• Patient reports satisfactory sleep.
• Patient sustains no injuries from drug-induced adverse CNS reactions.
• Patient and family state understanding of drug therapy.

pentostatin (2′-deoxycoformycin)
(pen-toh-STAH-tin)
Nipent

Pharmacologic class: antimetabolite (adenosine deaminase [ADA] inhibitor)
Therapeutic class: antineoplastic
Pregnancy risk category: D

Indications and dosages
▶ **Alpha-interferon–refractory hairy-cell leukemia.** *Adults:* 4 mg/m^2 I.V. every other week.

How supplied
Powder for injection: 10 mg/vial

Pharmacokinetics
Absorption: not applicable.
Distribution: plasma protein–binding is low (about 4%).
Metabolism: unknown.
Excretion: over 90% excreted in urine. *Half-life:* about 6 hours.

Route	Onset	Peak	Duration
I.V.	Unknown	Unknown	Unknown

Pharmacodynamics
Chemical effect: inhibits ADA, causing increase in intracellular levels of deoxyadenosine triphosphate. This leads to cell damage and death. Greatest activity of ADA is in cells of lymphoid system (especially malignant T cells).
Therapeutic effect: kills certain leukemic cells.

Adverse reactions
CNS: asthenia, malaise, *headache, neurologic symptoms, anxiety, confusion, depression, dizziness, insomnia, nervousness, paresthesia, somnolence, abnormal thinking, fatigue*.
CV: chest pain, ***arrhythmias,*** abnormal ECG, thrombophlebitis, peripheral edema, ***hemorrhage.***
EENT: abnormal vision, conjunctivitis, ear pain, eye pain, epistaxis, pharyngitis, rhinitis, sinusitis.

GI: abdominal pain, nausea, vomiting, anorexia, diarrhea, constipation, flatulence, stomatitis.
GU: *hematuria, dysuria, increased BUN and creatinine levels.*
Hematologic: ***myelosuppression,*** **LEUKOPENIA,** anemia, **THROMBOCYTOPENIA,** ***lymphocytopenia,*** lymphadenopathy.
Hepatic: *elevated liver enzyme levels,* increased LD level.
Metabolic: weight loss.
Musculoskeletal: back pain, myalgia, arthralgia.
Respiratory: *cough, bronchitis, dyspnea,* ***pulmonary edema,*** *pneumonia.*
Skin: photosensitivity, contact dermatitis, ecchymosis, petechiae, rash, eczema, dry skin, herpes simplex or zoster, maculopapular rash, vesiculobullous rash, pruritus, seborrhea, discoloration.
Other: fever, diaphoresis, **INFECTION,** pain, **HYPERSENSITIVITY REACTIONS,** ***neoplasm,*** chills, sepsis, flulike syndrome.

Interactions

Drug-drug. *Cytarabine, vidarabine:* increased adverse reactions to either drug. Avoid concomitant use.
Fludarabine: risk of fatal pulmonary toxicity. Don't use together.

Contraindications and precautions

- Contraindicated in patients hypersensitive to drug.
- Drug isn't recommended for pregnant or breast-feeding women.
- Safety of drug hasn't been established in children.

NURSING CONSIDERATIONS

Assessment
- Assess patient's condition before therapy and regularly thereafter.
- Be alert for adverse reactions and drug interactions.
- Evaluate patient's and family's knowledge of drug therapy.

Nursing diagnoses
- Ineffective health maintenance related to leukemia
- Ineffective protection related to drug-induced adverse hematologic reactions
- Deficient knowledge related to drug therapy

Planning and implementation
- Use drug only under supervision of prescriber qualified and experienced in use of chemotherapy drugs. Adverse reactions after therapy are common.
- Make sure patient is well hydrated before therapy. Administer 500 to 1,000 ml of dextrose 5% in half-normal saline solution for injection, as ordered, for hydration.
- Follow facility policy to reduce risks. Preparation and administration of parenteral form are linked to mutagenic, teratogenic, and carcinogenic risks for staff.
- Add 5 ml of sterile water for injection to vial containing pentostatin powder for injection. Mix thoroughly to make solution of 5 mg/ml. Drug may be administered by I.V. bolus injection or diluted further in 25 or 50 ml of D_5W or normal saline solution for injection and infused over 20 to 30 minutes.
- Use reconstituted solution within 8 hours; it contains no preservatives.
- Treat all spills and waste products with 5% sodium hypochlorite (household bleach).
- Give additional 500 ml of D_5W, as ordered, for hydration after drug is administered.
- Optimal duration of therapy is unknown. Current recommendations suggest two additional courses of therapy after complete response. If partial response isn't evident after 6 months, drug will be discontinued. If partial response is evident, drug will be continued for another 6 months or for two courses of therapy after complete response.
- Withhold drug in patients with CNS toxicity, severe rash, or active infection and notify prescriber. Drug may be resumed when infection clears. Avoid use in patients with renal damage (creatinine clearance of 60 ml/minute or less).
- Temporarily withhold drug and notify prescriber if absolute neutrophil count falls below 200/mm^3 and pretreatment level was over 500/mm^3. No recommendations exist for

dosage adjustments in patients with anemia, neutropenia, or thrombocytopenia.
- Use drug only in patients with hairy-cell leukemia refractory to alpha-interferon (disease that progresses after minimum of 3 months of treatment with alpha-interferon or disease that doesn't respond after 6 months of therapy).

ALERT Don't confuse pentostatin with pentosan.

Patient teaching
- Teach patient how to take infection-control and bleeding precautions.
- Tell patient to notify prescriber of adverse reactions.

Evaluation
- Patient responds well to therapy.
- Patient doesn't develop serious complications from adverse reactions.
- Patient and family state understanding of drug therapy.

pentoxifylline
(pen-tok-SIH-fi-lin)
Trental

Pharmacologic class: xanthine derivative
Therapeutic class: hemorrheologic
Pregnancy risk category: C

Indications and dosages
▶ **Intermittent claudication caused by chronic occlusive vascular disease.** *Adults:* 400 mg P.O. t.i.d. with meals.

How supplied
Tablets (extended-release): 400 mg

Pharmacokinetics
Absorption: absorbed almost completely but slowed by food. Undergoes first-pass hepatic metabolism.
Distribution: bound by erythrocyte membrane.
Metabolism: metabolized extensively by erythrocytes and liver.
Excretion: excreted primarily in urine; less than 4% of drug is excreted in feces. *Half-life:* about 30 to 45 minutes.

Route	Onset	Peak	Duration
P.O.	Unknown	2-4 hr	Unknown

Pharmacodynamics
Chemical effect: unknown; thought to increase RBC flexibility and lower blood viscosity.
Therapeutic effect: improves capillary blood flow.

Adverse reactions
CNS: headache, dizziness.
GI: dyspepsia, nausea, vomiting.

Interactions
Drug-drug. *Anticoagulants:* increased anticoagulant effect. Adjust anticoagulant dosage as ordered.
Antihypertensives: increased hypotensive effect. Dosage adjustments may be necessary.
Drug-lifestyle. *Smoking:* vasoconstriction may result. Advise patient to avoid smoking because it may worsen his condition.

Contraindications and precautions
- Contraindicated in patients who are intolerant of methylxanthines, such as caffeine and theophylline, and in those with recent cerebral or retinal hemorrhage.
- Drug isn't recommended for breast-feeding women.
- Use cautiously in pregnant women.
- Safety of drug hasn't been established in children.

NURSING CONSIDERATIONS

Assessment
- Assess patient's condition before therapy and regularly thereafter.
- Be alert for adverse reactions and drug interactions.
- Be aware that elderly patients may be more sensitive to drug's effects.
- Monitor patient's hydration status if adverse GI reactions occur.

• Evaluate patient's and family's knowledge of drug therapy.

Nursing diagnoses

• Ineffective peripheral tissue perfusion related to condition
• Risk for deficient fluid volume related to drug-induced adverse GI reactions
• Deficient knowledge related to drug therapy

Planning and implementation

• Drug is useful in patients who aren't good surgical candidates.
• Report adverse reactions to prescriber; dosage may need to be reduced.
ALERT Don't confuse Trental with Trendar or Trandate.

Patient teaching

• Advise patient to take drug with meals to minimize GI upset.
• Instruct patient to swallow drug whole, without breaking, crushing, or chewing.
• Tell patient to report adverse GI or CNS reactions.
• Advise patient to avoid smoking because nicotine causes vasoconstriction that can worsen his condition.
• Tell patient not to stop drug during first 8 weeks of therapy unless directed by prescriber.

Evaluation

• Patient has adequate peripheral tissue perfusion.
• Patient maintains adequate hydration throughout therapy.
• Patient and family state understanding of drug therapy.

pergolide mesylate

(PER-goh-lighd MES-ih-layt)
Permax

Pharmacologic class: dopaminergic agonist
Therapeutic class: antiparkinsonian
Pregnancy risk category: B

Indications and dosages

▶ **Adjunct treatment with levodopa-carbidopa in management of symptoms caused by Parkinson's disease.** *Adults:* initially, 0.05 mg P.O. daily for first 2 days followed by increased dosage of 0.1 to 0.15 mg every third day over 12 days. Subsequent dosage increased by 0.25 mg every third day until optimum response is seen if needed. Drug usually is administered in divided doses t.i.d. Gradual reductions in levodopa-carbidopa dosage could be made during dosage adjustment.

How supplied

Tablets: 0.05 mg, 0.25 mg, 1 mg

Pharmacokinetics

Absorption: well absorbed.
Distribution: drug is about 90% protein-bound.
Metabolism: metabolized to at least 10 different compounds, some of which retain pharmacologic activity.
Excretion: excreted mainly by kidneys.

Route	Onset	Peak	Duration
P.O.	Unknown	Unknown	Unknown

Pharmacodynamics

Chemical effect: directly stimulates dopamine receptors in nigrostriatal system.
Therapeutic effect: helps to relieve signs and symptoms of Parkinson's disease.

Adverse reactions

CNS: headache, asthenia, *dyskinesia, dizziness, hallucinations,* dystonia, confusion, *somnolence,* insomnia, anxiety, depression, tremor, abnormal dreams, personality disorder, psychosis, abnormal gait, akathisia, extrapyramidal syndrome, incoordination, akinesia, hypertonia, neuralgia, speech disorder, twitching paresthesia.
CV: chest pain; *orthostatic hypotension;* vasodilation; palpitations; hypotension; syncope; hypertension; ***arrhythmias; MI;*** facial, peripheral, or generalized edema.
EENT: *rhinitis,* epistaxis, abnormal vision, diplopia, eye disorder.

GI: dry mouth, dysgeusia, abdominal pain, *nausea, constipation,* diarrhea, dyspepsia, anorexia, vomiting.
GU: urinary frequency, urinary tract infection, hematuria.
Metabolic: weight gain.
Musculoskeletal: neck and back pain, arthralgia, bursitis, myalgia.
Skin: diaphoresis, rash.
Other: flulike syndrome, chills, infection.

Interactions

Drug-drug. *Butyrophenones, metoclopramide, other dopamine antagonists, phenothiazines, thioxanthenes:* may antagonize effects of pergolide. Avoid concomitant use.

Contraindications and precautions

- Contraindicated in patients hypersensitive to drug or ergot alkaloids.
- Use cautiously in pregnant women and patients prone to arrhythmias.
- Safety of drug hasn't been established in children and in breast-feeding women.

NURSING CONSIDERATIONS

Assessment

- Assess patient's condition before therapy. Monitor drug effectiveness by regularly checking patient's body movements for improvement.
- Monitor blood pressure and heart rate and rhythm. Symptomatic orthostatic or sustained hypotension may occur in some patients, especially at start of therapy. Drug also may induce arrhythmias.
- Be alert for adverse reactions and drug interactions.
- Evaluate patient's and family's knowledge of drug therapy.

Nursing diagnoses

- Impaired physical mobility related to Parkinson's disease
- Decreased cardiac output related to drug-induced adverse CV reactions
- Deficient knowledge related to drug therapy

Planning and implementation

- Dosage is gradually increased according to patient's response and tolerance.
- Notify prescriber if patient has significant changes in vital signs or mental status.

Patient teaching

- Inform patient of potential adverse reactions, especially hallucinations and confusion (27% risk).
- Warn patient to avoid activities that could result in injury from orthostatic hypotension and syncope.

Evaluation

- Patient has improved mobility.
- Patient maintains cardiac output.
- Patient and family state understanding of drug therapy.

perindopril erbumine

(PER-in-doh-pril ER-buh-mighn)
Aceon

Pharmacologic class: ACE inhibitor
Therapeutic class: antihypertensive
Pregnancy risk category: C (first trimester), D (second and third trimesters)

Indications and dosages

▶ **Treatment of essential hypertension.**
Adults: initially, 4 mg P.O. once daily. Increased until blood pressure is controlled or a maximum of 16 mg/day is reached. Usual maintenance dosage 4 to 8 mg once daily; may be divided into two doses.
Adults over age 65: initially, 4 mg P.O. daily as one dose or two divided doses. Dosage increases exceeding 8 mg/day should occur only under close medical supervision.
Renally impaired patients (creatinine clearance above 30 ml/minute): initially, 2 mg P.O. daily with a maximum maintenance dosage of 8 mg/day.
Patients taking diuretics: initially, 2 to 4 mg P.O. daily as one dose or divided into two doses with close medical supervision for several hours and until blood pressure has stabilized.

Adjust dosage based on patient's blood pressure response.

How supplied

Tablets: 2 mg, 4 mg, 8 mg

Pharmacokinetics

Absorption: rapidly absorbed following P.O. administration; levels peak at about 1 hour. Absolute P.O. bioavailability of perindopril is around 75%. Plasma perindopril and perindoprilat levels are about doubled in elderly patients.
Distribution: perindopril and perindoprilat are about 60% and 10% to 20% bound to plasma proteins, respectively. Drug interaction resulting from effects on protein-binding isn't anticipated.
Metabolism: extensively metabolized by the liver to the active ACE inhibitor, perindoprilat.
Excretion: about 4% to 12% of drug is excreted in the urine as unchanged drug. Clearance is reduced in elderly patients and patients with heart failure or renal insufficiency.

Route	Onset	Peak	Duration
P.O.	Unknown	1 hour	Unknown

Pharmacodynamics

Chemical effect: this is a prodrug converted by the liver to the active metabolite perindoprilat. Perindoprilat probably inhibits ACE activity, thereby preventing conversion of angiotensin I to angiotensin II, a potent vasoconstrictor. ACE inhibition results in decreased vasoconstriction and decreased aldosterone, thus reducing sodium and water retention.
Therapeutic effect: lowers blood pressure.

Adverse reactions

CNS: dizziness, asthenia, sleep disorder, paresthesia, depression, somnolence, nervousness, *headache.*
CV: palpitations, edema, chest pain, abnormal ECG.
EENT: rhinitis, sinusitis, ear infection, pharyngitis, tinnitus.
GI: dyspepsia, diarrhea, abdominal pain, nausea, vomiting, flatulence.
GU: proteinuria, urinary tract infection, sexual dysfunction in men, menstrual disorder.
Hepatic: increased ALT level.
Metabolic: triglyceride increase, hyperkalemia.
Musculoskeletal: back pain, hypertonia, neck pain, joint pain, myalgia, arthritis, leg or arm pain.
Respiratory: *cough,* upper respiratory infection.
Skin: rash.
Other: viral infection, fever, injury, seasonal allergy.

Interactions

Drug-drug. *Diuretics:* additive hypotensive effect. Monitor patient closely.
Lithium: increased lithium levels and possible lithium toxicity. Use together cautiously, and monitor serum lithium levels. Use of a diuretic may further increase the risk of lithium toxicity.
Potassium supplements, potassium-sparing diuretics (spironolactone, amiloride, triamterene), other drugs capable of increasing serum potassium (indomethacin, heparin, cyclosporine): additive hyperkalemic effect. Use together cautiously, and monitor serum potassium levels frequently.
Drug-herb. *Licorice:* can cause sodium retention and increase blood pressure, interfering with therapeutic effects of ACE inhibitors. Discourage concomitant use.
Drug-food. *Salt substitutes containing potassium:* may increase risk of hyperkalemia. Use together cautiously.

Contraindications and precautions

• Contraindicated in patients hypersensitive to perindopril or any other ACE inhibitor. Also contraindicated in patients with a history of angioedema secondary to ACE inhibitors. Don't use this drug in pregnant patients.
• Use cautiously in patients with a history of angioedema unrelated to ACE inhibitor therapy. Also use cautiously in patients with impaired renal function, heart failure, ischemic heart disease, cerebrovascular disease, renal artery stenosis, or collagen vascular disease,

such as systemic lupus erythematosis or scleroderma.

NURSING CONSIDERATIONS

Assessment

- Obtain complete medical history before therapy.
- Monitor CBC with differential before therapy, especially in renally impaired patients with systemic lupus erythematosis or scleroderma. Other ACE inhibitors have been linked to agranulocytosis and neutropenia.
- Monitor renal function before and periodically throughout therapy. Drug shouldn't be used in patients with a creatinine clearance less than 30 ml/minute.
- Assess patient for volume or sodium depletion as a result of prolonged diuretic therapy, dietary salt restriction, dialysis, diarrhea, or vomiting.
- Monitor serum potassium levels closely.
- If patient is at risk for hypotension, watch closely during first dose, for the first 2 weeks of treatment, and whenever the dose of perindopril or concomitant diuretic is increased. If severe hypotension occurs, place patient in supine position and treat symptomatically, as ordered.
- Evaluate patient's and family's knowledge of drug therapy.

Nursing diagnoses

- Risk for injury related to presence of hypertension
- Risk for activity intolerance related to drug-induced adverse effects
- Deficient knowledge related to drug therapy

Planning and implementation

- Correct volume and salt depletion before starting drug.

ALERT Angioedema of the face, limbs, lips, tongue, glottis, and larynx has been reported in patients treated with perindopril. Angioedema involving the tongue, glottis, or larynx may cause fatal airway obstruction. Appropriate therapy, such as S.C. epinephrine solution, should be promptly administered, as ordered. Discontinue drug, notify prescriber, and observe patient until the swelling resolves.

- Swelling confined to the face and lips will probably resolve without treatment, but antihistamines may help relieve symptoms.
- Patients with a history of angioedema unrelated to ACE inhibitor therapy may be at increased risk of angioedema while receiving an ACE inhibitor.
- Excessive hypotension can occur when drug is given with diuretics. If possible, diuretic therapy should be stopped 2 to 3 days before starting perindopril, as ordered. If diuretic can't be stopped, prescriber may consider starting perindopril at a reduced dosage, decreasing the diuretic dosage, or both.
- ACE inhibitors rarely are linked to a fatal syndrome of cholestatic jaundice and fulminant hepatic necrosis. Notify prescriber and stop drug, as ordered, if patient develops jaundice or marked elevation of hepatic enzyme levels during therapy.

Patient teaching

- Inform patient that angioedema, including laryngeal edema, can occur during therapy, especially with the first dose. Advise patient to stop taking the drug and immediately report any signs or symptoms that suggest angioedema (swelling of face, limbs, eyes, lips, tongue; hoarseness or difficulty in swallowing or breathing).
- Advise patient to report promptly any sign of infection (sore throat, fever) or jaundice (yellowing of eyes or skin).
- Advise patient to avoid salt substitutes containing potassium unless instructed otherwise by prescriber.
- Caution patient that light-headedness may occur, especially during the first few days of therapy. Advise patient to report light-headedness and, if fainting occurs, to discontinue the drug and consult prescriber promptly.
- Caution patient that inadequate fluid intake or excessive perspiration, diarrhea, or vomiting can lead to an excessive drop in blood pressure.
- Warn woman of childbearing age about the consequences of second and third trimester exposure to drug. Advise patient to notify prescriber immediately if she suspects pregnancy.

Evaluation

- Patient's blood pressure is controlled and he remains free of injury.
- Patient has no adverse effects that limit mobility.
- Patient and family state understanding of drug therapy.

perphenazine

(per-FEN-uh-zeen)

Apo-Perphenazine ♦, PMS Perphenazine ♦, Trilafon, Trilafon Concentrate

Pharmacologic class: phenothiazine (piperazine derivative)
Therapeutic class: antipsychotic, antiemetic
Pregnancy risk category: NR

Indications and dosages

▶ **Psychosis in nonhospitalized patients.** *Adults:* initially, 4 to 8 mg P.O. t.i.d., reduced as soon as possible to minimum effective dosage.
Children over age 12: lowest adult dose.
▶ **Psychosis in hospitalized patients.** *Adults:* initially, 8 to 16 mg P.O. b.i.d., t.i.d., or q.i.d., increased to 64 mg daily as needed. Or, 5 to 10 mg I.M. q 6 hours p.r.n. Maximum I.M. dose shouldn't exceed 30 mg/day.
Children over age 12: lowest limit of adult dosage.
▶ **Severe nausea and vomiting.** *Adults:* 5 to 10 mg I.M. p.r.n.

How supplied

Tablets: 2 mg, 4 mg, 8 mg, 16 mg
Oral concentrate: 16 mg/5 ml
Syrup: 2 mg/5 ml ♦
Injection: 5 mg/ml

Pharmacokinetics

Absorption: rate and extent vary. P.O. tablet absorption is erratic and variable; P.O. concentrate absorption is much more predictable. I.M. drug is rapidly absorbed from injection site.
Distribution: distributed widely; 91% to 99% of drug is protein-bound.
Metabolism: metabolized extensively by liver.
Excretion: most of drug excreted in urine; some in feces.

Route	Onset	Peak	Duration
P.O., I.M.	Varies	Unknown	Unknown

Pharmacodynamics

Chemical effect: unknown; probably blocks postsynaptic dopamine receptors in brain and inhibits medullary chemoreceptor trigger zone.
Therapeutic effect: relieves signs and symptoms of psychosis; also relieves nausea and vomiting.

Adverse reactions

CNS: *extrapyramidal reaction, tardive dyskinesia,* sedation, pseudoparkinsonism, EEG changes, dizziness, ***seizures, neuroleptic malignant syndrome.***
CV: *orthostatic hypotension,* tachycardia, ECG changes, ***cardiac arrest.***
EENT: ocular changes, blurred vision.
GI: dry mouth, constipation.
GU: *urine retention,* dark urine, menstrual irregularities, inhibited ejaculation.
Hematologic: transient ***leukopenia***, hyperprolactinemia, ***agranulocytosis, hemolytic anemia, thrombocytopenia.***
Hepatic: cholestatic jaundice, abnormal liver function test results.
Metabolic: weight gain, increased appetite.
Skin: *mild photosensitivity,* allergic reactions, pain at I.M. injection site, sterile abscess.
Other: gynecomastia.

Interactions

Drug-drug. *Antacids:* inhibited oral phenothiazine absorption. Administer separately.
Barbiturates: may decrease phenothiazine effect. Observe patient closely.
Other CNS depressants: increased CNS depression. Avoid concomitant use.
Drug-herb. *Dong quai, St. John's wort:* increased photosensitivity reactions. Discourage concomitant use.
Kava: increased risk of dystonic reactions. Discourage concomitant use.
Milk thistle: decreased liver toxicity caused by phenothiazines. Monitor liver enzyme levels.
Yohimbe: increased risk of yohimbe toxicity. Discourage concomitant use.

Drug-lifestyle. *Alcohol use:* increased CNS depression. Discourage concomitant use.
Sun exposure: increased photosensitivity reaction. Urge patient to take precautions.

Contraindications and precautions

- Contraindicated in patients hypersensitive to drug; patients experiencing coma; those with CNS depression, blood dyscrasia, bone marrow depression, liver damage, or subcortical damage; and those receiving large doses of CNS depressants.
- Use cautiously with other CNS depressants or anticholinergics. Also use cautiously in elderly patients, debilitated patients, pregnant women, and breast-feeding women.
- Use cautiously in patients with alcohol withdrawal, psychic depression, suicidal tendency, severe adverse reactions to other phenothiazines, impaired renal function, or respiratory disorders.
- Safety of drug hasn't been established in children age 12 and under.

NURSING CONSIDERATIONS

Assessment

- Assess patient's condition before therapy and regularly thereafter.
- Obtain baseline blood pressure before therapy, and monitor regularly. Watch for orthostatic hypotension, especially with I.M. administration.
- Monitor weekly bilirubin tests during first month; periodic blood tests (CBC and liver function); and ophthalmic tests (long-term use) as ordered.
- Be alert for adverse reactions and drug interactions.
- Monitor patient for tardive dyskinesia. It may occur after prolonged use. It may not appear until months or years later and may disappear spontaneously or persist for life despite discontinuation of drug.
- Monitor patient's hydration status if drug is used for nausea and vomiting.
- Evaluate patient's and family's knowledge of drug therapy.

Nursing diagnoses

- Disturbed thought processes related to psychosis
- Risk for deficient fluid volume related to nausea or vomiting
- Deficient knowledge related to drug therapy

Planning and implementation

P.O. use: Dilute liquid concentrate with fruit juice, milk, carbonated beverage, or semisolid food just before giving.
– Concentrate causes turbidity or precipitation in colas, black coffee, grape or apple juice, or tea. Don't mix with them.
I.M. use: Inject drug deep in upper outer quadrant of buttocks. Injection may sting.
– Massage slowly afterward to prevent sterile abscess.
– Keep patient supine for 1 hour after injection because of risk of hypotension.
- Prevent contact dermatitis by keeping drug away from skin and clothes. Wear gloves when preparing liquid forms.
- Protect drug from light. Slight yellowing of injection or concentrate doesn't affect potency. Discard markedly discolored solutions.
- Don't stop drug abruptly unless severe adverse reactions demand it. After abrupt withdrawal of long-term therapy, patient may experience gastritis, nausea, vomiting, dizziness, tremors, feeling of warmth or cold, diaphoresis, tachycardia, headache, or insomnia.
- Withhold dose and notify prescriber if patient develops jaundice, symptoms of blood dyscrasia (fever, sore throat, infection, cellulitis, weakness), or persistent extrapyramidal reactions (longer than a few hours).
- Acute dystonic reactions may be treated with diphenhydramine.

Patient teaching

- Advise patient to change positions slowly to minimize effects of orthostatic hypotension.
- Teach patient which fluids are appropriate for dilution of concentrate (see above).
- Warn patient to avoid hazardous activities until CNS effects of drug are known. Drowsiness and dizziness usually subside after a few weeks.
- Tell patient to avoid alcohol during drug therapy.

• Advise patient to report urine retention or constipation.
• Tell patient to use sunblock and to wear protective clothing to avoid photosensitivity reactions.
• Tell patient to relieve dry mouth with sugarless gum or hard candy.

Evaluation
• Patient's thought processes are normal.
• Patient maintains adequate hydration throughout drug therapy.
• Patient and family state understanding of drug therapy.

phenazopyridine hydrochloride (phenylazo diamino pyridine hydrochloride)
(fen-eh-soh-PEER-eh-deen high-droh-KLOR-ighd)

Azo-Standard†, Baridium†, Eridium†, Geridium†, Phenazo♦, Phenazodine†, Prodium†, Pyridiate†, Pyridium, Urodine†, Urogesic†, Viridium†

Pharmacologic class: azo dye
Therapeutic class: urinary analgesic
Pregnancy risk category: B

Indications and dosages
▶ **Urinary tract irritation or infection.** *Adults:* 200 mg P.O. t.i.d.
Children: 12 mg/kg P.O. daily divided into three equal doses.

How supplied
Tablets: 95 mg†, 100 mg†, 200 mg

Pharmacokinetics
Absorption: unknown.
Distribution: unknown.
Metabolism: metabolized in liver.
Excretion: excreted in urine.

Route	Onset	Peak	Duration
P.O.	Unknown	Unknown	Unknown

Pharmacodynamics
Chemical effect: unknown; has local anesthetic effect on urinary mucosa.
Therapeutic effect: relieves urinary tract pain.

Adverse reactions
CNS: headache, vertigo.
GI: nausea.
Skin: rash.

Interactions
None significant.

Contraindications and precautions
• Contraindicated in patients with glomerulonephritis, severe hepatitis, uremia, pyelonephritis during pregnancy, or renal insufficiency.
• Use cautiously in children.
• Safety of drug hasn't been established in breast-feeding women.

NURSING CONSIDERATIONS

Assessment
• Assess patient's pain before and after drug administration.
• Be alert for adverse reactions.
• Monitor patient's hydration status if nausea occurs.
• Evaluate patient's and family's knowledge of drug therapy.

Nursing diagnoses
• Acute pain related to underlying urinary tract condition
• Risk for deficient fluid volume related to drug-induced nausea
• Deficient knowledge related to drug therapy

Planning and implementation
• Administer drug with food to minimize nausea.
• Drug may alter Diastix results but doesn't affect Chemstrip uG used to test urine glucose.
ALERT Don't confuse Pyridium with pyridoxine.

Patient teaching
• Advise patient that taking drug with meals may minimize nausea.

• Caution patient to stop taking drug and to notify prescriber if skin or sclera becomes yellow-tinged.
• Alert patient that drug colors urine red or orange. It may stain fabrics and contact lenses.
• Tell patient to notify prescriber if urinary tract pain persists. Drug isn't for long-term therapy.

Evaluation
• Patient is free from pain.
• Patient maintains adequate hydration.
• Patient and family state understanding of drug therapy.

phenobarbital (phenobarbitone)
(feen-oh-BAR-bih-tol)
Ancalixir♦, Barbita, Solfoton

phenobarbital sodium (phenobarbitone sodium)
Luminal Sodium

Pharmacologic class: barbiturate
Therapeutic class: anticonvulsant, sedative-hypnotic
Controlled substance schedule: IV
Pregnancy risk category: D

Indications and dosages
▶ **All forms of epilepsy except absence seizures; febrile seizures in children.** *Adults:* 60 to 250 mg P.O. daily, in divided doses t.i.d. or as single dose h.s.
Children: 1 to 6 mg/kg P.O. daily, divided q 12 hours for total of 100 mg; can be given once daily, usually h.s.
▶ **Status epilepticus.** *Adults:* 10 to 20 mg/kg I.V.; repeat if necessary.
Children: 15 to 20 mg/kg I.V. Don't exceed 50 mg/minute.
▶ **Sedation.** *Adults:* 30 to 120 mg P.O. daily in two or three divided doses.
Children: 3 to 5 mg/kg P.O. daily in divided doses t.i.d.
▶ **Insomnia.** *Adults:* 100 to 200 mg P.O. or I.M. h.s.
▶ **Preoperative sedation.** *Adults:* 100 to 200 mg I.M. 60 to 90 minutes before surgery.
Children: 1 to 3 mg/kg I.V. or I.M. 60 to 90 minutes before surgery.

How supplied
Tablets: 15 mg, 16 mg, 30 mg, 32 mg, 60 mg, 65 mg, 100 mg
Capsules: 16 mg
Elixir*: 15 mg/5 ml, 20 mg/5 ml
Injection: 30 mg/ml, 60 mg/ml, 65 mg/ml, 130 mg/ml

Pharmacokinetics
Absorption: absorbed well after P.O. administration. Absorption from I.M. injection site is 100%.
Distribution: distributed widely throughout body. Drug is about 25% to 30% protein-bound.
Metabolism: metabolized in liver.
Excretion: excreted in urine. *Half-life:* 5 to 7 days.

Route	Onset	Peak	Duration
P.O.	20-60 min	Unknown	10-12 hr
I.V.	5 min	≥ 15 min	10-12 hr
I.M.	> 60 min	Unknown	10-12 hr

Pharmacodynamics
Chemical effect: unknown; may depress CNS synaptic transmission and increase seizure activity threshold in motor cortex. As sedative, may interfere with transmission of impulses from thalamus to brain cortex.
Therapeutic effect: prevents and stops seizure activity; promotes calmness and sleep.

Adverse reactions
CNS: drowsiness, lethargy, hangover, paradoxical excitement in elderly patients.
CV: ***bradycardia,*** hypotension.
GI: nausea, vomiting.
Hematologic: exacerbation of porphyria.
Respiratory: ***respiratory depression, apnea.***
Skin: rash; ***erythema multiforme; Stevens-Johnson syndrome;*** urticaria; pain, swelling, thrombophlebitis, necrosis, nerve injury at injection site.
Other: ***angioedema.***

Interactions

Drug-drug. *Chloramphenicol, MAO inhibitors, valproic acid:* potentiated barbiturate effect. Monitor patient for increased CNS and respiratory depression.
CNS depressants, including narcotic analgesics: excessive CNS depression. Use together cautiously.
Corticosteroids, digitoxin, doxycycline, estrogens and oral contraceptives, oral anticoagulants, tricyclic antidepressants: phenobarbital may enhance metabolism of these drugs. Monitor patient for decreased effect.
Diazepam: increased effects of both drugs. Use together cautiously.
Griseofulvin: decreased griseofulvin absorption. Administer separately.
Mephobarbital, primidone: excessive phenobarbital blood levels. Monitor patient closely.
Rifampin: may decrease barbiturate levels. Monitor patient for decreased effect.
Valproic acid: increased phenobarbital levels. Monitor patient for toxicity.
Drug-lifestyle. *Alcohol use:* excessive CNS depression. Discourage concomitant use.

Contraindications and precautions

• Contraindicated in patients with barbiturate hypersensitivity, history of manifest or latent porphyria, hepatic dysfunction, respiratory disease with dyspnea or obstruction, and nephritis.
• Drug isn't recommended for pregnant or breast-feeding women.
• Use cautiously in elderly patients, debilitated patients, and patients with acute or chronic pain, depression, suicidal tendencies, history of drug abuse, altered blood pressure, CV disease, shock, or uremia.

NURSING CONSIDERATIONS

Assessment

• Assess patient's condition before therapy and regularly thereafter.
• Monitor blood levels closely. Therapeutic level is 15 to 40 mcg/ml.
• Be alert for adverse reactions and drug interactions.
• Evaluate patient's and family's knowledge of drug therapy.

Nursing diagnoses

• Risk for trauma related to seizures
• Risk for injury related to drug-induced adverse CNS reactions
• Deficient knowledge related to drug therapy

Planning and implementation

P.O. use: Follow normal protocol.
I.V. use: I.V. injection is reserved for emergency treatment. Monitor respirations closely.
– Don't give more than 60 mg/minute. Have resuscitation equipment available.
I.M. use: Give drug by deep I.M. injection. Superficial injection may cause pain, sterile abscess, and tissue sloughing.
• Don't mix parenteral form with acidic solutions.
• Don't use injectable solution if it contains precipitate.
• Don't stop drug abruptly; seizures may worsen. Call prescriber immediately if adverse reactions occur.
ALERT Don't confuse pentobarbital with phenobarbital.

Patient teaching

• Make sure patient knows that phenobarbital is available in different strengths and sizes. Advise him to check prescription and refills closely.
• Inform him that full effects don't occur for 2 to 3 weeks except when loading dose is used.
• Advise him to avoid hazardous activities until CNS effects of drug are known.
• Warn patient and parents not to stop drug abruptly.
• Advise patient using oral contraceptives to consider other birth control methods.

Evaluation

• Patient is free from seizure activity.
• Patient has no injury from drug-induced adverse CNS reactions.
• Patient and family state understanding of drug therapy.

phentermine hydrochloride

(FEN-ter-meen high-droh-KLOR-ighd)

Adipex-P, Duromine♦, Fastin, OBY-CAP, Obe-Nix, Obephen, Panshape M, Phentercot, Phentride, Phentride Caplets, Phentrol, Phentrol-2, Phentrol-4, Phentrol-5, T-Diet, Teramine, Zantryl

Pharmacologic class: amphetamine congener
Therapeutic class: short-term adjunct anorexigenic
Controlled substance schedule: IV
Pregnancy risk category: C

Indications and dosages

▶ **Short-term adjunct in exogenous obesity.** *Adults:* 8 mg P.O. t.i.d. 15 minutes before meals. Or, 15 to 30 mg (resin complex) daily 2 hours before breakfast or 1 to 2 hours after breakfast.

How supplied

Tablets: 8 mg, 30 mg, 37.5 mg
Capsules: 15 mg, 18.75 mg, 30 mg, 37.5 mg
Capsules (resin complex, sustained-release): 15 mg, 30 mg

Pharmacokinetics

Absorption: absorbed readily from GI tract.
Distribution: distributed throughout body.
Metabolism: unknown.
Excretion: excreted in urine. *Half-life:* 19 to 24 hours.

Route	Onset	Peak	Duration
P.O.	Unknown	Unknown	12-14 hr

Pharmacodynamics

Chemical effect: unknown; probably promotes nerve impulse transmission by releasing stored norepinephrine from nerve terminals in brain. Main sites appear to be cerebral cortex and reticular activating system.
Therapeutic effect: depresses appetite.

Adverse reactions

CNS: overstimulation, headache, euphoria, dysphoria, dizziness, *insomnia.*
CV: palpitations, tachycardia, increased blood pressure.
EENT: mydriasis, eye irritation, blurred vision.
GI: dry mouth, dysgeusia, constipation, diarrhea, other GI disturbances.
GU: impotence.
Skin: urticaria.
Other: altered libido.

Interactions

Drug-drug. *Acetazolamide, antacids, sodium bicarbonate:* increased renal reabsorption. Monitor patient.
Ammonium chloride, ascorbic acid: decreased plasma levels and increased renal excretion of phentermine. Monitor patient for decreased effects.
Guanethidine: may decrease hypotensive effect. Monitor patient closely.
Haloperidol, phenothiazines, tricyclic antidepressants: increased CNS effects. Avoid concomitant use.
Insulin, oral antidiabetics: may alter antidiabetic requirements. Monitor blood glucose levels.
MAO inhibitors: severe hypertension and possible hypertensive crisis. Don't use together or within 14 days of MAO inhibitor.
Drug-food. *Caffeine:* may increase CNS stimulation. Discourage concurrent use.

Contraindications and precautions

- Contraindicated in agitated patients, patients hypersensitive to sympathomimetic amines, patients who have idiosyncratic reactions to them, patients who have taken an MAO inhibitor within 14 days, and patients with hyperthyroidism, moderate to severe hypertension, advanced arteriosclerosis, symptomatic CV disease, or glaucoma.
- Drug isn't recommended for pregnant or breast-feeding women.
- Use cautiously in patients with mild hypertension.
- Safety of drug hasn't been established in children.

NURSING CONSIDERATIONS

Assessment
- Weigh patient before therapy and regularly thereafter.
- Be alert for adverse reactions and drug interactions.
- Monitor patient for habituation and tolerance.
- Evaluate patient's and family's knowledge of drug therapy.

Nursing diagnoses
- Imbalanced nutrition: more than body requirements related to food intake
- Disturbed sleep pattern related to drug-induced insomnia
- Deficient knowledge related to drug therapy

Planning and implementation
- Give drug at least 6 hours before bedtime to avoid insomnia.
- Make sure patient is following a weight-reduction program.

ALERT Don't confuse phentermine with phentolamine.

Patient teaching
- Instruct patient to take drug at least 6 hours before bedtime to avoid sleep interference.
- Warn patient to avoid hazardous activities until CNS effects of drug are known.
- Tell patient to avoid caffeine because it increases the effects of amphetamines and related amines.
- Tell patient to report signs of excessive stimulation.
- Inform patient that fatigue may result as drug effects wear off.

Evaluation
- Patient loses weight.
- Patient doesn't have insomnia.
- Patient and family state understanding of drug therapy.

phentolamine mesylate
(fen-TOH-luh-meen MES-ih-layt)
Regitine, Rogitine♦

Pharmacologic class: alpha-adrenergic blocker
Therapeutic class: antihypertensive for pheochromocytoma, cutaneous vasodilator
Pregnancy risk category: C

Indications and dosages

▶ **To aid in diagnosis of pheochromocytoma; to control or prevent hypertension before or during pheochromocytomectomy.** *Adults:* I.V. diagnostic dose is 5 mg, with close monitoring of blood pressure. Before surgical removal of tumor, 5 mg I.M. or I.V. During surgery, patient may need 5 mg I.V.
Children: I.V. diagnostic dose is 1 mg with close monitoring of blood pressure. Before surgical removal of tumor, 1 mg, 0.1 mg/kg, or 3 mg/m^2 I.V. or I.M. During surgery, patient may need 1 mg I.V.

▶ **Dermal necrosis and sloughing after I.V. extravasation of norepinephrine.** *Adults and children:* infiltrate area with 5 to 10 mg phentolamine in 10 ml normal saline solution or give half dosage through infiltrated I.V. and other half around site. Must be done within 12 hours.

How supplied

Injection: 5 mg/ml in 1-ml vial, 10 mg/ml♦

Pharmacokinetics

Absorption: unknown.
Distribution: unknown.
Metabolism: unknown.
Excretion: about 10% of drug is excreted unchanged in urine; excretion of remainder is unknown. *Half-life:* 19 minutes after I.V. administration; unknown for I.M. administration.

Route	Onset	Peak	Duration
I.V., I.M.	Unknown	Unknown	Unknown

Pharmacodynamics

Chemical effect: competitively blocks effects of catecholamines on alpha-adrenergic receptors.
Therapeutic effect: lowers blood pressure; minimizes dermal damage from norepinephrine infiltration.

Adverse reactions

CNS: dizziness, weakness, flushing, ***cerebrovascular occlusion.***
CV: hypotension, ***shock,*** arrhythmias, palpitations, tachycardia, angina pectoris, ***MI.***
EENT: nasal congestion.
GI: *diarrhea,* abdominal pain, *nausea, vomiting,* hyperperistalsis.
Metabolic: hypoglycemia.

Interactions

Drug-drug. *Epinephrine:* excessive hypotension. Use cautiously and monitor patient closely.
Narcotics, rauwolfia alkaloids, sedatives: false-positive test results for pheochromocytoma. Don't give within 24 hours before phentolamine is used as diagnostic test. Withdraw rauwolfia alkaloids at least 4 weeks before such testing.

Contraindications and precautions

- Contraindicated in patients hypersensitive to drug and in those with angina, coronary artery disease, MI, or history of MI.
- Drug isn't recommended for breast-feeding women.
- Use cautiously in pregnant women and in patients with gastritis or peptic ulcer.

NURSING CONSIDERATIONS

Assessment

- Assess patient's condition before therapy and regularly thereafter.
- Before giving drug as diagnostic test for pheochromocytoma, check patient's blood pressure. Monitor it frequently during administration.
- Test is positive for pheochromocytoma if I.V. test dose causes severe hypotension.
- Be alert for adverse reactions and drug interactions.
- Evaluate patient's and family's knowledge of drug therapy.

Nursing diagnoses

- Ineffective health maintenance related to underlying condition
- Decreased cardiac output related to adverse CV reactions
- Deficient knowledge related to drug therapy

Planning and implementation

- Drug is supplied as powder. Use it immediately after reconstitution.

I.V. use: Dilute 5 to 10 mg of drug in 500 ml of normal saline solution.
– Use infusion pump to control rate.
I.M. use: Follow normal protocol.
Local use: To treat extravasation, infiltrate area with 5 to 10 mg of drug in 10 ml normal saline solution or give half dosage through infiltrated I.V. and other half around site. Must be done within 12 hours of infiltration.

- Don't administer epinephrine to treat phentolamine-induced hypotension because it may cause blood pressure to fall farther ("epinephrine reversal"). Use norepinephrine instead.

ALERT Don't confuse phentolamine with phentermine.

Patient teaching

- Explain if drug will be used as diagnostic test.
- Tell patient to report adverse reactions immediately.

Evaluation

- Patient responds well to therapy.
- Patient maintains adequate cardiac output.
- Patient and family state understanding of drug therapy.

phenylephrine hydrochloride

(fen-il-EF-rin high-droh-KLOR-ighd)

Neo-Synephrine

Pharmacologic class: adrenergic
Therapeutic class: vasoconstrictor
Pregnancy risk category: C

Indications and dosages

▶ **Hypotensive emergencies during spinal anesthesia.** *Adults:* initially, 0.1 to 0.2 mg I.V., followed by 0.1 to 0.2 mg, p.r.n.

▶ **Maintenance of blood pressure during spinal or inhalation anesthesia.** *Adults:* 2 to 3 mg S.C. or I.M. 3 or 4 minutes before anesthesia.
Children: 0.044 to 0.088 mg/kg S.C. or I.M.

▶ **Prolongation of spinal anesthesia.** *Adults:* 2 to 5 mg added to anesthetic solution.

▶ **Vasoconstrictor for regional anesthesia.** *Adults:* 1 mg phenylephrine added to 20 ml local anesthetic.

▶ **Mild to moderate hypotension.** *Adults:* 2 to 5 mg S.C. or I.M.; repeated in 1 to 2 hours as needed and tolerated. Initial dose shouldn't exceed 5 mg. Or, 0.1 to 0.5 mg slow I.V., no more than q 10 to 15 minutes.
Children: 0.1 mg/kg I.M. or S.C.; repeated in 1 to 2 hours as needed and tolerated.

▶ **Severe hypotension and shock (including drug-induced).** *Adults:* 10 mg in 250 to 500 ml of D_5W or normal saline solution for injection. Start I.V. infusion at 100 to 180 mcg/minute, then decrease to maintenance infusion of 40 to 60 mcg/minute when blood pressure stabilizes.

▶ **Paroxysmal supraventricular tachycardia.** *Adults:* initially, 0.5 mg rapid I.V. Subsequent doses may be increased by 0.1 to 0.2 mg. Maximum dose shouldn't exceed 1 mg.

How supplied

Injection: 10 mg/ml

Pharmacokinetics

Absorption: unknown after I.M. and S.C. administration.
Distribution: unknown.
Metabolism: metabolized in liver and intestine.
Excretion: unknown.

Route	Onset	Peak	Duration
I.V.	Immediate	Unknown	15-20 min
I.M.	10-15 min	Unknown	0.5-2 hr
S.C.	10-15 min	Unknown	50-60 min

Pharmacodynamics

Chemical effect: mainly stimulates alpha-adrenergic receptors in sympathetic nervous system.
Therapeutic effect: raises blood pressure and stops paroxysmal supraventricular tachycardia.

Adverse reactions

CNS: *headache, restlessness, light-headedness, weakness.*
CV: palpitations, ***bradycardia, arrhythmias,*** hypertension, angina, decreased cardiac output.
EENT: blurred vision.
GI: vomiting.
Respiratory: ***asthma attacks.***
Skin: pilomotor response, feeling of coolness.
Other: tachyphylaxis, decreased organ perfusion with prolonged use, tissue sloughing with extravasation, ***anaphylaxis.***

Interactions

Drug-drug. *Alpha-adrenergic blockers, phenothiazines:* decreased vasopressor response. Monitor patient closely.
Beta blockers: block cardiostimulatory effects. Monitor patient closely.
MAO inhibitors: may cause severe hypertension (hypertensive crisis). Monitor patient and blood pressure closely.
Oxytocics, tricyclic antidepressants: increased pressor response. Monitor patient.

Contraindications and precautions

- Contraindicated in patients hypersensitive to drug and patients with severe hypertension or ventricular tachycardia.
- Use with extreme caution in elderly patients and patients with heart disease, hyperthyroidism, severe atherosclerosis, bradycardia,

partial heart block, myocardial disease, or sulfite sensitivity.
- Use cautiously in pregnant or breast-feeding women.

NURSING CONSIDERATIONS

Assessment
- Assess patient's condition before therapy and regularly thereafter.
- Monitor blood pressure frequently; avoid severe increase. Maintain blood pressure slightly below patient's normal level, as ordered. In previously normotensive patient, maintain systolic pressure at 80 to 100 mm Hg; in previously hypertensive patient, maintain systolic pressure at 30 to 40 mm Hg below usual level.
- Monitor ECG throughout therapy.
- Be alert for adverse reactions and drug interactions.
- Evaluate patient's and family's knowledge of drug therapy.

Nursing diagnoses
- Ineffective tissue perfusion (cerebral, cardiopulmonary, peripheral, GI, renal) related to underlying condition
- Decreased cardiac output related to drug-induced adverse reaction
- Deficient knowledge related to drug therapy

Planning and implementation
I.V. use: For direct injection, dilute 10 mg (1 ml) with 9 ml sterile water for injection to provide solution containing 1 mg/ml. Prepare I.V. infusions by adding 10 mg of drug to 500 ml of D_5W or normal saline solution for injection.
– Initial infusion rate is usually 100 to 180 mcg/minute; maintenance rate is usually 40 to 60 mcg/minute.
– Use continuous infusion pump to regulate flow rate.
– During infusion, frequently monitor ECG, blood pressure, cardiac output, central venous pressure, pulmonary capillary wedge pressure, pulse rate, urine output, and color and temperature of limbs. Titrate infusion rate according to findings and prescriber's guidelines.
– Use central venous catheter or large vein, as in antecubital fossa, to minimize risk of extravasation.
– After prolonged I.V. infusion, avoid abrupt withdrawal.
– To treat extravasation, infiltrate site promptly with 10 to 15 ml of normal saline solution for injection that contains 5 to 10 mg phentolamine. Use a fine needle.
– Drug is incompatible with butacaine sulfate, alkalis, ferric salts, and oxidizing agents.
I.M. and S.C. use: Follow normal protocol.

Patient teaching
- Tell patient to report discomfort at infusion site immediately.

Evaluation
- Patient maintains tissue perfusion and cellular oxygenation.
- Patient maintains adequate cardiac output.
- Patient and family state understanding of drug therapy.

phenylephrine hydrochloride
(fen-il-EF-rin high-droh-KLOR-ighd)
Alconefrin 12†, Alconefrin 25†, Alconefrin 50†, Duration†, Neo-Synephrine†, Nōstril†, Rhinall†, Rhinall-10†, Sinex†

Pharmacologic class: adrenergic
Therapeutic class: vasoconstrictor
Pregnancy risk category: NR

Indications and dosages
▶ **Nasal congestion.** *Adults and children age 12 and older:* 2 to 3 gtt or 1 to 2 sprays in each nostril, p.r.n.
Children ages 6 to 12: 2 to 3 gtt or 1 to 2 sprays of 0.25% solution in each nostril q 3 to 4 hours, p.r.n.
Children under age 6: 2 to 3 gtt of 0.125% solution q 4 hours, p.r.n.

How supplied
Nasal solution: 0.125%, 0.16%, 0.25%, 0.5%, 1%

Pharmacokinetics

Absorption: small amounts may be absorbed.
Distribution: distributed locally to nasal tissue.
Metabolism: metabolized in liver.
Excretion: excreted in urine.

Route	Onset	Peak	Duration
Intranasal	Rapid	Unknown	0.5-4 hr

Pharmacodynamics

Chemical effect: causes local vasoconstriction of dilated arterioles, reducing blood flow.
Therapeutic effect: relieves nasal congestion.

Adverse reactions

CNS: headache, tremor, dizziness, nervousness.
CV: *palpitations, tachycardia, **PVCs,*** hypertension, pallor.
EENT: transient burning or stinging, dry nasal mucosa, rebound nasal congestion with continued use.
GI: nausea.

Interactions

None significant.

Contraindications and precautions

- Contraindicated in patients hypersensitive to drug.
- Use cautiously in children with low body weight, elderly patients, pregnant or breast-feeding women, and patients with hyperthyroidism, marked hypertension, type 1 diabetes mellitus, cardiac disease, or advanced arteriosclerotic changes.

NURSING CONSIDERATIONS

Assessment

- Assess patient's condition before therapy and regularly thereafter.
- Be alert for adverse reactions.
- Evaluate patient's and family's knowledge of drug therapy.

Nursing diagnoses

- Ineffective health maintenance related to nasal congestion
- Impaired tissue integrity related to adverse effect on nasal tissue
- Deficient knowledge related to drug therapy

Planning and implementation

- To administer drug, have patient hold head upright while you insert nozzle; have patient sniff spray briskly.

Patient teaching

- Teach patient how to administer drug.
- Tell patient not to share drug to prevent spread of infection.
- Warn patient not to exceed recommended dosage.
- Advise patient to contact prescriber if symptoms persist beyond 3 days.

Evaluation

- Patient's nasal congestion is relieved with phenylephrine therapy.
- Patient maintains normal nasal tissue integrity.
- Patient and family state understanding of drug therapy.

phenytoin (diphenylhydantoin)

(FEN-uh-toyn)

Dilantin, Dilantin-30♦, Dilantin-125, Dilantin Infatabs

phenytoin sodium

Dilantin, Phenytex♦

phenytoin sodium (extended)

Dilantin Kapseals

Pharmacologic class: hydantoin derivative
Therapeutic class: anticonvulsant
Pregnancy risk category: NR

Indications and dosages

▶ **Control of tonic-clonic (grand mal) and complex partial (temporal lobe) seizures, post–head trauma, Reye's syndrome.** *Adults:* highly individualized. Initially, 100 mg P.O. t.i.d., increased in increments of 100 mg P.O. q 2 to 4 weeks until desired response is obtained. Usual range is 300 to 600 mg daily.

Maintenance dose is 300 mg P.O. (extended-release capsule).
Children: 5 mg/kg or 250 mg/m^2 P.O. daily b.i.d. or t.i.d. Maximum daily dosage is 300 mg.
▶ **For patient who needs loading dose.** *Adults:* initially, 1 g P.O. daily divided into three doses and administered at 2-hour intervals. Or, 10 to 15 mg/kg I.V. at rate not exceeding 50 mg/minute. Begin maintenance dosage 24 hours later.
Children: 5 mg/kg/day P.O. in two or three equally divided doses. Subsequent dosage individualized to maximum of 300 mg daily.
▶ **Prevention and treatment of seizures occurring during neurosurgery.** *Adults:* 100 to 200 mg I.M. q 4 hours during surgery and postoperative period.
▶ **Status epilepticus.** *Adults:* loading dose of 10 to 15 mg/kg I.V. (1 to 1.5 g may be needed) at no more than 50 mg/minute followed by maintenance dosage (once controlled) of 300 mg P.O. daily.
Children: loading dose of 15 to 20 mg/kg I.V. at no more than 1 to 3 mg/kg/minute followed by highly individualized maintenance dosages.

How supplied

phenytoin
Tablets (chewable): 50 mg
Oral suspension: 30 mg/5 ml♦, 125 mg/5 ml
phenytoin sodium
Capsules: 30 mg (27.6-mg base), 100 mg (92-mg base)
Injection: 50 mg/ml (46-mg base)
phenytoin sodium (extended)
Capsules: 30 mg (27.6-mg base), 100 mg (92-mg base)

Pharmacokinetics

Absorption: absorbed slowly from small intestine after P.O. administration. Absorption is formulation-dependent and bioavailability may differ among products. Absorbed erratically from I.M. site.
Distribution: distributed widely throughout body. Drug is about 90% protein-bound.
Metabolism: metabolized by liver.
Excretion: excreted in urine; exhibits dose-dependent (zero-order) elimination kinetics. Above certain dosage level, small increases in dosage disproportionately increase serum levels. *Half-life:* varies with dose and serum concentration changes.

Route	Onset	Peak	Duration
P.O.	Unknown	1.5-12 hr	Unknown
I.V.	Immediate	1-2 hr	Unknown
I.M.	Unknown	Unknown	Unknown

Pharmacodynamics

Chemical effect: unknown; probably stabilizes neuronal membranes and limits seizure activity by either increasing efflux or decreasing influx of sodium ions across cell membranes in motor cortex during generation of nerve impulses.
Therapeutic effect: prevents and stops seizure activity.

Adverse reactions

CNS: *ataxia, slurred speech, confusion,* dizziness, insomnia, nervousness, twitching, headache.
CV: hypotension.
EENT: nystagmus, diplopia, blurred vision, gingival hyperplasia.
GI: nausea, vomiting.
Hematologic: ***thrombocytopenia, leukopenia, agranulocytosis, pancytopenia,*** macrocythemia, megaloblastic anemia.
Hepatic: ***toxic hepatitis.***
Metabolic: hyperglycemia.
Musculoskeletal: osteomalacia.
Skin: scarlatiniform or morbilliform rash; bullous, ***exfoliative,*** or purpuric dermatitis; ***Stevens-Johnson syndrome;*** lupus erythematosus; *hirsutism;* ***toxic epidermal necrolysis;*** photosensitivity; pain, necrosis, or inflammation at injection site; discoloration (purple glove syndrome) if given by I.V. push in back of hand; hypertrichosis.
Other: periarteritis nodosa, lymphadenopathy.

Interactions

Drug-drug. *Amiodarone, antihistamines, chloramphenicol, cimetidine, cycloserine, diazepam, disulfiram, influenza vaccine, isoniazid, phenylbutazone, salicylates, sulfamethizole, valproate:* increased therapeutic effects of phenytoin. Monitor patient for toxicity.

Dexamethasone, diazoxide, folic acid: decreased phenytoin activity. Monitor patient closely.
Drug-herb. *Milk thistle:* may decrease risk of liver toxicity. Monitor patient.
Drug-food. *Oral tube feedings with Osmolite or Isocal:* may interfere with absorption of oral phenytoin. Schedule feedings as far as possible from drug administration.
Drug-lifestyle. *Alcohol use:* decreased phenytoin activity. Discourage concomitant use.

Contraindications and precautions

- Contraindicated in patients hypersensitive to hydantoin and patients with sinus bradycardia, SA block, second- or third-degree AV block, or Adams-Stokes syndrome.
- Drug isn't recommended for pregnant or breast-feeding women.
- Use cautiously in elderly patients, debilitated patients, patients receiving other hydantoin derivatives, and patients with hepatic dysfunction, hypotension, myocardial insufficiency, diabetes, or respiratory depression.

NURSING CONSIDERATIONS

Assessment

- Assess patient's condition before therapy and regularly thereafter.
- Monitor blood levels as ordered. Therapeutic level is 10 to 20 mcg/ml.
- Monitor CBC and serum calcium level every 6 months, and periodically monitor hepatic function as ordered.
- Check vital signs, blood pressure, and ECG during I.V. administration.
- Be alert for adverse reactions and drug interactions.
- Mononucleosis may decrease phenytoin levels. Monitor patient for increased seizure activity.
- Evaluate patient's and family's knowledge of drug therapy.

Nursing diagnoses

- Risk for trauma related to seizures
- Impaired oral mucous membrane related to gingival hyperplasia
- Deficient knowledge related to drug therapy

Planning and implementation

- Elderly patients tend to metabolize phenytoin slowly and may need lower dosages.
- Use only clear or slightly yellow solution for injection. Don't refrigerate.

P.O. use: Divided doses given with or after meals may decrease adverse GI reactions.
– Dilantin capsule is only P.O. form that can be given once daily. Toxic levels may result if any other brand or form is given once daily. Dilantin tablets and P.O. suspension shouldn't be taken once daily.
I.V. use: If giving as infusion, don't mix drug with D_5W because it will precipitate. Clear I.V. tubing first with normal saline solution. May mix with normal saline solution if necessary and infuse over 30 to 60 minutes when possible.
– Infusion must begin within 1 hour after preparation and should run through in-line filter.
– Administer drug slowly (50 mg/minute) as I.V. bolus.
– Check patency of I.V. catheter before administering. Extravasation has caused severe local tissue damage.
– Never use cloudy solution.
– Discard 4 hours after preparation.
– Avoid giving phenytoin by I.V. push into veins on back of hand to avoid discoloration known as purple glove syndrome. Inject into larger veins or central venous catheter if available.
I.M. use: Don't give drug I.M. unless dosage adjustments are made. Drug may precipitate at site, cause pain, and be erratically absorbed.

- Discontinue drug if rash appears. If rash is scarlatiniform or morbilliform, drug may be resumed after rash clears. If rash reappears, therapy should be discontinued. If rash is exfoliative, purpuric, or bullous, drug won't be resumed.
- Don't withdraw drug suddenly; seizures may worsen. Call prescriber at once if adverse reactions develop.
- Phenytoin may cause altered laboratory test results, including reduced serum protein–bound iodine and free thyroxine levels without clinical signs of hypothyroidism; slight decrease in urinary 17-hydroxysteroid and 17-

ketosteroid levels; increased urine 6-hydroxycortisol excretion and serum levels of alkaline phosphatase or GGT; and decreased values for dexamethasone suppression or metyrapone tests.

• If patient has megaloblastic anemia, prescriber may order folic acid and vitamin B_{12}.

ALERT Don't confuse phenytoin with mephyton or Dilantin with Dilaudid.

Patient teaching

• Advise patient to avoid hazardous activities until CNS effects of drug are known.
• Advise patient not to change brands or dosage forms.
• Warn patient and parents not to stop drug abruptly.
• Promote oral hygiene and regular dental examinations. Gingivectomy may be necessary periodically if dental hygiene is poor.
• Caution patient that drug may color urine pink, red, or red-brown.
• Inform patient that heavy alcohol use may diminish drug's benefits.

Evaluation

• Patient is free from seizure activity.
• Patient expresses importance of good oral hygiene and regular dental examinations.
• Patient and family state understanding of drug therapy.

physostigmine salicylate (eserine salicylate)

(fiz-oh-STIG-meen sa-LIS-il-ayt)
Antilirium

Pharmacologic class: cholinesterase inhibitor
Therapeutic class: antimuscarinic antidote
Pregnancy risk category: C

Indications and dosages

▶ **To reverse CNS toxicity caused by clinical or toxic dosages of drugs capable of producing anticholinergic syndrome.**
Adults: 0.5 to 2 mg I.M. or I.V. (1 mg/minute I.V.) repeated q 10 minutes as necessary if life-threatening signs recur (coma, seizures, arrhythmias).
Children: 0.02 mg/kg I.M. or slow I.V. repeated q 5 to 10 minutes until response is obtained. Maximum dosage is 2 mg. Drug is reserved for life-threatening situations.

How supplied

Injection: 1 mg/ml

Pharmacokinetics

Absorption: absorbed well from injection site when administered I.M.
Distribution: distributed widely and crosses blood-brain barrier.
Metabolism: cholinesterase hydrolyzes physostigmine relatively quickly.
Excretion: primary mode of excretion unknown; small amount excreted in urine.

Route	Onset	Peak	Duration
I.V.	3-5 min	≤ 5 min	30-60 min
I.M.	3-5 min	20-30 min	30-60 min

Pharmacodynamics

Chemical effect: inhibits destruction of acetylcholine released from parasympathetic and somatic efferent nerves. Acetylcholine accumulates, promoting increased stimulation of receptor.
Therapeutic effect: reverses anticholinergic signs and symptoms.

Adverse reactions

CNS: ***seizures,*** hallucinations, muscle twitching, muscle weakness, ataxia, *restlessness, excitability, sweating.*
CV: irregular pulse, palpitations, ***bradycardia,*** hypotension.
EENT: miosis.
GI: nausea, vomiting, epigastric pain, *diarrhea, excessive salivation.*
GU: urinary urgency.
Respiratory: ***bronchospasm,*** bronchial constriction, dyspnea.

Interactions

Drug-drug. *Anticholinergics, atropine, procainamide, quinidine:* may reverse cholinergic effects. Observe patient for lack of drug effect.

Ganglionic blockers: may decrease blood pressure. Avoid concomitant use.
Drug-herb. *Jaborandi tree, pill-bearing spurge:* may have additive effect. Discourage concomitant use to avoid the risk of toxicity.

Contraindications and precautions

- Contraindicated in patients receiving choline esters or depolarizing neuromuscular blockers and in patients with mechanical obstruction of intestine or urogenital tract, asthma, gangrene, diabetes, CV disease, or vagotonia.
- Use cautiously in patients with sensitivity or allergy to sulfites.
- Use cautiously in pregnant women.
- Safety of drug hasn't been established in breast-feeding women.

NURSING CONSIDERATIONS

Assessment

- Assess patient's condition before therapy and regularly thereafter. Effectiveness is often immediate and dramatic, but may be transient and require repeated doses.
- Monitor vital signs frequently, especially respirations.
- Be alert for adverse reactions and drug interactions.
- Evaluate patient's and family's knowledge of drug therapy.

Nursing diagnoses

- Ineffective health maintenance related to underlying condition
- Risk for injury related to drug-induced adverse CNS reactions
- Deficient knowledge related to drug therapy

Planning and implementation

I.V. use: Give drug I.V. at controlled rate; use direct injection at no more than 1 mg/minute.
I.M. use: Follow normal protocol.

- Use only clear solution. Darkening of solution may indicate loss of potency.
- Position patient to ease breathing. Have atropine injection available and be prepared to give 0.5 mg S.C. or slow I.V. push as ordered. Provide respiratory support as needed. Best administered in presence of prescriber.
- Raise side rails of bed if patient becomes restless or hallucinates. Adverse reactions may indicate drug toxicity. Notify prescriber.

Patient teaching

- Tell patient to report adverse reactions especially pain at the I.V. site.

Evaluation

- Patient responds well to therapy.
- Patient doesn't experience injury from adverse CNS reactions.
- Patient and family state understanding of drug therapy.

phytonadione (vitamin K_1)

(figh-toh-neh-DIGH-ohn)
AquaMEPHYTON, Konakion, Mephyton

Pharmacologic class: vitamin K
Therapeutic class: blood coagulation modifier
Pregnancy risk category: C

Indications and dosages

▶ **RDA.** *Neonates and infants to age 6 months:* 5 mcg.
Infants ages 6 months to 1 year: 10 mcg.
Children ages 1 to 3: 15 mcg.
Children ages 4 to 6: 20 mcg.
Children ages 7 to 10: 30 mcg.
Children ages 11 to 14: 45 mcg.
Men ages 15 to 18: 65 mcg.
Men ages 19 to 24: 70 mcg.
Men age 25 and over: 80 mcg.
Women ages 15 to 18: 55 mcg.
Women ages 19 to 24: 60 mcg.
Women age 25 and over, pregnant or breast-feeding women: 65 mcg.

▶ **Hypoprothrombinemia secondary to vitamin K malabsorption, drug therapy, or excessive vitamin A.** *Adults:* depending on severity, 2 to 25 mg P.O., S.C., or I.M. repeated and increased up to 50 mg if necessary.
Children: 5 to 10 mg P.O. or parenterally. I.V. injection rate for infants and children shouldn't exceed 3 mg/m^2/minute or total of 5 mg.
Infants: 2 mg P.O. or parenterally.

▶ **Hypoprothrombinemia secondary to effect of oral anticoagulants.** *Adults:* 2.5 to 10 mg P.O., S.C., or I.M. based on PT, repeated if necessary within 12 to 48 hours after P.O. dose or within 6 to 8 hours after parenteral dose. In emergency, 10 to 50 mg slow I.V., maximum rate 1 mg/minute, repeated q 4 hours, p.r.n.

▶ **Prevention of hemorrhagic disease of newborn.** *Neonates:* 0.5 to 1 mg I.M. or S.C. within 1 hour after birth.

▶ **Treatment of hemorrhagic disease of newborn.** *Neonates:* 1 mg S.C. or I.M. based on laboratory tests. Higher doses may be necessary if mother has been receiving anticoagulants P.O.

▶ **To differentiate between hepatocellular disease or biliary obstruction as source of hypoprothrombinemia.** *Adults and children:* 10 mg I.M. or S.C.

▶ **Prevention of hypoprothrombinemia related to vitamin K deficiency in long-term parenteral nutrition.** *Adults:* 5 to 10 mg I.M. weekly.

Children: 2 to 5 mg I.M. weekly.

▶ **Prevention of hypoprothrombinemia in infants receiving less than 0.1 mg/L vitamin K in breast milk or milk substitutes.** *Infants:* 1 mg I.M. monthly.

How supplied

Tablets: 5 mg

Injection (aqueous colloidal solution): 2 mg/ml, 10 mg/ml

Injection (aqueous dispersion): 2 mg/ml, 10 mg/ml

Pharmacokinetics

Absorption: drug requires presence of bile salts for GI tract absorption after P.O. administration. Absorption unknown after I.M. or S.C. administration.

Distribution: concentrates in liver for short time.

Metabolism: metabolized rapidly by liver.

Excretion: not clearly defined.

Route	Onset	Peak	Duration
P.O.	6-12 hr	Unknown	12-14 hr
I.V., I.M., S.C.	1-2 hr	Unknown	12-14 hr

Pharmacodynamics

Chemical effect: an antihemorrhagic factor that promotes hepatic formation of active prothrombin.

Therapeutic effect: controls abnormal bleeding.

Adverse reactions

CNS: dizziness, seizure-like movements.

CV: transient hypotension after I.V. administration, rapid and weak pulse, cardiac irregularities.

Skin: diaphoresis, flushing, erythema.

Other: cramp-like pain; ***anaphylaxis and anaphylactoid reactions*** (usually after rapid I.V. administration); pain, swelling, and hematoma at injection site.

Interactions

Drug-drug. *Anticoagulants:* temporary resistance to prothrombin-depressing anticoagulants may result, especially when larger doses of phytonadione are used. Monitor patient closely.

Cholestyramine resin, mineral oil: inhibited GI absorption of oral vitamin K. Administer separately.

Contraindications and precautions

- Contraindicated in patients hypersensitive to drug.
- Use cautiously in pregnant or breast-feeding women.

NURSING CONSIDERATIONS

Assessment

- Assess patient's condition before therapy and regularly thereafter.
- Monitor PT to determine dosage effectiveness, as ordered.
- Failure to respond to vitamin K may indicate coagulation defects.
- Be alert for adverse reactions and drug interactions.
- Phytonadione therapy for hemorrhagic disease in infants causes fewer adverse reactions than other vitamin K analogues.
- Monitor patient's hydration status if adverse GI reactions occur.

• Evaluate patient's and family's knowledge of drug therapy.

Nursing diagnoses

• Ineffective protection related to underlying vitamin K deficiency
• Risk for deficient fluid volume related to adverse GI reactions
• Deficient knowledge related to drug therapy

Planning and implementation

• Check brand name labels for administration route restrictions.
P.O. and S.C. use: Follow normal protocol. S.C. is the preferred route of administration.
I.V. use: Dilute drug with normal saline solution for injection, D_5W, or dextrose 5% in normal saline solution for injection.
– Give I.V. by slow infusion over 2 to 3 hours. Maximum infusion rate 1 mg/minute in adult or 3 mg/m^2/minute in child.
– Protect parenteral products from light. Wrap infusion container with aluminum foil.
– Anticipate order for weekly addition of 5 to 10 mg of phytonadione to total parenteral nutrition solutions.
I.M. use: Administer drug in upper outer quadrant of buttocks in adult or older child; inject in anterolateral aspect of thigh or deltoid region in infant.
• If severe bleeding occurs, don't delay other treatments, such as fresh frozen plasma or whole blood.

Patient teaching

• Explain drug's purpose.
• Instruct patient to report adverse reactions.

Evaluation

• Patient achieves normal PT levels with drug therapy.
• Patient maintains adequate hydration throughout drug therapy.
• Patient and family state understanding of drug therapy.

pimozide

(PIH-mih-zighd)
Orap

Pharmacologic class: diphenylbutylpiperidine
Therapeutic class: antipsychotic
Pregnancy risk category: C

Indications and dosages

▶ **Suppression of motor and phonic tics in patients with Tourette syndrome refractory to first-line therapy.** *Adults and children over age 12:* initially, 1 to 2 mg P.O. daily in divided doses. Increased every other day, as needed. Maximum dosage is 20 mg daily.

How supplied

Tablets: 2 mg, 4 mg ♦, 10 mg ♦

Pharmacokinetics

Absorption: absorbed slowly and incompletely from GI tract.
Distribution: distributed widely into body.
Metabolism: metabolized by liver; significant first-pass effect.
Excretion: about 40% of drug is excreted in urine as parent drug and metabolites; about 15% is excreted in feces. *Half-life:* about 29 hours.

Route	Onset	Peak	Duration
P.O.	Unknown	4-12 hr	Unknown

Pharmacodynamics

Chemical effect: may block dopamine nonselectively at presynaptic and postsynaptic receptors on neurons in CNS.
Therapeutic effect: stops tics linked to Tourette syndrome.

Adverse reactions

CNS: *parkinsonian-like symptoms,* other extrapyramidal symptoms (dystonia, akathisia, hyperreflexia, opisthotonos, oculogyric crisis), *tardive dyskinesia, sedation.*
CV: ***ECG changes (prolonged QT interval),*** hypotension.
EENT: visual disturbances.

GI: dry mouth, constipation.
GU: impotence.
Musculoskeletal: muscle rigidity, ***neuroleptic malignant syndrome.***

Interactions

Drug-drug. *Antiarrhythmics, phenothiazines, tricyclic antidepressants:* increased risk of ECG abnormalities. Monitor patient closely.
CNS depressants: increased CNS depression. Avoid concomitant use.
Drug-lifestyle. *Alcohol use:* increased CNS depression. Discourage concomitant use.

Contraindications and precautions

- Contraindicated in patients hypersensitive to drug, patients with simple tics or tics other than those caused by Tourette syndrome, patients receiving concurrent therapy with drugs known to cause motor and phonic tics, and patients with congenital long-QT syndrome, history of arrhythmias, severe toxic CNS depression, or coma.
- Use cautiously in patients with hepatic or renal dysfunction, glaucoma, prostatic hyperplasia, seizure disorder, or EEG abnormalities.
- Safety of drug hasn't been established in breast-feeding women.

NURSING CONSIDERATIONS

Assessment

- Assess patient's tics before therapy and regularly thereafter.
- Perform ECG before therapy and periodically thereafter as directed. Check for prolonged QT interval.
- Monitor patient for tardive dyskinesia. It may occur after prolonged use. It may not appear until months or years later and may disappear spontaneously or persist for life despite discontinuing drug.
- Monitor patient who also is taking anticonvulsants for increased seizure activity. Pimozide may lower seizure threshold.
- Be alert for adverse reactions and drug interactions.
- Evaluate patient's and family's knowledge of drug therapy.

Nursing diagnoses

- Disturbed body image related to presence of tics
- Impaired physical mobility related to adverse reactions
- Deficient knowledge related to drug therapy

Planning and implementation

- Acute dystonic reactions may be treated with diphenhydramine.

ALERT Avoid concurrent administration of other drugs that prolong QT interval, such as antiarrhythmics.

Patient teaching

- Warn patient not to stop taking drug abruptly and not to exceed prescribed dosage.
- Tell patient to avoid alcohol during drug therapy.
- Tell patient to use sugarless hard candy, gum, and liquids to relieve dry mouth.

Evaluation

- Patient states positive feelings about self with absence of tics.
- Patient is able to perform activities of daily living.
- Patient and family state understanding of drug therapy.

pindolol

(PIN-duh-lol)
Novo-Pindol ♦, Syn-Pindolol ♦, Visken

Pharmacologic class: beta blocker
Therapeutic class: antihypertensive
Pregnancy risk category: B

Indications and dosages

▶ **Hypertension.** *Adults:* initially, 5 mg P.O. b.i.d. Increase as needed and tolerated to maximum of 60 mg daily.

How supplied

Tablets: 5 mg, 10 mg, 15 mg ♦

Pharmacokinetics

Absorption: absorbed rapidly from GI tract. Food doesn't reduce bioavailability but may increase rate of GI absorption.
Distribution: distributed widely throughout body and is 40% to 60% protein-bound.
Metabolism: about 60% to 65% of drug is metabolized in liver.
Excretion: 35% to 50% of dose excreted unchanged in urine. *Half-life:* about 3 to 4 hours.

Route	Onset	Peak	Duration
P.O.	Unknown	1-2 hr	24 hr

Pharmacodynamics

Chemical effect: unknown; possible mechanisms include reduced cardiac output, decreased sympathetic outflow to peripheral vasculature, and inhibition of renin release by kidneys.
Therapeutic effect: lowers blood pressure.

Adverse reactions

CNS: insomnia, fatigue, dizziness, nervousness, vivid dreams, hallucinations, lethargy.
CV: *edema, **bradycardia, heart failure,*** peripheral vascular disease, hypotension.
EENT: visual disturbances.
GI: *nausea,* vomiting, diarrhea.
Metabolic: hypoglycemia without tachycardia.
Musculoskeletal: *muscle pain, joint pain.*
Respiratory: increased airway resistance.
Skin: rash.

Interactions

Drug-drug. *Cardiac glycosides, diltiazem, verapamil:* excessive bradycardia and additive depression of AV node. Use together cautiously.
Epinephrine: severe vasoconstriction. Monitor blood pressure and observe patient carefully.
Indomethacin: decreased antihypertensive effect. Monitor blood pressure and adjust dosage.
Insulin, oral antidiabetics: may alter requirements for these drugs in previously stabilized diabetic patients. Monitor patient for hypoglycemia.

Contraindications and precautions

- Contraindicated in patients hypersensitive to drug and in those with bronchial asthma, severe bradycardia, heart block greater than first degree, cardiogenic shock, or overt cardiac failure.
- Drug isn't recommended for breast-feeding women.
- Use cautiously in pregnant women and in patients with heart failure, nonallergic bronchospastic disease, diabetes, hyperthyroidism, or impaired renal or hepatic function.
- Safe use of drug hasn't been established in children.

NURSING CONSIDERATIONS

Assessment

- Assess patient's blood pressure before therapy and regularly thereafter.
- Always check patient's apical pulse rate before giving drug.
- Be alert for adverse reactions and drug interactions.
- Evaluate patient's and family's knowledge of drug therapy.

Nursing diagnoses

- Risk for injury related to presence of hypertension
- Fatigue related to drug's adverse effect
- Deficient knowledge related to drug therapy

Planning and implementation

- If you detect extreme pulse rates, withhold medication and call prescriber immediately.
- Notify prescriber if severe hypotension occurs.
- Abrupt discontinuation can worsen angina and precipitate MI. Withdraw over 1 to 2 weeks after long-term administration, as ordered.

ALERT Don't confuse pindolol with Parlodel, Panadol, or Plendil.

Patient teaching

- Teach patient how to take his pulse, and tell him to do so before taking each pindolol dose. Tell him to notify prescriber before taking any more doses if his pulse rate varies significantly from its usual level.

• Tell patient not to stop drug suddenly even if he has unpleasant adverse reactions; urge him to discuss them with prescriber. Explain that stopping drug abruptly can worsen angina and increase the risk of MI.
• Instruct patient to check with prescriber before taking OTC medications.
• Teach patient and family caregiver to take blood pressure measurements. Tell them to notify prescriber of any significant change.
• Advise patient to monitor blood glucose levels closely. Drug may mask signs of hypoglycemia.

☑ Evaluation

• Patient's blood pressure is normal.
• Patient states energy-conserving measures to combat fatigue.
• Patient and family state understanding of drug therapy.

pioglitazone hydrochloride

(pigh-oh-GLIH-tah-zohn high-droh-KLOR-ighd)
Actos

Pharmacologic class: thiazolidinedione
Therapeutic class: antidiabetic
Pregnancy risk category: C

Indications and dosages

▶ **Monotherapy adjunct to diet and exercise to improve glycemic control in patients with type 2 diabetes mellitus, or combination therapy with a sulfonylurea, metformin, or insulin when diet and exercise plus the single drug doesn't yield adequate glycemic control.** *Adults:* initially, 15 or 30 mg P.O. once daily. For patients who respond inadequately to initial dose, it may be increased in increments; maximum is 45 mg/day. If used in combination therapy, dosage shouldn't exceed 30 mg/day.

How supplied

Tablets: 15 mg, 30 mg, 45 mg

Pharmacokinetics

Absorption: when taken on an empty stomach, pioglitazone is rapidly absorbed and is measurable in serum within 30 minutes; levels peak within 2 hours. Food slightly delays time to peak serum levels (to 3 to 4 hours), but doesn't affect the overall extent of absorption.
Distribution: drug and its metabolites are extensively protein-bound (more than 98%), primarily to serum albumin.
Metabolism: extensively metabolized by the liver. Three metabolites, M-II, M-III and M-IV, are pharmacologically active.
Excretion: about 15% to 30% of dose is recovered in urine, primarily as metabolites and their conjugates. Most of P.O. dose is excreted in bile and eliminated in feces. *Half-life:* 3 to 7 hours.

Route	Onset	Peak	Duration
P.O.	Unknown	Within 2 hr	Unknown

Pharmacodynamics

Chemical effect: lowers blood glucose levels by decreasing insulin resistance in the periphery and in the liver, resulting in increased insulin-dependent glucose disposal and decreased glucose output by the liver. A potent and highly selective agonist for receptors found in insulin-sensitive tissues, such as adipose tissue, skeletal muscle, and liver. Activation of these receptors modulates the transcription of a number of insulin-responsive genes involved in the control of glucose and lipid metabolism.
Therapeutic effect: lowers blood glucose levels.

Adverse reactions

CNS: headache.
CV: *edema (in combination with insulin).*
EENT: sinusitis, pharyngitis.
Hematologic: anemia.
Metabolic: hypoglycemia with combination therapy, aggravated diabetes mellitus, weight gain, decreased triglyceride levels, increased high-density lipoprotein cholesterol levels.
Musculoskeletal: myalgia.
Respiratory: upper respiratory tract infection.
Other: tooth disorder.

Interactions

Drug-drug. *Ketoconazole:* may inhibit pioglitazone metabolism. Monitor patient's blood glucose levels more frequently.
Oral contraceptives: may reduce plasma levels of oral contraceptives, resulting in less effective contraception. Advise patients taking pioglitazone and oral contraceptives to consider additional birth control measures.
Drug-herb. *Aloe, bitter melon, bilberry leaf, burdock, dandelion, fenugreek, garlic, ginseng:* may improve blood glucose control and allow reduction of antidiabetic dosage. Advise patient to discuss herbal remedies with prescriber before using them.

Contraindications and precautions

- Contraindicated in patients hypersensitive to pioglitazone or its components.
- Drug shouldn't be used in patients with type 1 diabetes mellitus or diabetic ketoacidosis, patients with clinical evidence of active liver disease, patients with serum ALT levels more than two and one-half times the upper limit of normal, patients who experienced jaundice while taking troglitazone, and patients with New York Heart Association Class III or IV heart failure.
- Use cautiously in patients with edema or heart failure.

NURSING CONSIDERATIONS

Assessment

- Obtain history of patient's underlying condition before therapy, and reassess regularly thereafter.
- Assess patients for excessive fluid volume. Patients with heart failure should be monitored for increased edema during pioglitazone therapy.
- Measure liver enzymes at start of therapy, every 2 months for the first year of therapy, and periodically thereafter. Obtain liver function tests in patients who develop evidence of liver dysfunction, such as nausea, vomiting, abdominal pain, fatigue, anorexia, or dark urine.
- Monitor hemoglobin level and hematocrit, especially during the first 4 to 12 weeks of therapy.
- Monitor blood glucose levels regularly, especially during situations of increased stress, such as infection, fever, surgery, and trauma.
- Check glycosylated hemoglobin periodically, as ordered, to evaluate therapeutic response to drug.
- Evaluate patient's and family's knowledge about drug therapy.

Nursing diagnoses

- Ineffective health maintenance related to hyperglycemia
- Risk for injury related to drug-induced hyperglycemia
- Deficient knowledge related to drug therapy

Planning and implementation

- Notify prescriber and discontinue drug, as ordered, if patient develops jaundice or if results of liver function tests show ALT elevations greater than three times the upper limit of normal.
- Management of type 2 diabetes should include diet control. Because calorie restrictions, weight loss, and exercise help improve insulin sensitivity and help make drug therapy more effective, these measures are essential for proper diabetes management.
- Watch for hypoglycemia in patients receiving pioglitazone with insulin or a sulfonylurea. Dosage adjustments of these drugs may be needed.
- Because ovulation may resume in premenopausal, anovulatory women with insulin resistance, contraceptive measures may need to be considered.
- Drug should be used in pregnancy only if benefit justifies risk to fetus. Insulin is the preferred antidiabetic for use during pregnancy.

Patient teaching

- Instruct patient to adhere to dietary instructions and to have blood glucose levels and glycosylated hemoglobin tested regularly.
- Inform patient taking pioglitazone with insulin or an oral antidiabetic about the signs and symptoms of hypoglycemia.
- Advise patient to notify prescriber about periods of stress, such as fever, trauma, infec-

tion, or surgery, because medication requirements may change.
• Notify patient that blood tests for liver function will be performed before the start of therapy, every 2 months for the first year, and periodically thereafter.
• Tell patient to report unexplained nausea, vomiting, abdominal pain, fatigue, anorexia, or dark urine immediately because these signs and symptoms may indicate liver problems.
• Inform patient that pioglitazone can be taken with or without meals.
• If patient misses a dose, caution against doubling the dose the following day.
• Advise premenopausal, anovulatory woman with insulin resistance that pioglitazone may restore ovulation; recommend that she consider contraception as needed.

✓ Evaluation

• Patient's blood glucose level is normal with drug therapy.
• Patient doesn't experience hypoglycemia.
• Patient and family state understanding of drug therapy.

pipecuronium bromide

(pigh-peh-kyoor-OH-nee-um BROH-mighd)
Arduan

Pharmacologic class: nondepolarizing neuromuscular blocker
Therapeutic class: skeletal muscle relaxant
Pregnancy risk category: C

Indications and dosages

▶ **To provide skeletal muscle relaxation during surgery as adjunct to general anesthesia.** Dosage is highly individualized. The following dosages may serve as a guide for use in nonobese patients with normal renal function.
Adults and children: initially, 70 to 85 mcg/kg I.V. provides conditions considered ideal for endotracheal intubation and maintains paralysis for 1 to 2 hours. If succinylcholine is used for endotracheal intubation, initial dose of 50 mcg/kg I.V. provides relaxation for 45 minutes or more. Maintenance dose of 10 to 15 mcg/kg provides relaxation for about 50 minutes.

How supplied

Powder for injection: 10 mg/vial

Pharmacokinetics

Absorption: not applicable.
Distribution: volume of distribution is about 0.25 L/kg and increases in patients with renal failure. Other conditions linked to increased volume of distribution (including edema, old age, and CV disease) may delay onset.
Metabolism: about 20% to 40% of drug is metabolized, probably in liver.
Excretion: excreted primarily in urine. *Half-life:* about 1¾ hours.

Route	Onset	Peak	Duration
I.V.	1-2 min	≤ 5 min	About 24 min

Pharmacodynamics

Chemical effect: competes with acetylcholine for receptor sites at motor end plate. Because this action may be antagonized by cholinesterase inhibitors, drug is considered a competitive antagonist.
Therapeutic effect: relaxes skeletal muscles.

Adverse reactions

CV: hypotension, ***bradycardia,*** hypertension, myocardial ischemia, ***CVA,*** thrombosis, atrial fibrillation, ***ventricular extrasystole.***
GU: anuria, increased creatinine levels.
Musculoskeletal: prolonged muscle weakness.
Respiratory: dyspnea, respiratory depression, ***respiratory insufficiency or apnea.***

Interactions

Drug-drug. *Aminoglycosides (gentamicin, kanamycin, neomycin, streptomycin), bacitracin, colistimethate, colistin, polymyxin B sulfate, tetracyclines:* potentiated neuromuscular blockade, leading to increased skeletal muscle relaxation and prolonged effect. Use together cautiously.
Inhaled anesthetics, quinidine: enhanced activity (or prolonged action) of nondepolarizing neuromuscular blocking agents. Monitor patient.

Magnesium salts: may enhance neuromuscular blockade. Monitor patient for excessive weakness.

Contraindications and precautions

- Contraindicated in patients hypersensitive to drug.
- Use cautiously and adjust dosage as directed in patients with renal failure because drug is excreted by kidneys. No information is available about use of drug in patients with hepatic disease.
- Use cautiously in pregnant or breast-feeding women.
- Drug isn't recommended for patients who need prolonged mechanical ventilation in intensive care unit, patients who received or will receive other nondepolarizing neuromuscular blockers, and patients undergoing cesarean section.
- Drug isn't recommended for neonates and infants younger than 3 months. Limited evidence suggests that infants and children (ages 1 to 14) under balanced anesthesia or halothane anesthesia may be less sensitive than adults.

NURSING CONSIDERATIONS

Assessment

- Assess patient's condition before therapy and regularly thereafter.
- Monitor respirations closely until patient is fully recovered from neuromuscular blockade, as evidenced by tests of muscle strength (hand grip, head lift, and ability to cough).
- Monitor patient for bradycardia during anesthesia because drug has minimal vagolytic action.
- Nerve stimulator and train-of-four monitoring are recommended to document antagonism of neuromuscular blockade and recovery of muscle strength. Before attempting pharmacologic reversal with neostigmine, some evidence of spontaneous recovery should be evident.
- Be alert for adverse reactions and drug interactions.
- Evaluate patient's and family's knowledge of drug therapy.

Nursing diagnoses

- Ineffective health maintenance related to underlying condition
- Ineffective breathing pattern related to drug's effect on respiratory muscles
- Deficient knowledge related to drug therapy

Planning and implementation

- Use drug under direct medical supervision by personnel skilled in use of neuromuscular blockers and techniques for maintaining patent airway. Don't use drug unless facilities and equipment for artificial respiration, mechanical ventilation, oxygen therapy, and intubation are available and antagonist is within reach.
- Give pipecuronium after succinylcholine when latter is used to facilitate intubation. No evidence exists to support safe use of pipecuronium before succinylcholine to decrease adverse effects of latter drug.

ALERT Give patient sedatives or general anesthetics before neuromuscular blockers, as directed. Neuromuscular blockers don't obtund consciousness or alter pain threshold.

- Reconstitute drug with 10 ml of sterile water for injection or other compatible I.V. solution (such as normal saline solution for injection, D_5W, lactated Ringer's injection, or dextrose 5% in normal saline solution), to yield solution of 1 mg/ml. Don't use large volume of diluent or add drug to hanging I.V. solution.
- If reconstituted with bacteriostatic water for injection, drug is stable for up to 5 days without refrigeration. If reconstituted with other solutions, drug is stable for 24 hours under refrigeration. Single use only; discard unused portion.
- Patients with myasthenia gravis or myasthenic syndrome (Eaton-Lambert syndrome) are particularly sensitive to nondepolarizing relaxants. Shorter-acting agents are recommended.
- Adjust dosage to ideal body weight in obese patients (30% or more over their ideal weight) to avoid prolonged neuromuscular blockade.
- Experimental evidence suggests that acid-base and electrolyte balances may influence actions of nondepolarizing neuromuscular blockers. Alkalosis may counteract paralysis and acidosis may enhance it.

ALERT Don't confuse pipercuronium with pancuronium.

Patient teaching
- Inform patient and family that drug will be given as part of anesthesia.
- Reassure patient that he will be monitored continuously.

Evaluation
- Patient responds well to therapy.
- Patient maintains adequate breathing pattern with mechanical assistance.
- Patient and family state understanding of drug therapy.

piperacillin sodium
(pigh-PER-uh-sil-in SOH-dee-um)
Pipracil, Pipril ♦

Pharmacologic class: extended-spectrum penicillin, acyclaminopenicillin
Therapeutic class: antibiotic
Pregnancy risk category: B

Indications and dosages
▶ **Systemic infections caused by susceptible strains of gram-positive and especially gram-negative organisms (including *Proteus* and *Pseudomonas aeruginosa*).** *Adults and children over age 12:* 12 to 18 g/day in divided doses q 4 to 6 hours I.V. Dosage for children under age 12 hasn't been established.
▶ **Prophylaxis of surgical infections.** *Adults:* 2 g I.V. 30 to 60 minutes before surgery. Dose may be repeated during surgery and once or twice after surgery.

How supplied
Injection: 2 g, 3 g, 4 g

Pharmacokinetics
Absorption: unknown after I.M. administration.
Distribution: distributed widely in body. It penetrates minimally into uninflamed meninges and slightly into bone and sputum. Drug is 16% to 22% protein-bound.
Metabolism: unknown.
Excretion: excreted mainly in urine (42% to 90%); some excreted in bile. *Half-life:* 30 to 90 minutes.

Route	Onset	Peak	Duration
I.V.	Immediate	Immediate	Unknown
I.M.	Unknown	30-50 min	Unknown

Pharmacodynamics
Chemical effect: inhibits cell wall synthesis during microorganism multiplication; bacteria resist penicillins by producing penicillinases, enzymes that convert penicillins to inactive penicilloic acid. Piperacillin sodium resists these enzymes.
Therapeutic effect: kills susceptible bacteria. Spectrum of activity includes many gram-negative aerobic and anaerobic bacilli, many gram-positive and gram-negative cocci, and some gram-positive aerobic and anaerobic bacilli. Drug may be effective against some strains of carbenicillin-resistant and ticarcillin-resistant gram-negative bacilli.

Adverse reactions
CNS: neuromuscular irritability, ***seizures,*** headache, dizziness.
GI: nausea, diarrhea.
Hematologic: bleeding with large doses, ***neutropenia,*** eosinophilia, ***leukopenia, thrombocytopenia.***
Metabolic: *hypokalemia.*
Other: hypersensitivity reactions (edema, fever, chills, rash, pruritus, urticaria, ***anaphylaxis***), overgrowth of nonsusceptible organisms, pain at injection site, vein irritation, phlebitis.

Interactions
Drug-drug. *Probenecid:* increased blood levels of piperacillin. Probenecid may be used for this purpose.

Contraindications and precautions
- Contraindicated in patients hypersensitive to drug or other penicillins.
- Use cautiously in patients with other drug allergies, especially to cephalosporins (possible cross-sensitivity); in those with bleeding tendencies, uremia, or hypokalemia; and in pregnant or breast-feeding women.

• Safety of drug hasn't been established in children under age 12.

NURSING CONSIDERATIONS

Assessment

• Assess patient's infection before therapy and regularly thereafter.
• Before giving drug, ask patient about allergic reactions to penicillin. However, negative history is no guarantee against future reaction.
• Obtain specimen for culture and sensitivity tests before first dose. Therapy may begin pending results.
• Check CBC and platelet counts frequently, as ordered. Drug may cause thrombocytopenia.
• Monitor serum potassium level.
• Be alert for adverse reactions and drug interactions.
• Cystic fibrosis patients tend to be most susceptible to fever or rash.
• Monitor patient's hydration status if adverse GI reactions occur.
• Evaluate patient's and family's knowledge of drug therapy.

Nursing diagnoses

• Infection related to presence of susceptible bacteria
• Risk for deficient fluid volume related to adverse GI reactions
• Deficient knowledge related to drug therapy

Planning and implementation

• Dosage should be altered in patient with impaired renal function.
• Drug is typically used with another antibiotic, such as gentamicin.

I.V. use: Reconstitute each gram of drug with 5 ml of diluent, such as sterile or bacteriostatic water for injection, normal saline solution for injection (with or without preservative), D_5W, or dextrose 5% in normal saline solution for injection. Shake until dissolved.
– Inject reconstituted solution directly into vein or into I.V. line of free-flowing solution over 3 to 5 minutes. Or, dilute with at least 50 ml of compatible I.V. solution and give by intermittent infusion over 30 minutes.
– Avoid continuous infusions to prevent vein irritation. Change site every 48 hours.
– Aminoglycoside antibiotics (such as gentamicin and tobramycin) are chemically incompatible with drug. Don't mix in same I.V. container.

I.M. use: Reconstitute drug with sterile or bacteriostatic water for injection, normal saline solution for injection (with or without preservative), or 0.5% to 1% lidocaine hydrochloride. Add 2 ml of diluent for each gram of drug. Final solution will contain 1 g/2.5 ml.
• Give drug at least 1 hour before bacteriostatic antibiotics.
• Institute seizure precautions. Patients with high serum levels of this drug may have seizures.

Patient teaching

• Tell patient to report pain or discomfort at I.V. site.
• Instruct patient to limit salt intake while taking piperacillin because drug contains 1.98 mEq sodium per gram.
• Tell patient to report adverse reactions.

Evaluation

• Patient is free from infection.
• Patient maintains adequate hydration throughout drug therapy.
• Patient and family state understanding of drug therapy.

piperacillin sodium and tazobactam sodium

(pigh-PER-uh-sil-in SOH-dee-um and taz-oh-BAK-tem SOH-dee-um)
Zosyn

Pharmacologic class: extended-spectrum penicillin/beta-lactamase inhibitor
Therapeutic class: antibiotic
Pregnancy risk category: B

Indications and dosages

▶ **Appendicitis (complicated by rupture or abscess) and peritonitis caused by *Escherichia coli, Bacteroides fragilis, B. ovatus, B.***

thetaiotaomicron,* or *B. vulgatus;* skin and skin-structure infections caused by *Staphylococcus aureus;* postpartum endometritis or pelvic inflammatory disease caused by *E. coli;* moderately severe community-acquired pneumonia caused by *Haemophilus influenzae. *Adults:* 3 g piperacillin and 0.375 g tazobactam I.V. q 6 hours.
Adults with renal impairment: if creatinine clearance is 20 to 40 ml/minute, 2 g piperacillin and 0.25 g tazobactam I.V. q 6 hours. If creatinine clearance is below 20 ml/minute, 2 g piperacillin and 0.25 g tazobactam I.V. q 8 hours.

How supplied

Powder for injection: 2 g piperacillin and 0.25 g tazobactam per vial, 3 g piperacillin and 0.375 g tazobactam per vial, 4 g piperacillin and 0.5 g tazobactam per vial

Pharmacokinetics

Absorption: not applicable.
Distribution: both drugs are about 30% protein-bound.
Metabolism: piperacillin is metabolized to a minor, microbiologically active desethyl metabolite. Tazobactam is metabolized to a single metabolite that lacks pharmacologic and antibacterial activities.
Excretion: excreted in urine and bile. *Half-life:* piperacillin, 40 minutes; tazobactam, 70 minutes.

Route	Onset	Peak	Duration
I.V.	Immediate	Immediate	Unknown

Pharmacodynamics

Chemical effect: piperacillin inhibits cell wall synthesis during microorganism multiplication; tazobactam increases piperacillin effectiveness by inactivating beta-lactamases, which destroy penicillins.
Therapeutic effect: kills susceptible bacteria. Spectrum of activity includes *E. coli, B. fragilis, B. ovatus, B. thetaiotaomicron, B. vulgatus, S. aureus,* and *H. influenzae.*

Adverse reactions

CNS: *headache, insomnia,* agitation, dizziness, anxiety.
CV: hypertension, tachycardia, chest pain, edema.
EENT: rhinitis.
GI: *diarrhea, nausea, constipation,* vomiting, dyspepsia, stool changes, abdominal pain.
Hematologic: ***thrombocytopenia.***
Respiratory: dyspnea.
Skin: rash (including maculopapular, bullous, urticarial, and eczematoid), pruritus.
Other: fever; pain, ***anaphylaxis,*** candidiasis, inflammation and phlebitis at I.V. site.

Interactions

Drug-drug. *Probenecid:* increased blood levels of piperacillin. Probenecid may be used for this purpose.
Vecuronium: prolongation of neuromuscular blockage. Monitor patient closely.

Contraindications and precautions

- Contraindicated in patients hypersensitive to drug or other penicillins.
- Use cautiously in patients with other drug allergies, especially to cephalosporins (possible cross-sensitivity); in those with bleeding tendencies, uremia, or hypokalemia; and in pregnant or breast-feeding women.
- Safety of drug hasn't been established in children under age 12.

NURSING CONSIDERATIONS

Assessment

- Before giving drug, ask patient about previous allergic reactions to this drug or other penicillins. However, negative history of penicillin allergy doesn't guarantee future safety.
- Assess patient's infection before therapy and regularly thereafter.
- Obtain specimen for culture and sensitivity tests before first dose. Therapy may begin pending results.
- Be alert for adverse reactions and drug interactions.
- Monitor patient's hydration status if adverse GI reactions occur.
- Evaluate patient's and family's knowledge of drug therapy.

Nursing diagnoses

- Infection related to presence of bacteria

• Risk of deficient fluid volume related to adverse GI reactions
• Deficient knowledge related to drug therapy

Planning and implementation

• Reconstitute each gram of piperacillin with 5 ml of diluent, such as sterile or bacteriostatic water for injection, normal saline solution for injection, bacteriostatic normal saline solution for injection, D_5W, dextrose 5% in normal saline solution for injection, or dextran 6% in normal saline solution for injection. Don't use lactated Ringer's injection. Shake until dissolved. Further dilute to final volume of 50 ml before infusion.

ALERT Infuse drug over at least 30 minutes. Stop other primary infusions during administration if possible. Aminoglycoside antibiotics (such as gentamicin and tobramycin) are chemically incompatible with drug. Don't mix in same I.V. container.

• Don't mix with other drugs.
• Use drug immediately after reconstitution. Discard unused drug after 24 hours if held at room temperature, after 48 hours if refrigerated. Once diluted, drug is stable in I.V. bags for 24 hours at room temperature or 1 week if refrigerated.
• Change I.V. site every 48 hours.
• Because hemodialysis removes 6% of piperacillin dose and 21% of tazobactam dose, supplemental doses may be needed after hemodialysis.

Patient teaching

• Tell patient to report pain or discomfort at I.V. site.
• Advise patient to limit salt intake while taking drug because piperacillin contains 1.98 mEq of sodium per gram.
• Tell patient to report adverse reactions.

Evaluation

• Patient is free from infection.
• Patient maintains adequate hydration.
• Patient and family state understanding of drug therapy.

pirbuterol acetate

(pir-BYOO-teh-rol AS-ih-tayt)
Maxair

Pharmacologic class: beta-adrenergic agonist
Therapeutic class: bronchodilator
Pregnancy risk category: C

Indications and dosages

▶ **Prevention and reversal of bronchospasm, asthma.** *Adults and children age 12 and over:* 1 or 2 inhalations (0.2 to 0.4 mg) repeated q 4 to 6 hours. Maximum, 12 inhalations daily.

How supplied

Inhaler: 0.2 mg/metered dose

Pharmacokinetics

Absorption: negligible serum levels after inhalation.
Distribution: distributed locally.
Metabolism: metabolized in liver.
Excretion: about 50% of inhaled dose is excreted in urine as parent drug and metabolites.

Route	Onset	Peak	Duration
Inhalation	≤ 5 min	30-60 min	5 hr

Pharmacodynamics

Chemical effect: relaxes bronchial smooth muscle by acting on $beta_2$-adrenergic receptors.
Therapeutic effect: improves breathing ability.

Adverse reactions

CNS: tremor, nervousness, dizziness, insomnia, headache.
CV: tachycardia, palpitations, increased blood pressure.
EENT: dry or irritated throat.

Interactions

Drug-drug. *MAO inhibitors, tricyclic antidepressants:* may potentiate action of beta-adrenergic agonist on vascular system. Use together cautiously.

Propranolol, other beta blockers: decreased bronchodilating effects. Avoid concomitant use.

Contraindications and precautions

- Contraindicated in patients hypersensitive to drug.
- Use cautiously in pregnant or breast-feeding women, in patients who are unusually responsive to sympathomimetic amines, and in patients with CV disorders, hyperthyroidism, diabetes, or seizure disorders.
- Safety of drug hasn't been established in children under age 12.

NURSING CONSIDERATIONS

Assessment

- Assess patient's condition before therapy.
- Monitor effectiveness by checking respiratory rate, auscultating lung fields frequently, and following laboratory studies (such as arterial blood gases) as ordered.
- Be alert for adverse reactions and drug interactions.
- Evaluate patient's and family's knowledge of drug therapy.

Nursing diagnoses

- Impaired gas exchange related to presence of bronchospasms
- Disturbed sleep pattern related to drug-induced insomnia
- Deficient knowledge related to drug therapy

Planning and implementation

- Shake canister well before each use.
- Store drug away from heat and direct sunlight.
- If patient also uses a corticosteroid inhaler, always administer pirbuterol first, and then wait about 5 minutes before giving the corticosteroid inhaler.
- Notify prescriber if patient's condition doesn't improve or worsens.

Patient teaching

- Give these instructions for using metered-dose inhaler: Clear nasal passages and throat. Breathe out, expelling as much air from lungs as possible. Place mouthpiece well into mouth and inhale deeply as you release a dose from inhaler. Hold breath for several seconds, remove mouthpiece, and exhale slowly.
- If more than one inhalation is ordered, tell patient to wait at least 2 minutes before repeating procedure.
- If patient also uses a corticosteroid inhaler, tell him to use the bronchodilator first and then wait about 5 minutes before using the corticosteroid. This allows the bronchodilator to open air passages for maximum effectiveness.
- Tell patient to notify prescriber if bronchospasm increases after drug use.
- Advise patient to seek medical attention if previously effective dosage no longer controls symptoms; this change may signify worsening of disease.

Evaluation

- Patient has improved gas exchange, as demonstrated by improved lung sounds and arterial blood gas measurements.
- Patient doesn't have insomnia.
- Patient and family state understanding of drug therapy.

piroxicam

(peer-OK-sih-cam)

Apo-Piroxicam ♦, Feldene, Novo-Pirocam ♦

Pharmacologic class: NSAID
Therapeutic class: nonnarcotic analgesic, antipyretic, anti-inflammatory
Pregnancy risk category: NR

Indications and dosages

▶ **Osteoarthritis, rheumatoid arthritis.** *Adults:* 20 mg P.O. daily. If desired, dosage may be divided b.i.d.

How supplied

Capsules: 10 mg, 20 mg

Pharmacokinetics

Absorption: absorbed rapidly from GI tract. Food delays absorption.
Distribution: drug is highly protein-bound.

Metabolism: metabolized in liver.
Excretion: excreted in urine. *Half-life:* about 50 hours.

Route	Onset	Peak	Duration
P.O.	15-30 min	3-5 hr	About 24 hr

Pharmacodynamics

Chemical effect: unknown; produces anti-inflammatory, analgesic, and antipyretic effects, possibly by inhibiting prostaglandin synthesis.
Therapeutic effect: relieves pain, fever, and inflammation.

Adverse reactions

CNS: headache, drowsiness, dizziness, paresthesia, somnolence.
CV: peripheral edema.
EENT: auditory disturbances.
GI: *epigastric distress, nausea, occult blood loss,* ***peptic ulceration, severe GI bleeding.***
GU: ***nephrotoxicity,*** elevated BUN level.
Hematologic: prolonged bleeding time, anemia, ***leukopenia, aplastic anemia, agranulocytosis, thrombocytopenia.***
Hepatic: elevated liver enzyme levels.
Metabolism: ***hyperkalemia, acidosis,*** dilutional hypernatremia.
Respiratory: ***bronchospasm.***
Skin: pruritus, rash, urticaria, *photosensitivity.*

Interactions

Drug-drug. *Aspirin, corticosteroids:* increased risk of GI toxicity. Decreased plasma piroxicam levels. Monitor patient closely.
Lithium: increased plasma lithium levels. Monitor patient for toxicity.
Oral anticoagulants: enhanced risk of bleeding. Monitor patient closely.
Oral antidiabetics: enhanced antidiabetic effects. Monitor patient.
Drug-herb. *Dong quai, feverfew, garlic, ginger, horse chestnut, red clover:* possible increased risk of bleeding. Monitor patient closely.
St. John's wort: increased risk of photosensitivity. Advise patient to avoid unprotected exposure to sunlight.
Drug-lifestyle. *Alcohol use:* increased risk of GI toxicity. Decreased plasma piroxicam levels. Discourage concomitant use.
Sun exposure: risk of photosensitivity reaction. Advise patient to take precautions.

Contraindications and precautions

- Contraindicated in pregnant or breast-feeding women, patients hypersensitive to drug, and patients with bronchospasm or angioedema caused by aspirin or NSAIDs.
- Use cautiously in elderly patients and those with GI disorders, history of renal or peptic ulcer disease, cardiac disease, hypertension, or conditions predisposing to fluid retention.
- Safety of drug hasn't been established in children.

NURSING CONSIDERATIONS

Assessment

- Assess patient's condition before therapy and regularly thereafter. Effects don't occur for at least 2 weeks after therapy begins. Evaluate response to drug by assessing for reduced symptoms.
- Check CBC and renal, hepatic, and auditory function periodically during prolonged therapy.
- Be alert for adverse reactions and drug interactions.
- Evaluate patient's and family's knowledge of drug therapy.

Nursing diagnoses

- Chronic pain related to arthritis
- Impaired tissue integrity related to adverse effect on GI mucosa
- Deficient knowledge related to drug therapy

Planning and implementation

- Give drug with milk, antacids, or food if adverse GI reactions occur.
- Stop drug and notify prescriber if laboratory abnormalities occur.

Patient teaching

- Tell patient that full therapeutic effects may be delayed for 2 to 4 weeks.
- Teach patient to recognize and report signs and symptoms of GI bleeding.

• Advise patient to use sunblock, wear protective clothing, and avoid prolonged exposure to sunlight.
• Warn patient to not take any NSAIDs during therapy.

Evaluation
• Patient is free from pain.
• Patient maintains normal GI tissue integrity.
• Patient and family state understanding of drug therapy.

plasma protein fraction
(PLAZ-muh PROH-teen FRAK-shun)
Plasmanate, Plasma-Plex, Plasmatein, Protenate

Pharmacologic class: blood derivative
Therapeutic class: plasma volume expander
Pregnancy risk category: C

Indications and dosages
▶ **Shock.** *Adults:* varies with patient's condition and response, but usual dose is 250 to 500 ml I.V. (12.5 to 25 g protein), usually no faster than 10 ml/minute.
Infants and young children: 6.6 to 33 ml/kg (0.33 to 1.65 g/kg of protein) I.V., 5 to 10 ml/minute.
▶ **Hypoproteinemia.** *Adults:* 1,000 to 1,500 ml I.V. daily. Maximum infusion rate is 8 ml/minute.

How supplied
Injection: 5% solution in 50-ml, 250-ml, 500-ml vials

Pharmacokinetics
Absorption: not applicable.
Distribution: distributed into intravascular space and extravascular sites, including skin, muscle, and lungs.
Metabolism: unknown.
Excretion: unknown.

Route	Onset	Peak	Duration
I.V.	Immediate	Immediate	Unknown

Pharmacodynamics
Chemical effect: supplies colloid to blood and expands plasma volume.
Therapeutic effect: raises serum protein levels and expands plasma volume.

Adverse reactions
CNS: headache.
CV: various effects on blood pressure after rapid infusion or intra-arterial administration, ***vascular overload*** after rapid infusion.
GI: nausea, vomiting, hypersalivation.
Musculoskeletal: back pain.
Respiratory: dyspnea, ***pulmonary edema.***
Skin: erythema, urticaria.
Other: flushing, chills, fever.

Interactions
None significant.

Contraindications and precautions
• Contraindicated in patients with severe anemia or heart failure and in those having undergone cardiac bypass surgery.
• Use cautiously in patients with hepatic or renal failure, low cardiac reserve, or restricted sodium intake.
• Also use cautiously in pregnant or breast-feeding women.

NURSING CONSIDERATIONS

Assessment
• Assess patient's condition before therapy and regularly thereafter.
• Monitor vital signs at least hourly.
• Be alert for adverse reactions.
• Evaluate patient's and family's knowledge of drug therapy.

Nursing diagnoses
• Decreased cardiac output related to underlying condition
• Acute pain related to headache
• Deficient knowledge related to drug therapy

Planning and implementation
• Check expiration date before using. Don't use solutions that are cloudy, contain sediment, or have been frozen. Discard container

that's been open for more than 4 hours because solution contains no preservatives.
- If patient is dehydrated, give additional fluids P.O. or I.V., as ordered.
- Don't give more than 250 g or 5,000 ml in 48 hours.
- Be prepared to slow or stop infusion if hypotension occurs. Vital signs should return to normal gradually.
- Drug contains 130 to 160 mEq sodium/L.
- Administer mild analgesic as ordered for drug-induced headache.

Patient teaching
- Tell patient and family the purpose of plasma protein fraction, and keep them informed of drug effectiveness.
- Instruct patient to report adverse reactions.

Evaluation
- Patient regains normal cardiac output.
- Patient is free from pain.
- Patient and family state understanding of drug therapy.

plicamycin (mithramycin)
(pligh-keh-MIGH-sin)
Mithracin

Pharmacologic class: antibiotic antineoplastic (not specific to cell cycle)
Therapeutic class: antineoplastic, hypocalcemic agent
Pregnancy risk category: X

Indications and dosages
Dosage and indications may vary. Check protocol with prescriber.

▶ **Hypercalcemia linked to advanced malignancy.** *Adults:* 15 to 25 mcg/kg/day I.V. for 3 to 4 days. Dosage repeated at weekly intervals until desired response is obtained.

▶ **Testicular cancer.** *Adults:* 25 to 30 mcg/kg/day I.V. for 8 to 10 days or until toxicity occurs.

How supplied
Injection: 2.5-mg vials

Pharmacokinetics
Absorption: not applicable.
Distribution: distributes mainly into Kupffer's cells of liver, into renal tubular cells, and along formed bone surfaces. Also crosses blood-brain barrier and reaches appreciable levels in CSF.
Metabolism: unknown.
Excretion: excreted mainly in urine.

Route	Onset	Peak	Duration
I.V.	1-2 days	3 days	7-10 days

Pharmacodynamics
Chemical effect: unknown; may form a complex with DNA, thus inhibiting RNA synthesis. Also inhibits osteocytic activity, blocking calcium and phosphorus resorption from bone.
Therapeutic effect: hinders growth of testicular cancer cells and lowers blood calcium levels.

Adverse reactions
CNS: drowsiness, weakness, lethargy, headache, dizziness, nervousness, depression.
GI: *nausea, vomiting,* anorexia, diarrhea, stomatitis, metallic taste.
GU: proteinuria, increased BUN and serum creatinine levels.
Hematologic: ***leukopenia, thrombocytopenia, bleeding syndrome from epistaxis to generalized hemorrhage.***
Hepatic: elevated liver enzymes levels, ***hepatotoxicity.***
Metabolic: ***decreased serum calcium,*** potassium, and phosphorus levels.
Skin: *facial flushing.*
Other: vein irritation, cellulitis with extravasation.

Interactions
None significant.

Contraindications and precautions
- Contraindicated in women who are or may become pregnant, in breast-feeding patients, and in patients with thrombocytopenia, bone marrow suppression, or bleeding disorder.
- Use with extreme caution in patients who have significant renal or hepatic impairment.

• Safety of drug hasn't been established in children.

NURSING CONSIDERATIONS

Assessment
• Assess patient's condition before therapy and regularly thereafter.
• Obtain baseline platelet count and PT before therapy, and monitor them during therapy, as ordered.
• Facial flushing is an early indicator of bleeding.
• Monitor LD, AST, ALT, alkaline phosphatase, BUN, creatinine, potassium, calcium, and phosphorus levels, as ordered.
• Monitor patient for tetany, carpopedal spasm, Chvostek's sign, and muscle cramps; check serum calcium level. Precipitous drop is possible.
• Be alert for adverse reactions.
• Evaluate patient's and family's knowledge of drug therapy.

Nursing diagnoses
• Ineffective health maintenance related to underlying condition
• Ineffective protection related to adverse hematologic reactions
• Deficient knowledge related to drug therapy

Planning and implementation
• Give antiemetic before administering drug, as ordered.
• Follow facility policy to reduce risks. Preparation and administration of parenteral form are related to carcinogenic, mutagenic, and teratogenic risks for personnel.
• To prepare solution, add 4.9 ml of sterile water for injection to vial and shake to dissolve. Then dilute for I.V infusion in 1,000 ml of D_5W or normal saline solution. Infuse over 4 to 6 hours. Discard unused drug.
• Slow infusion reduces nausea that develops with I.V. push.
• Avoid extravasation. Drug is a vesicant. If I.V. solution infiltrates, stop immediately, notify prescriber, and use ice packs. Restart I.V. line.
• Avoid contact with skin or mucous membranes.
• Discontinue drug and notify prescriber if WBC count is less than 4,000/mm^3, platelet count falls to less than 150,000/mm^3, or PT is prolonged to more than 4 seconds longer than control.
• Store lyophilized powder in refrigerator and protect from light.

Patient teaching
• Warn patient to watch for signs of infection (fever, sore throat, fatigue) and bleeding (easy bruising, nosebleeds, bleeding gums, melena). Have patient take temperature daily. Instruct patient and family on infection-control and bleeding precautions.
• Tell patient to use salicylate-free medication for pain or fever.
• Warn patient to protect against pregnancy during therapy. If she thinks she has become pregnant, tell her to contact her prescriber immediately.

Evaluation
• Patient responds well to therapy.
• Patient doesn't develop serious complications from adverse hematologic reactions.
• Patient and family state understanding of drug therapy.

polyethylene glycol and electrolyte solution
(pol-ee-ETH-ih-leen GLIGH-kohl and ee-LEK-troh-light soh-LOO-shun)
Colovage, CoLyte, Glycoprep ♦, GoLYTELY, NuLYTELY, OCL

Pharmacologic class: polyethylene glycol (PEG) 3350 nonabsorbable solution
Therapeutic class: laxative and bowel evacuant
Pregnancy risk category: C

Indications and dosages
▶ **Bowel preparation before GI examination.** *Adults:* 240 ml P.O. q 10 minutes until 4 L are consumed. Typically, give 4 hours before examination, allowing 3 hours for drinking and 1 hour for bowel evacuation.

How supplied

Powder for oral solution: PEG 3350 (6 g), anhydrous sodium sulfate (568 mg), saline solution (146 mg), potassium chloride (74.5 mg) per 100 ml (Colovage); PEG 3350 (120 g), sodium sulfate (3.36 g), saline solution (2.92 g), potassium chloride (1.49 g) per 2 L (CoLyte); PEG 3350 (60 g), saline solution (1.46 g), potassium chloride (745 mg), sodium bicarbonate (1.68 g), sodium sulfate (5.68 g) per liter (Glycoprep ♦); PEG 3350 (236 g), sodium sulfate (22.74 g), sodium bicarbonate (6.74 g), saline solution (5.86 g), potassium chloride (2.97 g) per 4.8 L (GoLYTELY); PEG 3350 (420 g), sodium bicarbonate (5.72 g), saline solution (11.2 g), potassium chloride (1.48 g) per 4 L (NuLYTELY); PEG 3350 (6 g), sodium sulfate decahydrate (1.29 g), saline solution (146 mg), potassium chloride (75 mg), polysorbate-80 (30 mg) per 100 ml (OCL)

Pharmacokinetics

Absorption: not absorbed.
Distribution: not applicable because drug isn't absorbed.
Metabolism: not applicable because drug isn't absorbed.
Excretion: excreted via GI tract.

Route	Onset	Peak	Duration
P.O.	≤ 1 hr	Varies	Varies

Pharmacodynamics

Chemical effect: PEG 3350, a nonabsorbable solution, acts as osmotic agent. Sodium sulfate greatly reduces sodium absorption. The electrolyte concentration causes virtually no net absorption or secretion of ions.
Therapeutic effect: cleanses bowel.

Adverse reactions

GI: nausea, bloating, cramps, vomiting.

Interactions

Drug-drug. *Oral drugs:* decreased absorption if given within 1 hour of starting therapy. Don't give with other oral drugs.

Contraindications and precautions

- Contraindicated in patients with GI obstruction or perforation, gastric retention, toxic colitis, or megacolon.
- Use cautiously in pregnant or breast-feeding women.

NURSING CONSIDERATIONS

Assessment

- Assess patient's condition before therapy and regularly thereafter.
- Be alert for adverse reactions and drug interactions.
- Evaluate patient's and family's knowledge of drug therapy.

Nursing diagnoses

- Health-seeking behavior (testing) related to need to determine cause of underlying GI problem
- Risk for deficient fluid volume related to adverse GI reactions
- Deficient knowledge related to drug therapy

Planning and implementation

- Use tap water to reconstitute powder. Shake vigorously to make sure all powder is dissolved. Refrigerate solution but use within 48 hours.

ALERT Don't add flavoring or additional ingredients to solution or administer chilled solution. Hypothermia has developed after ingestion of large amounts of chilled solution.

- Administer solution early in morning if patient is scheduled for midmorning examination. Orally administered solution induces diarrhea (onset 30 to 60 minutes) that rapidly cleans bowel, usually within 4 hours.
- When used as preparation for barium enema, administer solution the evening before examination, to avoid interfering with barium coating of colonic mucosa.
- If given to semiconscious patient or to patient with impaired gag reflex, take care to prevent aspiration.
- No major shifts in fluid or electrolyte balance have been reported.

Patient teaching

- Tell patient to fast for 4 hours before taking solution and to ingest only clear fluids until examination is complete.
- Warn patient about adverse GI reactions to drug.

Evaluation

- Patient is able to have examination.
- Patient maintains adequate fluid volume.
- Patient and family state understanding of drug therapy.

polysaccharide iron complex

(pol-ee-SAK-uh-righd IGH-ern KOM-pleks)

Hytinic, Niferex, Niferex-150, Nu-Iron, Nu-Iron 150

Pharmacologic class: oral iron supplement
Therapeutic class: hematinic
Pregnancy risk category: NR

Indications and dosages

▶ **Treatment of uncomplicated iron deficiency anemia.** *Adults and children age 12 and over:* 150 to 300 mg P.O. as capsules or tablets daily or 1 to 2 teaspoonfuls of elixir P.O. daily.
Children ages 6 to 12: 150 mg to 300 mg P.O. as tablets or 1 teaspoonful of elixir P.O. daily.
Children ages 2 to 6: ½ teaspoonful P.O. daily.

How supplied

Capsules: 150 mg
Solution: 100 mg/5 ml
Tablets (film-coated): 50 mg

Pharmacokinetics

Absorption: iron is absorbed from entire length of GI tract, but primary absorption sites are duodenum and proximal jejunum. Up to 10% of iron is absorbed by healthy people; people with iron-deficiency anemia may absorb up to 60%.
Distribution: iron is transported through GI mucosal cells directly into blood, where it's immediately bound to carrier protein, transferrin, and transported to bone marrow for incorporation into hemoglobin. Iron is highly protein-bound.
Metabolism: iron is liberated by destruction of hemoglobin, but is conserved and reused by body.
Excretion: men and postmenopausal women lose about 1 mg/day; premenopausal women, about 1.5 mg/day. Loss usually occurs in nails, hair, feces, and urine; trace amounts lost in bile and sweat.

Route	Onset	Peak	Duration
P.O.	≤ 3 days	5-30 days	2 mo

Pharmacodynamics

Chemical effect: provides elemental iron, an essential component in formation of hemoglobin.
Therapeutic effect: restores normal iron levels in body.

Adverse reactions

Although nausea, constipation, black stools, and epigastric pain are common adverse reactions linked to iron therapy, few, if any, occur with polysaccharide iron complex.

Interactions

Drug-drug. *Antacids, cholestyramine resin, cimetidine, tetracycline, vitamin E:* decreased iron absorption. Separate doses by 2 to 4 hours.
Chloramphenicol: delayed response to iron therapy. Monitor patient.
Fluoroquinolones, levodopa, methyldopa, penicillamine: decreased GI absorption, possibly resulting in decreased serum levels or efficacy. Administer separately.
Vitamin C: may increase iron absorption. Can be used for this effect.
Drug-food. *Cereals, cheese, coffee, eggs, milk, teas, whole-grain breads, yogurt:* may impair iron absorption. Don't administer together.

Contraindications and precautions

• Contraindicated in patients hypersensitive to drug or its components and in those with hemochromatosis or hemosiderosis.

NURSING CONSIDERATIONS

Assessment

• Assess patient's condition before therapy and regularly thereafter.
• Be alert for adverse reactions and drug interactions.
• Evaluate patient's and family's knowledge of drug therapy.

Nursing diagnoses

• Fatigue related to anemia
• Deficient knowledge related to drug therapy

Planning and implementation

• Give drug with juice (preferably orange juice) or water but not with milk or antacids.

Patient teaching

• Inform patient that drug may turn stools black.
• Advise patient to avoid foods that may impair absorption, including yogurt, cheese, eggs, milk, whole-grain breads and cereals, tea, and coffee. Tell him to take drug with juice or water.
• Inform parents that as few as three tablets can cause iron poisoning in children. Warn them to store drug out of reach of children.
• If patient misses a dose, tell him to take it as soon as he remembers but not to double the dose.

Evaluation

• Patient states that fatigue is relieved as hemoglobin and reticulocyte count return to normal.
• Patient and family state understanding of drug therapy.

potassium acetate

(puh-TAS-ee-um AS-ih-tayt)

Pharmacologic class: potassium supplement
Therapeutic class: therapeutic agent for electrolyte balance
Pregnancy risk category: C

Indications and dosages

▶ **Treatment of hypokalemia.** *Adults:* no more than 20 mEq I.V. hourly at concentration of 40 mEq/L or less. Potassium replacement should be done with ECG monitoring and frequent serum potassium tests. Use I.V. route only for life-threatening hypokalemia or when oral replacement isn't feasible.

▶ **Prevention of hypokalemia.** *Adults:* dosage is individualized to patient's needs. Usual dosage is 20 mEq P.O. daily.
Children: individualized dosage not to exceed 3 mEq/kg/day. Given as additive to I.V. infusions.

How supplied

Injection: 2 mEq/ml in 20-ml, 30-ml vials

Pharmacokinetics

Absorption: not applicable.
Distribution: distributed throughout body.
Metabolism: none significant.
Excretion: excreted largely by kidneys; small amounts may be excreted via skin and intestinal tract, but intestinal potassium is usually reabsorbed.

Route	Onset	Peak	Duration
I.V.	Immediate	Immediate	Unknown

Pharmacodynamics

Chemical effect: aids in transmitting nerve impulses, contracting cardiac and skeletal muscle, and maintaining intracellular tonicity, cellular metabolism, acid-base balance, and normal renal function.
Therapeutic effect: replaces and maintains potassium level.

Adverse reactions

CNS: paresthesia of limbs, listlessness, mental confusion, weakness or heaviness of legs, flaccid paralysis.
CV: ***arrhythmias, possible cardiac arrest, heart block,*** ECG changes.
GI: nausea, vomiting, abdominal pain, diarrhea, bowel ulceration.
GU: oliguria.
Respiratory: ***respiratory paralysis.***
Skin: cold skin, gray pallor.
Other: pain, redness at infusion site.

Interactions

Drug-drug. *ACE inhibitors, potassium-sparing diuretics:* increased risk of hyperkalemia. Use with extreme caution.
Drug-food: *Salt substitutes*: risk of hyperkalemia. Don't use together.

Contraindications and precautions

- Contraindicated in patients with severe renal impairment with oliguria, anuria, or azotemia; those with untreated Addison's disease; and those with acute dehydration, heat cramps, hyperkalemia, hyperkalemic form of familial periodic paralysis, and conditions related to extensive tissue breakdown.
- Use cautiously in pregnant women, breast-feeding women, and patients with cardiac disease or renal impairment.

NURSING CONSIDERATIONS

Assessment
- Assess patient's condition before therapy and regularly thereafter.
- During therapy, monitor ECG, renal function, fluid intake and output, and serum potassium, serum creatinine, and BUN levels.
- Be alert for adverse reactions and drug interactions.
- Evaluate patient's and family's knowledge of drug therapy.

Nursing diagnoses
- Ineffective health maintenance related to presence of hypokalemia
- Risk for injury related to drug-induced hyperkalemia
- Deficient knowledge related to drug therapy

Planning and implementation
- Give drug only by I.V. infusion, never by I.V. push or I.M. route.
- Watch for pain and redness at infusion site. Large-bore needle reduces local irritation.
- Administer drug slowly as diluted solution; life-threatening hyperkalemia may result from too-rapid infusion.
- Don't give potassium postoperatively until urine flow is established.

ALERT Potassium preparations aren't interchangeable. Verify preparation before administration.

Patient teaching
- Inform patient of need for potassium supplementation.
- Tell patient that drug will be given through an I.V. line.
- Instruct patient to report adverse reactions.

Evaluation
- Patient's potassium level returns to normal with drug therapy.
- Patient doesn't develop hyperkalemia as result of drug therapy.
- Patient and family state understanding of drug therapy.

potassium bicarbonate
(puh-TAS-ee-um bigh-KAR-buh-nayt)
K+Care ET, K-Ide, Klor-Con/EF, K-Lyte

Pharmacologic class: potassium supplement
Therapeutic class: therapeutic agent for electrolyte balance
Pregnancy risk category: C

Indications and dosages

▶ **Hypokalemia.** *Adults:* 25 to 50 mEq dissolved in 4 to 8 oz (120 to 240 ml) of water and given once daily to b.i.d.

How supplied

Effervescent tablets: 6.5 mEq, 25 mEq

Pharmacokinetics

Absorption: well absorbed from GI tract.
Distribution: distributed throughout body.

Metabolism: none significant.
Excretion: excreted largely by kidneys; small amounts may be excreted via skin and intestinal tract, but intestinal potassium is usually reabsorbed.

Route	Onset	Peak	Duration
P.O.	Unknown	≤ 4 hr	Unknown

Pharmacodynamics

Chemical effect: aids in transmitting nerve impulses, contracting cardiac and skeletal muscle, and maintaining intracellular tonicity, cellular metabolism, acid-base balance, and normal renal function.
Therapeutic effect: replaces and maintains potassium level.

Adverse reactions

CNS: paresthesia of limbs, listlessness, mental confusion, weakness or heaviness of legs, flaccid paralysis.
CV: ***arrhythmias, cardiac arrest, heart block,*** ECG changes (prolonged PR interval, widened QRS complex, ST-segment depression, and tall, tented T waves).
GI: *nausea, vomiting, abdominal pain,* diarrhea, ulcerations, hemorrhage, obstruction, perforation.

Interactions

Drug-drug. *ACE inhibitors, potassium-sparing diuretics:* risk of hyperkalemia. Use with extreme caution.
Drug-food. *Salt substitutes*: risk of hyperkalemia. Don't use together.

Contraindications and precautions

- Contraindicated in patients with untreated Addison's disease, acute dehydration, heat cramps, hyperkalemia, hyperkalemic form of familial periodic paralysis, other conditions linked to extensive tissue breakdown, and severe renal impairment with oliguria, anuria, or azotemia.
- Use cautiously in patients with cardiac disease or renal impairment and in pregnant or breast-feeding women.
- Safety of drug hasn't been established in children.

NURSING CONSIDERATIONS

Assessment

- Assess patient's condition before therapy and regularly thereafter.
- During therapy, monitor ECG, renal function, fluid intake and output, and serum potassium, serum creatinine, and BUN levels.
- Be alert for adverse reactions and drug interactions.
- Evaluate patient's and family's knowledge of drug therapy.

Nursing diagnoses

- Ineffective health maintenance related to presence of hypokalemia
- Risk for injury related to potassium-induced hyperkalemia
- Deficient knowledge related to drug therapy

Planning and implementation

- Dissolve potassium bicarbonate tablets completely in 6 to 8 oz of cold water to minimize GI irritation.
- Ask patient's flavor preference. Available in lime, fruit punch, and orange flavors.
- Have patient take with meals and sip slowly over 5 to 10 minutes.
- Don't give potassium supplements postoperatively until urine flow has been established.

ALERT Potassium preparations aren't interchangeable. Verify preparation before administration.

Patient teaching

- Inform patient about need for potassium supplementation.
- Teach patient how to prepare and take drug.
- Instruct patient to report adverse reactions.

Evaluation

- Patient's potassium level returns to normal.
- Patient doesn't develop hyperkalemia as result of drug therapy.
- Patient and family state understanding of drug therapy.

potassium chloride

(puh-TAS-ee-um KLOR-ighd)

Cena-K, K+10, Kaochlor 10%*, Kaochlor S-F 10%*, Kaon-Cl, Kaon-Cl 20%*, Kato Powder, Kay Ciel*, K+Care, K-Dur, K-Lease, K-Lor, Klor-Con, Klor-Con 10, Klorvess, Klotrix, K-Lyte/Cl, K-Norm, K-Tab, Micro-K Extencaps, Rum-K, Slow-K, Ten-K

Pharmacologic class: potassium supplement
Therapeutic class: therapeutic agent for electrolyte balance
Pregnancy risk category: C

Indications and dosages

▶ **Hypokalemia.** Use I.V. route only when P.O. replacement isn't feasible or when hypokalemia is life-threatening. Give up to 20 mEq/hr at concentration up to 60 mEq/L. Subsequent dosage based on serum potassium levels.
Adults: 40 to 100 mEq P.O. daily in three or four divided doses for treatment; 20 mEq for prevention.
Children: 3 mEq/kg daily. Maximum, 40 mEq/m^2/day.

How supplied

Tablets: 1.22 mEq (99 mg), 8 mEq (600 mg), 10 mEq (750 mg), 20 mEq (1,500 mg), 25 mEq (1,875 mg)
Tablets (controlled-release): 6.7 mEq (500 mg), 8 mEq (600 mg), 10 mEq (750 mg), 20 mEq (1,500 mg)
Tablets (enteric-coated): 4 mEq (300 mg), 13.4 mEq (1,000 mg)
Capsules (controlled-release): 8 mEq (600 mg), 10 mEq (750 mg)
Oral liquid: 5% (10 mEq/15 ml), 7.5% (15 mEq/15 ml), 10% (20 mEq/15 ml), 15% (30 mEq/15 ml), 20% (40 mEq/15 ml)
Powder for oral use: 15 mEq/packet, 20 mEq/packet, 25 mEq/packet, 25 mEq/dose
Injection: 20-mEq, 40-mEq ampules; additive syringes containing 30 mEq or 40 mEq; 10-mEq, 20-mEq, 30-mEq, 40-mEq, 45-mEq, 60-mEq, 100-mEq, 200-mEq, 400-mEq, or 1,000-mEq vials

Pharmacokinetics

Absorption: well absorbed from GI tract when administered P.O.
Distribution: distributed throughout body.
Metabolism: none significant.
Excretion: excreted largely by kidneys; small amounts may be excreted via skin and intestinal tract, but intestinal potassium is usually reabsorbed.

Route	Onset	Peak	Duration
P.O.	Unknown	≤ 4 hr	Unknown
I.V.	Immediate	Immediate	Unknown

Pharmacodynamics

Chemical effect: aids in transmitting nerve impulses, contracting cardiac and skeletal muscle, and maintaining intracellular tonicity, cellular metabolism, acid-base balance, and normal renal function.
Therapeutic effect: replaces and maintains potassium level.

Adverse reactions

CNS: paresthesia of limbs, listlessness, mental confusion, weakness or heaviness of limbs, flaccid paralysis.
CV: ***arrhythmias, heart block, possible cardiac arrest,*** ECG changes (prolonged PR interval, widened QRS complex, ST-segment depression, and tall, tented T waves).
GI: *nausea, vomiting, abdominal pain,* diarrhea, GI ulcerations (possible stenosis, hemorrhage, obstruction, perforation).
GU: oliguria.
Respiratory: ***respiratory paralysis.***
Skin: cold skin, gray pallor.
Other: postinfusion phlebitis.

Interactions

Drug-drug. *ACE inhibitors, potassium-sparing diuretics:* risk of hyperkalemia. Use with extreme caution.
Drug-food. *Salt substitutes*: risk of hyperkalemia. Don't use together.

Contraindications and precautions

• Contraindicated in patients with untreated Addison's disease, acute dehydration, heat cramps, hyperkalemia, hyperkalemic form of familial periodic paralysis, other conditions

linked to extensive tissue breakdown, and severe renal impairment with oliguria, anuria, or azotemia.
- Use cautiously in patients with cardiac disease or renal impairment and in pregnant or breast-feeding women.

NURSING CONSIDERATIONS

Assessment
- Assess patient's condition before therapy and regularly thereafter.
- During therapy, monitor ECG, renal function, fluid intake and output, and serum potassium, serum creatinine, and BUN levels.
- Be alert for adverse reactions and drug interactions.
- Evaluate patient's and family's knowledge of drug therapy.

Nursing diagnoses
- Ineffective health maintenance related to presence of hypokalemia
- Risk for injury related to drug-induced hyperkalemia
- Deficient knowledge related to drug therapy

Planning and implementation
P.O. use: Give with extreme caution because different potassium supplements deliver varying amounts of potassium. Never switch products without prescriber's order.
– Make sure powders are completely dissolved before administering.
– Don't crush sustained-release potassium products.
– Give potassium with or after meals with full glass of water or fruit juice to lessen GI distress.
– Use sugar-free liquid (Kaochlor S-F 10%) if tablet or capsule passage is likely to be delayed, as in GI obstruction. Have patient sip slowly to minimize GI irritation.
– Enteric-coated tablets aren't recommended because of increased risk of GI bleeding and small-bowel ulcerations.
– Tablets in wax matrix sometimes lodge in esophagus and cause ulceration in cardiac patients who have esophageal compression from enlarged left atrium. Use liquid form in such patients and in those with esophageal stasis or obstruction.
– Drug is commonly given with potassium-wasting diuretics to maintain potassium levels.
I.V. use: Give drug only by infusion; never by I.V. push or I.M. route.
– Give slowly as dilute solution; life-threatening hyperkalemia may result from too-rapid infusion.
ALERT Potassium preparations aren't interchangeable. Verify preparation before administration.
- Don't give potassium postoperatively until urine flow is established.

Patient teaching
- Inform patient of need for potassium supplement.
- Teach patient how to prepare and take supplement.
- Instruct patient to report adverse reactions and pain at the I.V. site.

Evaluation
- Patient's potassium level returns to normal.
- Patient doesn't develop hyperkalemia.
- Patient and family state understanding of drug therapy.

potassium gluconate
(puh-TAS-ee-um GLOO-kuh-nayt)
Glu-K, Kaon Liquid*, Kaon Tablets, Kaylixir*, K-G Elixir*, Potassium-Rougier♦

Pharmacologic class: potassium supplement
Therapeutic class: therapeutic agent for electrolyte balance
Pregnancy risk category: C

Indications and dosages
▶ **Hypokalemia.** *Adults:* 40 to 100 mEq P.O. daily in three or four divided doses for treatment; 20 mEq P.O. daily for prevention. Further dosage based on serum potassium determinations.

How supplied

Tablets: 500 mg (2 mEq K+), 1,170 mg (5 mEq K+)
Elixir*♦*: 4.68 g (20 mEq K+)/15 ml*

Pharmacokinetics

Absorption: well absorbed from GI tract.
Distribution: distributed throughout body.
Metabolism: none significant.
Excretion: excreted largely by kidneys; small amounts may be excreted via skin and intestinal tract, but intestinal potassium is usually reabsorbed.

Route	Onset	Peak	Duration
P.O.	Unknown	≤ 4 hr	Unknown

Pharmacodynamics

Chemical effect: aids in transmitting nerve impulses, contracting cardiac and skeletal muscle, and maintaining intracellular tonicity, cellular metabolism, acid-base balance, and normal renal function.
Therapeutic effect: replaces and maintains potassium level.

Adverse reactions

CNS: paresthesia of limbs, listlessness, mental confusion, weakness or heaviness of legs, flaccid paralysis.
CV: ***arrhythmias,*** ECG changes (prolonged PR interval, widened QRS complex, ST-segment depression, and tall, tented T waves).
GI: *nausea and vomiting; abdominal pain;* diarrhea; GI ulcerations that may be accompanied by stenosis, ***hemorrhage***, obstruction, or perforation (with oral products, especially enteric-coated tablets).

Interactions

Drug-drug. *ACE inhibitors, potassium-sparing diuretics:* risk of hyperkalemia. Use with extreme caution.
Drug-food: *Salt substitutes*: risk of hyperkalemia. Don't use together.

Contraindications and precautions

- Contraindicated in patients with untreated Addison's disease, acute dehydration, heat cramps, hyperkalemia, hyperkalemic form of familial periodic paralysis, other conditions related to extensive tissue breakdown, and severe renal impairment with oliguria, anuria, or azotemia.
- Use cautiously in patients with cardiac disease or renal impairment and in pregnant or breast-feeding women.
- Safety of drug hasn't been established in children.

NURSING CONSIDERATIONS

Assessment

- Assess patient's condition before therapy and regularly thereafter.
- During therapy, monitor ECG, renal function, fluid intake and output, and serum potassium, serum creatinine, and BUN levels.
- Be alert for adverse reactions and drug interactions.
- Evaluate patient's and family's knowledge of drug therapy.

Nursing diagnoses

- Ineffective health maintenance related to presence of hypokalemia
- Risk for injury related to potassium-induced hyperkalemia
- Deficient knowledge related to drug therapy

Planning and implementation

- Give oral potassium supplements with extreme caution because differing forms deliver varying amounts of potassium. Never switch products without prescriber's order.
- Give drug with or after meals with glass of water or fruit juice.
- Have patient sip liquid potassium slowly to minimize GI irritation.
- Enteric-coated tablets aren't recommended because of increased risk of GI bleeding and small-bowel ulcerations.

ALERT Potassium preparations aren't interchangeable. Verify preparation before administration.

- Don't give potassium supplements postoperatively until urine flow is established.

Patient teaching
- Inform patient of need for potassium supplementation.
- Teach patient how to take drug.
- Instruct patient to report adverse reactions.

Evaluation
- Patient's potassium level returns to normal.
- Patient doesn't develop hyperkalemia as result of drug therapy.
- Patient and family state understanding of drug therapy.

potassium iodide
(puh-TAS-ee-um IGH-uh-dighd)
Iosat, Pima, Thyro-Block

potassium iodide, saturated solution (SSKI)

strong iodine solution (Lugol's Solution)

Pharmacologic class: electrolyte
Therapeutic class: antihyperthyroid agent, expectorant
Pregnancy risk category: D

Indications and dosages
▶ **Preparation for thyroidectomy. Strong iodine solution, USP.** *Adults and children:* 0.1 to 0.3 ml P.O. t.i.d.
SSKI. *Adults and children:* 1 to 5 gtt in water P.O. t.i.d., after meals for 10 to 14 days before surgery.
▶ **Thyrotoxic crisis.** *Adults and children:* 500 mg P.O. q 4 hours (about 10 gtt of SSKI).
▶ **Radiation protectant for thyroid gland.** *Adults:* 130 mg P.O. immediately before and for 3 to 14 days after radiation exposure.

How supplied
potassium iodide
Tablets: 130 mg
Oral solution: 500 mg/15 ml
Syrup: 325 mg/5 ml
potassium iodide, saturated solution
Oral solution: 1 g/ml
strong iodine solution
Oral solution: iodine 50 mg/ml and potassium iodide 100 mg/ml

Pharmacokinetics
Unknown.

Route	Onset	Peak	Duration
P.O.	≤ 24 hr	10-15 days	Unknown

Pharmacodynamics
Chemical effect: inhibits thyroid hormone formation by blocking iodotyrosine and iodothyronine synthesis, limits iodide transport into thyroid gland, and blocks thyroid hormone release.
Therapeutic effect: lowers thyroid hormone levels.

Adverse reactions
CNS: frontal headache.
EENT: acute rhinitis, inflammation of salivary glands, periorbital edema, conjunctivitis, hyperemia.
GI: burning, irritation, *nausea,* vomiting, diarrhea (sometimes bloody), *metallic taste.*
Skin: acneiform rash, mucous membrane ulceration.
Other: fever, ***hypersensitivity reactions, potassium toxicity*** (confusion, irregular heart beat, numbness, tingling, pain or weakness in hands and feet, tiredness), tooth discoloration.

Interactions
Drug-drug. *ACE inhibitors, potassium-sparing diuretics:* risk of hyperkalemia. Avoid concomitant use.
Antithyroid medications: potassium iodide may potentiate hypothyroid or goitrogenic effects. Monitor effects closely.
Lithium carbonate: possible hypothyroidism. Use together cautiously.
Drug-food. *Salt substitutes*: risk of hyperkalemia. Don't use together.

Contraindications and precautions
- Contraindicated in patients with tuberculosis, acute bronchitis, iodide hypersensitivity, or hyperkalemia. Some forms contain sulfites, which may precipitate allergic reactions in hypersensitive people.

• Drug isn't recommended for pregnant or breast-feeding women.
• Use cautiously in patients with hypocomplementemic vasculitis, goiter, or autoimmune thyroid disease.

NURSING CONSIDERATIONS

Assessment
• Assess patient's condition before therapy and regularly thereafter.
• Be alert for adverse reactions and drug interactions.
• Earliest signs of delayed hypersensitivity reactions caused by iodides are irritation and swelling of eyelids.
• Evaluate patient's and family's knowledge of drug therapy.

Nursing diagnoses
• Ineffective health maintenance related to underlying thyroid condition
• Ineffective protection related to hypersensitivity reactions
• Deficient knowledge related to drug therapy

Planning and implementation
• Potassium iodide is usually given with other antithyroid drugs.
• Prescriber may avoid prescribing enteric-coated tablets, which have been linked to small bowel lesions and can lead to serious complications, including perforation, hemorrhage, or obstruction.
• Dilute oral doses in water, milk, or fruit juice to hydrate patient and mask salty taste; give drug after meals to prevent gastric irritation.
• Give iodide through straw to prevent tooth discoloration.
• Store drug in light-resistant container.

Patient teaching
• Teach patient how to administer drug.
• Warn patient that sudden withdrawal may cause thyroid crisis.
• Tell patient to ask prescriber about using iodized salt and eating shellfish.
• Tell him to report adverse reactions.

Evaluation
• Patient's thyroid hormone level is lower with potassium iodide therapy.
• Patient doesn't experience hypersensitivity reactions.
• Patient and family state understanding of drug therapy.

pralidoxime chloride (pyridine-2-aldoxime methochloride; 2-PAM chloride)
(pral-ih-DOKS-eem KLOR-ighd)
Protopam Chloride

Pharmacologic class: quaternary ammonium oxime
Therapeutic class: antidote
Pregnancy risk category: C

Indications and dosages
▶ **Antidote for organophosphate poisoning.** *Adults:* 1 to 2 g in 100 ml of saline solution by I.V. infusion over 15 to 30 minutes. If patient has pulmonary edema, give by slow I.V. push over at least 5 minutes. Repeat in 1 hour if muscle weakness persists; may give further doses cautiously. I.M. or S.C. injection may be used if I.V. route isn't feasible.
Children: 20 to 40 mg/kg I.V. administered as for adults.
▶ **Anticholinesterase overdose.** *Adults:* 1 to 2 g I.V., followed by 250 mg I.V. q 5 minutes, p.r.n.

How supplied
Injection: 1 g/20 ml in 20-ml vial without diluent or syringe; 1 g/20 ml in 20-ml vial with diluent, syringe, needle, and alcohol swab (emergency kit); 600 mg/2 ml auto-injector, parenteral

Pharmacokinetics
Absorption: absorption unknown after I.M. or S.C. administration.
Distribution: distributed throughout extracellular fluid; it isn't appreciably bound to plasma protein. It doesn't readily pass into CNS.

Metabolism: unknown but hepatic metabolism is considered likely.
Excretion: excreted rapidly in urine.

Route	Onset	Peak	Duration
I.V.	Unknown	5-15 min	Unknown
I.M.	Unknown	10-20 min	Unknown
S.C.	Unknown	Unknown	Unknown

Pharmacodynamics

Chemical effect: reactivates cholinesterase that has been inactivated by organophosphorus pesticides and related compounds, permitting degradation of accumulated acetylcholine and facilitating normal functioning of neuromuscular junctions.
Therapeutic effect: alleviates signs and symptoms of organophosphate poisoning and cholinergic crisis in myasthenia gravis.

Adverse reactions

CNS: dizziness, headache, drowsiness, excitement, manic behavior after recovery of consciousness.
CV: tachycardia.
EENT: blurred vision, diplopia, impaired accommodation, ***laryngospasm.***
GI: nausea.
Musculoskeletal: muscle weakness, muscle rigidity.
Respiratory: hyperventilation.

Interactions

None significant.

Contraindications and precautions

- No known contraindications.
- Use with extreme caution in patients with myasthenia gravis (overdose may cause myasthenic crisis).
- Use cautiously in pregnant women.
- Safety of drug hasn't been established in breast-feeding women.

NURSING CONSIDERATIONS

Assessment

- Assess patient's condition before therapy and regularly thereafter. Drug relieves paralysis of respiratory muscles but is less effective in relieving depression of respiratory center.
- Drug isn't effective against poisoning caused by phosphorus, inorganic phosphates, or organophosphates that have no anticholinesterase activity.
- Observe patient for 48 to 72 hours if poison was ingested. Delayed absorption may occur from lower bowel. It's difficult to distinguish between toxic effects produced by atropine or organophosphate compounds and those resulting from pralidoxime.
- Watch for signs of rapid weakening in patient with myasthenia gravis who was treated for overdose of cholinergic drugs. Patient can pass quickly from cholinergic crisis to myasthenic crisis and may need more cholinergic drugs to treat myasthenia. Keep edrophonium (Tensilon) available in such situations for establishing differential diagnosis.
- Be alert for adverse reactions.
- Evaluate patient's and family's knowledge of drug therapy.

Nursing diagnoses

- Ineffective health maintenance related to underlying condition
- Risk for injury related to adverse CNS reactions
- Deficient knowledge related to drug therapy

Planning and implementation

- Remove secretions, maintain patent airway, and start artificial ventilation if needed. After dermal exposure to organophosphate, remove patient's clothing and wash his skin and hair with sodium bicarbonate, soap, water, and alcohol as soon as possible. A second washing may be necessary. When washing patient, wear protective gloves and clothes to avoid exposure.
- Draw blood for cholinesterase levels before giving drug.
- Use drug only in hospitalized patients; have respiratory and other supportive measures available. If possible, obtain accurate medical history and chronology of poisoning. Give drug as soon as possible after poisoning; treatment is most effective if started within 24 hours after exposure.

I.V. use: Give I.V. preparation slowly as diluted solution. Dilute with unpreserved sterile water.
– To ameliorate muscarinic effects and block accumulation of acetylcholine related to organophosphate poisoning, give atropine 2 to 6 mg I.V. along with pralidoxime if cyanosis isn't present, as ordered. (If cyanosis is present, atropine should be given I.M.) Give atropine every 5 to 60 minutes in adults, as ordered, until muscarinic signs and symptoms disappear; if they reappear, repeat the dose. Maintain atropinization for at least 48 hours.
I.M. and S.C. use: Follow normal protocol.
ALERT Don't confuse pralidoxime with pramoxine or pyridoxine.

Patient teaching

- Tell patient to report adverse reactions immediately.
- Caution patient treated for organophosphate poisoning to avoid contact with insecticides for several weeks.

Evaluation

- Patient responds well to therapy.
- Patient sustains no injury from adverse CNS reactions.
- Patient and family state understanding of drug therapy.

pramipexole dihydrochloride
(pram-ih-PEKS-ohl digh-high-droh-KLOR-ighd)
Mirapex

Pharmacologic class: dopamine agonist
Therapeutic class: antiparkinsonian
Pregnancy risk category: C

Indications and dosages

▶ **Treatment of signs and symptoms of idiopathic Parkinson's disease.** *Adults:* initially, 0.375 mg P.O. daily in three divided doses; don't increase more often than q 5 to 7 days. Maintenance dosage range is 1.5 to 4.5 mg/day in three divided doses.

In patients with normal renal function to mild impairment (creatinine clearance over 60 ml/minute), initial dose is 0.125 mg P.O. t.i.d., up to 1.5 mg t.i.d. In patients with moderate impairment (creatinine clearance 35 to 59 ml/minute), initial dose is 0.125 mg P.O. b.i.d. up to 1.5 mg b.i.d. In patients with severe impairment (creatinine clearance 15 to 34 ml/minute), initial dose is 0.125 mg P.O. daily, up to 1.5 mg daily.

How supplied

Tablets: 0.125 mg, 0.25 mg, 1 mg, 1.5 mg

Pharmacokinetics

Absorption: rapid. Absolute bioavailability exceeds 90%.
Distribution: extensively distributed throughout body.
Metabolism: 90% of dose is excreted unchanged in urine.
Excretion: primary route of elimination is urinary. *Half-life:* 8 to 12 hours.

Route	Onset	Peak	Duration
P.O.	Rapid	2 hr	8-12 hr

Pharmacodynamics

Chemical effect: precise mechanism is unknown, but drug probably stimulates dopamine receptors in striatum.
Therapeutic effect: relieves symptoms of idiopathic Parkinson's disease.

Adverse reactions

CNS: malaise, akathisia, amnesia, *asthenia, confusion,* delusions, *dizziness, dream abnormalities, dyskinesia,* dystonia, *extrapyramidal syndrome,* gait abnormalities, *hallucinations,* hypoesthesia, hypertonia, *insomnia,* myoclonus, paranoid reaction, *somnolence,* sleep disorders, thought abnormalities.
CV: chest pain, peripheral edema, general edema, *orthostatic hypotension.*
EENT: accommodation abnormalities, diplopia, rhinitis, vision abnormalities.
GI: dry mouth, anorexia, *constipation,* dysphagia, *nausea.*
GU: impotence, urinary frequency, urinary tract infection, urinary incontinence.
Metabolic: weight loss.
Musculoskeletal: arthritis, bursitis, twitching, myasthenia.
Respiratory: dyspnea, pneumonia.

Skin: skin disorders.
Other: decreased libido, *accidental injury,* fever.

Interactions

Drug-drug. *Butyrophenones, metoclopramide, phenothiazines, thiothixenes:* may diminish pramipexole effectiveness. Monitor patient closely.
Cimetidine, diltiazem, quinidine, quinine, ranitidine, triamterene, verapamil: decreased pramipexole clearance. Adjust dosage as directed.
Levodopa: increased adverse effects of levodopa. Adjust levodopa dosage as directed.

Contraindications and precautions

• Contraindicated in patients hypersensitive to drug or its components.
• Use cautiously in elderly patients and patients with renal impairment; dosage may need adjustment.
• Use cautiously in breast-feeding women because it isn't known if drug appears in breast milk.

NURSING CONSIDERATIONS

Assessment

• Monitor vital signs carefully because drug may cause orthostatic hypotension, especially during dose escalation.
• Assess patient's risk for physical injury from adverse CNS effects of drug (dyskinesia, dizziness, hallucinations, and somnolence).
• Assess patient's response to drug therapy and adjust dose, as ordered.
• Evaluate patient's and family's knowledge of drug therapy.

Nursing diagnoses

• Impaired physical mobility related to underlying Parkinson's disease
• Disturbed thought processes related to drug-induced CNS adverse reactions
• Deficient knowledge related to drug therapy

Planning and implementation

• Institute safety precautions.

ALERT Don't withdraw drug abruptly. Adjust dosage gradually, as ordered, according to patient's response and tolerance.
• Provide ice chips, drinks, or hard, sugarless candy to relieve dry mouth. Increase fluid and fiber intake to prevent constipation as appropriate.

Patient teaching
• Instruct patient not to rise rapidly after sitting or lying down because of risk of orthostatic hypotension.
• Caution patient to avoid hazardous activities until CNS effects of drug are known
• Tell patient to use caution before taking drug with other CNS depressants.
• Tell patient—especially elderly patient—that hallucinations may occur.
• Advise patient to take drug with food if nausea develops.
• Tell woman to notify prescriber if she is breast-feeding or intends to do so.

Evaluation

• Patient has improved mobility and reduced muscle rigidity and tremor.
• Patient remains mentally alert.
• Patient and family state understanding of drug therapy.

pravastatin sodium (eptastatin)

(PRAH-vuh-stat-in SOH-dee-um)
Pravachol

Pharmacologic class: HMG-CoA reductase inhibitor
Therapeutic class: antilipemic
Pregnancy risk category: X

Indications and dosages

▶ **Adjunct to diet to reduce low-density lipoprotein (LDL), total cholesterol, and triglyceride levels in patients with primary hypercholesterolemia and mixed dyslipidemia (Frederickson types IIa and IIb); primary prevention of coronary events in hypercholesterolemic patients without clinical evidence of heart disease; reduction of risk of acute coronary events or slowing**

progression of coronary atherosclerosis in hypercholesterolemic patients with clinical evidence of coronary artery disease, including previous MI; reduction of risk of undergoing myocardial revascularization procedure; reduction of risk of recurrent MI, CVA, or transient ishcemic attacks in post-MI patients with normal cholesterol.
Adults: initially, 10 or 20 mg P.O. daily h.s. Dosage adjusted q 4 weeks based on patient tolerance and response; maximum daily dosage is 40 mg. Elderly patients respond to daily dosage of 20 mg or less. If patient takes an immunosuppressant, start at 10 mg P.O. daily; maximum daily dosage is 20 mg P.O.

How supplied

Tablets: 10 mg, 20 mg, 40 mg

Pharmacokinetics

Absorption: rapidly absorbed. Although food reduces bioavailability, drug effects are same if drug is taken with or 1 hour before meals.
Distribution: about 50% bound to plasma proteins. Drug undergoes extensive first-pass extraction, possibly because of active transport system into hepatocytes.
Metabolism: metabolized in liver; at least six metabolites have been identified. Some are active.
Excretion: excreted by liver and kidneys.
Half-life: 1¼ to 2½ hours.

Route	Onset	Peak	Duration
P.O.	Unknown	1 hr	Unknown

Pharmacodynamics

Chemical effect: inhibits 3-hydroxy-3-methylglutaryl coenzyme A reductase. This enzyme is an early (and a rate-limiting) step in synthetic pathway of cholesterol.
Therapeutic effect: lowers LDL and total cholesterol levels in some patients.

Adverse reactions

CNS: headache, fatigue, dizziness.
CV: chest pain.
EENT: rhinitis.
GI: vomiting, diarrhea, heartburn, nausea.
GU: ***renal failure*** secondary to myoglobinuria.
Musculoskeletal: myositis, myopathy, localized muscle pain, myalgia, ***rhabdomyolysis.***
Respiratory: cough.
Skin: rash.
Other: flulike symptoms.

Interactions

Drug-drug. *Cholestyramine, colestipol:* decreased plasma pravastatin levels. Give pravastatin 1 hour before or 4 hours after these drugs.
Drugs that decrease levels or activity of endogenous steroids (such as cimetidine, ketoconazole, spironolactone): may increase risk of endocrine dysfunction. No intervention appears necessary. Take complete drug history in patients who develop endocrine dysfunction.
Erythromycin, fibric acid derivatives (such as clofibrate, gemfibrozil), high doses of niacin (nicotinic acid; 1 g or more daily), immunosuppressants (such as cyclosporine): may increase risk of rhabdomyolysis. Monitor patient closely if concomitant use can't be avoided.
Gemfibrozil: decreases protein-binding and urinary clearance of pravastatin. Avoid concomitant use.
Hepatotoxic drugs: increased risk of hepatotoxicity. Avoid concomitant use.
Drug-herb. *Red yeast rice:* contains components similar to those of statin drugs, increasing the risk of adverse events or toxicity. Discourage concomitant use.
Drug-lifestyle. *Alcohol use:* increased risk of hepatotoxicity. Discourage concomitant use.

Contraindications and precautions

- Contraindicated in patients hypersensitive to drug, in women of childbearing age unless they have no risk of pregnancy, in pregnant and breast-feeding women, and in patients with active liver disease or unexplained persistent elevations of serum transaminase levels.
- Use cautiously in patients who consume large quantities of alcohol or have history of liver disease.
- Safety of drug hasn't been established in children.

NURSING CONSIDERATIONS

Assessment
- Assess patient's condition before therapy and regularly thereafter.
- Obtain liver function tests at start of therapy and periodically thereafter, as directed. A liver biopsy may be performed if elevations persist.
- Be alert for adverse reactions and drug interactions.
- Monitor patient's hydration status if adverse GI reactions occur.
- Evaluate patient's and family's knowledge of drug therapy.

Nursing diagnoses
- Risk for injury related to elevated cholesterol levels
- Risk for deficient fluid volume related to adverse GI reactions
- Deficient knowledge related to drug therapy

Planning and implementation
- Drug therapy should begin only after diet and other nondrug therapies have proved ineffective. Patient should follow a standard low-cholesterol diet during therapy.
- Dosage is adjusted about every 4 weeks. If cholesterol level falls below target range, dosage may be reduced.

Patient teaching
- Instruct patient to take recommended dosage in evening, preferably at bedtime.
- Teach patient about proper dietary management of serum lipids (restricting total fat and cholesterol intake), as well as measures to control other cardiac disease risk factors. When appropriate, recommend weight control, exercise, and smoking cessation programs.
- Inform woman that drug is contraindicated during pregnancy. Advise her to notify prescriber immediately if she becomes pregnant.

Evaluation
- Patient's LDL and total cholesterol levels are within normal range.
- Patient maintains adequate hydration.
- Patient and family state understanding of drug therapy.

prazosin hydrochloride
(PRAH-zoh-sin high-droh-KLOR-ighd)
Minipress

Pharmacologic class: alpha-adrenergic blocker
Therapeutic class: antihypertensive
Pregnancy risk category: C

Indications and dosages
▶ **Mild to moderate hypertension, alone or in combination with diuretic or other antihypertensive.** *Adults:* initial dosage is 1 mg P.O. t.i.d. Increased slowly; maximum daily dosage is 20 mg. Maintenance dosage is 6 to 15 mg daily in three divided doses. Some patients need larger dosages (up to 40 mg daily). If other antihypertensives or diuretics are added to this drug, prazosin is decreased to 1 to 2 mg t.i.d. and readjusted.

How supplied
Capsules: 1 mg, 2 mg, 5 mg

Pharmacokinetics
Absorption: variable.
Distribution: distributed throughout body; highly protein-bound (about 97%).
Metabolism: metabolized extensively in liver.
Excretion: over 90% excreted in feces via bile; remainder excreted in urine. *Half-life:* 2 to 4 hours.

Route	Onset	Peak	Duration
P.O.	30-90 min	2-4 hr	7-10 hr

Pharmacodynamics
Chemical effect: unknown; effects probably stem from alpha-adrenergic blocking activity.
Therapeutic effect: lowers blood pressure.

Adverse reactions
CNS: *dizziness,* headache, drowsiness, weakness, *first-dose syncope,* depression.
CV: orthostatic hypotension, *palpitations.*
EENT: blurred vision.
GI: vomiting, diarrhea, abdominal cramps, constipation, *nausea,* dry mouth.
GU: priapism, impotence.

Interactions

Drug-drug. *Diuretics, propranolol and other beta blockers:* increased frequency of syncope with loss of consciousness. Advise patient to sit or lie down if dizziness occurs.

Contraindications and precautions

- No known contraindications.
- Drug isn't recommended for breast-feeding women.
- Use cautiously in pregnant women and in patients taking other antihypertensives.
- Safety of drug hasn't been established in children.

NURSING CONSIDERATIONS

Assessment

- Assess patient's condition before therapy and regularly thereafter.
- Monitor patient's blood pressure and pulse rate frequently.
- Elderly patients may be more sensitive to hypotensive effects of drug.
- Be alert for adverse reactions and drug interactions.
- Evaluate patient's and family's knowledge of drug therapy.

Nursing diagnoses

- Risk for injury related to presence of hypertension
- Sexual dysfunction related to drug-induced impotence
- Deficient knowledge related to drug therapy

Planning and implementation

- If first dose is larger than 1 mg, severe syncope with loss of consciousness may occur (first-dose syncope).

ALERT Don't stop therapy abruptly.

- Twice-daily dosing may improve compliance. Discuss this dosing change with prescriber if you suspect compliance problems.

Patient teaching

- Tell patient not to stop taking drug abruptly, but to call prescriber if unpleasant adverse reactions occur.
- Advise patient to minimize effects of orthostatic hypotension by rising slowly and avoiding sudden position changes. Dry mouth can be relieved with sugarless chewing gum, sour hard candy, or ice chips.

Evaluation

- Patient's blood pressure is normal.
- Patient seeks counseling for alternative methods of sexual gratification because of drug-induced impotence.
- Patient and family state understanding of drug therapy.

prednisolone

(pred-NIS-uh-lohn)

Delta-Cortef, Deltasolone ♦, Panafcortelone ♦, Prelone, Solone ♦

prednisolone acetate

Articulose-50, Key-Pred 25, Key-Pred 50, Predaject-50, Predalone 50, Predate 50, Predcor-25, Predcor-50, Predicort-50

prednisolone sodium phosphate

Hydeltrasol, Key-Pred-SP, Pediapred, Predate S, Predicort-RP, Predsol Retention Enema ♦, Predsol Suppositories ♦

prednisolone steaglate

Sintisone ♦

prednisolone tebutate

Hydeltra-T.B.A., Nor-Pred T.B.A., Predalone T.B.A., Predate TBA, Predcor TBA

Pharmacologic class: glucocorticoid, mineralocorticoid
Therapeutic class: anti-inflammatory, immunosuppressant
Pregnancy risk category: NR

Indications and dosages

▶ **Severe inflammation or immunosuppression.** *Adults:* 2.5 to 15 mg P.O. b.i.d., t.i.d., or q.i.d. Or, 2 to 30 mg I.M. (acetate, phosphate) or I.V. (phosphate) q 12 hours. Or, 2 to 30 mg (phosphate) into joints, lesions, or soft tissue. Or, 4 to 40 mg (tebutate) into joints and lesions. Or, 0.25 to 1 ml (sodium phosphate-acetate suspension) into joints weekly, p.r.n.

▶ **Proctitis** ◇. *Adults:* 1 suppository b.i.d., preferably in morning and h.s.
▶ **Ulcerative colitis** ◇. *Adults:* 1 retention enema h.s. nightly for 2 to 4 weeks. The contents of enema should be retained overnight.

How supplied

prednisolone
Tablets: 1 mg ♦, 5 mg, 25 mg ♦
Syrup: 15 mg/5 ml
prednisolone acetate
Injection (suspension): 25 mg/ml, 50 mg/ml, 100 mg/ml
prednisolone acetate and prednisolone sodium phosphate
Injection (suspension): 80 mg acetate and 20 mg sodium phosphate/ml
prednisolone sodium phosphate
Oral solution: 5 mg/5 ml
Injection: 20 mg/ml
Retention enema: 20 mg/100 ml ♦
Suppositories: 5 mg ♦
prednisolone steaglate
Tablets: 6.65 mg (equal to 3.5 mg prednisolone) ♦
prednisolone tebutate
Injection (suspension): 20 mg/ml

Pharmacokinetics

Absorption: absorbed readily after P.O. administration; variable with other routes.
Distribution: distributed to muscle, liver, skin, intestine, and kidneys. Drug is extensively bound to plasma proteins. Only unbound portion is active.
Metabolism: metabolized in liver.
Excretion: inactive metabolites and small amounts of unmetabolized drug are excreted in urine; insignificant amount excreted in feces. *Half-life:* 18 to 36 hours.

Route	Onset	Peak	Duration
P.O.	Rapid	1-2 hr	30-36 hr
I.V.	Rapid	< 1 hr	Unknown
I.M.	Rapid	< 1 hr	< 4 wk
P.R.	Unknown	Unknown	Unknown
Intralesional, intra-articular	1-2 days	Unknown	3 days-4 wk

Pharmacodynamics

Chemical effect: not clearly defined; decreases inflammation, mainly by stabilizing leukocyte lysosomal membranes; suppresses immune response; stimulates bone marrow; and influences protein, fat, and carbohydrate metabolism.
Therapeutic effect: relieves inflammation and induces immunosuppression.

Adverse reactions

Most reactions to corticosteroids are dose- or duration-dependent.
CNS: *euphoria, insomnia,* psychotic behavior, pseudotumor cerebri, ***seizures.***
CV: ***heart failure, thromboembolism,*** hypertension, edema.
EENT: cataracts, glaucoma.
GI: *peptic ulceration,* GI irritation, increased appetite, pancreatitis.
Metabolic: hypokalemia, hyperglycemia, carbohydrate intolerance.
Musculoskeletal: muscle weakness, osteoporosis, growth suppression in children.
Skin: hirsutism, delayed wound healing, acne, various skin eruptions.
Other: susceptibility to infections, ***acute adrenal insufficiency with increased stress (infection, surgery, or trauma) or abrupt withdrawal after long-term therapy.***

Interactions

Drug-drug. *Aspirin, indomethacin, other NSAIDs:* increased risk of GI distress and bleeding. Avoid concomitant use.
Barbiturates, phenytoin, rifampin: decreased corticosteroid effect. Increase corticosteroid dosage, as ordered.
Oral anticoagulants: altered dosage requirements. Monitor PT and INR closely.
Potassium-depleting drugs (such as thiazide diuretics): enhanced potassium-wasting effects of prednisolone. Monitor serum potassium levels.
Skin-test antigens: decreased response. Defer skin testing until therapy is completed.
Toxoids, vaccines: decreased antibody response and increased risk of neurologic complications. Check with prescriber about when to reschedule vaccine if possible.

Contraindications and precautions

- Contraindicated in patients hypersensitive to drug or its ingredients and in those with fungal infections.
- High doses aren't recommended for breast-feeding women.
- Use with extreme caution in pregnant women and in patients with recent MI.
- Use cautiously in patients with GI ulcer, renal disease, hypertension, osteoporosis, diabetes mellitus, hypothyroidism, cirrhosis, diverticulitis, nonspecific ulcerative colitis, recent intestinal anastomoses, thromboembolic disorders, seizures, myasthenia gravis, heart failure, tuberculosis, ocular herpes simplex, emotional instability, and psychotic tendencies.

NURSING CONSIDERATIONS

Assessment

- Assess patient's condition before therapy and regularly thereafter.
- Monitor patient's weight, blood pressure, and serum electrolyte levels.
- Watch for depression or psychotic episodes, especially at high doses.
- Diabetic patient may need increased insulin; monitor blood glucose levels.
- Monitor patient's stress level; dosage adjustment may be needed.
- Be alert for adverse reactions and drug interactions.
- Evaluate patient's and family's knowledge of drug therapy.

Nursing diagnoses

- Ineffective health maintenance related to underlying condition
- Ineffective protection related to drug-induced adverse reactions
- Deficient knowledge related to drug therapy

Planning and implementation

- Always adjust to lowest effective dosage, as ordered. However, expect to increase dosage as specified during times of physiologic stress (such as surgery, trauma, or infection).
- Prednisolone salts (acetate, sodium phosphate, and tebutate) are used parenterally less often than other corticosteroids that have more potent anti-inflammatory action.
- Drug may be used for alternate-day therapy.

P.O. use: Give dose with food when possible to reduce GI irritation.

I.V. use: Use only prednisolone sodium phosphate; never give acetate form by I.V. route.

– When administering drug as direct injection, inject undiluted over at least 1 minute.

– When administering drug as intermittent or continuous infusion, dilute solution according to manufacturer's instructions and give over prescribed duration.

– D_5W and normal saline solution are recommended as diluents for I.V. infusions.

I.M. use: Inject drug deep into gluteal muscle.

– Alternate injection sites to prevent muscle atrophy.

P.R. use: Follow normal protocol.

Intralesional and intra-articular use: Assist prescriber with administration as directed.

- Avoid S.C. injection because atrophy and sterile abscesses may occur.
- Unless contraindicated, give low-sodium diet high in potassium and protein. Administer potassium supplements as needed.
- Notify prescriber immediately if serious adverse reactions occur, and be prepared to give supportive care.
- After long-term therapy, reduce dosage gradually as ordered. Abrupt withdrawal may cause rebound inflammation, fatigue, weakness, arthralgia, fever, dizziness, lethargy, depression, fainting, orthostatic hypotension, dyspnea, anorexia, or hypoglycemia. Sudden withdrawal after prolonged use may be fatal.

ALERT Don't confuse prednisolone with prednisone.

Patient teaching

- Tell patient not to stop drug without prescriber's knowledge.
- Tell patient to take drug as ordered. Tell patient what to do if he misses a dose.
- Advise patient to take oral form with meals to minimize GI reactions.
- Warn patient receiving long-term therapy about cushingoid symptoms.
- Teach signs of early adrenal insufficiency: fatigue, muscle weakness, joint pain, fever,

anorexia, nausea, dyspnea, dizziness, and fainting.

- Instruct patient to wear or carry medical identification that indicates his need for systemic glucocorticoids during stress.
- Tell patient to report sudden weight gain, swelling, or slow healing.
- Advise patient receiving long-term therapy to consider exercise or physical therapy and to ask prescriber about vitamin D or calcium supplements.

Evaluation
- Patient responds well to therapy.
- Patient has no serious adverse reactions.
- Patient and family state understanding of drug therapy.

prednisone
(PRED-nih-sohn)

Apo-Prednisone♦, Deltasone, Liquid Pred*, Meticorten, Novo-prednisone♦, Orasone, Panafcort♦, Panasol-S, Prednicen-M, Prednisone Intensol*, Sone♦, Sterapred, Winpred♦

Pharmacologic class: adrenocorticoid
Therapeutic class: anti-inflammatory, immunosuppressant
Pregnancy risk category: NR

Indications and dosages

▶ **Severe inflammation or immunosuppression.** *Adults:* 5 to 60 mg/day P.O. in single or divided doses. Maximum, 250 mg/day. Maintenance dosage given once daily or every other day. Dosage must be individualized.

▶ **Acute exacerbations of multiple sclerosis.** *Adults:* 200 mg P.O. daily for 1 week; then 80 mg P.O. every other day for 1 month.

How supplied

Tablets: 1 mg, 2.5 mg, 5 mg, 10 mg, 20 mg, 25 mg, 50 mg
Oral solution: 5 mg/5 ml*, 5 mg/ml (concentrate)*
Syrup: 5 mg/5 ml*

Pharmacokinetics

Absorption: absorbed readily after P.O. administration.
Distribution: distributed to muscle, liver, skin, intestine, and kidneys. Drug is extensively bound to plasma proteins. Only unbound portion is active.
Metabolism: metabolized in liver.
Excretion: inactive metabolites and small amounts of unmetabolized drug are excreted in urine; insignificant amounts excreted in feces. *Half-life:* 18 to 36 hours.

Route	Onset	Peak	Duration
P.O.	Varies	Varies	Varies

Pharmacodynamics

Chemical effect: not clearly defined; decreases inflammation; suppresses immune response; stimulates bone marrow; and influences protein, fat, and carbohydrate metabolism.
Therapeutic effect: relieves inflammation and induces immunosuppression.

Adverse reactions

Most reactions are dose- or duration-dependent.
CNS: *euphoria, insomnia,* psychotic behavior, pseudotumor cerebri, ***seizures.***
CV: ***heart failure, thromboembolism,*** hypertension, edema.
EENT: cataracts, glaucoma.
GI: *peptic ulceration,* GI irritation, increased appetite, pancreatitis.
Metabolic: hypokalemia, hyperglycemia, carbohydrate intolerance.
Musculoskeletal: muscle weakness, osteoporosis, growth suppression in children.
Skin: hirsutism, delayed wound healing, acne, various skin eruptions.
Other: susceptibility to infections.

Interactions

Drug-drug. *Aspirin, indomethacin, other NSAIDs:* increased risk of GI distress and bleeding. Give together cautiously.
Barbiturates, phenytoin, rifampin: decreased corticosteroid effect. Increase corticosteroid dosage, as ordered.
Oral anticoagulants: altered dosage requirements. Monitor PT and INR closely.

Potassium-depleting drugs (such as thiazide diuretics): enhanced potassium-wasting effects of prednisone. Monitor serum potassium levels.
Skin-test antigens: decreased response. Defer skin testing until therapy is completed.
Toxoids, vaccines: decreased antibody response and increased risk of neurologic complications. Avoid concomitant use.

Contraindications and precautions

- Contraindicated in patients hypersensitive to drug and in those with systemic fungal infections.
- Use of high doses isn't recommended in breast-feeding women.
- Use with extreme caution in pregnant women.
- Use cautiously in patients with GI ulcer, renal disease, hypertension, osteoporosis, diabetes mellitus, hypothyroidism, cirrhosis, diverticulitis, nonspecific ulcerative colitis, recent intestinal anastomoses, thromboembolic disorders, seizures, myasthenia gravis, heart failure, tuberculosis, ocular herpes simplex, emotional instability, and psychotic tendencies.

NURSING CONSIDERATIONS

Assessment

- Assess patient's condition before therapy and regularly thereafter.
- Monitor patient's weight, blood pressure, and serum electrolyte levels.
- Watch for depression or psychotic episodes, especially at high doses.
- Diabetic patient may need increased insulin; monitor blood glucose levels.
- Monitor patient's stress level; dosage adjustment may be needed.
- Be alert for adverse reactions and drug interactions.
- Evaluate patient's and family's knowledge of drug therapy.

Nursing diagnoses

- Ineffective health maintenance related to underlying condition
- Ineffective protection related to drug-induced adverse reactions
- Deficient knowledge related to drug therapy

Planning and implementation

- Always adjust to lowest effective dosage, as ordered. Expect to increase dosage as ordered during times of physiologic stress (such as surgery, trauma, or infection).
- Drug may be used for alternate-day therapy.
- For better results and less toxicity, give once-daily dose in morning.
- Give oral dose with food when possible to reduce GI irritation.
- After long-term therapy, reduce dosage gradually as ordered. Abrupt withdrawal may cause rebound inflammation, fatigue, weakness, arthralgia, fever, dizziness, lethargy, depression, fainting, orthostatic hypotension, dyspnea, anorexia, or hypoglycemia. After long-term therapy, increased stress or abrupt withdrawal may cause acute adrenal insufficiency. Sudden withdrawal after prolonged use may be fatal.
- Unless contraindicated, give low-sodium diet high in potassium and protein. Administer potassium supplements as needed.
- Notify prescriber immediately if serious adverse reactions occur; be prepared to give supportive care.

ALERT Don't confuse prednisone with prednisolone.

Patient teaching

- Tell patient not to stop drug without prescriber's knowledge.
- Tell patient to take drug as ordered. Tell patient what to do if he misses a dose.
- Advise patient to take oral form with meals to minimize GI reactions.
- Tell patient to report sudden weight gain, swelling, or slow healing.
- Advise patient receiving long-term therapy to consider exercise or physical therapy, to ask prescriber about vitamin D or calcium supplements, and to have periodic eye examinations.
- Instruct patient to wear or carry medical identification that indicates his need for systemic glucocorticoids during stress.
- Warn patient receiving long-term therapy about cushingoid symptoms.
- Teach signs of early adrenal insufficiency: fatigue, muscular weakness, joint pain, fever,

anorexia, nausea, dyspnea, dizziness, and fainting.

Evaluation
- Patient responds well to therapy.
- Patient doesn't experience serious adverse reactions.
- Patient and family state understanding of drug therapy.

primaquine phosphate
(PRIH-muh-kwin FOS-fayt)

Pharmacologic class: 8-aminoquinoline
Therapeutic class: antimalarial
Pregnancy risk category: C

Indications and dosages

▶ **Radical cure of relapsing *Plasmodium vivax* malaria, eliminating symptoms and infection completely; prevention of relapse.** *Adults:* 15 mg (base) P.O. daily for 14 days. (26.3-mg tablet = 15 mg of base.)

How supplied

Tablets: 7.5 mg (base)♦, 15 mg (base)

Pharmacokinetics

Absorption: well absorbed from GI tract.
Distribution: distributed widely into liver, lungs, heart, brain, skeletal muscle, and other tissues.
Metabolism: metabolized in liver.
Excretion: small amount excreted unchanged in urine. *Half-life:* 4 to 10 hours.

Route	Onset	Peak	Duration
P.O.	Unknown	2-3 hr	Unknown

Pharmacodynamics

Chemical effect: unknown; it may be effective because it can bind to and alter properties of DNA.
Therapeutic effect: prevents or treats relapsing *P. vivax* malaria.

Adverse reactions

GI: nausea, vomiting, epigastric distress, abdominal cramps.
Hematologic: ***leukopenia, hemolytic anemia in G6PD deficiency,*** methemoglobinemia in NADH methemoglobin reductase deficiency.

Interactions

Drug-drug. *Magnesium and aluminum salts:* decreased GI absorption. Separate administration times.
Quinacrine: enhanced primaquine toxicity. Don't use together.

Contraindications and precautions

- Contraindicated in patients with systemic diseases in which granulocytopenia may develop (such as lupus erythematosus or rheumatoid arthritis) and in those taking bone marrow suppressants and potentially hemolytic drugs.
- Use cautiously in patients with previous idiosyncratic reaction (hemolytic anemia, methemoglobinemia, or leukopenia), in those with family or personal history of favism, and in those with erythrocytic G6PD deficiency or NADH methemoglobin reductase deficiency. Also use cautiously in pregnant women.
- Safety of drug hasn't been established in children and in breast-feeding women.

NURSING CONSIDERATIONS

Assessment
- Assess patient's condition before therapy and regularly thereafter.
- Obtain frequent blood studies and urine examinations as ordered in light-skinned patients taking more than 30 mg (base) daily, dark-skinned patients taking more than 15 mg (base) daily, and patients with severe anemia or suspected sensitivity.
- Monitor patient for sudden drop in hemoglobin level, decreased erythrocyte or leukocyte count, or marked darkening of urine, each of which suggests impending hemolytic reactions.
- Be alert for adverse reactions and drug interactions.
- Evaluate patient's and family's knowledge of drug therapy.

Nursing diagnoses
- Infection related to malaria

• Ineffective protection related to adverse hematologic reactions
• Deficient knowledge related to drug therapy

Planning and implementation
• Administer drug with meals.
• A fast-acting antimalarial (such as chloroquine) is usually given with primaquine to reduce possibility of drug-resistant strains.
• Stop drug immediately and notify prescriber about abnormal CBC results or pronounced darkening of urine.

Patient teaching
• Instruct patient to take drug with meals.
• Tell patient to notify prescriber if adverse reactions occur, especially a marked darkening of urine.
• Tell patient to avoid hazardous activities if visual disturbances occur.

Evaluation
• Patient is free from malaria.
• Patient doesn't develop serious adverse hematologic reactions.
• Patient and family state understanding of drug therapy.

primidone
(PRIH-mih-dohn)
Apo-Primidone ♦, Mysoline, PMS Primidone ♦, Sertan ♦

Pharmacologic class: barbiturate analogue
Therapeutic class: anticonvulsant
Pregnancy risk category: NR

Indications and dosages
▶ **Generalized tonic-clonic, focal, and complex-partial (psychomotor) seizures.** *Adults and children age 8 and over:* initially, 100 to 125 mg P.O. h.s. on days 1 to 3; then 100 to 125 mg P.O. b.i.d. on days 4 to 6; then 100 to 125 mg P.O. t.i.d. on days 7 to 9; followed by maintenance dosage of 250 mg P.O. t.i.d.; maintenance dosage increased to 250 mg q.i.d. if needed.
Children under age 8: initially, 50 mg P.O. h.s. for 3 days; then 50 mg P.O. b.i.d. for 4 to 6 days; then 100 mg P.O. b.i.d. for 7 to 9 days followed by maintenance dosage of 125 to 250 mg P.O. t.i.d.
▶ **Benign familial tremor (essential tremor).** *Adults:* 750 mg P.O. daily.

How supplied
Tablets: 50 mg, 250 mg
Oral suspension: 250 mg/5 ml

Pharmacokinetics
Absorption: absorbed readily from GI tract.
Distribution: distributed widely throughout body.
Metabolism: metabolized slowly by liver to phenylethylmalonamide (PEMA) and phenobarbital; PEMA is the major metabolite.
Excretion: excreted in urine.

Route	Onset	Peak	Duration
P.O.	Unknown	3-4 hr	Unknown

Pharmacodynamics
Chemical effect: unknown; some activity may be caused by PEMA and phenobarbital.
Therapeutic effect: prevents seizures.

Adverse reactions
CNS: *drowsiness, ataxia,* emotional disturbances, vertigo, hyperirritability, fatigue.
CV: edema.
EENT: *diplopia,* nystagmus, edema of eyelids.
GI: anorexia, nausea, vomiting, thirst.
GU: impotence, polyuria.
Hematologic: ***leukopenia,*** eosinophilia, ***thrombocytopenia.***
Skin: morbilliform rash, alopecia.

Interactions
Drug-drug. *Carbamazepine:* increased primidone levels. Observe patient for toxicity.
Phenytoin: increased conversion of primidone to phenobarbital. Observe patient for increased phenobarbital effect.

Contraindications and precautions
• Contraindicated in pregnant or breast-feeding women and in patients with phenobarbital hypersensitivity or porphyria.

NURSING CONSIDERATIONS

Assessment
- Assess patient's condition before therapy and regularly thereafter.
- Monitor blood levels as ordered. Therapeutic primidone level is 5 to 12 mcg/ml. Therapeutic phenobarbital level is 15 to 40 mcg/ml.
- Monitor CBC and routine blood chemistry every 6 months, as ordered.
- Monitor patient's hydration status throughout drug therapy.
- Evaluate patient's and family's knowledge of drug therapy.

Nursing diagnoses
- Risk for trauma related to seizures
- Risk for deficient fluid volume related to adverse reactions
- Deficient knowledge related to drug therapy

Planning and implementation
- Shake liquid suspension well.
- Don't withdraw drug suddenly because seizures may worsen.
- Call prescriber immediately if adverse reactions develop.

ALERT Don't confuse primidone with prednisone.

Patient teaching
- Advise patient to avoid hazardous activities until CNS effects of drug are known.
- Warn patient and parents not to stop drug suddenly.
- Tell patient that full therapeutic response may take 2 weeks or more.

Evaluation
- Patient is free from seizure activity.
- Patient maintains adequate hydration throughout drug therapy.
- Patient and family state understanding of drug therapy.

probenecid
(proh-BEN-uh-sid)
Benemid, Benuryl♦, Probalan

Pharmacologic class: sulfonamide-derivative
Therapeutic class: uricosuric agent
Pregnancy risk category: NR

Indications and dosages
▶ **Adjunct to penicillin therapy.** *Adults and children over age 14 or weighing more than 50 kg (110 lb):* 500 mg P.O. q.i.d.
Children ages 2 to 14 weighing 50 kg or less: initially, 25 mg/kg P.O.; then 40 mg/kg in divided doses q.i.d.

▶ **Gonorrhea.** *Adults:* 3.5 g ampicillin P.O. with 1 g probenecid P.O. given together. Or, 1 g probenecid P.O. 30 minutes before 4.8 million units of aqueous penicillin G procaine I.M., injected at two different sites.

▶ **Hyperuricemia of gout, gouty arthritis.** *Adults:* 250 mg P.O. b.i.d. for first week; then 500 mg b.i.d., to maximum of 3 g daily. Maintenance dosage should be reviewed q 6 months and reduced by increments of 500 mg if indicated.

How supplied
Tablets: 500 mg

Pharmacokinetics
Absorption: completely absorbed.
Distribution: distributed throughout body; about 75% protein-bound.
Metabolism: metabolized in liver to active metabolites, with some uricosuric effect.
Excretion: drug and metabolites excreted in urine; probenecid is actively reabsorbed but metabolites aren't. *Half-life:* 3 to 8 hours after 500-mg dose, 6 to 12 hours after larger doses.

Route	Onset	Peak	Duration
P.O.	Unknown	2-4 hr	About 8 hr

Pharmacodynamics
Chemical effect: blocks renal tubular reabsorption of uric acid, increasing excretion, and inhibits active renal tubular secretion of many

weak organic acids, such as penicillins and cephalosporins.
Therapeutic effect: lowers uric acid and prolongs penicillin action.

Adverse reactions

CNS: *headache,* dizziness.
CV: flushing, hypotension.
GI: anorexia, nausea, vomiting, sore gums, *gastric distress.*
GU: urinary frequency, renal colic.
Hematologic: hemolytic anemia, ***aplastic anemia.***
Hepatic: ***hepatic necrosis.***
Skin: alopecia, dermatitis, pruritus.
Other: fever, ***hypersensitivity reaction, anaphylaxis.***

Interactions

Drug-drug. *Indomethacin:* decreased indomethacin excretion. Lower indomethacin dosages may be needed.
Methotrexate: decreased methotrexate excretion. Lower methotrexate dosage may be needed. Serum levels should be determined.
Oral antidiabetics: enhanced hypoglycemic effect. Monitor blood glucose levels closely. Dosage adjustment may be needed.
Salicylates: inhibited uricosuric effect of probenecid, causing urate retention. Don't use together.
Drug-lifestyle. *Alcohol use:* increased urate levels. Discourage concomitant use.

Contraindications and precautions

- Contraindicated in patients hypersensitive to drug, children under age 2, and patients with uric acid kidney stones, blood dyscrasias, or acute gout attack.
- Use cautiously in pregnant or breast-feeding women and patients with peptic ulcer or renal impairment.

NURSING CONSIDERATIONS

Assessment

- Assess patient's condition before therapy and regularly thereafter.
- Monitor periodic BUN and renal function tests in long-term therapy, as ordered.
- Drug is ineffective in patients with chronic renal insufficiency (GFR less than 30 ml/minute).
- Be alert for adverse reactions and drug interactions.
- Monitor patient's hydration status if adverse GI reactions occur.
- Evaluate patient's and family's knowledge of drug therapy.

Nursing diagnoses

- Ineffective health maintenance related to underlying condition
- Risk for deficient fluid volume related to adverse GI reactions
- Deficient knowledge related to drug therapy

Planning and implementation

- Give drug with milk, food, or antacids to minimize GI distress. Continued disturbances may indicate need to lower dosage.
- Force fluids to maintain minimum daily output of 2 L of water a day. Alkalinize urine with sodium bicarbonate or potassium citrate, as ordered. These measures will prevent hematuria, renal colic, urate stone development, and costovertebral pain.
- Keep in mind that therapy doesn't start until acute attack subsides. Drug contains no analgesic or anti-inflammatory agent and isn't useful during acute gout attacks.
- Drug may increase frequency, severity, and duration of acute gout attacks during first 6 to 12 months of therapy. Prophylactic colchicine or another anti-inflammatory is given during first 3 to 6 months.
- Drug may produce false-positive glucose tests with Benedict's solution or Clinitest, but not with glucose oxidase method (Diastix).
- Drug interferes with laboratory procedures by decreasing urinary excretion of 17-ketosteroids, bromsulphalein, aminohippuric acid, and iodine-related organic acids.

ALERT Don't confuse probenecid with Procanbid or Benemid with Beminal.

Patient teaching

- Instruct patient to take drug with food or milk to minimize GI distress.

• Advise patient with gout to avoid all drugs that contain aspirin, which may precipitate gout. Acetaminophen may be used for pain.
• Tell patient with gout to avoid alcohol during drug therapy; it increases urate level.
• Tell patient with gout to limit intake of foods high in purine, such as anchovies, liver, sardines, kidneys, sweetbreads, peas, and lentils.
• Instruct patient and family that drug must be taken regularly as ordered or gout attacks may result. Tell him to visit prescriber regularly so uric acid can be monitored and dosage adjusted, if necessary. Lifelong therapy may be required in patients with hyperuricemia.

Evaluation
• Patient responds positively to therapy.
• Patient maintains adequate hydration.
• Patient and family state understanding of drug therapy.

procainamide hydrochloride
(proh-KAYN-uh-mighd high-droh-KLOR-ighd)
Procainamide Durules◆, Procan SR, Promine, Pronestyl**, Pronestyl-SR

Pharmacologic class: procaine derivative
Therapeutic class: ventricular antiarrhythmic, supraventricular antiarrhythmic
Pregnancy risk category: C

Indications and dosages
▶ **Life-threatening ventricular arrhythmias.** *Adults:* 50 to 100 mg by slow I.V. push q 5 minutes, no faster than 25 to 50 mg/minute until arrhythmias disappear, adverse reactions develop, or 500 mg has been given. Usual effective dose is 500 to 600 mg. When arrhythmias disappear, give continuous infusion of 2 to 6 mg/minute. If arrhythmias recur, repeat bolus as above and increase infusion rate. Or, 50 mg/kg I.M. given in divided doses q 3 to 6 hours until oral therapy begins. For oral therapy, 50 mg/kg daily q 3 hours; average 250 to 500 mg q 3 hours.
Patients with renal or hepatic dysfunction: decreased dosages or longer dosing intervals may be needed.

How supplied
Tablets: 250 mg, 375 mg, 500 mg
Tablets (sustained-release): 250 mg, 500 mg, 750 mg
Capsules: 250 mg, 375 mg, 500 mg
Injection: 100 mg/ml, 500 mg/ml

Pharmacokinetics
Absorption: rate and extent of drug's absorption from intestine vary; usually 75% to 95% of P.O. dose is absorbed. Unknown after I.M. administration.
Distribution: distributed widely in most body tissues, including CSF, liver, spleen, kidneys, lungs, muscles, brain, and heart. About 15% binds to plasma proteins.
Metabolism: metabolized in liver.
Excretion: excreted in urine. *Half-life:* about 2½ to 4¾ hours.

Route	Onset	Peak	Duration
P.O.	2 hr	1-1.5 hr	Unknown
I.V.	Immediate	Immediate	Unknown
I.M.	10-30 min	15-60 min	Unknown

Pharmacodynamics
Chemical effect: class Ia antiarrhythmic that decreases excitability, conduction velocity, automaticity, and membrane responsiveness with prolonged refractory period. Larger doses may induce AV block.
Therapeutic effect: restores normal sinus rhythm.

Adverse reactions
CNS: hallucinations, confusion, depression, dizziness.
CV: hypotension, ***ventricular asystole,*** *bradycardia,* AV block, ***ventricular fibrillation*** after parenteral use, ***heart failure.***
GI: nausea, vomiting, anorexia, diarrhea, bitter taste with large doses.
Hematologic: ***thrombocytopenia, neutropenia*** (especially with sustained-release forms), ***agranulocytosis,*** hemolytic anemia, *increased antinuclear antibody titer.*
Musculoskeletal: *myalgia.*
Skin: maculopapular rash.

Other: *fever, lupuslike syndrome* (especially after prolonged administration).

Interactions

Drug-drug. *Amiodarone:* increased procainamide levels and toxicity; additive effects on QT interval and QRS complex. Avoid concomitant use.
Anticholinergics: additive anticholinergic effects. Monitor patient closely.
Anticholinesterases: decreased anticholinesterase effect. Anticholinesterase dosage may need to be increased.
Cimetidine: may increase procainamide blood levels. Monitor levels closely.
Neuromuscular blockers: increased skeletal muscle relaxant effects. Monitor patient.
Drug-herb. *Jimson weed:* may adversely affect CV function. Discourage concomitant use.
Licorice: may prolong QT interval and be additive. Discourage concomitant use.

Contraindications and precautions

- Contraindicated in patients hypersensitive to procaine and related drugs; in those with complete, second-, or third-degree heart block in absence of artificial pacemaker; and in those with myasthenia gravis or systemic lupus erythematosus. Also contraindicated in patients with atypical ventricular tachycardia (torsades de pointes) because procainamide may aggravate this condition.
- Drug isn't recommended for breast-feeding women.
- Use extreme caution when giving drug to treat ventricular tachycardia during coronary occlusion.
- Use cautiously in pregnant women and patients with hepatic or renal insufficiency, blood dyscrasias, bone marrow suppression, heart failure, or other conduction disturbances, such as bundle-branch heart block, sinus bradycardia, or cardiac glycoside intoxication.
- Safety of drug hasn't been established in children.

NURSING CONSIDERATIONS

Assessment

- Assess patient's condition before therapy and regularly thereafter.
- Monitor plasma levels of procainamide and its active metabolite NAPA. To suppress ventricular arrhythmias, therapeutic serum levels of procainamide are 4 to 8 mcg/ml; therapeutic levels of NAPA are 10 to 30 mcg/ml.
- Monitor QT interval closely in patient with renal failure.
- Hypokalemia predisposes patient to arrhythmias; monitor serum electrolytes, especially potassium level.
- Monitor blood pressure and ECG continuously during I.V. administration. Watch for prolonged QT intervals and QRS complexes, heart block, or increased arrhythmias.
- Monitor CBC frequently during first 3 months, particularly in patient taking sustained-release form.
- Be alert for adverse reactions and drug interactions.
- Evaluate patient's and family's knowledge of drug therapy.

Nursing diagnoses

- Decreased cardiac output related to presence of arrhythmia
- Ineffective protection related to adverse hematologic reactions
- Deficient knowledge related to drug therapy

Planning and implementation

P.O. and I.M. use: Follow normal protocol.
I.V. use: Patient receiving infusions must be attended at all times.
– Use infusion control device to administer infusion precisely.
– Vials for I.V. injection contain 1 g of drug: 100 mg/ml (10 ml) or 500 mg/ml (2 ml).
– Keep patient in supine position during I.V. administration. If drug is given too rapidly, hypotension can occur. Watch closely for adverse reactions during infusion, and notify prescriber if they occur.
– If procainamide solution becomes discolored, check with pharmacy and expect to discard.

ALERT If blood pressure changes significantly or ECG changes occur, withhold drug, obtain rhythm strip, and notify prescriber immediately.
- Positive antinuclear antibody titer occurs in about 60% of patients without lupuslike symptoms. This response seems to be related to prolonged use, not to dosage. May progress to systemic lupus erythematosus if drug isn't discontinued.

Patient teaching
- Instruct patient to report fever, rash, muscle pain, diarrhea, bleeding, bruises, or pleuritic chest pain.
- Stress importance of taking drug exactly as prescribed. This may require use of alarm clock for nighttime doses.
- Inform patient taking extended-release form that wax-matrix "ghost" from tablet may be passed in stool. Assure patient that drug is completely absorbed before this occurs.
- Tell patient not to crush or break sustained-release tablets.

Evaluation
- Patient regains normal cardiac output after drug stops abnormal heart rhythm.
- Patient maintains normal CBC.
- Patient and family state understanding of drug therapy.

procarbazine hydrochloride
(proh-KAR-buh-zeen high-droh-KLOR-ighd)
Matulane, Natulan

Pharmacologic class: antibiotic antineoplastic (specific to S phase of cell cycle)
Therapeutic class: antineoplastic
Pregnancy risk category: D

Indications and dosages
Dosage and indications may differ. Check with prescriber for treatment protocol.
▶ **Hodgkin's disease; lymphoma; brain and lung cancer.** *Adults:* 2 to 4 mg/kg P.O. daily in single dose or divided doses for first week. Then, 4 to 6 mg/kg/day until WBC count decreases to below 4,000/mm³ or platelet count decreases to below 100,000/mm³. After bone marrow recovers, maintenance dosage of 1 to 2 mg/kg/day resumed.
Children: 50 mg/m² P.O. daily for first week; then 100 mg/m² until response or toxicity occurs. Maintenance dosage is 50 mg/m² P.O. daily after bone marrow recovery.

How supplied
Capsules: 50 mg

Pharmacokinetics
Absorption: rapidly and completely absorbed.
Distribution: distributes widely into body tissues, with highest levels in liver, kidneys, intestinal wall, and skin. Drug crosses blood-brain barrier.
Metabolism: extensively metabolized in liver; some metabolites have cytotoxic activity.
Excretion: drug and metabolites excreted primarily in urine. *Half-life:* about 10 minutes.

Route	Onset	Peak	Duration
P.O.	Unknown	Unknown	Unknown

Pharmacodynamics
Chemical effect: unknown; thought to inhibit DNA, RNA, and protein synthesis.
Therapeutic effect: kills selected cancer cells.

Adverse reactions
CNS: nervousness, depression, insomnia, nightmares, paresthesia, neuropathy, *hallucinations,* confusion, ***seizures, coma.***
EENT: retinal hemorrhage, nystagmus, photophobia.
GI: *nausea, vomiting,* anorexia, stomatitis, dry mouth, dysphagia, diarrhea, constipation.
Hematologic: ***bleeding tendency, thrombocytopenia, leukopenia,*** anemia.
Hepatic: ***hepatotoxicity.***
Respiratory: *pleural effusion,* pneumonitis.
Skin: dermatitis, reversible alopecia.

Interactions
Drug-drug. *CNS depressants:* additive depressant effects. Avoid concomitant use.
Digoxin: may decrease serum digoxin levels. Monitor levels closely.
Local anesthetics, sympathomimetics, tricyclic antidepressants: possible tremors, palpita-

tions, increased blood pressure. Monitor patient closely.
Meperidine: may cause severe hypotension and possible death. Don't give together.
Drug-food. *Caffeine:* concurrent use may result in arrhythmias, severe hypertension. Discourage caffeine intake.
Foods high in tyramine (cheese, Chianti wine): possible tremors, palpitations, increased blood pressure. Monitor patient closely.
Drug-lifestyle. *Alcohol use:* mild disulfiram-like reaction. Warn patient to avoid alcohol.

Contraindications and precautions

- Contraindicated in patients hypersensitive to drug and those with inadequate bone marrow reserve as shown by bone marrow aspiration.
- Drug isn't recommended for pregnant or breast-feeding women.
- Use cautiously in patients with impaired hepatic or renal function.

NURSING CONSIDERATIONS

Assessment
- Assess patient's condition before therapy and regularly thereafter.
- Monitor CBC and platelet counts.
- Be alert for adverse reactions and drug interactions.
- Evaluate patient's and family's knowledge of drug therapy.

Nursing diagnoses
- Ineffective health maintenance related to presence of neoplastic disease
- Ineffective protection related to adverse hematologic reactions
- Deficient knowledge related to drug therapy

Planning and implementation
- Give drug at bedtime to lessen nausea.

ALERT Be prepared to stop drug and notify prescriber if patient becomes confused or if paresthesia or other neuropathies develop.

Patient teaching
- Advise patient to take drug at bedtime and in divided doses.
- Warn patient to watch for signs of infection (fever, sore throat, fatigue) and bleeding (easy bruising, nosebleeds, bleeding gums, melena). Tell him to take his temperature daily.
- Warn patient to avoid alcohol during drug therapy.
- Tell patient to stop drug and check with prescriber immediately if disulfiram-like reaction occurs (chest pains, rapid or irregular heartbeat, severe headache, stiff neck).
- Warn patient to avoid hazardous activities until CNS effects of drug are known.
- Advise woman of childbearing age not to become pregnant during therapy and to consult with prescriber before becoming pregnant.

Evaluation
- Patient responds well to therapy.
- Patient develops no serious adverse hematologic reactions.
- Patient and family state understanding of drug therapy.

prochlorperazine
(proh-klor-PER-ah-zeen)
Compazine, PMS Prochlorperazine♦, Prorazin♦, Stemetil

prochlorperazine edisylate
Compa-Z, Compazine Syrup, Cotranzine, Ultrazine-10

prochlorperazine maleate
Anti-Naus♦, Compazine Spansule, PMS Prochlorperazine♦, Prorazin♦, Stemetil

Pharmacologic class: phenothiazine (piperazine derivative)
Therapeutic class: antipsychotic, antiemetic, antianxiety agent
Pregnancy risk category: NR

Indications and dosages

▶ **Preoperative nausea control.** *Adults:* 5 to 10 mg I.M. 1 to 2 hours before induction of anesthesia; repeat once in 30 minutes, if necessary. Or, 5 to 10 mg I.V. 15 to 30 minutes before induction of anesthesia; repeat once if necessary. Or, 20 mg/L D_5W or normal saline solution by I.V. infusion. Begin infusion 15 to 30 minutes before induction of anesthesia.

▶ **Severe nausea and vomiting.** *Adults:* 5 to 10 mg P.O., t.i.d. or q.i.d. Or, 15 mg sustained-release form P.O. on arising. Or, 10 mg sustained-release form P.O. q 12 hours. Or, 25 mg P.R., b.i.d. Or, 5 to 10 mg I.M. repeated q 3 to 4 hours, p.r.n. Or, 5 to 10 mg may be given I.V. Maximum I.M. dosage is 40 mg daily.

Children weighing 18 to 39 kg (40 to 86 lb): 2.5 mg P.O. or P.R., t.i.d. Or, 5 mg P.O. or P.R., b.i.d. Maximum dosage is 15 mg daily. Or, give 0.132 mg/kg by deep I.M. injection. Control usually is obtained with one dose.

Children weighing 14 to 17 kg (30 to 38 lb): 2.5 mg P.O. or P.R., b.i.d. or t.i.d. Maximum dosage is 10 mg daily. Or give 0.132 mg/kg by deep I.M. injection. Control usually is obtained with one dose.

Children weighing 9 to 13 kg (20 to 29 lb): 2.5 mg P.O. or P.R. once daily or b.i.d. Maximum dosage is 7.5 mg daily. Or give 0.132 mg/kg by deep I.M. injection. Control usually is obtained with one dose.

▶ **To manage symptoms of psychotic disorders.** *Adults:* 5 to 10 mg P.O., t.i.d. or q.i.d. *Children ages 2 to 12:* 2.5 mg P.O. or P.R., b.i.d. or t.i.d. Don't exceed 10 mg on day 1. Increase dosage gradually to recommended maximum (if necessary). In children ages 2 to 5, maximum daily dosage is 20 mg. In children ages 6 to 10, maximum daily dosage is 25 mg.

▶ **To manage symptoms of severe psychoses.** *Adults:* 10 to 20 mg I.M. repeated in 1 to 4 hours, if needed. Rarely, patients may receive 10 to 20 mg q 4 to 6 hours. Institute P.O. therapy after symptoms are controlled.

Children ages 2 to 12: 0.13 mg/kg I.M.

▶ **Nonpsychotic anxiety.** *Adults:* 5 to 10 mg by deep I.M. injection q 3 to 4 hours, not to exceed 40 mg daily; or 5 to 10 mg P.O., t.i.d. or q.i.d. Or, give 15-mg extended-release capsule once daily or 10-mg extended-release capsule q 12 hours.

How supplied

prochlorperazine
Tablets: 5 mg, 10 mg
Injection: 5 mg/ml
Suppositories: 2.5 mg, 5 mg, 25 mg

prochlorperazine edisylate
Syrup: 1 mg/ml

prochlorperazine maleate
Tablets: 5 mg, 10 mg, 25 mg
Capsules (sustained-release): 10 mg, 15 mg, 30 mg

Pharmacokinetics

Absorption: erratic and variable with P.O. tablet; more predictable with P.O. concentrate. Unknown for P.R. administration. Rapid absorption with I.M. administration.
Distribution: distributed widely into body; 91% to 99% protein-bound.
Metabolism: metabolized extensively by liver, but no active metabolites are formed.
Excretion: excreted primarily in urine; some excreted in feces.

Route	Onset	Peak	Duration
P.O.	30-40 min	Unknown	3-12 hr
I.V.	Immediate	Immediate	Unknown
I.M.	10-20 min	Unknown	3-4 hr
P.R.	60 min	Unknown	3-4 hr

Pharmacodynamics

Chemical effect: acts on chemoreceptor trigger zone to inhibit nausea and vomiting; in larger doses, partially depresses vomiting center.
Therapeutic effect: relieves nausea and vomiting, signs and symptoms of psychosis, and anxiety.

Adverse reactions

CNS: *extrapyramidal reactions,* sedation, pseudoparkinsonism, EEG changes, dizziness.
CV: *orthostatic hypotension,* tachycardia, ECG changes.
EENT: *ocular changes, blurred vision.*
GI: *dry mouth, constipation.*
GU: *urine retention,* dark urine, menstrual irregularities, inhibited ejaculation.
Hematologic: ***transient leukopenia, agranulocytosis.***
Hepatic: cholestatic jaundice.
Metabolic: weight gain, increased appetite.

Skin: *mild photosensitivity,* ***allergic reactions, exfoliative dermatitis.***
Other: hyperprolactinemia, gynecomastia.

Interactions

Drug-drug. *Antacids:* inhibited absorption of oral phenothiazines. Separate antacid doses by at least 2 hours.
Anticholinergics, including antidepressants and antiparkinsonian agents: increased anticholinergic activity and aggravated parkinsonian symptoms. Use together cautiously.
Barbiturates: may decrease phenothiazine effect.
Drug-herb. *Dong quai, St. John's wort:* increased photosensitivity reactions. Discourage concomitant use.
Ginkgo: possible decreased adverse effects of phenothiazines. Monitor patient.
Kava: increased risk of dystonic reactions. Discourage concomitant use.
Milk thistle: decreased liver toxicity caused by phenothiazines. Monitor liver enzyme levels if used together.
Yohimbe: increased risk for yohimbe toxicity when used together. Discourage concomitant use.
Drug-lifestyle. *Sun exposure:* potential photosensitivity reaction. Urge patient to take precautions.

Contraindications and precautions

- Contraindicated in children under age 2, patients hypersensitive to phenothiazines, patients with CNS depression (including coma), patients undergoing pediatric surgery, and patients receiving spinal or epidural anesthetics, adrenergic blockers, or alcohol.
- Use cautiously in patients who have been exposed to extreme heat and patients with impaired CV function, glaucoma, or seizure disorders. Also use cautiously in breast-feeding women and acutely ill children.
- Safety of drug hasn't been established in pregnant women.

NURSING CONSIDERATIONS

Assessment

- Assess patient's condition before therapy and regularly thereafter.
- Watch for orthostatic hypotension, especially when giving drug I.V.
- Monitor CBC and liver function studies during prolonged therapy.
- Be alert for adverse reactions and drug interactions.
- Evaluate patient's and family's knowledge of drug therapy.

Nursing diagnoses

- Risk for deficient fluid volume related to nausea and vomiting
- Disturbed thought processes related to presence of psychosis
- Deficient knowledge related to drug therapy

Planning and implementation

P.O. use: Dilute solution with tomato or fruit juice, milk, coffee, carbonated beverage, tea, water or soup; or mix with pudding.
I.V. use: Drug may be given undiluted or diluted in an isotonic solution. Administration rate shouldn't exceed 5 mg/minute. Don't give by bolus injection.
I.M. use: Inject deep into upper outer quadrant of gluteal region.
P.R. use: Follow normal protocol.

- Don't give S.C. or mix in syringe with another drug.
- Avoid getting concentrate or injection solution on hands or clothing.
- Drug is used only if vomiting can't be otherwise controlled or if only a few doses are needed. If more than four doses are needed in 24 hours, notify prescriber.
- Store drug in light-resistant container. Slight yellowing doesn't affect potency; discard extremely discolored solutions.

Patient teaching

- Tell patient to mix oral solution with flavored liquid to mask taste.
- Advise patient to wear protective clothing when exposed to sunlight.
- Tell patient to notify prescriber about adverse reactions.

Evaluation

- Patient's nausea and vomiting are relieved.
- Patient behavior and communication show better thought processes.

• Patient and family state understanding of drug therapy.

progesterone
(proh-JES-teh-rohn)
Crinone 4%, Crinone 8%, Gesterol 50, PMS-Progesterone ♦, Progestasert, Prometrium

Pharmacologic class: progestin
Therapeutic class: hormonal agent
Pregnancy risk category: X

Indications and dosages

▶ **Amenorrhea.** *Adults:* 5 to 10 mg I.M. daily for 6 to 8 days usually beginning 8 to 10 days before anticipated start of menstruation.

▶ **Secondary amenorrhea:** *Adults:* 400 mg P.O. in the evening for 10 days. Or, Crinone 4% gel given intravaginally every other day up to 6 doses. Those who fail may try Crinone 8% gel given intravaginally every other day up to 6 doses.

▶ **Prevention of endometrial hyperplasia:** *Adult women with intact uterus:* 200 mg P.O. in the evening for 12 contiguous days per 28-day cycle, given with conjugated estrogen tablets.

▶ **Dysfunctional uterine bleeding.** *Adults:* 5 to 10 mg I.M. daily for six doses.

▶ **Contraception (as an intrauterine device [IUD]).** *Adults:* Progestasert system inserted into uterine cavity; replaced annually.

▶ **Infertility:** *Adults:* 90 mg (gel) administered intravaginally daily to b.i.d. May use up to 12 weeks after pregnancy to maintain placental autonomy.

How supplied

Injection (in oil): 50 mg/ml
IUD: 38 mg (with barium sulfate, dispersed in silicone fluid)
Capsules: 100 mg
Gel: 4%, 8%

Pharmacokinetics

Absorption: unknown.
Distribution: unknown.
Metabolism: metabolized in liver.
Excretion: excreted in urine. *Half-life:* several minutes.

Route	Onset	Peak	Duration
P.O., I.M., intravaginal	Unknown	Unknown	Unknown

Pharmacodynamics

Chemical effect: suppresses ovulation and forms thick cervical mucus.
Therapeutic effect: alleviates amenorrhea and dysfunctional uterine bleeding.

Adverse reactions

CNS: dizziness, migraine, lethargy, depression.
CV: hypertension, thrombophlebitis, ***thromboembolism, pulmonary embolism, CVA,*** edema.
GI: nausea, vomiting, abdominal cramps.
GU: breakthrough bleeding, dysmenorrhea, amenorrhea, cervical erosion, abnormal secretions, uterine fibromas, vaginal candidiasis.
Hepatic: cholestatic jaundice.
Metabolic: hyperglycemia.
Skin: melasma, rash.
Other: breast tenderness, enlargement, or secretion; decreased libido; pain at injection site.

Interactions

Drug-drug. *Barbiturates, carbamazepine, rifampin:* decreased progestin effects. Avoid concomitant use.
Bromocriptine: may cause amenorrhea. Monitor patient.

Contraindications and precautions

• Contraindicated in pregnant or breast-feeding women; patients hypersensitive to drug; patients with thromboembolic disorders, cerebral apoplexy, or a history of these conditions; and patients with breast cancer, undiagnosed abnormal vaginal bleeding, severe hepatic disease, or missed abortion.
• Use cautiously in patients with diabetes mellitus, seizure disorder, migraine, cardiac or renal disease, asthma, and depression.

• Safety of drug hasn't been established in children.

NURSING CONSIDERATIONS

Assessment
• Assess patient's condition before therapy and regularly thereafter.
• Be alert for adverse reactions and drug interactions.
• Evaluate patient's and family's knowledge of drug therapy.

Nursing diagnoses
• Risk for deficient fluid volume related to excessive uterine bleeding
• Risk for injury related to dizziness
• Deficient knowledge related to drug therapy

Planning and implementation
• Preliminary estrogen treatment is usually needed in menstrual disorders.
• Give peanut or sesame oil solutions by deep I.M. injection. Check sites frequently for irritation. Rotate injection sites.

Patient teaching
• Make sure patient reads package insert explaining possible adverse effects of progestins before taking first dose. Also, provide verbal explanation.
• Tell patient not to perform hazardous activities if dizziness occurs.
• Tell patient to report any unusual symptoms immediately and to stop drug and call prescriber if visual disturbances or migraine occurs.
• Teach patient how to perform routine breast self-examination.

Evaluation
• Patient's uterine bleeding ceases.
• Patient doesn't experience injury from drug-induced dizziness.
• Patient and family state understanding of drug therapy.

promethazine hydrochloride
(proh-METH-uh-zeen high-droh-KLOR-ighd)
Anergan 25, Anergan 50, Histantil♦, Pentazine, Phenazine 50, Phencen-50, Phenergan*, Phenergan Fortis*, Phenergan Plain*, Phenoject-50, PMS-Promethazine♦, Pro-50, Promethegan, Prorex-25, Prorex-50, Prothazine*, Prothazine Plain, V-Gan-25, V-Gan-50

promethazine theoclate
Avomine♦

Pharmacologic class: phenothiazine derivative
Therapeutic class: antiemetic, antivertigo agent, antihistamine (H_1-receptor antagonist), sedative
Pregnancy risk category: C

Indications and dosages
▶ **Motion sickness.** *Adults:* 25 mg P.O. b.i.d. *Children:* 12.5 to 25 mg P.O., I.M., or P.R. b.i.d.
▶ **Nausea.** *Adults:* 12.5 to 25 mg P.O., I.M., or P.R. q 4 to 6 hours, p.r.n.
Children: 0.25 to 0.5 mg/kg I.M. or P.R. q 4 to 6 hours, p.r.n.
▶ **Rhinitis, allergy symptoms.** *Adults:* 12.5 to 25 mg P.O. q.i.d. Or, 25 mg P.O. h.s.
Children: 6.25 to 12.5 mg P.O. t.i.d. or 25 mg P.O. or P.R. h.s.
▶ **Sedation.** *Adults:* 25 to 50 mg P.O. or I.M. h.s. or p.r.n.
Children: 12.5 to 25 mg P.O., I.M., or P.R. h.s.
▶ **Routine preoperative or postoperative sedation or adjunct to analgesics.** *Adults:* 25 to 50 mg I.M., I.V., or P.O.
Children: 12.5 to 25 mg I.M., I.V., or P.O.

How supplied
promethazine hydrochloride
Tablets: 12.5 mg, 25 mg, 50 mg
Syrup: 5 mg/5 ml†*, 6.25 mg/5 ml*, 10 mg/5 ml*, 25 mg/5 ml*
Injection: 25 mg/ml, 50 mg/ml
Suppositories: 12.5 mg, 25 mg, 50 mg
promethazine theoclate
Tablets: 25 mg†

Pharmacokinetics

Absorption: well absorbed from GI tract after P.O. use; absorbed fairly rapidly after P.R. or I.M. use.
Distribution: distributed widely throughout body.
Metabolism: metabolized in liver.
Excretion: excreted in urine and feces.

Route	Onset	Peak	Duration
P.O.	15-60 min	Unknown	≤ 12 hr
I.V.	3-5 min	Unknown	≤ 12 hr
I.M., P.R.	20 min	Unknown	≤ 12 hr

Pharmacodynamics

Chemical effect: competes with histamine for H_1-receptor sites on effector cells. Prevents, but doesn't reverse, histamine-mediated responses.
Therapeutic effect: prevents motion sickness and relieves nausea, nasal congestion, and allergy symptoms. Also promotes calmness.

Adverse reactions

CNS: *sedation,* confusion, restlessness, tremors, *drowsiness* (especially elderly patients).
CV: hypotension.
EENT: transient myopia, nasal congestion.
GI: anorexia, nausea, vomiting, constipation, *dry mouth.*
GU: urine retention.
Hematologic: ***leukopenia*, *agranulocytosis, thrombocytopenia.***
Other: photosensitivity.

Interactions

Drug-drug. *CNS depressants:* increased sedation. Use together cautiously.
Epinephrine: promethazine may block or reverse effects of epinephrine. Other vasopressors should be used.
Levodopa: promethazine may decrease antiparkinsonian action of levodopa. Avoid concomitant use.
Lithium: promethazine may reduce GI absorption or enhance renal elimination of lithium. Avoid concomitant use.
MAO inhibitors: increased extrapyramidal effects. Don't use together.
Protease inhibitors, selective serotonin reuptake inhibitors: increased serum levels of these drugs and serious adverse cardiac effects. Avoid concomitant use.
Drug-herb. *Dong quai, St. John's wort:* increased photosensitivity reactions. Discourage concomitant use.
Kava: increased risk of dystonic reactions. Discourage concomitant use.
Yohimbe: increased risk for yohimbe toxicity when used together. Discourage concomitant use.
Drug-lifestyle. *Alcohol use:* increased sedation. Discourage concomitant use.
Sun exposure: possible photosensitivity reaction. Urge patient to take precautions.

Contraindications and precautions

- Contraindicated in patients hypersensitive to drug and in those with intestinal obstruction, prostatic hyperplasia, bladder-neck obstruction, seizure disorders, coma, CNS depression, or stenosing peptic ulcerations. Also contraindicated in newborns, premature neonates, breast-feeding women, and acutely ill or dehydrated children.
- Use cautiously in patients with pulmonary, hepatic, or CV disease or asthma.
- Safety of drug hasn't been established in pregnant women.

NURSING CONSIDERATIONS

Assessment
- Assess patient's condition before therapy and regularly thereafter.
- Be alert for adverse reactions and drug interactions.
- Evaluate patient's and family's knowledge of drug therapy.

Nursing diagnoses
- Ineffective health maintenance related to underlying condition
- Risk for injury related to drug's sedating effects
- Deficient knowledge related to drug therapy

Planning and implementation
- Pronounced sedative effect limits use in many ambulatory patients.

• Drug is used as adjunct to analgesics (usually to increase sedation); it has no analgesic activity.
P.O. use: Give drug with food or milk to reduce GI distress.
I.V. use: Don't give in concentration greater than 25 mg/ml or at rate exceeding 25 mg/minute. Shield I.V. infusion from direct light.
I.M. use: Inject deep into large muscle mass. Rotate injection sites.
P.R. use: Follow normal protocol.
• Don't administer S.C.
• Drug may be safely mixed with meperidine (Demerol) in same syringe.
• In patient scheduled for myelogram, discontinue drug 48 hours before procedure and don't resume drug until 24 hours after procedure, as ordered, because of risk of seizures.
• Drug may cause false-positive immunologic urine pregnancy test using Gravindex and false-negative using Prepurex or Dap tests. Also may interfere with blood typing of ABO group.

Patient teaching
• When treating for motion sickness, tell patient to take first dose 30 to 60 minutes before travel. On succeeding days of travel, he should take dose after rising and with evening meal.
• Warn patient to avoid alcohol and hazardous activities until drug's CNS effects are known.
• Tell patient that coffee or tea may reduce drowsiness. Sugarless gum, sugarless sour hard candy, or ice chips may relieve dry mouth.
• Warn patient about possible photosensitivity and precautions to avoid it.
• Advise patient to stop drug 4 days before allergy skin tests.

☑ Evaluation
• Patient responds well to therapy.
• Patient doesn't experience injury from adverse reactions.
• Patient and family state understanding of drug therapy.

propafenone hydrochloride
(proh-puh-FEE-nohn high-droh-KLOR-ighd)
Rythmol

Pharmacologic class: sodium channel antagonist
Therapeutic class: antiarrhythmic (class IC)
Pregnancy risk category: C

Indications and dosages
▶ **Suppression of life-threatening ventricular arrhythmias, such as sustained ventricular tachycardia.** *Adults:* initially, 150 mg P.O. q 8 hours. Dosage may be increased at 3- to 4-day intervals to 225 mg q 8 hours. If necessary, increase dosage to 300 mg q 8 hours. Maximum daily dosage is 900 mg. Manufacturer recommends dosage reduction of 20% to 30% in patients with hepatic failure.

How supplied
Tablets: 150 mg, 300 mg

Pharmacokinetics
Absorption: well absorbed from GI tract. Because of significant first-pass effect, bioavailability is limited; however, it increases with dosage.
Distribution: 97% protein-bound.
Metabolism: metabolized in liver.
Excretion: excreted mainly in feces; some in urine. *Half-life:* 2 to 32 hours.

Route	Onset	Peak	Duration
P.O.	Unknown	≤ 3.5 hr	Unknown

Pharmacodynamics
Chemical effect: reduces inward sodium current in Purkinje and myocardial cells. Decreases excitability, conduction velocity, and automaticity in AV nodal, His-Purkinje, and intraventricular tissue; causes slight but significant prolongation of refractory period in AV nodal tissue.
Therapeutic effect: restores normal sinus rhythm.

Adverse reactions

CNS: anxiety, ataxia, dizziness, drowsiness, fatigue, headache, insomnia, syncope, tremor, weakness.
CV: atrial fibrillation, ***bradycardia,*** bundle branch block, ***heart failure,*** chest pain, edema, first-degree AV block, hypotension, increased QRS duration, intraventricular conduction delay, palpitations, ***proarrhythmic events (ventricular tachycardia, PVCs).***
EENT: blurred vision.
GI: abdominal pain or cramps, constipation, diarrhea, dyspepsia, flatulence, nausea, vomiting, dry mouth, unusual taste, anorexia.
Musculoskeletal: joint pain.
Respiratory: dyspnea.
Skin: rash, diaphoresis.

Interactions

Drug-drug. *Antiarrhythmics:* increased risk of heart failure. Monitor patient closely.
Cardiac glycosides, oral anticoagulants: propafenone may increase serum levels of these drugs by about 35% to 85%, resulting in toxicity. Monitor patient closely.
Cimetidine: decreased metabolism of propafenone. Monitor patient closely.
Local anesthetics: increased risk of CNS toxicity. Monitor patient closely.
Metoprolol, propranolol: propafenone slows metabolism of these drugs. Monitor patient for toxicity.
Quinidine: slowed propafenone metabolism. Avoid concomitant use.
Rifampin: increased propafenone clearance. Monitor patient closely.

Contraindications and precautions

- Contraindicated in patients hypersensitive to drug and in those with severe or uncontrolled heart failure, cardiogenic shock, bradycardia, marked hypotension, bronchospastic disorders, electrolyte imbalance, or SA, AV, or intraventricular disorders of impulse conduction in absence of pacemaker.
- Drug isn't recommended for breast-feeding women.
- Use cautiously in patients with heart failure because propafenone can have negative inotropic effect. Also use cautiously in patients taking other cardiac depressant drugs and in those with hepatic or renal failure.
- Safety of drug hasn't been established in children or pregnant women.

NURSING CONSIDERATIONS

Assessment

- Assess patient's condition before therapy and regularly thereafter.
- Continuous cardiac monitoring is recommended at start of therapy and during dosage adjustments.
- Be alert for adverse reactions and drug interactions.
- Evaluate patient's and family's knowledge of drug therapy.

Nursing diagnoses

- Decreased cardiac output related to presence of arrhythmia
- Ineffective protection related to drug-induced proarrhythmias
- Deficient knowledge related to drug therapy

Planning and implementation

- Administer drug with food to minimize adverse GI reactions.

ALERT If PR interval or QRS complex increases by more than 25%, notify prescriber because reduction in dosage may be necessary.

- During concomitant use with digoxin, monitor ECG and serum digoxin levels frequently.

Patient teaching

- Tell patient to take drug with food.
- Stress importance of taking drug exactly as ordered.
- Warn patient to avoid hazardous activities if adverse CNS disturbances occur.

Evaluation

- Patient regains adequate cardiac output when arrhythmia is corrected.
- Patient doesn't develop any proarrhythmic events.
- Patient and family state understanding of drug therapy.

propantheline bromide

(proh-PAN-thuh-leen BROH-mighd)
Pro-Banthine, Propanthel ♦

Pharmacologic class: anticholinergic
Therapeutic class: antimuscarinic, GI antispasmodic
Pregnancy risk category: C

Indications and dosages

▶ **Adjunct treatment of peptic ulcer, irritable bowel syndrome, and other GI disorders; reduction of duodenal motility during diagnostic radiologic procedures.** *Adults:* 15 mg P.O. t.i.d. before meals, and 30 mg h.s. *Elderly patients:* 7.5 mg P.O. t.i.d. before meals.

How supplied

Tablets: 7.5 mg, 15 mg

Pharmacokinetics

Absorption: about 10% to 25% absorbed (varies among patients).
Distribution: unknown.
Metabolism: appears to undergo considerable metabolism in upper small intestine and liver.
Excretion: absorbed drug is excreted in urine. *Half-life:* 1.6 hours.

Route	Onset	Peak	Duration
P.O.	Unknown	2 hr	6 hr

Pharmacodynamics

Chemical effect: blocks acetylcholine, which decreases GI motility and inhibits gastric acid secretion.
Therapeutic effect: relieves peptic ulcer pain.

Adverse reactions

CNS: headache, insomnia, drowsiness, dizziness, *confusion or excitement in elderly patients,* nervousness, weakness.
CV: palpitations, tachycardia.
EENT: *blurred vision,* mydriasis, increased intraocular pressure, cycloplegia, photophobia.
GI: *dry mouth,* dysphagia, constipation, heartburn, loss of taste, nausea, vomiting, paralytic ileus.
GU: urinary hesitancy, urine retention, impotence.
Skin: urticaria, decreased sweating or possible anhidrosis, other dermal manifestations.
Other: fever, ***allergic reactions***, ***anaphylaxis.***

Interactions

Drug-drug. *Amantadine, antihistamines, antiparkinsonians, disopyramide, glutethimide, meperidine, phenothiazines, procainamide, quinidine, tricyclic antidepressants:* additive adverse effects. Avoid concomitant use.
Antacids: decreased absorption of oral anticholinergics. Separate administration times by 2 to 3 hours.
Digoxin: increased serum digoxin levels. Monitor patient for cardiac toxicity.
Ketoconazole: anticholinergics may interfere with ketoconazole absorption. Avoid concomitant use.
Methotrimeprazine: anticholinergics may enhance risk of extrapyramidal reactions. Monitor patient closely.

Contraindications and precautions

- Contraindicated in patients hypersensitive to anticholinergics and in those with angle-closure glaucoma, obstructive uropathy, obstructive disease of GI tract, severe ulcerative colitis, myasthenia gravis, paralytic ileus, intestinal atony, toxic megacolon, or unstable CV status caused by acute hemorrhage.
- Use cautiously in patients with autonomic neuropathy, hyperthyroidism, coronary artery disease, arrhythmias, heart failure, hypertension, hiatal hernia linked to reflux esophagitis, hepatic or renal disease, or ulcerative colitis. Also use cautiously in pregnant or breast-feeding women and in patients in hot or humid environments (drug-induced heatstroke can develop).
- Safety of drug hasn't been established in children.

NURSING CONSIDERATIONS

Assessment

- Assess patient's condition before therapy and regularly thereafter.
- Monitor patient's vital signs and urine output carefully.

• Evaluate patient's and family's knowledge of drug therapy.

Nursing diagnoses

• Acute pain related to peptic ulcer
• Constipation related to drug's adverse effect on GI tract
• Deficient knowledge related to drug therapy

Planning and implementation

• Give drug 30 minutes to 1 hour before meals and at bedtime. Bedtime doses can be larger; give at least 2 hours after last meal of day.
• Overdose may cause curare-like effects, such as respiratory paralysis.

Patient teaching

• Tell patient when drug should be taken throughout day and at bedtime.
• Instruct patient to avoid driving and other hazardous activities if he's drowsy, dizzy, or has blurred vision
• Tell patient to drink plenty of fluids to help prevent constipation.
• Urge patient to report any rash or skin eruption.
• Advise him to use sugarless gum or hard candy to relieve dry mouth.

Evaluation

• Patient is free from pain.
• Patient states measures used to prevent constipation.
• Patient and family state understanding of drug therapy.

propoxyphene hydrochloride (dextropropoxyphene hydrochloride)

(proh-POK-sih-feen high-droh-KLOR-ighd)
Darvon, 642♦

propoxyphene napsylate (dextropropoxyphene napsylate)

Darvon-N

Pharmacologic class: opioid
Therapeutic class: analgesic
Controlled substance schedule: IV
Pregnancy risk category: C

Indications and dosages

▶ **Mild to moderate pain. Propoxyphene hydrochloride.** *Adults:* 65 mg P.O. q 4 hours p.r.n. Maximum, 390 mg/day.
Propoxyphene napsylate. *Adults:* 100 mg P.O. q 4 hours p.r.n. Maximum, 600 mg/day.

How supplied

propoxyphene hydrochloride
Capsules: 32 mg, 65 mg
propoxyphene napsylate
Tablets: 100 mg
Oral suspension: 10 mg/ml

Pharmacokinetics

Absorption: absorbed primarily in upper small intestine.
Distribution: drug enters CSF.
Metabolism: metabolized in liver; about one-quarter of dose is metabolized to norpropoxyphene, an active metabolite.
Excretion: excreted in urine. *Half-life:* 6 to 12 hours.

Route	Onset	Peak	Duration
P.O.	15-60 min	2-2.5 hr	4-6 hr

Pharmacodynamics

Chemical effect: binds with opioid receptors in CNS, altering both perception of and emotional response to pain through unknown mechanism.
Therapeutic effect: relieves pain.

Adverse reactions

CNS: *dizziness,* headache, *sedation,* euphoria, paradoxical excitement, insomnia.
GI: nausea, vomiting, constipation.
Respiratory: ***respiratory depression.***
Other: psychological and physical dependence.

Interactions

Drug-drug. *Barbiturate anesthetics:* may increase respiratory and CNS depression. Use together cautiously.
Carbamazepine: may increase carbamazepine levels. Monitor levels closely.

CNS depressants: additive effects. Use together cautiously.
Warfarin: increased anticoagulant effect. Monitor PT and INR.
Drug-lifestyle. *Alcohol use:* additive effects. Discourage concomitant use.

Contraindications and precautions

- Contraindicated in patients hypersensitive to drug.
- Use cautiously in pregnant or breast-feeding women and in patients with hepatic or renal disease, emotional instability, or history of drug or alcohol abuse.
- Safety of drug hasn't been established in children.

NURSING CONSIDERATIONS

Assessment
- Assess patient's pain before and after drug administration.
- Be alert for adverse reactions and drug interactions.
- Monitor patient's hydration status if adverse GI reactions occur.
- Evaluate patient's and family's knowledge of drug therapy.

Nursing diagnoses
- Acute pain related to underlying condition
- Risk for deficient fluid volume related to GI reactions
- Deficient knowledge related to drug therapy

Planning and implementation
- Administer with food to minimize adverse GI reactions.
- Drug can be considered a mild narcotic analgesic, but pain relief is equivalent to that provided by aspirin. Tolerance and physical dependence have been observed. Typically used with aspirin or acetaminophen to maximize analgesia.

ALERT A dose of 65 mg of propoxyphene hydrochloride equals 100 mg of propoxyphene napsylate.
- Drug may cause false decreases in urinary steroid excretion tests.

Patient teaching
- Advise patient to take drug with food or milk to minimize GI upset.
- Warn patient not to exceed recommended dosage. Respiratory depression, hypotension, profound sedation, and coma may result if used in excessive amounts or with other CNS depressants. Propoxyphene-containing products alone or in combination with other drugs are major cause of drug-related overdose and death.
- Advise patient to avoid alcohol during drug therapy.
- Caution ambulatory patient about getting out of bed or walking. Warn outpatient to avoid driving and other hazardous activities until drug's CNS effects are known.

Evaluation
- Patient is free from pain.
- Patient maintains adequate hydration.
- Patient and family state understanding of drug therapy.

propranolol hydrochloride
(proh-PRAH-nuh-lohl high-droh-KLOR-ighd)
Apo-Propranolol♦, Detensol♦, Inderal, Inderal LA, Novopranolol♦, PMS Propranolol♦

Pharmacologic class: beta blocker
Therapeutic class: antihypertensive, antianginal, antiarrhythmic, adjunct therapy for migraine, adjunct therapy for MI
Pregnancy risk category: C

Indications and dosages

▶**Angina pectoris.** *Adults:* total daily doses of 80 to 320 mg P.O. when given b.i.d, t.i.d., or q.i.d. Or one 80-mg extended-release capsule daily. Dosage increased at 7- to 10-day intervals.

▶**Mortality reduction after MI.** *Adults:* 180 to 240 mg P.O. daily in divided doses beginning 5 to 21 days after MI. Usually administered t.i.d. or q.i.d.

▶**Supraventricular, ventricular, and atrial arrhythmias; tachyarrhythmias caused by excessive catecholamine action during anes-**

thesia, hyperthyroidism, or pheochromocytoma. *Adults:* 0.5 to 3 mg by slow I.V. push, not to exceed 1 mg/minute. After 3 mg have been given, another dose may be given in 2 minutes; subsequent doses, no sooner than q 4 hours. May be diluted and infused slowly. Usual maintenance dosage is 10 to 30 mg P.O. t.i.d. or q.i.d.

▶ **Hypertension.** *Adults:* initially, 80 mg P.O. daily in two to four divided doses or extended-release form once daily. Increased at 3- to 7-day intervals to maximum daily dosage of 640 mg. Usual maintenance dosage is 160 to 480 mg daily.

▶ **Prevention of frequent, severe, uncontrollable, or disabling migraine or vascular headache.** *Adults:* initially, 80 mg P.O. daily in divided doses or one extended-release capsule daily. Usual maintenance dosage is 160 to 240 mg daily, t.i.d. or q.i.d.

▶ **Essential tremor.** *Adults:* 40 mg (tablets, solution) P.O. b.i.d. Usual maintenance dosage is 120 to 320 mg daily in three divided doses.

▶ **Hypertrophic subaortic stenosis.** *Adults:* 10 to 20 mg P.O. t.i.d. or q.i.d. before meals and h.s.

▶ **Adjunct therapy in pheochromocytoma.** *Adults:* 60 mg P.O. daily in divided doses with alpha-adrenergic blocker 3 days before surgery.

How supplied

Tablets: 10 mg, 20 mg, 40 mg, 60 mg, 80 mg, 90 mg
Capsules (extended-release): 60 mg, 80 mg, 120 mg, 160 mg
Oral solution: 4 mg/ml, 8 mg/ml, 80 mg/ml (concentrate)
Injection: 1 mg/ml

Pharmacokinetics

Absorption: absorbed almost completely from GI tract after P.O. administration. Absorption is enhanced when given with food.
Distribution: distributed widely throughout body. Drug is more than 90% protein-bound.
Metabolism: metabolized almost totally in liver. P.O. form undergoes extensive first-pass metabolism.
Excretion: about 96% to 99% excreted in urine as metabolites; remainder excreted in feces as unchanged drug and metabolites.
Half-life: about 4 hours.

Route	Onset	Peak	Duration
P.O.	30 min	60-90 min	About 12 hr
I.V.	≤ 1 min	≤ 1 min	< 5 min

Pharmacodynamics

Chemical effect: reduces cardiac oxygen demand by blocking catecholamine-induced increases in heart rate, blood pressure, and force of myocardial contraction. Depresses renin secretion and prevents vasodilation of cerebral arteries.
Therapeutic effect: relieves anginal and migraine pain, lowers blood pressure, restores normal sinus rhythm, and helps limit MI damage.

Adverse reactions

CNS: *fatigue, lethargy,* vivid dreams, hallucinations, mental depression.
CV: ***bradycardia,*** *hypotension,* ***heart failure,*** intermittent claudication.
GI: nausea, vomiting, diarrhea.
Hematologic: ***agranulocytosis.***
Musculoskeletal: arthralgia.
Respiratory: increased airway resistance.
Skin: rash.
Other: fever.

Interactions

Drug-drug. *Aminophylline:* antagonized beta-blocking effects of propranolol. Use together cautiously.
Cardiac glycosides, diltiazem, verapamil: hypotension, bradycardia, and increased depressant effect on myocardium. Use together cautiously.
Cimetidine: inhibits propranolol's metabolism. Monitor patient for increased beta-blocking effect.
Epinephrine: severe vasoconstriction. Monitor blood pressure and observe patient carefully.
Glucagon, isoproterenol: antagonized propranolol effect. May be used therapeutically and in emergencies.
Insulin, oral antidiabetics: can alter requirements for these drugs in previously stabilized

diabetic patients. Monitor patient for hypoglycemia.

Drug-lifestyle. *Cocaine use:* increases angina-inducing potential of cocaine. Inform patient of this potentially dangerous combination.

Contraindications and precautions

- Contraindicated in patients with bronchial asthma, sinus bradycardia, heart block greater than first-degree, cardiogenic shock, and heart failure (unless failure is secondary to tachyarrhythmia that can be treated with propranolol).
- Drug isn't recommended for breast-feeding women.
- Use cautiously in patients taking other antihypertensives; in those with renal impairment, nonallergic bronchospastic diseases, hepatic disease, diabetes mellitus (drug blocks some symptoms of hypoglycemia), or thyrotoxicosis (drug may mask some signs of that disorder); and in pregnant women.
- Safety of drug hasn't been established in children.

NURSING CONSIDERATIONS

Assessment

- Assess patient's condition before therapy and regularly thereafter.
- Monitor blood pressure, ECG, and heart rate and rhythm frequently, especially during I.V. administration.
- Be alert for adverse reactions and drug interactions.
- Evaluate patient's and family's knowledge of drug therapy.

Nursing diagnoses

- Ineffective health maintenance related to underlying condition
- Impaired gas exchange related to airway resistance
- Deficient knowledge related to drug therapy

Planning and implementation

- Check patient's apical pulse before giving drug. If you detect extremes in pulse rate, withhold drug and call prescriber immediately.

ALERT Don't confuse Inderal with Inderide or Isordil.

- Double-check dose and route. I.V. doses are much smaller than oral doses.

P.O. use: Give drug with meals. Food may increase absorption of propranolol.

I.V. use: Give drug by direct injection into large vessel or I.V. line containing free-flowing, compatible solution; continuous I.V. infusion generally isn't recommended.

– Or, dilute drug with normal saline solution and give by intermittent infusion over 10 to 15 minutes in 0.1- to 0.2-mg increments.

– Drug is compatible with D_5W, half-normal and normal saline solutions, and lactated Ringer's solution.

- Don't stop drug before surgery for pheochromocytoma. Before any surgical procedure, notify anesthesiologist that patient is receiving propranolol.
- Notify prescriber if patient develops severe hypotension; vasopressor may be prescribed.
- Elderly patient may have increased adverse reactions and may need dosage adjustment.
- Don't discontinue drug abruptly.
- For overdose, give I.V. isoproterenol, I.V. atropine, or glucagon; refractory cases may require pacemaker.

Patient teaching

- Teach patient how to check pulse rate, and tell him to do so before each dose. Tell him to notify prescriber if rate changes significantly.
- Tell patient that taking drug twice daily or as extended-release capsule may improve compliance. Advise him to check with prescriber.
- Advise patient to continue taking drug as prescribed, even when he's feeling well. Tell him not to stop drug suddenly because doing so can worsen angina and MI.

Evaluation

- Patient responds well to therapy.
- Patient maintains adequate gas exchange.
- Patient and family state understanding of drug therapy.

propylthiouracil (PTU)

(proh-pil-thigh-oh-YOOR-uh-sil)
Propyl-Thyracil ♦

Pharmacologic class: thyroid hormone antagonist
Therapeutic class: antihyperthyroid agent
Pregnancy risk category: D

Indications and dosages

▶ **Hyperthyroidism.** *Adults:* 100 to 150 mg P.O. t.i.d.; up to 1,200 mg daily have been used in severe cases. Maintenance dosage is 100 to 150 mg once daily in divided doses t.i.d.
Children over age 10: 150 to 300 mg P.O. daily in divided doses t.i.d. Maintenance dosage is determined by patient response.
Children ages 6 to 10: 50 to 150 mg P.O. daily in divided doses t.i.d. Maintenance dosage is determined by patient response.
▶ **Thyrotoxic crisis.** *Adults and children:* 200 to 400 mg P.O. q 4 to 6 hours on first day; after symptoms are under control, dosage is gradually reduced to usual maintenance levels.

How supplied

Tablets: 50 mg, 100 mg ♦

Pharmacokinetics

Absorption: about 80% of drug is absorbed rapidly and readily from GI tract.
Distribution: drug appears to be concentrated in thyroid gland. About 75% to 80% of drug is protein-bound.
Metabolism: metabolized rapidly in the liver.
Excretion: about 35% excreted in urine. *Half-life:* 1 to 2 hours.

Route	Onset	Peak	Duration
P.O.	Unknown	1-1.5 hr	Unknown

Pharmacodynamics

Chemical effect: inhibits oxidation of iodine in thyroid gland, blocking iodine's ability to combine with tyrosine to form T_4, and may prevent coupling of monoiodotyrosine and diiodotyrosine to form T_4 and T_3.
Therapeutic effect: lowers thyroid hormone level.

Adverse reactions

CNS: headache, drowsiness, vertigo.
CV: vasculitis.
EENT: visual disturbances.
GI: diarrhea, *nausea, vomiting* (may be dose-related), salivary gland enlargement, loss of taste.
Hematologic: ***agranulocytosis, thrombocytopenia, aplastic anemia, leukopenia.***
Hepatic: jaundice, ***hepatotoxicity.***
Metabolic: dose-related hypothyroidism (mental depression; cold intolerance; hard, nonpitting edema).
Musculoskeletal: arthralgia, myalgia.
Skin: rash, urticaria, skin discoloration, pruritus.
Other: drug-induced fever, lymphadenopathy.

Interactions

Drug-drug. *Aminophylline, oxtriphylline, theophylline:* decreased clearance. Dosage may need adjustment.
Anticoagulants: anticoagulants may be increased. Monitor PT, PTT, or INR.
Cardiac glycosides: increased serum glycoside levels. May need to decrease dose.
Potassium iodide: may decrease response to drug. May need to increase dose of antithyroid drug.

Contraindications and precautions

- Contraindicated in patients hypersensitive to drug and in breast-feeding women.
- Use cautiously in pregnant women.

NURSING CONSIDERATIONS

Assessment

- Assess patient's condition before therapy and regularly thereafter.
- Watch for signs of hypothyroidism (depression; cold intolerance; hard, nonpitting edema); adjust dosage as directed.
- Monitor CBC as directed to detect impending leukopenia, thrombocytopenia, and agranulocytosis.
- Be alert for adverse reactions.

• Monitor patient's hydration status if adverse GI reactions occur.
• Evaluate patient's and family's knowledge of drug therapy.

Nursing diagnoses
• Ineffective health maintenance related to thyroid condition
• Risk for deficient fluid volume related to adverse GI reactions
• Deficient knowledge related to drug therapy

Planning and implementation
• Give drug with meals to reduce adverse GI reactions.
• Pregnant woman may need less drug as pregnancy progresses. Monitor thyroid function studies closely. Thyroid may be added to regimen. Drug may be stopped during last few weeks of pregnancy.
• Discontinue drug and notify prescriber if patient develops severe rash or enlarged cervical lymph nodes.
• Store drug in light-resistant container.

Patient teaching
• Warn patient to report skin eruptions (sign of hypersensitivity), fever, sore throat, or mouth sores (early signs of agranulocytosis).
• Tell patient to ask prescriber about using iodized salt and eating shellfish.
• Warn patient against OTC cough medicines because many contain iodine.

Evaluation
• Patient's thyroid hormone level is normal.
• Patient maintains adequate hydration.
• Patient and family state understanding of drug therapy.

protamine sulfate
(PROH-tuh-meen SUL-fayt)

Pharmacologic class: antidote
Therapeutic class: heparin antagonist
Pregnancy risk category: C

Indications and dosages
▶ **Heparin overdose.** *Adults:* dosage based on venous blood coagulation studies, usually 1 mg for each 90 to 115 units of heparin. Give by slow I.V. injection over 1 to 3 minutes, not to exceed 50 mg in any 10-minute period.

How supplied
Injection: 10 mg/ml

Pharmacokinetics
Absorption: not applicable.
Distribution: unknown.
Metabolism: unknown, although it appears to be partially degraded, with release of some heparin.
Excretion: unknown.

Route	Onset	Peak	Duration
I.V.	30-60 sec	Unknown	2 hr

Pharmacodynamics
Chemical effect: forms inert complex with heparin sodium.
Therapeutic effect: blocks heparin's effects.

Adverse reactions
CV: drop in blood pressure, ***bradycardia***, ***circulatory collapse.***
Respiratory: dyspnea, ***pulmonary edema, acute pulmonary hypertension.***
Other: transitory flushing, feeling of warmth, ***anaphylaxis, anaphylactoid reactions.***

Interactions
None significant.

Contraindications and precautions
• Contraindicated in patients hypersensitive to drug.
• Use cautiously after cardiac surgery and in pregnant or breast-feeding women.
• Safety of drug hasn't been established in children.

NURSING CONSIDERATIONS

Assessment
• Assess patient's heparin overdose before therapy.

• Monitor patient continually. Check vital signs frequently.
• Watch for spontaneous bleeding (heparin rebound), especially in patients undergoing dialysis and in those who have undergone cardiac surgery. Protamine sulfate may act as anticoagulant in very high doses.
• Evaluate patient's and family's knowledge of drug therapy.

Nursing diagnoses
• Ineffective protection related to heparin overdose
• Risk for injury related to anaphylaxis
• Deficient knowledge related to drug therapy

Planning and implementation
• Calculate dosage carefully. One mg of protamine neutralizes 90 to 115 units of heparin depending on salt (heparin calcium or heparin sodium) and source of heparin (beef or pork).
• Give drug slowly by direct injection. Be prepared to treat shock.
ALERT Don't confuse protamine with Protopam.

Patient teaching
• Instruct patient to report adverse reactions immediately.

Evaluation
• Patient doesn't experience injury.
• Patient and family state understanding of drug therapy.

pseudoephedrine hydrochloride
(soo-doh-eh-FED-rin high-droh-KLOR-ighd)
Cenafed†, Children's Sudafed Liquid†, Deco-fed†, DeFed-60†, Dorcol Children's Decongestant†, Drixoral Non-Drowsy Formula†, Efidac/24†, Eltor 120♦†, Genaphed†, Halofed†, Halofed Adult Strength†, Maxenal♦†, Myfedrine†, Novafed†, PediaCare Infants' Oral Decongestant Drops†, Pseudo†, Pseudo-frin♦, Pseudogest†, Robidrine♦†, Sudafed†, Sudafed 12 Hour†, Sudafed-60†, Sufedrin†

pseudoephedrine sulfate
Afrin†, Drixoral♦

Pharmacologic class: adrenergic
Therapeutic class: decongestant
Pregnancy risk category: C

Indications and dosages
▶ **Nasal and eustachian tube decongestion.** *Adults and children age 12 and older:* 60 mg P.O. q 4 to 6 hours. Maximum, 240 mg daily. Or, 120 mg extended-release tablet P.O. q 12 hours or 240 mg extended-release (Efidac/24) once daily.
Children ages 6 to 11: 30 mg P.O. regular-release form q 4 to 6 hours. Maximum, 120 mg/day.
Children ages 2 to 5: 15 mg P.O. regular-release form q 4 to 6 hours. Maximum, 60 mg/day.

How supplied
pseudoephedrine hydrochloride
Tablets: 30 mg†, 60 mg†
Tablets (extended-release): 120 mg†, 240 mg†
Capsules: 60 mg†
Capsules (extended-release): 20 mg†
Oral solution: 15 mg/5 ml†, 30 mg/5 ml†, 7.5 mg/0.8 ml†
Syrup: 30 mg/5 ml
pseudoephedrine sulfate
Tablets (extended-release): 120 mg (60 mg immediate-release, 60 mg delayed-release)

Pharmacokinetics
Absorption: unknown.
Distribution: widely distributed throughout body.
Metabolism: incompletely metabolized in liver to inactive compounds.
Excretion: excreted in urine; rate is accelerated with acidic urine.

Route	Onset	Peak	Duration
P.O.	15-30 min	30-60 min	3-12 hr

Pharmacodynamics

Chemical effect: stimulates alpha-adrenergic receptors in respiratory tract, resulting in vasoconstriction.
Therapeutic effect: acts to relieve congestion of nasal and eustachian tube.

Adverse reactions

CNS: *anxiety,* transient stimulation, tremor, dizziness, headache, insomnia, *nervousness.*
CV: ***arrhythmias****, palpitations,* tachycardia.
GI: anorexia, nausea, vomiting, dry mouth.
GU: difficulty urinating.
Respiratory: respiratory difficulty.
Skin: pallor.

Interactions

Drug-drug. *Antihypertensives:* may attenuate hypotensive effect. Monitor patient closely.
MAO inhibitors: may cause severe hypertension (hypertensive crisis). Avoid concomitant use.

Contraindications and precautions

- Contraindicated in breast-feeding women, patients taking MAO inhibitors, and patients with severe hypertension or severe coronary artery disease. Extended-release forms are contraindicated in children under age 12.
- Use cautiously in patients with hypertension, cardiac disease, diabetes, glaucoma, hyperthyroidism, and prostatic hyperplasia.

NURSING CONSIDERATIONS

Assessment

- Assess patient's condition before therapy and regularly thereafter.
- Be alert for adverse reactions and drug interactions.
- Elderly patients are more sensitive to drug's effects.
- Evaluate patient's and family's knowledge of drug therapy.

Nursing diagnoses

- Ineffective health maintenance related to congestion
- Disturbed sleep pattern related to drug-induced insomnia
- Deficient knowledge related to drug therapy

Planning and implementation

- Don't crush or break extended-release forms.
- Give last dose at least 2 hours before bedtime to minimize insomnia.

Patient teaching

- Warn patient against using OTC products containing other sympathomimetics.
- Caution patient not to take drug within 2 hours of bedtime because it can cause insomnia.
- Tell patient to relieve dry mouth with sugarless gum or hard candy.
- Urge patient to stop drug if he becomes unusually restless and to notify prescriber promptly.

Evaluation

- Patient's congestion is relieved.
- Patient and family state understanding of drug therapy.

psyllium

(SIL-ee-um)

Alramucil†, Cillium†, Fiberall†, Hydrocil Instant†, Konsyl†, Metamucil†, Metamucil Instant Mix†, Metamucil Sugar Free†, Modane Bulk†, Naturacil†, Perdiem, Prodiem Plain♦†, Pro-Lax†, Reguloid†, Serutan†, Siblin†, Syllact†, V-Lax†

Pharmacologic class: adsorbent
Therapeutic class: bulk laxative
Pregnancy risk category: NR

Indications and dosages

▶ **Constipation, bowel management, irritable bowel syndrome.** *Adults:* 1 to 2 rounded teaspoonfuls P.O. in full glass of liquid once daily, b.i.d., or t.i.d., followed by second glass of liquid. Or, 1 packet dissolved in water once daily, b.i.d., or t.i.d. Or, 2 wafers b.i.d. or t.i.d. *Children over age 6:* 1 level teaspoonful P.O. in a half-glass of liquid h.s.

How supplied

Chewable pieces: 1.7 g/piece†

Effervescent powder: 3.4 g/packet†, 3.7 g/packet†
Granules: 2.5 g/tsp†, 4.03 g/tsp†
Powder: 3.3 g/tsp†, 3.4 g/tsp†, 3.5 g/tsp†, 4.94 g/tsp†
Wafers: 3.4 g/wafer†

Pharmacokinetics

Absorption: none.
Distribution: distributed locally in GI tract.
Metabolism: none.
Excretion: excreted in feces.

Route	Onset	Peak	Duration
P.O.	12-24 hr	≤ 3 days	Varies

Pharmacodynamics

Chemical effect: absorbs water and expands to increase bulk and moisture content of stool, thus encouraging peristalsis and bowel movement.
Therapeutic effect: relieves constipation.

Adverse reactions

GI: nausea, vomiting, and diarrhea with excessive use; esophageal, gastric, small intestinal, or colonic strictures with dry form; abdominal cramps in severe constipation.

Interactions

None significant.

Contraindications and precautions

- Contraindicated in patients hypersensitive to drug and those with intestinal obstruction or ulceration, disabling adhesions, difficulty swallowing, or symptoms of appendicitis, such as abdominal pain, nausea, and vomiting.
- Use cautiously in pregnant or breast-feeding women.

NURSING CONSIDERATIONS

Assessment

- Assess patient's condition before therapy and regularly thereafter.
- Before giving drug for constipation, determine if patient has adequate fluid intake, exercise, and diet.
- Be alert for adverse reactions.
- Evaluate patient's and family's knowledge of drug therapy.

Nursing diagnoses

- Constipation related to underlying condition
- Acute pain related to abdominal cramps
- Deficient knowledge related to drug therapy

Planning and implementation

- Mix drug with at least 8 oz (240 ml) of cold, pleasant-tasting liquid such as orange juice to mask grittiness. Stir only a few seconds. Have patient drink mixture immediately, before it congeals. Follow with another glass of liquid.
- For dosages in children under age 6, consult prescriber.
- Drug may reduce appetite if taken before meals.
- Drug isn't absorbed systemically and is nontoxic. It's especially useful in debilitated patients and those with postpartum constipation, irritable bowel syndrome, and diverticular disease. Also useful to treat chronic laxative abuse and with other laxatives to empty colon before barium enema examinations.

Patient teaching

- Teach patient how to properly mix drug. To enhance effect and prevent intestinal obstruction, tell him to take drug with plenty of water. Advise him that inhaling powder may cause allergic reactions.
- Tell patient that laxative effect usually occurs in 12 to 24 hours but may be delayed up to 3 days.
- Advise diabetic patient to check label and use brand of drug that doesn't contain sugar.
- Teach patient about dietary sources of bulk, including bran and other cereals, fresh fruit, and vegetables.

Evaluation

- Patient's constipation is relieved.
- Patient's abdominal cramping is minimal and tolerable.
- Patient and family state understanding of drug therapy.

pyrantel embonate

(peer-AN-tul EM-boh-nayt)
Anthel♦, Combantrin♦, Early Bird♦

pyrantel pamoate

Antiminth, Combantrin♦, Pin-Rid†, Pin-X, Reese's Pinworm Medicine

Pharmacologic class: pyrimidine derivative
Therapeutic class: anthelmintic
Pregnancy risk category: C

Indications and dosages

▶ **Roundworm and pinworm.** *Adults and children over age 2:* 11 mg/kg P.O. given as single dose. Maximum dosage is 1 g. For pinworm, dosage should be repeated in 2 weeks.

How supplied

pyrantel embonate
Tablets: 125 mg♦, 250 mg♦
Oral suspension: 50 mg/ml♦
Granules: 100 mg/g♦
Squares (chocolate-flavored): 100 mg♦
pyrantel pamoate
Tablets: 125 mg♦
Capsules: 180 mg†
Oral suspension: 50 mg/ml

Pharmacokinetics

Absorption: poorly absorbed.
Distribution: unknown.
Metabolism: small amount partially metabolized in liver.
Excretion: over 50% excreted in feces; about 7% excreted in urine.

Route	Onset	Peak	Duration
P.O.	Varies	1-3 hr	Varies

Pharmacodynamics

Chemical effect: blocks neuromuscular action, paralyzing worm and causing its expulsion by normal peristalsis.
Therapeutic effect: relieves roundworm and pinworm infestation. Spectrum of activity includes *Ancylostoma duodenale, Ascaris lumbricoides, Enterobius vermicularis, Necator americanus,* and *Trichostrongylus orientalis.*

Adverse reactions

CNS: headache, dizziness, drowsiness, insomnia, weakness.
GI: anorexia, nausea, vomiting, gastralgia, cramps, diarrhea, tenesmus.
Hepatic: transient elevation of AST levels.
Skin: rash.
Other: fever.

Interactions

Drug-drug. *Piperazine salts:* possible antagonism. Don't give together.

Contraindications and precautions

- Contraindicated in patients hypersensitive to drug.
- Use cautiously in pregnant women and patients with hepatic dysfunction or severe malnutrition or anemia.
- Safety of drug hasn't been established in breast-feeding women.

NURSING CONSIDERATIONS

Assessment

- Assess patient's condition before therapy and regularly thereafter.
- Be alert for adverse reactions and drug interactions.
- Monitor patient's hydration status if adverse GI reactions occur.
- Evaluate patient's and family's knowledge of drug therapy.

Nursing diagnoses

- Infection related to worm infestation
- Risk for deficient fluid volume related to adverse GI reactions
- Deficient knowledge related to drug therapy

Planning and implementation

- No dietary restrictions, laxatives, or enemas are needed.
- Drug should be administered to all family members, as prescribed, to prevent risk of spreading infection.
- Drug may be taken with food, milk, or fruit juices. Shake suspension well.

Patient teaching

- Tell patient to shake suspension well before taking it. Inform patient that drug may be taken with food or beverages.
- Teach patient about personal hygiene, especially good hand-washing technique. To avoid reinfection, teach him to wash perianal area daily, to change undergarments and bedclothes daily, and to wash hands and clean fingernails before meals and after bowel movements. Advise patient to refrain from preparing food for others during infestation.

Evaluation

- Patient is free from infestation.
- Patient maintains adequate hydration.
- Patient and family state understanding of drug therapy.

pyrazinamide

(peer-uh-ZIN-uh-mighd)

pms-Pyrazinamide ◆, Tebrazid ◆, Zinamide ◆

Pharmacologic class: synthetic pyrazine analogue of nicotinamide
Therapeutic class: antituberculotic
Pregnancy risk category: C

Indications and dosages

▶ **Adjunct treatment of tuberculosis when primary and secondary antituberculotics can't be used or have failed.** *Adults:* 15 to 30 mg/kg P.O. once daily, not to exceed 3 g/day. Or, twice-weekly dose of 50 to 70 mg/kg (based on lean body weight) to promote compliance. Dosage adjustment recommended in renal failure.

How supplied

Tablets: 500 mg

Pharmacokinetics

Absorption: absorbed well.
Distributed: distributed widely into body tissues and fluids, including lungs, liver, and CSF. Drug is 50% protein-bound.
Metabolism: hydrolyzed in liver and in stomach.
Excretion: excreted almost completely in urine. *Half-life:* 9 to 10 hours.

Route	Onset	Peak	Duration
P.O.	Unknown	1-2 hr	Unknown

Pharmacodynamics

Chemical effect: unknown.
Therapeutic effect: helps eradicate tuberculosis. Spectrum of activity is only *Mycobacterium tuberculosis*.

Adverse reactions

CNS: malaise.
GI: anorexia, nausea, vomiting, diarrhea.
GU: dysuria.
Hematologic: sideroblastic anemia, ***thrombocytopenia.***
Hepatic: ***hepatitis.***
Metabolic: *hyperuricemia.*
Musculoskeletal: arthralgia.
Other: fever.

Interactions

None significant.

Contraindications and precautions

- Contraindicated in patients hypersensitive to drug and patients with severe hepatic disease.
- Use cautiously in pregnant women and patients with diabetes mellitus, renal failure, or gout.
- Safety hasn't been established in children or in breast-feeding women.

NURSING CONSIDERATIONS

Assessment

- Assess patient's condition before therapy and regularly thereafter.
- Monitor hematopoietic studies and serum uric acid levels, as ordered.
- Monitor liver function studies; examine patient for jaundice and liver tenderness or enlargement before and frequently during therapy.
- Watch closely for signs of gout and liver impairment.
- Monitor patient's hydration status if adverse GI reactions occur.

• Evaluate patient's and family's knowledge of drug therapy.

Nursing diagnoses
• Infection related to tuberculosis
• Risk for deficient fluid volume related to adverse GI reactions
• Deficient knowledge related to drug therapy

Planning and implementation
• Drug should always be given with other antituberculotics to prevent development of resistant organisms.
• Reduced dosage is needed in patients with renal impairment because nearly all of drug is excreted in urine.
• Question doses that exceed 35 mg/kg; they may cause liver damage.
• Notify prescriber at once if you suspect liver dysfunction.
• When drug is used with surgical management of tuberculosis, it's started 1 to 2 weeks before surgery and continued for 4 to 6 weeks after.
• Patients with concomitant HIV infection may need longer course.

Patient teaching
• Stress importance of taking drug exactly as prescribed; warn patient against discontinuing drug without prescriber's approval.
• Teach patient to watch for and immediately report signs of gout and hepatic impairment.

Evaluation
• Patient is free from infection.
• Patient maintains adequate hydration.
• Patient and family state understanding of drug therapy.

pyridostigmine bromide
(peer-ih-doh-STIG-meen BROH-mighd)
Mestinon*, Mestinon-SR♦, Mestinon Timespans, Regonol

Pharmacologic class: cholinesterase inhibitor
Therapeutic class: muscle stimulant
Pregnancy risk category: NR

Indications and dosages
▶ **Antidote for nondepolarizing neuromuscular blocking agents.** *Adults:* 10 to 20 mg I.V. preceded by atropine sulfate 0.6 to 1.2 mg I.V.
▶ **Myasthenia gravis.** *Adults:* 60 to 120 mg P.O. t.i.d. Usual dosage is 600 mg daily but higher dosage may be needed (up to 1,500 mg daily). For I.M. or I.V. use, 1/30 of oral dosage is given. Dosage must be adjusted for each patient, depending on response and tolerance. Or, 180 to 540 mg timed-release tablets (1 to 3 tablets) P.O. b.i.d., with at least 6 hours between doses.
Children: 7 mg/kg or 200 mg/m^2 daily in five or six divided doses.
▶ **Supportive treatment of neonates born to myasthenic mothers.** *Neonates:* 0.05 to 0.15 mg/kg I.M. q 4 to 6 hours. Dosage decreased daily until drug can be withdrawn.

How supplied
Tablets: 60 mg
Tablets (extended-release): 180 mg
Syrup: 60 mg/5 ml
Injection: 5 mg/ml in 2-ml ampules or 5-ml vials

Pharmacokinetics
Absorption: poorly absorbed from GI tract.
Distribution: unknown.
Metabolism: unknown.
Excretion: excreted in urine.

Route	Onset	Peak	Duration
P.O.	20-60 min	1-2 hr	3-12 hr
I.V.	2-5 min	Unknown	2-3 hr
I.M.	15 min	Unknown	2-3 hr

Pharmacodynamics
Chemical effect: inhibits destruction of acetylcholine released from parasympathetic and somatic efferent nerves. Acetylcholine accumulates, promoting increased stimulation of receptor.
Therapeutic effect: reverses effect of nondepolarizing neuromuscular blockers and myasthenia gravis.

Adverse reactions

CNS: headache with large doses, weakness, sweating, ***seizures.***
CV: ***bradycardia,*** hypotension, thrombophlebitis.
EENT: miosis.
GI: abdominal cramps, nausea, vomiting, diarrhea, excessive salivation.
Musculoskeletal: muscle cramps, muscle fasciculations.
Respiratory: ***bronchospasm, bronchoconstriction,*** increased bronchial secretions.
Skin: rash.

Interactions

Drug-drug. *Aminoglycosides, anesthetics:* may decrease response to drug. Use together cautiously.
Anticholinergics, atropine, corticosteroids, magnesium, procainamide, quinidine: may antagonize cholinergic effects. Observe patient for lack of drug effect.
Ganglionic blockers: increased risk of hypotension. Monitor patient closely.

Contraindications and precautions

- Contraindicated in patients hypersensitive to anticholinesterase agents and in those with mechanical obstruction of intestine or urinary tract.
- Use cautiously in patients with bronchial asthma, bradycardia, or arrhythmias.
- Safety of drug hasn't been established in pregnant or breast-feeding women.

NURSING CONSIDERATIONS

Assessment

- Assess patient's condition before therapy and regularly thereafter.
- Monitor and document patient's response after each dose; optimum dosage is difficult to judge.
- Monitor patient's vital signs, especially respirations.
- Be alert for adverse reactions and drug interactions.
- Evaluate patient's and family's knowledge of drug therapy.

Nursing diagnoses

- Impaired physical mobility related to underlying condition
- Ineffective breathing pattern related to adverse respiratory reactions
- Deficient knowledge related to drug therapy

Planning and implementation

- Stop all other cholinergics before giving drug, as ordered.

P.O. use: Don't crush extended-release tablets.
– When using sweet syrup for patient who has difficulty swallowing, give over ice chips if he can't tolerate flavor.
I.V. use: Administer I.V. injection no faster than 1 mg/minute. If I.V. administration is too rapid, bradycardia and seizures may result.
I.M. use: Follow normal protocol.

- Position patient to ease breathing. Have atropine injection readily available, and provide respiratory support as needed.
- If patient's muscle weakness is severe, prescriber will determine if it's caused by drug-induced toxicity or worsening of myasthenia gravis. Test dose of edrophonium I.V. will aggravate drug-induced weakness but will temporarily relieve weakness caused by disease.
- The U.S. formulation of Regonol contains benzyl alcohol preservative that may cause toxicity in neonates if administered in large doses. The Canadian formulation of this drug doesn't contain benzyl ethanol.
- If appropriate, obtain prescriber's order for hospitalized patient to have bedside supply of tablets. Patients with long-standing disease often insist on self-administration.

ALERT Don't confuse Mestinon with Mesantoin or Metatensin.

Patient teaching

- When giving drug for myasthenia gravis, stress the importance of taking it exactly as ordered, on time, in evenly spaced doses. If prescriber has ordered extended-release tablets, tell patient to take tablets at same time each day, at least 6 hours apart. Tell him that he may have to take drug for life.
- Advise patient to wear or carry medical identification at all times.

Evaluation
- Patient has improved physical mobility.
- Patient maintains adequate respiratory pattern.
- Patient and family state understanding of drug therapy.

pyridoxine hydrochloride (vitamin B_6)

(peer-ih-DOKS-een high-droh-KLOR-ighd)
Beesix, Nestrex†, Rodex

Pharmacologic class: water-soluble vitamin
Therapeutic class: nutritional supplement
Pregnancy risk category: A

Indications and dosages

▶ **RDA.** *Men age 15 and over:* 2 mg.
Men ages 11 to 14: 1.7 mg.
Women age 19 and over: 1.6 mg.
Women ages 15 to 18: 1.5 mg.
Women ages 11 to 14: 1.4 mg.
Pregnant women: 2.2 mg.
Breast-feeding women: 2.1 mg.
Children ages 7 to 10: 1.4 mg.
Children ages 4 to 6: 1.1 mg.
Children ages 1 to 3: 1 mg.
Infants ages 6 months to 1 year: 0.6 mg.
Neonates and infants up to age 6 months: 0.3 mg.

▶ **Dietary vitamin B_6 deficiency.** *Adults:* 2.5 to 10 mg P.O., I.M., or I.V. daily for 3 weeks; then 2 to 5 mg daily as supplement to proper diet.

▶ **Seizures related to vitamin B_6 deficiency or dependency.** *Adults and children:* 10 to 100 mg I.M. or I.V. in single dose.

▶ **Vitamin B_6-responsive anemias or dependency syndrome (inborn errors of metabolism).** *Adults:* up to 600 mg/day I.M., P.O., or I.V. until symptoms subside; then 30 mg/day for life.

▶ **Prevention of vitamin B_6 deficiency during drug therapy.** *Adults:* 6 to 100 mg P.O. daily for isoniazid therapy.

▶ **Drug-induced vitamin B_6 deficiency.** *Adults:* 100 to 200 mg P.O. daily for 3 weeks, followed by 25 to 100 mg P.O. daily to prevent relapse.

▶ **Antidote for isoniazid poisoning.** *Adults:* 4 g I.V., followed by 1 g I.M. q 30 minutes until amount of pyridoxine administered equals amount of isoniazid ingested.

How supplied

Tablets: 10 mg†, 25 mg†, 50 mg†, 100 mg†, 200 mg†, 250 mg†, 500 mg†
Tablets (timed-release): 100 mg
Capsules: 500 mg
Capsules (timed-release): 100 mg
Injection: 100 mg/ml

Pharmacokinetics

Absorption: drug and its substituents are absorbed readily from GI tract. Absorption may be diminished in patients with malabsorption syndromes or following gastric resection.
Distribution: drug is stored mainly in liver.
Metabolism: metabolized in liver.
Excretion: in erythrocytes, pyridoxine is converted to pyridoxal phosphate and pyridoxamine is converted to pyridoxamine phosphate. The phosphorylated form of pyridoxine is transaminated to pyridoxal and pyridoxamine, which is phosphorylated rapidly. Conversion of pyridoxine phosphate to pyridoxal phosphate requires riboflavin. *Half-life:* 15 to 20 days.

Route	Onset	Peak	Duration
P.O, I.V., I.M.	Unknown	Unknown	Unknown

Pharmacodynamics

Chemical effect: acts as coenzyme that stimulates various metabolic functions, including amino acid metabolism.
Therapeutic effect: raises pyridoxine levels, prevents and relieves seizure activity related to pyridoxine deficiency or dependency, and blocks effects of isoniazid poisoning.

Adverse reactions

CNS: drowsiness, paresthesia, unstable gait.

Interactions

Drug-drug. *Levodopa:* decreased levodopa effect. Avoid concomitant use.
Phenobarbital, phenytoin: decreased anticonvulsant serum levels, increasing risk of seizures. Monitor serum levels closely.
Drug-lifestyle. *Alcohol use:* risk of possible delirium and lactic acidosis. Discourage concomitant use.

Contraindications and precautions

- Contraindicated in patients hypersensitive to pyridoxine.

NURSING CONSIDERATIONS

Assessment

- Assess patient before therapy and regularly thereafter.
- Be alert for adverse CNS reactions and drug interactions. Patient taking high doses (2 to 6 g/day) may have difficulty walking because of reduced proprioceptive and sensory function.
- Monitor patient's diet and snack habits. Excessive protein intake increases daily drug requirements.
- Evaluate patient's and family's knowledge of drug therapy.

Nursing diagnoses

- Ineffective health maintenance related to underlying condition
- Risk for injury related to drug-induced adverse CNS reactions
- Deficient knowledge related to drug therapy

Planning and implementation

P.O. and I.M. use: Follow normal protocol.
I.V. use: Inject undiluted drug into I.V. line containing free-flowing compatible solution. Or, infuse diluted drug over prescribed duration for intermittent infusions. Don't use for continuous infusion.

- Protect drug from light. Don't use solution if it contains precipitate, although slight darkening is acceptable.
- When using drug to treat isoniazid toxicity, expect to administer anticonvulsants.
- If sodium bicarbonate is required to control acidosis in isoniazid toxicity, don't mix in same syringe with pyridoxine.

ALERT Don't confuse pyridoxine with pralidoxime or pyridium.

Patient teaching

- Advise patient taking levodopa alone to avoid multivitamins containing pyridoxine because of decreased levodopa effect.
- Stress importance of compliance and good nutrition if prescribed for maintenance therapy to prevent recurrence of deficiency. Explain that pyridoxine in combination therapy with isoniazid has specific therapeutic purpose and isn't just a vitamin.

Evaluation

- Patient responds well to therapy.
- Patient doesn't experience injury from adverse CNS reactions.
- Patient and family state understanding of drug therapy.

pyrimethamine

(peer-ih-METH-uh-meen)
Daraprim

pyrimethamine with sulfadoxine

Fansidar

Pharmacologic class: aminopyrimidine derivative (folic acid antagonist)
Therapeutic class: antimalarial
Pregnancy risk category: C

Indications and dosages

▶ **Malaria prophylaxis and transmission control. Pyrimethamine.** *Adults and children over age 10:* 25 mg P.O. weekly.
Children ages 4 to 10: 12.5 mg P.O. weekly.
Children under age 4: 6.25 mg P.O. weekly.
Continued in all age groups at least 10 weeks after leaving endemic area.

▶ **Acute attacks of malaria. Fansidar.** *Adults:* 2 to 3 tablets as single dose, either alone or in sequence with quinine.
Children ages 9 to 14: 2 tablets.
Children ages 4 to 8: 1 tablet.

Children under age 4: ½ tablet.

▶ **Malaria prophylaxis. Fansidar.** *Adults:* 1 tablet weekly, or 2 tablets q 2 weeks.
Children ages 9 to 14: ¾ tablet weekly, or 1½ tablets q 2 weeks.
Children ages 4 to 8: ½ tablet weekly, or 1 tablet q 2 weeks.
Children under age 4: ¼ tablet weekly, or ½ tablet q 2 weeks.

▶ **Acute attacks of malaria. Pyrimethamine.** *Adults and children over age 10:* 25 mg P.O. daily for 2 days when used with faster-acting antimalarials; when used alone, 50 mg P.O. daily for 2 days.
Children ages 4 to 10: 25 mg P.O. daily for 2 days.

▶ **Toxoplasmosis. Pyrimethamine.** *Adults:* initially, 50 to 75 mg P.O. daily for 1 to 3 weeks; then 25 mg P.O. daily for 4 to 5 weeks along with 1 g sulfadiazine P.O. q 6 hours.
Children: initially, 1 mg/kg P.O. (not to exceed 100 mg) in two equally divided doses for 2 to 4 days; then 0.5 mg/kg daily for 4 weeks along with 100 mg sulfadiazine/kg P.O. daily, divided q 6 hours.

How supplied

pyrimethamine
Tablets: 25 mg
pyrimethamine with sulfadoxine
Tablets: pyrimethamine 25 mg, sulfadoxine 500 mg

Pharmacokinetics

Absorption: well absorbed from intestinal tract.
Distribution: distributed to kidneys, liver, spleen, and lungs. About 80% bound to plasma proteins.
Metabolism: metabolized to several unidentified compounds.
Excretion: excreted in urine. *Half-life:* 2 to 6 hours.

Route	Onset	Peak	Duration
P.O.	Unknown	1.5-8 hr	Unknown

Pharmacodynamics

Chemical effect: inhibits enzyme dihydrofolate reductase, thereby impeding reduction of dihydrofolic acid to tetrahydrofolic acid. Sulfadoxine competitively inhibits use of PABA.
Therapeutic effect: prevents malaria and treats malaria and toxoplasmosis infections. Spectrum of activity includes asexual erythrocytic forms of susceptible plasmodia and *Toxoplasma gondii.*

Adverse reactions

CNS: stimulation, ***seizures.***
GI: anorexia, vomiting, diarrhea, atrophic glossitis.
Hematologic: ***agranulocytosis, aplastic anemia,*** megaloblastic anemia, ***bone marrow suppression, leukopenia, thrombocytopenia, pancytopenia.***
Skin: rash, erythema multiforme, ***Stevens-Johnson syndrome, toxic epidermal necrolysis.***

Interactions

Drug-drug. *Co-trimoxazole, methotrexate, sulfonamides:* increased risk of bone marrow suppression. Don't use together.
Folic acid, PABA: decreased antitoxoplasmic effects. May require dosage adjustment.

Contraindications and precautions

- Contraindicated in patients hypersensitive to drug and in those with megaloblastic anemia caused by folic acid deficiency. Fansidar is contraindicated in patients with porphyria because it contains sulfadoxine, a sulfonamide.
- Repeated use of Fansidar is contraindicated in infants under age 2 months, pregnant women at term, breast-feeding women, patients hypersensitive to pyrimethamine or sulfonamides, and patients with severe renal insufficiency, marked liver parenchymal damage or blood dyscrasias, or megaloblastic anemia caused by folate deficiency.
- Use cautiously in patients with impaired hepatic or renal function, severe allergy or bronchial asthma, or G6PD deficiency; in those with seizure disorders (smaller doses may be needed); and in those treated with chloroquine.

NURSING CONSIDERATIONS

Assessment
- Assess patient's condition before therapy and regularly thereafter.
- Obtain twice-weekly blood counts, including platelets, as ordered, for patients with toxoplasmosis because dosages used approach toxic levels.
- Be alert for adverse reactions and drug interactions.
- Evaluate patient's and family's knowledge of drug therapy.

Nursing diagnoses
- Infection related to presence of susceptible organism
- Ineffective protection related to adverse hematologic reactions
- Deficient knowledge related to drug therapy

Planning and implementation
- Give drug with meals to minimize GI distress.
- If signs of folic acid or folinic acid deficiency develop, dosage should be reduced or discontinued while patient receives parenteral folinic acid (leucovorin) until blood counts become normal.
- When used to treat toxoplasmosis in patients with AIDS, therapy may be lifelong. Long-term suppressive therapy for patient's lifetime may also be necessary.

ALERT Because of possibly severe skin reactions, Fansidar should be used only in regions where chloroquine-resistant malaria is prevalent and only when traveler plans to stay in region longer than 3 weeks.

Patient teaching
- Advise patient to take drug with food.
- Teach patient to watch for and immediately report signs of folic or folinic acid deficiency and acute toxicity.
- Warn patient taking Fansidar to stop drug and notify prescriber at first sign of rash.
- Instruct patient to take first prophylactic dose of Fansidar 1 to 2 days before traveling to endemic area.

Evaluation
- Patient is free from infection.
- Patient maintains normal hematologic parameters.
- Patient and family state understanding of drug therapy.

Q

quetiapine fumarate
(KWET-ee-uh-peen FYOO-muh-rayt)
Seroquel

Pharmacologic class: dibenzothiazepine derivative
Therapeutic class: antipsychotic
Pregnancy risk category: C

Indications and dosages
▶**Management of the symptoms of psychotic disorders.** *Adults:* initially, 25 mg b.i.d.; increased in increments of 25 to 50 mg b.i.d. or t.i.d. on days 2 and 3, as tolerated. Target dosage range is 300 to 400 mg daily, divided into two or three daily doses by day 4. Further dosage adjustments, if indicated, usually occur at intervals of not less than 2 days. Dosages can be increased or decreased by 25 to 50 mg b.i.d. Antipsychotic efficacy typically occurs at 150 to 750 mg/day. Safety of doses above 800 mg/day hasn't been evaluated. Dosage adjustment may be required in patients with hepatic impairment.

How supplied
Tablets: 25 mg, 100 mg, 200 mg

Pharmacokinetics
Absorption: rapid following P.O. administration; 100% bioavailable.
Distribution: widely distributed throughout body; 83% bound to plasma protein.
Metabolism: extensively metabolized by liver to inactive metabolites.

Excretion: about 73% excreted in urine, 20% in feces. *Half-life:* 6 hours.

Route	Onset	Peak	Duration
P.O.	Unknown	1.5 hr	Unknown

Pharmacodynamics

Chemical effect: unknown, but drug is thought to exert antipsychotic activity by blocking dopamine D-2 receptors and serotonin 5-HT_2 receptors in the brain. It also may act at histamine H_1 receptors and adrenergic $alpha_1$ receptors.
Therapeutic effect: reduces symptoms of psychotic disorders.

Adverse reactions

CNS: asthenia, *dizziness, headache, somnolence,* hypertonia, dysarthria.
CV: orthostatic hypotension, tachycardia, palpitations, peripheral edema.
EENT: pharyngitis, rhinitis, ear pain.
GI: dry mouth, dyspepsia, abdominal pain, constipation, anorexia.
GU: urine retention.
Hematologic: ***leukopenia.***
Metabolic: *weight gain.*
Musculoskeletal: back pain.
Respiratory: increased cough, dyspnea.
Skin: rash, sweating.
Other: fever, flu syndrome.

Interactions

Drug-drug. *Antihypertensives:* increased effects. Monitor blood pressure.
Carbamazepine, glucocorticoids, phenobarbital, phenytoin, rifampin: increased quetiapine clearance. Adjust dosage as directed.
CNS depressants: increased CNS effects. Use together cautiously.
Erythromycin, fluconazole, itraconazole, ketoconazole: decreased quetiapine clearance. Use cautiously.
Lorazepam: reduced lorazepam clearance. Monitor patient.
Drug-lifestyle. *Alcohol use:* increased CNS effects. Discourage concurrent use.

Contraindications and precautions

- Contraindicated in patients hypersensitive to drug or its ingredients.
- Use cautiously in patients with CV or cerebrovascular disease or conditions that predispose them to hypotension; in those with history of seizures or conditions that lower seizure threshold; and in those who could experience conditions in which core body temperature may be elevated. Use cautiously in elderly patients; they may be more sensitive to adverse effects.

NURSING CONSIDERATIONS

Assessment

- Monitor patient for tardive dyskinesia. Condition may not appear until months or years after starting drug and may disappear spontaneously or persist for life, despite discontinuation of drug.
- Monitor patient's vital signs carefully, especially during the 3- to 5-day period of initial dosage adjustment and when restarting treatment or increasing dosage.
- Assess patient's risk of physical injury from adverse CNS effects.
- Be alert for adverse reactions and drug interactions.
- Evaluate patient's and family's knowledge of drug therapy.

Nursing diagnoses

- Risk for imbalanced body temperature related to drug-induced hyperpyrexia
- Impaired physical mobility related to drug-induced adverse CNS effects
- Deficient knowledge related to drug therapy

Planning and implementation

- Elderly or debilitated patients or patients with hepatic impairment or predisposition to hypotensive reactions usually require lower initial doses and more gradual dosage adjustment.

ALERT Withhold drug and notify prescriber if symptoms of neuroleptic malignant syndrome (hyperpyrexia, muscle rigidity, altered mental status, and autonomic instability) occur.

- Provide ice chips, drinks, or sugarless hard candy to help relieve dry mouth.

Patient teaching

- Caution patient about risk of orthostatic hypotension. Risk is greatest during 3- to 5-day period of initial dosage adjustment and when restarting treatment or increasing dosage.
- Tell patient to avoid becoming overheated or dehydrated during therapy.
- Warn patient to avoid activities that require mental alertness until CNS effects of drug are known.
- Remind patient to have eye examination before starting drug therapy and every 6 months during therapy to check for cataract formation.
- Tell patient to notify prescriber of other medications (prescription or OTC) he is taking or plans to take.
- Tell woman to notify prescriber if she becomes pregnant or intends to become pregnant during drug therapy. Advise her not to breast-feed during therapy.
- Advise patient to avoid alcohol during therapy.

☑ Evaluation

- Patient maintains normal body temperature.
- Patient maintains physical mobility and doesn't experience extrapyramidal effects of drug.
- Patient and family state understanding of drug therapy.

quinapril hydrochloride

(KWIN-eh-pril high-droh-KLOR-ighd)

Accupril, Asig ◇

Pharmacologic class: ACE inhibitor
Therapeutic class: antihypertensive
Pregnancy risk category: C (D in second and third trimesters)

Indications and dosages

▶ **Hypertension.** *Adults:* initially, 10 mg P.O. daily. Dosage adjusted based on patient response at intervals of about 2 weeks. Most patients are controlled at 20, 40, or 80 mg daily as single dose or in two divided doses.

▶ **Heart failure.** *Adults:* initially, 5 mg P.O. b.i.d. if patient is taking a diuretic and 10 mg P.O. b.i.d. if patient isn't taking a diuretic. Dosage increased at weekly intervals. Usual effective dosage is 20 to 40 mg b.i.d. in equally divided doses.

▶ **First dose in patients with renal impairment.** *Adults:* 10 mg P.O. if creatinine clearance is over 60 ml/minute, 5 mg if it's 30 to 60 ml/minute, and 2.5 mg if it's 10 to 30 ml/minute; no dose recommendations available for level below 10 ml/minute.

How supplied

Tablets: 5 mg, 10 mg, 20 mg, 40 mg

Pharmacokinetics

Absorption: at least 60% absorbed; rate and extent drop by 25% to 30% when taken with high-fat meals.
Distribution: about 97% of drug and active metabolite are bound to plasma proteins.
Metabolism: 38% of dose de-esterified in liver to active metabolite.
Excretion: excreted primarily in urine. *Half-life:* about 25 hours.

Route	Onset	Peak	Duration
P.O.	≤ 1 hr	1-2 hr	About 24 hr

Pharmacodynamics

Chemical effect: unknown; may inhibit transition of angiotensin I to angiotensin II, which lowers peripheral arterial resistance and decreases aldosterone secretion.
Therapeutic effect: lowers blood pressure.

Adverse reactions

CNS: somnolence, vertigo, light-headedness, syncope, malaise, nervousness, depression.
CV: palpitations, vasodilation, tachycardia, ***hypertensive crisis***, angina, orthostatic hypotension, *rhythm disturbances.*
EENT: dry throat.
GI: dry mouth, abdominal pain, constipation, hemorrhage.
Hepatic: elevated liver enzyme levels.
Metabolic: ***hyperkalemia***.
Musculoskeletal: back pain.
Respiratory: dry, persistent, tickling, nonproductive cough.

Skin: pruritus, ***exfoliative dermatitis,*** *photosensitivity,* diaphoresis.
Other: ***angioedema.***

Interactions

Drug-drug. *Diuretics, other antihypertensives:* risk of excessive hypotension. Expect to stop diuretic or lower dosage.
Lithium: increased serum lithium levels and lithium toxicity. Avoid concomitant use.
Potassium-sparing diuretics: risk of hyperkalemia. Monitor patient and serum potassium levels during concomitant use.
Drug-herb. *Licorice:* may cause sodium retention and increase blood pressure, interfering with the therapeutic effects of ACE inhibitors. Discourage concomitant use.
Drug-food. *High-fat foods:* may impair absorption. Discourage concurrent consumption.
Sodium substitutes containing potassium: risk of hyperkalemia. Monitor patient during concomitant use.

Contraindications and precautions

- Contraindicated in patients hypersensitive to ACE inhibitors, in those with a history of angioedema during previous ACE inhibitor treatment, and in those with renal artery stenosis.
- Drug isn't recommended for pregnant women in their second or third trimester.
- Use cautiously in breast-feeding women and in patients with impaired kidney function.
- Safety of drug hasn't been established in children.

NURSING CONSIDERATIONS

Assessment

- Assess patient's blood pressure before therapy and regularly thereafter. Take blood pressure when drug levels are at their peak (2 to 6 hours after dose) and at their trough (just before dose) to verify adequate blood pressure control.
- Assess kidney and liver function before and throughout therapy.
- Monitor serum potassium levels. Risk factors for development of hyperkalemia include renal insufficiency, diabetes, and concomitant use of drugs that raise potassium level.
- Other ACE inhibitors have been linked to agranulocytosis and neutropenia. Monitor CBC with differential before therapy, every 2 weeks for first 3 months of therapy, and periodically thereafter.
- Be alert for adverse reactions and drug interactions.
- Evaluate patient's and family's knowledge of drug therapy.

Nursing diagnoses

- Risk for injury related to presence of hypertension
- Disturbed sleep pattern related to drug-induced cough
- Deficient knowledge related to drug therapy

Planning and implementation

- Dosage adjustment is necessary if patient has renal impairment.
- Give drug on empty stomach; high-fat meals can impair absorption.

Patient teaching

- Advise patient to report signs of infection, such as fever and sore throat.
- Tell patient to report signs of angioedema, such as breathing difficulty and swelling of face, eyes, lips, or tongue, especially after first dose.
- Warn patient that light-headedness can occur, especially at first. Tell him to rise slowly and to stop drug and notify prescriber if he experiences syncope.
- Inadequate fluid intake, vomiting, diarrhea, and excessive perspiration can lead to light-headedness and syncope. Tell patient to use caution in hot weather and during exercise.
- Warn patient to avoid potassium supplements and sodium substitutes that contain potassium during therapy.
- Tell women to notify prescriber about suspected or confirmed pregnancy. Drug will need to be stopped.

Evaluation

- Patient's blood pressure is normal.
- Patient's sleep patterns are undisturbed throughout therapy.
- Patient and family state understanding of drug therapy.

quinidine bisulfate
(KWIN-eh-deen bigh-SUL-fayt)
(66.4% quinidine base)
Biquin Durules◆, Kinidin Durules◇

quinidine gluconate
(62% quinidine base)
Quinaglute Dura-Tabs, Quinalan, Quinate◆

quinidine polygalacturonate
(60.5% quinidine base)
Cardioquin

quinidine sulfate
(83% quinidine base)
Apo-Quinidine◆, Cin-Quin, Novoquinidin◆, Quinidex Extentabs, Quinora

Pharmacologic class: cinchona alkaloid
Therapeutic class: antiarrhythmic
Pregnancy risk category: C

Indications and dosages

▶ **Atrial flutter or fibrillation.** *Adults:* 200 mg of quinidine sulfate or equivalent base P.O. q 2 to 3 hours for five to eight doses, with subsequent daily increases until sinus rhythm is restored or toxic effects develop. Quinidine is given only after digitalization to avoid increasing AV conduction. Maximum dosage is 3 to 4 g daily.

▶ **Paroxysmal supraventricular tachycardia.** *Adults:* 400 to 600 mg of quinidine sulfate P.O. q 2 to 3 hours until toxic adverse reactions develop or arrhythmia subsides.

▶ **Premature atrial and ventricular contractions; paroxysmal AV junctional rhythm; paroxysmal atrial tachycardia; paroxysmal ventricular tachycardia; maintenance after cardioversion of atrial fibrillation or flutter.** *Adults:* quinidine sulfate or equivalent base 200 to 400 mg P.O. q 4 to 6 hours. Or, quinidine gluconate 400 mg I.M. q 2 hours, adjusting each dose by the effect of the previous. Or, quinidine gluconate infused I.V. at up to 0.25 mg/kg/minute (1 ml/kg/hour).

Children: test dose is 2 mg/kg; then 30 mg/kg/day P.O. or 900 mg/m²/day P.O. in five divided doses.

▶ **Severe *Plasmodium falciparum* malaria.** *Adults:* 10 mg/kg quinidine gluconate I.V. diluted in 250 ml of normal saline solution and infused over 1 to 2 hours; then continuous maintenance infusion of 0.02 mg/kg/minute for 72 hours or until parasitemia is reduced to less than 1%. Patients with heart failure or impaired liver function need reduced dosage.

How supplied

quinidine bisulfate
Tablets (extended-release): 250 mg◆ ◇
quinidine gluconate
Tablets (extended-release): 324 mg, 325 mg◆, 330 mg
Injection: 80 mg/ml
quinidine polygalacturonate
Tablets: 275 mg
quinidine sulfate
Tablets: 200 mg, 300 mg
Tablets (extended-release): 300 mg
Capsules: 200 mg, 300 mg
Injection: 200 mg/ml

Pharmacokinetics

Absorption: although all quinidine salts are well absorbed from GI tract after P.O. administration, serum drug levels vary greatly among individuals.
Distribution: well distributed in all tissues except brain; about 80% bound to plasma proteins.
Metabolism: about 60% to 80% metabolized in liver to two metabolites that may have some pharmacologic activity.
Excretion: 10% to 30% excreted in urine. Urine acidification increases excretion; alkalinization decreases it. *Half-life:* 5 to 12 hours.

Route	Onset	Peak	Duration
P.O.	1-3 hr	1-2 hr	6-8 hr
I.V.	Immediate	Immediate	Unknown
I.M.	Unknown	Unknown	Unknown

Pharmacodynamics

Chemical effect: class Ia antiarrhythmic that has direct and indirect (anticholinergic) effects

on cardiac tissue. Automaticity, conduction velocity, and membrane responsiveness are decreased. The effective refractory period is prolonged. Anticholinergic action reduces vagal tone.
Therapeutic effect: restores normal sinus rhythm and relieves signs and symptoms of malaria infection.

Adverse reactions

CNS: *vertigo, headache, light-headedness,* confusion, restlessness, cold sweats, pallor, fainting, dementia.
CV: ***PVCs, ventricular tachycardia, atypical ventricular tachycardia (torsades de pointes), severe hypotension, SA and AV block, ventricular fibrillation,*** tachycardia, ***aggravated heart failure,*** ECG changes (widening of QRS complex, notched P waves, widened QT interval, ST-segment depression).
EENT: *tinnitus,* blurred vision.
GI: *diarrhea, nausea, vomiting,* excessive salivation, anorexia, petechial hemorrhage of buccal mucosa, abdominal pain.
Hematologic: ***hemolytic anemia, thrombocytopenia, agranulocytosis.***
Hepatic: ***hepatotoxicity.***
Respiratory: ***acute asthma attack, respiratory arrest.***
Skin: rash, pruritus.
Other: ***angioedema,*** fever, cinchonism.

Interactions

Drug-drug. *Acetazolamide, antacids, sodium bicarbonate, thiazide diuretics:* may increase quinidine blood levels because of alkaline urine. Monitor patient for increased effect.
Amiodarone, cimetidine: increased serum quinidine levels. Monitor patient for increased effect.
Barbiturates, phenytoin, rifampin: may lower blood levels of quinidine. Monitor patient for decreased quinidine effect.
Digoxin: increased serum digoxin levels after quinidine therapy starts. Monitor patient closely.
Nifedipine: may decrease quinidine blood levels. Monitor patient carefully.
Other antiarrhythmics (such as lidocaine, phenytoin, procainamide, propranolol): increased risk of toxicity. Use together cautiously.
Verapamil: may result in hypotension, bradycardia, or AV block. Monitor blood pressure and heart rate.
Warfarin: increased anticoagulant effect. Monitor patient closely.
Drug-herb. *Jimson weed:* may adversely effect CV function. Discourage concomitant use.
Licorice: may prolong the QT interval. Discourage concomitant use.

Contraindications and precautions

- Contraindicated in patients hypersensitive to quinidine or related cinchona derivatives, in patients with idiosyncratic reactions to them, and in patients with intraventricular conduction defects, digitalis toxicity with grossly impaired AV conduction, or abnormal rhythms caused by escape mechanisms.
- Drug isn't recommended for breast-feeding women.
- Use cautiously in patients with asthma, muscle weakness, or infection with fever (hypersensitivity reactions to drug may be masked); patients with hepatic or renal impairment; and pregnant women.

NURSING CONSIDERATIONS

Assessment

- Assess patient's arrhythmia before therapy and regularly thereafter.
- Monitor serum quinidine levels. Therapeutic plasma levels for antiarrhythmic effects are 2 to 5 mcg/ml.
- Check apical pulse rate and blood pressure before starting therapy.
- Monitor liver function test results during first 4 to 8 weeks of therapy.
- Be alert for adverse reactions and drug interactions.
- Evaluate patient's and family's knowledge of drug therapy.

Nursing diagnoses

- Decreased cardiac output related to presence of arrhythmia

- Risk for deficient fluid volume related to drug-induced adverse GI reactions
- Deficient knowledge related to drug therapy

Planning and implementation

- Anticoagulant therapy is commonly advised before quinidine therapy in long-standing atrial fibrillation because restoration of normal sinus rhythm may dislodge thrombi from atrial wall, causing thromboembolism.

P.O. use: Don't crush extended-release tablets.

I.V. use: I.V. route should only be used for treating acute arrhythmias.

– Mix 10 ml of quinidine gluconate with 40 ml of D_5W and infuse at an initial rate of up to 0.25 mg/minute (1 ml/kg/hr).

– Never use discolored (brownish) quinidine solution.

I.M. use: Follow normal protocol.

ALERT Don't confuse quinidine with clonidine.

Patient teaching

- Tell patient to take drug with meals.
- Tell patient to report signs of toxicity.
- Stress importance of follow-up care.

Evaluation

- Patient regains normal cardiac output with resolution of arrhythmia.
- Patient maintains adequate hydration throughout therapy.
- Patient and family state understanding of drug therapy.

quinupristin/dalfopristin

(QUIN-uh-pris-tin DALF-oh-pris-tin)
Synercid

Pharmacologic class: streptogramin
Therapeutic class: antibiotic
Pregnancy risk category: B

Indications and dosages

▶ **Serious or life-threatening infections linked to vancomycin-resistant *Enterococcus faecium* (VREF) bacteremia.** *Adults and children age 16 and older:* 7.5 mg/kg I.V. infusion over 1 hour q 8 hours. Length of treatment determined by site and severity of infection.

▶ **Complicated skin and skin-structure infections caused by *Staphylococcus aureus* (methicillin susceptible) or *Streptococcus pyogenes*.** *Adults and children age 16 and older:* 7.5 mg/kg by I.V. infusion over 1 hour q 12 hours for at least 7 days.

How supplied

Injection: 500 mg/10 ml (150 mg quinupristin and 350 mg dalfopristin)

Pharmacokinetics

Absorption: not applicable.
Distribution: protein-binding is moderate.
Metabolism: quinupristin and dalfopristin are converted to several active major metabolites by nonenzymatic reactions.
Excretion: About 75% of both drugs and their metabolites in feces. About 15% of quinupristin and 19% of dalfopristin in urine. *Half-life:* about 0.85 hours for quinupristin and 0.7 hours for dalfopristin.

Route	Onset	Peak	Duration
I.V.	Unknown	Unknown	Unknown

Pharmacodynamics

Chemical effect: the two antibiotics work together to inhibit or destroy susceptible bacteria through combined inhibition of protein synthesis in bacterial cells. Dalfopristin inhibits the early phase of protein synthesis in the bacterial ribosome, and quinupristin inhibits the late phase of protein synthesis. Without the ability to manufacture new proteins, bacterial cells become inactive or die.

Therapeutic effect: inactivation or death of bacterial cells.

Adverse reactions

CNS: headache.
CV: thrombophlebitis.
GI: nausea, diarrhea, vomiting.
Hepatic: *elevated total and conjugated bilirubin level,* altered liver function studies.

Musculoskeletal: arthralgia, myalgia.
Skin: *inflammation, pain, and edema at infusion site;* rash; pruritus.
Other: *infusion site reaction,* pain.

Interactions

Drug-drug: *Cyclosporine:* metabolism of cyclosporine is reduced and levels may be increased. Monitor cyclosporine levels.
Drugs metabolized by cytochrome P-450 3A4 (carbamazepine, delavirdine, diazepam, diltiazem, disopyramide, docetaxel, indinavir, lidocaine, lovastatin, methylprednisolone, midazolam, nevirapine, nifedipine, paclitaxel, ritonavir, tacrolimus, verapamil, vinblastine, and others): increased plasma levels could increase therapeutic effects and adverse reactions of these drugs. Use together cautiously.
Drugs metabolized by cytochrome P-450 3A4 that may prolong the QTc interval (such as quinidine): decreased metabolism of these drugs, resulting in prolongation of QTc interval. Avoid concomitant use.

Contraindications and precautions

- Contraindicated in patients hypersensitive to drug or other streptogramin antibiotics.

NURSING CONSIDERATIONS

Assessment

- Obtain history of patient's underlying condition before therapy, and reassess regularly thereafter.
- Overgrowth of nonsusceptible organisms may occur; monitor patient closely for signs and symptoms of superinfection.
- Monitor liver function during therapy, as ordered.
- Evaluate patient's and family's knowledge of drug therapy.

Nursing diagnoses

- Risk for infection related to presence of bacteria
- Diarrhea related to drug-induced adverse effect
- Deficient knowledge related to drug therapy

Planning and implementation

- Reconstitute powder for injection by adding 5 ml of sterile water for injection or D_5W. Gently swirl vial to ensure dissolution; avoid shaking to limit foaming. Reconstituted solutions must be further diluted within 30 minutes.
- The dose of reconstituted solution should be added to 250 ml of D_5W; maximum concentration 2 mg/ml. This diluted solution is stable for 5 hours at room temperature or 54 hours refrigerated.

ALERT Quinupristin/dalfopristin is incompatible with saline and heparin solutions. Don't dilute drug with saline-containing solutions or infuse into lines that contain saline or heparin. Flush line with D_5W before and after each dose.

- Fluid-restricted patient with a central venous catheter may receive dose in 100 ml of D_5W. This concentration isn't recommended for peripheral venous administration.
- Administer all doses by I.V. infusion over 1 hour. Use an infusion pump or device to control rate of infusion.
- If moderate to severe peripheral venous irritation occurs, consider increasing infusion volume to 500 or 750 ml, changing injection site, or infusing by central venous catheter.

ALERT Quinupristin/dalfopristin isn't active against *Enterococcus faecalis*. Appropriate blood cultures are needed to avoid misidentifying *E. faecalis* as *E. faecium*.

- Adverse reactions, such as arthralgia and myalgia, may be reduced by decreasing dosage interval to every 12 hours.
- Notify prescriber if patient develops diarrhea during or following therapy because mild to life-threatening pseudomembranous colitis has been reported with use of quinupristin/dalfopristin.

Patient teaching

- Advise patient to immediately report irritation at I.V. site, pain in joints or muscles, and diarrhea.
- Tell patient about importance of reporting persistent or worsening signs and symptoms of infection, such as pain and erythema.

Evaluation
- Patient is free from infection.
- Patient doesn't experience diarrhea.
- Patient and family state understanding of drug therapy.

R

rabeprazole sodium
(rah-BEH-pruh-zohl SOH-dee-um)
Aciphex

Pharmacologic class: proton pump inhibitor
Therapeutic class: antiulcerative
Pregnancy risk category: B

Indications and dosages
▶ **Healing of erosive or ulcerative gastroesophageal reflux disease (GERD).** *Adults:* 20 mg P.O. daily for 4 to 8 weeks. Additional 8-week course may be considered, if necessary.
▶ **Maintenance of healing of erosive or ulcerative GERD.** *Adults:* 20 mg P.O. daily.
▶ **Healing of duodenal ulcers.** *Adults:* 20 mg P.O. daily after morning meal for up to 4 weeks.
▶ **Treatment of pathological hypersecretory conditions including Zollinger-Ellison syndrome.** *Adults:* 60 mg P.O. daily; increase p.r.n. to 100 mg P.O. daily or 60 mg P.O. twice daily.

How supplied
Tablets (delayed-release): 20 mg

Pharmacokinetics
Absorption: acid labile; enteric coating allows drug to pass through the stomach relatively intact. Plasma levels peak over a period of 2 to 5 hours.
Distribution: 96.3% plasma protein-bound.
Metabolism: extensively metabolized by the liver to inactive compounds.
Excretion: 90% eliminated in urine as metabolites. Remaining 10% of metabolites eliminated in feces. *Half-life:* 1 to 2 hours.

Route	Onset	Peak	Duration
P.O.	Within 1 hr	2-5 hr	> 24 hr

Pharmacodynamics
Chemical effect: blocks activity of the acid (proton) pump by inhibiting gastric hydrogen-potassium adenosine triphosphatase at the secretory surface of gastric parietal cells, thereby blocking gastric acid secretion.
Therapeutic effect: promotes healing of erosive or ulcerative conditions.

Adverse reactions
CNS: headache.

Interactions
Drug-drug. *Cyclosporine:* may inhibit cyclosporine metabolism. Use together cautiously.
Digoxin, ketoconazole, other gastric pH-dependent drugs: decreased or increased drug absorption at increased pH values. Monitor patient closely during concurrent therapy.
Drug-herb. *St. John's wort:* may increase risk of sunburn. Discourage concomitant use.

Contraindications and precautions
- Contraindicated in patients hypersensitive to rabeprazole, other benzimidazoles (lansoprazole, omeprazole), or components in these formulations. Use cautiously in patients with severe hepatic impairment.

NURSING CONSIDERATIONS

Assessment
- Obtain history of patient's underlying condition before therapy, and reassess regularly thereafter.
- Be alert for adverse reactions and drug interactions.
- Evaluate patient's and family's knowledge of drug therapy.

Nursing diagnoses
- Acute pain related to underlying condition

• Risk for injury related to drug-induced adverse reactions
• Deficient knowledge related to drug therapy

Planning and implementation
• Don't crush, split, or allow patient to chew tablets.
• Prescriber may consider additional courses of therapy when duodenal ulcer or GERD isn't healed after first course of therapy.
ALERT Symptomatic response to therapy doesn't rule out presence of gastric malignancy.

Patient teaching
• Explain importance of taking drug exactly as prescribed.
• Advise patient that delayed-release tablets should be swallowed whole and not crushed, chewed, or split.
• Advise patient that drug may be taken without regard to meals.

Evaluation
• Patient experiences decreased pain with drug therapy.
• Patient sustains no injury as a result of drug-induced adverse reactions.
• Patient and family state understanding of drug therapy.

rabies immune globulin, human
(RAY-bees ih-MYOON GLOH-byoo-lin, HYOO-mun)
Hyperab, Imogam

Pharmacologic class: immune serum
Therapeutic class: rabies prophylaxis agent
Pregnancy risk category: C

Indications and dosages
▶ **Rabies exposure.** *Adults and children:* 20 IU/kg I.M. at time of first dose of rabies vaccine. Use half of dose to infiltrate wound area. Give remainder I.M.

How supplied
Injection: 150 IU/ml in 2-ml, 10-ml vials

Pharmacokinetics
Absorption: absorption is slow after I.M. administration.
Distribution: unknown.
Metabolism: unknown.
Excretion: unknown. *Half-life:* about 24 days.

Route	Onset	Peak	Duration
I.M.	Unknown	24 hr	Unknown

Pharmacodynamics
Chemical effect: provides passive immunity to rabies.
Therapeutic effect: prevents rabies.

Adverse reactions
GU: ***nephrotic syndrome.***
Skin: *rash,* pain, redness, induration at injection site.
Other: slight fever, ***anaphylaxis, angioedema.***

Interactions
Drug-drug. *Corticosteroids, immunosuppressive drugs:* interfere with the active antibody response, predisposing patient to rabies. Avoid these drugs during postexposure immunization period.
Live-virus vaccines (measles, mumps, polio, rubella): interferes with response to vaccine. Delay immunization if possible.

Contraindications and precautions
• No known contraindications.
• Use cautiously in patients hypersensitive to thimerosal, in pregnant women, in patients with a history of systemic allergic reactions after administration of human immunoglobulin preparations, and in patients with immunoglobulin A deficiency.
• Safety of drug hasn't been established in breast-feeding women.

NURSING CONSIDERATIONS

Assessment
• Obtain history of animal bites, allergies, and immunization reactions.
• Ask patient when he last received a tetanus immunization; prescriber may order booster.

• Be alert for adverse reactions and drug interactions.
• Evaluate patient's and family's knowledge of drug therapy.

Nursing diagnoses
• Risk for injury related to rabies exposure
• Ineffective protection related to drug-induced hypersensitivity reaction
• Deficient knowledge related to drug therapy

Planning and implementation
• Use only with rabies vaccine and immediate local treatment of wound. Don't give in same syringe or at same site as rabies vaccine. Give drug regardless of interval between exposure and start of therapy.
• Don't administer live-virus vaccines within 3 months of rabies immune globulin.
ALERT Drug provides passive immunity. Don't confuse with rabies vaccine, which is suspension of attenuated or killed microorganisms used to confer active immunity. The two drugs usually are given together for prophylaxis after exposure to known or suspected rabid animals.
• Have epinephrine 1:1,000 available to treat anaphylaxis.
• Don't give more than 5 ml at one I.M. injection site; divide I.M. doses larger than 5 ml, and give at different sites. Use a large muscle, such as the gluteus.

Patient teaching
• Explain that patient may develop a slight fever and pain and redness at injection site.
• Advise patient that tetanus booster may be necessary.
• Instruct patient to report signs of hypersensitivity immediately.

Evaluation
• Patient has passive immunity to rabies.
• Patient shows no signs of hypersensitivity after receiving drug.
• Patient and family state understanding of drug therapy.

radioactive iodine (sodium iodide) ^{131}I

(ray-dee-oh-AK-tiv IGH-oh-dighn)
Iodotope, Sodium Iodide ^{131}I Therapeutic

Pharmacologic class: thyroid hormone antagonist
Therapeutic class: antihyperthyroid agent
Pregnancy risk category: X

Indications and dosages
▶ **Hyperthyroidism.** *Adults:* usual dosage is 4 to 10 millicuries (mCi) P.O. Dosage based on estimated weight of thyroid gland and thyroid uptake. Treatment repeated after 6 weeks, according to serum T_4 level.
▶ **Thyroid cancer.** *Adults:* 50 to 150 mCi P.O. Dosage based on estimated malignant thyroid tissue and metastatic tissue as determined by total body scan. Treatment repeated according to clinical status.

How supplied
All radioactivity concentrations are determined at time of calibration.
Iodotope
Capsules: radioactivity range is 1 to 50 mCi/capsule
Oral solution: radioactivity concentration is 7.05 mCi/ml; in vials containing about 7, 14, 28, 70, or 106 mCi
Sodium Iodide ^{131}I Therapeutic
Capsules: radioactivity range is 0.8 to 100 mCi/capsule
Oral solution: radioactivity range is 3.5 to 150 mCi/vial

Pharmacokinetics
Absorption: readily absorbed from GI tract.
Distribution: distributed in extracellular fluid. Selectively concentrated and bound to tyrosyl residues of thyroglobulin in thyroid gland. Also concentrated in stomach, choroid plexus, and salivary glands.
Metabolism: converted readily to protein-bound iodine by thyroid.

Excretion: excreted by kidneys. *Half-life:* 138 days; effective radioactive half-life is 7.6 days.

Route	Onset	Peak	Duration
P.O.	2-4 wk	2-4 mo	Unknown

Pharmacodynamics

Chemical effect: limits thyroid hormone secretion by destroying thyroid tissue. The affinity of radioactive iodine for thyroid tissue facilitates uptake of drug by cancerous thyroid tissue that has metastasized to other sites in body.
Therapeutic effect: decreases thyroid function.

Adverse reactions

CV: chest pain, tachycardia.
EENT: *fullness in neck,* pain with swallowing, sore throat.
Hematologic: anemia, blood dyscrasia, ***leukopenia, thrombocytopenia.***
Metabolic: hypothyroidism.
Respiratory: cough.
Skin: temporary thinning of hair.
Other: radiation-induced thyroiditis, radiation sickness (nausea, vomiting), allergic-type reactions, possible increased risk of leukemia later in life or birth defects in offspring after ^{131}I dosage sufficient for thyroid ablation after cancer surgery.

Interactions

Drug-drug. *Lithium carbonate:* hypothyroidism may occur. Use cautiously.
The following drugs can interfere with action of ^{131}I and should be withheld for specified time before administering ^{131}I dose:
Adrenocorticoids: 1 week.
Benzodiazepines: 1 month.
Cholecystographic drugs: 6 to 9 months.
Iodine-containing contrast media: 1 to 2 months.
Iodine-containing products, including antitussives, expectorants, topical agents, and vitamins: 2 weeks.
Salicylates: 1 to 2 weeks.

Contraindications and precautions

- Contraindicated in pregnant women, except to treat thyroid cancer, and in breast-feeding women.
- Drug isn't recommended for use in patients under age 30, unless other treatments are precluded.

NURSING CONSIDERATIONS

Assessment

- Assess patient's thyroid condition before therapy and regularly thereafter.
- Monitor thyroid function via serum T_4 levels, as ordered.
- Be alert for adverse reactions and drug interactions.
- Evaluate patient's and family's knowledge of drug therapy.

Nursing diagnoses

- Ineffective health maintenance related to presence of thyroid dysfunction
- Risk for injury related to drug's possible long-term effects
- Deficient knowledge related to drug therapy

Planning and implementation

- All antithyroid drugs and thyroid preparations should be stopped 1 week before ^{131}I dose. If not, patient may receive thyroid-stimulating hormone for 3 days before ^{131}I dose. When treating woman of childbearing age, give dose during or within 7 days after menstruation.
- Institute full radiation precautions. Have patient use appropriate disposal methods when coughing and expectorating. After dose for hyperthyroidism, urine and saliva are slightly radioactive for 24 hours; vomitus is highly radioactive for 6 to 8 hours.
- After dose for thyroid cancer, urine, saliva, and perspiration are radioactive for 3 days. Isolate patient. Don't allow pregnant personnel to care for patient. Instruct patient to use disposable eating utensils and linens and to save all urine in lead containers for 24 to 48 hours so amount of radioactive material excreted can be determined. Tell patient to drink as much fluid as possible for 48 hours after dose to fa-

cilitate excretion. Limit patient contact to 30 minutes per shift per person on first day and increase time, as needed, to 1 hour on second day and longer on third day.

Patient teaching

- Tell patient to fast overnight before dose; food may delay absorption.
- Inform patient that after therapy for hyperthyroidism, he shouldn't resume antithyroid drugs but should continue propranolol or other drugs used to treat symptoms of hyperthyroidism until onset of full ^{131}I effect (usually 6 weeks).
- Review safety precautions to take after radioactive iodine dose. If patient is discharged less than 7 days after ^{131}I dose for thyroid cancer, warn him to avoid close, prolonged contact with young children and to avoid sleeping in the same room with another person for 7 days after treatment. Tell patient he can use same bathroom as the rest of the family.
- Review symptoms of hypothyroidism and hyperthyroidism. Have patient contact his prescriber if these occur.

☑ Evaluation

- Patient's thyroid function returns to normal.
- Patient doesn't develop complications as result of therapy.
- Patient and family state understanding of drug therapy.

raloxifene hydrochloride

(rah-LOKS-ih-feen high-droh-KLOR-ighd)
Evista

Pharmacologic class: selective estrogen receptor modulator of the benzothiophene class
Therapeutic class: antiosteoporotic
Pregnancy risk category: X

Indications and dosages

▶ **Prevention and treatment of osteoporosis in postmenopausal women.** *Adults:* 60 mg P.O. daily.

How supplied

Tablets: 60 mg

Pharmacokinetics

Absorption: rapid, with about 60% of dose absorbed after P.O. administration.
Distribution: widely distributed and highly bound to plasma proteins.
Metabolism: extensive first-pass metabolism to glucuronide conjugates.
Excretion: primarily excreted in feces, with less than 0.2% excreted unchanged in urine.
Half-life: 27½ hours.

Route	Onset	Peak	Duration
P.O.	Unknown	Unknown	24 hr

Pharmacodynamics

Chemical effect: reduces resorption of bone and decreases overall bone turnover. These effects on bone are revealed as reduced serum and urine levels of bone turnover markers and increased bone mineral density.
Therapeutic effect: prevents bone breakdown in postmenopausal women.

Adverse reactions

CNS: depression, insomnia, migraine.
CV: *hot flushes,* chest pain, peripheral edema.
EENT: *sinusitis,* pharyngitis, laryngitis.
GI: nausea, dyspepsia, vomiting, flatulence, GI disorder, gastroenteritis, abdominal pain.
GU: vaginitis, urinary tract infection, cystitis, leukorrhea, endometrial disorder, vaginal bleeding.
Metabolic: weight gain.
Musculoskeletal: *arthralgia,* myalgia, arthritis, leg cramps.
Respiratory: increased cough, pneumonia.
Skin: rash, sweating.
Other: *infection, flu syndrome,* breast pain, fever.

Interactions

Drug-drug. *Cholestyramine:* significantly reduced raloxifene absorption. Don't give these drugs concurrently.
Highly protein-bound drugs (such as clofibrate, diazepam, diazoxide, ibuprofen, indomethacin, naproxen): may interfere with binding sites. Use together cautiously.

Warfarin: may cause a decrease in PT. Monitor PT and INR closely.

Contraindications and precautions

- Contraindicated in children, breast-feeding women, and women who are pregnant or planning to become pregnant.
- Also contraindicated in women hypersensitive to drug or its constituents and in women with current or past venous thromboembolic events, including deep vein thrombosis (DVT), pulmonary embolism, and retinal vein thrombosis.
- Use cautiously in patients with severe hepatic impairment.

NURSING CONSIDERATIONS

Assessment

- Obtain history of patient's condition, and reassess during therapy.
- Monitor patient for signs of blood clots. The greatest risk of thromboembolic events occurs during first 4 months of treatment.
- Monitor patient for breast abnormalities that occur during treatment.
- Monitor serum lipid levels, blood pressure, body weight, and liver function, as ordered.
- Evaluate patient's and family's knowledge of drug therapy.

Nursing diagnoses

- Ineffective peripheral tissue perfusion related to potential DVT formation
- Imbalanced nutrition: less than body requirements related to drug-induced adverse GI reactions
- Deficient knowledge related to drug therapy

Planning and implementation

ALERT Discontinue drug at least 72 hours before prolonged immobilization, and resume only after patient is fully mobile.

- Withhold drug and notify prescriber if you suspect thromboembolic event.
- Unexplained uterine bleeding should be reported to prescriber.
- Safety and efficacy haven't been evaluated in men.
- Effect on bone mineral density with more than 2 years of drug treatment isn't known.
- Concomitant use of drug with hormone replacement therapy or systemic estrogen isn't recommended.

Patient teaching

- Advise patient to avoid long periods of restricted movement (such as during traveling) because it increases the risk of venous thromboembolic events.
- Inform patient that hot flashes or flushing may occur and that drug doesn't aid in reducing them.
- Instruct patient to take other bone-loss prevention measures, including taking supplemental calcium and vitamin D if dietary intake is inadequate, performing weight-bearing exercises, and stopping alcohol consumption and smoking.
- Tell patient that drug may be taken without regard to food.
- Advise patient to report any unexplained uterine bleeding or breast abnormalities that occur during treatment.
- Explain adverse effects of drug. Instruct patient to read package insert before starting therapy and to read it again each time prescription is renewed.

Evaluation

- Patient doesn't develop pain, redness, or swelling in legs.
- Patient maintains normal dietary intake.
- Patient and family state understanding of drug therapy.

ramipril

(reh-MIH-pril)

Altace, Ramace ◇, Tritace ◇

Pharmacologic class: ACE inhibitor
Therapeutic class: antihypertensive
Pregnancy risk category: C (D in second and third trimesters)

Indications and dosages

▶ **Hypertension.** *Adults:* initially, 2.5 mg P.O. once daily for patients not taking a diuretic and 1.25 mg P.O. once daily for patients taking a diuretic. Dosage increased as needed based on patient response. Maintenance dosage is 2.5 to 20 mg daily as single dose or divided doses.

Patients with renal insufficiency: if creatinine clearance is less than 40 ml/minute, 1.25 mg P.O. daily. Dosage adjusted gradually based on response. Maximum, 5 mg daily.

▶ **Heart failure after MI.** *Adults:* 2.5 mg P.O. b.i.d. Adjust to target dose of 5 mg P.O. b.i.d.

How supplied

Capsules: 1.25 mg, 2.5 mg, 5 mg, 10 mg

Pharmacokinetics

Absorption: 50% to 60% absorbed from GI tract.

Distribution: 73% serum protein-bound; ramiprilat (metabolite), 58%.

Metabolism: almost completely converted to ramiprilat, which is six times more potent than parent drug.

Excretion: 60% in urine; 40% in feces. *Half-life:* ramipril, 5 hours; ramiprilat, 13 to 17 hours.

Route	Onset	Peak	Duration
P.O.	1-2 hr	< 1 hr	About 24 hr (ramipril); 3 hr (ramiprilat)

Pharmacodynamics

Chemical effect: unknown; may inhibit change from angiotensin I to angiotensin II, a potent vasoconstrictor. This decreases peripheral arterial resistance, thus decreasing aldosterone secretion.

Therapeutic effect: lowers blood pressure.

Adverse reactions

CNS: headache, dizziness, fatigue, asthenia, malaise, light-headedness, anxiety, amnesia, ***seizures,*** depression, insomnia, nervousness, neuralgia, neuropathy, paresthesia, somnolence, tremors, vertigo.

CV: orthostatic hypotension, syncope, angina, ***arrhythmias,*** chest pain, palpitations, ***MI,*** edema.

EENT: epistaxis, tinnitus.

GI: nausea, vomiting, abdominal pain, anorexia, constipation, diarrhea, dyspepsia, dry mouth, gastroenteritis.

GU: impotence.

Metabolic: ***hyperkalemia***, weight gain.

Musculoskeletal: arthralgia, arthritis, myalgia.

Respiratory: *dry, persistent, tickling, nonproductive cough;* dyspnea.

Skin: rash, dermatitis, pruritus, photosensitivity, increased diaphoresis.

Other: hypersensitivity reactions, ***angioedema***.

Interactions

Drug-drug. *Diuretics:* excessive hypotension, especially at start of therapy. Discontinue diuretic at least 3 days before starting ramipril, increase sodium intake, or reduce starting dose of ramipril.

Insulin, oral antidiabetics: risk of hypoglycemia, especially at start of ramipril therapy. Monitor patient closely.

Lithium: increased serum lithium levels. Use together cautiously, and monitor serum lithium levels.

Potassium-sparing diuretics, potassium supplements: increased risk of hyperkalemia because ramipril attenuates potassium loss. Monitor plasma potassium levels closely.

Drug-herb. *Licorice:* may cause sodium retention and increase blood pressure, interfering with therapeutic effects of ACE inhibitors. Discourage concomitant use.

Drug-food. *Salt substitutes containing potassium:* increased risk of hyperkalemia because ramipril attenuates potassium loss. Monitor plasma potassium levels closely.

Contraindications and precautions

- Contraindicated in patients hypersensitive to ACE inhibitors, those with history of angioedema during previous treatment with ACE inhibitor, and those with renal stenosis.
- Drug isn't recommended for pregnant or breast-feeding women.
- Use cautiously in patients with renal impairment.
- Safety of drug in children hasn't been established.

NURSING CONSIDERATIONS

Assessment

- Assess patient's blood pressure before therapy and regularly thereafter.
- Closely assess kidney function during first few weeks of therapy. Regular assessment (serum creatinine and BUN levels) is advisable. Patients with severe heart failure whose kidney function depends on angiotensin-aldosterone system have experienced acute renal failure during ACE inhibitor therapy. Hypertensive patient with renal artery stenosis also may show signs of worsening kidney function at start of therapy.
- Monitor CBC with differential before therapy, every 2 weeks for first 3 months of therapy, and periodically thereafter.
- Monitor serum potassium levels. Risk factors for development of hyperkalemia include renal insufficiency, diabetes, and concomitant use of drugs that raise potassium levels.
- Be alert for adverse reactions and drug interactions.
- Evaluate patient's and family's knowledge of drug therapy.

Nursing diagnoses

- Risk for injury related to presence of hypertension
- Disturbed sleep pattern related to drug-induced cough
- Deficient knowledge related to drug therapy

Planning and implementation

- Diuretic therapy should be stopped 2 to 3 days before start of ramipril therapy, if possible.

Patient teaching

- Warn patient to avoid sodium substitutes during therapy.
- If patient has trouble swallowing, tell him to open capsules and sprinkle contents on food.
- Tell patient to rise slowly to avoid initial light-headedness. If syncope occurs, he should stop drug and call prescriber.
- Tell patient not to stop therapy abruptly.
- Advise patient to report signs of angioedema and laryngeal edema, which may occur after first dose.
- Tell patient to report signs of infection.
- Tell woman to report pregnancy. Drug will need to be stopped.

Evaluation

- Patient's blood pressure is normal.
- Patient's sleep patterns are undisturbed throughout therapy.
- Patient and family state understanding of drug therapy.

ranitidine hydrochloride

(ruh-NIH-tuh-deen high-droh-KLOR-ighd)
Zantac*, Zantac-C ♦, Zantac EFFERdose, Zantac 75†

Pharmacologic class: H_2-receptor antagonist
Therapeutic class: antiulcer agent
Pregnancy risk category: B

Indications and dosages

▶ **Duodenal and gastric ulcer (short-term treatment); pathologic hypersecretory conditions, such as Zollinger-Ellison syndrome.** *Adults:* 150 mg P.O. b.i.d. or 300 mg daily h.s. Or, 50 mg I.V. or I.M. q 6 to 8 hours. Patients with Zollinger-Ellison syndrome may need up to 6 g P.O. daily.

▶ **Maintenance therapy for duodenal ulcer.** *Adults:* 150 mg P.O. h.s.

▶ **Gastroesophageal reflux disease.** *Adults:* 150 mg P.O. b.i.d.

▶ **Erosive esophagitis.** *Adults:* 150 mg P.O. q.i.d.

▶ **Relief of occasional heartburn, acid indigestion, and sour stomach.** *Adults and children age 12 and older:* 75 mg once or twice daily; maximum dosage is 150 mg/day.

How supplied

Tablets: 75 mg†, 150 mg, 300 mg
Tablets (dispersible): 150 mg†
Tablets (effervescent): 150 mg
Granules (effervescent): 150 mg
Syrup: 15 mg/ml*
Injection: 25 mg/ml
Infusion: 0.5 mg/ml in 100-ml containers

Pharmacokinetics

Absorption: about 50% to 60% of P.O. dose absorbed; absorbed rapidly from parenteral sites after I.M. dose.
Distribution: distributed to many body tissues and appears in CSF; about 10% to 19% protein-bound.
Metabolism: metabolized in liver.
Excretion: excreted in urine and feces. *Half-life:* 2 to 3 hours.

Route	Onset	Peak	Duration
P.O.	≤ 1 hr	1-3 hr	≤ 13 hr
I.V., I.M.	Unknown	Unknown	≤ 13 hr

Pharmacodynamics

Chemical effect: competitively inhibits action of H_2 at receptor sites of parietal cells, decreasing gastric acid secretion.
Therapeutic effect: relieves GI discomfort.

Adverse reactions

CNS: vertigo, malaise.
EENT: blurred vision.
Hematologic: ***reversible leukopenia, pancytopenia.***
Hepatic: elevated liver enzyme levels, jaundice.
Other: burning and itching at injection site, ***anaphylaxis, angioedema.***

Interactions

Drug-drug. *Antacids:* may interfere with ranitidine absorption. Stagger doses if possible.
Diazepam: decreased diazepam absorption. Monitor patient for decreased effectiveness.
Glipizide: possible increased hypoglycemic effect. Adjust glipizide dosage as directed.
Procainamide: possible decreased renal clearance of procainamide. Monitor patient for procainamide toxicity.
Warfarin: possible interference with warfarin clearance. Monitor patient closely.
Drug-lifestyle. *Smoking:* may increase gastric acid secretion and worsen disease. Discourage concomitant use.

Contraindications and precautions

• Contraindicated in patients hypersensitive to drug.
• Use cautiously in patients with hepatic dysfunction and in pregnant or breast-feeding women. Adjust dosage in patients with impaired kidney function, as ordered.

NURSING CONSIDERATIONS

Assessment

• Assess patient's GI condition before therapy and regularly thereafter.
• Be alert for adverse reactions and drug interactions.
• Evaluate patient's and family's knowledge of drug therapy.

Nursing diagnoses

• Impaired tissue integrity related to underlying GI condition
• Risk for injury related to drug-induced adverse CNS reactions
• Deficient knowledge related to drug therapy

Planning and implementation

• Don't use aluminum-based needles or equipment when mixing or giving drug parenterally because drug is incompatible with aluminum.
P.O. use: Administer once-daily dosage at bedtime.
I.V. use: When administering by I.V. push, dilute to total volume of 20 ml and inject over 5 minutes.
– When giving by intermittent I.V. infusion, dilute 50 mg ranitidine in 100 ml of D_5W and infuse over 15 to 20 minutes. Or, give by continuous I.V. infusion: 150 mg in 250 ml of compatible solution. Administer at 6.25 mg/hour using infusion pump.
– For premixed I.V. infusion, give by slow I.V. drip (over 15 to 20 minutes). Don't add other drugs to solution. If used with primary I.V. fluid system, stop primary solution during infusion.
I.M. use: Follow normal protocol. No dilution is needed when giving drug I.M.
ALERT Don't confuse ranitidine with ritodrine or rimantadine; don't confuse Zantac with Xanax.

Patient teaching

• Remind patient taking drug once daily to take it at bedtime.

• Instruct patient to take drug without regard to meals.
• Urge patient to avoid cigarette smoking because it may increase gastric acid secretion and worsen disease.

Evaluation
• Patient states that GI discomfort is relieved.
• Patient sustains no injury as result of drug-induced adverse CNS reactions.
• Patient and family state understanding of drug therapy.

rapacuronium bromide
(rah-pah-kyoo-ROH-nee-um BROH-mighd)
Raplon

Pharmacologic class: nondepolarizing neuromuscular blocker
Therapeutic class: skeletal muscle relaxant
Pregnancy risk category: C

Indications and dosages
▶ **Adjunct to general anesthesia to facilitate tracheal intubation and provide skeletal muscle relaxation during short surgical procedures.** Dosage is highly individualized; the following dosages should serve only as a guide.
Adults: initially, 1.5 mg/kg I.V. provides conditions considered ideal for tracheal intubation within 60 to 90 seconds and maintains paralysis for about 15 minutes. After intubating dose, up to three maintenance doses of 0.5 mg/kg I.V. may be administered as needed. Repeat doses are based on duration of previous dose and shouldn't be administered until recovery of neuromuscular function is evident.
Adults undergoing cesarean section with thiopental induction: 2.5 mg/kg I.V. is recommended intubating dose.
Children ages 13 to 17: individualize dosage considering physical maturity, height, and weight and using the other recommendations as a guide.
Children ages 1 month to 12 years: 2 mg/kg I.V. bolus will produce acceptable intubating conditions within 60 to 90 seconds; muscle paralysis should last about 15 minutes.

How supplied
Injection: 20 mg/ml

Pharmacokinetics
Absorption: begins within 90 seconds of administration and peaks in about 90 seconds. Duration is about 15 minutes for recommended adult dose.
Distribution: about 50% to 88% protein-bound.
Metabolism: undergoes hydrolysis to the 3-hydroxy metabolite, the major and active metabolite.
Excretion: about 28% of drug is excreted in both urine and feces.

Route	Onset	Peak	Duration
I.V.	60-90 sec	90 sec	15 min

Pharmacodynamics
Chemical effect: competes with acetylcholine for cholinergic receptors at the motor end plate, thus blocking depolarization. Action can be reversed by neostigmine, an acetylcholinesterase inhibitor.
Therapeutic effect: relaxes skeletal muscles.

Adverse reactions
CV: hypotension, tachycardia, ***bradycardia.***
GI: vomiting, nausea.
Respiratory: ***bronchospasm.***
Skin: rash.

Interactions
Drug-drug. *Anticonvulsants (carbamazepine, phenytoin):* may reduce duration of action of rapacuronium, resulting in higher infusion rates and development of resistance. Monitor patient.
Certain antibiotics (*aminoglycosides, bacitracin, polymyxin, tetracyclines, vancomycin*), *inhaled anesthetics (desflurane, enflurane, halothane, isoflurane, sevoflurane), lithium, local anesthetics, magnesium salts, procainamide, quinidine:* may enhance neuromuscular blocking action of rapacuronium. Use together cautiously; lower doses of rapacuronium should be considered.

Contraindications and precautions

• Contraindicated in patients hypersensitive to drug. Avoid repeated doses in children or adults who have been given intubating doses greater than 1.5 mg/kg.
• Use cautiously in patients with myasthenia gravis, myasthenic syndrome, renal or hepatic dysfunction, acid-base abnormalities, electrolyte disturbances, burns, disuse atrophy, cachexia, and carcinomatosis. Also use cautiously in debilitated patients and patients with neuromuscular disease.

NURSING CONSIDERATIONS

Assessment

• Obtain history of patient's underlying condition before therapy, and reassess regularly thereafter.
• Assess baseline electrolyte levels because electrolyte imbalance can potentiate neuromuscular blocking effects.
• Monitor vital signs, especially respirations and heart rate.
• In patients with end-stage renal disease, watch closely for return of neuromuscular function because condition increases drug clearance time.
• Evaluate patient's and family's knowledge of drug therapy.

Nursing diagnoses

• Ineffective health maintenance related to condition
• Ineffective breathing pattern related to drug's effect on respiratory muscles
• Deficient knowledge related to drug therapy

Planning and implementation

I.V. use: Use only under direct medical supervision by experienced clinician skilled in use of neuromuscular blockers and techniques of airway management. Don't administer unless an antagonist and equipment for artificial respiration, oxygen therapy, and intubation are within reach.
– Drug shouldn't be administered by infusion, particularly in long surgical procedures or ICU setting.
– Reconstitute drug with sterile water for injection or other compatible I.V. solutions, such as normal saline solution, D_5W, 5% dextrose in saline solution, lactated Ringer's solution, or bacteriostatic water for injection.
– Use within 24 hours of reconstitution. Prepared solutions may be stored at room temperature or refrigerated (36° to 77° F [2° to 25° C]). Don't use if particulates are present.
• Adequate anesthesic or sedating drugs must accompany rapacuronium, as ordered, because drug has no effect on consciousness or pain perception.
• Use a peripheral nerve stimulator to measure neuromuscular function during administration, monitor drug effect, determine need for additional doses, and confirm recovery from neuromuscular block.
• Don't administer additional doses until patient has a definite response to nerve stimulation.
• In morbidly obese patients (body mass index above 40 kg/m^2), initial dose is based on ideal body weight. In all other patients, dose is based on actual body weight.
ALERT Profound neuromuscular blockade can be reversed by neostigmine.

Patient teaching

• Explain all events and procedures to patient.
• Reassure patient and family that patient will be monitored at all times.

Evaluation

• Patient's condition improves.
• Patient maintains adequate ventilation with mechanical assistance.
• Patient and family state understanding of drug therapy.

repaglinide

(reh-PAG-lih-nighd)
Prandin

Pharmacologic class: meglitinide
Therapeutic class: antidiabetic
Pregnancy risk category: C

Indications and dosages

▶ Adjunct to diet and exercise in lowering blood glucose levels in patient with type 2

(non-insulin-dependent) diabetes mellitus whose hyperglycemia can't be controlled by diet and exercise alone. *Adults:* for patients not previously treated or whose glycosylated hemoglobin (HbA_{1c}) is below 8%, starting dose is 0.5 mg P.O. taken immediately to 30 minutes before each meal. For patients previously treated with glucose-lowering drugs and whose HbA_{1c} is 8% or more, initial dose is 1 to 2 mg P.O. taken immediately to 30 minutes before each meal. Recommended dosage range is 0.5 to 4 mg just before meals, divided b.i.d., t.i.d., or q.i.d. Maximum daily dosage is 16 mg.

How supplied

Tablets: 0.5 mg, 1 mg, 2 mg

Pharmacokinetics

Absorption: rapidly and completely absorbed from the GI tract. Absolute bioavailability is 56%.
Distribution: more than 98% bound to plasma proteins.
Metabolism: completely metabolized by oxidative biotransformation and direct conjugation with glucuronic acid.
Excretion: about 90% is recovered in feces and 8% in urine. *Half-life:* 1 hour.

Route	Onset	Peak	Duration
P.O.	Unknown	1 hr	Unknown

Pharmacodynamics

Chemical effect: stimulates the release of insulin from beta cells in the pancreas.
Therapeutic effect: lowers blood glucose levels.

Adverse reactions

CNS: *headache,* paresthesia.
CV: angina, chest pain.
EENT: rhinitis, sinusitis.
GI: constipation, diarrhea, dyspepsia, nausea, vomiting.
GU: urinary tract infection.
Metabolic: **HYPOGLYCEMIA,** hyperglycemia.
Musculoskeletal: arthralgia, back pain.
Respiratory: bronchitis, *upper respiratory infection.*
Other: tooth disorder.

Interactions

Drug-drug. *Barbiturates, carbamazepine, rifampin, troglitazone:* may increase repaglinide metabolism. Monitor glucose level.
Beta blockers, chloramphenicol, coumarins, MAO inhibitors, NSAIDs, other drugs that are highly protein-bound, probenecid, salicylates, sulfonamides: may potentiate hypoglycemic action of repaglinide. Monitor glucose level.
Calcium channel blockers, corticosteroids, estrogens, isoniazid, nicotinic acid, oral contraceptives, phenothiazines, phenytoin, sympathomimetics, thiazides and other diuretics, thyroid products: may produce hyperglycemia and loss of glycemic control. Monitor glucose level.
Erythromycin, inhibitors of P-450 cytochrome system 3A4, ketoconazole, miconazole: may inhibit repaglinide metabolism. Monitor glucose levels.
Drug-herb. *Aloe, bitter melon, bilberry leaf, burdock, dandelion, fenugreek, garlic, ginseng:* may improve blood glucose control and create a need to reduce antidiabetic dosage. Advise patient to discuss the use of herbal remedies before taking repaglinide.

Contraindications and precautions

- Contraindicated in patients hypersensitive to drug or its inactive ingredients and in those with insulin-dependent diabetes mellitus or diabetic ketoacidosis.
- Use cautiously in patients with hepatic insufficiency in whom reduced metabolism could increase blood repaglinide levels and cause hypoglycemia.
- Use cautiously in elderly, debilitated, or malnourished patients and in those with adrenal or pituitary insufficiency because they're more susceptible to the hypoglycemic effect of glucose-lowering drugs.

NURSING CONSIDERATIONS

Assessment

- Monitor blood glucose level before therapy and regularly thereafter.
- Be alert for adverse reactions and drug interactions.

• Monitor elderly patients and patients taking beta blockers carefully because hypoglycemia may be difficult to recognize in these patients.
• Evaluate patient's and family's knowledge of drug therapy.

Nursing diagnoses

• Imbalanced nutrition: more than body requirements related to patient's underlying condition
• Risk for injury related to drug-induced hypoglycemic episode
• Deficient knowledge related to drug therapy

Planning and implementation

• Increase dosage carefully in patients with impaired renal function or renal failure who need dialysis.
• Metformin may be added if repaglinide alone is inadequate.
• Loss of glycemic control can occur during stress, such as fever, trauma, infection, or surgery. Discontinue drug as ordered, and administer insulin.
• Administration of oral antidiabetics has been linked to increased CV mortality compared with diet treatment alone.
• Give drug immediately to 30 minutes before meals.

Patient teaching

• Teach patient about importance of diet and exercise in combination with drug therapy.
• Discuss symptoms of hypoglycemia with patient and family.
• Advise patient to monitor blood glucose periodically to determine minimum effective dose.
• Encourage patient to keep regular medical appointments and have glucose levels checked as ordered to monitor long-term glucose control.
• Tell patient to take drug before meals, usually 15 minutes before start of meal; however, time can vary from immediately to up to 30 minutes before meal.
• Tell patient to skip dose if he skips a meal and to add dose if he adds a meal.
• Teach patient how to monitor blood glucose carefully and what to do when he is ill, undergoing surgery, or under added stress.

Evaluation

• Patient's blood glucose is controlled and an adequate nutritional balance is maintained.
• Patient doesn't experience severe decreases in blood glucose levels.
• Patient and family state understanding of drug therapy.

reteplase, recombinant

(REE-teh-plays, ree-KUHM-buh-nent)
Retavase

Pharmacologic class: recombinant plasminogen activator, enzyme
Therapeutic class: thrombolytic enzyme
Pregnancy risk category: C

Indications and dosages

▶ **Management of acute MI.** *Adults:* double-bolus injection of 10 + 10 units. Give each bolus I.V. over 2 minutes. If complications don't occur after first bolus, give second bolus 30 minutes after start of first.

How supplied

Injection: 10.8 units (18.8 mg)/vial. Supplied in kit with components for reconstitution for 2 single-use vials.

Pharmacokinetics

Absorption: not applicable with I.V. administration.
Distribution: rapid distribution.
Metabolism: unknown.
Excretion: in urine and feces.

Route	Onset	Peak	Duration
I.V.	Unknown	Unknown	Unknown

Pharmacodynamics

Chemical effect: enhances cleavage of plasminogen to generate plasmin.
Therapeutic effect: fibrinolytic and thrombolytic action.

Adverse reactions

CNS: ***intracranial hemorrhage.***
CV: ***arrhythmias, cholesterol embolization, hemorrhage.***

GI: ***hemorrhage.***
GU: hematuria.
Hematologic: anemia, ***bleeding tendency.***
Other: bleeding at puncture sites.

Interactions

Drug-drug. *Heparin, oral anticoagulants, platelet inhibitors (abciximab, aspirin, dipyridamole):* may increase risk of bleeding. Use together cautiously.

Contraindications and precautions

- Contraindicated in patients with active internal bleeding, bleeding diathesis, history of CVA, recent intracranial or intraspinal surgery or trauma, severe uncontrolled hypertension, intracranial neoplasm, arteriovenous malformation, or aneurysm.
- Use cautiously in patients with recent (within 10 days) major surgery, obstetric delivery, organ biopsy, or trauma; previous puncture of noncompressible vessel; cerebrovascular disease; recent GI or GU bleeding; or heart disease.

NURSING CONSIDERATIONS

Assessment

- Monitor ECG during treatment.
- Monitor patient for bleeding. Avoid I.M. injections, invasive procedures, and unnecessary handling of patient.
- Evaluate patient's and family's knowledge of drug therapy.

Nursing diagnoses

- Ineffective cardiopulmonary tissue perfusion related to underlying condition
- Risk for injury related to adverse effects of drug
- Deficient knowledge related to drug therapy

Planning and implementation

- Reteplase is administered I.V. as double-bolus injection. If bleeding or anaphylactoid reaction occurs after first bolus, notify prescriber.
- Reconstitute drug according to manufacturer's instructions.

ALERT Don't administer drug with other I.V. medications through the same line. Heparin and reteplase are incompatible in solution.
- Avoid noncompressible pressure sites during therapy. If an arterial puncture is needed, use an arm vessel that can be compressed manually. Apply pressure for at least 30 minutes; then apply a pressure dressing. Check site often for bleeding.

Patient teaching
- Tell patient and family about drug.
- Tell patient to report adverse reactions immediately.

Evaluation

- Patient's cardiopulmonary assessment findings show improved perfusion.
- Patient is free from serious adverse reactions caused by therapy.
- Patient and family state understanding of drug therapy.

Rh_o(D) immune globulin, human

(R H O D ih-MYOON GLOH-byoo-lin, HYOO-mun)
Gamulin Rh, HypRho-D, MICRhoGAM, Mini-Gamulin Rh, RhoGAM

Pharmacologic class: immune serum
Therapeutic class: anti-Rh_o(D)-positive prophylaxis agent
Pregnancy risk category: C

Indications and dosages

▶ **Rh exposure (postabortion, postmiscarriage, ectopic pregnancy, postpartum, or threatened abortion 13 weeks or beyond).** *Women:* transfusion unit or blood bank determines fetal packed RBC volume entering patient's blood; then give one vial I.M. if fetal packed RBC volume is below 15 ml. More than one vial I.M. may be required if large fetomaternal hemorrhage occurs. Must be given within 72 hours after delivery or miscarriage.

▶ **Transfusion accident.** *Adults and children:* consult blood bank or transfusion unit at once. Must be given within 72 hours.

▶ **Postabortion or postmiscarriage to prevent Rh antibody formation up to and including 12 weeks' gestation.** *Women:* consult transfusion unit or blood bank. One microdose vial suppresses immune reaction to 2.5 ml Rh_o(D)-positive RBCs. Should be given within 3 hours but may be given up to 72 hours after abortion or miscarriage.

▶ **Amniocentesis or abdominal trauma during pregnancy.** *Women:* dose based on extent of fetomaternal hemorrhage.

How supplied

Injection: 300 mcg of Rh_o(D) immune globulin/vial (standard dose); 50 mcg of Rh_o(D) immune globulin/vial (microdose)

Pharmacokinetics

Unknown.

Route	Onset	Peak	Duration
I.M.	Unknown	Unknown	Unknown

Pharmacodynamics

Chemical effect: suppresses active antibody response and formation of anti-Rh_o(D) in Rh_o(D)-negative, D^u-negative people exposed to Rh-positive blood.

Therapeutic effect: blocks adverse effects of Rh-positive exposure.

Adverse reactions

Skin: discomfort at injection site.

Other: slight fever, ***anaphylaxis.***

Interactions

Drug-drug. *Live-virus vaccines:* may interfere with response to Rh_o(D) immune globulin. Delay immunization for 3 months if possible.

Contraindications and precautions

- Contraindicated in Rh_o(D)-positive or D^u-positive patients, those previously immunized to Rh_o(D) blood factor, and those with anaphylactic or severe systemic reaction to human globulin.
- Use cautiously in pregnant or breast-feeding women.

NURSING CONSIDERATIONS

Assessment

- Obtain history of Rh-negative patient's Rh-positive exposure, allergies, and reactions to immunizations.
- Evaluate patient's and family's knowledge of drug therapy.

Nursing diagnoses

- Risk for injury related to Rh-positive exposure
- Ineffective protection related to drug-induced anaphylaxis
- Deficient knowledge related to drug therapy

Planning and implementation

- Make sure epinephrine 1:1,000 is available in case of anaphylaxis.
- After delivery, have neonate's cord blood typed and crossmatched; confirm if mother is Rh_o(D)-negative and D^u-negative. Administer to mother, as ordered, only if infant is Rh_o(D)-positive or D^u-positive.
- Drug gives passive immunity to patient exposed to Rh_o(D)-positive fetal blood during pregnancy; it prevents formation of maternal antibodies, which would endanger future Rh_o(D)-positive pregnancies.
- Defer vaccination with live-virus vaccines for 3 months after administration of drug.
- MICRhoGAM is recommended for every patient undergoing abortion or miscarriage up to 12 weeks' gestation unless she is Rh_o(D)-positive or D^u-positive, she has Rh antibodies, or father or fetus is Rh-negative.
- Refrigerate drug at 36° to 46° F (2° to 8° C).

Patient teaching

- Explain how drug protects future Rh_o(D)-positive fetuses.

Evaluation

- Patient shows evidence of passive immunity to exposure to Rh_o(D)-positive blood.
- Patient doesn't develop anaphylaxis after drug administration.
- Patient and family state understanding of drug therapy.

ribavirin

(righ-beh-VIGH-rin)
Virazole

Pharmacologic class: synthetic nucleoside
Therapeutic class: antiviral
Pregnancy risk category: X

Indications and dosages

▶ **Hospitalized infants and young children infected by RSV.** *Infants and young children:* 20-mg/ml solution delivered by small particle aerosol generator (SPAG-2) and mechanical ventilator or oxygen hood, face mask, or oxygen tent at about 12.5 L of mist per minute. Treatment lasts 12 to 18 hours/day for 3 to 7 days.

How supplied

Powder to be reconstituted for inhalation: 6 g in 100-ml glass vial

Pharmacokinetics

Absorption: some ribavirin is absorbed systemically.
Distribution: concentrates in bronchial secretions.
Metabolism: metabolized to 1,2,4-triazole-3-carboxamide (deribosylated ribavirin).
Excretion: most of drug excreted in urine.
Half-life: first phase, 9½ hours; second phase, 40 hours.

Route	Onset	Peak	Duration
Inhalation	Immediate	Immediate	Unknown

Pharmacodynamics

Chemical effect: inhibits viral activity by unknown mechanism, possibly by inhibiting RNA and DNA synthesis by depleting intracellular nucleotide pools.
Therapeutic effect: inhibits RSV activity.

Adverse reactions

CV: ***cardiac arrest,*** hypotension.
EENT: conjunctivitis, rash or erythema of eyelids.
Hematologic: reticulocytosis.
Hepatic: elevated bilirubin, AST, ALT levels.
Respiratory: worsening of respiratory state, ***apnea,*** bacterial pneumonia, ***pneumothorax.***

Interactions

Drug-drug. *Acetaminophen, aspirin, cimetidine:* may affect plasma drug levels. Monitor patient.

Contraindications and precautions

- Contraindicated in patients hypersensitive to drug and women who are or may become pregnant during treatment.
- Drug isn't indicated for breast-feeding women.

NURSING CONSIDERATIONS

Assessment

- Assess patient's respiratory infection before therapy and regularly thereafter.
- Monitor ventilator function. Drug may precipitate in ventilator apparatus, causing equipment malfunction with serious consequences.
- Watch for anemia in patient receiving drug longer than 1 to 2 weeks.
- Be alert for adverse reactions.
- Evaluate patient's and family's knowledge of drug therapy.

Nursing diagnoses

- Infection related to presence of RSV
- Risk for injury related to drug-induced adverse CV reactions
- Deficient knowledge related to drug therapy

Planning and implementation

- Ribavirin aerosol is indicated only for severe lower respiratory tract infection caused by RSV. Treatment may start pending test results, but existence of RSV infection must be documented.
- Most infants and children with RSV infection don't need treatment. Infants with underlying conditions, such as prematurity or cardiopulmonary disease, benefit most from treatment with ribavirin aerosol.
- Give drug by SPAG-2 only. Don't use any other aerosol generator.
- Use sterile USP water for injection, not bacteriostatic water, for reconstitution. Water used to reconstitute this drug must not contain an antimicrobial agent.

• Discard solutions placed in SPAG-2 unit at least every 24 hours before adding newly reconstituted solution.
• Avoid unnecessary occupational exposure to drug. Adverse effects reported in health care personnel exposed to aerosolized ribavirin include eye irritation and headache.
• Store reconstituted solutions at room temperature for 24 hours.
• Continue providing supportive respiratory and fluid management.
ALERT Don't confuse ribavarin with riboflavin.

Patient teaching
• Inform parents of need for drug therapy, and answer their questions.
• Advise patient to use correct device.

Evaluation
• Patient is free from infection.
• Patient doesn't develop adverse CV reactions after drug administration.
• Parents state understanding of drug therapy.

riboflavin (vitamin B_2)†
(righ-boh-FLAY-vin)

Pharmacologic class: water-soluble vitamin
Therapeutic class: vitamin B complex vitamin
Pregnancy risk category: A (C in doses that exceed RDA)

Indications and dosages
▶ **RDA.** *Men age 51 and over:* 1.4 mg.
Men ages 19 to 50: 1.7 mg.
Men ages 15 to 18: 1.8 mg.
Men ages 11 to 14: 1.5 mg.
Women age 51 and over: 1.2 mg.
Women ages 11 to 50: 1.3 mg.
Pregnant women: 1.6 mg.
Breast-feeding women (first 6 months): 1.8 mg.
Breast-feeding women (second 6 months): 1.7 mg.
Children ages 7 to 10: 1.2 mg.
Children ages 4 to 6: 1.1 mg.
Children ages 1 to 3: 0.8 mg.
Infants ages 6 months to 1 year: 0.5 mg.
Neonates and infants to age 6 months: 0.4 mg.
▶ **Riboflavin deficiency or adjunct to thiamine treatment for polyneuritis or cheilosis caused by pellagra.** *Adults and children age 12 and over:* 5 to 30 mg P.O. daily, depending on severity.
Children under age 12: 3 to 10 mg P.O. daily, depending on severity. For maintenance, increase nutritional intake and supplement with vitamin B complex.
▶ **Microcytic anemia linked to splenomegaly and glutathione reductase deficiency.** *Adults:* 10 mg P.O. daily for 10 days.

How supplied
Tablets: 10 mg†, 25 mg†, 50 mg†, 100 mg†
Tablets (sugar-free): 50 mg†, 100 mg†

Pharmacokinetics
Absorption: absorbed readily from GI tract, although extent of absorption is limited. Absorption occurs at specialized segment of mucosa; riboflavin absorption is limited by duration of drug's contact with this area. Before being absorbed, riboflavin 5-phosphate is rapidly dephosphorylated in GI lumen. GI absorption increases when drug is given with food and decreases when hepatitis, cirrhosis, biliary obstruction, or probenecid administration is present.
Distribution: riboflavin, a coenzyme, functions in forms of flavin adenine dinucleotide (FAD) and flavin mononucleotide (FMN). FAD and FMN are distributed widely to body tissues. Riboflavin is stored in limited amounts in liver, spleen, kidneys, and heart, mainly in form of FAD. FAD and FMN are about 60% protein-bound in blood.
Metabolism: riboflavin is metabolized to FMN in erythrocytes, GI mucosal cells, and liver. FMN is converted to FAD in liver.
Excretion: excreted in urine. *Half-life:* 66 to 84 minutes.

Route	Onset	Peak	Duration
P.O.	Unknown	Unknown	Unknown

Pharmacodynamics
Chemical effect: converts to two other coenzymes needed for normal tissue respiration.

Therapeutic effect: relieves riboflavin deficiency.

Adverse reactions

GU: bright yellow urine.

Interactions

Drug-drug. *Probenecid:* reduced urinary excretion of riboflavin. Use together cautiously. *Propantheline, other anticholinergics:* decreased rate and extent of absorption. Avoid concomitant use.

Contraindications and precautions

- No known contraindications.

NURSING CONSIDERATIONS

Assessment

- Assess patient's riboflavin deficiency before and during therapy.
- Be alert for change in urine color.
- Evaluate patient's and family's knowledge of drug therapy.

Nursing diagnoses

- Imbalanced nutrition: less than body's needs, related to drug deficiency
- Deficient knowledge related to drug therapy

Planning and implementation

- Drug may be given I.M. or I.V. as component of multiple vitamins.
- Riboflavin deficiency usually accompanies other vitamin B–complex deficiencies and may require multivitamin therapy.
- Protect drug from air and light.

ALERT Don't confuse riboflavin with ribavarin.

Patient teaching

- Encourage patient to take with meals to increase absorption.
- Stress proper nutritional habits to prevent return of deficiency.
- Inform patient that urine will likely turn to bright yellow or orange.

Evaluation

- Patient's drug deficiency is resolved.
- Patient and family state understanding of drug therapy.

rifabutin

(rif-uh-BYOO-tin)
Mycobutin

Pharmacologic class: semisynthetic ansamycin
Therapeutic class: antibiotic
Pregnancy risk category: B

Indications and dosages

▶ **Prevention of disseminated *Mycobacterium avium* complex (MAC) in patients with advanced HIV infection.** *Adults:* 300 mg P.O. daily as single dose or divided b.i.d. taken with food.

How supplied

Capsules: 150 mg

Pharmacokinetics

Absorption: readily absorbed from GI tract.
Distribution: because of its high lipophilicity, rifabutin demonstrates high propensity for distribution and intracellular tissue uptake. About 85% of drug is bound to plasma proteins independent of concentration.
Metabolism: metabolized in liver.
Excretion: excreted primarily in urine; about 30% excreted in feces. *Half-life:* 45 hours.

Route	Onset	Peak	Duration
P.O.	Unknown	1.5-4 hr	Unknown

Pharmacodynamics

Chemical effect: inhibits DNA-dependent RNA polymerase in susceptible bacteria, blocking bacterial protein synthesis.
Therapeutic effect: prevents disseminated MAC in patients with advanced HIV infection.

Adverse reactions

CNS: headache.
GI: dyspepsia, eructation, flatulence, diarrhea, nausea, vomiting, abdominal pain.
GU: discolored urine.

Hematologic: eosinophilia, LEUKOPENIA, NEUTROPENIA, ***thrombocytopenia.***
Musculoskeletal: myalgia.
Skin: rash.
Other: fever.

Interactions

Drug-drug: *Drugs metabolized by the liver, zidovudine:* decreased serum zidovudine levels. Because rifabutin, like rifampin, induces liver enzymes, it may lower serum levels of many other drugs as well. Although dosage adjustments may be necessary, further study is needed.
Oral contraceptives: decreased effectiveness. Instruct patient to use nonhormonal forms of birth control.
Drug-food. *High-fat foods:* slows absorption of drug. Avoid taking drug with high-fat meals.

Contraindications and precautions

- Contraindicated in patients hypersensitive to drug or other rifamycin derivatives (such as rifampin) and in those with active tuberculosis because single-agent therapy with rifabutin increases risk of bacterial resistance to both rifabutin and rifampin.
- Drug isn't recommended for use in breast-feeding women.
- Use cautiously in patients with neutropenia and thrombocytopenia.
- Safety of drug hasn't been established in children.

NURSING CONSIDERATIONS

Assessment

- Assess patient's condition before therapy and regularly thereafter.
- Perform baseline hematologic studies and repeat periodically, as ordered.
- Be alert for adverse reactions and drug interactions.
- Evaluate patient's and family's knowledge of drug therapy.

Nursing diagnoses

- Infection related to advanced HIV infection
- Ineffective protection related to drug-induced adverse hematologic reactions
- Deficient knowledge related to drug therapy

Planning and implementation

- High-fat meals slow rate but not extent of absorption.
- Mix with soft foods for patient who has difficulty swallowing.
- No evidence exists that drug will provide effective prophylaxis against *Mycobacterium tuberculosis*. Patients requiring prophylaxis against both *M. tuberculosis* and MAC may require rifampin and rifabutin.

ALERT Don't confuse rifampin, rifapentine and rifabutin.

Patient teaching

- Tell patient that drug may turn urine, feces, sputum, saliva, tears, and skin brownish-orange. Tell him not to wear soft contacts because they may be permanently stained.
- Instruct patient to report photophobia, excessive lacrimation, or eye pain. Drug may rarely cause uveitis.

Evaluation

- Patient doesn't develop disseminated MAC.
- Patient maintains normal hematologic values throughout therapy.
- Patient and family state understanding of drug therapy.

rifampin (rifampicin)

(rih-FAM-pin)

Rifadin, Rifadin IV, Rimactane, Rimycin ◇, Rofact ♦

Pharmacologic class: semisynthetic rifamycin B derivative (macrocytic antibiotic)
Therapeutic class: antituberculotic
Pregnancy risk category: C

Indications and dosages

▶ **Pulmonary tuberculosis.** *Adults:* 600 mg P.O. or I.V. daily in single dose.
Children over age 5: 10 to 20 mg/kg P.O. or I.V. daily in single dose. Maximum, 600 mg daily. Concomitant use with other antituberculotics is recommended.

▶ **Meningococcal carriers.** *Adults:* 600 mg P.O. or I.V. b.i.d. for 2 days.
Children ages 1 month to 12 years: 10 mg/kg P.O. or I.V. b.i.d. for 2 days, maximum 600 mg/day.
Neonates: 5 mg/kg P.O. or I.V. b.i.d. for 2 days.
▶ **Prophylaxis of *Haemophilus influenzae* type b.** *Adults and children:* 20 mg/kg P.O. daily for 4 days; maximum 600 mg/day.
Note: Reduce dosage in patients with liver dysfunction.

How supplied

Capsules: 150 mg, 300 mg
Injection: 600 mg

Pharmacokinetics

Absorption: absorbed completely from GI tract after P.O. administration. Food delays absorption.
Distribution: distributed widely in body tissues and fluids, including CSF; ascitic, pleural, and seminal fluids; tears; saliva; and liver, prostate, lungs, and bone. It's 84% to 91% protein-bound.
Metabolism: metabolized extensively in liver. Drug undergoes enterohepatic circulation.
Excretion: drug and metabolite excreted primarily in bile; drug, but not metabolite, is reabsorbed. Some of drug and its metabolite are excreted in urine. *Half-life:* 1½ to 5 hours.

Route	Onset	Peak	Duration
P.O.	Unknown	2-4 hr	Unknown
I.V.	Unknown	Unknown	Unknown

Pharmacodynamics

Chemical effect: inhibits DNA-dependent RNA polymerase, thus impairing RNA synthesis (bactericidal).
Therapeutic effect: kills susceptible bacteria. Spectrum of activity includes *Mycobacterium bovis, M. kansasii, M. marinum, M. tuberculosis* and some strains of *M. avium-intracellulare* and *M. fortuitum* as well as many gram-positive and some gram-negative bacteria.

Adverse reactions

CNS: ataxia, behavioral changes, confusion, dizziness, fatigue, headache, drowsiness, generalized numbness.
EENT: visual disturbances, exudative conjunctivitis.
GI: epigastric distress, anorexia, nausea, vomiting, abdominal pain, diarrhea, flatulence, sore mouth and tongue, pseudomembranous colitis, ***pancreatitis.***
GU: hemoglobinuria, hematuria, ***acute renal failure,*** menstrual disturbances.
Hematologic: eosinophilia, ***transient leukopenia, thrombocytopenia,*** hemolytic anemia.
Hepatic: ***hepatotoxicity,*** *transient abnormalities in liver function test results,* worsening of porphyria.
Metabolic: hyperuricemia.
Musculoskeletal: osteomalacia.
Respiratory: shortness of breath, wheezing.
Skin: pruritus, urticaria, rash.
Other: flu syndrome, discoloration of body fluids, ***shock.***

Interactions

Drug-drug. *Analgesics, anticoagulants, anticonvulsants, barbiturates, beta blockers, cardiac glycosides, chloramphenicol, clofibrate, corticosteroids, cyclosporine, dapsone, diazepam, disopyramide, methadone, mexiletine, narcotics, oral contraceptives, progestins, quinidine, sulfonylureas, theophylline, verapamil:* reduced effectiveness of these drugs. Avoid concomitant use.
Halothane: may increase risk of hepatotoxicity in both drugs. Monitor liver function closely.
Ketoconazole, para-aminosalicylate sodium: may interfere with absorption of rifampin. Give these drugs 8 to 12 hours apart.
Probenecid: may increase rifampin levels. Use cautiously.
Drug-lifestyle. *Alcohol use:* may increase risk of hepatotoxicity. Discourage concomitant use.

Contraindications and precautions

- Contraindicated in patients hypersensitive to drug.
- Use cautiously in patients with liver disease and in pregnant or breast-feeding women.

NURSING CONSIDERATIONS

Assessment
- Assess patient's infection before therapy and regularly thereafter.
- Monitor liver function, hematopoiesis, and serum uric acid levels.
- Be alert for adverse reactions and drug interactions.
- Drug may cause hemorrhage in neonates of rifampin-treated mothers.
- Watch closely for signs of hepatic impairment.
- Monitor patient's hydration status if adverse GI reactions occur.
- Evaluate patient's and family's knowledge of drug therapy.

Nursing diagnoses
- Infection related to presence of susceptible bacteria
- Risk for deficient fluid volume related to drug-induced adverse reactions
- Deficient knowledge related to drug therapy

Planning and implementation
P.O. use: Give drug 1 hour before or 2 hours after meals for optimal absorption; if GI irritation occurs, patient may take rifampin with meals.
I.V. use: Reconstitute vial with 10 ml of sterile water for injection to make solution containing 60 mg/ml.
– Add to 100 ml of D_5W and infuse over 30 minutes, or add to 500 ml of D_5W and infuse over 3 hours.
– When dextrose is contraindicated, drug may be diluted with normal saline solution for injection. Don't use other I.V. solutions.
- Concomitant treatment with at least one other antituberculotic is recommended.
- Report hepatic impairment.

ALERT Don't confuse rifampin, rifapentine and rifabutin.

Patient teaching
- Warn patient about drowsiness and possible red-orange discoloration of urine, feces, saliva, sweat, sputum, and tears. Soft contact lenses may be permanently stained.
- Advise patient to avoid alcoholic beverages while taking this drug.

Evaluation
- Patient is free from infection.
- Patient maintains adequate hydration throughout therapy.
- Patient and family state understanding of drug therapy.

rifapentine
(rif-ah-PEN-tin)
Priftin

Pharmacologic class: rifamycin derivative antibiotic
Therapeutic class: antituberculotic
Pregnancy risk category: C

Indications and dosages
▶ **Pulmonary tuberculosis, with at least one other antituberculotic to which the isolate is susceptible.** *Adults:* during intensive phase of short-course therapy, 600 mg P.O. twice weekly for 2 months, with an interval between doses of not less than 3 days (72 hours). During the continuation phase of short-course therapy, 600 mg P.O. once weekly for 4 months in combination with isoniazid or another drug to which the isolate is susceptible.

How supplied
Tablets (film-coated): 150 mg

Pharmacokinetics
Absorption: relative bioavailability is 70%.
Distribution: about 98% bound to plasma proteins.
Metabolism: hydrolyzed by an esterase enzyme to the microbiologically active 25-desacetyl rifapentine. Rifapentine contributes 62% to drug's activity and 25-desacetyl contributes 38%.
Excretion: about 17% is excreted in urine and 70% in feces. *Half-life:* 13 hours.

Route	Onset	Peak	Duration
P.O.	Unknown	5-6 hr	Unknown

Pharmacodynamics

Chemical effect: inhibits DNA-dependent RNA polymerase in susceptible strains of *Mycobacterium tuberculosis*. It has intracellular and extracellular bactericidal activity. Rifapentine and rifampin share similar antimicrobial action.
Therapeutic effect: kills susceptible bacteria.

Adverse reactions

CNS: headache, dizziness.
CV: hypertension.
GI: anorexia, nausea, vomiting, dyspepsia, diarrhea, ***pseudomembranous colitis.***
GU: pyuria, proteinuria, hematuria, urinary casts.
Hematologic: ***neutropenia,*** lymphopenia, anemia, ***leukopenia,*** thrombocytosis.
Hepatic: elevated AST and ALT levels.
Metabolic: *hyperuricemia.*
Musculoskeletal: arthralgia.
Respiratory: hemoptysis.
Skin: rash, pruritus, acne, maculopapular rash.
Other: pain.

Interactions

Drug-drug. *Antiarrhythmics (disopyramide, mexiletine, quinidine, tocainide), antibiotics (chloramphenicol, clarithromycin, dapsone, doxycycline, fluoroquinolones), anticonvulsants (phenytoin), antifungals (fluconazole, itraconazole, ketoconazole), barbiturates, benzodiazepines (diazepam), beta blockers, calcium channel blockers (diltiazem, nifedipine, verapamil), cardiac glycosides, clofibrate, corticosteroids, haloperidol, HIV protease inhibitors (indinavir, nelfinavir, ritonavir, saquinavir), immunosuppressants (cyclosporine, tacrolimus), levothyroxine, narcotic analgesics (methadone), oral anticoagulants (warfarin), oral hypoglycemics (sulfonylureas), oral or other systemic hormonal contraceptives, progestins, quinine, reverse transcriptase inhibitors (delavirdine, zidovudine), sildenafil, theophylline, tricyclic antidepressants (amitriptyline, nortriptyline):* induces metabolism of hepatic cytochrome P-450 enzyme system, decreasing the activity of these drugs. Dosage adjustments may be needed.

Contraindications and precautions

- Contraindicated in patients hypersensitive to rifamycin (rifapentine, rifampin, or rifabutin).
- Use drug cautiously and with frequent monitoring in patients with liver disease.

NURSING CONSIDERATIONS

Assessment

- Assess patient's condition before therapy and regularly thereafter.
- Assess patient's understanding of disease and stress importance of strict compliance with drug and daily companion medications, as well as necessary follow-up visits and laboratory tests.
- Monitor liver function, CBC, and serum uric acid levels.
- Monitor patient for persistent or severe diarrhea and notify prescriber if it occurs.
- Evaluate patient's and family's knowledge of drug therapy.

Nursing diagnoses

- Infection related to patient's underlying condition
- Noncompliance related to long-term therapeutic regimen
- Deficient knowledge related to drug therapy

Planning and implementation

- Concomitant administration of pyridoxine (vitamin B_6) is recommended in malnourished patients, those predisposed to neuropathy (alcoholics, diabetics), and adolescents.
- Drug must be given with appropriate daily companion drugs. Compliance with all drugs, especially with daily companion drugs on the days when rifapentine isn't given, is crucial for early sputum conversion and protection from tuberculosis relapse.
- Administration of drug during last 2 weeks of pregnancy may lead to postnatal hemorrhage in mother or infant. Monitor clotting parameters closely.

ALERT Don't confuse rifampin, rifapentine, and rifabutin.

Patient teaching

- Stress importance of strict compliance with drug and daily companion drugs, as well as necessary follow-up visits and laboratory tests.
- Advise patient to use nonhormonal methods of birth control.
- Tell patient to take drug with food if nausea, vomiting, or GI upset occurs.
- Instruct patient to notify prescriber if any of the following occur: fever, loss of appetite, malaise, nausea, vomiting, darkened urine, yellowish discoloration of skin and eyes, pain or swelling of joints, and excessive loose stools or diarrhea.
- Instruct patient to protect pills from excessive heat.
- Tell patient that drug can turn body fluids red-orange. Contact lenses can become permanently stained.

☑ Evaluation

- Patient experiences sputum conversion and recovers from tuberculosis.
- Patient is compliant with therapeutic regimen.
- Patient and family state understanding of drug therapy.

riluzole

(RIGH-loo-zohl)
Rilutek

Pharmacologic class: benzothiazole
Therapeutic class: neuroprotector
Pregnancy risk category: C

Indications and dosages

▶ **Amyotrophic lateral sclerosis (ALS).**
Adults: 50 mg P.O. q 12 hours on empty stomach.

How supplied

Tablets: 50 mg

Pharmacokinetics

Absorption: well absorbed from GI tract, with average absolute oral bioavailability of about 60%. High-fat meal decreases absorption.
Distribution: 96% protein-bound.
Metabolism: extensively metabolized in liver.
Excretion: excreted primarily in urine, with small amount in feces. *Half-life:* 12 hours with repeated doses.

Route	Onset	Peak	Duration
P.O.	Unknown	Unknown	Unknown

Pharmacodynamics

Chemical effect: unknown.
Therapeutic effect: improves signs and symptoms of ALS.

Adverse reactions

CNS: headache, aggravation reaction, *asthenia,* hypertonia, depression, dizziness, insomnia, malaise, somnolence, vertigo, circumoral paresthesia.
CV: hypertension, tachycardia, palpitations, orthostatic hypotension, peripheral edema.
EENT: *rhinitis, sinusitis.*
GI: abdominal pain, *nausea,* vomiting, dyspepsia, anorexia, diarrhea, flatulence, stomatitis, dry mouth, oral candidiasis.
GU: urinary tract infection, dysuria.
Hematologic: neutropenia.
Metabolic: weight loss.
Musculoskeletal: back pain, arthralgia.
Respiratory: *decreased lung function,* increased cough.
Skin: pruritus, eczema, alopecia, exfoliative dermatitis.
Other: tooth disorder, phlebitis.

Interactions

Drug-drug. *Allopurinol, methyldopa, sulfasalazine:* increased risk of hepatotoxicity. Monitor patient closely.
Inducers of CVP 1A2 (omeprazole, rifampicin): may increase riluzole elimination. Monitor patient for loss of therapeutic effect.
Potential inhibitors of CYP 1A2 (amitriptyline, phenacetin, quinolones, theophylline): may decrease riluzole elimination. Monitor patient closely for toxicity.
Drug-food. *Any food:* decreased bioavailability. Administer 1 hour before or 2 hours after meals.
Caffeine: may decrease riluzole elimination. Monitor patient for adverse reactions.

Charbroiled foods: may increase riluzole elimination. Avoid concomitant use.
Drug-lifestyle. *Alcohol use:* may increase risk of hepatotoxicity. Discourage excessive use.
Smoking: may increase riluzole elimination. Advise patient to refrain from smoking.

Contraindications and precautions

- Contraindicated in patients severely hypersensitive to drug or components of the tablets.
- Drug isn't recommended for use in breast-feeding women.
- Use cautiously in patients with hepatic or renal dysfunction, elderly patients, and women and Japanese patients (who may have a lower metabolic capacity to eliminate riluzole compared to men and to white patients, respectively).
- Safety of drug hasn't been established in children.

NURSING CONSIDERATIONS

Assessment
- Obtain history of patient's ALS.
- Obtain liver and renal function studies and CBC before and during therapy.
- Evaluate patient's and family's knowledge of drug therapy.

Nursing diagnoses
- Impaired physical mobility related to ALS
- Risk for deficient fluid volume related to adverse GI reactions
- Deficient knowledge related to drug therapy

Planning and implementation
- Baseline elevations in liver function studies (especially elevated bilirubin level) should preclude use of riluzole. In many patients, drug may increase serum aminotransferase level. If level exceeds 10 times upper limit of normal range, or if jaundice develops, notify prescriber.
- Give drug at least 1 hour before or 2 hours after a meal to avoid a food-related decrease in bioavailability.

Patient teaching
- Tell patient to take drug at same time each day. If he misses a dose, tell him to take the next tablet as scheduled.
- Instruct patient to report febrile illness; his WBC count should be checked.
- Warn patient to avoid hazardous activities until drug's CNS effects are known.
- Advise patient to limit alcohol intake during therapy.
- Tell patient to store drug at room temperature, protected from bright light and out of children's reach.

Evaluation
- Patient responds well to therapy.
- Patient maintains adequate hydration.
- Patient and family state understanding of drug therapy.

rimantadine hydrochloride
(righ-MAN-tuh-deen high-droh-KLOR-ighd)
Flumadine

Pharmacologic class: adamantine
Therapeutic class: antiviral
Pregnancy risk category: C

Indications and dosages

▶ **Prevention of influenza A virus.** *Adults and children age 10 and over:* 100 mg P.O. b.i.d.
Elderly patients, patients with severe hepatic or renal dysfunction: 100 mg P.O. daily.
Children under age 10: 5 mg/kg (not to exceed 150 mg/day) P.O. once daily.
▶ **Treatment of influenza A virus infection.** *Adults:* 100 mg P.O. b.i.d. for 7 days from onset of symptoms.
Elderly patients, patients with severe hepatic or renal dysfunction: 100 mg P.O. daily.

How supplied

Tablets: 100 mg
Syrup: 50 mg/5 ml

Pharmacokinetics

Absorption: well absorbed from GI tract.

Distribution: plasma protein–binding is about 40%.
Metabolism: metabolized extensively in liver.
Excretion: excreted in urine. *Half-life:* 25½ to 32 hours.

Route	Onset	Peak	Duration
P.O.	Unknown	1-4 hr	Unknown

Pharmacodynamics

Chemical effect: unknown; appears to prevent viral uncoating, an early step in viral reproductive cycle.
Therapeutic effect: inhibits viral reproduction. Spectrum of activity is influenza A virus.

Adverse reactions

CNS: insomnia, headache, dizziness, nervousness, fatigue, asthenia.
GI: nausea, vomiting, anorexia, dry mouth, abdominal pain.

Interactions

Drug-drug. *Acetaminophen, aspirin:* reduced rimantadine level. Monitor patient for decreased rimantadine effectiveness.
Cimetidine: may decrease rimantadine clearance. Monitor patient for adverse reactions.

Contraindications and precautions

- Contraindicated in breast-feeding women and patients hypersensitive to drug or amantadine.
- Use cautiously in pregnant women, patients with renal or hepatic impairment, and patients with a history of seizures.

NURSING CONSIDERATIONS

Assessment

- Obtain history of patient's exposure to influenza A virus before therapy, and reassess regularly thereafter.
- Monitor patient's hydration status throughout rimantadine therapy.
- Evaluate patient's and family's knowledge of drug therapy.

Nursing diagnoses

- Infection related to exposure to influenza A virus
- Risk for deficient fluid volume related to drug-induced adverse GI reactions
- Deficient knowledge related to drug therapy

Planning and implementation

- Give within 48 hours of onset of influenza symptoms and continue for 7 days after signs and symptoms appeared.
- Consider risk to contacts of treated patients, who may be subject to morbidity from influenza A. Influenza A–resistant strains can emerge during therapy. Patients taking drug may still be able to spread disease.

ALERT Don't confuse rimantadine with amantadine.

Patient teaching

- Instruct patient to take drug several hours before bedtime to prevent insomnia.

Evaluation

- Patient is free from infection.
- Patient maintains adequate hydration throughout therapy.
- Patient and family state understanding of drug therapy.

Ringer's injection

(RING-erz in-JEK-shun)

Pharmacologic class: electrolyte solution
Therapeutic class: electrolyte and fluid replenishment
Pregnancy risk category: NR

Indications and dosages

▶ **Fluid and electrolyte replacement.** *Adults and children:* dosage highly individualized; usually 1.5 to 3 L (2% to 6% body weight) infused I.V. over 18 to 24 hours.

How supplied

Injection: 250 ml, 500 ml, 1,000 ml

Pharmacokinetics

Absorption: not applicable with I.V. administration.
Distribution: widely distributed.
Metabolism: not significant.

Excretion: excreted primarily in urine and minimally in feces.

Route	Onset	Peak	Duration
I.V.	Immediate	Immediate	Unknown

Pharmacodynamics

Chemical effect: replaces fluids and electrolytes.
Therapeutic effect: restores normal fluid and electrolyte balance.

Adverse reactions

CV: fluid overload.
Metabolic: electrolyte imbalance.

Interactions

None significant.

Contraindications and precautions

- Contraindicated in patients with renal failure, except as emergency volume expander.
- Use cautiously in pregnant women and patients with heart failure, circulatory insufficiency, renal dysfunction, hypoproteinemia, or pulmonary edema.

NURSING CONSIDERATIONS

Assessment

- Obtain history of patient's fluid and electrolyte status before therapy, and reassess regularly thereafter.
- Be alert for fluid overload.
- Evaluate patient's and family's knowledge of drug therapy.

Nursing diagnoses

- Deficient fluid volume related to underlying condition
- Deficient knowledge related to drug therapy

Planning and implementation

- Drug contains sodium, 147 mEq/L; potassium, 4 mEq/L; calcium, 4.5 mEq/L; and chloride, 155.5 mEq/L.
- Electrolyte content isn't enough to treat severe electrolyte deficiencies, but it does provide electrolytes in levels approximating those of blood.

ALERT Don't confuse Ringer's injection with Ringer's lactate solutions.

Patient teaching
- Inform patient of need for drug, and instruct him to report signs of fluid overload, such as difficulty breathing.

Evaluation

- Patient regains normal fluid and electrolyte balance.
- Patient and family state understanding of drug therapy.

Ringer's injection, lactated (Hartmann's solution, Ringer's lactate solution)

(RING-erz in-JEK-shun, LAK-tayt-ed)

Pharmacologic class: electrolyte-carbohydrate solution
Therapeutic class: electrolyte and fluid replenishment
Pregnancy risk category: NR

Indications and dosages

▶ **Fluid and electrolyte replacement.** *Adults and children:* dosage highly individualized according to patient's size and clinical condition.

How supplied

Injection: 150 ml, 250 ml, 500 ml, 1,000 ml

Pharmacokinetics

Absorption: not applicable with I.V. administration.
Distribution: widely distributed.
Metabolism: not significant for electrolytes. Lactate is oxidized to bicarbonate.
Excretion: excreted primarily in urine and minimally in feces.

Route	Onset	Peak	Duration
I.V.	Immediate	Immediate	Unknown

Pharmacodynamics

Chemical effect: replaces fluids and electrolytes.
Therapeutic effect: restores normal fluid and electrolyte balance.

Adverse reactions

CV: fluid overload.
Metabolic: electrolyte imbalance.

Interactions

None significant.

Contraindications and precautions

- Contraindicated in patients with renal failure, except as emergency volume expander.
- Use cautiously in pregnant women and patients with heart failure, circulatory insufficiency, renal dysfunction, hypoproteinemia, or pulmonary edema.

NURSING CONSIDERATIONS

Assessment
- Obtain history of patient's fluid and electrolyte status before therapy, and reassess regularly thereafter.
- Be alert for fluid overload.
- Evaluate patient's knowledge of drug therapy.

Nursing diagnoses
- Deficient fluid volume related to underlying condition
- Deficient knowledge related to drug therapy

Planning and implementation
- Drug contains sodium, 130 mEq/L; potassium, 4 mEq/L; calcium, 3 mEq/L; chloride, 109.7 mEq/L; and lactate, 28 mEq/L.
- Lactated Ringer's injection approximates electrolyte concentration in blood plasma.

ALERT Don't confuse Ringer's lactate solutions with Ringer's injection.

Patient teaching
- Inform patient of need for drug. Instruct him to report signs of fluid overload, such as difficulty breathing.

Evaluation
- Patient regains normal fluid and electrolyte balance.
- Patient and family state understanding of drug therapy.

risperidone
(ris-PER-ih-dohn)
Risperdal

Pharmacologic class: benzisoxazole derivative
Therapeutic class: antipsychotic
Pregnancy risk category: C

Indications and dosages

▶ **Psychosis.** *Adults:* initially, 1 mg P.O. b.i.d. Increased in increments of 1 mg b.i.d. on days 2 and 3 of treatment to target dose of 3 mg b.i.d. At least 1 week must pass before dosage is adjusted further.
Elderly or debilitated patients, hypotensive patients, patients with severe renal or hepatic impairment: initially, 0.5 mg P.O. b.i.d. Increased in increments of 0.5 mg b.i.d. on days 2 and 3 of treatment to target dosage of 1.5 mg P.O. b.i.d. At least 1 week must pass before dosage is increased further.

How supplied

Tablets: 1 mg, 2 mg, 3 mg, 4 mg
Oral solution: 1 mg/ml

Pharmacokinetics

Absorption: well absorbed; absolute oral bioavailability is 70%.
Distribution: plasma protein–binding is about 90% for risperidone and 77% for its major active metabolite.
Metabolism: extensively metabolized in liver.
Excretion: metabolite excreted in urine.

Route	Onset	Peak	Duration
P.O.	Unknown	About 1 hr	Unknown

Pharmacodynamics

Chemical effect: blocks dopamine and serotonin receptors as well as $alpha_1$, $alpha_2$, and H_1 receptors in CNS.

Therapeutic effect: relieves signs and symptoms of psychosis.

Adverse reactions

CNS: *somnolence, extrapyramidal symptoms,* headache, *insomnia, agitation, anxiety,* tardive dyskinesia, aggressiveness, sedation, ***neuroleptic malignant syndrome.***
CV: tachycardia, chest pain, orthostatic hypotension, ***prolonged QT interval.***
EENT: *rhinitis,* sinusitis, pharyngitis, abnormal vision.
GI: *constipation, nausea, vomiting, dyspepsia.*
Metabolic: weight gain.
Musculoskeletal: arthralgia, back pain.
Respiratory: coughing, upper respiratory tract infection.
Skin: rash, dry skin, photosensitivity.
Other: fever.

Interactions

Drug-drug. *Carbamazepine:* increased risperidone clearance, leading to decreased effectiveness. Monitor patient closely.
Clozapine: decreased risperidone clearance, increasing toxicity. Monitor patient closely.
CNS depressants: additive CNS depression. Avoid concomitant use.
Levodopa: antagonized effects. Don't use together.
Drug-lifestyle. *Alcohol use:* additive CNS depression. Discourage concomitant use.
Sun exposure: increased photosensitivity reactions. Discourage prolonged or unprotected sun exposure.

Contraindications and precautions

- Contraindicated in patients hypersensitive to drug and in breast-feeding women.
- Use with extreme caution in pregnant women.
- Use cautiously in patients with prolonged QT interval, CV disease, cerebrovascular disease, dehydration, hypovolemia, history of seizures, exposure to extreme heat, or conditions that could affect metabolism or hemodynamic responses.
- Safety of drug hasn't been established in children.

NURSING CONSIDERATIONS

Assessment

- Assess patient's psychosis before therapy and regularly thereafter.
- Assess blood pressure before therapy, and monitor regularly. Watch for orthostatic hypotension, especially during dosage adjustment.
- Be alert for adverse reactions and drug interactions.

ALERT Watch for tardive dyskinesia. It may occur after prolonged use; it may not appear until months or years later and may disappear spontaneously or persist for life despite stopping drug.

- Evaluate patient's and family's knowledge of drug therapy.

Nursing diagnoses

- Disturbed thought processes related to presence of psychosis
- Risk for injury related to drug-induced adverse CNS reactions
- Deficient knowledge related to drug therapy

Planning and implementation

- When restarting therapy for patient who has been off drug, follow 3-day dose initiation schedule.
- When switching patient to drug from another antipsychotic, stop other drug immediately when risperidone therapy starts, as directed.

Patient teaching

- Warn patient to rise slowly, avoid hot showers, and use extra caution during first few days of therapy to avoid fainting.
- Warn patient to avoid activities that require alertness until CNS effects of drug are known. Drowsiness and dizziness usually subside after a few days.
- Tell patient to avoid alcohol during therapy.
- Advise patient to use caution in hot weather to prevent heatstroke; drug may affect thermoregulation.
- Tell patient to use sunblock and to wear protective clothing.
- Tell woman to notify prescriber if she is or plans to become pregnant.

Evaluation
- Patient behavior and communication indicate improved thought processes.
- Patient doesn't experience injury as result of drug-induced adverse CNS reactions.
- Patient and family state understanding of drug therapy.

ritodrine hydrochloride
(RIGH-toh-dreen high-droh-KLOR-ighd)
Yutopar

Pharmacologic class: beta-receptor agonist
Therapeutic class: adjunct agent in suppression of preterm labor
Pregnancy risk category: B

Indications and dosages
▶ **Preterm labor.** *Adults:* usual initial dose is 0.05 mg/minute I.V., gradually increased by 0.05 mg/minute q 10 minutes until desired result is obtained or maternal heart rate is 130 beats/minute. Effective dosage is usually 0.15 to 0.35 mg/minute. Oral maintenance: 10 mg P.O. about 30 minutes before I.V. therapy stopped. Usual dosage for first 24 hours of maintenance is 10 mg P.O. q 2 hours. Then, 10 to 20 mg P.O. q 4 to 6 hours. Maximum daily dosage is 120 mg.

How supplied
Tablets: 10 mg
Injection: 10 mg/ml, 15 mg/ml

Pharmacokinetics
Absorption: 30% absorbed after P.O. dose. Food may inhibit absorption and effectiveness of oral drug.
Distribution: distributed to tissues; protein binding is low.
Metabolism: metabolized in liver.
Excretion: about 70% to 90% excreted in urine.

Route	Onset	Peak	Duration
P.O.	30-60 min	Unknown	Unknown
I.V.	5 min	Unknown	Unknown

Pharmacodynamics
Chemical effect: stimulates $beta_2$-adrenergic receptors in uterine smooth muscle, inhibiting contractility.
Therapeutic effect: stops uterine contractions.

Adverse reactions
CNS: nervousness, anxiety, *headache, tremors,* emotional upset, malaise.
CV: dose-related alterations in blood pressure, palpitations, ***pulmonary edema,*** *tachycardia.*
GI: *nausea, vomiting.*
Hematologic: ***leukopenia, agranulocytosis.***
Metabolic: *hyperglycemia,* hypokalemia.
Other: *erythema,* ***anaphylactic shock.***

Interactions
Drug-drug. *Atropine:* may potentiate systemic hypertension. Monitor blood pressure.
Beta blockers: may inhibit action of ritodrine. Avoid concurrent use.
Corticosteroids: may produce pulmonary edema in mother. Monitor patient closely.
Inhaled anesthetics: potentiated adverse cardiac effects, arrhythmias, and hypotension. Monitor patient.
Sympathomimetics: additive sympathomimetic effects. Use together cautiously.

Contraindications and precautions
- Contraindicated in patients hypersensitive to drug; pregnant women before week 20 of gestation; women with maternal medical conditions that would be seriously affected by pharmacologic properties of drug, such as hypovolemia, pheochromocytoma, or uncontrolled hypertension; and women with antepartum hemorrhage, eclampsia, intrauterine fetal death, chorioamnionitis, maternal cardiac disease, pulmonary hypertension, maternal hyperthyroidism, or uncontrolled maternal diabetes mellitus.
- Use cautiously in patients with sulfite sensitivity.

NURSING CONSIDERATIONS

Assessment
- Assess patient's uterine contractions before therapy and regularly thereafter.

• Because CV responses are common and more pronounced during I.V. administration, monitor CV effects, including maternal pulse rate and blood pressure and fetal heart rate. Maternal tachycardia of over 140 beats/minute or persistent respiratory rate of over 20 breaths/minute may signal impending pulmonary edema.
• Monitor blood glucose levels during infusion, especially in diabetic mother.
• Monitor amount of fluids given I.V. to prevent circulatory overload.
• Be alert for adverse reactions and drug interactions.
• Evaluate patient's and family's knowledge of drug therapy.

Nursing diagnoses

• Acute pain related to uterine contractions
• Risk for deficient fluid volume related to drug-induced adverse GI reactions
• Deficient knowledge related to drug therapy

Planning and implementation

P.O. use: Follow normal protocol. Start therapy about 30 minutes before I.V. therapy stops.
I.V. use: Dilute 150 mg (3 ampules) in 500 ml of fluid (final concentration is 0.3 mg/ml).
– Continue I.V. infusion for 12 hours after contractions have stopped.
– Don't use ritodrine I.V. if solution is discolored or contains precipitate.
– Use solution within 48 hours of preparation.
• Discontinue drug and notify prescriber if pulmonary edema develops.
ALERT Don't confuse ritodrine with ranitidine.

Patient teaching
• Caution patient not to stop taking oral drug without medical approval.
• Advise patient to keep scheduled follow-up appointments and to report adverse reactions promptly.

Evaluation

• Patient's uterine contractions cease.
• Patient maintains adequate fluid balance throughout therapy.
• Patient and family state understanding of drug therapy.

ritonavir

(rih-TOH-nuh-veer)
Norvir

Pharmacologic class: protease inhibitor
Therapeutic class: antiviral
Pregnancy risk category: B

Indications and dosages

▶ **Treatment of HIV infection in combination with nucleoside analogues or as monotherapy when antiretroviral therapy is warranted.** *Adults:* 600 mg P.O. b.i.d with meals. If nausea occurs, dosage escalation may provide relief: 300 mg b.i.d. for 1 day, 400 mg b.i.d. for 2 days, 500 mg b.i.d. for 1 day, and 600 mg b.i.d. thereafter.

How supplied

Capsules: 100 mg
Oral solution: 80 mg/ml

Pharmacokinetics

Absorption: food enhances absorption.
Distribution: absolute bioavailability unknown; 98% to 100% bound to serum albumin.
Metabolism: in liver and kidneys.
Excretion: in urine and feces.

Route	Onset	Peak	Duration
P.O.	Unknown	2-4 hr	Unknown

Pharmacodynamics

Chemical effect: HIV protease inhibitor with activity against HIV-1 and HIV-2 proteases; binds to protease-active site and inhibits enzyme activity.
Therapeutic effect: prevents cleavage of viral polyproteins, resulting in formation of immature noninfectious viral particles.

Adverse reactions

CNS: *asthenia,* headache, malaise, circumoral paresthesia, dizziness, insomnia, paresthesia,

peripheral paresthesia, somnolence, thinking abnormality, migraine headache.
CV: vasodilation.
EENT: local throat irritation, diplopia, blepharitis, pharyngitis, photophobia.
GI: abdominal pain, anorexia, constipation, *diarrhea, nausea, vomiting, taste perversion,* dyspepsia, flatulence.
Hematologic: decreased hemoglobin level, decreased hematocrit, ***leukopenia, thrombocytopenia.***
Hepatic: elevated transaminase levels.
Metabolic: increased CK level, hyperlipidemia.
Musculoskeletal: myalgia.
Skin: rash, sweating.
Other: fever.

Interactions

Drug-drug. *Drugs that increase CYP3A activity (carbamazepine, dexamethasone, phenobarbital, phenytoin, rifabutin, rifampin):* may increase ritonavir clearance and decrease plasma ritonavir levels. Monitor patient closely.
Alprazolam, clorazepate, diazepam, estazolam, flurazepam, midazolam, triazolam, zolpidem: significantly increased levels of these drugs. Because of potential for extreme sedation and respiratory depression, don't administer these drugs concurrently with ritonavir.
Amiodarone, bepridil, bupropion, clozapine, encainide, flecainide, meperidine, piroxicam, propafenone, propoxyphene, quinidine, rifabutin: significantly increased plasma levels of these drugs, which increases patient's risk of arrhythmias, hematologic abnormalities, seizures, or other potentially serious adverse effects. Don't administer drugs concurrently.
Clarithromycin: reduced creatinine clearance. Patients with impaired renal function receiving drug with ritonavir need 50% reduction in clarithromycin if creatinine clearance is 30 to 60 ml/minute and a 75% reduction if it's below 30 ml/minute.
Desipramine: increased serum desipramine levels. Monitor patient.
Disulfiram or other drugs that produce disulfiram-like reactions (metronidazole): increased risk of disulfiram-like reactions (alcohol in ritonavir formulation). Monitor patient closely.
Glucuronosyltransferases: may increase activity of these drugs and decrease therapeutic effects. If used concomitantly, monitor drug levels. Dosage reduction greater than 50% may be required for drugs extensively metabolized by CYP3A.
Oral contraceptives that contain ethinyl estradiol: decreased serum contraceptive levels. Concomitant therapy may require higher oral contraceptive dosage or alternative method.
Saquinavir: inhibited saquinavir metabolism, resulting in increased plasma levels. Monitor patient for toxicity.
Theophylline: decreased serum theophylline levels. Monitor theophylline level.
Drug-herb. *St. John's wort:* substantially reduced blood drug levels, which could cause loss of therapeutic effects. Discourage concomitant use.
Drug-food. *Any food:* increased absorption. Give drug with food.
Drug-lifestyle. *Smoking:* decreased serum levels of drug. Advise against tobacco use.

Contraindications and precautions

- Contraindicated in patients hypersensitive to drug.

NURSING CONSIDERATIONS

Assessment

- Use cautiously in patients with hepatic insufficiency.
- Evaluate patient's and family's understanding of drug therapy.

Nursing diagnoses

- Infection related to presence of virus
- Deficient knowledge related to drug therapy

Planning and implementation

- It's unclear if drug appears in breast milk.

Patient teaching

- Inform patient that drug isn't a cure for HIV infection and that illnesses caused by HIV infection may occur. Drug doesn't reduce risk of HIV transmission.
- Tell patient that the taste of oral solution may be improved by mixing with flavored milk within 1 hour of dose.

• Tell patient to take drug with meal.
• If a dose is missed, instruct patient to take next dose at once; he shouldn't double doses.
• Advise patient to report use of other drugs, including OTC drugs.
• Tell patient to stop breast-feeding to prevent transmission of HIV.

☑ Evaluation
• Patient's infection is eradicated.
• Patient and family state understanding of drug therapy.

rizatriptan benzoate

(rih-zah-TRIP-tin BEN-zoh-ayt)
Maxalt, Maxalt-MLT

Pharmacologic class: selective 5-hydroxytryptamine (5-HT_1) receptor agonist
Therapeutic class: antimigraine agent
Pregnancy risk category: C

Indications and dosages

▶ **Treatment of acute migraine headaches with or without aura.** *Adults:* initially, 5 to 10 mg P.O. If first dose is ineffective, another dose can be given at least 2 hours after first dose. Maximum, 30 mg daily. For patients taking propranolol, 5 mg P.O., up to maximum of three doses (15 mg total) in 24 hours.

How supplied

Tablets: 5 mg, 10 mg
Tablets (disintegrating): 5 mg, 10 mg

Pharmacokinetics

Absorption: completely absorbed with an absolute bioavailability of 45%.
Distribution: widely distributed, 14 % bound to plasma proteins.
Metabolism: primarily by oxidative deamination by MAO-A.
Excretion: excreted primarily in the urine (82%). *Half-life:* 2 to 3 hours.

Route	Onset	Peak	Duration
P.O.	Unknown	1-1.5 hr	Unknown

Pharmacodynamics

Chemical effect: believed to exert its effect by acting as an agonist at serotonin receptors on extracerebral intracranial blood vessels, which results in vasoconstriction of the affected vessels, inhibition of neuropeptide release, and reduction of pain transmission in the trigeminal pathways.
Therapeutic effect: relieves migraine pain.

Adverse reactions

CNS: dizziness, headache, somnolence, paresthesia, asthenia, fatigue, hypesthesia, decreased mental acuity, euphoria, tremor.
CV: chest pain, pressure or heaviness, palpitations, ***coronary artery vasospasm.***
EENT: neck, throat, and jaw pain, pressure, or heaviness.
GI: dry mouth, nausea, diarrhea, vomiting.
Respiratory: dyspnea.
Skin: flushing.
Other: pain, warm or cold sensations, hot flushes.

Interactions

Drug-drug. *Ergot-containing or ergot-type drugs (dihydroergotamine, methysergide), other 5-HT_1 agonists:* prolonged vasospastic reactions. Don't use within 24 hours of rizatriptan.
MAO inhibitors (moclobemide), nonselective MAO inhibitors (types A and B; isocarboxazid, pargyline, phenelzine, tranylcypromine): increased plasma rizatriptan levels. Avoid concurrent use, and allow at least 14 days between stopping an MAO inhibitor and taking rizatriptan.
Propranolol: increased rizatriptan levels. Reduce rizatriptan dose to 5 mg.
Selective serotonin reuptake inhibitors (fluoxetine, fluvoxamine, paroxetine, sertraline): weakness, hyperreflexia, incoordination may occur. Monitor patient.

Contraindications and precautions

• Contraindicated in patients with ischemic heart disease (angina pectoris, history of MI, or documented silent ischemia) or those with evidence of ischemic heart disease, coronary artery vasospasm (Prinzmetal's variant angina), or other significant underlying CV dis-

ease. Also contraindicated in patients with uncontrolled hypertension and within 24 hours of treatment with another 5-HT_1 agonist or with ergotamine-containing or ergot-type drugs such as dihydroergotamine or methysergide.
• Don't use within 2 weeks of an MAO inhibitor.
• Also contraindicated in patients hypersensitive to drug or its inactive ingredients.
• Use cautiously in patients with hepatic or renal impairment.
• Use cautiously in patients with risk factors for coronary artery disease (hypertension, hypercholesterolemia, smoking, obesity, diabetes, strong family history of coronary artery disease, women with surgical or physiologic menopause, or men over age 40), unless a cardiac evaluation provides evidence that patient is free from cardiac disease.

NURSING CONSIDERATIONS

Assessment
• Use drug only after a definite diagnosis of migraine is established.
• Assess patient for history of coronary artery disease, hypertension, arrhythmias, or presence of risk factors for coronary artery disease.
• Perform baseline and periodic CV evaluation in patients who develop risk factors for coronary artery disease during treatment.
• Monitor renal and liver function tests before starting drug therapy, and report abnormalities.
• Evaluate patient's and family's knowledge of drug therapy.

Nursing diagnoses
• Acute pain related to presence of migraine headache
• Risk for activity intolerance related to adverse drug reactions
• Deficient knowledge related to drug therapy

Planning and implementation
• Don't administer to patients with hemiplegic migraine, basilar migraine, or cluster headaches.
ALERT Don't administer drug within 24 hours of an ergot-containing drug or 5-HT_1 agonist or within 2 weeks of an MAO inhibitor.
• For patients with cardiac risk factors who have had a satisfactory cardiac evaluation, give first dose while monitoring ECG and have emergency equipment readily available.
• Withhold drug and notify prescriber if patient develops palpitations or neck, throat, or jaw pain, pressure, or heaviness.
• Safety of treating, on average, more than four headaches in a 30-day period hasn't been established.
• Safety and effectiveness haven't been evaluated in children under age 18.
• Drug contains phenylalanine.

Patient teaching
• Inform patient that drug doesn't prevent headache.
• For Maxalt-MLT, tell patient to remove blister pack from sachet and to remove drug from blister pack immediately before use. Tell him not to pop tablet out of blister pack but to carefully peel pack away with dry hands, place tablet on tongue, and let it dissolve. Tablet is then swallowed with saliva. No water is needed or recommended. Tell patient that dissolving tablet doesn't provide more rapid headache relief.
• Advise patient that if headache returns after first dose, a second dose may be taken with medical approval at least 2 hours after the first dose. Don't take more than 30 mg in a 24-hour period.
• Tell patient that food may delay onset of drug action.
• Advise patient to notify prescriber if pregnancy occurs or is suspected.
• Instruct patient not to breast-feed because the effects on the infant are unknown.

Evaluation
• Patient has relief from migraine headache.
• Patient maintains baseline activity level.
• Patient and family state understanding of drug therapy.

rocuronium bromide
(roh-kyoo-ROH-nee-um BROH-mighd)
Zemuron

Pharmacologic class: nondepolarizing neuromuscular blocker
Therapeutic class: skeletal muscle relaxant
Pregnancy risk category: B

Indications and dosages

▶ **Adjunct to general anesthesia, to facilitate endotracheal intubation, and to provide skeletal muscle relaxation during surgery or mechanical ventilation.** Dosage depends on anesthetic used, individual needs, and response. Dosages are representative and must be adjusted.
Adults and children age 3 months or older: initially, 0.6 mg/kg (adults, up to 1.2 mg/kg) I.V. bolus. In most patients, perform tracheal intubation within 2 minutes; muscle paralysis should last about 31 minutes. A maintenance dosage of 0.1 mg/kg should provide additional 12 minutes of muscle relaxation, 0.15 mg/kg will add 17 minutes, and 0.2 mg/kg will add 24 minutes to duration of effect.

How supplied

Injection: 10 mg/ml

Pharmacokinetics

Absorption: not applicable.
Distribution: about 30% bound to human plasma proteins.
Metabolism: unknown, although hepatic clearance may be significant.
Excretion: about 33% excreted in urine.

Route	Onset	Peak	Duration
I.V.	≤ 1 min	≤ 2 min	Dose-dependent

Pharmacodynamics

Chemical effect: prevents acetylcholine from binding to receptors on motor end plate, thus blocking depolarization.
Therapeutic effect: relaxes skeletal muscles.

Adverse reactions

CV: tachycardia, abnormal ECG, ***arrhythmias,*** transient hypotension, hypertension.
GI: nausea, vomiting.
Respiratory: hiccups, asthma, ***respiratory insufficiency, apnea.***
Skin: rash, edema, pruritus.

Interactions

Drug-drug. *Aminoglycoside antibiotics (including amikacin, gentamicin, kanamycin, neomycin, streptomycin), anticonvulsants, clindamycin, general anesthetics (such as enflurane, halothane, isoflurane), opioid analgesics, polymyxin antibiotics (colistin, polymyxin B sulfate), quinidine, succinylcholine, tetracyclines:* potentiated neuromuscular blockade, leading to increased skeletal muscle relaxation and potentiation of effect. Use cautiously during surgical and postoperative periods.

Contraindications and precautions

- Contraindicated in patients hypersensitive to bromides.
- Use cautiously in pregnant women and patients with hepatic disease, severe obesity, bronchogenic carcinoma, electrolyte disturbances, neuromuscular disease, and altered circulation time caused by CV disease, old age, or edema.
- Safety of drug hasn't been established in breast-feeding women.

NURSING CONSIDERATIONS

Assessment

- Assess patient's condition before therapy and regularly thereafter.
- Be alert for adverse reactions and drug interactions.
- Monitor patients with liver disease; they may need higher doses to achieve adequate muscle relaxation and may exhibit prolonged effects from drug.
- Monitor respirations closely until patient is fully recovered from neuromuscular blockade, as evidenced by tests of muscle strength (hand grip, head lift, and ability to cough).

• Evaluate patient's and family's knowledge of drug therapy.

Nursing diagnoses
• Ineffective health maintenance related to underlying condition
• Ineffective breathing pattern related to drug's effect on respiratory muscles
• Deficient knowledge related to drug therapy

Planning and implementation
• Drug should be used only by personnel skilled in airway management.
• Administer sedatives or general anesthetics before neuromuscular blockers, as ordered, because neuromuscular blockers don't obtund consciousness or alter pain perception.
• Give analgesics, as ordered, for pain.
• Keep airway clear. Have emergency respiratory support equipment (endotracheal equipment, ventilator, oxygen, atropine, edrophonium, epinephrine, and neostigmine) on hand.
• Give drug by rapid I.V. injection or continuous I.V. infusion. Infusion rates are highly individualized but range from 0.004 to 0.16 mg/kg/minute. Compatible solutions include D_5W, normal saline solution for injection, dextrose 5% in normal saline solution for injection, sterile water for injection, and lactated Ringer's injection.
• Store reconstituted solution in refrigerator. Discard after 24 hours.
• Nerve stimulator and train-of-four monitoring are recommended to confirm antagonism of neuromuscular blockade and recovery of muscle strength. Before attempting pharmacologic reversal with neostigmine, some evidence of spontaneous recovery should be evident.
• Prior administration of succinylcholine may enhance neuromuscular blocking effect and duration of action.

Patient teaching
• Explain all events and happenings to patient because he can still hear.
• Reassure patient that he is being monitored and that muscle use will return when drug has worn off.

Evaluation
• Patient has positive response to drug therapy.
• Patient maintains adequate breathing pattern with mechanical assistance throughout therapy.
• Patient and family state understanding of drug therapy.

rofecoxib
(roh-feh-COKS-ib)
Vioxx

Pharmacologic class: cyclooxygenase-2 (COX-2) inhibitor
Therapeutic class: nonnarcotic analgesic, anti-inflammatory
Pregnancy risk category: C

Indications and dosages
▶ **Relief of signs and symptoms of osteoarthritis.** *Adults:* initially, 12.5 mg P.O. once daily, increased as needed to maximum of 25 mg P.O. once daily.
▶ **Management of acute pain, treatment of primary dysmenorrhea.** *Adults:* 50 mg P.O. once daily as needed for up to 5 days.

How supplied
Tablets: 12.5 mg, 25 mg
Oral suspension: 12.5 mg/5 ml, 25 mg/5 ml

Pharmacokinetics
Absorption: well absorbed, with a mean bioavailability of 93%. Serum levels peak in 2 to 3 hours (median); range is 2 to 9 hours.
Distribution: about 87% of drug binds to proteins.
Metabolism: metabolized in liver to inactive metabolites.
Excretion: eliminated mainly through hepatic metabolism. Less than 1% of drug is eliminated via the kidneys as unchanged drug. *Half-life:* about 17 hours.

Route	Onset	Peak	Duration
P.O.	Unknown	2-3 hr	Unknown

Pharmacodynamics

Chemical effect: unknown; anti-inflammatory, analgesic, and antipyretic effects may stem from inhibited prostaglandin synthesis caused by inhibited COX-2 isoenzyme. At therapeutic serum levels, rofecoxib doesn't inhibit cyclooxygenase-1 (COX-1) isoenzyme.
Therapeutic effect: relieves inflammation and pain.

Adverse reactions

CNS: headache, asthenia, fatigue, dizziness.
CV: hypertension, leg edema.
EENT: sinusitis.
GI: diarrhea, dyspepsia, epigastric discomfort, heartburn, nausea, abdominal pain.
GU: urinary tract infection.
Musculoskeletal: back pain.
Respiratory: bronchitis, upper respiratory tract infection.
Other: flu syndrome.

Interactions

Drug-drug. *ACE inhibitors:* decreased antihypertensive effects of ACE inhibitors. Monitor patient closely.
Aspirin: increased rate of GI ulceration and other complications. Don't use together, if possible. If used together, monitor patient closely for GI bleeding.
Furosemide, thiazide diuretics: potentially reduced efficacy of these drugs. Monitor patient closely.
Lithium: increased plasma lithium levels and decreased lithium clearance. Monitor patient closely for toxic reaction to lithium.
Methotrexate: increased plasma methotrexate levels. Monitor patient closely for toxic reaction to methotrexate.
Rifampin: decreased rofecoxib levels by about 50%. Start therapy with a higher dosage of rofecoxib.
Warfarin: increased effects of warfarin. Monitor INR frequently for a few days after therapy starts or dosage changes.
Drug-lifestyle. *Chronic alcohol use, smoking:* increased risk of GI bleeding. Discourage concurrent use, and assess patient for bleeding.

Contraindications and precautions

- Contraindicated in patients hypersensitive to rofecoxib or any of its components and in patients who have experienced asthma, urticaria, or allergic-type reactions after taking aspirin or other NSAIDs.
- Drug should be avoided in patients with advanced kidney disease or moderate or severe hepatic insufficiency and in pregnant patients because it may cause the ductus arteriosus to close prematurely.
- Use cautiously in patients with asthma, renal disease, liver dysfunction, or abnormal liver function tests. Also use cautiously in patients with a history of ulcer disease or GI bleeding.
- Use cautiously in patients being treated with oral corticosteroids or anticoagulants, patients with a history of smoking or alcoholism, and elderly or debilitated patients because of the increased risk of GI bleeding.
- Use cautiously in patients with considerable dehydration. Rehydration is recommended before therapy begins.
- Use cautiously and start therapy at the lowest recommended dosage in patients with fluid retention, hypertension, or heart failure.

NURSING CONSIDERATIONS

Assessment

- Obtain history of patient's underlying condition before therapy, and reassess regularly thereafter.
- Ask patient if he has allergies to aspirin or other NSAIDs.
- Ask patient if he has asthma. Don't give drug if patient has had severe, potentially fatal bronchospasm after taking aspirin or other NSAIDs.
- Assess patient for dehydration.
- Monitor kidney function closely in patients with renal disease. Drug isn't recommended for patients with advanced kidney disease.
- Monitor patient closely for GI bleeding, which can occur any time, with or without warning.
- Monitor patient for signs and symptoms of liver toxicity. Discontinue drug as ordered if signs and symptoms consistent with liver disease develop.

• Check hemoglobin level and hematocrit, as ordered, in patients undergoing long-term treatment if they experience signs or symptoms of anemia or blood loss.
• Evaluate patient's and family's knowledge about drug therapy.

Nursing diagnoses

• Acute pain related to underlying condition
• Risk for injury related to drug-induced adverse reactions
• Deficient knowledge related to drug therapy

Planning and implementation

• Shake oral suspension well before giving it. Patient may take drug with food to decrease GI upset.
ALERT If patient has fluid retention, hypertension, or heart failure, use cautiously and start therapy at lowest recommended dosage, as ordered. Monitor blood pressure and check patient for fluid retention or worsening heart failure.
• In patients older than age 65, drug therapy should start at lowest recommended dosage.
• NSAIDs may cause serious GI toxicity. To minimize the risk of an adverse GI event, use lowest effective rofecoxib dosage for shortest possible duration.
• If patient is dehydrated, rehydrate him as directed before therapy begins.

Patient teaching

• Tell patient that drug may be taken without regard to food, although taking it with food may decrease GI upset.
• Tell patient that the most common adverse effects are dyspepsia, epigastric discomfort, heartburn, and nausea. Taking drug with food may help minimize these effects.
• Tell patient to avoid aspirin, products that contain aspirin, and OTC anti-inflammatories such as ibuprofen (Advil) unless his prescriber has instructed him otherwise.
• Warn patient that he may experience GI bleeding. Signs and symptoms include bloody vomitus, blood in urine and stool, and black, tarry stools. Advise patient to seek medical advice if he experiences any of these signs or symptoms.
• Advise patient to report to prescriber rash, unexplained weight gain, or edema.
• Tell patient that all NSAIDs, including rofecoxib, may adversely affect the liver. Explain that signs and symptoms of liver toxicity include nausea, fatigue, lethargy, itching, jaundice, right upper quadrant tenderness, and flulike symptoms. Advise patient to stop therapy and seek immediate medical advice if he experiences any of these signs or symptoms.
• Instruct patient to inform her prescriber if she becomes pregnant or plans to become pregnant while taking drug.

Evaluation

• Patient is free from pain.
• Patient sustains no injury from drug-induced adverse reactions.
• Patient and family state understanding of drug therapy.

ropinirole hydrochloride

(roh-PIN-er-ohl high-droh-KLOR-ighd)
Requip

Pharmacologic class: nonergoline dopamine agonist
Therapeutic class: antiparkinsonian
Pregnancy risk category: C

Indications and dosages

▶ **Idiopathic Parkinson's disease.** *Adults:* initially, 0.25 mg P.O. t.i.d. Dosages can be adjusted weekly. After week 4, dosage may be increased by 1.5 mg/day on a weekly basis up to dosage of 9 mg/day and then increased weekly by up to 3 mg/day to maximum of 24 mg/day.

How supplied

Tablets: 0.25 mg, 0.5 mg, 1 mg, 2 mg, 5 mg

Pharmacokinetics

Absorption: rapid, with an absolute bioavailability of 55%.
Distribution: widely distributed, with about 40% bound to plasma protein.
Metabolism: extensively metabolized by the liver to inactive metabolites.

Excretion: less than 10% excreted unchanged in urine. *Half-life:* 6 hours.

Route	Onset	Peak	Duration
P.O.	Unknown	1-2 hr	6 hr

Pharmacodynamics

Chemical effect: unknown. A nonergoline dopamine agonist thought to stimulate postsynaptic dopamine D_2 receptors in the caudate-putamen in the brain.

Therapeutic effect: improves physical mobility in patients with parkinsonism.

Adverse reactions

Early Parkinson's disease (without levodopa)—

CNS: asthenia, *fatigue,* malaise, hallucinations, *dizziness,* aggravated Parkinson's disease, *somnolence,* headache, confusion, hyperkinesia, hypesthesia, vertigo, amnesia, impaired concentration.

CV: hypotension, orthostatic symptoms, hypertension, *syncope,* edema, chest pain, extrasystoles, ***atrial fibrillation,*** palpitations, tachycardia.

EENT: pharyngitis, abnormal vision, eye abnormality, xerophthalmia, rhinitis, sinusitis.

GI: dry mouth, *nausea, vomiting, dyspepsia,* flatulence, abdominal pain, anorexia, constipation, abdominal pain.

GU: urinary tract infection, impotence (male).

Respiratory: bronchitis, dyspnea.

Skin: flushing.

Other: *viral infection*, pain, increased sweating, yawning, peripheral ischemia.

Advanced Parkinson's disease (with levodopa)—

CNS: *dizziness,* aggravated parkinsonism, *somnolence, headache,* insomnia, *hallucinations,* abnormal dreaming, confusion, tremor, anxiety, nervousness, amnesia, paresthesia.

CV: hypotension, syncope.

EENT: diplopia, increased saliva.

GI: *nausea,* abdominal pain, dry mouth, vomiting, constipation, diarrhea, dysphagia, flatulence.

GU: urinary tract infection, pyuria, urinary incontinence.

Hematologic: anemia.

Metabolic: weight loss.

Musculoskeletal: *dyskinesia,* hypokinesia, paresis, arthralgia, arthritis.

Respiratory: upper respiratory infection, dyspnea.

Skin: increased sweating.

Other: injury, *falls,* viral infection, pain.

Interactions

Drug-drug. *CNS depressants:* increased CNS effects. Use together cautiously.

Dopamine antagonists (bretyrophenones, metoclopramide, phenothiazines, thioxanthenes): may decrease ropinirole effectiveness. Monitor patient closely.

Estrogens: reduced ropinirole clearance. Adjust ropinirole dosage as directed if estrogens are started or stopped during ropinirole therapy.

Inhibitors or substrates of cytochrome P-450: altered ropinirole clearance. Adjust ropinirole dosage if drugs are started or stopped during ropinirole therapy.

Drug-lifestyle. *Alcohol use:* increased sedative effects. Discourage concurrent use.

Smoking: may increase drug clearance. Advise against concurrent use.

Contraindications and precautions

- Contraindicated in patients hypersensitive to drug.
- Use cautiously in patients with severe hepatic or renal impairment.

NURSING CONSIDERATIONS

Assessment

- Assess patient before and during therapy to evaluate effectiveness.
- Monitor patient carefully for orthostatic hypotension, especially during dose escalation.
- Assess patient for adequate nutritional intake.
- Evaluate patient's and family's knowledge of drug therapy.

Nursing diagnoses

- Impaired physical mobility related to underlying Parkinson's disease
- Disturbed thought processes related to drug-induced CNS adverse reactions

• Deficient knowledge related to drug therapy.

Planing and implementation
• Give drug with food to decrease nausea.
• Clearance is reduced in patients over age 65; dosage is individually adjusted to response.
• BUN and alkaline phosphatase levels may be increased during therapy.
• Drug can potentiate dopaminergic adverse effects of levodopa and may cause or worsen dyskinesia. Levodopa dosage may need to be decreased.
• Don't abruptly stop drug. Withdraw gradually over 7 days to avoid hyperpyrexia and confusion.

Patient teaching
• Tell patient to take drug with food if nausea occurs.
• Explain that hallucinations may occur, particularly in elderly patients.
• To minimize effects of orthostatic hypotension, instruct patient not to rise rapidly after sitting or lying down, especially when therapy starts or dosage changes,.
• Advise patient to avoid hazardous activities until CNS effects of drug are known.
• Tell patient to avoid alcohol during drug therapy.
• Tell woman to notify prescriber if pregnancy is suspected or is planned; also tell her to inform prescriber if she is breast-feeding.

Evaluation
• Patient has improved mobility and reduced muscle rigidity and tremor.
• Patient remains mentally alert.
• Patient and family state understanding of drug therapy.

rosiglitazone maleate
(roh-sih-GLIH-tah-zohn MAL-ee-ayt)
Avandia

Pharmacologic class: thiazolidinedione
Therapeutic class: antidiabetic
Pregnancy risk category: C

Indications and dosages
▶ **Monotherapy adjunct to diet and exercise to improve glycemic control in patients with type 2 diabetes mellitus; with metformin when diet, exercise, and rosiglitazone alone or diet, exercise, and metformin alone don't provide adequate glycemic control in patients with type 2 diabetes mellitus.** *Adults:* initially, 4 mg P.O. daily in the morning or in divided doses b.i.d. in the morning and evening. Dosage may be increased to 8 mg P.O. daily or in divided doses b.i.d. if fasting plasma glucose level doesn't improve after 12 weeks of treatment.
▶ **Adjunct to sulfonylureas, diet, and exercise in patients with type 2 diabetes mellitus.** *Adults:* 4 mg P.O. once daily or in two divided doses.

How supplied
Tablets: 2 mg, 4 mg, 8 mg

Pharmacokinetics
Absorption: plasma levels peak about 1 hour after a dose. Absolute bioavailability is 99%.
Distribution: about 99.8% of rosiglitazone binds to plasma proteins, primarily albumin.
Metabolism: extensively metabolized, with no unchanged drug excreted in the urine. Primarily metabolized through N-demethylation and hydroxylation.
Excretion: after oral administration, about 64% and 23% of the dose is eliminated in urine and feces, respectively. *Half-life:* 3 to 4 hours.

Route	Onset	Peak	Duration
P.O.	Unknown	1 hr	Unknown

Pharmacodynamics
Chemical effect: lowers blood glucose levels by improving insulin sensitivity. Highly selective and potent agonist for receptors in key target areas for insulin action, such as adipose tissue, skeletal muscle, and liver.
Therapeutic effect: lowers blood glucose levels.

Adverse reactions
CNS: headache, fatigue.
CV: edema.

EENT: sinusitis.
GI: diarrhea.
Hematologic: anemia.
Metabolic: hyperglycemia.
Musculoskeletal: back pain.
Respiratory: upper respiratory tract infection.
Other: injury.

Interactions

Drug-herb. *Aloe, bitter melon, bilberry leaf, burdock, dandelion, fenugreek, garlic, ginseng:* may improve blood glucose control. Patient may need reduced antidiabetic dosage. Advise against concurrent use.

Contraindications and precautions

- Contraindicated in patients hypersensitive to rosiglitazone or any of its components and in patients with New York Heart Association Class III and IV cardiac status unless expected benefits outweigh risks.
- Contraindicated in patients who developed jaundice while taking troglitazone and in patients with active liver disease, increased baseline liver enzyme levels (ALT level is greater than 2½ times the upper limit of normal), type 1 diabetes, or diabetic ketoacidosis.
- Combination therapy with metformin and rosiglitazone is contraindicated in patients with renal impairment. Rosiglitazone can be used as monotherapy in patients with renal impairment.
- Use cautiously in patients with edema or heart failure.

NURSING CONSIDERATIONS

Assessment

- Obtain history of patient's underlying condition before therapy, and reassess regularly thereafter.
- Check liver enzyme levels before therapy starts. Don't use drug in patients with increased baseline liver enzyme levels. In patients with normal baseline liver enzyme levels, these levels should be monitored every 2 months for the first 12 months of treatment and periodically afterward. If ALT level is elevated during treatment, recheck levels as soon as possible. Notify prescriber because drug should be stopped if levels remain elevated.
- Monitor blood glucose level regularly and glycosylated hemoglobin level periodically to determine therapeutic response to drug.
- If patient has heart failure, watch for increased edema during rosiglitazone therapy.
- Evaluate patient's and family's knowledge about drug therapy.

Nursing diagnoses

- Ineffective health maintenance related to hyperglycemia
- Risk for injury related to drug-induced hypoglycemia
- Deficient knowledge related to drug therapy

Planning and implementation

- Before starting rosiglitazone, patient should be treated for other causes of poor glycemic control, such as infection.
- Management of type 2 diabetes should include diet control. Because calorie restriction, weight loss, and exercise help improve insulin sensitivity and help make drug therapy effective, these measures are essential to proper diabetes treatment.
- For patients whose blood glucose levels are inadequately controlled with metformin, rosiglitazone should be added to, not substituted for, metformin.
- Hemoglobin level and hematocrit may decrease while patient is receiving this drug, usually during the first 4 to 8 weeks of therapy. Total cholesterol, low-density lipoprotein, and high-density lipoprotein levels may increase, and free fatty acid levels may decrease.
- Because ovulation may resume in premenopausal, anovulatory women with insulin resistance, contraceptive measures may need to be considered.

Patient teaching

- Advise patient that rosiglitazone can be taken with or without food.
- Notify patient that blood will be tested to check liver function before therapy starts,

every 2 months for the first 12 months, and periodically thereafter.
• Tell patient to immediately report unexplained signs and symptoms—such as nausea, vomiting, abdominal pain, fatigue, anorexia, or dark urine—because they may indicate liver problems.
• Inform premenopausal, anovulatory women with insulin resistance that ovulation may resume and that she may want to consider contraceptive measures.
• Advise patient that diabetes management should include diet control. Because calorie restriction, weight loss, and exercise help improve insulin sensitivity and help make drug therapy effective, these measures are essential to proper diabetes treatment.

Evaluation

• Patient's blood glucose level is normal with drug therapy.
• Patient doesn't experience hypoglycemia.
• Patient and family state understanding of drug therapy.

S

salmeterol xinafoate

(sal-MEE-ter-ohl zee-neh-FOH-ayt)
Serevent, Serevent Diskus

Pharmacologic class: selective $beta_2$-adrenergic agonist
Therapeutic class: bronchodilator
Pregnancy risk category: C

Indications and dosages

▶ **Long-term maintenance treatment of asthma; prevention of bronchospasm in patients with nocturnal asthma or reversible obstructive airway disease who need regular treatment with short-acting beta agonists. Inhalation aerosol.** *Adults and children over age 12:* 2 inhalations b.i.d., one in morning and one in evening. Drug shouldn't be used to treat acute symptoms.

Inhalation powder. *Adults and children over age 4:* 1 inhalation q 12 hours, one in the morning and one in the evening.

▶ **Prevention of exercise-induced bronchospasm. Inhalation aerosol.** *Adults and children age 12 and over:* 2 inhalations at least 30 to 60 minutes before exercise.

Inhalation powder. *Adults and children age 4 and older:* 1 inhalation at least 30 minutes before exercise.

▶ **Maintenance treatment of bronchospasm with COPD (including emphysema and chronic bronchitis).** *Adults:* 2 inhalations (42 mcg; inhalation aerosol) q 12 hours, in the morning and evening.

How supplied

Inhalation aerosol: 21 mcg per metered spray
Inhalation powder: 50 mcg/blister

Pharmacokinetics

Absorption: because of low therapeutic dose, systemic levels of drug are low or undetectable after inhalation of recommended doses.
Distribution: distributed locally to lungs; 94% to 99% bound to plasma proteins.
Metabolism: extensively metabolized by hydroxylation.
Excretion: excreted primarily in feces.

Route	Onset	Peak	Duration
Inhalation	10-20 min	About 3 hr	About 12 hr

Pharmacodynamics

Chemical effect: not clearly defined; selectively activates $beta_2$-adrenergic receptors, which results in bronchodilation. Drug also blocks release of allergic mediators from mast cells lining the respiratory tract.
Therapeutic effect: improves breathing ability.

Adverse reactions

CNS: *headache,* sinus headache, tremors, nervousness, dizziness.
CV: tachycardia, palpitations, ***ventricular arrhythmias.***
EENT: *upper respiratory tract infection, nasopharyngitis,* nasal cavity or sinus disorder.
GI: nausea, vomiting, diarrhea, heartburn.
Musculoskeletal: joint and back pain, myalgia.

Respiratory: cough, lower respiratory tract infection, ***bronchospasm.***
Other: ***hypersensitivity reactions.***

Interactions

Drug-drug. *Beta-adrenergic agonists, methylxanthines, theophylline:* possible adverse cardiac effects with excessive use. Monitor patient closely.
MAO inhibitors: risk of severe adverse CV effects. Avoid use within 14 days of MAO therapy.
Tricyclic antidepressants: risk of moderate to severe adverse CV effects. Use with extreme caution.

Contraindications and precautions

- Contraindicated in patients hypersensitive to drug or its components.
- Use cautiously in patients who are unusually responsive to sympathomimetics and patients with coronary insufficiency, arrhythmias, hypertension or other CV disorders, thyrotoxicosis, or seizure disorders. Also use cautiously in pregnant women.
- Safety of drug hasn't been established in breast-feeding women and in children age 12 or younger for inhalation aerosol (children younger than age 4 for inhalation powder).

NURSING CONSIDERATIONS

Assessment

- Assess patient's respiratory condition before therapy and regularly thereafter.
- Assess peak flow readings before starting treatment and periodically thereafter.
- Be alert for adverse reactions and drug interactions.
- Evaluate patient's and family's knowledge of drug therapy.

Nursing diagnoses

- Ineffective breathing pattern related to respiratory condition
- Acute pain related to drug-induced headache
- Deficient knowledge related to drug therapy

Planning and implementation

- Don't give drug for acute bronchospasm.
- Report insufficient relief or worsening condition.
- Obtain order for mild analgesic if drug-induced headache occurs.

ALERT Don't confuse Serevent with Serentil.

Patient teaching

- Tell patient to take drug at about 12-hour intervals and to take even when feeling better.
- Tell patient taking drug to prevent exercise-induced bronchospasm to take it 30 to 60 minutes before exercise.

ALERT Instruct patient not to take drug to treat acute bronchospasm. Patient must be provided with short-acting beta agonist (such as albuterol) to treat such exacerbations.

- Tell patient to contact prescriber if short-acting agonist no longer provides sufficient relief or if he needs more than four inhalations daily. This may be a sign that asthma symptoms are worsening. Tell patient not to increase dosage of drug.
- If patient is taking inhaled corticosteroid, he should continue to use it. Warn him not to take other drugs without prescriber's consent.

Evaluation

- Patient exhibits normal breathing pattern.
- Patient states that drug-induced headache is relieved after analgesic administration.
- Patient and family state understanding of drug therapy.

saquinavir
(sah-KWIN-ah-veer)
Fortovase

saquinavir mesylate
Invirase

Pharmacologic class: HIV-1 and HIV-2 protease inhibitor
Therapeutic class: antiviral
Pregnancy risk category: B

Indications and dosages

▶ **Adjunct treatment of advanced HIV infection in selected patients.** *Adults:* 600-mg capsule (Invirase) or 1,200 mg (Fortovase)

P.O. t.i.d. within 2 hours after full meal and with a nucleoside analogue, such as zalcitabine (0.75 mg P.O. t.i.d.) or zidovudine (200 mg P.O. t.i.d.).

How supplied

saquinavir
Capsules (soft gelatin): 200 mg
saquinavir mesylate
Capsules (hard gelatin): 200 mg

Pharmacokinetics

Absorption: poorly absorbed from GI tract.
Distribution: more than 98% bound to plasma proteins.
Metabolism: rapidly metabolized.
Excretion: excreted mainly in feces. *Half-life:* 1 to 2 hours.

Route	Onset	Peak	Duration
P.O.	Unknown	Unknown	Unknown

Pharmacodynamics

Chemical effect: inhibits activity of HIV protease and prevents cleavage of HIV polyproteins, which are essential for HIV maturation.
Therapeutic effect: hinders HIV activity.

Adverse reactions

CNS: asthenia, paresthesia, headache, dizziness.
CV: chest pain.
GI: diarrhea, ulcerated buccal mucosa, abdominal pain, nausea, ***pancreatitis.***
Hematologic: ***pancytopenia, thrombocytopenia.***
Musculoskeletal: musculoskeletal pain.
Respiratory: bronchitis, cough.
Skin: rash.

Interactions

Drug-drug. *Ketoconazole, ritonavir:* increased serum saquinavir levels. Monitor patient closely.
Phenobarbital, phenytoin, rifabutin, rifampin: reduces steady-state saquinavir level. Use together cautiously.
Drug-herb. *St. John's wort:* serum levels of protease inhibitors decreased up to 50%. Discourage concurrent use.
Drug-food. *Any food:* increased absorption. Give drug with food.

Contraindications and precautions

- Contraindicated in patients hypersensitive to drug or components of capsule.
- Safety of drug hasn't been established in pregnant or breast-feeding women and in children under age 16.

NURSING CONSIDERATIONS

Assessment

- Obtain history of patient's HIV infection.
- Evaluate CBC, platelet count, and electrolyte, uric acid, liver enzyme, and bilirubin levels before therapy and at appropriate intervals during therapy, as ordered.
- Be alert for adverse reactions and interactions, including those caused by adjunct therapy (zidovudine or zalcitabine).
- Monitor patient's hydration status if adverse GI reactions occur.
- Evaluate patient's and family's knowledge of drug therapy.

Nursing diagnoses

- Infection related to presence of HIV
- Risk for deficient fluid volume related to adverse GI reactions
- Deficient knowledge related to drug therapy

Planning and implementation

ALERT Don't confuse the two forms of this drug because dosages are different.
- If severe toxicity occurs during treatment, drug should be discontinued until cause is identified or toxicity resolves. Therapy may resume with no dosage modifications.
- Notify prescriber of adverse reactions, and obtain an order for a mild analgesic, antiemetic, or antidiarrheal, if necessary.

Patient teaching

- Tell patient to take drug within 2 hours after a full meal.
- Urge patient to notify prescriber of adverse reactions.
- Inform patient that drug is usually administered with other AIDS-related antiviral drugs.

• Tell patient that a change from Invirase to Fortovase capsules should be made only under a prescriber's supervision.

Evaluation
• Patient responds well to therapy.
• Patient maintains adequate hydration.
• Patient and family state understanding of drug therapy.

sargramostim (granulocyte macrophage colony–stimulating factor, GM-CSF)
(sar-GRAH-moh-stim)
Leukine

Pharmacologic class: biological response modifier
Therapeutic class: colony-stimulating factor
Pregnancy risk category: C

Indications and dosages
▶ **Acceleration of hematopoietic reconstitution after autologous bone marrow transplantation in patients with malignant lymphoma or acute lymphoblastic leukemia or during autologous bone marrow transplantation in patients with Hodgkin's disease.** *Adults:* 250 mcg/m^2 daily for 21 consecutive days given as 2-hour I.V. infusion beginning 2 to 4 hours after bone marrow transplantation.
▶ **Bone marrow transplantation failure or engraftment delay.** *Adults:* 250 mcg/m^2/day for 14 days as 2-hour I.V. infusion. Dose may be repeated after 7 days off therapy. If engraftment still hasn't occurred, a third course of 500 mcg/m^2/day I.V. for 14 days may be tried after another 7 days off therapy.
▶ **Acute myelogenous leukemia.** *Adults:* 250 mcg/m^2/day I.V. infusion over 4 hours. Start therapy about day 11 or 4 days after end of induction therapy.

How supplied
Powder for injection: 250 mcg, 500 mcg

Pharmacokinetics
Absorption: not applicable.
Distribution: bound to specific receptors on target cells.
Metabolism: unknown.
Excretion: unknown. *Half-life:* about 2 hours.

Route	Onset	Peak	Duration
I.V.	≤ 30 min	2 hr	Unknown

Pharmacodynamics
Chemical effect: glycoprotein manufactured by recombinant DNA technology in yeast expression system; differs from natural human GM-CSF. Drug induces cellular responses by binding to specific receptors on surfaces of target cells.
Therapeutic effect: stimulates formation of granulocytes (neutrophils, eosinophils) and macrophages.

Adverse reactions
CNS: *malaise, CNS disorders, asthenia.*
CV: *edema,* ***supraventricular arrhythmia,*** pericardial effusion.
EENT: *mucous membrane disorder.*
GI: *nausea, vomiting, diarrhea, anorexia,* ***hemorrhage,*** *GI disorder, stomatitis.*
GU: *urinary tract disorder,* abnormal kidney function.
Hemotologic: *blood dyscrasias,* ***hemorrhage.***
Hepatic: ***liver damage.***
Respiratory: *dyspnea, lung disorders,* pleural effusion.
Skin: *alopecia, rash.*
Other: *fever,* **SEPSIS.**

Interactions
Drug-drug. *Corticosteroids, lithium:* may potentiate myeloproliferative effects of sargramostim. Use together cautiously.

Contraindications and precautions
• Contraindicated in patients hypersensitive to drug or its components or to yeast-derived products. Also contraindicated in patients with excessive leukemic myeloid blasts in bone marrow or peripheral blood.
• Use cautiously in pregnant or breast-feeding women and patients with cardiac disease, hypoxia, fluid retention, pulmonary infiltrates, heart failure, or impaired kidney or liver function.

• Safety of drug hasn't been established in children.

NURSING CONSIDERATIONS

Assessment
• Assess patient's condition before therapy and regularly thereafter.
• Drug effect may be limited in patient who has received extensive radiotherapy to hematopoietic sites for treatment of primary disease in abdomen or chest or who has been exposed to multiple drugs (alkylating, anthracycline antibiotics, antimetabolites) before autologous bone marrow transplantation.
• Drug is effective in accelerating myeloid recovery in patients receiving bone marrow purged from monoclonal antibodies.
• Drug can act as growth factor for tumors, particularly myeloid cancers.
• Blood counts return to normal or baseline levels within 3 to 7 days after stopping treatment.
• Monitor CBC with differential, including examination for presence of blast cells, biweekly, as ordered.
• Be alert for adverse reactions and drug interactions.
• Monitor patient's hydration status throughout drug therapy.
• Evaluate patient's and family's knowledge of drug therapy.

Nursing diagnoses
• Ineffective health maintenance related to underlying condition
• Risk for deficient fluid volume related to drug-induced adverse effects
• Deficient knowledge related to drug therapy

Planning and implementation
• Reconstitute drug with 1 ml of sterile water for injection. Direct stream of sterile water against side of vial and gently swirl contents to minimize foaming. Avoid excessive or vigorous agitation or shaking. Dilute in normal saline solution. If final concentration is below 10 mcg/ml, add human albumin at final concentration of 0.1% to saline solution before adding sargramostim to prevent adsorption to components of delivery system. For final concentration of 0.1% human albumin, add 1 mg human albumin/1 ml saline solution. Administer as soon as possible after mixing and no later than 6 hours after reconstituting.
• Discard unused portion. Vials are for single-dose use and contain no preservatives. Don't reenter vial.
ALERT Don't add other drugs to infusion solution because no data exist on solution compatibility and stability.
• Notify prescriber and anticipate reducing dose by half or discontinuing drug temporarily if severe adverse reactions occur. Therapy may be resumed when reactions abate. Transient rashes and local reactions at injection site may occur; no serious allergic or anaphylactic reactions have been reported.
ALERT Don't give drug within 24 hours of last dose of chemotherapy or within 12 hours of last dose of radiotherapy; rapidly dividing progenitor cells may be sensitive to these cytotoxic therapies and drug would be ineffective.
• Stimulation of marrow precursors may result in rapid rise of WBC count. If blast cells appear or increase to 10% or more of WBC count or if underlying disease progresses, therapy should be discontinued. If absolute neutrophil count is above 20,000/mm^3 or if platelet count is above 50,000/mm^3, drug is temporarily discontinued or dose is reduced by half.
• Refrigerate sterile powder, reconstituted solution, and diluted solution for injection. Don't freeze or shake.

Patient teaching
• Inform patient and family about need for therapy.
• Advise patient to report adverse reactions immediately.

Evaluation
• Patient exhibits positive response to sargramostim therapy.
• Patient maintains adequate hydration throughout therapy.
• Patient and family state understanding of drug therapy.

scopolamine (hyoscine)

(skoh-POL-uh-meen)

Scop ◇, Transderm Scōp, Transderm-V ♦

scopolamine butylbromide (hyoscine butylbromide)

Buscopan ♦ ◇

scopolamine hydrobromide (hyoscine hydrobromide)

Pharmacologic class: anticholinergic
Therapeutic class: antimuscarinic, antiemetic, antivertigo agent, antiparkinsonian
Pregnancy risk category: C

Indications and dosagess

▶ **Spastic states.** *Adults:* 10 to 20 mg P.O. t.i.d. or q.i.d. Dosage adjusted, p.r.n. Or, 10 to 20 mg (butylbromide) S.C., I.M., or I.V. t.i.d. or q.i.d.

▶ **Preoperatively to reduce secretions. Scopolamine hydrobromide.** *Adults:* 0.2 to 0.6 mg I.M. 30 to 60 minutes before induction of anesthesia.
Children ages 8 to 12: 300 mcg I.M. 45 minutes before induction of anesthesia.
Children ages 3 to 8: 200 mcg I.M. 45 minutes before induction of anesthesia.
Children ages 7 months to 3 years: 150 mcg I.M. 45 minutes before induction of anesthesia.
Infants ages 4 to 7 months: 100 mcg I.M. 45 minutes before induction of anesthesia.

▶ **Prevention of nausea and vomiting from motion sickness. Scopolamine.** *Adults:* one Transderm Scōp or Transderm-V patch (a circular flat unit) programmed to deliver 0.5 mg daily over 3 days (72 hours), applied to skin behind ear several hours before antiemetic is required.
Scopolamine hydrobromide. *Adults:* 300 to 600 mcg S.C., I.M., or I.V.
Children: 6 mcg/kg or 200 mcg/m^2 of body surface S.C., I.M., or I.V.

How supplied

scopolamine
Transdermal patch: 1.5 mg
scopolamine butylbromide
Capsules: 0.25 mg
Suppositories: 10 mg ♦
Tablets: 10 mg ♦
scopolamine hydrobromide
Injection: 0.3, 0.4, 0.5, 0.6, and 1 mg/ml in 1-ml vials and ampules; 0.86 mg/ml in 0.5-ml ampules

Pharmacokinetics

Absorption: well absorbed percutaneously from behind ear with transdermal patch application. Well absorbed from GI tract when given P.O. or P.R. Absorbed rapidly when given I.M. or S.C.
Distribution: distributed widely throughout body tissues; probably crosses blood-brain barrier.
Metabolism: thought to be metabolized completely in liver.
Excretion: may be excreted in urine as metabolites. *Half-life:* 8 hours.

Route	Onset	Peak	Duration
P.O.	30-60 min	Unknown	4-6 hr
I.V., I.M., S.C.	30 min	Unknown	4 hr
P.R.	Unknown	Unknown	Unknown
Transdermal	Unknown	Unknown	≤ 72 hr

Pharmacodynamics

Chemical effect: inhibits muscarinic actions of acetylcholine on autonomic effectors innervated by postganglionic cholinergic neurons. Scopolamine also may affect neural pathways originating in labyrinth (inner ear) to inhibit nausea and vomiting.
Therapeutic effect: relieves spasticity, nausea, and vomiting; reduces secretions; and blocks cardiac vagal reflexes.

Adverse reactions

Adverse reactions may be caused by pending atropine-like toxicity and are dose-related. Individual tolerance varies greatly. Many adverse reactions (such as dry mouth, constipation) are expected extensions of drug's pharmacologic activity.

CNS: disorientation, restlessness, irritability, dizziness, drowsiness, headache, confusion, hallucinations, delirium.
CV: palpitations, tachycardia, ***paradoxical bradycardia.***
EENT: dilated pupils, blurred vision, photophobia, increased intraocular pressure, difficulty swallowing.
GI: *constipation, dry mouth, nausea, vomiting, epigastric distress.*
GU: urinary hesitancy, urine retention.
Respiratory: bronchial plugging, depressed respirations.
Skin: rash, flushing, dryness, contact dermatitis with transdermal patch.
Other: fever.

Interactions

Drug-drug. *Centrally acting anticholinergics (antihistamines, phenothiazines, tricyclic antidepressants):* increased risk of adverse CNS reactions. Monitor patient closely.
CNS depressants: increased risk of CNS depression. Monitor patient closely.
Digoxin: increased digoxin levels. Monitor patient for cardiac toxicity.
Drug-herb. *Squaw vine:* tannic acid may decrease metabolic breakdown. Discourage concomitant use.
Jaborandi tree: effects of these drugs may be decreased with concomitant administration. Discourage concomitant use.
Pill-bearing spurge: choline may decrease the effect of scopalamine. Discourage concomitant use.
Drug-lifestyle. *Alcohol use:* increased risk of CNS depression. Discourage concomitant use.

Contraindications and precautions

- Contraindicated in patients with angle-closure glaucoma, obstructive uropathy, obstructive disease of GI tract, asthma, chronic pulmonary disease, myasthenia gravis, paralytic ileus, intestinal atony, unstable CV status in acute hemorrhage, or toxic megacolon.
- Drug shouldn't be used in breast-feeding women.
- Use cautiously in patients with autonomic neuropathy, hyperthyroidism, coronary artery disease, arrhythmias, heart failure, hypertension, hiatal hernia with reflux esophagitis, hepatic or renal disease, or ulcerative colitis; in pregnant women; in children under age 6; and in patients in hot or humid environments (drug-induced heatstroke is possible).

NURSING CONSIDERATIONS

Assessment

- Assess patient's condition before therapy and regularly thereafter.
- Be alert for adverse reactions and drug interactions.
- Evaluate patient's and family's knowledge of drug therapy.

Nursing diagnoses

- Risk for deficient fluid volume related to nausea and vomiting
- Risk for injury related to drug-induced adverse CNS reactions
- Deficient knowledge related to drug therapy

Planning and implementation

P.O., I.M., S.C., and P.R. use: Follow normal protocol.
I.V. use: Intermittent and continuous infusions aren't recommended.
– For direct injection, dilute with sterile water and inject diluted drug at ordered rate through patent I.V. line.
– Protect I.V. solutions from freezing and light, and store at room temperature.
Transdermal patch use: Apply patch the night before patient's expected travel.
- Raise bed's side rails as precaution because some patients become temporarily excited or disoriented. Symptoms disappear when sedative effect is complete.
- In therapeutic doses, scopolamine may produce amnesia, drowsiness, and euphoria; patient may need to be reoriented.
- Tolerance may develop when scopolamine is given over a long time.

ALERT Overdose may cause curare-like effects such as respiratory paralysis.

Patient teaching

- Advise patient to apply patch the night before planned trip. Transdermal method releases controlled therapeutic amount of drug. Transderm Scōp is effective if applied 2 to 3 hours before experiencing motion but is more effective if applied 12 hours before.

- Advise patient to wash and dry hands thoroughly before and after applying transdermal patch on dry skin behind ear and before touching eye because pupil may dilate. After removing system, he should discard it and wash hands and application site thoroughly.
- Tell patient that if patch becomes displaced, he should remove it and replace it with another patch on fresh skin site behind ear.
- Alert patient about risk of withdrawal symptoms (nausea, vomiting, headache, dizziness) if transdermal system is used longer than 72 hours.
- Have patient ask pharmacist for brochure that comes with transdermal product.
- Instruct patient about P.O. or P.R. administration, if applicable.
- Advise patient to refrain from activities that require alertness until drug's CNS effects are known.
- Instruct patient to report signs of urinary hesitancy or urine retention.
- Recommend use of sugarless gum or hard candy to help minimize dry mouth.

☑ Evaluation

- Patient responds well to therapy.
- Patient doesn't experience injury from adverse CNS reactions.
- Patient and family state understanding of drug therapy.

secobarbital sodium

(sek-oh-BAR-bih-tohl SOH-dee-um)

Novosecobarb♦, Seconal Sodium

Pharmacologic class: barbiturate
Therapeutic class: sedative-hypnotic, anticonvulsant
Controlled substance schedule: II
Pregnancy risk category: D

Indications and dosages

▶ **Preoperative sedation.** *Adults:* 100 to 300 mg P.O. 1 to 2 hours before surgery. *Children:* 50 to 100 mg P.O. 1 to 2 hours before surgery. Maximum single dose is 100 mg.

▶ **Insomnia.** *Adults:* 100 mg P.O., 100 to 200 mg I.M., or 50 to 250 mg I.V.

▶ **Acute tetanus seizure.** *Adults:* 5.5 mg/kg I.M. or slow I.V., repeated q 3 to 4 hours, if needed; I.V. injection rate not to exceed 50 mg/15 seconds.

▶ **Status epilepticus.** *Children:* 15 to 20 mg/kg I.V. over 15 minutes.

How supplied

Capsules: 50 mg, 100 mg
Injection: 50 mg/ml

Pharmacokinetics

Absorption: 90% of drug absorbed rapidly after P.O. administration; unknown after I.M. administration.
Distribution: distributed rapidly throughout body tissues and fluids; about 30% to 45% protein-bound.
Metabolism: oxidized in liver to inactive metabolites.
Excretion: excreted in urine. *Half-life:* about 30 hours.

Route	Onset	Peak	Duration
P.O.	≤ 15 min	5-30 min	1-4 hr
I.V.	Almost immediate	1-3 min	15 min
I.M.	Unknown	7-10 min	Unknown

Pharmacodynamics

Chemical effect: unknown; probably interferes with transmission of impulses from thalamus to cortex of brain.
Therapeutic effect: promotes pain relief and calmness and relieves acute seizures.

Adverse reactions

CNS: *drowsiness, lethargy, hangover,* paradoxical excitement in elderly patients, somnolence.
CV: hypotension with I.V. use.
GI: nausea, vomiting.
Hematologic: exacerbation of porphyria.
Respiratory: ***respiratory depression.***
Skin: rash, urticaria, ***Stevens-Johnson syndrome,*** tissue reactions and injection-site pain.
Other: ***angioedema,*** physical and psychological dependence.

Interactions

Drug-drug. *Acidic solutions, lactated Ringer's solution:* incompatible with I.V. form of drug. Don't mix together.
Chloramphenicol, MAO inhibitors, valproic acid: inhibited metabolism of barbiturates; may cause prolonged CNS depression. Reduce barbiturate dosage.
CNS depressants, including narcotic analgesics: excessive CNS and respiratory depression. Use together cautiously.
Corticosteroids, digitoxin, doxycycline, estrogens and oral contraceptives, oral anticoagulants, theophylline, tricyclic antidepressants, verapamil: secobarbital may enhance metabolism of these drugs. Monitor patient for decreased effect.
Griseofulvin: decreased absorption of griseofulvin. Monitor patient for decreased griseofulvin effectiveness.
Rifampin: may decrease barbiturate levels. Monitor patient for decreased effect.
Drug-lifestyle. *Alcohol use:* excessive CNS and respiratory depression. Discourage concomitant use.

Contraindications and precautions

- Contraindicated in patients hypersensitive to barbiturates and patients with marked liver impairment, respiratory disease in which dyspnea or obstruction is evident, or porphyria.
- Drug isn't recommended for pregnant or breast-feeding women.
- Use cautiously in patients with acute or chronic pain, depression, suicidal tendencies, history of drug abuse, or hepatic impairment.

NURSING CONSIDERATIONS

Assessment

- Assess patient's condition before therapy and regularly thereafter.
- Assess mental status before therapy. Elderly patients are more sensitive to adverse CNS effects of drug.
- Be alert for adverse reactions and drug interactions.
- Evaluate patient's and family's knowledge of drug therapy.

Nursing diagnoses

- Disturbed sleep pattern related to underlying condition
- Risk for injury related to drug-induced adverse CNS reactions
- Deficient knowledge related to drug therapy

Planning and implementation

P.O. use: Prevent hoarding or intentional overdosing by patient who is depressed, suicidal, or drug-dependent or who has history of drug abuse.
I.V. use: I.V. injection is reserved for emergencies and given by direct injection under close supervision. Give slowly at no more than 50 mg/15 seconds. Drug may be given as supplied or diluted.
– Local tissue reactions and injection-site pain have been noted. Assess patency of I.V. site before and during administration.
– I.V. administration of barbiturates may cause severe respiratory depression, laryngospasm, or hypotension. Keep emergency resuscitation equipment readily available.
– Secobarbital sodium injection isn't compatible with lactated Ringer's solution but is compatible with Ringer's solution, sterile water for injection, and normal saline solution. Don't mix with acidic solutions.
– Use injection solution within 30 minutes after opening container to minimize deterioration. Don't use cloudy solution.
I.M. use: Give I.M. injection deeply. Superficial injection may cause pain, sterile abscess, and sloughing.
- Skin eruptions may precede potentially fatal reactions to barbiturate therapy. Discontinue drug if skin reactions occur, and notify prescriber. In some patients, high fever, stomatitis, headache, or rhinitis may precede skin reactions.
- Long-term use isn't recommended; drug loses its efficacy in promoting sleep after 14 days of continued use.

Patient teaching

- Caution patient to avoid activities that require mental alertness or physical coordination. For inpatient, supervise walking and raise bed rails, particularly for elderly patient.

• Inform patient that morning hangover is common after hypnotic dose, which suppresses REM sleep. Patient may experience increased dreaming after drug is discontinued.
• Advise patient who uses oral contraceptives to consider a different birth control method; drug may enhance contraceptive hormone metabolism and decrease its effect.

Evaluation
• Patient states that drug effectively induces sleep.
• Patient doesn't experience injury from adverse CNS reactions.
• Patient and family state understanding of drug therapy.

selegiline hydrochloride (L-deprenyl hydrochloride)
(see-LEJ-eh-leen high-droh-KLOR-ighd)
Atapryl, Carbex, Eldepryl, Selpak

Pharmacologic class: MAO inhibitor
Therapeutic class: antiparkinsonian
Pregnancy risk category: C

Indications and dosages
▶ **Adjunct treatment with levodopa-carbidopa in managing symptoms of Parkinson's disease.** *Adults:* 10 mg P.O. daily, taken as 5 mg at breakfast and 5 mg at lunch. After 2 or 3 days of therapy, gradual decrease of levodopa-carbidopa dosage is attempted.

How supplied
Tablets: 5 mg

Pharmacokinetics
Absorption: unknown.
Distribution: unknown.
Metabolism: three metabolites have been detected in serum and urine: *N*-desmethyldeprenyl, L-amphetamine, and L-methamphetamine.
Excretion: 45% excreted in urine as metabolite. *Half-life:* selegiline, 2 to 10 hours; *N*-desmethyldeprenyl, 2 hours; L-amphetamine, 17.7 hours; L-methamphetamine, 20.5 hours.

Route	Onset	Peak	Duration
P.O.	Unknown	0.5-2 hr	Unknown

Pharmacodynamics
Chemical effect: unknown; probably acts by selectively inhibiting MAO type B (found mostly in brain). At higher-than-recommended doses, it is nonselective inhibitor of MAO, including MAO type A (found in GI tract). It also may directly increase dopaminergic activity by decreasing reuptake of dopamine into nerve cells. Its active metabolites, amphetamine and methamphetamine, may contribute to this effect.
Therapeutic effect: improves physical mobility.

Adverse reactions
CNS: *dizziness,* increased tremors, chorea, loss of balance, restlessness, increased bradykinesia, facial grimacing, stiff neck, dyskinesia, involuntary movements, twitching, increased apraxia, behavioral changes, fatigue, headache, confusion, hallucinations, vivid dreams, malaise.
CV: orthostatic hypotension, hypertension, hypotension, ***arrhythmias,*** palpitations, new or increased anginal pain, tachycardia, peripheral edema, syncope.
EENT: blepharospasm.
GI: dry mouth, *nausea,* vomiting, constipation, weight loss, abdominal pain, anorexia or poor appetite, dysphagia, diarrhea, heartburn.
GU: slow urination, transient nocturia, prostatic hyperplasia, urinary hesitancy, urinary frequency, urine retention, sexual dysfunction.
Skin: rash, hair loss, diaphoresis.

Interactions
Drug-drug. *Adrenergics:* possible increased pressor response, particularly in patients who have taken overdose of selegiline. Use together cautiously.
Meperidine: may cause stupor, muscle rigidity, severe agitation, and elevated temperature. Avoid concomitant use.
Drug-herb. *Cacao tree:* potential vasopressor effects. Advise against concomitant use.

Ginseng: adverse reactions including headache, tremors, mania. Advise against concomitant use.
Drug-food. *Foods high in tyramine:* possible hypertensive crisis. Monitor blood pressure.

Contraindications and precautions

- Contraindicated in patients hypersensitive to drug and in those receiving meperidine.
- Use cautiously in pregnant women.
- Safety of drug hasn't been established in children and in breast-feeding women.

NURSING CONSIDERATIONS

Assessment

- Assess patient's condition before therapy and regularly thereafter.
- Be alert for adverse reactions and drug interactions.
- Evaluate patient's and family's knowledge of drug therapy.

Nursing diagnoses

- Impaired physical mobility related to underlying condition
- Risk for injury related to drug-induced adverse CNS reactions
- Deficient knowledge related to drug therapy

Planning and implementation

- Some patients experience increased adverse reactions related to levodopa and need a 10% to 30% reduction of levodopa-carbidopa dosage.

ALERT Don't confuse selegiline with Stelazine or Eldepryl with enalapril.

Patient teaching

- Warn patient to move cautiously at start of therapy because dizziness may occur.
- Advise patient not to take more than 10 mg daily because greater amount of drug won't improve efficacy and may increase adverse reactions.

Evaluation

- Patient exhibits improved physical mobility.
- Patient doesn't experience injury from adverse CNS reactions.
- Patient and family state understanding of drug therapy.

senna

(SEN-uh)

Black-Draught†, Fletcher's Castoria†, Senexon†, Senokot†, Senolax†, X-Prep*†

Pharmacologic class: anthraquinone derivative
Therapeutic class: stimulant laxative
Pregnancy risk category: C

Indications and dosages

▶ **Acute constipation; preparation for bowel examination. Black-Draught.** *Adults:* 2 tablets or ¼ to ½ tsp of granules mixed with water.
Other preparations. *Adults and children age 12 and over:* usual dose is 2 tablets, 1 tsp of granules dissolved in water, 1 suppository, or 10 to 15 ml syrup h.s. Maximum dosage varies with preparation used.
Children ages 6 to 11: 1 tablet, ½ tsp of granules dissolved in water, ½ suppository h.s., or 5 to 10 ml syrup. Maximum dosage is 2 tablets b.i.d. or 1 tsp of granules b.i.d.
Children ages 2 to 5: ½ tablet or ¼ tsp of granules dissolved in water. Maximum, 1 tablet b.i.d. or ½ tsp of granules b.i.d.
Children ages 1 to 5: 2.5 to 5 ml syrup h.s.
Children ages 1 month to 12 months: consult prescriber.

How supplied

Dosages expressed as sennosides (active principle)
Tablets†: 6 mg, 8.6 mg, 17 mg
Granules†: 15 mg/tsp, 20 mg/tsp
Liquid†: 3 mg/ml
Suppositories†: 30 mg
Syrup†: 8.8 mg/5 ml

Pharmacokinetics

Absorption: absorbed minimally from GI tract after P.O. or P.R. use.
Distribution: distributed in bile, saliva, colonic mucosa.

Metabolism: absorbed portion metabolized in liver.
Excretion: unabsorbed senna excreted mainly in feces; absorbed drug excreted in urine and feces.

Route	Onset	Peak	Duration
P.O.	6-10 hr	Varies	Varies
P.R.	30 min-2 hr	Varies	Varies

Pharmacodynamics

Chemical effect: unknown; increases peristalsis, probably by direct effect on smooth muscle of intestine. Senna may either irritate musculature or stimulate colonic intramural plexus. It also promotes fluid accumulation in colon and small intestine.
Therapeutic effect: relieves constipation and cleanses bowel.

Adverse reactions

GI: *nausea;* vomiting; diarrhea; malabsorption of nutrients; yellow or yellow-green cast to feces; *abdominal cramps,* especially in severe constipation; "cathartic colon" (syndrome resembling ulcerative colitis radiologically) with long-term misuse; possible constipation after catharsis; diarrhea in breast-feeding infants of mothers receiving senna; darkened pigmentation of rectal mucosa with long-term use (usually reversible within 4 to 12 months after stopping drug); laxative dependence; loss of normal bowel function with excessive use.
GU: red-pink discoloration in alkaline urine; yellow-brown color to acidic urine.
Metabolic: protein-losing enteropathy, electrolyte imbalance.

Interactions

None significant.

Contraindications and precautions

- Contraindicated in patients with ulcerative bowel lesions; nausea, vomiting, abdominal pain, or other symptoms of appendicitis or acute surgical abdomen; fecal impaction; or intestinal obstruction or perforation.
- Use cautiously in pregnant or breast-feeding women.

NURSING CONSIDERATIONS

Assessment

- Assess patient's condition before therapy and regularly thereafter.
- Before giving drug for constipation, determine if patient has adequate fluid intake, exercise, and diet.
- Be alert for adverse reactions.
- Evaluate patient's and family's knowledge of drug therapy.

Nursing diagnoses

- Constipation related to underlying condition
- Diarrhea related to drug-induced adverse GI reactions
- Deficient knowledge related to drug therapy

Planning and implementation

P.O. use: Limit diet to clear liquids after patient takes X-Prep Liquid.
P.R. use: Follow normal protocol.
- Avoid exposing drug to excessive heat or light.
- Drug is used for short-term treatment.
- Senna is one of the most effective laxatives for counteracting constipation caused by narcotic analgesics.

Patient teaching

- Teach patient about dietary sources of bulk, which include bran and other cereals, fresh fruit, and vegetables.
- Tell patient to maintain adequate fluid intake of at least 6 to 8 glasses of water or juices unless contraindicated.

Evaluation

- Patient's constipation is relieved.
- Patient states that diarrhea doesn't occur.
- Patient and family state understanding of drug therapy.

sertraline hydrochloride
(SER-truh-leen high-droh-KLOR-ighd)
Zoloft

Pharmacologic class: serotonin uptake inhibitor

Therapeutic class: antidepressant
Pregnancy risk category: B

Indications and dosages

▶ **Depression.** *Adults:* 50 mg P.O. daily. Dosage adjusted as tolerated and needed; clinical trials involved dosage of 50 to 200 mg daily. Dosage adjustments should be made at intervals of no less than 1 week.

▶ **Posttraumatic stress disorder**. *Adults:* initially, 25 mg P.O. once daily. Increase dosage to 50 mg P.O. once daily after 1 week of therapy. Dosage may be increased at weekly intervals to a maximum of 200 mg daily. Maintain patient on lowest effective dosage.

How supplied

Tablets: 25 mg, 50 mg, 100 mg

Pharmacokinetics

Absorption: well absorbed from GI tract. Absorption rate and extent are enhanced when taken with food.
Distribution: highly protein-bound (greater than 98%).
Metabolism: metabolism is probably hepatic.
Excretion: excreted mostly as metabolites in urine and feces. *Half-life:* 26 hours.

Route	Onset	Peak	Duration
P.O.	2-4 wk	4.5-8.5 hr	Unknown

Pharmacodynamics

Chemical effect: unknown; may be linked to inhibited neuronal uptake of serotonin in CNS.
Therapeutic effect: relieves depression.

Adverse reactions

CNS: *headache, tremors, dizziness, insomnia, somnolence,* paresthesias, hypoesthesia, hyperesthesia, *fatigue,* twitching, hypertonia, nervousness, anxiety, confusion.
CV: palpitations, chest pain, hot flushes.
GI: *dry mouth, nausea, diarrhea, loose stools, dyspepsia,* vomiting, constipation, thirst, flatulence, anorexia, abdominal pain, increased appetite.
GU: *male sexual dysfunction,* decreased libido.
Musculoskeletal: myalgia.
Skin: *diaphoresis,* rash, pruritus.
Other: flushing.

Interactions

Drug-drug. *Benzodiazepines (except lorazepam and oxazepam), tolbutamide:* decreased clearance of these drugs. Clinical significance unknown; monitor patient for increased drug effects.
Cimetidine: decreased sertraline clearance. Monitor patient for toxicity.
MAO inhibitors: may cause serious, sometimes fatal, reactions including myoclonus rigidity, mental status changes, hyperthermia, autonomic nervous system instability, rapid fluctuations of vital signs, delirium, coma, and death. Avoid concomitant use.
Warfarin, other highly protein-bound drugs: may increase plasma levels of sertraline or other highly bound drug. Small (8%) increases in PT and INR have been noted with concomitant use of warfarin. Monitor patient closely.
Drug-herb. *Ginkgo:* herb may decrease adverse sexual effects of drug. Advise patient to speak to presriber before taking any herbal remedy.
St. John's wort: increased serotonin levels and possible serotonin syndrome. Discourage concomitant use.

Contraindications and precautions

- No known contraindications.
- Use cautiously in patients at risk for suicide and in those with seizure disorder, major affective disorder, or diseases or conditions that affect metabolism or hemodynamic responses. Also use cautiously in pregnant or breast-feeding women.
- Safety of drug hasn't been established in children.

NURSING CONSIDERATIONS

Assessment

- Assess patient's depression before therapy, and reassess regularly thereafter.
- Assess patient for risk factors for suicide.
- Be alert for adverse reactions and drug interactions.
- Evaluate patient's and family's knowledge of drug therapy.

Nursing diagnoses
- Disturbed thought processes related to presence of depression
- Risk for injury related to drug-induced adverse CNS reactions
- Deficient knowledge related to drug therapy

Planning and implementation
- Administer drug once daily, either in morning or evening. Drug may be given with or without food.
- Drug shouldn't be given within 14 days of MAO inhibitor therapy. Allow 14 days after stopping drug before starting an MAO inhibitor, as ordered.
- Drug may change several laboratory values—increases in serum cholesterol and triglyceride levels, decreases in uric acid levels, and elevations in AST and ALT levels (usually within first 9 weeks of therapy). AST and ALT values return to normal after discontinuing drug; clinical significance is unknown.

Patient teaching
- Advise patient to use caution when performing hazardous tasks that require alertness and to avoid alcohol while taking this drug. Drugs that influence CNS may impair judgment.
- Caution patient to check with prescriber or pharmacist before taking OTC medications.

Evaluation
- Patient behavior and communication indicate improved thought processes.
- Patient doesn't experience injury from adverse CNS reactions.
- Patient and family state understanding of drug therapy.

sevelamer hydrochloride

(seh-VEL-ah-mer high-droh-KLOR-ighd)

Renagel

Pharmacologic class: polymeric phosphate binder
Therapeutic class: hyperphosphatemia agent
Pregnancy risk category: C

Indications and dosages

▶ **Reduction of serum phosphorus in patients with endstage renal disease.** *Adults:* initially, 2 to 4 capsules P.O. t.i.d. with meals, depending on severity of hyperphosphatemia. Gradually adjust dosage based on serum phosphorus level with goal of lowering serum phosphorus to 6 mg/dl or less. If serum phosphorus level is 9 mg/dl or more, 4 capsules P.O. t.i.d. with meals; if serum phosphorus level is between 7.5 and 9 mg/dl, 3 capsules P.O. t.i.d. with meals; if serum phosphorus level is between 6 and 7.5 mg/dl, 2 capsules P.O. t.i.d. with meals.

How supplied

Capsules: 403 mg

Pharmacokinetics

Absorption: drug isn't systemically absorbed.
Distribution: unknown.
Metabolism: unknown.
Excretion: unknown.

Route	Onset	Peak	Duration
P.O.	Unknown	Unknown	Unknown

Pharmacodynamics

Chemical effect: inhibits intestinal phosphate absorption.
Therapeutic effect: decreases serum phosphorus level.

Adverse reactions

CNS: *headache, pain.*
CV: hypertension, *hypotension,* ***thrombosis.***
GI: *vomiting,* nausea, constipation, *diarrhea,* flatulence, *dyspepsia.*
Respiratory: cough.
Other: *infection.*

Interactions

None significant.

Contraindications and precautions

- Contraindicated in patients hypersensitive to drug or its components and in those with hypophosphatemia or bowel obstruction.
- Use cautiously in patients with dysphagia, swallowing disorders, severe GI motility disorders, or major GI tract surgery.

NURSING CONSIDERATIONS

Assessment
- Obtain history of patient's underlying condition before therapy, and reassess regularly thereafter.
- Monitor serum calcium, bicarbonate, and chloride levels, as ordered.
- Watch for symptoms of thrombosis (numbness or tingling of limbs, chest pain, shortness of breath), and notify prescriber if they occur.
- Evaluate patient's and family's knowledge of drug therapy.

Nursing diagnoses
- Ineffective tissue perfusion (cardiopulmonary or peripheral) related to potential drug-induced thrombosis
- Imbalanced nutrition: less than body requirements related to drug-induced adverse GI effects
- Deficient knowledge related to drug therapy

Planning and implementation
- Don't crush or break capsules, and administer only with meals.
- Although no known drug interactions have been studied, drug may bind to concomitantly administered drugs and decrease their bioavailability. Administer other drugs 1 hour before or 3 hours after sevelamer.

ALERT Drug may reduce vitamins D, E, and K and folic acid; patient should take a multivitamin supplement.

Patient teaching
- Instruct patient to take with meals and adhere to prescribed diet.
- Inform patient that capsules must be taken whole because contents expand in water; caution him not to open or chew capsules.
- Tell patient to take other drugs as directed, but they must be taken either 1 hour before or 3 hours after sevelamer.
- Inform patient about common adverse reactions and instruct him to report them immediately. Teach patient signs and symptoms of thrombosis (numbness, tingling limbs, chest pain, changes in level of consciousness).

Evaluation
- Patient doesn't develop a thrombus.
- Patient maintains adequate nutrition.
- Patient and family state understanding of drug therapy.

sibutramine hydrochloride monohydrate
(sigh-BYOO-truh-meen high-droh-KLOR-ighd muh-noh-HIGH-drayt)
Meridia

Pharmacologic class: serotonin, norepinephrine, and dopamine reuptake inhibitor
Therapeutic class: antiobesity
Controlled substance schedule: IV
Pregnancy risk category: C

Indications and dosages
▶ **Management of obesity.** *Adults:* 10 mg P.O. once daily with or without food. May increase dosage to 15 mg P.O. daily after 4 weeks if weight loss is inadequate. Patients who don't tolerate the 10-mg dose may receive 5 mg P.O. daily. Doses above 15 mg daily aren't recommended.

How supplied
Capsules: 5 mg, 10 mg, 15 mg

Pharmacokinetics
Absorption: rapid; about 77% of administered dose is absorbed.
Distribution: rapid and extensive. Active metabolites are extensively bound to plasma proteins.
Metabolism: extensive first-pass metabolism by the liver to two active metabolites, M_1 and M_2.
Excretion: about 77% is excreted in urine.
Half-life: M_1 is 14 hours and M_2 is 16 hours.

Route	Onset	Peak	Duration
P.O.	Unknown	3-4 hr	Unknown

Pharmacodynamics

Chemical effect: inhibits reuptake of norepinephrine, serotonin, and dopamine.
Therapeutic effect: facilitates weight loss.

Adverse reactions

CNS: asthenia, *headache, insomnia,* dizziness, nervousness, anxiety, depression, paresthesia, somnolence, CNS stimulation, emotional lability, migraine.
CV: tachycardia, vasodilation, hypertension, palpitations, chest pain, generalized edema.
EENT: thirst, *rhinitis, pharyngitis,* sinusitis, ear disorder, ear pain, laryngitis.
GI: *dry mouth,* taste perversion, *anorexia, constipation,* increased appetite, nausea, dyspepsia, gastritis, vomiting, abdominal pain, rectal disorder.
GU: dysmenorrhea, UTI, vaginal candidiasis, metrorrhagia.
Hepatic: elevated liver enzyme levels.
Musculoskeletal: arthralgia, myalgia, tenosynovitis, joint disorder, neck or back pain.
Respiratory: cough.
Skin: rash, sweating, herpes simplex, acne.
Other: flu syndrome, injury, accident, ***allergic reaction***.

Interactions

Drug-drug. *CNS depressants:* may enhance CNS depression. Use cautiously.
Dextromethorphan, dihydroergotamine, fentanyl, fluoxetine, fluvoxamine, lithium, MAO inhibitors, meperidine, paroxetine, pentazocine, sertraline, sumatriptan, tryptophan, venlafaxine: may cause hyperthermia, tachycardia, loss of consciousness. Avoid concomitant use.
Ephedrine, pseudoephedrine: may increase blood pressure or heart rate. Use cautiously.
Drug-lifestyle. *Alcohol use:* enhanced CNS depression. Discourage concomitant use.

Contraindications and precautions

- Contraindicated in patients hypersensitive to drug or its active ingredients, those taking MAO inhibitors or other centrally acting appetite suppressants, and those with anorexia nervosa.
- Don't use drug in patients with severe renal or hepatic dysfunction, history of hypertension, seizures, coronary artery disease, heart failure, arrhythmias, or CVA.
- Use cautiously in patients with narrow-angle glaucoma.

NURSING CONSIDERATIONS

Assessment

- Monitor patient for adverse reactions and drug interactions.
- Assess patient for organic causes of obesity before starting therapy.
- Assess patient's dietary intake.
- Measure blood pressure and pulse before starting therapy, with dosage changes, and at regular intervals during therapy.
- Evaluate patient's and family's knowledge of drug therapy.

Nursing diagnoses

- Imbalanced nutrition: more than body requirements related to increased caloric intake
- Disturbed sleep pattern related to drug-induced insomnia
- Deficient knowledge related to drug therapy

Planning and implementation

- At least 2 weeks should elapse between stopping an MAO inhibitor and starting drug therapy, and vice versa.
- Give patient ice chips or sugarless hard candy to relieve dry mouth.
- Make sure patient follows appropriate diet regimen.
- Safety and effectiveness in children under age 16 haven't been established.

Patient teaching

- Advise patient to report rash, hives, or other allergic reactions immediately.
- Instruct patient to inform prescriber if he is taking or plans to take prescription or OTC drugs.
- Advise patient to have blood pressure and pulse monitored at regular intervals. Stress importance of regular follow-up visits with prescriber.

• Advise patient to use drug with reduced calorie diet.
• Tell patient that weight loss can precipitate gallstone formation. Teach patient about signs and symptoms and the need to report them to prescriber promptly.

Evaluation

• Patient achieves nutritional balance with the use of medication and a reduced calorie diet.
• Patient experiences normal sleep patterns.
• Patient and family state understanding of drug therapy.

sildenafil citrate

(sil-DEN-ah-fil SIGH-trayt)
Viagra

Pharmacologic class: selective inhibitor of cyclic guanosine monophosphate-specific phosphodiesterase type 5
Therapeutic class: therapy for erectile dysfunction
Pregnancy risk category: B

Indications and dosages

▶ **Treatment of erectile dysfunction.** *Men under age 65:* 50 mg P.O., p.r.n., about 1 hour before sexual activity. Dosage range is 25 mg to 100 mg based on effectiveness and tolerance. Maximum of 1 dose per day.
Men age 65 and older: 25 mg P.O., p.r.n. about 1 hour before sexual activity. Dose may be adjusted based on patient response. Maximum of 1 dose per day.

How supplied

Tablets: 25 mg, 50 mg 100 mg

Pharmacokinetics

Absorption: rapidly absorbed following P.O. administration. Absolute bioavailability is 40%.
Distribution: extensively into body tissues. About 96% bound to plasma proteins.
Metabolism: primarily metabolized in the liver to an active metabolite with properties similar to those of parent drug.
Excretion: following P.O. administration, about 80% is excreted in feces and 13% in urine. *Half-life:* 4 hours.

Route	Onset	Peak	Duration
P.O.	Unknown	0.5-2 hr	4 hr

Pharmacodynamics

Chemical effect: drug has no direct relaxant effect on isolated human corpus cavernosum, but enhances the effect of nitric oxide (NO) by inhibiting phosphodiesterase type 5 (PDE5), which is responsible for degradation of cyclic guanosine monophosphate (cGMP) in the corpus cavernosum. When sexual stimulation causes local release of NO, inhibition of PDE5 by sildenafil causes increased levels of cGMP in the corpus cavernosum, resulting in smooth muscle relaxation and inflow of blood to the corpus cavernosum.
Therapeutic effect: patient achieves an erection.

Adverse reactions

CNS: anxiety, *headache,* dizziness, ***seizures,*** somnolence, vertigo.
CV: ***MI, sudden cardiac death, ventricular arrhythmia, cerebrovascular hemorrhage, transient ischemic attack***, hypertension, *flushing.*
EENT: diplopia, temporary vision loss, decreased vision, ocular redness or bloodshot appearance, increased intraocular pressure, retinal vascular disease, retinal bleeding, vitreous detachment or traction, paramacular edema, abnormal vision (photophobia, color tinged vision, blurred vision), ocular burning, ocular swelling or pressure.
GI: dyspepsia, diarrhea.
GU: hematuria, prolonged erection, priapism, UTI.
Musculoskeletal: arthralgia, back pain.
Respiratory: respiratory tract infection.
Skin: rash.
Other: flu syndrome.

Interactions

Drug-drug. *Beta blockers, loop and potassium-sparing diuretics:* increased blood levels of major metabolite of sildenafil. Clinical significance of this interaction not known.

CYP3A4 inducers, rifampin: reduced sildenafil plasma levels. Monitor drug effect.
Hepatic isoenzyme inhibitors (such as cimetidine, erythromycin, itraconazole, ketoconazole): may reduce clearance of sildenafil. Avoid concomitant use.
Nitrates: sildenafil enhances hypotensive effects. Don't use together.
Drug-food. *High-fat meals:* reduced rate of absorption and decreased peak serum levels. Separate administration time from meals.

Contraindications and precautions

- Contraindicated in patients hypersensitive to drug or its components, those with underlying CV disease, and those using organic nitrates at any frequency and in any form.
- Use cautiously in patients age 65 or older; those with hepatic or severe renal impairment; those with anatomic deformation of the penis; those with conditions that may predispose them to priapism (such as sickle-cell anemia, multiple myeloma, leukemia), retinitis pigmentosa, bleeding disorders, or active peptic ulcer disease; those who have had an MI, CVA, or life-threatening arrhythmia during previous 6 months; and those with history of cardiac failure, coronary artery disease, or uncontrolled high or low blood pressure.

NURSING CONSIDERATIONS

Assessment
- Discuss patient's history of erectile dysfunction to establish need for drug versus other therapies.
- Discuss with patient his response to drug and if he is experiencing adverse effects.
- Assess patient for CV risk factors because serious events have been reported with drug use, and report risk factors to prescriber.
- Evaluate patient's and family's knowledge of drug therapy.

Nursing diagnoses
- Sexual dysfunction related to patient's underlying condition
- Ineffective tissue perfusion (cardiopulmonary) related to drug-induced effects on blood pressure and cardiac output
- Deficient knowledge related to drug therapy

Planning and implementation
- Dosage for adults with hepatic or severe renal impairment is 25 mg P.O. about 1 hour before sexual activity. Dose may be adjusted based on patient response. Maximum of 1 dose per day.

ALERT Drug's systemic vasodilatory properties cause transient decreases in supine blood pressure and cardiac output (about 2 hours postingestion). Together with the potential cardiac risk of sexual activity, the risk for patients with underlying CV disease is increased.
ALERT Serious CV events, including MI, sudden cardiac death, ventricular arrhythmia, cerebrovascular hemorrhage, transient ischemic attack, and hypertension, have occurred in patients during or shortly after sexual activity.

Patient teaching
- Advise patient that drug is contraindicated with regular or intermittent use of nitrates.
- Caution patient about cardiac risk with sexual activity, especially if patient has CV risk factors. If patient has symptoms (such as angina pectoris, dizziness, or nausea) at the start of sexual activity, instruct him to notify prescriber and refrain from further sexual activity.
- Warn patient that erections lasting more than 4 hours and priapism (painful erections more than 6 hours) can occur and should be reported immediately. Penile tissue damage and permanent loss of potency may result if priapism isn't treated immediately.
- Inform patient that drug doesn't offer protection against sexually transmitted diseases and that protective measures such as condoms should be used.
- Instruct patient to take drug 30 minutes to 4 hours before sexual activity; maximum benefit can be expected less than 2 hours after ingesting drug.
- Advise patient that drug is most rapidly absorbed if taken on an empty stomach.
- Inform patient to avoid potentially hazardous activities that rely on color discrimination because blue/green discrimination may be impaired.

• Instruct patient to notify prescriber if visual changes occur.
• Advise patient that drug is effective only in the presence of sexual stimulation.
• Caution patient to take drug only as prescribed.

Evaluation
• Sexual activity improves with drug therapy.
• Patient doesn't experience adverse CV events.
• Patient and family state understanding of drug therapy.

simethicone
(sigh-METH-ih-kohn)
Extra Strength Gas-X†, Gas Relief†, Gas-X†, Maximum Strength Gas Relief†, Maximum Strength Phazyme†, Mylanta Gas†, Mylanta Gas Maximum Strength†, Mylanta Gas Regular Strength†, Mylicon-80†, Mylicon-125†, Ovol♦, Ovol-40♦, Ovol-80♦, Phazyme†, Phazyme 95†, Phazyme 125†

Pharmacologic class: dispersant
Therapeutic class: antiflatulent
Pregnancy risk category: NR

Indications and dosages
▶ **Flatulence, functional gastric bloating.** *Adults and children over age 12:* 40 to 125 mg P.O. after each meal and h.s.

How supplied
Tablets: 40 mg†, 50 mg†, 60 mg†, 80 mg†, 95 mg†, 125 mg†
Capsules: 125 mg
Drops: 40 mg/0.6 ml†

Pharmacokinetics
Absorption: none.
Distribution: none.
Metabolism: none.
Excretion: excreted in feces.

Route	Onset	Peak	Duration
P.O.	Immediate	Immediate	Unknown

Pharmacodynamics
Chemical effect: by its defoaming action, disperses or prevents formation of mucus-surrounded gas pockets in GI tract.
Therapeutic effect: relieves gas.

Adverse reactions
GI: expulsion of excessive liberated gas as belching, rectal flatus.

Interactions
None significant.

Contraindications and precautions
• Contraindicated in patients hypersensitive to drug.
• Use cautiously in pregnant or breast-feeding women.
• Safety of drug hasn't been established in children age 12 and younger.

NURSING CONSIDERATIONS

Assessment
• Assess patient's condition before therapy and regularly thereafter.
• Be alert for adverse GI reactions.
• Evaluate patient's and family's knowledge of drug therapy.

Nursing diagnoses
• Acute pain related to gas in GI tract
• Deficient knowledge related to drug therapy

Planning and implementation
• Make sure patient chews tablet before swallowing.
ALERT Don't confuse simethicone with cimetidine.

Patient teaching
• Advise patient that medication doesn't prevent formation of gas.
• Encourage patient to change position frequently and ambulate to aid in passing flatus.

Evaluation
• Patient's gas pain is relieved.
• Patient and family state understanding of drug therapy.

simvastatin (synvinolin)

(sim-vuh-STAT-in)

Lipex◇, Zocor

Pharmacologic class: HMG-CoA reductase inhibitor
Therapeutic class: antilipemic, cholesterol-lowering agent
Pregnancy risk category: X

Indications and dosages

▶ **Adjunct to diet for reduction of low-density lipoprotein (LDL) and total cholesterol levels in patients with primary hypercholesterolemia (types IIa and IIb) and mixed dyslipidemia and in patients with coronary heart disease and hypercholesterolemia to reduce the risk of coronary death, nonfatal MI, CVA, transient ischemic attack, and myocardial revascularization procedures; to increase high-density lipoprotein cholesterol in patients with primary hypercholesterolemia and mixed dyslipidemia (Frederickson types IIa and IIb).** *Adults:* initially, 20 mg P.O. daily in the evening. Dosage adjusted q 4 weeks based on patient tolerance and response; maximum daily dose is 80 mg.
Elderly patients: initially, 5 mg P.O. daily in the evening. Maximum daily dose is 20 mg.
▶ **Hypertriglyceridemia (Fredrickson type IV hyperlipidemia), primary dysbetalipoproteinemia (Fredrickson type III hyperlipidemia).** *Adults:* initially, 20 mg P.O. daily in the evening. Adjust dosage q 4 weeks based on patient response and tolerance. Dosage range is 5 to 80 mg daily as single dose in the evening. Elderly patients may be adequately treated with daily dosage of 20 mg or less.
Patients taking cyclosporine: begin with 5 mg P.O. daily; don't exceed 10 mg P.O. daily. In patients taking fibrates or niacin, maximum dose is 10 mg P.O. daily. In patients with severe renal insufficiency, begin with 5 mg P.O. daily.
▶ **Reduction of total cholesterol and LDL levels in patients with homozygous familial hypercholesterolemia.** *Adults:* 40 mg P.O. daily in the evening or 80 mg P.O. daily given in 3 divided doses of 20 mg, 20 mg, and 40 mg in the evening.

How supplied

Tablets: 5 mg, 10 mg, 20 mg, 40 mg, 80 mg

Pharmacokinetics

Absorption: readily absorbed; however, extensive hepatic extraction limits plasma availability of active inhibitors to 5% of dose or less. Individual absorption varies considerably.
Distribution: parent drug and active metabolites are more than 95% bound to plasma proteins.
Metabolism: hydrolysis occurs in plasma; at least three major metabolites have been identified.
Excretion: excreted primarily in bile. *Half-life:* 3 hours.

Route	Onset	Peak	Duration
P.O.	Unknown	1.3-2.4 hr	Unknown

Pharmacodynamics

Chemical effect: inhibits 3-hydroxy-3-methylglutaryl coenzyme A reductase. This enzyme is early (and rate-limiting) step in synthetic pathway of cholesterol.
Therapeutic effect: lowers LDL and total cholesterol levels.

Adverse reactions

CNS: headache, asthenia.
GI: abdominal pain, constipation, diarrhea, dyspepsia, flatulence, nausea.
Hepatic: elevated liver enzyme levels.
Respiratory: upper respiratory tract infection.

Interactions

Drug-drug. *Digoxin:* simvastatin may elevate digoxin levels slightly. Closely monitor plasma digoxin levels at start of simvastatin therapy.
Drugs that decrease levels or activity of endogenous steroids (such as cimetidine, ketoconazole, spironolactone): may increase risk of developing endocrine dysfunction.
Erythromycin, fibric acid derivatives (such as clofibrate, gemfibrozil), high doses of niacin (nicotinic acid; 1 g or more daily), immuno-

suppressants (such as cyclosporine): may increase risk of rhabdomyolysis. Monitor patient closely if concomitant use can't be avoided. Limit daily dosage of simvastatin to 10 mg if patient must take cyclosporine.
Hepatotoxic drugs: increased risk of hepatotoxicity. Avoid concomitant use.
Warfarin: anticoagulant effect may be slightly enhanced. Monitor PT at start of therapy and during dosage adjustments.
Drug-lifestyle. *Alcohol use:* increased risk of hepatotoxicity. Discourage concomitant use.

Contraindications and precautions

- Contraindicated in patients hypersensitive to drug, pregnant or breast-feeding women, women of childbearing age unless they have no risk of pregnancy, and those with active liver disease or conditions that have unexplained persistent elevations of serum transaminase levels.
- Use cautiously in patients who consume substantial quantities of alcohol or have history of liver disease.
- Safety of drug hasn't been established in children.

NURSING CONSIDERATIONS

Assessment

- Obtain history of patient's LDL and total cholesterol levels before therapy, and reassess regularly thereafter.
- Liver function tests should be performed at start of therapy and periodically thereafter. A liver biopsy may be performed if enzyme level elevations persist.
- Be alert for adverse reactions and drug interactions.
- Assess patient's dietary fat intake.
- Evaluate patient's and family's knowledge of drug therapy.

Nursing diagnoses

- Risk for injury related to presence of elevated cholesterol levels
- Constipation related to drug-induced adverse GI reactions
- Deficient knowledge related to drug therapy

Planning and implementation

- Drug therapy starts only after diet and other nondrug therapies have proven ineffective. Patient should follow a standard low-cholesterol diet during therapy.
- Give drug with evening meal for enhanced effectiveness.
- If cholesterol level falls below target range, dosage may be reduced.
- Make sure patient follows an appropriate diet.

ALERT Don't confuse Zocor with Cozaar.

Patient teaching

- Tell patient to take drug with evening meal because absorption and cholesterol biosynthesis are enhanced.
- Teach patient dietary management of serum lipids (restricting total fat and cholesterol intake) and measures to control other cardiac disease risk factors. If appropriate, suggest weight control, exercise, and smoking cessation programs.
- Tell patient to inform prescriber about adverse reactions, particularly muscle aches and pains.

ALERT Inform woman that drug is contraindicated during pregnancy. Advise her to notify prescriber immediately if pregnancy occurs.

Evaluation

- Patient's LDL and total cholesterol levels are within normal limits.
- Patient regains and maintains normal bowel pattern throughout therapy.
- Patient and family state understanding of drug therapy.

sirolimus

(sir-AH-lih-mus)
Rapamune

Pharmacologic class: macrocyclic lactone
Therapeutic class: immunosuppressant
Pregnancy risk category: C

Indications and dosages

▶ **Prophylaxis, with cyclosporine and corticosteroids, of organ rejection in patients receiving renal transplants.** *Adults and adolescents ages 13 and older who weigh 40 kg (88 lb) or more:* initially, 6 mg P.O. as a one-time loading dose as soon as possible after transplantation; then maintenance dose of 2 mg P.O. once daily.
Adolescents ages 13 and older who weigh less than 40 kg: initially, 3 mg/m² P.O. as a one-time loading dose after transplantation; then maintenance dose of 1 mg/m² P.O. once daily.

How supplied

Oral solution: 1 mg/ml

Pharmacokinetics

Absorption: rapidly absorbed from GI tract, with mean peak levels occurring in about 1 to 3 hours. Oral bioavailability is about 14%. Food decreases peak plasma levels and increased time to peak level.
Distribution: extensively partitioned into formed blood elements. Drug is extensively bound to plasma proteins (about 92%).
Metabolism: extensively metabolized by the mixed function oxidase system, primarily cytochrome P-450 3A4. Seven major metabolites have been identified in whole blood.
Excretion: excreted in feces (91%) and in urine (2.2%). *Half-life:* about 62 hours.

Route	Onset	Peak	Duration
P.O.	Unknown	1-3 hr	Unknown

Pharmacodynamics

Chemical effect: an immunosuppressant that inhibits T-lymphocyte activation and proliferation that occur in response to antigenic and cytokine stimulation. Also inhibits antibody formation.
Therapeutic effect: immunosuppression in patients receiving renal transplants.

Adverse reactions

CNS: *headache, insomnia, tremor, anxiety, depression, asthenia,* malaise, syncope, confusion, dizziness, emotional lability, hypertonia, hypoesthesia, hypotonia, neuropathy, paresthesia, somnolence.
CV: *hypertension,* ***heart failure, atrial fibrillation,*** tachycardia, hypotension, *chest pain, edema,* ***hemorrhage,*** palpitations, peripheral vascular disorder, thrombophlebitis, thrombosis, vasodilation.
EENT: facial edema, *pharyngitis,* epistaxis, rhinitis, sinusitis, abnormal vision, cataract, conjunctivitis, deafness, ear pain, otitis media, tinnitus.
GI: *diarrhea, nausea, vomiting, constipation, abdominal pain, dyspepsia,* enlarged abdomen, hernia, ascites, peritonitis, anorexia, dysphagia, eructation, esophagitis, flatulence, gastritis, gastroenteritis, gingivitis, gum hyperplasia, ileus, mouth ulceration, oral candidiasis, stomatitis.
GU: dysuria, hematuria, albuminuria, ***kidney tubular necrosis****, increased creatinine level, urinary tract infection,* pelvic pain, glycosuria, increased BUN level, bladder pain, hernia, hydronephrosis, impotence, kidney pain, nocturia, oliguria, pyuria, scrotal edema, testis disorder, ***toxic nephropathy***, urinary frequency, urinary incontinence, urine retention.
Hematologic: *anemia,* THROMBOCYTOPENIA, ***leukopenia,*** thrombotic thrombocytopenic purpura, ecchymosis, leukocytosis, polycythemia, lymphadenopathy.
Hepatic: elevation in liver enzyme levels.
Metabolic: *hypercholesteremia, hyperlipidemia, hypokalemia, weight gain, hypophosphatemia, hyperkalemia,* hypervolemia, Cushing's syndrome, diabetes mellitus, acidosis, dehydration, hypercalcemia, hyperglycemia, hyperphosphatemia, hypocalcemia, hypoglycemia, hypomagnesemia, hyponatremia, weight loss.
Musculoskeletal: *back pain, arthralgia,* myalgia, arthrosis, bone necrosis, leg cramps, osteoporosis, tetany.
Respiratory: *dyspnea, cough, atelectasis, upper respiratory tract infection,* asthma, bronchitis, hypoxia, lung edema, pleural effusion, pneumonia.
Skin: *rash, acne,* hirsutism, fungal dermatitis, pruritus, skin hypertrophy, skin ulcer, sweating.

Other: *fever, pain, peripheral edema,* abscess, cellulitis, chills, flu syndrome, infection, ***sepsis,*** lymphadenopathy, abnormal healing.

Interactions

Drug-drug. *Aminoglycosides, amphotericin, other nephrotoxic drugs:* increased risk of nephrotoxicity. Use cautiously.
Bromocriptine, cimetidine, clarithromycin, clotrimazole, danazol, erythromycin, fluconazole, indinavir, itraconazole, metoclopramide, nicardipine, ritonavir, verapamil, other drugs that inhibit CYP3A4: may decrease sirolimus metabolism, thereby increasing sirolimus levels. Monitor patient for loss of therapeutic effect.
Carbamazepine, phenobarbital, phenytoin, rifabutin, rifapentine, other drugs that induce CYP3A4: may increase sirolimus metabolism, thereby decreasing sirolimus blood levels. Monitor patient closely.
Cyclosporine (oral solution and capsules): increased sirolimus levels. Give sirolimus 4 hours after cyclosporine. After long-term use, sirolimus may reduce cyclosporine clearance, leading to need for reduction in cyclosporine dosage.
Diltiazem: increased sirolimus levels. Monitor and reduce dosage of sirolimus as necessary.
Ketoconazole: increased rate and extent of sirolimus absorption. Avoid concomitant use.
Live virus vaccines (BCG, measles, mumps, oral polio, rubella, TY21a typhoid, varicella, yellow fever): reduced effectiveness of vaccines. Avoid concomitant use.
Rifampin: decreased sirolimus levels. Consider alternatives to rifampin as directed.
Drug-food. *Grapefruit juice:* decreased metabolism of sirolimus. Avoid concomitant use.

Contraindications and precautions

- Contraindicated in patients hypersensitive to active drug or its derivatives or components. Use cautiously in patients with hyperlipidemia or impaired liver or renal function.

NURSING CONSIDERATIONS

Assessment

- Obtain history of patient's organ transplant before therapy, and reassess regularly thereafter.
- Monitor patient's liver and renal function and serum triglycerides before therapy.
- Monitor sirolimus levels in children, patients 13 or older who weigh less than 40 kg (88 lb); patients with hepatic impairment; patients receiving concurrent administration of drugs that induce or inhibit CYP3A4; and patients whose cyclosporine dosage is markedly reduced or discontinued.
- Monitor patient for infection and development of lymphoma, which may result from immunosuppression.
- Watch for development of rhabdomyolysis if patient is receiving sirolimus and cyclosporine is started as an HMG-CoA reductase inhibitor.
- Evaluate patient's and family's knowledge about drug therapy.

Nursing diagnoses

- Risk for injury related to potential for organ rejection
- Ineffective protection related to drug-induced immunosuppression
- Deficient knowledge related to drug therapy

Planning and implementation

- Drug should be taken consistently with or without food.

ALERT In patients with mild to moderate hepatic impairment, reduce maintenance dose by about one-third. It isn't necessary to reduce loading dose.

- Drug must be diluted before administration. After dilution, it should be used immediately.
- When diluting drug, empty correct amount into glass or plastic container filled with at least 2 oz (60 ml) of water or orange juice. Don't use grapefruit juice or any other liquid. Stir vigorously and have patient drink immediately. Refill container with at least 4 oz (120 ml) of water or orange juice, stir again, and have patient drink all contents.
- After opening bottle, use contents within 1 month. If necessary, bottles and pouches can be stored at room temperature (up to 77° F

[25° C]) for several days. Drug can be kept in oral dosing syringe for 24 hours at room temperature or refrigerated at 36° to 46° F.
- The syringe should be discarded after one use.
- A slight haze may develop during refrigeration, but this won't affect quality of drug. If haze develops, bring drug to room temperature and shake gently until haze disappears.
- Drug should be used in a regimen with cyclosporine and corticosteroids. Sirolimus should be taken 4 hours after cyclosporine dose.
- After transplantation, give antimicrobials for 1 year as directed to prevent *Pneumocystis carinii* and for 3 months as directed to prevent *Cytomegalovirus*.
- Vaccination may be less effective during sirolimus treatment. Avoid concomitant use of vaccines.
- If patient has hyperlipidemia, additional interventions, such as diet, exercise, and lipid-lowering drugs, should start, as ordered. Treatment with lipid-lowering drugs during therapy isn't uncommon.

Patient teaching
- Show patient how to properly store, dilute, and administer drug.
- Tell patient to take drug consistently with or without food to minimize absorption variability.
- Advise patient to take drug 4 hours after taking cyclosporine.
- Tell patient to wash area with soap and water if solution touches skin or mucous membranes; tell him to rinse eyes with plain water if solution gets in eyes.
- Inform woman of childbearing age of risks during pregnancy. Tell her to use effective contraception before, during, and for 12 weeks after stopping drug.

☑ Evaluation
- Patient doesn't experience organ rejection.
- Patient is free from infection and serious bleeding episodes throughout drug therapy.
- Patient and family state understanding of drug therapy.

sodium bicarbonate
(SOH-dee-um bigh-KAR-buh-nayt)
Arm and Hammer Pure Baking Soda, Bell/ans, Citrocarbonate, Soda Mint

Pharmacologic class: alkalinizing agent
Therapeutic class: systemic and urinary alkalinizer, systemic hydrogen ion buffer, oral antacid
Pregnancy risk category: C

Indications and dosages
▶ **Cardiac arrest.** *Adults and children:* 1 mEq/kg I.V. of 7.5% or 8.4% solution, followed by 0.5 mEq/kg I.V. every 10 minutes, depending on blood gases. Further dosages based on results of blood gas analysis. If blood gas analysis is unavailable, give 0.5 mEq/kg I.V. every 10 minutes until spontaneous circulation returns.
Infants up to age 2: not to exceed 8 mEq/kg I.V. daily of 4.2% solution.
▶ **Metabolic acidosis.** *Adults and children:* dosage depends on blood CO_2 content, pH, and patient's clinical condition. Generally, 2 to 5 mEq/kg I.V. infused over 4- to 8-hour period.
▶ **Systemic or urinary alkalinization.** *Adults:* initially, 4 g P.O., followed by 1 to 2 g q 4 hours.
Children: 84 to 840 mg/kg P.O. daily.
▶ **Antacid.** *Adults:* 300 mg to 2 g P.O. up to q.i.d. taken with glass of water.

How supplied
Tablets†: 300 mg, 325 mg, 520 mg, 600 mg, 650 mg
Injection: 4% (2.4 mEq/5 ml), 4.2% (5 mEq/10 ml), 5% (297.5 mEq/500 ml), 7.5% (8.92 mEq/10 ml and 44.6 mEq/50 ml), 8.4% (10 mEq/10 ml and 50 mEq/50 ml)

Pharmacokinetics
Absorption: well absorbed after P.O. administration.
Distribution: bicarbonate is confined to systemic circulation.
Metabolism: none.

Excretion: bicarbonate is filtered and reabsorbed by kidneys; less than 1% of filtered bicarbonate is excreted.

Route	Onset	Peak	Duration
P.O.	Unknown	Unknown	Unknown
I.V.	Immediate	Immediate	Unknown

Pharmacodynamics

Chemical effect: restores body's buffering capacity and neutralizes excess acid.
Therapeutic effect: restores normal acid-base balance and relieves acid indigestion.

Adverse reactions

GI: gastric distention, belching, flatulence.
Metabolic: ***metabolic alkalosis,*** hypernatremia, hypokalemia, hyperosmolarity (with overdose).
Other: pain and irritation at injection site.

Interactions

Drug-drug. *Anorexigenics, flecainide, mecamylamine, quinidine, sympathomimetics:* increased urine alkalinization causes increased renal clearance and reduced effectiveness of these drugs. Monitor patient closely.
Chlorpropamide, lithium, methotrexate, salicylates, tetracycline: urine alkalinization causes decreased renal clearance of these drugs and increased risk of toxicity. Monitor patient closely.
Enteric-coated drugs: may be released prematurely in stomach. Avoid concomitant use.
Ketoconazole: concurrent use may decrease absorption. Use with caution.

Contraindications and precautions

• Contraindicated in patients with metabolic or respiratory alkalosis, patients who are losing chlorides from vomiting or continuous GI suction, patients receiving diuretics known to produce hypochloremic alkalosis, and patients with hypocalcemia in which alkalosis may produce tetany, hypertension, seizures, or heart failure. Oral sodium bicarbonate is contraindicated in patients with acute ingestion of strong mineral acids.
• Use with extreme caution in patients with heart failure or other edematous or sodium-retaining conditions or renal insufficiency.
• Use cautiously in pregnant or breast-feeding women.

NURSING CONSIDERATIONS

Assessment

• Assess patient's condition before therapy and regularly thereafter.
• To avoid risk of alkalosis, obtain blood pH, Pa_{O_2}, Pa_{CO_2}, and serum electrolyte levels.
• If sodium bicarbonate is being used to produce alkaline urine, monitor urine pH (should be greater than 7) every 4 to 6 hours.
• Be alert for adverse reactions and drug interactions.
• Evaluate patient's and family's knowledge of drug therapy.

Nursing diagnoses

• Ineffective health maintenance related to underlying condition
• Risk for injury related to drug-induced adverse reactions
• Deficient knowledge related to drug therapy

Planning and implementation

• Drug isn't routinely recommended for use in cardiac arrest because it may produce paradoxical acidosis from CO_2 production. It shouldn't be routinely administered during early stages of resuscitation unless acidosis is clearly present. Drug may be used at team leader's discretion after such interventions as defibrillation, cardiac compression, and administration of first-line drugs.
P.O. use: Give drug with water, not milk.
I.V. use: Drug is usually given by I.V. infusion. When immediate treatment is needed, drug may be given by direct, rapid I.V. injection. However, in neonates and children younger than age 2, slow I.V. administration is preferred to avoid hypernatremia, decreased CSF pressure, and possible intracranial hemorrhage.
ALERT Sodium bicarbonate inactivates such catecholamines as norepinephrine and dopamine and forms precipitate with calcium.

Don't mix sodium bicarbonate with I.V. solutions of these drugs, and flush I.V. line adequately.
- Keep prescriber informed of laboratory results.

Patient teaching
- Tell patient not to take with milk. Drug may cause hypercalcemia, alkalosis or, possibly, renal calculi.
- Discourage use as antacid. Offer nonabsorbable alternate antacid if it is to be used repeatedly.

Evaluation
- Patient regains normal acid-base balance in body.
- Patient doesn't experience injury from drug-induced adverse reactions.
- Patient and family state understanding of drug therapy.

sodium chloride
(SOH-dee-um KLOR-ighd)

Pharmacologic class: electrolyte
Therapeutic class: sodium and chloride replacement
Pregnancy risk category: C

Indications and dosages

▶ **Fluid and electrolyte replacement in hyponatremia caused by electrolyte loss, severe salt depletion.** *Adults:* dosage is highly individualized. The 3% and 5% solutions are used only with frequent electrolyte determination and given only slow I.V. With 0.45% solution: 3% to 8% of body weight, according to deficiencies, over 18 to 24 hours. With 0.9% solution: 2% to 6% of body weight, according to deficiencies, over 18 to 24 hours.

▶ **Management of heat cramp caused by excessive perspiration.** *Adults:* 1 g P.O. with every glass of water.

How supplied

Tablets (enteric-coated): 650 mg, 1 g, 2.25 g
Tablets (slow-release): 600 mg
Injection: 0.45% saline solution 500 ml, 1,000 ml; 0.9% saline solution 50 ml, 100 ml, 150 ml, 250 ml, 500 ml, 1,000 ml; 3% saline solution 500 ml; 5% saline solution 500 ml; 14.6% saline solution 20 ml, 40 ml, 200 ml; 23.4% saline solution 30 ml, 50 ml, and 200 ml

Pharmacokinetics

Absorption: absorbed readily from GI tract after P.O. administration.
Distribution: distributed widely in body.
Metabolism: none significant.
Excretion: excreted primarily in urine; some excreted in sweat, tears, and saliva.

Route	Onset	Peak	Duration
P.O.	Unknown	Unknown	Unknown
I.V.	Immediate	Immediate	Unknown

Pharmacodynamics

Chemical effect: replaces and maintains sodium and chloride levels.
Therapeutic effect: restores normal sodium and chloride levels.

Adverse reactions

CV: aggravation of heart failure, edema if given too rapidly or in excess, thrombophlebitis.
Metabolic: hypernatremia, aggravation of existing metabolic acidosis with excessive infusion, electrolyte disturbances, hypokalemia.
Respiratory: ***pulmonary edema*** if given too rapidly or in excess.
Other: local tenderness, abscess, tissue necrosis at injection site.

Interactions

None significant.

Contraindications and precautions

- Contraindicated in patients with conditions in which sodium and chloride administration is detrimental. The 3% and 5% saline solution injections are contraindicated in patients with increased, normal, or only slightly decreased serum electrolyte levels.
- Use cautiously in elderly patients, postoperative patients, pregnant women, breast-feeding

women, and patients with heart failure, circulatory insufficiency, renal dysfunction, or hypoproteinemia.

NURSING CONSIDERATIONS

Assessment

- Obtain history of patient's sodium and chloride levels before therapy, and reassess regularly thereafter.
- Monitor other serum electrolyte levels.
- Assess patient's fluid status.
- Be alert for adverse reactions.
- Evaluate patient's and family's knowledge of drug therapy.

Nursing diagnoses

- Imbalanced nutrition: less than body requirements related to subnormal levels of sodium and chloride
- Excessive fluid volume related to saline solution's water-drawing power
- Deficient knowledge related to drug therapy

Planning and implementation

P.O. use: Give tablet with glass of water.
I.V. use: Infuse 3% and 5% solutions very slowly and cautiously to avoid pulmonary edema. Use only for critical situations, and observe patient continually.
ALERT Don't confuse concentrates (14.6% and 23.4%) available to add to parenteral nutrient solutions with normal saline solution injection, and never give without diluting. Read label carefully.

Patient teaching

- Tell patient to report adverse reactions promptly.

Evaluation

- Patient's sodium and chloride levels are normal.
- Patient doesn't exhibit signs and symptoms of fluid retention.
- Patient and family state understanding of drug therapy.

sodium ferric gluconate complex

(SOH-dee-um FEH-rik GLOO-kuh-nayt KOM-pleks)
Ferrlecit

Pharmacologic class: macromolecular iron complex
Therapeutic class: hematinic
Pregnancy risk category: B

Indications and dosages

▶ **Treatment of iron deficiency anemia in patients undergoing long-term hemodialysis who are receiving supplemental erythropoietin therapy.** *Adults:* Before starting therapeutic doses, give a test dose of 2 ml sodium ferric gluconate complex (25 mg elemental iron) diluted in 50 ml normal saline solution I.V. over 1 hour. If test dose is tolerated, give therapeutic dose of 10 ml (125 mg elemental iron) diluted in 100 ml normal saline solution I.V. over 1 hour. Most patients need a minimum cumulative dose of 1 g elemental iron given at more than eight sequential dialysis treatments to achieve a favorable hemoglobin or hematocrit response.

How supplied

Injection: 62.5 mg elemental iron (12.5 mg/ml) in 5-ml ampules

Pharmacokinetics

Unknown.

Route	Onset	Peak	Duration
I.V.	Unknown	Unknown	Unknown

Pharmacodynamics

Chemical effect: drug restores total body iron content, which is critical for normal hemoglobin synthesis and oxygen transport. Iron deficiency in hemodialysis patients can result from increased iron utilization (such as from erythropoietin therapy), blood loss (such as from fistula, retention in dialyzer, hematologic testing, menses), decreased dietary intake or absorption, surgery, iron sequestration because of inflammatory process, and malignancy.

Therapeutic effect: restores total body iron content.

Adverse reactions

CNS: asthenia, headache, fatigue, malaise, dizziness, paresthesia, agitation, insomnia, somnolence, syncope.
CV: hypotension, hypertension, tachycardia, ***bradycardia,*** angina, chest pain, ***MI,*** edema, flushing.
EENT: conjunctivitis, abnormal vision, rhinitis.
GI: nausea, vomiting, diarrhea, rectal disorder, dyspepsia, eructation, flatulence, melena, abdominal pain.
GU: UTI.
Hematologic: abnormal erythrocytes, anemia.
Metabolic: hyperkalemia, hypoglycemia, hypokalemia, hypervolemia.
Musculoskeletal: myalgia, arthralgia, back pain, arm pain, cramps.
Respiratory: dyspnea, coughing, upper respiratory tract infections, pneumonia, pulmonary edema.
Skin: pruritus, increased sweating, rash.
Other: injection site reaction, pain, fever, infection, rigors, chills, flulike syndrome, sepsis, ***carcinoma, hypersensitivity reactions,*** lymphadenopathy.

Interactions

None reported.

Contraindications and precautions

- Contraindicated in patients hypersensitive to sodium ferric gluconate complex or its components (such as benzyl alcohol). Also contraindicated in patients with anemias not linked to iron deficiency. Don't give to patients with iron overload.
- Use cautiously in elderly patients.

NURSING CONSIDERATIONS

Assessment

- Obtain history of patient's underlying condition before therapy, and reassess regularly thereafter.
- Check with patient about other possible sources of iron, such as nonprescription iron preparations and iron-containing multiple vitamins with minerals.
- Monitor hematocrit and hemoglobin, serum ferritin, and iron saturation levels during therapy, as ordered.
- Evaluate patient's and family's knowledge of drug therapy.

Nursing diagnoses

- Risk for injury related to drug-induced adverse reactions
- Activity intolerance related to underlying condition
- Deficient knowledge related to drug therapy

Planning and implementation

- Dilute test dose of sodium ferric gluconate complex in 50 ml normal saline solution and give over 1 hour. Dilute therapeutic doses of drug in 100 ml normal saline solution and give over 1 hour.
- Don't mix sodium ferric gluconate complex with other drugs or add to parenteral nutrition solutions for I.V. infusion. Use immediately after dilution in normal saline solution.

ALERT Patient may develop profound hypotension with flushing, light-headedness, malaise, fatigue, weakness, or severe chest, back, flank, or groin pain after rapid I.V. administration of iron. These reactions don't indicate hypersensitivity and may result from too-rapid administration of drug. Don't exceed recommended rate of administration (2.1 mg/minute). Monitor patient closely during infusion.

- Dosage is expressed in mg of elemental iron.
- Don't give drug to patients with iron overload, which commonly occurs in hemoglobinopathies and other refractory anemias.
- Potentially life-threatening hypersensitivity reactions may occur during infusion (characterized by CV collapse, cardiac arrest, bronchospasm, oral or pharyngeal edema, dyspnea, angioedema, urticaria, or pruritus sometimes linked with pain and muscle spasm of chest or back). Have adequate supportive measures readily available. Monitor patient closely during infusion.
- Some adverse reactions in hemodialysis patients may be related to dialysis itself or to chronic renal failure.

Patient teaching

- Abdominal pain, diarrhea, vomiting, drowsiness, or hyperventilation may indicate iron poisoning. Advise patient to report any of these symptoms immediately.

Evaluation

- Patient doesn't experience injury as a result of drug-induced adverse reactions.
- Patient experiences improved activity tolerance.
- Patient and family state understanding of drug therapy.

sodium fluoride

(SOH-dee-um FLOR-ighd)

Fluor-A-Day ♦, Fluoritab, Fluorodex, Fluotic ♦, Flura, Flura-Drops, Flura-Loz, Karidium, Luride, Luride Lozi-Tabs, Luride-SF, Luride-SF Lozi-Tabs, Pediaflor, Pedi-Dent ♦, Pharmaflur, Pharmaflur df, Pharmaflur 1.1, Phos-Flur, Solu-Flur ♦

sodium fluoride, topical

ACT†, Fluorigard†, Fluorinse, Gel-Kam, Gel-Tin†, Karigel, Karigel-N, Listermint with Fluoride, Minute-Gel, Point-Two, Prevident, Thera-Flur, Thera-Flur-N

Pharmacologic class: trace mineral
Therapeutic class: dental caries prophylactic
Pregnancy risk category: NR

Indications and dosages

▶ **Prevention of dental caries.** *Adults and children over age 12:* 10 ml of rinse or thin ribbon of gel applied to teeth with toothbrush or mouth trays for at least 1 minute h.s.
Children ages 6 to 12: 5 ml of rinse or thin ribbon of gel applied to teeth with toothbrush or mouth trays for at least 1 minute h.s.
Children ages 6 to 16: 1 mg P.O. (tablet or lozenge) daily.
Children ages 3 to 6: 0.5 mg P.O. (tablet or gtt) daily.
Children ages 6 months to 3 years: 0.25 mg P.O. (tablet or gtt) daily.

How supplied

sodium fluoride
Tablets: 1 mg
Tablets (chewable): 0.5 mg, 1 mg
Drops: 0.125 mg/drop, 0.25 mg/drop, 0.2 mg/ml, 0.5 mg/ml
Lozenges: 1 mg
sodium fluoride, topical
Gel: 0.1%, 0.5%, 1.23%
Gel drops: 0.5%
Rinse: 0.01%†, 0.02%†, 0.09%

Pharmacokinetics

Absorption: absorbed readily and almost completely from GI tract. A large amount may be absorbed in stomach, and rate of absorption may depend on gastric pH. Oral fluoride absorption may be decreased by simultaneous ingestion of aluminum or magnesium hydroxide. Simultaneous ingestion of calcium also may decrease absorption of large doses.
Distribution: stored in bones and developing teeth after absorption. Skeletal tissue also has high storage capacity for fluoride ions. Because of storage-mobilization mechanism in skeletal tissue, constant fluoride supply may be provided. Although teeth have small mass, they also serve as storage sites. Fluoride deposited in teeth isn't released readily. Fluoride has been found in all organs and tissues with low accumulation in noncalcified tissues. Fluoride is distributed into sweat, tears, hair, and saliva.
Metabolism: none.
Excretion: excreted rapidly, mainly in urine.

Route	Onset	Peak	Duration
P.O.	Unknown	30-60 min	Unknown

Pharmacodynamics

Chemical effect: stabilizes apatite crystal of bone and teeth.
Therapeutic effect: prevents dental caries.

Adverse reactions

CNS: headache, weakness.
GI: gastric distress.
Skin: hypersensitivity reactions.
Other: staining of teeth.

Interactions

Drug-drug. *Aluminum hydroxide, calcium, iron, magnesium:* may decrease absorption. Administer separately.
Drug-food. *Dairy products:* incompatibility may occur because of formation of calcium fluoride, which is poorly absorbed. Avoid ingestion during sodium fluoride therapy.

Contraindications and precautions

- Contraindicated in patients hypersensitive to fluoride and in those whose drinking water exceeds 0.7 parts per million of flouride.
- Use cautiously in pregnant or breast-feeding women.

NURSING CONSIDERATIONS

Assessment
- Obtain history of patient's dental history and fluoride intake before therapy, and reassess regularly thereafter.
- Be alert for adverse reactions and drug interactions.
- Chronic toxicity (fluorosis) may result from prolonged use of higher-than-recommended doses.
- Evaluate patient's and family's knowledge of drug therapy.

Nursing diagnoses
- Health-seeking behavior related to desire for good dental care
- Risk for deficient fluid volume related to drug-induced adverse GI reactions
- Deficient knowledge related to drug therapy

Planning and implementation
- Administer oral drops undiluted or mixed with fluids or food.
- Fluoride in prenatal vitamins has produced healthier teeth in infants.

ALERT Chronic toxicity (fluorosis) may result from prolonged use of higher-than-recommended doses.

Patient teaching
- Tell patient that tablets may be dissolved in mouth, chewed, or swallowed whole.
- Advise parents that topical rinses and gels shouldn't be swallowed by children under age 3 or used if water supply is fluorinated.
- Tell patient that sodium fluoride is most effective when used immediately after brushing teeth. Tell patient to rinse around and between teeth for 1 minute, and then spit fluid out.
- Tell patient to dilute drops or rinses in plastic rather than glass containers.
- Advise patient to notify dentist of tooth mottling.

Evaluation
- Patient is free from dental caries.
- Patient maintains adequate hydration throughout therapy.
- Patient and family state understanding of drug therapy.

sodium lactate
(SOH-dee-um LAK-tayt)

Pharmacologic class: alkalinizing agent
Therapeutic class: systemic alkalizer
Pregnancy risk category: NR

Indications and dosages

▶ **Urine alkalinization.** *Adults:* 30 ml of 1/6 molar solution per kilogram of body weight P.O. given in divided doses over 24 hours.
▶ **Metabolic acidosis.** *Adults*: 1/6 molar injection (167 mEq lactate/L) I.V.; dosage depends on degree of bicarbonate deficit.

How supplied

Injection: 1/6 molar solution (167 mEq/L)
Injection: 5 mEq/ml

Pharmacokinetics

Absorption: not applicable.
Distribution: lactate ion occurs naturally throughout body.
Metabolism: metabolized in liver.
Excretion: none.

Route	Onset	Peak	Duration
I.V.	Immediate	Immediate	Unknown

Pharmacodynamics

Chemical effect: metabolized to sodium bicarbonate, producing buffering effect.
Therapeutic effect: restores normal acid-base balance.

Adverse reactions

CV: thrombophlebitis at injection site.
Metabolic: ***metabolic alkalosis,*** hypernatremia, hyperosmolarity with overdose.
Other: fever; infection.

Interactions

None significant.

Contraindications and precautions

- Contraindicated in patients with hypernatremia, lactic acidosis, or conditions in which sodium administration is detrimental.
- Use with extreme caution in patients with metabolic or respiratory alkalosis, severe hepatic or renal disease, shock, hypoxia, or beriberi.
- Use cautiously in pregnant or breast-feeding women.

NURSING CONSIDERATIONS

Assessment

- Obtain history of patient's underlying acid-base imbalance before therapy, and reassess regularly thereafter.
- Monitor serum electrolyte levels.
- Evaluate patient's and family's knowledge of drug therapy.

Nursing diagnoses

- Ineffective health maintenance related to underlying condition
- Ineffective protection related to drug-induced adverse reactions
- Deficient knowledge related to drug therapy

Planning and implementation

- Add drug to other I.V. solutions or give as isotonic 1/6 molar solution. Drug is compatible with most common I.V. solutions.
- Don't mix with sodium bicarbonate because drugs are physically incompatible.

Patient teaching

- Instruct patient to report discomfort at I.V. site immediately.

Evaluation

- Patient regains normal acid-base balance.
- Patient doesn't experience serious adverse reactions.
- Patient and family state understanding of drug therapy.

sodium phosphates

(SOH-dee-um FOS-fayts)
Fleet Phospho-soda†

Pharmacologic class: acid salt
Therapeutic class: saline laxative
Pregnancy risk category: NR

Indications and dosages

▶ **Constipation.** *Adults:* 20 to 30 ml of solution mixed with 120 ml of cold water P.O. Or, 120 ml P.R. (as enema).
Children: 5 to 10 ml of solution mixed with 120 ml of cold water P.O. Or, 60 ml P.R. in children over age 2.
▶ **Purgative action.** *Adults:* 45 ml solution mixed with 120 ml cold water.

How supplied

Liquid: 2.4 g/5 ml sodium phosphate and 900 mg sodium biphosphate/5 ml
Enema: 160 mg/ml sodium phosphate and 60 mg/ml sodium biphosphate

Pharmacokinetics

Absorption: about 1% to 20% of P.O. dose absorbed; unknown after P.R. administration.
Distribution: unknown.
Metabolism: unknown.
Excretion: unknown.

Route	Onset	Peak	Duration
P.O.	0.5-3 hr	Varies	Varies
P.R.	5-10 min	Varies	Ends with evacuation

Pharmacodynamics

Chemical effect: produces osmotic effect in small intestine by drawing water into intestinal lumen.
Therapeutic effect: relieves constipation.

Adverse reactions

GI: *abdominal cramping.*
Metabolic: fluid and electrolyte disturbances (such as hypernatremia or hyperphosphatemia) with daily use.
Other: laxative dependence with long-term or excessive use.

Interactions

None significant.

Contraindications and precautions

- Contraindicated in patients on sodium-restricted diets and patients with intestinal obstruction or perforation, edema, heart failure, megacolon, impaired renal function, or symptoms of appendicitis or acute surgical abdomen, such as abdominal pain, nausea, and vomiting.
- Use cautiously in patients with large hemorrhoids or anal excoriations and in pregnant or breast-feeding women.

NURSING CONSIDERATIONS

Assessment

- Assess patient's condition before therapy and regularly thereafter.
- Before giving drug for constipation, determine if patient has adequate fluid intake, exercise, and diet.
- Be alert for adverse reactions.

ALERT Up to 10% of sodium content of drug may be absorbed.

- Evaluate patient's and family's knowledge of drug therapy.

Nursing diagnoses

- Constipation related to underlying condition
- Acute pain related to drug-induced abdominal cramping
- Deficient knowledge related to drug therapy

Planning and implementation

P.O. use: Dilute drug with water before giving (add 30 ml of drug to 120 ml of cold water). Follow administration with full glass of water.
P.R. use: Follow normal protocol.
Make sure that patient has easy access to bathroom facilities, commode, or bedpan.
ALERT Severe electrolyte imbalances may occur if recommended dosage is exceeded.

Patient teaching

- Teach patient about dietary sources of bulk, which include bran and other cereals, fresh fruit, and vegetables.
- Tell patient to maintain adequate fluid intake of at least 6 to 8 glasses of water or juices unless contraindicated.

Evaluation

- Patient's constipation is relieved.
- Patient's abdominal cramping ceases.
- Patient and family state understanding of drug therapy.

sodium polystyrene sulfonate

(SOH-dee-um pol-ee-STIGH-reen SUL-fuh-nayt)
Kayexalate, SPS

Pharmacologic class: cation-exchange resin
Therapeutic class: potassium-removing resin
Pregnancy risk category: C

Indications and dosages

▶ **Hyperkalemia.** *Adults:* 15 g P.O. daily to q.i.d. in water or sorbitol (3 to 4 ml/g of resin). Or, mix powder with appropriate medium—aqueous suspension or diet appropriate for renal failure—and instill into NG tube. Or 30 to 50 g q 6 hours as warm emulsion deep into sigmoid colon (20 cm). In persistent vomiting or paralytic ileus, high-retention enema of sodium polystyrene sulfonate (30 g) suspended in 200 ml of 10% methylcellulose, 10% dextrose, or 25% sorbitol solution may be given.
Children: 1 g of resin P.O. or P.R. for each milliequivalent of potassium to be removed.

P.O. route preferred because drug should stay in intestine for at least 6 hours.

How supplied

Powder: 1-pound jar (3.5 g/teaspoon)
Suspension: 60 ml*, 120 ml*, 200 ml*, 480 ml*, 500 ml*

Pharmacokinetics

Absorption: not absorbed.
Distribution: none.
Metabolism: none.
Excretion: excreted unchanged in feces.

Route	Onset	Peak	Duration
P.O., P.R.	Unknown	Unknown	Unknown

Pharmacodynamics

Chemical effect: exchanges sodium ions for potassium ions in intestine: 1 g of sodium polystyrene sulfonate is exchanged for 0.5 to 1.0 mEq of potassium. The resin is then eliminated. Much of exchange capacity is used for cations other than potassium (calcium and magnesium) and, possibly, fats and proteins.
Therapeutic effect: lowers serum potassium level.

Adverse reactions

GI: *constipation,* fecal impaction in elderly patients, anorexia, gastric irritation, nausea, vomiting, *diarrhea* with sorbitol emulsions.
Metabolic: hypokalemia, hypocalcemia, sodium retention.

Interactions

Drug-drug. *Antacids and laxatives (nonabsorbable cation-donating types, including magnesium hydroxide):* systemic alkalosis and reduced potassium exchange capability. Don't use together.

Contraindications and precautions

- Contraindicated in patients hypersensitive to drug and in those with hypokalemia.
- Use cautiously in pregnant or breast-feeding women and patients with severe heart failure, severe hypertension, or marked edema.

NURSING CONSIDERATIONS

Assessment

- Obtain history of patient's serum potassium level before therapy.
- Monitor serum potassium level at least once daily, as ordered. Treatment may result in potassium deficiency. Treatment usually stops when potassium level declines to 4 or 5 mEq/L.

ALERT Watch for other signs of hypokalemia, such as irritability, confusion, arrhythmias, ECG changes, severe muscle weakness and paralysis, and cardiac toxicity in digitalized patients.

- Monitor patient for symptoms of other electrolyte deficiencies (magnesium, calcium) because drug is nonselective. Monitor serum calcium level in patient receiving sodium polystyrene therapy for more than 3 days. Supplementary calcium may be needed.
- Watch for sodium overload. Drug contains about 100 mg of sodium/g. About one-third of sodium in resin is retained.
- Be alert for adverse reactions and drug interactions.
- Watch for constipation with P.O. or NG administration.
- Evaluate patient's and family's knowledge of drug therapy.

Nursing diagnoses

- Ineffective health maintenance related to presence of hyperkalemia
- Constipation related to drug-induced adverse GI reactions
- Deficient knowledge related to drug therapy

Planning and implementation

- Don't heat resin; doing so will impair drug's effectiveness.

P.O. use: Mix resin only with water or sorbitol for P.O. administration. Never mix with orange juice (high potassium content) to disguise taste.
– Chill oral suspension for greater palatability.
– If sorbitol is given, mix with resin suspension.
– Consider solid form. Resin cookie and candy recipes are available; ask pharmacist or dietitian to supply.

– To prevent constipation, use sorbitol (10 to 20 ml of 70% syrup every 2 hours, as needed) to produce one or two watery stools daily.
P.R. use: Premixed forms are available (SPS and others).
– If preparing manually, mix polystyrene resin only with water and sorbitol for P.R. use. Don't use mineral oil for P.R. administration to prevent impaction; ion exchange requires aqueous medium. Sorbitol content prevents impaction.
– Prepare P.R. dose at room temperature. Stir emulsion gently during administration.
– Use #28 French rubber tube. Insert tube 20 cm into sigmoid colon and tape in place. Or, consider Foley catheter with 30-ml balloon inflated distal to anal sphincter to aid in retention. This is especially helpful for patients with poor sphincter control (for example, after CVA). Use gravity flow. Drain returns constantly through Y-tube connection. Place patient in knee-chest position or with hips on pillow for a while if back leakage occurs.
– After P.R. administration, flush tubing with 50 to 100 ml of nonsodium fluid to ensure delivery of all drug. Flush rectum to remove resin.
– Prevent fecal impaction in elderly patient by administering resin P.R., as ordered. Give cleansing enema before P.R. administration. Explain to patient the need to retain enema—6 to 10 hours is ideal, but 30 to 60 minutes is acceptable.
• If hyperkalemia is severe, prescriber won't depend solely on polystyrene resin to lower serum potassium level. Dextrose 50% with regular insulin may be given by I.V. push.

Patient teaching
• Explain importance of following prescribed low-potassium diet.
• Explain necessity of retaining enema (6 to 10 hours is ideal, but 30 to 60 minutes is acceptable).
• Tell patient to report adverse reactions.

Evaluation
• Patient's serum potassium level is normal.
• Patient doesn't develop constipation.
• Patient and family state understanding of drug therapy.

somatrem
(SOH-muh-trem)
Protropin

Pharmacologic class: anterior pituitary hormone
Therapeutic class: human growth hormone (GH)
Pregnancy risk category: C

Indications and dosages
▶ **Long-term treatment of children who have growth failure because of lack of adequate endogenous GH secretion.** *Children (prepuberty):* highly individualized; up to 0.1 mg/kg I.M. or S.C. three times weekly.

How supplied
Injectable lyophilized powder: 5 mg (10 IU)/vial

Pharmacokinetics
Absorption: unknown.
Distribution: unknown.
Metabolism: about 90% metabolized in liver.
Excretion: about 0.1% excreted unchanged in urine. *Half-life:* 20 to 30 minutes.

Route	Onset	Peak	Duration
I.M., S.C.	Unknown	Unknown	12-48 hr

Pharmacodynamics
Chemical effect: purified GH of recombinant DNA origin that stimulates linear, skeletal muscle, and organ growth.
Therapeutic effect: stimulates growth in children.

Adverse reactions
Metabolic: hypothyroidism, hyperglycemia.
Other: antibodies to GH.

Interactions
Drug-drug. *Glucocorticoids:* may inhibit growth-promoting action of somatrem. Adjust glucocorticoid dosage as necessary.

Contraindications and precautions

- Contraindicated in patients hypersensitive to benzyl alcohol and in those with epiphyseal closure or active neoplasia.
- Use cautiously in patients with hypothyroidism and in those whose GH deficiency results from an intracranial lesion.
- Drug isn't indicated for pregnant or breast-feeding women.

NURSING CONSIDERATIONS

Assessment

- Assess child's growth before therapy and regularly thereafter.
- Be alert for adverse reactions and drug interactions.

ALERT Toxicity in neonates has occurred from exposure to benzyl alcohol used in drug as preservative.

- Monitor height and blood with regular checkups; radiologic studies are also necessary.
- Observe patient for signs of glucose intolerance and hyperglycemia.
- Monitor periodic thyroid function tests for hypothyroidism, as ordered, which may require treatment with thyroid hormone.
- Evaluate patient's and family's knowledge of drug therapy.

Nursing diagnoses

- Delayed growth and development related to lack of adequate endogenous GH
- Ineffective health maintenance related to adverse metabolic reactions
- Deficient knowledge related to drug therapy

Planning and implementation

- Check drug's expiration date.
- To prepare solution, inject supplied bacteriostatic water for injection into vial containing drug. Then swirl vial with gentle rotary motion until contents are dissolved. Don't shake vial.
- After reconstitution, vial solution should be clear. Don't inject if solution is cloudy or contains particles.
- If drug is given to neonate, reconstitute immediately before use with sterile water for injection (without bacteriostat). Use vial once, then discard.
- Store reconstituted vial in refrigerator; use within 7 days.

ALERT Don't confuse somatrem with somatropin.

Patient teaching

- Reassure patient and family members that somatrem is pure and safe. Drug replaces pituitary-derived human GH, which was removed from market in 1985 because of an association with rare but fatal viral infection (Creutzfeldt-Jakob disease).

Evaluation

- Patient exhibits growth.
- Patient's thyroid function studies and blood glucose level are normal.
- Patient and family state understanding of drug therapy.

somatropin

(soh-muh-TROH-pin)

Genotropin, Humatrope, Norditropin, Nutropin, Saizen, Serostim

Pharmacologic class: anterior pituitary hormone
Therapeutic class: human growth hormone (GH)
Pregnancy risk category: C

Indications and dosages

▶ **Long-term treatment of growth failure in children with inadequate secretion of endogenous GH. Humatrope.** *Children:* 0.18 mg/kg of body weight S.C. weekly, divided equally and given on 3 alternate days, six times weekly or daily.
Nutropin. *Children:* 0.30 mg/kg of body weight S.C. weekly in daily divided doses.
Saizen. *Children:* 0.06 mg/kg S.C. or I.M. three times weekly.
Norditropin. *Children:* 0.024 to 0.034 mg/kg S.C. six or seven times weekly.
Genotropin. *Children:* 0.16 to 0.24 mg/kg/week divided into six or seven S.C. injections.
Serostim. *Children:* About 0.1 mg/kg S.C. daily h.s. See manufacturer's dosing chart.

▶ **Growth failure in children related to chronic renal insufficiency up to time of renal transplantation. Nutropin.** *Children:* 0.35 mg/kg of body weight S.C. weekly in daily divided doses.
▶ **Replacement of endogenous growth hormone in adult patients with growth hormone deficiency.** *Adults:* initially, no more than 0.006 mg/kg S.C. daily. May be increased to maximum of 0.025 mg/kg daily in patients younger than age 35 or 0.0125 mg/kg daily in patients older than age 35.

How supplied

Injection: 1.5 mg/ml; 5 mg/5 ml; 4-mg, 5-mg, 8-mg, 10-mg vials

Pharmacokinetics

Absorption: unknown.
Distribution: unknown.
Metabolism: about 90% metabolized in liver.
Excretion: about 0.1% excreted unchanged in urine. *Half-life:* 20 to 30 minutes.

Route	Onset	Peak	Duration
I.M, S.C.	Unknown	7.5 hr	12-48 hr

Pharmacodynamics

Chemical effect: purified GH of recombinant DNA origin that stimulates linear, skeletal muscle, and organ growth.
Therapeutic effect: stimulates growth.

Adverse reactions

CNS: headache, weakness.
CV: mild, transient edema.
Hematologic: ***leukemia.***
Metabolic: mild hyperglycemia, hypothyroidism.
Musculoskeletal: localized muscle pain.
Other: injection site pain, antibodies to GH.

Interactions

Drug-drug. *Corticosteroids, corticotropin:* long-term use inhibits growth response to GH. Monitor patient.

Contraindications and precautions

• Contraindicated in patients with closed epiphyses or an active underlying intracranial lesion. Humatrope shouldn't be reconstituted with supplied diluent for patients with known sensitivity to either m-cresol or glycerin.
• Use cautiously in children with hypothyroidism and those whose GH deficiency is caused by an intracranial lesion. These children should be examined frequently for progression or recurrence of underlying disease.
• Drug isn't indicated for pregnant or breast-feeding women.

NURSING CONSIDERATIONS

Assessment

• Assess child's growth before therapy and regularly thereafter.
• Be alert for adverse reactions.
• Toxicity in neonates has occurred from exposure to benzyl alcohol used in drug as preservative.
• Regular checkups with monitoring of height and of blood and radiologic studies are necessary.
• Observe patient for signs of glucose intolerance and hyperglycemia.
• Monitor periodic thyroid function tests for hypothyroidism, as ordered, which may require treatment with thyroid hormone.
• Evaluate patient's and family's knowledge of drug therapy.

Nursing diagnoses

• Delayed growth and development related to lack of adequate endogenous GH
• Ineffective health maintenance related to adverse metabolic reactions
• Deficient knowledge related to drug therapy

Planning and implementation

• To prepare solution, inject supplied diluent into vial containing drug by aiming stream of liquid against glass wall of vial. Then swirl vial with gentle rotary motion until contents are completely dissolved. Don't shake vial.
• After reconstitution, solution should be clear. Don't inject solution if it's cloudy or contains particles.
• Store reconstituted vial in refrigerator; use within 14 days.
• If sensitivity to diluent should occur, vials may be reconstituted with sterile water for injection. When drug is reconstituted in this

manner, use only one reconstituted dose per vial, refrigerate solution if it isn't used immediately after reconstitution, use reconstituted dose within 24 hours, and discard unused portion.

• Excessive glucocorticoid therapy inhibits growth-promoting effect of somatropin. Patient with coexisting corticotropin deficiency should have glucocorticoid replacement dosage carefully adjusted to avoid an inhibitory effect on growth.

ALERT Don't confuse somatropin with somatrem or sumatriptan.

Patient teaching

• Inform parents that child with endocrine disorders (including GH deficiency) may develop slipped capital epiphyses more frequently. Tell them that if they notice their child limping, they should notify prescriber.

Evaluation

• Patient exhibits growth.
• Patient's thyroid function studies and blood glucose level are normal.
• Patient and family state understanding of drug therapy.

sotalol hydrochloride

(SOH-tuh-lol high-droh-KLOR-ighd)
Betapace, Sotacor ♦ ◇

Pharmacologic class: beta blocker
Therapeutic class: antiarrhythmic, antihypertensive, antianginal
Pregnancy risk category: B

Indications and dosages

▶ **Documented, life-threatening ventricular arrhythmias.** *Adults:* initially, 80 mg P.O. b.i.d. Dosage is increased q 2 to 3 days as needed and tolerated; most patients respond to 160 to 320 mg daily. A few patients with refractory arrhythmias have received as much as 640 mg daily.
Patients with renal failure: if creatinine clearance is over 60 ml/minute, dosage adjustment isn't necessary. If creatinine clearance is 30 to 60 ml/minute, interval is increased to q 24 hours; if 10 to 30 ml/minute, q 36 to 48 hours; if less than 10 ml/minute, individualized dosage.

▶ **Maintenance of normal sinus rhythm or delay in time to recurrence of atrial fibrillation or atrial flutter in patients with symptomatic atrial fibrillation or atrial flutter who are currently in sinus rhythm.** *Adults:* 80 mg P.O. b.i.d. Dosage may be increased as needed to 120 mg P.O. b.i.d. after 3 days if the QT interval is less than 500 msec. Maximum dose is 160 mg P.O. b.i.d.

How supplied

Tablets: 80 mg, 120 mg, 160 mg, 240 mg

Pharmacokinetics

Absorption: well absorbed with bioavailability of 90% to 100%. Food may interfere with absorption.
Distribution: unknown; doesn't bind to plasma proteins and crosses blood-brain barrier poorly.
Metabolism: not metabolized.
Excretion: excreted primarily in urine in unchanged form. *Half-life:* 12 hours.

Route	Onset	Peak	Duration
P.O.	Unknown	2.5-4 hr	Unknown

Pharmacodynamics

Chemical effect: depresses sinus heart rate, slows AV conduction, decreases cardiac output, and lowers systolic and diastolic blood pressure.
Therapeutic effect: restores normal sinus rhythm, lowers blood pressure, and relieves angina.

Adverse reactions

CNS: *asthenia, headache, dizziness, weakness, fatigue,* sleep problems, *light-headedness.*
CV: ***bradycardia, arrhythmias, heart failure, AV block, proarrhythmic events (ventricular tachycardia, PVCs, ventricular fibrillation),*** edema, *palpitations, chest pain,* ECG abnormalities, hypotension.
GI: *nausea,* vomiting, diarrhea, dyspepsia.
Respiratory: *dyspnea,* ***bronchospasm.***

Interactions

Drug-drug. *Antiarrhythmics:* additive effects. Avoid concomitant use.
Antihypertensives, catecholamine-depleting drugs (such as guanethidine, haloperidol, and reserpine): enhanced hypotensive effects. Monitor patient closely.
Calcium channel blockers: enhanced myocardial depression. Monitor patient carefully.
Clonidine: beta blockers may enhance rebound effect seen after withdrawal of clonidine. Discontinue sotalol several days before withdrawing clonidine.
General anesthetics: may cause additional myocardial depression. Monitor patient closely.
Insulin, oral antidiabetics: may cause hyperglycemia and may mask symptoms of hyperglycemia. Adjust dosage as directed.
Drug-food. *Any food:* increased absorption. Give drug on an empty stomach.

Contraindications and precautions

- Contraindicated in patients hypersensitive to drug and patients with severe sinus node dysfunction, sinus bradycardia, second- or third-degree AV block in absence of an artificial pacemaker, congenital or acquired long-QT syndrome, cardiogenic shock, uncontrolled heart failure, or bronchial asthma.
- Use cautiously in pregnant women and patients with renal impairment or diabetes mellitus.
- Safety of drug hasn't been established in children or breast-feeding women.

NURSING CONSIDERATIONS

Assessment

- Assess patient's condition before therapy and regularly thereafter.
- Monitor serum electrolyte levels and ECG regularly, especially if patient is receiving diuretics. Electrolyte imbalances, such as hypokalemia and hypomagnesemia, may enhance QT-interval prolongation and increase risk of serious arrhythmias such as torsades de pointes.
- Be alert for adverse reactions and drug interactions.
- Evaluate patient's and family's knowledge of drug therapy.

Nursing diagnoses

- Ineffective health maintenance related to underlying condition
- Fatigue related to adverse reactions
- Deficient knowledge related to drug therapy

Planning and implementation

- Because proarrhythmic events may occur at start of therapy and during dosage adjustments, patient should be hospitalized. Facilities and personnel should be available to monitor cardiac rhythm and interpret ECG.
- Although patients receiving I.V. lidocaine have started sotalol therapy without ill effect, other antiarrhythmic drugs should be withdrawn before therapy with sotalol. Sotalol therapy typically is delayed until two or three half-lives of withdrawn drug have elapsed. After withdrawal of amiodarone, sotalol shouldn't be administered until QT interval normalizes.

ALERT In patients with creatinine clearance of 40 to 60 ml/minute, increase dosage interval to every 24 hours.

- Dosage should be adjusted slowly, allowing 2 to 3 days between dosage increments for adequate monitoring of QT intervals and for plasma drug levels to reach steady-state level.

ALERT Don't confuse sotalol with Statrol or Stadol. Don't substitute Betapace AF for Betapace.

Patient teaching

- Explain importance of taking drug as prescribed, even when feeling well. Caution patient not to stop drug suddenly.
- Tell patient to take drug 1 hour before or 2 hours after meals.
- Teach patient how to check his pulse rate.

Evaluation

- Patient responds well to therapy.
- Patient states energy-conserving measures to combat fatigue.
- Patient and family state understanding of drug therapy.

spectinomycin hydrochloride

(spek-tih-noh-MIGH-sin high-droh-KLOR-ighd)
Trobicin

Pharmacologic class: aminocyclitol
Therapeutic class: antibiotic
Pregnancy risk category: B

Indications and dosages

▶ **Gonorrhea.** *Adults:* 2 to 4 g I.M. as single dose injected deep into upper outer quadrant of buttock.

How supplied

Injection: 2-g vial with 3.2-ml diluent; 4-g vial with 6.2-ml diluent
Powder for injection: 2 g, 4 g

Pharmacokinetics

Absorption: absorbed rapidly after I.M. injection.
Distribution: unknown.
Metabolism: unknown.
Excretion: most excreted unchanged in urine. *Half-life:* 1 to 3 hours.

Route	Onset	Peak	Duration
I.M.	Unknown	1-2 hr	Unknown

Pharmacodynamics

Chemical effect: inhibits protein synthesis by binding to 30S subunit of ribosome.
Therapeutic effect: hinders bacterial growth. Drug is bactericidal; its spectrum of activity includes many gram-positive and gram-negative organisms. However, spectinomycin hydrochloride is used mostly against penicillin-resistant *Neisseria gonorrhoeae.*

Adverse reactions

CNS: insomnia, dizziness.
GI: nausea.
GU: decreased urine output, decreased creatinine clearance, increased BUN level.
Hematologic: decreased hemoglobin level and hematocrit.
Hepatic: transient increases in liver enzyme levels.
Skin: urticaria.
Other: ***anaphylaxis,*** fever, chills (may mask or delay symptoms of incubating syphilis), pain at injection site.

Interactions

None significant.

Contraindications and precautions

- Contraindicated in patients hypersensitive to drug.
- Use cautiously in pregnant women.
- Safety of drug hasn't been established in children or breast-feeding women.

NURSING CONSIDERATIONS

Assessment

- Assess patient's infection before therapy and regularly thereafter.
- Drug isn't effective against syphilis. Serologic test for syphilis should be done before treatment and 3 months afterward.
- Be alert for adverse reactions and drug interactions.
- Monitor patient's hydration status if adverse GI reactions occur.
- Evaluate patient's and family's knowledge of drug therapy.

Nursing diagnoses

- Infection related to presence of susceptible bacteria
- Risk for deficient fluid volume related to drug-induced adverse GI reactions
- Deficient knowledge related to drug therapy

Planning and implementation

- Shake vial vigorously after reconstitution and before withdrawing dose. Store at room temperature after reconstitution, and use within 24 hours.
- Use 20G needle to administer drug. Divide 4-g dose (10 ml) into two 5-ml injections and give one in each buttock.

Patient teaching

- Inform patient that sexual partners must be treated.
- Teach the patient that condoms may be used to prevent transmission of sexually transmitted diseases.

☑ Evaluation

- Patient is free from infection.
- Patient maintains adequate hydration throughout therapy.
- Patient and family state understanding of drug therapy.

spironolactone

(spih-ron-uh-LAK-tohn)

Aldactone, Novospiroton♦, Spiractin◇

Pharmacologic class: potassium-sparing diuretic
Therapeutic class: management of edema, antihypertensive, diagnosis of primary hyperaldosteronism, treatment of diuretic-induced hypokalemia
Pregnancy risk category: NR

Indications and dosages

▶ **Edema.** *Adults:* 25 to 200 mg P.O. daily or in divided doses.
Children: 3.3 mg/kg P.O. daily or in divided doses.
▶ **Hypertension.** *Adults:* 50 to 100 mg P.O. daily or in divided doses.
▶ **Diuretic-induced hypokalemia.** *Adults:* 25 to 100 mg P.O. daily when P.O. potassium supplements are contraindicated.
▶ **Detection of primary hyperaldosteronism.** *Adults:* 400 mg P.O. daily for 4 days (short test) or 3 to 4 weeks (long test). If hypokalemia and hypertension are corrected, presumptive diagnosis of primary hyperaldosteronism is made.
▶ **Management of primary hyperaldosteronism.** *Adults:* 100 to 400 mg P.O. daily.

How supplied

Tablets: 25 mg, 50 mg, 100 mg

Pharmacokinetics

Absorption: about 90% absorbed from GI tract.
Distribution: more than 90% plasma protein–bound.
Metabolism: metabolized rapidly and extensively to canrenone, its major active metabolite.
Excretion: canrenone and other metabolites excreted primarily in urine, minimally in feces. *Half-life:* 13 to 24 hours.

Route	Onset	Peak	Duration
P.O.	1-2 days	2-3 days	2-3 days

Pharmacodynamics

Chemical effect: antagonizes aldosterone in distal tubule.
Therapeutic effect: promotes water and sodium excretion and hinders potassium excretion, lowers blood pressure, and helps to diagnose primary hyperaldosteronism.

Adverse reactions

CNS: headache, drowsiness, lethargy, confusion, ataxia.
GI: diarrhea, gastric bleeding, ulceration, cramping, gastritis, vomiting.
GU: transient elevation in BUN level, inability to maintain an erection, menstrual disturbances.
Hematologic: ***agranulocytosis.***
Metabolic: ***hyperkalemia,*** hyponatremia, mild acidosis, dehydration.
Skin: urticaria, hirsutism, maculopapular eruptions.
Other: drug fever, gynecomastia, breast soreness, ***anaphylaxis.***

Interactions

Drug-drug. *ACE inhibitors, indomethacin, other potassium-sparing diuretics, potassium supplements:* increased risk of hyperkalemia. Don't use together, especially in patients with renal impairment.
Aspirin: possible blocked diuretic effect of spironolactone. Watch for diminished spironolactone response.
Digoxin: may alter digoxin clearance, increasing risk of digoxin toxicity. Monitor digoxin levels.
Warfarin: decreased anticoagulant effect. Monitor PT and INR.
Drug-food. *Potassium-containing salt substitutes, potassium-rich foods (such as citrus fruits, tomatoes):* increased risk of hyperkalemia. Tell patient to use low-potassium salt substitutes and to eat high-potassium foods cautiously.

Contraindications and precautions

• Contraindicated in patients with anuria, acute or progressive renal insufficiency, or hyperkalemia.
• Use cautiously in pregnant women and in patients with fluid or electrolyte imbalances, impaired kidney function, or hepatic disease.
• Safety of drug hasn't been established in breast-feeding women.

NURSING CONSIDERATIONS

Assessment

• Assess patient's condition before therapy and regularly thereafter. Maximum antihypertensive response may be delayed up to 2 weeks.
• Monitor serum electrolyte levels, fluid intake and output, weight, and blood pressure.
• Be alert for adverse reactions and drug interactions.
• Evaluate patient's and family's knowledge of drug therapy.

Nursing diagnoses

• Excessive fluid volume related to presence of edema
• Impaired urinary elimination related to diuretic therapy
• Deficient knowledge related to drug therapy

Planning and implementation

• Give drug with meals to enhance absorption.
• Protect drug from light.
• Inform laboratory that patient is taking spironolactone because it may interfere with some laboratory tests that measure digoxin levels.
ALERT Don't confuse Aldactone with Aldactazide.

Patient teaching

ALERT Warn patient to avoid excessive ingestion of potassium-rich foods, potassium-containing salt substitutes, and potassium supplements to prevent serious hyperkalemia.
• Tell patient to take drug with meals and, if possible, early in day to avoid interruption of sleep by nocturia.

Evaluation

• Patient shows no signs of edema.
• Patient demonstrates adjustment of lifestyle to deal with altered patterns of urinary elimination.
• Patient and family state understanding of drug therapy.

stavudine (2,3-didehydro-3-deoxythymidine, d4T)

(stay-VYOO-deen)
Zerit

Pharmacologic class: synthetic thymidine nucleoside analogue
Therapeutic class: antiviral
Pregnancy risk category: C

Indications and dosages

▶ **Patients with advanced HIV infection who are intolerant of or unresponsive to other antivirals.** *Adults who weigh 60 kg (132 lb) or more:* 40 mg P.O. q 12 hours. *Adults who weigh less than 60 kg:* 30 mg P.O. q 12 hours.

How supplied

Capsules: 15 mg, 20 mg, 30 mg, 40 mg
Powder for oral solution: 1 mg/ml

Pharmacokinetics

Absorption: rapidly absorbed with mean absolute bioavailability of 86.4%.
Distribution: distributed equally between RBCs and plasma; binds poorly to plasma proteins.
Metabolism: not extensively metabolized.
Excretion: renal elimination accounts for about 40% of overall clearance. *Half-life:* 1 to 2 hours.

Route	Onset	Peak	Duration
P.O.	Unknown	≤ 1hr	Unknown

Pharmacodynamics

Chemical effect: prevents replication of HIV by inhibiting enzyme reverse transcriptase.
Therapeutic effect: inhibits HIV growth.

Adverse reactions

CNS: *asthenia, peripheral neuropathy, headache, malaise, insomnia, anxiety, depression, nervousness,* dizziness.
CV: chest pain.
EENT: conjunctivitis.
GI: *abdominal pain, diarrhea, nausea, vomiting, anorexia,* dyspepsia, constipation, weight loss.
Hematologic: ***neutropenia, thrombocytopenia,*** anemia.
Hepatic: ***hepatotoxicity.***
Musculoskeletal: myalgia, *back pain, arthralgia.*
Respiratory: *dyspnea.*
Skin: *rash, diaphoresis, pruritus,* maculopapular rash.
Other: *chills, fever.*

Interactions

Drug-drug. *Ketoconazole, ritonavir:* increased stavudine level. Monitor patient closely.
Myelosuppressants: additive myelosuppression. Avoid concomitant use.

Contraindications and precautions

- Contraindicated in patients hypersensitive to drug.
- Use cautiously in pregnant women and patients with renal impairment or a history of peripheral neuropathy.
- Safety of drug hasn't been established in children or breast-feeding women.

NURSING CONSIDERATIONS

Assessment

- Assess patient's condition before therapy and regularly thereafter.
- Periodically monitor CBC and serum levels of creatinine, AST, ALT, and alkaline phosphatase, as ordered.
- Be alert for adverse reactions and drug interactions.
- Evaluate patient's and family's knowledge of drug therapy.

Nursing diagnoses

- Infection related to presence of HIV
- Disturbed sensory perception (peripheral) related to drug-induced peripheral neuropathy
- Deficient knowledge related to drug therapy

Planning and implementation

ALERT Peripheral neuropathy appears to be major dose-limiting adverse effect; it may or may not resolve after drug is discontinued.
- Dosage is calculated based on patient's weight.

ALERT Don't confuse drug with other antivirals that may use initials for identification.

Patient teaching

- Tell patient that drug may be taken without regard to meals.
- Advise patient that he can't take drug if he experienced peripheral neuropathy while taking other nucleoside analogues or if his treatment plan includes cytotoxic antineoplastics.
- Warn patient not to take any other drugs for HIV or AIDS (especially street drugs) unless prescriber has approved them.
- Teach patient signs and symptoms of peripheral neuropathy—pain, burning, aching, weakness, or pins and needles in limbs—and tell him to report these immediately.

Evaluation

- Patient's infection is controlled.
- Patient maintains normal peripheral neurologic function.
- Patient and family state understanding of drug therapy.

streptokinase

(strep-toh-KIGH-nayz)
Kabikinase, Streptase

Pharmacologic class: plasminogen activator
Therapeutic class: thrombolytic enzyme
Pregnancy risk category: C

Indications and dosages

▶ **Arteriovenous cannula occlusion.** *Adults:* 250,000 IU in 2 ml I.V. solution by I.V. pump infusion into each occluded limb of cannula over 25 to 35 minutes. Clamp cannula for 2 hours. Then aspirate contents of cannula; flush with saline solution and reconnect.

▶ **Venous thrombosis, pulmonary embolism, arterial thrombosis and embolism.** *Adults:* loading dose is 250,000 IU by I.V. infusion over 30 minutes. Sustaining dose is 100,000 IU/hour by I.V. infusion for 72 hours for deep vein thrombosis and 100,000 IU/hour over 24 hours by I.V. infusion pump for pulmonary embolism.

▶ **Lysis of coronary artery thrombi after acute MI.** *Adults:* The total dose for intracoronary infusion is 140,000 IU. Loading dose is 20,000 IU by coronary catheter, followed by infusion of maintenance dose of 2,000 IU/minute for 60 minutes. Or, may be administered as an I.V. infusion. Usual adult dose is 1,500,000 IU infused over 60 minutes.

How supplied

Injection: 100,000 IU, 250,000 IU, 600,000 IU, 750,000 IU, 1.5 million IU in vials for reconstitution

Pharmacokinetics

Absorption: not applicable.
Distribution: unknown.
Metabolism: insignificant.
Excretion: removed from circulation by antibodies and reticuloendothelial system. *Half-life:* first phase, 18 minutes; second phase, 83 minutes.

Route	Onset	Peak	Duration
I.V.	Immediate	20 min-2 hr	About 4 hr

Pharmacodynamics

Chemical effect: activates plasminogen in two steps. Plasminogen and streptokinase form a complex that exposes plasminogen-activating site. Plasminogen is then converted to plasmin by cleavage of peptide bond.
Therapeutic effect: dissolves blood clots.

Adverse reactions

CNS: polyradiculoneuropathy, headache.
CV: *hypotension,* vasculitis, ***reperfusion arrhythmias.***
EENT: periorbital edema.
GI: nausea.
Hematologic: ***bleeding.***
Musculoskeletal: musculoskeletal pain.
Respiratory: minor breathing difficulty, ***bronchospasm, pulmonary edema.***
Skin: urticaria, pruritus, flushing.
Other: phlebitis at injection site, hypersensitivity reactions ***(anaphylaxis), delayed hypersensitivity reactions*** (interstitial nephritis, vasculitis, serum sickness–like reactions), ***angioedema,*** fever.

Interactions

Drug-drug. *Anticoagulants:* increased risk of bleeding. Monitor patient closely.
Antifibrinolytic drugs: streptokinase activity is inhibited and reversed by antifibrinolytic drugs such as aminocaproic acid. Use only when indicated during streptokinase therapy.
Aspirin, dipyridamole, drugs that affect platelet activity, indomethacin, phenylbutazone: increased risk of bleeding. Monitor patient closely. Combined therapy with low-dose aspirin (162.5 mg) or dipyridamole has improved acute and long-term results.

Contraindications and precautions

- Contraindicated in patients with ulcerative wounds, active internal bleeding, recent CVA, recent trauma with possible internal injuries, visceral or intracranial malignant neoplasms, ulcerative colitis, diverticulitis, severe hypertension, acute or chronic hepatic or renal insufficiency, uncontrolled hypocoagulation, chronic pulmonary disease with cavitation, subacute bacterial endocarditis or rheumatic valvular disease, or recent cerebral embolism, thrombosis, or hemorrhage.
- Also contraindicated within 10 days after intra-arterial diagnostic procedure or any surgery, including liver or kidney biopsy, lumbar puncture, thoracentesis, paracentesis, or extensive or multiple cutdowns.
- I.M. injections and other invasive procedures are contraindicated during streptokinase therapy.
- Use cautiously when treating arterial embolism that originates from left side of heart because of danger of cerebral infarction. Also use cautiously in pregnant women.
- Safety of drug hasn't been established in children or breast-feeding women.

NURSING CONSIDERATIONS

Assessment
- Assess patient's condition before therapy and regularly thereafter.
- Assess patient for increased risk of bleeding (as from recent surgery, CVA, trauma, or hypertension) before starting therapy.
- Before starting therapy, draw blood to determine aPTT and PT. Rate of I.V. infusion depends on thrombin time and streptokinase resistance. Then repeat studies often, as ordered, and keep laboratory flow sheet on patient's chart to monitor aPTT, PT, and hemoglobin and hematocrit levels.
- Monitor patient for excessive bleeding every 15 minutes for first hour, every 30 minutes for second through eighth hours, then once every shift.
- Monitor pulse rates, color, and sensation of limbs every hour.
- Be alert for adverse reactions and drug interactions.
- Evaluate patient's and family's knowledge of drug therapy.

Nursing diagnoses
- Ineffective cardiopulmonary tissue perfusion related to condition
- Risk for deficient fluid volume related to potential for bleeding
- Deficient knowledge related to drug therapy

Planning and implementation
- Drug should be used only by prescriber with wide experience in thrombotic disease management and in a setting where clinical and laboratory monitoring can be performed.
- Before using streptokinase to clear an occluded arteriovenous cannula, try flushing with heparinized saline solution, as ordered.

ALERT To check for hypersensitivity reactions, give 100 IU I.D., as ordered; wheal and flare response within 20 minutes means patient is probably allergic. Monitor vital signs frequently.
- If patient has had either recent streptococcal infection or recent treatment with streptokinase, higher loading dose may be necessary.
- Reconstitute each vial with 5 ml of normal saline solution for injection. Further dilute to 45 ml. Don't shake; roll gently to mix. Some flocculation may be present; discard if large amounts appear. Filter solution with 0.8-micron or larger filter. Use within 24 hours. Store powder at room temperature and refrigerate after reconstitution.
- If bleeding occurs, stop therapy and notify prescriber. Pretreatment with heparin or drugs affecting platelets causes high risk of bleeding but may improve long-term results.
- Keep aminocaproic acid available to treat bleeding, and corticosteroids to treat allergic reactions.
- Have typed and crossmatched packed RBCs and whole blood ready to treat possible hemorrhage.
- Keep involved limb in straight alignment to prevent bleeding from infusion site.
- Avoid unnecessary handling of patient, and pad side rails. Bruising is more likely during therapy.
- Keep venipuncture sites to minimum; use pressure dressing on puncture sites for at least 15 minutes.

ALERT Notify prescriber immediately if hypersensitivity occurs. Antihistamines or corticosteroids may be used to treat mild reactions. If severe reaction occurs, infusion should be stopped and prescriber notified immediately.
- Heparin by continuous infusion is usually started within 1 hour after stopping streptokinase. Use infusion pump to administer heparin.
- Keep in mind that thrombolytic therapy in patient with acute MI may decrease infarct size, improve ventricular function, and decrease risk of heart failure. Drug must be administered within 6 hours of onset of symptoms for optimal effect.

Patient teaching
- Tell patient to report oozing, bleeding, or signs of hypersensitivity immediately.

Evaluation
- Patient responds well to therapy.
- Patient maintains adequate fluid balance.
- Patient and family state understanding of drug therapy.

streptomycin sulfate
(strep-toh-MIGH-sin SUL-fayt)

Pharmacologic class: aminoglycoside
Therapeutic class: antibiotic
Pregnancy risk category: D

Indications and dosages

▶ **Streptococcal endocarditis.** *Adults:* 1 g I.M. q 12 hours for 1 week, and then 500 mg q 12 hours for 1 week, given with penicillin.
Adults over age 60: 500 mg I.M. q 12 hours for entire 2 weeks.

▶ **Primary and adjunct treatment in tuberculosis.** *Adults:* 1 g or 15 mg/kg I.M. daily for 2 to 3 months, and then 1 g two or three times weekly.
Children: 20 to 40 mg/kg I.M. daily in divided doses injected deep into large muscle mass. Given with other antituberculotics but not with capreomycin. Continued until sputum specimen becomes negative.

▶ **Enterococcal endocarditis.** *Adults:* 1 g I.M. q 12 hours for 2 weeks, and then 500 mg q 12 hours for 4 weeks, given with penicillin.

▶ **Tularemia.** *Adults:* 1 to 2 g I.M. daily in divided doses injected deep into upper outer quadrant of buttocks. Continued for 5 to 7 days until patient is afebrile.

▶ **Dosage in renal failure.** *Adults and children:* initial dosage same for normal renal function. Subsequent doses and frequency determined by renal function study results and blood levels.

How supplied

Injection: 400 mg/ml, 1-g/2.5 ml ampules

Pharmacokinetics

Absorption: unknown after I.M. administration.
Distribution: wide distribution although CSF penetration is low; 36% protein-bound.
Metabolism: none.
Excretion: mainly in urine; less so in bile.
Half-life: 2 to 3 hours.

Route	Onset	Peak	Duration
I.M.	Unknown	1-2 hr	Unknown

Pharmacodynamics

Chemical effect: inhibits protein synthesis by binding directly to 30S ribosomal subunit. Drug is generally bactericidal.
Therapeutic effect: kills bacteria. Spectrum of activity includes many aerobic gram-negative organisms and some aerobic gram-positive organisms. Drug is also active against *Brucella* and *Mycobacterium.*

Adverse reactions

CNS: ***neuromuscular blockade.***
EENT: *ototoxicity (tinnitus, vertigo, hearing loss).*
GI: vomiting, nausea.
GU: some ***nephrotoxicity*** (not as much as other aminoglycosides).
Hematologic: eosinophilia, ***leukopenia, thrombocytopenia.***
Respiratory: ***apnea.***
Skin: ***exfoliative dermatitis.***
Other: ***hypersensitivity reactions, angioedema, anaphylaxis.***

Interactions

Drug-drug. *Cephalosporins:* increased nephrotoxicity. Use together cautiously.
Dimenhydrinate: may mask symptoms of streptomycin-induced ototoxicity. Use together cautiously.
General anesthetics, neuromuscular blockers: may potentiate neuromuscular blockade. Monitor patient.
I.V. loop diuretics (such as furosemide): increased ototoxicity. Use cautiously.
Other aminoglycosides, acyclovir, amphotericin B, cisplatin, methoxyflurane, vancomycin: increased nephrotoxicity. Monitor patient.

Contraindications and precautions

- Contraindicated in patients hypersensitive to drug or other aminoglycosides, pregnant women, and patients with labyrinthine disease. Never give I.V.
- Use cautiously in patients with impaired kidney function or neuromuscular disorders, elderly patients, and breast-feeding women.

NURSING CONSIDERATIONS

Assessment
- Assess patient's infection before therapy and regularly thereafter.
- Obtain specimen for culture and sensitivity tests before first dose except when treating tuberculosis. Therapy may begin pending results.

ALERT Obtain blood for peak streptomycin level 1 to 2 hours after I.M. injection; for trough levels, draw blood just before next dose. Don't use heparinized tube because heparin is incompatible with aminoglycosides.
- Evaluate patient's hearing before beginning therapy, during therapy, and 6 months after therapy.
- Be alert for adverse reactions and drug interactions.
- Evaluate patient's and family's knowledge of drug therapy.

Nursing diagnoses
- Infection related to presence of susceptible bacteria
- Disturbed sensory perception (auditory) related to drug-induced adverse reactions
- Deficient knowledge related to drug therapy

Planning and implementation
- Protect hands when preparing because drug is irritating.
- Inject drug deep into upper outer quadrant of buttocks. Rotate injection sites.

ALERT Never administer streptomycin I.V.
- Encourage adequate fluid intake; patient should be well hydrated while taking drug to minimize chemical irritation of renal tubules.
- In primary treatment of tuberculosis, drug is discontinued when sputum becomes negative.

Patient teaching
- Warn patient that injection may be painful.
- Emphasize the need to drink at least 2,000 ml daily (if not contraindicated) during therapy.
- Instruct patient to report hearing loss, roaring noises, or fullness in ears immediately.

Evaluation
- Patient is free from infection.
- Patient's auditory function remains normal.
- Patient and family state understanding of drug therapy.

streptozocin
(strep-tuh-ZOH-sin)
Zanosar

Pharmacologic class: antibiotic antineoplastic nitrosourea (not specific to phase of cell cycle)
Therapeutic class: antineoplastic
Pregnancy risk category: C

Indications and dosages
▶ **Metastatic islet cell carcinoma of pancreas.** *Adults and children:* 500 mg/m² I.V. for 5 consecutive days q 6 weeks until maximum benefit or toxicity is observed. Alternatively, 1,000 mg/m² at weekly intervals for first 2 weeks. Not to exceed single dose of 1,500 mg/m². Because of renal toxicity, drug should only be used in patients with symptomatic or progressive metastatic disease.

How supplied
Injection: 1-g vials

Pharmacokinetics
Absorption: not applicable.
Distribution: distributed mainly in liver, kidneys, intestines, and pancreas. Drug doesn't cross blood-brain barrier; however, its metabolites achieve CSF levels equivalent to plasma level.
Metabolism: extensively metabolized in liver and kidneys.
Excretion: excreted primarily in urine, minimally in exhaled air. *Half-life:* first phase, 5 minutes; second phase, 35 to 40 minutes.

Route	Onset	Peak	Duration
I.V.	Unknown	Unknown	Unknown

Pharmacodynamics
Chemical effect: unknown; probably cross-links strands of cellular DNA and interferes with RNA transcription, causing an imbalance of growth that leads to cell death.
Therapeutic effect: kills certain cancer cells.

Adverse reactions

CNS: confusion, lethargy, depression.
GI: *nausea, vomiting,* diarrhea.
GU: ***renal toxicity,*** mild proteinuria.
Hematologic: ***anemia, leukopenia, thrombocytopenia.***
Hepatic: *elevated liver enzyme levels, liver dysfunction.*
Metabolic: hyperglycemia, hypoglycemia, diabetes mellitus.

Interactions

Drug-drug. *Doxorubicin:* prolonged elimination half-life of doxorubicin. Doxorubicin dosage should be reduced.
Other potentially nephrotoxic drugs (such as aminoglycosides): increased risk of nephrotoxicity. Use cautiously.
Phenytoin: may decrease effectiveness of streptozocin in patients with pancreatic cancer. Monitor patient.

Contraindications and precautions

- No known contraindications.
- Drug isn't recommended for pregnant or breast-feeding women.
- Use cautiously in patients with renal disease.

NURSING CONSIDERATIONS

Assessment

- Assess patient's condition before therapy and regularly thereafter.
- Obtain kidney function tests before therapy and after each course of therapy, as ordered. Nephrotoxicity from streptozocin therapy is dose-related and cumulative. Urinalysis; BUN, creatinine, and serum electrolyte levels; and creatinine clearance should be obtained at least weekly during therapy. Weekly monitoring should continue for 4 weeks after each course.
- Monitor CBC and liver function studies at least weekly, as ordered.
- Be alert for adverse reactions and drug interactions.
- Evaluate patient's and family's knowledge of drug therapy.

Nursing diagnoses

- Ineffective health maintenance related to presence of neoplastic disease
- Ineffective protection related to adverse nephrotoxic reactions
- Deficient knowledge related to drug therapy

Planning and implementation

- Follow facility policy to reduce risks. Preparation and administration of parenteral form are linked to carcinogenic, mutagenic, and teratogenic risks for personnel.
- Reconstitute streptozocin powder with 9.5 ml of D_5W or normal saline solution injection. This produces pale gold solution. Drug may be further diluted with D_5W or normal saline solution injection. Infuse over at least 15 minutes to minimize risk of phlebitis.

ALERT If extravasation occurs, stop infusion immediately and notify prescriber.

- Use within 12 hours of reconstitution. Product lacks preservatives and isn't intended as multiple-dose vial.
- To minimize risk of nephrotoxicity, ensure adequate hydration using oral or parenteral fluids, as ordered.
- Monitor urine protein and glucose levels each shift. Mild proteinuria is one of first signs of nephrotoxicity; notify prescriber if this occurs. Dosage reduction may be necessary.
- Make sure patient is being treated with an antiemetic. Nausea and vomiting occur in most patients.
- Store unopened and unreconstituted vials in refrigerator.

ALERT Don't confuse streptozocin with streptomycin.

Patient teaching

- Warn patient to watch for signs of infection (fever, sore throat, fatigue) and bleeding (easy bruising, nosebleeds, bleeding gums, melena). Have patient take temperature daily.
- Review other potential adverse reactions and explain how to prevent or decrease their severity and when to notify prescriber.

Evaluation

- Patient responds well to therapy.
- Patient maintains adequate kidney function.

• Patient and family state understanding of drug therapy.

succimer
(SUK-sih-mer)
Chemet

Pharmacologic class: heavy metal
Therapeutic class: chelating agent
Pregnancy risk category: C

Indications and dosages

▶ **Lead poisoning in children with blood lead levels above 45 mcg/dl.** *Children:* 10 mg/kg or 350 mg/m² q 8 hours for 5 days. Dosage rounded to nearest 100 mg (see table). Then, frequency is decreased to q 12 hours for an additional 2 weeks.

Weight (kg)	Dose (mg)
8 to 15	100
16 to 23	200
24 to 34	300
35 to 44	400
≥ 45	500

How supplied

Capsules: 100 mg

Pharmacokinetics

Absorption: rapid but variable.
Distribution: unknown.
Metabolism: rapid and extensive.
Excretion: 39% excreted in feces as nonabsorbed drug; remainder excreted mainly in urine. *Half-life:* 48 hours.

Route	Onset	Peak	Duration
P.O.	Unknown	1-2 hr	Unknown

Pharmacodynamics

Chemical effect: forms water-soluble complexes with lead and increases its excretion in urine.
Therapeutic effect: relieves signs and symptoms of lead poisoning.

Adverse reactions

CNS: *drowsiness, dizziness, sensory motor neuropathy, sleepiness, paresthesias, headache.*
CV: *arrhythmias.*
EENT: plugged ears, cloudy film in eyes, otitis media, watery eyes, sore throat, rhinorrhea, nasal congestion.
GI: *nausea, vomiting, diarrhea, loss of appetite, abdominal cramps, hemorrhoidal symptoms, metallic taste, loose stools.*
GU: decreased urination, difficult urination, proteinuria.
Hematologic: increased platelet count, intermittent eosinophilia.
Hepatic: *elevated serum AST, ALT, alkaline phosphatase, or cholesterol levels.*
Musculoskeletal: *leg, kneecap, back, stomach, rib, or flank pain.*
Respiratory: cough, head cold.
Skin: papular rash, herpetic rash, mucocutaneous eruptions, pruritus.
Other: *flulike symptoms,* candidiasis.

Interactions

None reported.

Contraindications and precautions

• Contraindicated in patients hypersensitive to drug.
• Use cautiously in patients with compromised kidney function.
• Drug isn't indicated for use in pregnant or breast-feeding women.

NURSING CONSIDERATIONS

Assessment

• Assess child's condition before therapy and regularly thereafter.
• Measure severity by initial blood lead level and by rate and degree of rebound of blood lead level. Severity should be used as guide for more frequent blood lead monitoring.
• Monitor serum transaminase level before and at least weekly during therapy, as ordered. Transient, mild elevations of serum transaminase level have been observed. Patient with history of hepatic disease should be monitored more closely.

• Monitor patient at least once weekly for rebound blood lead levels, as ordered. Elevated blood lead levels and associated symptoms may return rapidly after drug is discontinued because of redistribution of lead from bone to soft tissues and blood.
• Be alert for adverse reactions.
• Monitor patient's hydration status if adverse GI reactions occur.
• Evaluate parents' knowledge of drug therapy.

Nursing diagnoses
• Ineffective health maintenance related to presence of lead poisoning
• Risk for deficient fluid volume related to drug-induced adverse GI reactions
• Deficient knowledge related to drug therapy

Planning and implementation
• Course of treatment lasts 19 days. Repeated courses may be necessary if indicated by weekly monitoring of blood lead levels.
• A minimum of 2 weeks between courses is recommended unless high blood lead level indicates need for immediate therapy.
• False-positive results for ketones in urine using nitroprusside reagents (Ketostix) and falsely decreased levels of serum uric acid and CK have been reported.
ALERT Administration of succimer with other chelating agents isn't recommended. Patient who has received edetate calcium disodium with or without dimercaprol may use succimer as subsequent therapy after 4-week interval.

Patient teaching
• Tell parents of child who can't swallow capsule to open it and sprinkle contents on small amount of soft food. Or, medicated beads from capsule may be poured on spoon and followed with flavored beverage such as a fruit drink.
• Help parents identify and remove sources of lead in child's environment. Chelation therapy isn't a substitute for preventing further exposure.
• Tell parents to consult prescriber if rash occurs. Consider possibility of allergic or other mucocutaneous reactions each time drug is used.

Evaluation
• Patient responds well to therapy.
• Patient maintains adequate hydration.
• Parents state understanding of drug therapy.

succinylcholine chloride (suxamethonium chloride)

(SUK-seh-nil-KOH-leen KLOR-ighd)
Anectine, Anectine Flo-Pack, Quelicin, Scoline ◇, Sucostrin

Pharmacologic class: depolarizing neuromuscular blocker
Therapeutic class: skeletal muscle relaxant
Pregnancy risk category: C

Indications and dosages

▶ **Adjunct to anesthesia to induce skeletal muscle relaxation; to facilitate intubation and assist with mechanical ventilation or orthopedic manipulations (drug of choice); to lessen muscle contractions in pharmacologically or electrically induced seizures.** Dosage depends on anesthetic used, individual needs, and response.
Adults: 0.6 mg/kg I.V.; then 2.5 mg/minute, p.r.n. Or, 2.5 mg/kg I.M. up to maximum of 150 mg I.M. in deltoid muscle.
Children: 1 to 2 mg/kg I.M. or I.V. Maximum I.M. dosage is 150 mg. (Children may be less sensitive to succinylcholine than adults.)

How supplied

Injection: 20 mg/ml, 50 mg/ml, 100 mg/ml; 100 mg/vial, 500 mg/vial, 1 g/vial

Pharmacokinetics

Absorption: unknown after I.M. administration.
Distribution: distributed in extracellular fluid and rapidly reaches its site of action.
Metabolism: occurs rapidly by plasma pseudocholinesterase.

Excretion: about 10% excreted unchanged in urine.

Route	Onset	Peak	Duration
I.M.	2-3 min	Unknown	10-30 min
I.V.	0.5-1 min	1-2 min	4-10 min

Pharmacodynamics

Chemical effect: prolongs depolarization of muscle end plate.
Therapeutic effect: relaxes skeletal muscles.

Adverse reactions

CV: ***bradycardia,*** tachycardia, hypertension, hypotension, ***arrhythmias,*** flushing, ***cardiac arrest.***
EENT: increased intraocular pressure.
Musculoskeletal: muscle fasciculation, *postoperative muscle pain,* myoglobinemia.
Respiratory: ***prolonged respiratory depression, apnea, bronchoconstriction.***
Other: ***malignant hyperthermia,*** excessive salivation, allergic or idiosyncratic hypersensitivity reactions ***(anaphylaxis).***

Interactions

Drug-drug. *Aminoglycoside antibiotics, including amikacin, gentamicin, kanamycin, neomycin, streptomycin; cholinesterase inhibitors, such as echothiophate, edrophonium, neostigmine, physostigmine, or pyridostigmine; general anesthetics, such as enflurane, halothane, isoflurane; polymyxin antibiotics, such as colistin and polymyxin B sulfate:* potentiated neuromuscular blockade, leading to increased skeletal muscle relaxation and potentiation of effect. Use cautiously during surgical and postoperative periods.
Cardiac glycosides: may cause arrhythmias. Use together cautiously.
Cyclophosphamide, lithium, MAO inhibitors: prolonged apnea. Monitor patient closely.
Methotrimeprazine, opioid analgesics: potentiated neuromuscular blockade, leading to increased skeletal muscle relaxation and, possibly, respiratory paralysis. Use with extreme caution.
Parenteral magnesium sulfate: potentiated neuromuscular blockade, increased skeletal muscle relaxation and, possibly, respiratory paralysis. Use cautiously, preferably with reduced doses.
Drug-herb. *Melatonin:* potentiated blocking properties of succinylcholine. Avoid concomitant use.

Contraindications and precautions

- Contraindicated in patients hypersensitive to drug and patients with abnormally low plasma pseudocholinesterase level, angle-closure glaucoma, malignant hyperthermia, or penetrating eye injury.
- Use cautiously in elderly or debilitated patients; those receiving quinidine or cardiac glycoside therapy; and those with severe burns or trauma, electrolyte imbalances, hyperkalemia, paraplegia, spinal neuraxis injury, CVA, degenerative or dystrophic neuromuscular disease, myasthenia gravis, myasthenic syndrome of lung cancer, bronchogenic carcinoma, dehydration, thyroid disorders, collagen diseases, porphyria, fractures, muscle spasms, eye surgery, pheochromocytoma, respiratory depression, or hepatic, renal, or pulmonary impairment.
- Also, use large doses cautiously in breast-feeding women and in women undergoing cesarean delivery.

NURSING CONSIDERATIONS

Assessment

- Assess patient's condition before therapy and regularly thereafter.
- Monitor baseline electrolyte determinations and vital signs (check respiratory rate every 5 to 10 minutes during infusion).
- Monitor respiratory rate and pulse oximetry closely until patient is fully recovered from neuromuscular blockade, as evidenced by tests of muscle strength (hand grip, head lift, and ability to cough).
- Be alert for adverse reactions and drug interactions.
- Evaluate patient's and family's knowledge of drug therapy.

Nursing diagnoses

- Ineffective health maintenance related to underlying condition

• Ineffective breathing pattern related to drug's effect on respiratory muscles
• Deficient knowledge related to drug therapy

Planning and implementation

ALERT Drug should be used only by personnel skilled in airway management.
• Succinylcholine is drug of choice for short procedures (less than 3 minutes) and for orthopedic manipulations; use caution in fractures or dislocations.
• Administer sedatives or general anesthetics before neuromuscular blockers, as ordered. Neuromuscular blockers don't obtund consciousness or alter pain threshold.
• Keep airway clear. Have emergency respiratory support equipment immediately available.
ALERT Careful drug calculation is essential. Always verify with another professional.
I.V. use: To evaluate patient's ability to metabolize succinylcholine, give test dose (10 mg I.M. or I.V.) after patient has been anesthetized. Normal response (no respiratory depression or transient depression for up to 5 minutes) indicates drug may be given. Don't give subsequent doses if patient develops respiratory paralysis sufficient to permit endotracheal intubation. (Recovery within 30 to 60 minutes.)
I.M. use: Give deep I.M., preferably high into deltoid muscle.
• Store injectable form in refrigerator. Store powder form at room temperature in tightly closed container. Use immediately after reconstitution. Don't mix with alkaline solutions (thiopental sodium, sodium bicarbonate, or barbiturates).
• Administer analgesics, as ordered.
ALERT Reversing drugs shouldn't be used. Unlike what happens with nondepolarizing drugs, giving neostigmine or edrophonium with this depolarizing drug may worsen neuromuscular blockade.
• Repeated or continuous infusions of succinylcholine are not advised; they may reduce response or prolong muscle relaxation and apnea.

Patient teaching
• Explain all events and happenings to patient because he can still hear.
• Reassure patient that he is being monitored at all times.
• Inform him that postoperative stiffness is normal and will soon subside.

Evaluation

• Patient responds well to therapy.
• Patient maintains adequate respiratory patterns with mechanical assistance.
• Patient and family state understanding of drug therapy.

sucralfate
(SOO-krahl-fayt)
Carafate, SCF ◇, Sulcrate ♦

Pharmacologic class: pepsin inhibitor
Therapeutic class: antiulcer agent
Pregnancy risk category: B

Indications and dosages

▶ **Short-term (up to 8 weeks) treatment of duodenal ulcer.** *Adults:* 1 g P.O. q.i.d. 1 hour before meals and h.s.
▶ **Maintenance therapy for duodenal ulcer.** *Adults:* 1 g P.O. b.i.d.

How supplied

Tablets: 1 g
Suspension: 500 mg/5 ml

Pharmacokinetics

Absorption: only about 3% to 5% absorbed from GI tract.
Distribution: sucralfate acts locally at ulcer site. Absorbed drug is distributed to many body tissues.
Metabolism: none.
Excretion: about 90% excreted in feces; absorbed drug excreted unchanged in urine.

Route	Onset	Peak	Duration
P.O.	Unknown	≤ 6 hr	Unknown

Pharmacodynamics

Chemical effect: unknown; probably adheres to and protects ulcer's surface by forming barrier.

Therapeutic effect: aids in duodenal ulcer healing.

Adverse reactions

CNS: dizziness, sleepiness, headache, vertigo.
GI: constipation, nausea, gastric discomfort, diarrhea, bezoar formation, vomiting, flatulence, dry mouth, indigestion.
Musculoskeletal: back pain.
Skin: rash, pruritus.

Interactions

Drug-drug. *Antacids:* may decrease binding of drug to gastroduodenal mucosa, impairing effectiveness. Don't administer within 30 minutes of each other.
Cimetidine, digoxin, norfloxacin, phenytoin, fluroquinolones, ranitidine, tetracycline, theophylline: decreased absorption. Separate administration times by at least 2 hours.

Contraindications and precautions

- No known contraindications.
- Use cautiously in patients with chronic renal failure and in pregnant or breast-feeding women.
- Safety of drug hasn't been established in children.

NURSING CONSIDERATIONS

Assessment
- Assess patient's GI symptoms before therapy and regularly thereafter.
- Be alert for adverse reactions and drug interactions.
- Monitor patient for severe, persistent constipation.
- Evaluate patient's and family's knowledge of drug therapy.

Nursing diagnoses
- Impaired tissue integrity related to presence of duodenal ulcer
- Constipation related to drug-induced adverse GI reactions
- Deficient knowledge related to drug therapy

Planning and implementation
- Administer drug on an empty stomach for best results.

Patient teaching
- Instruct patient to take drug 1 hour before each meal and at bedtime.
- Tell patient to continue on prescribed regimen to ensure complete healing. Pain and ulcerative symptoms may subside within first few weeks of therapy.
- Urge patient to avoid cigarette smoking because it may increase gastric acid secretion and worsen disease. Also teach patient to avoid alcohol, chocolate, and spicy foods.
- Tell patient to elevate the head of the bed to sleep.
- Tell patient to avoid large meals within 2 hours before bedtime.

Evaluation
- Patient's ulcer pain is gone.
- Patient maintains normal bowel elimination patterns.
- Patient and family state understanding of drug therapy.

sufentanil citrate

(soo-FEN-tih-nil SIGH-trayt)
Sufenta

Pharmacologic class: opioid
Therapeutic class: analgesic, adjunct to anesthesia, anesthetic
Controlled substance schedule: II
Pregnancy risk category: C

Indications and dosages

▶ **Adjunct to general anesthetic.** *Adults:* 1 to 8 mcg/kg I.V. with nitrous oxide and oxygen.
▶ **As primary anesthetic.** *Adults:* 8 to 30 mcg/kg I.V. with 100% oxygen and muscle relaxant.

How supplied

Injection: 50 mcg/ml in 1-, 2-, 5-ml ampules

Pharmacokinetics

Absorption: not applicable.
Distribution: highly protein-bound and redistributed rapidly.

Metabolism: unknown, although appears to be metabolized mainly in liver and small intestine.
Excretion: drug and its metabolites excreted primarily in urine. *Half-life:* about 2½ hours.

Route	Onset	Peak	Duration
I.V.	1-2 min	1-2 min	0.7-5 min

Pharmacodynamics

Chemical effect: binds with opioid receptors in CNS, altering perception of and emotional response to pain through unknown mechanism.
Therapeutic effect: relieves pain and promotes loss of consciousness.

Adverse reactions

CNS: chills, somnolence.
CV: *hypotension,* hypertension, ***bradycardia,*** tachycardia, ***arrhythmias.***
GI: nausea, vomiting.
Musculoskeletal: intraoperative muscle movement.
Respiratory: ***chest wall rigidity, apnea, bronchospasm.***
Skin: *pruritus,* erythema.

Interactions

Drug-drug. *CNS depressants:* additive effects. Use together cautiously.
Drug-lifestyle. *Alcohol use:* additive effects. Use together cautiously.

Contraindications and precautions

- Contraindicated in patients hypersensitive to drug.
- Drug isn't recommended for prolonged use or use of high doses at term in pregnant women.
- Use with extreme caution in elderly or debilitated patients and in patients with head injury, decreased respiratory reserve, or pulmonary, hepatic, or renal disease.
- Safety of drug hasn't been established in breast-feeding women and in children.

NURSING CONSIDERATIONS

Assessment

- Assess patient's condition before therapy and regularly thereafter.
- Because drug decreases rate and depth of respirations, monitoring arterial oxygen saturation may aid in assessing respiratory depression.
- Monitor respiratory rate of neonates exposed to drug during labor.
- Monitor postoperative vital signs.
- Be alert for adverse reactions and drug interactions.
- Evaluate patient's and family's knowledge of drug therapy.

Nursing diagnoses

- Ineffective health maintenance related to underlying condition
- Ineffective breathing pattern related to respiratory depression
- Deficient knowledge related to drug therapy

Planning and implementation

- Drug should be given only by personnel specifically trained in use of I.V. anesthetics.
- Elderly and debilitated patients need a reduced dosage.
- For obese patient who exceeds 20% of ideal body weight, dosage calculations should be based on an estimate of ideal weight.
- Give drug by direct I.V. injection. Although drug has been given by intermittent I.V. infusion, its compatibility and stability in I.V. solutions haven't been fully investigated.
- When used at doses over 8 mcg/kg, postoperative mechanical ventilation and observation are essential because of prolonged respiratory depression.
- Keep narcotic antagonist (naloxone) and resuscitation equipment available.
- Notify prescriber if respiratory rate falls below 12 breaths/minute.

ALERT High doses can produce muscle rigidity reversible by neuromuscular blockers; however, patient must be artificially ventilated.

ALERT Don't confuse sufentanil with alfentanil or Sufenta with Survanta.

Patient teaching

- Inform patient and family that sufentanil will be used as part of patient's anesthesia. Answer questions patient or family may have.

Evaluation

- Patient responds well to therapy.
- Patient maintains adequate ventilation with mechanical support.
- Patient and family state understanding of drug therapy.

sulfadiazine
(sul-fuh-DIGH-uh-zeen)

Pharmacologic class: sulfonamide
Therapeutic class: antibiotic
Pregnancy risk category: C (contraindicated at term)

Indications and dosages

▶ **UTI.** *Adults:* initially, 2 to 4 g P.O.; then 2 to 4 g daily in three to six divided doses.
Children age 2 months and older: initially, 75 mg/kg or 2 g/m^2 P.O.; then 150 mg/kg or 4 g/m^2 P.O. in four to six divided doses daily. Maximum daily dosage 6 g.
▶ **Rheumatic fever prophylaxis, as an alternative to penicillin.** *Children who weigh 30 kg (66 lb) or more:* 1 g P.O. daily.
Children who weigh less than 30 kg: 500 mg P.O. daily.
▶ **Adjunct treatment in toxoplasmosis.** *Adults:* 2 to 8 g P.O. daily in divided doses q 6 hours. Usually given with pyrimethamine.
Children: 100 to 200 mg/kg P.O. daily. Usually given with pyrimethamine.

How supplied

Tablets: 500 mg

Pharmacokinetics

Absorption: absorbed from GI tract.
Distribution: distributed widely in most body tissues and fluids; 32% to 56% protein-bound.
Metabolism: metabolized partially in liver.
Excretion: excreted unchanged mainly in urine. Urine solubility of unchanged drug increases as urine pH increases. *Half-life:* about 10 hours.

Route	Onset	Peak	Duration
P.O.	Unknown	≤ 6 hr	Unknown

Pharmacodynamics

Chemical effect: inhibits formation of dihydrofolic acid from PABA, decreasing bacterial folic acid synthesis.
Therapeutic effect: hinders bacterial activity. Spectrum of activity includes many gram-positive bacteria, *Chlamydia trachomatis*, many enterobacteriaceae, and some strains of *Plasmodium falciparum* and *Toxoplasma gondii.*

Adverse reactions

CNS: headache, mental depression, ***seizures,*** hallucinations.
GI: *nausea, vomiting, diarrhea,* abdominal pain, anorexia, stomatitis.
GU: ***toxic nephrosis with oliguria and anuria,*** crystalluria, hematuria.
Hematologic: ***agranulocytosis, aplastic anemia,*** megaloblastic anemia, ***leukopenia, hemolytic anemia, thrombocytopenia.***
Hepatic: jaundice.
Skin: ***erythema multiforme, Stevens-Johnson syndrome,*** *generalized skin eruption,* ***epidermal necrolysis, exfoliative dermatitis,*** photosensitivity, urticaria, pruritus.
Other: hypersensitivity *(serum sickness, drug fever,* ***anaphylaxis****)*, local irritation, extravasation.

Interactions

Drug-drug. *Methotrexate:* may increase methotrexate levels. Use together cautiously.
Oral anticoagulants: increased anticoagulant effect. Monitor patient for bleeding.
Oral antidiabetics: increased hypoglycemic effect. Monitor blood glucose level.
Oral contraceptives: decreased contraceptive effectiveness and increased risk of breakthrough bleeding. Suggest nonhormonal contraceptive.

Drug-herb. *Dong quai, St. John's wort:* increased risk of photosensitivity. Discourage using together.
Drug-lifestyle. *Sun exposure:* photosensitivity reactions may occur. Urge patient to take precautions.

Contraindications and precautions

- Contraindicated in patients hypersensitive to sulfonamides, in pregnant women at term, in breast-feeding women, in infants under age 2 months (except in congenital toxoplasmosis), and in patients with porphyria.
- Use cautiously and in reduced doses in patients with impaired liver or kidney function, bronchial asthma, history of multiple allergies, G6PD deficiency, or blood dyscrasia.

NURSING CONSIDERATIONS

Assessment
- Assess patient's condition before therapy and regularly thereafter.
- Obtain specimen for culture and sensitivity tests before first dose. Therapy may begin pending results.
- Monitor urine cultures, CBCs, and urinalyses before and during therapy.
- Monitor urine pH daily.
- Be alert for adverse reactions and drug interactions.
- Monitor patient's hydration if adverse GI reactions occur.
- Evaluate patient's and family's knowledge of drug therapy.

Nursing diagnoses
- Infection related to presence of susceptible bacteria
- Risk for deficient fluid volume related to drug-induced adverse GI reactions
- Deficient knowledge related to drug therapy

Planning and implementation
- Give drug on schedule to maintain constant blood level.
- Folic or folinic acid may be used during rest periods in toxoplasmosis therapy to reverse hematopoietic depression or anemia related to pyrimethamine and sulfadiazine.
- Have adult patient drink between 3 and 4 L daily to prevent crystalluria. Sodium bicarbonate may be given to alkalinize urine.

ALERT Don't confuse sulfadiazine with sulfasalazine. Don't confuse sulfonamide drugs.

Patient teaching
- Tell patient to drink full glass of water with each dose and plenty of water throughout day.
- Tell patient to take entire amount of medication exactly as prescribed, even if he feels better.
- Warn patient to avoid direct sunlight and ultraviolet light to prevent photosensitivity reaction.

Evaluation
- Patient is free from infection.
- Patient maintains adequate hydration.
- Patient and family state understanding of drug therapy.

sulfamethoxazole (sulphamethoxazole)

(sul-fuh-meth-OKS-uh-zohl)
Apo-Sulfamethoxazole ♦, Gantanol

Pharmacologic class: sulfonamide
Therapeutic class: antibiotic
Pregnancy risk category: C (contraindicated at term)

Indications and dosages

▶ **Urinary tract and systemic infections.** *Adults:* initially, 2 g P.O.; then 1 g P.O. b.i.d. up to t.i.d. for severe infections.
Children and infants over age 2 months: initially, 50 to 60 mg/kg P.O.; then 25 to 30 mg/kg b.i.d. Maximum dosage 75 mg/kg daily.

How supplied

Tablets: 500 mg
Oral suspension: 500 mg/5 ml

Pharmacokinetics

Absorption: absorbed from GI tract.

Distribution: distributed widely in most body tissues and fluids; 50% to 70% protein-bound.
Metabolism: metabolized partially in liver.
Excretion: unchanged drug and metabolites excreted primarily in urine. Urine solubility of unchanged drug increases as urine pH increases. *Half-life:* 7 to 12 hours.

Route	Onset	Peak	Duration
P.O.	Unknown	≤ 2 hr	Unknown

Pharmacodynamics

Chemical effect: inhibits formation of dihydrofolic acid from PABA, decreasing bacterial folic acid synthesis.
Therapeutic effect: hinders bacterial activity. Spectrum of activity includes many gram-positive bacteria, *Chlamydia trachomatis*, many enterobacteriaceae, and some strains of *Plasmodium falciparum* and *Toxoplasma gondii*.

Adverse reactions

CNS: headache, mental depression, ***seizures,*** hallucinations, aseptic meningitis, apathy.
EENT: tinnitus.
GI: *nausea, vomiting, diarrhea,* abdominal pain, anorexia, stomatitis, ***pancreatitis,*** pseudomembranous colitis.
GU: ***toxic nephrosis with oliguria and anuria,*** crystalluria, hematuria, interstitial nephritis.
Hematologic: ***agranulocytosis, aplastic anemia,*** megaloblastic anemia, ***thrombocytopenia, leukopenia, hemolytic anemia.***
Hepatic: *jaundice.*
Skin: ***erythema multiforme, Stevens-Johnson syndrome,*** *generalized skin eruption,* ***epidermal necrolysis, exfoliative dermatitis,*** photosensitivity, urticaria, pruritus.
Other: hypersensitivity reactions *(serum sickness, drug fever,* ***anaphylaxis****).*

Interactions

Drug-drug. *Methotrexate:* may increase methotrexate levels. Use together cautiously.
Oral anticoagulants: increased anticoagulant effect. Monitor patient for bleeding.
Oral antidiabetics: increased hypoglycemic effect. Monitor blood glucose level.
Oral contraceptives: decreased contraceptive effectiveness and increased risk of breakthrough bleeding. Suggest nonhormonal form of contraception.
Phenytoin: may increase phenytoin effect. Monitor patient closely.
Drug-herb. *Dong quai, St. John's wort:* increased risk of photosensitivity. Discourage using together.
Drug-lifestyle. *Sun exposure:* may cause photosensitivity reactions. Urge patient to take precautions.

Contraindications and precautions

- Contraindicated in patients hypersensitive to sulfonamides, pregnant women at term, breast-feeding women, infants under age 2 months (except in congenital toxoplasmosis), and patients with porphyria.
- Use cautiously and in reduced dosages in patients with impaired liver or kidney function, severe allergy or bronchial asthma, G6PD deficiency, or blood dyscrasia.

NURSING CONSIDERATIONS

Assessment

- Assess patient's condition before therapy and regularly thereafter.
- Obtain specimen for culture and sensitivity tests before first dose. Therapy may begin pending results.
- Monitor urine cultures, CBCs, and urinalyses before and during therapy, as ordered.
- Monitor urine pH daily.
- Be alert for adverse reactions and drug interactions.
- Monitor patient's hydration if adverse GI reactions occur.
- Evaluate patient's and family's knowledge of drug therapy.

Nursing diagnoses

- Infection related to presence of susceptible bacteria
- Risk for deficient fluid volume related to drug-induced adverse GI reactions
- Deficient knowledge related to drug therapy

Planning and implementation

- Give drug on schedule to maintain constant blood level.
- Folic or folinic acid may be used during rest periods in toxoplasmosis therapy to reverse hematopoietic depression or anemia related to pyrimethamine and sulfamethoxazole.
- Have adult patient drink between 3,000 and 4,000 ml daily to prevent crystalluria. Sodium bicarbonate may be given to alkalinize urine.

ALERT Don't confuse sulfamethoxazole with sulfamethiazole. Don't confuse the combination products (such as Gantanol) with sulfamethoxazole alone.

Patient teaching

- Tell patient to drink full glass of water with each dose and to drink plenty of water throughout day to prevent crystalluria. Teach patient how to monitor fluid intake and output. Intake should be sufficient to produce output of 1,500 ml daily for children and between 3,000 and 4,000 ml daily for adults.
- Tell patient to take entire amount of drug exactly as prescribed.
- Warn patient to avoid direct sunlight and ultraviolet light to prevent photosensitivity reaction.

ALERT Tell patient to notify prescriber about early signs of blood dyscrasia (sore throat, fever, and pallor). Also tell patient to be alert for flulike symptoms, cough, and lesions of the iris, skin, and mucous membranes. These are early signs of erythema multiforme, which can progress to the sometimes fatal Stevens-Johnson syndrome.

Evaluation

- Patient is free from infection.
- Patient maintains adequate hydration.
- Patient and family state understanding of drug therapy.

sulfasalazine (salazosulfapyridine, sulphasalazine)

(sul-fuh-SAL-uh-zeen)

Azulfidine, Azulfidine EN-tabs, PMS Sulfasalazine E.C.♦, Salazopyrin♦◇, Salazopyrin EN-Tabs♦◇, S.A.S.-500♦, S.A.S. Enteric-500♦

Pharmacologic class: sulfonamide
Therapeutic class: anti-inflammatory
Pregnancy risk category: B

Indications and dosages

▶ **Mild to moderate ulcerative colitis, adjunct therapy in severe ulcerative colitis, Crohn's disease.** *Adults:* initially, 3 to 4 g P.O. daily in evenly divided doses; usual maintenance dosage is 2 g P.O. daily in divided doses q 6 hours. Dosage may be started with 1 to 2 g, with gradual increase to minimize adverse effects.

Children over age 2: initially, 40 to 60 mg/kg P.O. daily, divided into three to six doses; then 30 mg/kg daily in four doses. Dosage may be started at lower dose if GI intolerance occurs.

▶ **Rheumatoid arthritis in patients who have responded inadequately to salicylates or NSAIDs.** *Adults:* 2 g P.O. daily b.i.d. in evenly divided doses. Dosage may be started at 0.5 to 1 g daily and gradually increased over 3 weeks to reduce possible GI intolerance.

How supplied

Tablets (with or without enteric coating): 500 mg
Oral suspension: 250 mg/5 ml

Pharmacokinetics

Absorption: absorbed poorly from GI tract; 70% to 90% transported to colon, where intestinal flora metabolize drug to its active ingredients, which exert their effects locally. One metabolite, sulfapyridine, is absorbed from colon, but only small portion of metabolite 5-aminosalicytic acid is absorbed.
Distribution: distributed locally in colon. Distribution of absorbed metabolites is unknown.

Metabolism: cleaved by intestinal flora in colon.
Excretion: systemically absorbed sulfasalazine is excreted chiefly in urine. *Half-life:* 6 to 8 hours.

Route	Onset	Peak	Duration
P.O.	Unknown (parent drug); 12-24 hr (metabolites)	1.5-6 hr	Unknown

Pharmacodynamics

Chemical effect: unknown.
Therapeutic effect: relieves inflammation in GI tract.

Adverse reactions

CNS: headache, depression, ***seizures,*** hallucinations.
GI: *nausea, vomiting, diarrhea,* abdominal pain, anorexia, stomatitis.
GU: ***toxic nephrosis with oliguria and anuria,*** crystalluria, hematuria, oligospermia, infertility.
Hematologic: ***agranulocytosis, aplastic anemia,*** megaloblastic anemia, ***thrombocytopenia, leukopenia,*** hemolytic anemia.
Hepatic: jaundice, ***hepatotoxicity.***
Skin: ***erythema multiforme, Stevens-Johnson syndrome,*** *generalized skin eruption,* ***epidermal necrolysis, exfoliative dermatitis,*** photosensitivity, urticaria, pruritus.
Other: ***hypersensitivity reactions*** *(serum sickness, drug fever,* ***anaphylaxis****).*

Interactions

Drug-drug. *Antibiotics:* may alter action of sulfasalazine by altering internal flora. Monitor patient closely.
Digoxin: may reduce digoxin absorption. Monitor patient closely.
Folic acid: absorption may be decreased. No intervention necessary.
Iron: lowered blood sulfasalazine levels caused by iron chelation. Monitor patient closely.
Oral anticoagulants: increased anticoagulant effect. Monitor patient for bleeding.
Oral antidiabetics: increased hypoglycemic effect. Monitor blood glucose level.
Oral contraceptives: decreased contraceptive effectiveness and increased risk of breakthrough bleeding. Suggest nonhormonal contraceptive.
Drug-herb. *Dong quai, St. John's wort:* increased risk of photosensitivity. Discourage using together.

Contraindications and precautions

- Contraindicated in patients hypersensitive to drug or its metabolites, infants under age 2, and patients with porphyria or intestinal or urinary obstruction.
- Use cautiously and in reduced dosages in patients with impaired liver or kidney function, severe allergy, bronchial asthma, or G6PD deficiency. Also use cautiously in pregnant or breast-feeding women.

NURSING CONSIDERATIONS

Assessment

- Assess patient's condition before therapy and regularly thereafter.
- Be alert for adverse reactions and drug interactions.
- Monitor patient's hydration status throughout drug therapy.
- Evaluate patient's and family's knowledge of drug therapy.

Nursing diagnoses

- Acute pain related to inflammation of GI tract
- Risk for deficient fluid volume related to drug-induced adverse GI reactions
- Deficient knowledge related to drug therapy

Planning and implementation

- Minimize adverse GI symptoms by spacing doses evenly and administering after food intake.
- Drug colors alkaline urine orange-yellow.

ALERT Discontinue immediately and notify prescriber if patient shows evidence of hypersensitivity.

ALERT Don't confuse sulfasalazine with sulfisoxazole, salsalate, or sulfadiazine.

Patient teaching

- Instruct patient to take drug after meals and to space doses evenly.
- Warn patient that drug may cause skin and urine to turn orange-yellow and may permanently stain soft contact lenses yellow.
- Warn patient to avoid direct sunlight and ultraviolet light to prevent photosensitivity reaction.

Evaluation

- Patient is free from pain.
- Patient maintains adequate hydration.
- Patient and family state understanding of drug therapy.

sulfinpyrazone

(sul-fin-PEER-uh-zohn)

Anturan ♦, Anturane

Pharmacologic class: uricosuric agent
Therapeutic class: renal tubular-blocking agent, platelet aggregation inhibitor
Pregnancy risk category: NR

Indications and dosages

▶ **Intermittent or chronic gouty arthritis.** *Adults:* initially, 100 mg to 200 mg P.O. b.i.d. during the first week; then 200 mg to 400 mg P.O. b.i.d. Maximum dosage is 800 mg daily. After serum urate level is controlled, dosage can sometimes be reduced to 200 mg daily in divided doses.

How supplied

Tablets: 100 mg
Capsules: 200 mg

Pharmacokinetics

Absorption: absorbed completely from GI tract.
Distribution: 98% to 99% protein-bound.
Metabolism: metabolized rapidly in liver.
Excretion: excreted in urine; about 50% excreted unchanged. *Half-life:* 4 to 6 hours.

Route	Onset	Peak	Duration
P.O.	Unknown	1-2 hr	4-6 hr

Pharmacodynamics

Chemical effect: blocks renal tubular reabsorption of uric acid, increasing excretion, and inhibits platelet aggregation.
Therapeutic effect: relieves signs and symptoms of gouty arthritis.

Adverse reactions

GI: *nausea, dyspepsia,* epigastric pain, reactivation of peptic ulcerations.
Hematologic: ***blood dyscrasias*** (such as anemia, ***leukopenia, agranulocytosis, thrombocytopenia, aplastic anemia***).
Respiratory: ***bronchoconstriction*** in patients with aspirin-induced asthma.
Skin: rash.

Interactions

Drug-drug. *Aspirin, niacin, salicylates:* inhibited uricosuric effect of sulfinpyrazone. Don't use together.
Oral anticoagulants: increased anticoagulant effect and risk of bleeding. Use together cautiously.
Oral antidiabetics: increased effects. Monitor patient closely.
Probenecid: inhibited renal excretion of sulfinpyrazone. Use together cautiously.
Drug-lifestyle: *Alcohol use:* decreased drug effectiveness. Avoid concomitant use.

Contraindications and precautions

- Contraindicated in patients hypersensitive to pyrazole derivatives (including oxyphenbutazone and phenylbutazone) and patients with active peptic ulcer, symptoms of GI inflammation or ulceration, or blood dyscrasias.
- Use cautiously in pregnant women and patients with healed peptic ulcer.
- Safety of drug hasn't been established in breast-feeding women or children.

NURSING CONSIDERATIONS

Assessment

- Assess patient's condition before therapy and regularly thereafter.
- Monitor BUN level, CBC, and kidney function studies periodically during long-term use, as ordered.

- Monitor fluid intake and output. Therapy may lead to renal colic and formation of uric acid stones until acid levels are normal (about 6 mg/dl).
- Be alert for adverse reactions and drug interactions.
- Evaluate patient's and family's knowledge of drug therapy.

Nursing diagnoses

- Ineffective health maintenance related to presence of gouty arthritis
- Risk for injury related to drug-induced adverse CNS reactions
- Deficient knowledge related to drug therapy

Planning and implementation

- Give drug with milk, food, or antacids to minimize GI disturbances.
- Force fluids to maintain minimum daily output of 2 to 3 L. Alkalinize urine with sodium bicarbonate or other agent, as ordered. Keep in mind that alkalinizing agents are used therapeutically to increase drug activity, preventing urolithiasis.
- Drug is recommended for patients unresponsive to probenecid. Suitable for long-term use; neither cumulative effects nor tolerance develops.
- Drug contains no analgesic or anti-inflammatory agent and is of no value during acute gout attacks.
- Drug may increase frequency, severity, and length of acute gout attacks during first 6 to 12 months of therapy. Prophylactic colchicine or another anti-inflammatory drug is given during first 3 to 6 months.
- Lifelong therapy may be required in patient with hyperuricemia.
- Drug decreases urinary excretion of aminohippuric acid, interfering with laboratory test results.

ALERT Don't confuse Anturane with Artane or Antabuse.

Patient teaching

- Warn patient with gout not to take aspirin-containing drugs because they may precipitate gout. Acetaminophen may be used for pain.
- Tell patient to take drug with food, milk, or antacid. Also instruct him to drink plenty of water.
- Instruct patient with gout to avoid foods high in purine, such as anchovies, liver, sardines, kidneys, sweetbreads, peas, and lentils.
- Inform patient and family that drug must be taken regularly, as ordered, or gout attacks may result. Tell patient to visit prescriber regularly so blood levels can be monitored and dosage adjusted if necessary.

Evaluation

- Patient regains and maintains normal uric acid levels.
- Patient doesn't experience injury from adverse CNS reactions.
- Patient and family state understanding of drug therapy.

sulfisoxazole (sulfafurazole, sulphafurazole)

(sul-fih-SOKS-uh-zohl)

Azo-Sulfisoxazole, Gantrisin, Novo-Soxazole ♦

Pharmacologic class: sulfonamide
Therapeutic class: antibiotic
Pregnancy risk category: C

Indications and dosages

▶ **Urinary tract and systemic infections.** *Adults:* initially, 2 to 4 g P.O.; then 4 to 8 g daily divided in four to six doses.
Children over age 2 months: initially, 75 mg/kg P.O. daily or 2 g/m² P.O. daily in divided doses q 6 hours; then 150 mg/kg or 4 g/m² P.O. daily in divided doses q 6 hours.

How supplied

Tablets: 500 mg
Liquid: 500 mg/5 ml

Pharmacokinetics

Absorption: absorbed readily from GI tract.
Distribution: distributed widely in most body tissues and fluids; 85% protein-bound.
Metabolism: metabolized partially in liver.

Excretion: unchanged drug and metabolites excreted primarily in urine. Urine solubility of unchanged drug increases as urine pH increases. *Half-life:* 4½ to 8 hours.

Route	Onset	Peak	Duration
P.O.	Unknown	2-4 hr	Unknown

Pharmacodynamics

Chemical effect: decreases bacterial folic acid synthesis.
Therapeutic effect: hinders activity of some gram-positive bacteria, *Chlamydia trachomatis*, many enterobacteriaceae, and some strains of *Plasmodium falciparum* and *Toxoplasma gondii.*

Adverse reactions

CNS: headache, mental depression, ***seizures,*** hallucinations.
CV: tachycardia, palpitations, syncope, cyanosis.
GI: *nausea, vomiting, diarrhea,* abdominal pain, anorexia, stomatitis, pseudomembranous colitis, ***hepatitis.***
GU: ***toxic nephrosis with oliguria and anuria, acute renal failure,*** crystalluria, hematuria, ***acute renal failure.***
Hematologic: ***agranulocytosis, aplastic anemia, megaloblastic anemia, thrombocytopenia, leukopenia,*** hemolytic anemia.
Hepatic: jaundice.
Skin: ***erythema multiforme,*** *generalized skin eruption,* ***epidermal necrolysis, exfoliative dermatitis,*** photosensitivity, urticaria, pruritus.
Other: hypersensitivity reactions *(serum sickness, drug fever,* ***anaphylaxis).***

Interactions

Drug-drug. *Methotrexate:* may increase methotrexate levels. Use together cautiously.
Oral anticoagulants: increased anticoagulant effect. Monitor patient for bleeding.
Oral antidiabetics: increased hypoglycemic effect. Monitor blood glucose levels.
Oral contraceptives: decreased contraceptive effectiveness, increased risk of breakthrough bleeding. Suggest nonhormonal form of contraception.
Drug-herb. *Dong quai, St. John's wort:* increased risk of photosensitivity. Discourage using together.
Drug-lifestyle. *Sun exposure:* photosensitivity reactions may occur. Urge patient to take precautions.

Contraindications and precautions

- Contraindicated in patients hypersensitive to sulfonamides, pregnant women at term, breast-feeding women, and infants under age 2 months (except in congenital toxoplasmosis).
- Use cautiously in patients with impaired liver or kidney function, severe allergy or bronchial asthma, or G6PD deficiency.

NURSING CONSIDERATIONS

Assessment

- Assess patient's condition before therapy and regularly thereafter.
- Obtain specimen for culture and sensitivity tests before giving first dose. Therapy may begin pending results.
- Monitor urine cultures, CBCs, and urinalyses before and during therapy.
- Monitor urine pH daily.
- Be alert for adverse reactions and drug interactions.
- Monitor patient's hydration if adverse GI reactions occur.
- Evaluate patient's and family's knowledge of drug therapy.

Nursing diagnoses

- Infection related to presence of susceptible bacteria
- Risk for deficient fluid volume related to drug-induced adverse GI reactions
- Deficient knowledge related to drug therapy

Planning and implementation

- Give drug on schedule to maintain constant blood level.
- Have adult patient drink between 3,000 and 4,000 ml daily to prevent crystalluria. Sodium bicarbonate may be given to alkalinize urine.

ALERT Don't confuse sulfisoxazole with sulfasalazine. Don't confuse the combination products (such as Gantrisin) with sulfamethoxazole alone.

Patient teaching
- Teach patient how to monitor fluid intake and output.
- Tell patient to take entire amount of drug exactly as prescribed.
- Warn patient to avoid direct sunlight and ultraviolet light to prevent photosensitivity reaction.

ALERT Tell patient to notify prescriber about early signs of blood dyscrasia (sore throat, fever, pallor) and moderate to severe diarrhea.

Evaluation
- Patient is free from infection.
- Patient maintains adequate hydration.
- Patient and family state understanding of drug therapy.

sulindac
(SUL-in-dak)

Aclin ◇, Apo-Sulin ♦, Clinoril, Novo-Sundac ♦

Pharmacologic class: NSAID
Therapeutic class: nonnarcotic analgesic, antipyretic, anti-inflammatory
Pregnancy risk category: NR

Indications and dosages
▶ **Osteoarthritis, rheumatoid arthritis, ankylosing spondylitis.** *Adults:* initially, 150 mg P.O. b.i.d.; increased to 200 mg b.i.d., as necessary.

▶ **Acute subacromial bursitis or supraspinatus tendinitis, acute gouty arthritis.** *Adults:* 200 mg P.O. b.i.d. for 7 to 14 days. Dose reduced as symptoms subside.

How supplied
Tablets: 100 mg ◇, 150 mg, 200 mg

Pharmacokinetics
Absorption: absorbed rapidly and completely from GI tract.
Distribution: highly protein-bound.
Metabolism: drug is inactive and metabolized in liver to an active sulfide metabolite.
Excretion: excreted in urine. *Half-life:* parent drug, 8 hours; active metabolite, about 16 hours.

Route	Onset	Peak	Duration
P.O.	Unknown	2-4 hr	Unknown

Pharmacodynamics
Chemical effect: unknown; produces anti-inflammatory, analgesic, and antipyretic effects, possibly by inhibiting prostaglandin synthesis.
Therapeutic effect: relieves pain, fever, and inflammation.

Adverse reactions
CNS: dizziness, headache, nervousness, psychosis.
CV: hypertension, ***heart failure,*** palpitations, edema.
EENT: tinnitus, transient visual disturbances.
GI: *epigastric distress,* ***peptic ulceration, pancreatitis, GI bleeding,*** occult blood loss, nausea, constipation, dyspepsia, flatulence, anorexia.
GU: interstitial nephritis, ***nephrotic syndrome, renal failure.***
Hematologic: prolonged bleeding time, ***aplastic anemia, thrombocytopenia, neutropenia, agranulocytosis, hemolytic anemia.***
Hepatic: elevated liver enzyme levels.
Skin: *rash,* pruritus.
Other: drug fever, ***anaphylaxis, hypersensitivity syndrome, angioedema.***

Interactions
Drug-drug. *Anticoagulants:* increased risk of bleeding. Monitor PT closely.
Aspirin: decreased sulindac plasma level and increased risk of adverse GI reactions. Avoid concomitant use.
Cyclosporine: increased nephrotoxicity of cyclosporine. Monitor patient.
Diflunisal, dimethyl sulfoxide: decreased metabolism of sulindac to its active metabolite, reducing its effectiveness. Don't use together.
Methotrexate: increased methotrexate toxicity. Avoid concomitant use.

Probenecid: increased plasma levels of sulindac and its active metabolite. Monitor patient for toxicity.
Sulfonamides, sulfonylureas, other highly protein-bound drugs: possible displacement of these drugs from plasma protein–binding sites, leading to increased toxicity. Monitor patient closely.

Contraindications and precautions

• Contraindicated in patients hypersensitive to drug and patients for whom aspirin or NSAIDs precipitate acute asthmatic attacks, urticaria, or rhinitis.
• Drug isn't recommended for pregnant women.
• Use cautiously in patients with history of ulcers and GI bleeding, renal dysfunction, compromised cardiac function or hypertension, or conditions predisposing to fluid retention.
• Safety of drug hasn't been established in breast-feeding women and in children.

NURSING CONSIDERATIONS

Assessment

• Assess patient's condition before therapy and regularly thereafter.
• Periodically monitor liver and kidney function and CBC in patient receiving long-term therapy, as ordered.
• Be alert for adverse reactions and drug interactions.
• Evaluate patient's and family's knowledge of drug therapy.

Nursing diagnoses

• Acute pain related to presence of arthritis
• Impaired tissue integrity related to drug's adverse effect on GI mucosa
• Deficient knowledge related to drug therapy

Planning and implementation

• Notify prescriber of adverse reactions.

Patient teaching

• Tell patient to take drug with food, milk, or antacids to reduce adverse GI reactions.
• Advise patient to refrain from driving or performing other hazardous activities that require mental alertness until CNS effects are known.
• Teach patient signs and symptoms of GI bleeding, and tell him to contact prescriber immediately if they occur. Serious GI toxicity, including peptic ulceration and bleeding, can occur in patient taking NSAIDs despite absence of GI symptoms.
ALERT Tell patient to notify prescriber immediately about easy bruising or prolonged bleeding.
• Instruct patient to report edema and have blood pressure checked monthly. Drug causes sodium retention but is thought to have less effect on kidneys than other NSAIDs.
• Instruct patient not to take aspirin or aspirin-containing products with sulindac.
• Tell patient to notify prescriber and undergo complete eye examination if visual disturbances occur.

Evaluation

• Patient is free from pain.
• Patient doesn't experience adverse GI reactions.
• Patient and family state understanding of drug therapy.

sumatriptan succinate

(soo-muh-TRIP-ten SEK-seh-nayt)
Imitrex

Pharmacologic class: selective 5-hydroxytryptamine (5-HT_1) receptor agonist
Therapeutic class: antimigraine agent
Pregnancy risk category: C

Indications and dosages

▶ **Acute migraine attacks (with or without aura).** *Adults:* 6 mg S.C. Maximum recommended dosage is two 6-mg injections in 24 hours, separated by at least 1 hour. Or, 25 to 100 mg P.O. If headache returns or responds only partially, dose may be repeated after 2 hours. Maximum daily dosage is 300 mg P.O. Intranasally, 5 mg, 10 mg, or 20 mg in one nostril (for 10 mg dose, one spray of 5-mg concentration into each nostril); if headache returns, may repeat once after 2 hours. Maximum daily dosage is 40 mg.

How supplied

Tablets: 25 mg, 50 mg, 100 mg (base) ♦
Injection: 6 mg/0.5 ml (12 mg/ml) in 0.5-ml prefilled syringes and vials
Nasal spray: 5 mg/spray; 20 mg/spray

Pharmacokinetics

Absorption: rapidly absorbed after P.O. administration but with low absolute bioavailability (about 15%); absorbed well from injection site after S.C. administration.
Distribution: drug has low protein-binding of about 14% to 21%.
Metabolism: about 80% metabolized in liver.
Excretion: excreted primarily in urine. *Half-life:* about 2 hours.

Route	Onset	Peak	Duration
P.O.	30 min	2-4 hr	Unknown
S.C.	10-20 min	1-2 hr	Unknown
Intranasal	Rapid	1-2 hr	Unknown

Pharmacodynamics

Chemical effect: unknown; thought to selectively activate vascular serotonin (5-HT) receptors. Stimulation of specific receptor subtype 5-HT_1, present on cranial arteries and the dura mater, causes vasoconstriction of cerebral vessels but has minimal effects on systemic vessels, tissue perfusion, and blood pressure.
Therapeutic effect: relieves acute migraine pain.

Adverse reactions

CNS: *dizziness, vertigo,* drowsiness, headache, anxiety, malaise, fatigue.
CV: ***atrial fibrillation, ventricular fibrillation, ventricular tachycardia, MI,*** pressure or tightness in chest, ECG changes such as ischemic ST-segment elevation (rare).
EENT: discomfort of throat, nasal cavity or sinus, mouth, jaw, or tongue; altered vision.
GI: abdominal discomfort, dysphagia.
Musculoskeletal: neck pain, myalgia, muscle cramps.
Skin: flushing.
Other: *tingling; warm or hot sensation; burning sensation; heaviness, pressure, or tightness;* feeling of strangeness; tight feeling in head; cold sensation; diaphoresis; *injection site reaction.*

Interactions

Drug-drug. *Ergot, ergot derivatives:* prolonged vasospastic effects. Don't use these drugs within 24 hours of sumatriptan.
MAO inhibitors: increased sumatriptan effects. Avoid use within 2 weeks of an MAO inhibitor.
Drug-herb. *Horehound:* may enhance serotonergic effects. Avoid concomitant use.

Contraindications and precautions

- Contraindicated in patients hypersensitive to drug, patients taking ergotamine, patients who have taken an MAO inhibitor within 14 days, and patients with uncontrolled hypertension, ischemic heart disease (such as angina pectoris, Prinzmetal's angina, history of MI, or documented silent ischemia), or hemiplegic or basilar migraine.
- Use cautiously in women who are pregnant or intend to become pregnant. Also, use cautiously in patients who may have unrecognized coronary artery disease (CAD), such as postmenopausal women, men over age 40, and patients with risk factors for CAD, such as hypertension, hypercholesterolemia, obesity, diabetes, smoking, or family history of CAD.
- Safety of drug hasn't been established in children and in breast-feeding women.

NURSING CONSIDERATIONS

Assessment

- Assess patient's condition before therapy and regularly thereafter.
- Be alert for adverse reactions and drug interactions.
- Evaluate patient's and family's knowledge of drug therapy.

Nursing diagnoses
- Acute pain related to presence of acute migraine attack
- Risk for injury related to drug-induced adverse reactions
- Deficient knowledge related to drug therapy

Planning and implementation
- Consider giving first dose in prescriber's office if patient has risk of unrecognized CAD.

P.O. use: Give single tablet whole with fluids as soon as patient complains of migraine symptoms. Give second tablet if symptoms come back, but no sooner than 2 hours after first tablet.

S.C. use: Maximum recommended dosage in 24-hour period is two 6-mg injections separated by at least 1 hour. Notify prescriber if patient doesn't obtain relief.

– Most patients experience relief within 1 to 2 hours.

– Redness or pain at injection site should subside within 1 hour after injection.

ALERT Serious adverse cardiac effects can follow S.C. administration of this drug, but such events are rare.

Intranasal use: Follow normal protocol.

– Notify prescriber if patient doesn't feel relief.

ALERT Don't confuse sumatriptan with somatropin.

Patient teaching
- Make sure patient understands that drug is intended only to treat migraine attack, not to prevent or reduce number of attacks.
- Tell patient that drug may be given at any time during migraine attack but should be given as soon as symptoms appear.
- Drug is available in spring-loaded injector system that facilitates administration by patient. Review detailed information with patient. Make sure patient understands how to load injector, administer injection, and dispose of used syringes.
- Instruct patient taking P.O. form when and how often to take drug. Warn patient not to take more than 300 mg within 24 hours.
- Instruct patient to use intranasal spray in one nostril (if 10 mg dose is ordered, 1 spray into each nostril). A second spray may be used if headache returns, but not before 2 hours has elapsed from the first use.
- Tell patient who experiences persistent or severe chest pain to call prescriber immediately. Patient who experiences pain or tightness in throat, wheezing, heart throbbing, rash, lumps, hives, or swollen eyelids, face, or lips should stop using drug and call prescriber.
- Tell woman who is pregnant or intends to become pregnant not to take this drug. Advise her to discuss with prescriber the risks and benefits of using drug during pregnancy.

Evaluation
- Patient is free from pain.
- Patient doesn't experience injury from adverse CV reactions.
- Patient and family state understanding of drug therapy.

T

tacrine hydrochloride
(TAK-reen high-droh-KLOR-ighd)
Cognex

Pharmacologic class: centrally acting reversible cholinesterase inhibitor
Therapeutic class: psychotherapeutic agent for Alzheimer's disease
Pregnancy risk category: C

Indications and dosages
▶ **Mild to moderate dementia of Alzheimer's type.** *Adults:* initially, 10 mg P.O. q.i.d. After 6 weeks and if patient tolerates treatment and transaminase levels aren't elevated, dosage increased to 20 mg q.i.d. After another 6 weeks, dosage adjusted upward to 30 mg q.i.d. If still tolerated, increased to 40 mg q.i.d. after another 6 weeks.

How supplied
Capsules: 10 mg, 20 mg, 30 mg, 40 mg

Pharmacokinetics

Absorption: rapidly absorbed with absolute bioavailability of about 17%. Food reduces tacrine bioavailability by 30% to 40%.
Distribution: about 55% bound to plasma proteins.
Metabolism: undergoes first-pass metabolism, which is dose-dependent; extensively metabolized.
Excretion: excreted in urine. *Half-life:* 2 to 4 hours.

Route	Onset	Peak	Duration
P.O.	Unknown	0.5-3 hr	Unknown

Pharmacodynamics

Chemical effect: reversibly inhibits enzyme cholinesterase in CNS, allowing buildup of acetylcholine.
Therapeutic effect: improves thinking ability in patients with Alzheimer's disease.

Adverse reactions

CNS: agitation, ataxia, insomnia, abnormal thinking, somnolence, depression, anxiety, *headache,* fatigue, *dizziness,* confusion.
CV: chest pain.
EENT: rhinitis.
GI: *nausea, vomiting,* anorexia, *diarrhea,* dyspepsia, loose stools, changes in stool color, constipation.
Hepatic: jaundice.
Metabolic: weight loss.
Musculoskeletal: myalgia.
Respiratory: upper respiratory tract infection, cough.
Skin: rash, facial flushing.

Interactions

Drug-drug. *Anticholinergics:* drug may decrease effectiveness of anticholinergics. Monitor patient closely.
Cholinergics (such as bethanechol), cholinesterase inhibitors: additive effects. Monitor patient for toxicity.
Succinylcholine: enhanced neuromuscular blockade and prolonged duration of action. Monitor patient.
Theophylline: increased theophylline serum levels and prolonged theophylline half-life. Carefully monitor plasma theophylline levels and adjust dosage as directed.
Drug-food. *Any food:* decreased tacrine absorption. Tell patient to take drug on empty stomach.
Drug-lifestyle. *Smoking:* decreased plasma levels of drug. Monitor response.

Contraindications and precautions

- Contraindicated in patients hypersensitive to drug or acridine derivatives and in those who have previously developed tacrine-related jaundice and been confirmed with elevated total bilirubin level of more than 3 mg/dl.
- Drug isn't recommended for pregnant or breast-feeding women.
- Use cautiously in patients with sick sinus syndrome or bradycardia; those at risk for peptic ulceration (including patients taking NSAIDs or those with history of peptic ulcer); those with history of hepatic disease; and those with renal disease, asthma, prostatic hyperplasia, or other urinary outflow impairment.
- Drug isn't indicated for children.

NURSING CONSIDERATIONS

Assessment

- Assess patient's cognitive ability before therapy and regularly thereafter.
- Monitor serum ALT levels weekly during first 18 weeks of therapy. If ALT is modestly elevated after first 18 weeks (twice upper limit of normal range), continue weekly monitoring. If no problems occur, determinations decreased to every 3 months. Whenever dosage is increased, resume weekly monitoring for at least 6 weeks.
- Be alert for adverse reactions and drug interactions.
- Evaluate patient's and family's knowledge of drug therapy.

Nursing diagnoses

- Disturbed thought processes related to Alzheimer's disease
- Diarrhea related to drug-induced adverse GI reactions
- Deficient knowledge related to drug therapy

Planning and implementation

- Give drug between meals. If GI upset becomes a problem, give drug with meals, although plasma levels may drop by 30% to 40%.
- If drug is discontinued for 4 weeks or more, full dosage adjustment and monitoring schedule must be restarted.
- Obtain order for antidiarrheal, if indicated.

Patient teaching

- Help patient and family members understand that drug only alleviates symptoms. Effect of therapy depends on drug administration at regular intervals.

ALERT Instruct caregivers when to give drug. Explain that dosage adjustment is integral to safe use. Abrupt discontinuation or large reduction in daily dosage (80 mg or more per day) may trigger behavioral disturbances and cognitive decline.

- Advise patient and caregivers to report immediately significant adverse effects or changes in status.

Evaluation

- Patient exhibits improved cognitive ability.
- Patient or caregiver states that drug-induced diarrhea hasn't occurred.
- Patient and family state understanding of drug therapy.

tacrolimus

(tek-roh-LEE-mus)

Prograf

Pharmacologic class: bacteria-derived macrolide
Therapeutic class: immunosuppressant
Pregnancy risk category: C

Indications and dosages

▶ **Prophylaxis of organ rejection in allogenic liver transplantation.** *Adults:* 0.05 to 0.1 mg/kg/day I.V. as continuous infusion administered no sooner than 6 hours after transplantation. P.O. therapy should be substituted as soon as possible, with first dose given 8 to 12 hours after discontinuing I.V. infusion. Recommended initial P.O. dosage is 0.15 to 0.3 mg/kg/day in two divided doses q 12 hours. Dosage should be adjusted according to clinical response.
Children: initially, 0.1 mg/kg/day I.V., followed by 0.3 mg/kg/day P.O. on schedule similar to that for adults; adjust dosage as needed.

How supplied

Capsules: 1 mg, 5 mg
Injection: 5 mg/ml

Pharmacokinetics

Absorption: absorption of tacrolimus from GI tract varies. Food reduces absorption and bioavailability of drug.
Distribution: distribution between whole blood and plasma depends on several factors, such as hematocrit, temperature of separation of plasma, drug level, and plasma protein level. Drug is 75% to 99% protein-bound.
Metabolism: extensively metabolized.
Excretion: excreted primarily in bile; less than 1% excreted unchanged in urine.

Route	Onset	Peak	Duration
P.O., I.V.	Unknown	1.5-3.5 hr	Unknown

Pharmacodynamics

Chemical effect: precise mechanism unknown; inhibits T-lymphocyte activation, which results in immunosuppression.
Therapeutic effect: prevents organ rejection.

Adverse reactions

CNS: *asthenia, headache, tremors, insomnia, paresthesia, delirium,* ***coma.***
CV: *hypertension, peripheral edema.*
GI: *diarrhea, nausea, constipation, anorexia, vomiting, abdominal pain.*
GU: *abnormal kidney function,* increased creatinine or BUN level, urinary tract infection, oliguria.
Hematologic: *anemia,* leukocytosis, THROMBOCYTOPENIA.
Hepatic: *abnormal liver function test results.*
Metabolic: ***hyperkalemia,*** hypokalemia, *hyperglycemia, hypomagnesemia.*
Musculoskeletal: *back pain.*

Respiratory: *pleural effusion, atelectasis, dyspnea.*
Skin: *photosensitivity.*
Other: *pain, fever, ascites,* ***anaphylaxis.***

Interactions

Drug-drug. *Bromocriptine, cimetidine, clarithromycin, clotrimazole, cyclosporine, danazol, diltiazem, erythromycin, fluconazole, itraconazole, ketoconazole, methylprednisolone, metoclopramide, nicardipine, verapamil:* may increase tacrolimus level. Monitor patient for adverse effects.
Carbamazepine, phenobarbital, phenytoin, rifabutin, rifampin: may decrease tacrolimus level. Monitor effectiveness of tacrolimus.
Cyclosporine: increased risk of excess nephrotoxicity. Don't administer together.
Immunosuppressants (except adrenocorticosteroids): may oversuppress immune system. Monitor patient closely, especially during times of stress.
Inducers of cytochrome P-450 enzyme system: may increase tacrolimus metabolism and decrease plasma level. Dosage adjustment may be needed.
Inhibitors of cytochrome P-450 enzyme system: may decrease tacrolimus metabolism and increase plasma level. Dosage adjustment may be needed.
Nephrotoxic drugs (such as aminoglycosides, amphotericin B, cisplatin, cyclosporine): may cause additive or synergistic effects. Monitor patient closely.
Viral vaccines: tacrolimus may interfere with immune response to live virus vaccines.
Drug-food. *Any food:* inhibited drug absorption. Tell patient to take drug on an empty stomach.
Grapefruit juice: increased drug blood levels in liver transplant patients. Discourage concomitant use.

Contraindications and precautions

- Contraindicated in patients hypersensitive to drug. The I.V. form is contraindicated in patients hypersensitive to castor oil derivatives.
- Drug isn't recommended for pregnant or breast-feeding women.

NURSING CONSIDERATIONS

Assessment

- Obtain history of patient's organ transplant before therapy and reassess regularly thereafter.
- Monitor patient continuously during first 30 minutes of infusion; then monitor frequently for anaphylaxis.
- Monitor patient for signs of neurotoxicity and nephrotoxicity, especially in those receiving high dosage or with renal dysfunction.
- Obtain serum potassium and blood glucose levels regularly. Monitor patient for hyperglycemia.
- Drug increases risk for infections, lymphomas, and other cancers.
- Be alert for adverse reactions and drug interactions.
- Evaluate patient's and family's knowledge of drug therapy.

Nursing diagnoses

- Risk for injury related to potential organ transplant rejection
- Ineffective protection related to drug-induced immunosuppression
- Deficient knowledge related to drug therapy

Planning and implementation

- Child with normal kidney and liver function may need higher dosage than adult.
- Patient with hepatic or renal dysfunction needs lowest possible dosage.
- Expect to give adrenocorticosteroids with this drug.

P.O. use: Give drug on empty stomach.
I.V. use: Dilute drug with normal saline solution injection or D_5W injection to 0.004 to 0.02 mg/ml before use.
– Store diluted solution for no more than 24 hours in glass or polyethylene containers. Don't store drug in polyvinyl chloride container.
– Each required daily dose of diluted drug is infused continuously over 24 hours.
ALERT Because of risk of anaphylaxis, use injection only in patient who cannot take oral form.
– Keep epinephrine 1:1,000 readily available to treat anaphylaxis.

• Other immunosuppressants (except for adrenocorticosteroids) shouldn't be used during therapy.
• Avoid use of potassium-sparing diuretics during therapy.

Patient teaching
• Instruct patient to take drug on empty stomach and not to take it with grapefruit juice.
• Explain need for repeated tests during therapy to monitor for adverse reactions and drug effectiveness.
• Advise woman of childbearing age to notify prescriber if she becomes pregnant or plans to do so.
• Instruct patient to check with prescriber before taking other medications.

Evaluation
• Patient doesn't exhibit signs and symptoms of organ rejection.
• Patient doesn't develop serious complications as result of drug-induced adverse reactions.
• Patient and family state understanding of drug therapy.

tamoxifen citrate
(teh-MOKS-uh-fen SIGH-trayt)
Apo-Tamox♦, Nolvadex, Nolvadex-D♦◇, Novo-Tamoxifen♦, Tamofen♦, Tamone♦

Pharmacologic class: nonsteroidal antiestrogen
Therapeutic class: antineoplastic
Pregnancy risk category: D

Indications and dosages
▶ **Advanced postmenopausal breast cancer.** *Adults:* 10 to 20 mg P.O. b.i.d.
▶ **Adjunct treatment for breast cancer.** *Adults:* 10 mg P.O. b.i.d. to t.i.d. for no more than 2 years.
▶ **Reduction of breast cancer risk in high-risk women.** *Adults:* 20 mg P.O. daily for 5 years.

How supplied
Tablets: 10 mg, 20 mg
Tablets (enteric-coated)♦: 10 mg, 20 mg

Pharmacokinetics
Absorption: appears to be well absorbed across GI tract.
Distribution: distributed widely in total body water.
Metabolism: metabolized extensively in liver to several metabolites.
Excretion: drug and metabolites excreted mainly in feces, mostly as metabolites. *Half-life:* over 7 days.

Route	Onset	Peak	Duration
P.O.	4-10 wk	Unknown	Several wk

Pharmacodynamics
Chemical effect: exact antineoplastic action is unknown; acts as estrogen antagonist.
Therapeutic effect: hinders function of breast cancer cells.

Adverse reactions
CNS: confusion, weakness, headache, sleepiness.
CV: *hot flushes.*
EENT: corneal changes, cataracts, retinopathy.
GI: *nausea, vomiting, diarrhea.*
GU: *vaginal discharge* and bleeding, *irregular menses,* increased BUN, *amenorrhea.*
Hematologic: transient fall in WBC or platelet count, ***leukopenia, thrombocytopenia.***
Hepatic: changes in liver enzyme levels, fatty liver, cholestasis, ***hepatic necrosis.***
Metabolic: *hypercalcemia, weight changes, fluid retention.*
Musculoskeletal: brief exacerbation of pain from osseous metastases.
Skin: *skin changes,* rash.
Other: temporary bone or tumor pain.

Interactions
Drug-drug. *Antacids:* may affect absorption of enteric-coated tablet. Don't use within 2 hours of tamoxifen dose.
Bromocriptine: may elevate tamoxifen levels. Monitor patient for toxicity.

Coumadin-type anticoagulants: may cause significant increase in anticoagulant effect. Monitor patient, PT, and INR closely.

Contraindications and precautions

- Contraindicated in patients hypersensitive to drug.
- Contraindicated in women receiving coumarin-type anticoagulants or with history of deep vein thrombosis or pulmonary emboli.
- Drug isn't recommended for use in pregnant or breast-feeding women.
- Use cautiously in patients with leukopenia or thrombocytopenia.
- Safety of drug hasn't been established in children.

NURSING CONSIDERATIONS

Assessment

- Assess patient's breast cancer before therapy and regularly thereafter.
- Monitor CBC closely in patient with leukopenia or thrombocytopenia, as ordered.
- Monitor serum lipid levels during long-term therapy in patients with hyperlipidemia.
- Monitor serum calcium level, as ordered. Drug may compound hypercalcemia related to bone metastases during initiation of therapy.
- Be alert for adverse reactions.
- Monitor patient's hydration status if adverse GI reactions occur.
- Evaluate patient's and family's knowledge of drug therapy.

Nursing diagnoses

- Ineffective health maintenance related to presence of breast cancer
- Risk for deficient fluid volume related to drug-induced adverse GI reactions
- Deficient knowledge related to drug therapy

Planning and implementation

- Drug acts as an antiestrogen. Best results have been reported in patients with positive estrogen receptors.
- Make sure patient swallows enteric-coated tablets whole. Don't give antacids within 2 hours of dose.

Patient teaching

- Reassure patient that acute bone pain during drug therapy usually means that drug will produce good response. Tell her to take an analgesic for pain.
- Encourage patient who is taking or has taken drug to have regular gynecologic examinations because of increased risk of uterine cancer.
- If patient is taking drug to reduce risk of breast cancer, teach proper technique for self breast exam.
- Tell patient that annual mammograms are important.
- Advise patient to use barrier form of contraception because short-term therapy induces ovulation in premenopausal women.
- Advise woman of childbearing age to avoid becoming pregnant during therapy and to consult with prescriber before becoming pregnant.

Evaluation

- Patient responds well to drug.
- Patient maintains adequate hydration.
- Patient and family state understanding of drug therapy.

tamsulosin hydrochloride

(tam-soo-LOH-sin high-droh-KLOR-ighd)
Flomax

Pharmacologic class: alpha$_{1a}$-antagonist
Therapeutic class: BPH agent
Pregnancy risk category: B

Indications and dosages

▶ **Treatment of BPH.** *Adults:* 0.4 mg P.O. once daily, administered 30 minutes after same meal each day. If no response after 2 to 4 weeks, dose may be increased to 0.8 mg P.O. once daily.

How supplied

Capsules: 0.4 mg

Pharmacokinetics

Absorption: almost complete with over 90% absorbed following P.O. administration. Food increases bioavailability by 30%.

Distribution: distributed into extracellular fluids. Extensively bound to protein (94% to 99%).
Metabolism: primarily metabolized by cytochrome P-450 enzymes in the liver.
Excretion: 76% of drug eliminated in urine; 21% in feces. *Half-life:* 9 to 13 hours.

Route	Onset	Peak	Duration
P.O.	Unknown	4-5 hr	9-15 hr

Pharmacodynamics

Chemical effect: selectively blocks alpha receptors in the prostate, leading to relaxation of smooth muscles in the bladder neck and prostate, which improves urine flow and reduces symptoms of BPH.
Therapeutic effect: improves urine flow.

Adverse reactions

CNS: asthenia, *dizziness, headache,* insomnia, somnolence, syncope, vertigo.
CV: chest pain, orthostatic hypotension.
EENT: amblyopia, pharyngitis, *rhinitis,* sinusitis.
GI: diarrhea, nausea.
GU: abnormal ejaculation.
Musculoskeletal: back pain.
Respiratory: cough.
Other: decreased libido, *infection,* tooth disorder.

Interactions

Drug-drug. *Alpha-adrenergic blockers:* may interact with tamsulosin. Avoid concomitant use.
Cimetidine: decreased tamsulosin clearance. Use cautiously.

Contraindications and precautions

- Contraindicated in patients hypersensitive to drug or its components.

NURSING CONSIDERATIONS

Assessment

- Assess patient for signs of prostatic hypertrophy, including frequency of urination, nocturnal urination, and urinary hesitancy.
- Monitor patient for decreases in blood pressure and notify prescriber.
- Evaluate patient's and family's knowledge of drug therapy.

Nursing diagnoses

- Risk for injury related to decreased blood pressure and resulting syncope
- Impaired urinary elimination related to underlying prostatic hypertrophy
- Deficient knowledge related to drug therapy

Planning and implementation

- Symptoms of BPH and cancer of the prostate are similar; cancer should be ruled out before therapy starts.
- If treatment is interrupted for several days or more, restart therapy at one capsule daily as ordered.
- Drug may cause a sudden drop in blood pressure, especially after the first dose or when changing doses.

ALERT Don't confuse Flomax with Fosamax.

Patient teaching

- Instruct patient not to crush, chew, or open capsules.
- Tell patient to get up slowly from chair or bed during initiation of therapy and to avoid situations where injury could occur because of syncope. Advise him that drug may cause a sudden drop in blood pressure, especially after the first dose or when changing doses.
- Instruct patient not to drive or perform hazardous tasks for 12 hours following the initial dose or changes in dose until response can be monitored.
- Tell patient to take drug about 30 minutes following same meal each day.

Evaluation

- Patient doesn't experience sudden decreases in blood pressure.
- Patient experiences normal urinary elimination patterns.
- Patient and family state understanding of drug therapy.

telmisartan

(tel-mih-SAR-tan)
Micardis

Pharmacologic class: angiotensin II receptor antagonist
Therapeutic class: antihypertensive
Pregnancy risk category: C (D in second and third trimesters)

Indications and dosages

▶ **Treatment of hypertension (used alone or with other antihypertensives).** *Adults:* 40 mg P.O. daily. Blood pressure response is dose-related between 20 to 80 mg daily.

How supplied

Tablets: 40 mg, 80 mg

Pharmacokinetics

Absorption: readily absorbed after P.O. administration.
Distribution: highly protein-bound; volume of distribution is about 500 L.
Metabolism: metabolized by conjugation to an inactive metabolite.
Excretion: mainly excreted unchanged in feces.

Route	Onset	Peak	Duration
P.O.	Unknown	0.5-1 hr	24 hr

Pharmacodynamics

Chemical effect: blocks the vasoconstricting and aldosterone-secreting effects of angiotensin II by selectively blocking the binding of angiotensin II to the AT_1 receptor in many tissues, such as vascular smooth muscle and the adrenal gland.
Therapeutic effect: lowers blood pressure.

Adverse reactions

CNS: dizziness, pain, fatigue, headache.
CV: chest pain, hypertension, peripheral edema.
EENT: pharyngitis, sinusitis.
GI: abdominal pain, diarrhea, dyspepsia, nausea.
GU: UTI.
Hepatic: elevated liver enzyme levels.
Musculoskeletal: back pain, myalgia.
Respiratory: cough, upper respiratory tract infection.
Other: flulike symptoms.

Interactions

Drug-drug. *Digoxin:* increased digoxin plasma levels. Monitor digoxin levels closely.
Warfarin: slightly decreased warfarin plasma levels. Monitor INR.

Contraindications and precautions

- Contraindicated in patients hypersensitive to drug or its components. Safety and effectiveness haven't been studied in patients age 18 or younger.
- Use cautiously in patients with renal and hepatic insufficiency and in those with an activated renin-angiotensin system, such as volume- or salt-depleted patients (such as those being treated with high doses of diuretics).
- Drugs that act directly on the renin-angiotensin system, such as telmisartan, can cause fetal and neonatal morbidity and death when given to pregnant women. These problems haven't been detected when exposure has been limited to the first trimester. If pregnancy is suspected, notify prescriber because drug should be discontinued.

NURSING CONSIDERATIONS

Assessment

- Monitor patient for hypotension after therapy starts. Place patient in supine position if hypotension occurs and administer normal saline solution I.V. if necessary.
- In patients whose renal function may depend on the activity of the renin-angiotensin-aldosterone system, such as those with severe heart failure, treatment with ACE inhibitors and angiotensin-receptor antagonists has been related to oliguria or progressive azotemia and (rarely) to acute renal failure or death.
- Drug levels may be increased in patients with biliary obstruction because of inability to excrete drug.

• Drug isn't removed by hemodialysis. Patients undergoing dialysis may develop orthostatic hypotension. Closely monitor blood pressure.
• Evaluate patient's and family's knowledge of drug therapy.

Nursing diagnoses
• Risk for injury related to presence of hypertension
• Ineffective cerebral and cardiopulmonary tissue perfusion related to drug-induced hypotension
• Deficient knowledge related to drug therapy

Planning and implementation
• Most of the antihypertensive effect is present within 2 weeks. Maximal blood pressure reduction is generally attained after 4 weeks. Diuretic may be added if blood pressure isn't controlled by drug alone.

Patient teaching
• Inform woman of childbearing age of consequences of second- and third-trimester exposure to drug. Instruct patient to report suspected pregnancy to prescriber immediately.
• Advise breast-feeding woman about risk for adverse effects on infant and need to stop breast-feeding or discontinue drug, taking into account importance of drug to patient.
• Tell patient that transient hypotension may occur. Instruct him to lie down if feeling dizzy and to climb stairs slowly and rise slowly to standing position.
• Instruct patient with heart failure to notify prescriber about decreased urine output.
• Tell patient that drug may be taken without regard to meals.
• Teach patient other means to reduce blood pressure, such as diet control, exercise, smoking cessation, and stress reduction.
• Inform patient that drug shouldn't be removed from blister-sealed packet until immediately before use.

Evaluation
• Patient doesn't experience injury from underlying disease.
• Patient doesn't experience hypotension and maintains adequate tissue perfusion.
• Patient and family state understanding of drug therapy.

temazepam
(teh-MAZ-ih-pam)
Euhypnos ◇, Normison ◇, Restoril, Temaze ◇

Pharmacologic class: benzodiazepine
Therapeutic class: sedative-hypnotic
Controlled substance schedule: IV
Pregnancy risk category: X

Indications and dosages
▶ **Insomnia.** *Adults up to age 65:* 7.5 to 30 mg P.O. 30 minutes before bedtime. *Adults over age 65:* 7.5 mg P.O. h.s.

How supplied
Capsules: 7.5 mg, 15 mg, 20 mg ◇, 30 mg

Pharmacokinetics
Absorption: well absorbed through GI tract.
Distribution: distributed widely throughout body; 98% protein-bound.
Metabolism: metabolized in liver to primarily inactive metabolites.
Excretion: metabolites excreted in urine. *Half-life:* 10 to 17 hours.

Route	Onset	Peak	Duration
P.O.	Unknown	1-2 hr	Unknown

Pharmacodynamics
Chemical effect: unknown; probably acts on limbic system, thalamus, and hypothalamus of CNS to produce hypnotic effects.
Therapeutic effect: promotes sleep.

Adverse reactions
CNS: *drowsiness, dizziness, lethargy,* disturbed coordination, daytime sedation, confusion, nightmares, vertigo, euphoria, weakness, headache, fatigue, nervousness, anxiety, depression.
EENT: blurred vision.
GI: diarrhea, nausea, dry mouth.
Other: physical and psychological dependence.

Interactions

Drug-drug. *CNS depressants, including narcotic analgesics:* increased CNS depression. Use together cautiously.
Drug-herb. *Ashwagandha, calendula, catnip, hops, lady's slipper, lemon balm, passion flower, sassafras, skullcap, valerian, yerba maté:* risk for increased sedative effects. Monitor patient closely.
Kava: excessive sedation. Advise against concomitant use.
Drug-lifestyle. *Alcohol use:* increased CNS depression. Discourage concurrent use.

Contraindications and precautions

- Contraindicated in pregnant women and patients hypersensitive to benzodiazepines.
- Drug isn't recommended for breast-feeding women.
- Use cautiously in patients with chronic pulmonary insufficiency, impaired liver or kidney function, severe or latent depression, suicidal tendencies, or history of drug abuse.
- Safety of drug hasn't been established in children.

NURSING CONSIDERATIONS

Assessment
- Assess patient's sleeping disorder before therapy and regularly thereafter.
- Assess mental status before therapy. Elderly patients are more sensitive to drug's adverse CNS effects.
- Be alert for adverse reactions and drug interactions.
- Evaluate patient's and family's knowledge of drug therapy.

Nursing diagnoses
- Disturbed sleep pattern related to presence of insomnia
- Risk for injury related to drug-induced adverse CNS reactions
- Deficient knowledge related to drug therapy

Planning and implementation
- Prevent hoarding or intentional overdosing by patient who is depressed, suicidal, or drug-dependent or who has history of drug abuse.
- Make sure patient has swallowed capsule before leaving bedside.
- Supervise walking and raise bed rails, particularly for elderly patient.

ALERT Don't confuse Restoril with Vistaril.

Patient teaching
- Warn patient to avoid activities that require mental alertness or physical coordination.

Evaluation
- Patient states that drug induces sleep.
- Patient doesn't experience injury from adverse CNS reactions.
- Patient and family state understanding of drug therapy.

temozolomide
(teh-moh-ZOHL-uh-mighd)
Temodar

Pharmacologic class: alkylating agent
Therapeutic class: antineoplastic
Pregnancy risk category: D

Indications and dosages

▶ **Refractory anaplastic astrocytoma that has relapsed following chemotherapy regimen containing a nitrosourea and procarbazine.** *Adults:* initial cycle: 150 mg/m^2 P.O. once daily for first 5 days of 28-day chemotherapy treatment cycle. Subsequent cycles: 100 to 200 mg/m^2 P.O. once daily for first 5 days of subsequent 28-day chemotherapy treatment cycles. Timing and dosage of subsequent cycles must be adjusted according to the absolute neutrophil count (ANC) and platelet count measured on cycle day 22 (expected nadir) and cycle day 29 (initiation of next cycle).

Dosage adjustments are based on the lowest of these ANC and platelet results. For ANC less than 1,000/mm^3 or platelets less than 50,000/mm^3: Hold therapy until ANC is above 1,500/mm^3 and platelets are above 100,000/mm^3. Reduce dose by 50 mg/m^2 for subsequent cycle. Minimum dose is 100 mg/m^2.

For ANC 1,000 to 1,500/mm^3 or platelets 50,000 to 100,000/mm^3: Hold therapy until ANC is above 1,500/mm^{3}and platelets are above 100,000/mm^3. Maintain prior dose for subsequent cycle.

For ANC greater than 1,500/mm^3 and platelets greater than 100,000/mm^3: Increase dose to, or maintain at, 200 mg/m^2 for first 5 days of subsequent cycle.

How supplied

Capsules: 5 mg, 20 mg, 100 mg, 250 mg

Pharmacokinetics

Absorption: Rapidly and completely absorbed from the GI tract following P.O. administration, with plasma levels peaking in 1 hour.
Distribution: 15% bound to plasma proteins.
Metabolism: Undergoes spontaneous hydrolysis to its active form and other metabolites. After 7 days, 38% of administered dose is recovered in urine and 0.8% in feces.
Excretion: Rapidly eliminated. *Half-life:* 1¾ hours.

Route	Onset	Peak	Duration
P.O.	Unknown	1 hr	Unknown

Pharmacodynamics

Chemical effect: temozolomide is a prodrug that is rapidly hydrolyzed to the active agent. It's thought to interfere with DNA replication in rapidly dividing tissues, primarily through alkylation (methylation) of guanine nucleotides in the DNA structure.
Therapeutic effect: hinders or kills certain cancer cells.

Adverse reactions

CNS: amnesia, anxiety, asthenia, ataxia, confusion, SEIZURES, coordination abnormality, depression, dizziness, dysphasia, fatigue, gait abnormality, headache, hemiparesis, insomnia, local seizures, paresis, paresthesia, somnolence.
CV: peripheral edema.
EENT: abnormal vision, diplopia, pharyngitis, sinusitis.
GI: abdominal pain, anorexia, constipation, diarrhea, nausea, vomiting.
GU: increased urinary frequency, urinary incontinence, UTI.
Hematologic: anemia, **LEUKOPENIA, NEUTROPENIA, THROMBOCYTOPENIA.**
Metabolic: weight increase.
Musculoskeletal: back pain, myalgia.
Respiratory: cough, upper respiratory tract infection.
Skin: pruritus, rash.
Other: hyperadrenocorticism, breast pain (women), fever, viral infection.

Interactions

Drug-drug. *Valproic acid:* decreases oral clearance of temozolomide by about 5%. Use cautiously.
Drug-food. *Any food:* reduces rate and extent of drug absorption; however, there are no dietary restrictions with drug administration. Give drug on an empty stomach to reduce nausea and vomiting.

Contraindications and precautions

- Contraindicated in patients hypersensitive to temozolomide or its components. Also contraindicated in patients allergic to dacarbazine, which is structurally similar to temozolomide.
- Use with caution in elderly patients and those with severe hepatic or renal impairment.

NURSING CONSIDERATIONS

Assessment

- Obtain history of patient's underlying condition before therapy and reassess regularly thereafter.
- Blood count should be drawn on days 22 and 29 of each treatment cycle. If the ANC falls below 1,500/mm^3 or the platelet count falls below 100,000/mm^3, obtain a weekly CBC until the counts have recovered.
- Be alert for adverse reactions and drug interactions.
- Evaluate patient's and family's knowledge of drug therapy.

Nursing diagnoses

- Ineffective health maintenance related to presence of neoplastic disease

• Risk for injury related to drug-induced adverse reactions
• Deficient knowledge related to drug therapy

Planning and implementation

• Nausea and vomiting, which may be self-limiting, are the most common adverse effects. Administering drug on an empty stomach or at bedtime may lessen these effects. Usual antiemetic medications effectively control nausea and vomiting linked to temozolomide administration.
• Women and elderly patients are at higher risk for developing myelosuppression.
ALERT Avoid skin contact with or inhalation of capsule contents if capsule is accidentally opened or damaged. Follow procedures for safe handling and disposal of antineoplastics.
• Store capsules at a controlled room temperature (59° to 86° F [15° to 30° C]).

Patient teaching

• Emphasize importance of taking dose exactly as prescribed, usually on an empty stomach or at bedtime.
• Stress importance of continuing medication despite nausea and vomiting.
• Tell patient to call immediately if vomiting occurs shortly after a dose is taken.
• Tell patient to promptly report sore throat, fever, unusual bruising or bleeding, rash, or seizures.
• Advise patient to avoid exposure to people with infections.
• Advise sexually active patient to use effective birth control measures during treatment because temozolomide may cause birth defects.
• Tell patient to swallow capsules whole and to not break open the capsules.

Evaluation

• Patient exhibits positive response to therapy, as noted on improvement of follow-up studies.
• Patient doesn't experience injury as a result of drug-induced adverse reactions.
• Patient and family state understanding of drug therapy.

teniposide (VM-26)

(teh-NIP-uh-sighd)
Vumon

Pharmacologic class: podophyllotoxin (specific to phase of cell cycle, G_2 and late S phase)
Therapeutic class: antineoplastic
Pregnancy risk category: D

Indications and dosages

▶ **Refractory childhood acute lymphoblastic leukemia.** *Children:* optimum dosage hasn't been established. One protocol reported by manufacturer is 165 mg/m^2 I.V. twice weekly for eight or nine doses. Usually used in combination with other agents.

How supplied

Injection: 50 mg/5 ml

Pharmacokinetics

Absorption: not applicable.
Distribution: distributed mainly in liver, kidneys, small intestine, and adrenals. Drug crosses blood-brain barrier to limited extent; highly bound to plasma proteins.
Metabolism: metabolized extensively in liver.
Excretion: about 40% eliminated through kidneys as unchanged drug or metabolites. *Half-life:* 5 hours.

Route	Onset	Peak	Duration
I.V.	Unknown	Unknown	Unknown

Pharmacodynamics

Chemical effect: acts in late S or early G_2 phase of cell cycle, thus preventing cells from entering mitosis.
Therapeutic effect: prevents reproduction of leukemic cells.

Adverse reactions

CV: hypotension from rapid infusion.
GI: *nausea, vomiting, mucositis, diarrhea.*
Hematologic: MYELOSUPPRESSION (dose-limiting), LEUKOPENIA, NEUTROPENIA, THROMBOCYTOPENIA, *anemia.*
Skin: alopecia.

Other: ***hypersensitivity reactions*** (chills, fever, urticaria, tachycardia, ***bronchospasm,*** dyspnea, hypotension, flushing), *phlebitis at injection site with extravasation.*

Interactions

Drug-drug. *Methotrexate:* may increase clearance and intracellular levels of methotrexate. Monitor patient closely.
Sodium salicylate, sulfamethizole, tolbutamide: may displace teniposide from protein-binding sites and increase toxicity. Monitor patient closely.

Contraindications and precautions

- Contraindicated in patients hypersensitive to drug or polyoxyethylated castor oil, an injection vehicle.
- Drug isn't recommended for use in pregnant or breast-feeding women.

NURSING CONSIDERATIONS

Assessment

- Assess patient's condition before therapy and regularly thereafter.
- Obtain baseline blood counts and kidney and liver function tests, as ordered, and then monitor periodically.
- Monitor blood pressure before therapy and at 30-minute intervals during infusion.
- Be alert for adverse reactions and drug interactions.
- Evaluate patient's and family's knowledge of drug therapy.

Nursing diagnoses

- Ineffective health maintenance related to presence of leukemia
- Ineffective protection related to drug-induced immunosuppression
- Deficient knowledge related to drug therapy

Planning and implementation

- Some prescribers may decide to use drug despite patient's history of hypersensitivity because therapeutic benefits may outweigh risks. Such patients should be treated with antihistamines and corticosteroids before infusion begins and be closely watched during drug administration.

ALERT Have diphenhydramine, hydrocortisone, epinephrine, and appropriate emergency equipment available to establish airway in case of anaphylaxis.

- Follow institutional policy to reduce risks. Preparation and administration of parenteral form are linked to carcinogenic, mutagenic, and teratogenic risks for personnel.
- Dilute drug in D_5W or normal saline solution injection to concentration of 0.1, 0.2, 0.4, or 1 mg/ml. Don't agitate vigorously; precipitation may occur. Discard cloudy solutions. Prepare and store in glass containers. Infuse over 45 to 90 minutes to prevent hypotension.
- Don't mix with other drugs or solutions.
- Heparin is physically incompatible with drug. Don't mix.
- Ensure careful placement of I.V. catheter. Extravasation can cause local tissue necrosis or sloughing.
- Don't administer drug through membrane-type in-line filter because diluent may dissolve filter.
- Solutions containing 0.5 to 1 mg/ml teniposide are stable for 4 hours; those containing 0.1 to 0.2 mg/ml are stable for 6 hours at room temperature.
- Report systolic blood pressure below 90 mm Hg and stop infusion.

Patient teaching

- Tell patient to report discomfort at I.V. site immediately.
- Encourage adequate fluid intake to increase urine output and facilitate excretion of uric acid.
- Review infection-control and bleeding precautions to take during therapy.
- Reassure patient that hair should grow back after treatment stops.
- Instruct patient and parents to notify prescriber if adverse reactions occur.

Evaluation

- Patient responds well to drug.
- Patient doesn't develop serious complications from immunosuppression.
- Patient and family state understanding of drug therapy.

terazosin hydrochloride
(ter-uh-ZOH-sin high-droh-KLOR-ighd)
Hytrin

Pharmacologic class: selective $alpha_1$-adrenergic blocker
Therapeutic class: antihypertensive
Pregnancy risk category: C

Indications and dosages

▶ **Hypertension.** *Adults:* initially, 1 mg P.O. h.s., increased gradually based on response. Usual dosage range is 1 to 5 mg daily. Maximum dosage is 20 mg/day.

▶ **Symptomatic BPH.** *Adults:* initially, 1 mg P.O. h.s. Dosage increased in stepwise manner to 2 mg, 5 mg, and 10 mg once daily to achieve optimal response. Most patients require 10 mg daily for optimal response.

How supplied

Capsules: 1 mg, 2 mg, 5 mg, 10 mg

Pharmacokinetics

Absorption: absorbed rapidly with about 90% of dose being bioavailable.
Distribution: about 90% to 94% plasma protein–bound.
Metabolism: metabolized in liver.
Excretion: about 40% excreted in urine, 60% in feces, mostly as metabolites. Up to 30% may be excreted unchanged. *Half-life:* about 12 hours.

Route	Onset	Peak	Duration
P.O.	≤ 15 min	2-3 hr	24 hr

Pharmacodynamics

Chemical effect: decreases blood pressure by vasodilation produced in response to blockade of $alpha_1$-adrenergic receptors. Improves urine flow in patients with BPH by blocking $alpha_1$-adrenergic receptors in smooth muscle of bladder neck and prostate, thus relieving urethral pressure and reestablishing urine flow.
Therapeutic effect: lowers blood pressure and relieves symptoms of BPH.

Adverse reactions

CNS: *asthenia, dizziness, headache,* nervousness, paresthesia, somnolence.
CV: palpitations, orthostatic hypotension, tachycardia, *peripheral edema.*
EENT: nasal congestion, sinusitis, blurred vision.
GI: nausea.
GU: impotence.
Musculoskeletal: back pain, muscle pain.
Respiratory: dyspnea.
Other: decreased libido.

Interactions

Drug-drug. *Antihypertensives:* excessive hypotension. Use together cautiously.
Clonidine: clonidine's antihypertensive effect may be decreased. Monitor patient.
Drug-herb. *Butcher's broom:* possible diminished effect. Advise against concomitant use.

Contraindications and precautions

- Contraindicated in patients hypersensitive to drug.
- Use cautiously in pregnant or breast-feeding women.
- Safety of drug hasn't been established in children.

NURSING CONSIDERATIONS

Assessment

- Assess patient's condition before therapy and regularly thereafter.
- Monitor blood pressure frequently.
- Be alert for adverse reactions and drug interactions.
- Evaluate patient's and family's knowledge of drug therapy.

Nursing diagnoses

- Risk for injury related to presence of hypertension
- Sexual dysfunction related to drug-induced impotence
- Deficient knowledge related to drug therapy

Planning and implementation

ALERT If drug is stopped for several days, dosage will need to be readjusted to initial dosing regimen.

Patient teaching

• Tell patient not to stop drug but to call prescriber if adverse reactions occur.
• Tell patient to take the first dose at bedtime. If he must get up, he should do so slowly to prevent syncope.
• Warn patient to avoid activities that require mental alertness for 12 hours after first dose.
• Teach patient other means to reduce blood pressure, such as diet control, exercise, smoking cessation, and stress reduction.

Evaluation

• Patient's blood pressure is normal.
• Patient develops and maintains positive attitude toward his sexuality despite impotence.
• Patient and family state understanding of drug therapy.

terbutaline sulfate

(ter-BYOO-tuh-leen SUL-fayt)

Brethaire, Brethine, Bricanyl

Pharmacologic class: beta$_2$-adrenergic agonist
Therapeutic class: bronchodilator
Pregnancy risk category: B

Indications and dosages

▶ **Bronchospasm in patients with reversible obstructive airway disease.** *Adults and children age 15 and older:* 5 mg P.O. t.i.d. at 6-hour intervals. Or, 0.25 mg S.C. may be repeated in 15 to 30 minutes; maximum 0.5 mg q 4 hours. Or, 2 inhalations q 4 to 6 hours, with 1 minute between inhalations.
Children ages 12 to 15: 2.5 mg P.O. t.i.d. Or, 2 inhalations q 4 to 6 hours with 1 minute between inhalations.

How supplied

Tablets: 2.5 mg, 5 mg
Aerosol inhaler: 200 mcg/metered spray
Injection: 1 mg/ml

Pharmacokinetics

Absorption: 33% to 50% of P.O. dose absorbed through GI tract; unknown after inhalation or S.C. administration.
Distribution: widely distributed throughout body.
Metabolism: partially metabolized in liver to inactive compounds.
Excretion: excreted primarily in urine.

Route	Onset	Peak	Duration
P.O.	30 min	2-3 hr	4-8 hr
S.C.	≤ 15 min	30-60 min	1.5-4 hr
Inhalation	5-30 min	1-2 hr	3-6 hr

Pharmacodynamics

Chemical effect: relaxes bronchial smooth muscle by acting on beta$_2$-adrenergic receptors.
Therapeutic effect: improves breathing ability.

Adverse reactions

CNS: *nervousness, tremors, headache, drowsiness, dizziness,* weakness.
CV: *palpitations,* tachycardia, ***arrhythmias,*** flushing.
EENT: dry and irritated nose and throat with inhaled form.
GI: *vomiting, nausea,* heartburn.
Metabolic: hypokalemia.
Respiratory: ***paradoxical bronchospasm,*** dyspnea.
Skin: diaphoresis.

Interactions

Drug-drug. *Cardiac glycosides, cyclopropane, halogenated inhaled anesthetics, levodopa:* increased risk of arrhythmias. Monitor patient closely.
CNS stimulants: increased CNS stimulation. Avoid concomitant use.
MAO inhibitors: when given with sympathomimetics, may cause severe hypertension (hypertensive crisis). Avoid concomitant use.
Propranolol, other beta blockers: blocked bronchodilating effects of terbutaline. Avoid concomitant use.

Contraindications and precautions

• Contraindicated in patients hypersensitive to drug or sympathomimetic amines.
• Use cautiously in patient with CV disorders, hyperthyroidism, diabetes, or seizure disorders and in pregnant or breast-feeding women.

• Safety of drug hasn't been established in children age 11 and younger.

NURSING CONSIDERATIONS

Assessment
• Assess patient's respiratory condition before therapy and regularly thereafter.
• Monitor patient closely for toxicity, especially if patient is using both tablets and aerosol.
• Evaluate patient's and family's knowledge of drug therapy.

Nursing diagnoses
• Ineffective breathing pattern related to underlying respiratory condition
• Pain related to drug-induced headache
• Deficient knowledge related to drug therapy

Planning and implementation
P.O. use: Follow normal protocol.
S.C. use: Inject in lateral deltoid area.
– Protect injection from light. Don't use if discolored.
Inhalation use: Follow normal protocol. If patient is also to receive corticosteroid by inhalation, administer terbutaline first, wait 5 minutes, and then administer corticosteroid inhaler. Encourage patient to use a spacer to assist with medication delivery.
• Patient may use tablets and aerosol concomitantly.
• Notify prescriber immediately if bronchospasms develop during therapy.
• Obtain order for mild analgesic to treat drug-induced headache.
ALERT Don't confuse terbutaline with tolbutamide or terbinafine.

Patient teaching
• Make sure patient and family understand why drug is needed.
• Teach patient to use metered-dose inhaler by giving these instructions: Clear nasal passages and throat. Breathe out, expelling as much air from lungs as possible. Place mouthpiece well into mouth and inhale deeply as you release a dose from inhaler. Hold breath for several seconds, remove mouthpiece, and exhale slowly.
• If more than one inhalation is ordered, tell patient to wait at least 2 minutes before repeating procedure.
• Tell patient also using corticosteroid inhaler to use bronchodilator first, and then wait about 5 minutes before using corticosteroid.
• Warn patient to report paradoxical bronchospasm and stop drug.
• Warn patient that tolerance may develop with prolonged use.

Evaluation
• Patient's breathing is improved.
• Patient's headache is relieved with mild analgesic.
• Patient and family state understanding of drug therapy.

terconazole
(ter-KON-uh-zohl)
Terazol 3, Terazol 7

Pharmacologic class: triazole derivative
Therapeutic class: antifungal
Pregnancy risk category: C

Indications and dosages
▶ **Vulvovaginal candidiasis.** *Women:* 1 applicatorful of cream or 1 suppository inserted into vagina h.s.; 0.4% cream used for 7 consecutive days; 0.8% cream or 80-mg suppository used for 3 consecutive days. Repeat course, if necessary, after reconfirmation by smear or culture.

How supplied
Vaginal cream: 0.4%, 0.8%
Vaginal suppositories: 80 mg

Pharmacokinetics
Absorption: minimal absorption may range from 5% to 16%.
Distribution: mainly local.
Metabolism: unknown.
Excretion: unknown.

Route	Onset	Peak	Duration
Intravaginal	Unknown	Unknown	Unknown

Pharmacodynamics

Chemical effect: unknown; may increase fungal cell membrane permeability (*Candida* species only).
Therapeutic effect: impairs fungus function. Spectrum of activity is *Candida* species only.

Adverse reactions

CNS: *headache.*
GI: abdominal pain.
GU: dysmenorrhea, vulvovaginal pain or burning.
Skin: irritation, photosensitivity, *pruritus.*
Other: fever, chills, body aches.

Interactions

None significant.

Contraindications and precautions

- Contraindicated in patients hypersensitive to drug or inactive ingredients in formulation.
- Drug isn't recommended for breast-feeding women.
- Use cautiously in pregnant women.

NURSING CONSIDERATIONS

Assessment

- Assess patient's infection before therapy and regularly thereafter.
- Be alert for adverse reactions.
- Evaluate patient's and family's knowledge of drug therapy.

Nursing diagnoses

- Risk for infection related to presence of susceptible fungi
- Acute pain related to drug-induced burning
- Deficient knowledge related to drug therapy

Planning and implementation

- Insert cream using applicator supplied.
- If vaginal suppository is used, have patient remain supine for about 30 minutes after insertion.
- Report fever, chills, other flulike symptoms, or sensitivity, and stop drug.

ALERT Don't confuse terconazole with tioconazole.

Patient teaching

- Instruct patient how to insert cream or suppository.
- Advise patient to continue treatment during menstrual period. Tell her not to use tampons.
- Tell patient to use for full treatment period prescribed. Explain how to prevent reinfection.

Evaluation

- Patient is free from infection.
- Patient states that drug-induced burning is tolerable.
- Patient and family state understanding of drug therapy.

testolactone

(tes-tuh-LAK-tohn)
Teslac

Pharmacologic class: androgen
Therapeutic class: antineoplastic
Controlled substance schedule: III
Pregnancy risk category: C

Indications and dosages

▶ **Advanced postmenopausal breast cancer.**
Women: 250 mg P.O. q.i.d.

How supplied

Tablets: 50 mg

Pharmacokinetics

Absorption: absorbed well across GI tract.
Distribution: widely distributed in total body water.
Metabolism: extensively metabolized in liver.
Excretion: testolactone and its metabolites excreted primarily in urine.

Route	Onset	Peak	Duration
P.O.	6-12 wk	Unknown	Unknown

Pharmacodynamics

Chemical effect: exact antineoplastic action unknown; probably changes tumor's hormonal environment and alters neoplastic process.
Therapeutic effect: hinders breast cancer cell activity.

Adverse reactions

CNS: paresthesia, peripheral neuropathy.
CV: increased blood pressure, edema.
GI: nausea, vomiting, diarrhea, anorexia, glossitis.
Skin: erythema, nail changes, alopecia.

Interactions

Drug-drug. *Oral anticoagulants:* increased pharmacologic effects. Monitor patient carefully.

Contraindications and precautions

- Contraindicated in patients hypersensitive to drug and in men with breast cancer.
- Drug isn't recommended for breast-feeding women.
- Use cautiously in pregnant women.
- Drug isn't indicated for children.

NURSING CONSIDERATIONS

Assessment

- Assess patient's breast cancer before therapy and regularly thereafter.
- Monitor fluid and electrolyte levels, especially calcium level.
- Be alert for adverse reactions and drug interactions.
- Evaluate patient's and family's knowledge of drug therapy.

Nursing diagnoses

- Ineffective health maintenance related to presence of breast cancer
- Disturbed sensory perception (tactile) related to drug-induced paresthesia and peripheral neuropathy
- Deficient knowledge related to drug therapy

Planning and implementation

- Force fluids to aid calcium excretion, and encourage exercise to prevent hypercalcemia. Immobilized patients are prone to hypercalcemia.
- Higher-than-recommended doses do not promote remission.

Patient teaching

- Inform patient that therapeutic response isn't immediate; it may take up to 3 months for benefit to be noted.
- Encourage patient to exercise and drink plenty of fluids to help prevent hypercalcemia.
- Tell patient to report adverse effects.

Evaluation

- Patient responds well to drug.
- Patient lists ways to protect against risk of injury caused by diminished tactile sensation.
- Patient and family state understanding of drug therapy.

testosterone

(tes-TOS-teh-rohn)

Andronaq-50, Histerone-50, Histerone 100, Testamone 100, Testaqua, Testoject-50

testosterone cypionate

Andronate 100, Andronate 200, depAndro 100, depAndro 200, Depotest, Depo-Testosterone, Duratest-100, Duratest-200, T-Cypionate, Testred Cypionate 200, Virilon IM

testosterone enanthate

Andro L.A. 200, Andropository 200, Andryl 200, Delatest, Delatestryl, Durathate-200, Everone 200, Testrin-P.A.

testosterone propionate

Malogen in Oil♦, Testex

Pharmacologic class: androgen
Therapeutic class: androgen replacement, antineoplastic
Controlled substance schedule: III
Pregnancy risk category: X

Indications and dosages

▶ **Male hypogonadism. Testosterone.** *Adults:* 10 to 25 mg I.M. two to three times weekly.
Testosterone cypionate, testosterone enanthate. *Adults:* 50 to 400 mg I.M. q 2 to 4 weeks.

Testosterone propionate. *Adults:* 10 to 25 mg I.M. two to three times weekly.

▶ **Delayed puberty in boys. Testosterone, testosterone propionate.** *Children:* 25 to 50 mg I.M. two or three times weekly for up to 6 months.

▶ **Metastatic breast cancer in women 1 to 5 years postmenopausal. Testosterone.** *Adults:* 100 mg I.M. three times weekly.

Testosterone propionate. *Adults:* 50 to 100 mg I.M. three times weekly.

Testosterone cypionate, testosterone enanthate. *Adults:* 200 to 400 mg I.M. q 2 to 4 weeks.

▶ **Postpartum breast pain and engorgement. Testosterone, testosterone propionate.** *Adults:* 25 to 50 mg I.M. daily for 3 to 4 days.

How supplied

testosterone

Injection (aqueous suspension): 25 mg/ml, 50 mg/ml, 100 mg/ml

testosterone cypionate

Injection (in oil): 100 mg/ml, 200 mg/ml

testosterone enanthate

Injection (in oil): 100 mg/ml, 200 mg/ml

testosterone propionate

Injection (in oil): 100 mg/ml

Pharmacokinetics

Absorption: unknown.

Distribution: 98% to 99% plasma protein–bound, primarily to testosterone-estradiol–binding globulin.

Metabolism: metabolized in liver.

Excretion: excreted in urine. *Half-life:* 10 to 100 minutes.

Route	Onset	Peak	Duration
I.M.	Unknown	Unknown	Unknown

Pharmacodynamics

Chemical effect: stimulates target tissues to develop normally in androgen-deficient men. Drug may have some antiestrogen properties, making it useful to treat certain estrogen-dependent breast cancers. Its action in postpartum breast engorgement isn't known because drug doesn't suppress lactation.

Therapeutic effect: increases testosterone levels, inhibits some estrogen activity, and relieves postpartum breast pain and engorgement.

Adverse reactions

CNS: headache, anxiety, depression, paresthesia, sleep apnea syndrome.

CV: edema.

GI: nausea.

GU: hypoestrogenic effects in women (*acne; edema; oily skin; hirsutism; hoarseness; weight gain;* clitoral enlargement; decreased or increased libido; flushing; diaphoresis; vaginitis, including itching, drying, and burning; vaginal bleeding; menstrual irregularities), excessive hormonal effects in men (prepubertal—premature epiphyseal closure, *acne,* priapism, *growth of body and facial hair,* phallic enlargement; postpubertal—testicular atrophy, oligospermia, decreased ejaculatory volume, impotence, gynecomastia, epididymitis), bladder irritability.

Hematologic: polycythemia, suppression of clotting factors.

Hepatic: reversible jaundice, cholestatic hepatitis, abnormal liver enzyme levels.

Metabolic: hypercalcemia.

Skin: pain and induration at injection site, local edema, hypersensitivity skin manifestations.

Other: androgenic effects in women.

Interactions

Drug-drug. *Hepatotoxic drugs:* increased risk of hepatotoxicity. Monitor patient closely.

Insulin, oral antidiabetics: altered dosage requirements. Monitor blood glucose level in diabetic patients.

Oral anticoagulants: altered dosage requirements. Monitor PT and INR.

Contraindications and precautions

- Contraindicated in men with breast or prostate cancer; patients with hypercalcemia; those with cardiac, hepatic, or renal decompensation; and pregnant or breast-feeding women.
- Use cautiously in elderly patients.

NURSING CONSIDERATIONS

Assessment
- Assess patient's condition before therapy and regularly thereafter.
- Periodically monitor calcium level and liver function test results.
- Monitor lab studies for polycythemia.
- Monitor prepubertal boys by X-ray for rate of bone maturation.
- Be alert for adverse reactions and drug interactions.
- Evaluate patient's and family's knowledge of drug therapy.

Nursing diagnoses
- Ineffective health maintenance related to underlying condition
- Disturbed body image related to drug-induced adverse androgenic reactions
- Deficient knowledge related to drug therapy

Planning and implementation
- Avoid use in women of childbearing age until pregnancy is ruled out.
- Administer daily dosage requirement in divided doses for best results.
- Store preparations at room temperature. If crystals appear, warm and shake bottle to disperse them.
- Inject deep into upper outer quadrant of gluteal muscle. Rotate sites to prevent muscle atrophy. Report soreness at site because of possibility of postinfection furunculosis.
- Unless contraindicated, use with diet high in calories and protein. Give small, frequent feedings.
- Report signs of virilization in woman.
- Edema generally can be controlled with sodium restriction or diuretics.

ALERT Therapeutic response in breast cancer usually appears within 3 months. Therapy should be stopped if signs of disease progression appear. In metastatic breast cancer, hypercalcemia usually signals progression of bone metastases. Report signs of hypercalcemia.
- Androgens may alter results of laboratory studies during therapy and for 2 to 3 weeks after therapy ends.

ALERT Testosterone and methyltestosterone aren't interchangeable. Don't confuse testosterone with testolactone.

Patient teaching
- Make sure patient understands importance of using effective nonhormonal contraceptive during therapy.
- Instruct man to report priapism, reduced ejaculatory volume, and gynecomastia. Drug may need to be discontinued.
- Inform woman that virilization may occur. Tell her to report androgenic effects immediately. Stopping drug will prevent further androgenic changes but probably won't reverse those already present.
- Teach patient to recognize and report signs of hypoglycemia.
- Instruct patient to follow dietary measures to combat drug-induced adverse reactions.

Evaluation
- Patient responds well to drug.
- Patient states acceptance of altered body image.
- Patient and family state understanding of drug therapy.

testosterone transdermal system
(tes-TOS-teh-rohn tranz-DER-mal SIHS-tum)
Androderm, Testoderm

Pharmacologic class: androgen
Therapeutic class: androgen replacement
Controlled substance schedule: III
Pregnancy risk category: X

Indications and dosages

▶ **Primary or hypogonadotropic hypogonadism in men age 18 and older. Testoderm.** *Adults:* one 6-mg/day patch applied to scrotal area daily. If scrotal area is too small for 6-mg/day patch, start with 4-mg/day patch. Patch worn for 22 to 24 hours daily.
Androderm. *Adults:* 5 mg/day either as two 2.5 mg/day systems or one 5 mg/day system applied h.s. to clean, dry skin on back, abdomen, upper arms, or thighs.

How supplied

Transdermal system: 2.5 mg/day, 4 mg/day, 5 mg/day, 6 mg/day

Pharmacokinetics

Absorption: absorbed from scrotal skin after application.
Distribution: chiefly bound in serum to sex hormone–binding globulin.
Metabolism: metabolized in liver.
Excretion: excreted in urine. *Half-life:* 10 to 100 minutes.

Route	Onset	Peak	Duration
Transdermal	Unknown	2-4 hr	2 hr after removal

Pharmacodynamics

Chemical effect: stimulates target tissues to develop normally in androgen-deficient men.
Therapeutic effect: increases testosterone in androgen-deficient men.

Adverse reactions

CV: ***CVA,*** headache, depression.
GI: ***GI bleeding.***
GU: prostatitis, prostate abnormalities, urinary tract infection.
Skin: acne, *pruritus,* irritation, *blister under system,* allergic contact dermatitis; burning, induration (at application site).
Other: gynecomastia, breast tenderness.

Interactions

Drug-drug. *Antidiabetics:* altered antidiabetic dosage requirements. Monitor blood glucose level.
Oral anticoagulants: altered anticoagulant dosage requirements. Monitor PT and INR.
Oxyphenbutazone: may elevate serum level of oxyphenbutazone. Monitor patient for adverse reactions.

Contraindications and precautions

- Contraindicated in patients hypersensitive to drug, women, and men with known or suspected breast or prostate cancer.
- Use cautiously in elderly men because they may be at greater risk for prostatic hyperplasia or prostate cancer and in patients with renal, hepatic, or cardiac disease.
- Drug isn't indicated for children.

NURSING CONSIDERATIONS

Assessment

- Assess patient's condition before therapy and regularly thereafter.
- Because long-term use of systemic androgens is linked to polycythemia, monitor hematocrit and hemoglobin values periodically in patient on long-term therapy, as ordered.
- Periodically assess liver function tests, serum lipid profiles, and prostatic acid phosphatase and prostate-specific antigen levels, as ordered.
- Be alert for adverse reactions and drug interactions.
- Evaluate patient's and family's knowledge of drug therapy.

Nursing diagnoses

- Sexual dysfunction related to androgen deficiency
- Risk for impaired skin integrity related to drug-induced irritation at application site
- Deficient knowledge related to drug therapy

Planning and implementation

- Apply Testoderm system on clean, dry scrotal skin. Dry shave scrotal hair (don't use chemical depilatories).
- Apply Androderm to clean, dry skin on back, abdomen, upper arms, or thighs.

ALERT Don't confuse Testoderm with Estraderm.

Patient teaching

- Teach patient how to apply transdermal system.
- Tell patient that topical testosterone preparations can cause virilization in female partners. These women should report acne or changes in body hair.
- Advise patient to report to prescriber persistent erections, nausea, vomiting, changes in skin color, or ankle edema.

Evaluation

- Patient states that he can resume normal sexual activity.
- Patient maintains normal skin integrity.

• Patient and family state understanding of drug therapy.

tetanus immune globulin, human
(TET-uh-nus ih-MYOON GLOH-byoo-lin, HYOO-mun)
Hyper-Tet

Pharmacologic class: immune serum
Therapeutic class: tetanus prophylaxis
Pregnancy risk category: C

Indications and dosages

▶ **Tetanus exposure.** *Adults and children over age 7:* 250 units I.M.
Children age 7 and under: 4 units/kg I.M.
▶ **Tetanus treatment.** *Adults and children:* single doses of 3,000 to 6,000 units I.M. Optimal dosage hasn't been established.

How supplied

Injection: 250 units per vial or syringe

Pharmacokinetics

Absorption: absorbed slowly.
Distribution: unknown.
Metabolism: unknown.
Excretion: unknown. *Half-life:* about 28 days.

Route	Onset	Peak	Duration
I.M.	Unknown	2-3 days	4 wk

Pharmacodynamics

Chemical effect: provides passive immunity to tetanus.
Therapeutic effect: prevents tetanus.

Adverse reactions

GU: nephrotic syndrome.
Skin: pain, stiffness, erythema at injection site.
Other: slight fever, ***hypersensitivity reactions, anaphylaxis, angioedema.***

Interactions

Drug-drug. *Live-virus vaccines:* may interfere with response. Defer administration of live-virus vaccines for 3 months after administration of tetanus immune globulin.

Contraindications and precautions

• Contraindicated in patients with thrombocytopenia or coagulation disorders that would contraindicate I.M. injection unless potential benefits outweigh risks.
• Use cautiously in pregnant or breast-feeding women.

NURSING CONSIDERATIONS

Assessment

• Obtain history of injury, tetanus immunizations, last tetanus toxoid injection, allergies, and reaction to immunizations.
• Antibodies remain at effective level for about 4 weeks (several times the duration of antitoxin-induced antibodies), which protects patient for incubation period of most tetanus cases.
• Be alert for adverse reactions and drug interactions.
• Evaluate patient's and family's knowledge of drug therapy.

Nursing diagnoses

• Risk for injury related to potential for tetanus to occur
• Deficient knowledge related to drug therapy

Planning and implementation

ALERT Have epinephrine 1:1,000 available to treat hypersensitivity reactions.
• Drug is used only if wound is more than 24 hours old or if patient has had fewer than two tetanus toxoid injections.
• Thoroughly clean wound and remove all foreign matter.
• Inject drug into deltoid muscle for adult and child age 3 and older and into anterolateral aspect of thigh in neonate and child under age 3.
ALERT Don't confuse drug with tetanus toxoid. Tetanus immune globulin isn't a substitute for tetanus toxoid, which should be given at same time to produce active immunization. Don't give at same site as toxoid.

Patient teaching

• Warn patient that pain and tenderness at injection site may occur. Suggest use of mild analgesic for pain relief.

• Tell patient to document date of tetanus immunization and encourage him to keep immunization current.

☑ Evaluation

• Patient doesn't develop tetanus.
• Patient and family state understanding of drug therapy.

tetracycline hydrochloride

(tet-ruh-SIGH-kleen high-droh-KLOR-ighd)
Achromycin V, Apo-Tetra♦, Mysteclin 250◇, Nor-Tet, Novo-Tetra♦, Panmycin**, Panmycin P◇, Robitet, Sumycin, Tetracap, Tetralan, Tetrex◇

Pharmacologic class: tetracycline
Therapeutic class: antibiotic
Pregnancy risk category: NR

Indications and dosages

▶ **Infections caused by sensitive gram-negative and gram-positive organisms, including *Chlamydia, Mycoplasma, Rickettsia,* and organisms that cause trachoma.** *Adults:* 1 to 2 g P.O. divided into two to four doses. *Children over age 8:* 25 to 50 mg/kg P.O. daily divided into four doses.

▶ **Uncomplicated urethral, endocervical, or rectal infection caused by *Chlamydia trachomatis.*** *Adults:* 500 mg P.O. q.i.d. for at least 7 days.

▶ **Brucellosis.** *Adults:* 500 mg P.O. q 6 hours for 3 weeks combined with 1 g of streptomycin I.M. q 12 hours first week and daily the second week.

▶ **Gonorrhea in patients sensitive to penicillin.** *Adults:* initially, 1.5 g P.O.; then 500 mg q 6 hours for 4 days.

▶ **Syphilis in nonpregnant patients sensitive to penicillin.** *Adults:* 500 mg P.O. q.i.d. for 15 days.

▶ **Acne.** *Adults and adolescents:* initially, 125 to 250 mg P.O. q 6 hours; then 125 to 500 mg daily or every other day.

How supplied

Tablets: 250 mg, 500 mg
Capsules: 100 mg, 250 mg, 500 mg
Oral suspension: 125 mg/5 ml

Pharmacokinetics

Absorption: 75% to 80% absorbed. Food or milk products significantly reduce P.O. absorption.
Distribution: distributed widely in body tissues and fluids. CSF penetration is poor. Drug is 20% to 67% protein-bound.
Metabolism: not metabolized.
Excretion: excreted primarily unchanged in urine. *Half-life:* 6 to 11 hours.

Route	Onset	Peak	Duration
P.O.	Unknown	2-4 hr	Unknown

Pharmacodynamics

Chemical effect: unknown; thought to exert bacteriostatic effect by binding to 30S ribosomal subunit of microorganisms, thus inhibiting protein synthesis.
Therapeutic effect: hinders bacterial activity. Spectrum of activity includes such gram-negative and gram-positive organisms as *Chlamydia, Mycoplasma, Rickettsia,* and spirochetes.

Adverse reactions

CNS: dizziness, headache, ***intracranial hypertension (pseudotumor cerebri).***
CV: pericarditis.
EENT: sore throat, glossitis, dysphagia.
GI: anorexia, *epigastric distress, nausea,* vomiting, *diarrhea,* esophagitis, oral candidiasis, stomatitis, enterocolitis, inflammatory lesions in anogenital region.
GU: *increased BUN level.*
Hematologic: ***neutropenia, thrombocytopenia,*** eosinophilia.
Hepatic: elevated liver enzyme levels.
Musculoskeletal: *retardation of bone growth if used in children under age 9.*
Skin: candidal superinfection, maculopapular and erythematous rashes, urticaria, photosensitivity, increased pigmentation.
Other: *permanent discoloration of teeth, enamel defects,* ***hypersensitivity reactions.***

Interactions

Drug-drug. *Antacids (including sodium bicarbonate); antidiarrheals containing bismuth*

subsalicylate, kaolin, or pectin; laxatives containing aluminum, calcium, or magnesium: decreased antibiotic absorption. Give tetracyclines 1 hour before or 2 hours after these drugs.
Ferrous sulfate, other iron products, zinc: decreased antibiotic absorption. Give tetracyclines 3 hours after or 2 hours before iron.
Lithium carbonate: may alter serum lithium level. Monitor patient.
Methoxyflurane: may cause severe nephrotoxicity with tetracyclines. Monitor patient carefully.
Oral anticoagulants: potentiated anticoagulant effects. Monitor PT and adjust anticoagulant dosage.
Oral contraceptives: decreased contraceptive effectiveness and increased risk of breakthrough bleeding. Recommend use of nonhormonal form of birth control.
Penicillins: may interfere with bactericidal action of penicillins. Avoid using together.
Drug-food. *Milk, dairy products, other foods:* decreased antibiotic absorption. Give tetracycline 1 hour before or 2 hours after these products.
Drug-lifestyle. *Sun exposure:* photosensitivity reactions may occur. Urge patient to take precautions.

Contraindications and precautions

- Contraindicated in patients hypersensitive to tetracyclines.
- Drug isn't recommended for breast-feeding women.
- Use with extreme caution in patients with impaired kidney or liver function. Also use with extreme caution (if at all) during last half of pregnancy and in children under age 8 because drug may cause permanent discoloration of teeth, enamel defects, and bone growth retardation.

NURSING CONSIDERATIONS

Assessment

- Assess patient's infection before therapy and regularly thereafter.
- Obtain specimen for culture and sensitivity tests before first dose. Therapy may begin pending results.
- Monitor patient's hydration status if adverse GI reactions occur.
- Be alert for adverse reactions and drug interactions.
- Evaluate patient's and family's knowledge of drug therapy.

Nursing diagnoses

- Risk for infection related to presence of susceptible bacteria
- Risk for deficient fluid volume related to drug-induced adverse GI reactions
- Deficient knowledge related to drug therapy

Planning and implementation

ALERT Check expiration date. Outdated or deteriorated tetracyclines have been linked to reversible nephrotoxicity (Fanconi's syndrome).
- Administer drug on empty stomach.
- Don't expose drug to light or heat.
- Drug may cause false-negative reading with glucose enzymatic tests (Diastix).

Patient teaching

- Explain that effectiveness of drug is reduced when taken with milk or other dairy products, food, antacids, or iron products. Tell patient to take drug with full glass of water on empty stomach, at least 1 hour before or 2 hours after meals. Also, tell him to take drug at least 1 hour before bedtime to prevent esophagitis.
- Tell patient to take drug exactly as prescribed, even after he feels better, and to take entire amount prescribed.
- Warn patient to avoid direct sunlight and ultraviolet light. Recommend use of sunscreen to help prevent photosensitivity reactions. Tell him that photosensitivity persists after drug is stopped.

Evaluation

- Patient is free from infection.
- Patient maintains adequate hydration.
- Patient and family state understanding of drug therapy.

theophylline

(thee-OF-ih-lin)

Immediate-release liquids
Accurbron*, Aquaphyllin, Asmalix*, Bronkodyl*, Elixomin*, Elixophyllin*, Lanophyllin*, Slo-Phyllin, Theolair

Immediate-release tablets and capsules
Bronkodyl, Elixophyllin, Nuelin ◇, Slo-Phyllin

Timed-release tablets
Quibron-T/SR Dividose, Respbid, Sustaire, Theo-Dur, Theolair-SR, Theo-Time, Theo-X, Uniphyl

Timed-release capsules
Elixophyllin SR, Nuelin-SR ◇, Slo-bid Gyrocaps, Slo-Phyllin, Theo-24, Theobid Duracaps, Theochron, Theospan-SR, Theovent Long-Acting

theophylline sodium glycinate

Pharmacologic class: xanthine derivative
Therapeutic class: bronchodilator
Pregnancy risk category: C

Indications and dosages

▶ **Oral theophylline for acute bronchospasm in patients not receiving theophylline.** *Adults (nonsmokers):* loading dose of 6 mg/kg P.O.; then 3 mg/kg q 6 hours for two doses. Maintenance dosage is 3 mg/kg q 8 hours.
Children ages 9 to 16 and young adult smokers: loading dose of 6 mg/kg P.O.; then 3 mg/kg q 4 hours for three doses; then 3 mg/kg q 6 hours.
Children ages 6 months to 9 years: loading dose of 6 mg/kg P.O.; then 4 mg/kg q 4 hours for three doses; then 4 mg/kg q 6 hours.
Older adults or those with cor pulmonale: loading dose of 6 mg/kg P.O.; then 2 mg/kg q 6 hours for two doses; then 2 mg/kg q 8 hours.
Adults with heart failure or liver disease: loading dose of 6 mg/kg P.O.; then 2 mg/kg q 8 hours for two doses; then 1 to 2 mg/kg q 12 hours.
Note: Extended-release preparations shouldn't be used for treatment of acute bronchospasm.

▶ **Parenteral theophylline for patients not receiving theophylline.** *Adults (nonsmokers):* loading dose of 4.7 mg/kg given slow I.V.; then maintenance infusion of 0.55 mg/kg/hour I.V. for 12 hours; then 0.39 mg/kg/hour.
Adults (otherwise healthy smokers): loading dose of 4.7 mg/kg given slow I.V.; then maintenance infusion of 0.79 mg/kg/hr I.V. for 12 hrs; then 0.63 mg/kg/hr.
Older adults or those with cor pulmonale: loading dose of 4.7 mg/kg given slow I.V.; then maintenance infusion of 0.47 mg/kg/hour I.V. for 12 hours; then 0.24 mg/kg/hour.
Adults with heart failure or liver disease: loading dose of 4.7 mg/kg given slow I.V.; then maintenance infusion of 0.39 mg/kg/hour I.V. for 12 hours; then 0.08 to 0.16 mg/kg/hour.
Children ages 9 to 16: loading dose of 4.7 mg/kg given slow I.V.; then maintenance infusion of 0.79 mg/kg/hour I.V. for 12 hours; then 0.63 mg/kg/hour.
Children ages 6 months to 9 years: loading dose of 4.7 mg/kg given slow I.V.; then maintenance infusion of 0.95 mg/kg/hour I.V. for 12 hours; then 0.79 mg/kg/hour.

▶ **Oral and parenteral theophylline for acute bronchospasm in patients receiving theophylline.** *Adults and children:* each 0.5 mg/kg I.V. or P.O. (loading dose) increases plasma level by 1 mcg/ml. Ideally, dose is based on current theophylline level. In emergencies, some clinicians recommend 2.5 mg/kg P.O. dose of rapidly absorbed form if no obvious signs of theophylline toxicity are present.

▶ **Chronic bronchospasm.** *Adults and children:* 16 mg/kg or 400 mg P.O. daily (whichever is less) given in three or four divided doses at 6- to 8-hour intervals. Or, 12 mg/kg or 400 mg P.O. daily (whichever is less) using extended-release preparation given in two or three divided doses at 8- or 12-hour intervals. Dosage increased as tolerated at 2- to 3-day intervals to maximum dosage as follows—
Adults and children age 16 and over: 13 mg/kg or 900 mg P.O. daily (whichever is less) in divided doses.
Children ages 12 to 16: 18 mg/kg P.O. daily in divided doses.

Children ages 9 to 12: 20 mg/kg P.O. daily in divided doses.
Children under age 9: 24 mg/kg P.O. daily in divided doses.

How supplied

theophylline
Tablets: 100 mg, 125 mg, 200 mg, 250 mg, 300 mg
Tablets (chewable): 100 mg
Tablets (extended-release): 100 mg, 200 mg, 250 mg, 300 mg, 400 mg, 450 mg, 500 mg
Capsules: 100 mg, 200 mg
Capsules (extended-release): 50 mg, 60 mg, 65 mg, 75 mg, 100 mg, 125 mg, 130 mg, 200 mg, 250 mg, 260 mg, 300 mg
Elixir: 27 mg/5 ml, 50 mg/5 ml*
Oral solution: 27 mg/5 ml, 50 mg/5 ml
Syrup: 27 mg/5 ml, 50 mg/5 ml
D_5W injection: 200 mg in 50 ml or 100 ml; 400 mg in 100 ml, 250 ml, 500 ml, or 1,000 ml; 800 mg in 500 ml or 1,000 ml
theophylline sodium glycinate
Elixir: 110 mg/5 ml (equivalent to 55 mg of anhydrous theophylline/5 ml)

Pharmacokinetics

Absorption: well absorbed after P.O.administration. Food may further alter rate of absorption, especially of some extended-release preparations.
Distribution: distributed throughout extracellular fluids; equilibrium between fluid and tissues occurs within 1 hour of I.V. loading dose.
Metabolism: metabolized in liver to inactive compounds.
Excretion: about 10% excreted unchanged in urine. *Half-life:* adults, 7 to 9 hours; smokers, 4 to 5 hours; children, 3 to 5 hours; premature infants, 20 to 30 hours.

Route	Onset	Peak	Duration
P.O.			
regular	15-60 min	1-2 hr	Unknown
enteric-coated	15-60 min	1-2 hr	5 hr
extended-release	15-60 min	1-2 hr	4-7 hr
I.V.	15 min	15-30 min	Unknown

Pharmacodynamics

Chemical effect: inhibits phosphodiesterase, the enzyme that degrades cAMP, and relaxes smooth muscle of bronchial airways and pulmonary blood vessels.
Therapeutic effect: improves breathing ability.

Adverse reactions

CNS: *restlessness, dizziness,* headache, *insomnia,* irritability, ***seizures,*** muscle twitching.
CV: *palpitations, sinus tachycardia,* extrasystoles, flushing, marked hypotension, ***arrhythmias.***
GI: *nausea, vomiting,* diarrhea, epigastric pain.
Respiratory: increased respiratory rate, ***respiratory arrest.***

Interactions

Drug-drug. *Adenosine:* decreased antiarrhythmic effectiveness. Higher doses of adenosine may be necessary.
Barbiturates, carbamazepine, phenytoin, rifampin: enhanced metabolism and decreased theophylline blood level. Monitor patient for decreased effect.
Beta blockers: antagonism. Propranolol and nadolol, especially, may cause bronchospasm in sensitive patients. Use together cautiously.
Cimetidine, fluoroquinolone (such as ciprofloxacin), influenza virus vaccine, macrolide antibiotics (such as erythromycin), oral contraceptives: decreased hepatic clearance of theophylline; elevated theophylline level. Monitor patient for toxicity.
Drug-herb. *Cacao tree:* possible inhibition of theophylline metabolism. Advise against ingesting large amounts of cocoa concomitantly with theophylline.
Cayenne: oral cayenne may increase the absorption of theophylline. Monitor patient for toxicity.
St. John's wort: potential for decreased effectiveness of theophylline. Advise against concomitant use.
Drug-food. *Any food:* accelerated absorption. Give drug on an empty stomach.
Caffeine: decreased hepatic clearance of theophylline; elevated theophylline level. Monitor patient for toxicity.

Drug-lifestyle. *Smoking:* increased elimination of theophylline, increasing dosage requirements. Monitor theophylline response and serum levels.

Contraindications and precautions

- Contraindicated in patients with active peptic ulcer, seizure disorders, or hypersensitivity to xanthine compounds (caffeine, theobromine).
- Use cautiously in young children, infants, and neonates; elderly patients; pregnant women; and those with COPD, cardiac failure, cor pulmonale, renal or hepatic disease, peptic ulceration, hyperthyroidism, diabetes mellitus, glaucoma, severe hypoxemia, hypertension, compromised cardiac or circulatory function, angina, acute MI, or sulfite sensitivity.
- Drug appears in breast milk and may cause irritability, insomnia, or fretting in breast-fed infant.

NURSING CONSIDERATIONS

Assessment

- Assess patient's condition before therapy and regularly thereafter.
- Monitor vital signs; measure fluid intake and output. Expected clinical effects include improvement in quality of pulse and respirations.
- Xanthine metabolism rate varies among individuals; dosage is determined by monitoring response, tolerance, pulmonary function, and serum theophylline level. Serum theophylline level should range from 10 to 20 mcg/ml in adults and 5 to 15 mcg/ml in children.
- Be alert for adverse reactions and drug interactions.

ALERT Monitor patient for signs and symptoms of toxicity including tachycardia, anorexia, nausea, vomiting, diarrhea, restlessness, irritability, and headache. The presence of any of these signs in patients taking theophylline warrants checking theophylline levels and adjusting dose as indicated and ordered.

- Monitor patient's hydration status if adverse GI reactions occur.
- Evaluate patient's and family's knowledge of drug therapy.

Nursing diagnoses

- Impaired gas exchange related to presence of bronchospasms
- Risk for deficient fluid volume related to drug-induced adverse GI reactions
- Deficient knowledge related to drug therapy

Planning and implementation

P.O. use: Give drug around-the-clock, using sustained-release product at bedtime.

ALERT Don't confuse sustained-release forms with standard-release forms.

I.V. use: Use commercially available infusion solution, or mix drug in D_5W. Use infusion pump for continuous infusion.

- Dosage may need to be increased in cigarette smokers and in habitual marijuana smokers; smoking causes drug to be metabolized faster.
- Daily dosage may need to be decreased in patients with heart failure or hepatic disease and in elderly patients because metabolism and excretion may be decreased.

ALERT Don't confuse Theolair with Thyrolar.

Patient teaching

- Warn patient not to dissolve, crush, or chew slow-release products. For child unable to swallow capsules, sprinkle contents of capsules over soft food and tell patient to swallow without chewing.
- Supply instructions for home care and dosage schedule.
- Tell patient to relieve GI symptoms by taking oral drug with full glass of water after meals, although food in stomach delays absorption.
- Warn patient to take drug regularly, as directed. Patients tend to want to take extra "breathing pills."
- Warn elderly patient that dizziness may occur start of therapy.
- Have patient change position slowly and avoid hazardous activities.
- Caution patient to check with prescriber about other drugs used. OTC drugs may contain ephedrine in combination with theophylline salts; excessive CNS stimulation may result.
- If patient's dosage is stabilized while he is smoking and then he quits smoking, tell him to

notify his prescriber; the dosage may need to be reduced.

Evaluation
- Patient demonstrates improved gas exchange, exhibited in arterial blood gas values and respiratory status.
- Patient maintains adequate hydration.
- Patient and family state understanding of drug therapy.

thiamine hydrochloride (vitamin B_1)

(THIGH-eh-min high-droh-KLOR-ighd)

Betamin ◇, Beta-Sol ◇, Biamine, Thiamilate†

Pharmacologic class: water-soluble vitamin
Therapeutic class: nutritional supplement
Pregnancy risk category: A

Indications and dosages

▶ **RDA.** *Men age 51 and over:* 1.2 mg.
Men ages 15 to 50: 1.5 mg.
Boys ages 11 to 14: 1.3 mg.
Women age 51 and over: 1 mg.
Women ages 11 to 50: 1.1 mg.
Pregnant women: 1.5 mg.
Breast-feeding women: 1.6 mg.
Children ages 7 to 10: 1 mg.
Children ages 4 to 6: 0.9 mg.
Children ages 1 to 3: 0.7 mg.
Infants age 6 months to 1 year: 0.4 mg.
Neonates and infants under age 6 months: 0.3 mg.

▶ **Beriberi.** *Adults:* depending on severity, 10 to 20 mg I.M. t.i.d. for 2 weeks, followed by dietary correction and multivitamin supplement containing 5 to 10 mg of thiamine daily for 1 month.
Children: depending on severity, 10 to 50 mg I.M. daily for several weeks with adequate diet.

▶ **Wet beriberi with myocardial failure.** *Adults and children:* 10 to 30 mg I.V. for emergency treatment.

▶ **Wernicke's encephalopathy.** *Adults:* initially, 100 mg I.V.; then 50 to 100 mg I.V. or I.M. daily until patient is consuming regular balanced diet.

How supplied

Tablets: 5 mg†, 10 mg†, 25 mg†, 50 mg†, 100 mg†, 250 mg†, 500 mg†
Tablets (enteric-coated): 20 mg
Elixir: 250 mcg/5 ml
Injection: 100 mg/ml, 200 mg/ml

Pharmacokinetics

Absorption: absorbed readily after small P.O. doses; after large P.O. dose, total amount absorbed is limited. In alcoholics and in patients with cirrhosis or malabsorption, GI absorption of thiamine is decreased. When given with meals, drug's GI rate of absorption decreases, but total absorption remains same. After I.M. dose, drug is absorbed rapidly and completely.
Distribution: distributed widely in body tissues. When intake exceeds minimal requirements, tissue stores become saturated.
Metabolism: metabolized in liver.
Excretion: excess thiamine excreted in urine.

Route	Onset	Peak	Duration
P.O., I.V., I.M.	Unknown	Unknown	Unknown

Pharmacodynamics

Chemical effect: combines with adenosine triphosphate to form coenzyme necessary for carbohydrate metabolism.
Therapeutic effect: restores normal thiamine level.

Adverse reactions

CNS: restlessness, weakness.
CV: ***CV collapse,*** cyanosis.
EENT: tightness of throat.
GI: nausea, ***hemorrhage.***
Respiratory: ***pulmonary edema.***
Skin: feeling of warmth, pruritus, urticaria, diaphoresis.
Other: tenderness and induration after I.M. administration, ***angioedema.***

Interactions

None significant.

Contraindications and precautions

- Contraindicated in patients hypersensitive to thiamine products.
- Use cautiously in pregnant women if dose exceeds RDA.

NURSING CONSIDERATIONS

Assessment

- Assess patient's condition before therapy and regularly thereafter.
- Be alert for adverse reactions.
- Evaluate patient's and family's knowledge of drug therapy.

Nursing diagnoses

- Imbalanced nutrition: less than body requirements related to presence of thiamine deficiency
- Diarrhea related to drug-induced adverse GI reactions
- Deficient knowledge related to drug therapy

Planning and implementation

- Use parenteral route only when P.O. route isn't feasible.

P.O. and I.M. use: Follow normal protocol.
I.V. use: Dilute drug before administration.
ALERT Give large I.V. doses cautiously; administer skin test before starting therapy if patient has history of hypersensitivity reactions. Have epinephrine on hand to treat anaphylaxis if it occurs.

- For treating alcoholic patient, give thiamine before dextrose infusions to prevent encephalopathy.
- Don't use with materials that yield alkaline solutions. Unstable in alkaline solutions.
- Drug malabsorption is most likely in patients with alcoholism, cirrhosis, and GI disease.
- Clinically significant deficiency can occur in about 3 weeks of thiamine-free diet. Thiamine deficiency usually requires concurrent treatment for multiple deficiencies.
- Doses larger than 30 mg t.i.d. may not be fully utilized. Tissues may become saturated with thiamine and drug is excreted in urine as pyrimidine.
- If breast-fed infant develops beriberi, both mother and child should be treated with thiamine.

ALERT Don't confuse thiamine with Thorazine.

Patient teaching

- Stress proper nutritional habits to prevent recurrence of deficiency.

Evaluation

- Patient regains normal thiamine level.
- Patient maintains normal bowel pattern.
- Patient and family state understanding of drug therapy.

thioguanine (6-thioguanine, 6-TG)

(thigh-oh-GWAH-neen)
Lanvis ♦

Pharmacologic class: antimetabolite (specific to S phase of cell cycle)
Therapeutic class: antineoplastic
Pregnancy risk category: D

Indications and dosages

▶ **Acute nonlymphocytic leukemia, chronic myelogenous leukemia.** *Adults and children:* initially, 2 mg/kg P.O. daily (usually calculated to nearest 20 mg). If necessary, dose is then increased gradually to 3 mg/kg/day, as tolerated.

How supplied

Tablets (scored): 40 mg

Pharmacokinetics

Absorption: incomplete and variable; average bioavailability is 30%.
Distribution: distributed well in bone marrow cells.
Metabolism: extensively metabolized to less active form in liver and other tissues.
Excretion: excreted in urine, mainly as metabolites. *Half-life:* initial phase, 15 minutes; terminal phase, 11 hours.

Route	Onset	Peak	Duration
P.O.	Unknown	Unknown	Unknown

Pharmacodynamics

Chemical effect: inhibits purine synthesis.
Therapeutic effect: inhibits selected leukemic cell reproduction.

Adverse reactions

GI: nausea, vomiting, stomatitis, diarrhea, anorexia.
Hematologic: ***leukopenia, anemia, thrombocytopenia*** (occurs slowly over 2 to 4 weeks).
Hepatic: ***hepatotoxicity,*** jaundice, hepatic fibrosis, toxic hepatitis.
Metabolic: hyperuricemia.

Interactions

Drug-drug. *Myelosuppressant drugs:* increased risk of toxicity, especially myelosuppression, hepatotoxicity, and bleeding. Use together cautiously.

Contraindications and precautions

- Contraindicated in patients whose disease has shown resistance to drug.
- Drug isn't recommended for pregnant or breast-feeding women.
- Use cautiously in patients with renal or hepatic dysfunction.

NURSING CONSIDERATIONS

Assessment

- Assess patient's condition before therapy and regularly thereafter.
- Monitor CBC daily during induction and then weekly during maintenance therapy, as ordered.
- Monitor serum uric acid level.
- Watch for jaundice.
- Be alert for adverse reactions and drug interactions.
- Evaluate patient's and family's knowledge of drug therapy.

Nursing diagnoses

- Ineffective health maintenance related to presence of leukemia
- Ineffective protection related to drug-induced immunosuppression
- Deficient knowledge related to drug therapy

Planning and implementation

- Dosage modification may be required in renal or hepatic dysfunction.
- Drug may be ordered as 6-thioguanine. The numeral 6 is part of drug name and doesn't signify dosage units.
- Report jaundice; it may be reversible if drug is stopped promptly. Also, drug must be stopped if hepatotoxicity or hepatic tenderness occurs.
- Force fluids to prevent hyperuricemia.

Patient teaching

- Warn patient to watch for signs of infection and bleeding, and teach him infection-control and bleeding precautions to use in daily living.
- Tell patient to increase fluid intake.
- Advise woman of childbearing age to avoid becoming pregnant during therapy. Also recommend that she consult with prescriber before becoming pregnant.

Evaluation

- Patient responds well to drug.
- Patient doesn't develop serious complications from drug-induced immunosuppression.
- Patient and family state understanding of drug therapy.

thioridazine hydrochloride

(thigh-oh-RIGH-duh-zeen high-droh-KLOR-ighd)
Aldazine ◇, Apo-Thioridazine ♦, Mellaril*, Mellaril Concentrate, Novo-Ridazine ♦, PMS Thioridazine ♦

Pharmacologic class: phenothiazine (piperidine derivative)
Therapeutic class: antipsychotic
Pregnancy risk category: NR

Indications and dosages

▶ **Psychosis.** *Adults:* initially, 50 to 100 mg P.O. t.i.d., with gradual, incremental increases up to 800 mg daily in divided doses, if needed. Dosage varies.

▶ **Short-term treatment of moderate to marked depression with variable degrees of anxiety; dementia in elderly patients; be-**

havioral problems in children. *Adults:* initially, 25 mg P.O. t.i.d. Maximum daily dosage is 200 mg.
Children ages 2 to 12: 0.5 to 3 mg/kg P.O. daily in divided doses. Give 10 mg b.i.d. to t.i.d. to children with moderate disorders and 25 mg b.i.d. to t.i.d. to hospitalized, severely disturbed, or psychotic children.

How supplied

Tablets: 10 mg, 15 mg, 25 mg, 50 mg, 100 mg, 150 mg, 200 mg
Oral suspension: 25 mg/5 ml, 100 mg/5 ml
Oral concentrate: 30 mg/ml, 100 mg/ml* (3% to 4.2% alcohol)

Pharmacokinetics

Absorption: erratic and variable, although P.O. concentrates and syrups are more predictable than tablets.
Distribution: distributed widely in body; 91% to 99% protein-bound.
Metabolism: metabolized extensively by liver.
Excretion: excreted mostly as metabolites in urine, some in feces.

Route	Onset	Peak	Duration
P.O.	Varies	Unknown	Unknown

Pharmacodynamics

Chemical effect: unknown; probably blocks postsynaptic dopamine receptors in brain.
Therapeutic effect: relieves signs of psychosis, depression, anxiety, stress, fears, and sleep disturbances.

Adverse reactions

CNS: extrapyramidal reactions, *tardive dyskinesia, sedation,* EEG changes, dizziness, ***neuroleptic malignant syndrome.***
CV: *orthostatic hypotension,* tachycardia, ECG changes.
EENT: *ocular changes, blurred vision,* retinitis pigmentosa.
GI: *dry mouth, constipation.*
GU: *urine retention,* dark urine, menstrual irregularities, inhibited ejaculation.
Hematologic: ***transient leukopenia, agranulocytosis,*** hyperprolactinemia.
Hepatic: cholestatic jaundice.
Metabolic: weight gain, increased appetite.
Skin: *mild photosensitivity,* ***allergic reactions.***
Other: gynecomastia.

Interactions

Drug-drug. *Antacids:* inhibited absorption of oral phenothiazines. Separate doses by at least 2 hours.
Barbiturates, lithium: may decrease phenothiazine effect. Monitor patient.
Centrally acting antihypertensives: decreased antihypertensive effect. Monitor blood pressure.
Other CNS depressants: increased CNS depression. Use together cautiously.
Drug-herb. *Dong quai, St. John's wort:* increased photosensitivity reactions. Discourage concomitant use.
Ginkgo: potential decreased adverse effects of thioridazine. Monitor patient.
Kava: increased risk of dystonic reactions. Discourage concomitant use.
Milk thistle: decreased liver toxicity caused by phenothiazines. Monitor liver enzymes if used together.
Yohimbe: increased risk for yohimbe toxicity when used together. Discourage concomitant use.
Drug-lifestyle. *Alcohol use:* increased CNS depression. Discourage concomitant use.
Sun exposure: increased photosensitivity reactions. Advise patient to avoid prolonged or unprotected sun exposure.

Contraindications and precautions

- Contraindicated in patients hypersensitive to drug and in those with CNS depression, severe hypertensive or hypotensive cardiac disease, or coma.
- Use cautiously in elderly or debilitated patients; pregnant or breast-feeding women; and patients with hepatic disease, CV disease, respiratory disorder, hypocalcemia, seizure disorder, severe reactions to insulin or electroconvulsive therapy, or exposure to extreme heat, cold (including antipyretic therapy), or organophosphate insecticides.

NURSING CONSIDERATIONS

Assessment
- Assess patient's condition before therapy and regularly thereafter.
- Monitor patient for tardive dyskinesia. It may occur after prolonged use, or may not appear until months or years later. It may disappear spontaneously or persist for life, despite discontinuation of drug.
- Monitor therapy with weekly bilirubin tests during first month, periodic blood tests (CBC and liver function), and ophthalmologic tests (long-term therapy), as ordered.

ALERT Monitor patient for symptoms of neuroleptic malignant syndrome (extrapyramidal effects, hyperthermia, autonomic disturbance), which is rare but can be fatal. It isn't necessarily related to length of drug use or type of neuroleptic; however, more than 60% of patients are men.
- Be alert for adverse reactions and drug interactions.
- Evaluate patient's and family's knowledge of drug therapy.

Nursing diagnoses
- Disturbed thought processes related to underlying condition
- Risk for injury related to drug-induced adverse CNS reactions
- Deficient knowledge related to drug therapy

Planning and implementation
ALERT Different liquid formulations have different concentrations. Check dosage.
- Prevent contact dermatitis by keeping drug away from skin and clothes. Wear gloves when preparing liquid forms.
- Dilute liquid concentrate with water or fruit juice just before giving.
- Shake suspension well before using.
- Don't withdraw drug abruptly unless required by severe adverse reactions. Abrupt withdrawal of long-term therapy may cause gastritis, nausea, vomiting, dizziness, tremors, feeling of warmth or cold, diaphoresis, tachycardia, headache, or insomnia.
- Report jaundice, symptoms of blood dyscrasia (fever, sore throat, infection, cellulitis, weakness), or persistent extrapyramidal reactions (longer than a few hours), especially in pregnant woman or in child, and withhold drug.
- Acute dystonic reactions may be treated with diphenhydramine.

ALERT Don't confuse thioridazine with Thorazine; don't confuse Mellaril with Elavil.

Patient teaching
- Warn patient to avoid activities that require alertness until CNS effects of drug are known. Drowsiness and dizziness usually subside after a few weeks.
- Tell patient to watch for orthostatic hypotension, especially with parenteral administration. Advise patient to change position slowly.
- Tell patient to avoid alcohol while taking drug.
- Instruct patient to report urine retention or constipation.
- Inform patient that drug may discolor urine.
- Tell patient to watch for and notify prescriber of blurred vision.
- Advise patient to relieve dry mouth with sugarless gum or hard candy.
- Tell patient to use sunblock and to wear protective clothing to avoid photosensitivity reactions.

Evaluation
- Patient's behavior and communication exhibit improved thought processes.
- Patient doesn't experience injury from adverse CNS reactions.
- Patient and family state understanding of drug therapy.

thiotepa
(thigh-oh-TEE-puh)
Thioplex

Pharmacologic class: alkylating agent (not specific to phase of cell cycle)
Therapeutic class: antineoplastic
Pregnancy risk category: D

Indications and dosages
▶ **Breast and ovarian cancers, lymphoma, Hodgkin's disease.** *Adults and children over*

age 12: 0.3 to 0.4 mg/kg I.V. q 1 to 4 weeks or 0.2 mg/kg for 4 to 5 days at intervals of 2 to 4 weeks.

▶ **Bladder tumor.** *Adults and children over age 12:* 60 mg in 30 to 60 ml of normal saline solution instilled in bladder for 2 hours once weekly for 4 weeks.

▶ **Neoplastic effusions.** *Adults and children over age 12:* 0.6 to 0.8 mg/kg intracavitarily or intratumor q 1 to 4 weeks.

How supplied

Injection: 15-mg vials

Pharmacokinetics

Absorption: absorption from bladder after instillation ranges from 10% to 100% of instilled dose; also variable after intracavitary administration; increased by certain pathologic conditions.

Distribution: crosses blood-brain barrier.

Metabolism: metabolized extensively in liver.

Excretion: thiotepa and its metabolites excreted in urine.

Route	Onset	Peak	Duration
I.V., bladder instillation, intracavitary	Unknown	Unknown	Unknown

Pharmacodynamics

Chemical effect: cross-links strands of cellular DNA and interferes with RNA transcription, causing growth imbalance that leads to cell death.

Therapeutic effect: kills certain cancer cells.

Adverse reactions

CNS: headache, dizziness, fatigue, weakness.
EENT: blurred vision, laryngeal edema, conjunctivitis.
GI: *nausea, vomiting,* abdominal pain, anorexia, stomatitis.
GU: amenorrhea, decreased spermatogenesis, dysuria, urine retention, hemorrhagic cystitis.
Hematologic: ***leukopenia*** (begins within 5 to 10 days), ***thrombocytopenia, neutropenia, anemia.***
Respiratory: asthma.
Skin: urticaria, rash, dermatitis, alopecia, pain at injection site.
Other: fever, ***hypersensitivity, anaphylaxis.***

Interactions

Drug-drug. *Anticoagulants, aspirin:* increased bleeding risk. Avoid concomitant use.
Neuromuscular blockers: may prolong muscular paralysis. Monitor patient closely.
Other alkylating agents, irradiation therapy: may intensify toxicity rather than enhance therapeutic response. Avoid concurrent use.
Succinylcholine: increased apnea with concomitant use. Monitor patient closely.

Contraindications and precautions

- Contraindicated in patients hypersensitive to drug and in those with severe bone marrow, hepatic, or renal dysfunction.
- Drug isn't recommended for pregnant or breast-feeding women.
- Use cautiously in patients with mild bone marrow suppression or renal or hepatic dysfunction.
- Safety of drug hasn't been established in children age 12 and younger.

NURSING CONSIDERATIONS

Assessment

- Assess patient's condition before therapy and regularly thereafter.
- Adverse GU reactions are reversible in 6 to 8 months.
- Monitor CBC weekly for at least 3 weeks after last dose, as ordered.
- Monitor serum uric acid levels.
- Be alert for adverse reactions and drug interactions.
- Evaluate patient's and family's knowledge of drug therapy.

Nursing diagnoses

- Ineffective health maintenance related to presence of neoplastic disease
- Ineffective protection related to drug-induced immunosuppression
- Deficient knowledge related to drug therapy

Planning and implementation

- Follow facility policy to minimize risks. Preparation and administration of parenteral

form are linked to mutagenic, teratogenic, and carcinogenic risks to personnel.
I.V. use: Reconstitute drug with 1.5 ml of sterile water for injection. Don't reconstitute with other solutions. Further dilute solution with normal saline solution injection, D_5W, dextrose %5 in normal saline solution injection, Ringer's injection, or lactated Ringer's injection.
– Drug may be given by rapid I.V. administration in doses of 0.3 to 0.4 mg/kg at intervals of 1 to 4 weeks. Solutions are stable for up to 5 days if refrigerated.
– Use local anesthetic at injection site, as ordered, if intense pain occurs.
– If pain occurs at insertion site, dilute further or use local anesthetic. Make sure drug doesn't infiltrate.
– Discard if solution appears grossly opaque or contains precipitate. Solutions should be clear to slightly opaque.
Intracavitary use: For neoplastic effusions, mix drug with 2% procaine hydrochloride or epinephrine hydrochloride 1:1,000, as ordered.
Bladder instillation use: Dehydrate patient 8 to 10 hours before therapy. Instill drug into bladder by catheter; ask patient to retain solution for 2 hours. Volume may be reduced to 30 ml if discomfort is too great with 60 ml. Reposition patient every 15 minutes for maximum area contact.
- Drug can be given by all parenteral routes, including direct injection into tumor.
- Refrigerate and protect dry powder from direct sunlight.
- Report WBC count below 3,000/mm^3 or platelet count below 150,000/mm^3 and stop drug, as ordered.
- To prevent hyperuricemia with resulting uric acid nephropathy, allopurinol may be used with adequate hydration.

Patient teaching
- Warn patient to watch for signs of infection (fever, sore throat, fatigue) and bleeding (easy bruising, nosebleeds, bleeding gums, melena). Tell patient to take temperature daily and to report even mild infections.
- Instruct patient to avoid OTC products containing aspirin.
- Advise woman to stop breast-feeding during therapy because of risk of toxicity to infant.
- Advise woman of childbearing age to avoid becoming pregnant during therapy and to consult with prescriber before becoming pregnant.

☑ Evaluation
- Patient responds well to drug.
- Patient doesn't develop serious complications from drug-induced immunosuppression.
- Patient and family state understanding of drug therapy.

thiothixene
(thigh-oh-THIKS-een)
Navane

thiothixene hydrochloride
Navane*

Pharmacologic class: thioxanthene
Therapeutic class: antipsychotic
Pregnancy risk category: C

Indications and dosages
▶ **Mild to moderate psychosis.** *Adults:* initially, 2 mg P.O. t.i.d. Increased gradually to 15 mg daily.
▶ **Severe psychosis.** *Adults:* initially, 5 mg P.O. b.i.d. Increased gradually to 20 to 30 mg daily. Maximum recommended dosage is 60 mg daily. Or, 4 mg I.M. b.i.d. or q.i.d. Maximum dosage is 30 mg I.M. daily. A P.O. form should supplant injectable form as soon as possible.

How supplied
thiothixene
Capsules: 1 mg, 2 mg, 5 mg, 10 mg, 20 mg
thiothixene hydrochloride
Oral concentrate: 5 mg/ml*
Injection: 2 mg/ml, 5 mg/ml

Pharmacokinetics
Absorption: rapid after P.O. and I.M. administration.
Distribution: distributed widely in body; 91% to 99% protein-bound.
Metabolism: minimal.

Excretion: most of drug excreted as parent drug in feces.

Route	Onset	Peak	Duration
P.O., I.M.	Several wk	Unknown	Unknown

Pharmacodynamics

Chemical effect: unknown; probably blocks postsynaptic dopamine receptors in brain.
Therapeutic effect: relieves signs and symptoms of psychosis.

Adverse reactions

CNS: *extrapyramidal reactions, tardive dyskinesia,* sedation, pseudoparkinsonism, EEG changes, dizziness, restlessness, agitation, insomnia, ***neuroleptic malignant syndrome.***
CV: *orthostatic hypotension,* tachycardia, ECG changes.
EENT: ocular changes, *blurred vision,* nasal congestion.
GI: *dry mouth, constipation.*
GU: *urine retention,* menstrual irregularities, inhibited ejaculation.
Hematologic: ***transient leukopenia,*** leukocytosis, ***agranulocytosis.***
Hepatic: jaundice.
Metabolic: weight gain.
Skin: *mild photosensitivity,* allergic reactions, pain at I.M. injection site, sterile abscess.
Other: gynecomastia.

Interactions

Drug-drug. *Other CNS depressants:* increased CNS depression. Avoid concomitant use.
Drug-herb. *Nutmeg*: herb may cause a loss of symptom control or interfere with therapy for psychiatric illnesses. Discourage concomitant use.
Drug-lifestyle. *Alcohol use:* increased CNS depression. Discourage concomitant use.
Sun exposure: increased photosensitivity reactions. Advise patient to avoid prolonged or unprotected sun exposure.

Contraindications and precautions

- Contraindicated in patients hypersensitive to drug and in those with circulatory collapse, coma, CNS depression, or blood dyscrasia.
- Use with extreme caution in patients with history of seizure disorder or during alcohol withdrawal.
- Use cautiously in pregnant or breast-feeding women, elderly or debilitated patients, and patients with CV disease (may cause sudden drop in blood pressure), glaucoma, or prostatic hyperplasia, or exposure to extreme heat.

NURSING CONSIDERATIONS

Assessment

- Assess patient's psychosis before therapy and regularly thereafter.
- Watch for orthostatic hypotension, especially with parenteral route.
- Monitor patient for tardive dyskinesia. It may occur after prolonged use or may not appear until months or years later. It may disappear spontaneously or persist for life, despite stopping drug.
- Monitor therapy with weekly bilirubin tests during first month, periodic blood tests (CBC and liver function), and ophthalmologic tests (long-term therapy), as ordered.

ALERT Monitor patient for symptoms of neuroleptic malignant syndrome (extrapyramidal effects, hyperthermia, autonomic disturbance), which is rare but can be fatal. It isn't necessarily related to length of drug use or type of neuroleptic; however, more than 60% of patients are men.

- Be alert for adverse reactions and drug interactions.
- Evaluate patient's and family's knowledge of drug therapy.

Nursing diagnoses

- Disturbed thought processes related to presence of psychosis
- Risk for injury related to drug-induced adverse CNS reactions
- Deficient knowledge related to drug therapy

Planning and implementation

P.O. use: Prevent contact dermatitis by keeping drug away from skin and clothes. Wear gloves when preparing liquid forms.
– Dilute liquid concentrate with water or fruit juice just before giving.

I.M. use: Give I.M. only in upper outer quadrant of buttocks or midlateral thigh. Massage slowly afterward to prevent sterile abscess. Injection may sting.
– Keep patient in supine position for 1 hour after drug administration.
• Slight yellowing of injection or concentrate is common and doesn't affect potency. Discard markedly discolored solutions.
• Don't withdraw drug abruptly unless required by severe adverse reactions. Abrupt withdrawal of long-term therapy may cause gastritis, nausea, vomiting, dizziness, tremors, feeling of warmth or cold, diaphoresis, tachycardia, headache, or insomnia.
• Report jaundice, symptoms of blood dyscrasia (fever, sore throat, infection, cellulitis, weakness), or persistent extrapyramidal reactions (longer than a few hours), especially in pregnant woman or in child, and withhold dose.
• Acute dystonic reactions may be treated with diphenhydramine.
ALERT Don't confuse Navane with Nubain or Norvasc.

Patient teaching
• Warn patient to avoid activities that require alertness until CNS effects of drug are known. Drowsiness and dizziness usually subside after a few weeks.
• Tell patient to avoid alcohol while taking drug.
• Instruct patient to notify prescriber if urine retention or constipation occurs.
• Tell patient to relieve dry mouth with sugarless gum or hard candy.
• Tell patient to use sunblock and to wear protective clothing to avoid photosensitivity reactions.
• Tell patient to watch for orthostatic hypotension, especially with parenteral administration. Advise patient to change position slowly.

Evaluation
• Patient's behavior and communication exhibit improved thought processes.
• Patient doesn't experience injury from adverse CNS reactions.
• Patient and family state understanding of drug therapy.

thyroid
(THIGH-royd)
Armour Thyroid, Thyroid USP

Pharmacologic class: thyroid hormone
Therapeutic class: thyroid agent
Pregnancy risk category: A

Indications and dosages
▶ **Adult hypothyroidism.** Initially, 30 mg P.O. daily, increased by 15 mg q 14 to 30 days, depending on disease severity until desired response is achieved. Usual maintenance dosage is 60 to 180 mg P.O. daily as a single dose.
▶ **Congenital hypothyroidism.** *Children over age 12:* may approach adult dosage (60 to 180 mg daily), depending on response.
Children ages 6 to 12: 60 to 90 mg P.O. daily.
Children ages 1 to 5: 45 to 60 mg P.O. daily.
Children ages 6 to 12 months: 30 to 45 mg P.O. daily.
Children up to age 6 months: 15 to 30 mg P.O. daily.

How supplied
Tablets: 15 mg, 30 mg, 60 mg, 65 mg, 90 mg, 120 mg, 130 mg, 180 mg, 240 mg, 300 mg
Tablets (enteric-coated): 60 mg, 120 mg

Pharmacokinetics
Absorption: absorbed from GI tract.
Distribution: highly protein-bound.
Metabolism: not fully understood.
Excretion: not fully understood. *Half-life:* T_4, 7 days; T_3, 2 days.

Route	Onset	Peak	Duration
P.O.	Unknown	Unknown	Unknown

Pharmacodynamics
Chemical effect: not clearly defined; stimulates metabolism of body tissues by accelerating cellular oxidation.
Therapeutic effect: raises thyroid hormone level in body.

Adverse reactions

Adverse reactions to thyroid hormones are extensions of their pharmacologic properties and reflect patient sensitivity to them.
CNS: *nervousness, insomnia,* tremors, headache.
CV: *tachycardia,* ***arrhythmias,*** angina pectoris, increased blood pressure, ***cardiac decompensation and collapse.***
GI: diarrhea, vomiting.
GU: menstrual irregularities.
Metabolic: weight loss, heat intolerance.
Musculoskeletal: accelerated rate of bone maturation in infants and children.
Skin: diaphoresis.
Other: ***allergic reactions.***

Interactions

Drug-drug. *Cholestyramine:* impaired thyroid absorption. Separate doses by 4 to 5 hours.
Insulin, oral antidiabetics: altered blood glucose level. Monitor level and adjust dosage as needed.
I.V. phenytoin: free thyroid released. Monitor patient for tachycardia.
Oral anticoagulants: altered PT. Monitor PT and INR; adjust dosage as needed.
Sympathomimetics (such as epinephrine): increased risk of coronary insufficiency. Monitor patient closely.

Contraindications and precautions

- Contraindicated in patients hypersensitive to drug and those with acute MI uncomplicated by hypothyroidism, untreated thyrotoxicosis, or uncorrected adrenal insufficiency.
- Use with extreme caution in elderly patients and those with renal insufficiency, an ischemic state, or angina pectoris, hypertension, or other CV disorder.
- Use cautiously in breast-feeding women and patients with myxedema, diabetes mellitus, or diabetes insipidus.

NURSING CONSIDERATIONS

Assessment

- Assess patient's thyroid condition before therapy and regularly thereafter.
- Monitor pulse rate and blood pressure.
- Sleeping pulse rate and basal morning temperature in children guide treatment.
- In patient with coronary artery disease who must receive drug, watch for possible coronary insufficiency.
- Be alert for adverse reactions and drug interactions.
- Evaluate patient's and family's knowledge of drug therapy.

Nursing diagnoses

- Ineffective health maintenance related to presence of hypothyroidism
- Disturbed sleep pattern related to drug-induced insomnia
- Deficient knowledge related to drug therapy

Planning and implementation

- Drug requirements are about 25% lower in patients over age 60 than in young adults.
- Thyroid hormones alter thyroid function test results.
- Patient taking drug usually requires decreased anticoagulant dosage.

ALERT Don't confuse Thyrolar with thyroid.

Patient teaching

- Tell patient to take drug at same time each day, preferably before breakfast, to maintain constant levels.
- Suggest that patient take drug in the morning to prevent insomnia.
- Advise patient who has achieved stable response not to change brands.
- Warn patient (especially elderly patient) to notify prescriber promptly if chest pain, palpitations, sweating, nervousness, or other signs of overdose occur or if chest pain, dyspnea, and tachycardia develop.
- Tell patient to report unusual bleeding and bruising.

Evaluation

- Patient regains normal thyroid function.
- Patient expresses importance of taking thyroid in morning if insomnia occurs.
- Patient and family state understanding of drug therapy.

thyrotropin (thyroid-stimulating hormone, or TSH)

(thigh-ROH-troh-pin)
Thytropar

Pharmacologic class: anterior pituitary hormone
Therapeutic class: thyrotropic hormone
Pregnancy risk category: C

Indications and dosages

▶ **Diagnosis of thyroid cancer remnant with ^{131}I after surgery.** *Adults:* 10 IU I.M. or S.C. for 3 to 7 days.
▶ **Differential diagnosis of primary and secondary hypothyroidism; to determine thyroid status of patient receiving thyroid hormone.** *Adults:* 10 IU I.M. or S.C. for 1 to 3 days.
▶ **In protein-bound iodine or ^{131}I uptake determinations for differential diagnosis of subclinical hypothyroidism or low thyroid reserve.** *Adults:* 10 IU I.M. or S.C.
▶ **Therapy for thyroid carcinoma (local or metastatic) with ^{131}I.** *Adults:* 10 IU I.M. or S.C. for 3 to 8 days.

How supplied

Powder for injection: 10 IU/vial

Pharmacokinetics

Absorption: within minutes from I.M. or S.C. injection site.
Distribution: distributed primarily in thyroid gland.
Metabolism: not fully understood.
Excretion: not fully understood.

Route	Onset	Peak	Duration
I.M., S.C.	Min	≤ 24 hr	Effects rapidly reverse after withdrawal

Pharmacodynamics

Chemical effect: stimulates uptake of radioactive iodine (^{131}I) in patients with thyroid carcinoma and promotes thyroid hormone production by anterior pituitary gland.
Therapeutic effect: evaluates thyroid function and inhibits thyroid cancer cell activity.

Adverse reactions

CNS: headache.
CV: *tachycardia,* atrial fibrillation, angina pectoris, ***heart failure,*** hypotension.
GI: nausea, vomiting.
GU: menstrual irregularities.
Other: thyroid hyperplasia (with large doses), fever, hypersensitivity reactions (postinjection flare, urticaria, ***anaphylaxis***).

Interactions

Drug-drug. *Insulin, oral antidiabetics:* altered blood glucose level. Monitor level. Dosage may need adjustment.
Oral anticoagulants: altered PT. Monitor PT and INR. Dosage adjustment may be necessary.
Sympathomimetics (such as epinephrine): increased risk of coronary insufficiency. Monitor patient closely.

Contraindications and precautions

• Contraindicated in patients hypersensitive to drug and those with coronary thrombosis or untreated Addison's disease.
• Use cautiously in pregnant or breast-feeding women and patients with angina pectoris, heart failure, hypopituitarism, or adrenocortical suppression.

NURSING CONSIDERATIONS

Assessment

• Assess patient's condition before therapy and regularly thereafter.
• Be alert for adverse reactions and drug interactions.
• Evaluate patient's and family's knowledge of drug therapy.

Nursing diagnoses

• Health-seeking behavior (desire to have thyroid problem diagnosed) related to thyroid dysfunction
• Ineffective protection related to drug-induced hypersensitivity reaction
• Deficient knowledge related to drug therapy

Planning and implementation

I.M. and S.C. use: Follow normal protocol.
- Three-day dosage schedule may be used in long-standing pituitary myxedema or with prolonged use of thyroid medication.

Patient teaching
- Warn patient to immediately report itching, redness, or swelling at injection site; rash; tightness of throat or wheezing chest pain; irritability; nervousness; rapid heartbeat; shortness of breath; or unusual sweating.

Evaluation

- Patient's thyroid dysfunction is diagnosed.
- Patient doesn't experience drug-induced hypersensitivity reaction.
- Patient and family state understanding of drug therapy.

tiagabine hydrochloride

(tigh-AG-ah-been high-droh-KLOR-ighd)
Gabitril

Pharmacologic class: gamma aminobutyric acid (GABA) uptake inhibitor
Therapeutic class: anticonvulsant
Pregnancy risk category: C

Indications and dosages

▶ **Adjunctive therapy in the treatment of partial seizures.** *Adults:* initially, 4 mg P.O. once daily. Total daily dosage may be increased by 4 to 8 mg at weekly intervals until clinical response or up to 56 mg/day. Daily dosage should be given in divided doses b.i.d. to q.i.d.
Adolescents ages 12 to 18: initially, 4 mg P.O. once daily. Total daily dosage may be increased by 4 mg at the beginning of week 2 and by 4 to 8 mg/week until clinical response or up to 32 mg/day. Daily dosage should be given in divided doses b.i.d. to q.i.d.

How supplied

Tablets: 4 mg, 12 mg, 16 mg, 20 mg

Pharmacokinetics

Absorption: drug is rapidly and nearly completely absorbed (more than 95%). Absolute bioavailability is 90%.
Distribution: about 96% bound to plasma protein.
Metabolism: likely to be metabolized by cytochrome P-450 3A isoenzymes.
Excretion: about 25% is excreted in urine (2% unchanged); 63% in feces. *Half-life:* 7 to 9 hours.

Route	Onset	Peak	Duration
P.O.	Rapid	45 min	7-9 hr

Pharmacodynamics

Chemical effect: unknown, but tiagabine may act by enhancing the activity of GABA, the major inhibitory neurotransmitter in the CNS. It binds to recognition sites related to the GABA uptake carrier and may thus permit more GABA to be available for binding to receptors on postsynaptic cells.
Therapeutic effect: prevents partial seizures.

Adverse reactions

CNS: generalized weakness, *dizziness, asthenia, somnolence, nervousness,* tremor, difficulty with concentration and attention, insomnia, ataxia, confusion, speech disorder, difficulty with memory, paresthesia, depression, emotional lability, abnormal gait, hostility, language problems, agitation.
CV: vasodilation.
EENT: nystagmus, pharyngitis.
GI: abdominal pain, *nausea,* diarrhea, vomiting, increased appetite, mouth ulceration.
Musculoskeletal: myasthenia.
Respiratory: increased cough.
Skin: rash, pruritus.
Other: pain.

Interactions

Drug-drug. *Carbamazepine, phenobarbital, phenytoin:* increased tiagabine clearance. Monitor patient for loss of therapeutic effect.
CNS depressants: enhanced CNS effects. Use cautiously.
Drug-lifestyle. *Alcohol use:* enhanced CNS effects. Advise cautious use.

Contraindications and precautions

• Contraindicated in patients hypersensitive to drug or its ingredients.
• Use cautiously in breast-feeding women.

NURSING CONSIDERATIONS

Assessment

• Assess patient's seizure disorder before therapy and regularly thereafter.
• Assess patient's compliance with therapy at each follow-up visit.
ALERT Monitor patient carefully for status epilepticus because sudden unexpected death has occurred in patients receiving antiepilepsy drugs, including tiagabine.
• Assess patient for adverse reactions and drug interactions.
• Evaluate patient's and family's knowledge of drug therapy.

Nursing diagnoses

• Risk for injury related to seizure disorder
• Impaired physical mobility related to drug-induced generalized weakness
• Deficient knowledge related to drug therapy

Planning and implementation

• Reduced initial and maintenance doses or longer dosing intervals may be required in patients with impaired liver function.
ALERT Never withdraw drug suddenly because seizure frequency may increase. Withdraw gradually unless safety concerns require a more rapid withdrawal.
• Patients who aren't receiving at least one enzyme-inducing antiepilepsy drug at the time of tiagabine initiation may require lower doses or slower dosage adjustments.
• Report breakthrough seizure activity to prescriber.

Patient teaching

• Advise patient to take drug only as prescribed.
• Advise patient to take tiagabine with food.
• Warn patient that drug may cause dizziness, somnolence, and other symptoms and signs of CNS depression. Advise patient to avoid driving and other potentially hazardous activities that require mental alertness until drug's CNS effects are known.
• Tell woman to call prescriber if she becomes pregnant or plans to become pregnant during therapy.
• Tell woman to notify prescriber if planning to breast-feed because drug may appear in breast milk.

Evaluation

• Patient is free from seizure activity.
• Patient receives therapeutic medication dose and doesn't experience muscle weakness.
• Patient and family state understanding of drug therapy.

ticarcillin disodium

(tigh-kar-SIL-in digh-SOH-dee-um)
Ticar, Ticillin ◊

Pharmacologic class: extended-spectrum penicillin, alpha-carboxypenicillin
Therapeutic class: antibiotic
Pregnancy risk category: B

Indications and dosages

▶ **Severe systemic infections caused by susceptible strains of gram-positive and especially gram-negative organisms (including *Pseudomonas* and *Proteus*).** *Adults and children over age 1 month:* 200 to 300 mg/kg I.V. daily in divided doses q 4 to 6 hours.
▶ **Uncomplicated UTI.** *Adults and children weighing 40 kg (88 lb) or more:* 1 g I.V. or I.M. q 6 hours.
Children over age 1 month and weighing less than 40 kg: 50 to 100 mg/kg I.V. or I.M. daily in divided doses q 6 to 8 hours.

How supplied

Injection: 1 g, 3 g, 6 g
I.V. infusion: 3 g

Pharmacokinetics

Absorption: unknown after I.M. administration.
Distribution: distributed widely. Penetrates minimally into CSF with uninflamed meninges; 45% to 65% protein-bound.

Metabolism: about 13% metabolized by hydrolysis to inactive compounds.
Excretion: excreted mostly in urine; also in bile. *Half-life:* about 1 hour.

Route	Onset	Peak	Duration
I.V.	Immediate	Immediate	Unknown
I.M.	Unknown	30-75 min	Unknown

Pharmacodynamics

Chemical effect: inhibits cell wall synthesis during microorganism multiplication; bacteria resist penicillins by producing penicillinases—enzymes that convert penicillins to inactive penicilloic acid. Ticarcillin resists these enzymes.
Therapeutic effect: kills bacteria. Activity includes many gram-negative aerobic and anaerobic bacilli, many gram-positive and gram-negative aerobic cocci, and some gram-positive aerobic and anaerobic bacilli. May be effective against some carbenicillin-resistant gram-negative bacilli.

Adverse reactions

CNS: ***seizures,*** neuromuscular excitability.
CV: vein irritation, phlebitis.
GI: nausea, diarrhea, vomiting.
Hematologic: ***leukopenia, neutropenia,*** eosinophilia, ***thrombocytopenia,*** hemolytic anemia.
Metabolic: hypokalemia.
Other: hypersensitivity reactions (rash, pruritus, urticaria, chills, fever, edema, ***anaphylaxis***), overgrowth of nonsusceptible organisms, pain at injection site.

Interactions

Drug-drug. *Lithium:* altered renal elimination of lithium. Monitor serum lithium level closely.
Oral contraceptives: efficacy of oral contraceptives may be decreased. Recommend an additional form of contraception during penicillin therapy.
Probenecid: increased blood levels of ticarcillin and other penicillins. Probenecid may be used for this purpose.

Contraindications and precautions

- Contraindicated in patients hypersensitive to penicillins.
- Use cautiously in pregnant or breast-feeding women; patients with other drug allergies, especially to cephalosporins (possible cross-sensitivity); and those with impaired kidney function, hemorrhagic conditions, hypokalemia, or sodium restrictions (contains 5.2 to 6.5 mEq sodium/g).

NURSING CONSIDERATIONS

Assessment

- Assess patient's infection before therapy and regularly thereafter.
- Before giving, ask patient if he is allergic to penicillin. Negative history of penicillin allergy is no guarantee against future allergic reaction.
- Obtain specimen for culture and sensitivity tests before giving first dose. Therapy may begin pending results.
- Monitor serum potassium level.
- Monitor CBC and platelet count.
- Monitor INR in patients receiving warfarin therapy because drug may prolong PT.
- Be alert for adverse reactions and drug interactions.
- Monitor patient's hydration status if adverse GI reactions occur.
- Evaluate patient's and family's knowledge of drug therapy.

Nursing diagnoses

- Risk for infection related to presence of susceptible bacteria
- Risk for deficient fluid volume related to drug-induced adverse GI reactions
- Deficient knowledge related to drug therapy

Planning and implementation

- Dosage should be decreased in patient with impaired kidney function.

I.V. use: Reconstitute vials using D_5W, normal saline solution injection, sterile water for injection, or other compatible solution. Add 4 ml of diluent for each gram of drug. Further dilute to maximum of 50 mg/ml, and inject slowly directly into vein or I.V. line containing free-flowing solution. Or, dilute to 10 to 100 mg/ml

and infuse intermittently over 30 minutes to 2 hours in adults or 10 to 20 minutes in neonates.
– Aminoglycoside antibiotics (such as gentamicin and tobramycin) are chemically incompatible. Don't mix in same I.V. container.
– Continuous infusion may cause vein irritation. Change site every 48 hours.
I.M. use: Reconstitute vials with sterile water for injection, normal saline solution injection, or lidocaine 1% (without epinephrine). Use 2 ml of diluent per gram of drug.
– Inject deep into large muscle. Don't exceed 2 g per injection.
• Give drug at least 1 hour before bacteriostatic antibiotics.
• Drug is typically used with another antibiotic, such as gentamicin.
ALERT Institute seizure precautions. Patient with high blood level of ticarcillin may develop seizures.

Patient teaching
• Instruct patient to report adverse reactions.

Evaluation
• Patient is free from infection.
• Patient maintains adequate hydration.
• Patient and family state understanding of drug therapy.

ticarcillin disodium/clavulanate potassium
(tigh-kar-SIL-in digh-SOH-dee-um/ KLAV-yoo-lan-nayt poh-TAH-see-um)
Timentin

Pharmacologic class: extended-spectrum penicillin, beta-lactamase inhibitor
Therapeutic class: antibiotic
Pregnancy risk category: B

Indications and dosages
▶ **Lower respiratory tract, urinary tract, bone and joint, skin, and skin-structure infections and septicemia when caused by beta-lactamase–producing strains of bacteria or by ticarcillin-susceptible organisms.** *Adults:* 3.1 g (3 g ticarcillin and 100 mg clavulanate acid) administered by I.V. infusion q 4 to 6 hours.

How supplied
Injection: 3 g ticarcillin and 100 mg clavulanic acid

Pharmacokinetics
Absorption: not applicable with I.V. administration.
Distribution: ticarcillin disodium distributed widely; penetrates minimally into CSF with uninflamed meninges. Clavulanic acid penetrates pleural fluid, lungs, and peritoneal fluid.
Metabolism: about 13% of ticarcillin dose metabolized by hydrolysis to inactive compounds; clavulanic acid is thought to undergo extensive metabolism but its fate is unknown.
Excretion: ticarcillin excreted primarily in urine; also excreted in bile. Clavulanate's metabolites are excreted in urine. *Half-life:* about 1 hour.

Route	Onset	Peak	Duration
I.V.	Immediate	Immediate	Unknown

Pharmacodynamics
Chemical effect: ticarcillin is an extended-spectrum penicillin that inhibits cell wall synthesis during microorganism replication; clavulanic acid increases ticarcillin's effectiveness by inactivating beta lactamases, which destroy ticarcillin.
Therapeutic effect: kills susceptible bacteria. Spectrum of activity for ticarcillin includes many gram-negative aerobic and anaerobic bacilli, many gram-positive and gram-negative aerobic cocci, and some gram-positive aerobic and anaerobic bacilli. The combination of ticarcillin and clavulanate potassium is also effective against many beta-lactamase–producing strains, including *Bacteroides fragilis, Escherichia coli, Haemophilus influenzae, Klebsiella, Neisseria gonorrhoeae, Providencia,* and *Staphylococcus aureus.*

Adverse reactions
CNS: ***seizures,*** neuromuscular excitability, headache, giddiness.
CV: vein irritation, phlebitis.

GI: nausea, diarrhea, stomatitis, vomiting, epigastric pain, flatulence, pseudomembranous colitis, taste and smell disturbances.
Hematologic: ***leukopenia, neutropenia,*** eosinophilia, ***thrombocytopenia,*** hemolytic anemia, anemia.
Metabolic: hypokalemia.
Other: hypersensitivity reactions (rash, pruritus, urticaria, chills, fever, edema, ***anaphylaxis***), overgrowth of nonsusceptible organisms, pain at injection site.

Interactions

Drug-drug. *Oral contraceptives:* efficacy of oral contraceptives may be decreased. Recommend an additional form of contraception during ticarcillin therapy.
Probenecid: increased blood levels of ticarcillin. Probenecid may be used for this purpose.

Contraindications and precautions

- Contraindicated in patients hypersensitive to penicillins.
- Use cautiously in pregnant or breast-feeding women; patients with other drug allergies, especially to cephalosporins (possible cross-sensitivity); and those with impaired kidney function, hemorrhagic condition, hypokalemia, or sodium restrictions (contains 4.5 mEq sodium/g).

NURSING CONSIDERATIONS

Assessment

- Assess patient's infection before therapy and regularly thereafter.
- Before giving drug, ask patient if he's allergic to penicillin. Negative history of penicillin allergy is no guarantee against future allergic reaction.
- Obtain specimen for culture and sensitivity tests before giving first dose. Therapy may begin pending results.
- Monitor CBC and platelet count.
- Be alert for adverse reactions and drug interactions.
- Monitor patient's hydration status if adverse GI reactions occur.
- Evaluate patient's and family's knowledge of drug therapy.

Nursing diagnoses

- Risk for infection related to presence of susceptible bacteria
- Risk for deficient fluid volume related to drug-induced adverse GI reactions
- Deficient knowledge related to drug therapy

Planning and implementation

- Dosage should be decreased in patient with impaired kidney function.
- Reconstitute drug with 13 ml of sterile water for injection or normal saline solution injection. Further dilute to maximum of 10 to 100 mg/ml (based on ticarcillin component) and infuse over 30 minutes. In fluid-restricted patient, dilute to maximum of 48 mg/ml if using D_5W, 43 mg/ml if using normal saline solution injection, or 86 mg/ml if using sterile water for injection.
- Aminoglycoside antibiotics (such as gentamicin and tobramycin) are chemically incompatible. Don't mix in same I.V. container.
- Give drug at least 1 hour before bacteriostatic antibiotics.

Patient teaching

- Instruct patient to report adverse reactions immediately.

Evaluation

- Patient is free from infection.
- Patient maintains adequate hydration.
- Patient and family state understanding of drug therapy.

ticlopidine hydrochloride

(tigh-KLOH-peh-deen high-droh-KLOR-ighd)
Ticlid

Pharmacologic class: platelet aggregation inhibitor
Therapeutic class: antithrombotic
Pregnancy risk category: C

Indications and dosages

▶ **To reduce risk of thrombotic CVA in patients with history of CVA or who have experienced CVA precursors.** *Adults:* 250 mg P.O. b.i.d. with meals.

How supplied

Tablets: 250 mg

Pharmacokinetics

Absorption: rapidly and extensively absorbed; enhanced by food.
Distribution: 98% bound to serum proteins and lipoproteins.
Metabolism: extensively metabolized by liver. More than 20 metabolites have been identified; unknown if parent drug or active metabolites are responsible for pharmacologic activity.
Excretion: 60% excreted in urine and 23% in feces.

Route	Onset	Peak	Duration
P.O.	Unknown	About 2 hr	Unknown

Pharmacodynamics

Chemical effect: unknown; probably blocks adenosine diphosphate–induced platelet-fibrinogen and platelet-platelet binding.
Therapeutic effect: prevents blood clots from forming.

Adverse reactions

CNS: dizziness, ***intracerebral bleeding.***
CV: vasculitis.
EENT: epistaxis, conjunctival hemorrhage.
GI: *diarrhea,* nausea, dyspepsia, vomiting, flatulence, anorexia, *abdominal pain,* bleeding.
GU: hematuria, ***nephrotic syndrome,*** dark-colored urine.
Hematologic: ***neutropenia, agranulocytosis, pancytopenia, immune thrombocytopenia.***
Hepatic: ***hepatitis,*** cholestatic jaundice, abnormal liver function test results.
Metabolic: ***hyponatremia.***
Musculoskeletal: arthropathy, myositis.
Respiratory: ***allergic pneumonitis.***
Skin: *rash,* purpura, pruritus, urticaria, ***thrombocytopenic purpura,*** ecchymosis.
Other: ***hypersensitivity reactions,*** postoperative bleeding, systemic lupus erythematosus, ***serum sickness.***

Interactions

Drug-drug. *Antacids:* decreased plasma ticlopidine level. Separate administration times by at least 2 hours.
Aspirin: potentiated aspirin effects on platelets. Don't use together.
Cimetidine: decreased clearance of ticlopidine and increased risk of toxicity. Avoid concomitant use.
Digoxin: slight decrease in serum digoxin level. Monitor level.
Theophylline: decreased theophylline clearance and risk of toxicity. Monitor patient closely and adjust theophylline dosage, as ordered.
Drug-herb. *Red clover:* possible increased risk of bleeding. Caution against concomitant use.

Contraindications and precautions

- Contraindicated in patients hypersensitive to drug and those with hematopoietic disorders (such as neutropenia, thrombocytopenia, or disorders of hemostasis), active pathologic bleeding (such as peptic ulceration or active intracranial bleeding), or severe hepatic impairment.
- Drug is reserved for patients intolerant to aspirin.
- Drug isn't recommended for breast-feeding women.
- Use cautiously in pregnant women.
- Safety of drug hasn't been established in children.

NURSING CONSIDERATIONS

Assessment

- Assess patient's condition before therapy and regularly thereafter.
- Obtain baseline liver function tests before therapy. Monitor closely, especially during first 4 months of treatment, and repeat when liver dysfunction is suspected.
- Determine baseline CBC and WBC differentials and then repeat at second week of therapy and every 2 weeks until end of third month. Test more frequently if patient shows signs of declining neutrophil count or if count falls 30% below baseline. After first 3 months, CBC and WBC differential determinations

should be performed only in patient showing signs of infection.
- Be alert for adverse reactions and drug interactions.
- Evaluate patient's and family's knowledge of drug therapy.

Nursing diagnoses
- Impaired cerebral tissue perfusion related to CVA potential or history
- Ineffective protection related to drug-induced adverse hematologic reactions
- Deficient knowledge related to drug therapy

Planning and implementation
- Thrombocytopenia has occurred rarely. Report platelet count of 80,000/mm^3 or less, and stop drug. If ordered, give 20 mg of methylprednisolone I.V. to normalize bleeding time within 2 hours. Platelet transfusions also may be used.
- When used preoperatively, drug may decrease risk of graft occlusion in patient receiving coronary artery bypass grafts and reduce severity of drop in platelet count in patient receiving extracorporeal hemoperfusion during open heart surgery.

Patient teaching
- Tell patient to take drug with meals; this substantially increases bioavailability and improves GI tolerance.
- Tell patient to avoid aspirin-containing products and to check with prescriber before taking OTC drugs.
- Explain that drug prolongs bleeding time but that patient should report unusual or prolonged bleeding. Advise him to tell dentist and other prescribers that he is taking this drug.
- Stress importance of regular blood tests. Because neutropenia can increase risk of infection, tell patient to promptly report such signs as fever, chills, and sore throat.
- If drug is substituted for fibrinolytic or anticoagulant, tell patient to discontinue those drugs before starting ticlopidine therapy, as ordered.
- Advise patient to stop drug 10 to 14 days before elective surgery.
- Tell patient to report yellow skin or sclera, severe or persistent diarrhea, rashes, S.C. bleeding, light-colored stools, and dark urine.

Evaluation
- Patient maintains adequate cerebral perfusion.
- Patient doesn't develop serious complications.
- Patient and family state understanding of drug therapy.

timolol maleate
(TIH-moh-lol MAL-ee-ayt)
Apo-Timol♦, Blocadren

Pharmacologic class: beta blocker
Therapeutic class: antihypertensive, adjunct in MI, antimigraine agent
Pregnancy risk category: C

Indications and dosages
▶ **Hypertension.** *Adults:* initially, 10 mg P.O. b.i.d. Usual daily maintenance dosage is 20 to 40 mg. Maximum daily dosage is 60 mg. Allow at least 7 days to elapse between increases in dosage.
▶ **MI (long-term prophylaxis in patients who have survived acute phase).** *Adults:* 10 mg P.O. b.i.d.
▶ **Prevention of migraine headache.** *Adults:* usual dose is 10 mg P.O. b.i.d. During maintenance therapy, 20-mg daily dose may be given once daily. Maximum daily dosage is 30 mg in divided doses (10 mg in morning, and 20 mg in evening). If maximum dosage for 6 to 8 weeks doesn't achieve an adequate response, another therapy should be instituted.

How supplied
Tablets: 5 mg, 10 mg, 20 mg

Pharmacokinetics
Absorption: about 90% absorbed from GI tract.
Distribution: distributed throughout body; depending on assay method, drug is 10% to 60% protein-bound.
Metabolism: about 80% metabolized in liver to inactive metabolites.

Excretion: drug and its metabolites excreted primarily in urine. *Half-life:* about 4 hours.

Route	Onset	Peak	Duration
P.O.	15-30 min	1-2 hr	6-12 hr

Pharmacodynamics

Chemical effect: mechanism of antihypertensive action unknown. In MI, drug may decrease myocardial oxygen requirements. It also prevents arterial dilation through beta blockade for migraine headache prophylaxis.
Therapeutic effect: lowers blood pressure and helps to prevent MI and migraine headaches.

Adverse reactions

CNS: fatigue, lethargy, dizziness.
CV: ***bradycardia,*** hypotension, peripheral vascular disease, ***arrhythmias, heart failure.***
GI: nausea, vomiting, diarrhea.
Respiratory: dyspnea, ***bronchospasm,*** *increased airway resistance.*
Skin: pruritus.

Interactions

Drug-drug. *Cardiac glycosides, diltiazem, verapamil:* excessive bradycardia and increased depressant effect on myocardium. Use together cautiously.
Catecholamine-depleting drugs (such as reserpine): may have additive effects when given with beta blockers. Monitor patient for hypotension and bradycardia.
Indomethacin: decreased antihypertensive effect. Monitor blood pressure and adjust dosage.
Insulin, oral antidiabetics: can alter requirements for these drugs in previously stabilized diabetic patients. Monitor patient for hypoglycemia.

Contraindications and precautions

- Contraindicated in patients hypersensitive to drug and in those with bronchial asthma, severe COPD, sinus bradycardia and heart block greater than first-degree, cardiogenic shock, or overt heart failure.
- Drug isn't recommended for breast-feeding women.
- Use cautiously in pregnant women and patients with compensated heart failure; hepatic, renal, or respiratory disease; diabetes; or hyperthyroidism.
- Safety of drug hasn't been established in children.

NURSING CONSIDERATIONS

Assessment

- Assess patient's condition before therapy and regularly thereafter.
- Monitor blood pressure frequently.
- Be alert for adverse reactions and drug interactions.
- Evaluate patient's and family's knowledge of drug therapy.

Nursing diagnoses

- Risk for injury related to history of hypertension or MI
- Acute pain related to migraine headache
- Deficient knowledge related to drug therapy

Planning and implementation

- Check patient's apical pulse rate before giving drug. Report extreme pulse rate, and withhold drug.
- Don't stop drug abruptly; this can exacerbate angina and precipitate MI. Dosage should be reduced gradually over 1 to 2 weeks.
- Teach patient other means to reduce blood pressure such as diet control, weight reduction, exercise, smoking cessation, and stress reduction.

ALERT Don't confuse timolol with atenolol.

Patient teaching

- Explain importance of taking drug exactly as prescribed.
- Tell patient not to discontinue drug abruptly because serious complications can occur. Instead, tell him to report adverse reactions.

Evaluation

- Patient doesn't experience injury from underlying disease.
- Patient doesn't develop migraine headaches.
- Patient and family state understanding of drug therapy.

tirofiban hydrochloride
(ty-roh-FYE-ban high-droh-KLOR-ighd)
Aggrastat

Pharmacologic class: GP IIb/IIIa receptor antagonist
Therapeutic class: inhibitor of platelet aggregation
Pregnancy risk category: B

Indications and dosages

▶ **Acute coronary syndrome, with heparin, aspirin, or both, including patients who are to be managed medically and those undergoing percutaneous transluminal coronary angioplasty (PTCA) or atherectomy.** *Adults:* I.V. loading dose of 0.4 mcg/kg/minute for 30 minutes; then continuous I.V. infusion of 0.1 mcg/kg/minute. Continue through angiography and for 12 to 24 hours after angioplasty or atherectomy.

How supplied

Injection: 50-ml vials (250 mcg/ml), 500-ml premixed vials (50 mcg/ml)

Pharmacokinetics

Absorption: not reported.
Distribution: drug is 65% protein-bound. Volume of distribution ranges from 22 to 42 liters.
Metabolism: drug's metabolism is limited. *Half-life:* 2 hours.
Excretion: renal clearance accounts for 39 to 69% of elimination; feces accounts for 25%.

Route	Onset	Peak	Duration
I.V.	Immediate	Immediate	4-8 hr after end of infusion

Pharmacodynamics

Chemical effect: reversibly binds to the glycoprotein IIb/IIIa (GP IIb/IIIa) receptor on human platelets and inhibits platelet aggregation.
Therapeutic effect: prevents clot formation.

Adverse reactions

CNS: dizziness, headache.
CV: ***bradycardia, coronary artery dissection,*** edema, vasovagal reaction.
GI: nausea, *occult bleeding.*
Hematologic: *bleeding,* ***thrombocytopenia,*** decreased hemoglobin level and hematocrit.
Musculoskeletal: pelvic pain, leg pain.
Skin: sweating.
Other: fever, bleeding at arterial access site.

Interactions

Drug-drug. *Clopidogrel, dipyridamole, NSAIDs, oral anticoagulants such as warfarin, thrombolytics, ticlopidine:* increased risk of bleeding. Monitor patient closely.
Levothyroxine, omeprazole: increased renal clearance of tirofiban. Monitor patient.
Drug-herb. *Dong quai, feverfew, garlic, ginger:* may increase the risk of bleeding. Tell patient to discontinue use before planned invasive procedures.

Contraindications and precautions

- Contraindicated in patients hypersensitive to drug or its ingredients, those with active internal bleeding or history of bleeding diathesis within the previous 30 days, and those with history of intracranial hemorrhage, intracranial neoplasm, arteriovenous malformation, aneurysm, thrombocytopenia following prior exposure to tirofiban, CVA within 30 days, or hemorrhagic CVA.
- Also contraindicated in those with history, symptoms, or findings suggestive of aortic dissection; severe hypertension (systolic blood pressure over 180 mm Hg or diastolic blood pressure over 110 mm Hg); acute pericarditis; those who have had major surgical procedure or severe physical trauma within previous month; or patients receiving another parenteral GP IIb/IIIa inhibitor.
- Use cautiously in patients with increased risk of bleeding, including those with hemorrhagic retinopathy or platelet count below 150,000/mm³.

NURSING CONSIDERATIONS

Assessment

- Obtain history of patient's underlying condition before therapy, and reassess regularly thereafter.

• Monitor hemoglobin level and hematocrit and platelet counts before starting therapy, 6 hours following loading dose, and at least daily during therapy.
• Monitor patient for bleeding.
• Notify prescriber if thrombocytopenia occurs.
• Evaluate patient's and family's knowledge of drug therapy.

Nursing diagnoses
• Ineffective cardiopulmonary tissue perfusion related to presence of acute coronary syndrome
• Risk for injury related to increased bleeding tendencies
• Deficient knowledge related to drug therapy

Planning and implementation
I.V. use: Dilute 50-ml injection vials (250 mcg/ml) to same strength as 500-ml premixed vials (50 mcg/ml) as follows: withdraw and discard 100 ml from a 500-ml bag of sterile saline solution or D_5W and replace this volume with 100 ml of tirofiban injection (from two 50-ml vials) or withdraw 50 ml from a 250-ml bag of sterile saline solution or D_5W and replace this volume with 50 ml of tirofiban injection, to achieve 50 mcg/ml.
• Inspect solution for particulate matter before administration, and check for leaks by squeezing the inner bag firmly. If particles are visible or if leaks occur, discard solution.
• Discard unused solution 24 hours following the start of infusion.
• Heparin and tirofiban can be administered through same I.V. catheter.
• Minimize injection and avoid noncompressible I.V. sites.
• Administer drug with aspirin and heparin, as ordered.
• The most common adverse effect is bleeding at the arterial access site for cardiac catheterization.
ALERT In patients with renal insufficiency (creatinine clearance below 30 ml/minute), give a loading dose of 0.2 mcg/kg/minute for 30 minutes; then continuous infusion of 0.05 mcg/kg/minute. Continue infusion through angiography and for 12 to 24 hours after angioplasty or atherectomy.
• Store drug at room temperature, and protect from light.

Patient teaching
• Explain that drug is a blood thinner used to prevent chest pain and heart attack.
• Explain that risk of serious bleeding is far outweighed by the benefits of drug.
• Instruct patient to report chest discomfort or other adverse events immediately.
• Inform patient that frequent blood sampling may be needed to evaluate therapy.

Evaluation
• Patient maintains adequate cardiopulmonary tissue perfusion.
• Patient doesn't experience life-threatening bleeding episode.
• Patient and family state understanding of drug therapy.

tizanidine hydrochloride
(tigh-ZAN-eh-deen high-droh-KLOR-ighd)
Zanaflex

Pharmacologic class: alpha$_2$-adrenergic agonist
Therapeutic class: antispasticity agent
Pregnancy risk category: C

Indications and dosages
▶ **Management of acute and intermittent increased muscle tone related to spasticity.** *Adults:* initially, 4 mg P.O. q 6 to 8 hours, p.r.n., to maximum of three doses in 24 hours. Dosage can be increased gradually in 2- to 4-mg increments. Maximum daily dosage is 36 mg.

How supplied
Tablets: 4 mg

Pharmacokinetics
Absorption: almost completely absorbed.
Distribution: distributed throughout body.
Metabolism: metabolized in liver.

Excretion: excreted in urine and feces. *Half-life:* 2.5 hours.

Route	Onset	Peak	Duration
P.O.	Unknown	1-2 hr	3-6 hr

Pharmacodynamics

Chemical effect: agonist at $alpha_2$-adrenergic receptor sites.
Therapeutic effect: reduces spasticity; reduces facilitation of spinal motor neurons.

Adverse reactions

CNS: *somnolence, sedation, asthenia, dizziness,* speech disorder, dyskinesia, nervousness, hallucinations.
CV: *hypotension,* ***bradycardia.***
EENT: amblyopia, pharyngitis, rhinitis.
GI: *dry mouth,* constipation, vomiting.
GU: *urinary tract infection,* urinary frequency.
Hepatic: elevation of liver function test results, hepatic injury.
Other: infection, flu syndrome.

Interactions

Drug-drug. *Acetaminophen:* delayed maximum absorption time of timolol. Avoid concomitant use.
Antihypertensives, other $alpha_2$-adrenergic agonists: may cause hypotension. Monitor patient closely. Don't use with other $alpha_2$-adrenergic agonists.
Baclofen, benzodiazepines, other CNS depressants: additive CNS depressant effects. Avoid concomitant use.
Oral contraceptives: decreased clearance of tizanidine. Dosage may be reduced.
Drug-lifestyle. *Alcohol use:* additive CNS depressant effects. Discourage concomitant use.

Contraindications and precautions

- Contraindicated in patients hypersensitive to drug.

NURSING CONSIDERATIONS

Assessment

- Use cautiously in patients who are taking antihypertensives, in those with renal or hepatic impairment, and in elderly patients.
- Obtain baseline liver function tests as ordered before treatment; during treatment at 1, 3, and 6 months; and then periodically thereafter.
- Evaluate patient's and family's knowledge of drug therapy.

Nursing diagnoses

- Risk for injury related to drug-induced adverse CNS reactions
- Disturbed body image related to spasticity
- Deficient knowledge related to drug therapy

Planning and implementation

- Dosage is reduced in patient with renal impairment. If higher dosage is needed, individual dose, not frequency, is increased.

Patient teaching

- Inform patient of limited clinical experience with drug.
- Warn patient that drug-induced drowsiness may occur and to avoid alcohol and activities that require alertness.
- Inform patient to rise slowly and avoid sudden position changes.

Evaluation

- Patient doesn't experience injury from adverse CNS reactions.
- Patient experiences decreased muscle spasticity and improved body image.
- Patient and family state understanding of drug therapy.

tobramycin sulfate

(toh-breh-MIGH-sin SUL-fayt)
Nebcin

Pharmacologic class: aminoglycoside
Therapeutic class: antibiotic
Pregnancy risk category: D

Indications and dosages

▶ **Serious infections caused by sensitive strains of *Citrobacter, Enterobacter, Escherichia coli, Klebsiella, Proteus, Providencia, Pseudomonas, Serratia, Staphylococcus aureus.*** *Adults and children with normal renal*

function: 3 mg/kg I.M. or I.V. daily divided q 8 hours. Up to 5 mg/kg daily divided q 6 to 8 hours for life-threatening infections.
Neonates under age 1 week or premature infants: up to 4 mg/kg I.V. or I.M. daily in two equal doses q 12 hours.

How supplied

Injection: 40 mg/ml, 10 mg/ml (pediatric)
Powder for injection: 30 mg/ml after reconstitution
Premixed parenteral injection for I.V. infusion: 60 mg or 80 mg in normal saline solution

Pharmacokinetics

Absorption: unknown after I.M. administration.
Distribution: distributed widely, although CSF penetration is low, even in patients with inflamed meninges. Protein-binding is minimal.
Metabolism: not metabolized.
Excretion: excreted primarily in urine; small amount may be excreted in bile. *Half-life:* 2 to 3 hours.

Route	Onset	Peak	Duration
I.V.	Immediate	Immediate	About 8 hr
I.M.	Unknown	30-90 min	About 8 hr

Pharmacodynamics

Chemical effect: inhibits protein synthesis by binding directly to 30S ribosomal subunit. Drug is generally bactericidal.
Therapeutic effect: kills susceptible bacteria. Spectrum of activity includes many aerobic gram-negative organisms, including most strains of *Pseudomonas aeruginosa* and some aerobic gram-positive organisms.

Adverse reactions

CNS: headache, lethargy, confusion, disorientation.
EENT: *ototoxicity.*
GI: nausea, vomiting, diarrhea.
GU: ***nephrotoxicity.***
Hematologic: anemia, eosinophilia, ***leukopenia, thrombocytopenia, agranulocytosis.***
Other: hypersensitivity reactions ***(anaphylaxis).***

Interactions

Drug-drug. *Acyclovir, amphotericin B, cisplatin, methoxyflurane, other aminoglycosides, vancomycin:* increased nephrotoxicity. Use together cautiously.
Cephalothin: increased nephrotoxicity. Use together cautiously.
Dimenhydrinate: may mask symptoms of ototoxicity. Use cautiously.
General anesthetics, neuromuscular blockers: may potentiate neuromuscular blockade. Monitor patient closely.
I.V. loop diuretics (such as furosemide): increased ototoxicity. Use together cautiously.
Parenteral penicillins (such as ticarcillin): tobramycin inactivation in vitro. Don't mix.

Contraindications and precautions

- Contraindicated in patients hypersensitive to aminoglycosides.
- Drug isn't recommended for pregnant or breast-feeding women.
- Use cautiously in elderly patients and patients with impaired kidney function or neuromuscular disorders.

NURSING CONSIDERATIONS

Assessment

- Assess patient's infection before therapy and regularly thereafter.
- Obtain specimen for culture and sensitivity tests before giving first dose. Therapy may begin pending results.
- Draw blood for peak tobramycin level 1 hour after I.M. injection and 30 minutes to 1 hour after infusion ends; draw blood for trough level just before next dose. Don't collect blood in heparinized tube because heparin is incompatible with drug.
- Weigh patient and review baseline kidney function studies before therapy.
- Evaluate patient's hearing before and during therapy. Report tinnitus, vertigo, or hearing loss.

ALERT Blood levels over 12 mcg/ml and trough levels over 2 mcg/ml may be linked to increased risk of toxicity.

- Monitor kidney function (output, specific gravity, urinalysis, BUN and creatinine levels, and creatinine clearance).

• Be alert for adverse reactions and drug interactions.
• Evaluate patient's and family's knowledge of drug therapy.

Nursing diagnoses
• Risk for infection related to susceptible bacteria
• Risk for injury related to potential for drug-induced nephrotoxicity
• Deficient knowledge related to drug therapy

Planning and implementation
I.M. use: Follow normal protocol.
I.V. use: Dilute in 50 to 100 ml of normal saline solution or D_5W for adults and in less volume for children. Infuse over 20 to 60 minutes. After I.V. infusion, flush line with normal saline solution or D_5W.
• Notify prescriber of signs of decreasing kidney function.
• Patient should be well hydrated while taking drug to minimize chemical irritation of renal tubules.
• If no response occurs in 3 to 5 days, therapy may be stopped and new specimens obtained for culture and sensitivity testing.
ALERT Don't confuse tobramycin with Tobicin.

Patient teaching
• Emphasize need to drink 2,000 ml of fluid each day.
• Instruct patient to report adverse reactions.

Evaluation
• Patient is free from infection.
• Patient maintains normal kidney function.
• Patient and family state understanding of drug therapy.

tocainide hydrochloride
(TOH-kay-nighd high-droh-KLOR-ighd)
Tonocard

Pharmacologic class: local anesthetic
Therapeutic class: ventricular antiarrhythmic
Pregnancy risk category: C

Indications and dosages
▶ **Suppression of symptomatic life-threatening ventricular arrhythmias, such as sustained ventricular tachycardia.**
Adults: initially, 400 mg P.O. q 8 hours. Usual dosage is between 1,200 and 1,800 mg daily in three divided doses.

How supplied
Tablets: 400 mg, 600 mg

Pharmacokinetics
Absorption: rapidly and completely absorbed from GI tract.
Distribution: not clearly defined, although drug appears to be widely distributed and apparently crosses blood-brain barrier. Only about 10% to 20% bound to plasma protein.
Metabolism: metabolized apparently in liver to inactive metabolites.
Excretion: excreted in urine. *Half-life:* about 11 to 23 hours.

Route	Onset	Peak	Duration
P.O.	Unknown	0.5-2 hr	8 hr

Pharmacodynamics
Chemical effect: class Ib antiarrhythmic that blocks fast sodium channel in cardiac tissues, especially Purkinje network, without involvement of autonomic nervous system. It reduces rate of rise and amplitude of action potential and decreases automaticity in Purkinje fibers. It shortens duration of action potential and, to lesser extent, decreases effective refractory period in Purkinje fibers.
Therapeutic effect: restores normal sinus rhythm.

Adverse reactions
CNS: *light-headedness, tremors,* restlessness, paresthesia, confusion, *dizziness, vertigo,* drowsiness, fatigue, confusion, headache.
CV: hypotension, ***new or worsened arrhythmias, heart failure, bradycardia,*** palpitations.
EENT: blurred vision, tinnitus.
GI: *nausea,* vomiting, diarrhea, anorexia.
Hematologic: ***blood dyscrasia.***
Hepatic: ***hepatitis.***
Respiratory: ***respiratory arrest, pulmonary fibrosis,*** pneumonitis, ***pulmonary edema.***

Skin: rash, diaphoresis.

Interactions

Drug-drug. *Beta blockers:* decreased myocardial contractility; increased CNS toxicity. Avoid concomitant use.
Cimetidine: may decrease peak tocainide level. Monitor cardiac rhythm closely.
Disopyramide, lidocaine, mexiletine, phenytoin, procainamide, quinidine: additive pharmacologic effect and CNS toxicity. Monitor patient closely.
Rifampin: increased clearance of tocainide. Monitor efficacy of tocainide.

Contraindications and precautions

- Contraindicated in patients hypersensitive to lidocaine or other amide-type local anesthetics and those with second- or third-degree AV block in absence of artificial pacemaker.
- Use cautiously in patients with heart failure or diminished cardiac reserve and those with hepatic or renal impairment. These patients often may be treated effectively with lower dose.
- Safety of drug hasn't been established in breast-feeding women and in children.

NURSING CONSIDERATIONS

Assessment

- Assess patient's condition before therapy and regularly thereafter.
- Monitor therapeutic blood level. Therapeutic blood levels range from 4 to 10 mcg/ml. Report deviations.

ALERT Monitor patient for tremors, which may indicate that maximum dosage has been reached.

- Monitor patient during transition from lidocaine to tocainide.
- Be alert for adverse reactions and drug interactions.
- Evaluate patient's and family's knowledge of drug therapy.

Nursing diagnoses

- Decreased cardiac output related to presence of cardiac arrhythmia
- Risk for injury related to drug-induced adverse reactions
- Deficient knowledge related to drug therapy

Planning and implementation

- Cardiologists commonly call drug "oral lidocaine." It may ease transition from I.V. lidocaine to oral antiarrhythmic therapy.

Patient teaching

- Instruct patient to take drug with food.
- Tell patient to report unusual bruising or bleeding or signs of infection. Agranulocytosis and bone marrow suppression have been reported in patients taking usual doses of drug. Most cases have been reported within first 12 weeks of therapy.
- Tell patient to report sudden onset of pulmonary symptoms, such as coughing, wheezing, and exertional dyspnea. Drug has been linked to serious pulmonary toxicity.
- Dizziness and falling are more likely to occur in elderly patient. Tell patient to take safety precautions.

Evaluation

- Patient exhibits normal cardiac output with abolishment of arrhythmia.
- Patient doesn't experience injury from adverse reactions.
- Patient and family state understanding of drug therapy.

tolazamide

(tohl-AZ-ah-mighd)
Tolinase

Pharmacologic class: sulfonylurea
Therapeutic class: antidiabetic
Pregnancy risk category: C

Indications and dosages

▶ **Adjunct to diet to lower blood glucose levels in patients with type 2 (non-insulin-dependent) diabetes mellitus.** *Adults:* initially, 100 mg P.O. daily with breakfast if fasting blood glucose is under 200 mg/dl, or 250 mg P.O. if fasting blood glucose is over 200 mg/dl. Dosage adjusted at weekly intervals by 100 to 250 mg, as necessary. To avoid hypoglycemia in underweight, undernourished, or elderly patients, increase dosage by 50 to 125 mg daily at weekly intervals, as needed. Maximum daily dosage is 500 mg b.i.d. before meals.

▶ **To change from insulin to oral therapy.** *Adults:* if insulin dosage is under 20 units daily, insulin may be stopped and oral therapy started at 100 mg P.O. daily with breakfast. If insulin dosage is 20 to 40 units daily, insulin may be stopped and oral therapy started at 250 mg P.O. daily with breakfast. If insulin dosage is over 40 units daily, insulin may be decreased by 50% and oral therapy started at 250 mg P.O. daily with breakfast. Dosage may be adjusted by 100 to 250 mg.

How supplied

Tablets: 100 mg, 250 mg, 500 mg

Pharmacokinetics

Absorption: absorbed slowly but well from GI tract.
Distribution: probably distributed in extracellular fluid.
Metabolism: metabolized to several mildly active metabolites.
Excretion: excreted in urine. *Half-life:* 7 hours.

Route	Onset	Peak	Duration
P.O.	4-6 hr	4-6 hr	12-24 hr

Pharmacodynamics

Chemical effect: unknown; probably stimulates insulin release from pancreatic beta cells and reduces glucose output by liver. An extrapancreatic effect increases peripheral sensitivity to insulin.
Therapeutic effect: lowers blood glucose levels.

Adverse reactions

GI: nausea, vomiting.
Hematologic: ***thrombocytopenia, aplastic anemia, agranulocytosis.***
Metabolic: ***hypoglycemia.***
Skin: rash, urticaria, facial flushing.
Other: ***hypersensitivity reactions.***

Interactions

Drug-drug. *Anabolic steroids, chloramphenicol, clofibrate, guanethidine, MAO inhibitors, phenylbutazone, salicylates, sulfonamides:* increased hypoglycemic activity. Monitor blood glucose levels carefully.
Beta blockers, clonidine: prolonged hypoglycemic effect and masked symptoms of hypoglycemia. Monitor patient closely.
Corticosteroids, glucagon, rifampin, thiazide diuretics: decreased hypoglycemic response. Monitor blood glucose level.
Hydantoins: increased blood level of hydantoins. Monitor blood level.
Oral anticoagulants: increased hypoglycemic activity or enhanced anticoagulant effect. Monitor blood glucose levels and PT and INR.
Drug-herb. *Aloe, bilberry leaf, bitter melon, dandelion, fenugreek, garlic, ginseng:* potential improved blood glucose control. Drug dosage may need adjustment.
Drug-lifestyle. *Alcohol use:* possible disulfiram-like reaction. Advise against use with moderate to large amounts of alcohol.

Contraindications and precautions

- Contraindicated in pregnant or breast-feeding women, patients hypersensitive to sulfonylureas, and patients with type 1 diabetes (insulin-dependent), diabetes that can be adequately controlled by diet, or uremia. Also contraindicated in type 2 diabetes complicated by ketosis, acidosis, coma, or other acute complications such as major surgery, severe infection, and severe trauma.
- Use cautiously in elderly, debilitated, or malnourished patients and in those with impaired liver or kidney function or porphyria.
- Safety of drug hasn't been established in children.

NURSING CONSIDERATIONS

Assessment

- Assess patient's blood glucose before therapy and regularly thereafter.
- Patient transferring from insulin therapy to oral antidiabetic requires blood glucose level testing at least three times a day before meals.
- Be alert for adverse reactions and drug interactions.
- Elderly patient may be more sensitive to drug's adverse effects.
- Evaluate patient's and family's knowledge of drug therapy.

Nursing diagnoses

- Ineffective health maintenance related to presence of hyperglycemia
- Risk for injury related to drug-induced hypoglycemia
- Deficient knowledge related to drug therapy

Planning and implementation

- Patient transferring from another oral antidiabetic agent usually needs no transition period.
- Administer drug with food if adverse GI reactions occur.
- Tablets may be crushed to ease administration.

Patient teaching

- Make sure patient knows that therapy relieves symptoms but doesn't cure disease.
- Teach patient about the disease. Stress importance of adhering to therapeutic regimen and diet, weight reduction, exercise, and personal hygiene programs. Emphasize need to avoid infection. Explain how and when to monitor blood glucose level, and teach recognition of and intervention for hypoglycemia and hyperglycemia.
- Tell patient not to change drug dosage without prescriber's consent and to report abnormal blood or urine glucose test results.
- Teach patient to carry candy or other simple sugars to treat mild hypoglycemic episodes. Severe episodes may require hospital treatment.
- Advise patient not to take other medications, including OTC drugs, without first checking with prescriber.
- Advise patient to avoid moderate to large intake of alcohol because of possible disulfiram-like reaction.
- Advise patient to wear or carry medical identification at all times.

Evaluation

- Patient's blood glucose level is normal.
- Patient doesn't experience hypoglycemia.
- Patient and family state understanding of drug therapy.

tolbutamide

(tole-BYOO-tah-mide)
Apo-Tolbutamide, Mobenol ♦, Novo-Butamide ♦, Orinase

Pharmacologic class: sulfonylurea
Therapeutic class: antidiabetic
Pregnancy risk category: C

Indications and dosages

▶ **Adjunct to diet to lower blood glucose levels in patients with type 2 diabetes mellitus (non-insulin-dependent).** *Adults:* initially, 1 to 2 g P.O. daily as single dose or in divided doses b.i.d. to t.i.d. Dosage adjusted, if necessary, to maximum of 3 g daily; manufacturer states that little benefit accrues from dosages above 2 g daily.

▶ **To change from insulin to oral therapy.** *Adults:* if insulin dosage is under 20 units daily, insulin may be stopped and oral therapy started at 1 to 2 g P.O. daily. If insulin dosage is 20 to 40 units daily, insulin may be reduced by 30% to 50% and oral therapy started as above. If insulin dosage is over 40 units daily, insulin may be reduced by 20% and oral therapy started as above. Further reductions in insulin are based on patient's response to oral therapy.

How supplied

Tablets: 250 mg, 500 mg

Pharmacokinetics

Absorption: absorbed well from GI tract.
Distribution: probably distributed in extracellular fluid.
Metabolism: metabolized in liver to inactive metabolites.
Excretion: excreted in urine and feces. *Half-life:* 4 to 5 hours.

Route	Onset	Peak	Duration
P.O.	≤ 1 hr	3-5 hr	6-12 hr

Pharmacodynamics

Chemical effect: unknown; probably stimulates insulin release from pancreatic beta cells and reduces glucose output by liver. An extra-

pancreatic effect increases peripheral sensitivity to insulin.
Therapeutic effect: lowers blood glucose levels.

Adverse reactions

GI: nausea, heartburn.
Hematologic: ***thrombocytopenia, aplastic anemia, agranulocytosis.***
Metabolic: ***hypoglycemia, dilutional hyponatremia.***
Skin: rash, pruritus, facial flushing.
Other: ***hypersensitivity reactions.***

Interactions

Drug-drug. *Anabolic steroids, chloramphenicol, clofibrate, guanethidine, MAO inhibitors, phenylbutazone, salicylates, sulfonamides:* increased hypoglycemic activity. Monitor blood glucose level.
Beta blockers, clonidine: prolonged hypoglycemic effect and masked symptoms of hypoglycemia. Use together cautiously.
Corticosteroids, glucagon, rifampin, thiazide diuretics: decreased hypoglycemic response. Monitor blood glucose level.
Hydantoins: increased blood levels of hydantoins. Monitor blood levels.
Oral anticoagulants: increased hypoglycemic activity or enhanced anticoagulant effect. Monitor blood glucose level, PT, and INR.
Drug-herb. *Aloe, bilberry leaf, bitter melon, dandelion, fenugreek, garlic, ginseng:* potential improved blood glucose control. Drug dosage may need adjustment.
Drug-lifestyle. *Alcohol use:* possible disulfiram-like reaction. Discourage concomitant use of moderate to large amounts of alcohol.

Contraindications and precautions

- Contraindicated in pregnant or breast-feeding women, patients hypersensitive to sulfonylureas, and patients with type 1 diabetes mellitus (insulin-dependent) or diabetes that can be adequately controlled by diet. Also contraindicated in patients with severe renal insufficiency or type 2 diabetes mellitus complicated by fever, ketosis, acidosis, coma, or other acute complications such as major surgery, severe infection, or severe trauma.
- Use cautiously in elderly, debilitated, or malnourished patients and patients with impaired liver or kidney function or porphyria.
- Safety of drug hasn't been established in children.

NURSING CONSIDERATIONS

Assessment

- Assess patient's blood glucose level before therapy and regularly thereafter.
- Patient transferring from insulin therapy to oral antidiabetic requires blood glucose level testing at least three times daily before meals.
- Be alert for adverse reactions and drug interactions.
- Elderly patient may be more sensitive to drug's adverse effects.
- Evaluate patient's and family's knowledge of drug therapy.

Nursing diagnoses

- Ineffective health maintenance related to presence of hyperglycemia
- Risk for injury related to drug-induced hypoglycemia
- Deficient knowledge related to drug therapy

Planning and implementation

- Patient transferring from another oral antidiabetic usually needs no transition period.
- To avoid GI intolerance for patient taking large doses and to improve control of hyperglycemia, give divided doses before morning and evening meals.
- Tablets may be crushed to ease administration.

Patient teaching

- Make sure patient knows that therapy relieves symptoms but doesn't cure disease.
- Teach patient about the disease. Stress the importance of adhering to therapeutic regimen and diet, weight reduction, exercise, and personal hygiene programs. Emphasize the need to avoid infection. Explain how and when to monitor blood glucose level, and teach recognition of and intervention for hypoglycemia and hyperglycemia.

• Tell patient not to change drug dosage without prescriber's consent and to report abnormal blood or urine glucose test results.
• Teach patient to carry candy or other simple sugars to treat mild hypoglycemic episodes. Severe episodes may require hospital treatment.
• Advise patient not to take other medication, including OTC drugs, without first checking with prescriber.
• Advise patient to avoid moderate to large intake of alcohol because of possible disulfiram-like reaction.
• Advise patient to wear or carry medical identification at all times.

☑ Evaluation

• Patient's blood glucose level is normal.
• Patient doesn't experience hypoglycemia.
• Patient and family state understanding of drug therapy.

tolcapone

(TOHL-cah-pohn)
Tasmar

Pharmacologic class: catechol-O-methyltransferase (COMT) inhibitor
Therapeutic class: antiparkinsonian
Pregnancy risk category: C

Indications and dosages

▶ **Adjunct to levodopa and carbidopa for treatment of signs and symptoms of idiopathic Parkinson's disease.** *Adults:* initially, 100 mg P.O. t.i.d. (with levodopa-carbidopa). Recommended daily dosage is 100 mg P.O. t.i.d. although 200 mg P.O. t.i.d. also can be given if the anticipated clinical benefit is justified. If starting treatment with 200 mg t.i.d. and dyskinesia occurs, reduced dosage of levodopa may be necessary. Maximum daily dosage is 600 mg.

How supplied

Tablets: 100 mg, 200 mg

Pharmacokinetics

Absorption: rapid. Absolute bioavailability is 65% following P.O. administration.
Distribution: not widely distributed into tissues; over 99.9% is bound to plasma proteins.
Metabolism: almost completely metabolized before excretion mainly by glucuronidation.
Excretion: following P.O. administration, 60% excreted in urine and 40% in feces. *Half-life:* 2 to 3 hours.

Route	Onset	Peak	Duration
P.O.	Unknown	2 hr	Unknown

Pharmacodynamics

Chemical effect: exact mechanism unknown. Thought to reversibly inhibit human erythrocyte COMT when given in combination with levodopa-carbidopa, resulting in a decrease in levodopa clearance and a twofold increase in levodopa bioavailability. Decreased clearance of levodopa prolongs elimination half-life of levodopa from 2 to 3.5 hours.
Therapeutic effect: improves physical mobility in patients with parkinsonism.

Adverse reactions

CNS: *dyskinesia, sleep disorder, dystonia, excessive dreaming, somnolence,* dizziness, *confusion, headache, hallucinations,* hyperkinesia, hypertonia, fatigue, falling, syncope, balance loss, depression, tremor, speech disorder, paresthesia, agitation, irritability, mental deficiency, hyperactivity, hypokinesia.
CV: *orthostatic complaints,* chest pain, chest discomfort, palpitations, hypotension.
EENT: pharyngitis, tinnitus, sinus congestion.
GI: *nausea, anorexia, diarrhea,* flatulence, *vomiting,* constipation, abdominal pain, dyspepsia, dry mouth.
GU: urinary tract infection, urine discoloration, hematuria, micturition disorder, urinary incontinence, impotence.
Musculoskeletal: *muscle cramps,* stiffness, arthritis, neck pain.
Respiratory: bronchitis, dyspnea, upper respiratory tract infection.
Skin: increased sweating, rash.
Other: bleeding, burning, fever, influenza.

Interactions

Drug-drug. *CNS depressants:* enhanced sedative effects. Use cautiously.
Desipramine: increased risk of adverse effects. Use cautiously.
Nonselective MAO inhibitors (phenelzine, tranylcypromine): possible hypertensive crisis. Avoid concomitant use.

Contraindications and precautions

- Contraindicated in patients hypersensitive to drug or its components and patients with liver disease or elevated ALT or AST values. Also contraindicated in patients withdrawn from tolcapone because of evidence of drug-induced hepatocellular injury and patients with history of nontraumatic rhabdomyolysis, hyperpyrexia, and confusion possibly related to drug.
- Use cautiously in patients with severe renal impairment and in breast-feeding women.

NURSING CONSIDERATIONS

Assessment

- Assess patient's history of Parkinson's disease, and reassess during therapy.
- Monitor liver enzyme levels before therapy, then every 2 weeks during first 3 and a half years of therapy, then every 8 weeks thereafter because of risk of liver toxicity. Stop drug if results are elevated or if patient appears jaundiced. Assess patient's risk for physical injury because of drug's CNS adverse effects.
- Monitor patient for orthostatic hypotension and syncope.
- Evaluate patient's and family's knowledge of drug therapy.

Nursing diagnoses

- Impaired physical mobility related to underlying Parkinson's disease
- Disturbed thought processes related to drug-induced CNS adverse reactions
- Deficient knowledge related to drug therapy

Planning and implementation

ALERT Patient should provide written informed consent before drug is used. Give drug only to patients receiving levodopa and carbidopa who don't respond to or who aren't appropriate candidates for other adjunctive therapies because of risk of liver toxicity.

- Administer first dose of day with first daily dose of levodopa-carbidopa.
- Patients with severe renal dysfunction may require a reduced dose.
- Withhold drug and notify prescriber if hepatic transaminases are elevated or if patient appears jaundiced.
- Because of risk of liver toxicity, stop treatment if patient shows no benefit within 3 weeks, as ordered.
- Because of highly protein-bound nature of tolcapone, drug isn't expected to be removed significantly during dialysis.
- Notify prescriber if severe diarrhea occurs that is linked to drug therapy.

Patient teaching

- Advise patient to take drug exactly as prescribed.
- Teach patient signs of liver injury (jaundice, fatigue, loss of appetite, persistent nausea, pruritus, dark urine or right upper quadrant tenderness) and instruct him to report them immediately.
- Warn patient about risk of orthostatic hypotension; tell him to use caution when rising from a seated or recumbent position.
- Caution patient to avoid hazardous activities until CNS effects of drug are known.
- Tell patient that nausea may occur at the start of therapy.
- Inform patient about risk of increased dyskinesia or dystonia.
- Tell patient to report planned, suspected, or known pregnancy during therapy.
- Instruct patient to report to prescriber adverse effects, including diarrhea and hallucinations.
- Inform patient that drug may be taken without regard to meals.

Evaluation

- Patient exhibits improved mobility with reduction of muscular rigidity and tremor.
- Patient remains mentally alert.
- Patient and family state understanding of drug therapy.

tolmetin sodium

(TOHL-meh-tin SOH-dee-um)
Tolectin 200, Tolectin 600, Tolectin DS

Pharmacologic class: NSAID
Therapeutic class: nonnarcotic analgesic, antipyretic, anti-inflammatory
Pregnancy risk category: C

Indications and dosages

▶ **Rheumatoid arthritis, osteoarthritis, juvenile rheumatoid arthritis.** *Adults:* 400 mg P.O. t.i.d. Maximum daily dosage is 1.8 g.
Children age 2 and over: 15 to 30 mg/kg P.O. daily in three or four divided doses.

How supplied

Tablets: 200 mg, 600 mg
Capsules: 400 mg

Pharmacokinetics

Absorption: absorbed rapidly from GI tract.
Distribution: highly protein-bound.
Metabolism: metabolized in liver.
Excretion: excreted in urine. *Half-life:* 1 to 2 hours.

Route	Onset	Peak	Duration
P.O.	Unknown	30-60 min	Unknown

Pharmacodynamics

Chemical effect: unknown; produces anti-inflammatory, analgesic, and antipyretic effects, possibly by inhibiting prostaglandin synthesis.
Therapeutic effect: relieves pain, fever, and inflammation.

Adverse reactions

CNS: headache, dizziness, drowsiness.
CV: edema.
EENT: tinnitus, visual disturbances.
GI: *epigastric distress, **peptic ulceration,*** occult blood loss, *nausea, **GI bleeding.***
GU: ***nephrotoxicity,*** pseudoproteinuria, ***renal failure.***
Hematologic: prolonged bleeding time, granulocytopenia, ***thrombocytopenia, agranulocytosis.***
Metabolic: sodium retention, weight gain.
Skin: rash, urticaria, pruritus.
Other: ***anaphylaxis.***

Interactions

Drug-drug. *Aspirin:* decreased tolmetin levels. Avoid concurrent use.
Methotrexate: increased risk of methotrexate toxicity. Monitor patient closely.
Oral anticoagulants: increased risk of bleeding. Monitor patient closely.
Drug-lifestyle. *Alcohol use:* increased risk of GI toxicity. Discourage concurrent use.

Contraindications and precautions

- Contraindicated in patients hypersensitive to drug; those whose acute asthmatic attacks, urticaria, or rhinitis is precipitated by aspirin or NSAIDs; and breast-feeding women.
- Drug isn't recommended for use during second half of pregnancy.
- Use cautiously in patients with cardiac or renal disease, GI bleeding, history of peptic ulcer disease, hypertension, or conditions predisposing to fluid retention.

NURSING CONSIDERATIONS

Assessment

- Assess patient's arthritis before therapy and regularly thereafter.
- During prolonged therapy, patient should have regular eye examinations, hearing tests, CBCs, and kidney function tests to check for toxicity.
- Be alert for adverse reactions and drug interactions.
- Evaluate patient's and family's knowledge of drug therapy.

Nursing diagnoses

- Acute pain related to presence of arthritis
- Impaired tissue integrity related to drug's adverse effect on GI mucosa
- Deficient knowledge related to drug therapy

Planning and implementation

- Drug may interfere with certain tests for urinary proteins; it doesn't interfere with dye-impregnated reagent strips.
- Report signs of serious GI toxicity.

Patient teaching

- Tell patient to take drug with food, milk, or antacids.
- Tell patient that therapeutic effect begins within 1 week but that full effect may be delayed 2 to 4 weeks.
- Advise patient to avoid activities that require alertness until drug's CNS effects are known.
- Teach patient signs of GI bleeding and tell him to report them promptly.
- Instruct patient to report immediately changes in vision or hearing.

Evaluation

- Patient has relief from pain.
- Patient doesn't exhibit signs of GI toxicity.
- Patient and family state understanding of drug therapy.

tolterodine tartrate

(tohl-TER-oh-deen TAR-trate)
Detrol

Pharmacologic class: muscarinic receptor antagonist
Therapeutic class: anticholinergic
Pregnancy risk category: C

Indications and dosages

▶ **Overactive bladder in patients with symptoms of urinary frequency, urgency, or urge incontinence.** *Adults:* 2 mg P.O. b.i.d. Dose may be lowered to 1 mg P.O. b.i.d. based on patient response and tolerance.

How supplied

Tablets: 1 mg, 2 mg

Pharmacokinetics

Absorption: drug is well absorbed with about 77% bioavailability. Peak serum levels occur within 1 to 2 hours after administration. Food increases bioavailability by 53%.
Distribution: volume of distribution is about 113 L. Drug is highly protein-bound (96%).
Metabolism: metabolized by the liver primarily by oxidation by the cytochrome P-450 2D6 pathway and leads to the formation of a pharmacologically active 5-hydroxymethyl metabolite.
Excretion: mostly recovered in urine; the rest in feces. Less than 1% of dose is recovered as unchanged drug, and 5% to 14% is recovered as the active metabolite. *Half-life:* 1¾ to 3½ hours.

Route	Onset	Peak	Duration
P.O.	Unknown	1-2 hr	Unknown

Pharmacodynamics

Chemical effect: a competitive muscarinic receptor antagonist. Both urinary bladder contraction and salivation are mediated via cholinergic muscarinic receptors.
Therapeutic effect: relieves symptoms of overactive bladder.

Adverse reactions

CNS: fatigue, paresthesia, vertigo, dizziness, *headache,* nervousness, somnolence.
CV: hypertension, chest pain.
EENT: abnormal vision, xerophthalmia, pharyngitis, rhinitis, sinusitis.
GI: *dry mouth,* abdominal pain, constipation, diarrhea, dyspepsia, flatulence, nausea, vomiting.
GU: dysuria, micturition frequency, urine retention, urinary tract infection.
Metabolic: weight gain.
Musculoskeletal: arthralgia, back pain.
Respiratory: bronchitis, cough, upper respiratory tract infection.
Skin: pruritus, rash, erythema, dry skin.
Other: flu syndrome, falls, infection fungal, infection.

Interactions

Drug-drug. *Antifungal drugs (itraconazole, ketoconazole, miconazole), cytochrome P-450 3A4 inhibitors (such as macrolide antibiotics clarithromycin and erythromycin):* effects haven't been studied. However, tolterodine doses above 1 mg b.i.d. shouldn't be given concurrently.

Fluoxetine: increased tolterodine levels. Avoid concomitant use.

Contraindications and precautions

- Contraindicated in patients hypersensitive to drug or its components and those with uncontrolled narrow-angle glaucoma or urine or gastric retention.
- Use with caution in patients with significant bladder outflow obstruction, GI obstructive disorders (such as pyloric stenosis), controlled narrow-angle glaucoma, and hepatic or renal impairment.

NURSING CONSIDERATIONS

Assessment

- Assess baseline bladder function and monitor therapeutic effects.
- Be alert for adverse reactions and drug interactions.
- Evaluate patient's and family's knowledge about drug therapy.

Nursing diagnoses

- Impaired urinary elimination related to underlying medical condition
- Urinary retention related to drug-induced adverse effects
- Deficient knowledge related to drug therapy

Planning and implementation

- Food increases the absorption of tolterodine, but no dosage adjustment is needed.
- In the case of urine retention, notify prescriber and prepare for urinary catheterization.
- Dry mouth is the most frequently reported adverse reaction.
- For adults with significantly reduced hepatic function or in those who are currently taking drug that inhibits cytochrome P-450 3A4 isoenzyme system, 1 mg P.O. b.i.d.

Patient teaching

- Tell patient that sugarless gum, hard candy, or saliva substitute may help relieve dry mouth.
- Advise patient to avoid driving or other potentially hazardous activities until visual effects of drug are known.
- Advise breast-feeding women to discontinue breast-feeding during therapy.
- Instruct patient to immediately report signs of infection, urine retention, or GI problems.

Evaluation

- Patient experiences improved bladder function with drug therapy.
- Patient doesn't experience urine retention.
- Patient and family state understanding of drug therapy.

topiramate

(toh-PEER-uh-mayt)

Topamax

Pharmacologic class: sulfamate-substituted monosaccharide

Therapeutic class: antiepileptic

Pregnancy risk category: C

Indications and dosages

▶ **Adjunctive therapy of partial-onset seizures.** *Adults:* adjust dosage up to maximum of 400 mg/day P.O. in divided doses b.i.d. Dosage adjustment schedule is as follows: Week 1, 50 mg P.O. in evening; week 2, 50 mg P.O. b.i.d.; week 3, 50 mg P.O. in morning and 100 mg P.O. in evening; week 4, 100 mg P.O. b.i.d.; week 5, 100 mg P.O. in morning and 150 mg P.O. in evening; week 6, 150 mg P.O. b.i.d.; week 7, 150 mg P.O. in morning and 200 mg P.O. in evening; week 8, 200 mg P.O. b.i.d.

▶ **Adjunctive therapy for partial onset seizures in children.** *Children ages 2 to 16:* initially, 25 mg (or less based on a range of 1 to 3 mg/kg/day) P.O. nightly for the first week. Increase dosage based on clinical response at 1- to 2-week intervals by increments of 1 to 3 mg/kg/day administered in two divided doses. The recommended total daily dosage is 5 to 9 mg/kg/day P.O. in two divided doses.

▶ **Adjunctive therapy for primary generalized tonic-clonic seizure.** *Adults:* 50 mg P.O. daily in the evening for the first week; then adjust to a maximum daily dosage of 400 mg given in two divided doses. Adjustment schedule is as follows: Week 1, 50 mg P.O. in the

evening; week 2, 50 mg P.O. twice daily (in the morning and evening); week 3, 50 mg P.O. in the morning and 100 mg P.O. in the evening; week 4, 100 mg P.O. twice daily (in the morning and evening); week 5, 100 mg P.O. in the morning and 150 mg P.O. in the evening; week 6, 150 mg P.O. twice daily (in the morning and evening); week 7, 150 mg P.O. in the morning and 200 mg P.O. in the evening; week 8, 200 mg P.O. twice daily (in the morning and evening).
Children ages 2 to 16: 1 to 3 mg/kg P.O. daily in the evening for the first week; then increase at 1- or 2-week intervals by increments of 1 to 3 mg/kg/day. Dosage range is 5 to 9 mg/kg/day given in two divided doses. Adjust dosage based on clinical response.

How supplied

Tablets: 25 mg, 100 mg, 200 mg
Capsules: 15 mg, 25 mg

Pharmacokinetics

Absorption: rapid absorption following P.O. dose.
Distribution: up to 17% bound to plasma proteins.
Metabolism: not extensively metabolized.
Excretion: primarily eliminated unchanged in urine. *Half-life:* 21 hours.

Route	Onset	Peak	Duration
P.O.	Unknown	2 hr	Unknown

Pharmacodynamics

Chemical effect: precise mechanism of action unknown. Thought to block action potential, suggestive of a sodium channel blocking action. Drug may also potentiate activity of gamma-aminobutyrate (GABA) and antagonize ability of kainate to activate the kainate/alpha-amino-3-hydroxy-5-methylisoxazole-4-proprionic acid subtype of excitatory amino acid (glutamate) receptor. Drug also has weak carbonic anhydrase inhibitor activity, which is unrelated to its antiepileptic properties.
Therapeutic effect: prevents partial-onset seizures.

Adverse reactions

CNS: *fatigue,* abnormal coordination, aggression, agitation, apathy, asthenia, *ataxia, confusion,* depression, depersonalization, *dizziness,* emotional lability, euphoria, ***generalized tonic-clonic seizures,*** hallucination, hyperkinesia, hypertonia, hypoesthesia, hypokinesia, insomnia, *nervousness, nystagmus, paresthesia,* personality disorder, *psychomotor slowing,* psychosis, *somnolence, speech disorders,* stupor, ***suicide attempts,*** *tremor,* vertigo, malaise, mood problems, difficulty with concentration, attention, language, or *memory.*
CV: chest pain, palpitations, edema.
EENT: *abnormal vision,* conjunctivitis, *diplopia,* eye pain, hearing problems, pharyngitis, sinusitis, tinnitus.
GI: taste perversion, abdominal pain, anorexia, constipation, diarrhea, dry mouth, dyspepsia, flatulence, gastroenteritis, gingivitis, *nausea,* vomiting.
GU: amenorrhea, decreased libido, dysuria, dysmenorrhea, hematuria, impotence, intermenstrual bleeding, menstrual disorder, menorrhagia, micturition frequency, renal calculus, urinary incontinence, urinary tract infection, vaginitis, leukorrhea.
Hematologic: anemia, epistaxis, ***leukopenia.***
Metabolic: weight changes.
Musculoskeletal: arthralgia, back or leg pain, muscle weakness, myalgia, rigors.
Respiratory: bronchitis, cough, dyspnea, *upper respiratory tract infection.*
Skin: acne, alopecia, increased sweating, pruritus, rash.
Other: body odor, fever, flulike symptoms, breast pain, hot flushes.

Interactions

Drug-drug. *Carbamazepine:* decreased topiramate levels. Monitor patient.
Carbonic anhydrase inhibitors (acetazolamide, dichlorphenamide): increased risk of renal calculus formation. Avoid concomitant use.
CNS depressants: possible topiramate-induced CNS depression, as well as other adverse cognitive and neuropsychiatric events. Use cautiously.
Oral contraceptives: decreased efficacy. Report changes in bleeding patterns.

Phenytoin: decreased topiramate levels and increased phenytoin levels. Monitor levels.
Valproic acid: decreased valproic acid and topiramate levels. Monitor patient.
Drug-lifestyle. *Alcohol use:* possible topiramate-induced CNS depression, as well as other adverse cognitive and neuropsychiatric events. Discourage concurrent use.

Contraindications and precautions

- Contraindicated in patients hypersensitive to drug or its components.
- Use cautiously in patients with hepatic impairment and in breast-feeding or pregnant women.

NURSING CONSIDERATIONS

Assessment

- Assess patient's seizure disorder before therapy and regularly thereafter.
- Carefully monitor patients taking topiramate in conjunction with other antiepileptic drugs; dosage adjustments may be needed to achieve optimal response.
- Assess patient's compliance with therapy at each follow-up visit.
- Evaluate patient's and family's knowledge of drug therapy.

Nursing diagnoses

- Risk for injury related to seizure disorder
- Acute pain related to increased risk of renal calculi formation
- Deficient knowledge related to drug therapy

Planning and implementation

- Renal insufficiency requires a reduced dose. For hemodialysis patients, supplemental doses may be required to avoid rapid drops in drug levels during prolonged dialysis treatment.
- Dosage will have to be adjusted according to patient's response.
- Initiate safety precautions as indicated.

Patient teaching

- Tell patient to maintain adequate fluid intake during therapy to minimize risk of forming renal calculi.
- Advise patient not to drive or operate hazardous machinery until CNS effects of drug are known.
- Tell patient that drug may decrease effectiveness of oral contraceptives and to use a barrier form of birth control.
- Tell patient to avoid crushing or breaking tablets because of bitter taste.
- Tell patient that drug can be taken without regard to food.

Evaluation

- Patient is free from seizure activity.
- Patient maintains adequate hydration to prevent renal calculus formation.
- Patient and family state understanding of drug therapy.

topotecan hydrochloride

(toh-poh-TEE-ken high-droh-KLOR-ighd)
Hycamtin

Pharmacologic class: antitumor agent
Therapeutic class: antineoplastic
Pregnancy risk category: NR

Indications and dosages

▶ **Metastatic carcinoma of ovary after failure of initial or subsequent chemotherapy; treatment of small cell lung cancer sensitive disease after failure of first-line chemotherapy.** *Adults:* 1.5 mg/m^2 by I.V. daily for 5 consecutive days, starting on day 1 of a 21-day cycle, for minimum of four cycles. For patients with creatinine clearance of 20 to 39 ml/minute, decrease dosage to 0.75 mg/m^2. If severe neutropenia occurs, reduce dosage by 0.25 mg/m^2 for subsequent courses. Or, in severe neutropenia, give granulocyte-colony stimulating factor (GSF) after subsequent course (before resorting to dosage reduction) starting from day 6 of the course (24 hours after topotecan administration).

How supplied

Injection: 4-mg single-dose vial

Pharmacokinetics

Absorption: proportional to dose.

Distribution: about 35% bound to plasma proteins.
Metabolism: metabolized by liver.
Excretion: 30% excreted in urine.

Route	Onset	Peak	Duration
I.V.	Unknown	Unknown	Unknown

Pharmacodynamics

Chemical effect: relieves torsional strain in DNA and prevents relegation of single-strand breaks.
Therapeutic effect: cytotoxicity is thought to result from double-strand DNA damage produced during DNA synthesis when replication enzymes interact with the complex formed.

Adverse reactions

CNS: *fatigue, asthenia, headache,* paresthesia.
GI: *nausea, vomiting, diarrhea, constipation, abdominal pain, stomatitis, anorexia.*
Hematologic: NEUTROPENIA, LEUKOPENIA, THROMBOCYTOPENIA, *anemia.*
Hepatic: transient elevation of AST, ALT, and bilirubin levels.
Respiratory: *dyspnea.*
Skin: *alopecia.*
Other: ***sepsis,*** *fever.*

Interactions

Drug-drug. *Cisplatin:* increases severity of myelosuppression. Use both drugs very cautiously.
GSF: prolongs duration of neutropenia. If GSF is used, don't start it until day 6 of course, 24 hours after completion of topotecan treatment.

Contraindications and precautions

- Contraindicated in patients hypersensitive to drug or its components, in pregnant or breast-feeding women, and in patients with severe bone marrow depression.

NURSING CONSIDERATIONS

Assessment

ALERT Patient must have a baseline neutrophil count above 1,500 cells/mm^3 and platelet count above 100,000 cells/mm^3 before therapy can start.

- Frequent monitoring of peripheral blood cell count is critical. Don't give repeated doses until neutrophil count is over 1,000 cells/mm^3, platelet count is over 100,000 cells/mm^3, and hemoglobin level over 9 mg/dl.
- Evaluate patient's and family's understanding of drug therapy.

Nursing diagnoses

- Ineffective health maintenance related to neoplastic disease
- Deficient knowledge related to drug therapy

Planning and implementation

- Prepare drug under a vertical laminar flow hood while wearing gloves and protective clothing. If drug contacts skin, wash immediately and thoroughly with soap and water. If mucous membranes are affected, flush with water.
- Reconstitute each 4-mg vial with 4 ml sterile water for injection. Dilute appropriate volume of reconstituted solution in normal saline solution or D_5W before use. Infuse over 30 minutes.
- Protect unopened vials of drug from light. Reconstituted vials stored at 68° to 77° F (20° to 25° C) and exposed to ambient lighting are stable for 24 hours.

Patient teaching

- Instruct patient to report promptly sore throat, fever, chills, or unusual bleeding or bruising.
- Advise woman of childbearing age to avoid pregnancy and breast-feeding during treatment.
- Tell patient and family about need for close monitoring of blood counts.

Evaluation

- Patient shows positive response to drug.
- Patient and family state understanding of drug therapy.

torsemide

(TOR-seh-mighd)
Demadex

Pharmacologic class: loop diuretic
Therapeutic class: diuretic, antihypertensive
Pregnancy risk category: B

Indications and dosages

▶ **Diuresis in patients with heart failure.** *Adults:* initially, 10 to 20 mg P.O. or I.V. once daily. If response is inadequate, dose is doubled until response is obtained. Maximum dosage is 200 mg daily.

▶ **Diuresis in patients with chronic renal failure.** *Adults:* initially, 20 mg P.O. or I.V. once daily. If response is inadequate, dose is doubled until response is obtained. Maximum dosage is 200 mg daily.

▶ **Diuresis in patients with hepatic cirrhosis.** *Adults:* initially, 5 to 10 mg P.O. or I.V. once daily with aldosterone antagonist or potassium-sparing diuretic. If response is inadequate, dose is doubled until response is obtained. Maximum dosage is 40 mg daily.

▶ **Hypertension.** *Adults:* initially, 5 mg P.O. daily. Increased to 10 mg in 4 to 6 weeks if needed and tolerated. If response is still inadequate, another antihypertensive agent should be added.

How supplied

Injection: 10 mg/ml
Tablets: 5 mg, 10 mg, 20 mg, 100 mg

Pharmacokinetics

Absorption: absorbed with little first-pass metabolism after P.O. administration.
Distribution: extensively bound to plasma protein.
Metabolism: metabolized in liver.
Excretion: 22% to 34% excreted unchanged in urine.

Route	Onset	Peak	Duration
P.O.	1 hr	1-2 hr	6-8 hr
I.V.	$\leq$ 10 min	$\leq$ 1 hr	6-8 hr

Pharmacodynamics

Chemical effect: enhances excretion of sodium, chloride, and water by acting on ascending portion of loop of Henle.
Therapeutic effect: promotes water and sodium excretion and lowers blood pressure.

Adverse reactions

CNS: asthenia; dizziness, headache, nervousness, insomnia, syncope.
CV: ECG abnormalities, chest pain, edema, ***dehydration,*** orthostatic hypertension.
EENT: rhinitis, sore throat.
GI: *excessive thirst,* diarrhea, constipation, nausea, dyspepsia, *hemorrhage.*
GU: *excessive urination,* impotence.
Hepatic: increased cholesterol level.
Metabolic: electrolyte imbalances, including *hypokalemia, hypomagnesemia,* hypocalcemia, hyperuricemia, gout, hyperglycemia; increased uric acid; hypochloremic alkalosis.
Musculoskeletal: arthralgia, myalgia.
Respiratory: cough.

Interactions

Drug-drug. *Cholestyramine:* decreased absorption of torsemide. Separate administration times by at least 3 hours.
Digoxin: decreased torsemide clearance. Dosage adjustments not needed.
Indomethacin: decreased diuretic effectiveness in sodium-restricted patients. Avoid concomitant use.
Lithium, ototoxic drugs (such as aminoglycosides, ethacrynic acid): possible increased toxicity of these drugs. Avoid concomitant use.
NSAIDs: may potentiate nephrotoxicity of NSAIDs. Use together cautiously.
Probenecid: decreased diuretic effectiveness. Avoid concomitant use.
Salicylates: decreased excretion, possibly leading to salicylate toxicity. Avoid concomitant use.
Spironolactone: decreased renal clearance of spironolactone. Dosage adjustments not necessary.
Drug-herb. *Licorice:* potential for rapid potassium loss. Discourage concomitant use.

Contraindications and precautions

• Contraindicated in patients hypersensitive to drug or other sulfonylurea derivatives and in those with anuria.
• Use cautiously in patients with hepatic disease, cirrhosis, and ascites; sudden changes in fluid and electrolyte balance may precipitate hepatic coma in these patients. Also use cautiously in pregnant or breast-feeding women.
• Safety of drug hasn't been established in children.

NURSING CONSIDERATIONS

Assessment

• Assess patient's condition before therapy and regularly thereafter.
• Monitor elderly patients, who are especially susceptible to excessive diuresis, with potential for circulatory collapse and thromboembolic complications.
• Monitor fluid intake and output, serum electrolyte levels, blood pressure, weight, and pulse rate during rapid diuresis and routinely with long-term use. Drug can cause profound diuresis and water and electrolyte depletion.
• Watch for signs of hypokalemia, such as muscle weakness and cramps.
• Be alert for adverse reactions and drug interactions.
• Evaluate patient's and family's knowledge of drug therapy.

Nursing diagnoses

• Excessive fluid volume related to presence of edema
• Risk for injury related to presence of hypertension
• Deficient knowledge related to drug therapy

Planning and implementation

P.O. use: Give drug in morning to prevent nocturia.
I.V. use: Inspect ampules for precipitate or discoloration before use.
– Drug may be given by direct injection over at least 2 minutes. Rapid injection may cause ototoxicity. Don't give more than 200 mg at a time.
• Consult prescriber and dietitian to provide high-potassium diet. Foods rich in potassium include citrus fruits, tomatoes, bananas, dates, and apricots.
ALERT Don't confuse torsemide with furosemide.

Patient teaching

• Tell patient to take drug in morning to prevent sleep interruption.
• Advise patient to change position slowly to prevent dizziness and to limit alcohol intake and strenuous exercise in hot weather to prevent orthostatic hypotension.
• Advise patient to immediately report ringing in ears because it may indicate toxicity.
• Tell patient to check with prescriber or pharmacist before taking other OTC medications.

Evaluation

• Patient shows no signs of edema.
• Patient's blood pressure is normal.
• Patient and family state understanding of drug therapy.

trace elements
(trays EL-uh-ments)

chromium (chromic chloride)
(KROH-mee-um)
Chroma-Pak, Chromic Chloride

copper (cupric sulfate)
(KAH-per)
Cupric Sulfate

iodine (sodium iodide)
(IGH-oh-dighn)
Iodopen

manganese (manganese chloride, manganese sulfate)
(MAN-geh-nees)

selenium (selenious acid)
(seh-LEHN-ee-um)
Sele-Pak, Selepen

zinc (zinc chloride, zinc sulfate)

(zink)

Zinca-Pak

Pharmacologic class: trace elements
Therapeutic class: nutritional agents
Pregnancy risk category: C

Indications and dosages

▶ **Prevention of individual trace element deficiencies in patients receiving long-term total parenteral nutrition (TPN). Chromium.** *Adults:* 10 to 15 mcg I.V. daily.
Children: 0.14 to 0.20 mcg/kg I.V. daily.
Copper. *Adults:* 0.5 to 1.5 mg I.V. daily.
Children: 20 mcg/kg I.V. daily.
Iodine. *Adults:* 1 to 2 mcg/kg I.V. daily.
Children: 2 to 3 mcg/kg I.V. daily.
Manganese. *Adults:* 0.15 to 0.8 mg I.V. daily.
Children: 2 to 10 mcg/kg I.V. daily.
Selenium. *Adults:* 20 to 40 mcg I.V. daily.
Children: 3 mcg/kg I.V. daily.
Zinc. *Adults:* 2.5 to 4 mg I.V. daily.
Children age 5 or younger: 100 mcg/kg I.V. daily.
Neonates: 300 mcg/kg/I.V. daily.

How supplied

chromium
Injection: 4 mcg/ml, 20 mcg/ml
copper
Injection: 0.4 mg/ml, 2 mg/ml
iodine
Injection: 100 mcg/ml
manganese
Injection: 0.1 mg/ml
selenium
Injection: 40 mcg/ml
zinc
Injection: 1 mg/ml, 5 mg/ml

Pharmacokinetics

Absorption: not applicable.
Distribution: unknown.
Metabolism: unknown.
Excretion: unknown.

Route	Onset	Peak	Duration
I.V.	Immediate	Immediate	Unknown

Pharmacodynamics

Chemical effect: participates in synthesis and stabilization of proteins and nucleic acids in subcellular and membrane transport systems.
Therapeutic effect: restores normal body levels of trace elements.

Adverse reactions

GI: nausea, vomiting.

Interactions

None significant at suggested dosages.

Contraindications and precautions

- No known contraindications.

NURSING CONSIDERATIONS

Assessment

- Obtain history of patient's underlying trace element deficiency before therapy and reassess regularly thereafter. Keep in mind that normal serum levels are 0.85 ng/ml chromium; 0.07 to 0.15 mg/ml copper; 4 to 20 mcg/dl manganese; 0.1 to 0.19 mcg/ml selenium; and 0.05 to 0.15 mg/dl zinc.
- Check serum levels of trace elements in patients who have received TPN for 2 months or longer, as ordered. Call prescriber's attention to low serum levels of these elements because supplement may be needed.
- Evaluate patient's and family's knowledge of drug therapy.

Nursing diagnoses

- Imbalanced nutrition: less than body requirements related to presence of deficiency of trace elements
- Deficient knowledge related to drug therapy

Planning and implementation

- Cautiously infuse diluted solution through patent I.V. line over ordered duration.

ALERT Don't administer undiluted because of potential for phlebitis.

- Solutions of trace elements are compounded by pharmacy for addition to TPN solutions according to various formulas. One common trace element solution is Shil's solution, which contains copper 1 mg/ml, iodide 0.06 mg/ml, manganese 0.4 mg/ml, and zinc 2 mg/ml.

Patient teaching
- Inform patient and family of need for trace elements.

☑ Evaluation
- Patient regains normal serum levels of trace elements.
- Patient and family state understanding of drug therapy.

tramadol hydrochloride
(TRAM-uh-dohl high-droh-KLOR-ighd)
Ultram

Pharmacologic class: synthetic analgesic
Therapeutic class: analgesic
Pregnancy risk category: C

Indications and dosages
▶ **Moderate to moderately severe pain.** *Adults:* 50 to 100 mg P.O. q 4 to 6 hours, p.r.n. Maximum dosage is 400 mg daily.

How supplied
Tablets: 50 mg

Pharmacokinetics
Absorption: rapidly and almost completely absorbed from GI tract.
Distribution: about 20% bound to plasma proteins.
Metabolism: extensively metabolized.
Excretion: 30% excreted in urine as unchanged drug and 60% as metabolites. *Half-life:* 6 to 7 hours.

Route	Onset	Peak	Duration
P.O.	Unknown	About 2 hr	Unknown

Pharmacodynamics
Chemical effect: unknown; centrally acting synthetic analgesic compound not chemically related to opioids that is thought to bind to opioid receptors and inhibit reuptake of norepinephrine and serotonin.
Therapeutic effect: relieves pain.

Adverse reactions
CNS: *dizziness, vertigo, headache, somnolence, CNS stimulation, asthenia,* anxiety, confusion, coordination disturbance, malaise, euphoria, nervousness, sleep disorder, ***seizures.***
CV: vasodilation.
EENT: visual disturbances.
GI: *nausea, constipation, vomiting,* dyspepsia, dry mouth, diarrhea, abdominal pain, anorexia, flatulence.
GU: urine retention, urinary frequency, menopausal symptoms.
Musculoskeletal: hypertonia.
Respiratory: ***respiratory depression.***
Skin: *pruritus,* sweating, rash.

Interactions
Drug-drug. *Carbamazepine:* increased tramadol metabolism. Patients receiving long-term carbamazepine therapy at dosage of up to 800 mg daily may require up to twice recommended dose of tramadol.
CNS depressants: additive effects. Use together cautiously. Dosage of tramadol may need to be reduced.
MAO inhibitors, neuroleptics: increased risk of seizures. Monitor patient closely.
Drug-herb. *5-hydroxytryptophan (5-HTP), SAMe, St John's wort:* increased serotonin levels. Advise against concurrent use.

Contraindications and precautions
- Contraindicated in patients hypersensitive to drug and in those with acute intoxication from alcohol, hypnotics, centrally acting analgesics, opioids, or psychotropic drugs.
- Drug isn't recommended for breast-feeding women.
- Use cautiously in patients at risk for seizures or respiratory depression; patients with increased intracranial pressure or head injury, acute abdominal conditions, or renal or hepatic impairment; and patients physically dependent on opioids.
- Safety hasn't been established in children or pregnant women.

NURSING CONSIDERATIONS

Assessment

- Assess patient's pain before therapy and regularly thereafter.
- Monitor CV and respiratory status.

ALERT Closely monitor patient at risk for seizures. Drug has been reported to reduce seizure threshold.

- Monitor patient for drug dependence. Tramadol can produce dependence similar to that of codeine or dextropropoxyphene and thus has potential to be abused.
- Be alert for adverse reactions and drug interactions.
- Evaluate patient's and family's knowledge of drug therapy.

Nursing diagnoses

- Acute pain related to underlying condition
- Risk for constipation related to drug-induced adverse GI reactions
- Deficient knowledge related to drug therapy

Planning and implementation

- For better analgesic effect, drug should be given before onset of intense pain.
- Withhold dose and notify prescriber if respiratory rate decreases or falls below 12 breaths/minute.
- Because constipation is a common adverse effect, anticipate need for laxative therapy.

Patient teaching

- Instruct patient to take drug only as prescribed and not to increase dosage or dosage interval unless instructed by prescriber.
- Caution ambulatory patient to be careful when getting out of bed and walking. Warn outpatient to refrain from driving and performing other potentially hazardous activities that require mental alertness until drug's CNS effects are known.
- Advise patient to check with prescriber before taking OTC medications; drug interactions can occur.

Evaluation

- Patient is free from pain.
- Patient regains normal bowel pattern.
- Patient and family state understanding of drug therapy.

trandolapril

(tran-DOH-luh-pril)

Mavik

Pharmacologic class: ACE inhibitor
Therapeutic class: antihypertensive
Pregnancy risk category: C (D in second and third trimesters)

Indications and dosages

▶ **Hypertension.** *Adults:* for patient not receiving a diuretic, initially 1 mg for a nonblack patient and 2 mg for a black patient P.O. once daily. If response isn't adequate, dosage may be increased at intervals of at least 1 week. Maintenance dosage range is 2 to 4 mg daily for most patients. Some patients receiving 4-mg once-daily doses may need b.i.d. doses. For patient also receiving diuretic, initial dose is 0.5 mg P.O. once daily. Subsequent dosages adjusted based on blood pressure response.

How supplied

Tablets: 1 mg, 2 mg, 4 mg

Pharmacokinetics

Absorption: food slows absorption.
Distribution: unknown.
Metabolism: metabolized in liver.
Excretion: excreted in urine and feces.

Route	Onset	Peak	Duration
P.O.	Unknown	1 hr	Unknown (drug); 4-10 hr (metabolite)

Pharmacodynamics

Chemical effect: inhibits circulating and tissue ACE activity, thus reducing angiotensin II formation, decreasing vasoconstriction, decreasing aldosterone secretion, and increasing plasma renin.

Therapeutic effect: decreases aldosterone secretion, leading to diuresis, natriuresis, and small increase in serum potassium.

Adverse reactions

CNS: dizziness, headache, fatigue, drowsiness, insomnia, paresthesia, vertigo, anxiety.
CV: chest pain, first-degree AV block, ***bradycardia,*** edema, flushing, hypotension, palpitations.
EENT: epistaxis, throat irritation.
GI: diarrhea, dyspepsia, abdominal distention, abdominal pain or cramps, constipation, vomiting, ***pancreatitis.***
GU: urinary frequency, impotence, decreased libido.
Hematologic: ***neutropenia, leukopenia.***
Metabolic: ***hyperkalemia***, hyponatremia.
Respiratory: dry, persistent, tickling, nonproductive cough; dyspnea; upper respiratory tract infection.
Skin: rash, pruritus, pemphigus.
Other: ***anaphylaxis, angioedema.***

Interactions

Drug-drug. *Diuretics:* increased risk of excessive hypotension. Monitor blood pressure closely.
Lithium: increased serum lithium levels and lithium toxicity. Avoid use together; monitor serum lithium levels.
Potassium-sparing diuretics, potassium supplements: increased risk of hyperkalemia. Monitor serum potassium closely.
Drug-herb. *Licorice:* herb may increase sodium retention and blood pressure. Discourage concomitant use.
Drug-food. *Salt substitutes containing potassium:* increased risk of hyperkalemia. Monitor serum potassium closely.

Contraindications and precautions

- Contraindicated in pregnant women, patients hypersensitive to drug, and patients with a history of angioedema with previous treatment with ACE inhibitor.
- Use cautiously in patients with impaired renal function, heart failure, or renal artery stenosis.

NURSING CONSIDERATIONS

Assessment

- Monitor patient's blood pressure and serum potassium levels before and during drug therapy.
- Monitor patient for hypotension. If possible, stop diuretic therapy 2 to 3 days before starting drug.
- Monitor patient for jaundice and alert prescriber immediately if occurs.
- Monitor patient's compliance with treatment.
- Evaluate patient's and family's knowledge of drug therapy.

Nursing diagnoses

- Risk for injury related to hypertension
- Deficient knowledge related to drug therapy

Planning and implementation

- Take steps to prevent or minimize orthostatic hypotension.
- Maintain patient's nondrug therapies, such as sodium restriction, stress management, smoking cessation, and exercise program.

ALERT Angioedema with involvement of the tongue, glottis, or larynx may be fatal because of airway obstruction. Appropriate therapy should be ordered, including epinephrine 1:1,000 (0.3 to 0.5 ml) S.C.; have resuscitation equipment for maintaining a patent airway readily available.

Patient teaching

- Advise patient to report infection and other adverse reactions.
- Tell patient to avoid salt substitutes.
- Tell patient to use caution in hot weather and during exercise.
- Tell woman to report suspected pregnancy immediately.
- Advise patient about to undergo surgery or anesthesia to inform prescriber about use of this drug.

Evaluation

- Patient's blood pressure is normal.
- Patient and family state understanding of drug therapy.

tranylcypromine sulfate
(tran-il-SIGH-proh-meen SUL-fayt)
Parnate

Pharmacologic class: MAO inhibitor
Therapeutic class: antidepressant
Pregnancy risk category: NR

Indications and dosages

▶ **Depression.** *Adults:* 10 mg P.O. t.i.d. Increased by 10 mg daily at 1- to 3-week intervals to maximum of 60 mg daily, if necessary, after 2 weeks of initial therapy.

How supplied

Tablets: 10 mg

Pharmacokinetics

Absorption: absorbed rapidly and completely from GI tract.
Distribution: unknown.
Metabolism: metabolized in liver.
Excretion: excreted primarily in urine; some excreted in feces. *Half-life:* 2½ hours.

Route	Onset	Peak	Duration
P.O.	Unknown	1-3.5 hr	≤ 10 days after drug stopped

Pharmacodynamics

Chemical effect: unknown; probably promotes accumulation of neurotransmitters by inhibiting MAO.
Therapeutic effect: relieves depression.

Adverse reactions

CNS: *dizziness, vertigo, headache,* anxiety, agitation, drowsiness, weakness, numbness, paresthesia, tremors, jitters, confusion.
CV: *orthostatic hypotension, tachycardia,* paradoxical hypertension, palpitations, *edema.*
EENT: blurred vision, tinnitus.
GI: dry mouth, *anorexia,* nausea, diarrhea, constipation, abdominal pain.
GU: impotence, SIADH, urine retention, impaired ejaculation.
Hematologic: anemia, ***leukopenia, agranulocytosis, thrombocytopenia.***
Hepatic: ***hepatitis.***
Musculoskeletal: muscle spasm, myoclonic jerks.
Skin: rash.
Other: chills.

Interactions

Drug-drug. *Amphetamines, antihistamines, ephedrine, levodopa, meperidine, metaraminol, methylphenidate, phenylephrine, sympathomimetics:* enhanced pressor effects of these drugs. Avoid concomitant use.
Antiparkinsonians, barbiturates, dextromethorphan, methotrimeprazine, narcotics, other sedatives, selective serotonin reuptake inhibitors, tricyclic antidepressants: enhanced adverse CNS effects. Use with caution and in reduced dosage.
Buspirone: may elevate blood pressure. Monitor patient closely.
Insulin, oral antidiabetics: increased risk of hypoglycemia. Use cautiously and in reduced dosages.
Drug-herb. *Cacao tree:* potential vasopressor effects. Advise against concurrent use.
Ginseng: headache, tremors, mania. Advise against concomitant use.
Green tea: contains caffeine. Advise against concurrent use.
Scotch broom: herb contains high levels of tyramine. Discourage concomitant use.
St. John's wort: herb has properties similar to those of selective serotonin reuptake inhibitors. Discourage use with this drug.
Drug-food. *Foods high in tryptophan, tyramine, caffeine:* may cause hypertensive crisis. Discourage concomitant consumption.
Drug-lifestyle. *Alcohol use:* enhanced adverse CNS effects. Discourage concomitant use.

Contraindications and precautions

- Contraindicated in patients receiving MAO inhibitors or dibenzazepine derivatives; sympathomimetics (including amphetamines); some CNS depressants (including alcohol); some serotonin reuptake inhibitors; antihypertensive, diuretic, antihistaminic, sedative, or anesthetic drugs; bupropion hydrochloride, buspirone hydrochloride, dextromethorphan, meperidine; foods high in tyramine or tryptophan; or excessive quantities of caffeine.

• Also contraindicated in patients with confirmed or suspected cerebrovascular defect, CV disease, hypertension, or history of headache and in those undergoing elective surgery.
• Drug isn't recommended for pregnant women.
• Use cautiously with antiparkinsonians or spinal anesthetics; in patients with renal disease, diabetes, seizure disorder, Parkinson's disease, or hyperthyroidism; and in patients at risk for suicide.
• Safety of drug hasn't been established in breast-feeding women and in children.

NURSING CONSIDERATIONS

Assessment
• Assess patient's condition before therapy and regularly thereafter.
• Assess patient for risk of self-harm.
• Obtain baseline blood pressure, heart rate, CBC, and liver function test results before beginning therapy; monitor throughout treatment.
• Be alert for adverse reactions and drug interactions.
• Evaluate patient's and family's knowledge of drug therapy.

Nursing diagnoses
• Disturbed thought processes related to presence of depression
• Risk for injury related to drug-induced adverse CNS reactions
• Deficient knowledge related to drug therapy

Planning and implementation
• Dosage usually is reduced to maintenance level as soon as possible.
ALERT Don't withdraw drug abruptly.
• In most patients, discontinue MAO inhibitors 14 days before elective surgery, as ordered, to avoid drug interactions that may occur during anesthetic procedure.
• If patient develops symptoms of overdose (palpitations, severe hypotension, or frequent headaches), withhold dose and notify prescriber.
ALERT Have phentolamine available to combat severe hypertension.
• Continue precautions for 10 days after stopping drug because it has long-lasting effects.

Patient teaching
• Warn patient to avoid foods high in tyramine or tryptophan and large amounts of caffeine. Tranylcypromine is the MAO inhibitor most often reported to cause hypertensive crisis with ingestion of foods high in tyramine, such as aged cheese, Chianti wine, beer, avocados, chicken livers, chocolate, bananas, soy sauce, meat tenderizers, salami, and bologna.
• Tell patient to avoid alcohol during drug therapy.
• Instruct patient to sit up for 1 minute before getting out of bed to avoid dizziness.
• Warn patient to avoid overexertion because MAO inhibitors may suppress angina.
• Advise patient to consult prescriber before taking other prescription or OTC medications. Severe adverse effects can occur if MAO inhibitors are taken with OTC cold, hay fever, or diet aids.
• Warn patient not to stop drug suddenly.

Evaluation
• Patient's behavior and communication exhibit improved thought processes.
• Patient doesn't experience injury from adverse CNS reactions.
• Patient and family state understanding of drug therapy.

trastuzumab
(trahs-TOO-zuh-mab)
Herceptin

Pharmacologic class: monoclonal antibody
Therapeutic class: antineoplastic
Pregnancy risk category: B

Indications and dosages

▶ **Single-agent treatment of patients with metastatic breast cancer whose tumors overexpress the human epidermal growth factor receptor 2 (HER2) protein and who have received one or more chemotherapy regimens for their metastatic disease; or in**

combination with paclitaxel for metastatic breast cancer in patients whose tumors overexpress the HER2 protein and who haven't received chemotherapy for their metastatic disease. *Adults:* initial loading dose of 4 mg/kg I.V. over 90 minutes. Maintenance dosage is 2 mg/kg I.V. weekly as a 30-minute I.V. infusion if the initial loading dose was well tolerated.

How supplied

Injection: lyophilized sterile powder containing 440 mg per vial

Pharmacokinetics

Absorption: no information available.
Distribution: drug's volume of distribution is 44 ml/kg.
Metabolism: no information available.
Excretion: no information available. *Half-life:* 5.8 days (range 1 to 32 days).

Route	Onset	Peak	Duration
I.V.	Unknown	Unknown	Unknown

Pharmacodynamics

Chemical effect: trastuzumab is a recombinant DNA–derived monoclonal antibody that selectively binds to HER2. Trastuzumab has been shown to inhibit the proliferation of human tumor cells that overexpress HER2.
Therapeutic effect: hinders function of specific breast cancer tumor cells that overexpress HER2.

Adverse reactions

CNS: *headache, asthenia, insomnia, dizziness,* paresthesia, depression, peripheral neuritis, neuropathy.
CV: tachycardia, ***heart failure,*** *peripheral edema.*
EENT: *rhinitis, pharyngitis,* sinusitis.
GI: *nausea, diarrhea, vomiting, anorexia, abdominal pain.*
GU: urinary tract infection.
Hematologic: anemia, ***leukopenia.***
Musculoskeletal: bone pain, arthralgia, *back pain.*
Respiratory: *cough, dyspnea.*
Skin: *rash,* acne.
Other: *pain, fever, chills, infection, flu syndrome,* ***allergic reaction,*** herpes simplex, edema.

Interactions

Drug-drug. *Anthracyclines:* increased potential for cardiotoxic effects. Monitor patient closely.
Paclitaxel: decreased clearance of trastuzumab. Monitor patient closely when used together.

Contraindications and precautions

- Use cautiously in patients with cardiac dysfunction, elderly patients, and patients hypersensitive to drug or its components.
- Safety and effectiveness in children haven't been established.

NURSING CONSIDERATIONS

Assessment

- Before beginning therapy, patient should undergo thorough baseline cardiac assessment, including history and physical examination and appropriate evaluation methods to identify those at risk of developing cardiotoxicity.
- Drug should be used only in patients with metastatic breast cancer whose tumors have HER2 protein overexpression.
- Assess patient for chills and fever, especially during the first infusion.
- Monitor patient closely for signs and symptoms of cardiac dysfunction, especially if also receiving anthracyclines and cyclophosphamide.
- Monitor patient for dyspnea, increased cough, paroxysmal nocturnal dyspnea, peripheral edema, and S3 gallop. Patients receiving chemotherapy concurrently should be monitored closely for cardiac dysfunction or failure, anemia and leukopenia, diarrhea, and infection.
- Evaluate patient's and family's understanding of drug therapy.

Nursing diagnoses

- Imbalanced nutrition: less than body requirements related to drug-induced GI adverse effects
- Decreased cardiac output related to drug-induced decreased left ventricular function
- Deficient knowledge related to drug therapy

Planning and implementation

- Treat first infusion-related symptoms with acetaminophen, diphenhydramine, and meperidine (with or without reducing the rate of infusion) as ordered.
- Notify prescriber if patient develops a clinically significant decrease in cardiac function.
- Reconstitute each vial with 20 ml of bacteriostatic water for injection, USP, 1.1% benzyl alcohol preserved, as supplied, to yield a multidose solution containing 21 mg/ml. Immediately after reconstitution, label vial for drug expiration 28 days from date of reconstitution.

ALERT If patient is hypersensitive to benzyl alcohol, drug must be reconstituted with sterile water for injection. Drug reconstituted with sterile water for injection must be used immediately; unused portion must be discarded. Avoid use of other reconstitution diluents.

ALERT Don't administer as an I.V. push or bolus.

- Determine dose (mg) of trastuzumab needed, based on loading dose of 4 mg/kg or maintenance dose of 2 mg/kg. Calculate volume of 21 mg/ml solution and withdraw amount from vial; add it to an infusion bag containing 250 ml of normal saline solution. D_5W solution shouldn't be used.
- Don't mix or dilute trastuzumab with other drugs.
- Vials of drug are stable at 36° to 46° F (2° to 8° C) before reconstitution. Discard reconstituted solution after 28 days. Store trastuzumab solution diluted in normal saline solution for injection at 36° to 46° F before use; it's stable for up to 24 hours.

Patient teaching

- Tell patient about possibility of first-dose, infusion-related adverse effects.
- Instruct patient to notify prescriber immediately if signs and symptoms of cardiac dysfunction develop, such as shortness of breath, increased cough, or peripheral edema.
- Instruct patient to report adverse effects to prescriber.
- Advise breast-feeding woman to discontinue breast-feeding during drug therapy and for 6 months after last dose.

Evaluation

- Patient doesn't experience adverse GI effects (nausea, vomiting, diarrhea).
- Patient doesn't exhibit dyspnea, increased cough, paroxysmal nocturnal dyspnea, peripheral edema, or S3 gallop as result of drug-induced cardiac dysfunction.
- Patient and family state understanding of drug therapy.

trazodone hydrochloride

(TRAYZ-oh-dohn high-droh-KLOR-ighd)
Desyrel

Pharmacologic class: triazolopyridine derivative
Therapeutic class: antidepressant
Pregnancy risk category: C

Indications and dosages

▶ **Depression.** *Adults:* initially, 150 mg P.O. daily in divided doses. Increased by 50 mg daily q 3 to 4 days, p.r.n. Average dosage ranges from 150 to 400 mg daily. Maximum daily dosage is 600 mg for hospitalized patients or 400 mg for outpatients.

How supplied

Tablets (film coated): 50 mg, 100 mg
Dividose tablets: 150 mg, 300 mg

Pharmacokinetics

Absorption: well absorbed from GI tract. Food delays absorption but increases amount of drug absorbed by 20%.
Distribution: distributed widely in body; isn't concentrated in any particular tissue.
Metabolism: metabolized by liver.
Excretion: about 75% excreted in urine; remainder excreted in feces. *Half-life:* first

phase, 3 to 6 hours; second phase, 5 to 9 hours.

Route	Onset	Peak	Duration
P.O.	Unknown	1-2 hr	Unknown

Pharmacodynamics

Chemical effect: unknown, although it inhibits serotonin uptake in brain; not a tricyclic derivative.
Therapeutic effect: relieves depression.

Adverse reactions

CNS: *drowsiness, dizziness,* nervousness, fatigue, confusion, tremors, weakness, hostility, anger, nightmares, vivid dreams, headache, insomnia.
CV: orthostatic hypotension, tachycardia, hypertension, syncope, shortness of breath.
EENT: blurred vision, tinnitus, nasal congestion.
GI: dry mouth, dysgeusia, constipation, nausea, vomiting, anorexia.
GU: urine retention; priapism, possibly leading to impotence; decreased libido; hematuria.
Hematologic: anemia.
Skin: rash, urticaria.
Other: diaphoresis.

Interactions

Drug-drug. *Antihypertensives:* increased hypotensive effect of trazodone. Monitor blood pressure; antihypertensive dosage may have to be decreased.
Clonidine, CNS depressants: enhanced CNS depression. Avoid concomitant use.
Digoxin, phenytoin: may increase serum levels of these drugs. Monitor patient for toxicity.
MAO inhibitors: no clinical experience. Use together with extreme caution.
Drug-herb. *St. John's wort:* serotonin syndrome may occur. Advise against concomitant use.
Drug-lifestyle. *Alcohol use:* enhanced CNS depression. Discourage concomitant use.

Contraindications and precautions

- Contraindicated in patients in initial recovery phase of MI and in patients hypersensitive to drug.
- Use cautiously in patients with cardiac disease and in those at risk for suicide.
- Safety of drug hasn't been established in pregnant or breast-feeding women and in children.

NURSING CONSIDERATIONS

Assessment

- Assess patient's condition before therapy and regularly thereafter.
- Be alert for adverse reactions and drug interactions.
- Evaluate patient's and family's knowledge of drug therapy.

Nursing diagnoses

- Disturbed thought processes related to presence of depression
- Risk for injury related to drug-induced adverse CNS reactions
- Deficient knowledge related to drug therapy

Planning and implementation

- Administer after meals or light snack for optimal absorption and to decrease risk of dizziness.
- Don't discontinue drug abruptly. However, it should be discontinued at least 48 hours before surgery.
- Notify prescriber if adverse reactions occur.

Patient teaching

- Instruct patient to take drug after meals or light snack.

ALERT Inform man that priapism is potential problem in patients taking trazodone. Advise him to notify prescriber immediately if it occurs; it may require surgical intervention.

- Warn patient to avoid activities that require alertness and good psychomotor coordination until CNS effects of drug are known. Drowsiness and dizziness usually subside after first few weeks.
- Teach patient's family how to recognize signs of suicidal tendency or suicidal ideation.

Evaluation

- Patient's behavior and communication exhibit improved thought processes.

- Patient doesn't experience adverse CNS reactions.
- Patient and family state understanding of drug therapy.

tretinoin

(TRET-ih-noyn)
Vesanoid

Pharmacologic class: retinoid
Therapeutic class: antineoplastic
Pregnancy risk category: D

Indications and dosages

▶ **Induction of remission in patients with acute promyelocytic leukemia (APL), French-American-British (FAB) classification M3 (including M3 variant), characterized by presence of the t(15,17) translocation or the PML/RAR alpha gene, who are refractory to or have relapsed from anthracycline chemotherapy or for whom anthracycline-based chemotherapy is contraindicated.** *Adults and children age 1 and older:* 45 mg/m^2 P.O. daily administered as two evenly divided doses until complete remission is documented. Therapy should be discontinued 30 days after achievement of complete remission or after 90 days of treatment, whichever occurs first.

How supplied

Capsules: 10 mg

Pharmacokinetics

Absorption: absorbed from GI tract.
Distribution: about 95% protein-bound.
Metabolism: drug induces its own metabolism.
Excretion: excreted in urine and feces.

Route	Onset	Peak	Duration
P.O.	Unknown	1-2 hr	Unknown

Pharmacodynamics

Chemical effect: unknown.
Therapeutic effect: induces remission in selected patients with certain types of leukemia.

Adverse reactions

CNS: hypothermia, weakness, fatigue, *malaise, headache,* dizziness, *paresthesia, anxiety, insomnia, depression, confusion,* ***cerebral hemorrhage, CVA,*** intracranial hypertension, agitation, hallucinations, abnormal gait, agnosia, aphasia, asterixis, cerebellar edema, cerebellar disorders, ***seizures, coma,*** CNS depression, dysarthria, encephalopathy, facial paralysis, hemiplegia, hyporeflexia, hypotaxia, no light reflex, neurologic reaction, spinal cord disorder, tremors, leg weakness, unconsciousness, dementia, forgetfulness, somnolence, slow speech.
CV: *chest discomfort,* **ARRHYTHMIAS,** *hypotension, hypertension, phlebitis, edema,* **HEART FAILURE, MI,** enlarged heart, heart murmur, ischemia, myocarditis, pericarditis, secondary cardiomyopathy, *pericardial effusions,* impaired myocardial contractility, *peripheral edema.*
EENT: *earache, ear fullness,* changed visual acuity, laryngeal edema, visual field defects, hearing loss, *visual disturbances, ocular disorders.*
GI: *GI hemorrhage, nausea, vomiting, anorexia, abdominal pain, GI disorders, diarrhea, constipation, dyspepsia, abdominal distention,* hepatosplenomegaly, ulcer.
GU: *renal insufficiency,* dysuria, ***acute renal failure,*** urinary frequency, renal tubular necrosis, enlarged prostate.
Hematologic: *leukocytosis,* **HEMORRHAGE,** ***disseminated intravascular coagulation.***
Hepatic: hepatitis, unspecified liver disorder, hypercholesterolemia, hypertriglyceridemia, abnormal liver function test results.
Metabolic: *weight changes,* fluid imbalance, ***acidosis.***
Musculoskeletal: *myalgia, bone pain,* flank pain, bone inflammation.
Respiratory: *pneumonia, upper respiratory tract disorders, dyspnea, respiratory insufficiency, pleural effusion, crackles, expiratory wheezing,* lower respiratory tract disorders, pulmonary infiltrates, bronchial asthma, ***pulmonary edema, progressive hypoxemia,*** unspecified pulmonary disease, pulmonary hypertension.

Skin: *flushing, skin and mucous membrane dryness, pruritus, increased sweating, alopecia, skin changes, rash.*
Other: ***retinoic acid-APL syndrome,*** *fever, infections, shivering, pain, injection site reactions, mucositis,* ***septicemia, multiorgan failure,*** cellulitis, facial edema, pallor, lymph disorder, ascites.

Interactions

None reported.

Contraindications and precautions

- Contraindicated in patients hypersensitive to retinoids or to parabens, which are used as preservatives in the gelatin capsule.
- Drug isn't recommended for pregnant or breast-feeding women.

NURSING CONSIDERATIONS

Assessment

- Assess patient's condition before therapy.
- Monitor CBC and platelet count regularly. Patients with elevated WBC counts at diagnosis have an increased risk of further rapid increase in WBC counts. Rapidly evolving leukocytosis is related to a higher risk of life-threatening complications.
- Monitor patient, especially a child, for signs and symptoms of pseudotumor cerebri. Early signs and symptoms include papilledema, headache, nausea, vomiting, and visual disturbances.
- Monitor cholesterol and triglyceride levels, coagulation profile, and liver function studies for abnormalities.
- Be alert for adverse reactions.
- Evaluate patient's knowledge of drug therapy.

Nursing diagnoses

- Ineffective health maintenance related to leukemia
- Risk for injury related to adverse reactions
- Deficient knowledge related to drug therapy

Planning and implementation

- Because patients with APL are at high risk in general and can have severe adverse reactions, drug should be given under supervision of a prescriber experienced in managing such patients and in a facility with laboratory and supportive services sufficient to monitor drug tolerance and to protect and maintain a patient compromised by toxicity.
- About 25% of patients treated during clinical studies have experienced a syndrome called retinoic acid-APL syndrome, which is characterized by fever, dyspnea, weight gain, radiographic pulmonary infiltrates, and pleural or pericardial effusion. Notify prescriber immediately if these signs and symptoms appear; this syndrome may be accompanied by impaired myocardial contractility and episodic hypotension with or without leukocytosis. Some patients have died of progressive hypoxemia and multiorgan failure. The syndrome generally occurs during the first month of therapy. Prompt treatment with high-dose steroids may reduce morbidity and mortality.
- Notify prescriber immediately if signs and symptoms of pseudotumor cerebri occur.
- Ensure that pregnancy testing and contraception counseling are repeated monthly throughout therapy and for 1 month after therapy.

ALERT Don't confuse tretinoin with trientine.

Patient teaching

- Inform woman that a pregnancy test is required within 1 week before therapy. When possible, therapy is delayed until a negative result is obtained. Also advise her to use two forms of effective contraception simultaneously during therapy and for 1 month after discontinuation, even with a history of infertility or menopause (unless hysterectomy has been performed), unless abstinence is the chosen method. Tell her to alert prescriber immediately of suspected pregnancy.
- Instruct patient about infection-control and bleeding precautions. Tell her to notify prescriber of signs of infection (fever, sore throat, fatigue) or bleeding (easy bruising, nosebleeds, bleeding gums, melena) and to take temperature daily.

Evaluation

- Patient responds well to therapy.

• Patient doesn't experience injury from adverse reactions.
• Patient and family state understanding of drug therapy.

triamcinolone

(trigh-am-SIN-oh-lohn)
Aristocort, Atolone, Kenacort**

triamcinolone acetonide

Cenocort A-40, Cinonide 40, Kenaject-40, Kenalog-10, Kenalog-40, Tac-3, Tac-40, Triam-A, Triamonide 40, Tri-Kort, Trilog

triamcinolone diacetate

Amcort, Aristocort, Aristocort Forte, Aristocort Intralesional, Articulose-L.A., Cenocort Forte, Cinalone 40, Kenacort Diacetate, Triam Forte, Triamolone 40, Trilone, Tristoject

triamcinolone hexacetonide

Aristospan Intra-Articular, Aristospan Intralesional

Pharmacologic class: glucocorticoid
Therapeutic class: anti-inflammatory, immunosuppressant
Pregnancy risk category: C

Indications and dosages

▶ **Severe inflammation or immunosuppression. Triamcinolone.** *Adults:* 8 to 16 mg P.O. daily, in a single or divided dose.
Triamcinolone diacetate. *Adults:* 40 mg I.M. weekly or 2 to 40 mg into lesions, joints, or soft tissue, or 4 to 48 mg P.O. divided q.i.d.
Triamcinolone hexacetonide. *Adults:* up to 0.5 mg per square inch of affected skin intralesionally, or 2 to 20 mg intra-articularly q 3 to 4 weeks, p.r.n.
Triamcinolone acetonide. *Adults:* initially, 2.5 to 60 mg I.M. Additional doses of 20 to 100 mg may be given, p.r.n., at 6-week intervals. Or, 2.5 to 15 mg intra-articularly, or up to 1 mg intralesionally, p.r.n.

How supplied

triamcinolone
Tablets: 1 mg, 2 mg, 4 mg, 8 mg
Syrup: 2 mg/ml, 4 mg/ml
triamcinolone acetonide
Injection (suspension): 3 mg/ml, 10 mg/ml, 40 mg/ml
triamcinolone diacetate
Injection (suspension): 25 mg/ml, 40 mg/ml
triamcinolone hexacetonide
Injection (suspension): 5 mg/ml, 20 mg/ml

Pharmacokinetics

Absorption: absorbed readily after P.O. administration. Absorption is variable after other routes of administration, depending on whether drug is injected into intra-articular space or muscle and on blood supply to that muscle.
Distribution: distributed to muscle, liver, skin, intestines, and kidneys. Drug is extensively bound to plasma proteins. Only unbound portion is active.
Metabolism: metabolized in liver.
Excretion: excreted in urine; insignificant quantities also excreted in feces. *Half-life:* 18 to 36 hours.

Route	Onset	Peak	Duration
P.O., I.M., intralesional, intra-articular, intrasynovial	Varies	Varies	Varies

Pharmacodynamics

Chemical effect: not clearly defined; decreases inflammation, mainly by stabilizing leukocyte lysosomal membranes; suppresses immune response; stimulates bone marrow; and influences protein, fat, and carbohydrate metabolism.
Therapeutic effect: relieves inflammation and suppresses immune system function.

Adverse reactions

Most adverse reactions to corticosteroids are dose- or duration-dependent.
CNS: *euphoria, insomnia,* psychotic behavior, pseudotumor cerebri, vertigo, headache, paresthesia, ***seizures.***

CV: ***heart failure,*** hypertension, edema, ***arrhythmias,*** thrombophlebitis, ***thromboembolism.***
EENT: cataracts, glaucoma.
GI: *peptic ulceration,* GI irritation, increased appetite, ***pancreatitis,*** nausea, vomiting.
GU: ***acute adrenal insufficiency*** may occur with increased stress (infection, surgery, or trauma) or abrupt withdrawal, menstrual irregularities.
Metabolic: hypokalemia, hyperglycemia, carbohydrate intolerance.
Musculoskeletal: muscle weakness, osteoporosis, growth suppression in children.
Skin: hirsutism, delayed wound healing, acne, various skin eruptions.
Other: susceptibility to infections, cushingoid state (moonface, buffalo hump, central obesity).

Interactions

Drug-drug. *Aspirin, indomethacin, other NSAIDs:* increased risk of GI distress and bleeding. Give together cautiously.
Barbiturates, phenytoin, rifampin: decreased corticosteroid effect. Increase corticosteroid, as ordered.
Oral anticoagulants: altered dosage requirements. Monitor PT closely.
Potassium-depleting drugs (such as thiazide diuretics): enhanced potassium-wasting effects of triamcinolone. Monitor serum potassium level.
Skin-test antigens: decreased response. Defer skin testing.
Toxoids, vaccines: decreased antibody response and increased risk of neurologic complications. Avoid concomitant use.

Contraindications and precautions

- Contraindicated in patients hypersensitive to drug or its components and in those with systemic fungal infections.
- Use cautiously in pregnant or breast-feeding women and patients with GI ulcer, renal disease, hypertension, osteoporosis, diabetes mellitus, hypothyroidism, cirrhosis, diverticulitis, nonspecific ulcerative colitis, recent intestinal anastomoses, thromboembolic disorders, seizures, myasthenia gravis, heart failure, tuberculosis, ocular herpes simplex, emotional instability, or psychotic tendencies.

NURSING CONSIDERATIONS

Assessment

- Assess patient before and after therapy; monitor weight, blood pressure, and serum electrolyte levels.
- Watch for adverse reactions, drug interactions, depression, or psychotic episodes, especially with high doses.
- Evaluate patient's and family's knowledge of drug therapy.

Nursing diagnoses

- Ineffective health maintenance related to underlying condition
- Risk for injury related to drug-induced adverse reactions
- Deficient knowledge related to drug therapy

Planning and implementation

- Drug isn't used for alternate-day therapy.
- Always adjust to lowest effective dose, as ordered.
- For better results and less toxicity, give once-daily dose in morning.

P.O. use: Give dose with food when possible to reduce GI irritation.
I.M. use: Give I.M. injection deep into gluteal muscle. Rotate injection sites to prevent muscle atrophy.
– Don't use 10 mg/ml strength for I.M. administration.
Intralesional, intra-articular, intrasynovial use: Assist prescriber with administration, as directed.
– Don't use 40 mg/ml strength for I.D. or intralesional administration.
ALERT Parenteral form isn't for I.V. use. Different salt formulations aren't interchangeable.
- Don't use diluents that contain preservatives; flocculation may occur.
- Unless contraindicated, give low-sodium diet high in potassium and protein. Administer potassium supplements, as needed.
- Gradually reduce drug dosage after long-term therapy, as ordered. After abrupt withdrawal, patient may experience rebound inflammation, fatigue, weakness, arthralgia,

fever, dizziness, lethargy, depression, fainting, orthostatic hypotension, dyspnea, anorexia, hypoglycemia; after prolonged use, sudden withdrawal may be fatal.

ALERT Don't confuse triamcinolone with Triaminicin or Triaminicol.

Patient teaching

- Tell patient not to discontinue drug abruptly or without prescriber's consent.
- Instruct patient to take oral drug with food.
- Teach patient signs of early adrenal insufficiency: fatigue, muscle weakness, joint pain, fever, anorexia, nausea, dyspnea, dizziness, and fainting.
- Instruct patient to wear or carry medical identification at all times.
- Warn patient receiving long-term therapy about cushingoid symptoms and to report sudden weight gain and swelling to prescriber.
- Tell patient to report slow healing.
- Advise patient receiving long-term therapy to consider exercise or physical therapy. Also tell patient to ask prescriber about vitamin D or calcium supplements.

Evaluation

- Patient responds well to drug.
- Patient doesn't experience injury from adverse reactions.
- Patient and family state understanding of drug therapy.

triamcinolone acetonide

(trigh-am-SIN-oh-lohn as-EE-tuh-nighd)
Azmacort

Pharmacologic class: glucocorticoid
Therapeutic class: anti-inflammatory, immunosuppressant
Pregnancy risk category: C

Indications and dosages

▶ **Corticosteroid-dependent asthma.** *Adults:* 2 inhalations t.i.d. to q.i.d. Maximum dosage is 16 inhalations daily. In some patients, maintenance can be accomplished when total daily dosage is given b.i.d.

Children ages 6 to 12: 1 or 2 inhalations t.i.d. to q.i.d. Maximum dosage is 12 inhalations daily.

How supplied

Inhalation aerosol: 100 mcg/metered spray

Pharmacokinetics

Absorption: absorbed slowly from lungs and GI tract.
Distribution: without use of spacer, about 10% to 25% of inhaled dose is deposited in airways; remainder is deposited in mouth and throat and swallowed. A greater percentage of inhaled dose may reach lungs with use of spacer device.
Metabolism: metabolized in liver. Some drug that reaches lungs may be metabolized locally.
Excretion: excreted in urine and feces. *Half-life:* 18 to 36 hours.

Route	Onset	Peak	Duration
Inhalation	1-4 wk	Unknown	Unknown

Pharmacodynamics

Chemical effect: unknown; probably decreases inflammation, mainly by stabilizing leukocyte lysosomal membranes.
Therapeutic effect: improves breathing ability.

Adverse reactions

EENT: dry or irritated nose or throat, hoarseness.
GI: *oral candidiasis,* dry or irritated tongue or mouth.
Respiratory: cough, wheezing.
Other: facial edema, ***hypothalamic-pituitary-adrenal function suppression,*** adrenal insufficiency.

Interactions

None significant.

Contraindications and precautions

- Contraindicated in patients hypersensitive to drug or its components and in those with status asthmaticus.
- Drug isn't recommended for breast-feeding women.

• Use with extreme caution, if at all, in patients with tuberculosis of respiratory tract; untreated fungal, bacterial, or systemic viral infections; or ocular herpes simplex.
• Use cautiously in patients receiving systemic corticosteroids and in pregnant women.

NURSING CONSIDERATIONS

Assessment
• Assess patient's asthma before therapy and regularly thereafter.
• Be alert for adverse reactions.
• Evaluate patient's and family's knowledge of drug therapy.

Nursing diagnoses
• Ineffective breathing pattern related to presence of asthma
• Impaired tissue integrity related to drug's adverse effect on oral mucosa
• Deficient knowledge related to drug therapy

Planning and implementation
• Patient who has recently been transferred to oral inhaled steroids from systemic administration of steroids may need to be placed back on systemic steroids during periods of stress or severe asthma attacks.
• Taper oral therapy slowly, as ordered.
• If patient is also to receive bronchodilator by inhalation, administer bronchodilator first, wait several minutes, then administer triamcinolone.
• If more than one inhalation of triamcinolone is ordered for each dose, allow 1 minute to elapse before repeat inhalations.
• Store drug between 36° and 86° F (2° and 30° C).
ALERT Don't confuse triamcinolone with Triaminicin or Triaminicol.

Patient teaching
• Inform patient that inhaled steroids don't provide relief for emergency asthma attacks.
• Teach patient to use medication as ordered, even when feeling well.
• Advise patient to ensure delivery of proper dose of medication by gently warming canister to room temperature before using. Patients can carry canister in pocket to keep it warm.
• Instruct patient requiring bronchodilator to use it several minutes before triamcinolone. Tell him to allow 1 minute to elapse before repeat inhalations and to hold breath for a few seconds to enhance drug action.
• Teach patient to check mucous membranes frequently for signs of fungal infection.
• Tell patient to prevent oral fungal infections by gargling or rinsing mouth with water after each use of inhaler but not to swallow water.
• Inform patient to keep inhaler clean and unobstructed by washing it with warm water and drying it thoroughly after use.
• Instruct patient to contact prescriber if response to therapy decreases; prescriber may need to adjust dosage. Tell patient not to exceed recommended dosage on his own.
• Instruct patient to wear or carry medical identification at all times.

Evaluation
• Patient exhibits improved breathing ability.
• Patient maintains normal oral mucosa integrity.
• Patient and family state understanding of drug therapy.

triamcinolone acetonide
(trigh-am-SIN-oh-lohn as-EE-tuh-nighd)
Nasacort

Pharmacologic class: glucocorticoid
Therapeutic class: anti-inflammatory
Pregnancy risk category: C

Indications and dosages

▶ **Relief of symptoms of seasonal or perennial allergic rhinitis.** *Adults and children age 12 and over:* initially, two sprays (110 mcg) in each nostril once daily. Increased as needed up to 220 mcg daily either as once-daily dosage or in divided doses up to four times daily. After desired effect is obtained, decrease dosage, if possible, to as little as one spray (55 mcg) in each nostril daily.

How supplied

Nasal aerosol: 55 mcg/metered spray

Pharmacokinetics

Absorption: minimally absorbed.
Distribution: distributed locally.
Metabolism: metabolized in liver.
Excretion: excreted primarily in feces. *Half-life:* 4 hours.

Route	Onset	Peak	Duration
Intranasal	≤ 12 hr	3-4 days	Several days after drug is stopped

Pharmacodynamics

Chemical effect: unknown.
Therapeutic effect: relieves signs and symptoms of nasal inflammation.

Adverse reactions

CNS: *headache.*
EENT: *nasal irritation,* dry mucous membranes, nasal and sinus congestion, irritation, burning, stinging, throat discomfort, sneezing, epistaxis.

Interactions

None known.

Contraindications and precautions

- Contraindicated in patients hypersensitive to drug or its components.
- Use with extreme caution, if at all, in patients with active or quiescent tuberculosis infection of respiratory tract and in patients with untreated fungal, bacterial, or systemic viral infection or ocular herpes simplex.
- Use cautiously in patients already receiving systemic corticosteroids because of increased likelihood of hypothalamic-pituitary-adrenal suppression compared with therapeutic dosage of either one alone. Also use cautiously in patients with recent nasal septal ulcers, nasal surgery, or trauma because of inhibitory effect on wound healing. Also use cautiously in pregnant or breast-feeding women.
- Safety of drug hasn't been established in children under age 12.

NURSING CONSIDERATIONS

Assessment

- Assess patient's condition before therapy and regularly thereafter.
- Be alert for adverse reactions.
- Evaluate patient's and family's knowledge of drug therapy.

Nursing diagnoses

- Ineffective health maintenance related to presence of allergic rhinitis
- Impaired tissue integrity related to drug's adverse effect on nasal mucosa
- Deficient knowledge related to drug therapy

Planning and implementation

ALERT When excessive doses are used, signs and symptoms of hyperadrenocorticism and adrenal suppression may occur; drug should be discontinued slowly.

- To administer drug, shake canister before each use and have patient blow his nose. To instill drug, tilt patient's head forward slightly and insert nozzle into nostril, pointing it away from septum. Have patient hold other nostril closed and then inhale gently when drug is sprayed. Repeat procedure for other nostril after shaking canister.

ALERT Don't confuse triamcinolone with Triaminicin or Triaminicol.

Patient teaching

- Urge patient to read instruction sheet in package before using drug for first time.
- To instill, instruct patient to shake canister before using; to blow nose to clear nasal passages; and to tilt head slightly forward and insert nozzle into nostril, pointing away from septum. Tell him to hold other nostril closed and then to inhale gently and spray. Next, have patient shake canister again and repeat this procedure in other nostril.
- Tell patient to discard canister after 100 actuations.
- Stress importance of using drug on regular schedule because its effectiveness depends on regular use. Caution patient not to exceed dosage prescribed because serious adverse reactions may occur.

• Tell patient to notify prescriber if symptoms don't improve within 2 to 3 weeks or if condition worsens.
• Warn patient to avoid exposure to chickenpox or measles and, if exposed to either, to obtain medical advice.
• Instruct patient to watch for signs and symptoms of nasal infection. If symptoms occur, tell patient to notify prescriber because drug may need to be discontinued and appropriate local therapy given.
• Advise patient not to break or incinerate canister or store it in extreme heat; contents are under pressure and may explode.

✓ Evaluation

• Patient's allergic rhinitis is visibly improved.
• Patient maintains normal tissue integrity in nasal passages.
• Patient and family state understanding of drug therapy.

triamterene

(trigh-AM-tuh-reen)
Dyrenium

Pharmacologic class: potassium-sparing diuretic
Therapeutic class: diuretic
Pregnancy risk category: B

Indications and dosages

▶ **Diuresis.** *Adults:* initially, 100 mg P.O. b.i.d. after meals. Total dosage shouldn't exceed 300 mg daily.

How supplied

Tablets: 50 mg, 100 mg
Capsules: 50 mg, 100 mg

Pharmacokinetics

Absorption: absorbed rapidly from GI tract but extent varies.
Distribution: about 67% protein-bound.
Metabolism: metabolized by hydroxylation and sulfation.
Excretion: excreted in urine. *Half-life:* 100 to 150 minutes.

Route	Onset	Peak	Duration
P.O.	2-4 hr	6-8 hr	7-9 hr

Pharmacodynamics

Chemical effect: inhibits sodium reabsorption and potassium and hydrogen excretion by direct action on distal tubule.
Therapeutic effect: promotes water and sodium excretion.

Adverse reactions

CNS: dizziness, weakness, fatigue, headache.
CV: hypotension.
GI: dry mouth, nausea, vomiting, diarrhea.
GU: interstitial nephritis, nephrolithiasis, transient elevation in BUN or creatinine level.
Hematologic: megaloblastic anemia related to low folic acid levels, ***thrombocytopenia, agranulocytosis.***
Hepatic: jaundice, increased liver enzyme abnormalities.
Metabolic: hyperkalemia, acidosis, hypokalemia, hyponatremia, hyperglycemia, azotemia.
Musculoskeletal: muscle cramps.
Skin: photosensitivity, rash.
Other: ***anaphylaxis.***

Interactions

Drug-drug. *ACE inhibitors, potassium supplements:* increased risk of hyperkalemia. Don't use together.
Amantadine: increased risk of amantadine toxicity. Don't use together.
Lithium: decreased lithium clearance, increasing risk of lithium toxicity. Monitor lithium level.
NSAIDs (indomethacin): may enhance risk of nephrotoxicity. Avoid concomitant use.
Quinidine: may interfere with some laboratory tests that measure quinidine levels. Inform laboratory that patient is taking triamterene.
Drug-food. *Potassium-containing salt substitutes, potassium-rich foods:* increased risk of hyperkalemia. Discourage concurrent use.
Drug-lifestyle. *Sun exposure:* photosensitivity reactions may occur. Urge patient to take precautions.

Contraindications and precautions

• Contraindicated in patients hypersensitive to drug and those with anuria, severe or progressive renal disease or dysfunction, severe hepatic disease, or hyperkalemia.
• Use cautiously in patients with impaired liver function or diabetes mellitus; elderly or debilitated patients; and pregnant women.
• Safe use of drug hasn't been established in breast-feeding women.

NURSING CONSIDERATIONS

Assessment

• Obtain history of patient's edema before therapy and reassess regularly thereafter. Full effect of triamterene is delayed 2 to 3 days when used alone.
• Monitor blood pressure and BUN and serum electrolyte levels.
• Watch for blood dyscrasia.
• Be alert for adverse reactions and drug interactions.
• Evaluate patient's and family's knowledge of drug therapy.

Nursing diagnoses

• Excessive fluid volume related to underlying condition
• Ineffective health maintenance related to drug-induced hyperkalemia
• Deficient knowledge related to drug therapy

Planning and implementation

• Give drug after meals to minimize nausea.
ALERT Withdraw drug gradually, as ordered, to minimize excessive rebound potassium excretion.
• Drug is less potent than thiazides and loop diuretics and is useful as adjunct to other diuretic therapy. Triamterene is usually used with potassium-wasting diuretics.
ALERT Don't confuse triamterene with trimipramine.

Patient teaching

• Tell patient to take drug after meals.
ALERT Warn patient to avoid excessive ingestion of potassium-rich foods, potassium-containing salt substitutes, and potassium supplements to prevent serious hyperkalemia.
• Teach patient to avoid direct sunlight, wear protective clothing, and use sunblock to prevent photosensitivity reactions.

Evaluation

• Patient exhibits no signs of edema.
• Patient's serum potassium level is normal.
• Patient and family state understanding of drug therapy.

triazolam

(trigh-AH-zoh-lam)
Alti-Triazolam ♦, Apo-Triazo ♦, Halcion, Novo-Triolam ♦

Pharmacologic class: benzodiazepine
Therapeutic class: sedative-hypnotic
Controlled substance schedule: IV
Pregnancy risk category: X

Indications and dosages

▶ **Insomnia.** *Adults:* 0.125 to 0.5 mg P.O. h.s. *Adults over age 65:* 0.125 mg P.O. h.s.; increased, p.r.n., to 0.25 mg P.O. h.s.

How supplied

Tablets: 0.125 mg, 0.25 mg

Pharmacokinetics

Absorption: well absorbed through GI tract.
Distribution: distributed widely throughout body; 90% protein-bound.
Metabolism: metabolized in liver.
Excretion: excreted in urine. *Half-life:* 1½ to 5½ hours.

Route	Onset	Peak	Duration
P.O.	Unknown	1-2 hr	Unknown

Pharmacodynamics

Chemical effect: unknown; probably acts on limbic system, thalamus, and hypothalamus of CNS to produce hypnotic effects.
Therapeutic effect: promotes sleep.

Adverse reactions

CNS: *drowsiness, dizziness, headache,* rebound insomnia, amnesia, light-headedness,

lack of coordination, confusion, depression, nervousness, ataxia.
GI: nausea, vomiting.
Other: physical or psychological abuse.

Interactions

Drug-drug. *Cimetidine, contraceptives, erythromycin, isoniazid, rantidine:* may cause prolonged triazolam blood levels. Monitor patient for increased sedation.
Other CNS depressants, including narcotic analgesics, other psychotropic medications, anticonvulsants, antihistamines: excessive CNS depression. Use together cautiously.
Potent CYP 3A inhibitors (itraconazole, ketoconazole, nefazodone): decreased clearance of triazolam. Don't use concomitantly.
Drug-herb. *Ashwagandha, calendula, catnip, hops, lady's slipper, lemon balm, passion flower, sassafras, skullcap, valerian, yerba maté:* potential for increased sedative effects. Monitor patient closely if used together.
Kava: excessive sedation. Discourage concomitant use.
Drug-food. *Grapefruit juice:* increased serum levels. Don't administer drug with grapefruit juice.
Drug-lifestyle. *Alcohol use:* excessive CNS depression. Discourage concurrent use.

Contraindications and precautions

- Contraindicated in patients hypersensitive to benzodiazepines and in pregnant women.
- Drug isn't recommended for use in breast-feeding women.
- Use cautiously in patients with impaired liver or kidney function, chronic pulmonary insufficiency, sleep apnea, depression, suicidal tendencies, or history of drug abuse.
- Safe use of drug hasn't been established in children.

NURSING CONSIDERATIONS

Assessment

- Assess patient's condition before therapy and regularly thereafter.
- Assess mental status before initiating therapy. Elderly patients are more sensitive to drug's CNS effects.
- Be alert for adverse reactions and drug interactions.
- Evaluate patient's and family's knowledge of drug therapy.

Nursing diagnoses

- Disturbed sleep pattern related to underlying disorder
- Risk for injury related to drug-induced adverse CNS reactions
- Deficient knowledge related to drug therapy

Planning and implementation

- Take precautions to prevent hoarding or intentional overdosing by patients who are depressed, suicidal, or drug-dependent, or who have a history of drug abuse.
- Store drug in cool, dry place away from light.
- Institute safety precautions once drug has been administered.

ALERT Don't confuse Halcion with Haldol or halcinonide.

Patient teaching

- Warn patient not to take more than prescribed amount because overdose can occur at total daily dosage of 2 mg (or four times the highest recommended amount).
- Caution patient about performing activities that require mental alertness or physical coordination. For inpatient, supervise walking and raise bed rails, particularly for elderly patient.
- Inform patient that drug is very short-acting and therefore has less tendency to cause morning drowsiness.
- Tell patient that rebound insomnia may develop for 1 or 2 nights after stopping therapy.

Evaluation

- Patient states that drug produces sleep.
- Patient doesn't experience injury from adverse CNS reactions.
- Patient and family state understanding of drug therapy.

trifluoperazine hydrochloride

(trigh-floo-oh-PER-eh-zeen high-droh-KLOR-ighd)
Apo-Trifluoperazine♦, Novo-Flurazine♦, PMS Trifluoperazine♦, Stelazine, Stelazine Concentrate

Pharmacologic class: phenothiazine (piperazine derivative)
Therapeutic class: antipsychotic, antiemetic
Pregnancy risk category: C

Indications and dosages

▶ **Anxiety.** *Adults:* 1 to 2 mg P.O. b.i.d. Maximum dosage is 6 mg/day. Drug shouldn't be used longer than 12 weeks for anxiety.

▶ **Schizophrenia and other psychotic disorders.** *Adult outpatients:* 1 to 2 mg P.O. b.i.d., increased as needed. Or 1 to 2 mg deep I.M. q 4 to 6 hours, p.r.n.
Hospitalized adults: 2 to 5 mg P.O. b.i.d.; may increase gradually to 40 mg daily.
Children ages 6 to 12 (hospitalized or under close supervision): 1 mg P.O. daily or b.i.d.; may increase gradually to 15 mg daily, if needed.

How supplied

Tablets (regular and film-coated): 1 mg, 2 mg, 5 mg, 10 mg
Oral concentrate: 10 mg/ml
Injection: 2 mg/ml

Pharmacokinetics

Absorption: variable with P.O. administration; rapid after I.M. use.
Distribution: distributed widely in body; 91% to 99% protein-bound.
Metabolism: metabolized extensively by liver.
Excretion: excreted primarily in urine; some excreted in feces.

Route	Onset	Peak	Duration
P.O., I.M.	Up to several wk	Unknown	Unknown

Pharmacodynamics

Chemical effect: unknown; probably blocks postsynaptic dopamine receptors in brain.
Therapeutic effect: relieves anxiety and signs and symptoms of psychotic disorders.

Adverse reactions

CNS: *extrapyramidal reactions, tardive dyskinesia,* pseudoparkinsonism, dizziness, drowsiness, insomnia, fatigue, headache, ***neuroleptic malignant syndrome.***
CV: *orthostatic hypotension,* tachycardia, ECG changes.
EENT: ocular changes, *blurred vision.*
GI: *dry mouth, constipation,* nausea.
GU: *urine retention,* menstrual irregularities, inhibited lactation.
Hematologic: ***transient leukopenia, agranulocytosis.***
Hepatic: cholestatic jaundice.
Metabolic: weight gain.
Skin: *photosensitivity,* ***allergic reactions,*** pain at I.M. injection site, sterile abscess, rash.
Other: gynecomastia.

Interactions

Drug-drug. *Antacids:* inhibited absorption of oral phenothiazines. Separate doses by at least 2 hours.
Barbiturates, lithium: may decrease phenothiazine effect. Monitor patient.
Centrally acting antihypertensives: decreased antihypertensive effect. Monitor blood pressure.
CNS depressants: increased CNS depression. Use together cautiously.
Propranolol: increased levels of both propranolol and trifluoperazine. Monitor patient closely.
Warfarin: decreased effect of oral anticoagulants. Monitor PT and INR.
Drug-herb. *Dong quai, St. John's wort:* increased photosensitivity reactions. Advise against concurrent use.
Ginkgo: potential decreased adverse effects of thioridazine. Monitor patient.
Kava: increased risk of dystonic reactions. Advise against concomitant use.
Milk thistle: decreased liver toxicity caused by phenothiazines. Monitor liver enzymes if used together.
Yohimbe: increased risk for yohimbe toxicity when used together. Advise against concurrent use.

Drug-lifestyle. *Alcohol use:* increased CNS depression. Discourage concurrent use.

Contraindications and precautions

- Contraindicated in patients hypersensitive to phenothiazines or in patients experiencing coma, CNS depression, bone marrow suppression, or liver damage.
- Use cautiously in patients with CV disease (may cause drop in blood pressure), exposure to extreme heat, seizure disorder, glaucoma, or prostatic hyperplasia and in elderly or debilitated patients.
- Safety of drug hasn't been established in pregnant or breast-feeding women and in children under age 6.

NURSING CONSIDERATIONS

Assessment

- Assess patient's condition before therapy and regularly thereafter.
- Watch for orthostatic hypotension, especially with parenteral use.
- Monitor patient for tardive dyskinesia, which may occur after prolonged use. It may not appear until months or years later and may disappear spontaneously or persist for life, despite discontinuation of drug.
- Monitor therapy with weekly bilirubin tests during first month; periodic blood tests (CBC and liver function); and ophthalmologic tests (long-term use), as ordered.

ALERT Monitor patient for symptoms of neuroleptic malignant syndrome (extrapyramidal effects, hyperthermia, autonomic disturbance), which is rare but can be fatal. It isn't necessarily related to length of drug use or type of neuroleptic; however, more than 60% of patients are men.

- Be alert for adverse reactions and drug interactions.
- Evaluate patient's and family's knowledge of drug therapy.

Nursing diagnoses

- Anxiety related to underlying condition
- Disturbed thought processes related to underlying psychotic disorder
- Deficient knowledge related to drug therapy

Planning and implementation

- Although there is little likelihood of contact dermatitis, people with known sensitivity to phenothiazine drugs should avoid direct contact. Wear gloves when preparing liquid forms.

P.O. use: Dilute liquid concentrate with 60 ml of tomato or fruit juice, carbonated beverages, coffee, tea, milk, water, or semisolid food.

I.M. use: Give deep I.M. only in upper outer quadrant of buttocks. Massage slowly afterward to prevent sterile abscess. Injection may sting.

– Protect drug from light. Slight yellowing of injection or concentrate is common; it doesn't affect potency. Discard markedly discolored solutions.

- Keep patient supine for 1 hour after drug administration, and advise him to change position slowly.
- Don't withdraw drug abruptly unless severe adverse reactions occur. Abrupt withdrawal of long-term therapy may cause gastritis, nausea, vomiting, dizziness, tremors, feeling of warmth or cold, diaphoresis, tachycardia, headache, insomnia, anorexia, muscle rigidity, altered mental status, or evidence of autonomic instability.
- Withhold dose and notify prescriber if patient develops jaundice, symptoms of blood dyscrasia (fever, sore throat, infection, cellulitis, weakness), or persistent extrapyramidal reactions (longer than a few hours), especially in pregnant woman or in child.
- Acute dystonic reactions may be treated with diphenhydramine.

ALERT Don't confuse trifluoperazine with triflupromazine.

Patient teaching

- Teach patient or caregiver how to prepare oral form of drug.
- Warn patient to avoid activities that require alertness or good psychomotor coordination until CNS effects of drug are known. Drowsiness and dizziness usually subside after a few weeks.
- Tell patient to avoid alcohol during drug therapy.

• Instruct patient to report urine retention or constipation.
• Tell patient to use sunblock and to wear protective clothing to avoid photosensitivity reactions.
• Tell patient to relieve dry mouth with sugarless gum or hard candy.

Evaluation
• Patient's anxiety is reduced.
• Patient's behavior and communication exhibit improved thought processes.
• Patient and family state understanding of drug therapy.

trihexyphenidyl hydrochloride
(trigh-heks-eh-FEEN-ih-dil high-droh-KLOR-ighd)

Apo-Trihex♦, Artane*, Artane Sequels, PMS Trihexyphenidyl, Trihexane, Trihexy-2, Trihexy-5

Pharmacologic class: anticholinergic
Therapeutic class: antiparkinsonian
Pregnancy risk category: C

Indications and dosages
▶ **All forms of parkinsonism and adjunct treatment to levodopa in management of parkinsonism.** *Adults:* 1 mg P.O. first day, 2 mg second day, then increased by 2 mg q 3 to 5 days until total of 6 to 10 mg is given daily. Usually given t.i.d. with meals. Sometimes given q.i.d. (last dose h.s.). Postencephalitic parkinsonism may require total daily dosage of 12 to 15 mg.

▶ **Drug-induced parkinsonism.** *Adults:* 5 to 15 mg P.O. daily.

How supplied
Tablets: 2 mg, 5 mg
Capsules (sustained-release): 5 mg
Elixir: 2 mg/5 ml

Pharmacokinetics
Absorption: readily absorbed from GI tract.
Distribution: unknown; crosses blood-brain barrier.
Metabolism: unknown.
Excretion: excreted in urine.

Route	Onset	Peak	Duration
P.O.	≤ 1 hr	2-3 hr	6-12 hr

Pharmacodynamics
Chemical effect: unknown; blocks central cholinergic receptors, helping to balance cholinergic activity in basal ganglia.
Therapeutic effect: improves physical mobility in patients with parkinsonism.

Adverse reactions
CNS: nervousness, dizziness, headache, hallucinations, drowsiness, weakness.
CV: tachycardia.
EENT: blurred vision, mydriasis, increased intraocular pressure.
GI: *dry mouth,* constipation, *nausea,* vomiting.
GU: urinary hesitancy, urine retention.

Interactions
Drug-drug. *Amantadine:* additive anticholinergic reactions, such as confusion and hallucinations. Reduce dosage of trihexyphenidyl before administering.
Levodopa: increased effect when used concomitantly with levodopa. May require lower doses of both drugs.
Drug-lifestyle. *Alcohol use:* increased sedative effects. Avoid concomitant use.

Contraindications and precautions
• Contraindicated in patients hypersensitive to drug.
• Drug isn't recommended for use in breastfeeding women.
• Use cautiously in patients with glaucoma; cardiac, hepatic, or renal disorders; obstructive disease of GI and GU tracts; or prostatic hyperplasia.
• Safety of drug hasn't been established in pregnant women and in children.

NURSING CONSIDERATIONS

Assessment
• Assess patient's condition before therapy and regularly thereafter.

ALERT Gonioscopic ocular evaluation and monitoring of intraocular pressure are needed, especially in patients over age 40.
- Be alert for adverse reactions and drug interactions. Adverse reactions are dose-related and usually transient.
- Monitor elderly patient for mental confusion or disorientation.
- Evaluate patient's and family's knowledge of drug therapy.

Nursing diagnoses
- Impaired physical mobility related to presence of parkinsonism
- Risk for injury related to drug-induced adverse CNS reactions
- Deficient knowledge related to drug therapy

Planning and implementation
- Dosage may need to be gradually increased in patient who develops tolerance to drug.
- Administer drug with meals.

ALERT Don't confuse Artane with Anturane or Altace.

Patient teaching
- Warn patient that drug may cause nausea if taken before meals.
- Tell patient to avoid activities that require alertness until CNS effects of drug are known.
- Advise patient to report urinary hesitancy or urine retention.
- Tell patient to relieve dry mouth with cool drinks, ice chips, or sugarless gum or hard candy.

Evaluation
- Patient exhibits improved physical mobility.
- Patient doesn't experience injury from adverse reactions.
- Patient and family state understanding of drug therapy.

trimethobenzamide hydrochloride
(trigh-meth-oh-BEN-zuh-mighd high-droh-KLOR-ighd)
Arrestin, Bio-Gan, Stemetic, Tebamide, T-Gen, Ticon, Tigan, Triban, Tribenzagan

Pharmacologic class: ethanolamine-related antihistamine
Therapeutic class: antiemetic
Pregnancy risk category: NR

Indications and dosages
▶ **Nausea, vomiting.** *Adults:* 250 mg P.O. t.i.d. or q.i.d.; or 200 mg I.M. or P.R. t.i.d. or q.i.d.
▶ **Prevention of postoperative nausea and vomiting.** *Adults:* 200 mg I.M. or P.R. as single dose before or during surgery; if needed, repeat 3 hours after termination of anesthesia. Limit use to prolonged vomiting from known cause.
Children weighing 13 to 40 kg (28 to 88 lb): 100 to 200 mg P.O. or P.R. t.i.d. or q.i.d.
Children weighing less than 13 kg: 100 mg P.R. t.i.d. or q.i.d.

How supplied
Capsules: 100 mg, 250 mg
Injection: 100 mg/ml
Suppositories: 100 mg, 200 mg

Pharmacokinetics
Absorption: about 60% absorbed after P.O. administration; unknown after P.R. or I.M. administration.
Distribution: unknown.
Metabolism: about 50% to 70% metabolized, probably in liver.
Excretion: excreted in urine and feces.

Route	Onset	Peak	Duration
P.O.	10-20 min	Unknown	3-4 hr
I.M.	15-30 min	Unknown	2-3 hr
P.R.	Unknown	Unknown	Unknown

Pharmacodynamics

Chemical effect: unknown; probably acts on chemoreceptor trigger zone to inhibit nausea and vomiting.
Therapeutic effect: prevents or relieves nausea and vomiting.

Adverse reactions

CNS: *drowsiness,* dizziness, headache, disorientation, depression, parkinsonian-like symptoms, ***coma, seizures.***
CV: hypotension.
EENT: blurred vision.
GI: diarrhea.
Hepatic: jaundice.
Musculoskeletal: muscle cramps.
Skin: hypersensitivity reaction (pain, stinging, burning, redness, swelling at I.M. injection site).

Interactions

Drug-drug. *CNS depressants:* additive CNS depression. Avoid concomitant use.
Drug-lifestyle. *Alcohol use:* additive CNS depression. Discourage concurrent use.

Contraindications and precautions

- Contraindicated in patients hypersensitive to drug. Suppositories are contraindicated in patients hypersensitive to benzocaine hydrochloride or similar local anesthetics.
- Use cautiously in children. Drug isn't recommended for use in children with viral illness because it may contribute to development of Reye's syndrome.
- Safety of drug hasn't been established in pregnant or breast-feeding women.

NURSING CONSIDERATIONS

Assessment

- Assess patient's condition before therapy and regularly thereafter.
- Be alert for adverse reactions and drug interactions.
- Evaluate patient's and family's knowledge of drug therapy.

Nursing diagnoses

- Risk for deficient fluid volume related to potential for or presence of nausea and vomiting
- Diarrhea related to drug-induced adverse GI reactions
- Deficient knowledge related to drug therapy

Planning and implementation

P.O. use: Follow normal protocol.
I.M. use: Inject deep into upper outer quadrant of gluteal region to reduce pain and local irritation.
P.R. use: Refrigerate suppositories.
- Withhold drug if skin hypersensitivity reaction occurs.

ALERT Don't confuse Tigan with Ticar.

Patient teaching

- Advise patient of possibility of drowsiness and dizziness, and caution against driving or performing other activities requiring alertness until CNS effects of drug are known.
- Warn patient that I.M. administration of drug may be painful.
- If patient will be using suppositories, instruct him to remove foil and, if necessary, moisten suppository with water for 10 to 30 seconds before inserting. Tell him to store suppositories in refrigerator.

Evaluation

- Patient maintains adequate hydration with cessation of nausea and vomiting.
- Patient maintains normal bowel pattern.
- Patient and family state understanding of drug therapy.

trimethoprim

(trigh-METH-uh-prim)
Alprim ◇, Proloprim, Trimpex, Triprim ◇

Pharmacologic class: synthetic folate antagonist
Therapeutic class: antibiotic
Pregnancy risk category: C

Indications and dosages

▶ **Uncomplicated urinary tract infections caused by susceptible strains of *Enterobacter, Escherichia coli, Klebsiella,* and *Proteus mirabilis.*** *Adults:* 200 mg P.O. daily as single dose or in divided doses q 12 hours for 10 days.

How supplied

Tablets: 100 mg, 200 mg

Pharmacokinetics

Absorption: absorbed quickly and completely.
Distribution: distributed widely; about 42% to 46% protein-bound.
Metabolism: less than 20% metabolized in liver.
Excretion: mostly excreted in urine. *Half-life:* 8 to 11 hours.

Route	Onset	Peak	Duration
P.O.	Unknown	1-4 hr	Unknown

Pharmacodynamics

Chemical effect: interferes with action of dihydrofolate reductase, inhibiting bacterial synthesis of folic acid.
Therapeutic effect: inhibits certain bacteria. Spectrum of activity includes many gram-positive and gram-negative organisms, including most enterobacteriaceae organisms (except *Pseudomonas*), *E. coli, Klebsiella,* and *P. mirabilis.*

Adverse reactions

GI: epigastric distress, nausea, vomiting, glossitis.
Hematologic: ***thrombocytopenia, leukopenia,*** megaloblastic anemia, methemoglobinemia.
Skin: *rash, pruritus,* ***exfoliative dermatitis.***
Other: fever.

Interactions

Drug-drug. *Phenytoin:* may decrease phenytoin metabolism and increase its serum level. Monitor patient for toxicity.

Contraindications and precautions

- Contraindicated in patients hypersensitive to drug and in those with documented megaloblastic anemia caused by folate deficiency.
- Drug isn't recommended for use in breast-feeding women.
- Use cautiously in patients with impaired liver function. Dosage should be decreased in patients with severely impaired kidney function. Also use cautiously in pregnant women.
- Safety of drug hasn't been established in children under age 12.

NURSING CONSIDERATIONS

Assessment

- Assess patient's infection before therapy and regularly thereafter.
- Obtain urine specimen for culture and sensitivity tests before giving first dose. Therapy may begin pending results.

ALERT Monitor CBC routinely. Signs and symptoms such as sore throat, fever, pallor, and purpura may be early indications of serious blood disorders. Prolonged use of trimethoprim at high doses may cause bone marrow suppression.

- Be alert for adverse reactions and drug interactions.
- Monitor patient's hydration status if adverse GI reactions occur.
- Evaluate patient's and family's knowledge of drug therapy.

Nursing diagnoses

- Infection related to presence of susceptible bacteria
- Risk for deficient fluid volume related to drug-induced adverse GI reactions
- Deficient knowledge related to drug therapy

Planning and implementation

- Because resistance to trimethoprim develops rapidly when administered alone, it's usually given with other drugs.

ALERT Trimethoprim is also used with sulfamethoxazole; don't confuse the two products.

- Drug isn't recommended for use in patient with creatinine clearance less than 15 ml/minute.

Patient teaching

- Instruct patient to take drug as prescribed, even if he feels better.

✓ Evaluation

- Patient is free from infection.
- Patient maintains adequate hydration.
- Patient and family state understanding of drug therapy.

trimipramine maleate

(trigh-MIH-pruh-meen MAL-ee-ayt)
Apo-Trimip ♦, Novo-Tripramine ♦, Rhotrimine ♦, Surmontil

Pharmacologic class: tricyclic antidepressant (TCA)
Therapeutic class: antidepressant
Pregnancy risk category: C

Indications and dosages

▶ **Depression.** *Adults:* 75 to 100 mg P.O. daily in divided doses, increased to 200 to 300 mg daily. Dosages over 300 mg daily aren't recommended in hospitalized patients; dosages over 200 mg aren't recommended in outpatients.

How supplied

Tablets: 25 mg ◊
Capsules: 25 mg, 50 mg, 100 mg

Pharmacokinetics

Absorption: absorbed rapidly from GI tract.
Distribution: distributed widely in body; 90% protein-bound.
Metabolism: metabolized in liver; significant first-pass effect may explain variability of serum level in different patients taking same dosage.
Excretion: most of drug excreted in urine; some excreted in feces. *Half-life:* 9 hours.

Route	Onset	Peak	Duration
P.O.	Unknown	2 hr	Unknown

Pharmacodynamics

Chemical effect: unknown; increases amount of norepinephrine, serotonin, or both in CNS by blocking their reuptake by presynaptic neurons.
Therapeutic effect: relieves depression.

Adverse reactions

CNS: *drowsiness, dizziness,* paresthesia, ataxia, hallucinations, delusions, anxiety, agitation, insomnia, tremors, weakness, confusion, headache, nervousness, EEG changes, ***seizures,*** extrapyramidal reactions.
CV: *orthostatic hypotension, tachycardia,* hypertension, ***arrhythmias, heart block, MI, CVA.***
EENT: *blurred vision,* tinnitus, mydriasis.
GI: *dry mouth, constipation,* nausea, vomiting, anorexia, paralytic ileus.
GU: *urine retention.*
Skin: rash, urticaria, photosensitivity, *diaphoresis.*
Other: ***hypersensitivity reaction.***

Interactions

Drug-drug. *Barbiturates:* decreased TCA blood level. Monitor patient for decreased antidepressant effect.
Cimetidine, methylphenidate: may increase drug serum level. Monitor patient for increased adverse reactions.
Clonidine, epinephrine, norepinephrine: increased hypertensive effect. Use cautiously.
CNS depressants: enhanced CNS depression. Avoid concomitant use.
MAO inhibitors: may cause severe excitation, hyperpyrexia, or seizures, usually with high dosage. Use cautiously.
Drug-herb. *5-HTP (5-hydroxytryptophan), SAMe, St. John's wort, yohimbe:* increased serotonin levels. Advise against concomitant use.
Drug-lifestyle. *Alcohol use:* enhanced CNS depression. Discourage concurrent use.
Sun exposure: increased risk of photosensitivity reactions. Urge patient to avoid unprotected or prolonged sun exposure.

Contraindications and precautions

- Contraindicated in patients in acute recovery phase of MI; patients hypersensitive to drug; and those receiving MAO inhibitor within 14 days.
- Use with extreme caution in patients with CV disease, increased intraocular pressure, hyperthyroidism, impaired liver function, or history of urine retention, angle-closure glaucoma, or seizures and in those receiving thy-

roid medications, guanethidine, or similar agents.
- Use cautiously in pregnant women.
- Safety of drug hasn't been established in children and in breast-feeding women.

NURSING CONSIDERATIONS

Assessment
- Assess patient's depression before therapy and regularly thereafter.
- Record patient's mood changes. Monitor patient for suicidal tendencies.
- Be alert for adverse reactions and drug interactions.
- Evaluate patient's and family's knowledge of drug therapy.

Nursing diagnoses
- Disturbed thought processes related to presence of depression
- Risk for injury related to drug-induced adverse CNS reactions
- Deficient knowledge related to drug therapy

Planning and implementation
- Administer full dose at bedtime if patient exhibits daytime sedation.
- Dosage should be reduced in elderly or debilitated patient.
- Don't withdraw drug abruptly. Abrupt withdrawal of long-term therapy may cause nausea, headache, malaise (doesn't indicate addiction).

ALERT Because hypertensive episodes may occur during surgery in patients receiving TCAs, dosage should be discontinued gradually several days before surgery.
- If signs of psychosis occur or increase, expect prescriber to reduce dosage.

ALERT Don't confuse trimipramine with triamterene or trimeprazine.

Patient teaching
- Tell patient to take full dosage at bedtime to avoid daytime sedation. Warn him about possible morning orthostatic hypotension.
- Warn patient to avoid hazardous activities that require alertness and good psychomotor coordination until CNS effects of drug are known. Drowsiness and dizziness usually subside after a few weeks.
- Tell patient to avoid alcohol during drug therapy.
- Warn patient not to stop taking drug suddenly. Advise him to consult prescriber before taking other prescription or OTC medications.
- Advise patient to use sunblock, wear protective clothing, and avoid prolonged exposure to sunlight to prevent photosensitivity reactions.

Evaluation
- Patient's behavior and communication exhibit improved thought processes.
- Patient doesn't experience injury from adverse CNS reactions.
- Patient and family state understanding of drug therapy.

tripelennamine citrate
(trigh-peh-LEN-uh-meen SIH-trayt)
PBZ*

tripelennamine hydrochloride
PBZ, PBZ-SR, Pelamine, Pyribenzamine

Pharmacologic class: ethylenediamine-derivative antihistamine
Therapeutic class: antihistamine (H_1-receptor antagonist)
Pregnancy risk category: NR

Indications and dosages
▶ **Rhinitis, allergy symptoms.** *Adults:* 25 to 50 mg P.O. q 4 to 6 hours (maximum dosage 600 mg daily); or 50 to 100 mg extended-release b.i.d. or t.i.d.
Children: 5 mg/kg P.O. daily in four to six divided doses. Maximum dosage is 300 mg daily. Don't use extended-release tablets in children.

How supplied
tripelennamine citrate
Elixir: 37.5 mg/5 ml (equivalent to 25 mg/5 ml of tripelennamine hydrochloride)*
tripelennamine hydrochloride
Tablets: 25 mg, 50 mg
Tablets (extended-release): 100 mg

Pharmacokinetics

Absorption: well absorbed from GI tract.
Distribution: distributed in high levels in liver.
Metabolism: appears to be almost completely metabolized.
Excretion: excreted almost entirely in urine.

Route	Onset	Peak	Duration
P.O.	15-60 min	Unknown	4-6 hr

Pharmacodynamics

Chemical effect: competes with histamine for H_1-receptor sites on effector cells. Drug prevents but doesn't reverse histamine-mediated responses.
Therapeutic effect: relieves allergy symptoms.

Adverse reactions

CNS: (especially in elderly patients) *drowsiness,* dizziness, confusion, restlessness, tremors, irritability, insomnia.
CV: palpitations.
GI: anorexia, diarrhea, constipation, *nausea, vomiting, dry mouth.*
GU: urinary frequency, urine retention.
Respiratory: thick bronchial secretions.
Skin: urticaria, rash.

Interactions

Drug-drug. *CNS depressants:* increased sedation. Use together cautiously.
MAO inhibitors: increased anticholinergic effects. Don't use together.

Contraindications and precautions

- Contraindicated in patients hypersensitive to drug or related compounds; those with angle-closure glaucoma, stenosing peptic ulcer, symptomatic prostatic hypertrophy, pyloroduodenal or bladder-neck obstruction, or lower respiratory tract symptoms, including asthma; and premature infants, neonates, or breast-feeding women.
- Use cautiously in elderly patients and patients with increased intraocular pressure, hyperthyroidism, CV disease, hypertension, or history of bronchial asthma.
- Safety of drug hasn't been established in pregnant women.

NURSING CONSIDERATIONS

Assessment

- Assess patient before and after therapy. Be alert for adverse reactions and drug interactions.
- Evaluate patient's and family's knowledge of drug therapy.

Nursing diagnoses

- Ineffective health maintenance related to allergies
- Risk for injury related to drug-induced adverse CNS reactions
- Deficient knowledge related to drug therapy

Planning and implementation

- Extended-release preparations shouldn't be used in children.
- Give drug with food or milk to reduce likelihood of GI distress.

Patient teaching

- Tell patient to take drug with food or milk and to use ice chips or sugarless gum or hard candy to relieve dry mouth.
- Warn patient to avoid alcohol, driving, and other activities that require alertness until CNS effects are known; coffee or tea may reduce drowsiness.
- Advise patient to stop drug 4 days before allergy skin tests.
- Tell patient to notify prescriber if tolerance develops.
- Tell patient that extended-release tablets shouldn't be crushed or chewed.

Evaluation

- Patient responds well to drug.
- Patient doesn't experience injury from adverse CNS reactions.
- Patient and family state understanding of drug therapy.

tromethamine

(troh-METH-eh-meen)

Tham

Pharmacologic class: sodium-free organic amine
Therapeutic class: systemic alkalinizer
Pregnancy risk category: C

Indications and dosages

▶ **Metabolic acidosis linked to cardiac bypass surgery or cardiac arrest.** *Adults:* dosage depends on bicarbonate deficit. Calculate as follows: each ml of 0.3 M tromethamine solution required = weight in kg^2 base deficit (mEq/L).

How supplied

Injection: 18 g/500 ml

Pharmacokinetics

Absorption: not applicable.
Distribution: at pH of 7.4 about 25% of drug is unionized; this portion may enter cells to neutralize acidic ions of intracellular fluid.
Metabolism: none.
Excretion: rapidly excreted in urine as bicarbonate salt. *Half-life:* 7 to 40 minutes.

Route	Onset	Peak	Duration
I.V.	Immediate	Immediate	Unknown

Pharmacodynamics

Chemical effect: combines with hydrogen ions and associated acid anions; resulting salts are excreted. Drug also has osmotic diuretic effect.
Therapeutic effect: restores normal acid-base balance in body.

Adverse reactions

CV: venospasm, I.V. thrombosis.
Hepatic: ***hemorrhagic hepatic necrosis.***
Metabolic: hypoglycemia, ***hyperkalemia*** (with decreased urine output).
Respiratory: ***respiratory depression.***
Other: inflammation, necrosis, sloughing (if extravasation occurs); fever.

Interactions

None significant.

Contraindications and precautions

- Contraindicated in patients with anuria, uremia, or chronic respiratory acidosis and in pregnant women (except in acute, life-threatening situations).
- Use cautiously in patients with renal disease and poor urine output.

NURSING CONSIDERATIONS

Assessment

- Assess patient's condition before therapy and regularly thereafter.
- Monitor ECG and serum potassium level in patient with renal disease and poor urine output.
- Make the following determinations before, during, and after therapy: blood pH; carbon dioxide tension; bicarbonate, glucose, and electrolyte levels.
- Be alert for adverse reactions.
- Evaluate patient's and family's knowledge of drug therapy.

Nursing diagnoses

- Ineffective health maintenance related to presence of acid-base imbalance
- Impaired tissue integrity related to tromethamine extravasation
- Deficient knowledge related to drug therapy

Planning and implementation

- Give slowly through 18G to 20G needle into largest antecubital vein or by indwelling I.V. catheter.
- Total dosage should be administered over at least 1 hour and shouldn't exceed 500 mg/kg. Additional therapy based on serial determinations of existing bicarbonate deficit.

ALERT Drug shouldn't be used longer than 1 day except in life-threatening situations.

- Have mechanical ventilation available for patients with associated respiratory acidosis.
- To prevent blood pH from rising above normal, be prepared to adjust dosage carefully, as ordered.

• If extravasation occurs, infiltrate area with 1% procaine and 150 units hyaluronidase, as ordered; this may reduce vasospasm and dilute remaining drug locally.

Patient teaching

• Inform patient and family of need for drug, and be prepared to answer their questions.

Evaluation

• Patient regains normal acid-base balance.
• Patient doesn't exhibit signs and symptoms of extravasation.
• Patient and family state understanding of drug therapy.

trovafloxacin mesylate

(troh-vah-FLOKS-ah-sin MES-eh-layt)
Trovan

alatrofloxacin mesylate

Trovan I.V.

Pharmacologic class: fluoroquinolone
Therapeutic class: antibiotic
Pregnancy risk category: C

Indications and dosages

▶ **Nosocomial pneumonia caused by *Escherichia coli, Pseudomonas aeruginosa, Haemophilus influenzae*, or *Staphylococcus aureus;* gynecologic and pelvic infections caused by *E. coli, Bacteroides fragilis,* viridans group streptococci, *Enterococcus faecalis, Streptococcus agalactiae, Peptostreptococcus* species, *Prevotella* species, or *Gardnerella vaginalis;* complicated intra-abdominal infections including postsurgical infections caused by *E. coli, B. fragilis,* viridans group streptococci, *P. aeruginosa, Klebsiella pneumoniae, Peptostreptococcus* species, *or Prevotella* species.** *Adults:* 300 mg I.V. daily followed by 200 mg P.O. daily for 7 to 14 days; 10 to 14 days for pneumonia.

▶ **Community-acquired pneumonia caused by *Streptococcus pneumoniae, H. influenzae, K. pneumoniae, S. aureus, Mycoplasma pneumoniae, Moraxella catarrhalis, Legionella pneumophila,* or *Chlamydia pneumoniae;* complicated skin and skin-structure infections including diabetic foot infections caused by *S. aureus, S. agalactiae, P. aeruginosa, E. faecalis, E. coli,* or *Proteus mirabilis* (not for treatment of osteomyelitis).** *Adults:* 200 mg P.O. or I.V. daily followed by 200 mg P.O. daily for 7 to 14 days; 10 to 14 days for complicated skin and skin-structure infections.

▶ **Prophylaxis of infection related to elective colorectal surgery or vaginal and abdominal hysterectomy.** *Adults:* 200 mg P.O. or I.V as a single dose 30 minutes to 4 hours before surgery.

▶ **Acute sinusitis caused by *H. influenzae, M. catarrhalis,* or *S. pneumoniae;* chronic prostatitis caused by *E. coli, E. faecalis,* or *Staphylococcus epidermis;* cervicitis caused by *Chlamydia trachomatis;* and pelvic inflammatory disease (mild to moderate) caused by *Neisseria gonorrhoeae* or *C. trachomatis*.** *Adults:* 200 mg P.O. daily for 5 days (cervicitis), 10 days (acute sinusitis), 14 days (pelvic inflammatory disease), or 28 days (chronic prostatitis).

▶ **Uncomplicated urinary tract infections caused by *E. coli;* uncomplicated skin and skin-structure infections caused by *S. aureus, Streptococcus pyogenes,* or *S. agalactiae;* acute bacterial exacerbation of chronic bronchitis caused by *H. influenzae, M. catarrhalis, S. pneumoniae, S. aureus,* or *Haemophilus parainfluenzae;* and uncomplicated gonorrhea caused by *N. gonorrhoeae.*** *Adults:* 100 mg P.O. daily for 3 days (urinary tract infections), 7 to 10 days (skin and skin structure infections, bronchitis), or single dose for treatment of gonorrhea.

How supplied

Trovan
Tablets (trovafloxacin): 100 mg, 200 mg
Trovan I.V.
Injection (alatrofloxacin): 5 mg/ml in 40-ml (200 mg) and 60-ml (300 mg) vials

Pharmacokinetics

Absorption: well absorbed following P.O. administration. Absolute bioavailability is about 88%.

Distribution: distributed widely and rapidly throughout body with about 76% bound to plasma proteins.
Metabolism: metabolized by conjugation.
Excretion: about 43% of drug excreted unchanged in feces and 6% unchanged in urine following oral administration. *Half-life:* 9 to 12 hours.

Route	Onset	Peak	Duration
P.O., I.V.	Unknown	1 hr	Unknown

Pharmacodynamics

Chemical effect: trovafloxacin is related to the fluoroquinolones with in vitro activity against a wide range of gram-positive and gram-negative aerobic and anaerobic microorganisms. Bactericidal action results from inhibition of DNA gyrase and topoisomerase IV, two enzymes involved in bacterial replication.
Therapeutic effect: hinders a wide range of gram-positive and gram-negative bacterial activity.

Adverse reactions

CNS: *dizziness,* light-headedness, headache, ***seizures,*** psychosis.
GI: diarrhea, nausea, vomiting, abdominal pain, pseudomembranous colitis.
GU: vaginitis, increased BUN and creatinine.
Hematologic: bone marrow aplasia (anemia, ***thrombocytopenia, leukopenia***), decreased hemoglobin and hematocrit, increased platelets.
Hepatic: increased ALT and AST.
Musculoskeletal: arthralgia, arthropathy, myalgia.
Skin: pruritus, rash, injection-site reaction, photosensitivity.

Interactions

Drug-drug. *Antacids containing aluminum, magnesium, or citric acid buffered with sodium citrate (Bicitra), sucralfate, iron-containing preparations, and I.V. morphine:* bioavailability of trovafloxacin is significantly reduced following concomitant use with these agents. Give these drugs 2 hours before or 2 hours after trovafloxacin. Avoid morphine I.V. for 4 hours if trovafloxacin is taken with food.

Drug-lifestyle. *Sun exposure:* photosensitivity reactions may occur. Urge patient to take precautions.

Contraindications and precautions

- Contraindicated in patients hypersensitive to drug, alatrofloxacin, other quinolone antimicrobials, or other components of these products.
- Use cautiously in patients with CNS disorders (such as cerebral atherosclerosis or epilepsy) and in those at increased risk for seizures. As with other quinolones, drug may cause neurologic complications such as seizures, psychosis, or increased intracranial pressure. Monitor patient with condition closely.

NURSING CONSIDERATIONS

Assessment

- Assess patient's infection before therapy and regularly thereafter.
- Obtain specimen for culture and sensitivity tests before giving first dose, as ordered. Therapy may begin pending test results.
- Assess patient for history of CNS disorders or increased risk for seizures, and monitor patient with condition closely.
- Perform periodic assessment of liver function because of potential for increases in ALT, AST, and alkaline phosphatase levels. Report abnormalities to prescriber.
- Patients with mild to moderate cirrhosis will require reduced dosages.
- Evaluate patient's and family's knowledge of drug therapy.

Nursing diagnoses

- Infection related to bacteria susceptible to drug
- Risk for injury related to drug-induced neurologic complications
- Deficient knowledge related to drug therapy

Planning and implementation

P.O. use: Drug can be given as a single daily dose without regard to food.
- No dosage adjustment is necessary when switching from I.V. to oral form. Give drug

with meals or at bedtime if patient experiences dizziness.

I.V. use: Alatrofloxacin mesylate is supplied in single-use vials which must be further diluted with an appropriate solution (D_5W, half-normal saline solution) before administration. Don't dilute drug with normal saline solution or lactated Ringer's solution. Follow package insert for specific instructions regarding preparation of desired dosage.

– After dilution, administer by I.V. infusion over 60 minutes. Avoid rapid bolus or infusion. Don't administer drug with solutions containing multivalent cations (such as magnesium) through same I.V. line.

• If *P. aeruginosa* is the known or presumed pathogen, combination therapy with either an aminoglycoside or aztreonam may be indicated.

ALERT Using drug for longer than 2 weeks greatly increases the risk of serious liver injury. Liver injury also has been reported following reexposure to the drug. Drug should be limited to patients with life- or limb-threatening infections who received their initial treatment as an inpatient in a hospital or a long-term care nursing facility. Don't use drug if effective and safer alternative antimicrobial therapy is available.

Patient teaching

• Inform patient that drug may be taken without regard to meals; however, advise patient to take drug with meals or at bedtime if lightheadedness or dizziness occurs.

• Warn patient to avoid excessive sunlight or artificial ultraviolet light and to use an effective sunscreen to prevent sunburn.

• Instruct patient to discontinue treatment, refrain from exercise, and seek medical advice if pain, inflammation, or rupture of a tendon occurs.

• Advise patient to discontinue treatment and seek medical help immediately at first sign of rash, hives, difficulty swallowing or breathing, or other symptoms suggesting an allergic reaction.

• Instruct patient to notify prescriber if severe diarrhea occurs.

Evaluation

• Patient is free from infection.

• Patient doesn't experience neurologic complications such as seizures or psychosis.

• Patient and family state understanding of drug therapy.

tubocurarine chloride

(too-boh-kyoo-RAH-reen KLOR-ighd)

Tubarine♦

Pharmacologic class: nondepolarizing neuromuscular blocker

Therapeutic class: skeletal muscle relaxant

Pregnancy risk category: C

Indications and dosages

▶ **Adjunct to general anesthesia.** Dosage depends on anesthetic used, individual needs, and response. Dosages listed are representative and must be adjusted. *Adults:* 1 unit/kg or 0.165 mg/kg I.V. slowly over 60 to 90 seconds. Average dose is initially 6 to 9 mg I.V. or I.M., followed by 3 to 4.5 mg in 3 to 5 minutes, if needed. Additional doses of 3 mg may be given if needed during prolonged anesthesia.

Children: 0.6 mg/kg I.V or I.M.

▶ **To assist with mechanical ventilation.** *Adults and children:* initially, 0.0165 mg/kg I.V. (average 1 mg), then adjust subsequent doses to patient response.

▶ **To lessen muscle contractions in pharmacologically or electrically induced seizures.** *Adults and children:* 1 unit/kg or 0.165 mg/kg I.V. over 60 to 90 seconds. Initial dose is 3 mg less than calculated dose.

▶ **Diagnosis of myasthenia gravis.** *Adults:* 0.004 to 0.033 mg/kg as single I.V. or I.M. dose.

How supplied

Injection: 3 mg (20 units)/ml; 10 mg/ml

Pharmacokinetics

Absorption: not applicable.

Distribution: distributed in extracellular fluid and rapidly reaches its site of action; 40% to

45% bound to plasma proteins, mainly globulins.
Metabolism: undergoes *N*-demethylation in liver.
Excretion: about 33% to 75% excreted unchanged in urine in 24 hours; up to 11% excreted in bile.

Route	Onset	Peak	Duration
I.V., I.M.	≤ 1 min	2-5 min	20-40 min

Pharmacodynamics

Chemical effect: prevents acetylcholine from binding to receptors on muscle end plate, thus blocking depolarization.
Therapeutic effect: relaxes skeletal muscles; diagnostic aid for myasthenia gravis.

Adverse reactions

CV: hypotension, ***arrhythmias, bradycardia, cardiac arrest.***
GI: increased salivation.
Musculoskeletal: profound and prolonged muscle relaxation, residual muscle weakness.
Respiratory: ***respiratory depression or apnea, bronchospasm.***
Other: ***hypersensitivity reactions, anaphylaxis.***

Interactions

Drug-drug. *Aminoglycoside antibiotics (including amikacin, gentamicin, kanamycin, neomycin, streptomycin), general anesthetics (such as enflurane, halothane, isoflurane), polymyxin antibiotics (colistin, polymyxin B sulfate):* potentiated neuromuscular blockade, leading to increased skeletal muscle relaxation and potentiation of effect. Use cautiously during surgical and postoperative periods.
Amphotericin B, ethacrynic acid, furosemide, methotrimeprazine, opioid analgesics, propranolol, thiazide diuretics: potentiated neuromuscular blockade, leading to increased skeletal muscle relaxation and, possibly, respiratory paralysis. Use with extreme caution during surgical and postoperative periods.
Quinidine: prolonged neuromuscular blockade. Use together cautiously. Monitor patient closely.

Contraindications and precautions

- Contraindicated in patients hypersensitive to drug and in those for whom histamine release is hazardous (such as asthmatic patients).
- Use cautiously in elderly or debilitated patients and in those with hepatic or pulmonary impairment, hypothermia, respiratory depression, myasthenia gravis, myasthenic syndrome of lung cancer or bronchogenic carcinoma, dehydration, thyroid disorders, collagen diseases, porphyria, electrolyte disturbances, fractures, or muscle spasms. Also use large doses cautiously in women undergoing cesarean delivery and in breast-feeding women.

NURSING CONSIDERATIONS

Assessment

- Assess patient's condition before therapy and regularly thereafter.
- Monitor baseline electrolyte determinations (imbalance can potentiate neuromuscular blocking effects).
- Check vital signs every 15 minutes.
- Measure fluid intake and output; renal dysfunction prolongs duration of action because much of drug is unchanged before excretion.
- Monitor respiratory rate closely until patient is fully recovered from neuromuscular blockade, as evidenced by tests of muscle strength (hand grip, head lift, and ability to cough).
- Be alert for adverse reactions and drug interactions.
- Evaluate patient's and family's knowledge of drug therapy.

Nursing diagnoses

- Ineffective health maintenance related to underlying condition
- Ineffective breathing pattern related to drug-induced respiratory depression
- Deficient knowledge related to drug therapy

Planning and implementation

- Allow succinylcholine effects to subside before giving tubocurarine.
- Administer sedatives or general anesthetics before neuromuscular blockers, as ordered. Neuromuscular blockers don't obtund consciousness or alter pain threshold.

• Only personnel skilled in airway management should administer tubocurarine.
• Keep airway clear. Have emergency respiratory support equipment immediately available.
I.V. use: Give drug I.V. over 60 to 90 seconds.
– Don't mix drug with barbiturates (precipitate will form). Use only fresh solutions and discard if discolored.
I.M. use: Follow normal protocol.
• Notify prescriber at once if changes in vital signs occur.
ALERT Nerve stimulator and train-of-four monitoring are recommended to confirm antagonism of neuromuscular blockade and recovery of muscle strength. Before attempting pharmacologic reversal with neostigmine, some evidence of spontaneous recovery should be evident.
• Administer analgesics, as ordered.
ALERT Careful drug calculation is essential. Always verify dosage with another health care professional.

Patient teaching
• Explain all events and happenings to patient because he still can hear.
• Reassure patient that he is being monitored at all times.

Evaluation
• Patient responds well to drug.
• Patient maintains adequate breathing patterns with or without mechanical assistance.
• Patient and family state understanding of drug therapy.

U

urea (carbamide)
(yoo-REE-eh)
Ureaphil

Pharmacologic class: carbonic acid salt
Therapeutic class: osmotic diuretic
Pregnancy risk category: C

Indications and dosages
▶ **Elevated intracranial or intraocular pressure.** *Adults:* 1 to 1.5 g/kg as 30% solution by slow I.V. infusion over 1 to 2½ hours. Maximum dosage is 120 g daily.
Children: 0.5 to 1.5 g/kg slow I.V. infusion or 35 g/m² in 24 hours. Children under age 2 may receive as little as 0.1 g/kg slow I.V. infusion.

How supplied
Injection: 40 g/150 ml

Pharmacokinetics
Absorption: not applicable.
Distribution: distributed in intracellular and extracellular fluid, including lymph, bile, and CSF.
Metabolism: hydrolyzed in GI tract by bacterial uridase.
Excretion: excreted by kidneys.

Route	Onset	Peak	Duration
I.V.	30-45 min	1-2 hr	3-10 hr

Pharmacodynamics
Chemical effect: increases osmotic pressure of glomerular filtrate, inhibiting tubular reabsorption of water and electrolytes. Drug also elevates blood plasma osmolality, resulting in enhanced water flow into extracellular fluid.
Therapeutic effect: promotes water excretion, which in turn reduces intracranial and intraocular pressure.

Adverse reactions
CNS: *headache,* syncope, disorientation.
CV: hypotension, tachycardia, dizziness, ECG changes.
GI: *nausea, vomiting.*
Metabolic: ***hyponatremia,*** hypokalemia, fluid overload.
Other: irritation, necrotic sloughing (with extravasation), hemolysis (with rapid administration).

Interactions
Drug-drug. *Lithium:* increased lithium clearance and decreased lithium effectiveness. Monitor lithium level.

Contraindications and precautions

• Contraindicated in patients with severely impaired kidney function, marked dehydration, frank hepatic failure, active intracranial bleeding, or sickle cell disease with CNS involvement.
• Use cautiously in patients with cardiac disease or hepatic or renal impairment and in pregnant or breast-feeding women.

NURSING CONSIDERATIONS

Assessment

• Assess patient's condition before therapy and regularly thereafter.
• Assess breath sounds for crackles, indicating pulmonary edema.
• Watch for signs of hyponatremia (nausea, vomiting, tachycardia) or hypokalemia (muscle weakness, lethargy); they may indicate electrolyte depletion before serum levels are reduced.
• Monitor blood pressure, fluid intake and output, and serum electrolyte levels.
• In patient with renal disease, monitor BUN level.
• Be alert for adverse reactions and drug interactions.
• Evaluate patient's and family's knowledge of drug therapy.

Nursing diagnoses

• Excessive fluid volume related to presence of water retention
• Acute pain related to drug-induced headache
• Deficient knowledge related to drug therapy

Planning and implementation

• To prepare 135 ml of 30% solution, mix contents of 40-g vial of urea with 105 ml of D_5W or dextrose 10% in water or 10% invert sugar in water. Each ml of 30% solution provides 300 mg of urea.
• Use only freshly reconstituted urea for I.V. infusion; solution becomes ammonia on standing. Use within minutes of reconstitution and discard within 24 hours.
ALERT Avoid rapid I.V. infusion; it may cause hemolysis or increased capillary bleeding. Maximum infusion rate is 4 ml/minute. Avoid extravasation; it may cause reactions ranging from mild irritation to necrosis.
• Don't give drug through same infusion set as blood or blood derivatives.
• Don't infuse drug into leg veins; doing so may cause phlebitis or thrombosis, especially in elderly patients.
• Maintain adequate hydration.
• To ensure bladder emptying in comatose patient, use indwelling urinary catheter. Use hourly urometer collection bag for accurate evaluation of diuresis.
• If satisfactory diuresis doesn't occur in 6 to 12 hours, urea should be discontinued and kidney function reevaluated.
• Administer mild analgesic if drug-induced headache occurs.

Patient teaching

• Inform patient and family of need for urea therapy, and answer any questions.

Evaluation

• Patient exhibits decreased intracranial or intraocular pressure.
• Patient states that drug-induced headache is relieved with mild analgesic.
• Patient and family state understanding of drug therapy.

urokinase

(yoo-roh-KIGH-nays)
Abbokinase Open-Cath, Ukidan ◇

Pharmacologic class: thrombolytic enzyme
Therapeutic class: thrombolytic enzyme
Pregnancy risk category: B

Indications and dosages

▶ **Lysis of acute massive pulmonary embolism or of pulmonary embolism accompanied by unstable hemodynamics.** *Adults:* priming dose: 4,400 IU/kg I.V. given over 10 minutes, followed by 4,400 IU/kg hourly for 12 hours. Total volume should not exceed 200 ml. Therapy followed with continuous I.V. infusion of heparin, then oral anticoagulants.
▶ **Coronary artery thrombosis.** *Adults:* after bolus dose of heparin ranging from 2,500 to

10,000 units, 6,000 IU/minute of urokinase is infused into occluded artery for up to 2 hours. Average total dosage is 500,000 IU.

▶ **Venous catheter occlusion.** *Adults:* 5,000 IU instilled into occluded line and aspirated after 5 minutes. Aspiration attempts repeated q 5 minutes for 30 minutes. If not patent after 30 minutes, line is capped and urokinase left to work for 30 to 60 minutes before aspirating again. May require second instillation.

How supplied

Injection: 5,000 units (IU) per unit-dose vial; 9,000 units (IU) per unit-dose vial; 250,000-IU vial

Pharmacokinetics

Absorption: not applicable.
Distribution: rapidly cleared from circulation; most of drug accumulates in kidneys and liver.
Metabolism: rapidly metabolized in liver.
Excretion: small amount excreted in urine and bile. *Half-life:* 10 to 20 minutes.

Route	Onset	Peak	Duration
I.V.	Immediate	20 min-2 hr	About 4 hr

Pharmacodynamics

Chemical effect: activates plasminogen by directly cleaving peptide bonds at two sites.
Therapeutic effect: dissolves blood clots in lungs, coronary arteries, and venous catheters.

Adverse reactions

CV: ***reperfusion arrhythmias,*** hypotension.
Hematologic: *bleeding.*
GI: nausea, vomiting.
Respiratory: ***bronchospasm,*** minor breathing difficulties.
Other: phlebitis at injection site, hypersensitivity reactions, ***anaphylaxis,*** fever, chills.

Interactions

Drug-drug. *Anticoagulants:* increased risk of bleeding. Monitor patient closely.
Aspirin, dipyridamole, indomethacin, phenylbutazone, other drugs affecting platelet activity: increased risk of bleeding. Monitor patient closely.

Contraindications and precautions

- Contraindicated in pregnant women and in patients with active internal bleeding; history of CVA; aneurysm; arteriovenous malformation; bleeding diathesis; recent trauma with possible internal injuries; visceral or intracranial cancer; ulcerative colitis; diverticulitis; severe hypertension; hemostatic defects, including those secondary to severe hepatic or renal insufficiency; uncontrolled hypocoagulation; chronic pulmonary disease with cavitation; subacute bacterial endocarditis or rheumatic valvular disease; or recent cerebral embolism, thrombosis, or hemorrhage.
- Also contraindicated during the first 10 days postpartum; within 10 days after intra-arterial diagnostic procedure or surgery (liver or kidney biopsy, lumbar puncture, thoracentesis, paracentesis, or extensive or multiple cutdowns); and within 2 months after intracranial or intraspinal surgery.
- I.M. injections and other invasive procedures are contraindicated during urokinase therapy.
- Safety of drug hasn't been established in children.

NURSING CONSIDERATIONS

Assessment

- Assess patient's condition before therapy and regularly thereafter.
- Assess patient for any contraindications to the therapy.
- Monitor patient for excessive bleeding every 15 minutes for first hour; every 30 minutes for second through eighth hours; then once every shift. Pretreatment with drugs affecting platelets places patient at high risk for bleeding.
- Monitor pulse rates, color, and sensation of limbs every hour.
- Although risk of hypersensitivity is low, watch for signs of this reaction.
- Keep laboratory flowsheet on patient's chart to monitor PTT, PT, INR, and hemoglobin and hematocrit levels.
- Monitor vital signs.
- Be alert for adverse reactions and drug interactions.
- Evaluate patient's and family's knowledge of drug therapy.

Nursing diagnoses

- Ineffective tissue perfusion (cardiopulmonary, peripheral) related to presence of blood clot(s)
- Ineffective protection related to drug-induced bleeding
- Deficient knowledge related to drug therapy

Planning and implementation

- Have typed and crossmatched RBCs, whole blood, and aminocaproic acid available to treat bleeding and corticosteroids to treat allergic reactions.
- Add 5 ml of sterile water for injection to vial. Dilute further with normal saline solution or D_5W solution before infusion. Total volume of fluid administered shouldn't exceed 200 ml. Don't use bacteriostatic water for injection to reconstitute; it contains preservatives. Urokinase solutions may be filtered through 0.45-mcg or smaller cellulose membrane filter before administration. Administer by infusion pump.
- Keep venipuncture sites to a minimum; use pressure dressing on puncture sites for at least 15 minutes.
- Keep limb being treated in straight alignment to prevent bleeding from infusion site.
- Avoid unnecessary handling of patient; pad side rails. Bruising is more likely during therapy.
- Heparin by continuous infusion should be started when patient's thrombin time has decreased to less than twice the normal control value after urokinase has been stopped to prevent recurrent thrombosis.

Patient teaching

- Instruct patient to report symptoms of bleeding and other adverse reactions.

Evaluation

- Patient regains normal tissue perfusion with dissolution of blood clots.
- Patient doesn't experience serious complications from drug-induced bleeding.
- Patient and family state understanding of drug therapy.

ursodiol

(ur-sih-DIGH-al)
Actigall

Pharmacologic class: bile acid
Therapeutic class: gallstone solubilizing agent
Pregnancy risk category: B

Indications and dosages

▶ **Dissolution of gallstones smaller than 20 mm in diameter in patients who are poor candidates for surgery or who refuse surgery.** *Adults:* 8 to 10 mg/kg P.O. daily in two or three divided doses.

How supplied

Capsules: 300 mg

Pharmacokinetics

Absorption: about 90% of therapeutic dose absorbed in small intestine after administration.
Distribution: after absorption, ursodiol enters portal vein and is extracted from portal blood by liver (first-pass effect), where it's conjugated and then secreted into hepatic bile ducts. Ursodiol in bile is concentrated in gallbladder and expelled into duodenum in gallbladder bile. A small amount appears in systemic circulation.
Metabolism: metabolized in liver. A small amount undergoes bacterial degradation with each cycle of enterohepatic circulation.
Excretion: excreted primarily in feces. Very small amount excreted in urine. Reabsorbed free ursodiol reconjugated by liver.

Route	Onset	Peak	Duration
P.O.	Unknown	1-3 hr	Unknown

Pharmacodynamics

Chemical effect: unknown; probably suppresses hepatic synthesis and secretion of cholesterol as well as intestinal cholesterol absorption. After long-term administration, ursodiol can solubilize cholesterol from gallstones.
Therapeutic effect: dissolves cholesterol gallstones.

Adverse reactions

CNS: *headache,* fatigue, anxiety, depression, *dizziness,* sleep disorders.
EENT: rhinitis.
GI: *nausea, vomiting, dyspepsia,* metallic taste, *abdominal pain,* biliary pain, cholecystitis, *diarrhea, constipation,* stomatitis, flatulence.
GU: urinary tract infection.
Musculoskeletal: arthralgia, myalgia, back pain.
Respiratory: cough.
Skin: pruritus, rash, dry skin, urticaria, hair thinning, diaphoresis.

Interactions

Drug-drug. *Aluminum-containing antacids, cholestyramine, colestipol:* bind ursodiol and prevent its absorption. Avoid concomitant use. *Clofibrate, estrogens, oral contraceptives:* increased hepatic cholesterol secretion; may counteract effects of ursodiol. Avoid concomitant use.

Contraindications and precautions

- Contraindicated in patients hypersensitive to ursodiol or other bile acids.
- Also contraindicated in patients with chronic hepatic disease, unremitting acute cholecystitis, cholangitis, biliary obstruction, gallstone-induced pancreatitis, or biliary fistula.
- Use cautiously in pregnant or breast-feeding women.
- Safety of drug hasn't been established in children.

NURSING CONSIDERATIONS

Assessment

- Assess patient's condition before therapy and regularly thereafter.
- Usually therapy is long-term and requires ultrasound images of gallbladder taken at 6-month intervals. If partial stone dissolution doesn't occur within 12 months, eventual success is unlikely. Safety of use for longer than 24 months hasn't been established.

ALERT Monitor liver function test results, including AST and ALT levels, at beginning of therapy and after 1 month, 3 months, and then every 6 months during ursodiol therapy, as ordered. Abnormal test results may indicate worsening of disease. A theoretical risk exists that hepatotoxic metabolite of ursodiol may form in some patients.

- Be alert for adverse reactions and drug interactions.
- Monitor patient's hydration status if adverse GI reactions occur.
- Evaluate patient's and family's knowledge of drug therapy.

Nursing diagnoses

- Risk for injury related to presence of gallstones
- Risk for deficient fluid volume related to drug-induced adverse GI reactions
- Deficient knowledge related to drug therapy

Planning and implementation

- Drug won't dissolve calcified cholesterol stones, radiolucent bile pigment stones, or radiopaque stones.

Patient teaching

- Tell patient about alternative therapies, including watchful waiting (no intervention) and cholecystectomy because relapse rate after bile acid therapy may be as high as 50% after 5 years.

Evaluation

- Patient is free from gallstones.
- Patient maintains adequate hydration.
- Patient and family state understanding of drug therapy.

V

valacyclovir hydrochloride

(val-ay-SIGH-kloh-veer high-droh-KLOR-ighd)
Valtrex

Pharmacologic class: synthetic purine nucleoside
Therapeutic class: antiviral
Pregnancy risk category: B

Indications and dosages

▶ **Treatment of herpes zoster (shingles) in immunocompetent patients.** *Adults:* 1 g P.O. t.i.d. daily for 7 days. Dosage is adjusted for patients with impaired kidney function, based on creatinine clearance levels.

How supplied

Caplets: 500 mg, 1 gm

Pharmacokinetics

Absorption: rapidly absorbed from GI tract; absolute bioavailability of about 54.5%.
Distribution: protein-binding ranges from 13.5% to 17.9%.
Metabolism: rapidly and nearly completely converted to acyclovir and L-valine by first-pass intestinal or hepatic metabolism.
Excretion: excreted in urine and feces. *Half-life:* averages 2.5 to 3.3 hours.

Route	Onset	Peak	Duration
P.O.	About 30 min	Unknown	Unknown

Pharmacodynamics

Chemical effect: rapidly converted to acyclovir, which becomes incorporated into viral DNA and inhibits viral DNA polymerase, thereby inhibiting viral replication.
Therapeutic effect: inhibits susceptible viral growth of herpes zoster.

Adverse reactions

CNS: *headache,* dizziness, asthenia.
GI: *nausea,* vomiting, diarrhea, constipation, abdominal pain, anorexia.

Interactions

Drug-drug. *Cimetidine, probenecid:* reduces rate (but not extent) of conversion from valacyclovir to acyclovir and reduces renal clearance of acyclovir, thereby increasing acyclovir blood levels. Monitor patient for possible toxicity.

Contraindications and precautions

- Contraindicated in patients hypersensitive to or intolerant of valacyclovir, acyclovir, or components of their formulations.
- Drug isn't recommended for immunocompromised patients. Thrombotic thrombocytopenic purpura and hemolytic uremic syndrome have been fatal in some patients with advanced HIV disease and in bone marrow transplant and renal transplant recipients.
- Use cautiously in patients with renal impairment and in those receiving other nephrotoxic drugs.
- Safety and efficacy haven't been established in children and in breast-feeding women. Drug should be given to pregnant women only if potential benefits outweigh risk to the fetus.

NURSING CONSIDERATIONS

Assessment

- Assess patient's infection before therapy.
- Evaluate patient's and family's knowledge of drug therapy.

Nursing diagnoses

- Risk for infection related to herpes zoster
- Deficient fluid volume related to adverse GI reactions
- Deficient knowledge related to drug therapy

Planning and implementation

- Follow-up studies haven't shown an increased risk of birth defects for infants born to patients exposed to the drug during pregnancy.
- Dosage adjustment may be necessary in elderly patient, depending on underlying renal status.
- Although overdose hasn't been reported, precipitation of acyclovir in renal tubules may occur when solubility (2.5 mg/ml) is exceeded in the intratubular fluid. In the event of acute renal failure and anuria, the patient may benefit from hemodialysis until kidney function is restored.

Patient teaching

- Inform patient that drug may be taken without regard to meals.
- Review signs and symptoms of herpes infection (rash, tingling, itching, and pain), and advise patient to notify prescriber immediately if they occur. Treatment should begin as soon as possible after symptoms appear, preferably within 48 hours.

Evaluation
- Patient is free from infection.
- Patient maintains adequate hydration.
- Patient and family state understanding of drug therapy.

valproate sodium
(val-PROH-ayt SOH-dee-um)
Depacon, Depakene Syrup, Epilim ◊

valproic acid
Depakene, Myproic Acid

divalproex sodium
Depakote, Depakote Sprinkle, Epival ♦

Pharmacologic class: carboxylic acid derivative
Therapeutic class: anticonvulsant
Pregnancy risk category: D

Indications and dosages
▶ **Simple and complex absence seizures, mixed seizure types (including absence seizures).** *Adults and children:* initially, 15 mg/kg P.O. daily; then increased by 5 to 10 mg/kg daily at weekly intervals up to maximum of 60 mg/kg daily. When dosage exceeds 250 mg daily, drug should be divided into two or more equal doses. Or, 10 to 15 mg/kg/day I.V., increased by 5 to 10 mg/kg/week to clinical response. Maximum I.V.dosage is 60 mg/kg/day.

How supplied
valproate sodium
Syrup: 250 mg/ml
Injection: 100 mg/ml
valproic acid
Tablets (enteric-coated): 200 mg ◊, 500 mg ◊
Crushable tablets: 100 mg ◊
Capsules: 250 mg
Syrup: 200 mg/5 ml ◊
divalproex sodium
Capsules (delayed-release): 125 mg
Tablets (enteric-coated): 125 mg, 250 mg, 500 mg

Pharmacokinetics
Absorption: valproate sodium and divalproex sodium quickly convert to valproic acid after administration.
Distribution: distributed rapidly throughout body; 80% to 95% protein-bound.
Metabolism: metabolized by liver.
Excretion: excreted primarily in urine; some excreted in feces and exhaled air. *Half-life:* 6 to 16 hours (may be considerably longer in patient with liver function impairment, in elderly patient, and in child up to age 18 months; may be considerably shorter in patient receiving hepatic enzyme-inducing anticonvulsants).

Route	Onset	Peak	Duration
P.O.	Unknown	1-4 hr	Unknown
I.V.	Unknown	Unknown	Unknown

Pharmacodynamics
Chemical effect: unknown; probably increases brain levels of gamma-aminobutyric acid, which transmits inhibitory nerve impulses in CNS.
Therapeutic effect: prevents and treats certain types of seizure activity.

Adverse reactions
Because drug typically is used with other anticonvulsants, adverse reactions reported may not be caused by valproic acid alone.
CNS: *sedation,* emotional upset, depression, psychosis, aggressiveness, hyperactivity, behavioral deterioration, muscle weakness, tremors, ataxia, headache, dizziness, incoordination.
EENT: nystagmus, diplopia.
GI: *nausea, vomiting, indigestion,* diarrhea, abdominal cramps, constipation, increased appetite and weight gain, anorexia, ***pancreatitis.***
Hematologic: petechiae, bruising, eosinophilia, ***hemorrhage, leukopenia, bone marrow suppression, thrombocytopenia,*** increased bleeding time.
Hepatic: *elevated liver enzyme levels,* ***toxic hepatitis.***
Skin: rash, alopecia, pruritus, photosensitivity, ***erythema multiforme.***

Interactions

Drug-drug. *Aspirin, chlorpromazine, cimetidine, felbamate:* may cause valproic acid toxicity. Use together cautiously and monitor blood levels.
Benzodiazepines, other CNS depressants: excessive CNS depression. Avoid concomitant use.
Erythromycin: increased serum valproate levels. Monitor patient for toxicity.
Lamotrigine: increased or decreased lamotrigine levels. Monitor levels closely.
Phenobarbital: increased phenobarbital levels. Monitor patient closely.
Phenytoin: increased or decreased phenytoin level. Monitor patient closely.
Rifampin: may decrease valproate levels. Monitor levels.
Warfarin: valproic acid may displace warfarin from binding sites. Monitor PT and INR.
Drug-herb. *Glutamine:* increased risk of seizures. Discourage concomitant use.
White willow: herb contains substances similar to aspirin. Discourage concomitant use.
Drug-lifestyle. *Alcohol use:* excessive CNS depression. Discourage concurrent use.

Contraindications and precautions

- Contraindicated in patients hypersensitive to drug.
- Drug isn't recommended for pregnant or breast-feeding women.
- Use with extreme caution in patients with history of hepatic dysfunction.

NURSING CONSIDERATIONS

Assessment

- Assess patient's condition before therapy and regularly thereafter.
- Monitor blood levels, as ordered. Therapeutic blood level is 50 to 100 mcg/ml.
- Monitor liver function studies, platelet counts, and PT before starting drug and periodically thereafter, as ordered.
- Be alert for adverse reactions and drug interactions.
- Evaluate patient's and family's knowledge of drug therapy.

Nursing diagnoses

- Risk for trauma related to seizure activity
- Disturbed thought processes related to drug-induced adverse CNS reactions
- Deficient knowledge related to drug therapy

Planning and implementation

P.O. use: Don't administer syrup to patient who needs sodium restriction. Check with prescriber.
– Administer drug with food or milk to minimize adverse GI reactions.
I.V. use: Dilute with at least 50 ml of a compatible diluent (D_5W, saline solution, lactated Ringer's injection) and administer I.V. over 1 hour. Don't exceed 20 mg/minute.

- Sudden withdrawal may worsen seizures. Call prescriber at once if adverse reactions develop.

ALERT Serious or fatal hepatotoxicity may follow nonspecific symptoms, such as malaise, fever, and lethargy. Notify prescriber at once if patient has suspected or apparently substantial hepatic dysfunction because drug will need to be discontinued.

- Patients at high risk for developing hepatotoxicity include those with congenital metabolic disorders, mental retardation, or organic brain disease; those taking other anticonvulsants; and children under age 2.
- Divalproex sodium carries a lower risk of adverse GI effects than other drug forms.
- Notify prescriber if tremors occur. Dosage may need to be reduced.
- Drug may produce false-positive test results for ketones in urine.

Patient teaching

- Tell patient that drug may be taken with food or milk to reduce adverse GI effects.
- Advise patient not to chew capsules.
- Tell patient and parents that syrup shouldn't be mixed with carbonated beverages.
- Tell patient and parents to keep drug out of children's reach.
- Warn patient and parents not to stop drug therapy abruptly.
- Advise patient to refrain from driving or performing other potentially hazardous activities that require mental alertness until drug's CNS effects are known.

Evaluation
- Patient is free from seizure activity.
- Patient maintains normal thought processes.
- Patient and family state understanding of drug therapy.

valrubicin
(val-ROO-buh-sin)
Valstar

Pharmacologic class: anthracycline
Therapeutic class: antineoplastic
Pregnancy risk category: C

Indications and dosages
▶ **Intravesical therapy of BCG-refractory carcinoma in situ of the urinary bladder in patients for whom immediate cystectomy would be linked to unacceptable morbidity or mortality.** *Adults:* 800 mg intravesically once weekly for six weeks.

How supplied
Solution for intravesical instillation: 200 mg/5 ml

Pharmacokinetics
Absorption: unknown.
Distribution: penetrates into the bladder wall after intravesical administration. Systemic exposure depends on the condition of the bladder wall.
Metabolism: metabolites found in the blood.
Excretion: drug is almost completely excreted by voiding the instillate.

Route	Onset	Peak	Duration
Intravesical	Unknown	Unknown	Unknown

Pharmacodynamics
Chemical effect: drug is an anthracycline that exerts cytotoxic activity by penetrating into cells, inhibiting the incorporation of nucleosides into nucleic acids, causing extensive chromosomal damage, and arresting the cell cycle in G_2. It also interferes with the normal DNA breaking-resealing action of DNA topoisomerase II, thereby inhibiting DNA synthesis.
Therapeutic effect: kills certain cancer cells.

Adverse reactions
CNS: asthenia, headache, malaise, dizziness.
CV: vasodilation, chest pain, peripheral edema.
GI: diarrhea, flatulence, nausea, vomiting, abdominal pain.
GU: urine retention, *urinary tract infection, urinary frequency, dysuria, urinary urgency, bladder spasm, hematuria, bladder pain, urinary incontinence,* pelvic pain, urethral pain, nocturia, *cystitis,* local burning.
Hematologic: anemia.
Metabolic: hyperglycemia.
Musculoskeletal: myalgia, back pain.
Respiratory: pneumonia.
Skin: rash.
Other: fever.

Interactions
None reported.

Contraindications and precautions
- Contraindicated in patients hypersensitive to drug, other anthracyclines, or Cremophor EL (polyoxyethyleneglycol triricinoleate). Also contraindicated in patients with urinary tract infections, patients with a small bladder capacity (unable to tolerate a 75-ml instillation), and patients with a perforated bladder or those in whom the integrity of the bladder mucosa has been compromised.
- Use cautiously in patients with severe irritable bladder symptoms.

NURSING CONSIDERATIONS

Assessment
- Obtain history of patient's underlying condition before therapy and reassess regularly thereafter.
- For patients undergoing transurethral resection of the bladder, evaluate the status of the bladder before intravesical instillation of drug in order to avoid dangerous systemic exposure. For bladder perforation, delay administration until bladder integrity has been restored.

• Monitor patient for myelosuppression, which begins during the first week, with the nadir by the second week and recovery by the third week.
• Monitor patient closely for disease recurrence or progression by cystoscopy, biopsy, and urine cytology every 3 months.
• Monitor complete blood counts every 3 weeks if valrubicin is administered when bladder rupture or perforation is suspected.
• Evaluate patient's and family's knowledge about drug therapy.

Nursing diagnoses

• Impaired urinary elimination related to drug-induced adverse effects
• Imbalanced nutrition: less than body requirements related to drug-induced adverse GI effects
• Deficient knowledge related to drug therapy

Planning and implementation

• Procedures for proper handling and disposal of antineoplastic drugs should be used.
• Use caution when handling and preparing solution. Use gloves during dose preparation and administration. Prepare and store solution in glass, polypropylene, or polyolefin containers and tubing, and use polyethylene-lined administration sets. Don't use polyvinyl chloride I.V. bags and tubing.
• Use aseptic techniques during administration to avoid introducing contaminants into the urinary tract or traumatizing the urinary mucosa.
• To prepare, slowly warm four vials of the drug to room temperature. Withdraw a total of 20 ml from the four vials (200 mg valrubicin in each 5-ml vial), and dilute with 55 ml of normal saline solution for injection, providing 75 ml of a diluted valrubicin solution.
• Refigerate unopened vials at 2° to 8° C (36° to 46° F). Diluted valrubicin is stable for 12 hours at temperatures up to 25° C (77° F).
ALERT Don't mix valrubicin with other drugs. No compatability data are available.
ALERT Drug should be administered intravesically only under the supervision of clinicians experienced in the use of intravesical antineoplastic drugs. Don't give I.V. or I.M.
• To give drug, first drain the bladder by inserting a urethral catheter into the patient's bladder under aseptic conditions. Then, instill the solution slowly via gravity flow over a period of several minutes. Withdraw the catheter. The patient should retain the drug for two hours before voiding. At the end of two hours, have the patient void. (Some patients will be unable to retain the drug for the full two hours.)
• In patients with severe irritable bladder symptoms, bladder spasm and spontaneous discharge of the intravesical instillate may occur. Clamping of the urinary catheter isn't advised and, if performed, should be executed cautiously under medical supervision.
• If carcinoma in situ (CIS) doesn't show a complete response to valrubicin treatment after 3 months, or if it recurs, cystectomy must be reconsidered because, if delayed, the patient could develop metastatic bladder cancer.

Patient teaching

• Inform patient that drug has been shown to induce complete response in only about 1 in 5 patients with refractory CIS. If there isn't a complete response of CIS to treatment after 3 months, or if CIS recurs, tell patient to discuss with health care provider the risks of cystectomy versus the risks of metastatic bladder cancer.
• Advise patient to retain the drug for two hours before voiding, if possible. Instruct patient to void at the end of two hours.
• Instruct patient to maintain adequate hydration following treatment.
• Inform patient that the major adverse reactions are related to irritable bladder symptoms that may occur during instillation and retention of the drug and for a limited period following voiding. For the first 24 hours following administration, red-tinged urine is typical. Tell patient to immediately report prolonged irritable bladder symptoms or prolonged passage of red-colored urine.
• Advise women of childbearing age to avoid pregnancy during treatment. Advise men to avoid procreative activities while receiving treatment. Effective contraception should be used by all patients during the treatment period.

Evaluation
- Patient maintains adequate urinary elimination.
- Patient doesn't experience adverse GI effects.
- Patient and family state understanding of drug therapy.

valsartan
(val-SAR-tin)
Diovan

Pharmacologic class: angiotensin II receptor blocker
Therapeutic class: antihypertensive
Pregnancy risk category: C (D in second and third trimesters)

Indications and dosages
▶ **Hypertension, used alone or with other antihypertensives.** *Adults:* initially, 80 mg P.O. once daily. Expect a reduction in blood pressure in 2 to 4 weeks. If additional antihypertensive effect is needed, dosage may be increased to 160 or 320 mg daily, or a diuretic may be added. (Addition of a diuretic has a greater effect than dosage increases beyond 80 mg.) Usual dosage range is 80 to 320 mg daily.

How supplied
Capsules: 80 mg, 160 mg

Pharmacokinetics
Absorption: bioavailability about 25%; food decreases absorption.
Distribution: not distributed into tissues extensively; 95% bound to serum proteins.
Metabolism: metabolized in liver and kidneys.
Excretion: excreted in urine and feces.

Route	Onset	Peak	Duration
P.O.	Within 2 hr	2-4 hr	24 hr

Pharmacodynamics
Chemical effect: blocks binding of angiotensin II to receptor sites in vascular smooth muscle and adrenal gland.
Therapeutic effect: inhibits pressor effects of renin-angiotensin system.

Adverse reactions
CNS: headache, dizziness, fatigue.
CV: edema.
EENT: rhinitis, sinusitis, pharyngitis.
GI: abdominal pain, diarrhea, nausea.
Hematologic: ***neutropenia.***
Metabolic: hyperkalemia.
Musculoskeletal: arthralgia.
Respiratory: upper respiratory tract infection, cough.
Other: viral infection.

Interactions
Drug-drug. *Diuretics:* risk of hypotension. Assess fluid status before starting concomitant therapy. Monitor patient closely.
Drug-food. *Any food:* decreased peak drug levels. Give drug on an empty stomach.

Contraindications and precautions
- Contraindicated in patients hypersensitive to drug.

NURSING CONSIDERATIONS

Assessment
- Use cautiously in patients with severe renal or hepatic disease.
- Monitor patient for hypotension. Correct volume and sodium depletions as ordered before starting drug therapy.

Nursing diagnoses
- Risk for injury related to presence of hypertension
- Deficient knowledge related to drug therapy

Planning and implementation
- Don't give drug during second or third trimester of pregnancy or to breast-feeding women.
- Safety and effectiveness in children haven't been established.

Patient teaching
- Tell woman to notify prescriber if she becomes pregnant.

• Teach patient other means of reducing blood pressure, including proper diet, exercise, smoking cessation, and decreasing stress.

☑ Evaluation

• Patient's blood pressure becomes normal.
• Patient and family state understanding of drug therapy.

vancomycin hydrochloride

(van-koh-MIGH-sin high-droh-KLOR-ighd)
Vancocin, Vancoled

Pharmacologic class: glycopeptide
Therapeutic class: antibiotic
Pregnancy risk category: C

Indications and dosages

▶ **Severe staphylococcal infections when other antibiotics are ineffective or contraindicated.** *Adults:* 500 mg I.V. q 6 hours, or 1 g q 12 hours.
Children: 40 mg/kg I.V. daily in divided doses q 6 hours.
Neonates: initially, 15 mg/kg; then 10 mg/kg I.V. daily, divided q 12 hours for first week after birth; then q 8 hours up to age 1 month.
▶ **Antibiotic-related pseudomembranous and staphylococcal enterocolitis.** *Adults:* 125 to 500 mg P.O. q 6 hours for 7 to 10 days.
Children: 40 mg/kg P.O. daily in divided doses q 6 to 8 hours for 7 to 10 days. Maximum, 2 g daily.
▶ **Endocarditis prophylaxis for dental procedures.** *Adults:* 1 g I.V. slowly over 1 hour, starting 1 hour before procedure.
Children: 20 mg/kg I.V. over 1 hour, starting 1 hour before procedure.

How supplied

Capsules: 125 mg, 250 mg
Powder for oral solution: 1-g, 10-g bottles
Powder for injection: 500-mg, 1-g vials

Pharmacokinetics

Absorption: minimal systemic absorption with P.O. administration. (Drug may accumulate in patients with colitis or renal failure.)
Distribution: distributed in body fluids; achieves therapeutic levels in CSF if meninges inflamed.
Metabolism: unknown.
Excretion: excreted in urine with parenteral administration; excreted in feces with P.O. administration. *Half-life:* 6 hours.

Route	Onset	Peak	Duration
P.O.	Unknown	Unknown	Unknown
I.V.	Immediate	Immediate	Unknown

Pharmacodynamics

Chemical effect: hinders bacterial cell wall synthesis, damaging bacterial plasma membrane and making cell more vulnerable to osmotic pressure.
Therapeutic effect: kills susceptible bacteria. Spectrum of activity includes many gram-positive organisms, including those resistant to other antibiotics. It's useful for *Staphylococcus epidermidis*, methicillin-resistant *Staphylococcus aureus,* and penicillin-resistant *Streptococcus pneumoniae.*

Adverse reactions

CV: hypotension.
EENT: tinnitus, ototoxicity.
GI: nausea.
GU: ***nephrotoxicity,*** pseudomembranous colitis.
Hematologic: eosinophilia, ***leukopenia.***
Respiratory: wheezing, dyspnea.
Skin: "red-neck" or "red-man" syndrome (maculopapular rash on face, neck, trunk, and limbs with rapid I.V. infusion; pruritus and hypotension with histamine release).
Other: chills, fever, ***anaphylaxis,*** superinfection, pain, thrombophlebitis at injection site.

Interactions

Drug-drug. ***Aminoglycosides, amphotericin B, cisplatin, pentamidine:*** increased risk of nephrotoxicity and ototoxicity. Monitor patient closely.

Contraindications and precautions

• Contraindicated in patients hypersensitive to drug.
• Use cautiously in patients receiving other neurotoxic, nephrotoxic, or ototoxic drugs; pa-

tients over age 60; those with impaired liver or kidney function, hearing loss, or allergies to other antibiotics; and pregnant women.
• Safety of drug hasn't been established in breast-feeding women.

NURSING CONSIDERATIONS

Assessment
• Assess patient's infection before therapy and regularly thereafter.
• Obtain urine specimen for culture and sensitivity tests before giving first dose. Therapy may begin pending test results.
• Obtain hearing evaluation and kidney function studies before therapy and repeat, as ordered, during therapy.
• Check serum levels regularly, especially in elderly patients, premature infants, and those with decreased renal function.
• Be alert for adverse reactions and drug interactions.
• Evaluate patient's and family's knowledge of drug therapy.

Nursing diagnoses
• Risk for infection related to presence of susceptible bacteria
• Risk for injury related to drug-induced adverse reactions
• Deficient knowledge related to drug therapy

Planning and implementation
• Patient with renal dysfunction needs dosage adjustment.
ALERT Oral administration is ineffective for systemic infections, and I.V. administration is ineffective for pseudomembranous (*Clostridium difficile*) diarrhea.
P.O. use: Oral form is stable for 2 weeks if refrigerated.
I.V. use: For I.V. infusion, dilute in 200 ml of saline solution injection or D_5W and infuse over 60 minutes.
– Check site daily for phlebitis and irritation. Report pain at infusion site. Avoid extravasation; severe irritation and necrosis can result.
– If red-neck or red-man syndrome occurs because drug is infused too rapidly, stop infusion and report to prescriber.
– Refrigerate I.V. solution after reconstitution and use within 96 hours.
• Don't give drug I.M.
• When using drug to treat staphylococcal endocarditis, give for at least 4 weeks.

Patient teaching
• Tell patient to take entire amount of drug exactly as directed, even after he feels better.
• Tell patient to stop drug immediately and report adverse reactions, especially fullness or ringing in ears.

Evaluation
• Patient is free from infection.
• Patient doesn't experience injury from adverse reactions.
• Patient and family state understanding of drug therapy.

vasopressin (ADH)
(VAY-soh-preh-sin)
Pitressin

Pharmacologic class: posterior pituitary hormone
Therapeutic class: ADH, peristaltic stimulant
Pregnancy risk category: D

Indications and dosages
▶ **Nonnephrogenic, nonpsychogenic diabetes insipidus.** *Adults:* 5 to 10 units I.M. or S.C. b.i.d. to q.i.d., p.r.n. Or, intranasally (aqueous solution used as spray or applied to cotton balls) in individualized dosages, based on response.
Children: 2.5 to 10 units I.M. or S.C. b.i.d. to q.i.d., p.r.n. Or, intranasally (aqueous solution used as spray or applied to cotton balls) in individualized doses.
▶ **Postoperative abdominal distention.** *Adults:* initially, 5 units (aqueous) I.M.; then q 3 to 4 hours, dose increased to 10 units, if needed. Dosage reduced proportionately for children.
▶ **To expel gas before abdominal X-ray.** *Adults:* 5 to 15 units S.C. 2 hours before X-ray; then again 90 minutes later.

How supplied

Injection: 0.5-ml and 1-ml ampules, 20 units/ml

Pharmacokinetics

Absorption: unknown.
Distribution: distributed throughout extracellular fluid without evidence of protein-binding.
Metabolism: most of drug is destroyed rapidly in liver and kidneys.
Excretion: excreted in urine. *Half-life:* 10 to 20 minutes.

Route	Onset	Peak	Duration
S.C., I.M., intranasal	Unknown	Unknown	2-8 hr

Pharmacodynamics

Chemical effect: increases permeability of renal tubular epithelium to adenosine monophosphate and water; epithelium promotes reabsorption of water and produces concentrated urine (ADH effect).
Therapeutic effect: promotes water reabsorption and stimulates GI motility.

Adverse reactions

CNS: tremors, vertigo, headache.
CV: angina in patients with vascular disease, vasoconstriction, ***arrhythmias, cardiac arrest,*** myocardial ischemia, circumoral pallor, decreased cardiac output.
GI: abdominal cramps, nausea, vomiting, flatulence.
Skin: cutaneous gangrene, diaphoresis.
Other: water intoxication (drowsiness, listlessness, headache, confusion, weight gain, ***seizures, coma***), hypersensitivity reactions (urticaria, ***angioedema, bronchoconstriction, anaphylaxis***).

Interactions

Drug-drug. *Carbamazepine, chlorpropamide, clofibrate, fludrocortisone, tricyclic antidepressants:* increased antidiuretic response. Use together cautiously.
Demeclocycline, heparin, lithium, norepinephrine: reduced antidiuretic activity. Use together cautiously.
Drug-lifestyle. *Alcohol use:* reduced antidiuretic activity. Discourage concurrent use.

Contraindications and precautions

- Contraindicated in patients with chronic nephritis accompanied by nitrogen retention.
- Use cautiously in children, elderly patients, pregnant or breast-feeding women, preoperative and postoperative polyuric patients, and those with seizure disorders, migraine headache, asthma, CV disease, heart failure, renal disease, goiter with cardiac complications, arteriosclerosis, or fluid overload.

NURSING CONSIDERATIONS

Assessment

- Assess patient's condition before therapy and regularly thereafter.
- Monitor specific gravity of urine and fluid intake and output to aid evaluation of drug effectiveness.
- To prevent possible seizures, coma, and death, observe patient closely for early signs of water intoxication.
- Monitor blood pressure of patient on vasopressin frequently. Watch for excessively elevated blood pressure or lack of response to drug, which may be indicated by hypotension. Also monitor daily weight.
- Be alert for adverse reactions and drug interactions.
- Evaluate patient's and family's knowledge of drug therapy.

Nursing diagnoses

- Risk for deficient fluid volume related to polyuria from diabetes insipidus
- Diarrhea related to drug-induced increased GI motility
- Deficient knowledge related to drug therapy

Planning and implementation

- Drug may be used for transient polyuria resulting from ADH deficiency related to neurosurgery or head injury.
- Minimum effective dosage should be used to reduce adverse reactions.
- Give drug with one to two glasses of water to reduce adverse reactions and to improve therapeutic response.
- A rectal tube facilitates gas expulsion after vasopressin injection.

I.M. and S.C. use: Follow normal protocol.

⚠ **ALERT** Never inject during first stage of labor; doing so may cause uterus to rupture.
Intranasal use: Aqueous solution can be used as a spray or applied to cotton balls. Follow manufacturer's guidelines for intranasal use.
⚠ **ALERT** Don't confuse vasopressin with desmopressin.

Patient teaching
- Instruct patient how to administer drug. Tell patient taking drug S.C. to rotate injection sites to prevent tissue damage.
- Stress importance of monitoring fluid intake and output.
- Tell patient to notify prescriber immediately if adverse reactions occur.

☑ Evaluation
- Patient maintains adequate hydration.
- Patient doesn't experience diarrhea.
- Patient and family state understanding of drug therapy.

vecuronium bromide
(veh-kyoo-ROH-nee-um BROH-mighd)
Norcuron

Pharmacologic class: nondepolarizing neuromuscular blocker
Therapeutic class: skeletal muscle relaxant
Pregnancy risk category: C

Indications and dosages

▶ **Adjunct to general anesthesia; to facilitate endotracheal intubation; to provide skeletal muscle relaxation during surgery or mechanical ventilation.** Dosage depends on anesthetic used, individual needs, and response. Dosages are representative and must be adjusted.
Adults and children over age 9: initially, 0.08 to 0.1 mg/kg I.V. bolus. Maintenance doses of 0.01 to 0.015 mg/kg within 25 to 40 minutes of initial dose should be administered during prolonged surgical procedures. Maintenance doses may be given q 12 to 15 minutes in patients receiving balanced anesthesia.
Children under age 9: may require slightly higher initial dose as well as supplementation slightly more often than adults. Or, drug may be given by continuous I.V. infusion of 1 mcg/kg/minute initially, then 0.8 to 1.2 mcg/kg/minute.

How supplied

Injection: 10 mg/vial; 20 mg/vial

Pharmacokinetics

Absorption: not applicable.
Distribution: distributed in extracellular fluid and rapidly reaches its site of action (skeletal muscles); 60% to 90% plasma protein–bound.
Metabolism: undergoes rapid and extensive hepatic metabolism.
Excretion: excreted in feces and urine. *Half-life:* 20 minutes.

Route	Onset	Peak	Duration
I.V.	≤ 1 min	3-5 min	25-30 min

Pharmacodynamics

Chemical effect: prevents acetylcholine from binding to receptors on motor end plate, thus blocking depolarization.
Therapeutic effect: relaxes skeletal muscle.

Adverse reactions

Musculoskeletal: skeletal muscle weakness.
Respiratory: ***prolonged, dose-related respiratory insufficiency or apnea.***

Interactions

Drug-drug. *Aminoglycoside antibiotics, including amikacin, gentamicin, kanamycin, neomycin, streptomycin; bacitracin; clindamycin; general anesthetics, such as enflurane, halothane, isoflurane; other skeletal muscle relaxants; polymyxin antibiotics such as colistin, polymyxin B sulfate; quinidine; tetracyclines:* potentiated neuromuscular blockade, leading to increased skeletal muscle relaxation and potentiation of effect. Use cautiously during surgical and postoperative periods.
Opioid analgesics: potentiated neuromuscular blockade, leading to increased skeletal muscle relaxation and possible respiratory paralysis. Use with extreme caution, and reduce vecuronium dosage as directed.

Contraindications and precautions

- Contraindicated in patients hypersensitive to bromides.
- Use cautiously in elderly patients; patients with altered circulation caused by CV disease and edematous states; and patients with hepatic disease, severe obesity, bronchogenic carcinoma, electrolyte disturbances, or neuromuscular disease.
- Also use cautiously in pregnant or breast-feeding women.

NURSING CONSIDERATIONS

Assessment

- Assess patient's condition before therapy and regularly thereafter.
- Monitor respiratory rate closely until patient is fully recovered from neuromuscular blockade as evidenced by tests of muscle strength (hand grip, head lift, and ability to cough).
- Be alert for adverse reactions and drug interactions.
- Evaluate patient's and family's knowledge of drug therapy.

Nursing diagnoses

- Ineffective health maintenance related to underlying condition
- Ineffective breathing pattern related to drug's effect on respiratory muscles
- Deficient knowledge related to drug therapy

Planning and implementation

- Keep airway clear. Have emergency respiratory support equipment available immediately.
- Drug should be used only by personnel skilled in airway management.
- Previous administration of succinylcholine may enhance neuromuscular blocking effect and duration of action.
- Administer sedatives or general anesthetics before neuromuscular blockers, as ordered. Neuromuscular blockers don't obtund consciousness or alter pain threshold.
- Administer drug by rapid I.V. injection. Or, 10 to 20 mg may be added to 100 ml of compatible solution and given by I.V. infusion. Compatible solutions include D_5W, normal saline solution for injection, dextrose 5% in normal saline solution for injection, and lactated Ringer's injection.
- Don't mix drug with alkaline solutions.
- Store reconstituted solution in refrigerator. Discard after 24 hours.
- Administer analgesics, as ordered, for pain.
- Nerve stimulator and train-of-four monitoring are recommended to confirm antagonism of neuromuscular blockade and recovery of muscle strength. Before attempting pharmacologic reversal with neostigmine, some evidence of spontaneous recovery should be seen.

ALERT Careful dosage calculation is essential. Always verify with another health care professional.

Patient teaching

- Explain all events and happenings to patient because he can still hear.
- Reassure patient that he is being monitored at all times.

Evaluation

- Patient responds well to drug.
- Patient maintains effective breathing pattern with mechanical assistance.
- Patient and family state understanding of drug therapy.

venlafaxine hydrochloride

(ven-leh-FAKS-een high-droh-KLOR-ighd)
Effexor

Pharmacologic class: neuronal serotonin, norepinephrine, and dopamine reuptake inhibitor
Therapeutic class: antidepressant
Pregnancy risk category: C

Indications and dosages

▶ **Depression.** *Adults:* initially, 75 mg P.O. daily in two or three divided doses with food. Dosage increased as tolerated and needed in increments of 75 mg/day at intervals of no less than 4 days. For moderately depressed outpatients, usual maximum dosage is 225 mg/day; in certain severely depressed patients, dosage may be as high as 350 mg/day.

How supplied

Tablets: 25 mg, 37.5 mg, 50 mg, 75 mg, 100 mg

Pharmacokinetics

Absorption: about 92% absorbed after P.O. administration.
Distribution: about 25% to 29% protein-bound in plasma.
Metabolism: extensively metabolized in liver.
Excretion: excreted in urine.

Route	Onset	Peak	Duration
P.O.	Unknown	Unknown	Unknown

Pharmacodynamics

Chemical effect: blocks reuptake of norepinephrine and serotonin into neurons in CNS.
Therapeutic effect: relieves depression.

Adverse reactions

CNS: *asthenia, headache, somnolence, dizziness, nervousness, insomnia,* anxiety, tremors, abnormal dreams, paresthesia, agitation.
CV: hypertension.
EENT: blurred vision.
GI: *nausea, constipation,* vomiting, *dry mouth, anorexia,* diarrhea, dyspepsia, flatulence.
GU: *abnormal ejaculation,* impotence, urinary frequency, impaired urination.
Metabolic: weight loss.
Skin: *diaphoresis,* rash.
Other: yawning, chills, infection.

Interactions

Drug-drug. *MAO inhibitors:* may precipitate syndrome similar to neuroleptic malignant syndrome (myoclonus, hyperthermia, seizures, and death). Don't start venlafaxine within 14 days of stopping an MAO inhibitor, and don't start MAO inhibitor within 7 days of stopping venlafaxine.
Drug-herb. *Yohimbe:* additive stimulation. Encourage cautious concomitant use.

Contraindications and precautions

- Contraindicated in patients hypersensitive to drug and those who took an MAO inhibitor within 14 days.
- Use cautiously in patients with renal impairment or diseases, those with conditions that could affect hemodynamic responses or metabolism, and those with a history of mania or seizures.
- Also use cautiously in pregnant or breast-feeding women.
- Safety of drug hasn't been established in children.

NURSING CONSIDERATIONS

Assessment

- Assess patient's depression before therapy and regularly thereafter.
- Carefully monitor blood pressure. Venlafaxine therapy is linked to sustained, dose-dependent increases in blood pressure. Greatest increases (averaging about 7 mm Hg above baseline) occur in patients taking 375 mg daily.
- Be alert for adverse reactions and drug interactions.
- Evaluate patient's and family's knowledge of drug therapy.

Nursing diagnoses

- Disturbed thought processes related to presence of depression
- Risk for injury related to drug-induced adverse CNS reactions
- Deficient knowledge related to drug therapy

Planning and implementation

- Total daily dosage should be reduced by 50% in patient with hepatic impairment. In patient with moderate renal impairment (GFR of 10 to 70 ml/minute), reduce total daily dosage by 25% as directed. In patient undergoing hemodialysis, dose should be withheld until dialysis session is completed; reduce daily dosage by 50%.
- Administer drug with food.

ALERT Don't discontinue drug abruptly if administered for 6 weeks or more. Stop drug by tapering dosage over a 2-week period, as directed.

Patient teaching

- Instruct patient to take with food.

• Caution patient to avoid hazardous activities until full effects of drug are known.
• Tell patient it may take several weeks before the full antidepressant effect is seen.
• Tell patient to avoid alcohol while taking drug and to notify prescriber before taking other medications, including OTC preparations, because of possible interactions.
• Instruct patient to notify prescriber if adverse reactions occur.

☑ Evaluation

• Patient's behavior and communication exhibit improved thought processes.
• Patient doesn't experience injury from adverse CNS reactions.
• Patient and family state understanding of drug therapy.

verapamil

(veh-RAP-uh-mil)

Apo-Verap ♦, Calan, Isoptin, Novo-Veramil ♦, Nu-Verap ♦

verapamil hydrochloride

Anpec ◇, Calan, Calan SR, Cordilox ◇, Cordilox SR ◇, Covera-HS, Isoptin, Isoptin SR, Veracaps SR ◇, Verelan

Pharmacologic class: calcium channel blocker
Therapeutic class: antianginal, antihypertensive, antiarrhythmic
Pregnancy risk category: C

Indications and dosages

▶ **Vasospastic angina; classic chronic, stable angina pectoris; chronic atrial fibrillation.** *Adults:* starting dose is 80 to 120 mg P.O. t.i.d. Increased at weekly intervals as needed. Some patients may need up to 480 mg daily.
▶ **Supraventricular arrhythmias.** *Adults:* 0.075 to 0.15 mg/kg (5 to 10 mg) by I.V. push over 2 minutes with ECG and blood pressure monitoring. If no response occurs, give a second dose of 10 mg (0.15 mg/kg) 15 to 30 minutes after the initial dose.
Children ages 1 to 15: 0.1 to 0.3 mg/kg as I.V. bolus over 2 minutes.
Children under age 1: 0.1 to 0.2 mg/kg as I.V. bolus over 2 minutes with continuous ECG monitoring. Repeat in 30 minutes if no response.
▶ **Hypertension.** *Adults:* start therapy with sustained-release capsules at 180 mg (240 mg for Verelan) P.O. daily in the morning. Adjust dosage based on clinical effectiveness 24 hours after dosing. Increase in increments of 120 mg daily to a maximum daily dosage of 480 mg.

How supplied

verapamil
Tablets: 40 mg, 80 mg, 120 mg
verapamil hydrochloride
Tablets: 40 mg ◇, 80 mg ◇, 120 mg ◇, 160 mg ◇
Tablets (extended-release): 120 mg, 180 mg, 240 mg
Capsules (extended-release): 120 mg, 160 mg ◇, 180 mg, 240 mg, 360 mg
Injection: 2.5 mg/ml

Pharmacokinetics

Absorption: absorbed rapidly and completely from GI tract after P.O. administration; only about 20% to 35% reaches systemic circulation.
Distribution: about 90% of circulating drug is bound to plasma proteins.
Metabolism: metabolized in liver.
Excretion: excreted in urine as unchanged drug and active metabolites. *Half-life:* 6 to 12 hours.

Route	Onset	Peak	Duration
P.O.	1-2 hr	1-9 hr	8-24 hr
I.V.	Rapid	Immediate	1-6 hr

Pharmacodynamics

Chemical effect: not clearly defined; inhibits calcium ion influx across cardiac and smooth-muscle cells, thus decreasing myocardial contractility and oxygen demand. Drug also dilates coronary arteries and arterioles.
Therapeutic effect: relieves angina, lowers blood pressure, and restores normal sinus rhythm.

Adverse reactions

CNS: dizziness, headache, asthenia.
CV: transient hypotension, ***heart failure, bradycardia, AV block, ventricular asystole, ventricular fibrillation,*** peripheral edema.
GI: constipation, nausea.
Hepatic: elevated liver enzyme levels.
Respiratory: ***pulmonary edema.***
Skin: rash.

Interactions

Drug-drug. *Antihypertensives, quinidine:* may cause hypotension. Monitor blood pressure.
Carbamazepine, cardiac glycosides: may increase serum levels of these drugs. Monitor patient for toxicity.
Cyclosporine: may increase serum cyclosporine level. Monitor cyclosporine level.
Disopyramide, flecainide, propranolol, other beta blockers: may cause heart failure. Use together cautiously.
Lithium: may decrease serum lithium level. Monitor patient closely.
Rifampin: may decrease oral bioavailability of verapamil. Monitor patient for lack of effect.
Drug-herb. *Black catechu:* additive effects. Tell patient to use together cautiously.
Yerba maté: may decrease clearance of yerba maté methylxanthines and cause toxicity. Tell patient to use together cautiously.
Drug-food. *Any food:* increased absorption. Tell patient to take drug with food.
Drug-lifestyle. *Alcohol use:* may enhance effects of alcohol. Discourage concurrent use.

Contraindications and precautions

- Contraindicated in patients hypersensitive to drug and those with severe left ventricular dysfunction; cardiogenic shock; second- or third-degree AV block or sick sinus syndrome, except in presence of functioning pacemaker; atrial flutter or fibrillation and accessory bypass tract syndrome; severe heart failure (unless secondary to verapamil therapy); or severe hypotension. I.V. verapamil contraindicated in patients with ventricular tachycardia and in those receiving I.V. beta blockers.
- Drug isn't recommended for breast-feeding women.
- Use cautiously in elderly patients, pregnant women, and patients with increased intracranial pressure or hepatic or renal disease.

NURSING CONSIDERATIONS

Assessment

- Assess patient's condition before therapy and regularly thereafter.
- All patients receiving I.V. verapamil should receive cardiac monitoring. Monitor R-R interval.
- Monitor blood pressure at start of therapy and during dosage adjustments.
- Monitor liver function studies during prolonged treatment, as ordered.
- Be alert for adverse reactions and drug interactions.
- Evaluate patient's and family's knowledge of drug therapy.

Nursing diagnoses

- Acute pain related to presence of angina
- Decreased cardiac output related to presence of arrhythmia
- Deficient knowledge related to drug therapy

Planning and implementation

- Patient with severely compromised cardiac function or patient taking beta blockers should receive lower doses of verapamil.

P.O. use: Drug should be taken with food, but keep in mind that taking extended-release tablets with food may decrease rate and extent of absorption. It also produces smaller fluctuations of peak and trough blood levels.
I.V. use: Give drug by direct injection into vein or into tubing of free-flowing, compatible I.V. solution. Compatible solutions include D_5W, half-normal and normal saline solutions, and Ringer's and lactated Ringer's solutions.
– Administer I.V. doses slowly over at least 2 minutes (3 minutes for elderly patients) to minimize risk of adverse reactions.
– Perform continuous ECG and blood pressure monitoring during administration.

- If verapamil is being used to terminate supraventricular tachycardia, prescriber may have patient perform vagal maneuvers after receiving drug.

• Assist patient with walking because dizziness may occur.
• Notify prescriber if patient has signs of heart failure, such as swelling of hands and feet or shortness of breath.
ALERT Don't confuse Isoptin with Intropin; don't confuse Verelan with Vivarin, Voltaren, Ferralyn, or Virilon.

Patient teaching
• Instruct patient to take drug with food.
• If patient is kept on nitrate therapy during adjustment of oral verapamil dosage, urge continued compliance. S.L. nitroglycerin, especially, may be taken as needed when angina is acute.
• Encourage patient to increase fluid and fiber intake to combat constipation. Administer stool softener, as ordered.
• Instruct patient to report adverse reactions, especially swelling of hands and feet and shortness of breath.

Evaluation
• Patient has reduced severity or frequency of angina.
• Patient regains normal cardiac output with restoration of normal sinus rhythm.
• Patient and family state understanding of drug therapy.

vinblastine sulfate (VLB)
(vin-BLAH-steen SUL-fayt)
Velban, Velbe ♦ ◇

Pharmacologic class: vinca alkaloid (specific to M phase of cell cycle)
Therapeutic class: antineoplastic
Pregnancy risk category: D

Indications and dosages
▶ **Breast or testicular cancer, Hodgkin's and non-Hodgkin's lymphoma, choriocarcinoma, lymphosarcoma, mycosis fungoides, Kaposi's sarcoma, histiocytosis.** *Adults:* 0.1 mg/kg or 3.7 mg/m² I.V. weekly or q 2 weeks. May be increased to maximum dosage of 0.5 mg/kg or 18.5 mg/m² weekly according to response. Dosage shouldn't be repeated if WBC count is less than 4,000/mm³.
Children: 2.5 mg/m² I.V. as a single dose every week, increased weekly in increments of 1.25 mg/m² to a maximum of 7.5 mg/m².

How supplied
Injection: 10-mg vials (lyophilized powder), 1 mg/ml in 10-ml vials

Pharmacokinetics
Absorption: not applicable.
Distribution: distributed widely in body tissues; crosses blood-brain barrier but doesn't achieve therapeutic levels in CSF.
Metabolism: metabolized partially in liver to active metabolite.
Excretion: excreted primarily in bile as unchanged drug; smaller portion excreted in urine. *Half-life:* alpha phase, 3.7 minutes; beta phase, 1.6 hours; terminal phase, 25 hours.

Route	Onset	Peak	Duration
I.V.	Unknown	Unknown	Unknown

Pharmacodynamics
Chemical effect: arrests mitosis in metaphase, blocking cell division.
Therapeutic effect: inhibits replication of certain cancer cells.

Adverse reactions
CNS: depression, *paresthesia, peripheral neuropathy and neuritis, numbness, loss of deep tendon reflexes,* ***seizures, CVA,*** headache.
CV: hypertension, ***MI,*** *phlebitis.*
EENT: pharyngitis.
GI: *nausea, vomiting,* ulcer, bleeding, *constipation, ileus, anorexia,* diarrhea, abdominal pain, *stomatitis.*
GU: oligospermia, aspermia, urine retention.
Hematologic: anemia, ***leukopenia*** (nadir on days 4 to 10; lasts another 7 to 14 days), ***thrombocytopenia.***
Respiratory: ***acute bronchospasm,*** shortness of breath.
Metabolic: hyperuricemia, *weight loss.*
Musculoskeletal: uric acid nephropathy, *muscle pain and weakness.*
Skin: reversible alopecia, vesiculation, cellulitis, necrosis with extravasation.

Interactions

Drug-drug. *Erythromycin, other drugs that inhibit cytochrome P-450 pathway:* may increase toxicity of vinblastine. Monitor patient closely.
Mitomycin: increased risk of bronchospasm and shortness of breath. Monitor patient closely.
Phenytoin: decreased plasma phenytoin level. Monitor patient closely.

Contraindications and precautions

- Contraindicated in patients with severe leukopenia or bacterial infection.
- Drug isn't recommended for pregnant or breast-feeding women.
- Use cautiously in patients with hepatic dysfunction.

NURSING CONSIDERATIONS

Assessment

- Assess patient's condition before therapy and regularly thereafter.

ALERT After administering drug, monitor patient for development of life-threatening acute bronchospasm. Reaction is most likely if patient also receives mitomycin.

- Be alert for adverse reactions and drug interactions.
- Assess for numbness and tingling in hands and feet. Assess gait for early evidence of footdrop. Drug is less neurotoxic than vincristine.
- Evaluate patient's and family's knowledge of drug therapy.

Nursing diagnoses

- Ineffective health maintenance related to presence of neoplastic disease
- Ineffective protection related to drug-induced adverse hematologic reactions
- Deficient knowledge related to drug therapy

Planning and implementation

- Give antiemetic before administering drug, as ordered.
- Follow facility policy to reduce risks. Preparation and administration of parenteral form are linked to carcinogenic, mutagenic, and teratogenic risks for personnel.
- Reconstitute 10-mg vial with 10 ml of saline solution injection or sterile water. This yields 1 mg/ml. Refrigerate reconstituted solution. Discard after 30 days.
- Inject drug directly into vein or running I.V. line over 1 minute. Drug also may be given in 50 ml of D_5W or normal saline solution infused over 15 minutes.
- If extravasation occurs, stop infusion immediately and notify prescriber. Manufacturer recommends that moderate heat be applied to area of leakage. Local injection of hyaluronidase may help disperse drug. Some clinicians prefer to apply ice packs on and off every 2 hours for 24 hours, with local injection of hydrocortisone or normal saline solution.
- Don't administer drug into limb with compromised circulation.

ALERT Drug is fatal if given intrathecally; it's for I.V. use only.

- If acute bronchospasm occurs after administration, notify prescriber immediately.
- Make sure patient maintains adequate fluid intake to facilitate excretion of uric acid.
- Be prepared to stop drug and notify prescriber if stomatitis occurs.
- Dosage shouldn't be repeated more frequently than every 7 days or severe leukopenia will develop.

ALERT Don't confuse vinblastine with vincristine or vindesine.

- Anticipate decrease in dosage by 50% if bilirubin level is greater than 3 mg/dl.

Patient teaching

- Teach patient about infection-control and bleeding precautions.
- Warn patient that alopecia may occur, but that it's usually reversible.
- Tell patient to report adverse reactions promptly.
- Encourage adequate fluid intake to increase urine output and facilitate excretion of uric acid.

Evaluation

- Patient responds well to drug.
- Patient doesn't develop serious complications from adverse hematologic reactions.
- Patient and family state understanding of drug therapy.

vincristine sulfate
(vin-KRIH-steen SUL-fayt)
Oncovin, Vincasar PFS

Pharmacologic class: vinca alkaloid (specific to M phase of cell cycle)
Therapeutic class: antineoplastic
Pregnancy risk category: D

Indications and dosages

▶**Acute lymphoblastic and other leukemias, Hodgkin's disease, non-Hodgkin's lymphoma, neuroblastoma, rhabdomyosarcoma, Wilms' tumor.** *Adults:* 1.4 mg/m² I.V. weekly. Maximum weekly dosage is 2 mg. *Children weighing over 10 kg (22 lb):* 2 mg/m² I.V. weekly. Maximum single dose is 2 mg. *Children weighing 10 kg and less:* 0.05 mg/kg I.V. once weekly.

How supplied

Injection: 1 mg/ml in 1-ml, 2-ml, 5-ml multiple-dose vials; 1 mg/ml in 1-ml, 2-ml preservative-free vials

Pharmacokinetics

Absorption: not applicable.
Distribution: distributed widely in body tissues and bound to erythrocytes and platelets; crosses blood-brain barrier but doesn't achieve therapeutic levels in CSF.
Metabolism: metabolized extensively in liver.
Excretion: excreted primarily in bile; smaller portion excreted in urine. *Half-life:* first phase, 4 minutes; second phase, 2¼ hours; terminal phase, 85 hours.

Route	Onset	Peak	Duration
I.V.	Unknown	Unknown	Unknown

Pharmacodynamics

Chemical effect: arrests mitosis in metaphase, blocking cell division.
Therapeutic effect: inhibits replication of certain cancer cells.

Adverse reactions

CNS: *peripheral neuropathy,* sensory loss, *loss of deep tendon reflexes, paresthesia, wristdrop and footdrop,* headache, ataxia, cranial nerve palsies, *jaw pain,* hoarseness, vocal cord paralysis, ***seizures, coma,*** permanent neurotoxicity.
CV: hypotension, hypertension, *phlebitis.*
EENT: visual disturbances, diplopia, optic and extraocular neuropathy, ptosis.
GI: diarrhea, *constipation, cramps,* ileus that mimics surgical abdomen, *nausea, vomiting,* anorexia, dysphagia, ***intestinal necrosis,*** *stomatitis.*
GU: urine retention, SIADH, dysuria, acute uric acid neuropathy, polyuria.
Hematologic: anemia, ***leukopenia, thrombocytopenia.***
Metabolic: hyponatremia, hyperuricemia, weight loss.
Musculoskeletal: *muscle weakness and cramps.*
Respiratory: ***acute bronchospasm.***
Skin: rash, *reversible alopecia,* cellulitis at injection site, severe local reaction with extravasation.
Other: fever.

Interactions

Drug-drug. *Asparaginase:* decreased hepatic clearance of vincristine. Monitor patient closely for toxicity.
Calcium channel blockers: enhanced vincristine accumulation. Monitor patient for toxicity.
Digoxin: decreased digoxin effects. Monitor serum digoxin level.
Mitomycin: possible increased frequency of bronchospasm and acute pulmonary reactions. Monitor patient closely.
Phenytoin: may reduce phenytoin levels. Monitor patient closely.

Contraindications and precautions

- Contraindicated in patients hypersensitive to drug and in those with demyelinating form of Charcot-Marie-Tooth syndrome. Don't give drug to patients who are concurrently receiving radiation therapy through ports that include liver.
- Drug isn't recommended for pregnant or breast-feeding women.
- Use cautiously in patients with hepatic dysfunction, neuromuscular disease, or infection.

NURSING CONSIDERATIONS

Assessment

- Assess patient's condition before therapy and regularly thereafter.

ALERT After giving drug, monitor patient for development of life-threatening acute bronchospasm. Reaction is most likely to occur if patient also receives mitomycin.

- Monitor patient for hyperuricemia, especially if he has leukemia or lymphoma.
- Be alert for adverse reactions and drug interactions.
- Check for depression of Achilles tendon reflex, numbness, tingling, footdrop or wristdrop, difficulty in walking, ataxia, and slapping gait. Also check ability to walk on heels.
- Monitor bowel function. Constipation may be early sign of neurotoxicity.
- Evaluate patient's and family's knowledge of drug therapy.

Nursing diagnoses

- Ineffective health maintenance related to presence of neoplastic disease
- Ineffective protection related to drug-induced adverse hematologic reactions
- Deficient knowledge related to drug therapy

Planning and implementation

- Give antiemetic before drug, as ordered.
- All vials (1-mg, 2-mg, 5-mg) contain 1 mg/ml solution and should be refrigerated.
- Follow facility policy to reduce risks. Preparation and administration of parenteral form are linked to carcinogenic, mutagenic, and teratogenic risks for personnel.
- Inject drug directly into vein or running I.V. line slowly over 1 minute. Drug also may be given in 50 ml of D_5W or normal saline solution infused over 15 minutes.
- If drug extravasates, stop infusion immediately and notify prescriber. Apply heat on and off every 2 hours for 24 hours. Administer 150 units of hyaluronidase, as ordered, to area of infiltrate.
- Don't administer drug to one patient as single dose. The 5-mg vials are for multiple-dose use.

ALERT Drug is fatal if given intrathecally; it's for I.V. use only.

- Because of risk of neurotoxicity, drug shouldn't be given more than once a week. Children are more resistant to neurotoxicity than adults. Neurotoxicity is dose-related and usually reversible.
- If acute bronchospasm occurs after administration, notify prescriber immediately.
- Maintain good hydration and give allopurinol, as ordered, to prevent uric acid nephropathy.
- Fluid restriction may be necessary if SIADH develops.
- Give stool softener or laxative, as ordered, or water before dosing to help prevent constipation.

ALERT Don't confuse vincristine with vinblastine or vindesine.

Patient teaching

- Instruct patient on infection-control and bleeding precautions.
- Warn patient that alopecia may occur, but that it's usually reversible.
- Tell patient to report adverse reactions promptly.
- Encourage fluid intake to facilitate excretion of uric acid.
- Advise woman of childbearing age to avoid becoming pregnant during therapy. Also recommend that she consult with prescriber before becoming pregnant.

Evaluation

- Patient responds well to drug.
- Patient doesn't develop serious complications from adverse hematologic reactions.
- Patient and family state understanding of drug therapy.

vinorelbine tartrate

(vin-oh-REL-been TAR-trayt)
Navelbine

Pharmacologic class: semisynthetic vinca alkaloid
Therapeutic class: antineoplastic
Pregnancy risk category: D

Indications and dosages

▶ **Alone or as adjunct therapy with cisplatin for first-line treatment of ambulatory patients with nonresectable advanced non-small-cell lung cancer (NSCLC); alone or with cisplatin in stage IV of NSCLC; with cisplatin in stage III of NSCLC.** *Adults:* 30 mg/m² I.V. weekly. In combination treatment, same dosage used along with 120 mg/m² of cisplatin, given on days 1 and 29, and then every 6 weeks.

How supplied

Injection: 10 mg/ml, 50 mg/5 ml

Pharmacokinetics

Absorption: not applicable.
Distribution: distributed widely in body tissues and bound to lymphocytes and platelets.
Metabolism: metabolized extensively in liver.
Excretion: excreted primarily in bile; smaller portion excreted in urine. *Half-life:* 27.7 to 43.6 hours.

Route	Onset	Peak	Duration
I.V.	Unknown	Unknown	Unknown

Pharmacodynamics

Chemical effect: arrests mitosis in metaphase, blocking cell division.
Therapeutic effect: inhibits replication of selected cancer cells.

Adverse reactions

CNS: *peripheral neuropathy, asthenia, fatigue.*
GI: *nausea, vomiting, anorexia, diarrhea, constipation, stomatitis.*
Hematologic: ***bone marrow suppression*** (***agranulocytosis,*** **LEUKOPENIA,** ***thrombocytopenia,*** anemia).
Hepatic: *abnormal liver function test results, bilirubinemia.*
Musculoskeletal: jaw pain, chest pain, myalgia, arthralgia, loss of deep tendon reflexes.
Respiratory: dyspnea.
Skin: *alopecia,* rash, *injection site pain or reaction.*
Other: SIADH.

Interactions

Drug-drug. *Cisplatin:* increased risk of bone marrow suppression when given with cisplatin. Monitor patient's hematologic status closely.
Mitomycin: may cause pulmonary reactions. Monitor patient's respiratory status closely.

Contraindications and precautions

- Contraindicated in patients with pretreatment granulocyte counts below 1,000 cells/mm³.
- Drug isn't recommended for pregnant or breast-feeding women.
- Use with extreme caution in patients whose bone marrow may have been compromised by previous exposure to radiation therapy or chemotherapy or whose bone marrow is still recovering from previous chemotherapy.
- Use cautiously in patients with hepatic impairment.
- Safety of drug hasn't been established in children.

NURSING CONSIDERATIONS

Assessment

- Assess patient's condition before therapy and regularly thereafter.
- Monitor patient closely for hypersensitivity reactions.
- To judge effects of therapy, monitor patient's peripheral blood count and bone marrow, as ordered.
- Be alert for adverse reactions and drug interactions.
- Assess for numbness and tingling in hands and feet. Assess gait for early evidence of footdrop.

ALERT Monitor patient's deep tendon reflexes; loss may indicate cumulative toxicity.

- Evaluate patient's and family's knowledge of drug therapy.

Nursing diagnoses

- Ineffective health maintenance related to presence of neoplastic disease
- Ineffective protection related to drug-induced adverse hematologic reactions
- Deficient knowledge related to drug therapy

Planning and implementation

- Give antiemetic before administering drug, as ordered.
- Check patient's granulocyte count before administration. It should be 1,000 cells/mm³ or more for drug to be administered. Withhold drug and notify prescriber if count is less.
- Drug must be diluted before administration. Administer drug I.V. over 6 to 10 minutes into side port of free-flowing I.V. line that is closest to I.V. bag. Afterward, flush with 75 to 125 ml of D_5W or normal saline solution.
- Take care to avoid extravasation during administration because drug can cause considerable irritation, localized tissue necrosis, and thrombophlebitis. If extravasation occurs, stop drug immediately and inject remaining portion of dose into a different vein.

ALERT Drug is fatal if given intrathecally; it's for I.V. use only.

- Dosage adjustments are made according to hematologic toxicity or hepatic insufficiency, whichever results in lower dosage. Expect dosage to be halved if patient's granulocyte count falls between 1,000 and 1,500 cells/mm³. If three consecutive doses are skipped because of agranulocytosis, discontinue vinorelbine, as directed.
- Drug may be a contact irritant, and solution must be handled and administered with care. Gloves are recommended. Avoid inhaling vapors and allowing drug to contact skin or mucous membranes, especially those of eyes. In case of contact, wash with copious amounts of water for at least 15 minutes.

Patient teaching

- Instruct patient on infection-control and bleeding precautions.
- Warn patient that alopecia may occur, but that it's usually reversible.
- Instruct patient not to take other drugs, including OTC preparations, unless approved by prescriber.
- Instruct patient to tell prescriber about signs and symptoms of infection (fever, chills, malaise) because drug may have immunosuppressant activity.

Evaluation

- Patient responds well to drug.
- Patient doesn't develop serious complications from adverse hematologic reactions.
- Patient and family state understanding of drug therapy.

vitamin A (retinol)

(VIGH-tuh-min ay)

Aquasol A

Pharmacologic class: fat-soluble vitamin
Therapeutic class: vitamin
Pregnancy risk category A (C at higher-than-recommended doses)

Indications and dosages

▶ **RDA.** *Note:* RDAs have been converted to retinol equivalents (RE). One RE has activity of 1 mcg of all-*trans* retinol, 6 mcg of beta carotene, or 12 mcg of carotenoid provitamins.
Men over age 11: 1,000 mcg RE or 5,000 IU.
Pregnant women and women over age 11: 800 mcg RE or 4,000 IU.
Breast-feeding women (first 6 months): 1,300 mcg RE or 6,500 IU.
Breast-feeding women (second 6 months): 1,200 mcg RE or 6,000 IU.
Children ages 7 to 10: 700 mcg RE or 3,500 IU.
Children ages 4 to 6: 500 mcg RE or 2,500 IU.
Children ages 1 to 3: 400 mcg RE or 2,000 IU.
Neonates and infants to age 1: 375 mcg RE or 1,875 IU.

▶ **Severe vitamin A deficiency.** *Adults and children over age 8:* 100,000 IU I.M. or P.O. daily for 3 days, followed by 50,000 IU I.M. or P.O. daily for 2 weeks; then 10,000 to 20,000 IU P.O. daily for 2 months. Follow with adequate dietary nutrition and RE vitamin A supplements.
Children ages 1 to 8: 17,500 to 35,000 IU I.M. daily for 10 days.
Infants under age 1: 7,500 to 15,000 IU I.M. daily for 10 days.

▶ **Maintenance dosage to prevent recurrence of vitamin A deficiency.** *Children ages 1 to 8:* 5,000 to 10,000 IU P.O. daily for 2 months; then adequate dietary nutrition and RE vitamin A supplements.

How supplied

Tablets: 5,000 IU, 10,000 IU
Capsules: 10,000 IU, 25,000 IU, 50,000 IU
Drops: 30 ml with dropper (50,000 IU/0.1 ml)
Injection: 2-ml vials (50,000 IU/ml with 0.5% chlorobutanol, polysorbate 80, butylated hydroxyanisol, and butylated hydroxytoluene)

Pharmacokinetics

Absorption: in normal doses, absorbed readily and completely if fat absorption is normal; larger doses or regular dose in patients with fat malabsorption, low protein intake, or hepatic or pancreatic disease may be absorbed incompletely. Because vitamin A is fat-soluble, absorption requires bile salts, pancreatic lipase, and dietary fat.
Distribution: stored (primarily as palmitate) in Kupffer's cells of liver. Normal adult liver stores are sufficient to provide vitamin A requirements for 2 years. Lesser amounts of retinyl palmitate are stored in kidneys, lungs, adrenal glands, retinas, and intraperitoneal fat. Vitamin A circulates bound to specific alpha, protein, retinol-binding protein.
Metabolism: metabolized in liver.
Excretion: retinol (fat-soluble) combines with glucuronic acid and is metabolized to retinal and retinoic acid. Retinoic acid undergoes biliary excretion in feces. Retinal, retinoic acid, and other water-soluble metabolites are excreted in urine and feces.

Route	Onset	Peak	Duration
P.O., I.M.	Unknown	3-5 hr	Unknown

Pharmacodynamics

Chemical effect: stimulates retinal function, bone growth, reproduction, and integrity of epithelial and mucosal tissues.
Therapeutic effect: raises vitamin A levels in body.

Adverse reactions

Adverse reactions are usually seen only with toxicity.
CNS: irritability, headache, ***increased intracranial pressure,*** fatigue, lethargy, malaise.
EENT: papilledema, exophthalmos.
GI: anorexia, epigastric pain, vomiting, polydipsia.
GU: hypomenorrhea, polyuria.
Hepatic: jaundice, hepatomegaly, ***cirrhosis,*** elevated liver enzyme levels.
Metabolic: slow growth, decalcification of bone, hypercalcemia, periostitis, premature closure of epiphyses, migratory arthralgia, cortical thickening over radius and tibia.
Skin: alopecia; drying, cracking, scaling of skin; pruritus; lip fissures; erythema; inflamed tongue, lips, and gums; massive desquamation; increased pigmentation; night sweating.
Other: splenomegaly, ***anaphylactic shock.***

Interactions

Drug-drug. *Cholestyramine resin, mineral oil:* reduced GI absorption of fat-soluble vitamins. If needed, give mineral oil at bedtime.
Isotretinoin, multivitamins containing vitamin A: increased risk of toxicity. Avoid concomitant use.
Neomycin (oral): decreased vitamin A absorption. Avoid concomitant use.
Oral contraceptives: may increase plasma vitamin A levels. Monitor patient.
Warfarin: increased risk of bleeding. Monitor PT and INR closely.

Contraindications and precautions

- Contraindicated for oral administration in patients with malabsorption syndrome; if malabsorption is from inadequate bile secretion, oral route may be used with concurrent administration of bile salts (dehydrocholic acid). Also contraindicated in patients hypersensitive to other ingredients in product and in those with hypervitaminosis A.
- I.V. administration contraindicated except for special water-miscible forms intended for infusion with large parenteral volumes. I.V. push of vitamin A of any type is also contraindicated (anaphylaxis or anaphylactoid reactions and death have resulted).
- Use cautiously in pregnant or breast-feeding women, avoiding doses exceeding RE.

NURSING CONSIDERATIONS

Assessment

- Assess patient's vitamin A intake from fortified foods, dietary supplements, self-administered drugs, and prescription drug sources before therapy and reassess regularly thereafter.
- Be alert for adverse reactions (if dose is high). Acute toxicity has resulted from single doses of 25,000 IU/kg; 350,000 IU in infants and over 2 million IU in adults also have proved acutely toxic. Doses that don't exceed RE are usually nontoxic.
- Chronic toxicity in infants (3 to 6 months) has resulted from doses of 18,500 IU daily for 1 to 3 months. In adults, chronic toxicity has resulted from doses of 50,000 IU daily for more than 18 months; 500,000 IU daily for 2 months, and 1 million IU daily for 3 days.
- Be alert for drug interactions.
- Evaluate patient's and family's knowledge of drug therapy.

Nursing diagnoses

- Imbalanced nutrition: less than body requirements related to inadequate intake
- Ineffective health maintenance related to vitamin A toxicity caused by excessive intake
- Deficient knowledge related to drug therapy

Planning and implementation

- Adequate vitamin A absorption requires suitable protein, vitamin E, and zinc intake and bile secretion; give supplemental salts, if necessary and ordered. Zinc supplements may be necessary in patient receiving long-term total parenteral nutrition.

P.O. use: Follow normal protocol.

– Liquid preparations available if NG administration is necessary. They may be mixed with cereal or fruit juice.

I.M. use: Absorption is fastest and most complete with water-miscible preparations, intermediate with emulsions, and slowest with oil suspensions.

ALERT Give parenteral form by I.M. route or continuous I.V infusion in total parenteral nutrition. Never give as I.V. bolus.

- Protect drug from light.

Patient teaching

- Warn patient against taking megadoses of vitamins without specific indications. Also stress that he not share prescribed vitamins with others.
- Explain importance of avoiding prolonged use of mineral oil while taking this drug because mineral oil reduces vitamin A absorption.
- Review the signs and symptoms of vitamin A toxicity, and tell patient to report them immediately.
- Advise patient to consume adequate protein, vitamin E, and zinc, which, along with bile, are necessary for vitamin A absorption.
- Instruct patient to store vitamin A in tight, light-resistant container.

Evaluation

- Patient regains normal vitamin A levels.
- Patient doesn't exhibit signs and symptoms of vitamin A toxicity.
- Patient and family state understanding of drug therapy.

vitamin C (ascorbic acid)

(VIGH-tuh-min see)

Ascorbicap†, Cebid Timecelles†, Cecon†, Cenolate†, Cetane†, Cevalin†, Cevi-Bid, Ce-Vi-Sol*, Dull-C†, Flavorcee†, N'ice Vitamin C Drops†, Penta-Vite ◇, Redoxon♦, Vita-C†

Pharmacologic class: water-soluble vitamin
Therapeutic class: vitamin
Pregnancy risk category: A (C at higher-than-recommended doses)

Indications and dosages

▶ **RDA.** *Adults and children age 15 and over:* 60 mg.
Pregnant women: 70 mg.
Breast-feeding women (first 6 months): 95 mg.
Breast-feeding women (second 6 months): 90 mg.
Children ages 11 to 14: 50 mg.
Children ages 4 to 10: 45 mg.
Children ages 1 to 3: 40 mg.
Infants ages 6 months to 1 year: 35 mg.

Neonates and infants to age 6 months: 30 mg.

▶ **Frank and subclinical scurvy.** *Adults:* depending on severity, 300 mg to 1 g P.O., S.C., I.M., or I.V. daily; then at least 50 mg daily for maintenance.
Children: depending on severity, 100 to 300 mg P.O., S.C., I.M., or I.V. daily, then at least 30 mg daily for maintenance.
Premature infants: 75 to 100 mg P.O., I.M., I.V., or S.C. daily.

▶ **Extensive burns, delayed fracture or wound healing, postoperative wound healing, severe febrile or chronic disease states.** *Adults:* 300 to 500 mg P.O., S.C., I.M., or I.V. daily for 7 to 10 days. For extensive burns, 1 to 2 g daily.
Children: 100 to 200 mg P.O., S.C., I.M., or I.V. daily.

▶ **Prevention of vitamin C deficiency in patients with poor nutritional habits or increased requirements.** *Adults:* 70 to 150 mg P.O., S.C., I.M., or I.V. daily.
Pregnant or breast-feeding women: 70 to 150 mg P.O., S.C., I.M., or I.V. daily.
Children: at least 40 mg P.O., S.C., I.M., or I.V. daily.
Infants: at least 35 mg P.O., S.C., I.M., or I.V. daily.

▶ **Potentiation of methenamine in urine acidification.** *Adults:* 4 to 12 g P.O. daily in divided doses.

How supplied

Tablets: 25 mg†, 50 mg†, 100 mg†, 250 mg†, 500 mg†, 1,000 mg†
Tablets (chewable): 50 mg, 100 mg†, 250 mg†, 500 mg†, 1,000 mg†
Tablets (effervescent): 1,000 mg sugar-free†
Tablets (timed-release): 500 mg†, 1,000 mg†, 1,500 mg
Capsules (timed-release): 500 mg†
Crystals: 100 g (4 g/tsp)†, 500 g (4 g/tsp)†
Lozenges: 60 mg†
Oral liquid: 50 ml (35 mg/0.6 ml)*†
Oral solution: 60 mg/ml†, 100 mg/ml†
Powder: 100 g (4 g/tsp)†, 500 g (4 g/tsp)†
Syrup: 20 mg/ml in 120 ml, 480 ml†; 500 mg/5 ml in 5 ml†, 120 ml†, 480 ml†
Injection: 100 mg/ml; 250 mg/ml; 500 mg/ml

Pharmacokinetics

Absorption: after P.O. administration, ascorbic acid is absorbed readily from GI tract. After very large doses, absorption may be limited because absorption is an active process. Absorption also may be reduced in patients with diarrhea or GI diseases. Degree of absorption unknown after I.M. or S.C. administration.
Distribution: distributed widely in body with high levels found in liver, leukocytes, platelets, glandular tissues, and lens of eyes. Protein-binding is low.
Metabolism: metabolized in liver.
Excretion: excreted in urine. Renal excretion is directly proportional to blood concentrations.

Route	Onset	Peak	Duration
All routes	Unknown	Unknown	Unknown

Pharmacodynamics

Chemical effect: stimulates collagen formation and tissue repair; involved in oxidation-reduction reactions throughout body.
Therapeutic effect: raises vitamin C levels in body.

Adverse reactions

CNS: faintness, dizziness with too-fast I.V. administration.
GI: diarrhea.
GU: acid urine, oxaluria, renal calculi.
Other: discomfort at injection site.

Interactions

Drug-drug. *Aspirin (high doses):* increased risk of ascorbic acid deficiency. Monitor patient closely.
Contraceptives, estrogen: increased serum levels of estrogen. Monitor patient.
Oral iron supplements: increased iron absorption. A beneficial drug interaction. Encourage concomitant use.
Warfarin: decreased anticoagulant effect. Monitor patient closely.
Drug-herb. *Bearberry:* inactivation of bearberry in urine. Caution patient about lack of effect.

Contraindications and precautions

No known contraindications.

NURSING CONSIDERATIONS

Assessment
- Assess patient's condition before therapy and regularly thereafter.
- When administering for urine acidification, check urine pH to ensure efficacy.
- Be alert for adverse reactions and drug interactions.
- Monitor patient's hydration status if adverse GI reactions occur.
- Evaluate patient's and family's knowledge of drug therapy.

Nursing diagnoses
- Imbalanced nutrition: less than body requirements related to inadequate intake
- Risk for deficient fluid volume related to drug-induced adverse GI reactions
- Deficient knowledge related to drug therapy

Planning and implementation
P.O. use: Administer P.O. solution directly into mouth or mix with food.
– Effervescent tablets should be dissolved in glass of water immediately before ingestion.
I.V. use: Administer I.V. infusion cautiously in patients with renal insufficiency.
ALERT Avoid rapid I.V. administration. It may cause faintness or dizziness.
I.M. use: Utilization of vitamin may be better with I.M. route, the preferred parenteral route.
S.C. use: Follow normal protocol.
- Protect solution from light, and refrigerate ampules.

Patient teaching
- Stress proper nutritional habits to prevent recurrence of deficiency.
- Advise patient with vitamin C deficiency to decrease or stop smoking.

Evaluation
- Patient regains normal vitamin C levels.
- Patient maintains adequate hydration.
- Patient and family state understanding of drug therapy.

vitamin D

cholecalciferol (vitamin D_3)
(koh-lih-kal-SIF-eh-rol)
Delta-D†, Vitamin D_3†

ergocalciferol (vitamin D_2)
(er-goh-kal-SIF-er-ohl)
Calciferol, Drisdol, Radiostol Forte♦, Vitamin D

Pharmacologic class: fat-soluble vitamin
Therapeutic class: vitamin
Pregnancy risk category: C

Indications and dosages
▶ **RDA for cholecalciferol.** *Adults age 25 and over:* 200 IU.
Pregnant or breast-feeding women: 400 IU.
Adults under age 25 and children age 6 months and over: 400 IU.
Neonates and infants to age 6 months: 300 IU.
▶ **Rickets and other vitamin D deficiency diseases.** *Adults:* initially, 12,000 IU P.O. or I.M. daily, usually increased according to response up to 500,000 IU daily. After correction of deficiency, maintenance includes adequate diet and RDA supplements.
▶ **Hypoparathyroidism.** *Adults and children:* 50,000 to 200,000 IU P.O. or I.M. daily with calcium supplement.
▶ **Familial hypophosphatemia.** *Adults:* 10,000 to 80,000 IU P.O. or I.M. daily with phosphorus supplement.

How supplied
Tablets: 1.25 mg (50,000 IU)
Capsules: 1.25 mg (50,000 IU)
Oral liquid: 8,000 IU/ml in 60-ml dropper bottle†
Injection: 12.5 mg (500,000 IU)/ml

Pharmacokinetics
Absorption: absorbed from small intestine with P.O. administration; unknown for I.M. administration.
Distribution: widely distributed throughout body; bound to proteins stored in liver.
Metabolism: metabolized in liver and kidneys.

Excretion: excreted primarily in bile; small amount excreted in urine. *Half-life*: 24 hours.

Route	Onset	Peak	Duration
P.O., I.M.	2-24 hr	3-12 hr	Varies

Pharmacodynamics

Chemical effect: promotes absorption and utilization of calcium and phosphate, helping to regulate calcium homeostasis.
Therapeutic effect: helps to maintain normal calcium and phosphate levels in body.

Adverse reactions

Adverse reactions listed are usually seen only in vitamin D toxicity.
CNS: headache, weakness, somnolence, overt psychosis, irritability.
CV: ***calcifications of soft tissues including heart, arrhythmias;*** hypertension.
EENT: rhinorrhea, conjunctivitis (calcific), photophobia.
GI: anorexia, nausea, vomiting, constipation, dry mouth, metallic taste, polydipsia.
GU: polyuria, albuminuria, hypercalciuria, nocturia, impaired kidney function, reversible azotemia.
Metabolic: ***hypercalcemia,*** hyperthermia, weight loss.
Musculoskeletal: bone and muscle pain, bone demineralization.
Skin: pruritus.
Other: decreased libido.

Interactions

Drug-drug. *Cardiac glycosides:* increased risk of arrhythmias. Monitor serum calcium level.
Cholestyramine resin, mineral oil: inhibited GI absorption of oral vitamin D. Space doses. Use together cautiously.
Corticosteroids: antagonized effect of vitamin D. Monitor vitamin D level closely.
Phenobarbital, phenytoin: increased vitamin D metabolism, which decreases half-life as well as drug's effectiveness. Monitor patient closely.
Thiazide diuretics: may cause hypercalcemia in patients with hypoparathyroidism. Monitor patient closely.
Verapamil: atrial fibrillation has occurred because of increased calcium. Monitor patient closely.

Contraindications and precautions

- Contraindicated in patients with hypercalcemia, hypervitaminosis A, or renal osteodystrophy with hyperphosphatemia.
- Administer ergocalciferol with extreme caution, if at all, to patients with impaired kidney function, heart disease, renal calculi, or arteriosclerosis.
- Use cautiously in cardiac patients, especially those receiving cardiac glycosides; patients with increased sensitivity to these drugs; and pregnant or breast-feeding women.

NURSING CONSIDERATIONS

Assessment

- Assess patient's condition before therapy and regularly thereafter.

ALERT Monitor patient's eating and bowel habits; dry mouth, nausea, vomiting, metallic taste, and constipation may be early evidence of toxicity.

- Monitor serum and urine calcium, potassium, and urea levels when high therapeutic dosages are used.
- Be alert for adverse reactions and drug interactions.
- Evaluate patient's and family's knowledge of drug therapy.

Nursing diagnoses

- Imbalanced nutrition: less than body requirements related to inadequate intake
- Ineffective health maintenance related to vitamin D toxicity
- Deficient knowledge related to drug therapy

Planning and implementation

P.O. use: Follow normal protocol.
I.M. use: Use I.M. injection of vitamin D dispersed in oil for patient unable to absorb P.O. form, as ordered.

- Dosages of 60,000 IU/day can cause hypercalcemia.

• Malabsorption from inadequate bile or hepatic dysfunction may require addition of exogenous bile salts with oral form.
• Patient with hyperphosphatemia requires dietary phosphate restrictions and binding agents to avoid metastatic calcifications and renal calculus formation.

Patient teaching
• Warn patient of dangers of increasing dosage without consulting prescriber. Vitamin D is fat-soluble.
• Tell patient taking vitamin D to restrict his intake of magnesium-containing antacids.

Evaluation
• Patient regains normal vitamin D level.
• Patient doesn't develop vitamin D toxicity.
• Patient and family state understanding of drug therapy.

vitamin E (tocopherol)

(VIGH-tuh-min ee)
Amino-Opti-E†, Aquasol E†, E-Complex-600†, E-200 I.U. Softgels†, E-400 I.U. Softgels†, E-Vitamin Succinate†, Vita-Plus E Softgels†

Pharmacologic class: fat-soluble vitamin
Therapeutic class: vitamin
Pregnancy risk category: A

Indications and dosages

▶ **RDA.** *Note:* RDAs for vitamin E have been converted to α-tocopherol equivalents (α-TE). One α-TE equals 1 mg of D-α tocopherol or 1.49 IU.
Men age 11 and over: 10 α-TE or 15 IU.
Women age 11 and over: 8 α-TE or 12 IU.
Pregnant women: 10 α-TE or 15 IU.
Breast-feeding women (first 6 months): 12 α-TE or 18 IU.
Breast-feeding women (second 6 months): 11 α-TE or 16 IU.
Children ages 4 to 10: 7 α-TE or 10 IU.
Children over age 1 to age 3: 6 α-TE or 9 IU.
Infants ages 6 months to 1 year: 4 α-TE or 6 IU.
Neonates and infants to age 6 months: 3 α-TE or 4 IU.

▶ **Vitamin E deficiency in adults and in children with malabsorption syndrome.**
Adults: depending on severity, 60 to 75 IU P.O. daily. *Children:* 1 IU/kg P.O. daily.

How supplied

Tablets (chewable): 200 IU†, 400 IU†
Capsules: 200 IU†, 400 IU†, 500 IU†, 600 IU†, 1,000 IU†, 73.5 mg, 147 mg, 330 mg
Oral solution: 50 mg/ml†

Pharmacokinetics

Absorption: GI absorption depends on presence of bile. Only 20% to 60% of vitamin obtained from dietary sources is absorbed. As dosage increases, fraction of vitamin E absorbed decreases.
Distribution: distributed to all tissues and stored in adipose tissues.
Metabolism: metabolized in liver.
Excretion: excreted primarily in bile; small amount excreted in urine.

Route	Onset	Peak	Duration
P.O.	Unknown	Unknown	Unknown

Pharmacodynamics

Chemical effect: unknown; thought to act as an antioxidant and protect RBC membranes against hemolysis.
Therapeutic effect: raises vitamin E level in body.

Adverse reactions

None reported with recommended dosages.

Interactions

Drug-drug. *Cholestyramine resin, mineral oil:* inhibited GI absorption of oral vitamin E. Space doses. Use together cautiously.
Iron: may catalyze oxidation and increase daily requirements. Administer separately.
Oral anticoagulants: hypoprothrombinemic effects may be increased, possibly causing bleeding. Monitor patient closely.
Vitamin K: antagonized effects of vitamin K possible with large doses of vitamin E. Avoid concurrent use.

Contraindications and precautions

No known contraindications.

NURSING CONSIDERATIONS

Assessment
- Assess patient's condition before therapy and regularly thereafter.
- Monitor patient with liver or gallbladder disease for response to therapy. Adequate bile is essential for vitamin E absorption.
- Be alert for drug interactions.
- Evaluate patient's and family's knowledge of drug therapy.

Nursing diagnoses
- Imbalanced nutrition: less than body requirements related to inadequate intake
- Deficient knowledge related to drug therapy

Planning and implementation
- Requirements increase with rise in dietary polyunsaturated acids.
- Make sure patient swallows tablets or capsules whole.
- Store drug in tightly closed light-resistant container.
- Vitamin E should be given with bile salts if patient has malabsorption caused by lack of bile.
- Hypervitaminosis E symptoms include fatigue, weakness, nausea, headache, blurred vision, flatulence, diarrhea.

Patient teaching
- Tell patient not to crush tablets or open capsules. An oral solution and chewable tablets are commercially available.
- Discourage patient from taking megadoses, which can cause thrombophlebitis. Vitamin E is fat-soluble.

Evaluation
- Patient regains normal vitamin E level.
- Patient and family state understanding of drug therapy.

W

warfarin sodium
(WAR-feh-rin SOH-dee-um)
Coumadin, Warfilone ♦

Pharmacologic class: coumarin derivative
Therapeutic class: anticoagulant
Pregnancy risk category: X

Indications and dosages

▶ **Pulmonary embolism related to deep vein thrombosis, MI, rheumatic heart disease with heart valve damage, prosthetic heart valves, chronic atrial fibrillation.**
Adults: initially, 2 to 5 mg P.O.; then daily PT and INR are used to establish optimal dose. Usual maintenance dosage is 2 to 10 mg daily.

How supplied

Tablets: 1 mg, 2 mg, 2.5 mg, 4 mg, 5 mg, 7.5 mg, 10 mg

Pharmacokinetics

Absorption: rapidly and completely absorbed from GI tract.
Distribution: highly bound to plasma proteins, especially albumin.
Metabolism: metabolized in liver.
Excretion: metabolites reabsorbed from bile and excreted in urine. *Half-life:* 1 to 3 days.

Route	Onset	Peak	Duration
P.O.	0.5-3 days	Unknown	2-5 days

Pharmacodynamics

Chemical effect: inhibits vitamin K–dependent activation of clotting factors II, VII, IX, and X, formed in liver.
Therapeutic effect: reduces ability of blood to clot.

Adverse reactions

CNS: headache.
GI: anorexia, nausea, vomiting, cramps, *diarrhea,* mouth ulcerations, sore mouth, melena.

GU: hematuria, excessive menstrual bleeding.
Hematologic: ***hemorrhage*** with excessive dosage.
Hepatic: ***hepatitis,*** elevated liver function test results, jaundice.
Skin: dermatitis, urticaria, necrosis, gangrene, alopecia, *rash.*
Other: *fever.*

Interactions

Drug-drug. *Acetaminophen:* may increase bleeding with prolonged therapy (more than 2 weeks) with high doses (more than 2 g/day) of acetaminophen. Monitor patient very carefully.
Allopurinol, amiodarone, anabolic steroids, cephalosporins, chloramphenicol, cimetidine, ciprofloxacin, clofibrate, danazol, diazoxide, diflunisal, disulfiram, erythromycin, ethacrynic acid, fenoprofen calcium, fluoroquinolones, glucagon, heparin, ibuprofen, influenza virus vaccine, isoniazid, ketoprofen, lovastatin, meclofenamate, methimazole, methylthiouracil, metronidazole, miconazole, nalidixic acid, neomycin (oral), pentoxifylline, propafenone, propoxyphene, propylthiouracil, quinidine, streptokinase, sulfinpyrazone, sulfonamides, sulindac, tamoxifen, tetracyclines, thiazides, thyroid drugs, tricyclic antidepressants, urokinase, vitamin E: increased PT. Monitor patient for bleeding. Reduce anticoagulant dosage if directed.
Anticonvulsants: increased serum levels of phenytoin and phenobarbital. Monitor patient for toxicity.
Barbiturates, carbamazepine, corticosteroids, corticotropin, ethchlorvynol, griseofulvin, mercaptopurine, methaqualone, nafcillin, oral contraceptives containing estrogen, rifampin, spironolactone, sucralfate, trazodone: decreased PT with reduced anticoagulant effect. Monitor patient carefully.
Chloral hydrate, glutethimide, propylthiouracil, sulfinpyrazone: increased or decreased PT. Avoid use, if possible. Monitor patient carefully.
Cholestyramine: decreased response when given too close together. Administer 6 hours after oral anticoagulants.
NSAIDs, salicylates: increased PT; ulcerogenic effects. Don't use together.
Sulfonylureas (oral antidiabetics): increased hypoglycemic response. Monitor blood glucose level.
Drug-herb. *Angelica:* significantly prolonged PT when used together. Discourage concomitant use.
Motherwort, red clover: risk of increased bleeding. Discourage concomitant use.
Drug-food. *Foods or enteral products containing vitamin K:* may impair anticoagulation. Tell patient to maintain consistent daily intake of leafy green vegetables.
Drug-lifestyle. *Alcohol use:* enhanced anticoagulant effects. Discourage alcohol intake; however, one or two drinks daily are unlikely to affect warfarin response.

Contraindications and precautions

- Contraindicated in pregnant women; patients with bleeding or hemorrhagic tendencies, GI ulcerations, severe hepatic or renal disease, severe uncontrolled hypertension, subacute bacterial endocarditis, polycythemia vera, or vitamin K deficiency; and patients who had recent eye, brain, or spinal cord surgery.
- Use cautiously in breast-feeding women and patients with diverticulitis, colitis, mild or moderate hypertension, mild or moderate hepatic or renal disease, drainage tubes in any orifice, or regional or lumbar block anesthesia. Also use cautiously if patient has any condition that increases the risk of hemorrhage.
- Infants, especially neonates, may be more susceptible to anticoagulants because of vitamin K deficiency.

NURSING CONSIDERATIONS

Assessment

- Assess patient's condition before therapy and regularly thereafter.
- Draw blood to establish baseline coagulation parameters before therapy.

ALERT INR determinations are essential for proper control. Clinicians typically try to maintain INR at 2 to 3 times normal; risk of bleeding is high when INR exceeds 6 times normal.

- Be alert for adverse reactions and drug interactions. Elderly patients and patients with re-

nal or hepatic failure are especially sensitive to warfarin effect.
- Regularly inspect patient for bleeding gums, bruises on arms or legs, petechiae, nosebleeds, melena, tarry stools, hematuria, and hematemesis.
- Observe breast-feeding infant for unexpected bleeding if infant's mother takes drug.
- Evaluate patient's and family's knowledge of drug therapy.

Nursing diagnoses
- Risk for injury related to potential for blood clot formation from underlying condition
- Ineffective protection related to increased risk of bleeding
- Deficient knowledge related to drug therapy

Planning and implementation
- Give drug at same time daily.
- I.V. form may be obtained from manufacturer for rare patient who can't have oral therapy. Follow guidelines carefully for preparation and administration.
- Because onset of action is delayed, heparin sodium is commonly given during first few days of treatment. When heparin is being given simul-taneously, blood for PT shouldn't be drawn within 5 hours of intermittent I.V. heparin administration. However, blood for PT may be drawn at any time during continuous heparin infusion.
- Elderly patients have an increased risk of bleeding and usually receive lower dosages.

ALERT Withhold drug and call prescriber immediately if fever and rash occur; they may signal severe adverse reactions.
- The drug's anticoagulant effect can be neutralized by vitamin K injections.
- Drug is best oral anticoagulant for patient taking antacids or phenytoin.

Patient teaching
- Stress importance of compliance with prescribed dosage and follow-up appointments. Patient should wear or carry medical identification that indicates his increased risk of bleeding.
- Instruct patient and family to watch for signs of bleeding and to notify prescriber immediately if they occur.
- Warn patient to avoid OTC products containing aspirin, other salicylates, or drugs that may interact with warfarin.
- Tell patient to notify prescriber if menses is heavier than usual; dosage adjustment may be necessary.
- Tell patient to use electric razor when shaving to avoid scratching skin and to use soft toothbrush.
- Caution patient to read food labels. Food and enteral feedings that contain vitamin K may impair anticoagulation.
- Tell patient to eat a daily, consistent amount of leafy green vegetables that contain vitamin K. Eating varying amounts may alter anticoagulant effects.

Evaluation
- Patient doesn't develop blood clots.
- Patient states appropriate bleeding precautions to take.
- Patient and family state understanding of drug therapy.

X-Y

xylometazoline hydrochloride
(zigh-loh-met-uh-ZOH-leen high-droh-KLOR-ighd)
Otrivin

Pharmacologic class: sympathomimetic
Therapeutic class: decongestant, vasoconstrictor
Pregnancy risk category: NR

Indications and dosages
▶ **Nasal congestion.** *Adults and children age 12 and over:* 2 to 3 gtt or sprays of 0.1% solution in each nostril q 8 to 10 hours. *Children ages 6 months to 12 years:* 2 to 3 gtt of 0.05% solution in each nostril q 8 to 10 hours. *Children under 6 months:* 1 gtt of 0.05% solution in each nostril q 6 hours, p.r.n.

How supplied
Nasal solution: 0.05%, 0.1%.

Pharmacokinetics

Unknown.

Route	Onset	Peak	Duration
Intranasal	5-10 min	Unknown	5-6 hr

Pharmacodynamics

Chemical effect: unknown; thought to cause local vasoconstriction of dilated arterioles, reducing blood flow and nasal congestion.
Therapeutic effect: relieves nasal congestion.

Adverse reactions

EENT: transient burning, stinging; dryness or ulceration of nasal mucosa; sneezing; rebound nasal congestion or irritation (with excessive or long-term use).

Interactions

None significant.

Contraindications and precautions

- Contraindicated in patients hypersensitive to drug and in those with angle-closure glaucoma.
- Use cautiously in patients with hyperthyroidism, cardiac disease, hypertension, diabetes mellitus, or advanced arteriosclerosis.
- Safety of drug hasn't been established in pregnant or breast-feeding women.

NURSING CONSIDERATIONS

Assessment

- Assess patient's condition before therapy and regularly thereafter.
- Be alert for adverse reactions.
- Evaluate patient's and family's knowledge of drug therapy.

Nursing diagnoses

- Ineffective health maintenance related to presence of nasal congestion
- Impaired tissue integrity related to drug's adverse effect on nasal mucosa
- Deficient knowledge related to drug therapy

Planning and implementation

- When giving more than one spray, allow 3 to 5 minutes to elapse between sprays, and have patient clear his nose before each spray.

Patient teaching

- Teach patient how to use drug. Have him hold his head upright to minimize swallowing of the drug; tell him to sniff spray briskly. Instruct him to wait 3 to 5 minutes between sprays and to his clear nose before each spray.
- Tell patient not to share drug to prevent spread of infection.
- Tell patient not to exceed recommended dosage and to use only as needed and only for 3 to 5 days.

Evaluation

- Patient's nasal congestion is eliminated.
- Patient maintains normal intranasal mucosa.
- Patient and family state understanding of drug therapy.

Z

zafirlukast

(zay-FEER-loo-kast)
Accolate

Pharmacologic class: synthetic, selective peptide leukotriene receptor antagonist
Therapeutic class: antiasthma, bronchodilator
Pregnancy risk category: B

Indications and dosages

▶ **Prophylaxis and treatment of chronic asthma.** *Adults and children age 12 and older:* 20 mg P.O. b.i.d. taken 1 hour before or 2 hours after meals.
Children ages 7 to 11: 10 mg P.O. b.i.d.

How supplied

Tablets: 10 mg, 20 mg

Pharmacokinetics

Absorption: rapidly absorbed.
Distribution: unknown.

Metabolism: extensively metabolized.
Excretion: in feces; 10% in urine.

Route	Onset	Peak	Duration
P.O.	Unknown	3 hr	Unknown

Pharmacodynamics

Chemical effect: selectively competes for leukotriene receptor sites.
Therapeutic effect: blocks inflammatory action, inhibits bronchoconstriction, improves breathing.

Adverse reactions

CNS: *headache,* asthenia, dizziness.
GI: nausea, diarrhea, abdominal pain, vomiting, dyspepsia.
Hepatic: elevated liver enzyme levels.
Musculoskeletal: myalgia, back pain.
Other: infection, pain, accidental injury, fever.

Interactions

Drug-drug. *Aspirin:* increased plasma zafirlukast levels. Monitor patient.
Erythromycin, theophylline: decreased plasma zafirlukast levels. Monitor patient.
Warfarin: increased PT. Monitor PT and INR levels, and adjust dosage of anticoagulant, as ordered.
Drug-food. *Any food:* reduced rate and extent of drug absorption. Give drug 1 hour before or 2 hours after meals.

Contraindications and precautions

- Contraindicated in patients hypersensitive to drug.

NURSING CONSIDERATIONS

Assessment

- Use cautiously in patients with hepatic impairment and in elderly patients.
- Evaluate patient's and family's understanding of drug therapy.

Nursing diagnoses

- Impaired gas exchange related to bronchospasm
- Deficient knowledge related to drug therapy

Planning and implementation

- Don't use drug for reversing bronchospasm in acute asthma attack.

ALERT Reduction in oral steroid dose has been followed in rare cases by eosinophilia, vasculitic rash, worsening pulmonary symptoms, cardiac complications, or neuropathy, sometimes presenting as Churg-Strauss syndrome.

- Safety and effectiveness in patients under age 7 haven't been established.

Patient teaching

- Tell patient to keep taking drug even if symptoms disappear.
- Advise patient to continue taking other antiasthma drugs as ordered.
- Instruct patient to take drug 1 hour before or 2 hours after meals.

Evaluation

- Patient demonstrates improved gas exchange.
- Patient and family state understanding of drug therapy.

zalcitabine (ddC, dideoxycytidine)

(zal-SIGH-tuh-been)
Hivid

Pharmacologic class: nucleoside analogue
Therapeutic class: antiviral
Pregnancy risk category: C

Indications and dosages

▶ **Advanced HIV infection (CD4+ T-cell count below 300 cells/mm^3) in patients with significant clinical or immunologic deterioration.** *Adults and children age 13 or older weighing at least 30 kg (66 lb):* 0.75 mg P.O. q 8 hours. Drug must be taken with zidovudine 200 mg P.O. q 8 hours.

How supplied

Tablets: 0.375 mg, 0.75 mg

Pharmacokinetics

Absorption: mean absolute bioavailability is above 80%. Administering drug with food decreases rate and extent of absorption.
Distribution: enters CNS.
Metabolism: doesn't appear to undergo significant hepatic metabolism; phosphorylation to active form occurs within cells.
Excretion: excreted primarily in urine. *Half-life:* 2 hours.

Route	Onset	Peak	Duration
P.O.	Unknown	1-2 hr	Unknown

Pharmacodynamics

Chemical effect: inhibits replication of HIV by blocking viral DNA synthesis.
Therapeutic effect: reduces symptoms linked to advanced HIV infection.

Adverse reactions

CNS: *peripheral neuropathy, headache, fatigue,* dizziness, confusion, ***seizures,*** impaired concentration, amnesia, insomnia, depression, tremors, hypertonia, asthenia, agitation, abnormal thinking, anxiety.
CV: cardiomyopathy, ***heart failure,*** chest pain.
EENT: pharyngitis, ocular pain, abnormal vision, ototoxicity, nasal discharge.
GI: nausea, vomiting, diarrhea, abdominal pain, anorexia, constipation, stomatitis, esophageal ulcer, glossitis, ***pancreatitis.***
Hematologic: anemia, ***neutropenia, leukopenia, thrombocytopenia.***
Hepatic: increased liver function test results.
Metabolic: hypoglycemia.
Respiratory: cough.
Musculoskeletal: myalgia, arthralgia.
Skin: pruritus; night sweats; *erythematous, maculopapular, or follicular rash;* urticaria.
Other: *fever.*

Interactions

Drug-drug. *Aminoglycosides, amphotericin B, foscarnet, other drugs that may impair kidney function:* increased risk of nephrotoxicity. Avoid concomitant use.
Antacids: decreased zalcitabine absorption. Administer separately.
Antacids containing aluminum or magnesium: decreased bioavailability of zalcitabine. Don't use together.
Chloramphenicol, cisplatin, dapsone, disulfiram, ethionamide, glutethimide, gold salts, hydralazine, iodoquinol, isoniazid, metronidazole, nitrofurantoin, phenytoin, ribavirin, and vincristine as well as other drugs that can cause peripheral neuropathy: increased risk of peripheral neuropathy. Avoid concomitant use.
Cimetidine, probenecid: increased serum zalcitabine levels. Monitor patient carefully.
Pentamidine: increased risk of pancreatitis. Avoid concomitant use.
Drug-food. *Any food:* decreased rate of absorption. Give drug on empty stomach.

Contraindications and precautions

- Contraindicated in patients hypersensitive to drug or its components.
- Use with extreme caution in patients with peripheral neuropathy.
- Use cautiously in patients with renal impairment (creatinine clearance below 55 ml/minute) because they may be at increased risk for toxicity.
- Also use cautiously in patients with hepatic failure. In clinical trials, drug regimen (zalcitabine plus zidovudine) worsened hepatic dysfunction in patients with hepatic impairment.
- Also use cautiously in patients with history of pancreatitis. Rarely, pancreatitis has been fatal in patients receiving zalcitabine. In patients receiving zalcitabine as only treatment, pancreatitis was rare (less than 1%).
- Use cautiously in patients with baseline cardiomyopathy or history of heart failure.
- Safety of drug in children under age 13 and in pregnant women hasn't been established.

NURSING CONSIDERATIONS

Assessment

- Assess patient's condition before therapy and regularly thereafter.
- Assess patient for signs of peripheral neuropathy, characterized by numbness and burning in limbs, the major toxicity resulting from drug.

• Be alert for adverse reactions and drug interactions.
• Evaluate patient's and family's knowledge of drug therapy.

Nursing diagnoses
• Risk for infection related to presence of HIV
• Disturbed sensory perceptions (tactile) related to drug-induced peripheral neuropathy
• Deficient knowledge related to drug therapy

Planning and implementation
• Dosage adjustments are necessary in patient with moderate to severe renal failure.
• Don't administer drug with food because it decreases rate and extent of absorption.
• Notify prescriber if signs and symptoms of peripheral neuropathy occur. If drug isn't withdrawn, peripheral neuropathy can progress to sharp, shooting pain or severe continuous burning pain requiring opioid analgesics. It may or may not be reversible.
• If patient experiences symptoms that resemble peripheral neuropathy, prepare to withdraw drug. Drug should be discontinued if symptoms are bilateral and persist beyond 72 hours. If symptoms persist or worsen beyond 1 week, drug should be permanently discontinued. If all findings relevant to peripheral neuropathy have resolved to minor symptoms, drug may be reintroduced at 0.375 mg P.O. q 8 hours, as ordered.
• If zalcitabine is discontinued because of toxicity, patient should resume recommended dose for zidovudine (100 mg q 4 hours).
ALERT Don't confuse drug with other antivirals that use initials for identification.

Patient teaching
• Make sure patient understands that drug doesn't cure HIV infection and that opportunistic infections may occur despite continued use. Review safe sex practices with patient.
• Inform patient that peripheral neuropathy is the major toxicity linked to this drug and that pancreatitis is the major life-threatening toxicity. Review signs and symptoms of these adverse reactions, and instruct patient to call prescriber promptly if they appear.
• Instruct woman of childbearing age to use effective contraceptive during drug therapy.

Evaluation
• Patient responds well to drug.
• Patient doesn't develop peripheral neuropathy.
• Patient and family state understanding of drug therapy.

zaleplon
(ZAL-eh-plon)
Sonata

Pharmacologic class: pyrazolopyrimidine
Therapeutic class: hypnotic
Controlled substance schedule: IV
Pregnancy risk category: C

Indications and dosages
Short-term treatment of insomnia. *Adults:* 10 mg P.O. h.s.; may increase dose to 20 mg if needed. Low-weight adults may respond to 5-mg dose.
Elderly and debilitated patients: initially, 5 mg P.O. h.s.; doses over 10 mg aren't recommended.

How supplied
Capsules: 5 mg, 10 mg

Pharmacokinetics
Absorption: rapidly and almost completely absorbed. Levels peak within 1 hour. Dosing after a high-fat or heavy meal delays peak levels by about 2 hours.
Distribution: substantially distributed into extravascular tissues. Plasma protein–binding is about 60%.
Metabolism: extensively metabolized, primarily by aldehyde oxidase and, to a lesser extent, CYP 3A4 to inactive metabolites. Less than 1% of dose is excreted unchanged in urine.
Excretion: rapidly excreted. *Half-life:* 1 hour.

Route	Onset	Peak	Duration
P.O.	1 hr	1 hr	3-4 hr

Pharmacodynamics

Chemical effect: although zaleplon is a hypnotic with a chemical structure unrelated to benzodiazepines, it interacts with the gamma-aminobutyric acid BZ receptor complex in the CNS. Modulation of this complex is hypothesized to be responsible for sedative, anxiolytic, muscle relaxant, and anticonvulsant effects of benzodiazepines.
Therapeutic effect: promotes sleep.

Adverse reactions

CNS: *headache,* amnesia, dizziness, somnolence, depression, hypertonia, nervousness, depersonalization, hallucinations, vertigo, difficulty concentrating, anxiety, paresthesia, hypoesthesia, tremor, asthenia, migraine, malaise.
CV: chest pain, peripheral edema.
EENT: abnormal vision, conjunctivitis, eye pain, ear pain, hyperacusis, epistaxis, parosmia.
GI: constipation, dry mouth, anorexia, dyspepsia, nausea, abdominal pain, colitis.
GU: dysmenorrhea.
Musculoskeletal: arthritis, myalgia, back pain.
Respiratory: bronchitis.
Skin: pruritus, rash, photosensitivity reaction.
Other: fever.

Interactions

Drug-drug. *Carbamazepine, phenobarbital, phenytoin, rifampin, other drugs that induce CYP 3A4:* may reduce bioavailability and peak levels of zaleplon by about 80%. Consider a different hypnotic as directed.
CNS depressants (imipramine, thioridazine): may produce additive CNS effects. Use cautiously together.
Cimetidine: increases zaleplon bioavailability and peak levels by 85%. For patient taking cimetidine, use an initial zaleplon dose of 5 mg.
Drug-food. *High-fat foods, heavy meals:* prolonged absorption, delaying peak zaleplon levels by about 2 hours; sleep onset may be delayed. Separate administration from meals.
Drug-lifestyle. *Alcohol use:* may increase CNS effects. Discourage concurrent use.

Contraindications and precautions

- Don't use in patients with severe hepatic impairment. Use cautiously in elderly and debilitated patients, in those with compromised respiratory function, and in those with signs and symptoms of depression.

NURSING CONSIDERATIONS

Assessment

- Careful patient evaluation is necessary because sleep disturbances may be a symptom of an underlying physical or psychiatric disorder.
- Closely monitor elderly or debilitated patients and patients with compromised respiratory function because of illness.
- Monitor patient for drug abuse and dependence.
- Evaluate patient's and family's knowledge about drug therapy.

Nursing diagnoses

- Disturbed sleep pattern related to presence of insomnia
- Risk for injury related to drug-induced adverse CNS reactions
- Deficient knowledge related to drug therapy

Planning and implementation

- Don't give drug with or following a high-fat or heavy meal.
- Because zaleplon works rapidly, it should only be taken immediately before bedtime or after patient has gone to bed and has experienced difficulty falling asleep.
- Adverse reactions are usually dose-related. The lowest effective dose should be given, as ordered.
- Limit hypnotic use to 7 to 10 days. Patient should be reevaluated by a prescriber if hypnotics will be taken for more than 3 weeks.
- The potential for drug abuse and dependence exists. Zaleplon shouldn't be given as more than a 1-month supply.
- Patients with mild to moderate hepatic failure or those receiving cimetidine concomitantly should take 5 mg P.O. every day at bedtime.

Patient teaching

- Advise patient that zaleplon works rapidly and should be taken immediately before bedtime or after going to bed and having difficulty falling asleep.

- Advise patient to take drug only if he can sleep for at least 4 undisturbed hours.
- Caution patient that drowsiness, dizziness, light-headedness, and difficulty with coordination occur most often within 1 hour after taking drug.
- Advise patient to avoid performing activities that require mental alertness until CNS effects of drug are known.
- Advise patient to avoid alcohol while taking drug and to notify prescriber before taking any prescription or OTC drugs.
- Tell patient not to take drug after a high-fat or heavy meal.
- Advise patient to report any continued sleep problems despite use of drug.
- Notify patient that dependence can occur, and that drug is recommended for short-term use only.
- Warn patient not to abruptly discontinue drug because withdrawal symptoms, including unpleasant feelings, stomach and muscle cramps, vomiting, sweating, shakiness, and seizures, may occur.
- Notify patient that insomnia may recur for a few nights after stopping drug, but should resolve on its own.
- Advise patient that zaleplon may cause changes in behavior and thinking, including outgoing or aggressive behavior, loss of personal identity, confusion, strange behavior, agitation, hallucinations, worsening of depression, or suicidal thoughts. Tell patient to notify presciber immediately if any of these symptoms occur.

☑ Evaluation

- Patient states that drug effectively promotes sleep.
- Patient doesn't experience injury as a result of drug-induced adverse CNS reactions.
- Patient and family state understanding of drug therapy.

zanamivir

(zah-NAM-ah-veer)
Relenza

Pharmacologic class: neuraminidase inhibitor
Therapeutic class: antiviral
Pregnancy risk category: B

Indications and dosages

▶ **Treatment of uncomplicated acute illness caused by influenza A and B virus in patients who have been symptomatic for no more than 2 days.** *Adults and children age 7 and older:* 2 oral inhalations (one 5-mg blister per inhalation for a total dose of 10 mg) b.i.d. using the Diskhaler inhalation device for 5 days. Two doses should be taken on the first day of treatment provided there is at least 2 hours between doses. Subsequent doses should be about 12 hours apart (in the morning and evening) at about the same time each day.

How supplied

Powder for inhalation: 5 mg per blister

Pharmacokinetics

Absorption: about 4% to 17% of orally inhaled zanamivir is systemically absorbed, with peak serum levels occurring 1 to 2 hours following a 10-mg dose.
Distribution: drug has limited (less than 10%) plasma protein–binding.
Metabolism: not metabolized.
Excretion: excreted unchanged in the urine within 24 hours. Unabsorbed drug is excreted in the feces. *Half-life:* 2½ to 5¼ hours.

Route	Onset	Peak	Duration
Inhalation	Unknown	1-2 hr	Unknown

Pharmacodynamics

Chemical effect: Zanamivir most likely inhibits neuraminidase on the surface of the influenza virus, possibly altering virus particle aggregation and release. With the inhibition of neuraminidase, the virus cannot escape from its host cell to attack others, thereby inhibiting the process of viral proliferation.

Therapeutic effect: lessens the symptoms of influenza.

Adverse reactions

CNS: headache, dizziness.
EENT: nasal signs and symptoms; sinusitis; ear, nose, and throat infections.
GI: diarrhea, nausea, vomiting.
Respiratory: bronchitis, cough.

Interactions

None reported.

Contraindications and precautions

- Contraindicated in patients hypersensitive to zanamivir or its components. Use cautiously in patients with severe or decompensated chronic obstructive pulmonary disease, asthma, or other underlying respiratory disease.

NURSING CONSIDERATIONS

Assessment

- Obtain accurate patient medical history before starting therapy.
- Lymphopenia, neutropenia, and a rise in liver enzyme and CK levels have been reported during zanamivir treatment. Monitor patient appropriately.
- Monitor patient for bronchospasm and decline in lung function. Stop the drug, as ordered, in such situations.
- Evaluate patient's and family's knowledge about drug therapy.

Nursing diagnoses

- Risk for infection related to influenza virus
- Imbalanced nutrition: less than body requirements related to drug's adverse GI effects
- Deficient knowledge related to drug therapy

Planning and implementation

- Have patient exhale fully before putting the mouthpiece in his mouth. Then, keeping the Diskhaler level, have patient close his lips around the mouthpiece, and have him breathe in steadily and deeply. Advise patient to hold his breath for a few seconds after inhaling to help zanamivir stay in the lungs.
- Patients with underlying respiratory disease should have a fast-acting bronchodilator available in case of wheezing while taking zanamivir. Patients scheduled to use an inhaled bronchodilator for asthma should use their bronchodilator before taking zanamivir.
- Safety and efficacy of zanamivir haven't been established for influenza prophylaxis. Use of zanamivir should not affect the evaluation of patients for their annual influenza vaccination.
- No data are available to support safety and efficacy of zanamivir in patients who begin treatment after 48 hours of symptoms.

Patient teaching

- Tell patient to carefully read the instructions regarding how to use the Diskhaler inhalation device properly to administer zanamivir.
- Advise patient to keep the Diskhaler level when loading and inhaling zanamivir. Inform patient to always check inside the mouthpiece of the Diskhaler before each use to make sure it's free of foreign objects.
- Tell patient to exhale fully before putting the mouthpiece in his mouth, then, keeping the Diskhaler level, to close his lips around the mouthpiece and breathe in steadily and deeply. Advise patient to hold his breath for a few seconds after inhaling to help zanamivir stay in the lungs.
- Advise patient who has an impending scheduled dose of inhaled bronchodilator to take it before taking zanamivir. Tell patient to have a fast-acting bronchodilator available in case of wheezing while taking zanamivir.
- Advise patient that it's important to finish the entire 5-day course of treatment even if he starts to feel better and symptoms improve before the fifth day.
- Advise patient that the use of zanamivir hasn't been shown to reduce the risk of transmission of influenza virus to others.

Evaluation

- Patient recovers from influenza.
- Patient doesn't experience adverse GI effects.
- Patient and family state understanding of drug therapy.

zidovudine (azidothymidine, AZT)

(zigh-DOH-vyoo-deen)

Apo-Zidovudine ♦, Novo-AZT ♦, Retrovir

Pharmacologic class: thymidine analogue
Therapeutic class: antiviral
Pregnancy risk category: C

Indications and dosages

▶ **Symptomatic HIV infection, including AIDS.** *Adults and children age 12 and older:* 100 mg P.O. q 4 hours.
Children ages 3 months to 12 years: 180 mg/m² P.O. q 6 hours (720 mg/m²/day), not to exceed 200 mg q 6 hours.

▶ **Selected patients with AIDS or advanced AIDS-related complex (ARC) who have history of *Pneumocystis carinii* pneumonia or CD4+ lymphocyte count below 200 cells/mm³.** *Adults:* 1 to 2 mg/kg I.V. infused over 1 hour q 4 hours around the clock, followed by 200 mg P.O. q 4 hours around the clock when P.O. administration can replace parenteral administration.

▶ **Asymptomatic HIV infection.** *Adults and children age 12 and older:* 100 mg P.O. q 4 hours while awake (500 mg daily).
Children ages 3 months to 12 years: 180 mg/m² P.O. q 6 hours (720 mg/m²/day), not to exceed 200 mg q 6 hours.

▶ **To reduce risk of transmission of HIV to neonate from infected mother with baseline CD4+ lymphocyte counts greater than 200 cells/mm³.** *Adults:* 100 mg P.O. q 4 hours while awake (total of five doses daily) given initially between 14 and 34 weeks' gestation and continued throughout pregnancy. During labor, give loading dose of 2 mg/kg, followed by infusion of 1 mg/kg/hour until delivery.
Infants: 2 mg/kg P.O. (syrup) q 6 hours for 6 weeks starting 12 hours after birth.

How supplied

Capsules: 100 mg
Syrup: 50 mg/5 ml
Injection: 10 mg/ml

Pharmacokinetics

Absorption: absorbed rapidly from GI tract.
Distribution: preliminary data reveal good CSF penetration; about 36% plasma protein-bound.
Metabolism: metabolized rapidly to inactive compound.
Excretion: excreted in urine. *Half-life:* 1 hour.

Route	Onset	Peak	Duration
P.O.	Unknown	0.5-1.5 hr	Unknown
I.V.	Immediate	0.5-1.5 hr	Unknown

Pharmacodynamics

Chemical effect: prevents replication of HIV by inhibiting the enzyme reverse transcriptase.
Therapeutic effect: reduces symptoms of HIV infection.

Adverse reactions

CNS: *asthenia, headache, **seizures,*** paresthesia, *malaise,* insomnia, *dizziness,* somnolence.
GI: *nausea, anorexia, abdominal pain, vomiting,* constipation, *diarrhea,* dyspepsia, taste perversion.
Hematologic: ***severe bone marrow suppression (resulting in anemia), agranulocytosis, thrombocytopenia.***
Hepatic: increased liver enzyme levels.
Metabolic: ***lactic acidosis.***
Musculoskeletal: myalgia.
Skin: *rash,* diaphoresis.
Other: *fever.*

Interactions

Drug-drug. *Acetaminophen, aspirin, indomethacin:* may impair hepatic metabolism of zidovudine, increasing drug's toxicity. Avoid concomitant use.
Acyclovir: possible seizures, lethargy, and fatigue. Use together cautiously.
Amphotericin B, dapsone, flucytosine, pentamidine: increased risk of nephrotoxicity and bone marrow suppression. Monitor patient closely.
Fluconazole, methadone, valproic acid: increased zidovudine level. Monitor patient for toxicity.
Ganciclovir: increased risk of hematologic toxicity. Monitor patient.
Other cytotoxic drugs: additive adverse effects on bone marrow. Avoid concomitant use.

Probenecid: may decrease renal clearance of zidovudine. Avoid concomitant use.
Ribavirin: antagonizes antiviral activity of zidovudine against HIV. Use cautiously.

Contraindications and precautions

- Contraindicated in patients hypersensitive to drug.
- Use cautiously and with close monitoring in patients with advanced symptomatic HIV infection and in those with severe bone marrow depression.
- Use cautiously in patients with hepatomegaly, hepatitis, or other known risk factors for hepatic disease.

NURSING CONSIDERATIONS

Assessment

- Assess patient's condition before therapy and regularly thereafter.
- Monitor blood studies every 2 weeks, as ordered, to detect anemia or agranulocytosis.
- Be alert for adverse reactions and drug interactions.
- Evaluate patient's and family's knowledge of drug therapy.

Nursing diagnoses

- Infection related to presence of HIV
- Ineffective protection related to drug-induced adverse hematologic reactions
- Deficient knowledge related to drug therapy

Planning and implementation

- Zidovudine temporarily decreases morbidity and mortality in certain patients with AIDS or ARC.
- Optimum duration of treatment and optimum dosage for effectiveness with minimum toxicity aren't yet known.

P.O. use: Follow normal protocol.
I.V. use: Dilute drug before use. Remove calculated dose from vial; add to D_5W to yield no more than 4 mg/ml.
– Infuse drug over 1 hour at constant rate; give every 4 hours around the clock. Avoid rapid infusion or bolus injection.
– Adding mixture to biological or colloidal fluids (for example, blood products, protein solutions) isn't recommended.
– After drug is diluted, solution is physically and chemically stable for 24 hours at room temperature and for 48 hours if refrigerated at 36° to 46° F (2° to 8° C). Store undiluted vials at 59° to 77° F (15° to 25° C) and protect them from light.

- Notify prescriber of abnormal hematologic study results. Patient may require dosage reduction or temporary discontinuation of drug.

Patient teaching

- Advise patient that blood transfusions may be needed during treatment. Drug often causes low RBC count.
- Stress importance of compliance with every-4-hour dosage schedule. Suggest ways to avoid missing doses, perhaps by using an alarm clock.
- Warn patient not to take other drugs for AIDS (especially those available on street) unless approved by prescriber. Some purported AIDS cures may interfere with drug's effectiveness.
- Advise pregnant HIV-infected women that drug therapy only reduces risk of HIV transmission to neonates. Long-term risks to infants are unknown.
- Advise health care worker who considers zidovudine prophylaxis after occupational exposure (for example, after needle-stick injury) that drug's safety and efficacy haven't been proven.

Evaluation

- Patient exhibits reduced severity and frequency of symptoms linked to HIV infection.
- Patient doesn't develop complications from therapy.
- Patient and family state understanding of drug therapy.

zileuton

(zigh-LOO-tun)
Zyflo

Pharmacologic class: leukotriene inhibitor
Therapeutic class: antiasthma agent, bronchodilator
Pregnancy risk category: C

Indications and dosages

▶ **Prophylaxis and long-term treatment of asthma.** *Adults and children age 12 and older:* 600 mg P.O. q.i.d.

How supplied

Tablets: 600 mg

Pharmacokinetics

Absorption: rapidly absorbed.
Distribution: unknown; plasma protein–bound; well absorbed into systemic circulation.
Metabolism: metabolized by liver.
Excretion: excreted in feces and urine. *Half-life:* mean terminal half-life is 2½ hours.

Route	Onset	Peak	Duration
P.O.	Unknown	2 hr	Unknown

Pharmacodynamics

Chemical effect: inhibits enzyme that forms leukotrienes.
Therapeutic effect: reduces inflammatory response.

Adverse reactions

CNS: *headache,* asthenia, dizziness, insomnia, nervousness, somnolence, malaise.
CV: chest pain.
EENT: conjunctivitis.
GI: dyspepsia, nausea, abdominal pain, constipation, flatulence, vomiting.
GU: urinary tract infection, vaginitis.
Hematologic: ***leukopenia.***
Hepatic: elevated liver enzyme levels.
Musculoskeletal: myalgia, arthralgia, hypertonia, neck pain and rigidity.
Skin: pruritus.
Other: pain, accidental injury, fever, lymphadenopathy.

Interactions

Drug-drug. *Propranolol, other beta blockers:* increased beta blocker effect. Monitor patient and reduce dosage as needed.
Theophylline: lowers theophylline clearance. Reduce theophylline dose, as ordered, and monitor serum levels.
Warfarin: increased PT. Monitor PT and INR, and adjust dosage of anticoagulant, as ordered.

Contraindications and precautions

- Contraindicated in patients hypersensitive to drug and in those with active liver disease or transaminase levels at least three times the upper limit or normal.
- Use cautiously in patients with hepatic impairment or history of heavy alcohol use.

NURSING CONSIDERATIONS

Assessment

- Assess patient's disease process before and during therapy.
- Obtain baseline and periodic liver enzyme levels, as ordered.
- Evaluate patient's and family's understanding of drug therapy.

Nursing diagnoses

- Ineffective health maintenance related to underlying condition
- Deficient knowledge related to drug therapy

Planning and implementation

ALERT Drug isn't indicated for reversing bronchospasm in acute asthma attack.

- Safety and effectiveness in children under age 12 haven't been established.

Patient teaching

- Tell patient to keep taking drug even if symptoms disappear.
- Warn patient not to use drug for an acute asthma attack.
- Advise patient to continue taking other antiasthma drugs, as ordered.
- Instruct patient to notify prescriber if a short-acting bronchodilator doesn't relieve symptoms.
- Tell patient of need to regularly check liver enzyme levels.
- Tell patient to notify prescriber at once if signs of liver dysfunction occur.
- Tell patient to avoid alcohol during therapy and to consult prescriber before taking OTC or new prescription drugs.

Evaluation

- Patient exhibits improvement in underlying condition.

• Patient and family state understanding of drug therapy.

zolmitriptan

(zohl-muh-TRIP-tan)

Zomig

Pharmacologic class: selective 5-hydroxytryptamine receptor agonist
Therapeutic class: antimigraine agent
Pregnancy risk category: C

Indications and dosages

▶ **Treatment of acute migraine headaches.** *Adults:* initially, 2.5 mg or less P.O. increased to 5 mg per dose, p.r.n. If headache returns after initial dose, second dose may be administered after 2 hours. Maximum dosage is 10 mg in 24-hour period.

How supplied

Tablets: 2.5 mg, 5 mg

Pharmacokinetics

Absorption: well absorbed following P.O. administration with an absolute bioavailability of 40%.
Distribution: 25% bound to plasma protein.
Metabolism: converted to active N-desmethyl metabolite.
Excretion: about 65% of dose is recovered in urine (8% unchanged) and 30% in feces. *Half-life:* 3 hours.

Route	Onset	Peak	Duration
P.O.	Unknown	2 hr	3 hr

Pharmacodynamics

Chemical effect: selective serotonin receptor agonist that causes constriction of cranial blood vessels and inhibits pro-inflammatory neuropeptide release.
Therapeutic effect: relieves migraine headache pain.

Adverse reactions

CNS: somnolence, vertigo, *dizziness,* syncope, hyperesthesia, paresthesia, warm or cold sensations, asthenia, sweating.
CV: pain or heaviness in chest, ***arrhythmias,*** hypertension, *pain, tightness, or pressure in the neck, throat, or jaw.*
GI: dry mouth, dyspepsia, dysphagia, nausea.
Musculoskeletal: myalgia.

Interactions

Drug-drug. *Cimetidine:* doubles half-life of zolmitriptan. Monitor patient.
Ergot-type or ergot-containing drugs, 5-HT$_1$ agonists: may cause additive vasospastic reactions. Avoid concomitant use.
Fluoxetine, fluvoxamine, paroxetine, sertraline: may cause weakness, hyperreflexia, and incoordination. Use cautiously.
MAO inhibitors: increased effects of zolmitriptan. Avoid concomitant use.

Contraindications and precautions

• Contraindicated in patients hypersensitive to drug and in those with ischemic heart disease or other significant heart disease (including Wolff-Parkinson-White syndrome) or uncontrolled hypertension. Don't give drug within 24 hours of 5-HT$_1$ agonists, ergot-containing or ergot-type drugs. Use of zolmitriptan with MAO inhibitor or within 2 weeks of MAO inhibitor therapy is also contraindicated.
• Use cautiously in patients with liver disease.
• Drug isn't intended for preventing migraine headaches or treating hemiplegic or basilar migraines.
• Safety of drug hasn't been established for cluster headaches.
• Don't give drug to woman who is or may be pregnant or who is breast-feeding.

NURSING CONSIDERATIONS

Assessment

• Assess patient's history of migraine headaches and drug's effectiveness.
• Assess patient for history of known coronary artery disease, hypertension, arrhythmias, or presence of risk factors for coronary artery disease.
• Monitor liver function test results before starting drug therapy, and report abnormalities.
• Drug should be used only when a clear diagnosis of migraine has been established.

• Evaluate patient's and family's knowledge of drug therapy.

Nursing diagnoses

• Acute pain related to presence of migraine headache
• Impaired cardiopulmonary tissue perfusion related to drug-induced adverse cardiac events
• Deficient knowledge related to drug therapy

Planning and implementation

• Use a lower dose, as ordered, in patients with moderate to severe hepatic impairment.
• Don't give drug to prevent migraine headaches or to treat hemiplegic migraines, basilar migraines, or cluster headaches.
ALERT Don't give drug within 24 hours of ergot-containing drugs or within 2 weeks of MAO inhibitor.

Patient teaching

• Tell patient that drug is intended to relieve the symptoms of migraines, not to prevent them.
• Advise patient to take drug as prescribed. Caution against taking a second dose unless instructed by prescriber. Tell patient that if a second dose is indicated and permitted, he should take it at least 2 hours after initial dose.
• Advise patient to immediately report pain or tightness in chest or throat, heart throbbing, rash, skin lumps, or swelling of face, lips, or eyelids.
• Tell woman not to take drug if she plans or suspects pregnancy.

Evaluation

• Patient has relief from migraine headache.
• Patient doesn't experience pain or tightness in the chest or throat, arrhythmias, increases in blood pressure, or MI.
• Patient and family state understanding of drug therapy.

zolpidem tartrate

(ZOHL-peh-dim TAR-trayt)
Ambien

Pharmacologic class: imidazopyridine
Therapeutic class: hypnotic
Controlled substance schedule: IV
Pregnancy risk category: B

Indications and dosages

▶ **Short-term management of insomnia.**
Adults: 10 mg P.O. h.s.
Elderly or debilitated patients and patients with hepatic insufficiency: 5 mg P.O. h.s. Maximum daily dosage is 10 mg.

How supplied

Tablets: 5 mg, 10 mg

Pharmacokinetics

Absorption: absorbed rapidly from GI tract. Food delays drug absorption.
Distribution: protein-binding about 92.5%.
Metabolism: metabolized in liver.
Excretion: excreted primarily in urine. *Half-life:* 2½ hours.

Route	Onset	Peak	Duration
P.O.	Rapid	0.5-2 hr	Unknown

Pharmacodynamics

Chemical effect: interacts with one of three identified GABA-benzodiazepine receptor complexes but isn't a benzodiazepine. It exhibits hypnotic activity but no muscle relaxant or anticonvulsant properties.
Therapeutic effect: promotes sleep.

Adverse reactions

CNS: daytime drowsiness, light-headedness, abnormal dreams, amnesia, dizziness, *headache,* hangover effect, sleep disorder, lethargy, depression.
CV: palpitations.
EENT: sinusitis, pharyngitis.
GI: nausea, vomiting, diarrhea, dyspepsia, constipation, abdominal pain, dry mouth.
Musculoskeletal: back or chest pain, myalgia, arthralgia.

Skin: rash.
Other: flulike symptoms, ***hypersensitivity reactions.***

Interactions

Drug-drug. *CNS depressants:* enhanced CNS depression. Use together cautiously.
Drug-food. *Any food:* decreased rate and extent of absorption. Take drug on an empty stomach.
Drug-lifestyle. *Alcohol use:* excessive CNS depression. Discourage concurrent use.

Contraindications and precautions

- No known contraindications.
- Drug isn't recommended for use in breast-feeding women.
- Use cautiously in patients with diseases or conditions that could affect metabolism or hemodynamic responses and in those with compromised respiratory status because hypnotics may depress respiratory drive. Also use cautiously in pregnant women and patients with depression or history of alcohol or drug abuse.
- Safety of drug hasn't been established in children.

NURSING CONSIDERATIONS

Assessment

- Assess patient's condition before therapy and regularly thereafter.
- Be alert for adverse reactions and drug interactions.
- Evaluate patient's and family's knowledge of drug therapy.

Nursing diagnoses

- Disturbed sleep pattern related to presence of insomnia
- Risk for injury related to drug-induced adverse CNS reactions
- Deficient knowledge related to drug therapy

Planning and implementation

- Drug has a rapid onset of action and should be given when patient is ready to go to bed.
- Hypnotics should be used only for short-term management of insomnia, usually 7 to 10 days. Persistent insomnia may indicate primary psychiatric or medical disorder.
- Because most adverse reactions are dose-related, smallest effective dose should be used in all patients, especially those who are elderly or debilitated.
- Administer drug at least 1 hour before meals or 2 hours after meals.

ALERT Don't confuse Ambien with Amen.

Patient teaching

- Tell patient to take drug immediately before going to bed.
- For faster sleep onset, instruct patient not to take drug with or immediately after meals. Food decreases drug's absorption.
- Caution patient about performing activities that require mental alertness or physical coordination. For inpatient, supervise walking and raise bed rails, particularly for elderly patient.

Evaluation

- Patient states that drug effectively promotes sleep.
- Patient doesn't experience injury from adverse CNS reactions.
- Patient and family state understanding of drug therapy.

zonisamide

(zon-ISS-a-mide)
Zonegran

Pharmacologic class: sulfonamide
Therapeutic class: antiseizure drug
Pregnancy risk category: C

Indications and dosages

▶ **Adjunct therapy for partial seizures in adults with epilepsy.** *Adults:* Initially, 100 mg P.O. as a single daily dose for 2 weeks. After 2 weeks, the dose may be increased to 200 mg/day for at least 2 weeks. It can be increased to 300 mg and 400 mg P.O. daily, with the dose stable for at least 2 weeks to achieve steady state at each level. Doses larger than 100 mg can be divided. Can be taken with or without food.

How supplied

Capsules: 100 mg

Pharmacokinetics

Absorption: plasma levels peak in 2 to 6 hours; food delays but doesn't affect bioavailability.
Distribution: extensively binds to erythrocytes. The drug is about 40% bound to plasma proteins. Protein-binding is unaffected in the presence of therapeutic levels of phenytoin, phenobarbital, or carbamazepine.
Metabolism: metabolized by cytochrome P-450 3A4. Drug clearance increases in patients who are also taking enzyme-inducing drugs.
Excretion: Excreted primarily in urine as parent drug and as glucuronide of a metabolite. *Half-life:* about 63 hours.

Route	Onset	Peak	Duration
P.O.	Unknown	Unknown	Unknown

Pharmacodynamics

Chemical effect: the exact mechanism of action is unknown, but it's thought to produce antiseizure effects through action at the sodium and calcium channels, thereby stabilizing neuronal membranes and suppressing neuronal hypersynchronization. Other models suggest that synaptically driven electrical activity is suppressed without potentiation of GABA synaptic activity. The drug also may facilitate dopaminergic and serotonergic neurotransmission.
Therapeutic effect: prevents and stops seizure activity.

Adverse reactions

CNS: *headache, dizziness,* ataxia, nystagmus, paresthesia, confusion, difficulties in concentration and memory, mental slowing, agitation, irritability, depression, insomnia, anxiety, nervousness, schizophrenic or schizophreniform behavior, *somnolence,* fatigue, speech abnormalities, difficulties in verbal expression.
EENT: diplopiarhinitis.
GI: *anorexia,* nausea, diarrhea, dyspepsia, constipation, dry mouth, taste perversion, abdominal pain.
Hematologic: ecchymosis.
Metabolic: weight loss.
Skin: *rash.*
Other: flu syndrome.

Interactions

Drug-drug. *Drugs that induce or inhibit CYP 3A4:* altered serum zonisamide levels. Zonisamide clearance is increased by phenytoin, carbamazepine, phenobarbital, and valproate. Monitor patient closely.

Contraindications and precautions

- Contraindicated in patients hypersensitive to sulfonamides or zonisamide.
- Rare fatalities have occurred in patients receiving sulfonamides because of severe reactions such as Stevens-Johnson syndrome, fulminant hepatic necrosis, aplastic anemia, otherwise unexplained rashes, and agranulocytosis. If signs of hypersensitivity or other serious reactions occur, discontinue zonisamide immediately.
- Use cautiously in patients with renal and hepatic dysfunction. If GFR is less than 50 ml/minute, don't use drug. If patient develops acute renal failure or a clinically significant sustained increase in creatinine or BUN levels, the drug should be discontinued.

NURSING CONSIDERATIONS

Assessment

- Obtain history of patient's underlying condition before therapy, and reassess regularly thereafter.
- Monitor patient for symptoms of hypersensitivity.
- Monitor body temperature, especially in the summer, since decreased sweating has occurred (especially in patients 17 years old and younger) resulting in heatstroke and dehydration.
- Monitor renal function periodically.
- Evaluate patient's and family's knowledge about drug therapy.

Nursing diagnoses

- Risk for trauma related to seizures

• Risk for injury related to drug-induced adverse CNS effects
• Deficient knowledge related to drug therapy

Planning and implementation

• Drug may be taken with or without food. Don't bite or break the capsule.
• Use cautiously in patients with hepatic and renal disease; may need slower adjustment and more frequent monitoring. If GFR is less than 50 ml/minute, don't use drug.
• Abrupt zonisamide withdrawal may cause increased frequency of seizures or status epilepticus; reduce dose or discontinue drug gradually.
• Increase fluid intake and urine output to help prevent renal calculi, especially in patients with predisposing factors.

Patient teaching

• Tell patient to take medication with or without food. Caution against biting or breaking the capsule.
• Instruct patient to contact prescriber immediately if a skin rash develops or seizures worsen.
• Tell patient to contact prescriber immediately if he develops sudden back pain, abdominal pain, pain when urinating, bloody or dark urine, fever, sore throat, mouth sores, easy bruising, decreased sweating, increased body temperature, depression, or speech or language problems.
• Tell patient to drink 6 to 8 glasses of water a day.
• Tell patient to avoid hazardous activities until full effects of drug are known. It may cause drowsiness.
• Tell patient to not stop taking drug without prescriber's approval.
• Tell patient to notify prescriber about planned, suspected, or known pregnancy. Also tell her to notify prescriber if she's breastfeeding.
• Advise woman of child bearing potential to use contraception while taking drug.

Evaluation

• Patient is free from seizure activity.
• Patient doesn't experience adverse CNS effects.
• Patient and family state understanding of drug therapy

Herbal Medicines

aloe

(AH-loh)

aloe vera, Barbados aloe, Cape aloe, Curacao aloe, lily of the desert

Reported uses

Used externally as a topical gel for minor burns, sunburn, cuts, frostbite, skin irritation, and other wounds and abrasions.

Used internally as a stimulant laxative. Also to treat amenorrhea, asthma, colds, seizures, bleeding, and ulcers.

Aloe preparations are also used to treat acne, AIDS, arthritis, asthma, blindness, bursitis, cancer, colitis, depression, diabetes, glaucoma, hemorrhoids, multiple sclerosis, peptic ulcers, and varicose veins.

Common forms

In capsules or as cream, hair conditioner, jelly, juice, liniment, lotion, ointment, shampoo, skin cream, soap, sunscreen, and in facial tissues. Also as an ingredient in Benzoin Compound Tincture.

Capsules: 75 mg, 100 mg, 200 mg aloe vera extract or aloe vera powder.

Gel: 98%, 99.5%, 99.6% aloe vera gel.

Juice: 99.6%, 99.7% aloe vera juice.

Tincture*: 1:10, 50% alcohol.

Actions

When taken internally, aloin produces a metabolite that irritates the large intestine and stimulates colonic activity. It also causes active secretion of fluids and electrolytes and inhibits reabsorption of fluids from the colon, resulting in a feeling of distention and increased peristalsis. The cathartic effect occurs 8 to 12 hours after ingestion.

When taken externally, besides acting as a moisturizer on burns and other wounds, aloe reduces inflammation. Its antipruritic effect may result from blockage of the conversion of histidine to histamine. Wound healing may result from increased blood flow to the wound area.

Dosages

▶ **For pruritus, skin irritation, burns, and other wounds (external forms).** Applied liberally, p.r.n. Although internal use isn't recommended, some sources suggest 100 to 200 mg aloe or 50 to 100 mg aloe extract P.O., taken in the evening. Information about dosages for aloe juice is lacking.

Adverse reactions

CV: ***arrhythmias.***

GI: painful intestinal spasms, damage to intestinal mucosa, harmless brown discoloration of intestinal mucous membranes, ***severe hemorrhagic diarrhea.***

GU: kidney damage, red discoloration of urine, reflex stimulation of uterine musculature causing miscarriage or premature birth.

Metabolic: fluid and electrolyte loss, hypokalemia.

Musculoskeletal: muscle weakness, accelerated bone deterioration.

Skin: contact dermatitis, delayed healing of deep wounds.

Interactions

Herb-drug. *Antiarrhythmics, cardiac glycosides such as digoxin:* oral aloe may lead to toxic reaction. Monitor patient closely.

Corticosteroids, diuretics: increased potassium loss. Monitor patient for signs of hypokalemia.

Disulfiram: tincture contains alcohol and could precipitate a disulfiram reaction. Discourage concomitant use.

Herb-herb. *Licorice:* increased risk of potassium deficiency. Discourage using together.

Cautions

- External aloe preparations contraindicated in patients hypersensitive to aloe and in those with history of allergic reactions to plants in the *Liliaceae* family (such as garlic, onions, and tulips).
- Oral use is contraindicated in patients with cardiac or kidney disease (because of risk of hypokalemia and disturbance of cardiac rhythm); in those with intestinal obstruction; in those with Crohn's disease, ulcerative colitis, appendicitis, or abdominal pain of un-

* Liquid may contain alcohol.

known origin; in women who are pregnant or breast-feeding; and in children.

NURSING CONSIDERATIONS

- Oral use can cause severe abdominal discomfort and serious hypokalemia and electrolyte imbalance.
- Unapproved use of aloe vera injections for cancer has been linked to death.
- Use of injectable aloe vera preparations or chemical constituents of aloe vera isn't recommended.

Patient teaching

- Caution patient against use of aloe vera gel or aloe vera juice for internal use.
- Advise patient to consult health care provider before using an herbal preparation, because a treatment with proven efficacy may be available.
- Tell the patient that, when filling a new prescription, he should remind the pharmacist of any herbal or dietary supplement he's taking.
- Tell patient that if he uses aloe and delays in seeking medical diagnosis and treatment, his condition could worsen.
- Warn patient not to take aloe if he's also taking digoxin, another drug to control his heart rate, a diuretic, or a corticosteroid without medical advice.
- Aloe may cause feelings of dehydration, weakness, and confusion especially if used for a prolonged period. Caution patient to seek medical help immediately if any of these signs or symptoms appear.

angelica

(an-JEL-ih-kah)

angelica root, angelique, dong quai, garden angelica, tang-kuei, wild angelica

Reported uses

Used to treat gynecologic disorders, postmenopausal symptoms, menstrual discomfort, regulation of the menstrual cycle, and anemia. Also used to treat headaches and backaches, improve circulation in the limbs, and relieve osteoporosis, hay fever, asthma, and eczema.

Common forms

Fluidextract, tincture, essential oil, or cut, dried, or powdered root.

Actions

Root extracts may have antitumor properties in animals; also may have anti-inflammatory and analgesic actions.

Isolated substances extracted from the root inhibit platelet aggregation, exert antimicrobial action, and decrease myocardial injury and the risk of PVCs and arrhythmias induced by myocardial reperfusion.

Improved pulmonary function and decreased mean arterial pulmonary pressures occurred when compounds were used with nifedipine in patients with chronic obstructive pulmonary disease and pulmonary hypertension.

Dosages

No consensus exists.

Adverse reactions

CV: hypotension.
Skin: photodermatitis, phototoxicity.

Interactions

Herb-drug. *Antacids, H_2-receptor antagonists, proton pump inhibitors, sucralfate:* angelica may increase acid production in the stomach and so may interfere with absorption of these drugs. Discourage concomitant use. *Anticoagulants:* potentiated effects with excessive doses of angelica. Monitor patient for bleeding.
Herb-lifestyle. *Sun exposure:* photosensitivity reactions may occur. Advise patient to avoid unprotected exposure to sunlight.

Cautions

- Contraindicated in pregnant or breast-feeding women because of potential stimulant effects on the uterus.
- Urge caution in diabetic patients because various species of this plant contain polysaccharides that may disrupt blood glucose control.

NURSING CONSIDERATIONS

- Monitor patients taking angelica for signs of bleeding—especially those already taking anticoagulants.
- Find out why patient is using the herb.
- Monitor patient for persistent diarrhea, which may be a sign of something more serious.
- Monitor patient for dermatologic reactions.
- Photodermatosis is possible after contact with the plant juice or plant extract.

Patient teaching

- Tell the patient that, when filling a new prescription, he should remind the pharmacist of any herbal or dietary supplement he's taking.
- Warn patient not to treat symptoms with angelica before seeking appropriate medical evaluation because doing so may delay diagnosis of a potentially serious medical condition.
- Advise patient not to take angelica if pregnant or if taking an acid blocker or blood-thinning drug.
- Advise patient to report skin rash.

bilberry

(BIL-beh-ree)

bilberries, bog bilberries, European blueberries, huckleberries, whortleberries

Reported uses

Used to treat visual and circulatory problems, glaucoma, cataracts, diabetic retinopathy, macular degeneration, varicose veins, and hemorrhoids. Also used to improve night vision.

Common forms

Capsules: 60 mg, 80 mg, 120 mg, 450 mg. Also available in liquid, tincture, fluidextract, and dried root, leaves, and berries.

Actions

May reduce vascular permeability and tissue edema. Also may aid blood flow. Exerts potent antioxidant effects and a protective effect on low-density lipoproteins.

Chemical components of bilberry may exert changes in the retina, allowing better adaptation to darkness and light, decrease excessive platelet aggregation, and exert preventative and curative antiulcer actions.

Dosages

Suggested dosages vary considerably. Most herbalists recommend using standardized products consisting of 25% anthocyanoside content.

▶ **To improve night vision.** 60 to 120 mg of bilberry extract P.O. daily.

▶ **For visual and circulatory problems.** 240 to 480 mg P.O. daily in two or three divided doses.

Adverse reactions

Other: toxic reactions.

Interactions

Herb-drug. *Anticoagulants, other antiplatelet drugs:* inhibited platelet aggregation, possibly increasing the risk of bleeding. Monitor patient.

Disulfiram: disulfiram reaction if herb preparation contains alcohol. Avoid concurrent use.

Cautions

- Contraindicated in pregnant and breast-feeding women.
- Urge caution in patients taking anticoagulants. Herb may be unsuitable for those with a bleeding disorder.

NURSING CONSIDERATIONS

ALERT Long-term consumption of large doses of bilberry leaves can be poisonous. Dosages of 1.5 g/kg/day or higher may be fatal.

- Herb may reduce blood glucose level in diabetics. Dosage may need to be adjusted in those taking a conventional antidiabetic.
- For treatment of vascular and ocular conditions, consistent dosing is required.

Patient teaching

- Tell the patient that, when filling a new prescription, he should remind the pharmacist of any herbal or dietary supplement he's taking.

* Liquid may contain alcohol.

• Warn patient not to treat symptoms with bilberry before seeking appropriate medical evaluation because doing so may delay diagnosis of a potentially serious medical condition.
• Bilberry may be taken without regard to meals or food.
• Advise any patient using the dried fruit to take each dose with a full glass of water.

capsicum

(KAP-sih-kem)

bell pepper, capsaicin, cayenne pepper, chili pepper, hot pepper, paprika, red pepper, tabasco pepper

Reported uses

Used to treat bowel disorders, chronic laryngitis, and peripheral vascular disease. Various preparations of capsicum are applied topically as counterirritants and external analgesics. The FDA has approved topical capsaicin for temporary relief of pain from rheumatoid arthritis, osteoarthritis, postherpetic neuralgia (shingles), and diabetic neuropathy. It's being tested for treatment of psoriasis, intractable pruritus, vitiligo, phantom limb pain, mastectomy pain, Guillain-Barré syndrome, neurogenic bladder, vulvar vestibulitis, apocrine chromhidrosis, and reflex sympathetic dystrophy. It's also used in personal defense sprays. Also used to treat refractory pruritus and pruritus caused by renal failure.

Common forms

Cream: 0.025%, 0.075%, 0.25%.
Gel: 0.025%.
Lotion: 0.025%, 0.075%.
Roll-on: 0.075%.
Self-defense spray: 5%, 10%.
Also available as the vegetable, pepper.

Actions

Topical capsicum produces an extremely intense irritation at the contact point. Initial dose causes profound pain; however, repeated applications cause desensitization, with analgesic and anti-inflammatory effects.

Juices from the fruits may have antibacterial properties in vitro.

Dosages

Topical preparations range from 0.025% to 0.25%. Most effective when applied t.i.d. or q.i.d.; they have a duration of action of about 4 to 6 hours. Less frequent applications typically produce incomplete analgesia.

Adverse reactions

EENT: blepharospasm, extreme burning pain, lacrimation, conjunctival edema, hyperemia, burning pain in nose, sneezing, serous discharge.
GI: oral burning, diarrhea, gingival irritation, bleeding gums.
Respiratory: ***bronchospasm,*** cough, retrosternal discomfort.
Skin: transient skin irritation, itching, stinging, erythema without vesicular eruption, contact dermatitis.

Interactions

Herb-drug. *ACE inhibitors:* increased risk of cough when applied topically. Monitor patient closely.
Anticoagulants: may alter anticoagulant effects. Monitor PT and INR closely; tell patient to avoid using together.
Antiplatelet drugs, heparin and low-molecular-weight heparin, warfarin: increased risk of bleeding. Advise patient to avoid using together. If they must be used together, monitor patient for bleeding.
Aspirin, salicylic acid compounds: reduced bioavailability of these drugs. Discourage concurrent use.
Theophylline: increased absorption when given with capsicum. Discourage concurrent use.
Herb-herb. *Feverfew, garlic, ginger, ginkgo, ginseng:* increased anticoagulant effects of capsicum, and thus an increased risk of bleeding. Discourage concurrent use; if these herbs must be used together, monitor patient closely for bleeding.

Cautions

• Contraindicated in patients hypersensitive to capsicum or chili pepper products.

• Also contraindicated in pregnant women because of possible uterine stimulant effects. Patients with irritable bowel syndrome should avoid use because capsicum has irritant and peristaltic effects. Patients with asthma who use capsicum may experience more bronchospasms.

NURSING CONSIDERATIONS

• Find out why patient is using the herb.
• Topical product shouldn't be used on broken or irritated skin or covered with a tight bandage.
• Adverse skin reactions to topically applied capsicum are treated by washing the area thoroughly with soap and water. Soaking the area in vegetable oil after washing provides a slower onset but longer duration of relief than cold water. Vinegar water irrigation is moderately successful. Rubbing alcohol also may help.
• EMLA, an emulsion of lidocaine and prilocaine, provides pain relief in about 1 hour to skin that has been severely irritated by capsaicin.
• Capsicum shouldn't be taken orally for more than 2 days and shouldn't be used again for 2 weeks.
• After topical application, relief may occur in 3 days but may take as long as 14 to 28 days, depending on the condition requiring analgesia.

Patient teaching
• Tell patient to avoid contact with eyes, mucous membranes, and broken skin.
• If patient is using capsicum topically, instruct him to wash his hands before and immediately after applying it. Advise contact lens wearers to wash hands and to use gloves or an applicator if handling lenses after applying capsicum.
• If incidental contact occurs, inform patient to flush exposed area with cool running water for as long as necessary.
• Caution patient taking MAO inhibitors or centrally acting adrenergics against use of this herb.

cat's claw
(KATS klaw)
life-giving vine of Peru, samento, una de gato

Reported uses

Used to treat GI problems, including Crohn's disease, colitis, inflammatory bowel disease, diverticulitis, gastritis, dysentery, ulcerations and hemorrhoids—and to enhance immunity. Used to treat systemic inflammatory diseases (such as arthritis and rheumatism). Also used by cancer patients for its antimutagenic effects. Also used with zidovudine to stimulate the immune system by patients with HIV infection. Also used as a contraceptive.

Common forms

In tablets and capsules; also as teas or tinctures and the cut, dried, or powdered bark, roots, and leaves.
Tablets, capsules: 25 mg, 150 mg, 175 mg, 300 mg, 350 mg (standard extract); 400 mg, 500 mg, 800 mg, 1 g, 5 g (raw herb).

Actions

Some chemical components stimulate immune system function and exert antitumor activity. Other components may inhibit platelet aggregation and the sympathetic nervous system, reduce the heart rate, decrease peripheral vascular resistance, and lower blood pressure. They also may exhibit antiviral activity and antioxidant properties in vitro. One component has weak diuretic properties.

Dosages

No consensus exists. Herbal literature suggests 500 to 1,000 mg P.O. t.i.d. Other souces suggest different dosages depending on condition and form of herbal product.
Capsules: 2 capsules (175 mg/capsule) P.O. daily or 3 capsules P.O. t.i.d.; dosage varies by manufacturer.
Decoction: 2 to 3 cups/day made from 10 to 30 g inner stalk bark or root in 1 qt (1 L) of water for 30 to 60 minutes.

* Liquid may contain alcohol.

Extract (alcohol-free): 7 to 10 gtt t.i.d. up to 15 gtt five times a day.
Liquid or alcohol extract*: 10 to 15 gtt b.i.d. to t.i.d., to 1 to 3 ml t.i.d.
Powdered extract: 1 to 3 capsules (500 mg/capsule) P.O. b.i.d. to q.i.d.

Adverse reactions

CV: hypotension.

Interactions

Herb-drug. *Antihypertensives:* may potentiate hypotensive effects. Discourage concurrent use.
Immunosuppressants: may counteract the therapeutic effects because herb has immunostimulant properties. Advise patient to avoid using together.
Herb-food. *Food:* enhances absorption of herb. Patient can take herb with food.

Cautions

- Pregnant and breast-feeding patients, patients who have had transplant surgery, and patients who have autoimmune disease, multiple sclerosis, or tuberculosis should avoid use.
- Patients with coagulation disorders or receiving anticoagulants should avoid use.
- Those with a history of peptic ulcer disease or gallstones should use caution when taking this herb because it stimulates stomach acid secretion.

NURSING CONSIDERATIONS

- Find out why patient is using the herb.
- Some liquid extracts contain alcohol and may be unsuitable for children or patients with liver disease.
- This herb and its contents vary from manufacturer to manufacturer; the alkaloid concentration, from season to season.

Patient teaching

- Tell the patient that, when filling a new prescription, he should remind the pharmacist of any herbal or dietary supplement he's taking.
- Inform patient that herb shouldn't be used for more than 8 weeks without a 2- to 3-week rest period from the herb.
- Instruct patient to promptly report adverse reactions and new signs or symptoms.
- Recommend another method of contraception if herb is being used for this purpose.
- Tell patient to rise slowly from a sitting or lying position to avoid dizziness from possible hypotension.
- Advise patient to watch for signs of bleeding, especially if anticoagulants are also being taken.

chamomile

(KAH-meh-mighl)

common chamomile, English chamomile, German chamomile, Hungarian chamomile, sweet false chamomile

Reported uses

Used to treat stomach disorders, such as GI spasms, other GI inflammatory conditions, and insomnia because of chamomile's sedative properties. Also used to treat menstrual disorders, migraine, epidermolysis bullosa, eczema, eye irritation, throat discomfort, and hemorrhoids, and as a topical bacteriostat, and mouthwash. Teas are mainly used for sedation or relaxation.

Common forms

As capsules, liquid, tea, and in many cosmetic products.
Capsules: 354 mg, 360 mg

Actions

Exhibits anti-inflammatory, antiallergenic, antidiuretic, sedative, antibacterial, and antifungal properties. May lower serum urea levels. Some compounds may stimulate liver regeneration after oral use; others have in vitro antitumor activity. One component may have antiulcer effects.

Dosages

Usually taken as a tea, prepared by adding 1 tbs (3 g) of the flower head to hot water and steeping for 10 to 15 minutes; it is then taken up to q.i.d.

Adverse reactions

EENT: conjunctivitis, eyelid angioedema.
GI: nausea, vomiting.
Skin: eczema, contact dermatitis.
Other: ***anaphylaxis.***

Interactions

Herb-drug. *Anticoagulants:* may potentiate effects. Discourage concomitant use.
Other drugs: potential for decreased absorption of drugs because of antispasmodic activity of chamomile in the GI tract. Discourage concomitant use.

Cautions

- Discourage use by pregnant or breast-feeding women. Chamomile is believed to be an abortifacient, and some of its components have teratogenic effects in animals.
- Urge caution in patients hypersensitive to components of volatile oils and in those at risk for contact dermatitis. Chamomile shouldn't be used in teething babies or in children younger than age 2.
- Safety in patients with liver or kidney disorders hasn't been established, so these patients should avoid use.

NURSING CONSIDERATIONS

- Find out why patient is using the herb.

ALERT People sensitive to ragweed and chrysanthemums or other *Compositae* family members (arnica, yarrow, feverfew, tansy, artemisia) may be more susceptible to contact allergies and anaphylaxis. Those with hay fever or bronchial asthma caused by pollens are more susceptible to anaphylactic reactions.
- Signs and symptoms of anaphylaxis include shortness of breath, swelling of the tongue, rash, tachycardia, and hypotension.

Patient teaching

- Advise patient to consult health care provider before using an herbal preparation because a treatment with proven efficacy may be available.
- Tell the patient that, when filling a new prescription, he should remind the pharmacist of any herbal or dietary supplement he's taking.
- If patient is pregnant or is planning pregnancy, advise her not to use chamomile.
- If patient is taking an anticoagulant, advise him not to use chamomile because of possibly enhanced anticoagulant effects.
- Advise patient that chamomile may enhance an allergic reaction or make existing symptoms worse in susceptible individuals.
- Instruct parent not to give chamomile to any child before checking with a knowledgeable practitioner.

echinacea

(eh-kih-NAY-zyah)
American cone flower, black sampson, black susans, coneflower, echinacea care liquid, Indian head

Reported uses

Used as a wound-healing agent for abscesses, burns, eczema, varicose ulcers of the leg and other skin wounds, and as a nonspecific immunostimulant for the supportive treatment of upper respiratory tract infections, the common cold, and urinary tract infections.

Common forms

In capsules and tablets; also as hydroalcoholic extracts, fresh-pressed juice, glycerite, lozenges, and tinctures.
Capsules: 125 mg, 355 mg (85 mg herbal extract powder), 500 mg.
Tablets: 335 mg.

Actions

Extract stimulates the immune system and reduces growth of bacteria responsible for vaginal infections. Components may exert local anesthetic effects and anti-inflammatory activities. Essential oil components produce a tingling sensation on the tongue. Some compounds also exhibit direct antitumor activity and insecticidal activity. Conjugates in the plant activate adrenal cortex activity. The fresh-pressed juice of the aerial portion and the extract of the roots may inhibit influenza, herpes infections, and vesicular stomatitis virus.

* Liquid may contain alcohol.

Dosages

Expressed juice: 6 to 9 ml P.O. daily.
Capsules containing powdered herb: equivalent to 900 mg to 1 g P.O. t.i.d.; doses can vary.
Tea: 2 tsp (4 g) of coarsely powdered herb simmered in 1 cup of boiling water for 10 minutes. Avoid this method of administration because some active compounds are water-insoluble.
Tincture: 0.75 to 1.5 ml (15 to 30 gtt) P.O. two to five times daily. The tincture has been given as 60 gtt P.O. t.i.d.

Adverse reactions

GI: nausea, vomiting, unpleasant taste, minor GI symptoms.
GU: diuresis.
Other: tachyphylaxis, fever, allergic reactions in patients allergic to plants belonging to the daisy family.

Interactions

Herb-drug. *Disulfiram, metronidazole:* herbal products that contain alcohol may cause a disulfiram reaction. Discourage concurrent use.
Immunosuppressants such as cyclosporine: decreased effectiveness of these drugs. Discourage concurrent use.
Herb-lifestyle. *Alcohol:* echinacea preparations containing alcohol may enhance CNS depression. Discourage concurrent use.

Cautions

- Contraindicated in patients with severe illnesses such as HIV infection, collagen disease, leukosis, multiple sclerosis, and tuberculosis or other autoimmune diseases.
- Discourage use of herb by pregnant or breast-feeding women; effects are unknown.

NURSING CONSIDERATIONS

- Daily dose depends on the preparation and potency.
- Echinacea shouldn't be taken for more than 8 weeks.
- Echinacea is considered supportive treatment for infection; it shouldn't be use in place of antibiotic therapy.
- Echinacea is usually taken at the first sign of illness and continued for up to 14 days. Regular prophylactic use isn't recommended.
- Herbalists recommend using liquid preparations because it's believed that echinacea functions in the mouth and should have direct contact with the lymph tissues at the back of the throat.
- Some tinctures contain 15% to 90% alcohol, which may be unsuitable for children and adolescents, alcoholics, and patients with hepatic disease.

Patient teaching

- Tell the patient that, when filling a new prescription, he should remind the pharmacist of any herbal or dietary supplement he's taking.
- Advise patient not to delay seeking appropriate medical evaluation for a prolonged illness.

ALERT Advise patient taking herb for prolonged time that overstimulation of the immune system and possible immune suppression may occur.

- Advise woman to avoid use of herb during pregnancy or when breast-feeding.

eucalyptus

(yoo-kah-LIP-tes)
fevertree, gum tree, Tasmanian blue gum

Reported uses

Used internally and externally as an expectorant. Used to treat infections and fevers. Also used topically to treat sore muscles and rheumatism.

Common forms

As an oil and a lotion.

Actions

Produces a stimulant effect on nasal cold receptors. Acts as a counterirritant and causes an increase in cutaneous blood flow. Also exhibits antimicrobial, antifungal, and anti-inflammatory effects.

Dosages

Essential oil: Oil is used in massage blends for sore muscles and in foot baths or saunas, steam inhalations, chest rubs, room sprays, bath blends, and air diffusions. For external use only.
Leaf: Average daily dose is 4 to 16 g P.O. divided every 3 to 4 hours.
Oil: For internal use, average dose is 0.3 to 0.6 g P.O. daily. For external use, oil with 5% to 20% concentration or a semisolid preparation with 5% to 10% concentration.
Tea: Prepared using one of two methods. For the infusion method, 6 oz (180 ml) of dried herb is steeped in boiling water for 2 to 3 minutes, and then strained. For the decoction method, 6 to 8 oz (180 to 240 ml) of dried herb is placed in boiling water, boiled for 3 to 5 minutes, and then strained.
Tincture: 3 to 4 g P.O. daily.

Adverse reactions

CNS: delirium, dizziness, ***seizures.***
EENT: miosis.
GI: epigastric burning, nausea, vomiting.
Musculoskeletal: muscle weakness.
Respiratory: asthma-like attacks.

Interactions

Herb-drug. *Antidiabetics:* enhanced effects. Discourage concurrent use except under direct medical supervision.
Other drugs: eucalyptus oil induces detoxication enzyme systems in the liver; therefore, the oil may affect any drug metabolized in liver. Monitor patient for effect and toxic reaction.
Herb-herb. *Other herbs that cause hypoglycemia (basil, glucomannan, Queen Anne's lace):* decreased blood glucose level. Monitor patient for effect, and advise caution.

Cautions

- Patients who have had an allergic reaction to eucalyptus or its vapors should avoid use.
- Patients who are pregnant or breast-feeding, have liver disease, or have intestinal tract inflammation should avoid use.
- Essential oil preparations shouldn't be applied to an infant's or child's face because of risk of severe bronchial spasm.

NURSING CONSIDERATIONS

- In susceptible patients, particularly infants and children, application of eucalyptus to the face or the inhalation of vapors can cause asthma-like attacks.
- Monitor blood glucose level in diabetic patient taking eucalyptus.

ALERT The oil shouldn't be taken internally unless it has been diluted. As little as a few drops of oil for children and 4 to 5 ml of oil for adults can cause poisoning. Signs include hypotension, circulatory dysfunction, and cardiac and respiratory failure.

- If poisoning or overdose occurs, don't induce vomiting because of risk of aspiration. Administer activated charcoal and treat symptomatically.

Patient teaching

- Tell the patient that, when filling a new prescription, he should remind the pharmacist of any herbal or dietary supplement he's taking.
- Advise the patient to stop taking eucalyptus immediately and to check with his health care provider if he has hives, skin rash, or trouble breathing.
- Inform patient of potential adverse effects.
- Instruct caregiver not to apply to the face of a child or infant, especially around the nose.

fennel

(FEN-el)

bitter fennel, carosella, common fennel, fenchel, fenouil, fenouille, sweet fennel

Reported uses

Used to increase milk secretion, promote menses, facilitate birth, and increase libido. Used as an expectorant to manage cough and bronchitis. Also used to treat mild, spastic disorders of the GI tract, feelings of fullness, and flatulence. Fennel syrup has been used to treat upper respiratory tract infections in children.

* Liquid may contain alcohol.

Common forms

Volatile oil in water: 2% (sweet fennel), 4% (bitter fennel)

Actions

May exhibit stimulant and antiflatulent properties. Fennel oil with methylparaben inhibits the growth of *Salmonella enteritidis* and, to a lesser extent, *Listeria monocytogenes*.

Dosages

▶ **For GI complaints.** Herbalists recommend 0.1 to 0.6 ml P.O. of the oil daily; or 5 to 7 g of the fruit daily.

Adverse reactions

CNS: ***seizures,*** hallucinations.
GI: nausea, vomiting.
Respiratory: ***pulmonary edema.***
Skin: photodermatitis, contact dermatitis.
Other: allergic reaction.

Interactions

Herb-drug. *Drugs that lower the seizure threshold, anticonvulsants:* increased risk of seizure. Monitor patient very closely.
Herb-lifestyle. *Sun exposure:* increased risk of photosensitivity reaction. Advise patient to wear protective clothing and sunscreen and to limit exposure to direct sunlight.

Cautions

- Urge caution in patients allergic to other members of the *Umbelliferae* family, such as celery, carrots, or mugwort.
- Discourage use by pregnant women and those with a history of seizures.

NURSING CONSIDERATIONS

- Find out why patient is using the herb.
- Verify that the patient doesn't have an allergic response to celery, fennel, or similar spices and herbs.

Patient teaching

- Inform patient that herb cannot be recommended for any use because of insufficient evidence.
- Tell the patient that, when filling a new prescription, he should remind the pharmacist of any herbal or dietary supplement he's taking.

ALERT Don't mistake poison hemlock for fennel. Hemlock can cause vomiting, paralysis, and death. Know the source of preparation before taking fennel.

- Tell patient to stop taking this herb and contact health care provider immediately if he experiences hives, rash, or difficulty breathing.
- Advise patient to avoid sun exposure if photodermatitis occurs.

feverfew

(FEE-ver-fyoo)

altamisa, bachelors' button, chamomile grande, featherfew, featherfoil, midsummer daisy

Reported uses

Used as an antipyretic and to treat psoriasis, toothache, insect bites, rheumatism, asthma, stomachache, menstrual problems, and threatened miscarriage. Also used for migraine prophylaxis.

Common forms

Available as capsules, dried leaves, liquid, powder, seeds, and tablets.
Capsules: 250 mg (leaf extract), 380 mg (pure leaf).

Actions

Main active ingredients may inhibit serotonin release by human platelets. Extracts of feverfew contain chemicals that inhibit activation of leukocytes and the synthesis of leukotrienes and prostaglandins.

Dosages

Infusion: Prepared by steeping 2 tsp of feverfew in a cup of water for 15 minutes. For stronger infusion, double the amount feverfew and allow it to steep for 25 minutes. Infusion dose in folk medicine is 1 cup t.i.d.; stronger infusions are used for washes.
Powder: Daily dose recommended by herbalists is 50 mg to 1.2 g.

▶ **For migraine treatment.** Average dose of 543 mcg P.O. parthenolide (a component of feverfew) daily.
▶ **For migraine prophylaxis.** 25 mg of freeze-dried leaf extract P.O. daily, or 50 mg of leaf P.O. daily with food, or 50 to 200 mg of aerial parts of plant P.O. daily.

Adverse reactions

CNS: dizziness.
CV: tachycardia.
GI: GI upset, mouth ulcerations.
Skin: contact dermatitis.

Interactions

Herb-drug. *Anticoagulants, antiplatelet drugs including aspirin and thrombolytics:* feverfew inhibits prostaglandin synthesis and platelet aggregation. Monitor patient for increased bleeding.

Cautions

- Pregnant women should avoid use because of herb's potential abortifacient properties; breast-feeding women also should avoid use.
- Patients allergic to members of the daisy, or *Asteraceae,* family—including yarrow, southernwood, wormwood, chamomile, marigold, goldenrod, coltsfoot, and dandelion—and patients who have had previous reactions to feverfew shouldn't take it internally.
- Feverfew shouldn't be used in children.
- Those taking an anticoagulants such as warfarin and heparin should use cautiously.

NURSING CONSIDERATIONS

- Find out why patient is using the herb.
- Rash or contact dermatitis may indicate sensitivity to feverfew. Patient should discontinue use immediately.

Patient teaching

- Assure patient that several other strategies for migraine treatment and prophylaxis exist and that these should be attempted before taking products with unknown benefits and risks.
- Instruct patient not to withdraw herb abruptly, but to taper its use gradually because of risk of post-feverfew syndrome. Symptoms include tension headaches, insomnia, joint stiffness and pain, and lethargy.
- Remind patient to promptly report unusual signs and symptoms, such as mouth sores or skin ulcerations.
- Tell the patient that, when filling a new prescription, he should remind the pharmacist of any herbal or dietary supplement he's taking.
- Educate patient about risk of increased bleeding when combining herb with an anticoagulant, such as warfarin or heparin, or an antiplatelet, such as aspirin or an NSAID.
- Caution patient that a rash or abnormal skin condition may indicate an allergy to feverfew. Instruct patient to stop taking the herb if a rash appears.
- Feverfew potency is often based on the parthenolide content in the preparation, which varies.

flax

(flaks)
flaxseed, linseed, lint bells, linum

Reported uses

Used to treat constipation, functional disorders of the colon resulting from laxative abuse, irritable bowel syndrome, and diverticulitis. Also used as a supplement to decrease the risk of hypercholesterolemia and atherosclerosis. Externally, flax has been made into a poultice and used to treat areas of local inflammation.

Common forms

As a powder, capsules, softgel capsules, and an oil.
Softgel capsules: 1,000 mg.

Actions

Decreases total cholesterol and low-density lipoprotein levels. May decrease thrombin-mediated platelet aggregation. Flax contains lignans, which may have weak estrogenic, antiestrogenic, and steroidlike activity. Diets high in flax may lower the risk of breast and other hormone-dependent cancers. Linolenic acid supplement, derived from flax, arginine,

* Liquid may contain alcohol.

and yeast RNA, may improve weight gain in some patients with HIV.

Dosages

▶ **For all systemic uses.** 1 to 2 tbs of oil or mature seeds daily in two or three divided doses. Average dosage is 1 oz of oil or mature seeds daily.

▶ **For topical use.** 30 to 50 g of flax meal applied as a hot, moist poultice or compress as needed.

Adverse reactions

GI: diarrhea, flatulence, nausea.

Interactions

Herb-drug. *Laxatives, stool softeners:* possible increase in laxative actions of flax. Discourage concurrent use.

Oral medications: because of its fibrous content and binding potential, drug absorption may be altered or prevented. Advise patient to avoid using flax within 2 hours of a drug.

Cautions

- Those with an ileus, those with esophageal strictures, and those experiencing an acute inflammatory illness of the GI tract should avoid use.
- Pregnant and breast-feeding patients and those planning to become pregnant also should avoid use.

NURSING CONSIDERATIONS

- Find out why patient is using the herb.

ALERT Immature seedpods are especially poisonous. Overdose symptoms include, but aren't limited to, shortness of breath, tachypnea, cyanosis, weakness, and unstable gait, progressing to paralysis and seizures.

Patient teaching

- Encourage patient to drink plenty of fluids to minimize flatulence.
- Instruct patient to refrigerate flaxseed oil to prevent breakdown of essential fatty acids.
- Remind patient that other cholesterol-lowering therapies exist that have been proven to improve survival and lower the risk of cardiac disease; flax has no such clinical support.
- Warn patient not to treat chronic constipation or other GI disturbances or ophthalmic injury with flax before seeking appropriate medical evaluation because doing so may delay diagnosis of a potentially serious medical condition.
- Instruct patient never to ingest immature seeds and to keep flax away from children and pets.
- Tell patient to report decreased effects of other drugs being taken if patient continues to use the herb.

garlic

(GAR-lik)

allium, camphor of the poor, da-suan, la-suan, nectar of the gods, poor man's treacle, stinking rose

Reported uses

Used most commonly to decrease total cholesterol level, decrease triglyceride level, and increase high-density lipoprotein cholesterol level. Also used to help prevent atherosclerosis because of its effect on blood pressure and platelet aggregation. Used to decrease the risk of cancer, especially cancer of the GI tract. Used to decrease the risk of CVA and MI and to treat cough, colds, fevers, and sore throats.

Used to treat asthma, diabetes, inflammation, heavy metal poisoning, constipation, and athlete's foot. Also used as an antimicrobial and to reduce symptoms in patients with AIDS.

Common forms

In tablets; also as fresh bulb, antiseptic oil, fresh extract, powdered, freeze-dried garlic powder, and garlic oil (essential oil).

Tablets (garlic extract): 100 mg, 320 mg, 400 mg, 600 mg.

Tablets (allicin total potential): 2 to 5 mg.

Dried powder: 400 to 1,200 mg.

Fresh bulb: 2 to 5 g.

Actions

May exhibit antithrombotic, lipid-lowering, cholesterol-lowering, antitumor, and antimicrobial effects. May have hypoglycemic activity and hypotensive properties, as well as antibacterial, antifungal, larvicidal, insecticidal, amebicidal, and antiviral activities. A component in garlic oil may inhibit adenosine diphosphate–induced platelet aggregation. Also may decrease a type of carcinogen and nitrite accumulation.

Dosages

▶ **To lower cholesterol level.** 600 to 900 mg of dried power, 2 to 5 mg of allicin, or 2 to 5 g of fresh clove. Average dose is 4 g of fresh garlic or 8 mg of essential oil daily.

Adverse reactions

CNS: dizziness.
GI: halitosis; irritation of mouth, esophagus, and stomach; nausea; vomiting.
Hematologic: decreased hemoglobin production and lysis of RBCs (with long-term use or excessive dosages).
Skin: contact dermatitis, diaphoresis.
Other: allergic reactions, ***anaphylaxis,*** garlic odor.

Interactions

Herb-drug. *Anticoagulants, NSAIDs, prostacyclin:* may increase bleeding time. Discourage concurrent use.
Antidiabetics: blood glucose level may be further decreased. Advise caution if using together, and tell patient to monitor blood glucose level closely.
Drugs metabolized by the enzyme cytochrome P-2E1, a member of the cytochrome P-450 system (such as acetaminophen): decreased metabolism of these drugs. Monitor patient for clinical effects and toxic reaction.
Herb-herb. *Herbs with anticoagulant effects:* increased bleeding time. Discourage concurrent use.
Herbs with antihyperglycemic effects: blood glucose level may be further decreased. Tell patient to use caution and to monitor blood glucose level closely.

Cautions

• Contraindicated in patients sensitive to garlic or other members of the *Lilaceae* family and in those with GI disorders, such as peptic ulcer or reflux disease.
• Also contraindicated in pregnant women because of its oxytocic effects.

NURSING CONSIDERATIONS

• Garlic isn't recommended for patients with diabetes, insomnia, pemphigus, organ transplants, and rheumatoid arthritis, and in post-surgical patients.
• Garlic may lower blood glucose level. If patient is taking an antihyperglycemic, watch for signs and symptoms of hypoglycemia and monitor his serum glucose level.

Patient teaching

• Advise patient that cholesterol-lowering drugs are commonly used for hypercholesterolemia because of their proven survival data and ability to lower cholesterol levels more effectively than garlic.
• Instruct patient to watch for signs of bleeding (bleeding gums, easy bruising, tarry stools, petechiae) if garlic supplements are taken with antiplatelet agents.
• Tell the patient that, when filling a new prescription, he should remind the pharmacist of any herbal or dietary supplement he's taking.
• Advise patient not to delay seeking appropriate medical evaluation because doing so may delay diagnosis of a potentially serious medical condition.
• Discourage heavy use of garlic before surgery.
• If patient is using garlic to lower his serum cholesterol levels, advise him to notify his health care provider and to have his serum cholesterol levels monitored.
• If patient is using garlic as a topical antiseptic, tell him to avoid prolonged exposure to the skin because burns can occur.

ginger

(JIN-jer)
zingiber

Reported uses

Used as an antiemetic, GI protectant, anti-inflammatory agent useful for arthritis treat-

* Liquid may contain alcohol.

ment, CV stimulant, antitumor agent, antioxidant, and as a therapy for microbial and parasitic infestations. Also used to treat morning, motion, or sea sickness; postoperative nausea and vomiting; and to provide relief from pain and swelling caused by rheumatoid arthritis, osteoarthritis, or muscular discomfort.

Common forms

As root, extract, liquid, powder, capsules, tablets, and teas.
Root: 530 mg.
Extract: 250 mg.
Liquid, powder, capsules: 100 mg, 465 mg.
Tablets (chewable): 67.5 mg.

Actions

Inhibits platelet aggregation induced by adenosine diphosphate and epinephrine. May exhibit anti-inflammatory and positive inotropic effects. Specific components of ginger produce varying CV effects.

Dosages

Infusion: Prepared by steeping 0.5 to 1 g of herb in boiling water and then straining after 5 minutes. (1 tsp = 3 g of drug.)
Dosage forms and strengths vary with the condition.
▶ **As an antiemetic.** 500 to 1,000 mg powdered ginger P.O., or 1,000 mg fresh ginger root P.O.
▶ **For arthritis.** 1 to 2 g daily.
▶ **For nausea caused by chemotherapy.** 1 g before chemotherapy.
▶ **For migraine headache or arthritis.** Up to 2 g daily.
▶ **For motion sickness.** 1 g P.O. 30 minutes before travel, then 0.5 to 1 g q 4 hours. Also could begin 1 to 2 days before trip.

Adverse reactions

CNS: CNS depression.
CV: ***cardiac arrhythmias,*** increased bleeding time.
GI: heartburn.

Interactions

Herb-drug. *Anticoagulants and other drugs that can increase bleeding time:* May further increase bleeding time. Discourage concurrent use.
Herb-herb. *Herbs that may increase bleeding time:* May further increase bleeding time. Discourage concurrent use.

Cautions

- Patients with gallstones or with an allergy to ginger should avoid use.
- Pregnant women and those with bleeding disorders should avoid using large amounts of ginger.
- Patients taking a CNS depressant or an antiarrhythmic should use cautiously.

NURSING CONSIDERATIONS

- Find out why patient is taking herb.
- Ginger may interfere with the intended therapeutic effect of conventional drugs.
- If overdose occurs, monitor patient for arrhythmias and CNS depression.

Patient teaching

- Advise patient to consult health care provider before using an herbal preparation because a treatment with proven efficacy may be available.
- Tell the patient that, when filling a new prescription, he should remind the pharmacist of any herbal or dietary supplement he's taking.
- Advise pregnant patient to consult with a knowledgeable practitioner before using ginger medicinally.
- Educate patients to look for signs and symptoms of bleeding, such as nosebleeds or excessive bruising.

ginkgo
(GIN-koh)
EGB 761, GBE, GBE 24, GBX, ginkgo biloba, ginkogink, LI 1370, rokan, sophium, tanakan, tebonin

Reported uses

Primarily used to manage cerebral insufficiency, dementia, and circulatory disorders such as intermittent claudication. Also used to treat headaches, asthma, colitis, impotence, depression, altitude sickness, tinnitus, cochlear deafness, vertigo, premenstrual syndrome, macular degeneration, diabetic retinopathy, and allergies.

Used as an adjunctive treatment for pancreatic cancer and schizophrenia. Also used in addition to physical therapy for Fontaine stage IIb peripheral arterial disease to decrease pain during ambulation with a minimum of 6 weeks of treatment.

In Germany, standardized ginkgo extracts are required to contain 22% to 27% ginkgo flavonoids and 5% to 7% terpenoids.

Common forms

As ginkgo biloba extract in capsules, tablets, and sublingual sprays (standardized to contain 24% flavone glycosides and 6% terpenes) and as concentrated alcoholic extract of fresh leaf.
Tablets, capsules: 30 mg, 40 mg, 60 mg, 120 mg, 260 mg, 420 mg.
Capsules (ginkgo biloba extract [24% standardized extract] bound to phosphatidylcholine): 80 mg.
S.L. sprays: 15 mg/spray, 40 mg/spray.

Actions

Produces arterial and venous vasoactive changes that increase tissue perfusion and cerebral blood flow. Also produces arterial vasodilation, inhibits arterial spasms, decreases capillary permeability, reduces capillary fragility, decreases blood viscosity, and reduces erythrocyte aggregation. Ginkgo biloba extract acts as an antioxidant, and ginkgolide B (a component of gingko) may be a potent inhibitor of platelet activating factor.

Dosages

▶ **For dementia syndromes.** 120 to 240 mg P.O. daily in two or three divided doses.
▶ **For peripheral arterial disease, vertigo, and tinnitus.** 120 to 160 mg P.O. daily in two or three divided doses.

Adverse reactions

CNS: headache, ***seizures,*** subarachnoid hemorrhage.
GI: diarrhea, flatulence, nausea, vomiting.
Skin: contact hypersensitivity reactions, dermatitis.

Interactions

Herb-drug. *Anticoagulants, antiplatelets, high-dose vitamin E:* may increase the risk of bleeding. Discourage concurrent use.
MAO inhibitors: theoretically, ginkgo can potentiate the activity of these drugs. Advise caution.
Selective serotonin reuptake inhibitors: ginkgo extracts may reverse the sexual dysfunction caused by these drugs.
Warfarin: possibly increased INR when taken together. Monitor INR.
Herb-herb. *Garlic and other herbs that increase bleeding time:* potentiated anticoagulant effects. Advise patient to use together cautiously.

Cautions

- Patients with a history of an allergic reaction to gingko or any of its components should avoid use, as should patients with increased risk of intracranial hemorrhage (hypertension, diabetes).
- Patients receiving an antiplatelet or an anticoagulant should avoid use because of the increased risk of bleeding.
- Herb should be avoided in the perioperative period and before childbirth.

NURSING CONSIDERATIONS

- Ginkgo extracts are considered standardized if they contain 24% ginkgo flavonoid glycosides and 6% terpene lactones.
- Treatment period ranges from 6 to 8 weeks, but therapy beyond 3 months isn't recommended.

ALERT Seizures have been reported in children after ingestion of more than 50 seeds.

- Patients must be monitored for possible adverse reactions such as GI problems, headaches, dizziness, allergic reactions, and serious bleeding.

Patient teaching

- Inform patient that the therapeutic and toxic components of gingko can vary significantly from product to product. Advise him to obtain gingko from a reliable source.

- Advise patient to discontinue use at least 2 weeks before surgery.
- Advise patient to report unusual bleeding or bruising.
- Instruct patient to keep seeds out of reach of children because of potential risk of seizures with ingestion.
- Advise patient to avoid contact with the fruit pulp or seed coats because of the risk of contact dermatitis. More potent preparations may cause irritation or blistering of skin or mucous membranes if applied externally.

ginseng

(JIN-sehng)

American ginseng, Asiatic ginseng, Chinese ginseng, G115, Japanese ginseng, jintsam, Korean ginseng

Reported uses

Used to minimize or reduce the activity of the thymus gland. Also used as a sedative, demulcent (soothes irritated or inflamed internal tissues or organs), aphrodisiac, antidepressant, sleep aid, and diuretic. May be used to improve stamina, concentration, healing, stress-resistance, vigilance, and work efficiency and to improve well-being in elderly patients with debilitated or degenerative conditions.

Also used to decrease fasting blood glucose and hemoglobin A1c in diabetic and nondiabetic patients, and to treat hyperlipidemia, hepatic dysfunction, and impaired cognitive function.

Common forms

As capsules, teas, extract, root powder, whole root (by the pound), and oil.

Capsules: 100 mg, 250 mg, 500 mg.
Tea bags: 1,500 mg ginseng root.
Extract*: 2 oz root extract (in alcohol base).
Root powder: 1 oz, 4 oz.

Actions

Ginseng compounds may exert opposing effects. For example, one compound has CNS-depressant, anticonvulsant, analgesic, and antipsychotic effects and stress-ulcer preventing action. Another compound has CNS-stimulating, antifatigue, hypertensive, and stress-ulcer aggravating effects. Some components enhance cardiac performance, whereas others depress cardiac function.

Oral ginseng may reduce cholesterol and triglycerides, decrease platelet adhesiveness, impair coagulation, and increase fibrinolysis. It may also reduce stress by acting on the adrenal gland.

Extracts of ginseng may exhibit antioxidant activity.

Dosages

Dosages vary with the disease state; usually, 0.5 to 2 g dry ginseng root daily or 200 to 600 mg ginseng extract daily, in one or two equal doses.

▶ **For improved well-being in debilitated elderly patients.** 0.4 to 0.8 g root P.O. daily on a continual basis.

Adverse reactions

CNS: headache, insomnia, nervousness.
CV: chest pain, palpitations, hypertension.
EENT: epistaxis.
GI: diarrhea, nausea, vomiting.
GU: impotence, vaginal bleeding.
Skin: pruritus, skin eruptions (with ginseng abuse).
Other: breast pain.

Interactions

Herb-drug. *Anticoagulants, antiplatelet drugs:* may decrease the effects of these drugs. Monitor PT and INR.
Antidiabetics, insulin: Increased hypoglycemic effects. Monitor serum glucose level.
Drugs metabolized by CYP 3A4: ginseng may inhibit this enzyme system. Monitor patient for clinical effects and toxicity.
Phenelzine, other MAO inhibitors: headache, irritability, visual hallucinations, and other interactions possible. Discourage concurrent use.
Warfarin: ginseng may decrease warfarin effect. Discourage concomitant use.

Cautions

• Urge caution in patients with CV disease, hypertension, hypotension, or diabetes, and in those receiving steroid therapy.
• Discourage use by pregnant or breast-feeding women; effects are unknown.

NURSING CONSIDERATIONS

• Some debate exists concerning a possible ginseng abuse syndrome. It reportedly occurs when large doses of the herb are taken with other psychomotor stimulants, such as tea and coffee; symptoms include diarrhea, hypertension, restlessness, insomnia, skin eruptions, depression, appetite suppression, euphoria, and edema. However, some reputable herbal sources discredit such reports.
• Considering the high level of bioactivity found for ginseng components, ginseng may not be safe for patients with a serious or chronic medical condition.
• Monitor diabetic patient for signs and symptoms of hypoglycemia.

Patient teaching

• Tell patient with medical conditions to check with prescriber before taking ginseng.
• Advise diabetic patient to check glucose levels closely until effects on serum glucose are known.
• Instruct patient to watch for unusual symptoms (nervousness, insomnia, palpitations, diarrhea) because of risk of ginseng toxicity.
• Inform patient that the therapeutic and toxic components of ginseng can vary significantly from product to product. Advise him to obtain ginseng from a reliable source.

goldenseal

(GOHL-den-seel)

eye balm, eye root, goldsiegel, ground raspberry, Indian dye, Indian turmeric, jaundice root

Reported uses

Used to treat GI disorders, gastritis, peptic ulceration, anorexia, postpartum hemorrhage, dysmenorrhea, eczema, pruritus, tuberculosis, cancer, mouth ulcerations, otorrhea, tinnitus, and conjunctivitis; also used as a wound antiseptic, diuretic, laxative, and anti-inflammatory agent.

Used to shorten the duration of acute *Vibrio cholera* diarrhea and diarrhea caused by some species of *Giardia, Salmonella, Shigella,* and some *Enterobacteriaceae*. May be used to improve biliary secretion and function in patients with hepatic cirrhosis.

Common forms

In capsules and tablets; also as alcohol and water extracts, dried ground root powder, tinctures, and teas.
Capsules, tablets: 250 mg, 350 mg, 400 mg, 404 mg, 470 mg, 500 mg, 535 mg, 540 mg.

Actions

May have astringent, anti-inflammatory, oxytocic, antihemorrhagic, and laxative properties. Inhibits muscular contractions.

Decreases the anticoagulant effect of heparin and acts as a cardiac stimulant (at lower dosages), increases coronary perfusion, and inhibits cardiac activity (at higher dosages). May exhibit antipyretic activity (greater than aspirin) and antimuscarinic, antihistaminic, antitumor, antimicrobial, antiparasitic, and hypotensive effects.

Causes vasoconstriction and produces significant changes in blood pressure.

Dosages

Alcohol and water extract: 250 mg P.O. t.i.d.
Dried rhizome: 0.5 to 1 g t.i.d.

Adverse reactions

CNS: sedation, reduced mental alertness, hallucinations, delirium, paresthesia, paralysis.
CV: hypotension, hypertension, ***asystole, heart block.***
GI: nausea, vomiting, diarrhea, GI cramping, mouth ulceration.
Hematologic: megaloblastic anemia from decreased vitamin B absorption, ***leukopenia.***
Respiratory: ***respiratory depression.***
Skin: contact dermatitis.

* Liquid may contain alcohol.

Interactions

Herb-drug. *Anticoagulants:* may reduce anticoagulant effect. Discourage concurrent use.
Antidiabetics, insulin: increased hypoglycemic effects. Advise caution.
Antihypertensives: may reduce or enhance hypotensive effect. Discourage concurrent use.
Beta blockers, calcium channel blockers, digoxin: may interfere or enhance cardiac effects. Discourage concurrent use.
CNS depressants such as benzodiazepines: may enhance sedative effects. Discourage concurrent use.
Cephalosporins, disulfiram, metronidazole: disulfiram-like reaction when taken with liquid herbal preparations. Discourage concurrent use.
Herb-lifestyle. *Alcohol use:* may enhance sedative effects. Discourage concurrent use.

Cautions

- Patients with hypertension, heart failure, or arrhythmias should avoid use.
- Pregnant and breast-feeding patients and those with severe renal or hepatic disease should also avoid use.
- Goldenseal shouldn't be given to infants.

NURSING CONSIDERATIONS

- German Commission E hasn't endorsed the use of goldenseal for any condition because of its potential toxicity and lack of well-documented efficacy.
- Berberine, a chemical constitute of goldenseal, increases bilirubin levels in infants and thus shouldn't be given to them.
- Monitor patient for signs and symptoms of vitamin B deficiency such as megaloblastic anemia, paresthesia, seizures, cheilosis, glossitis, and seborrheic dermatitis.
- Monitor patient for adverse cardiovascular, respiratory, and neurologic effects. If patient has a toxic reaction, induce vomiting and perform gastric lavage. After lavage, instill activated charcoal and treat symptomatically.

Patient teaching

- Tell the patient that, when filling a new prescription, he should remind the pharmacist of any herbal or dietary supplement he's taking.
- Advise patient not to use goldenseal because of its toxicity and lack of documented efficacy, especially if the patient has CV disease.

ALERT High doses may lead to vomiting, bradycardia, hypertension, respiratory depression, exaggerated reflexes, seizures, and death.

grapeseed; pinebark

(GRAYP-seed; PIGHN-bahrk)
muskat, *Pinus maritima, Pinus nigra, Vitis coignetiae, Vitis vinifera*

Reported uses

Used as an antioxidant to treat circulatory disorders (hypoxia from atherosclerosis, inflammation, and cardiac or cerebral infarction). Also used to treat pain, limb heaviness, and swelling in patients with peripheral circulatory disorders and to treat inflammatory conditions, varicose veins, and cancer.

Common forms

Tablets, capsules: 25 mg to 300 mg.

Actions

Demonstrates antilipoperoxidant activity and xanthine oxidase inhibition. Inhibits enzymes responsible for skin turnover. Extract exhibits therapeutic effects in Ehrlich ascites carcinoma and inhibits growth of *Streptococcus mutans*.

Dosages

Tablets, capsules: 25 to 300 mg P.O. daily for up to 3 weeks; maintenance dosage of 40 to 80 mg P.O. once daily.

Adverse reactions

Hepatic: ***hepatotoxicity.***

Interactions

None reported.

Cautions

• Patients with liver dysfunction should use cautiously.

NURSING CONSIDERATIONS

• Grapeseed may interfere with the intended therapeutic effect of conventional drugs.
• Grapeseed extract may have antiplatelet effects. If a patient is having elective surgery, it may be prudent to stop the supplement 2 to 3 days before surgery. Monitor PT and INR.

Patient teaching
• Warn patient not to treat symptoms of venous insufficiency or circulatory disorders before seeking appropriate medical evaluation because doing so may delay diagnosis of a potentially serious medical condition.
• Tell the patient that, when filling a new prescription, he should remind the pharmacist of any herbal or dietary supplement he's taking.

kava

(KAH-veh)
ava, awa, kava-kava, kawa, kew, sakau, tonga, yagona

Reported uses

Used to treat nervous anxiety, stress, and restlessness. Used orally as a sedative, to promote wound healing, and to treat headaches, seizure disorders, the common cold, respiratory tract infection, tuberculosis, and rheumatism. Also used to treat urogenital infections, including chronic cystitis, venereal disease, uterine inflammation, menstrual problems, and vaginal prolapse. Some herbal practitioners consider kava an aphrodisiac. Kava juice is used to treat skin diseases, including leprosy. Also used as a poultice for intestinal problems, otitis, and abscesses.

Common forms

A drink from pulverized roots, tablets, capsules, or extract.

Actions

Components of the root may cause local anesthetic activity that is similar to cocaine but lasts longer than benzocaine. Some components show fungistatic properties against several fungi.

Induces muscular relaxation and inhibits the limbic system, an effect linked to suppression of emotional excitability and mood enhancement. Produces mild euphoria with no effect on thoughts and memory during the intoxication. Other effects include analgesia, sedation, hyporeflexia, impaired gait, and pupil dilation.

Dosages

▶ **Anxiety.** 50 to 70 mg purified kava lactones t.i.d., equivalent to 100 to 250 mg of dried kava root extract per dose. (By comparison, the traditional bowl of raw kava beverage contains about 250 mg of kava lactones.)
▶ **Restlessness.** 180 to 210 mg of kava lactones taken as a tea 1 hour before bedtime. The typical dose in this form is 1 cup t.i.d. Prepared by simmering 2 to 4 g of the root in 5 oz boiling water for 5 to 10 minutes and then straining.

Adverse reactions

CNS: mild euphoric changes characterized by feelings of happiness, fluent and lively speech, and increased sensitivity to sounds; morning fatigue.
EENT: visual accommodation disorders, pupil dilation, and disorders of oculomotor equilibrium.
GI: reduced levels of albumin, total protein, bilirubin and urea; increased HDL cholesterol, mild GI disturbances, mouth numbness.
GU: hematuria.
Hematologic: increased RBC count, decreased platelets and lymphocytes.
Respiratory: pulmonary hypertension.
Skin: scaly rash.

Interactions

Herb-drug. *Antiplatelet drugs, MAO type B inhibitors:* possible additive effects. Monitor patient closely.

* Liquid may contain alcohol.

Barbiturates, benzodiazepines: kava lactones potentiate the effects of CNS depressants, leading to toxicity. Discourage concurrent use.
Levodopa: possible reduced effectiveness of levodopa therapy in patients with Parkinson's disease, apparently because of dopamine antagonism. Advise patient to use cautiously.
Herb-herb. *Calamus, calendula, California poppy, capsicum, catnip, celery, couch grass, elecampane, German chamomile, goldenseal, gotu kola, hops, Jamaican dogwood, lemon balm, sage, sassafras, shepherd's purse, Siberian ginseng, skullcap, stinging nettle, St. John's wort, valerian, wild lettuce, yerba maté:* additive sedative effects may occur. Monitor patient closely.
Herb-lifestyle. *Alcohol:* increased risk of CNS depression and liver damage. Discourage concurrent use.

Cautions

- Patients hypersensitive to kava or any of its components should avoid this herb. Depressed patients should avoid the herb because of possible sedative activity; those with endogenous depression should avoid it because of possible increased risk of suicide. Pregnant women should avoid the herb because of possible loss of uterine tone; those who are breast-feeding also should avoid it. Children shouldn't use this herb.
- Patients with renal disease, thrombocytopenia, or neutropenia should use cautiously.

NURSING CONSIDERATIONS

- Heavy kava users are more likely to complain of poor health. About 20% are underweight with reduced levels of albumin, total protein, bilirubin, urea, platelets, and lymphocytes; increased HDL cholesterol and RBCs; hematuria; puffy faces; scaly rashes; and some evidence of pulmonary hypertension. These symptoms resolve several weeks after the herb is stopped. Toxic doses can cause progressive ataxia, muscle weakness, and ascending paralysis, all of which resolve when herb is stopped. Extreme use (more than 300 g/week) may increase gamma-glutamyl transferase levels.
- Patient shouldn't use kava with conventional sedative-hypnotics, anxiolytics, MAO inhibitors, other psychopharmacologic drugs, levodopa, or antiplatelet drugs without first consulting health care provider.
- Adverse effects of kava may occur at start of therapy but are usually transient.

Patient teaching

- Encourage patients to seek medical diagnosis before taking kava.
- Advise patient that usual doses can affect motor function; caution against performing hazardous activities.
- Warn patient to avoid taking herb with alcohol because of increased risk of CNS depression and liver damage.
- Tell the patient that, when filling a new prescription, he should remind the pharmacist of any herbal or dietary supplement he's taking.

milk thistle

(MILK THIH-sel)

Carduus marianus L., Cnicus marianus, holy thistle, Lady's thistle, Marian thistle, Mary thistle, St. Mary thistle

Reported uses

Used to treat dyspepsia, liver damage from chemicals, *Amanita* mushroom poisoning, supportive therapy for inflammatory liver disease and cirrhosis, loss of appetite, and gallbladder and spleen disorders. It's also used as a liver protectant.

Common forms

Available as capsules, tablets, and extract.
Capsules: 50 mg, 100 mg, 175 mg, 200 mg, 505 mg.
Tablets: 85 mg (standardized to contain 80% silymarin with the flavonoid silibinin).

Actions

Exerts hepatoprotective and antihepatotoxic actions over liver toxins by altering the outer liver membrane cell structure so that toxins cannot enter the cell. Also leads to activation of the regenerative capacity of the liver through cell development.

Dosages

Oral: Doses of milk thistle extract vary from 200 to 400 mg of silibinin (70% silymarin extract) P.O. daily.
Dried fruit or seed: 12 to 15 g P.O. daily.
Tea: 3 to 5 g freshly crushed fruit or seed steeped in 5 oz of boiling water for 10 to 15 minutes. One cup of tea P.O. t.i.d. to q.i.d., 30 minutes before meals.

Adverse reactions

Herb-drug. *Aspirin:* herb may improve aspirin metabolism in patients with liver cirrhosis. Advise patient to consult prescriber before use.
Cisplatin: herb may prevent kidney damage by cisplatin. Advise patient to consult prescriber before use.
Disulfiram: products that contain alcohol may cause a disulfiram-like reaction. Discourage concurrent use.
Hepatotoxic drugs: may prevent liver damage from butyrophenones, phenothiazines, phenytoin, acetaminophen, and halothane.
Tacrine: silymarin reduces adverse cholinergic effects when given together. Advise patient to consult prescriber before use.

Cautions

• Milk thistle shouldn't be used by women who are pregnant or breast-feeding or by patients hypersensitive to it or to plants in the *Asteraceae* family. Use in decompensated cirrhosis isn't recommended.

NURSING CONSIDERATIONS

• Warn patient not to take herb for liver inflammation or cirrhosis before seeking appropriate medical evaluation because doing so may delay diagnosis of a potentially serious medical condition.
• Mild allergic reactions may occur, especially in people allergic to members of the *Asteraceae* family, including ragweed, chrysanthemums, marigolds, and daisies.
• Don't confuse milk thistle seeds or fruit with other parts of the plant or with blessed thistle *(Cnictus benedictus)*.
• Silymarin has poor water solubility; therefore, efficacy when prepared as a tea is questionable.

Patient teaching

• Tell the patient that, when filling a new prescription, he should remind the pharmacist of any herbal or dietary supplement he's taking.
• Although no chemical interactions have been reported in clinical studies, advise patient that herb may interfere with therapeutic effect of conventional drugs.
• Warn patient not to take this herb while pregnant or breast-feeding.
• Tell patient to stay alert for possible allergic reactions, especially if allergic to ragweed, chrysanthemums, marigolds, or daisies.

nettle

(NEH-tel)
common nettle, greater nettle, stinging nettle

Reported uses

Used to treat allergic rhinitis, osteoarthritis, rheumatoid arthritis, kidney stones, asthma, and BPH. Also used as a diuretic, an expectorant, a general health tonic, a blood builder and purifier, a pain reliever and anti-inflammatory, and a lung tonic for ex-smokers. Also used for eczema, hives, bursitis, tendinitis, laryngitis, sciatica, and premenstrual syndrome. Nettle is being investigated for treatment of hay fever and irrigation of the urinary tract.

Common forms

Available as capsules and dried leaf and root extract or tincture.
Capsules: 150 mg, 300 mg.

Actions

Acts primarily as a diuretic by increasing urine volume and decreasing systolic blood pressure. May stimulate uterine contractions. Extract reduces urine flow, nocturia, and residual urine.

* Liquid may contain alcohol.

Dosages

▶ **Allergic rhinitis.** 600 mg freeze-dried leaf P.O. at onset of symptoms.
▶ **BPH.** 4 g root extract P.O. daily, or 600 to 1,200 mg P.O. encapsulated extract daily.
Fresh juice: 5 to 10 ml P.O. t.i.d.
Infusion: 1.5 g powdered nettle in cold water; heated to boiling for 1 minute, then steeped covered for 10 minutes and strained (1 tsp = 1.3 g herb).
Liquid extract (1:1 in 25% alcohol)*: 2 to 6 ml P.O. t.i.d.
▶ **Osteoarthritis.** 1 leaf applied to affected area daily.
▶ **Rheumatoid arthritis.** 8 to 12 g leaf extract P.O. daily.
Tea: 1 tbs fresh young plant steeped in 1 cup boiled water for 15 minutes. Three or more cups taken daily.
Tincture (1:5 in 45% alcohol)*: 2 to 6 ml P.O. t.i.d.

Adverse reactions

CV: edema.
GI: gastric irritation, gingivostomatitis.
GU: decreased urine formation; oliguria; increased diuresis in patients with arthritic conditions and those with myocardial or chronic venous insufficiency.
Skin: topical irritation, burning sensation.

Interactions

Herb-drug. *Disulfiram:* possible adverse reaction if taken with liquid extract or tincture. Discourage concurrent use.
Herb-lifestyle. *Alcohol:* possible additive effect from liquid extract and tincture. Discourage alcohol use.

Cautions

- Contraindicated in pregnant and breast-feeding women because of its diuretic and uterine stimulation properties.
- Also contraindicated in children.

NURSING CONSIDERATIONS

- Nettle is reported to be an abortifacient and may affect the menstrual cycle.
- Internal adverse effects are rare and allergic in nature.

Patient teaching

- Advise patient to consult prescriber before using an herbal preparation because a treatment with proven efficacy may be available.
- Tell patient that, when filling a new prescription, he should remind the pharmacist of any herbal or dietary supplement he's taking.
- Recommend caution if patient takes an antihypertensive or antidiabetic.
- Warn patient that external adverse effects result from skin contact and include burning and stinging that may persist for 12 hours or more.
- Advise patient to eat foods high in potassium, such as bananas and fresh vegetables, to replenish electrolytes lost through diuresis.
- Caution patient against using nettle for BPH or to relieve fluid accumulation caused by heart failure without medical approval and supervision.
- Tell patient to wash thoroughly with soap and water, use antihistamines and steroid creams, and wear heavy gloves if plant will be handled. If rubbed against the skin, nettles can cause intense burning for 12 hours or more.

passion flower

(PAH-shen FLOW-er)

apricot vine, granadilla, Jamaican honeysuckle, maypop, passion fruit, water lemon

Reported uses

Used as a sedative, a hypnotic, an analgesic, and an antispasmodic for treating muscle spasms caused by indigestion, menstrual cramping, pain, or migraines. Also used for neuralgia, generalized seizures, hysteria, nervous agitation, and insomnia. Crushed leaves and flowers are used topically for cuts and bruises.

Common forms

As liquid extract, crude extract, tincture, dried herb, and in several homeopathic remedies.
Liquid extract*: 1:1 in 25% alcohol.
Tincture*: 1:8 in 45% alcohol, or containing 0.7% flavonoids.

Bold italic type indicates that reaction may be life-threatening.

Actions

Obtained from leaves, fruits, and flowers of *Passiflora incarnata*. Contains indole alkaloids, including harman and harmine, flavonoids, and maltol. Indole alkaloids are the basis of many biologically active substances, such as serotonin and tryptophan. Exact effect of these alkaloids is unknown; however, they can cause CNS stimulation via MAO inhibition, thereby decreasing intracellular metabolism of norepinephrine, serotonin, and other biogenic amines. Flavonoids can reduce capillary permeability and fragility. Maltol can cause sedative effects and potentiate hexobarbital and anticonvulsive activity.

Dosages

Dried herb: 250 mg to 1 g P.O., two to three 100-mg capsules P.O. b.i.d., or one 400-mg capsule P.O. daily.
Extract in vegetable glycerin base (alcohol free): 10 to 15 gtt P.O., b.i.d. or t.i.d.
▶ **For cuts and bruises.** Crushed leaves and flowers are applied topically, p.r.n.
▶ **For hemorrhoids.** Prepared by soaking 20 g dried herb in 200 ml of simmering water, straining, then cooling before use. Applied topically, as indicated.
Infusion: 150 ml of hot water poured over 1 tsp of herb. Strained after standing for 10 minutes. Taken b.i.d. or t.i.d., with a final dose about 30 minutes before h.s.
Liquid extract (1:1 in 25% alcohol)*: 0.5 to 1 ml P.O. t.i.d.
Solid extract: Taken in doses of 150 to 300 mg/day P.O.
Tincture (1:8 in 45% alcohol)*: 0.5 to 2 ml P.O. t.i.d. or ½ to 1 tsp P.O. t.i.d.
▶ **For Parkinson's disease.** 10 to 30 gtt P.O. (0.7% flavonoids) t.i.d.
Dried herb: 0.25 to 1 g P.O. t.i.d.
Liquid extract: 0.5 to 1 ml P.O. t.i.d.
Tea: 4 to 8 g (3 to 6 tsp) daily in divided doses.
Tincture: 0.5 to 2 ml P.O. t.i.d.

Adverse reactions

CNS: drowsiness, headache, flushing, agitation, confusion, psychosis.
CV: tachycardia, hypotension, ***ventricular arrhythmias.***
GI: nausea, vomiting.
Respiratory: asthma.
Other: allergic reactions, ***shock.***

Interactions

Herb-drug. *Disulfiram, metronidazole:* herbal products that contain alcohol may cause a disulfiram-like reaction. Discourage concurrent use.
Hexobarbital: increased sleeping time and other barbiturate effects may be potentiated. Monitor patient's level of consciousness carefully.
Isocarboxazid, moclobemide, phenelzine, selegiline, and tranylcypromine: actions can be potentiated by passion flower. Discourage concurrent use.

Cautions

- Excessive doses may cause sedation and may potentiate MAO inhibitor therapy.
- Pregnant and breast-feeding women shouldn't take this herb.
- Those with liver disease or a history of alcoholism should avoid products that contain alcohol.

NURSING CONSIDERATIONS

- Monitor patient for possible adverse CNS effects.
- A disulfiram-like reaction may produce nausea, vomiting, flushing, headache, hypotension, tachycardia, and possibly ventricular arrhythmias and shock leading to death.
- Patients with liver disease or alcoholism shouldn't use herbal products that contain alcohol.

Patient teaching

- Warn patient not to take herb for chronic pain or insomnia before seeking medical attention because doing so may delay diagnosis of a potentially serious medical condition.
- Tell the patient that, when filling a new prescription, he should remind the pharmacist of any herbal or dietary supplement he's taking.
- Because sedation is possible, caution patient to avoid activities that require alertness and coordination until CNS effects are known.

* Liquid may contain alcohol.

primrose, evening
(PRIHM-rohz, EEV-ning)
king's-cure-all

Reported uses

Infusion used for sedative and astringent properties. Used to treat asthmatic coughs, GI disorders, whooping cough, psoriasis, multiple sclerosis, asthma, Raynaud's disease, and Sjögren's syndrome. Poultices made with evening primrose oil may be used to speed wound healing.

Used to treat pruritic symptoms of atopic dermatitis and eczema, breast pain and tenderness from premenstrual syndrome, benign breast disease, and diabetic neuropathy.

Used in rheumatoid arthritis to improve patients' symptoms and reduce the need for pain medication; also used to lower serum cholesterol, improve hypertension, and decrease platelet aggregation.

Also may be used to calm hyperactive children and to reduce mammary tumors from baseline size.

Common forms

Capsules: 50 mg, 500 mg, 1,300 mg.
Gelcaps: 500 mg, 1,300 mg.

Actions

Aids prostaglandin synthesis.

Dosages

The following dosages are based on a standardized gamma linoleic acid content of 8%.

▶ **For eczema.** *Adults:* 320 mg to 8 g P.O. daily.
Children ages 1 to 12: 160 mg to 4 g P.O. daily for 3 months.

▶ **For breast pain.** 3 to 4 g P.O. daily.

No consensus exists for all other disorders.

Adverse reactions

CNS: headache, temporal lobe epilepsy.
GI: nausea.
Skin: rash.
Other: inflammation, thrombosis, immunosuppression.

Interactions

Herb-drug. *Phenothiazines:* may increase risk of seizures. Discourage concomitant use.

Cautions

- Discourage use of herb by pregnant women; effects are unknown.
- Urge caution or discourage use in schizophrenic patients or in those taking seizure drugs.

NURSING CONSIDERATIONS

- Find out why patient is using the herb.
- Monitor patient for adverse effects, especially with long-term use.

Patient teaching

- Instruct patient with seizure disorders to reconsider need to use herb.
- Caution parents to use herb for a hyperactive child only under medical supervision.

Saint John's wort
(SAYNT JAHNS WART)
amber, devil's scourge, goatweed, grace of God, Hypericum, klamath weed, St. John's wort

Reported uses

Used to treat depression, bronchial inflammation, burns, cancer, enuresis, gastritis, hemorrhoids, hypothyroidism, insect bites and stings, insomnia, kidney disorders, and scabies, and has been used as a wound-healing agent. Saint John's wort can be used to treat HIV infection; also can be used topically for phototherapy of skin diseases, including psoriasis, cutaneous T-cell lymphoma, warts, and Kaposi's sarcoma.

Common forms

As capsules, sublingual capsules, and liquid tinctures.

Capsules: 100 mg, 300 mg, 500 mg (standardized to 0.3% hypericin); 250 mg (standardized to 0.14% hypericin).

Actions

Inhibits stress-induced increase in corticotropin-releasing hormone, corticotropin, and cortisol. Also has antiviral activity, including action against retroviruses.

Dosages

▶ **For depression.** 300 mg standardized extract preparations (standardized to 0.3% hypericin) P.O. t.i.d. for 4 to 6 weeks; or 2 to 4 g tea that has been steeped in 1 to 2 cups of water for about 10 minutes and taken P.O. daily for 4 to 6 weeks.

▶ **For burns and skin lesions.** Cream applied topically; strength isn't standardized.

Adverse reactions

CNS: fatigue, neuropathy, restlessness, headache.
GI: digestive complaints, fullness sensation, constipation, diarrhea, nausea, abdominal pain, dry mouth.
Skin: photosensitivity reaction, pruritus.
Other: delayed hypersensitivity.

Interactions

Herb-drug. *Amitriptyline, chemotherapy drugs, cyclosporine, digoxin, drugs metabolized by the cytochrome P-450 enzyme system, oral contraceptives, protease inhibitors, theophylline, and warfarin:* decreased effectiveness, requiring possible dosage adjustment. Monitor patient closely; discourage concurrent use.
Barbiturates: decreased sedative effects. Monitor patient closely.
Indinavir: substantially reduces blood levels of the drug that could cause loss of therapeutic effects. Discourage concomitant use.
MAO inhibitors, including phenelzine and tranylcypromine: may increase effects and cause possible toxicity and hypertensive crisis. Discourage concurrent use.
Narcotics: increased sedative effects. Discourage concurrent use.
Reserpine: antagonized effects of reserpine. Discourage concurrent use.
Selective serotonin reuptake inhibitors (SSRIs), such as citalopram, fluoxetine, paroxetine, sertraline: increased risk of serotonin syndrome. Discourage concurrent use.
Herb-herb. *Herbs with sedative effects, such as calamus, calendula, California poppy, capsicum, catnip, celery, couch grass, elecampane, German chamomile, goldenseal, gotu kola, Jamaican dogwood, kava, lemon balm, sage, sassafras, shepherd's purse, Siberian ginseng, skullcap, stinging nettle, valerian, wild carrot, and wild lettuce:* possible enhanced effects of herbs. Monitor patient closely, and discourage concurrent use.
Herb-food. *Tyramine-containing foods such as beer, cheese, dried meats, fava beans, liver, wine, and yeast:* may cause hypertensive crisis when used together. Advise patient to separate administration times.
Herb-lifestyle. *Alcohol use:* possible increased sedative effects. Discourage concurrent use.
Sun exposure: increased risk of photosensitivity reactions. Advise patient to avoid unprotected exposure to sunlight.

Cautions

• Pregnant patients and those planning pregnancy shouldn't take St. John's wort because of mutagenic risk to sperm cells and oocytes and adverse effects on reproductive cells. Transplant patients maintained on cyclosporine therapy should avoid this herb because of the risk of organ rejection.

NURSING CONSIDERATIONS

• Monitor patient for response to herbal therapy, as evidenced by improved mood and lessened depression.
• By using standardized extracts, patient can better control the dosage. Clinical studies have used formulations of standardized 0.3% hypericin as well as hyperforin-stabilized version of the extract.
• St. John's wort interacts with many other products; they must be considered before patient takes it with other prescription or OTC products.
• Signs and symptoms of serotonin syndrome include dizziness, nausea, vomiting, headache,

epigastric pain, anxiety, confusion, restlessness, and irritability.
- Because St. John's wort decreases the effect of certain prescription drugs, watch for signs of drug toxicity if patient stops herb. Drug dosage may need reduction.

Patient teaching
- Tell the patient that, when filling a new prescription, he should remind the pharmacist of any herbal or dietary supplement he's taking.
- Instruct patient to consult a health care provider for a thorough medical evaluation before using St. John's wort.
- If patient takes St. John's wort for mild to moderate depression, explain that several weeks may pass before effects occur. Tell patient that a new therapy may be needed if no improvement occurs in 4 to 6 weeks.

ALERT If patient wants to switch from an SSRI to St. John's wort, tell him he may need to wait a few weeks for the SSRI to leave his system before it's safe to start taking the herb. The exact time required depends on which SSRI he's taking.
- Inform patient that St. John's wort interacts with many other prescription and OTC products.

saw palmetto

(SAW pal-MEH-toh)

American dwarf palm tree, cabbage palm, IDS 89, LSESR, sabal

Reported uses

Used as a mild diuretic; also used to treat such GU problems as BPH and to increase sperm production, breast size, and sexual vigor.

Common forms

As tablets, capsules, teas, berries (fresh or dried), and liquid extract.

Actions

Has an anti-inflammatory effect and inhibits prolactin and growth factor–induced prostatic cell proliferation. May inhibit hormonally induced prostate enlargement.

Dosages

▶ **For BPH.** 320 mg P.O. daily in two divided doses for 3 months. Other recommendations include 1 to 2 g fresh saw palmetto berries or 0.5 to 1 g dried berry in decoction P.O. t.i.d.

Adverse reactions

CNS: headache.
CV: hypertension.
GI: abdominal pain, constipation, diarrhea, nausea.
GU: dysuria, impotence, urine retention.
Musculoskeletal: back pain.
Other: decreased libido.

Interactions

Herb-drug. *Adrenergics, hormones, hormone-like drugs:* possible estrogen, androgen, and alpha-blocking effects. Drug dosages may need adjustment if patient takes this herb. Monitor patient closely.

Cautions

- Pregnant or breast-feeding women and women of childbearing age shouldn't use this herb.
- Adults and children with hormone-dependent illnesses other than BPH or breast cancer should avoid this herb.

NURSING CONSIDERATIONS

- Find out why patient is using the herb.
- Herb should be used cautiously for conditions other than BPH because data about its effectiveness in other conditions is lacking.
- Obtain a baseline prostate-specific antigen (PSA) test before patient starts taking herb because it may cause a false-negative PSA result.
- Saw palmetto may not alter prostate size.

Patient teaching
- Tell the patient that, when filling a new prescription, he should remind the pharmacist of any herbal or dietary supplement he's taking.
- Warn patient not to take herb for bladder or prostate problems before seeking medical attention because doing so could delay diagnosis of a potentially serious medical condition.

• Tell patient to take herb with food to minimize GI effects.

valerian

(veh-LEHR-ee-ehn)

all heal, amantilla, herba benedicta, katzenwurzel, phu germanicum, phu parvum

Reported uses

Used to treat menstrual cramps, restlessness and sleep disorders from nervous conditions, and other symptoms of psychological stress, such as anxiety, nervous headaches, and gastric spasms. Used topically as a bath additive for restlessness and sleep disorders.

Common forms

As standardized capsules, tablets, and tinctures; also as tinctures and teas containing crude dried herb and in combination with other dietary supplements.

Standardized capsules, tablets (0.8% valerenic acid): 250 mg, 400 mg, 450 mg, 493 mg, 530 mg, 550 mg.

Standardized tinctures: 2% essential oil.

Actions

May exhibit a sedative effect and weak anticonvulsant and antidepressant properties. Also has antispasmodic effects on GI smooth muscle, produces coronary dilation, and has antiarrhythmic activity.

Dosages

Bath additive: 100 g of root mixed with 2 L of hot water and added to one full bath.

Tea: 1 cup P.O. b.i.d. to t.i.d., and h.s.

Tincture (1:5 in 45% to 50% alcohol)*: 15 to 20 gtt in water several times daily.

▶ **For hastening sleep and improving sleep quality.** 400 to 800 mg root P.O. up to 2 hours before h.s. Some patients need 2 to 4 weeks of use for significant improvement. Maximum, 15 g daily.

▶ **For restlessness.** 220 mg of extract P.O. t.i.d.

Adverse reactions

CNS: excitability, headache, insomnia.
CV: cardiac disturbance.
EENT: blurred vision.
GI: nausea.
Other: hypersensitivity reactions.

Interactions

Herb-drug. *Barbiturates, benzodiazepines:* possible additive effects. Monitor patient closely.
CNS depressants: potential additive effects. Discourage concomitant use.
Disulfiram: disulfiram reaction may occur if herbal extract or tincture contains alcohol. Discourage concomitant use.
Herb-herb. *Herbs with sedative effects, such as catnip, hops, kava, passion flower, skullcap:* may potentiate sedative effects. Monitor patient closely.
Herb-lifestyle. *Alcohol use:* May potentiate sedative effects. Advise patient to avoid using together.

Cautions

• Patients with history of allergy to valerian shouldn't use this herb.
• Patients with hepatic impairment shouldn't use this herb because of the risk of hepatotoxicity.
• Pregnant and breast-feeding women should avoid this herb; effects are unknown.
• Patients with acute or major skin injuries, fever, infectious diseases, cardiac insufficiency, or hypertonia shouldn't bathe with valerian products.

NURSING CONSIDERATIONS

• Valerian seems to have a more pronounced effect on those with disturbed sleep or sleep disorders.
• Evidence of valerian toxicity includes difficulty walking, hypothermia, and increased muscle relaxation.
• Withdrawal symptoms, such as increased agitation and decreased sleep, can occur if valerian is abruptly stopped after prolonged use.

* Liquid may contain alcohol.

Patient teaching

- Warn patient not to take herb for insomnia before seeking medical attention because doing so may delay diagnosis of a potentially serious medical condition.
- Tell the patient that, when filling a new prescription, he should remind the pharmacist of any herbal or dietary supplement he's taking.
- If patient takes valerian, explain that herb may take 2 to 4 weeks to take effect.
- Inform patient that many extract products contain 40% to 60% alcohol and may not be appropriate for all patients.
- Inform patient that most adverse effects occur only after long-term use.

Appendices and Index

Selected topical antibacterials

Drug	Indications	Dosages
bacitracin	▶Topical infections, impetigo, abrasions, cuts, and minor burns or wounds.	▶*Adults and children:* apply thin film b.i.d., t.i.d., or p.r.n., depending on severity.
chloramphenicol	▶Superficial skin infections.	▶*Adults and children:* after thoroughly cleaning the skin, rub into infected area b.i.d. or t.i.d.
clindamycin phosphate	▶Acne vulgaris. ▶Bacterial vaginosis.	▶*Adults and adolescents:* apply b.i.d., morning and evening. ▶*Adults:* 100 mg intravaginally h.s. for 7 consecutive days.
erythromycin	▶Inflammatory acne vulgaris.	▶*Adults and children:* apply to affected area b.i.d.
gentamicin sulfate	▶Superficial skin infections.	▶*Adults and children over age 1:* rub in small amount gently t.i.d. or q.i.d., with or without gauze dressing.
mafenide acetate	▶Adjunct treatment of second- and third-degree burns.	▶*Adults and children:* apply 1⁄16″ thickness of cream daily or b.i.d. to clean, debrided wounds. Reapply p.r.n. to keep burned area covered.
metronidazole	▶Acne rosacea. ▶Bacterial vaginosis.	▶*Adults:* apply a thin film to affected area b.i.d., a.m. and p.m. Frequency and duration of therapy is adjusted after response is seen. ▶*Adults:* 1 applicatorful b.i.d., a.m. and p.m., for 5 days.
mupirocin	▶Impetigo.	▶*Adults and children:* apply to affected areas t.i.d. for 1 to 2 weeks.
neomycin sulfate	▶Prevention or treatment of superficial bacterial infections.	▶*Adults and children:* rub into affected area one to three times daily.
nitrofurazone	▶Adjunctive treatment of second- and third-degree burns; prevention of skin allograft infection.	▶*Adults and children:* apply directly to lesion daily or every few days, depending on severity of burn. May also be applied to dressings used to cover affected area.
silver sulfadiazine	▶Prevention and treatment of wound infection in second-and third-degree burns.	▶*Adults and children:* apply 1⁄16″ thickness to clean debrided burn wound daily or b.i.d.
tetracycline hydrochloride	▶Acne vulgaris. ▶Superficial skin infections.	▶*Adults and children over age 12:* rub generously into affected areas b.i.d. until skin is thoroughly covered. ▶*Adults and children:* apply to affected area once to five times daily.

(continued)

Cautions	Special considerations
• Topical antibacterial drugs are contraindicated in patients hypersensitive to them. If patient shows signs of hypersensitivity, withhold drug and notify prescriber immediately. • Prolonged use of antibacterial drugs may result in overgrowth of nonsusceptible organisms. • Use mafenide cautiously in patients with acute renal failure. • Use metronidazole cautiously in patients with history or evidence of blood dyscrasia; chemically related compounds have caused blood dyscrasia. • Use mupirocin cautiously in patients with burns or impaired renal function. • Use neomycin cautiously in patients with extensive dermatologic conditions. • Use nitrofurazone cautiously in patients with known or suspected renal impairment. • Use mafenide and silver sulfadiazine cautiously in patients hypersensitive to sulfonamides. • Use tetracycline cautiously in patients with hepatic or renal impairment.	• As appropriate, clean the area before applying drug, especially if patient has crusted or suppurative lesions. • Some topical antibacterial drugs may need to be supplemented by appropriate systemic drugs for all but very superficial infections. • Teach the patient how to apply the prescribed drug. • Instruct the patient to avoid getting drug in eyes and mouth. • Tell patient to continue using drug for full prescribed treatment period, even if his condition improves. • Advise patient to store drug at room temperature and protect from excessive heat. • Tell patient not to share drug with anyone. • Tell patient to notify prescriber if condition gets worse or fails to improve.

Selected topical corticosteroids

Drug	Indications	Dosages
alclometasone dipropionate	▶ Inflammation associated with corticosteroid-responsive dermatoses.	▶ *Adults:* apply a thin film to affected areas b.i.d. or t.i.d. Gently massage until drug disappears.
amcinonide	▶ Inflammation associated with corticosteroid-responsive dermatoses.	▶ *Adults and children:* apply a light film to affected areas b.i.d. or t.i.d. Rub cream in gently and thoroughly until it disappears.
betamethasone benzoate	▶ Inflammation associated with corticosteroid-responsive dermatoses.	▶ *Adults and children:* clean area; apply sparingly daily to q.i.d.
clobetasol propionate	▶ Inflammation associated with corticosteroid-responsive dermatoses.	▶ *Adults:* apply a thin layer to affected skin areas b.i.d., in the morning and evening for a maximum of 14 days. Total dosage should not exceed 50 g weekly.
desonide	▶ Inflammation associated with corticosteroid-responsive dermatoses.	▶ *Adults and children:* clean area; apply sparingly b.i.d. to q.i.d.
desoximetasone	▶ Inflammation associated with corticosteroid-responsive dermatoses.	▶ *Adults and children:* clean area; apply sparingly b.i.d.
dexamethasone dexamethasone sodium phosphate	▶ Inflammation associated with corticosteroid-responsive dermatoses.	▶ *Adults and children:* clean area; apply sparingly t.i.d. to q.i.d.
diflorasone diacetate	▶ Inflammation associated with corticosteroid-responsive dermatoses.	▶ *Adults and children:* clean area; apply sparingly in a thin film. Apply daily to q.i.d. as determined by severity.
fluocinolone acetonide	▶ Inflammation associated with corticosteroid-responsive dermatoses.	▶ *Adults and children over age 2:* clean area; apply sparingly b.i.d. to q.i.d.
fluocinonide	▶ Inflammation associated with corticosteroid-responsive dermatoses.	▶ *Adults and children:* clean area; apply sparingly b.i.d. or t.i.d.
flurandrenolide	▶ Inflammation associated with corticosteroid-responsive dermatoses.	▶ *Adults and children:* clean area; apply sparingly daily to q.i.d. Apply Cordran tape q 12 hours.
fluticasone propionate	▶ Inflammation associated with corticosteroid-responsive dermatoses.	▶ *Adults:* apply sparingly to affected area b.i.d. and rub in gently and completely.
halcinonide	▶ Inflammation associated with corticosteroid-responsive dermatoses.	▶ *Adults and children:* clean area; apply sparingly b.i.d. or t.i.d.

(continued)

Drug	Indications	Dosages
halobetasol propionate	▶ Inflammation associated with corticosteroid-responsive dermatoses.	▶ *Adults:* apply sparingly to affected area once daily or b.i.d. and rub in gently and completely. Treatment beyond 2 consecutive weeks is not recommended. Total dosage should not exceed 50 g weekly.
hydrocortisone hydrocortisone acetate hydrocortisone butyrate hydrocortisone valerate	▶ Inflammation associated with corticosteroid-responsive dermatoses; adjunctive topical management of seborrheic dermatitis of scalp. ▶ Inflammation associated with proctitis.	▶ *Adults and children:* clean area; apply cream, gel, lotion, ointment, or topical solution sparingly daily to q.i.d. Spray aerosol onto affected area daily until acute phase is controlled; then reduce dosage to one to three times weekly as needed. ▶ *Adults:* 1 applicatorful of rectal foam P.R. daily or b.i.d. for 2 to 3 weeks, then every other day as necessary.
mometasone furoate	▶ Inflammation associated with corticosteroid-responsive dermatoses.	▶ *Adults:* apply to affected areas once daily.
triamcinolone acetonide	▶ Inflammation associated with corticosteroid-responsive dermatoses. ▶ Inflammation associated with oral lesions.	▶ *Adults and children:* clean area; apply cream, lotion, or ointment sparingly b.i.d. to q.i.d., or spray b.i.d. or q.i.d. ▶ *Adults and children:* apply paste h.s. and, if needed, b.i.d. or t.i.d., preferably after meals. Apply a small amount without rubbing and press to lesion in mouth until a thin film develops.

Cautions	Special considerations
• Topical corticosteroids are contraindicated in patients hypersensitive to them or other corticosteroids. • Fluticasone propionate is also contraindicated in patients with viral, fungal, herpetic, or tubercular skin lesions. • Children have an increased risk of adrenal suppression, Cushing's syndrome, intracranial hypertension, and growth retardation with improper use of drug. Make sure parents or patient fully understand correct use of drug. • Elderly patients have an increased risk of purpura and skin lacerations and should be monitored closely.	• Gently wash skin before applying drug. Rub drug in gently, leaving a thin coat. When treating hairy sites, part the hair and apply drug directly to lesions. • Avoid eyes, mucous membranes, and inside ear canal; topical corticosteroids may be safely used on the face, groin, armpits, and undersides of breasts. • If an occlusive dressing is ordered, don't leave it in place longer than 16 hours each day; don't use occlusive dressings on infected or exudative lesions. • For patients with eczematous dermatitis whose skin may be irritated by adhesive material, hold dressings in place with gauze, elastic bandages, stockings, or stockinette. • Notify prescriber and remove occlusive dressing if fever develops. • Change dressing as ordered. • Stop drug and notify prescriber if patient develops skin infection, striae, or atrophy.

Cautions	Special considerations
	• When using an aerosol form around the face, cover the patient's eyes and warn him not to inhale the spray. Aerosols contains alcohol and may cause irritation or burning in open lesions. Don't spray longer than 3 seconds or closer than 6" (15 cm) to avoid freezing of tissues. Apply to dry scalp after shampooing; no need to massage medication into scalp after spraying. • If antifungals or antibiotics are used concomitantly, stop corticosteroids until infection is controlled, as ordered. • Monitor patient for systemic adverse reactions. Systemic absorption is likely with use of occlusive dressings, prolonged treatment, or treatment of extensive body surface area. • Avoid using plastic pants or tight-fitting diapers on treated areas in young children. Children may absorb larger amounts of drug and be more prone to systemic toxicity. • To prevent recurrence, continue treatment for a few days after lesions clear, as ordered. • Repeated application of some topical corticosteroids leads to reduced effectiveness. • Stop drug and notify prescriber if the patient develops signs of systemic absorption, skin irritation or ulceration, hypersensitivity, or infection. • Teach patient how to apply the drug. • Teach the patient how to apply an occlusive dressing, if ordered. Tell the patient not to leave it on each day for longer than 16 hours and to stop the drug and notify the doctor if a fever occurs. • Tell the patient to stop the drug and notify the doctor if signs of systemic absorption, skin irritation or ulceration, hypersensitivity, or infection occur. • Stress importance of using the drug exactly as directed and not to exceed frequency of application or dosage. • Tell the breast-feeding woman not to apply a topical corticosteroid preparation to her breast before breast-feeding. • Instruct patient to apply a missed dose of drug as soon as possible. However, if it's almost time for the next dose, he should skip the missed dose and resume the normal schedule. Caution against doubling the dose. • Warn patient that some topical corticosteroids contain alcohol and may cause burning or irritation in open lesions. Tell patient to notify prescriber if burning and irritation persist. • If patient will be using Cordran tape, tell him to cut it with scissors rather than tearing it. • Instruct the patient on proper storage of the drug.

Selected ophthalmic anti-infectives

Drug	Indications	Dosages
bacitracin	▶ Ocular infections.	▶ *Adults and children:* small amount of ointment applied into conjunctival sac once daily to t.i.d.
chloramphenicol	▶ Surface bacterial infection involving conjunctiva or cornea.	▶ *Adults and children:* 2 drops of solution or a small amount of ointment to affected eye q 3 hours or more frequently, as instructed by the doctor, for the first 48 hours. Then, the interval between applications may be increased. Treatment should continue for 48 hours after the eye appears normal.
ciprofloxacin hydrochloride	▶ Corneal ulcers.	▶ *Adults and children over age 12:* 2 drops in the affected eye q 15 minutes for the first 6 hours; then 2 drops q 30 minutes for the remainder of the first day. On day 2, 2 drops hourly. On days 3 to 14, 2 drops q 4 hours.
	▶ Bacterial conjunctivitis.	▶ *Adults and children over age 12:* 1 or 2 drops into the conjunctival sac of the affected eye q 2 hours while awake, for the first 2 days. Then 1 or 2 drops q 4 hours while awake, for the next 5 days.
erythromycin	▶ Acute and chronic conjunctivitis, trachoma, other eye infections.	▶ *Adults and children:* 1 cm in length applied directly to the infected eye up to six times daily, depending on the severity of infection.
	▶ Ophthalmia neonatorum.	▶ *Neonates:* a ribbon of ointment about 1 cm long applied in the lower conjunctival sac of each eye shortly after birth.
gentamicin sulfate	▶ External ocular infections (conjunctivitis, keratoconjunctivitis, corneal ulcers, blepharitis, blepharoconjunctivitis, meibomianitis, and dacryocystitis).	▶ *Adults and children:* 1 or 2 drops instilled in eye q 4 hours. In severe infections, up to 2 drops q hour. Or, ointment applied to lower conjunctival sac b.i.d. or t.i.d.
idoxuridine	▶ Herpes simplex keratitis.	▶ *Adults and children:* 1 drop of solution into conjunctival sac q hour during day and q 2 hours at night until improvement; then decreased to 1 drop q 2 hours during day and q 4 hours at night. If no response occurs in 7 days, drug is discontinued.
natamycin	▶ Fungal keratitis.	▶ *Adults:* 1 drop in conjunctival sac q 1 to 2 hours. After 3 to 4 days, 1 drop six to eight times daily.
	▶ Blepharitis or fungal conjunctivitis.	▶ *Adults:* 1 drop q 4 to 6 hours.

Drug	Indications	Dosages
norfloxacin	▶ Conjunctivitis.	▶ *Adults and children 1 year and over:* 1 or 2 drops in affected eye q.i.d. for up to 7 days. If condition warrants, 2 drops q 2 hours during waking hours of first day of treatment.
ofloxacin 0.3%	▶ Conjunctivitis.	▶ *Adults and children over age 1:* 1 to 2 drops in conjunctival sac q 2 to 4 hours while awake for first 2 days, and then q.i.d. for 5 days.
polymyxin B sulfate	▶ Superficial eye infections involving the conjunctiva and cornea.	▶ *Adults and children:* 1 to 3 drops of 0.1% to 0.25% (10,000 to 25,000 units/ml) q hour until favorable response occurs. Not to exceed 2 million units daily. Or, apply small amount of ointment q 3 to 4 hours for 7 to 10 days depending on the severity of the infection.
silver nitrate 1%	▶ Gonorrheal ophthalmia neonatorum.	▶ *Neonates:* 2 drops of 1% solution into the lower conjunctival sac of each eye at angle of the nasal bridge and eyes, no later than 1 hour after delivery.
sulfacetamide sodium 10% sulfacetamide sodium 15% sulfacetamide sodium 30%	▶ Inclusion conjunctivitis, corneal ulcers, trachoma, prophylaxis to ocular infection.	▶ *Adults and children:* 1 to 2 drops of 10% solution instilled into lower conjunctival sac q 2 to 3 hours during day, less often at night; or 1 to 2 drops of 15% solution instilled into lower conjunctival sac q 1 to 2 hours initially. Interval increased as condition responds; or 1 drop of 30% solution instilled into lower conjunctival sac q 2 hours. 1.25 to 2.5 cm 10% ointment applied into conjunctival sac q.i.d. and h.s. Ointment may be used at night along with drops during the day.
sulfisoxazole diolamine	▶ Conjunctivitis, corneal ulcers, and other superficial ocular infections; adjunct in systemic sulfonamide therapy of trachoma.	▶ *Adults:* 1 to 2 drops instilled in the conjunctival sac q 1 to 4 hours daily.
tobramycin	▶ External ocular infections.	▶ *Adults and children:* in mild to moderate infections, 1 or 2 drops into affected eye q 4 to 6 hours. In severe infections, 2 drops into infected eye q hour until condition improves; then frequency reduced. Or, a thin strip of ointment applied into conjunctival sac t.i.d. or q.i.d.
trifluridine	▶ Primary keratoconjunctivitis and recurrent epithelial keratitis caused by herpes simplex virus, types I and II.	▶ *Adults:* 1 drop of solution into affected eye q 2 hours while patient is awake, to a maximum of 9 drops daily until corneal ulcer reepithelialization occurs; then 1 drop q 4 hours (minimum 5 drops daily) for an additional 7 days. Trifluridine should not be used for more than 21days continuously because of the risk of ocular toxicity.

(continued)

Drug	Indications	Dosages
vidarabine	▶ Acute keratoconjunctivitis, superficial keratitis, and recurrent epithelial keratitis resulting from herpes simplex type I and II.	▶ *Adults and children:* 1 cm ointment applied into lower conjunctival sac five times daily at 3-hour intervals.

Cautions	Special considerations
• Ophthalmic anti-infectives are contraindicated in patients hypersensitive to them. • Bacitracin is contraindicated in atopic patients. • Ciprofloxacin, norfloxacin, and ofloxacin 0.3% are contraindicated in patients with a history of hypersensitivity to other fluoroquinolone antibiotics. • Ofloxacin 0.3% is also contraindicated in breast-feeding women. • Sulfacetamide sodium and sulfisoxazole diolamine are contraindicated in children younger than age 2 months. • Sulfisoxazole diolamine is also contraindicated in pregnant women who are at term and in breast-feeding women. • Use ciprofloxacin cautiously in breast-feeding women. • Use gentamicin cautiously in patients with history of sensitivity to aminoglycosides; cross-sensitivity may occur. • Before giving, ask the patient about past allergic reactions to the drug.	• When using chloramphenicol, reconstitute powder for solution with supplied diluent. Use 5 ml of diluent to make a 0.5% solution, 10 ml to make a 0.25% solution, or 15 ml to make a 0.16% solution. • Shake suspensions well before using them. • Clean excessive exudate from eye area before application. • After instilling eye drops, apply light finger pressure on lacrimal sac for 1 minute to help prevent systemic absorption. • When instilling more than one drop, wait 2 to 3 minutes between drops to avoid losing a drop from tearing or blinking. • When using two different ophthalmic solutions, allow at least 5 minutes between instillations. • Don't mix idoxuridine with other topical ophthalmics. • When applying eye ointment, have patient look up while you pull the lower eyelid down. As patient continues to look up, apply a thin ribbon of ointment into the conjunctival sac, beginning at the inner canthus. • To avoid contamination, don't let tube touch patient's eye or conjunctiva. At the outer canthus, rotate the tube to detach the ointment. • Have the patient gently close the eye containing the ointment, but caution him not to squeeze it closed. • If the patient has more than a superficial infection, anticipate using systemic therapy as well. • Start appropriate therapy if superinfection develops. Prolonged use of some ophthalmic anti-infectives may result in overgrowth of nonsusceptible organisms, including fungi. • Store drug in tightly closed, light-resistant container at room temperature (except iodoxuridine and trifluridine which must be refrigerated) unless otherwise directed. • Tell patient to take drug as prescribed, even after he feels better; if the drug is stopped too soon, infection may return. • Teach patient how to clean eye area before and how to apply the prescribed drug. Tell him to wash his hands before and after administration, and caution him not to touch tip of tube to eye or surrounding tissue. • If patient uses ointment form, tell him that only a small amount is needed. • If patient uses eye drops, tell him to apply light finger pressure on the lacrimal sac for 1 minute after drops are instilled. • Tell patient to wait at least 5 minutes before administering other eye drops. • If patient uses suspension, tell him to shake container well before using.

Cautions	Special considerations
	• Caution patient not to use discolored solutions. • Tell patient to take a missed dose as soon as he remembers. However, if almost time for the next dose, he should skip the missed dose and resume regular dosing schedule. • Warn the patient that ophthalmic anti-infective drugs may blur vision temporarily. Remind him to take safety precautions until vision clears. • Advise patient to watch for signs of sensitivity, such as itching lids, swelling, or constant burning. If such signs develop, tell him to stop drug and notify prescriber immediately. • Caution patient not to use leftover ophthalmic anti-infective medication for a new eye infection. Adverse reactions may occur, or the drug may have lost potency. • Tell patient to discard medication when therapy has ended. • Advise patient not to share eye medications, washcloths, or towels with family members. • Warn patient to notify prescriber immediately if other family members develop similar ocular symptoms. • Stress the importance of compliance with recommended therapy, even when the patient is feeling better. • Instruct the patient to notify prescriber if eye condition worsens or fails to improve. • Tell patient that some eye medications cause photophobia; suggest that he wear sunglasses and avoid prolonged exposure to sunlight. • Instruct patient to store drug in a tightly closed, light-resistant container at room temperature (except idoxuridine and trifluridine), unless otherwise instructed. • Tell patient to keep eye medication out of the reach of children.

Selected ophthalmic anti-inflammatories

Drug	Indications	Dosages
dexamethasone dexamethasone sodium phosphate	▶ Uveitis; iridocyclitis; inflammatory conditions of eyelids, conjunctiva, cornea, anterior segment of globe; corneal injury from chemical or thermal burns, or penetration of foreign bodies; allergic conjunctivitis.	▶ *Adults and children:* 1 to 2 drops of suspension or solution or 1.25 to 2.5 cm of ointment into conjunctival sac. In severe disease, drops may be used hourly, tapering to discontinuation as condition improves. In mild conditions, drops may be used up to six times daily or ointment applied t.i.d. or q.i.d. As condition improves, dosage tapered to b.i.d., then once daily. Treatment may last up to several weeks.
diclofenac sodium 0.1%	▶ Postoperative inflammation following removal of cataract.	▶ *Adults:* 1 drop in conjunctival sac q.i.d., beginning 24 hours after surgery and continuing for 2 weeks.
fluorometholone	▶ Inflammation of cornea, conjunctiva, sclera, anterior uvea.	▶ *Adults and children:* 1 to 2 drops in conjunctival sac b.i.d. to q.i.d. May be given q hour during first 1 to 2 days or 1.25 cm of ointment to conjunctival sac q 4 hours, decreasing to once to three times daily as inflammation subsides.
flurbiprofen sodium	▶ Inhibition of intraoperative miosis.	▶ *Adults:* 1 drop into eye undergoing surgery about every ½ hour, beginning 2 hours before surgery. A total of 4 drops is given.
ketorolac tromethamine	▶ Relief of itching caused by allergic conjunctivitis. ▶ Treatment of postoperative inflammation in patients who have undergone cataract extraction.	▶ *Adults:* 1 drop into conjunctival sac q.i.d. ▶ *Adults:* 1 drop in the operative eye(s) q.i.d. starting 24 hours after cataract surgery and continued throughout the first 2 weeks.
medrysone	▶ Allergic conjunctivitis, vernal conjunctivitis, episcleritis, ophthalmic epinephrine sensitivity reaction.	▶ *Adults and children:* 1 drop in conjunctival sac b.i.d. to q.i.d. May use q hour during first 1 to 2 days.
prednisolone acetate prednisolone sodium phosphate (solution)	▶ Inflammation of palpebral and bulbar conjunctiva, cornea, and anterior segment of globe.	▶ *Adults and children:* 1 to 2 drops instilled in eye. In severe conditions, may be used hourly, tapering to discontinuation as inflammation subsides. In mild conditions, may be used up to six times daily.
rimexolone	▶ Postoperative inflammation following ocular surgery.	▶ *Adults:* 1 to 2 drops in the conjunctival sac q.i.d., beginning 24 hours after surgery and continuing throughout the first 2 weeks of the postoperative period.

Drug	Indications	Dosages
rimexolone *(continued)*	▶ Anterior uveitis.	▶ *Adults:* 1 to 2 drops in the conjunctival sac q hour during waking hours for the first week, 1 drop q 2 hours during waking hours of the second week, and then tapered until uveitis is resolved.
suprofen	▶ Inhibition of intraoperative miosis.	▶ *Adults:* 2 drops instilled into the conjunctival sac q 4 hours the day before surgery. On the day of surgery, 2 drops instilled 3 hours, 2 hours, and 1 hour before surgery.

Cautions	Special considerations
• Ophthalmic anti-inflammatory drugs have a variety of precautions. Check manufacturer's warnings before administering any of these drugs. • Ophthalmic anti-inflammatory drugs are contraindicated in patients hypersensitive to them. • Dexamethasone, dexamethasone sodium phosphate, fluorometholone, medrysone, prednisolone acetate, prednisolone sodium phosphate, and rimexolone are contraindicated in patients with acute superficial herpes simplex (dendritic keratitis), vaccinia, varicella, or other fungal or viral disease of cornea and conjunctiva; ocular tuberculosis; or acute, purulent, untreated infections of the eye. • Diclofenac sodium 0.1% and ketorolac tromethamine are contraindicated in patients wearing soft contact lenses. • Diclofenac sodium 0.1% is also contraindicated during late pregnancy. • Suprofen is contraindicated in patients with epithelial herpes simplex keratitis.	• Corneal viral and fungal infections may be worsened by use of an ophthalmic anti-inflammatory. • Ophthalmic anti-inflammatory drugs usually aren't intended for long-term use and may delay wound healing if used. • Check with prescriber to determine whether patient should wear an eye pad after ointment application. • When administering eye drops, apply light finger pressure on the lacrimal sac for about 1 minute after instillation. Tell patient to do so as well if he applies the drug. • Notify presciber immediately if patient complains of visual disturbance. Also notify prescriber if patient's ocular condition fails to improve or becomes worse. • Teach patient how to apply drug. Remind him to wash hands before and after administration, and caution him not to let tube or dropper tip contact eye or surrounding tissue. • Instruct the patient using a suspension to shake it well before use. • Warn patient not to use leftover medication for a new eye inflammation; it may cause serious problems. • Urge patient to stop drug and call prescriber immediately if visual acuity changes or visual field diminishes. • Tell patient not to share eye medications, washcloths, or towels with family members. If anyone develops similar symptoms, tell patient to notify prescriber.

Selected otic drugs

Drug	Indications	Dosages
acetic acid	▶ External ear canal infection.	▶ *Adults and children:* 4 to 6 drops into ear canal q 2 to 3 hours; or insert saturated wick for first 24 hours, then continue with instillations.
carbamide peroxide	▶ Impacted cerumen.	▶ *Adults and children age 12 and over:* 5 to 10 drops into ear canal b.i.d. for 3 to 4 days. Allow solution to remain in ear canal for 15 to 30 minutes; remove with warm water.
chloramphenicol	▶ External ear canal infection.	▶ *Adults and children:* 2 to 3 drops into ear canal t.i.d. or q.i.d.
triethanolamine polypeptide oleate-condensate	▶ Impacted cerumen.	▶ *Adults and children:* fill ear canal with solution and insert cotton plug. After 15 to 30 minutes, flush ear with warm water.

Cautions	Special considerations
• Otic drugs are contraindicated in patients with perforated eardrums. • Triethanolamine polypeptide oleate-condensate is also contraindicated in patients with otitis media and otitis externa.	• Reculture persistent drainage. • Watch for signs of superinfection (continual pain, inflammation, fever). • Teach patient or caregiver how to administer drug. • Warn patient or caregiver to avoid touching the ear with the dropper to prevent reinfection. • Tell patient using a cotton plug to moisten it with medication. • Instruct patient to keep container tightly closed and protected from moisture and heat.

Normal laboratory test values

Hematology

Activated partial thromboplastin time
25 to 36 seconds

Hematocrit
Males: 42% to 54%
Females: 38% to 46%

Hemoglobin, total
Males: 14 to 18 g/dl
Females: 12 to 16 g/dl

Platelet count
140,000 to 400,000/mm^3

Prothrombin time
10 to 14 seconds; INR for patients on warfarin therapy, 2 to 3 (those with pediatric heart valve, 2.5 to 3.5)

Red blood cell (RBC) count
Males: 4.5 to 6.2 million/mm^3 venous blood
Females: 4.2 to 5.4 million/mm^3 venous blood

RBC indices
Mean corpuscular volume: 84 to 99 femtoliter
Mean corpuscular hemoglobin: 26 to 32 picograms/cell
Mean corpuscular hemoglobin concentration: 30 to 36 grams/deciliter

Reticulocyte count
0.5% to 2% of total RBC count

White blood cell (WBC) count
4,100 to 10,900/mm^3

WBC differential, blood
Neutrophils: 47.6% to 76.8%
Lymphocytes: 16.2% to 43%
Monocytes: 0.6% to 9.6%
Eosinophils: 0.3% to 7%
Basophils: 0.3% to 2%

Blood chemistry

Alanine aminotransferase
Males: 10 to 35 units/L
Females: 9 to 24 units/L

Alkaline phosphatase, serum
Males ≥ age 19: 98 to 251 units/L
Females ages 24 to 65: 81 to 282 units/L
Females ≥ age 65: 119 to 309 units/L

Amylase, serum
Age ≥ 18: 35 to 115 units/L

Arterial blood gases
Pao_2: 75 to 100 mm Hg
$Paco_2$: 35 to 45 mm Hg
pH: 7.35 to 7.45
SaO_2: 94% to 100%
HCO_3^-: 22 to 26 mEq/L

Aspartate aminotransferase
Males: 8 to 20 units/L
Females: 5 to 40 units/L

Bilirubin, serum
Adults: direct, < 0.5 mg/dl; indirect, 1.1 mg/dl

Blood urea nitrogen
8 to 20 mg/dl

Calcium, serum
Males ≥ age 22, females ≥ age 19: 8.9 to 10.1 mg/dl

Carbon dioxide, total, blood
22 to 34 mEq/L

Chloride, serum
100 to 108 mEq/L

Creatine kinase (CK)
Total: Males ≥ age 18, 52 to 336 units/L; females ≥ age 18, 38 to 176 units/L
CK-BB: None
CK-MB: 0 to 7 units/L
CK-MM: 5 to 70 units/L

Creatine, serum
Males: 0.2 to 0.6 mg/dl
Females: 0.6 to 1 mg/dl

Creatinine, serum
Males: 0.8 to 1.2 mg/dl
Females: 0.6 to 0.9 mg/dl

Glucose, fasting, plasma
70 to 100 mg/dl

Lactate dehydrogenase (LD)
Total: 48 to 115 IU/L
LD_1: 14% to 26%
LD_2: 29% to 39%
LD_3: 20% to 26%
LD_4: 8% to 16%
LD_5: 6% to 16%

Magnesium, serum
1.5 to 2.5 mEq/L
Atomic absorption: 1.7 to 2.1 mg/dl

Phosphates, serum
1.8 to 2.6 mEq/L
Atomic absorption: 2.5 to 4.5 mg/dl

Potassium, serum
3.8 to 5.5 mEq/L

Protein, total, serum
26.6 to 7.9 g/dl
Albumin fraction: 3.3 to 4.5 g/dl

Sodium, serum
135 to 145 mEq/L

Uric acid, serum
Males: 4.3 to 8 mg/dl
Females: 2.3 to 6 mg/dl

Table of equivalents

Metric system equivalents

Metric weight

1 kilogram (kg or Kg)	=	1,000 grams (g or gm)
1 gram	=	1,000 milligrams (mg)
1 milligram	=	1,000 micrograms (µg or mcg)
0.6 g	=	600 mg
0.3 g	=	300 mg
0.1 g	=	100 mg
0.06 g	=	60 mg
0.03 g	=	30 mg
0.015 g	=	15 mg
0.001 g	=	1 mg

Metric volume

1 liter (l or L)	=	1,000 milliiters (ml)*
1 milliliter	=	1,000 microliters (µl)

Household		Metric
1 teaspoon (tsp)	=	5 ml
1 tablespoon (T or tbs)	=	15 ml
2 tablespoons	=	30 ml
8 ounces (oz)	=	240 ml
1 pint (pt)	=	473 ml
1 quart (qt)	=	946 ml
1 gallon (gal)	=	3,785 ml

Temperature conversions

Fahrenheit degrees	Centigrade degrees	Fahrenheit degrees	Centigrade degrees	Fahrenheit degrees	Centigrade degrees
106.0	41.1	100.6	38.1	95.2	35.1
105.8	41.0	100.4	38.0	95.0	35.0
105.6	40.9	100.2	37.9	94.8	34.9
105.4	40.8	100.0	37.8	94.6	34.8
105.2	40.7	99.8	37.7	94.4	34.7
105.0	40.6	99.6	37.6	94.2	34.6
104.8	40.4	99.4	37.4	94.0	34.4
104.6	40.3	99.2	37.3	93.8	34.3
104.4	40.2	99.0	37.2	93.6	34.2
104.2	40.1	98.8	37.1	93.4	34.1
104.0	40.0	98.6	37.0	93.2	34.0
103.8	39.9	98.4	36.9	93.0	33.9
103.6	39.8	98.2	36.8	92.8	33.8
103.4	39.7	98.0	36.7	92.6	33.7
103.2	39.6	97.8	36.5	92.4	33.6
103.0	39.4	97.6	36.4	92.2	33.4
102.8	39.3	97.4	36.3	92.0	33.3
102.6	39.2	97.2	36.2	91.8	33.2
102.4	39.1	97.0	36.1	91.6	33.1
102.2	39.0	96.8	36.0	91.4	33.0
102.0	38.9	96.6	35.9	91.2	32.9
101.8	38.8	96.4	35.8	91.0	32.8
101.6	38.7	96.2	35.7	90.8	32.7
101.4	38.6	96.0	35.6	90.6	32.6
101.2	38.4	95.8	35.4	90.4	32.4
101.0	38.3	95.6	35.3	90.2	32.3
100.8	38.2	95.4	35.2	90.0	32.2

Weight conversions

1 oz = 30 g   1 lb = 453.6 g   2.2 lb = 1 kg

*1 ml = 1 cubic centimeter (cc); however, ml is the preferred measurement term.

Estimating surface area in children

Pediatric drug dosages should be calculated on the basis of body surface area or body weight. If the child is of average size, find his weight and corresponding surface area in the box. Otherwise, to use the nomogram, lay a straightedge on the correct height and weight points for the patient, and observe the point where it intersects on the surface area scale. Note: Don't use drug dosages based on body surface area in premature or full-term newborns. Instead, use body weight.

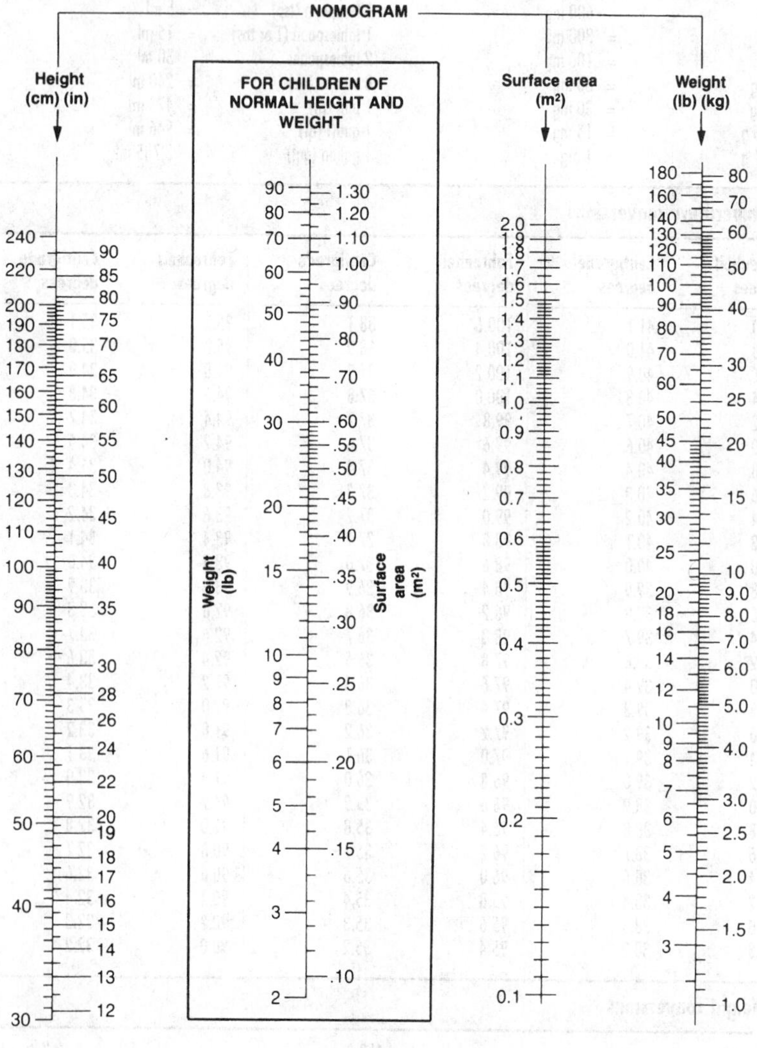

Behrman, R.E., et al. *Nelson Textbook of Pediatrics,* 15th edition.1996. Courtesy W.B.Saunders Co., Philadelphia.

Drugs that shouldn't be crushed

Many drug forms—such as slow-release, enteric-coated, encapsulated beads, wax-matrix, sublingual, and buccal forms—are made to release their active ingredients over a certain period of time or at preset points after administration. The disruptions caused by crushing these drug forms can dramatically affect the absorption rate and increase the risk of adverse reactions.

Other reasons not to crush these drug forms include such considerations as taste, tissue irritation, and unusual formulation—for example, a capsule within a capsule, a liquid within a capsule, or a multiple-compressed tablet. Avoid crushing the following drugs, listed by brand name, for the reasons noted beside them.

Accutane (mucous membrane irritant)

Aciphex (delayed release)

Acutrim (slow release)

Adalat (slow release)

Aggrenox (extended release)

Aller-Chlor (slow release)

Allerest 12-Hour (slow release)

Ammonium Chloride Enseals (enteric coated)

Artane Sequels (slow release)

Arthrotec (delayed release)

Asacol (delayed release)

Atrohist LA, Sprinkle (slow release)

Azulfidine EN-tabs (enteric coated)

Bellergal-S (slow release)

Betapen-VK (taste)

Bisacodyl (enteric coated)

Bisco-Lax (enteric coated)

Bontril Slow-Release (slow release)

Breonesin (liquid filled)

Brexin L.A. (slow release)

Bromfed (slow release)

Bromfed-PD (slow release)

Bromphen (slow release)

Bromphen TD (slow release)

Calan SR (slow release)

Carbatrol (extended release)

Carbiset-TR (slow release)

Cardizem CD, SR (slow release)

Ceftin (taste)

Charcoal Plus (enteric coated)

Chloral Hydrate (liquid within a capsule, taste)

Chlor-Trimeton Allergy 8-hour and 12-hour (slow release)

Choledyl SA (slow release)

Cipro (taste)

Codimal-L.A. (slow release)

Colace (liquid within a capsule, taste)

Colestid (protective coating)

Comhist LA (slow release)

Compazine Spansules (slow release)

Congess SR, JR (slow release)

Contac 12 Hour, Maximum Strength 12 Hour (slow release)

Control (slow release)

Cotazym-S (enteric coated)

Creon (enteric coated)

Dallergy (slow release)

Dallergy-D, JR (slow release)

Deconamine SR (slow release)

Deconsal, Sprinkle Capsules (slow release)

Demazin Repetabs (slow release)

Depakene (slow release, mucous membrane irritant)

Depakote (enteric coated)

Desoxyn Gradumets (slow release)

Desyrel (taste)

Dexatrim (slow release)

Dexedrine Spansule (slow release)

Diamox Sequels (slow release)

Dilacor XR (slow release)

Dilatrate-SR (slow release)

Dimetane Extentabs (slow release)

Dimetapp Extentabs (slow release)

Disobrom (slow release)

Donnatal Extentabs (slow release)

Donnazyme (slow release)

Drisdol (liquid filled)

Drixoral (slow release)

Drixoral Sinus (slow release)

Drize (slow release)

Dulcolax (enteric coated)

Easprin (enteric coated)

Ecotrin (enteric coated)

Ecotrin Maximum Strength (enteric coated)

E.E.S. 400 Filmtab (enteric coated)

Effexor XR (extended release)

E-Mycin (enteric coated)

Endafed (slow release)

Entex LA (slow release)

Equanil (taste)

Eryc (enteric coated)

Ery-Tab (enteric coated)

Erythrocin Stearate (enteric coated)

Erythromycin Base (enteric coated)

Eskalith CR (slow release)

Extendryl SR, JR (slow release)

Fedahist Gyrocaps, Timecaps (slow release)

Feldene (mucous membrane irritant)

Feocyte (slow release)

Feosol (enteric coated)

Feratab (enteric coated)

Fergon (slow release)

Fero-Grad-500 (slow release)

Ferro-Sequel (slow release)

Feverall Children's Capsules, Sprinkle (taste)

Fumatinic (slow release)

Geocillin (taste)

Gris-PEG (crushing may cause precipitation of larger particles)

Guaifed (slow release)

Guaifed-PD (slow release)

Humibid Sprinkle, DM, DM Sprinkle, LA (slow release)

Hydergine LC (liquid within a capsule)

Hytakerol (liquid filled)

Iberet (slow release)

Iberet-500 (slow release)

ICAPS Plus (slow release)

ICAPS Time Release (slow release)

Ilotycin (enteric coated)

Inderal LA (slow release)

Inderide LA (slow release)

Indocin SR (slow release)

Ionamin (slow release)

Isoptin SR (slow release)

Isordil Sublingual (sublingual)

Isordil Tembids (slow release)

Isosorbide Dinitrate Sublingual (sublingual)

Isuprel Glossets (sublingual)

Kaon-Cl (slow release)

K-Dur (slow release)

Klor-Con (slow release)

Klotrix (slow release)
K-Tab (slow release)
Levsinex Timecaps (slow release)
Lithobid (slow release)
Lodrane LD (slow release)
Mestinon Timespans (slow release)
Methylin ER (extended release)
Micro-K (slow release)
Micro-K Extencaps (slow release)
Motrin (taste)
MS Contin (slow release)
Naldecon (slow release)
Nitro-Bid (slow release)
Nitroglyn (slow release)
Nitrong (sublingual)
Nitrostat (sublingual)
Nolamine (slow release)
Norflex (slow release)
Norpace CR (slow release)
Novafed A (slow release)
Oramorph SR (slow release)
Ornade Spansules (slow release)
Pancrease (enteric coated)
Pancrease MT (enteric coated)
PBZ-SR (slow release)
PCE (slow release)
Pentasa (controlled release)
Perdiem (wax coated)
Phazyme (slow release)
Phazyme 95 (slow release)
Phenergan (taste)
Phyllocontin (slow release)
Plendil (slow release)
Polaramine Repetabs (slow release)
Poly-Histine-D (slow release)
Prelu-2 (slow release)
Prevacid (delayed release)
Prilosec (slow release)
Pro-Banthine (taste)
Procainamide HCl SR (slow release)
Procardia (delayed absorption)
Procardia XL (slow release)
Pronestyl-SR (slow release)
Protonix (delayed release)
Proventil Repetabs (slow release)
Prozac (slow release)
Quibron-T/SR (slow release)
Quinaglute Dura-Tabs (slow release)
Quinidex Extentabs (slow release)
Respaire SR (slow release)
Respbid (slow release)
Ritalin-SR (slow release)
Rondec-TR (slow release)
Ru-Tuss (slow release)
Ru-Tuss DE, II (slow release)
Sinemet CR (slow release)
Singlet (slow release)
Slo-bid Gyrocaps (slow release)
Slo-Niacin (slow release)
Slo-Phyllin GG, Gyrocaps (slow release)
Slow FE (slow release)
Slow-K (slow release)
Slow-Mag (slow release)
Sorbitrate SA (slow release)
Sparine (taste)
Sudafed 12 Hour (slow release)
Sustaire (slow release)
Tamine S.R. (slow release)

Tavist-D (multiple compressed tablet)
Tegretol-XR (extended release)
Teldrin (slow release)
Teldrin Spansules (slow release)
Ten-K (slow release)
Tenuate Dospan (slow release)
Tessalon Perles (slow release)
Theobid Duracaps (slow release)
Theochron (slow release)
Theoclear LA (slow release)
Theo-Dur (slow release)
Theolair-SR (slow release)
Theo-Sav (slow release)
Theospan-SR (slow release)
Theo-24 (slow release)
Theovent (slow release)
Theo-X (slow release)
Thorazine Spansules (slow release)
Tiazac (extended release)
Topamax (bitter taste)
Toprol XL (slow release)
T-Phyl (slow release)
Tranxene-SD (slow release)
Trental (slow release)
Triaminic (slow release)
Triaminic TR (slow release)
Triaminic-12 (slow release)
Trilafon Repetabs (slow release)
Trinalin Repetabs (slow release)
Triptone Caplets (slow release)
Tuss-LA (slow release)
Tuss-Ornade Spansules (slow release)
Tylenol Extended Relief (slow release)
ULR-LA (slow release)
Uniphyl (slow release)
Verelan (slow release)
Voltaren (enteric coated)
Voltaren-XR (enteric coated)
Wellbutrin SR (sustained release)
Wygesic (taste)
ZORprin (slow release)
Zyban (slow release)
Zymase (enteric coated)

Acknowledgments

We would like to thank the following companies for granting us permission to include their drugs in the full-color photoguide.

Abbott Laboratories
Biaxin®
Depakote®
Depakote® Sprinkle
E.E.S.®
Ery-Tab®
Erythrocin® Stearate
Filmtab®
Erythromycin Base Filmtab®
Hytrin®
PCE®

AstraZeneca LP
Nolvadex®
Prilosec®
Tenormin®
Toprol-XL®
Zestril®

Aventis Pharmaceuticals
Allegra®
Carafate®
DiaBeta®
Lasix®
Trental®

Bayer Corporation
Adalat® CC
Cipro®

Biovail Corporation
Cardizem®
Cardizem® CD

Bristol-Myers Squibb Company
BuSpar®
Capoten®
Cefzil®
Duricef®
Estrace®
Glucophage®
Monopril®
Pravachol®
Serzone®

DuPont Pharmaceuticals Company
Coumadin®

Elkins-Sinn Division of American Home Products Corporation
atenolol

Ethex Corporation
potassium chloride

Forest Pharmaceuticals, Inc.
Celexa®

Geneva Pharmaceuticals, Inc.
Sumycin®
Trimox®
Veetids®

GlaxoSmithKline
Amoxil®
Augmentin®
Compazine®
Coreg®
Paxil®
Relafen®
Tagamet®

Glaxo Wellcome, Inc.
Ceftin®
Lanoxin®
Wellbutrin®
Wellbutrin SR®
Zantac®
Zovirax®

Janssen Pharmaceutica, Inc.
Risperdal®

Jones Pharma
Levoxyl®

King Pharmaceuticals, Inc.
Altace®
Lorabid®

KV Pharmaceutical Company
Micro-K® Extencaps®

Eli Lilly and Company
Axid®
Ceclor®
Evista®
Prozac®

McNeil-PPC, Inc.
Motrin®

Medeva Pharmaceuticals
methylphenidate hydrochloride

Merck & Co., Inc.
Cozaar®
Fosamax®
Mevacor®
Pepcid®
Prinivil®
Sinemet®
Sinemet® CR
Singulair®
Vasotec®
Vioxx®
Zocor®

Mylan Pharmaceuticals, Inc.
amitriptyline hydrochloride
cimetidine
cyclobenzaprine hydrochloride
doxepin hydrochloride
furosemide
glipizide
naproxen
propoxyphene napsylate with acetaminophen

Novartis Pharma Corporation
Lotensin®
Pamelor®

Novopharm
amoxicillin trihydrate

Ortho-McNeil Pharmaceutical
Floxin®
Levaquin®
Ultram®

Pfizer, Inc.
Cardura®
Diflucan®
Glucotrol®
Glucotrol XL®
Norvasc®
Procardia XL®
Viagra®
Zithromax®
Zoloft®

Pharmacia Corporation
Deltasone®
Glynase® PresTab®
Micronase®
Provera®
Xanax®

Roche Laboratories, Inc.
Bumex®
Klonopin®
Naprosyn®
Ticlid®
Toradol®
Valium®

Schering Corporation and Key Pharmaceuticals, Inc.
Claritin®
K-Dur®
Theo-Dur®

Schwarz Pharma
Verelan®

G.D. Searle & Company
Ambien®
Calan®
Celebrex®
Daypro®

Tap Pharmaceuticals, Inc.
Prevacid®

Teva Pharmaceuticals, USA
cephalexin

Warner-Lambert Company
Accupril®
Dilantin® Infatabs®
Dilantin® Kapseals®
Lipitor®
Lopid®
Neurontin®
Nitrostat®

Watson Pharma, Inc.
Dilacor XR®
nortriptyline hydrochloride

Wyeth-Ayerst Laboratories
Ativan®
Cordarone®
Effexor®
Inderal®
Lodine®
Oruvail®
Premarin®

Zenith Goldline Pharmaceuticals
verapamil hydrochloride

Index

t refers to a table; **boldface** refers to full-color photographs

t refers to a table; **boldface** refers to full-color photographs

B

t refers to a table; **boldface** refers to full-color photographs

t refers to a table; **boldface** refers to full-color photographs

t refers to a table; **boldface** refers to full-color photographs

D

F

G

t refers to a table; **boldface** refers to full-color photographs

J

K

N

O

t refers to a table; **boldface** refers to full-color photographs

U

V

W

X

Y

Z

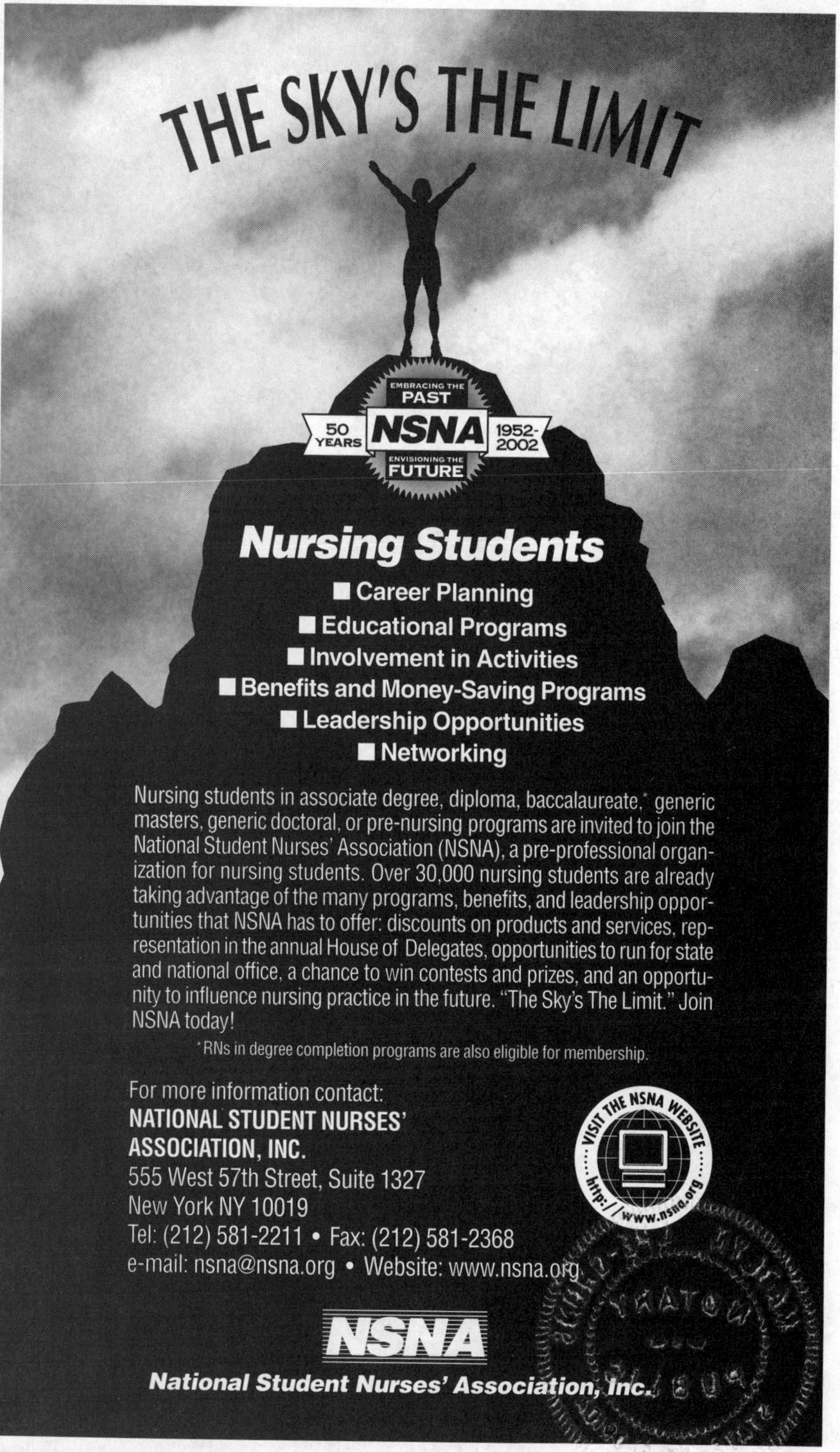
THE SKY'S THE LIMIT
EMBRACING THE PAST
50 YEARS
NSNA
1952-2002
ENVISIONING THE FUTURE
Nursing Students
Career Planning
Educational Programs
Involvement in Activities
Benefits and Money-Saving Programs
Leadership Opportunities
Networking
Nursing students in associate degree, diploma, baccalaureate,* generic masters, generic doctoral, or pre-nursing programs are invited to join the National Student Nurses' Association (NSNA), a pre-professional organization for nursing students. Over 30,000 nursing students are already taking advantage of the many programs, benefits, and leadership opportunities that NSNA has to offer: discounts on products and services, representation in the annual House of Delegates, opportunities to run for state and national office, a chance to win contests and prizes, and an opportunity to influence nursing practice in the future. "The Sky's The Limit." Join NSNA today!
*RNs in degree completion programs are also eligible for membership.
For more information contact:
NATIONAL STUDENT NURSES' ASSOCIATION, INC.
555 West 57th Street, Suite 1327
New York NY 10019
Tel: (212) 581-2211 • Fax: (212) 581-2368
e-mail: nsna@nsna.org • Website: www.nsna.org
VISIT THE NSNA WEBSITE
http://www.nsna.org
NSNA
National Student Nurses' Association, Inc.